DUBOIS'
Lupus Erythematosus and Related Syndromes

EIGHTH EDITION

DUBOIS'
Lupus Erythematosus and Related Syndromes

EIGHTH EDITION

Edited by

Daniel J. Wallace, MD, FACP, FACR
Associate Director, Rheumatology Fellowship Program
Cedars-Sinai Medical Center
Clinical Professor of Medicine
David Geffen School of Medicine at UCLA
Los Angeles, California

Bevra Hannahs Hahn, MD
Chief, Rheumatology and Arthritis Professor of Medicine
Department of Medicine
David Geffen School of Medicine
University of California at Los Angeles
Los Angeles, California

Associate Editors:

David Isenberg, MD, FRCP, FAMS
Consultant Rheumatologist
University College London
London, United Kingdom

Nan Shen, MD
Shanghai Institute of Rheumatology
Renji Hospital
Shanghai JiaoTong University School of Medicine
Shanghai, China
Division of Rheumatology
The Center for Autoimmune Genomics and Etiology (CAGE)
Cincinnati Children's Hospital Medical Center
Cincinnati, Ohio
Joint Molecular Rheumatology Laboratory
Institute of Health Sciences and Shanghai Renji Hospital
Shanghai Institutes for Biological Sciences
Chinese Academy of Sciences
Shanghai Jiaotong University School of Medicine
Shanghai, China

Ronald F. van Vollenhoven, MD, PhD
Professor and Chief
Unit for Clinical Therapy Research Inflammatory Diseases (ClinTRID)
The Karolinska Institute
Chief, Clinical Trials Unit
Department of Rheumatology
The Karolinska University Hospital
Stockholm, Sweden

Michael H. Weisman, MD
Attending Physician
Division of Rheumatology
Professor in Residence
Cedars-Sinai Medical Center
David Geffen School of Medicine
University of California at Los Angeles
Los Angeles, California

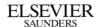
ELSEVIER
SAUNDERS

1600 John F. Kennedy Blvd.
Ste 1800
Philadelphia, PA 19103-2899

Library of Congress Cataloging-in-Publication Data
Dubois' lupus erythematosus and related syndromes / [edited by] Daniel J Wallace, Bevra Hannahs Hahn.—8th
ed.
  p. ; cm.
  Lupus erythematosus and related syndromes
  Rev. ed. of: Dubois' lupus erythematosus / editors, Daniel J. Wallace, Bevra Hannahs Hahn. 7th ed. c2007.
  Includes bibliographical references and index.
  ISBN 978-1-4377-1893-5 (hardcover)
  I. Wallace, Daniel J. (Daniel Jeffrey), 1949-   II. Hahn, Bevra.   III. Dubois, Edmund L. Lupus
erythematosus.   IV. Dubois' lupus erythematosus.   V. Title: Lupus erythematosus and related syndromes.
  [DNLM: 1. Lupus Erythematosus, Systemic.   2. Lupus Erythematosus, Cutaneous.   WD 380]
  616.7'72—dc23
                                                                              2012021186

Content Strategist: Pamela Hetherington
Content Development Manager: Maureen Iannuzzi
Publishing Services Manager: Hemamalini Rajendrababu
Project Manager: Saravanan Thavamani
Design Manager: Steven Stave

Printed in China

Last digit is the print number: 9 8 7 6 5 4 3 2 1

Contributors

Joseph M. Ahearn, MD
Chief Scientific Officer and Vice President, Allegheny Singer Research Institute, West Penn Allegheny Health System, Pittsburgh, Pennsylvania
Professor of Medicine, Temple University School of Medicine, Philadelphia, Pennsylvania
Chapter 14: Complement and Systemic Lupus Erythematosus

Cynthia Aranow, MD
Investigator, Feinstein Institute for Medical Research, Manhasset, New York
Chapter 28: Pathogenesis of the Nervous System

J. Antonio Aviña-Zubieta, MD, PhD
Assistant Professor of Medicine, University of British Columbia, British Columbia Lupus Society Scholar, Research Scientist, Arthritis Research Centre of Canada, Vancouver, British Columbia, Canada
Chapter 49: Antimalarial Medications

Andre Barkhuizen, MD, FCP(SA), FACR
Medical Director, Portland Rheumatology Clinic, LLC, Portland, Oregon
Chapter 31: Ocular, Aural, and Oral Manifestations

Sasha Bernatsky, MD
Associate Professor, Divisions of Clinical Epidemiology and Rheumatology, Research Institute of the McGill University Health Centre, Montreal, Quebec, Canada
Chapter 57: Mortality in Systemic Lupus Erythematosus

Celine Berthier, PhD
Department of Internal Medicine, Nephrology, University of Michigan, Ann Arbor, Michigan
Chapter 18: Pathogenetic Mechanisms in Lupus Nephritis

Hendrika Bootsma, MD
Professor of Rheumatology, Department of Rheumatology and Clinical Immunology, University of Groningen, University Medical Center Groningen, Groningen, The Netherlands
Chapter 32: Management of Sjögren Syndrome in Patients with Systemic Lupus Erythematosus

Lukas Bossaller, MD
Division of Infectious Diseases and Immunology, University of Massachusetts Medical School, Worcester, Massachusetts
Chapter 6: The Innate Immune System in Systemic Lupus Erythematosus

H. R. Bouma, MD, PhD
Professor in Residence, Department of Rheumatology and Clinical Immunology, University of Groningen, University Medical Center Groningen, Groningen, The Netherlands
Chapter 32: Management of Sjögren Syndrome in Patients with Systemic Lupus Erythematosus

Dimitrios T. Boumpas, MD, FACP
Professor of Medicine, University of Athens, Director, Divisions of Internal Medicine and Rheumatology, University Hospital, Heraklion, Greece
Chapter 48: Systemic Glucocorticoid Therapy in Systemic Lupus Erythematosus

Cherie L. Butts, PhD
Associate Director, Immunology Research, Biogen Idec, Cambridge, Massachusetts
Chapter 13: Neural Immune Interactions: Principles and Relevance to Systemic Lupus Erythematosus

Eliza F. Chakravarty, MD, MS
Associate Member, Arthritis and Clinical Immunology, Oklahoma Medical Research Foundation, Oklahoma City, Oklahoma
Chapter 38: Reproductive and Hormonal Issues in Women with Autoimmune Diseases

Benjamin F. Chong, MD
Assistant Professor, Department of Dermatology, University of Texas Southwestern Medical Center, Dallas, Texas
Chapter 24: Skin Disease in Cutaneous Lupus Erythematosus

Ann E. Clarke, MD, MSC
Professor of Medicine, Divisions of Clinical Epidemiology and Allergy/Clinical Immunology, McGill University Health Centre, Montreal, Quebec, Canada
Chapter 57: Mortality in Systemic Lupus Erythematosus

Megan E. B. Clowse, MD, MPH
Assistant Professor of Medicine, Division of Rheumatology and Immunology, Department of Medicine, Duke University Medical Center, Durham, North Carolina
Chapter 36: Pregnancy in Systemic Lupus Erythematosus
Chapter 37: Neonatal Lupus Erythematosus

José C. Crispín, MD
Instructor in Medicine, Department of Medicine, Division of Rheumatology, Beth Israel Deaconess Medical Center, Harvard Medical School, Boston, Massachusetts
Chapter 9: T Cells

Mary K. Crow, MD
Physician-in-Chief and Chair of the Division of Rheumatology, Hospital for Special Surgery, New York, New York
Chapter 7: Cytokines and Interferons in Lupus

Maria Dall'Era, MD
Associate Professor of Medicine, University of California, San Francisco, California
Chapter 1: Classification of Lupus and Lupus-Related Disorders

Anne Davidson, MBBS
Investigator, Center for Autoimmunity and Musculoskeletal Diseases, Feinstein Institute for Medical Research, Manhasset, New York
Chapter 18: Pathogenetic Mechanisms in Lupus Nephritis

Yun Deng, MD
Postdoctoral Research Fellow, Division of Rheumatology, Department of Medicine, David Geffen School of Medicine, University of California at Los Angeles, Los Angeles, California
Chapter 4: Genetics of Human Systemic Lupus Erythematosus

Betty Diamond, MD
Investigator and Head, North Shore Long Island Jewish Health System, The Center for Autoimmune and Musculoskeletal Disease, Manhasset, New York
Chapter 8: The Structure and Derivation of Antibodies and Autoantibodies
Chapter 28: Pathogenesis of the Nervous System

Mary Anne Dooley, MD, MPH
Associate Professor of Medicine, University of North Carolina School of Medicine, Chapel Hill, North Carolina
Chapter 35: Clinical and Epidemiologic Features of Lupus Nephritis

Christina Drenkard, MD, PhD
Assistant Professor of Medicine, Division of Rheumatology, Emory University School of Medicine, Atlanta, Georgia
Chapter 2: The Epidemiology of Lupus

Shweta Dubey, PhD
Assistant Professor, Amity Institute of Virology and Immunology, Amity University, Uttar Pradesh, Noida, India
Chapter 19: Immune Tolerance Defects in Lupus
Chapter 21: Autoantigenesis and Antigen-Based Therapy and Vaccination in Systemic Lupus Erythematosus

Jan P. Dutz, MD, FRCPC
Professor, Department of Dermatology and Skin Science, University of British Columbia, Vancouver, British Columbia, Canada
Chapter 23: Pathomechanisms of Cutaneous Lupus Erythematosus

Keith B. Elkon, MD
Professor of Medicine and Immunology, Division of Rheumatology, University of Washington, Seattle, Washington
Chapter 11: Apoptosis, Necrosis, and Autophagy

John M. Esdaile, MD, MPH, FRCPC, FCAHS
Scientific Director, Arthritis Research Centre of Canada, Vancouver, British Columbia, Canada
Chapter 49: Antimalarial Medications

John D. Fisk, PhD
Psychologist, Queen Elizabeth II Health Sciences Centre, Associate Professor, Department of Psychiatry, Assistant Professor, Department of Medicine, Adjunct Professor, Department of Psychology, Dalhousie University, Halifax, Nova Scotia, Canada
Chapter 30: Psychopathology, Neurodiagnostic Testing, and Imaging

Giovanni Franchin, MD, PhD
Investigator, North Shore Long Island Jewish Health System, The Center for Autoimmune and Musculoskeletal Disease, Manhasset, New York
Chapter 8: The Structure and Derivation of Antibodies and Autoantibodies

Serene Francis, MD
Central Dupage Hospital, Wheaton, Illinois
Chapter 44: Differential Diagnosis and Disease Associations

Dafna D. Gladman, MD, FRCPC
Professor of Medicine, University of Toronto, Senior Scientist, Toronto Western Research Institute, Co-Director, University of Toronto Lupus Clinic, Centre for Prognosis Studies in the Rheumatic Diseases, Toronto Western Hospital, University of Toronto, Toronto, Ontario, Canada
Chapter 46: Clinical Measures, Metrics, and Indices

Tania Gonzalez-Rivera, MD
Clinical Instructor in Internal Medicine, Division of Rheumatology, Department of Internal Medicine, University of Michigan, Ann Arbor, Michigan
Chapter 50: Immunosuppressive Drug Therapy

Caroline Gordon, MD, FRCP
Consultant Rheumatologist, Rheumatology Research Group, College of Medical and Dental Sciences, School of Immunity and Infection, University of Birmingham, Edgbaston, Birmingham, United Kingdom
Chapter 57: Mortality in Systemic Lupus Erythematosus

Eric L. Greidinger, MD
Associate Professor of Medicine, Chief, Division of Rheumatology and Immunology, University of Miami Miller School of Medicine, Miami, Florida
Chapter 41: Mixed Connective Tissue Disease and Undifferentiated Connective Tissue Disease

Jennifer Grossman, MD
Associate Clinical Professor of Medicine, Division of Rheumatology, David Geffen School of Medicine, University of California at Los Angeles, Los Angeles, California
Chapter 26: Pathogenesis and Treatment of Atherosclerosis in Lupus

Bevra H. Hahn, MD
Chief, Rheumatology and Arthritis, Professor of Medicine, Department of Medicine, David Geffen School of Medicine, University of California at Los Angeles, Los Angeles, California
Chapter 3: The Pathogenesis of Systemic Lupus Erythematosus
Chapter 17: Animal Models of Systemic Lupus Erythematosus

David S. Hallegua, MD
Assistant Professor of Medicine, Internal Medicine, Rheumatology, Cedars-Sinai Medical Center, Los Angeles, California
Chapter 33: Gastrointestinal and Hepatic Manifestations

John G. Hanly, MD, FRCPC
Professor of Medicine and Pathology, Attending staff RheumatologistDivision of Rheumatology, Department of Medicine, Nova Scotia Rehabilitation Center, Dalhousie University and Capital Health Halifax, Nova Scotia, Canada
Chapter 30: Psychopathology, Neurodiagnostic Testing, and Imaging

Falk Hiepe, MD, PhD
Professor of Rheumatology, Charité Campus Virchow, Charité University Hospital, Berlin, Germany
Chapter 20 (Part E): Antibodies Against the Extractable Nuclear Antigens, RNP, Sm, Ro/SSA, and La/SSB

Andrea Hinojosa-Azaola, MD
Staff Rheumatologist, Instituto Nacional de Ciencias Médicas y Nutrición Salvador Zubirán, México, Distrito Federal, México
Chapter 22: Overview and Clinical Presentation

Robert W. Hoffman, DO
Senior Medical Director, Translational Medicine, Lilly Research Laboratories, Eli Lilly and Company, Indianapolis, Indiana
Chapter 41: Mixed Connective Tissue Disease and Undifferentiated Connective Tissue Disease

David Isenberg, MD, FRCP, FAMS
Consultant Rheumatologist, University College London, London, United Kingdom
Chapter 20 (Part A): Autoantibodies to DNA, Histones, and Nucleosomes

Mariko L. Ishimori, MD
Assistant Professor of Medicine, Cedars-Sinai Medical Center, Assistant Health Sciences Clinical Professor of Medicine, David Geffen School of Medicine, University of California at Los Angeles, Los Angeles, California
Chapter 47: Principles of Therapy, Local Measures, and Nonsteroidal Medications

Judith A. James, MD, PhD
Lou Kerr Chain in Biomedical Research, Oklahoma Medical Research Foundation, University of Oklahoma Health Sciences Center, Oklahoma City, Oklahoma
Chapter 45: Systemic Lupus Erythematosus and Infections

Meenakshi Jolly, MD
Associate Professor of Medicine, Rush University Medical School, Chicago, Illinois
Chapter 44: Differential Diagnosis and Disease Associations

J. Michelle Kahlenberg, MD, PhD
Associate Professor of Internal Medicine, Division of Rheumatology, Department of Internal Medicine, University of Michigan, Ann Arbor, Michigan
Chapter 15: Mechanisms of Acute Inflammation and Vascular Injury in Systemic Lupus Erythematosus

C. G. M. Kallenberg, MD, PhD
Department of Rheumatology and Clinical Immunology, University of Groningen, University Medical Center Groningen, Groningen, the Netherlands
Chapter 20 (Part D): Anti-C1q Antibodies

Diane L. Kamen, MD, MSCR
Associate Professor of Medicine, Division of Rheumatology, Medical University of South Carolina, Charleston, South Carolina
Chapter 52: Adjunctive and Preventive Measures

Mariana J. Kaplan, MD
Associate Professor of Internal Medicine, Division of Rheumatology, Department of Internal Medicine, University of Michigan Medical School, Ann Arbor, Michigan
Chapter 15: Mechanisms of Acute Inflammation and Vascular Injury in Systemic Lupus Erythematosus

George A. Karpouzas, MD
Associate Professor of Medicine, David Geffen School of Medicine, University of California at Los Angeles, Los Angeles, California
Chief, Division of Rheumatology, Harbor–UCLA Medical Center, Torrance, California
Chapter 34: Hematologic and Lymphoid Abnormalities in Systemic Lupus Erythematosus

Munther A. Khamashta, MD, FRCP, PhD
Professor of Medicine and Lupus Research, Director, Graham Hughes Lupus Research Unit, Division of Women's Health, The Rayne Institute, St. Thomas' Hospital, King's College, London, United Kingdom
Chapter 27: Cardiopulmonary Disease in Systemic Lupus Erythematosus

Robert P. Kimberly, MD
Professor of Medicine, Department of Medicine, University of Alabama at Birmingham School of Medicine, Birmingham, Alabama
Chapter 12: Abnormalities in Immune Complex Clearance and Fcγ Receptor Function

Kyriakos A. Kirou, MD, FACP
Assistant Professor of Clinical Medicine, Department of Medicine, Weill Medical College of Cornell University, Clinical Co-Director, Mary Kirkland Center for Lupus Care, Hospital for Special Surgery, New York, New York
Chapter 7: Cytokines and Interferons in Lupus
Chapter 48: Systemic Glucocorticoid Therapy in Systemic Lupus Erythematosus

Dwight Kono, MD
Professor of Immunology, Department of Immunology and Microbial Science, The Scripps Research Institute, La Jolla, California
Chapter 17: Animal Models of Systemic Lupus Erythematosus

Matthias Kretzler, MD
Professor of Internal Medicine, Department of Internal Medicine, Nephrology, University of Michigan, Ann Arbor, Michigan
Chapter 18: Pathogenetic Mechanisms in Lupus Nephritis

Frans G. M. Kroese, MD
Professor of Immunology, Department of Rheumatology and Clinical Immunology, University of Groningen, University Medical Center Groningen, Groningen, the Netherlands
Chapter 32: Management of Sjögren Syndrome in Patients with Systemic Lupus Erythematosus

Biji T. Kurien, PhD
Associate Professor of Research, Department of Medicine, University of Oklahoma Health Sciences Center, Arthritis and Clinical Immunology Program, Oklahoma Medical Research Foundation, Department of Veterans Affairs Medical Center, Oklahoma City, Oklahoma
Chapter 16: Mechanisms of Tissue Damage—Free Radicals and Fibrosis

Antonio La Cava, MD, PhD
Division of Rheumatology, Department of Medicine, David Geffen School of Medicine, University of California at Los Angeles, Los Angeles, California
Chapter 10: Regulatory Cells in Systemic Lupus Erythematosus

Aisha Lateef, MBBS, M. Med, MRCP, FAMS
Consultant, University Medicine Cluster, National University Health System, Singapore, Singapore
Chapter 42: Clinical Aspects of the Antiphospholipid Syndrome

Thomas J. A. Lehman, MD
Chief, Division of Pediatric Rheumatology, Senior Scientist Hospital for Special Surgery, Professor of Clinical Pediatrics, Weill Medical College of Cornell University, New York, New York
Chapter 40: Systemic Lupus Erythematosus in Childhood and Adolescence

Deborah Levy, MD, FRCPC, MSC
Assistant Professor of Pediatrics, Division of Rheumatology, Hospital for Sick Children and University of Toronto, Toronto, Ontario, Canada
Chapter 57: Mortality in Systemic Lupus Erythematosus

Dong Liang, PhD
Research Associate, Division of Rheumatology, The Center for Autoimmune Genomics and Etiology (CAGE), Cincinnati Children's Hospital Medical Center, Cincinnati, Ohio
Chapter 5: Epigenetics of Lupus

Lyndell Lim, MBBS, FRANZCO
Senior Research Fellow, Consultant Ophthalmologist, Centre for Eye Research Australia, Royal Victorian Eye and Ear Hospital, University of Melbourne, East Melbourne, Victoria, Australia
Chapter 31: Ocular, Aural, and Oral Manifestations

S. Sam Lim, MD, MPH
Associate Professor of Medicine, Division of Rheumatology, Emory University School of Medicine, Atlanta, Georgia
Chapter 2: The Epidemiology of Lupus

Chau-Ching Liu, MD, PhD
Research Scientist, AlleghenySinger Research Institute, West Penn Allegheny Health System, Pittsburgh, Pennsylvania
Associate Professor of Medicine, Temple University School of Medicine, Philadelphia, Pennsylvania
Chapter 14: Complement and Systemic Lupus Erythematosus

Meggan Mackay, MD
Associate Investigator, Feinstein Institute for Medical Research, The Center for Autoimmune and Musculoskeletal Disease, Manhasset, New York
Chapter 28: Pathogenesis of the Nervous System

Jessica Manson, PhD, MRCP
Consultant Rheumatologist, Department of Rheumatology, University College Hospital, London, United Kingdom
Chapter 20 (Part A): Autoantibodies to DNA, Histones, and Nucleosomes
Chapter 20 (Part C): Antibody Structure, Function, and Production

Susan Manzi, MD, MPH
System Chair, Department of Medicine, West Penn Allegheny Health System, Pittsburgh, Pennsylvania
Vice Chair and Professor of Medicine, Temple University School of Medicine, Philadelphia, Pennsylvania
Chapter 14: Complement and Systemic Lupus Erythematosus

Ann Marshak-Rothstein, PhD
Professor of Medicine, Division of Rheumatology, University of Massachusetts Medical School, Worcester, Massachusetts
Chapter 6: The Innate Immune System in Systemic Lupus Erythematosus

Maureen McMahon, MD
Assistant Clinical Professor of Medicine, Division of Rheumatology, David Geffen School of Medicine, University of California at Los Angeles, Los Angeles, California
Chapter 26: Pathogenesis and Treatment of Atherosclerosis in Lupus

W. Joseph McCune, MD
Professor of Internal Medicine, Medical School, Michael H. and Marcia S. Klein Professor of Rheumatic Diseases, University of Michigan, Ann Arbor, Michigan
Chapter 50: Immunosuppressive Drug Therapy

Chandra Mohan, MBBS, PhD
Professor of Medicine, Internal Medicine Rheumatic Diseases, UT Southwestern Medical Center, Dallad, Texas
Chapter 16: Mechanisms of Tissue Damage—Free Radicals and Fibrosis

Sandra V. Navarra, MD
Professor of Medicine and Rheumatology, Section of Rheumatology, Clinical Immunology and Osteoporosis, University of Santo Tomas, Manila, Philippines
Chapter 25: The Musculoskeletal System and Bone Metabolism

Timothy B. Niewold, MD
Assistant Professor of Medicine, Division of Biological Sciences, Rheumatology, The University of Chicago, Chicago, Illinois
Chapter 7: Cytokines and Interferons in Lupus

Antonina Omisade, PhD
Psychologist, Queen Elizabeth II Health Sciences Centre, Halifax, Nova Scotia, Canada
Chapter 30: Psychopathology, Neurodiagnostic Testing, and Imaging

Jenny Thorn Palter
Director of Publications, Publications Department, Lupus Foundation of America, Inc., Northwest, Washington
Appendix: Resources

Dipak Patel, MD, PhD
Clinical Lecturer in Internal Medicine, Department of Internal Medicine, Division of Rheumatology, University of Michigan Medical School, Ann Arbor, Michigan
Chapter 39: Drug-Induced Lupus: Etiology, Pathogenesis, and Clinical Aspects

Michelle Petri, MD, MPH
Professor, Division of Rheumatology, School of Medicine, Johns Hopkins Lupus Center, Johns Hopkins University, Baltimore, Maryland
Chapter 42: Clinical Aspects of the Antiphospholipid Syndrome

Julia Pinkhasov, PhD
Assistant Researcher, Division of Rheumatology, David Geffen School of Medicine, University of California at Los Angeles, Los Angeles, California
Chapter 19: Immune Tolerance Defects in Lupus
Chapter 21: Autoantigenesis and Antigen-Based Therapy and Vaccination in Systemic Lupus Erythematosus

Priti Prasad, MS
Graduate Student, Division of Rheumatology, David Geffen School of Medicine, University of California at Los Angeles, Los Angeles, California
Chapter 21: Autoantigenesis and Antigen-Based Therapy and Vaccination in Systemic Lupus Erythematosus

Yuting Qin
PhD candidate, Joint Molecular Rheumatology Laboratory, Institute of Health Sciences and Shanghai Renji Hospital, Shanghai Institutes for Biological Sciences, Chinese Academy of Sciences, Shanghai Jiaotong University School of Medicine, Shanghai, China
Chapter 5: Epigenetics of Lupus

Francisco P. Quismorio, Jr., MD
Professor of Medicine and Pathology, Division of Rheumatology,
University of Southern California, Keck School of Medicine,
Los Angeles County Medical Center, Los Angeles, California
Chapter 43: Clinical Application of Serologic Tests, Serum Protein Abnormalities, and Other Clinical Laboratory Tests in Systemic Lupus Erythematosus

Anisur Rahman, PhD, FRCP
Professor of Rheumatology, Department of Rheumatology,
University College London, London, United Kingdom
Chapter 20 (Part A): Autoantibodies to DNA, Histones, and Nucleosomes
Chapter 20 (Part B): Antilipoprotein and Antiendothelial Cell Antibodies
Chapter 57: Mortality in Systemic Lupus Erythematosus

Rosalind Ramsey-Goldman, MD, DrPh
Professor of Medicine, Division of Rheumatology, Feinberg School
of Medicine, Northwestern University, Chicago, Illinois
Chapter 57: Mortality in Systemic Lupus Erythematosus

Bruce C. Richardson, MD, PhD
Professor of Internal Medicine, Department of Internal Medicine,
Division of Rheumatology, University of Michigan Medical
School, Ann Arbor, Michigan
Chapter 39: Drug-Induced Lupus: Etiology, Pathogenesis, and Clinical Aspects

Gabriela Riemekasten, MD
Group leader, German Rheumatism Research Centre, Charité
Campus Virchow, Charité University Hospital, Berlin, Germany
Chapter 20 (Part E): Antibodies Against the Extractable Nuclear Antigens, RNP, Sm, Ro/SSA, and La/SSB

James Rosenbaum, AB, MD
Professor, Ophthalmology, Medicine, and Cell Biology, Oregon
Health and Science University, Portland, Oregon
Chapter 31: Ocular, Aural, and Oral Manifestations

Guillermo Ruiz-Irastorza, MD, PhD
Professor of Medicine, Department of Internal Medicine,
Autoimmune Diseases Research Unit, Hospital Universitario
Cruces, University of the Basque Country, Bizkaia, Spain
Chapter 27: Cardiopulmonary Disease in Systemic Lupus Erythematosus

Jane E. Salmon, MD
Collette Kean Research Professor, Hospital for Special Surgery,
Professor of Medicine, Weill Cornell Medical College, New York,
New York
Chapter 12: Abnormalities in Immune Complex Clearance and Fcγ Receptor Function

Jorge Sánchez-Guerrero, MD, MS
Professor of Medicine, Head, Division of Rheumatology, University
Health Network, Mount Sinai Hospital, Onatario, Canada
Chapter 22: Overview and Clinical Presentation

Robert Hal Scofield, MD
Professor of Medicine, Department of Medicine, University of
Oklahoma Health Sciences Center, Arthritis and Clinical
Immunology Program, Oklahoma Medical Research Foundation,
Department of Veterans Affairs Medical Center, Oklahoma City,
Oklahoma
Chapter 16: Mechanisms of Tissue Damage—Free Radicals and Fibrosis

Winston Sequeira, MD
Professor of Medicine, Rush University Medical School, Chicago,
Illinois
Chapter 44: Differential Diagnosis and Disease Associations

Andrea L. Sestak, MD, PhD
Clinical Assistant Professor, Department of Pediatric
Rheumatology, University of Oklahoma Health Sciences Center,
Oklahoma City, Oklahoma
Chapter 45: Systemic Lupus Erythematosus and Infections

Katy Setoodeh, MD
Attending Physician, Division of Rheumatology, Cedars-Sinai
Medical Center, Los Angeles, California
Chapter 47: Principles of Therapy, Local Measures, and Nonsteroidal Medications

Nan Shen, MD
Professor of Medicine, Shanghai Institute of Rheumatology, Renji
Hospital, Shanghai JiaoTong University School of Medicine,
Shanghai, China
Division of Rheumatology, The Center for Autoimmune Genomics
and Etiology (CAGE), Cincinnati Children's Hospital Medical
Center, Cincinnati, Ohio
Joint Molecular Rheumatology Laboratory, Institute of Health
Sciences and Shanghai Renji Hospital, Shanghai Institutes for
Biological Sciences, Chinese Academy of Sciences, Shanghai
Jiaotong University School of Medicine, Shanghai, China
Chapter 5: Epigenetics of Lupus

Ram Raj Singh, MD
Professor of Medicine and Pathology, Division of Rheumatology,
David Geffen School of Medicine, Jonsson Comprehensive
Cancer Center, University of California at Los Angeles,
Los Angeles, California
Chapter 17: Animal Models of Systemic Lupus Erythematosus
Chapter 19: Immune Tolerance Defects in Lupus
Chapter 21: Autoantigenesis and Antigen-Based Therapy and Vaccination in Systemic Lupus Erythematosus

Brian Skaggs, PhD
David Geffen School of Medicine, University of California at Los
Angeles, Los Angeles, California
Chapter 26: Pathogenesis and Treatment of Atherosclerosis in Lupus

Josef S. Smolen, MD, FRCP
Professor of Internal Medicine, Department of Rheumatology,
Medical University of Vienna, Vienna, Austria
Chapter 56: Investigational Agents and Future Therapy for Systemic Lupus Erythematosus

Sven-Erik Sonesson, MD, PhD
Pediatric Cardiology Unit, Department of Women's and Children's
Health, Karolinska Institute, Stockholm, Sweden
Chapter 37: Neonatal Lupus Erythematosus

Esther M. Sternberg, MD
Chief, Section on Neuroendocrine Immunology and Behavior,
National Institute of Mental Health, Bethesda, Maryland
Chapter 13: Neural Immune Interactions: Principles and Relevance to Systemic Lupus Erythematosus

George H. Stummvoll, MD
Professor of Internal Medicine, Department of Rheumatology,
Medical University of Vienna, Vienna, Austria
Chapter 56: Investigational Agents and Future Therapy for Systemic Lupus Erythematosus

Yuajia Tang, PhD
Associate Professor, Joint Molecular Rheumatology Laboratory, Institute of Health Sciences and Shanghai Renji Hospital, Shanghai Institutes for Biological Sciences, Chinese Academy of Sciences, Shanghai Jiaotong University School of Medicine, Shanghai, China
Chapter 5: Epigenetics of Lupus

Karina D. Torralba, MD
Assistant Professor of Medicine, Division of Rheumatology, Keck School of Medicine, University of Southern California, Los Angeles County Medical Center, Los Angeles, California
Chapter 43: Clinical Application of Serologic Tests, Serum Protein Abnormalities, and Other Clinical Laboratory Tests in Systemic Lupus Erythematosus

Tito P. Torralba, MD
Professor Emeritus, Faculty of Medicine and Surgery, Section of Rheumatology, Clinical Immunology and Osteoporosis, University of Santo Tomas, Manila, Philippines
Chapter 25: The Musculoskeletal System and Bone Metabolism

Zahi Touma, MD, PhD, FACP
Clinical Research Fellow of Rheumatology, Institute of Medical Science, University of Toronto Lupus Clinic, Centre for Prognosis Studies in the Rheumatic Diseases, Toronto Western Hospital, Toronto, Ontario, Canada
Chapter 46: Clinical Measures, Metrics, and Indices

Dennis R. Trune, PhD
Professor, Oregon Hearing Research Center, Department of Otolaryngology, Head and Neck Surgery, Oregon Health and Science University, Portland, Oregon
Chapter 31: Ocular, Aural, and Oral Manifestations

Betty P. Tsao, MD, PhD
Professor of Medicine, Division of Rheumatology, Department of Medicine, David Geffen School of Medicine, University of California at Los Angeles, Los Angeles, California
Chapter 4: Genetics of Human Systemic Lupus Erythematosus

George C. Tsokos, MD
Professor of Medicine, Department of Medicine, Division of Rheumatology, Beth Israel Deaconess Medical Center, Harvard Medical School, Boston, Massachusetts
Chapter 9: T Cells

Murray B. Urowitz, MD, FRCPC
Professor of Medicine, University of Toronto, Senior Scientist, Toronto Western Research Institute, Director, University of Toronto Lupus Clinic, Centre for Prognosis Studies in the Rheumatic Diseases, Toronto Western Hospital, University of Toronto, Toronto, Ontario, Canada
Chapter 46: Clinical Measures, Metrics, and Indices

Ronald F. van Vollenhoven, MD, PhD
Professor and Chief, Unit for Clinical Therapy Research Inflammatory Diseases (ClinTRID), The Karolinska Institute, Chief, Clinical Trials Unit, Department of Rheumatology, The Karolinska University Hospital, Stockholm, Sweden
Chapter 53: Novel Therapies for Systemic Lupus Erythematosus—Biological Agents Available in Practice Today
Chapter 54: Critical Issues in Drug Development for Systemic Lupus Erythematosus

Swamy Venuturupalli, MD
Clinical Chief of Rheumatology, Cedars-Sinai Medical Center, Assistant Clinical Prof. Of Medicine, University of California at Los Angeles, Los Angeles, California
Chapter 33: Gastrointestinal and Hepatic Manifestations

Arjan Vissink, MD
Department of Oral and Maxillofacial Surgery, University of Groningen, University Medical Center Groningen, Groningen, the Netherlands
Chapter 32: Management of Sjögren Syndrome in Patients with Systemic Lupus Erythematosus

Evan S. Vista, MD
Associate Professor of Medicine, University of Santo Tomas Hospital, St. Luke's Medical Center College of Medicine, Manila, Philippines
Chapter 45: Systemic Lupus Erythematosus and Infections

Marie Wahren-Herlenius, MD, PhD
Rheumatology Unit, Department of Medicine, Karolinska Institute, Stockholm, Sweden
Chapter 37: Neonatal Lupus Erythematosus

Daniel J. Wallace, MD, FACP, FACR
Associate Director, Rheumatology Fellowship Program, Clinical Professor of Medicine, Cedars-Sinai Medical Center, David Geffen School of Medicine, University of California at Los Angeles, Los Angeles, California
Chapter 32: Management of Sjögren Syndrome in Patients with Systemic Lupus Erythematosus
Chapter 47: Principles of Therapy, Local Measures, and Nonsteroidal Medications
Chapter 51: Specialized Treatment Approaches and Niche Therapies for Lupus Subsets

Michael M. Ward, MD, MPH
Senior Investigator, National Institute of Arthritis and Musculoskeletal and Skin Diseases, National Institutes of Health, Bethesda, Maryland
Chapter 55: Socioeconomic and Disability Aspects

Michael H. Weisman, MD
Attending Physician, Division of Rheumatology, Professor in Residence, Cedars-Sinai Medical Center, David Geffen School of Medicine, University of California at Los Angeles, Los Angeles, California
Chapter 47: Principles of Therapy, Local Measures, and Nonsteroidal Medications

Victoria P. Werth, MD
Professor of Dermatology and Medicine, Department of Dermatology, University of Pennsylvania and Philadelphia VAMC, Philadelphia, Pennsylvania
Chapter 24: Skin Disease in Cutaneous Lupus Erythematosus

Sterling G. West, MD, MACP, FACR
Division of Rheumatology, University of Colorado School of Medicine, Aurora, Colorado
Chapter 29: Clinical Aspects of the Nervous System

Jinoos Yazdany, MD, MPH
Assistant Professor of Medicine, University of California, San Francisco, California
Chapter 1: Classification of Lupus and Lupus-Related Disorders

Yong-Rui Zou, PhD
Investigator, North Shore Long Island Jewish Health System, The Center for Autoimmune and Musculoskeletal Disease, Manhasset, New York
Chapter 8: The Structure and Derivation of Antibodies and Autoantibodies

Preface

HISTORIOGRAPHY, LUPUS AND ADVANCES IN RHEUMATIC DISEASE PUBLISHING (1966-2012)

In 1948, Edmund Dubois finished a pathology fellowship at the Los Angeles County General Hospital and was looking for a job. Although he had trained at Johns Hopkins, Parkland Hospital in Dallas and in Salt Lake City, he recently had married a local woman whose family was tied to the community, and knew that he could not leave Southern California. After several fits and starts in private practice settings, in 1950 Ed had a momentous meeting with Paul Starr, the chief of Internal Medicine at the general hospital. "We have 8 patients with a newly positive blood test known as the LE cell prep who have interesting clinical features, and it would be great if you could look into this" was all that he needed to know before accumulating 500 lupus patients by the mid-1960s.

First edition (1966): Dubois signed a contract with McGraw-Hill to publish the first monograph devoted to lupus erythematosus that appeared in 1966 and sold for $20. It was 479 pages with 183 figures and had 1500 references. He wrote 70% of the text, with Ian Mackay and Naomi Rothfield (who are still active in teaching and research) along with Peter Miescher covering most of the basic science sections.

Second edition (1974): After unsuccessful negotiations with McGraw-Hill to put out a second edition and an eight-year time lapse, with the permission of the university Ed established the University of Southern California Press and paid the Jeffries Banknote Company (which printed checks for banks) to publish the second edition. His wife and family bought booth space at medical meetings and sold the book, which was titled "Lupus Erythematosus: a Review of the Current Status of Discoid and Systemic Lupus Erythematosus and their Variants". It had 798 pages and 2975 alphabetized references and 11 of the 16 chapters were written by Dubois. Other notable authors included Ian Mackay, Larry Shulman, Sam Rapaport and Victor Pollack.

Second edition, revised (1976): Also self published, this edition included the 1974 edition unchanged and tagged on a supplement to each chapter with two year updates. It now had 3145 alphabetized references and over 200 black and white illustrations.

Third edition (1985): Dubois was diagnosed with myeloma in 1977 and Dan Wallace joined his practice in 1979. With the assistance of Larry Shulman, Lea &Febiger was signed on to publish the third edition after a 9-year interval. Dubois passed away just before this edition appeared, and the title was changed to "Dubois' Lupus Erythematosus". It was 770 pages long with alphabetized references (compiled by Mavis Cox who raised chickens and goats in urban Los Angeles and was a whiz with an Apple IIe computer) and new chapter authors included Bevra Hahn, Frank Arnett, and Peter Schur. Dubois insisted on being the sole author of 60% of the text which included all the clinical and treatment chapters, and its completion fell on Dr. Wallace's shoulders as he became increasingly impaired. Instructions to the authors were to include every peer review article ever written on their subject.

Fourth edition (1993): Bevra Hahn's arrival at UCLA and the cooperation of James Klinenberg and Frank Quismorio facilitated the first edition without any input from Ed Dubois. Now 955 pages (of which 320 were alphabetized references at the end), this Lea & Febiger publication had 64 chapters and 80 authors (all from North America and only 8 were women). Wallace and Hahn wrote 30% of the text.

Fifth edition (1997): The Lea's and Febiger's traced their bloodline to Marquis de Lafayette but the passing of their last descendents resulted in the family owned publishing company to be sold to Williams & Wilkins which published the fifth edition. Now containing 69 chapters and 1289 pages, the book was the first with color plates and without alphabetized references.

Sixth edition (2002): Lippincott purchased Williams & Wilkins and moved production back to Philadelphia from Baltimore. Containing 64 chapters, color plate and 1348 pages, this was the last edition where authors were encouraged to include every peer review article on the subject in their contributions. Although a solely North American effort, the number of female authors tripled from previous editions.

Seventh edition (2007): The internet, color printing, power point and on-line references (e.g. Pub Med) was starting to change the way physicians used medical textbooks. Wolters Kluwer purchased Lippincott and published the last "standard" type medical textbook of this revered genre. 1414 pages with 73 chapters, the 7th edition was the most comprehensive of all published ones, but trends toward shorter text, more illustrations and tables, and availability for quick reading online were increasingly driving the acquisition of medical information.

Eighth and current edition (2012): The editors were fortunate to partner with Elsevier and enter this reference into the 21st century. Significant changes in *Dubois* in this edition include the following:

a) internationalization of the text with authors outside of the United States and Canada representing a significant percentage of the monograph as well as the addition of an editor from China and two Europeans. The majority of authors are women.

b) availability of color figures and tables throughout the text and elimination of color plates;

c) Electronic access through Expert Consult and e-book platforms (www.expertconsult.com);

d) chapters represent a "current state of the art" (rather than a comprehensive compilation of every article published on the subject) written by experts in their field who can put the principal take home points into a reader-friendly, engaging context

e) "on-line" supplements not part of the print edition that contain additional references, tables and figures for readers interested in more erudite aspects of lupus

f) Dubois has now been renamed "Dubois Lupus Erythematosus and Related Disorders" to include sections on antiphospholipid syndrome, Sjogren's syndrome and related topics.

We hope that Dubois' will be a relevant and valuable resource to its loyal constituency which has supported disseminating information on lupus through 8 editions for 46 years.

Daniel J. Wallace MD
Bevra H. Hahn MD
Los Angeles, CA

Contents

Online Content (www.expertconsult.com)

Historical Background of Discoid and SLE

Patient Guide to Lupus Erythematosus

Worksheet for Lupus Metrics

WHAT IS LUPUS?

Definition and Classification of Lupus and Lupus-Related Disorders

Jinoos Yazdany and Maria Dall'Era

The goal of this chapter is to introduce the reader to the terminology and classification criteria associated with systemic lupus erythematosus (SLE) and lupus-related disorders. Classification criteria were originally developed as a means of defining a group of patients who could be studied in a systematic fashion. Criteria have provided a consistent way of classifying patients on the basis of descriptive characteristics and have improved the ability of researchers to categorize patients for the purpose of enrollment into clinical trials and observational studies. Criteria also serve as useful reminders of the wide variety of clinical features that can be seen in patients with SLE and lupus-related disorders and have helped organize the thinking of clinicians. Most sets of criteria are developed from a combination of expert opinion and statistical modeling, using the best evidence available at the time. As new information becomes available through research, criteria are often expanded upon and updated. Thus, one would expect criteria to evolve over time.

Importantly, classification criteria were never intended to be utilized for the diagnosis of individual patients. All of the criteria discussed within this chapter have imperfect sensitivity and specificity, and therefore should be used only as a guide in clinical practice. For example, a person without SLE but with an active viral infection might fulfill the classification criteria for SLE and, conversely, a patient with a positive ANA titer result and biopsy-proven lupus nephritis might not fulfill the criteria. If the criteria had been relied upon for the diagnosis of SLE, both of these patients would have been misdiagnosed. Experienced clinicians not uncommonly observe that some patients can evolve from meeting one set of classification criteria to another over the passage of time. In addition, some patients can have features of more than one connective tissue disease and are then believed to have an overlap syndrome.

Despite these caveats, the introduction and use of standardized classification criteria represent a significant scientific advance that has enabled high-quality clinical research. Moreover, as long as the caveats are noted, criteria can also be very useful for clinicians in systematically documenting key disease features. Here we review classification criteria for systemic lupus erythematosus and several related conditions, including cutaneous lupus, drug-induced lupus, mixed connective tissue disease, undifferentiated connective tissue disease, antiphospholipid antibody syndrome, and neonatal lupus.

SYSTEMIC LUPUS ERYTHEMATOSUS
Definition of SLE
Systemic lupus erythematosus is the prototypic systemic autoimmune disease characterized by heterogeneous, multisystem involvement and the production of an array of autoantibodies. Clinical features in individual patients can be quite variable, ranging from mild joint and skin involvement to severe, life-threatening internal organ disease. Lupus might be confined to the skin, without the presence of systemic involvement. There is no gold standard test for the diagnosis of SLE. Instead, the diagnosis rests on the judgment of an experienced clinician who recognizes the constellation of characteristic symptoms, signs, and laboratory findings in the appropriate clinical context, all other reasonable diagnoses having been excluded.

Development of the SLE Classification Criteria
The first classification criteria for SLE were developed by the American Rheumatism Association (ARA) in 1971.[1] The criteria were derived from a group of 245 patients with SLE contributed by 52 rheumatologists in the United States and Canada. The patients with SLE were compared with 234 patients who had rheumatoid arthritis (RA) and 217 patients without rheumatic disease. Out of 74 SLE manifestations reviewed, 14 were decided upon as the final criteria. Four or more of the 14 criteria had to be fulfilled in order for a person to be classified as having SLE. Importantly, the criteria could occur simultaneously or serially over any period. The final criteria heavily emphasized mucocutaneous features by including malar rash, discoid rash, photosensitivity, and oral ulcers as independent criteria. Notably, the criteria incorporated the presence of LE cells and a false-positive syphilis test result, but did not include tests for autoantibodies such as an antinuclear antibody (ANA) test and anti–double stranded DNA antibody (anti-dsDNA) because these tests were not widely in use at the time the criteria were developed. When tested in the population from which they were derived, the criteria were determined to have a sensitivity of 90% and a specificity of 99% against rheumatoid arthritis. After publication, the 1971 criteria became widely utilized. It has been estimated that approximately 90% of articles on SLE incorporated the criteria by 1978.[2]

In an effort to improve upon the 1971 criteria and incorporate new immunologic tests, the ARA commissioned a subcommittee in 1979 to update the 1971 criteria. The revised criteria for the classification of SLE were published in 1982.[3] As part of the revision process, the subcommittee scrutinized each of the original criteria, and new potential variables were put forward, such as serologic tests and skin and kidney histopathology. In the end, 30 potential variables were assessed. Eighteen academic investigators contributed 177 patients with SLE along with 162 age-, race-, and sex-matched controls with various other connective tissue diseases. The majority of the control patients had RA, with scleroderma being the second most common diagnosis. Cluster analysis and other techniques were used to analyze relationships between variables. Potential sets of criteria were tested on random subsets of patients from the case and control groups. After completion of the process, the final criteria were composed of 11 elements. Consistent with the 1971 criteria, a patient had to fulfill 4 out of 11 criteria in order to be classified as having SLE. Five of the elements were composites of more than one variable: serositis, renal disorder, neurologic disorder, hematologic disorder, and immunologic disorder. Repeated analyses determined that the four original mucocutaneous variables (malar rash, discoid rash, photosensitivity, and oral ulcerations) should remain as independent variables. Raynaud's phenomenon and alopecia were eliminated from the original criteria because of low sensitivity and specificity. The decision was made not to include skin and renal histopathology because it was the opinion of the investigators that those tests were infrequently performed. The arthritis criterion was revised to include the descriptor "nonerosive" and the necessity for more than two involved joints rather than more than one joint. The definition of proteinuria was altered from a threshold of >3.5 g/day in the 1971 criteria to >0.5 g/day in the revised criteria. The serologic tests for ANA, anti-DNA, and anti-Smith antibody (anti-Sm) were incorporated into the revised criteria. ANA was thought to be the strongest addition to the criteria because of its very high sensitivity, despite a relatively low specificity of 50%. The investigators decided not to include serum complement components because they did not improve accuracy. When tested in the population from which they were derived, the criteria had sensitivity and specificity values of 96%. When the criteria were tested against a separate population of patients with SLE, scleroderma, and dermato/polymyositis, the sensitivity was 83% and the specificity was 89%.

Over the years, several groups have studied the revised classification criteria in other patient populations. When studied in 156 patients with SLE from the University of Connecticut, the sensitivities of the original and revised criteria were 88% and 83%, respectively.[4] When the "nonerosive" aspect of the arthritis criterion was removed because hand radiographs were not available for all patients, the sensitivity of the revised criteria increased to 91%. The investigators of this study determined that both sets of criteria were more likely to be met in patients with a longer duration of disease. The same group later determined that the specificities of the preliminary and revised criteria were 98% and 99%, respectively, when tested in a group of 207 patients with other rheumatic diseases.[5] When the revised criteria were tested in SLE and control groups of Japanese patients, the sensitivity was 97% and specificity was 89%.[6] A study of 135 patients with SLE from Tehran demonstrated a sensitivity of 90% for the revised criteria.[7] Lastly, in a Zimbabwean study of 18 patients with the disease, the sensitivity of the revised criteria was 94%. When serologic elements were excluded, the sensitivity declined to 78%.[8]

In 1997, the criteria for the classification of SLE were revised for a second time in order to incorporate advancing knowledge about the association of antiphospholipid antibodies with SLE. Under the criterion "immunologic disorder," the decision was made to exclude LE cells and insert antiphospholipid antibodies. Antiphospholipid antibodies were defined as the presence of immunoglobulin (Ig) G or IgM anticardiolipin antibodies, a positive lupus anticoagulant test result, or a false-positive serologic syphilis test result (Table 1-1).[9] The changes reflected in the updated 1997 criteria were studied in an

TABLE 1-1 The 1997 Update of the 1982 Revised American College of Rheumatology Classification Criteria for SLE

CRITERION	DEFINITION
Malar rash	Fixed erythema, flat or raised, over the malar eminences, sparing the nasolabial folds
Discoid rash	Erythematous raised patches with adherent keratotic scale and follicular plugging; atrophic scarring may occur in older lesions
Photosensitivity	Skin rash as a result of unusual reaction to sunlight, by patient history or physician observation
Oral ulcers	Oral or nasopharyngeal ulceration, usually painless, observed by a physician
Arthritis	Nonerosive arthritis involving 2 or more peripheral joints, characterized by tenderness, swelling, or effusion
Serositis	Pleuritis—convincing history of pleuritic chest pain or rub heard by a physician or evidence of pleural effusions *or* Pericarditis—documented by electrocardiogram or rub or evidence of pericardial effusion
Renal disorder	Persistent proteinuria, either >0.5 g/day or >3+ if quantification not performed, *or* Cellular casts—may be red blood cell, hemoglobin, granular tubular, or mixed
Neurologic disorder	(a) Seizures—in the absence of offending drugs or known metabolic derangements (e.g., uremia, acidosis, or electrolyte imbalance) *or* (b) Psychosis—in the absence of offending drugs or known metabolic derangements (e.g., uremia, acidosis, or electrolyte imbalance)
Hematologic disorder	(a) Hemolytic anemia with reticulocytosis *or* (b) Leukopenia <4000/mm^3 *or* (c) Lymphopenia <1500/mm^3 *or* (d) Thrombocytopenia <100,000/mm^3 in the absence of offending drugs
Immunologic disorder	(a) Anti-DNA antibody—antibody to native DNA in abnormal titer *or* (b) Anti-Smith antibody—presence of antibody to Sm nuclear antigen *or* (c) Finding of antiphospholipid antibodies based on (1) abnormal serum concentration of immunoglobulin (Ig) G or IgM anticardiolipin antibodies, (2) positive test result for lupus anticoagulant using a standard method, or (3) false-positive serologic test result for syphilis known to be positive for at least 6 mo and confirmed by *Treponema pallidum* immobilization or fluorescent treponemal antibody absorption test
Positive antinuclear antibody test result	An abnormal titer of antinuclear antibody by immunofluorescence or an equivalent assay at any point in time and in the absence of drugs known to be associated with drug-induced lupus syndromes

The presence of 4 or more criteria is required for SLE classification. All other reasonable diagnoses must be excluded.

inception cohort of 154 patients with SLE in order to determine whether the replacement of LE cells with antiphospholipid antibodies would result in the selection of different groups of patients for inclusion in clinical studies.[10] From the cohort of 154 patients, 36 patients were selected who met four criteria, one of which was the immunologic disease element. When the LE cell criterion was removed from the patients, 2 of 36 were no longer classified as having SLE. Both of these patients tested negative for anticardiolipin antibodies and lupus anticoagulant. To assess the impact of the addition of the anticardiolipin antibodies and lupus anticoagulant criteria, the investigators evaluated those patients who tested positive for anticardiolipin antibodies or lupus anticoagulant, but negative for LE cells. Only 1 patient was identified. Thus, the investigators determined that this alteration in the immunologic criterion would not result in a significant change in the patients classified as having SLE in their cohort. Going forward, it will be important to more fully study and validate the 1997 revised criteria in other cohorts of patients with SLE and related rheumatologic diseases.

Constraints of the Current SLE Classification Criteria

Despite the fact that the 1997 revised criteria are widely accepted and utilized, several limitations affect their use in clinical practice. SLE can involve virtually any organ system with heterogeneous manifestations; however, only a relatively few potential manifestations are represented in the criteria. In addition, some of the manifestations might be confused with common mimickers. For example, the criteria of malar rash and photosensitivity can be troublesome for clinicians because several common conditions closely mimic these findings. Acne rosacea and flushing can appear similar to a lupus malar rash, and polymorphous light eruption can simulate photosensitivity. The potential difficulty in interpreting malar rash and photosensitivity might lead to decreased specificity of those criteria. The serositis criterion includes pleuritis and pericarditis but not peritonitis. Arthritis is defined as "nonerosive," implying that a radiograph has been taken. In routine clinical evaluations for SLE, however, hand radiographs are rarely performed. Proteinuria, defined as serum protein higher than 0.5 g/day, and urinary cellular casts are the only two renal criteria. Because many clinical laboratories do not routinely report cellular casts, the usefulness of this criterion is unclear. Notably, a positive renal biopsy result is not included in the criteria. It is possible for a patient with biopsy-proven lupus nephritis to not meet the necessary four criteria for classification as having SLE. Although there are a variety of ways in which SLE can affect the central and peripheral nervous system, psychosis and seizures are the only two manifestations included in the classification criteria. The hematologic criterion is categorized into the four subcomponents of hemolytic anemia, leukopenia, lymphopenia, and thrombocytopenia. Leukopenia and lymphopenia must be present on at least two occasions. The criteria do not specify how leukopenia and lymphopenia secondary to medications should be differentiated from those due to SLE.

Future Directions

Because of the limitations of the criteria as previously described, there has been a concerted effort by the Systemic Lupus International Collaborative Clinics (SLICC) group to further revise the ACR classification criteria.[11] During this process, patient scenarios from 716 patients with SLE and control patients were submitted by the SLICC members, and a consensus diagnosis was established for each scenario. The group identified those variables that were most predictive of SLE, and a classification rule was derived on the basis of multiple potential predictor variables. Although this effort is still a work in progress, 11 clinical and 6 immunologic elements have been selected for inclusion in the SLICC revision of the classification criteria. A patient is classified as having SLE if he or she (1) has biopsy-proven lupus nephritis with a positive ANA or anti–double-stranded DNA antibody test result or (2) fulfills four of the criteria including at least

one clinical criterion and one immunologic criterion. Thus, one of the ways in which the classification of SLE by the SLICC criteria differs from that of the ACR criteria is by allowing for the stand-alone criterion biopsy-proven lupus nephritis. This alteration corrects a notable problem with the ACR criteria, in which a patient with biopsy-proven lupus nephritis might not meet enough criteria to be classified as having SLE. Also, counter to the ACR criteria, the SLICC criteria require at least one clinical element and one immunologic element for this classification. A patient cannot be classified as having SLE on the basis of purely clinical features. The SLICC criteria significantly expand upon the dermatologic elements by including various types of acute, subacute, and chronic cutaneous lupus lesions, as opposed to the ACR criteria inclusion of only malar rash and discoid rash. Photosensitivity has been removed, and nonscarring alopecia has been added. In the arthritis criterion, the term "inflammatory synovitis" has been substituted for "nonerosive arthritis." In addition to the original seizures and psychosis elements, the new neurologic criterion incorporates several other neurologic manifestations of SLE, such as mononeuritis multiplex, myelitis, peripheral or cranial neuropathy, and acute confusional state. Within the group of immunologic criteria, low complement levels and positive direct Coombs test result in the absence of hemolytic anemia have been added. At the time of the writing of this chapter, the SLICC criteria were undergoing finalization and validation. It remains to be seen whether these criteria will eventually replace the ACR classification criteria.

CHRONIC CUTANEOUS LUPUS

Cutaneous lupus lesions have traditionally been divided into two broad categories: lupus-specific lesions and lupus-nonspecific lesions.[12] Lupus-specific lesions are distinguished from lupus-nonspecific lesions by the presence in the former of the histopathologic finding of interface dermatitis, which is defined as inflammatory cell infiltrates in the dermoepidermal junction. Chronic cutaneous lupus erythematosus (CCLE) is a type of lupus-specific lesion lasting for months to years that can lead to scar and atrophy. The most common subtype of CCLE is discoid lupus erythematosus (DLE), which can occur either in the context of SLE or as a process limited to the skin. DLE lesions are characterized by discrete, erythematous, hyperkeratotic plaques that are coin shaped, or *discoid,* in appearance. With progression of the lesions, follicular plugging (dilated follicles filled with keratin) and scarring alopecia can occur. By definition, localized DLE is confined to the head and neck, and generalized DLE occurs above and below the neck. CCLE can occur as a distinct isolated entity or as a manifestation of systemic lupus. One study of 161 patients demonstrated that the classification criteria for SLE were present in 28% of patients with any form of discoid lupus and in 6% with localized discoid lupus confined to the head and neck.[13]

DRUG-INDUCED LUPUS ERYTHEMATOSUS

Drug-induced lupus erythematosus (DIL) is a subset of lupus defined as a lupus-like syndrome that develops in temporal relation to exposure to a drug and resolves after cessation of the drug exposure. DIL was initially described in 1945 following treatment with sulfadiazine.[14] Since that time, DIL has been associated with more than 80 different medications, the best known being hydralazine and procainamide. Minocycline, hydrochlorothiazide, angiotensin converting enzyme inhibitors, and anti–tumor necrosis factor agents have also been implicated. The presentation of DIL varies from systemic involvement to disease limited to the skin. Clinical features of DIL with systemic involvement differ from those that occur in SLE. Notably, DIL is characterized by the presence of fever, arthralgia/arthritis, myalgia, and serositis; internal organ involvement, such as lupus nephritis and central nervous system disease, is rare. Classic cutaneous lesions of SLE such as malar rash and discoid rash are rare in DIL. Lastly, although SLE has a striking female predominance, DIL has a more equal female-to-male distribution. Antinuclear antibodies are universally present and antihistone antibodies are detectable in

TABLE 1-2 Comparison of Diagnostic Criteria Proposed for Mixed Connective Tissue Disease (MCTD)

	Proposed Criteria			
	ALARCON-SEGOVIA AND VILLAREAL[19]	**KAHN AND APPELBOOM**[20]	**KASUKAWA ET AL.**[21]	**SHARP**[22]
Serologic criteria(on)	Anti-RNP antibodies with titer ≥1:1600	High titer anti-RNP corresponding to a speckled-pattern ANA titer ≥1:2000	Presence of anti–U1-RNP	Highest observed anti-ENA titer ≥1:10,000, and anti–U1-RNP positive and anti-Smith negative responses (major criteria)
Clinical criteria	Edema of hands Synovitis Myositis Raynaud's phenomenon Acrosclerosis	Swollen fingers Synovitis Myositis Raynaud's phenomenon	**Common Symptoms** • Raynaud's phenomenon • Swollen fingers or hands **Mixed Findings** **A. *SLE-Like*** • Polyarthritis • Pericarditis/pleuritis • Lymphadenopathy • Malar rash • Leukopenia/thrombocytopenia **B. *Scleroderma-Like*** • Sclerodactyly • Pulmonary fibrosis • Esophageal dysmotility **C. *Polymyositis-Like*** • Muscle weakness • High creatinine phosphokinase • Myogenic pattern on electromyogram	**Major Criteria** • Myositis, severe • Pulmonary involvement • Raynaud's phenomenon or esophageal hypomotility • Swollen hands (observed) or sclerodactyly • Serologic criteria above **Minor Criteria** • Alopecia • Leukopenia • Anemia • Pleuritis • Pericarditis • Arthritis • Trigeminal neuropathy • Malar rash • Thrombocytopenia • Myositis, mild • Swollen hands or history of swollen hands
Diagnosis	Serologic criteria plus 3 of 5 clinical criteria required; *if hand edema, Raynaud's phenomenon, and acrosclerosis present, at least one of the other two criteria is also required*	Serologic criterion plus 3 of 4 clinical criteria (which must include Raynaud's phenomenon) required	Serologic criterion plus at least one common symptom and one or more findings in at least two of three clinical categories (A, B, or C)	*Definite MCTD:* 4 major criteria and serologic criteria *Probable MCTD:* 3 major criteria and serologic criteria *or* 2 major criteria and 2 minor criteria *Possible MCTD:* 3 major criteria *or* 2 major criteria and serologic criteria *or* 1 major and 3 minor and serologic criteria

ANA, antinuclear antibody; ENA, extractable nuclear antigen; MCTD, mixed connective tissue disease; RNP, ribonucleoprotein.

75% of patients with DIL. In contrast, anti-DNA and/or anti-Smith antibodies rarely occur.

Although there are no formal criteria for the diagnosis or classification of DIL, the following features should be present:
• Treatment with the suspected drug for at least 1 month's duration.
• Symptoms such as arthralgia, myalgia, fever, and serositis should be present.
• ANA and antihistone antibodies are present in the absence of other subserologic findings.
• Symptoms should improve within days to weeks of drug discontinuation.

MIXED CONNECTIVE TISSUE DISEASE

In 1972, Sharp and colleagues[15] published a report describing a series of patients with features of SLE, systemic sclerosis, and polymyositis who were found to have high titers of a distinct autoantibody to ribonucleoprotein. This antibody was later found to be anti–U1-RNP[16] and was present universally in those patients the researchers defined as having the clinical syndrome mixed connective tissue disease (MCTD) but also present in approximately 30% of the patients with SLE.

In the ensuing decades, several attempts to develop diagnostic criteria for MCTD were undertaken, although there remains no universally agreed-upon definition. Moreover, whether MCTD should be thought of as a distinct clinical entity, or merely a subcategory of another condition such as SLE or systemic sclerosis, remains a matter of debate.[17,18] Despite this controversy, identifying patients with MCTD can be useful in clinical practice because of the higher

incidence in this disorder of important end-organ manifestations that may require monitoring, including pulmonary hypertension, interstitial lung disease, and esophageal hypomotility.

Several sets of criteria for MCTD have been proposed, and those reported by Alarcon-Segovia and Villareal,[19] Kahn and Apelboom,[20] Kasukawa and associates,[21] and Sharp[22] are presented in Table 1-2. Common to all of the criteria are the following features:
• Presence of anti–U1-RNP antibodies
• Swelling of the hands or fingers
• Synovitis
• Myalgia or myositis
• Raynaud's phenomenon

Although the presence of anti–U1-RNP antibodies is key for all proposed criteria (and mandatory in all but Sharp's[22] criteria), the numbers and types of clinical features required differ. For example, the criteria proposed by Alarcon-Segovia and Villareal,[19] which are the most widely used, require assessment of only five clinical features. These criteria are therefore efficient for use in clinical practice. In contrast, the criteria described by Kasukawa and associates[21] are more detailed, and 13 separate clinical features are listed. To some extent, the multiple sets of conflicting criteria reflect how difficult it has been to precisely define the disease. Several groups have attempted to compare the sensitivity and specificity of the different criteria.[23-25] In 1989, Alarcon-Segovia and Cardiel[23] compared different sets of criteria for MCTD (Alarcon-Segovia, Kasukawa, and Sharp) in a large population of patients with various connective tissue diseases, including MCTD (n = 80), rheumatoid arthritis (n = 100), scleroderma (n = 80), dermato/polymyositis (n = 53), and Sjögren syndrome (n = 80). The Alarcon-Segovia criteria outperformed the others, but this study was limited because it involved the same cohort of patients on which the original Alarcon-Segovia criteria had been developed. In 1996, Amigues and colleagues[25] reported that in their clinical cohort of 45 patients with anti–U1-RNP antibodies in Toulouse, the Alarcon-Segovia and Kahn criteria had better specificity (86.2%) for identifying MCTD than the two other criteria examined (Sharp and Kasukawa) but that the Sharp criteria had better sensitivity (100% versus 62.5%).[25] Sensitivity of the Alarcon-Segovia criteria increased to 81.3% with no decrease in specificity if "myalgia" was substituted for "myositis."

Regardless of the criteria used, it is important to note that early in the course of their disease, patients with MCTD may be difficult to identify because the characteristic clinical features of SLE, systemic sclerosis, and polymyositis are rarely present.[26] Instead, most patients present with less specific features of connective tissue disease, such as fatigue, arthralgias, and Raynaud's phenomenon. Vigilance for the development of additional disease features, particularly in patients with high titers of speckled-pattern ANA, puffy hands, and anti–U1-RNP antibodies, is therefore required. The timely identification of patients with MCTD can assist in directing appropriate clinical monitoring, such as periodic echocardiography and pulmonary function testing.

UNDIFFERENTIATED CONNECTIVE TISSUE DISEASE AND OVERLAP SYNDROMES

Many patients fulfill one discrete set of classification criteria for connective tissue disease, but others may have features of two or more diseases. Alternatively, some may not meet criteria for any specific disease. Those meeting criteria for two or more diseases are described as having an *overlap syndrome,* such as the overlap of rheumatoid arthritis and SLE, sometimes referred to as *rhupus.*[27] Those who have some features of connective tissue disease but who cannot be definitively classified are designated as having undifferentiated connective tissue disease (UCTD).

Overlap syndromes involving almost all connective tissue diseases have been described; patients may simultaneously fulfill two or more classification criteria for conditions such as SLE, systemic sclerosis, dermato/polymyositis, rheumatoid arthritis, Sjögren syndrome and antiphospholipid antibody syndrome. In patients meeting two or more sets of classification criteria, the primary importance of designating an overlap syndrome is to direct clinical evaluation and management for each of the identified conditions. For example, a patient with features of SLE and rheumatoid arthritis will need careful monitoring for important features of SLE, such as renal disease, and for features of rheumatoid arthritis, such as progression of erosive joint disease.

In contrast, the primary importance of noting that a patient's clinical presentation remains undifferentiated is to ensure that a diagnosis is not assigned prematurely. This strategy prevents heuristic clinical decision making, avoids unnecessary psychological distress for patients because in many patients UCTD does not progress over time, and alerts the clinician to maintain vigilance for the development of new signs and symptoms during follow-up. Most studies suggest that only one third of patients with UCTD demonstrate a defined syndrome over time. SLE is the most common syndrome that evolves, but a variety of others, including rheumatoid arthritis, systemic sclerosis, dermato/polymyositis, MCTD, and vasculitis, have been described.[28-32] In general, studies suggest that those cases that progress do so early after presentation, most often in the first 3 to 5 years.[33] In the remaining 70% of patients, UCTD remains stable over time, and they are generally thought to have mild disease and a good prognosis.

Preliminary classification criteria for this latter group of patients, referred to as having "stable" UCTD, have been proposed as follows[34]:
- Signs and symptoms suggestive of a connective tissue disease, but not fulfilling criteria for a defined disease
- Presence of ANAs
- Disease duration of at least 3 years

These criteria attempt to delineate the large group of patients whose disease is likely to remain undifferentiated and who therefore might be distinguished from those with very early undifferentiated disease (<3 years) who require close monitoring for progression, and those with overlap syndromes. Although these criteria require further study, their application in research studies may further elucidate the epidemiology, prognosis, and proper clinical monitoring of patients with stable UCTD.

ANTIPHOSPHOLIPID ANTIBODY SYNDROME

Antiphospholipid antibody syndrome (APS) is an autoimmune syndrome with heterogeneous clinical and serologic manifestations. It may occur as an isolated entity (primary APS) or may be associated with another autoimmune disease such as SLE (secondary APS). The major manifestations of primary and secondary APS are similar, and the two subtypes are characterized in a similar manner. An international consensus conference held in Sapporo, Japan, in 1999 developed the initial classification criteria for APS.[35] These criteria were then revised during a second consensus conference in Sydney, Australia, and were subsequently published in 2006 (Box 1-1).[36] The criteria defined APS as the presence of one clinical criterion and one laboratory criterion. The clinical criterion includes evidence of a vascular thrombosis (arterial, venous, or small vessel) or pregnancy morbidity (fetal loss). Pregnancy morbidly is defined as (1) one or more unexplained deaths of a morphologically normal fetus at more than 10 weeks' gestation, (2) one or more premature births before the 34th week of gestation due to preeclampsia/eclampsia or placental insufficiency, or (3) three or more consecutive spontaneous abortions before the 10th week of gestation. The laboratory criterion includes the presence of (1) anticardiolipin antibodies of IgG or IgM isotype, (2) lupus anticoagulant, or (3) anti–β_2 glycoprotein I antibodies of IgG or IgM isotype. All antibodies must be present on two or more occasions at least 12 weeks apart. It is important to note that several clinical manifestations and serologic findings that have been associated with APS are not included in the classification criteria. Such clinical manifestations include, but are not limited to, thrombocytopenia, cardiac valvular disease, livedo reticularis, and seizures. Examples of laboratory abnormalities not included in the criteria are IgA anticardiolipin antibodies and antibodies to prothrombin and annexin.

NEONATAL LUPUS

Antibodies to SSA/Ro and ssB/La are common in women with SLE, with estimated lifetime incidences of 67% and 49%, respectively. The transit of these antibodies passively through the placenta can induce a neonatal lupus syndrome. Manifestations can include congenital heart block in the fetus and photosensitive rash, cytopenias, or hepatic abnormalities in the newborn. The incidence of congenital heart block in offspring of seropositive women has been estimated to be between 2% and 5%, and the risk increases to approximately 16% to 25% when a seropositive mother has previously given birth to a child with congenital heart block.[37-42]

There are currently no specific diagnostic criteria for neonatal lupus. The diagnosis is made when characteristic manifestations occur in the fetus or infant and the mother is found to have anti-SSA/Ro (anti–Sjögren syndrome antigen A) and/or anti-SSB/La (anti–Sjögren syndrome antigen B) antibodies. In women with known anti-SSA/Ro and/or anti-ssB/La antibodies, careful screening during pregnancy and in the postpartum period can ensure timely diagnosis. Often, however, neonatal diagnosis is made when characteristic manifestations occur in a fetus or infant whose mother was not previously known to have an autoimmune disease but on testing is found to have anti-SSA/Ro and/or anti-SSB/La antibodies.

SUMMARY

The definitions of SLE and lupus-related disorders presented in this chapter lay the foundation for the extensive discussion of these disorders throughout the remainder of this textbook. Although initially

Box 1-1 Revised Classification Criteria for the Antiphospholipid Antibody Syndrome

Antiphospholipid antibody syndrome (APS) is present if at least one of the clinical criteria and one of the laboratory criteria that follow are met:*

Clinical Criteria

1. Vascular thrombosis[†]: One or more clinical episodes[‡] of arterial, venous, or small vessel thrombosis,[§] in any tissue or organ. Thrombosis must be confirmed by objective validated criteria (i.e., unequivocal findings of appropriate imaging studies or histopathology). For histopathologic confirmation, thrombosis should be present without significant evidence of inflammation in the vessel wall.
2. Pregnancy morbidity:
   (a) One or more instances of unexplained death of a morphologically normal fetus at or beyond the 10th week of gestation, with normal fetal morphology documented by ultrasound or by direct examination of the fetus, *or*
   (b) One or more instances of premature birth of a morphologically normal neonate before the 34th week of gestation because of: (i) eclampsia or severe preeclampsia defined according to standard definitions, or (ii) recognized features of placental insufficiency,[‖] *or*
   (c) Three or more unexplained consecutive spontaneous abortions before the 10th week of gestation, with maternal

anatomic or hormonal abnormalities and paternal and maternal chromosomal causes excluded.

In studies of populations of patients who have more than one type of pregnancy morbidity, investigators are strongly encouraged to stratify groups of subjects according to *a, b,* or *c* above.

Laboratory Criteria[¶]

1. Lupus anticoagulant (LA) present in plasma, on two or more occasions at least 12 weeks apart, detected according to the guidelines of the International Society on Thrombosis and Haemostasis, Scientific Subcommittee on Lupus Anticoagulant/Antiphospholipid Antibody.
2. Anticardiolipin (aCL) antibody of immunoglobulin (Ig) G and/or IgM isotype in serum or plasma, present in medium or high titer (i.e., >40 G or M, or >99th percentile), on two or more occasions, at least 12 weeks apart, measured by a standardized enzyme-linked immunosorbent assay (ELISA).
3. Anti–β_2 glycoprotein I antibody of IgG and/or IgM isotype in serum or plasma (in titer >99th percentile), present on two or more occasions, at least 12 weeks apart, measured by a standardized ELISA, according to recommended procedures.

*Classification of APS should be avoided if less than 12 weeks or more than 5 years separate the positive antiphospholipid antibody (aPL) test result and the clinical manifestation.

[†]Coexisting inherited or acquired factors for thrombosis are not reasons for excluding patients from APS trials. However, two subgroups of patients with APS should be recognized, according to (a) the presence and (b) the absence of additional risk factors for thrombosis. Indicative (not an exhaustive list) factors include: age (>55 yr in men and >65 yr in women) and the presence of any of the established risk factors for cardiovascular disease (hypertension, diabetes mellitus, elevated low-density lipoprotein LDL or low high-density lipoprotein cholesterol value, cigarette smoking, family history of premature cardiovascular disease, body mass index ≥30 kg m^{-2}, microalbuminuria, estimated glomerular filtration rate <60 mL min^{-1}), inherited thrombophilias, oral contraceptives, nephritic syndrome, malignancy, immobilization, and surgery. Thus, patients who fulfill criteria for APS trials should be stratified according to contributing causes of thrombosis.

[‡]A thrombotic episode in the past could be considered a clinical criterion, provided that thrombosis is proved by appropriate diagnostic means and that no alternative diagnosis or cause of thrombosis is found.

[§]Superficial venous thrombosis is not included in the clinical criteria.

[‖]Generally accepted features of placental insufficiency include: (i) abnormal or nonreassuring fetal surveillance test result(s), e.g., a nonreactive non-stress test response, suggestive of fetal hypoxemia, (ii) abnormal Doppler flow velocimetry waveform analysis suggestive of fetal hypoxemia, e.g., absence of end-diastolic flow in the umbilical artery, (iii) oligohydramnios, e.g., an amniotic fluid index of 5 cm or less, or (iv) a postnatal birth weight less than the 10th percentile for the gestational age.

[¶]Investigators are strongly advised to classify patients with APS in studies into one of the following categories: I, more than one laboratory criterion present (any combination); IIa, LA present alone; IIb, aCL antibody present alone; IIc, anti–β_2 glycoprotein I antibody present alone.

Modified from Miyakis S, Lockshin, MD, Atsumi T, et al: International consensus statement on an update of the classification criteria for definite antiphospholipid syndrome (APS). *J Thromb Haemost* 4:295-306, 2006.

designed for the goal of categorizing patients for enrollment into clinical studies, the formulation of classification criteria for SLE and related disorders has served to organize the thinking of clinicians and students as they encounter patients with potential connective tissue disorders. Although these various sets of criteria should not be relied upon for the diagnosis of individual patients, they can serve as useful guides as clinicians grapple with the complexity of these disorders.

References

1. Cohen AS, Reynolds WE, Franklin EC, et al: Preliminary criteria for the classification of systemic lupus erythematosus. *Bull Rheum Dis* 21:643–648, 1971.
2. Canoso JJ, Cohen AS: A review of the use, evaluations, and criticisms of the preliminary criteria for the classification of systemic lupus erythematosus. *Arthritis Rheum* 22:917–921, 1979.
3. Tan EM, Cohen AS, Fries J, et al: The 1982 revised criteria for the classification of systemic lupus erythematosus. *Arthritis Rheum* 25:1271–1277, 1982.
4. Levin RE, Weinstein A, Peterson M, et al: A comparison of the sensitivity of the 1971 and 1982 American Rheumatism Association criteria for the classification of systemic lupus erythematosus. *Arthritis Rheum* 27:530–528, 1984.
5. Passas CM, Wong RL, Peterson M, et al: A comparison of the specificity of the 1971 and 1982 American Rheumatism Association criteria for the classification of systemic lupus erythematosus. *Arthritis Rheum* 28:620–623, 1985.
6. Yokohari R, Tsunematsu T: Application, to Japanese patients, of the 1982 American Rheumatism Association revised criteria for the classification of systemic lupus erythematosus. *Arthritis Rheum* 28:693–698, 1985.
7. Davatchi F, Chams C, Akbarian M: Evaluation of the 1982 American Rheumatism Association revised criteria for the classification of systemic lupus erythematosus (letter). *Arthritis Rheum* 28:715, 1985.
8. Davis P, Stein M: Evaluation of criteria for the classification of SLE in Zimbabwean patients (letter). *Br J Rheum* 28:546–547, 1989.
9. Hochberg MC, for the Diagnostic and Therapeutic Criteria Committee of the American College of Rheumatology: Updating the American College of Rheumatology revised criteria for the classification of systemic lupus erythematosus letter. *Arthritis Rheum* 40:1725, 1997.
10. Feletar M, Ibanez D, Urowitz MB, et al: Concise communications: the impact of the 1997 update of the American College of Rheumatology revised criteria for the classification of systemic lupus erythematosus: what has been changed? *Arthritis Rheum* 48:2067–2068, 2003.
11. Petri M, Systemic Lupus International Collaborating Clinic (SLICC): SLICC revision of the ACR classification criteria for SLE [abstract]. *Arthritis Rheum Abstract* 60(Suppl 10):895, 2009.
12. Sontheimer RD: The lexicon of cutaneous lupus erythematosus—a review and personal perspective on the nomenclature and classification of the cutaneous manifestations of lupus erythematosus. *Lupus* 6:84–95, 1997.
13. Watanabe T, Tsuchida T: Classification of lupus erythematosus based upon cutaneous manifestations. Dermatologic, systemic, and laboratory features in 191 patients. *Dermatology* 190(4):277–283, 1995.
14. Katz U, Zandman-Goddard G: Drug-induced lupus: an update. *Autoimmun Rev* 10:46–50, 2010.
15. Sharp GC, Irvin WS, Tan EM, et al: Mixed connective tissue disease–an apparently distinct rheumatic disease syndrome associated with a specific

antibody to an extractable nuclear antigen (ENA). *Am J Med* 52(2):148–159, 1972 Feb.

16. Pettersson I, Wang G, Smith EI, et al: The use of immunoblotting and immunoprecipitation of (U) small nuclear ribonucleoproteins in the analysis of sera of patients with mixed connective tissue disease and systemic lupus erythematosus: a cross-sectional, longitudinal study. *Arthritis Rheum* 29:986–996, 1986.

17. Aringer M, Steiner G, Smolen JS: Does mixed connective tissue disease exist? Yes. *Rheum Dis Clin North Am* 31:411–420, 2005.

18. Swanton J, Isenberg D: Mixed connective tissue disease: still crazy after all these years. *Rheum Dis Clin North Am* 31:421–436, 2005.

19. Alarcon-Segovia D, Villareal M: Classification and diagnostic criteria for mixed connective tissue disease. In Kasukawa R, Sharp GC, editors: *Mixed connective tissue disease and antinuclear antibodies*, Amsterdam, 1987, Elsevier, pp 33–40.

20. Kahn MF, Appelboom T: Syndrome de Sharp. In Kahn MF, Peltier AP, Mayer O, Piette JC, editors: *Les maladies systémiques*, ed 3, Paris, 1991, Flammarion, pp 545–556.

21. Kasukawa R, Tojo T, Miyawaki S: Preliminary diagnostic criteria for classification of mixed connective tissue disease. In Kasukawa R, Sharp GC, editors: *Mixed connective tissue disease and antinuclear antibodies*, Amsterdam, 1987, Elsevier, pp 41–47.

22. Sharp GC: Diagnostic criteria for classification of MCTD. In Kasukawa R, Sharp GC, editors: *Mixed connective tissue disease and antinuclear antibodies*, Amsterdam, 1987, Elsevier, pp 23–30.

23. Alarcon-Segovia D, Cardiel MH: Comparison between 3 diagnostic criteria for mixed connective tissue disease. Study of 593 patients. *J Rheumatol* 16(3):328–334, 1989.

24. Doria A, Ghirardello A, de Zambiasi P, et al: Japanese diagnostic criteria for mixed connective tissue disease in Caucasian patients. *J Rheumatol* 19(2):259–264, 1992 Feb.

25. Amigues JM, Cantagrel A, Abbal M, et al: Comparative study of 4 diagnosis criteria sets for mixed connective tissue disease in patients with anti-RNP antibodies. Autoimmunity Group of the Hospitals of Toulouse. *J Rheumatol* 23(12):2055–2062, 1996.

26. Sullivan WD, Hurst DJ, Harmon CE, et al: A prospective evaluation emphasizing pulmonary involvement in patients with mixed connective tissue disease. *Medicine Baltimore* 63:92–107, 1984.

27. Panush RS, Edwards NL, Longley S, et al: "Rhupus" syndrome. *Arch Intern Med* 148(7):1633, 1988.

28. Williams HJ, Alarcon GS, Joks R, et al: Early undifferentiated tissue disease. VI. An inception cohort after 10 years: disease remissions and changes in diagnoses in well established and undifferentiated CTD. *J Rheumatol* 26:816–825, 1999.

29. Mosca M, Neri R, Bencivelli W, et al: Undifferentiated connective tissue disease: analysis of 83 patients with a minimum follow up of 5 years. *J Rheumatol* 29:2345–2349, 2002.

30. Calvo-Alen J, Alarcon GS, Burgard SL, et al: Systemic lupus erythematosus: predictors of its occurrence among a cohort of patients with early undifferentiated connective tissue disease: multivariate analyses and identification of risk factors. *J Rheumatol* 23:469–475, 1996.

31. Bodolay E, Csiki Z, Szekanecz Z, et al: Five-year follow-up of 665 Hungarian patients with undifferentiated connective tissue disease (UCTD). *Clin Exp Rheumatol* 21:313–320, 2003.

32. Danieli MG, Fraticelli P, Franceschini F, et al: Five- year follow-up of 165 Italian patients with undifferentiated connective tissue diseases. *Clin Exp Rheumatol* 17:585–591, 1999.

33. Mosca M, Tani C, Bombardieri S: Undifferentiated connective tissue diseases (UCTD): a new frontier for rheumatology. *Best Pract Res Clin Rheumatol* 21(6):1011, 2007.

34. Mosca M, Neri R, Bombardieri S: Undifferentiated connective tissue diseases (UCTD): a review of the literature and a proposal for preliminary classification criteria. *Clin Exp Rheumatol* 17:615–620, 1999.

35. Wilson WA, Gharavi AE, Koike T, et al: International consensus statement on preliminary classification criteria for definite antiphospholipid syndrome: report of an international workshop. *Arthritis Rheum* 42(7):1309–1311, 1999.

36. Miyakis S, Lockshin, MD, Atsumi T, et al: International consensus statement on an update of the classification criteria for definite antiphospholipid syndrome APS. *J Thromb Haemost* 4:295–306, 2006.

37. Brucato A, Frassi M, Franceschini F, et al: Risk of congenital complete heart block in newborns of mothers with anti-Ro/SSA antibodies detected by counterimmunoelectropho resis: a prospective study of 100 women. *Arthritis Rheum* 44:1832–1835, 2001.

38. Buyon JP, Hiebert R, Copel J, et al: Autoimmune-associated congenital heart block: mortality, morbidity, and recurrence rates obtained from a national neonatal lupus registry. *J Am Coll Cardiol* 31:1658–1666, 1998.

39. Cimaz R, Spence DL, Hornberger L, et al: Incidence and spectrum of neonatal lupus erythematosus: a prospective study of infants born to mothers with anti-Ro autoantibodies. *J Pediatr* 142:678–683, 2003.

40. Julkunen H, Eronen M: The rate of recurrence of isolated congenital heart block: a population-based study. *Arthritis Rheum* 44:487–488, 2001.

41. Motta M, Rodriguez-Perez C, Tincani A, et al: Outcome of infants from mothers with anti-SSA/Ro antibodies. *J Perinatol* 27:278–283, 2007.

42. Gerosa M, Cimaz R, Stramba-Badiale M, et al: Electrocardiographic abnormalities in infants born from mothers with autoimmune diseases—a multicentre prospective study. *Rheumatology* 46:1285–1289, 2007.

Chapter 2

The Epidemiology of Lupus

S. Sam Lim and Cristina Drenkard

Epidemiology is the study of the frequency and distribution of disease and the determinants associated with disease occurrence and outcome in populations. The term "epidemiology" is used in a variety of descriptive settings. However, epidemiology is, at its core, an exercise in counting. It seeks to thoroughly identify and count people with a disease in a particular place at a particular time, a true population-based assessment. This chapter focuses primarily on the epidemiology of SLE and cutaneous lupus as defined by incidence and prevalence rates, which vary greatly. In order to interpret these disparate rates, this chapter first reviews the fundamentals of epidemiologic methods as they particularly pertain to lupus. It concludes with an overview of environmental studies using various epidemiologic techniques.

THE FUNDAMENTALS OF EPIDEMIOLOGY

The earliest reports on SLE were based on clinical and pathologic experiences from relatively small numbers that distinguished the disorder from other connective tissue diseases and established a relationship to such factors as age and sex, photosensitivity, trauma, surgery, infection, and chemotherapy.[1] Population studies of SLE were felt to be more feasible in the early 1950s with the advent of the LE cell test, a serologic test that was hoped to have the ability to identify cases uniformly or without characteristic features. Reliance on the LE cell test to diagnose SLE began to diminish after a few years as its poor specificity was better appreciated[2] and its lack of sensitivity to identify the broad spectrum of SLE patients became evident. To this day, a widely available test that is both sensitive and specific for SLE on a population level does not exist. Nevertheless, many studies have attempted to define the frequency of disease.

Discrepancies in rates are in part due to the inherent disparities of SLE (i.e., higher rates in certain ethnic groups). However, interpretation of rates should also take into account differences in the methodology used to determine these rates. These differences exist not only across different countries and health care systems but also within the same country. In the determination and comparison of incidence and prevalence rates, three fundamental issues must be addressed:
1. Case definition
2. Case ascertainment
3. Population at risk

Case Definition

How cases are defined is essential to a study's interpretation and comparability to other studies. The "gold standard" for diagnosing SLE is by clinical assessment from an experienced clinician (i.e., a rheumatologist), which is often impractical for population-based studies. However, relatively smaller geographical areas with a unified health care system are particularly amenable to this type of approach.

Classification criteria are designed to provide consistency across study populations and are appropriate for epidemiologic purposes. Several exist for SLE.[3] The most universally accepted criteria have been those endorsed by the American College of Rheumatology (ACR). The former American Rheumatism Association, now known

as the ACR, established the first classification criteria for SLE in 1971. These criteria, which included the LE cell test, allowed for standardized classification of patients. The earliest studies adhered generally to the 1971 criteria but did not strictly apply them.[4] In 1982, the criteria were revised to include further advances in serologic testing—for antinuclear antibody (ANA) and anti–double-stranded DNA (anti-dsDNA)—as well as improved biostatistical techniques. In 1997, the Diagnostic and Therapeutic Criteria Committee of the ACR reviewed the 1982 criteria and recommended that a positive result of LE cell preparation be removed and replaced with the finding of antiphospholipid antibodies. These updates were based on committee consensus but were never subjected to rigorous validation testing.

Although the use of ACR criteria enhances the comparability of research studies, there are also drawbacks. Notably, the sensitivity of the 1982 criteria has been shown to be only 83% in an external population compared with 96% in the test population. Additionally, the criteria tend to be skewed toward limited detection of mild cases of SLE, or incident cases at early stages of their prodrome. Not only would the population size be underestimated with the criteria but the cases would also be biased toward those of longer disease duration and greater severity. Four of the 11 ACR criteria are overly biased toward cutaneous manifestations of SLE, even though every other organ system has one. The Systemic Lupus International Collaborating Clinics (SLICC) group has revised the ACR SLE classification criteria and validated alternative criteria in order to improve clinical relevance, meet more stringent methodology requirements, and incorporate new knowledge in SLE immunology since 1982.[4a] It will be important to externally compare these and any new criteria with the existing ACR criteria. Cutaneous lupus does not have classification criteria. Biopsies of the skin may not be available and are not specific.

Each scientific advance that leads to improved laboratory techniques and/or any greater public awareness of the disease can make a profound impact on our ability to define and ascertain cases and, therefore, the rates of disease. Comparisons of earlier studies with later ones are difficult. Therefore, epidemiologic studies utilizing case definitions prior to the 1982 ACR criteria are presented separately (see Table 2-1).

Case Ascertainment

Patients with SLE interact with the health care system at a variety of different points. So that the full spectrum of disease can be assessed, ascertainment of cases should come from a range of sources. A unified health care system with centralized health information has a potential advantage in that several different sources across a health system can be queried with relative efficiency, thereby improving case ascertainment. Furthermore, because lupus manifestations change over time for a particular patient or certain types of damage predominate, patients with SLE may be more likely to be captured at different types of facilities.

Administrative data are often used to find patients with potential lupus. Using such information can be an efficient way to ascertain cases throughout large health systems and different levels of care.

TABLE 2-1 Early Population-Based Studies of Incidence and Prevalence of SLE

FIRST AUTHOR (YEAR)	STUDY LOCATION/ COUNTRY	STUDY YEARS	POPULATION AT RISK (RACES)	CASE DEFINITION	CASE ASCERTAINMENT SOURCES	NUMBER OF SLE CASES	INCIDENCE*	PREVALENCE[†]
Siegel (1970)[4]	New York City and Jefferson County, AL/US	1956-1965	1,165,700 (white and black)	Clinical suspicion, characteristic serologic and pathologic findings	Hospital files, selected clinics and rheumatologists, LE cell tests	Total: 193 White: 124 Black: 69	2.0[‡] overall	19[‡] overall
Fessel (1974)[46]	San Francisco, CA/US	1965-1973	121,444 members of Kaiser (all races)	≥4 1971 ARA criteria by chart review	Outpatient diagnoses from internists and dermatologists	Total: 74	7.6 overall	51 overall
Hochberg (1985)[15]	Baltimore, MD/US	1970-1977	Not given	≥4 1971 ARA criteria by chart review	Hospital discharge (SLE)	Total: 302 White: 79 Black: 223	4.6[‡] overall	Not determined

ARA, American Rheumatism Association.
*Per 100,000 per year.
[†]Per 100,000.
[‡]Age adjusted to national or regional population.

However, the validity and accuracy of the data need to be better determined in different health systems. This can be achieved by utilizing multiple sources and adjusting for error in each.[5] Self-reported physician diagnosis of SLE has been used but was found to be unreliable after a review of a sample of available medical records or asking whether the patients take lupus medications.[6,7] With the advent of electronic medical records in certain countries, there may be ways to query large systems with improved accuracy.

Rheumatologists and hospitals have been the common sources for many studies. However, nephrologists and dermatologists may potentially see high numbers of cases. Unless a study takes advantage of a relatively closed health system or administrative data, there is little consistency with regard to ascertaining cases from these physician groups. Cutaneous manifestations of SLE are quite common and may be addressed by dermatologists. Other specialists, such as hematologists, cardiologists, and obstetricians, may also encounter patients with SLE. But it is unclear how many new cases or additional clinical information could be derived from these specialists. University databases, though an important source of cases, can be biased toward patients with more severe disease. Access to clinical and pathology (particularly skin and renal) laboratories would be a high-yield source of locating additional patients. Those with end-stage renal disease are an important group but pose a unique challenge in epidemiologic studies. These patients often have less active systemic disease activity and can spend several years having other important comorbidities addressed. Therefore, their lupus-related information may be less likely to be found at a rheumatologist's or outpatient nephrologist's office, particularly as time goes by. Identifying presumably milder cases of SLE that are located in the primary care arena or that have not yet been diagnosed is challenging to address on a population-based level and requires different methodology.

Although a number of different sources may be utilized to find cases, the final result is likely to be an underestimate. Capture-recapture methodology of data analysis aims to correct for this by taking advantage of duplicate cases to mathematically determine the degree of overlap between the sources. The result is an alternative estimate that includes potentially missed cases and should be incorporated whenever possible.[8]

Although much of the epidemiologic data have been from the more developed Western nations, relatively little has been known about other countries (Tables 2-2 to 2-6). An enduring epidemiologic question is how African, Asian, and Hispanic ancestry influences the risk for SLE. There are no reports of significant rates of SLE in rural Africa or Asia, a situation that could, in part, be the result of underreporting due to a lack of health resources and expertise as well as other, more prevalent competing health issues. Further confirmation of the underlying indigenous rates of disease in these ethnic groups is needed. The strikingly increased rate in Americans of African ancestry has suggested that an SLE "prevalence gradient" exists,[9] whereby genetic admixture and environmental factors are thought to raise the risk of SLE in people of African descent living in industrialized nations.

The Community Oriented Program for the Control of Rheumatic Diseases (COPCORD) strategy was designed to be cost effective and has been implemented in various regions throughout the world in the past three decades. This validated method utilizes multistage random probability sampling to select participants, who are visited in their households by trained staff and administered a survey. Rheumatologists then examine and confirm the diagnosis in participants with suspected rheumatic disease. This strategy has the advantage of being able to compare prevalence rates in various parts of the country where it has been performed. It also engages participation of community lay workers and brings rheumatologists out in the field to experience the burden of disease at the community level.

Population at Risk

The population from which incidence and prevalence rates are being determined and the geographic area they live in should be well defined. Significant numbers of people at risk for the disease should be captured. It would not be appropriate for countries with a heterogeneous mix of ethnicities, like the United States, to extrapolate national rates on the basis of a single study, particularly those with few cases and large confidence intervals. Multiple studies are needed in areas that contain different high-risk ethnic populations. This "sampling" of rates could be used to determine more accurate national estimates.

Special attention should be given to different ethnic groups with appropriate stratified rates. Data summarized in the mid-2000s showed that some of the lowest rates are seen among Caucasian Americans, Canadians, and Spaniards with incident rates of 1.4, 1.6, and 2.2 cases per 100,000 people, respectively.[10] In predominantly Caucasian populations, who tend to have less severe and longer duration of disease, prevalence rates may be underestimated if milder cases or patients in remission are not ascertained. The data from Northern European countries are excellent resources for understanding the burden of SLE in this group. Incident and prevalence rates

Text continued on p. 15

TABLE 2-2 Population-Based Studies of the Incidence and Prevalence of SLE in North America, Including the Caribbean and Puerto Rico

FIRST AUTHOR (YEAR)	STUDY LOCATION/ COUNTRY	STUDY YEAR(S)	POPULATION AT RISK (RACES)	CASE DEFINITION	CASE ASCERTAINMENT SOURCES	NUMBER OF SLE CASES	INCIDENCE*	PREVALENCE†
Nossent (1992)[47]	Island of Curacao/ Netherlands Antilles	1980-1990	146,500 (≈95% African Caribbean, <5% white)	≥4 1982 ACR criteria by chart review	Hospital discharge records, all internal medicine and dermatology specialists by physician report, death certificates in Public Health Department	Total: 94 (1980-1990, all African Caribbean) Prevalent: 69 (1990) Incident: 68 (1980-1989)	4.6 overall 7.9 females 1.1 males	48 overall 84 females 9 males
McCarty (1995)[8]	Allegheny County, PA/US	1985-1990	1,336,449 (all races)	≥4 ACR criteria validated by chart review	Rheumatologists, hospitals, university database (SLE)	Total: 191 White: 141 Black: 48 Other: 2	2.4 overall	ND
Uramoto (1999)[19]	Rochester, MN/US	1950-1992	Rochester population (white)	≥4 1982 ACR criteria by review of 430 medical records	Community diagnostic retrieval system (SLE, ANA, LE cell, false-positive syphilis test result)	Total: 48	3.1§ overall 5.6§ 1980-1992 1.5§ 1950-1979	122‡ (Jan 1992)
Peschken (2000)[48]	Province of Manitoba/ Canada	1980-1996	≈1,100,000 (NAI and NI)	≥4 1982 ACR criteria validated by chart review	Regional arthritis center DB and the MRs of all rheumatologists, hematologists, nephrologists, and general internists	Total: 257 NAI: 49 NI: 208	2.0-7.4 NAI 0.9-2.3 NI	42.3 NAI 20.6 NI
Walsh (2001)[42]	Nogales, AZ/ US	1997	19,489 (92% Mexican American)	≥4 1982 ACR revised criteria (definite) or 3 ACR revised criteria (probable) by chart review & exam	Community referrals to lupus evaluation center, practice DB search (SLE)	Total: 26 Definite: 19 Probable: 7	ND	94 overall
Deligny (2002)[49]	Martinique Island/ French West Indies	1990-1999	381,427 (mostly African Caribbean)	≥4 1982 revised ACR criteria by investigator chart review	Hospital electronic records (university and community hospitals), practitioners and software of specialists, independent practitioners, files of antinuclear antibodies and antiphospholipids, filings for Social Security, mortality DB	Total: 286	4.7 overall	64.2 overall

Study	Location	Year	Sample/Population	Case definition	Data source	No. of cases	Incidence	Prevalence
Ward (2004)[6]	NHANES III (sample of US population)	2000	20,050 (all races)	Self-reported MD diagnosis ± SLE drugs	Self-reported physician diagnosis from NHANES III	Self-report: 40 Taking SLE drugs: 12	ND	241 self-reported 54 taking SLE drugs
Naleway (2005)[50]	Rural area North Central Wisconsin/US	1991-2001	77,280 (97% white)	≥4 1982 ACR revised criteria (definite) or 1-3 ACR criteria (incomplete) by chart review	Community clinic electronic records (SLE)	Total: 174 Definite: 117 Incomplete: 57	5.1‡ definite 8.2‡ definite females 1.9‡ definite males	79‡ definite 132‡ definite females 25‡ definite males
Molina (2007)[51]	Puerto Rico/US	2003	552,733 private insured people (race ND)	ICD-9 code 710.0	All insurance claims submitted by health care providers (physicians, dentists, laboratories, pharmacies, and hospitals)	Total: 877 Females: 812 Males: 65	ND	159 overall 277 females 25 males
Bernatsky (2007)[52]	Quebec/Canada	1994-2003	≈7.5 million (all races)	>2 claims of SLE (>2 months & <2 yr apart)	Administrative data: billing codes, hospitalization data, and procedure code data	Total: 3825 (2003)	3.0 PB 2.8 HDD	33 PB 33 HDD 51 composite 45 Bayesian model
Pelaez-Ballestas (2011)[53]	Mexico City, Nuevo Leon, Yucatan, Sinaloa, Chihuahua/Mexico	2008-2010 depending on region	Sample of 19,213 people age 18 yr and older (race ND)	≥4 1982 revised ACR criteria by study rheumatologist assessment	Community-Oriented Program for the Control of Rheumatic Diseases (COPCORD) methodology	Not available	ND	60† overall 80 females 40 males 90 Mexico City 40 N. Leon 70 Yucatan 40 Sinaloa 40 Chihuahua

ACR, American College of Rheumatology; DB, database; HDD, hospital discharge data; ICD-9, *International Classification of Diseases*, 9th edition; MR, medical record; ND, not determined; NAI, North American Indian; NHANES, National Health and Nutrition Examination Survey; NI, Non-Indian; PB, physician billing.

*Per 100,000 per year.

†Per 100,000.

‡Age adjusted to national or regional population.

§Age- and sex-adjusted.

TABLE 2-3 Population-Based Studies of the Incidence and Prevalence of SLE in South America

FIRST AUTHOR (YEAR)	STUDY LOCATION/ COUNTRY	STUDY YEAR(S)	POPULATION AT RISK (RACES)	CASE DEFINITION	CASE ASCERTAINMENT SOURCES	NUMBER OF SLE CASES	INCIDENCE*	PREVALENCE†
Vilar (2002)[54]	Natal city, Rio Grande do Norte/ Brazil	2000	493,239 people age >15 yr (race ND)	≥4 1982 revised ACR criteria by study rheumatologist assessment	University hospital, public health network hospitals, community specialists (nephrologists, hematologists, rheumatologists, dermatologists) and laboratories	Total: 43 White: 33 Black: 6 Mulatto: 4	8.7‡ overall 14.1 females 2.2 males	ND
Senna (2004)[55]	Montes Claros, Minas Gerais/ Brazil	ND	Sample of 3,038 people age >16 yr (38% white, 62% nonwhite)	≥4 1982 revised ACR criteria by rheumatologist assessment	Community-Oriented Program for the Control of Rheumatic Diseases (COPCORD) methodology§	Total: 3 (1 white, 2 nonwhite)	ND	98 overall 90 male 110 female

ACR, American College of Rheumatology; ND, not determined.
*Per 100,000 per year.
†Per 100,000.
‡Sex-adjusted.
§COPCORD questionnaire to screen for rheumatic disease, rheumatologist assessment of individuals with pain and/or functional disability.

TABLE 2-4 Population-Based Studies of the Incidence and Prevalence of SLE in Asia

FIRST AUTHOR (YEAR)	STUDY LOCATION/ COUNTRY	STUDY YEAR(S)	POPULATION AT RISK (RACES)	CASE DEFINITION	CASE ASCERTAINMENT SOURCES	NUMBER OF SLE CASES	INCIDENCE*	PREVALENCE†
Huang (2004)[14]	Nationwide/ Taiwan	1999	5.78 million children age <16 yr	ICD-9 code 710.0	National health insurance registry	365	ND	6.3 overall 11.2 girls 1.8 boys
Mok (2003)[56]	Hong Kong/ China	2001	1.49 million (Hong Kong Chinese)	≥4 ACR criteria	Medical clinics at 2 hospitals	876	ND	58.8
Mok (2008)[57]	Hong Kong/ China	2000-2006	1 million (Hong Kong Chinese)	≥4 1982 revised ACR criteria by rheumatologist assessment	Cohort database from large regional public hospital	272 (2000) 442 (2006) prevalent only	3.1 (2000) 2.8 (2006)	ND
Chiu (2010)[58]	Nationwide/ Taiwan	2000-2007	22.28 million (in 2000) 22.96 million (in 2007)	ICD-9 code 710.0	National health insurance registry	22,182 (incident in 2001-2007 + prevalent in 2000)	8.1 (2001-2007)	42.2 (2000) 67.4 (2007)

ACR, American College of Rheumatology; ICD-9, *International Classification of Diseases*, 9th edition; ND, not determined.
*Per 100,000 per year.
†Per 100,000.

TABLE 2-5 Population-Based Studies of the Incidence and Prevalence of SLE in Australia

FIRST AUTHOR (YEAR)	STUDY LOCATION/ COUNTRY	STUDY YEARS	POPULATION AT RISK (RACES)	CASE DEFINITION	CASE ASCERTAINMENT SOURCES	NUMBER OF SLE CASES	INCIDENCE*	PREVALENCE†
Bossingham (2003)[59]	Far North Queensland/ Australia	1996-1998	238,000 (mostly Caucasian, 11.8% aboriginal)	≥4 1982 revised ACR criteria by study rheumatologist assessment or chart review	Survey of all specialists, family doctors, medical staff of peripheral hospitals, and staff of the Aboriginal Health Services	Total: 108 European and mixed: 82 Aboriginal: 26	ND	45.3 overall 92.8 aborigines
Segasothy (2001)[60]	Alice Springs and Barkly regions/ Australia	1990-1999	19,000 aboriginal 31,000 Caucasian	Medical	Record review from all major medical facilities, including renal dialysis unit	14 aborigine 6 Caucasian	ND	73.5 aborigine 19.3 Caucasian

ACR, American College of Rheumatology; ND, not determined.
*Per 100,000 per year.
†Per 100,000.

TABLE 2-6 Population-Based Studies of the Incidence and Prevalence of SLE in Europe

AUTHOR (YEAR)	STUDY LOCATION/ COUNTRY	STUDY YEAR(S)	POPULATION AT RISK (RACES)	CASE DEFINITION	CASE ASCERTAINMENT SOURCES	NUMBER OF SLE CASES	ANNUAL INCIDENCE*	PREVALENCE†
Hopkinson (1994)[11]	Nottingham/ UK	1989-1990	601,693 (all races)	≥4 1982 revised ACR criteria by rheumatologist assessment of patients	Hospital physicians surveys, CTD registry in immunology dept, immunology lab, renal unit DB, inpatient MRs, acute psychiatric admissions	Total: 147 White: 117 Afro-Car: 21 Asian: 7 Chinese: 2	4.0‡ overall 3.4‡ white 31.9‡ black 4.1‡ Asian ND Chinese	24.7‡ overall 20.3‡ white 207.0‡ black 48.8‡ Asian 92.9‡ Chinese
Johnson (1995)[12]	Birmingham and Solihull Districts/ UK	1991-1992	872,877 (all races)	≥4 1982 revised ACR criteria or 3 criteria with strong suspicion upon review of charts assessed by study rheumatologist	National and private attending physicians, GPs, lupus patient group, university database, 4 immunology labs, HDD	Total: 242 White: 155 Afro-Car: 50 Asian: 36 Chinese: 1	3.8§ overall	27.7§ overall 20.7§ white 111.8§ Afro-Car 46.7§ Asian ND Chinese
Voss (1998)[61]	Funen County/ Denmark	1980-1994	387,841 (white)	≥4 1982 revised ACR criteria (definite) or <4 criteria (incomplete) by rheumatologist assessment of patients	Central inpatient registry (1980-1994), outpatient registry (1993-1994), private specialists and GPs, university autoimmune test DB	Definite: 107 Incomplete: 20	1.0 (1980) 3.6 (1994)	Definite: 22.2‡ Incomplete: 5.2
Stahl-Hallengren (2000)[62]	Lund and Orup districts/ South Sweden	1986-1991	174,952 (mostly white)	≥4 1982 revised ACR criteria by rheumatologist assessment	Hospital registry, private clinics network, primary health care registry, private practitioners, university laboratory	Incident 1987-1991: 41 Prevalent 1986: 121	4.8 (1987-1991); 4.5 if patients with >4 ACR are assessed	42.0 (1986) 68.0 (1991)
Nossent (2001)[63]	Finnmark and Troms counties/ Norway	1978-1996	224,403 (mostly white)	≥4 1982 revised ACR criteria by medical record review	Community and tertiary hospitals registry, national mortality DB, general practitioners	Total 105	2.9§ (overall) 2.4 (1978-1986) 2.7 (1987-1995)	49.7§ (1996)
Lopez (2003)[64]	Asturias, North Spain	1998-2002	1,073,971 (mostly white)	≥4 1982 revised ACR criteria by rheumatologist assessment	One centralized immunology lab DB with registry of SLE patients operating since 1992	Total 367	2.15 (overall)	34.1 (2002)
Alamanos (2003)[65]	6 districts of northwest Greece	1982-2001	488,435	≥4 1982 revised ACR criteria by medical record review	Inpatients and outpatients from 2 hospitals, 8 private rheumatologists in study area	Total 178	1.41§ (1982-1986) 1.95§ (1987-1991) 2.19§ (1997-2001)	38.12§ (2001)

Continued

TABLE 2-6 Population-Based Studies of the Incidence and Prevalence of SLE in Europe—cont'd

AUTHOR (YEAR)	STUDY LOCATION/ COUNTRY	STUDY YEAR(S)	POPULATION AT RISK (RACES)	CASE DEFINITION	CASE ASCERTAINMENT SOURCES	NUMBER OF SLE CASES	ANNUAL INCIDENCE*	PREVALENCE†
Benucci (2005)[66]	Scandicci-Le Signe (Florence)/ Italy	2002	71,204 (>18 yr old)	≥4 1982 revised ACR criteria by rheumatologist assessment of patients	20 GPs screened 32,521 using Lupus Screening Questionnaire	Total: 23	ND	71
Govoni (2006)[67]	Ferrara District/ Italy	1996-2002	≈346,000 (mostly White)	>4 ACR criteria validated by MR review	HDD code 710.0. Outpatient rheumatology clinic DB, National Health Care System	Total: 201	2.01 (2000) 1.15 (2001) 2.60 (2002)	57.9 overall
Nightingale (2006),[68] (2007)[69]	Nationwide/ UK	1992-1998	12,911,216 person-years (all races)	Systemic disease and 4 ACR criteria, or SLE stated in MR, or use of drugs to treat SLE after diagnosis	General practice research DBs, medical and prescription records	Incident: 390 Prevalent: 1538 (no racial assessment)	3.0 overall	25.0 (1992) 40.7 (1998)
Somers (2007)[45]	Nationwide/ UK	1990-1999	33,666,320 person-years (all races)	GP, SLE diagnosis codes	General practice research DBs	Total: 1638 (no racial assessment)	4.7‡ (overall)	ND
Laustrup (2009)[70]	Funen County/ Denmark	1995-2003	386,884 (mostly white, ≥15 yr old)	≥4 1982 revised ACR criteria (definite) or <4 criteria (incomplete) by rheumatologist assessment of patients	Central inpatient registry (1980-1994), outpatient registry (1993-1994), private specialists and GPs, university autoimmune test DBs	Definite: 109 Incomplete: 29	1.04 definite 0.36 incomplete	28.3 definite 7.53 incomplete
Anagnostopoulos (2010)[39]	Prefecture of Magnesia/ Greece	2007-2008	176,433	≥4 1982 revised ACR criteria by rheumatologist assessment of patients	Postal questionnaire to random sample of individuals	Total: 2	ND	110

ACR, American College of Rheumatology; Afro-Car, Afro-Caribbean; CTD, connective tissue disease; GP, general practitioners; HDD, hospital discharge data; MR, medical record; ND, not determined.
*Per 100,000 per year.
†Per 100,000.
‡Age standardized to European population.
§Age standardized to national or regional population.

are consistently higher among those of African, Hispanic, or Asian descent in studies from different countries. In England, for example, the annual incidence rate in people of Afro-Caribbean ethnicity has been reported to be 31.9/100,000 for both genders in Nottingham, and 25.8/100,000 for females in Birmingham, whereas whites showed rates of 3.4/100,000 and 4.3/100,000, respectively.[11,12]

Recent migration patterns may also introduce biases that are rarely accounted for in population-based studies. In most European countries, where the net migration rate is usually ±1% per year, the overall prevalence estimates may not appear to be affected significantly by migration. However, they may be susceptible to the "healthy migrant effect."[13] An area of south London showed much higher prevalence of SLE in recent immigrants from West Africa (110/100,000) than in European women (35/100,000), although the prevalence in West African women was lower than in Afro-Caribbean women living in the same area (177/100,000). Because most West Africans migrated as adults, individuals with SLE are thought to have been less likely to leave their countries. On the other hand, Afro-Caribbeans were predominantly either born in the United Kingdom or had migrated as children and so their migration patterns were less likely to have been influenced by the disease. Continued epidemiologic evaluation and surveillance of the prevalence rate of SLE in the second generation of West African immigrants could help confirm this migration bias. In the United States, the undocumented Hispanic population is mobile and may move depending on a variety of different factors (economic, legislative, etc.). Immigrants with SLE may cluster in areas with better access to medical care. On the other hand, their numbers may be underestimated because they have more barriers to health care in general than the native population. Evaluation of migration rates should be considered and, when possible, adjusted for.

PEDIATRIC SYSTEMIC LUPUS ERYTHEMATOSUS

Although children have been identified in population-based epidemiologic studies of SLE, many have not been focused or consistent. Pediatric SLE represents an important subgroup of SLE that deserves special attention. One challenge is that there is no consensus age range. Depending on factors in each country, studies define pediatric patients anywhere from 14 to 18 years old. In general, they are found in pediatric hospitals and in specialist practices (pediatric rheumatologists, nephrologists, etc.). It is important that these sources are included in case ascertainment if pediatric rates are to be valid. Some studies from the United States and Europe included pediatric patients from a wide range of ages, whereas others only included those 15 years of age and older. A nationwide, prospective, population-based study from Taiwan reported a prevalence rate of 6.3/100,000 children younger than 16 years, and the at-risk population was 5.78 million.[14] Though some U.S. studies do report pediatric SLE rates, either case ascertainment efforts have not been broad enough or the numbers have been too small to be considered valid. An early study of Alabama and New York City reported an incidence of 6.3/1,000,000 during a 10-year period for white girls younger than 15 years.[4] This was based on only two hospitalized patients, with none being reported as black. A study of Allegheny County, Pennsylvania, determined an incident rate of 3.0 and 3.4/100,000/year among white and black females between the ages of 12 and 19 years, respectively. This rate was based on 12 white and 3 black children with the disease. In a rural region of Wisconsin, only 2 new patients younger than 19 years were identified between 1991 and 2001. The lowest annual incidence rate, 0.5/100,000/year, was reported in Baltimore, where 10 black patients younger than 15 years old were identified from hospital discharge records.[15]

CUTANEOUS LUPUS

Relative to SLE, research on cutaneous lupus erythematosus (CLE) with or without systemic manifestations has been sparse and limited mostly to clinical descriptions with little known about the epidemiology and disease burden. Studies conducted in dermatology settings suggested that the prevalence of CLE is three times higher than that of SLE,[16] whereas when rheumatology settings were assessed, the ratio between rates of CLE and SLE was 1:7.[17] Three population-based studies using different case definitions have attempted to ascertain all potential cases of CLE in well-defined geographic areas (Table 2-7). The first one was conducted between 1965 and 2005 in Olmsted County, Minnesota, using the Rochester Epidemiologic Project database.[18] The incidence and prevalence rates adjusted by age and sex were 4.3/100,000, and 73.2/100,000, respectively. These rates are similar to SLE estimates in the same population.[19] Potentially higher-risk individuals from minority groups were not represented in the Rochester population, making it impossible to generalize these rates to the rest of the U.S. population.

A nationwide study from Sweden with nonvalidated administrative data on cutaneous lupus estimated similar incidence rates for the years 2005 through 2007.[20] Almost 25% of the 1088 Swedish patients had systemic manifestations at the time of their CLE diagnosis. On the other hand, the probability of progression to SLE was 18% at 3 years. Despite similar racial background of the two populations, the progression to systemic phenotypes was much slower in Rochester (5% at 5 years), pointing out potential differences in case definition, access to health care, and diagnosis bias. Whether environmental exposures or biological factors might play a role in the progression from limited to skin to systemic phenotypes was not addressed in these population studies.

The only study of the incidence of CLE in a higher-risk ethic group is from French Guiana, which has a predominantly African descendant population. This study found lower annual incidence of chronic CLE (CCLE) (2.6/100,000) than the two studies performed among Caucasian persons.[21] It is likely that the lower rate in Guiana is a consequence of under-ascertainment of potential cases.

OTHER CONSIDERATIONS

The most profound change in the epidemiologic description of SLE occurred during the 1950s with the availability of the LE cell preparation and the greater awareness throughout the medical community that was associated with it. Advances in technologies due to a better understanding of the pathophysiology of lupus and changes in awareness will continue to be factors that could influence the reported rates of the disease. Belimumab was approved for the treatment of moderate to severe SLE in the United States in March 2011, more than 50 years after the last drug approved for use in the disease by the U.S. Food and Drug Administration. This approval marked the culmination of a period of unprecedented investment in lupus drug development. Associated with those efforts have been equally remarkable efforts to increase awareness of lupus by various organizations, including private and governmental groups. More patients, especially those in high-risk groups or those with milder disease, may be diagnosed. Heightened awareness of physicians may lead to greater administrative coding of patients with undifferentiated or mixed connective tissue disease or lupus-like disease as having SLE. Insurance companies may require an SLE diagnosis code for coverage of newer and more expensive treatments.

Five ongoing population-based lupus registries in the United States funded by the Centers for Disease Control and Prevention are currently addressing many of the issues outlined in this chapter using methods that take advantage of novel federal, state, and local partnerships with academic centers.[22] Two of these registries (Georgia–Emory University, Michigan–University of Michigan) have finished their data collection and are currently analyzing their results. The other three (California–University of California, San Francisco, New York–New York University, and the Indian Health Service) have started data collection.

ENVIRONMENTAL EPIDEMIOLOGY IN LUPUS

The pathogenesis of lupus is thought to involve complex interactions between genetic and environmental factors. Many exogenous factors, such as drugs, chemicals, ultraviolet (UV) light, hormones, infections

TABLE 2-7 Incidence of Cutaneous Lupus Erythematosus and Progression to SLE in Population-Based Studies

FIRST AUTHOR (YEAR)	STUDY LOCATION/ COUNTRY	STUDY YEARS	POPULATION AT RISK (RACES)	CASE DEFINITION	CASE ASCERTAINMENT SOURCES	NUMBER OF CLE CASES	INCIDENCE*	NUMBER OF CLE CASES THAT PROGRESSED TO SLE
Durosaro (2009)[18]	Minnesota/ US	1965-2005	Entire population of Olmsted County 1965-2005 (denominator and race not provided, 95% of population is white)	SCLE (Sontheimer definition), CCLE (Gilliam and Sontheimer classification criteria), and no fulfillment of 1982 ACR criteria for SLE by chart review	Community diagnostic retrieval system (classic DLE, lupus panniculitis, lupus bullous, SCLE)	Total: 156 DLE: 129 SCLE: 23 LEP: 3 Bullous LE: 1	4.0 (1966-1975) 3.0 (1976-1985) 5.5 (1986-1995) 4.0 (1996-2005)	Total: 19 LDLE: 9 GDLE: 4 LEP: 2 SCLE: 4
Deligny (2010)[21]	French Guiana	1995-1999	157,000 (data on race/ ethnicity was not provided, 90% of French Guianans are black)	Definite CCLE confirmed by biopsy, probable CCLE by chart review, SLE per 1982 ACR criteria excluded	Dermatology, rheumatology, and internal medicine practitioners, hospital administrative data	Total: 20 Definite: 15 Probable: 5 DLE: 18 LEP: 1 LET: 1	2.6† overall 1995-1999 4.7† women 0.5† men	ND
Gronhagen (2011)[20]	Sweden, nationwide	2005-2007	9,086,233 representing the whole Swedish population Data on race/ ethnicity was not provided; most of Swedish population is white	CLE, DLE, SCLE, other local LE based on administrative data (ICD-10 codes)	Swedish National Patient Registry (inpatients and outpatients from public and private caregivers—primary care not included)	Total: 1088 DLE: 868 SCLE: 171 Other CLE: 49	4.0 overall 3.2 DLE 0.6 SCLE	Total: 107 DLE: 73 SCLE: 30 Other: 4

ACR, American College of Rheumatology; CCLE, chronic cutaneous lupus; CLE, cutaneous lupus; DLE, discoid lupus erythematosus; GLDE, generalized discoid lupus erythematosus; ICD-10, *International Classification of Diseases*, 10th edition; LE, lupus erythematosus; LEP, lupus erythematosus profundus; LET, lupus erythematosus tumidus; LDLE, localized discoid lupus erythematosus; SCLE, subacute cutaneous lupus erythematosus.
*Per 100,000 persons, age- and sex-adjusted.
†Crude average annual rate.

and vaccines, are recognized to interact with the immune system and thereby may play a role in the development and progression of lupus.[23,24] Epidemiologic methods have been integrated into several other lines of research, including those determining the impact of environmental (nongenetic) exposures in SLE. In this section we discuss selected environmental exposures that have been investigated in epidemiologic studies of lupus (cigarette smoking, alcohol intake, chemicals, and UV light).

Population-based cohort studies have the advantage of analyzing the prospective assessment of exposures (Table 2-8). This issue is particularly relevant to the immunopathology of SLE, in which autoantibodies can be produced many years before the disease is clinically apparent. However, adequate sample size, representation of minority groups at risk, retention rates, and costs are major limitations of prospective cohort studies. On the other hand, case-control studies are less expensive and provide quicker results. Potential limitations of case-control studies include the length of disease duration when the questionnaire is applied, different recruitment and response rate for cases and controls, and recall bias for the exposure. Analysis of prevalent cases increases the possibility of exposure modification after the symptoms start or the disease is diagnosed. This last issue is particularly relevant for behavior-related exposures (e.g., smoking, alcohol intake) (Table 2-9). Assessing the role of occupational risk factors for SLE involves challenging methodologic issues in characterizing exposure histories, gene-environment interactions, and potential modification of effects by other exposures. An excellent review of the evidence and exposure assessment methods in clinical and population-based studies of SLE has been published.[25]

Smoking

The tar and gaseous phases of cigarette smoke contain many toxic components with multiple known and unknown effects on the immune system. Tobacco smoking activates macrophages in the alveoli, increasing myeloperoxidase activity and free-radical production. Long exposure may impair the production of proinflammatory cytokines and decrease the activity of natural killer cells. Three large population-based cohorts in the United States, two of predominantly Caucasian female nurses and one of black women, were unable to find an association between current smoking, past smoking, or early childhood exposure to cigarette smoking and development of SLE (see Table 2-8).[26-28] Only a few case-control studies have reported current or former smoking as a risk factor for SLE[29-31] or discoid lupus.[32] A meta-analysis found a weak but significant association between current smoking and development of SLE.[33] However, one of the

Text continued on p. 22

TABLE 2-8 Prospective Cohort and Cross-Sectional Studies on Smoking, Alcohol, Chemicals, and UV Light Exposures and Risk of SLE

FIRST AUTHOR (YEAR)	STUDY DESIGN/ CATCHMENT AREA	STUDY YEARS	POPULATION AT RISK AND DEMOGRAPHICS	CASE DEFINITION	EXPOSURE(S)	OUTCOME	NUMBER OF EVENTS (RACES)	STRENGTH OF ASSOCIATION, HAZARD RATIO (95% CI)
Sanchez-Guerrero (1996)[26]	Prospective population-based cohort/11 states in US	1976-1990	106,391 out of 121,701 female married registered nurses, ages 30-55 yr, >98% whites enrolled in the NHS	Definite SLE: 4 ACR criteria by chart review Probable SLE: 3 ACR criteria for SLE, and patients diagnosed as having SLE by their physicians even if they did not meet classification criteria by chart review	Cigarette smoking (never, past, current smokers of 1-14, 15-24, or >25 cigarettes/day) Hair dye use	Incident SLE	85	Smoking: 1.1[*] (0.7, 1.8) 0.9[†] (0.5, 1.6) Hair dye use: 1976-1990: 1.0 (0.6, 1.5) 1976-1982: 1.2 (0.6, 2.3)
Formica (2003)[28]	Prospective population-based cohort/ US nationwide	1995-1999	53,924 AA women ages <60 yr enrolled in the Black Women Health Study	Self-reported diagnosis of SLE and appropriate medication, validated, when possible, as "confirmed case" by chart review: ≥3 ACR criteria	Cigarette smoking (never, past, current smoking; never or ever passive smoking) Alcohol consumption (never, past, current, ever)	Incident SLE	Total: 67 Confirmed: 34	Smoking, all cases: 1.6[*] (0.8, 3.3) 1.6[†] (0.8, 3.3) 1.6[‡] (0.9, 2.9) Smoking, confirmed SLE: 1.5[‡] (0.6, 4.2) 1.9[†] (0.8, 4.8) 1.7[‡] (0.8, 3.9) Alcohol consumption, all cases: 1.1[*] (0.6, 1.0) 0.9[†] (0.4, 2.0) 1.0[‡] (0.6, 1.8)
Tsai (2007)[41]	Prospective follow-up study/central Taiwan	1979-2003	≈2000 Taiwanese	ICD-9 code for SLE in the national death registry	Rice oil contaminated with polychlorinated biphenyls/dibenzofurans (PCBs/PCDFs)	Death attributed to SLE	0-7 yr: 0 8-15 yr: 2 16-23 yr: 3	8-15 yr: SMR 19.8 16-23 yr: SMR 18.9

Continued

TABLE 2-8 Prospective Cohort and Cross-Sectional Studies on Smoking, Alcohol, Chemicals, and UV Light Exposures and Risk of SLE

FIRST AUTHOR (YEAR)	STUDY DESIGN/ CATCHMENT AREA	STUDY YEARS	POPULATION AT RISK AND DEMOGRAPHICS	CASE DEFINITION	EXPOSURE(S)	OUTCOME	NUMBER OF EVENTS (RACES)	STRENGTH OF ASSOCIATION, HAZARD RATIO (95% CI)
Karlson (2007)[43]	Population-based cross-sectional/ Roxbury, Dorchester, and Mattapan Boston neighborhoods/ US	1993-2002	88,210 women age >18 yr (75% AA, 15% Hispanic, 5% white)	≥4 1982 revised ACR criteria by study rheumatologist chart review	Proximity to 416 hazardous sites (petrochemicals) GST genotypes	Prevalent SLE Interaction between GST genotypes and environmental exposure to hazardous waste sites	Total: 209 AA: 167	Prevalence rate: 2.4/1000 overall female, 3.6/1000 AA female Significant interaction between GST genotypes and proximity to 67 sites with higher risk for exposure to volatile organic compounds
Simard (2009)[27]	Two prospective population-based cohorts of women from 17 states in the US	1976-2004, 1989-2003	93,054 out of 121,701 female nurses, ages 30-55 yr, >98% white, enrolled in the NHS, and 95,554 out of 116,608 females nurses, ages 25-42 yr, >97% white, enrolled in NHSII	Reviewer's consensus of SLE, 3 ACR criteria and 4 ACR criteria	Early childhood exposure to cigarette as proxy of maternal smoking	Incident SLE	142 from NHS 94 from NHSII	Early cigarette smoking exposure (mother): 0.9[§] (0.6, 1.4)
Parks (2011)[71]	Prospective population-based multicenter cohort/40 clinics US nationwide	1993-1998	76,861 out of 93,676 postmenopausal women, ages 50-79 yr, enrolled in the Women's Health Initiative Observational Study	Newly self-reported RA or SLE at yr 1, 2, or 3 plus DMARD use at yr 3	History of personal or indirect insecticide exposure (residential or work place) since age 21 yr Alcohol use Coffee use	Incident SLE and RA	SLE: 27 SLE and RA: 8 RA: 186	Personal pesticide exposure: ≥6 times/yr: 2.0[¶] (1.2, 3.6) For ≥20 yr 2.0[¶] (1.2, 3.2) Indirect pesticide exposure (by others): ≥6 times/yr: 1.0[¶] (0.5, 1.9) For ≥20 yr: 1.9[¶] (1.1, 3.2)

AA-, American; ACR, American College of Rheumatology; CI, confidence interval; DMARD, disease modifying anti-rheumatic drug; GTS, glutathione S-transferase; ICD-9, *International Classification of Diseases*, 9th ed; NHS, Nurses Health Study; RA, rheumatoid arthritis.

*Current vs. never exposed.

†Past vs. never exposed.

‡Ever vs. never exposed.

§Adjusted for age, time on study, race, parents' occupations (NHS only), preterm birth, birth weight (five categories), and exposure to father's smoking during childhood.

¶Adjusted for age, race, region, education, occupation, smoking, reproductive factors, asthma, other autoimmune diseases, and comorbidities.

TABLE 2-9 Case-Control Studies on Smoking, Alcohol, Chemicals, and Ultraviolet Light Exposures and Risk of SLE and CLE

FIRST AUTHOR (YEAR)	STUDY SETTING/ LOCATION/ COUNTRY	STUDY YEARS	SOURCES OF CASES AND CONTROLS	NUMBER OF CASES AND CONTROLS (RACES)	MAIN EXPOSURE(S)	STRENGTH OF ASSOCIATION, ODDS RATIO (95% CI)§	RESPONSE RATE (%)	TIME BETWEEN SLE DIAGNOSIS AND STUDY
Hardy (1998)[29]	Population-based/central urban Nottingham/ UK	1993-1995	Cases from the population-based Nottingham cohort Controls from the Nottingham Family Health Services Authority registry	150 prevalent SLE* cases (80% white) and 300 age-and sex-matched controls (97% white)	Cigarette smoking (current, former, never smokers) Alcohol consumption (units of alcohol, based on week before interview)	Current smoker[1]: 2.0 (1.1, 3.3)[2] Former smoker[1]: 1.2 (0.7, 2.2)[2] Units of alcohol: 1-2: 0.7 (0.4, 1.4) 3-5: 0.4 (0.2, 0.9) 6-10: 0.5 (0.2, 0.9) >10: 0.3 (0.1, 0.6)	Cases: 95% Controls: 39%	NR Analysis restricted to smoking history preceding diagnosis
Ghaussy (2001)[30]	University Center-based cohort, New Mexico/US		Cases from University of New Mexico Systemic Lupus DB Controls from University of New Mexico general medicine outpatient clinics	125 SLE† cases (42 white, 80 Hispanic, 3 other race) and 125 age- and sex-matched controls (41 white, 75 Hispanic, 10 other race)	Cigarette smoking (current, former, never smokers) Alcohol consumption	Current smoker[1]: 6.7 (2.3, 17.3) Former smoker[1]: 3.6 (1.2, 10.7)	Cases: 91% Controls: 95%	NR Smoking history preceding diagnosis age in cases and matched age in controls
Cooper (2001)[72]	Population-based in 60 contiguous counties of eastern and central North Carolina and South Carolina/US	SLE diagnosis between 1995 and 1999	Cases from the Carolina Lupus Study (community rheumatologists, university and community practices) Controls from driver's license registries in same geographic area as cases	265 SLE† cases (60% AA) and 355 controls (30% AA), age-, sex-, and state-matched	Hair dyes used >5 times Cigarette smoking (current, former, never; duration and pack-years)	Permanent hair dyes: 1.5 (1.0, 2.2) Current smoker[1]: 1.3 (0.6, 2.8) Former smoker[1]: 0.5 (0.2, 1.0)	93% of all cases and 75% of eligible screened controls	Median 13 months, 75% cases interviewed within 1.7 yr of diagnosis
Bengtsson (2002)[34]	Hospital-based in Lund-Orup Health Care District/ Sweden	SLE diagnosis between 1981 and 1999	92,962 females age >15 yr	91 incident SLE Caucasian female cases from the outpatient and inpatient computerized diagnosis registry at Lund University Hospital and 205 controls from the general population matched by year of birth	UVR Sun-reactive skin type Animals (pets and farm animals) Hair dyes Alfalfa sprouts Cigarette smoking (pack-year and duration) Alcohol intake (quantity) Silicone breast implants	Skin type: I-II (always burn, sometimes/ never tan) vs. III/IV (sometimes/never burn, always tan): 2.9 (1.6, 5.1) Smoking (pack-years vs. none): 1-10: 1.5 (0.8, 2.9) >10: 1.5 (0.8, 2.9) Alcohol consumption (g/month vs. none): 1-150: 0.7 (0.3, 1.3) >150: 0.4 (0.2, 0.8)	Cases: 93% Controls: 53%	Median 9 yr Only exposures preceding clinical diagnosis were analyzed in controls, and exposures before year of diagnosis of corresponding case in controls
Parks (2002)[36]	Population-based in 60 contiguous counties of eastern and central North Carolina and South Carolina/US	SLE diagnosis between 1995 and 1999	Cases from The Carolina Lupus Study (community rheumatologists, university and community practices) Controls from driver's license registries in same geographic area as cases	265 SLE† cases (60% AA) and 355 controls (30% AA), age-, sex-, and state-matched	Crystalline silica Expert review of occupational history	Occupational silica exposure: Any: • Low: 1.6 (0.8, 3.3) • Medium/high: 3.1 (1.4, 7.0) >1 year: • Low: 1.5 (0.7, 3.1) Medium/high: 1.9 (0.8, 4.7)	93% of all cases and 75% of eligible screened controls	Median 13 months, 75% cases interviewed within 1.7 yr of diagnosis

Continued

TABLE 2-9 Case-Control Studies on Smoking, Alcohol, Chemicals, and Ultraviolet Light Exposures and Risk of SLE and CLE—cont'd

FIRST AUTHOR (YEAR)	STUDY SETTING/ LOCATION/ COUNTRY	STUDY YEARS	SOURCES OF CASES AND CONTROLS	NUMBER OF CASES AND CONTROLS (RACES)	MAIN EXPOSURE(S)	STRENGTH OF ASSOCIATION, ODDS RATIO (95% CI)[9]	RESPONSE RATE (%)	TIME BETWEEN SLE DIAGNOSIS AND STUDY
Cooper (2004)[44]	Population-based in 60 contiguous counties of eastern and central North Carolina and South Carolina/US	SLE diagnosis between 1995 and 1999	Cases from the Carolina Lupus Study (community rheumatologists, university and community practices) Controls from driver's license registries in same geographic area as cases	265 SLE[†] cases (60% AA) and 355 controls (30% AA), age-, sex-, and state-matched	Occupational exposures to: • Solvents • Mercury • Pesticides • Shift work Expert review of occupational history	Occupational exposures: Mercury (yes) 3.6 (1.3, 10) Solvents (vs. none): • Indirect: 1.0 (0.5, 2.3) • Possible-low: 0.9 (0.5, 2.3) • Possible-mod: 1.0 (0.6, 1.9) • Likely-high mod: 1.0 (0.6, 1.6) Pesticides (vs. none): • Applying: 0.8 (0.3, 1.8) • Mixing: 7.4 (1.4, 40) Dental worker 7.1 (2.2, 23)	93% of all cases and 75% of eligible screened controls	Median 13 months, 75% cases interviewed within 1.7 yr of diagnosis Analysis limited to exposures before age of diagnosis in cases, and before reference age in controls
Miott (2005)[32]	Hospital-based/ Botucatu/ Brazil	7/02-10/03	Cases from the connective diseases outpatient clinic of Hospital das Clinicas, UNESP Medical School Controls from spouses, close relatives, and household members	57 DLE cases confirmed by biopsy 215 controls matched for sex, age, and city of origin	Cigarette smoking (current smoking of at least 4 cigarettes/day for 4 yr, nonsmokers)	Current smoker[1]: 14.4 (6.2, 33.8)[5]	NR	NR Smoking preceded diagnosis for mean 17 yr by patient recall
Washio (2006)[31]	Hospital-based Kyushu, southern Japan, and Hokkaido, northern Japan	2002-2005 (Kyushu) 2004-2005 (Hokkaido)	Cases from outpatients of university hospitals and collaborating hospitals Controls from nursing college students and care workers in nursing (Kyushu) or from participants in a health checkup in a local town (Hokkaido)	78 female SLE[†] cases and 329 female controls (Kyushu) 35 female SLE[†] cases and 188 female controls (Hokkaido)	Cigarette smoking (current, former, never smokers) Alcohol consumption (those who drank 1 day/week or more)	SLE <5 yr in Kyushu: Ever smoked[1]: 2.2 (1.0, 4.8)[3] Current smoker[1]: 2.5 (1.1, 5.5)[3] Former smoker[1]: 1.4 (0.3, 7.0)[3] SLE <5 yr in Hokkaido: Ever smoked[1]: 2.7 (0.9, 7.6)[3] Current smoker[1]: 2.5 (0.9, 73)[3] Former smoker[1]: 5.9 (0.7, 51)[3]	Cases: 54% in Kyushu and 49% in Hokkaido Controls: NR	<5 and <10 yr Smoking history preceding date of diagnosis in cases and at date of assessment in controls
Finckh (2006)[37]	Population-based in Boston neighborhoods of Roxbury, North Dorchester, and Mattapan, Massachusetts/ US	NR	Cases from the Roxbury Lupus Project (91% from hospitals and 9% from the community) Controls from female residents of the same study area who participated in one of the connective tissue disease screening events but had negative results for SLE on the Connective Tissue Disease Questionnaire	95 SLE[†] cases (84% AA) and 191 age- and ethnicity-matched controls (92% AA)	Occupational exposure to silica dust or solvents Cigarette smoking as potential modifier of the effect of occupational exposures Expert review of occupational history	Exposure to silica: >1 yr: 4.3 (1.7, 11.2) 1-5 yr: 4.0 (1.2, 12.9) >5 yr: 4.9 (1.1, 21.9) Exposure to organic solvents: 1.0 (0.3, 3.2)	47% of potentially eligible cases Controls: NR	NR

Study	Design/location	Time period	Cases/controls	Exposures assessed	Results (OR)	Participation	Time from diagnosis
Parks (2008)[73]	Population-based in 60 contiguous counties of eastern and central North Carolina and South Carolina/US	NR SLE diagnosis between 1995 and 1999	265 SLE[†] cases (60% AA) and 355 controls (30% AA), age-, sex-, and state-matched	Cases from the Carolina Lupus Study (community rheumatologists, university and community practices) Controls from driver's license registries in same geographic area as cases	Childhood and adult occupational exposure to organic dust. Occupational silica (used to adjust odds ratio). Expert review of occupational history	Childhood: 0.2 (0.06, 0.6)[6] and adult livestock. Adult organic dust occupational: 0.8 (0.5, 1.2)[6]	93% of all cases and 75% of eligible screened controls	Median 13 months, 75% cases interviewed within 1.7 yr of diagnosis
Nagata (2010)[35]	Population-based/13 prefectures in Japan	04/98-03/90	282 SLE[‡] female cases and 292 controls matched for age at registration	Cases from the Japanese government financial aid registry of intractable diseases. Controls from residents registered at same public health center (health checkup program)	Cigarette smoking (current, former, never smokers; number cigarettes/day, number years smoked, age when smoking started). Alcohol and milk intake/week	Current smoker[1]: 2.3 (1.3, 4.0)[4]. Former smoker[1]: 1.1 (0.4, 3.1)[4]. Alcohol drinking: Weekly: 0.5 (0.3, 1.1); Daily: 0.6 (0.2, 0.7). Ex-drinker: 4.5 (0.5, 39)	97% of eligible cases Controls: NR	NR, no difference when analyzed by < or >3 yr. Smoking history preceding date of diagnosis in cases and date of assessment in controls
Cooper (2010)[38]	Population-based/Canada	NR	258 SLE[†] cases for which parents were alive (82% white) and 263 controls matched for age, sex, and area of residence (86% white)	Cases from 11 rheumatology centers in Canada (Canadian Network for Improved Outcomes in SLE [CaNIOS]) Controls randomly selected from phone number listings	Cigarette smoking (current, former, never smokers; age began, number of cigarettes/day). UV light. Silica. Gasoline fumes. Stains, varnishes, paint strippers. Pesticides. Metal cleaning solvents. Mercury. Nail polish. Hair dyes. Expert review of occupational history	Ever smoked[1]: 0.9 (0.6, 1.3). Former smoker[1]: 1.2 (0.7, 2.3). Current smoker[1]: 0.8 (0.6, 1.2). Outdoor: 2.7 (1.0, 6.9)[7]. Work: 7.9 (1.0, 65)[8]. Any silica[9]: 1.6 (1.1, 2.3). Nail polish[10]: 10.2 (1.3, 82). Paints, dyes[10]: 3.9 (1.3, 12.3). Pottery or ceramic hobbies: 1.7 (1.1, 2.7)	65% of the eligible controls interested in the study, and 27% of total eligible controls per screening process Cases: NR	Median: 9 yr. Jobs or hobbies that occurred after diagnosis were not analyzed

AA, African American; ACR, American College of Rheumatology; DLE, discoid lupus erythematosus; NR, not reported; S, smoking; solv, solvents; UV, ultraviolet; W, white.

*SLE defined as >4 1982 ACR criteria.

†SLE defined as >4 1982 revised ACR criteria.

‡American Rheumatism Association SLE criteria.

§Superscript numbers indicate the following: 1, vs. never smoked; 2, adjusted by social class; 3, adjusted for age and drinking; 4, adjusted for age; 5, adjusted by sex, age, and UV index; 6, adjusted for age, sex, state, race, education, and silica exposure; 7, in the 12 months before SLE diagnosis and among people whose reaction to midday sun is sunburn; 8, in the 12 months before SLE diagnosis and among people whose reaction to midday sun is blistering, burn, or rash; 9, occupational and no occupational sources; 10, occupational sources.

case-control studies in the meta-analysis was an outlier with high odds ratios and was responsible for much of the study heterogeneity.[30] A dose-response effect between smoking and the outcome was not confirmed.

Alcohol Consumption

Moderate alcohol intake has been hypothesized to have beneficial effects on blood vessels and consequently to be protective against of lupus development. Several studies have assessed the potential effect of both smoking and alcohol intake, considering that these exposures may be correlated and therefore have confounder effects.[28,29,31,34,35] Inconsistent results and potential biases associated with retrospective assessment of the exposures and with selection of cases and controls do not permit the establishment of a clear association between alcohol and lupus (see Tables 2-8 and 2-9).

Occupational Exposures and Chemicals

A growing body of epidemiologic and experimental studies has addressed potential relationships between SLE and occupational and nonoccupational exposures to chemicals. Crystalline silica exposure can be high in rural farming communities and certain urban occupations, such as sandblasting. This substance is a known adjuvant resulting in increased production of proinflammatory cytokines (tumor necrosis factor and interleukin-1) and has been implicated in murine models of SLE and epidemiologic studies as a trigger of SLE. The Carolina Lupus Study is a population-based, case-control study in 60 contiguous counties of North Carolina and South Carolina that has greatly contributed to the research of occupational exposures in SLE. Patients were identified and referred through 30 community-based rheumatologists, four university rheumatology practices, public health clinics, and patient support groups. The findings suggested that crystalline silica might promote SLE in some patients.[36] The association was further confirmed in two population-based case-control studies of an urban area of Boston and 11 rheumatology centers in Canada.[37,38] Both studies also suggested an exposure-response gradient. The Michigan Silicosis Registry ascertained 1 SLE case among 1022 confirmed cases with silicosis (Table 2-10). The relative risk of the association was 2.5l.[40]

In 1979, 2000 people in Taiwan were victims of the ingestion of rice oil accidentally contaminated with chlorinated compounds (PCBs/PCDFs). After 24 years of follow-up, the frequency of SLE was found to be higher in this group.[41] The standardized mortality ratio attributed to SLE in these individuals was 20 times higher than in the Taiwan general population, with deaths starting 10 years after the exposure. The researchers concluded that the exposure to these toxins might have triggered abnormal immunologic responses. In the United States–Mexican border town of Nogales, Arizona, a study confirmed a community-reported excess prevalence of SLE and pointed to a possible connection to pollutants (air and water) and/or ethnicity.[42] Another study in Massachusetts identified the majority of SLE cases in three predominantly African-American neighborhoods that contained a large number of hazardous waste sites. As in the Nogales study, community concerns about a possible "cluster" of SLE cases from these neighborhoods initiated the investigation. No association was identified between proximity to one of the hazardous waste sites and earlier SLE diagnosis, although there was some suggestion that a genetic polymorphism may influence this risk.[43]

The Carolina Lupus Study and the Canadian Network for Improved Outcomes in SLE (CaNIOS) have assessed the role of occupational exposures to liquid solvents, mercury, and pesticides in the risk for SLE. Table 2-9 shows relatively strong associations of potential solvents with SLE in people who work with paints, dyes, or developing film, nail polish or nail applications, and pottery or ceramics work.[39] Self-reported occupational exposures to mercury in those mixing pesticides for agricultural work and among dental workers were significantly associated with SLE.[44] However, the prevalence of these exposures was very low and therefore the odds ratios were based on small numbers of cases and controls.

Ultraviolet Light Exposure and Lupus

Cutaneous and extracutaneous flares after sun exposure have been observed since the first descriptions of lupus erythematosus in the 19th century. The autoimmune pathways responsible for lupus exacerbation after exposure to UV radiation are not completely clear. Experimental studies have shown that UV light is a potent inhibitor of DNA methylation in CD4+ cells, causing autoreactivity of T cells. Sun exposure also induces apoptosis of keratinocytes and production of anti-Ro, anti-La, anti-Sm, and other lupus autoantibodies. Phagocytosis of apoptotic blebs by dendritic cells is considered an early step in the production of antinucleosomal antibody responses in lupus. Epidemiologic studies assessing the effect of sun exposure by geographic area or seasonal variation have shown inconsistent results. For instance, among 1437 cases of SLE ascertained from the General

TABLE 2-10 Prevalence of SLE in the Michigan Silicosis Registry

FIRST AUTHOR (YEAR)	STUDY LOCATION/ COUNTRY	STUDY YEARS	POPULATION AT RISK (RACES)	CASE DEFINITION	CASE ASCERTAINMENT SOURCES	NUMBER OF SLE CASES	INCIDENCE	PREVALENCE*
Makol (2011)[40]	State of Michigan/ US	1985 to 2006	1022 patients confirmed to have silicosis; 790 medical records available for review 41% African American	Available charts reviewed first by an internal medicine resident "Positive" charts reviewed by a physician board-certified in both internal medicine and occupational medicine who made the final determination whether the chart indicated a CTD Available records were insufficient to determine whether the patients met the American College of Rheumatology criteria for the respective CTDs	Michigan Silicosis Surveillance system: hospital discharge database, physician-reported known or suspected cases, death certificates and workers' compensation data are assessed annually to ascertain cases of silicosis or pneumoconiosis 790 medical records were reviewed to ascertain CTD	Total 1	ND	0.1/100 Risk ratio 2.53 (95% confidence interval 0.3, 21.64)

CTD, connective tissue disease.
*Relative risk estimated on the basis of the prevalence of 0.01% white men, 0.05% African-American men.[74]

Practice Research Data base in the United Kingdom, latitude was not associated with incidence of SLE, although regional differences were observed.[45]

Summary

Several observational studies around the world reveal the potential contributions of environmental exposures to the risk for lupus. A better understanding of the etiopathogenetic mechanisms of SLE is needed to clarify the complex interactions between environmental exposures and genetic factors in the development and progression of SLE.

CONCLUSION

The epidemiologic knowledge of lupus has grown significantly since the 1950s. It is a dynamic field that is influenced not only by the inherent waxing and waning of disease activity in a particular individual but also by the evolving and ever-changing landscape of lupus research. Solid epidemiologic evaluation of SLE will advance our knowledge of this complex, multifactorial disease in the hopes that it, too, will go the way of previous scourges to mankind that were conquered with scientific inquiry, international collaboration, patience, and determination.

References

1. Harvey AM, Shulman LE, Tumulty PA, et al. Systemic lupus erythematosus: Review of the literature and clinical analysis of 138 cases. *Medicine* 33:291–437, 1954.
2. Kievits JH, Goslings J, Schuit HR, et al: Rheumatoid arthritis and the positive LE-cell phenomenon. *Ann Rheum Dis* 15:211–216, 1956.
3. Petri M: Review of classification criteria for systemic lupus erythematosus. *Rheum Dis Clin North Am* 31(2):245–254, vi, 2005.
4. Siegel M, Holley HL, Lee SL: Epidemiologic studies on systemic lupus erythematosus. Comparative data for New York City and Jefferson County, Alabama, 1956-1965. *Arthritis Rheum* 13(6):802–811, 1970.
4a. Petri M, Orbai AM, Alarcon GS, et al: Derivation and validation of systemic lupus international collaborating clinics classification criteria for systemic lupus erythematosus. *Arthritis and rheumatism* 2012.
5. Bernatsky S, Linehan T, Hanly J: The Accuracy of Administrative Data Diagnoses of Systemic Autoimmune Rheumatic Diseases. *J Rheumatol* 38(8):1–5, 2011.
6. Ward MM: Prevalence of physician-diagnosed systemic lupus erythematosus in the United States: results from the third National Health and Nutrition Examination Survey. *J Womens Health (Larchmt)* 13(6):713–718, 2004.
7. Hochberg MC, Perlmutter DL, Medsger TA, et al: Prevalence of self-reported physician-diagnosed systemic lupus erythematosus in the USA. *Lupus* 4(6):454–456, 1995.
8. McCarty DJ, Manzi S, Medsger TA, Jr, et al: Incidence of systemic lupus erythematosus. Race and gender differences. *Arthritis Rheum* 38(9):1260–1270, 1995.
9. Bae SC, Fraser P, Liang MH: The epidemiology of systemic lupus erythematosus in populations of African ancestry: a critical review of the "prevalence gradient hypothesis." *Arthritis Rheum* 41(12):2091–2099, 1998.
10. Danchenko N, Satia JA, Anthony MS: Epidemiology of systemic lupus erythematosus: a comparison of worldwide disease burden. *Lupus* 15(5):308–318, 2006.
11. Hopkinson ND, Doherty M, Powell RJ: Clinical features and race-specific incidence/prevalence rates of systemic lupus erythematosus in a geographically complete cohort of patients. *Ann Rheum Dis* 53(10):675–680, 1994.
12. Johnson AE, Gordon C, Palmer RG, Bacon PA: The prevalence and incidence of systemic lupus erythematosus in Birmingham, England. Relationship to ethnicity and country of birth. *Arthritis Rheum* 38(4):551–558, 1995.
13. Molokhia M, McKeigue PM, Cuadrado M, Hughes G: Systemic lupus erythematosus in migrants from west Africa compared with Afro-Caribbean people in the UK. *Lancet* 357(9266):1414–1415, 2001.
14. Huang JL, Yao TC, See LC: Prevalence of pediatric systemic lupus erythematosus and juvenile chronic arthritis in a Chinese population: a nation-wide prospective population-based study in Taiwan. *Clin Exp Rheumatol* 22(6):776–780, 2004.
15. Hochberg MC: The incidence of systemic lupus erythematosus in Baltimore, Maryland, 1970–1977. *Arthritis Rheum* 28(1):80–86, 1985.
16. Tebbe B, Orfanos CE: Epidemiology and socioeconomic impact of skin disease in lupus erythematosus. *Lupus* 6(2):96–104, 1997.
17. Wallace DJ, Pistiner M, Nessim S, et al: Cutaneous lupus erythematosus without systemic lupus erythematosus: clinical and laboratory features. *Semin Arthritis Rheum* 21(4):221–226, 1992.
18. Durosaro O, Davis MD, Reed KB, et al: Incidence of cutaneous lupus erythematosus, 1965-2005: a population-based study. *Arch Dermatol* 145(3):249–253, 2009.
19. Uramoto KM, Michet CJ, Jr, Thumboo J, et al: Trends in the incidence and mortality of systemic lupus erythematosus, 1950-1992. *Arthritis Rheum* 42(1):46–50, 1999.
20. Gronhagen CM, Fored CM, Granath F, Nyberg F: Cutaneous lupus erythematosus and the association with systemic lupus erythematosus: a population-based cohort of 1088 patients in Sweden. *Br J Dermatol* 64:1335–1341, 2011.
21. Deligny C, Clyti E, Sainte-Marie D, et al: Incidence of chronic cutaneous lupus erythematosus in French Guiana: a retrospective population-based study. *Arthritis Care Res (Hoboken)* 62(2):279–282, 2010.
22. Lim SS, Drenkard C, McCune WJ, et al: Population-based lupus registries: advancing our epidemiologic understanding. *Arthritis Rheum* 61(10):1462–1466, 2009.
23. Cooper GS, Gilbert KM, Greidinger EL, et al: Recent advances and opportunities in research on lupus: environmental influences and mechanisms of disease. *Environ Health Perspect* 116(6):695–702, 2008.
24. Sarzi-Puttini P, Atzeni F, Iaccarino L, et al: Environment and systemic lupus erythematosus: an overview. *Autoimmunity* 38(7):465–472, 2005.
25. Parks CG, Cooper GS: Occupational exposures and risk of systemic lupus erythematosus: a review of the evidence and exposure assessment methods in population- and clinic-based studies. *Lupus* 15(11):728–736, 2006.
26. Sanchez-Guerrero J, Karlson EW, Colditz GA, et al: Hair dye use and the risk of developing systemic lupus erythematosus. *Arthritis Rheum* 39(4):657–662, 1996.
27. Simard JF, Costenbader KH, Liang MH, et al: Exposure to maternal smoking and incident SLE in a prospective cohort study. *Lupus* 18(5):431–435, 2009.
28. Formica MK, Palmer JR, Rosenberg L, et al: Smoking, alcohol consumption, and risk of systemic lupus erythematosus in the Black Women's Health Study. *J Rheumatol* 30(6):1222–1226, 2003.
29. Hardy CJ, Palmer BP, Muir KR, et al: Smoking history, alcohol consumption, and systemic lupus erythematosus: a case-control study. *Ann Rheum Dis* 57(8):451–455, 1998.
30. Ghaussy NO, Sibbitt WL, Jr, Qualls CR: Cigarette smoking, alcohol consumption, and the risk of systemic lupus erythematosus: a case-control study. *J Rheumatol* 28(11):2449–2453, 2001.
31. Washio M, Horiuchi T, Kiyohara C, et al: Smoking, drinking, sleeping habits, and other lifestyle factors and the risk of systemic lupus erythematosus in Japanese females: findings from the KYSS study. *Mod Rheumatol* 16(3):143–150, 2006.
32. Miot HA, Bartoli Miot LD, Haddad GR: Association between discoid lupus erythematosus and cigarette smoking. *Dermatology* 211(2):118–122, 2005.
33. Costenbader KH, Kim DJ, Peerzada J, et al: Cigarette smoking and the risk of systemic lupus erythematosus: a meta-analysis. *Arthritis Rheum* 50(3):849–857, 2004.
34. Bengtsson AA, Rylander L, Hagmar L, et al: Risk factors for developing systemic lupus erythematosus: a case-control study in southern Sweden. *Rheumatology (Oxford)* 41(5):563–571, 2002.
35. Nagata C, Fujita S, Iwata H, et al: Systemic lupus erythematosus: a case-control epidemiologic study in Japan. *Int J Dermatol* 34(5):333–337, 1995.
36. Parks CG, Cooper GS, Nylander-French LA, et al: Occupational exposure to crystalline silica and risk of systemic lupus erythematosus: a population-based, case-control study in the southeastern United States. *Arthritis Rheum* 46(7):1840–1850, 2002.
37. Finckh A, Cooper GS, Chibnik LB, et al: Occupational silica and solvent exposures and risk of systemic lupus erythematosus in urban women. *Arthritis Rheum* 54(11):3648–3654, 2006.
38. Cooper GS, Wither J, Bernatsky S, et al: Occupational and environmental exposures and risk of systemic lupus erythematosus: silica, sunlight, solvents. *Rheumatology (Oxford)* 49(11):2172–2180, 2010.
39. Anagnostopoulos I, Zinzaras E, Alexiou I, et al: The prevalence of rheumatic diseases in central Greece: a population survey. *BMC Musculoskelet Disord* 11:98, 2010.

40. Makol A, Reilly MJ, Rosenman KD: Prevalence of connective tissue disease in silicosis (1985–2006)—a report from the state of Michigan surveillance system for silicosis. *Am J Ind Med* 54(4):255–262, 2011.

41. Tsai PC, Ko YC, Huang W, et al: Increased liver and lupus mortalities in 24-year follow-up of the Taiwanese people highly exposed to polychlorinated biphenyls and dibenzofurans. *Sci Total Environ* 374(2-3):216–222, 2007.

42. Walsh BT, Pope C, Reid M, et al: SLE in a United States-Mexico border community. *J Clin Rheumatol* 7(1):3–9, 2001.

43. Karlson EW, Watts J, Signorovitch J, et al: Effect of glutathione S-transferase polymorphisms and proximity to hazardous waste sites on time to systemic lupus erythematosus diagnosis: results from the Roxbury lupus project. *Arthritis Rheum* 56(1):244–254, 2007.

44. Cooper GS, Parks CG, Treadwell EL, et al: Occupational risk factors for the development of systemic lupus erythematosus. *J Rheumatol* 31(10):1928–1933, 2004.

45. Somers EC, Thomas SL, Smeeth L, et al: Incidence of systemic lupus erythematosus in the United Kingdom, 1990-1999. *Arthritis Rheum* 57(4):612–618, 2007.

46. Fessel WJ: Systemic lupus erythematosus in the community. Incidence, prevalence, outcome, and first symptoms; the high prevalence in black women. *Arch Intern Med* 134(6):1027–1035, 1974.

47. Nossent JC: Systemic lupus erythematosus on the Caribbean island of Curacao: an epidemiological investigation. *Ann Rheum Dis* 51(11):1197–1201, 1992.

48. Peschken CA, Esdaile JM: Systemic lupus erythematosus in North American Indians: a population based study. *J Rheumatol* 27(8):1884–1891, 2000.

49. Deligny C, Thomas L, Dubreuil F, et al: [Systemic lupus erythematosus in Martinique: an epidemiologic study]. *Rev Med Interne* 23(1):21–29, 2002.

50. Naleway AL, Davis ME, Greenlee RT, et al: Epidemiology of systemic lupus erythematosus in rural Wisconsin. *Lupus* 14(10):862–866, 2005.

51. Molina MJ, Mayor AM, Franco AE, et al: Prevalence of systemic lupus erythematosus and associated comorbidities in Puerto Rico. *J Clin Rheumatol* 13(4):202–204, 2007.

52. Bernatsky S, Joseph L, Pineau CA, et al: A population-based assessment of systemic lupus erythematosus incidence and prevalence–results and implications of using administrative data for epidemiological studies. *Rheumatology (Oxford)* 46(12):1814–1818, 2007.

53. Pelaez-Ballestas I, Sanin LH, Moreno-Montoya J, et al: Epidemiology of the rheumatic diseases in Mexico. A study of 5 regions based on the COPCORD methodology. *J Rheumatol Suppl* 86:3–8, 2011.

54. Vilar MJ, Sato EI: Estimating the incidence of systemic lupus erythematosus in a tropical region (Natal, Brazil). *Lupus* 11(8):528–532, 2002.

55. Senna ER, De Barros AL, Silva EO, et al: Prevalence of rheumatic diseases in Brazil: a study using the COPCORD approach. *J Rheumatol* 31(3):594–597, 2004.

56. Mok CC, Lau CS: Lupus in Hong Kong Chinese. *Lupus* 12(9):717–722, 2003.

57. Mok CC, To CH, Ho LY, et al: Incidence and mortality of systemic lupus erythematosus in a southern Chinese population, 2000-2006. *J Rheumatol* 35(10):1978–1982, 2008.

58. Chiu YM, Lai CH: Nationwide population-based epidemiologic study of systemic lupus erythematosus in Taiwan. *Lupus* 19(10):1250–1255, 2010.

59. Bossingham D: Systemic lupus erythematosus in the far north of Queensland. *Lupus* 12(4):327–331, 2003.

60. Segasothy M, Phillips PA: Systemic lupus erythematosus in Aborigines and Caucasians in central Australia: a comparative study. *Lupus* 10(6):439–444, 2001.

61. Voss A, Green A, Junker P: Systemic lupus erythematosus in Denmark: clinical and epidemiological characterization of a county-based cohort. *Scand J Rheumatol* 27(2):98–105, 1998.

62. Stahl-Hallengren C, Jonsen A, Nived O, et al: Incidence studies of systemic lupus erythematosus in Southern Sweden: increasing age, decreasing frequency of renal manifestations and good prognosis. *J Rheumatol* 27(3):685–691, 2000.

63. Nossent HC: Systemic lupus erythematosus in the Arctic region of Norway. *J Rheumatol* 28(3):539–546, 2001.

64. Lopez P, Mozo L, Gutierrez C, Suarez A: Epidemiology of systemic lupus erythematosus in a northern Spanish population: gender and age influence on immunological features. *Lupus* 12(11):860–865, 2003.

65. Alamanos Y, Voulgari PV, Siozos C, et al: Epidemiology of systemic lupus erythematosus in northwest Greece 1982–2001. *J Rheumatol* 30(4):731–735, 2003.

66. Benucci M, Del Rosso A, Li Gobbi F, et al: Systemic lupus erythematosus (SLE) in Italy: an Italian prevalence study based on a two-step strategy in an area of Florence (Scandicci-Le Signe). *Med Sci Monit* 11(9):CR420–CR425, 2005.

67. Govoni M, Castellino G, Bosi S, et al: Incidence and prevalence of systemic lupus erythematosus in a district of north Italy. *Lupus* 15(2):110–113, 2006.

68. Nightingale AL, Farmer RD, de Vries CS: Incidence of clinically diagnosed systemic lupus erythematosus 1992-1998 using the UK General Practice Research Database. *Pharmacoepidemiol Drug Saf* 15(9):656–661, 2006.

69. Nightingale AL, Farmer RD, de Vries CS: Systemic lupus erythematosus prevalence in the UK: methodological issues when using the General Practice Research Database to estimate frequency of chronic relapsing-remitting disease. *Pharmacoepidemiol Drug Saf* 16(2):144–151, 2007.

70. Laustrup H, Voss A, Green A, et al: Occurrence of systemic lupus erythematosus in a Danish community: an 8-year prospective study. *Scand J Rheumatol* 38(2):128–132, 2009.

71. Parks CG, Walitt BT, Pettinger M, et al: Insecticide use and risk of rheumatoid arthritis and systemic lupus erythematosus in the Women's Health Initiative Observational Study. *Arthritis Care Res (Hoboken)* 63(2):184–194, 2011.

72. Cooper GS, Dooley MA, Treadwell EL, et al: Smoking and use of hair treatments in relation to risk of developing systemic lupus erythematosus. *J Rheumatol* 28(12):2653–2656, 2001.

73. Parks CG, Cooper GS, Dooley MA, et al: Childhood agricultural and adult occupational exposures to organic dusts in a population-based case-control study of systemic lupus erythematosus. *Lupus* 17(8):711–719, 2008.

74. Helmick CG, Felson DT, Lawrence RC, et al: Estimates of the prevalence of arthritis and other rheumatic conditions in the United States. Part I. *Arthritis Rheum* 58(1):15–25, 2008.

Chapter

3

The Pathogenesis of SLE

Bevra H. Hahn

The purpose of this brief chapter is to review how SLE evolves and is sustained. Ideas reflect the author's opinions, which are based largely on the information provided throughout this book. References are restricted to recent review articles, because each topic is addressed in detail in other chapters.

THE PHASES OF SLE: EVOLUTION OF DISEASE IN SUSCEPTIBLE PERSONS

As shown in Figure 3-1, the development of SLE occurs in a series of steps. There is a long period of predisposition to autoimmunity, conferred by genetic susceptibility, gender, and environmental exposures, and then (in a small proportion of those predisposed) development of autoantibodies, which usually precede clinical symptoms by months to years. A proportion of individuals with autoantibodies demonstrate clinical SLE, often starting with involvement of a small number of organ systems or abnormal laboratory values, and then evolving into enough clinical and laboratory abnormalities to be classified as SLE. Finally, over a period of many years, most individuals with clinical SLE experience intermittent disease flares and improvements (usually not complete remission), and compile organ damage and comorbidities related to genetic predisposition, chronic inflammation, activation of pathways that damage organs (such as renal tubules), and/or induce fibrosis, to therapies, and to aging.

OVERVIEW: THE MAJOR IMMUNE PATHWAYS FAVORING AUTOANTIBODY PRODUCTION

These pathways are summarized in Figure 3-2.

Stimulation of Innate and Adaptive Immune Responses by Autoantigens

The autoantigen stimulation of the innate and adaptive immune responses is provided by cells undergoing apoptosis (which present autoantigens such as nucleosome and Ro in surface blebs, and phosphatidyl serine on outer surfaces of membranes), by cells undergoing necrosis and releasing cell components which can form neoantigens under the influence of oxidation, phosphorylation, and cleavage, and by microorganisms that have antigenic sequences that cross-react with human autoantigens. Antigen-presenting cells—dendritic cells (DCs), monocytes/macrophages (M/Ms), and B lymphocytes process and present such antigens (Ags). In addition, cells of innate immunity (DC, M/M) are activated via internal Toll-like receptors (TLRs) by DNA/protein and RNA/protein that can be provided by dying cells, particularly polymorphonuclear neutrophils (PMNs) undergoing NETosis, by SLE immune complexes (ICs), and by infectious agents.

The net result of activation of DCs from tolerogenic to proinflammatory cells secreting inflammatory cytokines (including the lupus-promoting interferon alpha [IFN-α]), and of M/Ms to proinflammatory cells secreting tumor necrosis factor alpha (TNF-α), and interleukins IL-1, IL-12, and IL-23, is activation of effector T cells that help B cells make immunoglobulin (Ig) G autoantibodies, infiltrate tissues, and be cytotoxic for some tissue cells such as podocytes in the kidney. B lymphocytes, activated directly by DNA/protein and RNA/protein via their TLRs and by IFN-α, can also be helped in their secretion of autoantibodies by T cells, and in their survival and maturation to plasmablasts by BLyS (B-lymphocyte stimulator)/BAFF (B cell–activating factor), IL-6, and other cytokines. In patients with SLE these processes escape normal regulatory mechanisms, which are listed in Box 3-1. Thus, autoantibodies induce the first phase of clinical disease (organ inflammation of joints, skin, glomeruli, destruction of platelets, etc.) because (1) the autoantibodies and the ICs they form persist, (2) they are quantitatively high, (3) they contain subsets that bind target tissues, (4) they form immune complexes that are trapped in basement membranes or bound on cell surfaces, (5) charges on antibodies or ICs favor nonspecific binding to tissues, and (6) their complexes activate complement. And yet, in spite of this deluge of autoantibodies and ICs attacking tissue, mouse models suggest that susceptibility to clinical disease requires more—there are several examples of autoantibody formation, abundant Ig deposition in glomeruli, and complement fixation without development of clinical nephritis.

Autoantibodies and Immune Complexes of SLE

Autoantibodies are the main effectors of the onset of disease in SLE. In humans, they are probably necessary for disease, but not sufficient. That is, their deposition must be followed by activation of complement and/or other mediators of inflammation, and a series of events that include chemotaxis for lymphocytes and phagocytic mononuclear cells, and release of cytokines, chemokines, and proteolytic enzymes, as well as oxidative damage, must occur for organ inflammation and damage to be severe. In nearly 85% of patients with SLE, autoantibodies precede the first symptom of disease by an average of 2 to 3 years—sometimes as long as 9 years. The autoantibodies appear in a temporal hierarchy, with antinuclear antibodies (ANAs) first, then anti-DNA and antiphospholipid, and finally anti-Sm and anti-ribonucleoprotein (anti-RNP). These observations imply that immunoregulation of potentially pathogenic autoantibodies can occur for a sustained period, and that only in individuals whose regulation becomes "exhausted" does disease appear. Among autoantibodies,

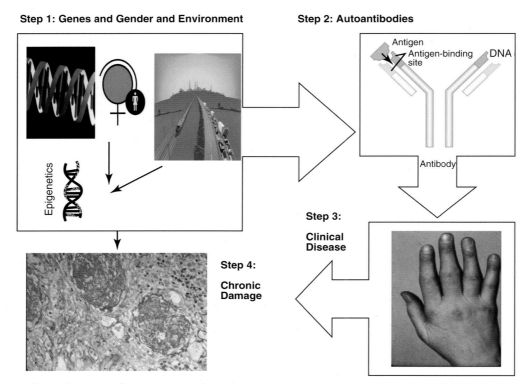

FIGURE 3-1 Overview of the pathogenesis of SLE. In a process that probably takes decades, SLE develops in an individual. At birth the individual is predisposed by multiple genes/gene copies/epigenetic changes and by a permissive gender (usually female). Exposure to environmental stimuli such as ultraviolet B (UVB) light and silica and infections such as Epstein-Barr virus (EBV) stimulate immune responses and probably additional epigenetic changes. Over time, persistent autoantibodies appear; they are usually present for several years before the first symptom of disease. In some autoantibody-positive individuals, clinical SLE develops, shown here as polyarthritis. Within that group, some have chronic irreversible damage; end-stage renal disease with sclerotic glomeruli is shown here.

some are clearly pathogenic, such as certain subsets of anti-DNA that cause nephritis upon transfer to healthy animals. Antibodies to neurons (anti-N-methyl-aspartate receptor, a subset of anti-DNA) can cause neuronal death. Antibodies to platelets and erythrocytes can cause the cells to be phagocytized and destroyed. Antibodies to Ro/La (SSA/SSB) can cause fetal cardiac conduction defects. Human antibodies to phospholipids can cause fetal loss in mice and probably in humans. In addition, autoantibodies generate self-perpetuating cycles; the autoantibodies contain amino acid sequences that are T-cell determinants; these peptides activate T helper cells to further expand autoantibody production. Mechanisms of pathogenicity are discussed in detail in other chapters, and for many autoantibodies the mechanisms are not entirely known. Pathogenic ICs in patients with SLE are dominated by soluble complexes that avoid clearance by phagocytic mononuclear cells, and both size and charge of the complexes can cause them to be trapped in tissue, rather than continuing to circulate. In addition, complement products in ICs are bound by complement receptors; Ig in ICs is bound by FcR, and thus the ICs can fix to cells and tissues by those interactions. Defects in clearing the complexes characteristic of SLE are probably major causes of their persistence and enhance their quantities and potentially harmful properties.

Regulatory Mechanisms Fail to Control Autoimmune Responses

As shown in Box 3-1, several mechanisms that downregulate active immune responses are defective in SLE.

Abnormalities in T and B Lymphocytes in SLE

B- and T-cell interactions in SLE play a major role in production of IgG and complement-fixing autoreactive antibodies. It is likely that

hyperactivation of T and/or B cells promotes SLE by making higher quantities of autoantibodies and proinflammatory cytokines, and that hypoactivation also promotes autoreactivity by allowing autoreactive B and T cells to escape apoptosis. Thus, tweaking of the T/B activation immunostat away from the "norm" promotes autoimmunity. B-cell surface antigen receptors (BCRs) are assembled from various combinations of Ig heavy and light chains in bone marrow; the vast majority of BCRs and their autoantibodies in people with SLE are assembled from a variety of Ig genes and combinations that do not differ from normal protective antibody assembly. The SLE autoantibody response has somewhat limited clonality (not different from antibody responses to external antigens), and somatic hypermutation, indicating that cells have been stimulated by antigens. A major difference between people with SLE and healthy individuals is abnormalities of B-cell tolerance. The end result is elevated quantities of activated B cells, of memory B cells, and of plasma cells in patients with active SLE.

There are several defects that permit survival of autoreactive B-cell subsets in SLE. The usual tolerance processes (apoptosis, anergy, ignorance, BCR editing) are blunted, allowing survival and maturation of dangerous autoreactive B cells. After normal B cells exit the bone marrow, they go through a series of checkpoints that normally remove autoreactive cells. There are defects in several of these checkpoints in SLE, including entry of early immature B to mature B and of transitional B to mature B, entry into germinal centers (GCs), and naïve B to activated B maturation. In addition, some patients have defective expression of FcγRIIB in memory B cells, a molecule that suppresses B-cell development. Thus, defects allow persistence of autoreactive cells that would be inactive or deleted in healthy individuals. Many patients with SLE have abnormally high levels of BLyS/BAFF cytokine, which promotes survival of B cells from the late

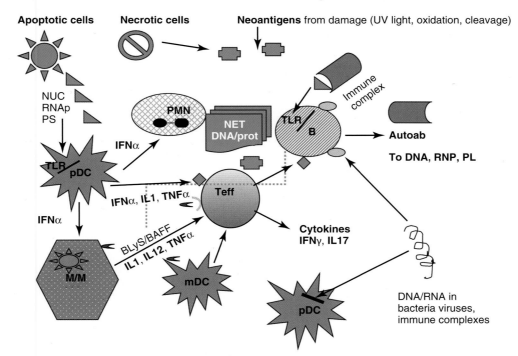

FIGURE 3-2 Interactions between innate and acquired immune systems. Antigen/cell interactions that drive autoimmune responses in SLE. Antigens containing nucleosomal DNA, RNA/protein, phospholipids presented by apoptotic cells, neoantigens generated from necrotic cells and inflammatory cell debris, and RNA/protein; DNA/protein in the neutrophil extracellular traps (NET) like structures of polymorphonuclear neutrophils (PMNs) and immune complexes set up immune responses that characterize human SLE. Plasmacytoid dendritic cells and B lymphocytes are activated upon engagement of these antigens by their Toll-like receptors (TLRs); plasmacytoid dendritic cells (pDCs) generate interferon alpha (IFN-α), and B cells produce autoantibodies and cytokines. The IFN-α activates PMNs to die by NETosis; the NETs they secrete contain DNA and DNA-binding proteins that further engage TLRs in B cells, with more B-cell activation. Both pDC and myeloid DC (mDC) subsets present autoantigens and cytokines to T lymphocytes, resulting in T-cell activation with pushing of T cells to helper/effector subsets that include IFN-γ–producing T helper 1 (Th1) and tissue-damaging Th17 cells (Teffectors). SLE T and B cells are intrinsically abnormal and hyperrespond to stimuli. Multiple "hits" drive B cells, which at this level of maturation are prone to hyperactivation. The hits include T-cell help, exposure to increased quantities of apoptotic materials and neoantigens recognized by their B cell receptors, and exposure to activated DCs and pools of activating cytokines. In the figure, *green* indicates molecules, antigens, and pathways that promote the hyperimmune responses of SLE. *Green diamonds* indicate cytokine receptors on cell surfaces. *Black bars* indicate TLRs in pDCs and B cells. *Red circles* or *crescents* indicate B-cell receptors or T-cell receptors, respectively. *Pink ovoids* are B cell receptors. B, B lymphocyte; M/M, monocyte/macrophage; NUC, DNA-containing nucleosome; PS, phosphatidylserine, the phospholipid presented to the immune system on the outer surface of cells undergoing apoptosis; RNAp, RNA bound to a protein that in complex can be recognized by the immune system; Teff, effector (helper) which can be CD4+ Th1 or Th2, or Th17, or follicular T cell helper (TFH) that secretes IL-17.

transitional stage through mature activated and memory B cells. Genetic polymorphisms predisposing to SLE include several that affect signaling through the BCR, such as PTPN22 and BLK. Abnormally high quantities of Ca++ are mobilized intracellularly after BCR activation in SLE. Overall, memory and activated B cells, as well as plasma cells, are increased in numbers in SLE, they require smaller-than-normal stimuli to be activated, and many pathways from BCR signaling to nuclear factor kappa B (NF-κB) activation may be altered.

Normally, in GCs, nonautoreactive B cells migrate into T zone areas, where they contact CD4+ T helper cells, which drive them into activated and memory subsets, with subsequent Ig class switching and plasma cell production. This process results in protective antibody responses. In SLE there is a blockade of whatever process prevents autoreactive B cells from travelling to T cell zones. Thus in GCs there is a tolerance defect that allows T-cell help for production of potentially harmful autoantibodies. Normal and SLE B cells can also produce autoantibodies with class switching and maturation independent of T-cell help, via activation of B-cell TLRs. In SLE this process may be enhanced, probably by autoantigens in ICs. This environmental exposure of B cells to autoantigens is probably influenced by the SLE genetic variants that promote activation of innate immunity and high IFN production by innate immune cells.

T cells in SLE are also abnormal. Like B cells, they respond to lesser stimuli than are required for healthy T cells. A major abnormality of

SLE CD4+ T cells is assembly of an abnormal signaling apparatus after T-cell receptor (TCR) activation. Figure 3-3 shows some of these abnormalities. In health, TCR stimulation results in assembly of the CD3ζ chain into the surface activation cluster. In SLE, the FcRγ chain is substituted for CD3ζ, resulting in a different activation pathway. The end results are increased release of intracellular calcium, which promotes translocation of calcium/calmodulin-dependent protein kinase IV (CaMK4) to the nucleus, and upregulation of transcription repressor cyclic adenosine monophosphate (AMP) response–element modulator alpha (CREM-α), which on binding to promoter regions of DNA suppresses IL-2 production and enhances IL-17 production. Abnormally low secretion of IL-2 by T cells impairs production of regulatory T cells, whereas increased production of IL-17 promotes inflammation. Causes of the downregulation of CD3ζ include antibodies to T lymphocytes and mTOR activation in T cells resulting from increased levels of nitric oxide (NO) and elevated transmembrane potentials in the mitochondria of SLE T cells. SLE T-cell subsets have many other abnormalities: CD8+ cytotoxic T cells may be defective, adding to the persistence of autoreactive B cells. Regulatory T cells of CD4+ and CD8+ phenotypes also are abnormal in quantities and/or functions. Double-negative (DN) T cells (CD3+CD4−CD8−), which probably derive from CD8+ T cells, infiltrate tissue and secrete IL-17.

Lupus nephritis biopsy specimens contain large numbers of B cells, plasma cells, CD4+ T cells and CD8+ T cells, and DN T cells, as well

Box 3-1 Mechanisms of Downregulation of the Immune Response That Are Defective in SLE

1. Disposal of immune complexes (ICs) and apoptotic cells (ACs): Defective phagocytosis, transport by complement receptors, and binding by Fcγ receptors. Can be due to macrophage defects intrinsic to SLE, low levels of complement-binding CR1 receptors—or occupied receptors, FcγRs that are occupied, downregulated, or genetically low-binding of the immunoglobulin (Ig) in ICs. Early components of complement or mannose-binding lectin/protein (MBL) also participate in solubilizing and transporting IC. They may be missing or defective.

2. Defective idiotypic networks: due to low production of anti-idiotypic antibodies, defective regulation of T helper cells by T-regulator cells that recognize idiotypes in their T-cell receptors (TCRs).

3. Inadequate production and/or function of regulatory cells that kill or suppress autoreactive B cells, T helper cells, other effector cells. This includes CD8⁺ cytotoxic cells that kill autoreactive B, regulatory CD4⁺CD25⁺Foxp3⁺ T cells that normally target both T helper cells and autoreactive B cells, inhibitory CD8⁺Foxp3⁺ T cells that suppress both T helper and B cells, regulatory B cells, and tolerogenic dendritic cells (DCs). Possibly natural killer (NK) cell defects.

4. Low production of interleukin-2 (IL-2) by T cells. Survival of regulatory T cells requires IL-2, and effector T cells in SLE make decreased quantities of IL-2. IL-2 is also required for activation-induced death in lymphocytes.

5. Defects in apoptosis that permit survival of effector T and autoreactive B cells, usually genetically determined.

as monocyte/macrophages and dendritic cells. These are discussed in more detail in the section on tissue damage.

Cytokines/Chemokines and SLE

Actions of cytokines and chemokines in SLE are complex, with some properties favoring autoimmunity and others opposing it. Table 3-1 lists some of these proteins that are thought to play a major role in the pathogenesis of SLE. The end of the table lists some of the proteins that are excreted in higher quantities in the urine of patients with SLE, especially those with nephritis, than in the urine of controls.

Genetics and Epigenetics

Genetic predisposition is probably the single most important factor in development and progression of SLE. The risk for SLE is approximately tenfold higher in monozygotic than in dizygotic twins, and 8- to 20-fold higher in siblings of patients with SLE, than the healthy population. However, concordance for SLE in monozygotic twins is approximately 40%, suggesting that nongenetic and epigenetic factors play a major role in disease susceptibility. Some of the gene polymorphisms or mutations associated with increased risk for SLE are shown in Figure 3-4, placed within the cellular networks they influence. The vast majority of patients with SLE inherit multiple predisposing genes that are common in the population, with each gene associated with odds ratios of 1.1 to 2.5. Rare exceptions in which 25% to 95% of people with single gene mutations go on to have SLE include homozygous deficiencies of early complement components (especially C1q), mutations in TREX1 or DNASE1 genes that regulate destruction of genomic DNA, and ACP5 polymorphisms, which result in overactivation of IFN-α. For SLE polygenic disease, our current knowledge of predisposing gene polymorphisms, copy numbers, mutations, and gene-gene interactions accounts for at best 50% of genetic predisposition to SLE.

This said, many predisposing genetic elements have been identified. The highest signal for genome-wide associations with SLE is in the HLA/MHC region. This is not surprising, since the extended major histocompatibility complex (MHC) region occupies 7.6 Mb of DNA, and the gene products are responsible for antigen presentation and for some components of complement. Within HLA, DR3 and DR2 have consistently strong associations with susceptibility to SLE in European and EuroAmerican Caucasians, each gene in a heterozygotic person conferring an odds ratio of 1.2 to 1.5, and in a homozygote of 1.8 to 2.8. Approximately 75% of patients with SLE in all ethnic groups have at least one HLA gene that increases risk (primarily subsets of DR2, DR3, DR4 or DR8). A stronger association for several SLE-predisposing genes is with autoantibody production, rather than disease. For example, there is a strong association with DR3 and DQ2 (which are in strong disequilibrium) and antibodies to Ro(SSA) and La(SSB), and of DR4 with antibodies to phospholipids. Many SLE-predisposing genes influence the pathways to disease shown in Figure 3-2. These include disposal of immune complexes/apoptotic cells (C1Q, C2, C4, CR2, FcγR-2A, -3A, -2B), activation/regulation of the innate immune pathway (TLR7 copy numbers, IRF5, STAT4, IRF7, TNFAIP3), regulation of adaptive immunity (PTPN22, TNFS4, BLK, BANK1, LYN, ETS1, IL-10, IL-21), and migration/adhesion to target tissues (ITGAM/CD11B). In some cases, altered copy numbers of a given gene, such as complement C4 and Tlr7, confer predisposition to SLE, rather than the gene itself. Many polymorphisms in predisposing genes differ between populations, particularly racial groups (e.g., HLA D3 in Caucasians), whereas others are found in patients with SLE of multiple races (e.g., IRF7,TLR7/8, TNFS4, IL-10 in Asians, Mexicans, African Americans, and Europeans). Gene-gene interactions are also known to increase susceptibility and/or disease severity, such as HLA+CTLA4+ITGAM +IRF5, or IRF5+STAT4.

Some of these genes and/or interactions are associated with earlier disease, anti-DNA, and nephritis, such as certain single nucleotide polymorphisms (SNPs) of STAT4. Some of the individual "lupus" genes/SNPs are also associated with other autoimmune diseases, such as inflammatory bowel disease, psoriasis, type 1 diabetes, and multiple sclerosis. Thus, it is possible that some individuals are predisposed genetically to autoimmunity, and other genes determine exactly which clinical autoimmune disease will develop. There is one report of a gene that confers protection from SLE—a polymorphism for TLR5—that reduces the levels of proinflammatory cytokines, such as TNF-αa, IL-1β, and IL-6, released from cells stimulated by bacterial flagellin.

One of the reasons that discovery of predisposing genes, gene copies, and gene interactions fails to fully account for susceptibility to SLE is the role of epigenetics in gene expression. Epigenetics refers to alterations in DNA that are inheritable. The ability to transcribe DNA into messenger RNA (mRNA) and then into proteins, or posttranslational modifications in mRNA, may be altered by DNA methylation, histone modulation (especially acetylation, but also ubiquination, phosphorylation, etc.). These epigenetic changes alter gene transcription into protein, as does binding of transcription regions by microRNA (miRNA, miR). All of these processes can be altered in people with SLE. Within DNA, islands of CpG are sites of methylation by methyltransferases, with 70% to 90% of somatic cell DNA being methylated in healthy individuals. DNA from T cells of patients with SLE is hypomethylated, resulting in upregulated expression of surface molecules, such as lymphocyte function–associated antigen 1 (LFA-1), that are associated with T-cell autoreactivity. Factors that promote hypomethylation of DNA include ultraviolet light, SLE-inducing drugs, aging, and altered expression of certain miRNAs. For example, increases in miR-148a and miR-21 inhibit expression of DNA methyltransferase 1 (DMNT1), with resultant hypomethylation of target DNA. Nucleosomal DNA exists as 146 base pairs of DNA wrapped around an octamer of histones. Alteration of the histones can change DNA transcription and repair. Deacetylation of histones seems to promote autoimmunity. There has been great interest in observations that histone deacetylase inhibitors alter TLR signaling as well as cytokine production in CD4⁺ T cells;

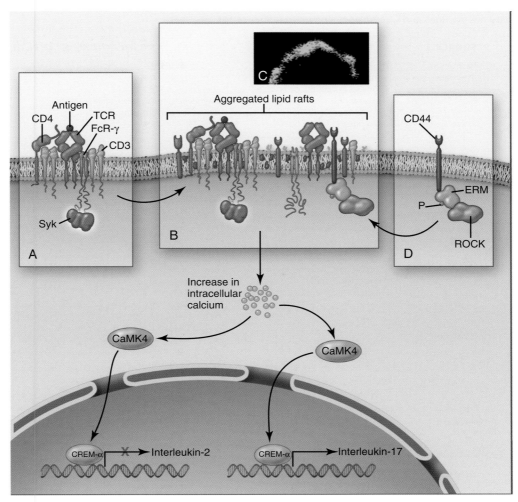

FIGURE 3-3 Abnormalities of T lymphocyte activation in patients with SLE. After T-cell stimulation, SLE T cells have abnormal signaling, with the net result that in comparison with healthy T cells, IL-2 production is decreased (IL-2 is required for production/maintenance of regulatory T cells) and proinflammatory IL-17 production is increased. The process starts with replacement of the usual CD3ζ chain with FcRγ (which signals via Syk) in the surface signaling complex (*panel A*). Aggregation of lipid rafts occurs (*panels B* and *C*). The rafts contain aggregated T-cell receptors (TCRs) and additional signaling molecules, including CD44, an adhesion molecule facilitating homing of T cells to target tissues, such as kidneys (*panel D*). CD44 signals via ERM (ezfin, radixin, moesin) and is phosphorylated by Rho kinase (ROCK). The increased intracellular calcium concentrations that result in activated SLE B cells and T cells promote translocation of protein kinase IV (CaMK4) to the nucleus. CaMK4 facilitates binding of the transcriptional repressor cyclic adenosine monophosphate (AMP) response–element modulator alpha (CREM-α) to the promoter for IL-2, suppressing its expression. At the same time, binding of CREM-α to the promoter for IL-17 enhances its transcription. (*From Tsokas GC: Systemic lupus erythematosus. N Eng J Med 365:2110–2121, 2011.*)

in animal models, treatment with these inhibitors prevents development of SLE.

MiRNAs are endogenous noncoding small RNAs (19-25 nucleotides in length) that regulate gene expression at posttranscriptional levels, primarily by binding to mRNA regions that encode proteins. At least 1000 unique miRNAs have been identified in humans, and approximately 45% of immune response genes contain miRNA binding sites. miRNAs can alter target gene expression or mRNA translation via levels of miRNA expression or via polymorphisms in the sequence of individual miRs. For example, miR-155 is an essential regulator of responses in both innate and adaptive immunity. Expression of miR-182 in T cells inhibits Foxo1 activation and thus decreases synthesis of IL-2. All the known lupus susceptibility genes in humans and mice can be targeted by miRNAs. In the early studies currently available, differential expression of miRNA in SLE in comparison with normal tissues has yielded different results. However, there is good evidence that activation of TLRs 2, 4, and 5 leads to upregulation of miR-146a, which increases expression of TRAF6, IRAK1, IRF5, and STAT1, with subsequent enhancement of innate immune

cell signaling and increase in production of IFN-α—a hallmark cytokine in many patients with SLE. Over the next few years, we can expect an explosion of information on how epigenetic influences influence susceptibility to SLE and its clinical severity.

Gender Influences

Gender influences on disease susceptibility must be of major importance, because there are nine women for every man with SLE. The most important impact may be hormonal, because sex differences in susceptibility are largest during reproductive years. Estradiol probably prolongs the life of autoreactive B and T lymphocytes. Women exposed to oral contraceptives, or to hormone replacement therapy regimens containing estrogenic compounds, have a small but statistically significant increased risk for the development of SLE. Prospective, randomized, blinded, controlled trials showed that administration of one hormone replacement therapy containing conjugated estrogens and a progesterone significantly raised the risk of mild/moderate disease flare in women with established SLE. There are many experiments in some murine SLE strains showing that an increase in levels

TABLE 3-1 Summary of Cytokines and Chemokines Known to Influence SLE

CYTOKINE/ CHEMOKINE	SOURCE	ACTIONS	OBSERVATIONS IN SLE PATIENTS
Interferon alpha	pDC (plasmacytoid dendritic cells)	Anti-viral Promotes DC maturation Stimulates B cell diff. to Ig-secreting plasma cells Increases expression of Toll-like receptors (TLRs) 7/9 Enhances CD8$^+$ T-cell production of granzyme B and perforin	IFN-α–inducible genes increased in many cell types in majority Serum IFN-α activity Increased in 40%-50% High levels are an inheritable trait Target for current clinical trials
Interferon gamma	NK, Th1	Expression enhanced by IL-12 + IL-27 Signature cytokine of Th1 cells	Present in renal tissue in human LN Induces apoptosis in renal parenchymal cells IL-27 levels low in SLE sera Necessary for nephritis in several murine lupus strains. Potential target for clinical trials
IL-1	Activated mononuclear phagocytic cells, T cells	Proinflammatory in tissues	High serum levels associated with disease activity Low levels associated with LN
IL-2	Lymphocytes, T cells	Growth factor for lymphocytes, especially T cells Required for generation of Tregs	Levels in PBMCs from SLE patients are low; low levels suppress activation-induced cell death in T helper cells (increasing apoptotic autoantigen load) and prevent generation of Tregs (allowing persistence of autoreactive T and B cells) Several murine lupus strains also develop low IL-2 levels in serum and PBMCs prior to disease onset Administration of low levels may suppress chronic graft-versus-host response in humans, and vasculitis associated with hepatitis C
IL-4	T cells	Signature cytokine of Th2 cells May protect from tissue fibrosis (mice)	IL4$^+$ T cells increased in PBMCs of SLE patients
IL-6	T and B lymphocytes, monocytes, fibroblasts, endothelial cells, epithelial cells	In combination with IL-2 and TGF-β promotes differentiation of Th17 cells Promotes differentiation of B cells to terminal cells secreting Ig	Increased serum levels in SLE patients Expressed in target tissues, including kidney
IL-10	Monocytes, T and B cells	Promotes Ig synthesis by B cells, also mediates suppression by some Tregs	Increased serum levels in many patients with SLE
IL-17	T follicular helper cells (TFH), DN (double-negative) T cells	Signature cytokine of Th17 cells Proinflammatory Cells also make IL-21 and IL-22 Th17 cells require IL-23 for maintenance	Found in target tissue in human and murine SLE, including kidneys Potential target for clinical trials
IL-12, IL-18	Activated macrophages	Required to generate Th1 and NK cells	Increased serum levels in patients with SLE
TNF-α	Macrophages, DCs	Proinflammatory in tissue and tissue fluids	Found in renal tissue of patients with LN Elevated serum levels in some patients Therapy with TNF inhibitors not yet proved to have good efficacy/toxicity ratio
TGF-β	NK and other cells	Required to generate regulatory T cells (with IL-2) Participates in generation of Th17 cells (with IL-2 + IL-6 or IL-1) Can downregulate autoimmune responses Also contributes to tissue fibrosis	PBMCs from SLE patients secrete abnormally low levels Serum levels are low in some patients
BLyS (B-lymphocyte stimulator)/ BAFF (B cell–activating factor)	Myeloid lineage cells	Maintains B cells and required for maturation to Ig-secreting cells	High serum levels in SLE patients; levels correlate positively with disease activity in some studies Found in target tissues, especially dermis, also in kidney Targeted by anti-BLyS (belumimab), which is approved for treatment of patients with SLE
Chemokines in Serum			
IL-8, IP-10, MCP-1, fractaline	Endothelial and other cells	Chemotactic for polymorphonuclear neutrophils (PMNs), T cells, monocytes	Increased in renal tissue in LN Increased in sera of patients, especially those with LN

TABLE 3-1 Summary of Cytokines and Chemokines Known to Influence SLE—cont'd

CYTOKINE/ CHEMOKINE	SOURCE	ACTIONS	OBSERVATIONS IN SLE PATIENTS
Chemokines and Other Molecules Increased in Urine			
TWEAK	Activated monocyte/ macrophages	TNF superfamily member, TWEAK-R binds Fn14 on endothelial cells and vascular smooth muscle. May mediate renal tissue damage by causing proliferation of mesangial cells, damage to podocytes and renal tubular cells. Induces IP-10, MCP-1, macrophage inflammatory protein (MIP), intercellular adhesion molecule 1 (ICAM-1), vascular cell adhesion molecule 1 (VCAM-1), MMP-1, and MMP-9. Induces apoptosis in human monocytes	Elevations in urine have 50% sensitivity and 90% specificity for active GN in LN. May come into use to predict flare and response to treatment in LN
Neutrophil gelatinase–associated lipocalin (NGAL)	Mesangial cells	Iron-bearing protein. Induces apoptosis via activation of caspase 3, increases expression of proinflammatory genes in renal tissue	Increase in urine excretion correlates with flare of LN. Knockout in mice protects from nephrotoxic nephritis
CXCL-16 (chemokine [C-X-C motif] ligand 16)	Expressed on DCs and monocytes	Recruits T and NK cells to tissues, mates with CXCR6	Increased urine excretion correlated with active GN and renal SLEDAI scores
IP-10	Endothelial cells, fibroblasts, monocytes	Interferon-gamma-inducible protein 10. Mates with CXCR3. Attracts lymphocytes	Increased urine excretion in some patients with LN

CXCR, receptor for C-X-C motif chemokine; DC, dendritic cell; GN, glomerulonephritis; IFN, interferon; Ig, immunoglobulin; IL, interleukin; IP, inducible protein; LN, lupus nephritis; MCP-1, monocyte chemotactic protein 1; MMP, matrix metalloproteinase; NK, natural killer; PBMC, peripheral blood mononuclear cell; SLE, systemic lupus erythematosus; SLEDAI, SLE Disease Activity Index; TGF, transforming growth factor; Th1/2/17, T helper 1/2/17; TNF, tumor necrosis factor; Treg, T-regulator cell; TWEAK, TNF-like weak inducer of apoptosis.

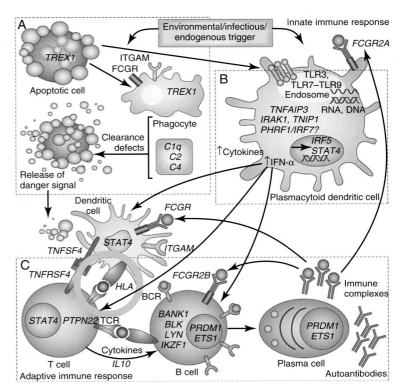

FIGURE 3-4 Summary of putative human genes with polymorphisms (or duplications or mutations) that increase susceptibility to SLE. Genes are presented in the cell networks known to be activated in patients with SLE. *Panel a* shows genes that affect cell apoptosis (or DNA breakdown) and genes that influence clearing of apoptotic cells, and immune complexes. *Panel b* shows genes that influence the response of plasmacytoid dendritic cells (pDCs) to binding of surface and endosomal TLRs by external danger signals and by RNA and DNA in infectious agents and in lupus immune complexes—with resultant increase in IFN-α. *Panel c* shows genes influencing the response of T cells, B cells, and plasma cells to activation by DC (and other antigen-presenting cells) with ultimate production of autoantibodies and the immune complexes they form with antigens. *(From Deng Y, Tsao BP: Genetic susceptibility to SLE in the genomic era. Nat Rev Rheumatol 20:683–692, 2010.)*

of estrogen or progesterone worsens disease, whereas male hormones are protective. However, other features of female gender may also be important in predisposing to SLE. For example, most women after pregnancy have circulating stem cells from their fetuses (microchimerism), which might set up lupus-like graft-versus-host–type immune reactions. The X chromosome and its loci and methylation status may be important in predisposing to SLE. Women may be predisposed to SLE because their inactive X chromosome is enriched in hypomethylated regions. The CpG in these regions can be bound by TLR9, thus activating innate immune responses and increasing risk for autoimmunity. Lupus-predisposing genes located on the X chromosome include *TLR7/9* (where copy number seems important), *IRAK1,* and *TREX1*. Whether their location on X in humans is important in their effects remains to be determined. Additional evidence for the importance of the X chromosome in SLE includes the observation that phenotypic men with an extra X (XXY, Klinefelter syndrome) have a significantly higher prevalence of SLE than men who are XY.

Environmental Factors

Environmental factors that predispose to SLE are undoubtedly important, although few have been identified in a definitive manner. Ultraviolet light (UVB in particular) exacerbates disease in a majority of people with SLE, and in some the clinical onset of disease is preceded by unusually large exposure. Mechanisms include alteration of the structure of DNA in the dermis to render it more immunogenic (i.e., neoantigen formation) and induction of apoptosis in keratinocytes and other dermal cells, presenting higher quantities of self-antigens to the immune system. Infections have long been suspect as inducers and enhancers of SLE. Work from several laboratories has linked infection with Ebstein-Barr virus (EBV) to SLE. EBV infection activates B lymphocytes, which might cause a genetically predisposed person to make large quantities of autoantibodies, overwhelming regulatory mechanisms. The EBNA-1 molecule of EBV has molecular mimicry with a sequence in the Ro particle; immunization with that sequence can induce multiple autoantibodies and lupus-like disease in animals. Evidence has now implicated exposure to silica dust as predisposing to SLE, especially in African-American women. Exposure can occur in agricultural or industrial settings. Many potential toxins in the environment may initiate and influence immune and inflammatory responses, but so far there is no consistent evidence for many that have been implicated, such as exposure to dogs and wearing of lipstick.

Tissue Damage in SLE

Initiation of SLE by tissue deposition/binding of pathogenic subsets of autoantibodies and ICs is only the beginning of the story. Many other processes are required to initiate inflammation and the tissue damage that ultimately destroys quantity and quality of life in this chronic disease. Inflammation and damage begin with complement activation. The 30 plasma and membrane-bound proteins in the complement system, through sequential serine protease–mediated cleavage events, release biologically active fragments. In the first stage early complement components are cleaved to ultimately form C3 convertases; in the second stage proinflammatory activation products such as C3a and C5a form, as well as a lytic complex containing terminal complement components C5b-9. Initiation of the cascade begins with (1) binding of the Fc portion of Ig in ICs by C1q (classical pathway), (2) binding of factors B, D, or properdin by interaction with carbohydrates, lipid, and proteins on surfaces of microbial pathogens or apoptotic cells, with subsequent C3 activation (the alternative pathway), and (3) binding of lectins such as mannose-binding lectin/protein (MBL) to carbohydrate moieties on microorganisms, with changes in MBL that cleave C4 and then C3 (the lectin pathways). Several other proteins control complement activation, including factor I carboxypeptidase, factor H (a membrane cofactor protein), and protease and convertase inhibitors (C1-inhibitor, C4-binding protein). A membrane protein, protectin (CD59), can prevent formation of the lytic complex within plasma membranes.

C3a, C4a, and C5a recruit leukocytes into sites of IC deposition, activate them, and cause inflammation. C4b and C3b bind to ICs and facilitate their clearance, including transport by CR1 on erythrocytes and phagocytosis by cells with FcR in the reticuloendothelial system. However, when CR1 transport systems are overloaded, as in SLE, IC clearance is impaired and the system tilts toward complement activation by persistent ICs, with resultant persistent inflammation. Thus, as in other systems, balance must be maintained between complement activation to remove pathogens, immune complexes, and apoptotic cells/debris, and dysregulated persistent activation that promotes inflammation.

Hereditary deficiencies of early complement components or MBL predispose to SLE. Some patients with SLE make antibodies to C1q, to C1-INH, or to the convertase BbC3b; each of these autoantibodies may promote SLE. In general, quantitatively low plasma levels of C3, C4, and C1q and functionally low quantities of total hemolytic complement have a statistically significant association with SLE disease activity, particularly with nephritis. Increased excretion of C3d in urine is associated with active disease, and rising levels of complement have correlated with clinical improvement in high-quality clinical trials, both in SLE and in lupus nephritis (LN). However, positive and negative predictive values for these measures in general clinical use are not strong. New testing methods identifying erythrocyte-bound C4d (high in active SLE) plus erythrocyte display of CR1 receptor (low in active SLE) have better positive and negative predictive values but are not yet in wide use.

The imperfect ability to correlate SLE activity with complement activation may reflect failure to reflect subsequent tissue damage initiated by post–complement fixation pathways. The extensive number of cells and structures that are assaulted in LN are illustrated in Figure 3-5. Some of the proteins excreted in the urine that reflect processes beyond immune complex/complement fixation are listed in Table 3-1. In Figure 3-5 (*insert*), the autoantibodies and ICs (shown as green Ys) binding to capillaries in glomeruli not only fix complement (shown as *black stars*) but also activate endothelial cells to secrete chemokines, such as monocyte chemotactic protein 1 (MCP-1), and mesangial cells to initiate proliferation pathways. The process also results in podocyte injury, initiating pathways that lead to the podocyte fusion characteristic of patients with membranous features of LN. During the nephritic process, endothelial cells are damaged in vessels outside glomeruli, leading to ischemia of renal tubules; pathways promoting thrombosis are initiated; and renal tubule epithelial cells are activated, initiating pathways that can lead to renal tubular atrophy. The soluble mediators released by tissue cells (such as metalloproteinases) and infiltrating cells activate tissue-resident mononuclear phagocytic cells (variably regarded as tissue-fixed macrophages or dendritic cells) attract circulating monocytes and T and B cells into tissues. Thus, damage is driven by immune pathway cells that we partially understand, and by nonimmune pathway cells that may take over the process of chronic inflammation and damage. In the most unfortunate patients, pathways that promote fibrosis (with known participation by TGF-βand IL-4 as well as many other growth factors), with resultant glomerulosclerosis and interstitial fibrosis, have the highest chance of progressing to renal failure. Although chronic inflammation may initiate the ischemia/endothelial cell damage/podocyte damage, and so on, other processes that occur in tissue, such as chronic oxidative damage and metalloproteinase release, probably continue to drive at least some of these pathways.

The accelerated atherosclerosis characteristic of patients with SLE is another example of a tissue in which an initial attack by the immune system leads to serious chronic disease mediated by nonimmune cells. Risk for atherosclerotic disease is fivefold to tenfold higher in SLE patients than in age-matched non-SLE populations. Immune complexes, complement split products, and some autoantibodies directly activate endothelial cells (ECs) in arteries. This activation sets in motion the release of chemokines and cytokines from the ECs and infiltration of the artery wall with monocytes and lymphocytes. As

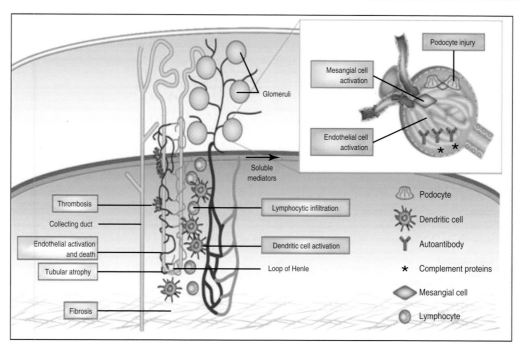

FIGURE 3-5 Cells and substrates in a target organ, the kidney, that are all subject to damage in patients with lupus nephritis. *(From Davidson A, Aranow C: Lupus nephritis: Lessons from murine models. Nat Rev Rheumatol 6:13–20, 2010.)*

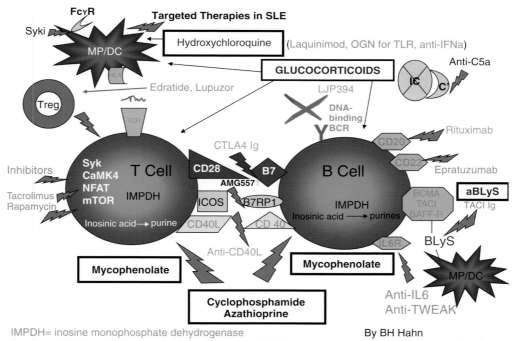

FIGURE 3-6 **Targets of current and experimental therapies for patients with SLE.** Treatments are presented as affecting specific cell types; many have multiple effects in addition to what is shown. Treatments that are standard of care in the management of SLE at the time of this writing (2012) are surrounded by *bold black boxes*. Others listed have either failed to be better than placebo in recent clinical trials (*red*) or are currently in active clinical trials (*black lettering*).

with lupus nephritis, monocyte infiltration and activation of mononuclear phagocytic cells is an initiator of tissue damage. In the arteries, the activated monocyte becomes the nidus of plaque formation, as it phagocytizes oxidized lipids, particularly oxLDL, to become a foam cell. The continuing process of simmering SLE with chronic oxidation, chronic inflammation, release of metalloproteinases, and long-term activation of ECs leads to plaque formation, to smooth

muscle proliferation, to activated cell surfaces that trap platelets, to fibrosis in late lesions, and to narrowing and occlusion that presage myocardial infarcts. Damage to ECs also results in altered pathways of repair; in SLE, replacement of damaged ECs with progenitor cells is impaired. This finding brings up the possibility that stem cells of patients with SLE have inherent abnormalities. It is equally possible that because of the local "toxic" environment in arteries, veins, glomeruli, pulmonary capillaries, synovium, and other vascular tissue assaulted by SLE, stem cells cannot support development of normal ECs, mesangial cells, and so on.

Currently, our therapies are directed primarily at suppressing the initiating autoantibody/immune attack on tissues. It is likely that we need to give more attention to other involved cells and processes that lead to tissue damage. For example, it is disappointing that one study has not shown a reduction in the rate of end-stage renal disease in lupus nephritis, in spite of the fact that we have better therapies for reducing disease activity, maintaining improvement, and reducing damage from hypertension and proteinuria. In later high-quality clinical trials, remission of LN in patients treated with cyclophosphamide or mycophenolate plus glucocorticoids plus antimalarials occurred in only a minority of patients over a period of 6 to 36 months. Our mandate is to move quickly to understand and inhibit these additional pathways and processes that lead to damage. It is hoped that the next edition of this text will be able to recommend such strategies.

CURRENT APPROVED AND INVESTIGATIONAL THERAPIES FOR SLE

Figure 3-6 illustrates therapies for SLE associated with their effects on various portions of innate/adaptive immunity.

Suggested Reading

1. Tsokas G: Systemic lupus erythematosus. *N Engl J Med* 365:2110–2121, 2011.
2. Rahman A, Isenberg DA: Systemic lupus erythematosus. *N Engl J Med* 28:929–939, 2008.
3. Davidson A, Aranow C: Lupus nephritis: lessons from murine models. *Nat Rev Rheumatol* 6:13–20, 2010.
4. Gualtierotti R, Biggioggero M, Penatti AE, et al: Updating on the pathogenesis of systemic lupus erythematosus. *Autoimmun Rev* 10:3–7, 2010.
5. Pisetsky D, Vrabie IA: Antibodies to DNA: infection or genetics? *Lupus* 18:1176–1180, 2009.
6. Sestak AL, Furnrohr BG, Harley JB, et al: The genetics of systemic lupus erythematosus and implications for targeted therapy. *Ann Rheum Dis* 70(Suppl 1):137–143, 2011.

Genetics of Human SLE

Yun Deng and Betty P. Tsao

The complex etiopathology of systemic lupus erythematosus (SLE) has been attributed to "cross talk" between multiple genetic predispositions and environmental factors. Traditional case-control candidate gene studies and genome-wide linkage scans, together with recent genome-wide association studies (GWASs) and large-scale replication studies, have identified and confirmed more than 30 disease-associated loci predisposing to SLE susceptibility. In parallel, evidence for important epigenetic contributions to SLE is emerging. In this chapter, we emphasize studies published after the last edition of this book (2007), summarizing established genetic risk loci and their potential effects on SLE manifestations as well as describe the current understanding of the impact of epigenetic changes on the initiation and progression of SLE.

MONOGENIC DEFICIENCIES AND RARE MUTATIONS WITH SLE

Most patients affected with SLE have no family history of this disease. In families with multiple affected members, the disease occurrence does not follow the classic mendelian inheritance model for a single-gene disorder. However, in a few cases, SLE is associated with rare but highly penetrant mutations (Table 4-1), resulting in deficiency of classical complement components and/or defective degradation of DNA.

Complement Deficiency

An extremely strong genetic risk for SLE is conferred by a complete deficiency in one of the classical complement pathway genes, such as *C1Q*, *C1R/S*, *C2*, *C4A*, and *C4B*, even though these deficiencies are relatively rare. The incidence of SLE or lupus-like manifestations has been identified in 93% of homozygous *C1Q*-deficient individuals, in 57% of *C1R/C1S*-deficient individuals, in 75% of *C4*-deficient individuals, and in 10% to 25% of *C2*-deficient individuals.[1] Patients with SLE and deficiency of *C1Q* or *C4* usually demonstrate disease at a young age without a female predominance and have an approximate 30% frequency of renal involvement (glomerulonephritis).[1] In contrast, patients with SLE and *C2* deficiency show a sex distribution similar to that seen in lupus in general (female/male 7:1) and demonstrate disease later in life.[2] The severity of disease in patients with SLE and *C2* deficiency does not differ from that in most patients with SLE; however, an increased rate of skin or cardiovascular involvement and a low frequency of glomerulonephritis is observed in *C2* deficiency (reviewed by Jonsson[3]). Complement is critical for the opsonization and clearance of autoantibody-containing immune complexes (ICs). Deficiencies of complement components in the classical pathway are involved in several key steps in the SLE; pathogenesis, including reduced tolerance of autoantigens, reduced handling of apoptotic cell debris and IC clearance, and dysregulation of TLR (Toll-like receptor)– or IC-induced cytokines.[1]

TREX1

Mutations in one of three genes encoding the intracellular nucleases, TREX1 (a major 3′-5′ DNA exonuclease), RNase H2 (degrades DNA:RNA hybrids), and SAMHD1 (a putative nuclease), cause the Aicardi-Goutières syndrome (AGS), which shares several features with SLE, such as hypocomplementemia and antinuclear autoantibodies.[4] Of note, missense mutations of *TREX1* are found in 0.5% to 2.7% of patients with SLE but are nearly absent in healthy controls.[5,6] A 2011 analysis of more than 8000 multiancestral patients with SLE has revealed a risk haplotype of *TREX1* associated with neurologic manifestations, especially seizures, in patients of European descent.[6] TREX1 serves as a cytosolic DNA sensor, preferentially binds to single-stranded DNA, and functions as a DNA-degrading enzyme in granzyme-A–mediated apoptosis.[7] TREX1 deficiency impairs DNA damage repair, leading to the accumulation of endogenous retroelement-derived DNA. Defective clearance of this DNA induces IFN production of interferon (IFN) and an immune-mediated inflammatory response, promoting systemic autoimmunity.[7]

TRAP

The immuno-osseous dysplasia spondyloenchondrodysplasia (SPENCD) has been regarded primarily as a skeletal dysplasia, but patients with the disease also show a high frequency of autoimmune phenotypes, including SLE, Sjögren syndrome, hemolytic anemia, thrombocytopenia, hypothyroidism, inflammatory myositis, Raynaud disease, and vitiligo.[8,9] Loss-of-function mutations in the acid phosphatase 5 gene (*ACP5*; encoding tartrate-resistant acid phosphatase, TRAP), which have been identified as causative of the disease,[8,9] result in an elevated serum IFN-α activity and an IFN signature in patients with SPENCD.[8] Because TRAP is responsible for dephosphorylating osteopontin (OPN; encoded by *SPP1*), a multifunctional cytokine involved in immune system signaling, it is possible that in the absence of TRAP, OPN would remain phosphorylated and maintain persistent activation of IFN-α through the TLR9/MyD88 pathway.[9] Of interest, *SPP1* genetic polymorphisms have been associated with SLE and enhanced IFN-α activity, and elevated OPN protein values are correlated with the inflammatory process and SLE development.[10,11]

DNASE 1

Deoxyribonuclease I (DNase I, encoded by *DNASE1*) is a specific endonuclease facilitating chromatin breakdown during apoptosis. DNase I activity is important to prevent immune stimulation, and reduced activity may result in an increased risk for production of antinucleosome antibodies, a hallmark of SLE.[12] Several studies have found a connection between low DNase I activity and the development of human or murine SLE.[13,14] By sequencing the *DNASE1* gene in 20 Japanese patients with SLE, Yasumoto[15] found two female patients with a mutation in exon 2; the mutation resulted in a replacement of lysine with a stop signal, so they had decreased DNase I activity and an extremely high immunoglobulin G (IgG) titer against nucleosomal antigens.[15] Although this mutation has not been confirmed in other patient populations, specific common single-nucleotide polymorphisms (SNPs) of *DNASE1* (e.g., Q244R) have been associated with SLE susceptibility but not with DNase I activity nor with autoantibody titers.[16,17]

TABLE 4-1 Rare Mutations and Susceptibility to SLE or Lupus-Like Manifestations

FUNCTION	CHR	GENE	GENETIC VARIANT	FREQUENCY (%) OR ODDS RATIO OF SLE	MAIN LUPUS CLINICAL FEATURES
Impaired clearance of immune complexes and apoptotic cells	1p36	C1Q	Deficiency	93%	Glomerulonephritis Photosensitivity Neurological disorder
	12p13	C1R/C1S	Deficiency	57%	Glomerulonephritis
	6p21.3	C4A&B	Deficiency	75%	Glomerulonephritis
	6p21.3	C2	Deficiency	10-25%	Photosensitivity Anticardiolipin antibodies (aCLs)and antibodies to the collagen-like region of C1q (anti-C1qCLRs) Articular and cardiovascular disorders
Impaired DNA degradation	3p21.31	TREX1	Missense mutation	~25	Neuropsychiatric SLE
	16p13.3	DNASE1	Nonsense mutation	2 case reports	High titer of immunoglobulin G against nucleosomal antigens
Overactivation of interferon alpha	19p13	ACP5	Missense mutation	24 patients with SPENCD	Antinuclear antibodies (ANAs) and antibodies to the double-stranded DNA (anti-dsDNAs) Thrombocytopenia Nephritis Nonerosive arthritis

POLYGENIC COMMON VARIANTS IN SLE

In the majority of cases, genetic susceptibility of SLE fits the common disease–common variant hypothesis, which predicts that risk variants are present in more than 1% to 5% of general populations and that each has a modest magnitude of risk, with an odds ratio in the range of 1.1 to 2.5 accounting for a fraction of the overall genetic risk. Genetic dissection of SLE has been approached by three main methods: (1) targeted and genome-wide linkage analysis in multiplex families, (2) candidate gene association studies, and (3) GWASs.

Genome-Wide Linkage Studies

Linkage analysis is a comprehensive and unbiased approach, in which a few hundred genetic markers (such as DNA polymorphisms) are screened at 10- to 15-kb (kilobase) genomic intervals to identify chromosomal regions cotransmitted with disease in families containing multiple affected members. A total of 12 genome-wide scans and eight targeted linkage analyses have established 9 loci reaching the threshold for significant linkage to SLE (1q23, 1q31-32, 1q41-43, 2q37, 4p16, 6p11-21, 10q22-23, 12q24, and 16q12-13).[18] An alternative approach, that of stratifying by the presence of a clinical symptom in multiplex pedigrees, has led to the identification of 11 significant loci linked to particular SLE manifestations (reviewed by Sestak[18]). Progress toward further localizations of underlying causal variants has met with limited success because linkage intervals usually span large genomic regions that contain hundreds, if not thousands, of potential candidate genes, and because some important genes (e.g., IRF5) associated with SLE are not located within established linkage regions.

Candidate Gene Studies

Candidate gene studies are traditionally used to assess whether a test genetic marker (usually SNPs are under investigation) is present at a higher frequency among patients with SLE than in ethnically matched healthy control individuals. Candidate genes are chosen on the basis of either their functional relevance to the disease pathogenesis or their locations within chromosomal regions implicated in linkage studies. The test SNP observed with greater than expected frequency in individuals with disease is either a functional, disease-causing variant (a direct association) or a nonfunctional variant that exhibits strong linkage disequilibrium (LD) with the functional variant (an indirect association).[19] Literally hundreds of association studies of SLE were published in the last century, which, however, uncovered a limited number of confirmed SLE susceptibility genes because of small sample collections and/or a lack of dense marker coverage (reviewed by Tsao[20]). These limitations in linkage and candidate gene studies have hindered our understanding of the pathways causally involved in disease pathogenesis. This situation changed dramatically with the advent of the GWAS.

Genome-Wide Association Studies

The GWAS, an important step beyond the two previously mentioned methods, is built on efforts to identify associations of common genetic variations across the entire human genome with disease susceptibility. Rapid advances in technology have enabled a simultaneous genotyping of up to 1 million SNPs in a single GWAS. A typical GWAS usually consists of the following four parts[21]: (1) selection of a large number of individuals with disease of interest and a well-matched comparison group, (2) genotyping and data review to ensure high genotyping quality, (3) statistical association tests of the SNPs passing quality thresholds, and (4) replication of identified associations in an independent population or assessment of their functional implications. Since 2007, six GWASs[22-27] and a series of subsequent large-scale replication studies in SLE using both European and Asian populations not only have confirmed associations at previously established loci but also, and more importantly, have identified a number of novel loci (Table 4-2). Many of the disease-specific genes can be grouped into three major immunologic pathways (Figure 4-1). A growing number of genes seem to predispose to multiple autoimmune disorders, including SLE, rheumatoid arthritis (RA), systemic sclerosis (SSc), type 1 diabetes (T1D), Crohn disease (CD), Graves disease (GD), and psoriasis, highlighting the shared immunologic mechanisms conferred by common genetic variants among some of these disease processes. A few genes that cannot be mapped to a known disease pathway are likely to reveal new paradigms for disease pathogenesis and may provide new therapeutic targets for disease management.

A role for gene copy number variation (CNV) in SLE has been appreciated through studies of the complement component 4 (C4), Fcγ receptor IIIB (FCGR3B), TLR 7 (TLR7), and later work in complement regulator factor H–related 3 and 1 (CFHR3 and CFHR1).[28,29] CNVs can be detected either through direct scoring or identification of SNP markers known to be in LD with CNVs. The availability of large SNP-based GWAS datasets and future genetic screens using more dense markers, including structural variants (known as CNVs), will facilitate the genome-wide analysis and identification of CNVs predisposing to SLE susceptibility.

Human Leukocyte Antigen
Major Histocompatibility Complex Structure

The classical major histocompatibility complex (MHC) (also referred as the human leukocyte antigen [HLA]) region encompasses approximately 3.6 Mb on 6p21.3 and is divided into the class I (telomeric),

TABLE 4-2 Common Genetic Variants in SLE*

CHROMOSOME	GENE	GENETIC VARIANT	ODDS RATIO	STUDY POPULATION	ASSOCIATED MANIFESTATION(S)†
1p13.2	PTPN22	rs2476601 (R620W)	1.4-2.4	EU, HS	
1p36	C1Q	SNPs	1.4-2.2	AA, HS	Nephritis Photosensitivity
1q23	FCGR2A	rs1801274 (H131R)	1.3-1.4	EU, EA, AA, AS	Nephritis APS Malar rash
	FCGR3A	rs396991 (F158V)	1.2-1.5	EU, AA	Nephritis
	FCGR2B	rs1050501 (I232T)	1.3-2.5	AS	
	FCGR3B	Low copy number	1.7-2.3	EU, AA	Glomerulonephritis
1q25	TNFSF4	SNPs	1.2-1.5	EU, EA, AS	Renal disorder
1q31-q32	IL10	Microsatellite SNPs	1.2-1.3	EU, EA, AS, HS	aCL–immunoglobulin M, anti-Sm, anti-SSa antibodies Discoid lesions Renal and neurologic disorders
1q32	CR2	SNPs	1.1-1.5	EA, EU, AS	
1q32	CFHR3&CFHR1	Deletion	1.5	EA, AA, AS	
2p25-p24	RASGRP3	rs13385731	1.2-1.4	AS	Malar rash Discoid rash Anti-ANA
2q32	STAT4	rs7574865	1.5-1.8	EU, EA, AS, HS	Early age at disease onset Renal disorder Anti-dsDNA APS Protection from oral ulcers
		rs7582694	1.4	EU	Anti-dsDNA
3p14.3	PXK	SNPs	1.2-1.3	EU	Photosensitivity
4q24	BANK1	SNPs	1.2-1.4	EU, EA, AS	
4q26-q27	IL21	SNPs	1.1-1.6	EA, AA	Hematologic disorder
5q32-q33	TNIP1	rs10036748	1.3-1.4	EU, AS	Photosensitivity Vasculitis
6p21.3	HLA-DR2&DR3		1.5-2.5	EU	Anti-Ro/La and anti-dsDNA antibodies
6p21.3	C4A	Low copy number	1.6-6.5	EU, EA, AS	Arthritis
6p21	UHRF1BP1	rs11755393 (Q454R)	1.2-1.3	EU, EA, AS	Immunologic disorder
6q21	PRDM1/ATG5	SNPs	1.2-1.3	EU, AS	
6q23	TNFAIP3	SNPs	1.7-2.3	EU, EA, AS	Renal and hematologic disorders
		TT → A dinucleotide	1.7-2.5	EU, AS	
7p13-p11	IKZF1	SNPs	1.2-1.4	EU, AS	Malar rash Renal disorder
7p15.2	JAZF1	rs849142	1.2	EU, EA	
7q32	IRF5	Four functional SNPs	1.3-1.9	EU, EA, AA, AS, HS	
		rs10488631	1.6-1.7	EU, EA	Anti-dsDNA
8p23	BLK	SNPs	1.2-1.6	EU, EA, AS	APS Anti-dsDNA
8p23.1	XKR6	SNPs	1.2-1.3	EU, EA	
8q13	LYN	SNPs	1.2-1.3	EU, EA	Discoid rash Hematologic disorder
10q11.23	LRCC18/WDFY4	SNPs	1.2-1.3	AS	
11p13	PDHX/CD44	Microsatellite SNPs	1.2-1.4	EA, AA, AS	Thrombocytopenia
11p15	PHRF1/IRF7	rs4963128	1.3-2.0	EU, AA	Anti-dsDNA, anti-Sm antibodies; Immunologic disorder
		rs702966	1.8	EA	Anti-dsDNA
		rs1131665 (Q412R)	1.3-1.8	EA, AA, AS	
11q23.3	ETS1	SNPs	1.3	AS	Early age at disease onset

Continued

TABLE 4-2 Common Genetic Variants in SLE—cont'd

CHROMOSOME	GENE	GENETIC VARIANT	ODDS RATIO	STUDY POPULATION	ASSOCIATED MANIFESTATION(S)[†]
12q24.32	SLC15A4	SNPs	1.1-1.3	EU, AS	Discoid rash
16p11.2	ITGAM	rs1143679 (R77H)	1.3-2.1	EA, EU, AA, AS, HS	Discoid rash Arthritis Renal, neurologic, hematologic, and immunologic disorders
		rs9888739	1.3-1.4	EA, EU	Anti-dsDNA Arthritis
16p11.2	PRKCB	rs16972959	1.2	AS	
19p13	C3	SNPs	1.2-1.4	EU, AS	Decreased serum C3 level
22q11.21	UBE2L3	SNPs	1.2-1.3	EU, AS	Anti-dsDNA
Xp22	TLR7/TLR8	rs3853839	1.2-2.3	AS	Anti-RBP antibodies
Xq28	IRAK1/MECP2	SNPs	1.1-1.6	EU, EA, AS, HS	

AA, African American; aCL, anticardiolipin antibodies; ANA, antinuclear antibodies; anti-dsDNA, antibodies to double-stranded DNA; APS, antiphospholipid syndrome; anti-RBP antibodies, presence of one or more autoantibodies to Ro/SSA, La/SSB, RNP, and/or Sm; AS, Asian; EA, European American; EU, European; HS, Hispanic; SNP, single-nucleotide polymorphism.
*These loci are identified through genome-wide association studies, genome-wide association meta-analysis studies, candidate gene studies, or replication papers.
†The association of genetic variant with clinical manifestation is identified in one or more studied populations.

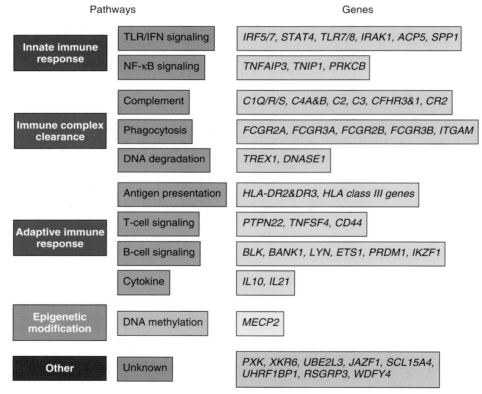

FIGURE 4-1 Important immunologic pathways in the pathogenesis of SLE as highlighted by the identified susceptibility genes. IFN, interferon; NF-κB, nuclear factor kappa B; TLR, Toll-like receptor.

class III, and class II (centromeric) regions. The class I and class II regions encode the classical HLA genes (HLA-A, -B, -C, -DR, -DQ, and -DP) involved in antigen presentation to T cells and transplant compatibility. The class I and class II molecules are the most polymorphic human proteins known to date. Because these molecules shape the immune repertoire of an individual, the extreme polymorphism is thought to have evolved in response to infectious pathogens. Perhaps that is the reason that the MHC is associated with more diseases than any other region of the human genome and is linked to most, if not all, autoimmune disorders. The class III region lies between the class I and class II regions and is the most gene-dense region in the genome, encoding a variety of molecules including the early complement components (e.g., C2, C4, and factor B), cytokines (e.g., tumor necrosis factor alpha [TNF-α] and lymphotoxin-α), the heat shock protein cluster, and proteins involved in growth and development. Given the existence of long-range LD- and MHC-related genes outside this classically defined locus, there comes to be a concept of the extended MHC (xMHC), spanning nearly 7.6 Mb of the genome, that consists of five subregions: the extended class I subregion (*HIST1H2AA* to *MOG*; 3.9 Mb), classical class I subregion (*C6orf40* to *MICB*; 1.9 Mb), classical class III subregion (*PPIP9* to *NOTCH4*; 0.7 Mb), classical class II subregion (*C6orf10* to *HCG24*; 0.9 Mb); and extended class II subregion (*COL11A2* to *RPL12P1*; 0.2 Mb);[30] Of the 421 genes within this extended region, 60% are expressed and approximately 22% have putative immunologic function.

HLA Class II Region and SLE

The association between SLE and variations in the HLA region has been extensively studied. Until 2005, most published disease association studies of HLA using small case-control panels of predominant European ancestries were restricted to a subset of about 20 genes, including the classical HLA loci (*HLA-A, -B, -C, -DRB, -DQA, -DQB, -DPA, -DPB*), *TNFA, LTA, LTB, TAP, MICA, MICB* and the complement loci (*C2, C4A, C4B,* and *CFB*) (reviewed by Fernando[30]). A pooled analysis of the past 30 years of research work regarding HLA genetics in SLE has pointed to the most consistent association with *HLA-DR3* (or *DRB1*0301*; one of the alleles from the previous DR3 specificity) and *HLA-DR2* (or *DRB1*1501*; one of the alleles from the previous DR2 specificity) and their respective haplotypes in predominantly European-derived populations.[31] In particular, the strongest associations were for the *HLA-DR3* haplotypes, *B8-DRB1*0301* and *B18-DRB1*0301*, with odds ratios (ORs) ranging from 1.5 to 2.5; whereas the associations of *DR2, DR15, DRB1*1501*, and *DQB1*0602*, which mapped to the *DR2/DRB1*1501* haplotype, exhibited an OR of 1.7.[31] Studies in non-European populations have revealed inconsistent results. For instance, the association with another *HLA-DR2* subtype, *DRB1*1503*, was only found in African Americans, who demonstrated no association with *DR2* or *DR3* alleles.[32] *HLA-DRB1*1602* has been observed in Mexican Mestizo, Thai, and Bulgarian populations; and *HLA-DRB1*0401* has been seen largely in Mexican Mestizo and Hispanic populations.[31] Two further class II alleles, *HLA-DQA1*0401* and *HLA-DQB1*0402*, reside on a *DR8* haplotype that is uncommon in European populations.[33]

Given the role for HLA class II molecules in T cell–dependent antibody responses, there is a close association of class II alleles, especially *HLA-DR* and *HLA-DQ* alleles with autoantibody subsets in patients with SLE of multiple ancestries (reviewed by Fernando[30]). The strongest associations have been demonstrated between anti-Ro/La antibodies and *DR3* and *DQ2* (*DQB1*0201*), which are in strong LD. Predominant associations with antiphospholipid antibodies—including anticardiolipin antibody (aCL), lupus anticoagulant (LA), and anti-β_2 glycoprotein I antibody (anti-β2GPI—are found for the *DR4* (*DRB1*04*)/*DQ8* (*DQB1*0302*) haplotype and other class II alleles. The HLA associations with other autoantibodies, including anti–double-stranded DNA (anti-dsDNA), anti-RNP, and anti-Sm, are much more complex, yielding inconclusive results.

HLA Class III Region and SLE

Despite a remarkably high gene density in the HLA class III region, only complement C4 CNVs and polymorphisms of tumor necrosis factor (*TNFA*) have been studied in detail in SLE (reviewed by Wu[34] and Postal[35]). It is concluded that a lower copy number of *C4* (due to increases in homozygous and heterozygous deficiencies of *C4A* but not *C4B*) increases risk and a higher copy number decreases risk for SLE. CNVs of *C4* genes determine the basal levels of circulating complement C4 proteins that function in the clearance of ICs, which can otherwise promote autoimmunity. Studies of *TNFA* polymorphisms have pointed to the promoter SNP-308A/G for its association with SLE either independently or as a part of an extended HLA haplotype, *HLA-A1-B8-DRB1*0301-DQ2*, in multiple ancestries. However, this association is not confirmed in other similar studies, so additional work is needed to clarify the role of genetic variants of *TNFA* in susceptibility to SLE.

With high-density genetic markers, GWASs and fine-mapping studies of SLE in populations of European and Asian ancestries have revolutionized our understanding of the *HLA* genetic contributions, which not only confirm predominant association signals at the class II region but also highlight the importance of class III genes in SLE susceptibility. For example, one SNP (rs3131379) of the HLA class III locus *MSH5* (mutS homolog 5) exhibited the highest association in a GWAS conducted in 2008.[23] A mapping study in 314 European families with SLE reported two distinct and independent signals[36]: one from a small, 180-kb class II region tagged by *HLA-DRB1*0301* allele and the other observed at an SNP marker (rs419788) in the class III gene *SKIV2L* (superkiller viralicidic activity 2–like [*Saccharomyces cerevisiae*]). Examination of LD structure around this marker (rs419788) showed this class III signal to be restricted to a 40-kb interval containing the genes *CFB*, *RDBP* (RD RNA binding protein), *DOM3Z* (dom-3 homolog Z [*Caenorhabditis elegans*]), and *STK19* (serine-threonine kinase 19). *CFB* encodes complement factor B, which is a vital component of the alternate complement pathway. The functions of *RDBP*, *SKIV2L*, *DOM3Z*, and *STK19* are not well characterized, although their products have been reported to play a role in messenger RNA (mRNA) processing. Of note, this study provided evidence against an independent effect of *TNFA*-308G/A polymorphism in SLE, which is inconsistent with results from another meta-analysis study.[37] Another collaborative study in multiple immune-mediated diseases indicated that the highest association signal for SLE was detected at SNP (rs1269852), located in the class III region between *TNXB* (tenascin XB) and *ATF6B* (activating transcription factor 6 beta) genes.[38] Other class III association signals were peaks centered on the *NOTCH4* gene and those on either side of the *RCCX* module (which contains *C4A* and *C4B* genes along with three neighboring genes). The influence of CNVs at the complement *C4/RCCX* locus in relation to the association signals revealed in this study remains to be established.[38]

Summary

In summary, GWASs and fine-mapping studies have confirmed genetic association with SLE in the *HLA* region, which exhibits complex and multilocus effects. In spite of these successes, there remains much work to further refine *HLA* association signals in SLE, including assessment of the effect of structural variations and localization of causal variants within this complex region.

Innate Immunity Genes

The role of innate immunity in SLE is widely recognized, in that immune complexes containing self-antigens/nucleic acids bind to endosomal TLR7 or TLR9, activate transcription factors of the IFN pathway (e.g., IRF5/7, nuclear factor kappa B [NF-κB], and STAT4) and finally lead to augmented production of IFN-α. Initial GWASs and follow-up studies provide convincing evidence for genetic association of the innate immunity pathway with SLE, highlighting the importance of innate immunity in SLE pathophysiology.

IRF5

IRF5 encodes for interferon regulatory factor 5 (IRF5), a pivotal transcription factor in the type I IFN pathway that regulates the expression of IFN-dependent genes, inflammatory cytokines, and genes involved in apoptosis. *IRF5* is one of the most strongly and consistently SLE-associated genes outside the HLA region, conferring a modest risk with an OR of 1.3 or more. Predominant associations of *IRF5* with SLE in populations of multiple ancestries are identified at four functional variants, a 5–base pair (bp) indel (insertion/deletion) near the 5′ untranslated region (UTR) rs2004640 in the first intron, a 30-bp indel in the sixth exon, and rs10954213 in the 3′ UTR.[39] Alleles of these functional variants in different combinations define various haplotypes that are associated with increased, decreased, or neutral levels of risk for SLE. The risk haplotypes have functional consequences, including greater expression of *IRF5* mRNA and IFN-inducible chemokines, as well as elevated IFN-α activity.[40,41] Indeed, a critical role for *IRF5* in mediating lupus pathogenesis is demonstrated in murine models of lupus-like disease using *Irf5*-deficient and *Irf5*-sufficient *FcγRIIB*[-/-] Yaa mice[42] or *Irf5*[-/-] MRL/lpr mice.[43]

STAT4

The signal transducer and activator of transcription 4 (encoded by *STAT4*) can transmit signals from the receptor for type I IFN, interleukin (IL) 12, and IL-23, and contribute to autoimmune responses by affecting the functions of several innate and adaptive immune cells. The SLE-associated SNP (rs7574865) in the third intron of *STAT4* was first identified in several case-control studies, exhibiting an OR of 1.5 to 1.7,[44] and was confirmed by GWASs using populations of European or Asian ancestry.[23,25-27,45] The risk allele of rs7574865 is associated with a more severe SLE phenotype, characterized by development of disease at an early age (<30 years), a high frequency of nephritis, the presence of antibodies against dsDNA, and an increased sensitivity to IFN-α signaling.[46-48] Fine-mapping studies led to the identification of several markers that are independently associated with SLE and/or with differential levels of *STAT4* expression,[47,49,50] and a 73-kb risk haplotype common to European Americans, Koreans, and Hispanic Americans.[50]

PHRF1/IRF7

Two independent studies in European populations have reported an SLE-associated SNP (rs4963128) in a gene of unknown function named PHD and RING-finger domains 1 (*PHRF1*, also known as *KIAA1542*).[23,45] Given that a strong LD ($r^2 = 0.94$) between this disease-associated SNP and the 3′UTR *PHRF1* SNP (rs702966) is within a 0.6-kb flanking region of the *IRF7* gene, this observed association might be attributable to its close proximity to *IRF7* (which codes interferon regulatory factor 7).[23] Like IRF5, IRF7 is a transcription factor that can activate transcription of IFN-α and IFN-α–inducible genes downstream of endosomal TLRs. Two studies support *PHRF1/IRF7* as an SLE susceptibility locus with the following findings: (1) patients with SLE carrying the risk allele of *PHRF1* SNP (rs702966) and expressing autoantibodies to dsDNA or Sm exhibit elevated serum IFN-α activity[51] and (2) the major allele of a nonsynonymous SNP (Q412R) in *IRF7* confers elevated IFN-stimulated response in vitro and predisposes to SLE in Asians, European Americans, and African Americans.[52] However, a complete assessment of this locus with dense genetic markers and/or sequencing to localize all possible causal variants is still pending.

TLR7/TLR8

TLR7 and its functionally related gene *TLR8*, located on the X chromosome, encode proteins that recognize endogenous RNA-containing autoantigens and induce the production of IFN-α, leading to autoimmunity. There is compelling evidence supporting the contribution of *TLR7* to the development of SLE. Transgenic mice with a two-fold overexpression of *Tlr7* have accelerated development of spontaneous autoimmunity,[53] whereas *Tlr7*-deficient mice have ameliorated lupus disease, decreased lymphocyte activation, and reduced serum IgG.[54] In addition, inhibitors of *Tlr7* can reduce a number of lupus-associated phenotypes both in the MRL and NZB/W lupus-prone strains.[55] However, studies of *TLR7* CNVs in human SLE have shown inconsistent results, with an increased copy number of *TLR7* observed in Mexicans with childhood-onset SLE but not in patients with adult-onset SLE who are of European and African American ancestries.[56,57] Differences in the study sample size, ethnicity, or genetic background between childhood-onset and adult-onset SLE may explain the discrepancies. Fine mapping the *TLR7/TLR8* genomic region in large-scale Eastern Asian population led to the identification of a functional SNP (rs3853839) in the 3′UTR of *TLR7* associated with SLE. The risk allele confers elevated *TLR7* expression and an increased IFN response in patients.[58] Similar studies in other populations are under way to elucidate variants within the *TLR7/TLR8* region for risk of SLE.

IRAK1 and MECP2

IRAK1, another X-linked gene, encodes a serine-threonine protein kinase named IL-1 receptor–associated kinase 1, which regulates multiple pathways in both innate and adaptive immune responses by linking several immune receptor complexes to TRAF6 (TNF receptor–associated factor 6). Studies by Jacob provide an important insight into *Irak1* function in murine models of SLE, as *Irak1* could play a role in the regulation of NF-κB in T-cell receptor (TCR) signaling and TLR activation, as well as in the induction of IFN-α and IFN-γ.[59] Additionally, in a study of approximately 5000 subjects in four different populations, five SNPs spanning the *IRAK1* gene were found to show disease association in patients with both adult-onset and childhood-onset SLE.[59] Located in the region of LD with *IRAK1* is another potential risk gene for SLE, methyl-CpG-binding protein 2 (*MECP2*), which has a critical role in the transcriptional suppression of methylation sensitive genes. A large replication study in a European population has confirmed the genetic contribution of the *IRAK1/MECP2* region to SLE, although further work is required to identify the causal variants.[45]

TNFAIP3 and TNIP1

The zinc finger A20 protein (encoded by *TNFAIP3*) is an ubiquitin-modifying enzyme critical for termination of NF-κB responses downstream of signal transduction through tumor necrosis factor–receptor (TNF-R), TLR, IL-1 receptor (IL-1R), and nucleotide-binding oligomerization domain containing 2 (NOD2). Reduced A20 expression predisposes to autoimmunity, as is demonstrated in mice with B lymphocyte–specific A20 ablation, which exhibit elevated numbers of germinal center B cells, autoantibodies, and glomerular immunoglobulin deposits.[60] In humans, *TNFAIP3* has been identified as a susceptibility gene for SLE.[25-27,61,62] Independent genetic associations with SLE in European populations are localized to a region 185 kb upstream of *TNFAIP3* that is also associated with RA, a region 249 kb downstream of *TNFAIP3*, and a 109-kb haplotype spanning the *TNFAIP3* coding region, which harbors a putative causal variant in exon 3 (rs2230926, F127C). By fine mapping and genomic resequencing, Adrianto[63] has further characterized the *TNFAIP3* risk haplotype and identified a TT→A dinucleotide (T deletion followed by a T-to-A transversion) as the best candidate polymorphism responsible for the association between *TNFAIP3* and SLE in subjects of European and Korean ancestries.[63] The TT→A dinucleotide variant, 42 kb downstream of the *TNFAIP3* promoter, is located in a region of high conservation and regulatory potential that may influence *TNFAIP3* expression by altering the binding of a nuclear protein complex composed of NF-κB subunits. An interacting protein of A20 named TNFAIP3-interacting protein 1 (encoded by *TNIP1*) is involved in inhibition of NF-κB activation. GWASs have also revealed a genetic association of *TNIP1* with SLE in both Chinese and European populations.[26,45]

PRKCB

Identification of a genetic association at rs16972959 in intron 2 of *PRKCB* in a Chinese population provides an example that some candidate loci not reaching genome-wide significance ($P < 5 \times 10^{-8}$) in the initial GWAS are confirmed in the subsequent replication study.[64] *PRKCB* (protein kinase C-β), a member of the *PKC* gene family, is involved in many different cellular functions, including B-cell activation, apoptosis induction, endothelial cell proliferation, and intestinal sugar absorption. The role for *PRKCB* in the pathogenesis of SLE is suggested by its involvement in apoptosis and in B-cell receptor (BCR)–mediated NF-κB activation.

Adaptive Immunity Genes

SLE is characterized by a loss of T- and B-cell tolerance, accounting for the formation of autoantibodies. GWASs have identified multiple susceptibility genes involved in T- and B-cell signal transduction pathways, illustrating the importance of the differentiation, activation, or function of various lymphocytes participating in SLE pathogenesis.

PTPN22

PTPN22 encodes the protein tyrosine–protein phosphatase nonreceptor type 22, which is a critical gatekeeper of T-cell receptor (TCR) signaling. The 620W allele of a nonsynonymous SNP (rs2476601) is associated with susceptibility to multiple autoimmune diseases (Table 4-3), providing evidence for shared mechanisms despite their diversely different clinical presentations.[65] The association between rs2476601 and SLE has been confirmed in European but not in Asian GWASs,[23,26,27,45] possibly as a result of a high variability in 620W allele frequencies among populations (European, 2%-15%; Asian, nearly absent). The substitution of arginine (R) with tryptophan (W) at the amino acid 620 occurs within a protein-protein interaction domain and results in a gain of function that inhibits TCR signaling and promotes the development of autoimmunity.[66] Supporting this notion, another loss-of-function polymorphism (rs33996649, R263Q) that leads to reduced phosphatase activity of PTPN22 and increased threshold for TCR signaling has been associated with protection against SLE in a European population.[67] The observation of higher serum IFN-α activity in patients with SLE carrying the 620W allele implicates a link between *PTPN22* and the type I IFN pathway.[68]

TNFSF4

Interaction of TNF ligand superfamily member 4 (encoded by *TNFSF4*, also known as *OX40L*) with TNF receptor superfamily member 4 (encoded by *TNFRSF4*, also known as *OX40*) can induce the production of co-stimulatory signals. OX40 plays a role in CD4⁺ T-cell responses, as well as T cell–dependent B-cell proliferation and differentiation. OX40L-mediated signaling induces B-cell activation and differentiation as well as IL-17 production but inhibits the generation and function of IL-10–producing T-regulator cells. A high expression of OX40 on CD4⁺ T cells and an elevated serum level of OX40L are observed in patients with SLE, especially in patients with nephritis, implicating a role for OX40-OX40L interaction in the pathogenesis of SLE.[69] From the genetic standpoint, a haplotype defined by tag SNPs in the upstream region of *TNFSF4* has been identified for association with SLE and greater expression of OX40L.[70] Subsequently, associations between *TNFSF4*-tagging SNPs and an increased risk for SLE have been confirmed in an Asian GWAS and two independent replication studies performed in populations of European ancestries.[26,45,71]

CD44

The chromosome region 11p13, which lies between two immune-related genes, *PDHX* and *CD44,* was first identified as linked to SLE through the study of families multiplex for SLE with thrombocytopenia.[72] In an association study using more than 15,000 multiethnic case-control samples in Europeans, African Americans, and Asians, one intergenic SNP rs2732552 was identified that exhibited robust and consistent disease association.[73] *CD44* encodes a cell-surface glycoprotein that plays an important role in lymphocyte activation, recirculation, apoptosis, hematopoiesis, and tumor metastasis. Although there is no direct genetic evidence of an association between *CD44 itself* and SLE susceptibility, the observation of elevations of CD44 protein and/or specific transcript isoforms (CD44v3 and CD44v6) in T cells from patients with SLE suggests a role for *CD44* in the pathogenesis of SLE.[74,75]

BLK, BANK1, and LYN

B lymphocyte–specific tyrosine kinase (encoded by *BLK*), a member of the Src family kinases, functions in intracellular signaling and regulates the proliferation, differentiation, and tolerance of B cells. Two *BLK* SNPs were first identified for association with SLE in GWASs of European populations[22,23]: One is rs13277113, located in the intergenic region between *FAM167A* and *BLK;* that risk allele is associated with reduced expression of *BLK* but increased expression of *FAM167A* in patients with SLE. The other is rs2248932 in the intron of *BLK,* 43 kb downstream of rs13277113. These two disease-associated variants have been subsequently confirmed in Asian populations.[27,76,77]

BANK1 encodes an adaptor/scaffold protein primarily expressed in B cells, which regulates direct coupling between the Src family of tyrosine kinases and the calcium channel IP3R, and facilitates the release of intracellular calcium, altering the B-cell activation threshold. Tyrosine-protein kinase Lyn (encoded by *LYN*), a binding partner of BANK1, plays an essential and rate-limiting role in mediating B-cell inhibition by phosphorylation of CD22 and recruitment of SHP-1. GWASs in European populations have implicated *BANK1* and *LYN* as susceptibility genes for SLE.[23,24] Three functional *BANK1* SNPs, including a nonsynonymous SNP in the IP3R binding domain (rs10516487; R61H), a branch point-site SNP (rs17266594; located in an intron), and another nonsynonymous SNP in the ankyrin domain (rs3733197; A383T), contribute to sustained B-cell receptor signaling and B-cell hyperactivity characteristic of SLE.[24] With the exception of one *BANK1* SNP (rs10516487), which showed a weak association with SLE, the remaining variants of *BANK1* and *LYN* have not been confirmed in Asian GWASs, partly owing to the low frequencies of the SNPs in Asian populations.[26,27]

ETS1 and PRDM1

E26 *ETS1* transformation–specific 1 (Ets-1, encoded by *ETS1*), a member of the ETS family of transcription factors, inhibits the function of PR domain zinc finger protein 1 (encoded by *PRDM1,* also known as *BLIMP1*) and negatively regulates B-cell and T-helper-17-cell differentiation. Of interest, *PRDM1/ATG5* has been identified as a risk locus for SLE in both European and Asian GWASs,[23,26,45] but genetic associations within the ETS1 region have been reported only in Asian GWAS.[26,27] The risk allele of *ETS1* 3′UTR SNP (rs1128334) predisposes to a decreased expression of *ETS1* in peripheral blood

TABLE 4-3 Genes Shared by SLE and Other Autoimmune Diseases

FUNCTION	GENE(S)	LOCATION	DISEASE
Immune complex clearance	FCGR2A	1q23	T1D, UC
	FCGR3A	1q23	RA
	ITGAM	16p11.2	SSc
Innate immune response	IRF5	7q32	RA, IBD, SSc
	STAT4	2q33	RA, SS, SSc, pAPS, CD
	TNFAIP3	6q23	RA, T1D, PsA, CeD
	TNIP1	5q33	PsA, SSc
Adaptive immune response	HLA Class II	6p21.3	RA, SSc, GD, IBD, T1D
	PTPN22	1p13	RA, T1D, SSc, GD, CD, PsA
	TNFSF4	1q25	SSc
	BANK1	4q24	SSc, RA
	BLK	8p23	SSc, pAPS, RA
	Intergenic (PRDM1)	6q21	RA, CD
	Intergenic (IKZF1)	7p12	CD
	IL10	1q31-q32	UC, T1D, Behçet disease
	IL21	4q26-q27	RA, T1D, psoriasis, IBD
Unknown	UBE2L3	22q11.21	RA, CD
	PXK	3p14.3	RA

CD, Crohn disease; CeD, celiac disease; GD, Graves disease; IBD, inflammatory bowel disease; pAPS, primary antiphospholipid syndrome; PsA, psoriatic arthritis; RA, rheumatoid arthritis; SLE, systemic lupus erythematosus; SS, primary Sjögren syndrome; SSc, systemic sclerosis; T1D, type 1 diabetes; UC, ulcerative colitis.

mononuclear cells (PBMCs).[27] The connection between *ETS1* and SLE is further supported by the development in *Ets1*-deficient mice of a lupus-like disease characterized by high titers of autoantibodies and local activation of complement.[78]

IKZF1

DNA-binding protein Ikaros (encoded by *IKZF1*) is a member of a family of lymphoid-restricted zinc finger transcription factors that regulates lymphocyte differentiation and proliferation, as well as self-tolerance through regulation of B cell–receptor signaling. *IKZF1* was identified as a novel SLE susceptibility gene in a GWAS using a Chinese population[26] and then confirmed in a replication study in a European population.[45] Decreased mRNA expression of *IKZF1* was observed in peripheral blood mononuclear cells from patients with SLE[79]; however, the role for *IKZF1* in the pathogenesis of SLE requires further study.

IL10

Interleukin-10 (encoded by *IL10*) is an important regulatory cytokine with both immunosuppressive and immunostimulatory properties. It can inhibit the functions of T cells and antigen presenting cells (APCs) but promotes B cell–mediated functions, enhancing survival, proliferation, differentiation, and antibody production. Of note, an increased IL-10 production by peripheral blood B cells and monocytes is observed in patients with SLE and is associated with disease activity, a finding that can explain B-cell hyperactivity in SLE.[80] Three SNPs in the *IL10* promoter region have been associated with variability in IL-10 production and confer a risk for SLE in European, Hispanic American, and Asian populations.[81] *IL10* has also been confirmed as an SLE susceptibility gene in a large-scale replication study of a European population.[45]

IL21

Interleukin-21 (encoded by *IL21*) is a newly discovered cytokine produced by activated CD4+ T cells that acts on natural killer cells, CD4+ cells, and B cells to induce and sustain antibody production and mediate antibody class switching.[82] A later series of studies has implicated the contribution of IL-21 in the pathogenesis of SLE. Evidence obtained from murine models of SLE (BXSB.B6-Yaa+/J mice) suggests the important role of IL-21 in the production of pathogenic autoantibodies and end-organ damage.[82] In humans, compared to healthy controls, patients with SLE show a higher plasma level of IL-21 and an enhanced *IL21* mRNA expression in skin biopsy specimens.[83,84] Genetic studies have identified the *IL2/IL21* region at chromosome 4q27 as a susceptibility locus in multiple autoimmune disorders, including inflammatory bowel disease (IBD), psoriasis, asthma, T1D, RA, and SLE.[82] With regard to SLE, the first study indicated the association between two *IL21* intronic SNPs (rs907715 and rs2221903) and SLE in European and African Americans. Further transethnic fine mapping of the *IL2/IL21* locus in two large independent lupus sets (European and African American ancestries) has localized the main genetic effect on the SNP rs907715 with a genome-wide significance ($P < 5 \times 10^{-8}$).[85] Functional consequences of the associated *IL21* SNPs need to be better characterized.

Immune Complex Clearance

Deficiencies of immune complex and apoptotic cell clearance lead to initiation and maintenance of autoimmune responses and ensuing chronic inflammation in SLE. Identifying disease association with genes involved in this pathway provides molecular support for immune complex processing as an important pathogenic theme in SLE.

Common Genetic Variants of Complement Components

The relationship between complement and SLE pathogenesis has long been noticed because low levels of complement are common immunologic features of SLE, particularly during disease flares. In addition to the rare complete deficiencies of classical complement pathway genes, common genetic variants, including gene deletion and SNPs, that result in low levels of complement components, and contribute to risk for SLE are (1) deletion of genes encoding two regulators of the alternative complement pathway, *CFHR3* and *CFHR1* (complement regulator factor H–related 3 and 1), which may lead to dysregulated complement activation and are associated with SLE susceptibility in European American, African American, and Asian populations[29] and (2) a common SNP of *C1Q*, *C3*, or *CR2* (complement receptor 2) gene, which either confers lower serum levels of C1q or C3 or alters transcriptional activity of CR2 and is associated with increased risk for SLE in multiple populations.[39,86,87]

Fcγ Receptor Genes

Five genes located at chromosome 1q23 (*FCGR2A*, *FCGR3A*, *FCGR2C*, *FCGR3B*, and *FCGR2B*) encode the low affinity Fcγ receptors (FcγRs), which play critical roles in regulating a variety of humoral and cellular immune responses, including IC clearance and antibody-dependent cellular cytotoxicity.[88] Functional SNPs of these genes, which may alter the binding affinities of the encoded receptors, leading to lower efficiency in IC clearance, have been reported to confer risk for SLE and/or lupus nephritis among multiple populations, as follows: rs1801274 (H131R) of *FCGR2A*, rs396991 (F158V) in the mature sequence of *FCGR3A*, and rs1050501 (I187T) of *FCGR2B*.[88] In addition, a decreased copy number of *FCGR3B*, which correlates with levels of protein expression and IC clearance, is observed in some patients with SLE.[89] However, the presence of high sequence homology among the *FCGR* genes, together with the presence of known segmental duplication and structural variation in this region, may preclude the assessment of specific SNPs in the *FCGR* gene complex on the currently available GWAS arrays. Further interpretations of the relative contribution of various *FCGR* variants to SLE must be made in the context of LD involving multiple functional variants.

ITGAM

ITGAM (also known as *CD11B*) encodes integrin αM, which combines with integrin β2 to form a leukocyte-specific integrin. The αMβ2 integrin plays a role in the regulation of leukocyte adhesion and emigration through interactions with a myriad of ligands that are potentially relevant to SLE (such as intercellular adhesion molecules 1 and 2 [ICAM-1 and ICAM-2], C3bi, and fibrinogen) and also in the phagocytosis of complement components and neutrophil apoptosis. Of note, the expression level of αMβ2 integrin is elevated in neutrophils from patients with SLE with active disease activity, which correlates with endothelial injury.[90] Two independent GWASs performed in European populations have reported genetic association at four SNPs in or very near the *ITGAM* gene,[22,23] which is located within the previously identified linkage interval 16p12.3-16q12.2. Consistently, a transethnic fine-mapping study shows a nonsynonymous SNP of *ITGAM* (rs1143679, R77H) with an effect on structural and functional changes of integrin αM, contributing to SLE susceptibility.[91] In a subsequent meta-analysis, this association and the role of rs1143679 were confirmed in various ethnicities, including Americans of European, Hispanic, or African ancestries as well as Mexican and Colombian populations.[92] Despite a low frequency of the 77H allele in Asian populations, it also displays a significant association with SLE risk and with severe manifestations (e.g., lupus nephritis, neurologic, hematologic, and immunologic disorders) in Hong Kong Chinese and Thai individuals.[93] However, the correlation between this variant and different clinical manifestations needs further replication studies using larger samples.

Other Genes

Application of GWAS and transethnic mapping study has revealed several SLE susceptibility genes that appear to be unique to a specific ethnic population, such as *PXK* (PX domain containing serine/threonine kinase), *XKR6* (XK, Kell blood group complex–related family member 6), and *JAZF1* (juxtaposed with another zinc finger gene 1) in European-derived populations,[23,45] but *RASGRP3* (RAS guanyl–releasing protein 3) and *WDFY4* (WDFY family member 4) in Asians.[26,27] Functions of these novel genes are neither fully characterized nor obviously connect to the known pathways contributing to SLE. Understanding how they increase the risk for SLE will provide exciting insights into the pathogenesis of this disease.

Correlation of Genotypes with Disease Phenotypes in SLE

SLE is a genetically complex disease with heterogeneous clinical manifestations. Following the GWASs that have greatly expanded the number of established SLE risk loci, later studies have begun to assess the relationship between specific disease-associated alleles and clinical symptoms of SLE, which support genetic profiling as a potentially useful tool to predict disease manifestations and direct personalized treatment in patients with SLE. In the first genome-wide genotype-phenotype study, 22 previously established SLE susceptibility loci were chosen for testing and composed a *genetic risk score* (GRS) for SLE, defined as the number of risk alleles with each weighted by the SLE risk OR.[94] This analysis categorized SLE subphenotypes into three groups: (1) those associated with GRSs (cumulative risk loci), including age at diagnosis, anti-dsDNA autoantibody, oral ulcers, and immunologic and hematologic disorders, (2) those associated with single risk loci, including renal involvement and arthritis, and (3) those with no known genetic associations, such as serositis, neurologic disorder, photosensitivity, and malar and discoid rashes. In the second genotype-phenotype study, 16 confirmed SLE susceptibility loci were tested in a large multiethnic set of patients with SLE, and statistically significant associations were found only in European populations, including correlation of *ITGAM* and *TNFSF4* with renal disease, *FCGR2A* with malar rash, *ITGAM* with discoid rash, *IL21* with hematologic disorders (specifically leukopenia), and *STAT4* with protection from oral ulcers.[95] Anti-dsDNA autoantibody, with diagnostic and clinical importance, was present in 40% to 60% of patients with SLE. A GWAS performed in European-derived populations has reported that SNPs of *STAT4, IRF5, ITGAM,* and *HLA* show stronger disease association in anti-dsDNA⁺ patients than in anti-dsDNA⁻ patients, and associations between SLE and SNPs of *BANK1*, *PHRF1*, and *UBE2L3* were observed only in anti-dsDNA⁺ patients.[96] These data suggest that many established SLE susceptibility loci may confer disease risk through their roles in autoantibody production. Ongoing genotype-phenotype association studies will produce a more detailed view of genetic markers associated with specific clinical manifestations, presenting important insights into the role of genetics in organ involvement.

GENE-GENE INTERACTIONS AMONG SUSCEPTIBILITY LOCI IN SLE

Despite the success in GWASs, the joint modest effects of these loci account for only a small proportion of the heritability of SLE. Three potential mechanisms may explain the missing heritability in SLE: common and rare genetic variants that have yet to be discovered, a heritable epigenetic component, and gene-gene interactions among known and/or yet to be identified loci for SLE susceptibility. Several studies have provided evidence for genetic interactions between the HLA region and *CTLA4*, *ITGAM* and *IRF5*, between *IL21* and *PDCD1*, between *BLK* and *BANK1* and *TNFSF4*, and between *IRF5* and *STAT4* in patients with SLE, again highlighting the importance of antigen presentation, T- and B-cell responses, and the IFN signaling pathway in disease pathogenesis.[49,97-99] However, investigating gene-gene interactions has proven difficult because of the computational burden of analysis. With advances in statistical developments, application of the interaction strategy to GWAS data will help uncover potential novel loci contributing to SLE. See Chapter 5 for discussion of the role of epigenetics in SLE.

COMMON LOCI AMONG AUTOIMMUNE DISEASES

Paralleling the GWASs in mapping SLE risk loci are the successes in identifying genetic associations with other autoimmune diseases, including RA, SSc, T1D, GD, CD, primary antiphospholipid syndrome (APS), Behçet disease (BD), inflammatory bowel disease, ulcerative colitis (UC), and psoriatic arthritis (PsA). Identifying risk loci shared by SLE and other autoimmune disorders suggests the existence of common immunologic mechanisms and furthers our understanding of the development and concomitance of these diseases (see Table 4-3). For example, a cluster of genes involved in T-cell activation may predict susceptibility to autoimmune disease generically[65]: *HLA class II* with multiple autoimmune diseases; *PTPN22* with SLE, RA, SSc, psoriatic arthritis, GD, CD, and T1D; and *TNFSF4* with SLE and SSc. The newly developed ImmunoChip genotyping microarray provides a powerful tool for immunogenetics gene mapping. The ImmunoChip contains 184 loci with more than 200,000 SNPs representing genetic associations identified from one or more of 12 different autoimmune inflammatory phenotypes, including SLE, RA, T1D, CD, ulcerative colitis, psoriasis, primary biliary cirrhosis, autoimmune thyroid disease, multiple sclerosis, celiac disease, IgA deficiency, and ankylosing spondylitis. The availability of this platform will accelerate the identification of variants shared by multiple autoimmune diseases and loci that promote disease-specific phenotypes.

CONCLUSION

Rapid advances in the human genome sequences and high-throughput genotyping technology have revolutionized our understanding of the genetic basis of SLE in GWASs. In spite of the tremendous progress, there remain several challenges for future studies: First, current GWASs are designed to identify disease-associated SNPs that are common in human populations (frequency >5%), and the accumulative genetic contribution of all identified risk loci probably represents less than half of the total genetic susceptibility to SLE. Ongoing investigations such as next-generation sequencing strategies are attempting to address the remaining genetic components (known as missing heritability), including rare SNPs with prevalence less than 1% and other structural polymorphisms (e.g., insertion/deletion, copy number, and repeat element variations). Second, it is of note that most of the reported disease associations have been identified in European or Asian populations. Similar studies using large samples of African and Hispanic ancestries are also required, which will help clarify the basis for disparities of SLE association between different populations. Third, a central goal of the ongoing characterization of SLE is to correlate the genetic profile with the clinical course of disease through generating knowledge of individual patterns of disease predisposition and identifying novel biological pathways and therapeutic targets, therefore facilitating personalized risk assessment and disease management.

References

1. Truedsson L, Bengtsson AA, Sturfelt G: Complement deficiencies and systemic lupus erythematosus. *Autoimmunity* 40:560–566, 2007.
2. Jonsson H, Nived O, Sturfelt G: Outcome in systemic lupus erythematosus: a prospective study of patients from a defined population. *Medicine (Baltimore)* 68(3):141–150, 1989.
3. Jonsson G, Sjoholm AG, Truedsson L, et al: Rheumatological manifestations, organ damage and autoimmunity in hereditary C2 deficiency. *Rheumatology (Oxford)* 46(7):1133–1139, 2007.
4. Ramantani G, Kohlhase J, Hertzberg C, et al: Expanding the phenotypic spectrum of lupus erythematosus in Aicardi-Goutieres syndrome. *Arthritis Rheum* 62(5):1469–1477, 2010.
5. Lee-Kirsch MA, Gong M, Chowdhury D, et al: Mutations in the gene encoding the 3′-5′ DNA exonuclease TREX1 are associated with systemic lupus erythematosus. *Nat Genet* 39(9):1065–1067, 2007.
6. Namjou B, Kothari PH, Kelly JA, et al: Evaluation of the TREX1 gene in a large multi-ancestral lupus cohort. *Genes Immun* 12(4):270–279, 2011.
7. Stetson DB, Ko JS, Heidmann T, et al: Trex1 prevents cell-intrinsic initiation of autoimmunity. *Cell* 134(4):587–598, 2008.

8. Briggs TA, Rice GI, Daly S, et al: Tartrate-resistant acid phosphatase deficiency causes a bone dysplasia with autoimmunity and a type I interferon expression signature. *Nat Genet* 43(2):127–131, 2011.

9. Lausch E, Janecke A, Bros M, et al: Genetic deficiency of tartrate-resistant acid phosphatase associated with skeletal dysplasia, cerebral calcifications and autoimmunity. *Nat Genet* 43(2):132–137, 2011.

10. Han S, Guthridge JM, Harley ITW, et al: Osteopontin and Systemic Lupus Erythematosus Association: a probable gene-gender interaction. *PLoS ONE* 3(3):e0001757, 2008.

11. Kariuki SN, Moore JG, Kirou KA, et al: Age- and gender-specific modulation of serum osteopontin and interferon-alpha by osteopontin genotype in systemic lupus erythematosus. *Genes Immun* 10(5):487–494, 2009.

12. Martinez Valle F, Balada E, Ordi-Ros J, et al: DNase 1 and systemic lupus erythematosus. *Autoimmun Rev* 7(5):359–363, 2008.

13. Sallai K, Nagy E, Derfalvy B, et al: Antinucleosome antibodies and decreased deoxyribonuclease activity in sera of patients with systemic lupus erythematosus. *Clin Diagn Lab Immunol* 12(1):56–59, 2005.

14. Napirei M, Karsunky H, Zevnik B, et al: Features of systemic lupus erythematosus in Dnase1-deficient mice. *Nat Genet* 25(2):177–181, 2000.

15. Yasutomo K, Horiuchi T, Kagami S, et al: Mutation of DNASE1 in people with systemic lupus erythematosus. *Nat Genet* 28(4):313–314, 2001.

16. Bodano A, Gonzalez A, Balada E, et al: Study of DNASE I gene polymorphisms in systemic lupus erythematosus susceptibility. *Ann Rheum Dis* 66(4):560–561, 2007.

17. Bodano A, Gonzalez A, Ferreiros-Vidal I, et al: Association of a non-synonymous single-nucleotide polymorphism of DNASEI with SLE susceptibility. *Rheumatology (Oxford)* 45(7):819–823, 2006.

18. Sestak AL, Nath SK, Sawalha AH, et al: Current status of lupus genetics. *Arthritis Res Ther* 9(3):210, 2007.

19. Rhodes B, Vyse TJ: The genetics of SLE: an update in the light of genome-wide association studies. *Rheumatology* 47(11):1603–1611, 2008.

20. Tsao BP, Deng Y: Constitutive genes and lupus. In Lahita RG, editor: *Systemic lupus erythematosus*, New York, 2011, pp 47–62.

21. Pearson TA, Manolio TA: How to interpret a genome-wide association study. *JAMA* 299(11):1335–1344, 2008.

22. Hom G, Graham RR, Modrek B, et al: Association of systemic lupus erythematosus with C8orf13-BLK and ITGAM-ITGAX. *N Engl J Med* 358(9):900–909, 2008.

23. Harley JB, Alarcon-Riquelme ME, Criswell LA, et al: Genome-wide association scan in women with systemic lupus erythematosus identifies susceptibility variants in ITGAM, PXK, KIAA1542 and other loci. *Nat Genet* 40(2):204–210, 2008.

24. Kozyrev SV, Abelson AK, Wojcik J, et al: Functional variants in the B-cell gene BANK1 are associated with systemic lupus erythematosus. *Nat Genet* 40(2):211–216, 2008.

25. Graham RR, Cotsapas C, Davies L, et al: Genetic variants near TNFAIP3 on 6q23 are associated with systemic lupus erythematosus. *Nat Genet* 40(9):1059–1061, 2008.

26. Han JW, Zheng HF, Cui Y, et al: Genome-wide association study in a Chinese Han population identifies nine new susceptibility loci for systemic lupus erythematosus. *Nat Genet* 41(11):1234–1237, 2009.

27. Yang W, Shen N, Ye DQ, et al: Genome-wide association study in Asian populations identifies variants in ETS1 and WDFY4 associated with systemic lupus erythematosus. *PLoS Genet* 6(2):e1000841, 2010.

28. Ptacek T, Li X, Kelley JM, et al: Copy number variants in genetic susceptibility and severity of systemic lupus erythematosus. *Cytogenet Genome Res* 123(1-4):142–147, 2008.

29. Zhao J, Wu H, Khosravi M, et al: Association of genetic variants in complement factor H and factor H-related genes with systemic lupus erythematosus susceptibility. *PLoS Genet* 7(5):e1002079, 2011.

30. Fernando MM, Vyse TJ: Major histocompatibility complex class II. In Lahita RG, editor: *Systemic lupus erythematosus*, New York, 2011, pp 3–20.

31. Fernando MM, Stevens CR, Walsh EC, et al: Defining the role of the MHC in autoimmunity: a review and pooled analysis. *PLoS Genet* 4(4):e1000024, 2008.

32. Uribe AG, McGwin G, Jr., Reveille JD, et al: What have we learned from a 10-year experience with the LUMINA (Lupus in Minorities; Nature vs. nurture) cohort? Where are we heading? *Autoimmun Rev* 3(4):321–329, 2004.

33. Fernando MMA, Stevens CR, Walsh EC, et al: Defining the role of the MHC in autoimmunity: a review and pooled analysis. *PLoS Genet* 4(4):e1000024, 2008.

34. Wu YL, Yang Y, Chung EK, et al: Phenotypes, genotypes and disease susceptibility associated with gene copy number variations: complement C4 CNVs in European American healthy subjects and those with systemic lupus erythematosus. *Cytogenet Genome Res* 123(1-4): 131–141, 2008.

35. Postal M, Appenzeller S: The role of tumor necrosis factor-alpha (TNF-alpha) in the pathogenesis of systemic lupus erythematosus. *Cytokine* 56(3):537–543, 2011.

36. Fernando MM, Stevens CR, Sabeti PC, et al: Identification of two independent risk factors for lupus within the MHC in United Kingdom families. *PLoS Genet* 3(11):e192, 2007.

37. Lee YH, Harley JB, Nath SK: Meta-analysis of TNF-alpha promoter-308 A/G polymorphism and SLE susceptibility. *Eur J Hum Genet* 14(3):364–371, 2006.

38. Rioux JD, Goyette P, Vyse TJ, et al: Mapping of multiple susceptibility variants within the MHC region for 7 immune-mediated diseases. *Proc Natl Acad Sci U S A* 106(44): 18680–18685, 2009.

39. Deng Y, Tsao BP: Genetic susceptibility to systemic lupus erythematosus in the genomic era. *Nat Rev Rheumatol* 6(12):683–692, 2010.

40. Niewold TB, Kelly JA, Flesch MH, et al: Association of the IRF5 risk haplotype with high serum interferon-alpha activity in systemic lupus erythematosus patients. *Arthritis Rheum* 58(8):2481–2487, 2008.

41. Rullo OJ, Woo JM, Wu H, et al: Association of IRF5 polymorphisms with activation of the interferon-alpha pathway. *Ann Rheum Dis* 69(3):611–617, 2010.

42. Richez C, Yasuda K, Bonegio RG, et al: IFN regulatory factor 5 is required for disease development in the FcgammaRIIB-/-Yaa and FcgammaRIIB-/- mouse models of systemic lupus erythematosus. *J Immunol* 184(2):796–806, 2010.

43. Tada Y, Kondo S, Aoki S, et al: Interferon regulatory factor 5 is critical for the development of lupus in MRL/lpr mice. *Arthritis Rheum* 63(3):738–748, 2011.

44. Yuan H, Feng JB, Pan HF, et al: A meta-analysis of the association of STAT4 polymorphism with systemic lupus erythematosus. *Mod Rheumatol* 20(3):257–262, 2010.

45. Gateva V, Sandling JK, Hom G, et al: A large-scale replication study identifies TNIP1, PRDM1, JAZF1, UHRF1BP1 and IL10 as risk loci for systemic lupus erythematosus. *Nat Genet* 41(11):1228–1233, 2009.

46. Taylor KE, Remmers EF, Lee AT, et al: Specificity of the STAT4 genetic association for severe disease manifestations of systemic lupus erythematosus. *PLoS Genet* 4(5):e1000084, 2008.

47. Sigurdsson S, Nordmark G, Garnier S, et al: A risk haplotype of STAT4 for systemic lupus erythematosus is over-expressed, correlates with anti-dsDNA and shows additive effects with two risk alleles of IRF5. *Hum Mol Genet* 17(18):2868–2876, 2008.

48. Kariuki SN, Kirou KA, MacDermott EJ, et al: Cutting edge: autoimmune disease risk variant of STAT4 confers increased sensitivity to IFN-alpha in lupus patients in vivo. *J Immunol* 182(1):34–38, 2009.

49. Abelson AK, Delgado-Vega AM, Kozyrev SV, et al: STAT4 associates with systemic lupus erythematosus through two independent effects that correlate with gene expression and act additively with IRF5 to increase risk. *Ann Rheum Dis* 68(11):1746–1753, 2009.

50. Namjou B, Sestak AL, Armstrong DL, et al: High-density genotyping of STAT4 reveals multiple haplotypic associations with systemic lupus erythematosus in different racial groups. *Arthritis Rheum* 60(4):1085–1095, 2009.

51. Salloum R, Franek BS, Kariuki SN, et al: Genetic variation at the IRF7/PHRF1 locus is associated with autoantibody profile and serum interferon-alpha activity in lupus patients. *Arthritis Rheum* 62(2):553–561, 2010.

52. Fu Q, Zhao J, Qian X, et al: Association of a functional IRF7 variant with systemic lupus erythematosus. *Arthritis Rheum* 63(3):749–754, 2011.

53. Deane JA, Pisitkun P, Barrett RS, et al: Control of Toll-like receptor 7 expression is essential to restrict autoimmunity and dendritic cell proliferation. *Immunity* 27(5):801–810, 2007.

54. Christensen SR, Shupe J, Nickerson K, et al: Toll-like receptor 7 and TLR9 dictate autoantibody specificity and have opposing inflammatory and regulatory roles in a murine model of lupus. *Immunity* 25(3):417–428, 2006.

55. Barrat FJ, Meeker T, Chan JH, et al: Treatment of lupus-prone mice with a dual inhibitor of TLR7 and TLR9 leads to reduction of autoantibody production and amelioration of disease symptoms. *Eur J Immunol* 37:3582–3586, 2007.

56. Kelley J, Johnson MR, Alarcon GS, et al: Variation in the relative copy number of the TLR7 gene in patients with systemic lupus erythematosus and healthy control subjects. *Arthritis Rheum* 56(10):3375–3378, 2007.

57. Garcia-Ortiz H, Velazquez-Cruz R, Espinosa-Rosales F, et al: Association of TLR7 copy number variation with susceptibility to childhood-onset

systemic lupus erythematosus in Mexican population. *Ann Rheum Dis* 69(10):1861–1865, 2010.

58. Shen N, Fu Q, Deng Y, et al: Sex-specific association of X-linked Toll-like receptor 7 (TLR7) with male systemic lupus erythematosus. *Proc Natl Acad Sci U S A* 107(36):15838–15843, 2010.

59. Jacob CO, Zhu J, Armstrong DL, et al: Identification of IRAK1 as a risk gene with critical role in the pathogenesis of systemic lupus erythematosus. *Proc Natl Acad Sci U S A* 106(15):6256–6261, 2009.

60. Tavares RM, Turer EE, Liu CL, et al: The ubiquitin modifying enzyme A20 restricts B cell survival and prevents autoimmunity. *Immunity* 33(2):181–191, 2010.

61. Musone SL, Taylor KE, Lu TT, et al: Multiple polymorphisms in the TNFAIP3 region are independently associated with systemic lupus erythematosus. *Nat Genet* 40(9):1062–1064, 2008.

62. Bates JS, Lessard CJ, Leon JM, et al: Meta-analysis and imputation identifies a 109 kb risk haplotype spanning TNFAIP3 associated with lupus nephritis and hematologic manifestations. *Genes Immun* 10(5):470–477, 2009.

63. Adrianto I, Wen F, Templeton A, et al: Association of a functional variant downstream of TNFAIP3 with systemic lupus erythematosus. *Nat Genet* 43(3):253–258, 2011.

64. Sheng YJ, Gao JP, Li J, et al: Follow-up study identifies two novel susceptibility loci PRKCB and 8p11.21 for systemic lupus erythematosus. *Rheumatology (Oxford)* 50(4):682–688, 2011.

65. Gregersen PK, Olsson LM: Recent advances in the genetics of autoimmune disease. *Annu Rev Immunol* 27:363–391, 2009.

66. Bottini N, Musumeci L, Alonso A, et al: A functional variant of lymphoid tyrosine phosphatase is associated with type I diabetes. *Nat Genet* 36(4):337–338, 2004.

67. Orru V, Tsai SJ, Rueda B, et al: A loss-of-function variant of PTPN22 is associated with reduced risk of systemic lupus erythematosus. *Hum Mol Genet* 18(3):569–579, 2009.

68. Kariuki SN, Crow MK, Niewold TB: The PTPN22 C1858T polymorphism is associated with skewing of cytokine profiles toward high interferon-alpha activity and low tumor necrosis factor alpha levels in patients with lupus. *Arthritis Rheum* 58(9):2818–2823, 2008.

69. Farres MN, Al-Zifzaf DS, Aly AA, et al: OX40/OX40L in systemic lupus erythematosus: association with disease activity and lupus nephritis. *Ann Saudi Med* 31(1):29–34, 2011.

70. Cunninghame Graham DS, Graham RR, Manku H, et al: Polymorphism at the TNF superfamily gene TNFSF4 confers susceptibility to systemic lupus erythematosus. *Nat Genet* 40(1):83–89, 2008.

71. Delgado-Vega AM, Abelson AK, Sanchez E, et al: Replication of the TNFSF4 (OX40L) promoter region association with systemic lupus erythematosus. *Genes Immun* 10(3):248–253, 2009.

72. Scofield RH, Bruner GR, Kelly JA, et al: Thrombocytopenia identifies a severe familial phenotype of systemic lupus erythematosus and reveals genetic linkages at 1q22 and 11p13. *Blood* 101(3):992–997, 2003.

73. Lessard CJ, Adrianto I, Kelly JA, et al: Identification of a systemic lupus erythematosus susceptibility locus at 11p13 between PDHX and CD44 in a multiethnic study. *Am J Hum Genet* 88(1):83–91, 2011.

74. Li Y, Harada T, Juang YT, et al: Phosphorylated ERM is responsible for increased T cell polarization, adhesion, and migration in patients with systemic lupus erythematosus. *J Immunol* 178(3):1938–1947, 2007.

75. Crispin JC, Keenan BT, Finnell MD, et al: Expression of CD44 variant isoforms CD44v3 and CD44v6 is increased on T cells from patients with systemic lupus erythematosus and is correlated with disease activity. *Arthritis Rheum* 62(5):1431–1437, 2010.

76. Zhang Z, Zhu KJ, Xu Q, et al: The association of the BLK gene with SLE was replicated in Chinese Han. *Arch Dermatol Res* 302(8):619–624, 2010.

77. Ito I, Kawasaki A, Ito S, et al: Replication of the association between the C8orf13-BLK region and systemic lupus erythematosus in a Japanese population. *Arthritis Rheum* 60(2):553–558, 2009.

78. Wang D, John SA, Clements JL, et al: Ets-1 deficiency leads to altered B cell differentiation, hyperresponsiveness to TLR9 and autoimmune disease. *Int Immunol* 17(9):1179–1191, 2005.

79. Hu W, Sun L, Gao J, et al: Down-regulated expression of IKZF1 mRNA in peripheral blood mononuclear cells from patients with systemic lupus erythematosus. *Rheumatol Int* 31(6):819–822, 2011.

80. Hagiwara E, Gourley MF, Lee S, et al: Disease severity in patients with systemic lupus erythematosus correlates with an increased ratio of interleukin-10:interferon-gamma-secreting cells in the peripheral blood. *Arthritis Rheum* 39(3):379–385, 1996.

81. Lopez P, Gutierrez C, Suarez A: IL-10 and TNFalpha genotypes in SLE. *J Biomed Biotechnol* 2010:838390, 2010.

82. Sarra M, Monteleone G: Interleukin-21: a new mediator of inflammation in systemic lupus erythematosus. *J Biomed Biotechnol* 2010:294582, 2010.

83. Wong CK, Wong PT, Tam LS, et al: Elevated production of B cell chemokine CXCL13 is correlated with systemic lupus erythematosus disease activity. *J Clin Immunol* 30(1):45–52, 2010.

84. Caruso R, Botti E, Sarra M, et al: Involvement of interleukin-21 in the epidermal hyperplasia of psoriasis. *Nat Med* 15(9):1013–1015, 2009.

85. Hughes T, Kim-Howard X, Kelly JA, et al: Fine-mapping and transethnic genotyping establish IL2/IL21 genetic association with lupus and localize this genetic effect to IL21. *Arthritis Rheum* 63(6):1689–1697, 2011.

86. Wu H, Boackle SA, Hanvivadhanakul P, et al: Association of a common complement receptor 2 haplotype with increased risk of systemic lupus erythematosus. *Proc Natl Acad Sci U S A* 104(10):3961–3966, 2007.

87. Douglas KB, Windels DC, Zhao J, et al: Complement receptor 2 polymorphisms associated with systemic lupus erythematosus modulate alternative splicing. *Genes Immun* 10(5):457–469, 2009.

88. Li X, Ptacek TS, Brown EE, et al: Fcgamma receptors: structure, function and role as genetic risk factors in SLE. *Genes Immun* 10(5):380–389, 2009.

89. Mamtani M, Anaya JM, He W, et al: Association of copy number variation in the FCGR3B gene with risk of autoimmune diseases. *Genes Immun* 11(2):155–160, 2010.

90. Molad Y, Buyon J, Anderson DC, et al: Intravascular neutrophil activation in systemic lupus erythematosus (SLE): dissociation between increased expression of CD11b/CD18 and diminished expression of L-selectin on neutrophils from patients with active SLE. *Clin Immunol Immunopathol* 71(3):281–286, 1994.

91. Nath SK, Han S, Kim-Howard X, et al: A nonsynonymous functional variant in integrin-alpha(M) (encoded by ITGAM) is associated with systemic lupus erythematosus. *Nat Genet* 40(2):152–154, 2008.

92. Han S, Kim-Howard X, Deshmukh H, et al: Evaluation of imputation-based association in and around the integrin-alpha-M (ITGAM) gene and replication of robust association between a non-synonymous functional variant within ITGAM and systemic lupus erythematosus (SLE). *Hum Mol Genet* 18(6):1171–1180, 2009.

93. Yang W, Zhao M, Hirankarn N, et al: ITGAM is associated with disease susceptibility and renal nephritis of systemic lupus erythematosus in Hong Kong Chinese and Thai. *Hum Mol Genet* 18(11):2063–2070, 2009.

94. Taylor KE, Chung SA, Graham RR, et al: Risk alleles for systemic lupus erythematosus in a large case-control collection and associations with clinical subphenotypes. *PLoS Genet* 7(2):e1001311, 2011.

95. Sanchez E, Nadig A, Richardson BC, et al: Phenotypic associations of genetic susceptibility loci in systemic lupus erythematosus. *Ann Rheum Dis* 70(10):1752–1757, 2011.

96. Chung SA, Taylor KE, Graham RR, et al: Differential genetic associations for systemic lupus erythematosus based on anti-dsDNA autoantibody production. *PLoS Genet* 7(3):e1001323, 2011.

97. Hughes T, Adler A, Kelly JA, et al: Evidence for gene-gene epistatic interactions among susceptibility loci for systemic lupus erythematosus. *Arthritis Rheum* 64(2):485–492, 2012.

98. Castillejo-Lopez C, Delgado-Vega AM, Wojcik J, et al: Genetic and physical interaction of the B-cell systemic lupus erythematosus-associated genes BANK1 and BLK. *Ann Rheum Dis* 71(1):136–142, 2012.

99. Zhou XJ, Lu XL, Nath SK, et al: Gene-gene interaction of BLK, TNFSF4, TRAF1, TNFAIP3, REL in systemic lupus erythematosus. *Arthritis Rheum* 64(1):222–231, 2012.

Epigenetics of Lupus

Chapter 5

Nan Shen, Dong Liang, Yuajia Tang, and Yuting Qin

For a long time, genetic variation has been thought to be the primary cause of systemic lupus erythematosus (SLE; also called lupus). This belief led to gene-hunting studies to identify a list of genes, such as the MHC region, *IRF5, ITGAM, STAT4, BLK, BANK1, PDCD1, PTPN22, TNFSF4, TNFAIP3, SPP1,* some of the Fcγ-receptors, and several complement components,[1] which are well-established risk factors predisposing to lupus. However, genetic variation could not fully explain the pathogenesis of SLE. Environmental factors also influence the pathogenic processes.[2] Now more evidence has emerged to support that epigenetic variation also plays a part in diseases in which environmental and genetic factors are both involved, for example, cancer and autoimmune diseases.[3]

Epigenetics refers to the inheritance of variation without changes in the DNA sequence.[4] Up to now, studies on the epigenetics of SLE have focused on DNA methylation, histone modification, and microRNA (miRNA) regulation.

DNA HYPOMETHYLATION IN SLE

DNA methylation usually occurs at the 5′ position of cytosine residues located in dinucleotide CpG sites that nonrandomly distribute in genomes.[5] CpG-rich regions called *CpG islands*, about 500 to 5000 base pairs (bp) long, usually extend in the promoter and the first exon of genes. Other lone CpG dinucleotides are located in the intergenic and intronic regions, particularly within repeat sequences and transposable elements.[5] DNA methylation patterns are regulated by particular methyltransferases, namely, DNA (cytosine-5)-methyltransferase 1 (DNMT1), DNMT3A, DNMT3B, and DNMT3L.[6,7] DNMT1 maintains DNA methylation by replicating existing methylation patterns. DNMT3A and DNMT3B establish de novo DNA methylation. DNMT3L assists the function of DNMT3A and DNMT3B[8,9] but does not contain any intrinsic DNA methyltransferase activity.[8] In normal somatic cells of humans, 70% to 90% of CpG dinucleotides are methylated.[10,11] Conversely, abnormalities in DNA methylation can lead to increased or decreased expression of genes and transposable elements, which may contribute to disease.[5]

It has been reported that the DNA methylation level is lower in thymus and axillary lymph nodes of diseased 20-week-old MRL/lpr mice.[12] In humans, DNA extracted from the T cells of patients with lupus is hypomethylated compared with the DNA from normal T cells.[13] Various environmental factors, such as procainamide, hydralazine, ultraviolet (UV) light, aging, and diet, can prevent the replication of DNA methylation patterns during mitosis, resulting in the DNA demethylation in T cells and lupus-like autoimmunity.[14-16] Such agents usually induce the overexpression of autoimmune-associated methylation-sensitive genes, such as *TNFSF7* (CD70) and *LFA-1,* which confer an autoreactive status to T cells.[17,18] Adoptive transfer of T cells made autoreactive by treatment with DNA methylation inhibitors or by transfection with *LFA-1* is sufficient to cause a lupus-like disease in unirradiated syngeneic mice.[19,20] All of these findings suggest that DNA hypomethylation plays a crucial role in the pathogenesis of SLE. However, mechanisms that may contribute to low levels of T-cell DNA methylation in SLE remain to be studied. It has also been reported that miRNAs, such as miR148a[21] and miR126,[22] and the ERK signaling pathway[15,23] can regulate DMNT1 levels in T cells from patients with SLE. Despite the regulation of DNMT1 expression, other observations suggest that DNA demethylation may also play a role.[24] The p53-effector gene *GADD45a,* which may participate in DNA demethylation, has a higher expression level in CD4⁺ T cells of patients with SLE than in normal people. Moreover, UV light can induce *GADD45a* expression, and GADD45a⁻/⁻ mice can demonstrate SLE-like autoimmunity disease.[25]

HISTONE MODIFICATION CHANGES IN SLE

The nucleosome, basic unit of chromatin, is composed of a histone octamer (H2A and H2B dimers and H3/H4 tetramers) surrounded by 146 bp of DNA. Tails in the *N* end of histones protruding outside the octamer have different posttranslational modification, including acetylation, methylation, ubiquitination, phosphorylation, sumoylation, and adenosine diphosphate (ADP) ribosylation. These modifications can change the interaction between histone and DNA so as to affect DNA replication, transcription, DNA repair, and chromatin relaxation or condensation.[26]

In general, some histone modifications have certain association with gene expression activation or repression. For example, H3 and H4 hyperacetylation (H3Ac, H4Ac), H3 trimethyl-lysine4 (H3K4me3), H3 trimethyl-lysine36, and H3 trimethyl-lysine72, are present in many active genes; while H3 and H4 hypoacetylation, H3 trimethyl-lysine9 (H3K9me3), H3 trimethyl-lysine[27] (H3K27me3), and H4 trimethyl-lysine 20 (H4K20me3), are characteristic of many repressed genes and heterochromatin.[28] Like DNA methylation, the balance of histone modifications is also established and maintained by a group of enzymes, such as for histone lysine acetyltransferases and demethylases, histone lysine and arginine methyltransferases and demethylases, histone serine phosphorylases. Now many of these enzymes are becoming potential targets for the development of new therapeutic compounds.

However, the role of histone modifications in the pathogenesis of SLE is not well understood. Although examination of the global histone modification pattern in both MRL⁻ˡᵖʳ/ˡᵖʳ mice splenocytes and CD4⁺ T cells from patients with SLE showed H3 and H4 hypoacetylation and site-specific histone methylation changes,[27,28] the roles of these modification variations in the process of SLE pathogenesis are not clear. One study reported that the histone deacetylase inhibitor trichostatin A (TSA) can restore skewed expression of CD154 (CD40L), interleukin (IL) 10, and interferon gamma (IFN-γ) in lupus T cells.[29] Similarly, treating MRL⁻ˡᵖʳ/ˡᵖʳ mice with TSA and suberoylanilide hydroxamic acid (SAHA), another histone deacetylase inhibitor, decreased expression of IL-6, IL-12, IL-10, and IFN-γ and modulated renal disease through reduction in proteinuria, glomerulonephritis, and spleen weight.[30,31] This finding suggests that histone modification variation can also play a role in lupus and offers a potential new way to treat this disease.

microRNAS IN SLE

microRNAs (miRNAs) are a novel class of endogenous, noncoding small RNAs 19 to 25 nucleotides in length. They are ubiquitous in a

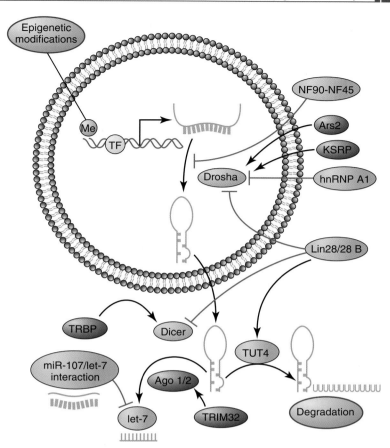

FIGURE 5-1 Biogenesis of human miRNAs. miRNA expression is first regulated by epigenetic and/or transcription factors. Primary miRNAs (pri-miRNAs), transcribed by polymerase II, are processed in the nucleus into precursor miRNAs (pre-miRNAs) by various factors, including Drosha, KSRP (KH-type splicing regulatory protein), and ARS2 (arsenate resistance protein 2). The pre-miRNAs are then exported to the cytoplasm and processed by the RNAse Dicer. Dicer, TRBP (TAR RNA-binding protein), and Argonaute1 through 4 (also known as EIF2C1 to 4) mediate the assembly of the RISC (RNA-induced silencing complex) in humans. One strand of the miRNA duplex remains on the RISC as the mature miRNA, but the other strand is degraded. Posttranscriptional controls of miRNA biogenesis are mediated by different mechanisms. For example, the protein Lin28 competes with Dicer for pre-let-7 and regulates the let-7 (a tumor suppressor miRNA) process. Upon binding by recognizing a specific sequence motif in the terminal loop, Lin28 also recruits TUT4 (terminal uridylyltransferase 4) to pre-let-7, leading to the 30-terminal uridylation and the degradation of pre-let-7. Stability of let-7 is also controlled by miR-107 through a direct interaction. hnRNA A1, heteronuclear ribonucleoprotein A1; Me, Methylation; TF, Transcription factor; TRIM32, Tripartite motif containing 32.

wide range of species, such as viruses, worms, flies, plants, and animals,[32,33] and function to negatively regulate gene expression at the posttranscriptional level. Although our current knowledge of miRNAs is still limited, it is being gradually accepted that miRNAs can modulate gene expression similarly as the transcription factors (TFs) in higher eukaryotes, representing a new layer of gene regulation. In parallel, mixed regulatory circuits are emerging in which close interplay between miRNAs and TFs cooperatively contributes to the formation of a complex posttranscriptional network.[34] It has been well established that miRNAs are involved in multiple physiologic and pathologic processes, including stem cell development, cell differentiation and organogenesis, proliferation and apoptosis, immune regulation, and disease development.[32,35-37]

miRNA Biogenesis
Genomic analysis of miRNA transcripts[38,39] revealed that a large proportion of miRNAs reside within introns of coding or noncoding regions, with a few in exons of long noncoding regions. Generally, miRNA genes are transcribed by RNA polymerase II to generate stem-loop primary miRNAs composed of one or several miRNA hairpin structures.[40] The primary miRNAs (also called pri-miRNAs) are sequentially recognized by DiGeorge syndrome–critical region gene 8 (DGCR8), which functions, by formation of a microprocessor complex with nuclear RNase III enzyme Drosha, to produce pre-miRNAs (or miRNA precursors). After being actively transported to cytoplasm via the exportin-5 pathway, the pre-miRNAs are further processed by RNase III Dicer to yield the miRNA duplex, the "mature" miRNA. One functional strand of this duplex is then recognized by Argonaute (Ago)–containing RNA-induced silencing complex (RISC) and loaded onto the messenger RNA (mRNA) target with imperfect complementarity.[40] This leads to either destabilization (most miRNA impact falls into this category[41]) or translational

repression of target mRNAs.[42-44] In some relatively rare cases, intronic miRNAs, called *mirtrons*, can bypass Drosha processing and be processed only by Dicer as pre-miRNAs.[45-47] In addition, it has been reported that maturation of the microRNA miR-451 can be directly processed by Ago2, an indispensable catalytic component of RISC, without the participation of Dicer.[48] Intriguingly, it has also been reported that anti-Su antibodies in sera from human patients with rheumatic diseases can recognize Ago2 and Dicer, two core catalytic enzymes in the miRNA pathway,[49] but the effect of these autoantibodies on miRNA biogenesis is not clear.

The biogenesis of miRNAs is a highly regulated process that involves participation of multiple proteins at various stages. The maturation of miRNAs might be the key regulatory step in miRNA biogenesis, which can be well exemplified by the deliberately controlled maturation of the tumor suppressor miRNA let-7 (Figure 5-1). By impairing the Drosha-mediated pri-miRNA processing step, the nuclear factor NF90-NF45 complex negatively regulates Let-7 biogenesis.[50] In contrast, the KH-type splicing regulatory protein (KSRP) promotes this processing by binding to the terminal loop of the pri-let-7.[51] Heteronuclear ribonucleoprotein A1 (hnRNP A1), another negative regulator, blocks the pri-let-7a processing through antagonizing KSRP-binding activity.[52] In addition, Lin-28/28B, as a highly conserved RNA-binding protein, exerts an inhibitory effect on let-7 maturation through inhibition of pri-let-7 processing and pre-let-7 cleavage mediated by Drosha and Dicer,[53-55] respectively. One study has reported that miR-107 regulates let-7 stability through direct interaction with it, thereby participating in cancer progression and metastasis.[56]

Novel Functions of miRNA in the Immune System
Table 5-1 summarizes the functions described here.

TABLE 5-1 Novel Functions of miRNA in the Immune System

MIRNAS	IMMUNE FUNCTION	CELL OR TISSUE	(POTENTIALLY) INVOLVED PATHWAY	TARGET(S)	CHAPTER REFERENCE(S)
miR-155	Regulates T helper cell differentiation and germinal center reaction	CD19$^+$ mature spleen B cells, CD4$^+$ T cells			62
	Increases lung airway remodeling; early-stage immunodeficiency	Lung, T helper 1/ hhelper 2 cells	Th2 pathway, etc.		63
	Modulates the IL-1 signaling pathway	Human monocyte–derived dendritic cells	TLR/IL-1 inflammatory pathway	TAB2	73
	Human dendritic cell maturation; involved in cellular immune response against foreign pathogens	Human dendritic cells; THP-1 monocytic cells	C/EBP-α–PU.1 pathway	PU.1	71
	Regulation of hematopoiesis; Akt kinase activation	Hematopoietic cells; macrophages	Akt pathway	SHIP1	69
	Maintains competitive fitness of Treg cells	Treg cells	IL-2 pathway	SOSC1	64
	Contributes to chronic skin inflammation	T (H) cells; PBMCs; skin	B7-CD28/CTLA-4 pathway	CTLA-4	76
	Regulates host antiviral innate immune response	Macrophages and dendritic cells	Type I IFN signaling	SOCS1	68
	Regulates M1/M2 phenotype balance in macrophages	Macrophages; THP-1 cells	IL-13 pathway	IL13Rα1	132
	Contributes to cellular response to TGF-β	Macrophages; THP-1 cells	TGF-β signaling	SMAD2	133
	Regulates inflammatory and immune reaction	Kidney; mesangial cells	TAB2/NF-κB pathway	TAB2	134
	Acute coronary syndrome; T17 helper cell differentiation	T17 helper cells; PBMCs			77
	Dendritic cell maturation and function; inhibits T cell–mediated immunity	Dendritic cells		c-Fos	72
	Inflammatory arthritis	Synovial macrophages and monocytes in rheumatoid arthritis; CD14$^+$ cells	miR-155/SHIP pathway	SHIP-1	78
	Regulates Treg cell phenotype	CD4$^+$CD25$^+$Foxp3$^+$ Treg cells (mouse)		CD62L	135
	Increases CD4$^+$ cell proliferation	CD2$^+$ T lymphocytes and CD4$^+$ T lymphocytes		PIK3R1, IRS2, IKBKE, FOS (targets of either miR-155 or miR-221)	136
miR-146a	In vitro monocytic cell–based endotoxin-induced tolerance and cross-tolerance	THP-1 monocytes	TLR4 signaling	IRAK-1 and TRAF6	81, 82
	Contributes to intestinal epithelial innate immune tolerance	m-ICcl2 and RAW-264.7 cell lines	TLR signaling	IRAK-1	83
	Epidermal Langerhans cell differentiation	Monocytes and neutrophil granulocytes	TLR2-dependent NF-κB signaling	PU.1	137
	Maintains HIV-mediated chronic inflammation of brain	Microglial cells (human fetal primary)		CCL8/MCP-2	85
	T-cell activation; modulates adaptive immunity, activation-induced cell death (AICD)	CD4$^+$ T lymphocytes	MEK/ERK pathway	FADD	86
	Bone destruction in rheumatoid arthritis, inhibition of osteoclastogenesis	PBMCs		c-Jun, NFATc1, PU.1, and TRAP	87
miR-106a	Regulates IL-10 production	A549, Raji, Jurkat, and THP-1 cells		IL-10	138
miR-124	Regulates microglia quiescence in central nervous system; modulates monocyte and macrophage activation	Macrophages, EAE mice	C/EBP-α–PU.1 pathway	C/EBP-α	100
miR-125b	Preferential differentiation of mouse HSCs to lymphoid lineage; lymphoid fate decision; early induction of progenitor B cells	HSCs		Bmf, KLF13	90
miR-126	Allergic asthma	Airway tissue, resident airway cells, lung T helper 2 cells	TLR signaling		99

TABLE 5-1 Novel Functions of miRNA in the Immune System—cont'd

MIRNAS	IMMUNE FUNCTION	CELL OR TISSUE	(POTENTIALLY) INVOLVED PATHWAY	TARGET(S)	CHAPTER REFERENCE(S)
miR-130/301	CD8+ T-cell survival and accumulation	CD8+ T cells		CD69	58
miR-132	Suppression of peripheral inflammation	Macrophages, RAW-264.7 and U937 cell lines	Cholinergic signaling	AChE	106
miR-142	Antigen-specific immunologic tolerance	Splenic and liver-derived CD8+ T cell			139
miR-142-3p	Regulates DC response to LPS, affects endotoxin-induced lethality	DCs	IL-6 pathway	IL-6	103
miR-148a/b, miR-152	Regulates innate response and antigen presentation of dendritic cells	DCs	CaM-CaMKII pathway	CaMKII α	105
miR-150	c-Myb–mediated lymphocyte development; B-cell differentiation	Progenitor B cells		c-Myb	95
miR-182	Promotes T helper lymphocyte expansion; induced by IL-2	T helper lymphocytes		Foxo 1	97
miR-181c	Modulates CD4+ T-cell activation and proliferation	Jurket cells, PBMCs CD4+		IL-2	94
miR-184	Early adaptive immune response; impacts umbilical cord blood CD4+ T-cell activation	Umbilical cord blood CD4+ T cells	NFAT/IL-2 pathway	NF-ATc2	96
miR-24	Cell cycle progression	HepG2, K562 cell lines		E2F2, etc.	91
miR-29	Suppresses immune response to intracellular bacterial infection	Natural killer cells, CD4+ and CD8+ T cells	IFN-γ pathway	IFN-γ	104
miR-375	Involved in gut homeostasis and mucosal immunity; induced by IL-13	HT-29 cells, colon	PI3K pathway	KLF5	61
miR-511	Positively regulates TLR4 in arrested cells; involved in immune response	Dendritic cells, macrophages	NF-κB pathway	TLR4, CD80	140
miR-663	Optimizes use of resveratrol as both an anti-inflammatory and anticancer agent	THP-1 monocytes		JunB, JunD	141
Let-7 family	Suppresses miR-155 expression in endotoxin-tolerant macrophages	Macrophages		miR-155	142
Let-7i	Regulates LPS-induced DC maturation and immune function	DCs	JAK/STAT pathway	SOCS1	102

AChE, acetylcholinesterase; Bmf, Bcl2-modifying factor; CAM, Ca2+-calmodulin; CaMKII, calcium/calmodulin-dependent protein kinase II; CCL8, chemokine (C-C motif) ligand 8; CD62L, L-selectin; C/EBP-α, CCAAT/enhancer-binding protein alpha; CLTA-4, cytotoxic T-lymphocyte–associated protein 4; E2F2, E2F transcription factor 2; DC, dendritic cell; EAE, encephalomyelitis; FACDD, Fas (TNFRSF6)–associated via death domain; IFN-γ, interferon gamma; Fos, FBJ osteosarcoma oncogene; FOS, FBJ murine osteosarcoma viral oncogene homolog; Foxo 1, forkhead box O1; HSC, hematopoietic stem cell; IKBKE, inhibitor of κ light polypeptide gene enhancer in B cells, kinase epsilon; IL, interleukin; IL13Rα1, IL-13 receptor alpha 1; IRAK, IL-1 receptor–associated kinase; IRS2, insulin receptor substrate 2; JAK, Janus kinase; JunB(D), jun B(D) proto-oncogene; KFC13, Kruppel-like factor 13; KLF, Kruppel-like factor; LPS, lipopolysaccharide; MCP-2, monocyte chemotactic protein 2; MEK/ERK, extracellular signal-regulated kinase (ERK) mitogen–activated protein kinase; Myb, myeloblastosis oncogene; NF-κB, nuclear factor kappa B; NF-ATc, nuclear factor of activated T cells, cytoplasmic, calcineurin-dependent; PBMC, peripheral blood mononuclear cell; PI3K, phosphoinositide 3-kinase; PIK3R1, regulatory subunit 1 of PI3K; PU.1, alias of ASPI1, spleen focus forming virus (SFFV) proviral integration oncogene spi1, DC-SIGN, alias of CD209, CD209 molecule; SHIP, alias of INPP5D, inositol polyphosphate-5-phosphatase D; SMAD2, SMAD family member 2; SOCS1, suppressor of cytokine signaling 1; STAT, signal transducer and activator of transcription; TAB2, TGF-β activated kinase 1/MAP3K7 binding protein 2; TGF-β, transforming growth factor beta; TLR4, Toll-like receptor 4; TRAF6, tumor necrosis factor (TNF) receptor–associated factor 6; TRAP, tartrate-resistant acid phosphatase; Treg cell, T regulatory cell.

Dicer−/−

Genetic ablation of the key component involved in miRNA biogenesis can severely impair immune development and response. Depletion of Dicer protein, a crucial miRNA-processing RNaseIII enzyme, causes disrupted Regulatory T (Treg) cell–mediated tolerance,[57] impaired CD8+ T-cell survival and accumulation,[58] and blocked progenitor B-cell differentiation.[59] In human leukemic cells deficient in Dicer, significantly enhanced apoptosis has also been observed.[60] Specific Dicer1 deletion in gut epithelium renders mice more susceptible to parasites as a result of ineffective immune response.[61] Mice deficient in Dicer in peripheral mature CD8+ T cells showed reduced T-cell expansion and immune response upon infection.[58] These findings indicate a pivotal role for Dicer and its mediated RNA interference (RNAi) machinery in normal immune system maintenance.

miR-155

Multiple lines of evidence are emerging that miR-155 operates, as an essential immune regulator, in both innate immunity and adaptive immunity at the center of immune regulation.

Depletion of miR-155 Causes Severe Immune Deficiency

A role of miR-155 in the immune system was first demonstrated in bic/miR-155−/− mice.[62,63] Through specific regulation of T-cell differentiation and germinal center response, miR-155 influences the T cell–dependent antibody generation and controls lymphocyte cytokine production—tumor necrosis factor alpha (TNF-α), lymphtoxins alpha and beta (LT-α/β, interleukins 4 and 10 (IL-4/10), interferon gamma (IFN-γ), and so on.[62] Although lymphoid cells from miR-155–deficient mice exhibited normal cell development, lymphocyte immune deficiencies such as altered T helper 1 cell (Th1) function, skewed Th2 differentiation, and defective B-cell class switching, were observed.[62,63] In addition to the effect of miR-155 on differentiation and immune function of T and B cells, recent studies extend its role in Treg cell regulation. It was reported that miR-155 regulates Treg cell homeostasis by specifically inhibiting expression of suppressor of cytokine signaling 1 (SOCS1), a key negative regulator of cytokine signaling.[64] This miRNA was also shown to be critically involved in Treg cell–mediated tolerance through regulation of CD4[+] Th cell activity, in which depletion of miR-155 resulted in enhanced cell sensitivity to natural Treg (nTreg)–mediated suppression.[65]

miR-155 Is a Multifunctional Regulator in Toll-Like Receptor Signaling

The robust upregulation of miR-155 upon stimulation of multiple Toll-like receptor (TLR) ligands[66,67] indicates the role of miR-155 in response to bacterial and viral infection. Indeed, numerous molecular targets have been identified for miR-155 in TLR signaling. In IFN-mediated antiviral response, SOCS1 is targeted by miR-155 in macrophages to attenuate viral propagation.[68] Inositol-5′-phosphatase SHIP1 (alias of INPP5D, inositol polyphosphate-5-phosphatase D), which negatively regulates TLR4 signaling, can be targeted for repression by miR-155 induced in response to lipopolysaccharide (LPS) stimulation.[69] miR-155 is also critical for dendritic cell (DC) maturation and its antigen-presenting cell (APC) function.[70] Transcription factors PU.1[71] and c-Fos[72] have been identified as direct targets of miR-155, the repression of which leads to functional defects in DCs. In LPS-activated DCs[73] and plasmacytoid DCs,[74] TAK1-binding protein 2 (TAB2), an essential molecule that regulates TLR-mediated nuclear factor kappa B (NF-κB) activation by recruiting TRAF6, has been confirmed as a direct target of miR-155. In addition, miR-155 was demonstrated to repress the expression of MyD88,[75] a vital adapter molecule in TLR signaling.

Involvement of miR-155 in Inflammation

miR-155 has been reported to be potentially implicated in the pathogenesis of multiple inflammatory disorders, including atopic dermatitis,[76] acute coronary syndrome,[77] and inflammatory arthritis.[78] miR-155[−/−] mice exhibit strong resistance to experimental autoimmune encephalomyelitis induced by myelin oligodendrocyte glycoprotein 35-55 (MOG$_{35-55}$), with defective inflammatory T-cell development, mass loss of Th17 cells, and markedly reduced production of Th17-relevant inflammatory cytokines.[79] In a study of skin inflammation, upregulation of miRN-155 was observed in activated T cells, resulting in repression of cytotoxic T-lymphocyte–associated protein 4 (CTLA-4) in T cells.[76] miR-155 is also required for the development of collagen-induced arthritis; stronger resistance to the disease was reported in miR-155 mutant mice that had reduced proinflammatory cytokine production.[78]

miR-146a: A Critical Immunomodulator

In 2006, Taganov first reported that miR-146a is highly induced upon LPS stimulation, as a strong negative regulator of TLR signaling, in human monocytes with targeted repression of TNF receptor–associated factor 6 (TRAF6) and interleukin-1 receptor–associated kinase 1 (IRAK1).[80] It was later shown that miR-146a can be induced by various inflammatory ligands in monocytic THP-1 cells, the expression of which is inversely correlated with TNF-α production, rendering cells tolerant[81] and cross-tolerant[82] to TLR stimulus. These results were further confirmed by an *in vivo* study demonstrating that the sustainably expressed miR-146a induces proteolytic degradation of IRAK1 during the neonatal period, contributing to innate immune tolerance of the intestinal epithelium.[83] miR-146a was also reported to be highly expressed in Treg cells and to selectively regulate Treg-mediated suppression, which inhibits IFN-γ–dependent Th1 activity and inflammation, by acting on transcription factor STAT-1 (signal transducer and activator of transcription 1).[84] Moreover, an elevation of miRNA-146a was observed in HIV-infected microglia cells and

brain specimens from patients with HIV encephalitis (HIVE), in which the chemokine CCL8/MCP-2 was identified as its specific target.[85]

Apart from its role in innate immune response, miR-146a has also been reported to function to modulate adaptive immunity and participate in disease pathogenesis. Curtale reported that the expression of miR-146a can be affected by T-cell receptor (TCR) signaling activation, and its induction leads to impairment of IL-2 production through modulation of AP-1 (activator protein 1) transcriptional activity.[86] In addition, high miR-146a induction was reported to reduce the expression of transcription factors Jun, NF-ATc1, PU.1, and TRAP in peripheral blood mononuclear cells (PBMCs), resulting in alleviation of bone destruction in rheumatoid arthritis (RA).[87]

Other miRNAs

miRNAs in Immune Cell Differentiation and Maturation

In mammals, it has been well established that miRNAs function as positive modulators for hematopoietic lineage differentiation.[88,89] One study has revealed that highly expressed miR-125b in hematopoietic stem cells (HSCs) promotes their differentiation toward lymphoid lineage.[90] It was also demonstrated that miR-24 is upregulated and functions in hematopoietic cell terminal differentiation by targeting E2F2[91] and H2AFx,[92] two key components regulating cell cycle progression.

It has been shown that miR-181, which is highly expressed in spleen and thymus, plays a crucial role in both B- and T-cell differentiation. Transplantation of lethally irradiated mice with bone marrow cells overexpressing miR-181a results in increased CD19[+] B-cell proliferation along with severe CD8[+] T-cell reduction.[88] When ectopically expressed in undifferentiated B-cell progenitors, miR-181a specifically promotes B-lymphocyte differentiation in mouse bone marrow,[88] whereas its upregulation in immature T cells is responsible for modulating TCR signaling (positive and negative selection) by inhibiting expression of multiple downstream phosphatases,[93] thereby negatively regulating the downstream signaling cascades. Another study has revealed that ectopic expression of miR-181c inhibits IL-2 expression and reduces cell proliferation in activated CD4[+] T cells.[94]

The roles of miRNAs in regulation of lymphocyte development are often achieved by posttranscriptional negative regulation of key transcription factors in corresponding signalings. For example, miR-150 is specifically expressed in mature B cells, but not in their progenitors. The ectopic expression of miR-150 in mice dramatically impairs B-cell development with a remarkable reduction in B1 cell numbers via targeted repression of c-Myb protein, a critical transcription factor required for pro–B-cell differentiation.[95] In the early adaptive immune response, miR-184 influences immune cell activation (umbilical cord blood CD4 T cells) and limits downstream IL-2 production by targeting NFAT1, a key transcription factor regulating the production of multiple proinflammatory cytokines.[96] Moreover, it was reported that during T helper lymphocyte development, miR-182 expression is induced by IL-2 to inhibit transcription factor Foxo 1 activity, resulting in T-cell clonal expansion.[97]

miRNAs in Immune Response

The roles of miRNA in regulation of immune response has been extensively investigated over the past several years.[32,35-37] Numerous miRNAs have been identified with functions intimately related to TLR signaling.[98] Later studies provide more evidence for the notion that miRNA plays an essential role in control of immune cell function through precise modulation of key molecules in TLR signaling for prevention and control of excessive inflammation.

For example, dust-induced TLR activation and the consequent inflammatory response in allergic asthma can be inhibited by miR-126, which indirectly reduces expression of the PU.1 and transcription activator OBF.1/BOB.1.[99] Also, miR-124 was shown to be involved in the inhibition of macrophage activation and attenuation of central nervous system (CNS) inflammation by repressing expression of transcription factor C/EBP-α (CCAAT/enhancer-binding protein alpha) and limiting the production of TNF-α in macrophages.[100] It is noteworthy that the same miRNAs, in different cellular contexts or under distinct pathologic conditions, may not act uniformly when immune cells develop immunity to foreign pathogens. In human cholangiocytes, for example, let-7i, which functions to negatively regulate TLR4 expression, is downregulated in response to LPS stimulation and bacterial infection.[101] In LPS-induced DC maturation, however, let-7i was reported to be upregulated to maintain LPS-induced production of proinflammatory cytokines (IL-12, IL-27, TNF-α, and IFN-γ) by translational repression of SOCS1 protein.[102] It would be interesting to examine whether different post-transcriptional gene regulatory machineries are employed for the let-7i expression in these two situations during the innate immune response, considering that its miRNA maturation is known to occur under complex control by a network of multiple regulatory factors. In addition to targeting TLR signaling pathways, multiple lines of evidence have unambiguously indicated that miRNAs can also exert a direct influence on inflammation via inhibition of the production of proinflammatory cytokines or their upstream regulators. In DCs, miR-142-3p was shown to be highly induced after LPS stimulation, resulting in targeted repression of both protein and mRNA levels of IL-6 to suppress inflammation that otherwise causes endotoxin-induced mortality.[103] Downregulation of miR-29 was observed in activated natural killer (NK) and T cells from *Listeria monocytogenes* or *Mycobacterium bovis bacillus Calmette-Guérin* (BCG)–infected mice, which promotes the production of its mRNA target IFN-γ, contributing to greater host resistance to bacterial infection.[104] By directly targeting CaMKII-α (calcium/calmodulin-dependent protein kinase II alpha) for repression, miR-148/152 was shown to inhibit LPS-induced major histocompatibility (MHC) II expression and limit cytokine production in DCs.[105] Interestingly, it was reported that excessive inflammation in the brain can be attenuated by induction of miR-132, which targets acetylcholinesterase (AChE), a crucial enzyme hydrolyzing acetylcholine (ACh), which in turn intercepts proinflammatory cytokine production,[106] bridging a link between cholinergic signaling and inflammation in neuroimmune disease.

Roles of miRNA in SLE

It is estimated that the human genome can encode at least 1000 unique miRNAs[107] that are predicted to target more than 30% of the total genome. Immune genes constitute an enriched source of miRNA targets, with more than 45% of them harboring potential miRNA-binding sites.[108] During the past several years, extensive investigation has been made to dissect how dysregulation of miRNA contributes to autoimmune diseases. Novel roles for miRNA have been unveiled in the pathogenesis of many autoimmune diseases, including multiple sclerosis (MS),[109] rheumatoid arthritis (RA),[110,111] and SLE.[112]

SLE, characterized by complex immunologic phenotypes, is regarded as a prototype systemic autoimmune disease[113] that affects multiple organs and systems. It has long been a "hot" field for research owing to its undefined etiology and complicated pathogenesis and to the unavailability of specific treatment for it. A computational target prediction revealed that all 72 of the tested lupus susceptibility genes in humans or mice can be potentially targeted by miRNAs, most of them possessing multiple binding sites for more than 140 conserved miRNAs.[114] Considering that miRNAs are known to function as modulators in several pathophysiologic processes in the immune system, it is reasonable to infer that miRNAs may also contribute to the pathogenesis of SLE.

miRNA Profiling in SLE

Studies of miRNA expression profiles in patients with SLE or lupus-like animal models reveal the biological and clinical relevance of miRNAs in SLE. Dai identified seven downregulated and nine upregulated miRNAs in patients with SLE, in comparison with levels of these miRNAs in healthy and diseased (idiopathic thrombocytopenic purpura) controls.[115] Through the use of TaqMan Array miRNA Assay (Applied Biosystems, Carlsbad, CA), our group has identified 42 differentially expressed miRNAs in PBMCs from patients with SLE. Among them, expression of 7 miRNAs (miR-31, miR-95, miR-99a, miR-130b, miR-10a, miR-134, and miR-146a) were more than sixfold lower in patients than in controls.[116] Using an miRNA microarray technique, another group investigated miRNA expression levels in Epstein-Barr virus (EBV)–transformed B-cell lines and frozen PMBCs obtained from patients with lupus nephritis and from unaffected controls in different racial groups (African American and European American), and identified 4 upregulated miRNAs (miR-371-5P, miR-423-5P, miR-638, and miR-663) and 1 downregulated miRNA (miR-1224-3P) in the lupus nephritis cells.[117] In a study of kidney biopsy specimen miRNA profiles, miRNA microarray chip analysis identified 66 miRNAs differentially expressed in the lupus nephritis cells.[118] Although miR-423, miR-638, and miR-663 were also present in the list of "positive" miRNAs, miR-423 and miR-663 were found to be downregulated in patients with lupus nephritis in comparison with normal controls.

Yet another group used TaqMan Low-Density Arrays to analyze the expression of 365 miRNAs in PBMCs from 34 patients with SLE and 20 healthy controls. Fourteen miRNAs were identified to be significantly downregulated, and 13 miRNAs upregulated, in patients with active SLE in comparison with controls.[119] This study also showed that miR-21, miR-25, and miR-106b are upregulated in both T and B lymphocytes from patients with SLE; 8 miRNAs (let-7a, let-7d, let-7g, miR-148a, miR-148b, miR-324-3p, miR-296, miR-196a) exhibited altered expression only in T cells of patients with SLE, whereas 4 miRNAs (miR-15a, miR-16, miR-150, miR-155) did so only in B cells from patients with SLE.[119] Another group also reported that 11 miRNAs are differentially expressed in CD4+ T cells from patients with SLE; 6 of them (miR-1246, miR-1308, miR-574-5p, miR-638, miR-126, miR-7) being upregulated and 5 (miR-142-3p, miR-142-59, miR-197, miR-155, miR-31) are down regulated.[120]

In a 2010 report, Dai profiled miRNA expressions in splenic lymphocytes from three spontaneous genetically lupus-prone murine models and found a common set of upregulated miRNAs (miR-182-96-183 cluster, miR-31, and miR-155).[121] This result, however, is partially inconsistent with data generated from human patients, in which miR-155 was identified to be downregulated in CD4+ T cells from patients with SLE[122] but up regulated in PBMCs and CD19+ B cells.[119] miR-31 was also found to be downregulated in PBMCs[116] and CD4+ T cells[120] from Chinese patients with SLE. The dysregulation of the miR-182-96-183 cluster was not reported in any miRNA expression profile studies in human patients with SLE.

Although numerous dysregulated miRNAs have been identified in human patients with lupus and lupus mouse models, relatively little overlap can be observed between the miRNA lists generated in these studies. This statement is also true for the studies of miRNA expression profile in multiple sclerosis (MS).[123] The inconsistency of the data generated in these studies could partially be explained by diversity in disease severity, medical history, and race of patients with SLE as well as differences in cell types, sample species, detection sensitivity, and miRNA quantification methods.

Dysfunction of miRNAs in Lupus Pathogenesis
miRNA-Mediated Hyperactivation of the Interferon Pathway in SLE

With the use of TaqMan miRNA Low-Density Arrays, a unique SLE signature was first characterized in our group's study of the roles of miRNA in SLE pathogenesis. We observed that miR-146a is considerably downregulated in patients with SLE in comparison with normal controls. This differential expression level is negatively correlated with disease activity and activation of the IFN pathway.[116] Abnormal activation of the type I IFN pathway is a key molecular phenotype of lupus. Delineation of its underlying molecular mechanism has become a hot and frontier research topic. Deficiency in the negative regulation of the type I IFN pathway is probably one of the causes of

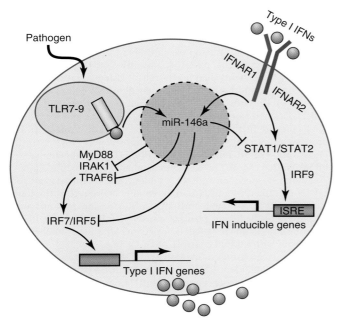

FIGURE 5-2 Roles of miRNA in abnormal activation of the type I interferon pathway in lupus. Under physiologic conditions, activation of Toll-like receptors (e.g., TLR7-TLR9) triggers sequential signaling and leads to the production of type I interferons (IFNs), which in turn bind to their receptors and induce downstream activation. In this scenario, various negative regulators, including miR-146a, are simultaneously induced. The mature miR-146a uses inhibitory machinery to reduce expression of its target genes, including *IRAK1, TRAF6, IRF5,* and *STAT1,* thereby attenuating the positive signaling. In lupus, owing to the miR-146a expression deficiency, the aberrant accumulation of its targeted proteins (TRAF6 [tumor necrosis factor (TNF) receptor–associated factor 6], IRAK1 [IL-1 receptor–associated kinase 1], IRF5, and STAT1 [signal transducer and activator of transcription]) leads to cascade signal amplification, contributing to the abnormal activation of the IFN pathway. IRF, interferon regulatory factor; ISRE, IFN-stimulated response element; MyD88, protein encoded by myeloid differentiation primary response gene 88.

its abnormal activation in cells from patients with lupus. In 2006, Taganov reported that miR-146a is negatively involved in the regulation of cellular signal transduction in innate immune response, through modulating expression of IRAK1 and TRAF6.[80] In line with this discovery, our data revealed that miR-146a can regulate production of type I IFN (IFN-α and IFN-β), and the INF-mediated downstream pathway as well. In patients with SLE, because of the miR-146a expression deficiency, the aberrant accumulation of its targeted proteins (STAT1, IRF5, TRAF6, and IRAK1) results in cascade signal amplification, contributing to the altered activation of the IFN pathway (Figure 5-2).[116] Of note, we also demonstrated that exogenous introduction of miR-146a into PBMCs from patients with SLE quite remarkably alleviates the coordinate activation of the type I interferon pathway, as indicated by a substantial reduction (≈75%) in mRNA levels of three selected IFN-inducible genes, IFN-induced protein with tetratricopeptide repeats 3 (IFIT3), myxovirus resistance 1 (MX1), and 2′,5′-oligoadenylate synthetase 1 (OAS1).[116] Our finding thus suggests that miR-146a can serve as a potential therapeutic target in SLE treatment.

Roles of miRNAs in DNA Hypomethylation in Lupus CD4⁺ T Cells

It is known that CD4⁺ T cells from patients with SLE have generally low levels of DNA methylation, a clinical symptom that is highly associated with lupus disease. However, the underlying cause remains largely undetermined. Our group has shown for the first time that miRNAs might be involved in DNA methylation abnormalities in patients with SLE. By using a high-throughput miRNA profiling technique, we identified miR-21 and miR-148a to be robustly upregulated in CD4⁺ T cells from both patients with lupus and lupus-prone MRL/lpr mice. The dysregulation of these two miRNAs (miR-21 and miR-148a) gives rise to DNA hypomethylation via inhibition of DNMT1 expression both indirectly and directly by respectively targeting RASGRP1, its upstream regulator, or DNMT1 itself.[21] In addition, another independent research group reported that DNA methylation status can be modulated in SLE CD4⁺ T cells by highly expressed miR-126, which specifically binds to the 3′ untranslated region (3′ UTR) of DNMT1.[122] It is becoming apparent that multiple miRNAs may contribute actively to mechanisms that underlie the low DNA methylation level in SLE (Figure 5-3).

Dysregulation of miRNAs as a Causal Factor of Abnormal Cytokine/Chemokine Production

It has been well documented that altered expression of cytokines such as IL-6, IL-10, RANTES (regulated upon activation, normal T-cell expressed, and secreted), and IL-2, plays a crucial role in SLE development. For example, RANTES, an inflammatory chemokine, is abnormally overexpressed in blood sera from patients with SLE, whereas the expression level of IL-2 is significantly lower in lupus T cells. In a first characterization of low expression of miRNAs in patients with SLE, our group found that miR-125a can reduce T-cell–mediated production of the inflammatory chemokine RANTES.[124] Further investigation revealed that miR-125a inhibited the T-cell–mediated secretion of RANTES by directly targeting its transcription factor, Kruppel-like factor 13 (KLF13) (Figure 5-4), as determined by a Dual-Luciferase Reporter Assay System. It is noteworthy to mention that introduction of exogenous miR-125a into T cells from patients with SLE resulted in a noticeable alleviation of raised RANTES expression, providing new insight into a potential strategy for therapeutic intervention in SLE.

Upregulation of miR-21 has been reported in patients with SLE, in whom the expression presents a positive correlation with disease activity. Inhibition of miR-21 expression in SLE CD4⁺ T cells increases expression of its target protein, programmed cell death protein 4 (PDCD4), resulting in impaired T-cell proliferation and reduced production of IL-10 and CD40L.[119] Our group dissected the role of another downregulated miRNA (miR-31) in lupus PBMCs[116] or T cells[120] and found that underexpression of miR-31 contributes to the decreased expression of IL-2 by targeting the guanosine triphosphatase RhoA in lupus T cells (unpublished data). These novel findings highlight an important but previously unappreciated contribution of dysregulated miRNAs in SLE development through modulation of key cytokine/chemokine production.

Interaction of miRNAs with Genetic Factors in Lupus

SLE is an autoimmune disease with a strong genetic disposition. Studies of the roles of miRNA in cancer pointed out that either altered miRNA expression or polymorphism in the sequence of miRNA or miRNA target sites can provide the intrinsic link between miRNA and the disease mechanism.[125] Our group's study indicated that expression deficiency of miR-146a in patients with lupus is involved in development of lupus through hyperactivation of the type I IFN pathway.[116] Using a candidate gene approach, we identified, in multiple independent cohorts, a novel genetic variant (rs57095329) in the promoter region of miRNA-146a to be highly associated with SLE susceptibility.[126] The individuals carrying the risk-associated G allele exhibit significantly reduced expression of miR-146a in comparison with those carrying the protective C allele. Further exploration showed an allelic difference of rs57095329 in miR-146a promoter activity, as revealed by altered binding affinity of Ets-1, a transcription factor identified in genome-wide association studies to be strongly associated with SLE susceptibility.

Some disease-related single-nucleotide polymorphisms (SNPs), located in the 3′ UTR or even in the coding sequence region can

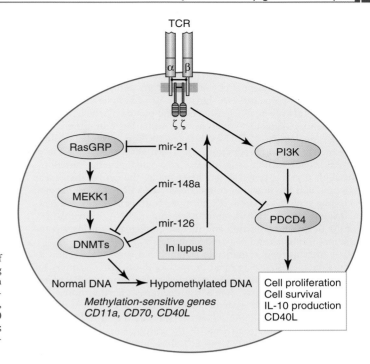

FIGURE 5-3 Roles of miRNA in lupus hypomethylation. Upregulation of miR-21 indirectly inhibits DNA methyltransferase 1 (DNMT1) by targeting the guanyl nucleotide–releasing protein RasGRP. MiR-148 and miR-126 can directly inhibit DNMT1. This inhibition in turn reduces the CpG methylation level and causes upregulation of autoimmune-associated genes in SLE, such as *CD70, CD11a,* and *CD40L.* MiR-21 can also increase interleukin-10 (IL-10) production by targeting PDCD4 in the lupus T cell. IL, interleukin; MEKK1, Mitogen-activated protein kinase kinase kinase1; P13K, phosphoinositide 3 kinase; TCR, T-cell receptor.

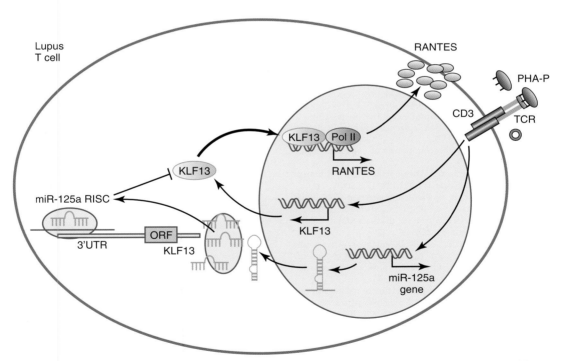

FIGURE 5-4 Role of miRNA in elevation of RANTES in lupus T cells. A regulatory feedback loop involves expression of miR-125a, the transcription factor KLF13 (Kruppel-like factor 13), and the inflammatory chemokine RANTES (regulated upon activation, normal T-cell expressed, and secreted) in activated T cells. RANTES induced after stimulation requires the binding of KLF13 to its promoter. This schematic representation shows that in patients with lupus, miR-125a acts as a negative regulator that reduces RANTES expression by targeting KLF13. In lupus T cells, decreased expression of miR-125a leads to the upregulation of the critical KLF13, which in turn contributes to the elevation of RANTES. ORF, Open reading frame; PHA-P, Phytohaemagglutinin-P; Pol II, Polymerase II; RISC, RNA-induced silencing complex; TCR, T-cell receptor; UTR, untranslated region.

regulate gene expression through introducing or abolishing miRNA binding sites. Patrick has reported that the risk allele of a synonymous SNP (rs10065172) in the *IRGM* gene can render higher susceptibility to Crohn's disease through alteration of the binding site for miR-196.[127] In line with this finding, Hikami demonstrated that a functional polymorphism (rs1057233) in the 3′ UTR of the *SPI1* gene is in strong linkage disequilibrium (LD) with SLE.[128] The disruption of the miR-569 binding site caused by the risk allele resulted in an elevation of SPI1 mRNA, contributing to SLE susceptibility.

CONCLUSIONS AND FUTURE PERSPECTIVES

miRNAs, as an important class of immunomodulators, are critically implicated in diverse aspects of immune system development and function. Moreover, novel cellular and molecular mechanisms by which miRNAs contribute to SLE pathogenesis are being formed and put forward. High-throughput miRNA expression profiling studies have revealed unique miRNA signatures for SLE. A series of *in vitro* studies have also given us a reasonably clear picture in which miRNAs play essential regulatory roles in SLE initiation and progression through mediation of IFN pathway activation, proinflammatory cytokine/chemokine production, and T-cell DNA methylation level as well as interaction with disease-associated genetic variations. Although exciting progress has been made, the provocative ideas proposed and the potential connections[129] between SLE risk factors, including genetic variation, sex hormone (estrogen) or environmental triggers (such as EBV infection), and miRNA dysregulation, require deeper investigation and further confirmation using a combination of *in vitro* and *in vitro* techniques.

Considering their remarkable stability and ease of detection in body fluids, miRNAs isolated from blood or urine samples of patients with SLE[130] have the potential to serve as novel clinical biomarkers, particularly for early diagnosis. Furthermore, one study has shown that systemic delivery of a seed-targeting tiny locked nucleic acid (LNA) efficiently silences the miR-21 in vivo and reverses splenomegaly, one of the cardinal manifestations of autoimmunity in B6.Sle123 mice,[131] shedding light on new drug design strategies. MiRNA can have long-lasting and accumulative effects on different facets of signaling pathways, distinct from biological behaviors of any single known SLE risk genes, thereby potentially providing a new layer of insight into SLE and holding great promise for the development of novel therapeutic targets in the future.

References

1. Moser KL, Kelly JA, Lessard CJ, et al: Recent insights into the genetic basis of systemic lupus erythematosus. *Genes Immun* 10(5):373–379, 2009.
2. Kotzin BL: Systemic lupus erythematosus. *Cell* 85(3):303–306, 1996.
3. Feinberg AP, Phenotypic plasticity and the epigenetics of human disease. *Nature* 447(7143):433–440, 2007.
4. Bonasio R, Tu S, Reinberg D, Molecular signals of epigenetic states. *Science* 330(6004):612–616, 2010.
5. Wilson AS, Power BE, Molloy PL, DNA hypomethylation and human diseases. *Biochimica et biophysica acta* 1775(1):138–162, 2007.
6. Feltus FA, Lee EK, Costello JF, et al: Predicting aberrant CpG island methylation. *Proc Natl Acad Sci U S A* 100(21):12253–12258, 2003.
7. Klose, RJ, Bird AP, Genomic DNA methylation: the mark and its mediators. *Trends in biochemical sciences* 31(2):89–97, 2006.
8. Chedin F, Lieber MR, Hsieh CL, The DNA methyltransferase-like protein DNMT3L stimulates de novo methylation by Dnmt3a. *Proceedings of the National Academy of Sciences of the United States of America* 99(26):16916–16921, 2002.
9. Chen ZX, Mann JR, Hsieh CL, et al: Physical and functional interactions between the human DNMT3L protein and members of the de novo methyltransferase family. *J Cell Biochem* 95(5):902–917, 2005.
10. Ehrlich M, Gama-Sosa MA, Huang LH, et al: Amount and distribution of 5-methylcytosine in human DNA from different types of tissues of cells. *Nucleic Acids Res* 10(8):2709–2721, 1982.
11. Tuck-Muller CM, Narayan A, Tsien F, et al: DNA hypomethylation and unusual chromosome instability in cell lines from ICF syndrome patients. *Cytogenet Cell Genet* 89(1–2):121–128, 2000.
12. Mizugaki M, Yamaguchi T, Ishiwata S, et al: Alteration of DNA methylation levels in MRL lupus mice. *Clin Exp Immunol* 110(2):265–269, 1997.
13. Ballestar E, Esteller M, Richardson BC: The epigenetic face of systemic lupus erythematosus. *Journal of immunology* 176(12):7143–7147, 2006.
14. Cornacchia E, Golbus J, Maybaum J, et al: Hydralazine and procainamide inhibit T cell DNA methylation and induce autoreactivity. *J Immunol* 140(7):2197–2200, 1988.
15. Deng C, Lu Q, Zhang Z, et al: Hydralazine may induce autoimmunity by inhibiting extracellular signal-regulated kinase pathway signaling. *Arthritis Rheum* 48(3):746–756, 2003.
16. Gorelik G, Fang JY, Wu A, et al: Impaired T cell protein kinase C delta activation decreases ERK pathway signaling in idiopathic and hydralazine-induced lupus. *J Immunol* 179(8):5553–5563, 2007.
17. Lu Q, Kaplan M, Ray D, et al: Demethylation of ITGAL (CD11a) regulatory sequences in systemic lupus erythematosus. *Arthritis Rheum* 46(5):1282–1291, 2002.
18. Lu Q, Wu A, Richardson BC: Demethylation of the same promoter sequence increases CD70 expression in lupus T cells and T cells treated with lupus-inducing drugs. *Journal of immunology* 174(10):6212–6219, 2005.
19. Quddus J, Johnson KJ, Gavalchin J, et al: Treating activated CD4+ T cells with either of two distinct DNA methyltransferase inhibitors, 5-azacytidine or procainamide, is sufficient to cause a lupus-like disease in syngeneic mice. *J Clin Invest* 92(1):38–53, 1993.
20. Yung R, Powers D, Johnson K, et al: Mechanisms of drug-induced lupus. II. T cells overexpressing lymphocyte function-associated antigen 1 become autoreactive and cause a lupuslike disease in syngeneic mice. *J Clin Invest* 97(12):2866–2871, 1996.
21. Pan W, Zhu S, Yuan M, et al: MicroRNA-21 and microRNA-148a contribute to DNA hypomethylation in lupus CD4+ T cells by directly and indirectly targeting DNA methyltransferase 1. *J Immunol* 184(12):6773–6781, 2010.
22. Zhao S, Wang Y, Liang Y, et al: MicroRNA-126 regulates DNA methylation in CD4+ T cells and contributes to systemic lupus erythematosus by targeting DNA methyltransferase 1. *Arthritis Rheum* 63(5):1376–1386, 2011.
23. MacLeod AR, Rouleau J, Szyf M: Regulation of DNA methylation by the Ras signaling pathway. *The Journal of biological chemistry* 270(19):11327–11337, 1995.
24. Li Y, Zhao M, Yin H, et al: Overexpression of the growth arrest and DNA damage-induced 45alpha gene contributes to autoimmunity by promoting DNA demethylation in lupus T cells. *Arthritis Rheum* 62(5):1438–1447, 2010.
25. Salvador JM, Hollander MC, Nguyen AT, et al: Mice lacking the p53-effector gene Gadd45a develop a lupus-like syndrome. *Immunity* 16(4):499–508, 2002.
26. Esteller M, Cancer epigenomics: DNA methylomes and histone-modification maps. Nature reviews. *Genetics* 8(4):286–298, 2007.
27. Garcia BA, Busby SA, Shabanowitz J, et al: Resetting the epigenetic histone code in the MRL-lpr/lpr mouse model of lupus by histone deacetylase inhibition. *J Proteome Res* 4(6):2032–2042, 2005.
28. Hu N, Long H, Zhao M, et al: Aberrant expression pattern of histone acetylation modifiers and mitigation of lupus by SIRT1-siRNA in MRL/lpr mice. *Scand J Rheumatol* 38(6):464–471, 2009.
29. Mishra N, Brown DR, Olorenshaw IM, et al: Trichostatin A reverses skewed expression of CD154, interleukin-10, and interferon-gamma gene and protein expression in lupus T cells. *Proc Natl Acad Sci U S A* 98(5):2628–2633, 2001.
30. Mishra N, Reilly CM, Brown DR, et al: Histone deacetylase inhibitors modulate renal disease in the MRL-lpr/lpr mouse. *J Clin Invest* 111(4):539–552, 2003.
31. Reilly CM, Mishra N, Miller JM, et al: Modulation of renal disease in MRL/lpr mice by suberoylanilide hydroxamic acid. *J Immunol* 173(6):4171–4178, 2004.
32. Bartel DP, MicroRNAs: genomics, biogenesis, mechanism, and function. *Cell* 116(2):281–297, 2004.
33. Carrington JC, Ambros V, Role of microRNAs in plant and animal development. *Science* 301(5631):336–338, 2003.
34. El Baroudi M, Cora D, Bosia C, et al: A curated database of miRNA mediated feed-forward loops involving MYC as master regulator. *PLoS One* 6(3):e14742, 2011.
35. Xiao C, Rajewsky K, MicroRNA control in the immune system: basic principles. *Cell* 136(1):26–36, 2009.
36. Inui M, Martello G, Piccolo S, MicroRNA control of signal transduction. *Nat Rev Mol Cell Biol* 11(4):252–263, 2010.
37. Luo X, Tsai LM, Shen N, et al: Evidence for microRNA-mediated regulation in rheumatic diseases. *Ann Rheum Dis* 69(Suppl 1):i30–i36, 2010.
38. Rodriguez A, Griffiths-Jones S, Ashurst JL, et al: Identification of mammalian microRNA host genes and transcription units. *Genome Res* 14(10A):1902–1910, 2004.
39. Saini HK, Griffiths-Jones S, Enright AJ, Genomic analysis of human microRNA transcripts. *Proc Natl Acad Sci U S A* 104(45):17719–11724, 2007.
40. Lee Y, Kim M, Han J, et al: MicroRNA genes are transcribed by RNA polymerase II. *EMBO J* 23(20):4051–4060, 2004.
41. Guo H, Ingolia NT, Weissman JS, et al: Mammalian microRNAs predominantly act to decrease target mRNA levels. *Nature* 466(7308): 835–840, 2010.
42. Diederichs S, Haber DA, Dual role for argonautes in microRNA processing and posttranscriptional regulation of microRNA expression. *Cell* 131(6):1097–1108, 2007.

43. Carthew RW, Sontheimer EJ, Origins and mechanisms of miRNAs and siRNAs. *Cell* 136(4):642–565, 2009.

44. Kim VN, Han J, Siomi MC, Biogenesis of small RNAs in animals. *Nat Rev Mol Cell Biol* 10(2):126–139, 2009.

45. Okamura K, Hagen JW, Duan H, et al: The mirtron pathway generates microRNA-class regulatory RNAs in *Drosophila*. *Cell* 130(1):89–100, 2007.

46. Ruby JG, Jan CH, Bartel DP: Intronic microRNA precursors that bypass Drosha processing. *Nature* 448(7149):83–86, 2007.

47. Yang JS, Lai EC: Alternative miRNA biogenesis pathways and the interpretation of core miRNA pathway mutants. *Molecular cell* 43(6):892–903, 2011.

48. Yang JS, Lai EC: Dicer-independent, Ago2-mediated microRNA biogenesis in vertebrates. *Cell Cycle* 9(22):4455–4460, 2010.

49. Jakymiw A, Ikeda K, Fritzler MJ, et al: Autoimmune targeting of key components of RNA interference. *Arthritis Res Ther* 8(4):R87, 2006.

50. Sakamoto S, Aoki K, Higuchi T, et al: The NF90-NF45 complex functions as a negative regulator in the microRNA processing pathway. *Mol Cell Biol* 29(13):3754–3769, 2009.

51. Trabucchi M, Briata P, Garcia-Mayoral M, et al: The RNA-binding protein KSRP promotes the biogenesis of a subset of microRNAs. *Nature* 459(7249):1010–1014, 2009.

52. Michlewski G, Caceres JF: Antagonistic role of hnRNP A1 and KSRP in the regulation of let-7a biogenesis. *Nature structural & molecular biology* 17(8):1011–1018, 2010.

53. Heo I, Joo C, Kim YK, et al: TUT4 in concert with Lin28 suppresses microRNA biogenesis through pre-microRNA uridylation. *Cell* 138(4):696–708, 2009.

54. Viswanathan SR, Daley GQ, Gregory RI: Selective blockade of microRNA processing by Lin28. *Science* 320(5872):97–100, 2008.

55. Heo I, Joo C, Cho J, et al: Lin28 mediates the terminal uridylation of let-7 precursor microRNA. *Mol Cell* 32(2):276–284, 2008.

56. Chen PS, Su JL, Cha ST, et al: miR-107 promotes tumor progression by targeting the let-7 microRNA in mice and humans. *J Clin Invest* 121(9):3442–3455, 2011.

57. Liston A, Lu LF, O'Carroll D, et al: Dicer-dependent microRNA pathway safeguards regulatory T cell function. *J Exp Med* 205(9):1993–2004, 2008.

58. Zhang N, Bevan MJ, Dicer controls CD8+ T-cell activation, migration, and survival. *Proceedings of the National Academy of Sciences of the United States of America* 107(50):21629–21634, 2010.

59. Koralov SB, Muljo SA, Galler GR, et al: Dicer ablation affects antibody diversity and cell survival in the B lymphocyte lineage. *Cell* 132(5):860–874, 2008.

60. Smith LK, Shah RR, Cidlowski JA, Glucocorticoids modulate microRNA expression and processing during lymphocyte apoptosis. *The Journal of biological chemistry* 285(47):36698–36708, 2010.

61. Biton M, Levin A, Slyper M, et al: Epithelial microRNAs regulate gut mucosal immunity via epithelium-T cell crosstalk. *Nat Immunol* 12(3):239–246, 2011.

62. Thai TH, Calado DP, Casola S, et al: Regulation of the germinal center response by microRNA-155. *Science* 316(5824):604–608, 2007.

63. Rodriguez A, Vigorito E, Clare S, et al: Requirement of bic/microRNA-155 for normal immune function. *Science* 316(5824):608–611, 2007.

64. Lu LF, Thai TH, Calado DP, et al: Foxp3-dependent microRNA155 confers competitive fitness to regulatory T cells by targeting SOCS1 protein. *Immunity* 30(1):80–91, 2009.

65. Stahl HF, Fauti T, Ullrich N, et al: miR-155 inhibition sensitizes CD4+ Th cells for TREG mediated suppression. *PloS One* 4(9):e7158, 2009.

66. O'Connell RM, Taganov KD, Boldin MP, et al: MicroRNA-155 is induced during the macrophage inflammatory response. *Proc Natl Acad Sci U S A* 104(5):1604–1609, 2007.

67. Tili E, Michaille JJ, Cimino A, et al: Modulation of miR-155 and miR-125b levels following lipopolysaccharide/TNF-alpha stimulation and their possible roles in regulating the response to endotoxin shock. *J Immunol* 179(8):5082–5089, 2007.

68. Wang P, Hou J, Lin L, et al: Inducible microRNA-155 feedback promotes type I IFN signaling in antiviral innate immunity by targeting suppressor of cytokine signaling 1. *J Immunol* 185(10):6226–6233, 2010.

69. O'Connell RM, Chaudhuri AA, Rao DS, et al: Inositol phosphatase SHIP1 is a primary target of miR-155. *Proc Natl Acad Sci U S A* 106(17):7113–7118, 2009.

70. Mao CP, He L, Tsai YC, et al: In vivo microRNA-155 expression influences antigen-specific T cell-mediated immune responses generated by DNA vaccination. *Cell & Biosci* 1(1):3, 2011.

71. Martinez-Nunez RT, Louafi F, Friedmann PS, et al: MicroRNA-155 modulates the pathogen binding ability of dendritic cells (DCs) by down-regulation of DC-specific intercellular adhesion molecule-3 grabbing non-integrin (DC-SIGN). *J Biol Chem* 284(24):16334–16342, 2009.

72. Dunand-Sauthier I, Santiago-Raber ML, Capponi L, et al: Silencing of c-Fos expression by microRNA-155 is critical for dendritic cell maturation and function. *Blood* 117(17):4490–4500, 2011.

73. Ceppi M, Pereira PM, Dunand-Sauthier I, et al: MicroRNA-155 modulates the interleukin-1 signaling pathway in activated human monocyte-derived dendritic cells. *Proc Natl Acad Sci U S A* 106(8):2735–2740, 2009.

74. Zhou H, Huang X, Cui H, et al: miR-155 and its star-form partner miR-155* cooperatively regulate type I interferon production by human plasmacytoid dendritic cells. *Blood* 116(26):5885–5894, 2010.

75. Tang B, Xiao B, Liu Z, et al: Identification of MyD88 as a novel target of miR-155, involved in negative regulation of *Helicobacter pylori*-induced inflammation. *FEBS Lett* 584(8):1481–1486, 2010.

76. Sonkoly E, Janson P, Majuri ML, et al: MiR-155 is overexpressed in patients with atopic dermatitis and modulates T-cell proliferative responses by targeting cytotoxic T lymphocyte-associated antigen 4. *J Allergy Clin Immunol* 126(3):581–589, 2010.

77. Yao R, Ma Y, Du Y, et al: The altered expression of inflammation-related microRNAs with microRNA-155 expression correlates with Th17 differentiation in patients with acute coronary syndrome. *Cellular & Modecular immunology* 8(6):486–495, 2011.

78. Kurowska-Stolarska M, Alivernini S, Ballantine LE, et al: MicroRNA-155 as a proinflammatory regulator in clinical and experimental arthritis. *Proc Natl Acad Sci U S A* 108(27):11193–11198, 2011.

79. O'Connell RM, Kahn D, Gibson WS, et al: MicroRNA-155 promotes autoimmune inflammation by enhancing inflammatory T cell development. *Immunity* 33(4):607–619, 2010.

80. Taganov KD, Boldin MP, Chang KJ, et al: NF-kappaB-dependent induction of microRNA miR-146, an inhibitor targeted to signaling proteins of innate immune responses. *Proc Natl Acad Sci U S A* 103(33):12481–12486, 2006.

81. Nahid MA, Pauley KM, Satoh M, et al: miR-146a is critical for endotoxin-induced tolerance: implication in innate immunity. *J Biol Chem* 284(50):34590–34599, 2009.

82. Nahid MA, Satoh M, Chan EK: Mechanistic role of microRNA-146a in endotoxin-induced differential cross-regulation of TLR signaling. *Journal of immunology* 186(3):1723–1734, 2011.

83. Chassin C, Kocur M, Pott J, et al: miR-146a mediates protective innate immune tolerance in the neonate intestine. *Cell Host & Microbe* 8(4):358–368, 2010.

84. Lu LF, Boldin MP, Chaudhry A, et al: Function of miR-146a in controlling Treg cell-mediated regulation of Th1 responses. *Cell* 142(6):914–929, 2010.

85. Rom S, Rom I, Passiatore G, et al: CCL8/MCP-2 is a target for mir-146a in HIV-1-infected human microglial cells. *Faseb J* 24(7):2292–2300, 2010.

86. Curtale G, Citarella F, Carissimi C, et al: An emerging player in the adaptive immune response: microRNA-146a is a modulator of IL-2 expression and activation-induced cell death in T lymphocytes. *Blood* 115(2):265–273, 2010.

87. Nakasa T, Shibuya H, Nagata Y, et al: The inhibitory effect of microRNA-146a expression on bone destruction in collagen-induced arthritis. *Arthritis Rheum* 63(6):1582–1590, 2011.

88. Chen CZ, Li L, Lodish HF, et al: MicroRNAs modulate hematopoietic lineage differentiation. *Science* 303(5654):83–86, 2004.

89. Chen CZ, Lodish HF: MicroRNAs as regulators of mammalian hematopoiesis. *Semin Immunol* 17(2):155–165, 2005.

90. Ooi AG, Sahoo D, Adorno M, et al: MicroRNA-125b expands hematopoietic stem cells and enriches for the lymphoid-balanced and lymphoid-biased subsets. *Proc Natl Acad Sci U S A* 107(50):21505–21510, 2010.

91. Lal A, Navarro F, Maher CA, et al: miR-24 inhibits cell proliferation by targeting E2F2, MYC, and other cell-cycle genes via binding to "seedless" 3′UTR microRNA recognition elements. *Molecular cell* 35(5):610–625, 2009.

92. Lal A, Pan Y, Navarro F, et al: miR-24-mediated downregulation of H2AX suppresses DNA repair in terminally differentiated blood cells. *Nat Struct Mol Biol* 16(5):492–498, 2009.

93. Li QJ, Chau J, Ebert PJ, et al: miR-181a is an intrinsic modulator of T cell sensitivity and selection. *Cell* 129(1):147–161, 2007.

94. Xue Q, Guo ZY, Li W, et al: Human activated CD4(+) T lymphocytes increase IL-2 expression by downregulating microRNA-181c. *Mol Immunol* 48(4):592–599, 2011.

95. Xiao C, Calado DP, Galler G, et al: MiR-150 controls B cell differentiation by targeting the transcription factor c-Myb. *Cell* 131(1):146–159, 2007.

96. Weitzel RP, Lesniewski ML, Haviernik P, et al: microRNA 184 regulates expression of NFAT1 in umbilical cord blood CD4+ T cells. *Blood* 113(26):6648–6657, 2009.

97. Stittrich AB, Haftmann C, Sgouroudis E, et al: The microRNA miR-182 is induced by IL-2 and promotes clonal expansion of activated helper T lymphocytes. *Nat Immunol* 11(11):1057–1062, 2010.

98. O'Neill LA, Sheedy FJ, McCoy CE, MicroRNAs: the fine-tuners of Toll-like receptor signalling. Nature reviews. *Immunology* 11(3):163–175, 2011.

99. Mattes J, Collison A, Plank M, et al: Antagonism of microRNA-126 suppresses the effector function of TH2 cells and the development of allergic airways disease. *Proc Natl Acad Sci U S A* 106(44):18704–18709, 2009.

100. Ponomarev ED, Veremeyko T, Barteneva N, et al: MicroRNA-124 promotes microglia quiescence and suppresses EAE by deactivating macrophages via the C/EBP-alpha-PU.1 pathway. *Nat Med* 17(1):64–70, 2011.

101. Chen XM, Splinter PL, O'Hara SP, et al: A cellular micro-RNA, let-7i, regulates Toll-like receptor 4 expression and contributes to cholangiocyte immune responses against *Cryptosporidium parvum* infection. *J Biol Chem* 282(39):28929–28938, 2007.

102. Zhang M, Liu F, Jia H, et al: Inhibition of microRNA let-7i depresses maturation and functional state of dendritic cells in response to lipopolysaccharide stimulation via targeting suppressor of cytokine signaling 1. *J Immunol* 187(4):1674–1683, 2011.

103. Sun Y, Varambally S, Maher CA, et al: Targeting of microRNA-142–3p in dendritic cells regulates endotoxin-induced mortality. *Blood* 117(23):6172–6183, 2011.

104. Ma F, Xu S, Liu X, et al: The microRNA miR-29 controls innate and adaptive immune responses to intracellular bacterial infection by targeting interferon-gamma. *Nat Immunol* 12(9):861–869, 2011.

105. Liu X, Zhan Z, Xu L, et al: MicroRNA-148/152 impair innate response and antigen presentation of TLR-triggered dendritic cells by targeting CaMKIIalpha. *J Immunol* 185(12):7244–7251, 2010.

106. Shaked I, Meerson A, Wolf Y, et al: MicroRNA-132 potentiates cholinergic anti-inflammatory signaling by targeting acetylcholinesterase. *Immunity* 31(6):965–973, 2009.

107. Bentwich I, Avniel A, Karov Y, et al: Identification of hundreds of conserved and nonconserved human microRNAs. *Nat Genet* 37(7):766–770, 2005.

108. Asirvatham AJ, Gregorie CJ, Hu Z, et al: MicroRNA targets in immune genes and the Dicer/Argonaute and ARE machinery components. *Mol Immunol* 45(7):1995–2006, 2008.

109. Junker A, Hohlfeld R, Meinl E, The emerging role of microRNAs in multiple sclerosis. *Nat Rev Neurol* 7(1):56–59, 2011.

110. Duroux-Richard I, Jorgensen C, Apparailly F: What do microRNAs mean for rheumatoid arthritis? *Arthritis Rheum* 64(1):11–20, 2012.

111. Alevizos I, Illei GG: MicroRNAs as biomarkers in rheumatic diseases. *Nat Rev Rheumatol* 6(7):391–398, 2010.

112. Ceribelli A, Yao B, Dominguez-Gutierrez PR, et al: MicroRNAs in systemic rheumatic diseases. *Arthritis Res Ther* 13(4):229, 2011.

113. Fairhurst AM, Wandstrat AE, Wakeland EK: Systemic lupus erythematosus: multiple immunological phenotypes in a complex genetic disease. *Adv Immunol* 92:1–69, 2006.

114. Vinuesa CG, Rigby RJ, Yu D: Logic and extent of miRNA-mediated control of autoimmune gene expression. *Int Rev Immunol* 28(3–4):112–138, 2009.

115. Dai Y, Huang YS, Tang M, et al: Microarray analysis of microRNA expression in peripheral blood cells of systemic lupus erythematosus patients. *Lupus* 16(12):939–946, 2007.

116. Tang Y, Luo X, Cui H, et al: MicroRNA-146A contributes to abnormal activation of the type I interferon pathway in human lupus by targeting the key signaling proteins. *Arthritis Rheum* 60(4):1065–1075, 2009.

117. Te JL, Dozmorov IM, Guthridge JM, et al: Identification of unique microRNA signature associated with lupus nephritis. *PloS One* 5(5):e10344, 2010.

118. Dai Y, Sui W, Lan H, et al: Comprehensive analysis of microRNA expression patterns in renal biopsies of lupus nephritis patients. *Rheumatol Int* 29(7):749–754, 2009.

119. Stagakis E, Bertsias G, Verginis P, et al: Identification of novel microRNA signatures linked to human lupus disease activity and pathogenesis: miR-21 regulates aberrant T cell responses through regulation of PDCD4 expression. *Ann Rheum Dis* 70(8):1496–1506, 2011.

120. Zhao S, Wang Y, Liang Y, et al: MicroRNA-126 regulates DNA methylation in CD4+ T cells and contributes to systemic lupus erythematosus by targeting DNA methyltransferase 1. *Arthritis Rheum.* 63(5):1376–1386, 2011.

121. Dai R, Zhang Y, Khan D, et al: Identification of a common lupus disease-associated microRNA expression pattern in three different murine models of lupus. *PLoS One* 5(12):e14302, 2010.

122. Zhao S, Wang Y, Liang Y, et al: MicroRNA-126 regulates DNA methylation in CD4(+) T cells and contributes to systemic lupus erythematosus by targeting DNA methyltransferase 1. *Arthritis Rheum* 63(5):1376–1386, 2011.

123. Junker A, Hohlfeld R, Meinl E: The emerging role of microRNAs in multiple sclerosis. *Nat Rev Neurol* 7(1):56–59, 2011.

124. Zhao X, Tang Y, Qu B, et al: MicroRNA-125a contributes to elevated inflammatory chemokine RANTES levels via targeting KLF13 in systemic lupus erythematosus. *Arthritis Rheum* 62(11):3425–3435, 2010.

125. Kloosterman WP, Plasterk RH: The diverse functions of microRNAs in animal development and disease. *Dev Cell* 11(4):441–450, 2006.

126. Luo X, Yang W, Ye DQ, et al: A functional variant in microRNA-146a promoter modulates its expression and confers disease risk for systemic lupus erythematosus. *PLoS Genet* 7(6):e1002128, 2011.

127. Brest P, Lapaquette P, Souidi M, et al: A synonymous variant in IRGM alters a binding site for miR-196 and causes deregulation of IRGM-dependent xenophagy in Crohn's disease. *Nat Genet* 43(3):242–245, 2011.

128. Hikami K, Kawasaki A, Ito I, et al: Association of a functional polymorphism in the 3′-untranslated region of SPI1 with systemic lupus erythematosus. *Arthritis Rheum* 63(3):755–763, 2010.

129. Vinuesa CG, Rigby RJ, Yu D: Logic and extent of miRNA-mediated control of autoimmune gene expression. *International reviews of immunology* 28(3–4):112–138, 2009.

130. Hanke M, Hoefig K, Merz H, et al: A robust methodology to study urine microRNA as tumor marker: microRNA-126 and microRNA-182 are related to urinary bladder cancer. *Urol Oncol* 28(6):655–661, 2010.

131. Garchow BG, Encinas OB, Leung YT, et al: Silencing of microR6–21 in vivo ameliorates autoimmune splenomegaly in lupus mice. *EMBO Mol Med* 3(10):605–615, 2011.

132. Martinez-Nunez RT, Louafi F, Sanchez-Elsner T: The interleukin 13 (IL-13) pathway in human macrophages is modulated by microRNA-155 via direct targeting of interleukin 13 receptor alpha1 (IL13Ralpha1). *The Journal of biological chemistry* 286(3):1786–1794, 2011.

133. Louafi F, Martinez-Nunez RT, Sanchez-Elsner T: MicroRNA-155 targets SMAD2 and modulates the response of macrophages to transforming growth factor-β. *The Journal of biological chemistry* 285(53):41328–41336, 2010.

134. Imaizumi T, Tanaka H, Tajima A, et al: IFN-gamma and TNF-alpha synergistically induce microRNA-155 which regulates TAB2/IP-10 expression in human mesangial cells. *Am J Nephrol* 32(5):462–468, 2010.

135. Divekar AA, Dubey S, Gangalum PR, et al: Dicer insufficiency and microRNA-155 overexpression in lupus regulatory T cells: an apparent paradox in the setting of an inflammatory milieu. *J Immunol* 186(2):924–930, 2011.

136. Grigoryev YA, Kurian SM, Hart T, et al: MicroRNA regulation of molecular networks mapped by global microRNA, mRNA, and protein expression in activated T lymphocytes. *J Immunol* 187(5):2233–2243, 2011.

137. Jurkin J, Schichl YM, Koeffel R, et al: miR-146a is differentially expressed by myeloid dendritic cell subsets and desensitizes cells to TLR2-dependent activation. *J Immunol* 184(9):4955–4965, 2010.

138. Sharma A, Kumar M, Aich J, et al: Posttranscriptional regulation of interleukin-10 expression by hsa-miR-106a. *Proc Natl Acad Sci U S A* 106(14):5761–5766, 2009.

139. Annoni A, Brown BD, Cantore A, et al: In vivo delivery of a microRNA-regulated transgene induces antigen-specific regulatory T cells and promotes immunologic tolerance. *Blood* 114(25):5152–5161, 2009.

140. Tserel L, Runnel T, Kisand K, et al: MicroRNA expression profiles of human blood monocyte-derived dendritic cells and macrophages reveal miR-511 as putative positive regulator of Toll-like receptor 4. *J Biol Chem* 286(30):26487–26495, 2011.

141. Tili E, Michaille JJ, Adair B, et al: Resveratrol decreases the levels of miR-155 by upregulating miR-663, a microRNA targeting JunB and JunD. *Carcinogenesis* 31(9):1561–1566, 2010.

142. Schulte LN, Eulalio A, Mollenkopf HJ, et al: Analysis of the host microRNA response to Salmonella uncovers the control of major cytokines by the let-7 family. *EMBO J* 30(10):1977–1989, 2011.

The Innate Immune System in SLE

Lukas Bossaller and Ann Marshak-Rothstein

Adaptive immunity and innate immunity can be distinguished from each other by the nature of the receptors involved in antigen recognition. At one end of the spectrum, we find the extreme heterogeneity of the classical T- and B-cell antigen receptors. Here, multiple gene segments are assembled through a mechanism that utilizes combinatorial diversity, junctional diversity, nontemplated base inserts, and even somatic mutation (in B cells) to generate repertoires that approximate 10^{13} to 10^{18} unique sequences and thereby allow the immune system to develop a highly tuned and sophisticated response to the world of pathogens. At the other extreme are the pattern recognition receptors (PRRs) used by dendritic cells, macrophages, neutrophils, and many other components of the innate immune system to target a broader category of molecular patterns. Importantly, lymphocytes, and especially B cells, can also express PRRs and can therefore be considered a component of the innate immune system as well as the adaptive immune system. These PRRs were originally conceived as a highly efficient surveillance system, designed to discriminate host from pathogen by detection of pathogen-associated molecular patterns (PAMPs) and thereby alert the immune system to the first signs of microbial infection.[1] However, it is becoming increasingly apparent that these same PRRs can detect endogenous ligands that can be released from dead or dying cells or can be expressed on the surfaces of apoptotic cells or bodies. Although the response to such danger-associated molecular patterns (DAMPs) presumably plays a critical role in tissue repair and/or the clearance of cell debris, the failure to appropriately regulate such self-recognition can lead to serious pathologic complications. A case in point are systemic autoimmune diseases such as SLE.

WHAT CONSTITUTES AN AUTOANTIGEN?

Autoantibodies in general target a remarkably small fraction of the general pool of mammalian proteins. This level of specificity has to be addressed by any theory that tries to explain the loss of tolerance so evident in systemic autoimmunity. Circumstantial data from a variety of studies have linked the onset and recurrence of SLE with various types of viral infections.[2,3] As alluded to previously, in this context, engagement of PRRs can activate innate immune system components to produce inflammatory cytokines and chemokines and to upregulate co-stimulatory molecules. Such events could theoretically enhance the presentation of self-peptides, as well as microbial peptides, and thereby lead to a loss of tolerance. However, if such a "revved-up" immune system were the major cause of SLE, autoreactivity would be much more common and would most likely target a much broader set of self-components than we know to be the case.

The concept of molecular mimicry constitutes a second potential link between infection and autoimmune disease. Cross-reactivity between viral peptides and specific autoantigen-associated peptides has been reported by a number of groups.[4] Weakly self-reactive T cells activated by the viral peptide could then further activate any antigen-presenting cells, including B cells, thereby extending the response to additional epitopes associated with a particular macromolecular complex or even to unrelated proteins located on apoptotic bodies or other aggregates of cell debris. Although attractive

conceptually, this molecular mimicry model cannot explain why the same autoantibody specificities are found in populations of patients with SLE, animal models of SLE, and even germ-free autoimmune-prone mice.

A third possible pathogen-linked explanation for the break in tolerance is the creation of neoepitopes by antiviral effector mechanisms. It has been shown that many of the common autoantigens are substrates for granzymes or caspases produced by activated cytotoxic effector populations.[5] The cleaved protein fragments theoretically could adopt novel conformations for which tolerance has not been established or could be processed by the antigen presentation machinery to reveal previously unavailable "cryptic" peptides. Other examples of protein modification that could result in neoepitopes are oxidation, phosphorylation, methylation, demethylation, and citrullination. Such modifications are commonly associated with tissue injury, inflammation, and various forms of cell death,[6-8] conditions that can again promote immune activation.

All the preceding possibilities may well contribute to the onset of autoimmunity and may depend directly or indirectly on an activated innate immune response. However, in all cases, they imply a relatively passive role for the autoantigen per se and still fail to explain why most of the major autoantigens are recurring targets in a wide range of autoimmune conditions, including SLE. Alternatively, growing evidence accumulated over the past decade points to a much more proactive role for the autoantigen in immune activation. In fact, it is now clear that many autoantigens can either directly engage PRRs or can activate components of the innate immune system through other mechanisms and thereby act as autoadjuvants.[9,10] Importantly, further identification of the relevant PRRs and their downstream signaling pathway components will point to less invasive therapeutic options than those currently available to patients.

THE ENDOSOMAL NUCLEIC ACID–SENSING PRRS

Viral replication is detected by an assortment of PRRs that sense the presence of viral nucleic acids, both RNA and DNA. These receptors trigger an antiviral response characterized by the production of type I interferon (IFN). As discussed elsewhere in this text, dysregulated IFN responses appear to be a common feature of SLE. A remarkably high percentage of SLE-associated autoantibodies react with DNA, DNA-binding proteins, RNA, or RNA-binding proteins, and consistent with the autoadjuvant concept, a variety of the "viral" nucleic acid–sensing receptors have now been linked to the pathogenesis of SLE and the recognition of endogenous nucleic acids.

The clearest association is with members of the Toll-like receptor (TLR) family. TLRs are class I transmembrane proteins consisting of an *N*-terminal region made up of a tandem array of leucine-rich repeats, a transmembrane domain, and a cytosolic Toll–interleukin-1 receptor (TIR) domain responsible for downstream signaling events.[11] TLRs are normally found as homodimers or heterodimers that characteristically form overlapping horseshoe-shaped ectodomains. TLRs can be divided into two categories, those that are normally expressed on the cell surface and those whose expression is predominantly limited to intracellular compartments—endoplasmic reticulum (ER), endosomes, and lysosomes. The endosomal receptors, TLR3, TLR7, TLR8, and TLR9, recognize either RNA or DNA, and are the TLRs primarily involved in viral immunity. In order for these endosomal receptors to traffic from the ER to the endosomal/lysosomal compartments, they need to associate with the chaperone protein Unc93b. Murine or human cells that express a nonfunctional form of Unc93b cannot respond to any of the ligands normally detected by the endosomal receptors.[12,13] Cathepsins active in low-pH compartments cleave TLR9 and TLR7, and this cleavage is thought to enhance ligand recognition.[14,15]

Because these TLRs are located in intracellular compartments, and not on the cell surface, one major factor that limits their activity is ligand accessibility—nucleic acids need to colocalize with the TLRs in the appropriate endosomal/lysosomal compartment in order to engage these receptors. Autoantigen trafficking to these compartments is mediated by cell type–specific cell surface receptors. Dendritic cells and neutrophils depend on Fc-gamma receptors (FcγR) to bind autoantigen/autoantibody immune complexes and then transport the complexes to endosomes. In B cells, this transport role is facilitated by the B-cell receptor (BCR).[16] Nucleic acid–associated cell debris, perhaps in the form of apoptotic bodies or microvesicles, can also be taken up by phagocytic cells via various scavenger receptors. In addition, delivery of nucleic acids to the right compartment can be facilitated by antimicrobial peptides such as LL37.[17]

TLR9 is the main sensor of DNA and was originally thought to distinguish microbial DNA from mammalian DNA, on the basis of reactivity with so-called hypomethylated CpG motifs, which are rarely found in mammalian DNA but are common in bacterial and viral DNA. Later studies have clearly demonstrated that under the appropriate circumstances, TLR9 can also detect mammalian DNA. Nevertheless, DNA sequence is still relevant because mammalian DNA sequences enriched for CpG dinucleotides are more potent activators of TLR9 than DNA sequences devoid of CpG dinucleotides.[18] Potential sources of immunostimulatory mammalian DNA include CpG islands, mitochondrial DNA, and retroelements.

TLR7, TLR8, and TLR3 are the RNA-sensing TLRs. TLR7 and TLR8 were initially identified by their ability to respond to synthetic antiviral compounds such as imidazoquinoline derivatives and guanine analogs with strong type I IFN–inducing activity. TLR3 was identified by its capacity to bind a synthetic analog of double-stranded RNA, polyinosinic-polycytidylic acid (poly(I:C)), another mimic of viral infection and a strong inducer of IFN. These receptors bind various forms of single-stranded (ss) or double-stranded (ds) viral RNAs, respectively, and failure to express functional forms of each of these RNA-sensing receptors is associated with susceptibility to very specific types of viral infections. As in the case of TLR9, the RNA-reactive TLRs can also detect mammalian RNAs.[19,20] Here again, sequence and structure are most likely key determinants of ligand avidity, because TLR7 and TLR8 preferentially bind unmodified uridine (U)–rich ssRNAs. Many of the small RNAs associated with the macromolecular structures that include common autoantibody targets fit this category.

Both TLR9 and TLR7 are constitutively expressed by plasmacytoid dendritic cells (pDCs). Although a relatively rare DC population, pDCs can produce extremely high levels of IFN-α in response to both exogenous (viral) and endogenous inducers. Importantly, TLR ligands also induce pDCs to make proinflammatory cytokines such as tumor necrosis factor alpha (TNF-α) and interleukin (IL) 6. B cells also express TLR9 and TLR7, although B-cell expression of TLR7 is markedly increased by type I IFNs. The role of TLR8 in mice is controversial, with data to suggest that it is relatively nonfunctional or a negative regulator of other TLRs. In humans, TLR8 is found predominantly on myeloid-derived cells, where it can also lead to the production of inflammatory cytokines. TLR7, TLR8, and TLR9 signaling pathways depend on the adaptor protein MyD88, on downstream components IRAK4, IRAK1, and IRAK2, and on TRAF6 (TNF-receptor associated factor 6) to activate interferon regulatory factors IRF7 and IRF5 as well as the nuclear factor kappa B (NF-κB)

pathway to promote both the production of IFN and proinflammatory cytokines, respectively. TLR3 is expressed by both hematopoietic and nonhematopoietic cells (fibroblasts) and works through the adaptor protein TRIF to activate the transcription factors IRF3 and NF-κB, also leading to the production of IFN and proinflammatory cytokines (Figure 6-1).

TLR7 AND TLR9 IN SLE

The critical connection among pDCs, type I interferons, B cells, and SLE was initially revealed in patients receiving IFN-α therapeutically. Some of these patients demonstrated autoantibody titers, and a significant fraction went on to have additional clinical features of systemic autoimmune disease.[21] In fact, elevated values of type I IFN can be detected in the serum of patients with SLE, and such patients frequently exhibit a gene expression profile consistent with an IFN signature.[22] Early studies by Ronnblom further demonstrated that pDCs were the major IFN-producing cell type and that SLE sera contained an IFN-α–inducing factor.[23] Importantly, this IFN-inducing activity turned out to be due to circulating ICs consisting of autoantibodies bound to DNA- and RNA-associated autoantigens.[24] These ICs were shown to bind the FcgRII (CD32) receptor on pDCs and trigger the release of very high levels of IFN-α. The pleiotropic effects of IFN-α promote many of the clinical aspects of SLE.

However, in order to form autoantigen-bound ICs, autoreactive B cells need to be activated and to differentiate to autoantibody-producing cells. It was in this context that the connection was first made to TLRs. The initial studies involved a BCR transgenic cell line that expressed a low-affinity receptor for autologous immunoglobulin (Ig) G2a, in essence a rheumatoid factor (RF), that was originally developed and characterized by Weigert.[25] Because these B cells recognize IgG2a with low affinity, they escape the negative selection mechanisms, such as receptor editing, that are known to eliminate high-affinity autoreactive B cells from the repertoire and successfully develop as naïve follicular B cells. The rheumatoid factor B cells are very efficiently activated by IgG2a ICs that incorporate DNA or RNA, but not by ICs that contain only proteins, through a mechanism that depends on either TLR9 or TLR7.[16,19] The associated nucleic acids are recognized by the IgG2a-reactive BCR and thereby transported to the endosomal/lysosomal compartments, where TLR engagement ensues, resulting in a robust proliferative response. Later studies have clearly demonstrated that this BCR/TLR paradigm most likely applies to peripheral B cells reactive with other common autoantigens; B cells that bind DNA, RNA, or any DNA/RNA-associated protein can deliver these molecules to the same TLR-associated compartments and thereby trigger TLR activation. Numerous in vitro studies implicate TLR9 in the detection of DNA, chromatin, and other DNA-associated proteins, and TLR7/8 in the detection of RNA and RNA-associated proteins. In addition to making autoantibodies, activated B cells produce cytokines and play an important role in antigen presentation.

IN VIVO SUPPORT FOR TLR ASSOCIATIONS WITH SLE

The connection between TLR detection of mammalian ligands and systemic autoimmune disease has been further tested in vivo in murine models of SLE. These studies have taken advantage of the existence of numerous spontaneous or targeted mutations of the TLRs and/or their associated proteins. Loss-of-function mutations in the chaperone protein Unc93B or the adaptor protein MyD88 result in complete deficiency of the TLR7 and TLR9 signaling cascades, and autoimmune mice that inherit these mutations produce little if any autoantibody, demonstrate much less severe clinical disease, and exhibit a dramatically improved survival rate. Mice deficient for only TLR7 do not make autoantibodies reactive with the common RNA-associated autoantigens but still make antibodies reactive with DNA and/or other chromatin components. Despite their antichromatin titers, they also have a markedly improved disease status with extended survival rates. By contrast, mice deficient for only TLR9 do

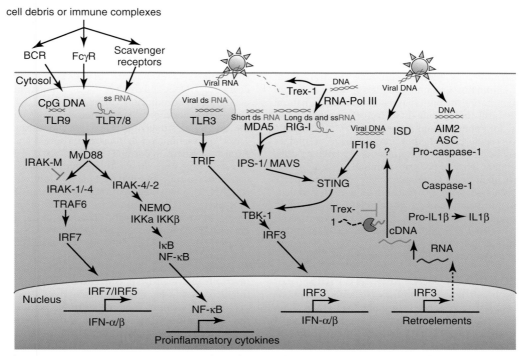

FIGURE 6-1 RNA and DNA sensing receptors activate a variety of signaling cascades to promote the production of type I interferon (IFN), proinflammatory cytokines, and interleukin IL-1β. The relevant Toll-like receptors, TLR9, TLR7, TLR8, and TLR3, are found in endosomal/lysosomal compartments (shown in yellow), where they detect both microbial and endogenous DNA (in red) and RNA (in blue). DNA presence in the cytosol can be detected by a group of interferon stimulatory DNA (ISD) receptors, such as IFI16. Cytosolic DNA can also activate AIM2, which together with ASC drives the processing of IL1β. In contrast to extrinsic DNA or RNA, that is shuttled to the endosomal TLRs, cell-intrinsic DNA or RNA from transcribed retroelements must be efficiently degraded by Trex-1 (DNAse III) or RNAseH2 (not shown) to prevent recognition by cytosolic nucleic acid sensors. Cytosolic RNA can be sensed by MDA-5 and/or RIG-I. IRAK-M is a negative regulator of TLR signaling. ASC, an adaptor molecule (apoptosis-associated specklike protein containing a caspase activation and recruitment domain); IκB, inhibitor of kappa B; IKK, IκB kinase; MDA5 (melanoma-differentiation-associated gene 5); NEMO, NF-κB essential modulator.

TABLE 6-1 Deficiencies in Toll-Like Receptor Pathways and Summary of Key Findings in Different Murine Lupus Models

GENETIC DEFICIENCY	AUTOANTIBODIES		CLINICAL DISEASE		
	Anti-DNA	Anti-RNA	Kidney	Mortality	References
TLR3	nc	nc	nc	nd	26
TLR7	↑	↓	↓	nd	27, 32, 35
TLR8	↑	↑	↑	↑	28
TLR9	↓↓	↑	↑	↑	26, 29-31, 36
TLR7+9	↓↓	↓	↓	nd	31
MyD88	↓↓	↓↓	↓↓	↓↓	19, 33
Unc93b1	↓↓	↓	↓↓	↓	34

↑↑, major increase; ↑, modest increase; nc, no change; ↓, modest decrease; ↓↓, major decrease; nd, not determined.

not make antichromatin antibodies but still produce antibodies reactive with RNA-associated autoantigens (Table 6-1).[19,26-36] Quite unexpectedly, these TLR9-deficient autoimmune-prone mice have more severe clinical disease and decreased survival rates. At this time it is not clear whether this pattern reflects (1) a unique property of the TLR7-deficient mice used for these studies, (2) a TLR9-dependent regulatory population, or (3) distinct outcomes of TLR7 and TLR9 downstream signaling events in B cells or another critical cell type.

POTENTIAL SOURCES OF AUTOANTIGEN

The autoantigens most commonly targeted in SLE are for the most part components of macromolecules normally found in the cell nucleus. The question is therefore how these cell constituents become available to the immune system. Pivotal studies from Rosen demonstrated that many of these autoantigens can be found clustered on the surfaces of apoptotic cells in what are now referred to as *apoptotic blebs.*[37] The relocation of nuclear antigens in this context suggests a potential route to immune activation. However, under normal circumstances, apoptotic cells are very efficiently cleared from the circulation by phagocytic cells that express an assortment of scavenger receptors on their surfaces, through noninflammatory mechanisms. Importantly, mutations that disrupt the normal processes required for the clearance of cell debris are frequently associated with the production of autoantibodies and a predisposition to development of systemic autoimmune disease. For example, the complement component C1q can directly bind to apoptotic cells, and patients or mice with an inherited deficiency in C1q fail to appropriately clear *apoptotic debris*. This connection most likely contributes to the fact that SLE develops in more than 80% of individuals with C1q deficiency.[38] Deficiencies in other molecules known to promote the clearance of apoptotic cells or chromatin immune complexes, such as serum amyloid P component (SAP), the protein tyrosine kinase mer, natural IgM, and MFG-E8 (milk fat globule–EGF factor 8 protein), also confer susceptibility to systemic autoimmune disease.[39-42] If apoptotic cells are not appropriately cleared, they may undergo secondary necrosis and/or may be taken up by nonprofessional scavenger cells, conditions that are more likely to promote immune activation.

Later studies have identified another potentially important source of immunogenic DNA associated with inflammation. Activated neutrophils undergo an unusual form of cell death, referred to as *netosis*, associated with the rapid extrusion of chromatin neutrophil extracellular traps (NETs). The NET DNA is associated with LL37 and other peptides that enhance delivery to the endosomal compartment, and NETs may therefore constitute major autoantigen depots.[43,44]

THE CYTOSOLIC NUCLEIC ACID–SENSING PRRS

DNA is normally sequestered away from the cytoplasm. Exceptions include instances of viral replication, cytosolic bacterial infection, tissue damage, and endogenous retroelements. Non-TLR elements of the innate immune system, present in the cytosol, are now known to also effectively activate downstream pathways leading to the production of IFN and inflammatory pathways. However, the detection of cytosolic DNA appears to involve multiple redundant receptors and mechanisms, and many of the details are still unclear. It is known that both viral dsDNA and experimentally delivered dsDNA fragments can be detected by cytosolic DNA sensors, often referred to as the *interferon stimulatory DNA (ISD) sensors*. Potential candidates include DAI (DNA-dependent activator of IFN regulatory factors) and IFI16 (interferon gamma–inducible factor 16), both of which sense DNA and trigger pathways that converge on an ER-associated protein, STING (stimulator of IFN genes), which then leads to the activation of TBK-1 (TANK-binding kinase 1) and IRF3 and the subsequent transcription of IFN-β.[45,46] Another cytosolic DNA receptor, designated AIM2 (absent in melanoma 2), is structurally related to IFI16. However, AIM2 does not induce IFN production; instead, it promotes the assembly of an inflammasome complex that leads to the processing and release of IL-1b.[47]

Another family of receptors, referred to as RLRs (RIG-I [retinoic acid–inducible gene I]–like receptors), are known to recognize viral dsRNA and ssRNA.[48] These receptors all appear to assemble with the mitochondrium-associated adaptor protein IPS (IFN-β promoter stimulator) or MAVS, which then feeds into the STING pathway mentioned previously. RIG-I also plays a role in the detection of cytosolic DNA through a mechanism that depends on DNA-dependent RNA polymerase III to convert dsDNA into dsRNA, which in turn is detected by RIG-I (see Figure 6-1).

DEFECTS IN DNA AND RNA DEGRADATION

Ineffective degradation of both extracellular and cytosolic DNA has been clearly implicated in autoimmunity and autoinflammation. *DNase I* is the major endonuclease found in the serum and urine, where it is responsible for degrading extracellular dsDNA. Mutations in DNase I have been found in patients with lupus[49] and parallel the phenotype seen in certain DNase I–deficient mice.[50] In addition, the serum of a subpopulation of patients with SLE has been reported to contain unidentified DNase I inhibitors or blocking antibodies,[43] such that DNA (or DNA ICs) persist in the serum for an extended period. *DNAse II* is a lysosome-associated enzyme, and DNAse II deficiency can also lead to autoimmunity. DNAse II deficiency in mice is an embryo-lethal mutation that results from the inability of macrophages to degrade nuclear debris. These engorged macrophages then produce extremely high levels of IFN, through a

TLR9-independent mechanism that presumably involves a cytosolic DNA receptor. DNAse II mice that do not express a type I IFN receptor survive to adulthood, but then systemic autoimmune disease develops through an IFN-independent mechanism.[51]

The cytosolic DNA exonuclease *DNAse III*, or Trex1, is the most abundant 3′→5′ exonuclease in the cell and plays a major role in degrading ssDNA and dsDNA that accumulate in the cytosol. Trex1-deficient cells accumulate cytosolic DNA, which is thought to initiate severe IFN-dependent autoimmune syndromes through one of the interferon stimulatory DNA receptors. Most individuals with Trex1 loss of function demonstrate a severe encephalitis known as Aicardi-Goutières syndrome (AGS).[52,53] Around 60% of patients with this syndrome were shown in one study to have autoimmune manifestations typically found in patients with lupus (antinuclear antibodies [ANAs], cytopenia, arthritis, oral ulcers, and skin lesions).[54] Moreover, certain mutations in Trex1 can cause familial chilblain lupus[55] or SLE.[56] Intriguingly, mutations in the human ribonuclease H2 enzyme complex can also result in AGS.[57] The endonuclease RNaseH2 degrades RNA : DNA hybrids, and RNaseH2 mutations can also cause AGS. This correlation points to a role for undegraded endogenous retroelements in patients with AGS. Intriguingly, reverse-transcribed DNA is a Trex1 substrate, and retroviral DNA fragments have been recovered from Trex1-deficient cells.[58]

Other associations between cytosolic sensors and SLE are less direct and based mainly on genetic associations with patient populations. These include polymorphisms in IPS-1, the downstream adaptor protein for the cytosolic RNA sensors and SNPs in IFI16. Interestingly, knockdown of AIM2 has been found to potentiate IFN-β induction,[47] and AIM2 is localized within a susceptibility locus for SLE.[59]

SUMMARY AND POTENTIAL THERAPIES: IMPLICATION FOR TARGETING PRR PATHWAYS

Over the past decade, tremendous progress has been made in the field of innate immunity and the identification of different categories of nucleic acid–sensing PRRs. These evolutionarily conserved receptors play a critical role in microbial immunity. However, on the downside, a variety of conditions can lead to dysregulated activation of these receptors and ensuing autoimmune consequences. Defining exactly how and why this imbalance becomes established in the individual patient will be a major challenge for the future physician, geneticist, and researcher in order to better treat a complex and mechanistically heterogeneous disease like SLE.

The important question is whether it will be possible to translate knowledge gained from murine lupus models into efficacious human therapeutics. Potential strategies include oligonucleotide-based inhibitors of TLR7 and TLR9, removal of undegraded extracellular or intracellular autoantigen stores, and modulation of the PRR-specific signaling cascades.

Finding the key to blocking or modulating nonpathogen activation of the innate immune system will require further large-scale screenings for TLR agonists/antagonists and the newly discovered intracellular DNA and RNA sensing pathways, which should eventually generate novel treatment options for autoimmune diseases.

References

1. Medzhitov R, Janeway CA, Jr: Innate immunity: the virtues of a nonclonal system of recognition. *Cell* 91:295–298, 1997.
2. Phillips PE: The virus hypothesis in systemic lupus erythematosus. *Ann Intern Med* 83:709–715, 1975.
3. Denman AM: Systemic lupus erythematosus—is a viral aetiology a credible hypothesis? *J Infect* 40:229–233, 2000.
4. McClain MT, Heinlen LD, Dennis GJ, et al: Early events in lupus humoral autoimmunity suggest initiation through molecular mimicry. *Nat Med* 11:85–89, 2005.
5. Casciola-Rosen L, Andrade F, Ulanet D, et al: Cleavage by granzyme B is strongly predictive of autoantigen status: implications for initiation of autoimmunity. *J Exp Med* 190:815–826, 1999.

6. Utz PJ, Gensler TJ, Anderson P: Death, autoantigen modifications, and tolerance. *Arthritis Res* 2:101–114, 2000.

7. Anderton SM: Post-translational modifications of self antigens: implications for autoimmunity. *Curr Opin Immunol* 16:753–758, 2004.

8. Hall JC, Casciola-Rosen L, Rosen A: Altered structure of autoantigens during apoptosis. *Rheum Dis Clin North Am* 30:455–471, vii, 2004.

9. Plotz PH: The autoantibody repertoire: searching for order. *Nat Rev Immunol* 3:73–78, 2003.

10. Busconi L, Lau CM, Tabor AS, et al: DNA and RNA autoantigens as autoadjuvants. *J Endotoxin Res* 12:379–384, 2006.

11. Kawai T, Akira S: The role of pattern-recognition receptors in innate immunity: update on Toll-like receptors. *Nat Immunol* 11:373–384, 2010.

12. Tabeta K, Hoebe K, Janssen EM, et al: The Unc93b1 mutation 3d disrupts exogenous antigen presentation and signaling via Toll-like receptors 3, 7 and 9. *Nat Immunol* 7:156–164, 2006.

13. Isnardi I, Ng YS, Srdanovic I, et al: IRAK-4–and MyD88-dependent pathways are essential for the removal of developing autoreactive B cells in humans. *Immunity* 29:746–757, 2008.

14. Kim YM, Brinkmann MM, Paquet ME, et al: UNC93B1 delivers nucleotide-sensing toll-like receptors to endolysosomes. *Nature* 452:234–238, 2008.

15. Ewald SE, Lee BL, Lau L, et al: The ectodomain of Toll-like receptor 9 is cleaved to generate a functional receptor. *Nature* 456:658–662, 2008.

16. Leadbetter EA, Rifkin IR, Hohlbaum AM, et al: Chromatin-IgG complexes activate B cells by dual engagement of IgM and Toll-like receptors. *Nature* 416:603–607, 2002.

17. Lande R, Gregorio J, Facchinetti V, et al: Plasmacytoid dendritic cells sense self-DNA coupled with antimicrobial peptide. *Nature* 449:564–569, 2007.

18. Uccellini MB, Busconi L, Green NM, et al: Autoreactive B cells discriminate CpG-rich and CpG-poor DNA and this response is modulated by IFN-alpha. *J Immunol* 181:5875–5884, 2008.

19. Lau CM, Broughton C, Tabor AS, et al: RNA-associated autoantigens activate B cells by combined B cell antigen receptor/Toll-like receptor 7 engagement. *J Exp Med* 202:1171–1177, 2005.

20. Vollmer J, Tluk S, Schmitz C, et al: Immune stimulation mediated by autoantigen binding sites within small nuclear RNAs involves Toll-like receptors 7 and 8. *J Exp Med* 202:1575–1585, 2005.

21. Ronnblom LE, Alm GV, Oberg KE: Possible induction of systemic lupus erythematosus by interferon-alpha treatment in a patient with a malignant carcinoid tumour. *J Intern Med* 227:207–210, 1990.

22. Baechler EC, Batliwalla FM, Karypis G, et al: Interferon-inducible gene expression signature in peripheral blood cells of patients with severe lupus. *Proc Natl Acad Sci U S A* 100:2610–2615, 2003.

23. Ronnblom L, Alm GV: A pivotal role for the natural interferon alpha-producing cells (plasmacytoid dendritic cells) in the pathogenesis of lupus. *J Exp Med* 194:F59–F63, 2001.

24. Bave U, Magnusson M, Eloranta ML, et al: Fc gamma RIIa is expressed on natural IFN-alpha-producing cells (plasmacytoid dendritic cells) and is required for the IFN-alpha production induced by apoptotic cells combined with lupus IgG. *J Immunol* 171:3296–3302, 2003.

25. Shlomchik MJ, Zharhary D, Saunders T, et al: A rheumatoid factor transgenic mouse model of autoantibody regulation. *Int Immunol* 5:1329–1341, 1993.

26. Christensen SR, Kashgarian M, Alexopoulou L, et al: Toll-like receptor 9 controls anti-DNA autoantibody production in murine lupus. *J Exp Med* 202:321–331, 2005.

27. Lee PY, Kumagai Y, Li Y, et al: TLR7-dependent and FcgammaR-independent production of type I interferon in experimental mouse lupus. *J Exp Med* 205:2995–3006, 2008.

28. Demaria O, Pagni PP, Traub S, et al: TLR8 deficiency leads to autoimmunity in mice. *J Clin Invest* 120:3651–3662, 2010.

29. Christensen SR, Shupe J, Nickerson K, et al: Toll-like receptor 7 and TLR9 dictate autoantibody specificity and have opposing inflammatory and regulatory roles in a murine model of lupus. *Immunity* 25:417–428, 2006.

30. Lartigue A, Courville P, Auquit I, et al: Role of TLR9 in anti-nucleosome and anti-DNA antibody production in lpr mutation-induced murine lupus. *J Immunol* 177:1349–1354, 2006.

31. Santiago-Raber ML, Dunand-Sauthier I, Wu T, et al: Critical role of TLR7 in the acceleration of systemic lupus erythematosus in TLR9-deficient mice. *J Autoimmun* 34:339–348, 2010.

32. Nickerson KM, Christensen SR, Shupe J, et al: TLR9 regulates TLR7- and MyD88-dependent autoantibody production and disease in a murine model of lupus. *J Immunol* 184:1840–1848, 2010.

33. Ehlers M, Fukuyama H, McGaha TL, et al: TLR9/MyD88 signaling is required for class switching to pathogenic IgG2a and 2b autoantibodies in SLE. *J Exp Med* 203:553–561, 2006.

34. Kono DH, Haraldsson MK, Lawson BR, et al: Endosomal TLR signaling is required for anti-nucleic acid and rheumatoid factor autoantibodies in lupus. *Proc Natl Acad Sci U S A* 106:12061–12066, 2009.

35. Savarese E, Steinberg C, Pawar RD, et al: Requirement of Toll-like receptor 7 for pristane-induced production of autoantibodies and development of murine lupus nephritis. *Arthritis Rheum* 58(4):1107–1115, 2008.

36. Yu P, Wellmann U, Kunder S, et al: Toll-like receptor 9-independent aggravation of glomerulonephritis in a novel model of SLE. *Int Immunol* 18(8):1211–1219, 2006.

37. Rosen A, Casciola-Rosen L, Ahearn J: Novel packages of viral and self-antigens are generated during apoptosis. *J Exp Med* 181:1557–1561, 1995.

38. Manderson AP, Botto M, Walport MJ: The role of complement in the development of systemic lupus erythematosus. *Annu Rev Immunol* 22:431–456, 2004.

39. Bickerstaff MC, Botto M, Hutchinson WL, et al: Serum amyloid P component controls chromatin degradation and prevents antinuclear autoimmunity. *Nat Med* 5:694–697, 1999.

40. Lu Q, Lemke G: Homeostatic regulation of the immune system by receptor tyrosine kinases of the Tyro 3 family. *Science* 293:306–311, 2001.

41. Boes M, Schmidt T, Linkemann K, et al: Accelerated development of IgG autoantibodies and autoimmune disease in the absence of secreted IgM. *Proc Natl Acad Sci U S A* 97:1184–1189, 2000.

42. Hanayama R, Tanaka M, Miyasaka K, et al: Autoimmune disease and impaired uptake of apoptotic cells in MFG-E8-deficient mice. *Science* 304:1147–1150, 2004.

43. Hakkim A, Furnrohr BG, Amann K, et al: Impairment of neutrophil extracellular trap degradation is associated with lupus nephritis. *Proc Natl Acad Sci U S A* 107:9813–9818, 2010.

44. Lande R, Ganguly D, Facchinetti V, et al: Neutrophils activate plasmacytoid dendritic cells by releasing self-DNA-peptide complexes in systemic lupus erythematosus. *Sci Transl Med* 3(73):73ra19, 2011.

45. Takaoka A, Wang Z, Choi MK, et al: DAI (DLM-1/ZBP1) is a cytosolic DNA sensor and an activator of innate immune response. *Nature* 448:501–505, 2007.

46. Unterholzner L, Keating SE, Baran M, et al: IFI16 is an innate immune sensor for intracellular DNA. *Nat Immunol* 11:997–1004, 2010.

47. Hornung V, Ablasser A, Charrel-Dennis M, et al: AIM2 recognizes cytosolic dsDNA and forms a caspase-1-activating inflammasome with ASC. *Nature* 458:514–518, 2009.

48. Myong S, Cui S, Cornish PV, et al: Cytosolic viral sensor RIG-I is a 5′-triphosphate-dependent translocase on double-stranded RNA. *Science* 323:1070–1074, 2009.

49. Yasutomo K, Horiuchi T, Kagami S, et al: Mutation of DNASE1 in people with systemic lupus erythematosus. *Nature Genetics* 28:313–314, 2001.

50. Napirei M, Karsunky H, Zevnik B, et al: Features of systemic lupus erythematosus in Dnase1-deficient mice. *Nature Genetics* 25:177–181, 2000.

51. Kawane K, Ohtani M, Miwa K, et al: Chronic polyarthritis caused by mammalian DNA that escapes from degradation in macrophages. *Nature* 443(7114):998–1002, 2006.

52. Crow YJ, Hayward BE, Parmar R, et al: Mutations in the gene encoding the 3′-5′ DNA exonuclease TREX1 cause Aicardi-Goutières syndrome at the AGS1 locus. *Nat Genet* 38:917–920, 2006.

53. Stetson DB, Ko JS, Heidmann T, et al: Trex1 prevents cell-intrinsic initiation of autoimmunity. *Cell* 134:587–598, 2008.

54. Ramantani G, Kohlhase J, Hertzberg C, et al: Expanding the phenotypic spectrum of lupus erythematosus in Aicardi-Goutieres syndrome. *Arthritis Rheum* 62:1469–1477, 2010.

55. Rice G, Newman WG, Dean J, et al: Heterozygous mutations in TREX1 cause familial chilblain lupus and dominant Aicardi-Goutieres syndrome. *Am J Hum Genet* 80:811–815, 2007.

56. Lee-Kirsch MA, Gong M, Chowdhury D, et al: Mutations in the gene encoding the 3′-5′ DNA exonuclease TREX1 are associated with systemic lupus erythematosus. *Nat Genet* 39:1065–1067, 2007.

57. Crow YJ, Leitch A, Hayward BE, et al: Mutations in genes encoding ribonuclease H2 subunits cause Aicardi-Goutières syndrome and mimic congenital viral brain infection. *Nature Genetics* 38:910–916, 2006.

58. Perl A, Fernandez D, Telarico T, et al: Endogenous retroviral pathogenesis in lupus. *Curr Opin Rheumatol* 22:483–492, 2010.

59. Roberts TL, Idris A, Dunn JA, et al: HIN-200 proteins regulate caspase activation in response to foreign cytoplasmic DNA. *Science* 323:1057–1060, 2009.

Cytokines and Interferons in Lupus

Mary K. Crow, Timothy B. Niewold, and Kyriakos A. Kirou

The immunopathology of systemic lupus erythematosus (SLE) has traditionally been attributed to the deposition in tissues and organs of immune complexes or autoantibodies with specificity for or cross-reactivity with locally expressed antigens. These mechanisms are likely to account for an important component of the inflammation that generates tissue damage in this disease, but accumulating data suggest that additional mechanisms should be considered. The complement of soluble mediators, particularly cytokines and chemokines, that are produced in the context of innate and adaptive immune system activation in patients with lupus is likely to be a product of whatever endogenous and exogenous triggers are inducing autoimmunity as well as the efforts of the immune system cells to gain control over its activated components. These molecules may shape the character of the immune system dysfunction and organ system involvement. In SLE, given the heterogeneity of the disease, distinct cytokine pathways may operate in different patients, and those pathways may, in part, determine the different organ systems affected. In addition, different cytokine pathways may be important at different stages of the disease. Understanding the balance of cytokines that are expressed in a given patient may ultimately guide medical management as new approaches to modulating cytokine pathways therapeutically become available.

PROPERTIES OF CYTOKINES AND THEIR RECEPTORS

Cytokines are small soluble proteins that are produced by immune system cells and mediate activation or functional regulation of nearby cells by binding to cell surface receptors.[1] In health, the immune system functions as a coordinated whole, with each cell type playing a carefully orchestrated role. These molecules mediate the communication between immune cells, which is critical for coordinated responses to pathogens. Cytokines are important at each stage of the immune response, from the initial activation of the innate immune system, through the maturation of T and B cells in the adaptive response, to the resolution of the immune response once the pathogen is cleared. Given these important roles, it is easy to imagine that inappropriate cytokine signaling could lead to autoimmunity. Both excessive inflammatory cytokine production and insufficient inhibitory cytokine production likely play a role in the chronic autoimmune inflammation that characterizes SLE. Abnormal cytokine signaling may participate in the initiation of SLE, and cytokines are also important in the progression and propagation of the illness.

Cytokines act in an autocrine or paracrine manner, in close proximity to their source, and have been considered to serve a similar function to that of neurotransmitters in the nervous system. Basal production of most cytokines is negligible, and activation of the producer cells, through pattern-recognition or antigen-specific receptors, results in either new gene transcription or translation of preexisting cytokine messenger RNAs (mRNA) and protein secretion. Many cytokines have been reported to be elevated or decreased in the sera of patients with SLE in comparison with healthy controls (Table 7-1). Cytokine protein is typically detected at low levels or not at all in serum from healthy individuals, but in patients with SLE, elevations of some cytokines are measurable and some vary with disease activity. These findings should reflect the immune dysregulation that characterizes the disease to some degree. Presumably the cytokines observed in the circulation come from the inflamed tissues, although some cytokines could be produced in the blood as well.

The level of cell surface expression of the receptors to which cytokines bind is also highly regulated and contributes to the impact of the cytokines on immune system activity. Once the receptors are engaged, complex multicomponent molecular pathways transduce a signal from cell surface to nucleus, resulting in new gene transcription. The Janus kinase (Jak)–signal transducer and activator of transcription (STAT) pathways are common mediators of cytokine-cytokine receptor interactions.[2] The strength of these signaling pathways can be affected by the state of activation of the target cell and the additional signals that it has received, with the mitogen-activated protein (MAP) kinase and other signaling systems modulating the function of the Jak-STAT pathway. In addition, negative regulators of cytokine signals, such as the suppressor of cytokine signaling (SOCS) proteins, further modulate the strength of target cell response to the cytokine.[3]

The degree of expression of individual cytokines or activation of their pathways is also regulated on that basis of genetic differences among individuals that translate into variable efficiency in cytokine production or response.[4] Great progress has been made in understanding the genetic basis of SLE, and many of the well-established genetic risk loci are genes that function in cytokine pathways.[5,6] Genetic variability can be localized to regulatory regions of genes, potentially modifying the level of expression, or can be in coding sequences, sometimes resulting in an altered amino acid sequence and modified conformational structure. Both of these types of genetic variations are represented in the list of genetic associations with SLE, and some of these SLE-associated variations are also associated with altered cytokine levels, supporting the idea that genetic variability in cytokine response is a component of SLE pathogenesis.[6]

ASSESSMENT OF CYTOKINE PRODUCTION

As small soluble proteins, cytokines are frequently measured in the serum or plasma of patients, and in experimental systems, cytokines can be measured in cell culture supernatants.

The expression of cytokines and the capacity to produce cytokines in an individual can be assessed using numerous distinct and complementary approaches.[7] Measurement of an mRNA encoding a cytokine can be used to provide a reasonable indication of the amount of cytokine protein produced. However, the variable stability of one or another mRNA must be considered, and the presence of an mRNA may not necessarily indicate that the mRNA is translated and the corresponding protein generated.

TABLE 7-1 Role of Cytokines and Interferons in Lupus Pathogenesis

MEDIATOR	ROLE IN PATHOGENESIS
Products of the Innate Immune Response	
Type I interferon: IFN-α, IFN-β, IFN-ω	Increased in active SLE
	Mediates multiple immune system alterations, including dendritic cell maturation, immunoglobulin (Ig) class switching, and induction of IL-10, IFN-γ, and other immunoregulatory molecules
	Accelerates disease in murine models. Inhibition of IFN-α is under study in lupus clinical trials
Tumor necrosis factor	Role in SLE not clear
	Serum values elevated in some patients
Interleukin-1 (IL-1)	Increased levels associated with active SLE
IL-10	Complex role in SLE
	Promotes B-cell expansion and Ig class switching
	Progenitor B-cell effects may dominate its anti-inflammatory effects
BLyS/BAFF (B-lymphocyte stimulator/B-cell–activating factor)	Increased levels in SLE
	Promotes B-cell survival and may contribute to Ig class switching
	Is therapeutic target of belimumab, approved by U.S. Food and Drug Administration for treatment of SLE
IL-6	Increased levels in active SLE
	Promotes terminal B-cell differentiation
	Being targeted by new anti–IL-6 receptor antibody in clinical trials
IL-12 and IL-18	Support expansion of T helper 1 (Th1) cells and natural killer (NK) cells
IL-8, IP-10, MIG (monokine induced by IFN-γ), MCP-1 (monocyte chemotactic protein 1), fractalkine	Chemokines that may be increased in active SLE and may recruit inflammatory cells to sites of organ inflammation, particularly in lupus nephritis
Products of the Adaptive Immune Response	
IL-2	Decreased production in SLE in in vitro studies
	Mediates T-cell proliferation and activation-induced cell death
IFN-γ	Produced by Th1 cells and NK cells
	Implicated in lupus nephritis in murine models and human SLE
IL-6 and IL-10	Produced by T and B lymphocytes as well as monocytes
TGF-β (tumor growth factor beta)	Produced by multiple cell types
	Role in SLE not clear, but may contribute to function of T regulatory cells and renal scarring
IL-17	Produced by Th17 cells
	Is proinflammatory
	Role in SLE is not clear
IL-21	Produced by T follicular helper cells
	Drives B-cell proliferation and differentiation
	Role in SLE not clear, but may be rational therapeutic target

Direct measurement of protein, as by enzyme-linked immunosorbent assay (ELISA), is a fairly reliable indicator of the presence of that protein, and this technique is one of the most common methods used to measure cytokines in solution. In ELISAs, antibodies are used to specifically detect the soluble protein, utilizing either fluorescence or a colorimetric enzyme reaction to reflect the amount of specific protein present in the sample. Results are read from a standard curve, and the presumption is made that the antibody binds only to the particular protein being measured. Multiplex assays capable of measuring a large number of cytokines simultaneously are also available and rely upon similar antibody-based recognition coupled with specific fluorescence indicating each cytokine. Issues of protein degradation and variable detection, based on the antibodies used and the availability of their corresponding epitopes, suggest that confirmation of protein concentration using alternative approaches can be valuable. Although ELISA determines quantity of protein per volume of fluid, usually serum or plasma, intracellular staining for cytokine protein and the enzyme-linked immunospot assay (ELISPOT) determine the percentage of cytokine-producing cells in a cell preparation and permit identification of those cells. The latter approach provides important information, because some of the pathogenic cytokines are products of multiple cell types. Knowing the major cell source can assist in development of therapeutic strategies to inhibit (or augment) production of the cytokine.

Living cells can be used to detect cytokines as well. In this type of assay, the characteristic impact of a cytokine upon cells is measured. For example, one assay for the antiviral type I interferons (IFN) involves applying the sample to cells that are infected with a virus and then examining the cells for visible signs of inhibition of the infection. Other methods that are currently more widely used involve measuring gene expression in cells from patients or in cells that are stimulated in culture. Cytokines induce typical patterns of gene expression, and these patterns can reveal the presence of the cytokine. Cell-based assays can involve exposing cells to the sample containing a cytokine and then using polymerase chain reaction (PCR) to measure the amount of characteristic downstream gene transcription attributable to ligation of a cytokine receptor. In an alternate strategy, samples are applied to cell lines containing a plasmid with a fluorescent protein under the control of a promoter, which is bound after characteristic downstream signaling from cytokine receptors. Ligation of the cytokine receptor induces activation of a characteristic transcription factor, which then induces the transcription of the fluorescent protein on the plasmid. Because any given gene target can usually be induced by multiple triggers, inhibition of gene expression with an antibody that neutralizes the activity of a specific cytokine can be used to demonstrate the relevance of that cytokine to the induction of the target mRNA (or protein) being measured.

USE OF MICROARRAY TO STUDY CYTOKINE EFFECTS

Microarray analysis, a system in which thousands of oligonucleotide sequences are spotted on a solid substrate, usually a glass slide, and RNA-derived material from a cell population is hybridized to the gene array, is an innovative technology that permits a global view of the profile of genes expressed in a cell population at a point in time, including genes in the cytokine pathways.[8] Applying microarray analysis to heterogeneous cell populations in peripheral blood from patients with autoimmune diseases raises technical challenges. The variable proportions of different cell populations in each subject, each making variable contributions to the mRNAs in the blood sample, adds complexity to the comparison of study groups. Additionally, the statistical analysis of thousands of gene sequences studied in multiple individuals is daunting. Investigations have now demonstrated that in spite of these technical challenges, significant and useful microarray data can be derived from complex cell samples, including peripheral blood mononuclear cells stimulated in vitro and peripheral blood preparations from patients with autoimmune disease. The view that IFN-α might play a central pathogenic role in SLE has only lately gained momentum with the completion of several large-scale studies of gene expression profiling with microarray technology. Multiple groups have used this powerful technology to demonstrate that mRNAs encoded by IFN-regulated genes are among the most prominent observed in peripheral blood cells of patients with lupus (Figure 7-1).[8-12] This coordinate overexpression of multiple IFN-α–induced

transcripts is what would be expected following ligation of the type I IFN receptor by IFN-α, and this molecular footprint has been called an "IFN-α signature."

It should be emphasized that microarray is a screen to identify genes potentially altered in expression in a cell preparation or disease state. Microarray data should be confirmed by more quantitative techniques, such as real-time PCR, and data derived from patient samples should be confirmed in additional patient cohorts.

ACTIVATION OF THE IMMUNE RESPONSE IN SLE

The mechanisms that account for aberrant production of autoantibodies, cytokines, and other soluble mediators in SLE can be modeled in parallel with the production of antibodies and mediators in a productive immune response to microbial pathogens in a healthy individual. The initial encounter with the microbe is mediated by cells of the innate immune response. Although those cells have traditionally been considered to initiate an immune response through nonspecific cell surface receptors, the elucidation of the Toll-like receptor (TLR) family has altered that picture.[13] Although the innate immune response does not have the fine level of specificity that characterizes the adaptive immune response generated by T and B lymphocytes, the members of the TLR family do recognize classes of stimuli with characteristic structural features. Among the TLR ligands are nucleic acids, including hypomethylated CpG DNA and single-stranded (ss) or double-stranded (ds) RNA. These nucleic acids are typical components of viruses and bacteria but might also be products of apoptotic or necrotic host cells. Whether microbe-derived in the setting of infection or self-derived, these oligonucleotides provide an adjuvant-like stimulus that can initiate a heightened level of immune system activity, including the production of cytokines.

It is the production of cytokines in the context of innate immune response activation that permits the activation and maturation of antigen-presenting cells (APCs), such that T cells of the adaptive, highly specific component of the immune response can become engaged. Whether the antigenic target is a viral or bacterial protein or a self-antigen concentrated in the cell surface blebs of apoptotic cells, antigen-specific T-cell receptors and T-cell surface co-stimulatory molecules, such as CD28, interact with the antigenic peptide–major histocompatibility (MHC) complex and the co-stimulatory ligand, CD80 or CD86, on the surface of an APC and stimulate biochemical signals, new gene transcription, and cell activation. The activated T cell is then able, through expression of new cell surface molecules that mediate cell-cell interactions with B cells and other target cells, along with production of cytokines, to drive the humoral immune response and activate effector cells. It is the nature of the cytokines produced by the APCs' T cells, and B cells that shape the quality of the adaptive immune response to a microbe. It is likely that parallel mechanisms account for the induction of immune responses to self-antigens, although genetic and other host factors must be important in setting a threshold for lymphocyte activation that favors an immune response to stimulation by self-antigens in a lupus-susceptible individual. In both innate and adaptive immune responses to foreign antigens and self-antigens, the antigens determine the specificity of the response but cytokines determine the quality of the response. The isotype of antibodies produced and the extent of amplification of an inflammatory response by chemokines and cells are determined by the particular cytokines generated.

CYTOKINES OF THE INNATE IMMUNE RESPONSE

The innate immune system functions in the initial recognition of pathogens, and cytokine production is critical in sounding the alarm. Cells of the innate immune system—macrophages, neutrophils, and dendritic cells (DCs)—are among the first cells to encounter pathogens in the setting of infection and are likely to be early players in the lupus autoimmune response. Initial responses by these cell types trigger the production of cytokines and chemotactic factors, resulting in the migration of cells into the area and the subsequent activation

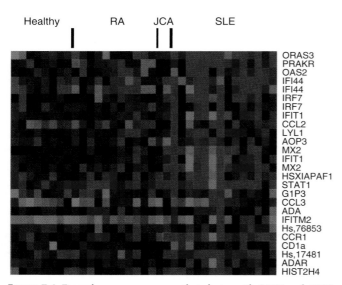

Healthy   RA   JCA   SLE

ORAS3
PRAKR
OAS2
IFI44
IFI44
IRF7
IRF7
IFIT1
CCL2
LYL1
AOP3
MX2
IFIT1
MX2
HSXIAPAF1
STAT1
G1P3
CCL3
ADA
IFITM2
Hs.76853
CCR1
CD1a
Hs.17481
ADAR
HIST2H4

FIGURE 7-1 Exemplary gene sequences that cluster with *PRKR* and *OAS3*. Hierarchical clustering was performed on the total study population to determine genes that cluster with *PRKR* and *OAS3*. A visual demonstration of the expression of a selection from those genes, comprising a partial IFN signature, is shown. Data are shown from a subset of samples from patients with SLE tested (*n* = 14), with rheumatoid arthritis (RA) (*n* = 11), and with juvenile, chronic arthritis (JCA) (*n* = 2) and control samples (*n* = 8). Relative expression compared with an internal control ranged from approximately −0.5 (*bright green*) to 0.5 (*bright red*). (*From Crow MK, Wohlgemuth J: Microarray analysis of gene expression in lupus. Arthritis Res Ther 5:279–287, 2003.*)

of APCs, T cells, and B cells. Microbial pattern recognition receptors are a group of receptors that allow for detection of conserved microbial epitopes, and activation of these receptors represents an important first warning system against pathogens. One such system is the TLR family of pattern recognition receptors. TLRs are found in the cell membrane and in the endosomal compartment. Different TLRs recognize different canonical microbe-associated patterns, including lipopolysaccharide (TLR4), ssRNA (TLR3), dsRNA (TLRs 7, 8), and demethylated DNA (TLR9). The endosomal TLRs 7 and 9, which sense nucleic acid, are involved in defense against viruses and induce type I IFN upon ligation. In addition to the membrane-bound TLRs, there are cytosolic pattern recognition receptors. The RIG-I (retinoic acid–inducible gene 1) and MDA5 (melanoma differentiation–associated protein 5) receptors can recognize nucleic acids in the cytosol, and they induce cytokine production upon ligation.

Later studies support a contribution of signals through TLRs to the activation of the innate immune response in lupus.[14-19] Among the documented triggers relevant to SLE are immune complexes containing DNA or RNA, along with specific antibodies.[16-19] A consequence of TLR ligation is production of type I IFN, predominantly IFN-α, which then mediates numerous functional effects on immune system cells. Plasmacytoid dendritic cells (PDCs), a rare cell type that is enriched in skin lesions of lupus patients, are presumed to be active producers of IFN-α.[20-24] Interaction of IFN with widely expressed cell surface receptors activates intracellular signaling pathways and induction of transcription of a large number of IFN-responsive genes, including those associated with maturation of myeloid dendritic cells. The result is predicted to be increased APC function and augmented capacity to trigger self-reactive T cells.[25]

In addition to plasmacytoid and myeloid dendritic cells, mononuclear phagocytes are essential for the inactivation of pathogenic infectious organisms and for the clearance of potentially pathogenic immune complexes and senescent or apoptotic cells. These cells are also important in SLE. Impaired clearance of apoptotic cells has been demonstrated in some studies of patients with SLE, and IFN-mediated maturation of monocytes into effective APCs has been shown in another study.[25,26] Macrophages bind, process, and present antigenic peptides to T cells; they physically interact with T cells, delivering secondary activation signals through cell surface adhesion and co-stimulatory molecules; and they secrete a panoply of soluble products, including tumor necrosis factor (TNF), interleukin-1 (IL-1), IL-6, IL-10, IL-12, and B-lymphocyte stimulator (BLyS), that provide important accessory and regulatory signals to both T and B cells. The roles of these products of innate immune system cells are highlighted here, with a particular emphasis on the type I IFNs.

Type I Interferons

Productive infection of host cells by a virus, leading to synthesis of RNA or DNA molecules of viral origin, induces production of host proteins, including the IFNs. The function of these proteins is to inhibit viral replication and to modulate the immune response to the virus, with the aim of controlling infection. The type I IFN locus on chromosome 9p21 comprises genes encoding 13 IFN-α subtypes as well as IFN-β, IFN-ω, IFN-κ, and IFN-ε, the last mostly restricted to trophoblast cells and produced early in pregnancy.[27,28] The IFN-α gene complex is likely to have been generated by repeated gene duplications and recombinations. Although the need for and function of each of the IFN-α genes are not clear, specific virus infections are associated with induction of one or another IFN-α.[29,30] Data have now identified additional IFNs that are encoded by a gene family related to the classic type I IFNs.[31,32] IFN-λs (IL-28 and IL-29) have only moderate sequence similarity to IFN-α, bind to a distinct receptor, yet induce genes similar to those induced by IFN-α. The relative functional roles of IFN-λ and the chromosome 9p–encoded IFNs are under study.[33]

IFNα can probably be produced by all leukocytes, but PDCs are the most active producers. Rapid progress in study of type I IFN regulation indicates that cell type (PDC vs. fibroblast), stimulus (dsRNA, ssRNA, DNA), and signaling pathway used (TLR3 vs. TLR7/8 vs. TLR9) all contribute to determining the specific IFN isoforms that are produced.[33-45] The TLR family of innate immune system receptors and their downstream signaling components play a central role in mediating activation of type I IFN gene transcription (Figure 7-2). TLRs 7, 8, and 9 signal through the MyD88 adaptor.

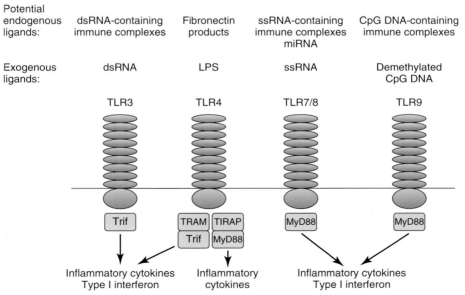

FIGURE 7-2 Induction of the type I interferon pathway through Toll-like receptors (TLRs). Both exogenous and endogenous stimuli can induce TLR activation, resulting in new gene transcription. Among potential endogenous ligands are immune complexes containing DNA or RNA or matrix-derived components. TLR ligands trigger activation of intracellular adaptors—including Trif (TIR [Toll/interleukin-1 receptor] domain–containing adapter inducing IFN-β), TRAM (Trif-related adaptor molecule), TIRAP, TIR-domain-containing adapter protein; or MyD88 (myeloid differentiation primary response protein 88)—and induce transcription of type I interferons or inflammatory cytokines. dsDNA, double-stranded DNA; LPS, lipopolysaccharide; ssDNA, single-stranded DNA.

IFN regulatory factors and additional transcription factors, including nuclear factor kappa B (NF-κB) and activating transcription factor 2 (ATF2), bind to and activate an IFN-stimulated response element (ISRE) present in the IFN-α and IFN-β gene promoters.[35-37] Tracking the specific intracellular factors that mediate transcription of specific IFN isoforms may provide clues to the innate immune system receptors and the relevant triggers that drive production of those IFNs.

Type I IFN production represents the first line of defense in response to viral infection. Following invasion of the host by a virus, IFN-α is secreted by PDCs, along with other immune system cells, and binds its receptor on many target cells, resulting in engagement of intracellular signaling molecules and induction of a gene transcription program.[46] The IFNs were used as model cytokines when Darnell's group defined the requirements for cytokine-mediated signal transduction.[47-49] Binding of IFN-α to its cell surface receptor was shown to activate Jak1 and then STAT1. Subsequently, it was shown that Tyk2, also a Jak kinase, is constitutively associated with the α subunit of the type I IFN receptor (IFNAR), whereas Jak1 is associated with the β subunit of the receptor. Cytokine binding leads to activation of Tyk2 and Jak1 and phosphorylation of the α receptor subunit and part of the β subunit. Subsequent events include activation of STATs 1, 2, and 3, the insulin receptor substrate proteins 1 and 2 (IRS1 and IRS2), and *vav* (a protein in guanine nucleotide exchange factor of cell signaling).[50] STAT1-to-STAT1 and STAT1-to-STAT2 dimers bind to the pIRE element and ISGF3 (interferon-stimulated gene factor 3), including STAT1 and STAT2, and a third protein, p48, binds the IFN-stimulated response element.[35,48] The Jak-STAT pathway seems to be sufficient to mediate the antiviral effect of IFN-α, whereas the IRS proteins, as well as other undefined factors, are also required for the antiproliferative effect of IFN-α.[50]

Activation of the type I IFN pathway has diverse and numerous functional effects on immune system cells. IFN-α matures DCs by inducing expression of intercellular adhesion molecule 1 (ICAM-1), CD86, MHC class I molecules, and IL-12p70, and promotes expression of some T-cell activation molecules.[51-53] However, IFN-α has antiproliferative effects on T cells, and it is generally described as a suppressor of T-cell immune activity. IFN-α inhibits expression of some proinflammatory cytokines, including IL-8, IL-1, and granulocyte-monocyte colony-stimulating factor (GM-CSF), and it preferentially promotes T helper 1 cell responses by decreasing IL-4 and increasing IFN-γ secretion.[54,55] In the setting of coculture of monocytes with lipopolysaccharide (LPS) or CD4⁺ T cells with anti-CD3 and anti-CD28 monoclonal antibodies, IFN-α augments IL-10 production.[54,56] IFN-γ does not have these effects and in fact inhibits IL-10 production. Although IL-10 has important suppressive effects on T-cell proliferative responses, its capacity to promote B-cell proliferation and immunoglobulin class switching suggests that IFN-α may favor antibody production.[57-63] Finally, IFN-α leads to increased natural killer (NK) and T-cell–mediated cytotoxicity.[64-66] This effect on cytotoxic T lymphocyte (CTL) function has been exploited in the treatment of several malignancies with IFN-α in order to augment tumor lysis, although the mechanism that accounts for the increased killing has not been elucidated fully. At least one such mechanism is the induction of FasL expression on natural killer (NK) cells and increased Fas-mediated apoptosis.[66] IFN-α can also promote an inflammatory response. Among IFN-α–inducible gene targets are several chemokines, soluble mediators that attract lymphocytes and inflammatory cells to tissues. In brief summary, IFN-α helps initiate an adaptive immune response that results in increases in cytotoxic T- and NK-cell activity, Fas-mediated apoptosis, and antibody production and inflammation but decreased T-cell proliferation. Many of these immune system effects are reminiscent of those observed in patients with SLE (Figure 7-3).

Several sets of compelling data suggest an important pathogenic role for IFNs in SLE. Papers published as early as 1979 described increased serum levels of IFN in patients with SLE, particularly those with active disease.[67-71] At that time, the distinct type I and type II IFNs had not yet been documented, but within several years IFN-α

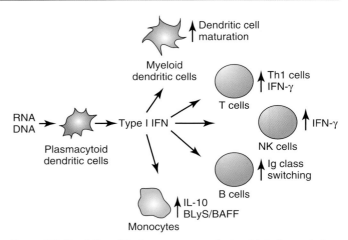

FIGURE 7-3 Regulation of the immune response by type I interferons. Activation of plasmacytoid dendritic cells through Toll-like receptors, perhaps triggered by endogenous DNA or RNA, results in production of type I interferon (IFN). Actions of type I IFN on the immune system include dendritic cell maturation; increased T helper 1 (Th1) cell production, particularly IFN-γ; activation and IFN-γ production by natural killer (NK) cells; augmented immunoglobulin (Ig) class switching by B cells; and increased interleukin-10 (IL-10) and BLyS/BAFF (B-lymphocyte stimulator/B-cell–activating factor) expression by monocytes. Many of these functions are among the features of the altered immune system that have been described in SLE.

was cloned, and it became clear that IFN-α was present in particularly high levels in SLE blood. Soon after, it was observed that tubuloreticular-like structures in the renal endothelial cells of patients with SLE and in murine lupus models were associated with IFN-α and that in vitro culture of cell line cells with IFN-α-induced similar intracellular structures.[72] These observations suggested not only that IFN-α was increased in concentration in SLE blood but also that it might have a functional impact on cells and perhaps contribute to disease. Another key observation was first reported in 1990 and has been noted many times subsequently. Therapeutic administration of IFN-α to patients with viral infection or malignancy occasionally results in induction of typical lupus autoantibodies and, in some cases, clinical lupus.[73-77] This demonstration of induction by IFN-α of SLE in some individuals indicated that given the appropriate genetic background and perhaps in the setting of concurrent stimuli, SLE could be induced by IFN-α. Twenty percent to 80% of patients treated with IFN-α have been noted to demonstrate autoantibodies specific for thyroid or nuclear antigens, including anti-DNA autoantibodies.[78] Clinically apparent disorders include autoimmune thyroiditis, inflammatory arthritis, and SLE. Hints regarding possible mechanisms of these IFN-α toxicities come from an animal model of autoimmune diabetes.[79] Expression of IFN-α by pancreatic islets correlates with development of type I diabetes, and transgenic mice overexpressing IFN-α acquire diabetes. These mice develop autoreactive CD4⁺ T cells that are Th1 and can kill islet cells. Blanco showed that IFN-α is one component in lupus serum that can promote maturation of blood monocytes to have increased antigen-presenting activity.[25] These data are consistent with the demonstration that IFN-α is one of several maturation factors for immature DCs, permitting efficient antigen-presenting function to T cells.[80,81] Generation by IFN-α of an APC functional phenotype competent for activation of autoantigen-specific T cells could be an important immune mechanism that incorporates many of these findings.[82] Murine studies have supported a role for type I IFN in SLE. Both NZB lupus mice and B6/lpr mice deficient in the IFN-α/β receptor show significant improvement in some manifestations of autoimmunity as well as improvement in clinical disease, and type I IFN promotes development of glomerular crescents and accelerated disease in lupus mice.[83-86]

In the early 1990s, the major cellular source of IFN-α had not yet been identified, but Ronnblom's group were able to demonstrate that immune complexes containing lupus autoantibodies and cellular material could induce production of IFN-α by peripheral blood mononuclear cells in vitro.[14,20,21,87,88] With the assignment of PDCs as the major source of IFN-α, lupus immune complexes were shown to be active inducers of IFN-α by those cells, and additional data implicate TLR7, TLR9, and the receptor FcγRIIa in the induction of IFN-α by some of those complexes.[18-20] Immune complexes containing RNA are particularly effective inducers of type I IFN, presumably through TLR7. Additionally, later data have implicated DNA-containing material derived from neutrophils, referred to as *neutrophil extracellular traps* (NETs), as stimuli for production of IFN by PDCs.[89,90] TLR9 is likely to be the receptor that interacts with those complexes and triggers new gene transcription. A similar scenario has been demonstrated, in a collaboration between two laboratories, in another system relevant to rheumatic diseases, the activation of rheumatoid factor–producing B cells by DNA enriched in CpG immunostimulatory sequences opsonized with anti-DNA antibody.[15,16] PDCs appear to be somewhat reduced in the blood, but they have been demonstrated in the skin lesions of patients with lupus.[24] It is possible, or likely, that the IFN-α–producing cells have also been recruited to other sites of active disease, including lymph nodes and kidney. Monoclonal antibody to BDCA-2, a cell surface C-type lectin that may contribute to internalization of immune complexes, has been used to identify PDCs.[91]

Several previous reports documented increased expression of IFN-α–induced genes in SLE, including dsRNA-dependent protein kinase (PRKR) and oligoadenylate synthase (OAS), as well as the protein Mx1, present in lupus-involved skin,[92-94] and microarray studies have reproducibly demonstrated that in SLE, IFN-induced genes are the most significantly overexpressed of all those assayed on the microarray.[8-12] The type I IFN-inducible gene transcripts are coordinately expressed in lupus peripheral blood, providing strong support for one or more type I IFNs, or a virus-like trigger, as upstream inducers of this gene expression pattern.[95] High expression of IFN-inducible genes is seen in approximately 40% to 60% of adult patients with SLE and in a higher proportion of pediatric patients with lupus.[10] Adult patients with the IFN signature are characterized by autoantibodies to RNA-binding proteins (Ro, La, Sm, and RNP), higher disease activity, and frequent renal involvement.[96] Additionally, younger patients with SLE have higher serum levels of IFN-α,[97] and patients of African-American and Hispanic-American ancestry have higher serum IFN-α levels on average than European-ancestry patients with SLE.[98] Expression of IFN-α or IFN-inducible gene transcripts or proteins in involved tissue supports the hypothesis that IFN-α contributes to disease pathogenesis in lupus. Of particular interest is the strong IFN gene expression signature observed in SLE synovial tissue in comparison with the pattern seen in rheumatoid arthritis tissue.[99]

A number of the genetic loci associated with risk of SLE are in or near genes that function in the type I IFN pathway, including *IRF5*, *IRF7,* and *STAT4*,[5,100] suggesting that genetic variability among individuals in production and signaling of IFN underlie SLE susceptibility. In fact, a heritable tendency toward high circulating levels of IFN-α has been demonstrated in families with SLE, supporting the idea that genetically determined differences in type I IFN production predispose to SLE.[101] Some of the well-established SLE risk genes have been shown to correlate with either higher circulating levels of IFN-α or with increased sensitivity to IFN-α in patients with SLE. For example, in those patients who have autoantibodies that can form immune complexes that trigger the TLR system, the SLE-associated polymorphisms of *IRF5*[102] and *IRF7*[103] result in higher circulating IFN-α levels. These data support the concept that these polymorphisms are gain-of-function in humans, resulting in greater output of IFN-α from the endosomal TLR pathway when this pathway is chronically stimulated by endogenous immune complexes. Other SLE-associated polymorphisms have been associated with a greater sensitivity to IFN signaling in patients with SLE,[104,105] resulting in a greater amount of IFN-induced gene expression for a given amount of IFN-α signaling. It is likely that combinations of these relatively common SLE-associated polymorphisms that increase IFN-α production or enhance cellular sensitivity to IFN-α would act in concert in many patients, contributing to the marked IFN pathway dysregulation observed in many patients with SLE. Rare genetic variations resulting in familial lupus may also result in IFN pathway dysregulation. Rare variants in the *TREX1* gene have been associated with familial chilblain lupus and SLE.[106-108] TREX1 is a nuclease, and the rare variations that are associated with disease are loss-of-function and are thought to result in decreased clearance of nucleic acid. This reduction could lead to activation of the type I IFN pathway via the cytoplasmic nucleic acid receptors or the TLR system, and in fact, the TREX1 deficiency syndromes are characterized by high IFN.[109] Given all of the described observations, there is strong support for the hypothesis that inhibition of the type I IFN pathway may benefit patients with lupus, particularly those with increased expression of IFN-inducible genes. However, IFN pathway blockade might weaken the innate and adaptive immune responses to viral infection. Potential approaches to inhibition of the type I IFN pathway could include antibodies specific for the IFN-α receptor or for one or more of the various IFN subtypes noted previously. Other approaches are inhibition of upstream (e.g., TLR pathways) or downstream (e.g., Jaks or STATs) signaling molecules.[110] Clinical trials of monoclonal antibodies to IFN-α are currently under way, and initial reports from early-phase studies show inhibition of the IFN signature in skin and blood and some effect on disease activity.[111,112]

Tumor Necrosis Factor

Tumor necrosis factor, the prototype member of the TNF family, is expressed as a trimer on the cell surface and in soluble form after activation of innate immune system cells, including macrophages and DCs, through TLRs, Fc receptors, and receptors for other cytokines. Like type I IFN, TNF is produced early during immune responses to microbes and is particularly effective in promoting influx of inflammatory cells into sites of microbial invasion and in stimulating granuloma formation. The important role of TNF in controlling microbial infections is demonstrated by the reactivation of *Mycobacterium tuberculosis* that can occur in the setting of TNF blockade.

The role of TNF as a central upstream inducer of inflammation has been clearly shown in rheumatoid arthritis, on the basis of in vitro studies and the impressive clinical response experienced by some patients treated with TNF inhibitors. The importance of TNF in lupus is still being debated. In murine lupus models, it has been described as both protective and harmful, depending on the mouse strain and stage of disease development.[113-116] In patients with SLE, data are variable, but at least some studies show high levels of TNF in sera and kidneys of such patients.[117-121] The observation that anti-TNF agents can sometimes induce anti-dsDNA antibodies and occasionally clinical lupus raises interesting questions about the mechanisms by which reducing TNF might promote autoimmunity as well as concern about TNF inhibitor treatment of patients with SLE.[122-124] Nevertheless, a report of 13 patients treated with infliximab indicated improvement in lupus nephritis, arthritis, and lung involvement after four infusions plus azathioprine, but 2 patients treated with a longer course had life-threatening complications (central nervous system lymphoma and *Legionella* pneumonia).[125,126]

A potential mechanistic relationship between TNF and type I IFN has been suggested, with some experimental support.[127] In some in vitro and in vivo settings, TNF can inhibit synthesis of type I IFN, and vice versa.[128,129] It is possible that when availability of TNF is reduced by anti-TNF agents, negative regulation of IFN production is abrogated, allowing increased activation of the type I IFN pathway and augmented immune system capacity to develop autoimmunity. An alternative mechanism is the induction of increased self-antigen, because serum nucleosome levels are increased by treatment with infliximab.[130]

Osteopontin

Osteopontin (OPN, also called secreted phosphoprotein 1) is a secreted protein with a variety of functions, including immunologic functions such as T-cell activation, Th1 differentiation, B-cell activation,[131] and macrophage activation and chemotaxis,[132] as well as roles in wound healing and bone formation and remodeling.[133] Studies have demonstrated high levels of OPN in biopsy specimens from inflamed tissues in SLE and other autoimmune diseases,[134] and variants of the *OPN* gene have been associated with SLE susceptibility.[135,136] In murine models, OPN is essential for IFN-α production downstream of the endosomal TLR-9 in PDCs, likely via interaction with the MyD88 adaptor protein.[137] In patients with SLE, OPN levels are high in serum in many patients and correlate with serum IFN-α levels.[138] Additionally, genetic variations in the *OPN* gene associated with SLE susceptibility are associated with higher levels of OPN in patients with SLE.[138] These genetic and serum protein measurement studies of OPN in patients with SLE suggest gender- and age-related effects[136,138] that are not well understood but are of interest given the particular age- and gender-related patterns in SLE incidence.

Interleukin-1

IL-1 and its physiologic inhibitor IL-1 receptor antagonist (IL-1ra) are produced by monocytes and macrophages in the early stages of an immune response and are also demonstrated at local sites of inflammation. High serum IL-1 levels have been associated with active SLE and correlate with serum C-reactive protein levels.[139] Interestingly, low serum IL-1ra levels correlated with renal flares.[139] Only limited clinical experience is available for therapy with recombinant IL-1ra in SLE. In one study of three patients, arthritic symptoms but not myositis improved.[140] Moreover, in another study of four patients with SLE and arthritis, IL-1ra therapy resulted in improvement in all.[141] However, two experienced relapse despite continued therapy. At this time, there is neither strong rational nor experimental support for a central role for IL-1 in SLE.

Interleukin-10

IL-10, a pleiotropic cytokine produced by monocytes and lymphocytes, is considered to have antiinflammatory effects in that it inhibits activation of APCs, reduces expression of co-stimulatory molecules on their cell surfaces, thereby blunting T-cell activation, and inhibits TNF production. However its functional effects are complex, because when it binds to activated monocytes, as may occur in autoimmune disease, IL-10 may not effectively generate intracellular signals. For example, in the presence of IFN-α, it can mediate proinflammatory effects on target monocytes.[142] Additionally, IL-10 augments B-cell proliferation and immunoglobulin class switching, resulting in greater secretion of antibodies with the capacity to enter extravascular compartments and promote inflammation and disease in SLE.[143]

Immune complexes, present at increased levels in many patients with SLE, can stimulate production of IL-10 after binding to FcγRII (CD32).[144] Indeed, IL-10 levels are increased in the serum of patients with active lupus.[145] Increased IL-10 has also been associated with greater activation-induced apoptosis of SLE T cells, an effect reduced by anti–IL-10 antibodies.[146] Increased burden of apoptotic cells could potentially contribute to a higher load of self-antigens that are ultimately targeted by autoantibodies.

When the diverse activities of IL-10 are considered in a host with an otherwise activated immune system, its overall effects may contribute to disease, on the basis of its less efficacious inhibition of activated, compared with unstimulated, monocytes and its positive actions on B cells.[143,144]

Interestingly, a previous study has demonstrated increased IL-10 production in patients with SLE from multiple-case families, possibly suggesting that increased IL-10 is involved in SLE pathogenesis.[147] In this study, unaffected spouses of the patients with SLE also showed higher IL-10 production than healthy controls, and thus, environmental factors were suggested as a potential cause of the observed increase in IL-10. In animal models of lupus there is evidence that

therapy with anti–IL-10 monoclonal antibodies, or IL-10 itself, might be beneficial.[148] In humans, treatment of six patients with SLE with a murine anti–IL-10 monoclonal antibody resulted in significant improvement in cutaneous lesions, joint symptoms, and the SLE Disease Activity Index (SLEDAI), even 6 months after the 21-day therapy.[149] Although this study showed benefit, additional studies with humanized reagents would be needed to assess the value of this therapy in SLE.

B-Lymphocyte Stimulator (BLyS)

B-lymphocyte stimulator (also called B-cell–activating factor [BAFF]) and a related molecule, "a proliferation inducing ligand" (APRIL), belong to the TNF ligand superfamily, and like TNF, they can exist in a soluble trimeric form.[150] These molecules are produced by myeloid lineage cells and act exclusively on B cells through several receptors, transmembrane activator and CAML (calcium-modulating cyclophilin ligand) interactor (TACI), BAFF receptor, and less so through B-cell maturation factor (BCMA), to induce B-cell maturation and survival.[150] BLyS supports survival of transitional and mature B cells and also supports immunoglobulin class switching to mature immunoglobulin isotypes, although with less activity than that provided by CD40 ligation.[151] In mice, BLyS is overexpressed in NZB × NZW F1 and MRL/lpr lupus mice, and BlyS inhibition ameliorates disease.[152] Patients with SLE express high levels of BLyS as well.[153,154] BlyS levels are correlated with IFN-α, are higher in African-American patients with SLE than in European-American patients with SLE, and BlyS levels are correlated with measures of SLE disease activity.[155] In a phase III study, LymphoStat-B (now known as belimumab, a humanized monoclonal antibody to BLyS) was well tolerated and showed clinical effects that met the primary end point[156]; and the 2011 approval by the U.S. Food and Drug Administration (FDA) of belimumab for the treatment of SLE marks the first new drug approved for the treatment of SLE in more than 50 years. Treatment with belimumab resulted in decreases in B-cell populations and a reduction in serologic disease activity.[157] Not all patients showed response to belimumab, and the degree of response to treatment was variable, as is the case with other SLE treatments. The successful development and phase 3 trial of belimumab represents a landmark in the development of cytokine inhibitors for the treatment of SLE. Atacicept, a soluble form of the TACI receptor that inhibits both BLyS and APRIL, provides an alternative approach to B-cell inhibition.

Interleukin-6

IL-6 is a pleiotropic cytokine secreted mainly by monocytes, fibroblasts, endothelial cells, and also B cells and T cells. It is induced by inflammatory signals (such as LPS) and cytokines (such as TNF and IL-1), as well as by anti-dsDNA antibodies.[158] Among the many properties of IL-6 is its ability to activate and mediate terminal differentiation of B cells to secrete immunoglobulin, as well as to induce synthesis of acute-phase proteins, including C-reactive protein.[159] Interestingly, although IL-6 is primarily thought of as a proinflammatory cytokine, it can inhibit TNF and IL-1 synthesis. With regard to kidney function, IL-6 can induce mesangial cell proliferation.

IL-6 has been implicated in lupus, both in animal models and in human disease.[159] Blockade of IL-6 ameliorates murine lupus and inhibits anti-dsDNA production.[160,161] Moreover, IL-6 has been noted to be present at increased levels in SLE sera and has been associated with active disease in some but not all studies.[162,163] Indeed, in one large cross-sectional study, IL-6 levels were associated only with hematologic disease activity (mainly reflected in an inverse correlation with hemoglobin levels) but not with any other organ disease activity, as measured by the British Isles Lupus Assessment Group (BILAG) index.[164] High levels of IL-6 have also been noted in the urine of active nephritis patients.

Inhibition of IL-6 by a humanized monoclonal antibody to IL-6 receptor (IL-6R) has been effective in rheumatoid arthritis and juvenile idiopathic arthritis, and this therapy is an FDA-approved treatment for rheumatoid arthritis.[165] The antibody, called tocilizumab, was tolerated well, but significant hypercholesterolemia and serious infections were significant reported adverse events. Tocilizumab binds soluble and membrane-bound IL-6R, blocking its binding to IL-6 and thereby inhibiting IL-6–mediated signaling. Signaling by other IL-6–like cytokines, such as IL-11, is spared.[166] In summary, there is some evidence that anti–IL-6 therapy could decrease anti-dsDNA levels and ameliorate disease activity, including renal disease, in patients with SLE. Results of a phase 1 trial of tocilizumab in SLE have been published in which safety appeared tolerable,[167] and we await further trial data regarding the efficacy of this agent in SLE.

Other Cytokines

In addition to the cytokine products of the innate immune response discussed previously, IL-12, IL-18, and IL-8 have also been found to be high in sera of patients with active SLE.[168-170] Both IL-12 and IL-18 are produced by activated macrophages and can promote the differentiation of IFN-γ–secreting T cells and NK cells. Inhibition of IL-18 in MRL/lpr lupus mice reduced renal damage and mortality, suggesting that the cytokine plays a pathogenic role in that model.[171] IL-8 is a chemokine with potent chemoattractant activity. IL-8, along with the chemokines IP-10 (IFN-γ–induced protein 10), MIG (monokine induced by gamma interferon), MCP-1 (monocyte chemotactic protein 1), and fractalkine, have been observed at high levels in SLE sera and are candidate markers of increased disease activity.[168,172] Although some of them may be attractive candidates to therapeutically target in patients with active end-organ disease, such as nephritis, there is as yet no significant clinical experience with inhibitors of those mediators in patients with lupus.

CYTOKINES OF THE ADAPTIVE IMMUNE RESPONSE

SLE is characterized by production of autoantibodies, and abundant data indicate that those autoantibodies both are antigen driven and depend on T-cell help. The T-cell–derived signals that drive B-cell expansion and immunoglobulin class switching to produce the potentially pathogenic isotypes immunoglobulin G (IgG) and IgA are those delivered by cell contact, such as signals mediated by the CD154 (CD40 ligand)/CD40 pathway as well as signals delivered by T-cell–derived cytokines.[173] The degree of activation of T cells and the effector pathways to which T-cell differentiation is directed depend on many factors, including the avidity of the interaction between antigenic peptide–MHC antigen and the T-cell antigen receptor, the level of expression of co-stimulatory ligands and receptors on APCs and T cells, and the cytokines produced by those APCs. Inherent features of T cells, including structure and expression of cell surface molecules, intracytoplasmic T-cell signaling pathways, and transcription factors, show variability among individuals based on genetic polymorphisms. These differences can contribute to variable T-cell function, including cytokine production. The nature of the cytokines produced by T cells has an important impact on the character of the B-cell immune response, particularly with regard to selection of immunoglobulin isotypes, and on induction or control of inflammation, through effects on mononuclear phagocyte Fc receptor expression, phagocytic activity, and production of effector cytokines.

Cytokines Generated in the Adaptive Immune Response: T-Cell–Derived Cytokines
The Th1/Th2 Paradigm

The concept that T lymphocytes differentiate along one of two possible vectors, termed T helper 1 (Th1) and T helper 2 (Th2), was presented by Mossman.[174] Each of these T-cell types was characterized by production of distinct cytokines (IL-2 and IFN-γ for Th1 and interleukins 4, 5, 6, 9, 10, and 13 for Th2). Subsequent studies elucidated some of the determinants of differentiation along one or the other pathway, including cytokines to which T cells were exposed (IL-12 supporting Th1 and IL-4 supporting Th2 development) and transcription factors expressed in the T cell (T-box expressed in T cells [T-bet] in Th1 cells and GATA3 in Th2 cells).[175-177] The two T-cell types have been generally associated with distinct functions, Th1 cells being viewed as promoting cell-mediated immunity and inflammation by supporting T-cell expansion and monocyte activation and Th2 considered to support humoral immunity, including immunoglobulin class switching to produce some IgG subclasses as well as IgE.

The classic Th1/Th2 paradigm might suggest that Th2 cytokines would predominate in SLE, because Th2 cytokines are thought to drive B-cell differentiation and production of pathologically significant autoantibodies is a central feature of lupus, but in fact, the cytokine picture in SLE is complex.[178] In murine lupus models, the IgG subclasses that make up a substantial proportion of the autoantibodies that are found in serum are IgG2a, a subclass supported by the Th1 cytokine IFN-γ.[179] Moreover, IFN-γ–deficient lupus mice are protected from nephritis, suggesting an important role for that cytokine in end-organ inflammation and tissue damage.[180] On the other hand, IL-10, a product of Th2 cells, is elevated in SLE as discussed. Careful measurement of T-cell, monocyte, and DC-derived cytokines, as well as definition of the cells that produce those cytokines, will be important for more complete characterization of the pathogenic mechanisms that contribute to disease in SLE and other autoimmune syndromes.

Interleukin-2

IL-2, a classic Th1 cytokine, is produced by T cells after activation through the T-cell antigen receptor and the co-stimulatory molecule CD28. The regulation of IL-2 occurs through activation of signaling pathways and transcription factors that act on the IL-2 promoter to generate new gene transcription, but also involves modulation of the stability of IL-2 mRNA. IL-2 binds to a multichain receptor, including a highly regulated α chain and β and γ chains that mediate signaling through the Jak-STAT pathway. IL-2 delivers activation, growth, and differentiation signals to T cells, B cells, and NK cells. IL-2 is also important in mediating activation-induced cell death of T cells, a function that provides an essential mechanism for terminating immune responses. Perhaps because IL-2 was among the first cytokines to be studied in detail by immunologists investigating basic mechanisms of T-cell and general immune function, the level of expression and functional role of IL-2 in the cellular alterations that characterize SLE were the focus of numerous studies over the past 25 years.

In general, the consistent observations were that IL-2 production by T cells stimulated in vitro was low in SLE.[181] However, among studies in which the process was studied in vivo, there are some reports of increased serum IL-2 protein and IL-2 mRNA transcripts in unstimulated SLE peripheral blood cells.[182] Regarding IL-2 receptors, in vitro studies have indicated impaired induction under conditions of cell activation, but serum levels of soluble IL-2 receptor are increased in patients with active disease.[183] T-regulator (Treg) cells are highly dependent on IL-2 for survival, and it is possible that the lower levels of IL-2 observed in SLE could relate to a quantitative or qualitative defect in Treg function.[184] Additionally, one study has implicated a genetic variation in *PPP2CA* that results in increased expression of PP2Ac, which should lead to decreased IL-2 production.[185] This genetic variation was associated with SLE susceptibility, suggesting that primary IL-2 pathway abnormalities are associated with risk of SLE. At this time there is no strong support for therapeutically manipulating the IL-2 pathway in SLE.

Interferon-γ

IFN-γ is the sole type II IFN. Early in an immune response, IFN-γ is mainly generated by NK cells, and once the adaptive immune response is engaged, it is a major product of Th1 cells activated by APCs that produce IL-12 or IL-18. IFN-γ implements a broad spectrum of effects on immune responses, including activation of monocytes, and when produced in excess can promote tissue injury.[186] Among its activities are the induction of other proinflammatory cytokines such as TNF and induction of apoptosis in renal parenchymal cells. The relationship between IFN- and IFN-γ is complex.[187] IFN-α inhibits the induction of IFN-γ by NK cells in the presence of STAT1. In contrast, in the absence of STAT1, IFN-α can stimulate production of IFN-γ by T cells. Like IFN-α, IFN-γ signals cell activation through STAT1 but can also utilize a poorly defined STAT1-independent pathway.[188]

The role of IFN-γ in the pathogenesis of SLE has been best illustrated in studies of murine lupus. Experiments using IFN-γ–deficient mice have demonstrated a requirement for IFN-γ in the development of significant nephritis and for expression of IgG2a anti-dsDNA antibodies in MRL/lpr and NZB × NZW F1 mice.[179,180,189,190] However, in pristane-induced lupus, the pristane treatment was sufficient to induce some IgG2a anti-Sm/RNP autoantibody, even in the absence of IFN-γ.[191] Additional approaches supporting a requirement for IFN-γ for most manifestations of lupus include administration of anti–IFN-γ antibody, soluble IFN-γ receptor, and study of IFN-γ receptor–deficient mice. Nephritis appears to be particularly dependent on IFN-γ.[179,190] It is likely that the different murine models will show variable dependence on either type I or type II IFN for the development of autoimmunity and disease, perhaps on the basis of their baseline relative expressions of those cytokines. Although murine studies support important roles for both type I and type II IFN in lupus, support for IFN-γ in human lupus is less well documented. Gene expression studies of peripheral blood cells do not show increased levels of CXCL9 mRNA, a gene product that is highly induced by IFN-γ.[95] However, IFN-γ may be more highly expressed in kidneys of patients with lupus nephritis and could play an important role in augmenting expression of chemokines that contribute to recruitment of inflammatory cells and tissue damage.

Th2 Cytokines in SLE

As previously described, IL-6 and IL-10, typical Th2 cytokines, are increased in the serum of patients with active lupus, but the production of those cytokines is more likely to be attributable to monocytes and B cells than to T cells.[192] IL-4 and IL-5 are additional Th2 cytokines, but the role for these mediators in SLE is less well supported than for others discussed. Increased production of IL-4 has not been consistently demonstrated in SLE.

TGF-β

TGF-β is a pleiotropic and multifunctional cytokine. Although it is produced by many cell types, it is included in the Th2 cytokine family. TGF-β is produced as a latent molecule that is then activated by plasmin-mediated cleavage and release of the biologically active fragment. When TGF-β binds to its receptor, SMAD proteins translocate from cytoplasm to nucleus and promote generation of new mRNAs. TGF-β plays an important role at each stage of an immune response and in the context of wound healing.[193] Early in an immune response, TGF-β promotes activation of innate immune system cells. Once an adaptive immune response is well under way, the cytokine inhibits activation and proliferation of T cells to provide regulation of cellular immunity. Finally, TGF-β is a central mediator of tissue repair.[194]

TGF-β plays an important role in the differentiation and the inhibitory activity of Tregs.[193] Treg function resides in the CD4+CD25+ T-cell population and is associated with production of TGF-β and IL-10 as well as with expression of a transcription factor, FOXP3.[195,196] TGF-β also appears to contribute to induction of Tregs from precursor T cells.

As is the case for other T-cell–derived cytokines, interpretation of data addressing the expression and function of TGF-β in SLE is challenging, particularly in view of the fact that most of the cytokine present in serum is present in the latent form. Most data indicate that production of TGF-β in peripheral blood cells is decreased in SLE, a finding that would be consistent with impaired regulation of T-cell

activation.[197] However, TGF-β may be expressed at sites of inflammation, such as the lupus kidney, and potentially contribute to renal scarring.[198] Intracellular pathways activated by TGF-β are well known to target genes, such as those encoding collagen and fibronectin, that are implicated in tissue fibrosis.

Additional T-Cell–Derived Cytokines

IL-17 is produced by some T cells (the Th17 subset), as well as NK cells and neutrophils, and contributes to inflammatory responses by inducing chemokines and proinflammatory cytokines and by promoting migration of lymphocytes into tissue.[199] A potential role for IL-17 in lupus pathogenesis has not yet been well defined, but there is evidence for increased serum IL-17 in patients with lupus that was associated with skin involvement and serositis.[200] T cells producing IL-17 have been observed in kidney tissue of patients with lupus nephritis, further supporting a potential pathogenic role for that cytokine.[199] An interesting connection between the type I IFN pathway and IL-17 is suggested by data indicating that PDCs activated through TLR7 promote differentiation of CD4+ precursor T cells into Th17 cells.[201] Moreover, expression of IL-17 is correlated with IFN-α expression in lupus skin lesions.[202]

IL-21, a cytokine in the IL-2 family, is synthesized by many T-cell populations, although its production by T follicular helper cells, important in the lymph node germinal center reaction, might be particularly significant for its roles in B-cell activation and differentiation. IL-21 acts along with B-cell receptor ligation and co-stimulatory signals, such as CD40 stimulation and TLR activation, to promote B-cell proliferation and differentiation to plasma cells.[203] IL-21 binds to a heterodimeric receptor on B cells and other target cells and triggers the Jak-STAT signaling pathway. Studies in patients with SLE have shown elevations of IL-21 but decreased expression of its receptor in the setting of lupus nephritis or elevated anti-dsDNA antibodies.[204] Of interest is an association of single-nucleotide polymorphisms in the IL-21 genomic region with SLE and other inflammatory diseases.[205] Although the biology of IL-21 is complex, the available data suggest that it could be an important therapeutic target in SLE.

Cytokines Generated in the Adaptive Immune Response: B-Cell–Derived Cytokines

B-lymphocyte function in SLE is most simply characterized as hyperactive. A high proportion of peripheral blood B cells are activated by morphologic criteria. SLE B cells in vitro proliferate and differentiate to antibody-secreting cells spontaneously, without the addition of traditional mitogens.[197] The spectrum of B cells that secrete antibody in patients with SLE represents a polyclonal assortment, but characteristic of SLE is the selective and high-level secretion of a restricted population of autoantibody specificities, including those reactive with nucleic acids and nucleic acid–associated proteins.

Studies of B lymphocytes have focused on their exclusive role in generating antibody-producing plasma cells, with some additional emphasis on the capacity of activated B cells to effectively present antigen to T cells. Current thinking has expanded the function of B cells to include production of soluble mediators, including cytokines. Most of the products of B cells are not exclusive to those cells, also being expressed by monocytes and T cells. Among those, IL-6 and IL-10 have been discussed. As noted, these cytokines have been demonstrated to be expressed at high levels in patients with active SLE, and both contribute to B-cell expansion and differentiation. Although it is likely that multiple cell types produce these cytokines in lupus, activated B cells may be particularly active in this function.

SUMMARY

The scope of immune system alterations in SLE is so extensive that it has been difficult for investigators to determine which of those altered functions is a primary contributor to lupus pathogenesis. The resurgence of interest in the type I IFN system and documentation of a prominent and broad activation of the IFN pathway in cells of patients with lupus, along with rapid progress in the elucidation of the TLR system, has helped reformulate the view of lupus pathogenesis to include an important role for innate immune system activation, by either exogenous or endogenous adjuvant-like triggers, in generating type I IFN and many of its downstream effects on immune function.[110] As in immune responses to microbes, the adaptive immune system is engaged subsequent to activation of the innate immune system, but in SLE it is focused on self-antigens. Activation of T and B lymphocytes results in production of a diverse complement of cytokines, along with autoantibodies, that contribute to the character of the disease. IFN-γ produced by T cells and NK cells is a potent inducer of chemokines that attract inflammatory cells to involved tissues and organs. IL-21, a product of T follicular helper cells, can contribute to B-cell proliferation and differentiation. BLyS/BAFF, IL-6, and IL-10 are products of the innate immune response but promote survival and differentiation of B cells, amplifying their production of pathogenic autoantibodies. Each of these cytokines represents a rational therapeutic target. The successful development program that resulted in FDA approval of belimumab, a BLyS inhibitor, provides a road map for additional future successes targeting other cytokines in lupus.

References

1. Vilcek J: The cytokines: an overview. In Thompson A, editor: *The cytokine handbook*, ed 3, San Diego, 1998, Academic Press, pp 1–20.
2. O'Shea JJ, Park H, Pesu M, et al: New strategies for immunosuppression: interfering with cytokines by targeting the Jak/Stat pathway. *Curr Opin Rheumatol* 17(3):305–311, 2005.
3. Yoshimur A: Negative regulation of cytokine signaling. *Clin Rev Allergy Immunol* 28(3):205–220, 2005.
4. Ollier WE: Cytokine genes and disease susceptibility. *Cytokine* 28(4–5):174–178, 2004.
5. Crow MK: Collaboration, genetic associations, and lupus erythematosus. *N Engl J Med* 358(9):956–961, 2008.
6. Kariuki SN, Niewold TB: Genetic regulation of serum cytokines in systemic lupus erythematosus. *Transl Res* 155(3):109–117, 2010.
7. Kirou KA, Lee C, Crow MK: Measurement of cytokines in autoimmune disease. *Methods Mol Med* 102:129–154, 2004.
8. Crow MK, Wohlgemuth J: Microarray analysis of gene expression in lupus. *Arthritis Res Ther* 5:279–287, 2003.
9. Baechler EC, Batliwalla FM, Karypis G, et al: Interferon-inducible gene expression signature in peripheral blood cells of patients with severe lupus. *Proc Natl Acad Sci USA* 100:2610–2615, 2003.
10. Bennett L, Palucka AK, Arce E, et al: Interferon and granulopoiesis signatures in systemic lupus erythematosus blood. *J Exp Med* 197:711–723, 2003.
11. Han G-M, Chen S-L, Shen N, et al: Analysis of gene expression profiles in human systemic lupus erythematosus using oligonucleotide microarray. *Genes Immun* 4:177–186, 2003.
12. Crow MK, Kirou KA, Wohlgemuth J: Microarray analysis of interferon-regulated genes in SLE. *Autoimmunity* 36(8):481–490, 2003.
13. Beutler B: The toll-like receptors: analysis by forward genetic methods. *Immunogenetics* 57:385–392, 2005.
14. Magnusson M, Magnusson S, Vallin H, et al: Importance of CpG dinucleotides in activation of natural IFN-alpha-producing cells by a lupus-related oligodeoxynucleotide. *Scand J Immunol* 54:543–550, 2001.
15. Leadbetter EA, Rifkin IR, Hohlbaum AM, et al: Chromatin-IgG complexes activate B cells by dual engagement of IgM and Toll-like receptors. *Nature* 416:603–607, 2002.
16. Viglianti GA, Lau CM, Hanley TM, et al: Activation of autoreactive B cells by CpG dsDNA. *Immunity* 19(6):837–847, 2003.
17. Means TK, Latz E, Hayashi F, et al: Human lupus autoantibody-DNA complexes activate DCs through cooperation of CD32 and TLR9. *J Clin Invest* 115(2):407–417, 2005.
18. Barrat F, Meeker T, Gregorio J, et al: Nucleic acids of mammalian origin can act as endogenous ligands for Toll-like receptors and may promote systemic lupus erythematosus. *J Exp Med* 202(8):1131–1139, 2005.
19. Kelly-Scumpia KM, Nacionales DC, Scumpia PO, et al: In vivo adjuvant activity of the RNA component of the Sm/RNP lupus autoantigen. *Arthritis Rheum* 56(10):3379–3386, 2007.
20. Blomberg S, Eloranta ML, Magnusson M, et al: Expression of the markers BDCA-2 and BDCA-4 and production of interferon-alpha by plasmacytoid dendritic cells in systemic lupus erythematosus. *Arthritis Rheum* 48(9):2524–2532, 2003.
21. Bave U, Vallin H, Alm GV, et al: Activation of natural interferon-alpha producing cells by apoptotic U937 cells combined with lupus IgG and its regulation by cytokines. *J Autoimmun* 17:71–80, 2001.
22. Siegel FP, Kadowaki N, Shodell M, et al: The nature of the principal type I interferon-producing cells in human blood. *Science* 284:1835–1837, 1999.
23. Ronnblom L, Alm GV: A pivotal role for the natural interferon α-producing cells (plasmacytoid dendritic cells) in the pathogenesis of lupus. *J Exp Med* 194:59–63, 2001.
24. Farkas L, Beiske K, Lund-Johansen F, et al: Plasmacytoid dendritic cells (natural interferon-alpha/beta-producing cells) accumulate in cutaneous lupus erythematosus lesions. *Am J Pathol* 159:237–243, 2001.
25. Blanco P, Palucha AK, Gill M, et al: Induction of dendritic cell differentiation by IFN-alpha in systemic lupus erythematosus. *Science* 294:1540–1543, 2001.
26. Herrmann M, Voll RE, Zoller OM, et al: Impaired phagocytosis of apoptotic cell material by monocyte-derived macrophages from patients with systemic lupus erythematosus. *Arthritis Rheum* 41(7):1241–1250, 1998.
27. Fountain JW, Karayiorgou M, Taruscio D, et al: Genetic and physical map of the interferon region on chromosome 9p. *Genomics* 14:105–112, 1992.
28. Martal JL, Chene NM, Huynh LP, et al: IFN-tau: A novel subtype I IFN1. Structural characteristics, non-ubiquitous expression, structure-function relationships, a pregnancy hormonal embryonic signal and cross-species therapeutic potentialities. *Biochimie* 80:755–777, 1998.
29. Lin R, Genin P, Mamane Y, et al: Selective DNA binding and association with the CREB binding protein coactivator contribute to differential activation of alpha interferon genes by interferon regulatory factors 3 and 7. *Mol Cell Biol* 20:6342–6354, 2000.
30. Barnes BJ, Moore PA, Pitha PM: Virus-specific activation of a novel interferon regulatory factor 5, results in the induction of distinct interferon alpha genes. *J Biol Chem* 276:23382–23390, 2001.
31. Kotenko SV, Gallagher G, Baurin VV, et al: IFN-lambdas mediate antiviral protection through a distinct class II cytokine receptor complex. *Nat Immunol* 4:69–77, 2003.
32. Sheppard P, Kindsvogel W, Xu W, et al: IL-28, IL-29 and their class II cytokine receptor IL-28R. *Nat Immunol* 4:63–68, 2003.
33. Coccia EM, Severa M, Giacomini E, et al: Viral infection and Toll-like receptor agonists induce a differential expression of type I and lambda interferons in human plasmacytoid and monocyte-derived dendritic cells. *Eur J Immunol* 34:796–805, 2004.
34. Greenway AL, Hertzog PJ, Devenish RJ, et al: Constitutive and virus-induced interferon production by peripheral blood leukocytes. *Exp Hematol* 23:229–235, 1995.
35. Daly C, Reich NC: Characterization of specific DNA-binding factors activated by double-stranded RNA as positive regulators of interferon alpha/beta-stimulated genes. *J Biol Chem* 279:23739–23746, 1995.
36. Bandyopadhyay SK, Leonard GT, Jr, Bandyopadhyay T, et al: Transcriptional induction by double-stranded RNA is mediated by interferon-stimulated response elements without activation of interferon-stimulated gene factor 3. *J Biol Chem* 270:19624–19629, 1995.
37. Nguyen H, Hiscott J, Pitha PM: The growing family of interferon regulatory factors. *Cytokine Growth Factor Rev* 8:293–312, 1997.
38. Juang Y-T, Lowther W, Kellum M, et al: Primary activation of interferon α and interferon β gene transcription by interferon regulatory factor 3. *Proc Natl Acad Sci USA* 95:9837–9842, 1998.
39. Barnes BJ, Kellum MJ, Field AE, et al: Multiple regulatory domains of IRF-5 control activation, cellular localization, and induction of chemokines that mediate recruitment of T lymphocytes. *Mol Cell Biol* 22(16):5721–5740, 2002.
40. Barnes BJ, Kellum MJ, Pinder KE, et al: Interferon regulatory factor 5, a novel mediator of cell cycle arrest and cell death. *Cancer Res* 63(19):6424–6431, 2003.
41. Barnes BJ, Field AE, Pitha-Rowe PM: Virus-induced heterodimer formation between IRF-5 and IRF-7 modulates assembly of the IFNA enhanceosome in vivo and transcriptional activity of IFNA genes. *J Biol Chem* 278(19):16630–16641, 2003.
42. Kawai T, Sato S, Ishii KJ, et al: Interferon-alpha induction through Toll-like receptors involves a direct interaction of IRF7 with MyD88 and TRAF6. *Nat Immunol* 5(10):1061–1068, 2004.
43. Barnes BJ, Richards J, Mancl M, et al: Global and distinct targets of IRF-5 and IRF-7 during innate response to viral infection. *J Biol Chem* 279(43):45194–45207, 2004.
44. Takaoka A, Yanai H, Kondo S, et al: Integral role of IRF-5 in the gene induction programme activated by Toll-like receptors. *Nature* 434:243–249, 2005.

45. Schoenemeyer A, Barnes BJ, Mancl ME, et al: The interferon regulatory factor, IRF5, is a central mediator of TLR7 signaling. *J Biol Chem* 280:21078–21090, 2005.

46. Belardelli F, Ferrantini M: Cytokines as a link between innate and adaptive antitumor immunity. *Trends Immunol* 23(4):201–208, 2002.

47. Reich NC, Darnell JE, Jr: Differential binding of interferon-induced factors to an oligonucleotide that mediates transcriptional activation. *Nucleic Acids Res* 17:3415–3424, 1989.

48. Veals SA, Schindler C, Leonard D, et al: Subunit of an alpha-interferon-responsive transcription factor is related to interferon regulatory factor and Myb families of DNA-binding proteins. *Mol Cell Biol* 12:3315–3324, 1992.

49. Darnell JE Jr, Kerr IM, Stark GR: Jak-STAT pathways and transcriptional activation in response to IFNs and other extracellular signaling proteins. *Science* 264:1415–1421, 1994.

50. Uddin S, Fish EN, Sher D, et al: The IRS-pathway operates distinctively from the Stat-pathway in hematopoietic cells and transduces common and distinct signals during engagement of the insulin or interferon-α receptors. *Blood* 90:2574–2582, 1997.

51. Luft T, Pang KC, Thomas E, et al: Type I IFNs enhance the terminal differentiation of dendritic cells. *J Immunol* 161:1947–1953, 1998.

52. Radvanyi LG, Banerjee A, Weir M, et al: Low levels of interferon-alpha induce CD86 (B7.2) and accelerate dendritic cell maturation from human peripheral blood mononuclear cells. *Scand J Immunol* 50:499–509, 1999.

53. Kayagaki N, Yamaguchi N, Nakayama M, et al: Type I interferons (IFNs) regulate tumor necrosis factor-related apoptosis-inducing ligand (TRAIL) expression on human T cells: a novel mechanism for the antitumor effects of type I IFNs. *J Exp Med* 189:1451–1460, 1999.

54. Aman MJ, Tretter T, Eisenbeis I, et al: Interferon-alpha stimulates production of interleukin-10 in activated CD4+ T cells and monocytes. *Blood* 87:4731–4736, 1996.

55. Brinkmann V, Geiger T, Alkan S, et al: Interferon alpha increases the frequency of interferon gamma-producing human CD4+ T cells. *J Exp Med* 178:1655–1663, 1993.

56. Hermann P, Rubio M, Nakajima T, et al: IFN-α priming of human monocytes differentially regulates gram-positive and gram-negative bacteria-induced IL-10 release and selectively enhances IL-12p70, CD80, and MHC class I expression. *J Immunol* 161:2011–2018, 1998.

57. Ding L, Shevach EM: IL-10 inhibits mitogen-induced T cell proliferation by selectively inhibiting macrophage costimulatory function. *J Immunol* 148:3133–3139, 1992.

58. Malefyt RDW, Yssel H, de Vries J: Direct effects of IL-10 on subsets of human CD4+ T cell clones and resting T cells. Specific inhibition of IL-2 production and proliferation. *J Immunol* 150:4754–4765, 1993.

59. Taga K, Mostowski H, Tosato G: Human interleukin-10 can directly inhibit T cell growth. *Blood* 81:2964–2971, 1993.

60. Itoh K, Hirohata S: The role of IL-10 in human B cell activation, proliferation, and differentiation. *J Immunol* 154:4341–4350, 1995.

61. Malisan F, Briere F, Bridon JM, et al: Interleukin-10 induces immunoglobulin G isotype switch recombination in human CD40-activated naive B lymphocytes. *J Exp Med* 183:937–947, 1996.

62. Le Bon A, Schiavoni G, D'Agostino G, et al: Type I interferons potently enhance humoral immunity and can promote isotype switching by stimulating dendritic cells in vivo. *Immunity* 14:461–470, 2001.

63. Jego G, Palucka AK, Blanck JP, et al: Plasmacytoid dendritic cells induce plasma cell differentiation through type I interferon and interleukin 6. *Immunity* 19(2):225–234, 2003.

64. Trinchieri G, Santoli D: Antiviral activity induced by culturing lymphocytes with tumor-derived or virus-transformed cells. Enhancement of natural killer cell activity by interferon and antagonistic inhibition of susceptibility of target cell to lysis. *J Exp Med* 147:1314–1333, 1978.

65. Djeu JY, Stocks N, Zoon K, et al: Positive self regulation of cytotoxicity in human natural killer cells by production of interferon upon exposure to influenza and herpes viruses. *J Exp Med* 156:1222–1234, 1982.

66. Kirou KA, Vakkalanka RK, Butler MJ, et al: Induction of Fas ligand-mediated apoptosis by interferon-alpha. *Clin Immunol* 95:218–226, 2000.

67. Hooks JJ, Moutsopoulos HM, Geis SA, et al: Immune interferon in the circulation of patients with autoimmune disease. *N Engl J Med* 301:5–8, 1979.

68. Hooks JJ, Jordan GW, Cupps T, et al: Multiple interferons in the circulation of patients with systemic lupus erythematosus and vasculitis. *Arthritis Rheum* 25:396–400, 1982.

69. Shi SN, Feng SF, Wen YM, et al: Serum interferon in systemic lupus erythematosus. *Br J Dermatol* 117:155–159, 1987.

70. Preble OT, Black RJ, Friedman RM, et al: Systemic lupus erythematosus: presence in human serum of an unusual acid-labile leukocyte interferon. *Science* 216:429–431, 1982.

71. Yee AM, Yip YK, Fischer HD, et al: Serum activity that confers acid lability to alpha-interferon in systemic lupus erythematosus: its association with disease activity and its independence from circulating alpha-interferon. *Arthritis Rheum* 33:563–568, 1990.

72. Rich SA: Human lupus inclusions and interferon. *Science* 213:772–775, 1981.

73. Ronnblom LE, Alm GV, Oberg KE: Possible induction of systemic lupus erythematosus by interferon-alpha treatment in a patient with a malignant carcinoid tumour. *J Intern Med* 227(3):207–210, 1990.

74. Wandl U, Nagel-Hiemke M, May D, et al: Lupus-like autoimmune disease induced by interferon therapy for myeloproliferative disorders. *Clin Immunol Immunopathol* 65:70–74, 1992.

75. Zhang ZX, Milich DR, Peterson DL, et al: Interferon-alpha treatment induces delayed CD4 proliferative responses to the hepatitis C virus nonstructural protein 3 regardless of the outcome of therapy. *J Infect Dis* 175:1294–1301, 1997.

76. Schilling PJ, Kurzrock R, Kantarjian H, et al: Development of systemic lupus erythematosus after interferon therapy for chronic myelogenous leukemia. *Cancer* 68:1536–1537, 1991.

77. Pittau E, Bogliolo A, Tinti A, et al: Development of arthritis and hypothyroidism during alpha-interferon therapy for chronic hepatitis C. *Clin Exp Rheumatol* 15:415–419, 1997.

78. Gota C, Calabrese L: Induction of clinical autoimmune disease by therapeutic interferon-alpha. *Autoimmunity* 36(8):511–518, 2003.

79. Chakrabarti D, Hultgren B, Stewart TA: IFN-alpha induces autoimmune T cells through induction of intracellular adhesion molecule-1 and B7.2. *J Immunol* 157:522–528, 1996.

80. Radvanyi LG, Banerjee A, Weir M, et al: Low levels of interferon-alpha induce CD86 (B7.2) expression and accelerates dendritic cell maturation from human peripheral blood mononuclear cells. *Scand J Immunol* 50:499–509, 1999.

81. Luft T, Pang KC, Thomas E, et al: Type I IFNs enhance the terminal differentiation of dendritic cells. *J Immunol* 161:1947–1953, 1998.

82. Crow MK: Interferon-alpha: a new target for therapy in SLE? *Arthritis Rheum* 48:2396–4001, 2003.

83. Santiago-Raber ML, Baccala R, Haraldsson KM, et al: Type-I interferon receptor deficiency reduces lupus-like disease in NZB mice. *J Exp Med* 197:777–788, 2003.

84. Braun D, Geraldes P, Demengeot J: Type I interferon controls the onset and severity of autoimmune manifestations in lpr mice. *J Autoimmun* 20:15–25, 2003.

85. Liu Z, Bethunaickan R, Huang W, et al: Interferon-α accelerates murine systemic lupus erythematosus in a T cell-dependent manner. *Arthritis Rheum* 63(1):219–229, 2011.

86. Triantafyllopoulou A, Franzke CW, Seshan SV, et al: Proliferative lesions and metalloproteinase activity in murine lupus nephritis mediated by type I interferons and macrophages. *Proc Natl Acad Sci USA* 107(7):3012–3017, 2010.

87. Vallin H, Peters A, Alm GV, et al: Anti-double-stranded DNA antibodies and immunostimulatory plasmid DNA in combination mimic the endogenous IFN-alpha inducer in systemic lupus erythematosus. *J Immunol* 163:6306–6313, 1999.

88. Bave U, Alm GV, Ronnblom L: The combination of apoptotic U937 cells and lupus IgG is a potent IFN-alpha inducer. *J Immunol* 165:3519–3526, 2000.

89. Lande R, Ganguly D, Facchinetti V, et al: Neutrophils activate plasmacytoid dendritic cells by releasing self-DNA-peptide complexes in systemic lupus erythematosus. *Sci Transl Med* 3(73):73ra19, 2011.

90. Garcia-Romo GS, Caielli S, Vega B, et al: Netting neutrophils are major inducers of type I IFN production in pediatric systemic lupus erythematosus. *Sci Transl Med* 3(73):73ra20, 2011.

91. Dzionek A, Sohma Y, Nagafune J, et al: BDCA-2, a novel plasmacytoid dendritic cell-specific type II C-type lectin, mediates antigen capture and is a potent inhibitor of interferon α/β induction. *J Exp Med* 194:1823–1834, 2001.

92. Grolleau A, Kaplan MJ, Hanash SM, et al: Impaired translational response and increased protein kinase PKR expression in T cells from lupus patients. *J Clin Invest* 106(12):1561–1568, 2000.

93. Preble OT, Rothko K, Klippel JH, et al: Interferon-induced 2′-5′ adenylate synthetase in vivo and interferon production in vitro by lymphocytes from systemic lupus erythematosus patients with and without circulating interferon. *J Exp Med* 157:2140–2146, 1983.

94. Grolleau A, Kaplan MJ, Hanash SM, et al: Impaired translational response and increased protein kinase R expression in T cells from lupus patients. *J Clin Invest* 106:1561–1568, 2000.

95. Kirou KA, Lee C, George S, et al: Coordinate overexpression of interferon-alpha-induced genes in systemic lupus erythematosus. *Arthritis Rheum* 50(12):3958–3967, 2004.

96. Kirou KA, Lee C, George S, et al: Activation of the interferon-alpha pathway identifies a subgroup of systemic lupus erythematosus patients with distinct serologic features and active disease. *Arthritis Rheum* 52(5):1491–1503, 2005.

97. Niewold TB, Adler JE, Glenn SB, et al: Age- and sex-related patterns of serum interferon-alpha activity in lupus families. *Arthritis Rheum* 58(7):2113–2119, 2008.

98. Weckerle CE, Franek BS, Kelly JA, et al: Network analysis of associations between serum interferon-alpha activity, autoantibodies, and clinical features in systemic lupus erythematosus. *Arthritis Rheum* 63(4):1044–1053, 2011.

99. Nzeusseu Toukap A, Galant C, Theate I, et al: Identification of distinct gene expression profiles in the synovium of patients with systemic lupus erythematosus. *Arthritis Rheum* 56(5):1579–1588, 2007.

100. Niewold TB: Interferon alpha as a primary pathogenic factor in human lupus. *J Interferon Cytokine Res* 31(12):887–892, 2011.

101. Niewold TB, Hua J, Lehman TJ, et al: High serum IFN-alpha activity is a heritable risk factor for systemic lupus erythematosus. *Genes Immun* 8:492–502, 2007.

102. Niewold TB, Kelly JA, Kariuki SN, et al: IRF5 haplotypes demonstrate diverse serological associations which predict serum interferon alpha activity and explain the majority of the genetic association with systemic lupus erythematosus. *Ann Rheum Dis* 71(3):463–469, 2012.

103. Salloum R, Franek BS, Kariuki SN, et al: Genetic variation at the IRF7/PHRF1 locus is associated with autoantibody profile and serum interferon-alpha activity in lupus patients. *Arthritis Rheum* 62(2):553–561, 2010.

104. Kariuki SN, Kirou KA, MacDermott EJ, et al: Cutting edge: autoimmune disease risk variant of STAT4 confers increased sensitivity to IFN-alpha in lupus patients in vivo. *J Immunol* 182(1):34–38, 2009.

105. Robinson T, Kariuki SN, Franek BS, et al: Autoimmune disease risk variant of IFIH1 is associated with increased sensitivity to IFN-alpha and serologic autoimmunity in lupus patients. *J Immunol* 187(3):1298–1303, 2011.

106. Rice G, Newman WG, Dean J, et al: Heterozygous mutations in TREX1 cause familial chilblain lupus and dominant Aicardi-Goutieres syndrome. *Am J Hum Genet* 80(4):811–815, 2007.

107. Lee-Kirsch MA, Gong M, Chowdhury D, et al: Mutations in the gene encoding the 3′-5′ DNA exonuclease TREX1 are associated with systemic lupus erythematosus. *Nat Genet* 39(9):1065–1067, 2007.

108. Namjou B, Kothari PH, Kelly JA, et al: Evaluation of the TREX1 gene in a large multi-ancestral lupus cohort. *Genes Immun* 12(4):270–279, 2011.

109. Crow YJ, Rehwinkel J: Aicardi-Goutieres syndrome and related phenotypes: linking nucleic acid metabolism with autoimmunity. *Hum Mol Genet* 18(R2):R130–R136, 2009.

110. Crow MK: Interferon-alpha: a therapeutic target in systemic lupus erythematosus. *Rheum Dis Clin North Am* 36:173–186, 2010.

111. Merrill JT, Wallace DJ, Petri M, et al: Safety profile and clinical activity of sifalimumab, a fully human anti-interferon alpha monoclonal antibody, in systemic lupus erythematosus: a phase I, multicentre, double-blind randomised study. *Ann Rheum Dis* 70(11):1905–1913, 2011.

112. Yao Y, Richman L, Higgs BW, et al: Neutralization of interferon-alpha/beta-inducible genes and downstream effect in a phase I trial of an anti-interferon-alpha monoclonal antibody in systemic lupus erythematosus. *Arthritis Rheum* 60(6):1785–1796, 2009.

113. Moore KJ, Yeh K, Naito T, et al: TNF-alpha enhances colony-stimulating factor-1-induced macrophage accumulation in autoimmune renal disease. *J Immunol* 157(1):427–432, 1996.

114. Jacob CO, McDevitt HO: Tumour necrosis factor-alpha in murine autoimmune "lupus" nephritis. *Nature* 331(6154):356–358, 1988.

115. Gordon C, Ranges GE, Greenspan JS, et al: Chronic therapy with recombinant tumor necrosis factor-alpha in autoimmune NZB/NZW F1 mice. *Clin Immunol Immunopathol* 52(3):421–434, 1989.

116. Brennan DC, Yui MA, Wuthrich RP, et al: Tumor necrosis factor and IL-1 in New Zealand Black/White mice. Enhanced gene expression and acceleration of renal injury. *J Immunol* 143(11):3470–3475, 1989.

117. Maury CP, Teppo AM: Tumor necrosis factor in the serum of patients with systemic lupus erythematosus. *Arthritis Rheum* 32(2):146–150, 1989.

118. Gabay C, Cakir N, Moral F, et al: Circulating levels of tumor necrosis factor soluble receptors in systemic lupus erythematosus are significantly higher than in other rheumatic diseases and correlate with disease activity. *J Rheumatol* 24(2):303–308, 1997.

119. Malide D, Russo P, Bendayan M: Presence of tumor necrosis factor alpha and interleukin-6 in renal mesangial cells of lupus nephritis patients. *Hum Pathol* 26(5):558–564, 1995.

120. Herrera-Esparza R, Barbosa-Cisneros O, Villalobos-Hurtado R, et al: Renal expression of IL-6 and TNFalpha genes in lupus nephritis. *Lupus* 7(3):154–158, 1998.

121. Studnicka-Benke A, Steiner G, Petera P, et al: Tumour necrosis factor alpha and its soluble receptors parallel clinical disease and autoimmune activity in systemic lupus erythematosus. *Br J Rheumatol* 35(11):1067–1074, 1996.

122. Postal M, Appenzeller S: The role of tumor necrosis factor-alpha (TNF-α) in the pathogenesis of systemic lupus erythematosus. *Cytokine* 56(3):537–543, 2011.

123. Charles PJ, Smeenk RJ, De Jong J, et al: Assessment of antibodies to double-stranded DNA induced in rheumatoid arthritis patients following treatment with infliximab, a monoclonal antibody to tumor necrosis factor alpha: findings in open-label and randomized placebo-controlled trials. *Arthritis Rheum* 43(11):2383–2390, 2000.

124. Shakoor N, Michalska M, Harris CA, et al: Drug-induced systemic lupus erythematosus associated with etanercept therapy. *Lancet* 359(9306):579–580, 2002.

125. Aringer M, Houssiau F, Gordon C, et al: Adverse events and efficacy of TNF-alpha blockade with infliximab in patients with systemic lupus erythematosus: long-term follow-up of 13 patients. *Rheumatology (Oxford)* 48(11):1451–1454, 2009.

126. Aringer M, Smolen JS: Therapeutic blockade of TNF in patients with SLE—Promising or crazy? *Autoimmun Rev* 11:321–325, 2011.

127. Banchereau J, Pascual V, Palucka AK: Cross-regulation of TNF and IFN-alpha in autoimmune diseases. *Immunity* 20(5):539–550, 2004.

128. Palucka AK, Blanck JP, Bennett L, et al: Autoimmunity through cytokine-induced dendritic cell activation. *Proc Natl Acad Sci U S A* 102(9):3372–3377, 2005.

129. Mavragani CP, Niewold TB, Moutsopoulos NM, et al: Augmented interferon-alpha pathway activation in patients with Sjögren's syndrome treated with etanercept. *Arthritis Rheum* 56(12):3995–4004, 2007.

130. Cantaert T, DeRycke L, Mavragani CP, et al: Exposure to nuclear antigens contributes to the induction of humoral autoimmunity during tumour necrosis factor alpha blockade. *Ann Rheum Dis* 68(6):1022–1029, 2009.

131. Lampe MA, Patarca R, Iregui MV, et al: Polyclonal B cell activation by the Eta-1 cytokine and the development of systemic autoimmune disease. *J Immunol* 147(9):2902–2906, 1991.

132. Scatena M, Liaw L, Giachelli CM: Osteopontin: a multifunctional molecule regulating chronic inflammation and vascular disease. *Arterioscler Thromb Vasc Biol* 27(11):2302–2309, 2007.

133. Denhardt DT, Noda M: Osteopontin expression and function: role in bone remodeling. *J Cell Biochem Suppl* 30–31:92–102, 1998.

134. Masutani K, Akahoshi M, Tsuruya K, et al: Predominance of Th1 immune response in diffuse proliferative lupus nephritis. *Arthritis Rheum* 44(9):2097–2106, 2001.

135. D'Alfonso S, Barizzone N, Giordano M, et al: Two single-nucleotide polymorphisms in the 5′ and 3′ ends of the osteopontin gene contribute to susceptibility to systemic lupus erythematosus. *Arthritis Rheum* 52(2):539–547, 2005.

136. Han S, Guthridge JM, Harley IT, et al: Osteopontin and systemic lupus erythematosus association: a probable gene-gender interaction. *PLoS ONE* 3(3):e0001757, 2008.

137. Shinohara ML, Lu L, Bu J, et al: Osteopontin expression is essential for interferon-alpha production by plasmacytoid dendritic cells. *Nat Immunol* 7(5):498–506, 2006.

138. Kariuki SN, Moore JG, Kirou KA, et al: Age- and gender-specific modulation of serum osteopontin and interferon-alpha by osteopontin genotype in systemic lupus erythematosus. *Genes Immun* 10(5):487–494, 2009.

139. Sturfelt G, Roux-Lombard P, Wollheim FA, et al: Low levels of interleukin-1 receptor antagonist coincide with kidney involvement in systemic lupus erythematosus. *Br J Rheumatol* 36(12):1283–1289, 1997.

140. Moosig F, Zeuner R, Renk C, et al: IL-1RA in refractory systemic lupus erythematosus. *Lupus* 13(8):605–606, 2004.

141. Ostendorf B, Iking-Konert C, Kurz K, et al: Preliminary results of safety and efficacy of the interleukin 1 receptor antagonist anakinra in patients with severe lupus arthritis. *Ann Rheum Dis* 64(4):630–633, 2005.

142. Sharif MN, Tassiulas I, Hu Y, et al: IFN-alpha priming results in a gain of proinflammatory function by IL-10: implications for systemic lupus erythematosus pathogenesis. *J Immunol* 172(10):6476–6481, 2004.

143. Llorente L, Zou W, Levy Y, et al: Role of interleukin 10 in the B lymphocyte hyperactivity and autoantibody production of human systemic lupus erythematosus. *J Exp Med* 181(3):839–844, 1995.

144. Ronnelid J, Tejde A, Mathsson L, et al: Immune complexes from SLE sera induce IL10 production from normal peripheral blood mononuclear cells by an FcgammaRII dependent mechanism: implications for a possible vicious cycle maintaining B cell hyperactivity in SLE. *Ann Rheum Dis* 62(1):37–42, 2003.

145. Park YB, Lee SK, Kim DS, et al: Elevated interleukin-10 levels correlated with disease activity in systemic lupus erythematosus. *Clin Exp Rheumatol* 16(3):283–288, 1998.

146. Georgescu L, Vakkalanka RK, Elkon KB, et al: Interleukin-10 promotes activation-induced cell death of SLE lymphocytes mediated by Fas ligand. *J Clin Invest* 100:2622–2633, 1997.

147. Grondal G, Traustadottir KH, Kristjansdottir H, et al: Increased T-lymphocyte apoptosis/necrosis and IL-10 producing cells in patients and their spouses in Icelandic systemic lupus erythematosus multicase families. *Lupus* 11(7):435–442, 2002.

148. Ravirajan CT, Wang Y, Matis LA, et al: Effect of neutralizing antibodies to IL-10 and C5 on the renal damage caused by a pathogenic human anti-dsDNA antibody. *Rheumatology (Oxford)* 43(4):442–447, 2004.

149. Llorente L, Richaud-Patin Y, Garcia-Padilla C, et al: Clinical and biologic effects of anti-interleukin-10 monoclonal antibody administration in systemic lupus erythematosus. *Arthritis Rheum* 43(8):1790–1800, 2000.

150. Stohl W: A therapeutic role for BLyS antagonists. *Lupus* 13(5):317–322, 2004.

151. He B, Raab-Traub N, Casali P, et al: EBV-encoded latent membrane protein 1 cooperates with BAFF/BLyS and APRIL to induce T cell-independent Ig heavy chain class switching. *J Immunol* 171(10):5215–5224, 2003.

152. Gross JA, Johnston J, Mudri S, et al: TACI and BCMA are receptors for a TNF homologue implicated in B-cell autoimmune disease. *Nature* 404(6781):995–999, 2000.

153. Zhang J, Roschke V, Baker KP, et al: Cutting edge: a role for B lymphocyte stimulator in systemic lupus erythematosus. *J Immunol* 166(1):6–10, 2001.

154. Cheema GS, Roschke V, Hilbert DM, et al: Elevated serum B lymphocyte stimulator levels in patients with systemic immune-based rheumatic diseases. *Arthritis Rheum* 44(6):1313–1319, 2001.

155. Ritterhouse LL, Crowe SR, Niewold TB, et al: B lymphocyte stimulator levels in systemic lupus erythematosus: higher circulating levels in African American patients and increased production after influenza vaccination in patients with low baseline levels. *Arthritis Rheum* 63(12):3931–3941, 2011.

156. Furie R, Petri M, Zamani O, et al: A phase III, randomized, placebo-controlled study of belimumab, a monoclonal antibody that inhibits B lymphocyte stimulator, in patients with systemic lupus erythematosus. *Arthritis Rheum* 63(12):3918–3930, 2011.

157. Stohl W, Hiepe F, Latinis KM, et al: Belimumab reduces autoantibodies, normalizes low complement, and reduces select B-cell populations in patients with systemic lupus erythematosus. *Arthritis Rheum* 2012; January 24. doi: 10.1002/art.34400.

158. Sun KH, Yu CL, Tang SJ, et al: Monoclonal anti-double-stranded DNA autoantibody stimulates the expression and release of IL-1beta, IL-6, IL-8, IL-10 and TNF-alpha from normal human mononuclear cells involving in the lupus pathogenesis. *Immunology* 99(3):352–360, 2000.

159. Tackey E, Lipsky PE, Illei GG: Rationale for interleukin-6 blockade in systemic lupus erythematosus. *Lupus* 13(5):339–343, 2004.

160. Finck BK, Chan B, Wofsy D: Interleukin 6 promotes murine lupus in NZB/NZW F1 mice. *J Clin Invest* 94(2):585–591, 1994.

161. Mihara M, Takagi N, Takeda Y, et al: IL-6 receptor blockage inhibits the onset of autoimmune kidney disease in NZB/W F1 mice. *Clin Exp Immunol* 112(3):397–402, 1998.

162. Linker-Israeli M, Deans RJ, Wallace DJ, et al: Elevated levels of endogenous IL-6 in systemic lupus erythematosus. A putative role in pathogenesis. *J Immunol* 147(1):117–123, 1991.

163. Grondal G, Gunnarsson I, Ronnelid J, et al: Cytokine production, serum levels and disease activity in systemic lupus erythematosus. *Clin Exp Rheumatol* 18(5):565–570, 2000.

164. Ripley BJ, Goncalves B, Isenberg DA, et al: Raised levels of interleukin 6 in systemic lupus erythematosus correlate with anaemia. *Ann Rheum Dis* 64(6):849–853, 2005.

165. Hushaw LL, Sawaqed R, Sweis G, et al: Critical appraisal of tocilizumab in the treatment of moderate to severe rheumatoid arthritis. *Ther Clin Risk Manag* 6:143–152, 2010.

166. Mihara M, Kasutani K, Okazaki M, et al: Tocilizumab inhibits signal transduction mediated by both mIL-6R and sIL-6R, but not by the receptors of other members of IL-6 cytokine family. *Int Immunopharmacol* 5(12):1731–1740, 2005.

167. Illei GG, Shirota Y, Yarboro CH, et al: Tocilizumab in systemic lupus erythematosus: data on safety, preliminary efficacy, and impact on circulating plasma cells from an open-label phase I dosage-escalation study. *Arthritis Rheum* 62(2):542–552, 2010.

168. Lit LC, Wong CK, Tam LS, et al: Raised plasma concentration and ex vivo production of inflammatory chemokines in patients with systemic lupus erythematosus. *Ann Rheum Dis* 65(2):209–215, 2006.

169. Park MC, Park YB, Lee SK: Elevated interleukin-18 levels correlated with disease activity in systemic lupus erythematosus. *Clin Rheumatol* 23(3):225–229, 2004.

170. Wong CK, Li EK, Ho CY, et al: Elevation of plasma interleukin-18 concentration is correlated with disease activity in systemic lupus erythematosus. *Rheumatology (Oxford)* 39(10):1078–1081, 2000.

171. Bossu P, Neumann D, Del Guidice E, et al: IL-18 cDNA vaccination protects mice from spontaneous lupus-like autoimmune disease. *Proc Natl Acad Sci USA* 100:14181–14186, 2003.

172. Yajima N, Kasama T, Isozaki T, et al: Elevated levels of soluble fractalkine in active systemic lupus erythematosus: potential involvement in neuropsychiatric manifestations. *Arthritis Rheum* 52(6):1670–1675, 2005.

173. Crow MK, Kirou KA: Regulation of CD40 ligand expression in systemic lupus erythematosus. *Curr Opin Rheumatol* 13:361–369, 2001.

174. Mosmann TR, Cherwinski H, Bond MW, et al: Two types of murine helper T cell clone. I. Definition according to profiles of activities and secreted proteins. *J Immunol* 136:2348–2357, 1986.

175. Crane IJ, Forrester JV: Th1 and Th2 lymphocytes in autoimmune disease. *Crit Rev Immunol* 25(2):75–102, 2005.

176. Zhou M, Ouyang W: The function role of GATA-3 in Th1 and Th2 differentiation. *Immunol Res* 28(1):25–37, 2003.

177. Harris DP, Goodrich S, Gerth AJ, et al: Regulation of IFN-gamma production by B effector 1 cells: essential roles for T-bet and the IFN-gamma receptor. *J Immunol* 174(11):6781–6790, 2005.

178. Kirou KA, Crow MK: New pieces to the SLE cytokine puzzle. *Clin Immunol* 91:1–5, 1999.

179. Peng SL, Moslehi J, Craft J: Roles of interferon-gamma and interleukin-4 in murine lupus. *J Clin Invest* 99(8):1936–1946, 1997.

180. Balomenos D, Rumold R, Theofilopoulos AN: Interferon-γ is required for lupus-like disease and lymphoaccumulation in MRL-lpr mice. *J Clin Invest* 101:364–371, 1998.

181. Linker-Israeli M, Bakke AC, Kitridou RC, et al: Defective production of interleukin 1 and interleukin 2 in patients with systemic lupus erythematosus (SLE). *J Immunol* 130:2651–2655, 1983.

182. Horwitz DA, Wang H, Gray JD: Cytokine gene profile in circulating blood mononuclear cells from patients with systemic lupus erythematosus: increased interleukin-2 but not interleukin-4 mRNA. *Lupus* 3:423–428, 1994.

183. Semenzato G, Bambara LM, Biasi D, et al: Increased serum levels of soluble interleukin-2 receptor in patients with systemic lupus erythematosus and rheumatoid arthritis. *J Clin Immunol* 8:447–452, 1988.

184. Crispin JC, Kyttaris VC, Terhorst C, et al: T cells as therapeutic targets in SLE. *Nat Rev Rheumatol* 6(6):317–325, 2010.

185. Tan W, Sunahori K, Zhao J, et al: Association of PPP2CA polymorphisms with systemic lupus erythematosus susceptibility in multiple ethnic groups. *Arthritis Rheum* 63(9):2755–2763, 2011.

186. Boehm U, Klamp T, Groot M, et al: Cellular responses to interferon-gamma. *Annu Rev Immunol* 15:749–795, 1997.

187. Nguyen KB, Cousens LP, Doughty LA, et al: Interferon α/β-mediated inhibition and promotion of interferon γ: STAT1 resolves a paradox. *Nat Immunol* 1:70–76, 2000.

188. Gil MP, Bohn E, O'Guin AK, et al: Biologic consequences of Stat1-independent IFN signaling. *Proc Natl Acad Sci U S A* 98:6680–6685, 2001.

189. Schwarting A, Wada T, Kinoshita K, et al: IFN-γ receptor signaling is essential for the initiation, acceleration, and destruction of autoimmune kidney disease in MRL-Fas(lpr) mice. *J Immunol* 161:494–503, 1998.

190. Ozmen L, Roman D, Fountoulakis M, et al: Experimental therapy of systemic lupus erythematosus: the treatment of NZB/W mice with mouse soluble interferon-gamma receptor inhibits the onset of glomerulonephritis. *Eur J Immunol* 25:6–12, 1995.

191. Richards HB, Satoh M, Jennette JC, et al: Interferon-γ is required for lupus nephritis in mice treated with the hydrocarbon oil pristane. *Kidney Int* 60:2173–2180, 2001.

192. Kitani A, Hara M, Hirose T, et al: Autostimulatory effects of IL-6 on excessive B cell differentiation in patients with systemic lupus erythematosus: analysis of IL-6 production and IL-6 receptor expression. *Clin Exp Immunol* 88:75–83, 1992.

193. Chen W, Wahl SM: TGF-beta: receptors, signaling pathways and autoimmunity. *Curr Dir Autoimmun* 5:62–91, 2002.

194. Del Giudice G, Crow MK: Role of transforming growth factor beta (TGF beta) in systemic autoimmunity. *Lupus* 2(4):213–220, 1993.

195. Shevach EM: Regulatory T cells in autoimmunity. *Annu Rev Immunol* 18:1303–1307, 2000.

196. Fu S, Zhang N, Yopp AC, et al: TGF-beta induces Foxp3 + T-regulatory cells from CD4 + CD25- precursors. *Am J Transplant* 4(10):1614–1627, 2004.

197. Ohtsuka K, Gray JD, Stimmler MM, et al: Decreased production of TGF-beta by lymphocytes from patients with systemic lupus erythematosus. *J Immunol* 160:2539–2545, 1998.

198. Yamamoto K, Loskutoff DJ: Expression of transforming growth factor-beta and tumor necrosis factor-alpha in the plasma and tissues of mice with lupus nephritis. *Lab Invest* 80:1561–1570, 2000.

199. Crispin JC, Tsokos GC: IL-17 in systemic lupus erythematosus. *J Biomed Biotechnol* 2010:943254, 2010.

200. Mok MY, Wu JJ, Lo Y, et al: The relation of interleukin 17 (IL-17) and IL-23 to Th1/Th2 cytokines and disease activity in systemic lupus erythematosus. *J Rheumatol* 37(10):2046–2052, 2010.

201. Yu CF, Peng WM, Oldenburg J, et al: Human plasmacytoid dendritic cells support Th17 cell effector function in response to TLR7 ligation. *J Immunol* 184(3):1159–1167, 2010.

202. Oh SH, Roh HJ, Kwon JE, et al: Expression of interleukin-17 is correlated with interferon-α expression in cutaneous lesions of lupus erythematosus. *Clin Exp Dermatol* 36(5):512–520, 2011.

203. Ettinger R, Sims GP, Fairfurst AM, et al: IL-21 induces differentiation of human naive and memory B cells into antibody-secreting plasma cells. *J Immunol* 175(12):7867–7879, 2005.

204. Dolff S, Abdulahad WH, Westra J, et al: Increase in IL-21 producing T-cells in patients with systemic lupus erythematosus. *Arthritis Res Ther* 13(5):R157, 2011.

205. Hughes T, Kim-Howard X, Kelly JA, et al: Fine-mapping and transethnic genotyping establish IL2/IL21 genetic association with lupus and localize this genetic effect to IL21. *Arthritis Rheum* 63(6):1689–1697, 2011.

Chapter 8

The Structure and Derivation of Antibodies and Autoantibodies

Giovanni Franchin, Yong-Rui Zou, and Betty Diamond

The humoral immune response protects an organism from environmental pathogens by producing antibodies (immunoglobulins) that mediate the destruction or inactivation of microbial organisms and their toxins. To perform this function, the immune system generates antibodies to a diverse and changing array of foreign antigens, yet it must do so without generating pathogenic antibodies to self. The production of high-affinity antibodies that bind to self-determinants is a prominent feature of systemic lupus erythematosus (SLE).[1] Some autoantibodies in SLE are considered markers for disease (anti-Sm/ribonucleoprotein [RNP], antinuclear antibody) because they have no established pathogenicity; others play a role in disease pathogenesis and cause tissue damage (anti-DNA, anticardiolipin, anti-Ro).[2-6]

Extensive investigations of autoantibodies in SLE have addressed the following specific questions:

1. Do polymorphisms of immunoglobulin variable region genes contribute to disease susceptibility?
2. Do B cells producing autoantibodies arise from an antigen-triggered and antigen-selected response? If so, are these triggering and selecting antigens self or foreign?
3. Are particular B-cell lineages or differentiation pathways responsible for autoantibody production?
4. What are the characteristics of pathogenic autoantibodies, and how do they mediate pathology?
5. What defects in immune regulation permit the sustained expression of pathogenic autoantibodies?

This chapter discusses autoantibody structure, assembly, and regulation. Novel potential therapeutic strategies based on new advances in our knowledge of autoantibody structure and regulation are also briefly addressed.

STRUCTURE OF THE ANTIBODY MOLECULE

Antibodies are glycoproteins produced by B lymphocytes in both membrane-bound and secreted forms. They are composed of two heavy chains and two light chains. In general, the two heavy chains are linked by disulfide bonds, and each heavy chain is linked to a light chain by a disulfide bond. The intact molecule has two functional regions: a constant region that determines its effector functions and a variable region that is involved in antigen binding and is unique to a given B-cell clone (Figure 8-1).[7] The light chains appear to contribute solely to antigen binding and are not known to mediate any other antibody function. In contrast, the heavy chains possess a constant region that determines the isotype (i.e., class: immunoglobulin M [IgM], IgD, IgG, IgA, or IgE) of the antibody molecule (Figure 8-2). Rarely, the same variable region associated with a different constant region may display an altered binding to antigen.[8,9] IgM is the first isotype produced by a B cell and the first to appear in the serum response to a newly encountered antigen. IgM antibodies normally polymerize into pentamers known as *macroglobulin,* thus conferring higher functional binding strength, or avidity. A 15-kd glycoprotein called the J chain is covalently associated with the pentameric IgM and mediates the polymerization process.[10,11] IgM antibodies can activate complement through the classical pathway and therefore cause lysis of cells expressing target antigens. Under the appropriate conditions, B cells producing IgM can switch to the production of the other isotypes. IgG is the predominant isotype of the secondary (also called memory) immune response. In humans, the IgG isotype is divided into four subclasses, IgG1, IgG2, IgG3, and IgG4, all of which possess different functional attributes. IgG1 is the most abundant in the serum. Antinuclear antibodies in SLE are mainly of IgG1 and IgG3 subclasses.[12] In addition to activating complement, IgG antibodies can promote Fc receptor (FcR)–mediated phagocytosis of antigen-antibody complexes. High concentrations of antigen-IgG complexes can downregulate an immune response by cross-linking membrane immunoglobulin and the receptor FcRII on antigen-specific B cells. This may be an important mechanism for turning off antibody production after all the available antigen is bound to antibody, and there is some evidence for defective FcRII function in some patients with lupus. The IgA constant region allows antibody translocation across epithelial cells into mucosal sites such as saliva, lung, intestine, and the genitourinary tract; IgA antibodies can be found as monomers in serum and as dimers in the mucous secretions. The J chain, implicated in IgM polymerization, is not required for IgA dimerization but does have a role in maintaining IgA dimer stability and is essential for transport of IgA by the hepatic polymeric Ig receptor.[13] IgE antibodies can trigger mast cells and eosinophils, which are important cellular mediators of the immune response to extracellular parasites and cause allergic reactions.

Every complete antibody has two identical antigen-binding sites, each of which is composed of the variable regions of a heavy and a light chain. Each variable region is divided into the highly polymorphic complementarity-determining regions (CDRs), and the more conserved framework regions (FRs). There are three distinct CDRs in both the heavy chain and the light chain, and the most variable portion of the antibody molecule is the CDR3.[14,15] There are four FRs. When the variable regions from the light and heavy chain pair, hypervariable CDRs come together and generate a unique antigen-binding site (see Figure 8-1). X-ray crystallographic studies have shown that the amino acids of the CDRs are arranged in flexible loops but the FRs have a more rigid structure that maintains the spatial orientation of the antigen-binding pocket[16]—a finding consistent with the fact that CDRs contain the contact amino acids for antigen binding and thus contribute more than the FRs to antigenic specificity.

Antibody molecules can be cleaved into functionally distinct fragments by papain and pepsin.[17,18] Limited digestion with papain cleaves the antibody into three fragments: two identical Fab (fragment antigen-binding) fragments and an Fc (fragment crystallizable) fragment. The Fab fragment consists of the entire light chain and the heavy-chain variable region with the CH1 domain. It contains the antigen-binding site, which is formed by the variable regions of the light and heavy chains. The Fc fragment is composed of the two carboxyterminal domains from the heavy chains, the hinge region, and CH2 and CH3, and interacts with soluble and cell membrane–bound effector molecules. The Fc fragment does not have antigen-binding activity. The Fab portions are linked to the Fc fragment at the hinge region, an arrangement that allows independent movement

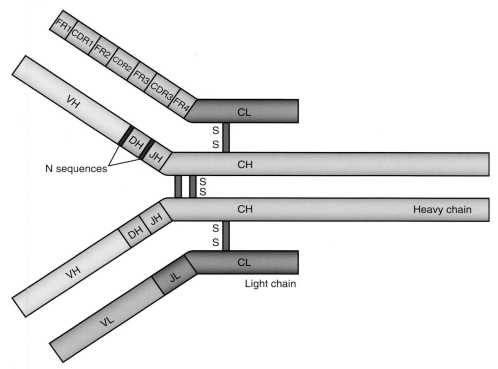

FIGURE 8-1 A prototypic antibody molecule. C, constant region; CDR, complementary-determining region; D, diversity region; FW, framework region; H, heavy chain; J, joining region; L, light chain; N, non–template-encoded nucleotide; V, variable region.

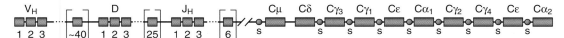

FIGURE 8-2 The heavy-chain immunoglobulin gene locus on chromosome 14. C, constant region; D, diversity gene locus; J, joining gene locus; S, switch region; V, variable gene locus.

of the two Fabs.[19] Another protease, pepsin, cleaves the antibody molecule on the carboxyterminal side of the heavy-chain disulfide bridges, producing several small fragments and an F(ab)2 fragment, which contains both Fabs linked to each other with an intact hinge region. F(ab)2 cannot be obtained from IgG2 by pepsin. However, lysyl endopeptidase digestion can generate F(ab)2 from IgG2.[20] On the basis of the fact that the F(ab)2 fragment has the same avidity for antigen as the intact antibody but does not possess any effector functions, this cleavage product may have therapeutic applications.

The variable region of an antibody may itself serve as an antigen, called an *idiotype*. *Antiidiotypes* are antibodies that bind to specific determinants in the CDRs or FRs of other antibodies.[21,22] Antibodies that have the same idiotype presumably have a high degree of structural homology and may be encoded by related variable region genes.[23] Idiotypes have been postulated to be important in the regulation of the immune response because they can be recognized by both T and B cells.[24-27] Antiidiotypic antibodies may therefore be useful reagents for tolerizing pathogenic autoantibody–producing B cells (see later).

ANTIBODY ASSEMBLY

The immunoglobulin light-chain and heavy-chain variable region genes are formed by a process of rearrangement of distinct gene segments in B cells through a process called *somatic recombination*. During this process, V (variable), D (diversity), and J (joining) segments are brought together to form a heavy-chain variable region gene, and V and J segments to form a light-chain variable region gene.[28-33]

In humans, heavy-chain V, D, and J gene segments each come from gene clusters that are arrayed on chromosome 14 (see Figure 8-2).[33,34] The 50 to 100 functional heavy-chain V segment genes are divided into seven families, which share 80% homology by DNA sequence primarily in FRs.[35-38] V gene family members are interspersed along the V locus. There are approximately 30 functional D gene segments and six known J gene segments for the human immunoglobulin heavy chain.[35]

Assembly of the complete heavy-chain gene begins with the joining of a D segment from the D cluster to a J segment in the J cluster, mediated by DNA cleavage and deletion of the intervening DNA. In a similar manner, a V gene segment is next rearranged to the DJ unit to form a complete VDJ variable region.[28,38] Each V, D, and J gene segment is flanked by conserved heptamer/nonamer consensus sequences known as *recombination signal sequences* (RSSs), which are crucial for the rearrangement process.[35] This process of variable region recombination is very elaborate and requires a complex of enzymes called V(D)J recombinase.[39] Most of these enzymes are also necessary for the maintenance of double-stranded DNA (dsDNA) and are present in all cells. However, for the first cleavage step, specialized enzyme products of the recombination-activating genes, RAG-1 and RAG-2, are required.[40] The proteins encoded by these genes are active in the early stages of lymphoid development. Signals from both stromal cells and the cytokines interleukin-3 (IL-3), IL-6, and IL-7 are necessary for induction of RAG expression in lymphoid progenitors.[41] RAGs initiate VDJ recombination by generating dsDNA breaks at the end of the RSS. Joining of the coding segments is mediated by the following enzymes involved in repair of dsDNA breaks: Ku70, Ku80, DNA-PKs, XRCC4, DNA ligase IV, Artemis, and Mre 11.[42] Members of the high-mobility group family of proteins, HMG1 and HMG2,[43] also play a significant role in the formation and stabilization of the precleavage and post-cleavage synaptic complex.[44,45]

Antibody diversification can be further generated by the addition of P and N nucleotides at the VD and DJ junctions. If the single-stranded DNA (ssDNA) that is present after the break can form a hairpin loop, the resulting double-stranded (palindromic [P]) sequences are added at the junction. Alternatively, N-nucleotides, or non–template-encoded nucleotides, are randomly inserted at the VD and DJ junctions by the enzyme terminal deoxynucleotidyl transferase (TdT).[46] Such N sequences are common in antibodies of the adult immunoglobulin repertoire but are less frequent early in the ontogeny of the B-cell repertoire.[47] These random modifications create unique junctions and increase the diversity of the antibody repertoire. Because VDJ joining is imprecise and includes P and N sequences, CDRs of variable length and sequence are generated.

After generation of a functional heavy chain, the light-chain gene segments can rearrange from either of two loci, κ or λ. The ratio of the two types of light chains varies in different species. For example, in mice the κ/λ ratio is 20 : 1 and in humans it is 2 : 1. The light-chain isotype has in general not been found to influence major properties of the antibody molecule. The light-chain variable region is composed of only two gene segments: V and J. Genes for the V and J segments of κ light chains are located on chromosome 2 in humans. The κ locus contains approximately 40 functional V gene segments, which are grouped into seven families, and five J segments.[48-52] The λ light-chain locus is on human chromosome 22 and contains at least seven V gene families with up to 70 members.[53-57] As with the heavy chain, V and J elements of the light-chain loci also rearrange by recombination at heptamer/nonamer consensus sites. Only rarely are N sequences inserted at the VJ junction of the light chain.[58]

The importance of the V(D)J recombination process has been demonstrated in animal studies as well as in some hereditary immune disorders. Mutations that abolish V(D)J recombination cause an early block in lymphoid development resulting in severe combined immune deficiency (SCID) with a complete lack of circulating B and T lymphocytes. Mice missing either RAG-1 or RAG-2 are unable to rearrange immunoglobulin genes or T-cell receptor genes.[59] In humans, a loss or marked reduction of V(D)J recombination activity can cause a T-B-SCID[60,61] or B-SCID phenotype.[62] Mutations that impair but do not completely abolish the function of RAG-1 or RAF-2 in humans result in Omenn syndrome, a form of combined immune deficiency characterized by lack of B cells and the presence of oligoclonal, activated T lymphocytes with a skewed T helper 2 (Th2) profile.[63] It is clear, however, from studies of immunodeficient mouse strains that additional gene products are needed for successful rearrangement to occur. Defects in any of the components of the dsDNA break repair machinery, such as Ku70, Ku80, DNA PKs, DNA ligase IV, Artemis, and XRCC4, lead to an immunodeficient phenotype with increased radiation sensitivity as a common feature.[64]

Although the rearranged heavy-chain VDJ segment is initially joined with an IgM constant region gene, it can undergo a second kind of gene rearrangement during the secondary response to recombine with the other downstream constant region genes (see Figure 8-2).[65-67] Switch sequences located upstream of each constant region gene mediate heavy-chain class switching.[68]

Although all somatic cells are endowed with two of each chromosome, only one rearranged heavy-chain gene and one rearranged light-chain gene normally are expressed by a B cell. This phenomenon is known as *allelic exclusion*. A productive rearrangement on one chromosome inhibits assembly of variable region genes on the other chromosome. Rearrangement of the first chromosome is often unproductive because of DNA reading frame shifts or because nonfunctional variable region gene segments called pseudogenes are used. If rearrangement on the first chromosome does not lead to the formation of a functional polypeptide chain, then the

immunoglobulin genes on the other chromosome undergo rearrangement. Monoallelic expression avoids potential expression of immunoglobulins or B-cell receptors (BCRs) with two different specificities on the same B cell, which could interfere with normal selection processes (see later). Regulation of allelic exclusion seems to occur at the recombination level, as suggested by the observation that transgenic mice allow the expression of two prearranged alleles at either the heavy- or light-chain locus.[69] Single-cell analysis of germ-line transcription in pro-B cells has shown transcription of Vκ genes on both chromosomes[70]; however, the earlier-expressed alleles are almost always the first to undergo rearrangement.[71] Methylation of DNA mediates gene repression and, when found in the proximity to recombination sites, decreases the probability of recombination.[72]

Although the heavy chain has a single locus of V, D, and J segments on each chromosome, the light chain has two. The κ locus is the first set of light-chain gene segments to rearrange. If these rearrangements are nonproductive on both chromosomes, however, then the V and J segments of the λ locus rearrange to produce an intact light chain.[73,74] Thus, the heavy chain has two loci from which to form a functional gene, but the light chain may rearrange at four loci. Moreover, additional or secondary rearrangements can occur in B cells already expressing an intact antibody molecule if that antibody has a forbidden autospecificity. These additional rearrangements, which are termed *receptor editing*, are important in allowing B cells to regulate autoreactivity.

Immune tolerance mediated by receptor editing occurs frequently in developing B cells.[75] High-affinity receptor binding to self-antigen induces a new gene recombination[76] and the replacement of the gene encoding a self-reactive receptor by a gene encoding a non–self-reactive receptor.[77,78] Receptor editing occurs at both light- and heavy-chain loci, but at a much lower frequency at the heavy-chain locus.[79] There is some debate about whether Ig gene rearrangement can occur also in mature B cells or only in immature B cells.[80] RAG protein expression in germinal centers, as well as after immunization,[81,82] has suggested that antibody genes may undergo modification not only in developing but also in mature B cells.[82-84] Immunization of BALB/c mice with a multimeric form of a peptide mimotope of dsDNA induces the generation of dsDNA-reactive B cells. Mature B cells that respond to peptide reexpress RAG for a short time only, suggesting that receptor editing can also participate in peripheral tolerance.[85] The regulation and function of secondary rearrangements of Ig genes in mature B cells remain incompletely understood, however, because some data suggest that rearrangement events can be initiated in germinal center B cells that fail to bind antigen.

GENERATION OF ANTIBODY DIVERSITY

The immune system has several mechanisms to ensure a large antibody repertoire. Before exposure to antigen, B-cell diversity results from (1) combinations of V, D, and J gene segments and V and J segments into heavy- and light-chain genes, respectively, (2) junctional diversity produced by N or P sequence insertion and/or imprecise joining of gene segments, and (3) the random pairing of heavy and light chains. These three mechanisms are consequences of the process of recombination used to create complete Ig variable regions. The fourth mechanism, called *somatic hypermutation* (SHM), occurs later on rearranged DNA. This mechanism introduces point mutations into rearranged variable region genes (Box 8-1). These mechanisms are potentially capable of producing a repertoire of 10^{11} different antibodies.[86]

Cross-linking of surface immunoglobulin on the B cell by a multivalent antigen is the first in a series of critical steps that eventually can lead to B-cell activation and antibody production. After cross-linking of membrane immunoglobulin, the antigen-antibody complexes are internalized, and the antigen is cleaved and processed in the cell. Peptide fragments of protein antigen bound to the major histocompatibility complex (MHC) class II molecules are then expressed on the cell surface, where they can be recognized by antigen-specific helper T cells (Figure 8-3). These T cells provide the

Box 8-1 Mechanisms of Antibody Diversity

Combinatorial diversity of V, D, and J gene segments for the heavy-chain variable region and V and J gene segments for the light-chain variable region
Junctional diversity of rearranged heavy- and light-chain variable regions:
  N-terminal addition
  Imprecise joining
Random association of heavy and light chains
Somatic point mutation

TABLE 8-1 Distinguishing Features of the Naïve and Antigen-Activated Antibody Repertoire

FEATURE	NAÏVE	ANTIGEN ACTIVATED
Isotype	Primarily immunoglobulin (Ig) M	Primarily IgG
Specificity	Polyreactive	Monospecific
Affinity	Low affinity	High affinity
Sequence	Germline gene encoded	Somatically mutated (high replacement–to–silent mutation [R:S] ratio)
Titer	Low titer	High titer

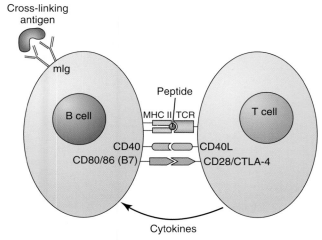

FIGURE 8-3 B-cell–T-cell cognate interactions. MHC II, class II major histocompatibility complex; mIg, membrane immunoglobulin; TCR, T-cell receptor.

co-stimulation and cytokines that are necessary for full B-cell activation.

On initial exposure to an antigen, naïve B cells recognizing the antigen proliferate and begin to secrete IgM. These B cells can belong to the B1, marginal zone, subset or the follicular B cell subset. The antibodies of this primary immune response generally are polyreactive and display low affinity for a multitude of antigens, even for antigens without obvious structural homology (Table 8-1). The amplification of antigen-specific B follicular cells occurs in specific regions of the lymphoid tissue called *germinal centers*. Somatic hypermutation (discussed later), leads to the selection of high-avidity B-cell clones. Within the germinal center, heavy-chain isotype switching and further differentiation to plasma cells and memory B cells also occur.

Studies using mice with targeted disruptions of particular genes have shown that in addition to a cognate interaction between the T-cell receptor and an MHC class II molecule, other pairs of B cell–T cell contacts are necessary for germinal center formation and function (see Figure 8-3). One important interaction is between CD40 on the B cell and CD40 ligand (CD40L, gp39) expressed on activated CD4+ T cells. Activation of CD40 is thought to be necessary for the formation of germinal centers and germinal center reactions.[87,88] Defective CD40L on T cells in humans and mice causes X-linked hyper-IgM syndrome type I, which is characterized by a defect in isotype switching and severe humoral immunodeficiency, leading to increased susceptibility to infections with extracellular bacteria.[89] After the primary immune response is complete, specific antibody secretion decreases. Reexposure to the antigen and activated T cells, however, can activate memory B cells, which arise in the germinal center response to initiate the secondary immune response. The

secondary serum response is characterized by rapidly produced high titers of IgG antibodies that have greater specificity and increased affinity for the antigen.[90-92] The increase in both affinity and specificity is a consequence of SHM and the selection process within the germinal center. Anti-dsDNA antibodies, which are the well-characterized pathogenic autoantibodies to date, possess all the features of secondary response antibodies (see Table 8-1; see Chapter 23).[93-96]

SOMATIC HYPERMUTATION

Somatic point mutations are single-nucleotide substitutions that can occur throughout the heavy- and light-chain variable region genes[97-99]; they represent a site-specific, differentiation stage–specific, and lineage-specific phenomenon.[100] Somatic mutation takes place in dividing centroblasts (noncleaved cells in the centers of lymphoid follicles), in which rearranged Ig variable region genes undergo a mutation rate of 1 base pair (bp) per 10^3 cell divisions, compared with 1 bp per 10^{10} cell divisions in all other somatic cells. The DNA mismatch repair system has been implicated in Ig gene mutation because it functions generally to correct point mutations in DNA. A genetic deficiency in a component of the mismatch repair system, PMS2, has been shown to enhance the rate of mutation, suggesting that the DNA mismatch repair system may be altered in hypermutating B cells.[101] Similarly, mice deficient in Msh6, a component of the mismatch repair system, have altered nucleotide targeting for mutations.[102] Because somatic mutation occurs concurrently with heavy-chain class switching, although by a different mechanism, mutation is more common in IgG than in IgM antibodies.

The generation of high-affinity antibodies through B-cell maturation with SHM and class switch recombination (CSR) critically depends on the action of activation-induced cytidine deaminase (AID).[103] AID is a member of a family of APOBEC (apolipoprotein B messenger RNA–editing, enzyme-catalytic, polypeptide-like 3G) cytidine deaminases that causes DNA conversions of cytosine to uracil, generating mutations in the immunoglobulin gene that can increase antibody affinity for the antigen.[104] AID deficiency in humans causes a disorder called hyper-IgM syndrome type 2, which is characterized by elevated serum values of IgM and undetectable levels of IgG, IgA, and IgE.[105] Mice with a homozygous deletion of AID display normal B-cell maturation but are deficient in SHM and CSR, whereas overexpression of AID is sufficient to induce SHM and CSR in B-cell lines or fibroblasts.[106,107] AID expression is tightly regulated and appears to be restricted to GC, although clearly CSR can occur outside GC. Genomic instability and higher mutation rates are likely to occur in the presence of poorly regulated AID expression, possibly leading to malignancies.[104]

Genealogies of B cells with serial mutations in their immunoglobulin gene sequences demonstrate how point mutations can lead to antibodies with altered affinity for antigen (Figure 8-4).[108-111] Although B cells producing antibodies with decreased affinity appear within the germinal center, progression of these cells to the plasma or memory cell compartment is rare, because they fail to expand further in the germinal center response. In contrast, B cells producing

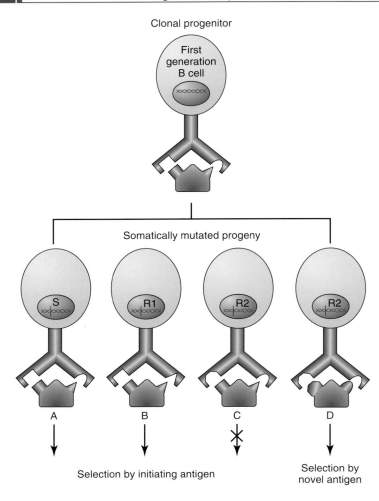

Clonal progenitor

First generation B cell

Somatically mutated progeny

S   R1   R2   R2

A   B   C   D

Selection by initiating antigen

Selection by novel antigen

FIGURE 8-4 B-cell genealogy. The progenitor B cell depicted at the *top* expresses an antibody that is encoded by germline immunoglobulin genes and has a low affinity for antigen. When antigen and T-cell factors trigger B-cell proliferation, class switching, and somatic mutation, numerous B-cell progeny are possible. Three examples are schematized here. *A,* A B cell with a silent (S) point mutation. This nucleotide substitution does not encode a new amino acid. Therefore, the antibody molecule is unaffected, and affinity for antigen does not change. *B,* A B cell whose point mutation encodes an amino acid replacement (R), leading to increased affinity for antigen. This mutated antibody exemplifies affinity maturation. *C,* A B cell with a replacement mutation that alters antigenic specificity. This antibody can no longer bind to the initial triggering antigen. *D,* The same antibody as in *C,* despite no longer being able to bind to the initial triggering antigen, can acquire specificity for a novel (perhaps self-) antigen.

antibodies of higher affinity continue to expand. SHM is an important process in the generation of high-affinity antibodies, and a suboptimal frequency of Ig V gene mutation leads to common variable immunodeficiency (CVID).[112] Mutated antibodies also can acquire novel antigenic specificities. In one in vitro system, a single amino acid change in a protective antipneumococcal antibody results in reduced binding to pneumococci and a newly acquired affinity for dsDNA.[113] Abundant evidence suggests that antibodies to foreign antigen also can acquire autospecificity in vivo through somatic point mutation.[114,115]

Because a given amino acid can be encoded by more than one DNA triplet, not every point mutation causes an amino acid substitution that can change antibody affinity for an antigen. It is possible to indirectly analyze antigen selection during the course of the germinal center response by calculating the ratio of replacement (R) mutations (mutations that lead to amino acid changes) to silent (S) mutations (mutations that do not lead to such changes) in rearranged antibody genes. Purely random point mutations within a DNA sequence containing equal numbers of each possible codon would result in a predicted random R:S ratio of approximately 3:1.[116,117] The random R:S ratio for a particular DNA sequence, however, might be lower or higher, depending on the actual codon usage.[118,119]

In an antigen-selected response, one might expect a higher than random R:S ratio, because B cells containing mutations leading to higher affinity for antigen would be favored to proliferate. Further, antigen selection would predict a higher frequency of R mutations in the CDRs, because these regions include the contact amino acids for antigen binding. This type of analysis has been performed to assess whether certain autoantibodies arise from antigen selected responses.[94-96] There are two concerns, however, with this analysis. First, the assumption of purely random mutation is incorrect; studies have now shown that bias for particular kinds of mutations occurs and that hot spots of mutation exist.[120] Second, although antibodies with a higher-than-random R:S ratio probably are part of an antigen-selected repertoire, the converse clearly is not true; a single amino acid substitution is capable of conferring a tenfold increase in affinity.[121,122] Thus, antigen selection may occur in the absence of a high R:S ratio.

B-CELL SUBSETS: IMPLICATIONS FOR SLE

B-1 cells (also CD5 or Ly-1) represent a distinct population of B cells.[123,124] B-1 cells are the only subset of B lymphocytes that constitutively express the pan–T-cell surface antigen CD5. B-1 cells are mainly found in the peritoneal and pleural cavities of mice (accounting for 35% to 70% of total B cells found in these sites) and are rare in lymphoid organs and blood.[125] They can be further divided into B-1a and B-1b cells and are usually recognized as having the following surface phenotype: $CD19^{hi}CD23^-D43^+gM^{hi}IgD^{variable}CD5^{\pm}$. Data showing that CD5 is implicated in the maintenance of tolerance in anergic B cells,[126] along with data demonstrating that CD5 mediates negative regulation of BCR signaling in B-1 cells,[127] support the hypothesis that the expression of CD5 may help inhibit autoimmune responses. The phenotype of B-1 cells in humans has been reported to be $CD27^+$, $CD43^+$, $CD70^-$; this subset contains DNA-reactive B cells.[128]

A two-pathway model of B-1 cell development has been proposed on the basis of the identification of a bone marrow and fetal liver precursor to mainly B-1b cells and the observation that B-1a cells can be differentiated from B-2 cell precursors under certain physiologic conditions.[125] B-1 cells are unique among mature B lymphocytes in that they appear to be a self-replenishing population that arises in the fetal liver.[129] Being a major source of natural autoantibodies,[130-132] the B-1 lineage is of particular interest to those studying autoimmunity. Elevated numbers of B-1 cells are present in the autoimmune New Zealand black (NZB) mouse strain,[129] and prevention of the autoimmune symptoms has been reported with their elimination.[133] B-1 cell expansion is found in some patients with rheumatoid arthritis and Sjögren' syndrome,[134] but an association with SLE is weaker.[135,136]

B-1 cells generally express germline-encoded, polyreactive IgM antibodies with limited V gene segment usage.[129-131] Much controversy exists about the physiologic function of the B-1 lymphocytes, although there is now growing evidence that many of the low-affinity autoantibodies made by this B-cell subset are important in the clearance of apoptotic debris. Adoptive transfer experiments have shown that B-1 cells are poor at forming germinal centers,[137] which are characteristic of a T-dependent B-cell response and are thought to be necessary for antigen selection and class switching; however, class-switched, somatically mutated B-1 antibodies that appear to show evidence of antigen selection have been isolated from humans.[138]

MZ (marginal zone) B cells share many features with B-1 B cells. They are phenotypically characterized by cell surface expression of $IgM^{hi}IgD^{lo}CD21^{hi}CD22^{hi}CD23^{lo}CD1^{hi}$ and reside in the marginal zones that girdle the follicles in spleen and tonsils.[139] Their hallmark functional characteristic is represented by early activation and rapid Ig secretion in response to T-independent (TI) antigens, which arrive via a hematogenous route in the spleen. Like B-1 cells, MZ B cells are key players of innate immunity because they respond rapidly to antigen and do not generate a memory response. Although it has been generally accepted that MZ B cells are a self-renewing and mostly nonrecirculating population,[140,141] later studies suggest that a large population of IgM-positive peripheral B cells correspond to circulating splenic MZ B cells.[142,143]

Both MZ and B-1 B cells have a high antigen presentation capacity and are strategically located to encounter and process foreign antigens. Both cells secrete polyreactive "natural" antibodies, including self-reactive ones that are generally germline encoded.[144] Low titers of low-affinity autoantibodies are part of the normal B-cell repertoire.[145-148] Such antibodies are not unique to any autoimmune disease, nor is there any evidence that they are pathogenic. These natural autoantibodies resemble the antibodies of a primary immune response, in that they are mainly IgM and polyreactive and bind to a wide variety of both autoantigens and foreign antigens that often have no apparent structural homology.[149-151] "Natural" antibodies have also been shown to bind to altered phospholipids expressed on the surfaces of cells undergoing apoptosis. The opsonization of apoptotic cells increases their clearance and routes them to nonimmunogenic pathways.[152] Although sequence analysis shows that the antibodies made by MZ B cells are encoded mainly by germline (i.e., unmutated) genes,[153-157] numerous exceptions exist.[158] Analysis of the variable regions of natural autoantibodies suggests that they may contain more flexible hydrophilic amino acid residues in their CDRs than somatically mutated, affinity-matured antibodies, as well as longer CDRs,[158] features that may explain their polyreactivity. It is thought that they present a shallow groove for antigen binding that can accommodate more diverse structures.

There are some indications that the B cells producing natural antibodies may be clonally related to pathogenic B cells. Idiotypic analyses of natural anti-DNA antibodies from normal individuals and of potentially pathogenic anti-DNA antibodies from patients with SLE demonstrate that cross-reactive idiotypes are present in both populations.[159,160] Some investigators have speculated that natural autoantibodies can be the precursors to pathogenic autoantibodies,[161,162] and other data suggest that the two classes of autoantibodies arise from distinct B-cell populations and that the SLE autoantibodies arise by

the somatic mutation of genes that encode protective antibodies.[93,163-168] Adoptive transfer experiments of MZ B cells, like those of B-1 cells, have demonstrated T-dependent class-switching and SHM, resulting in the production of high-affinity antibodies.[169,170] If one assumes that MZ B cells can undergo affinity maturation, it is conceivable that an enhanced differentiation of MZ B cells along this pathway could contribute to autoimmunity. Another potential role for MZ B cells in autoimmunity is as antigen-presenting cells for self-antigens, resulting in the activation of autoreactive CD4+ T cells. These T cells can then amplify an autoreactive B-cell response by activating additional autoreactive B cells.

Understanding of innate immune B cells in humans has been further advanced through the study of a population of B cells that can be identified using a monoclonal antibody (9G4) that binds to a unique epitope encoded by the human heavy-chain variable region gene V4-34.[171] These 9G4-positive B cells represent 5% to 10% of the mature naïve B-cell repertoire and recognize autoantigens and pathogens. In addition, these cells are present in the MZ B cell compartment and are normally excluded from the T-dependent IgG memory repertoire. However, in patients with SLE, 9G4-positive B cells are expanded in the IgG memory population, supporting the hypothesis that inappropriate positive selection of innate B cells into an adaptive immune phenotype is a feature of autoimmunity. Although 9G4-positive antibodies have not been demonstrated to have a direct pathogenic effect, they are elevated in up to 75% of patients with active SLE.

Follicular B cells have the most diverse immunoglobulin repertoire. These are the B cells that participate in T-cell–dependent antibody responses. Follicular B cells, when they encounter antigen and T-cell help, can become short-lived plasma cells or can enter into a germinal center response in which long-lived plasma cells and memory cells are generated. Because the recognition of an increased expression of type I interferon–inducible genes, and an interferon signature in mononuclear cells of patients with SLE, several investigators have studied a mouse model of SLE in which disease is accelerated through the administration of type I interferon. Interestingly, this interferon-accelerated model is characterized by the presence of short-lived plasma cells as opposed to germinal center–matured cells,[172] perhaps related to interferon induction of IL-12.[173] During the germinal center response, heavy-chain class switching and SHM of Ig variable region genes occur. The process of SHM can clearly generate autoreactivity. Studies of both MRL-lpr/lpr and NZB/W mice have shown that many anti-DNA antibodies display extensive somatic mutation, which is responsible in some cases for increasing affinity for DNA and in other cases for the acquisition of autoreactivity. In these models there are clearly impairments in both central tolerance and peripheral tolerance, with defects in negative selection of antigen-naïve and antigen-activated B cells, respectively. There are now a number of mouse models of SLE in which all the DNA-reactive B cells appear to be generated in the germinal center response, through the process of SHM.[174] These models are of particular interest because B-cell autoreactivity appears to be regulated appropriately at early stages of B-cell development but not in germinal center B cells.

TOLL-LIKE RECEPTORS IN B-CELL FUNCTION

B cells express Toll-like receptors (TLRs), which recognize specific molecular determinants common to many pathogens. In mouse B cells, coengagement of TLRs and the BCR acts synergistically to induce activation; in humans, TLR expression appears to be induced following BCR activation.[175]

TLRs have been shown to bind exogenous ligands, such as lipopolysaccharides (LPSs), single- and double-stranded RNA and dsDNA derived from bacteria, and neutrophils undergoing NETosis, or from apoptotic debris.[176-178] Inducible TLR expression and B-cell activation from a wide range of self-ligands and foreign ligands may provide a link between innate immune dysregulation and autoimmunity. Interestingly TLR-dependent activation of B cells expressing antichromatin antibodies leads to isotype switching and SHM in the absence of T-cell co-stimulation.[179] A number of additional factors have been found to promote T-independent isotype switching, including B-cell–activating factor (BAFF) and type I IFN. In addition, CpG binding to TLR9 in B cells from several lupus mouse strains increases the secretion of IL-10 and results in the suppression of IL-12 production.[180] IL-10 has been shown to be elevated in patients with SLE, and serum levels can correlate with disease activity.[181,182] In an uncontrolled study, a small number of patients with active SLE were given anti–IL-10 antibody and experienced an improvement of disease activity.[183] Similarly, anti–IL-10 treatment of NZB/W mice resulted in delayed onset of lupus-like disease.[184] However, MRL-Fas(lpr) IL-10$^{-/-}$ mice showed an increased severity of lupus and higher concentrations of anti-dsDNA antibodies.[185] An IL-10–producing B-cell subset (regulatory B cells [Bregs]) has now been identified that can suppress immune responses to foreign antigen and self-antigen.[186] Transitional (CD19$^+$CD21^{hi}CD23^{hi}CD1d^{hi}) are able to suppress mouse models of inflammatory arthritis, experimental allergic encephalitis, and lupus in an IL-10–dependent fashion.[187] A better understanding of the impact of Bregs in lupus may lead to new therapeutic targets.

PATHOGENIC AUTOANTIBODIES

Indirect evidence for the pathogenicity of several autoantibodies present in SLE includes their association with clinical manifestations in SLE and their presence in affected tissue. There is growing evidence to directly support the pathogenic potential of several lupus-associated autoantibodies. Glomerulonephritis has been shown to develop in a transgenic mouse expressing the heavy and light chains of the secreted form of an anti-DNA antibody, thereby confirming that anti-DNA antibodies cause renal disease.[188] Support for the pathogenic role of anti-DNA antibodies in nephritis can also be found in autoimmune disease models displaying high titers of anti-DNA antibodies together with immunoglobulin deposition in the kidney and histologic nephritis.[189-192] Perfusion of monoclonal mouse and polyclonal human IgG anti-DNA antibodies through isolated rat kidney induces significant proteinuria and decreased clearance of inulin.[193] Addition of plasma as a source of complement markedly increases proteinuria, whereas preincubation of the antibodies with DNA can abolish binding to renal tissue.[193] It is still unknown, however, whether pathogenic anti-DNA antibodies form immune complexes with antigen in situ or the antibodies bind to a target antigen that is actually some component of glomerular tissue and/or tubular components. A decrease in binding of anti-DNA antibodies to glomerular elements with DNase treatment occurred in some experimental models[194] but not in others,[195] suggesting that both models pertain; some anti-DNA antibodies directly cross-react with glomerular antigens, whereas other anti-DNA antibodies may bind via a DNA-containing bridge. A number of investigators have administered monoclonal anti-DNA antibodies to nonautoimmune mice, either intraperitoneally in the form of ascites-producing hybridomas or intravenously as purified immunoglobulins.[196,197] In these models, it is possible to demonstrate that anti-DNA antibodies differ with respect to pathogenicity,[197,198] with some antibodies depositing in the kidney and others not. Moreover, those antibodies that are deposited in the kidney may differ with respect to the localization of deposition. In studies performed with the congenic mouse strain NZM2328.C57Lc4, chronic glomerulonephritis and severe proteinuria develop despite the fact that the mice do not generate autoantibodies to dsDNA or other nuclear antigens,[199] consistent with the clinical observation that kidney disease can arise in individuals with no DNA-reactive antibodies.

Studies have also elegantly demonstrated the arrhythmogenic potential of anti-Ro antibodies. Affinity-purified anti-Ro antibodies from mothers with lupus whose babies have congenital heart block have been reported to inhibit calcium currents and induce complete heart block in an ex vivo perfused human fetal heart system.[200] In another study, immunization of female BALB/c mice with recombinant La and Ro particles led to first-degree atrioventricular block in 6 of 20 pups born to immunized mothers and rarely to more advanced conduction defects.[201] Finally, passive transfer of purified human IgG containing anti-Ro and anti-La antibodies to pregnant BALB/c mice was found to result in fetal bradycardia and first-degree atrioventricular block.[202]

Experimental evidence also supports the close epidemiologic association between antiphospholipid antibodies and thrombosis. Following experimental induction of vascular injury in mice, injection of affinity-purified immunoglobulin from patients with antiphospholipid syndrome was found to result in a significant increase in thrombus size and a delay in disappearance of the thrombus.[203] Injecting human monoclonal anticardiolipin antibodies into pregnant BALB/c mice was reported to lead to fetal resorption and a significant decrease in placental and fetal weight.[204] Similar results have been obtained with passive transfer of monoclonal murine and polyclonal human anticardiolipin antibodies.[205]

The combination of the epidemiologic and experimental data makes it clear that the importance of several lupus-associated autoantibodies lies not only in their diagnostic significance as markers for the disease but also in their pathogenic role in tissue damage in affected target organs in SLE. Treating disease with the end point of lowering the titer of specific autoantibodies then becomes a therapeutic goal with a clear pathophysiologic rationale.

Heavy-chain isotype appears to be important in determining the pathogenicity of autoantibodies. For example, marked differences in the severity of induced hemolysis exist among IgG isotype switch variants of an antierythrocytic antibody that are related to the capacity of each isotype to bind to Fc receptors.[206] In murine lupus, the switch from serum IgM anti-DNA activity to IgG anti-DNA activity heralds the onset of renal disease.[207] Similarly, human IgG antibodies present in the immune complex deposits within the kidneys of patients with SLE appear to trigger mesangial cell proliferation and subsequent tissue damage to a greater extent than IgM antibodies, perhaps because mesangial cells or infiltrating mononuclear cells have Fc receptors for IgG.[208] The importance of isotype for anticardiolipin antibodies is intriguing[2]; several groups have noted that IgG antiphospholipid and beta 2–glycoprotein antibodies correlate better with clinical thrombosis than other isotypes do (see Chapter 27). Nevertheless, pathogenicity has been shown also for IgM and IgA antibodies.[203] IgM and IgA anticardiolipin antibodies also correlate with specific disease phenotypes. For example, IgM antiphospholipid antibodies are associated with hemolytic anemia.[209]

It was formerly widely believed that antibodies could not penetrate live cells and that nuclear staining of sectioned tissues was an artifact of tissue preparation. There is now evidence that some anti-DNA and anti–ribosomal P autoantibodies bind to the cell surface, traverse the cytoplasm, and reach the nucleus. Furthermore, data demonstrate a pathogenic effect from cellular penetration by autoantibodies.[210-212] Although antigen translocation to the cell membrane may explain the accessibility of normally intranuclear antigens to interaction with autoantibodies,[213,214] the capability to penetrate live cells and interact with cytoplasmic or nuclear components may be an additional pathogenic characteristic of some autoantibodies.

This chapter discusses aspects of autoantibody production, but it is increasingly evident that autoantibody-mediated tissue damage requires not just the presence of autoantibodies with particular pathogenic features but also the display of a specific antigen in the target organ.[215] Differential display of antigen at the level of the target organ may contribute to genetic susceptibility to autoimmune disease. Evidence for such a hypothesis comes, in part, from a murine model of autoimmune myocarditis, in which differential susceptibility to antimyosin antibody–induced disease in different mouse strains depends on differences in the composition of cardiac extracellular matrix.[216] Similarly, in a rat model for tubular nephritis, antibody-mediated disease depends on genetically determined antigen display in the renal tubules.[217]

GENETIC AND MOLECULAR ANALYSIS OF ANTI-DNA ANTIBODIES

Genetic analyses of anti-DNA antibodies in both human and murine lupus have provided important information regarding the production of autoantibodies. There is currently no evidence that a distinct set of disease-associated, autoreactive V region genes is present only in individuals with a familial susceptibility to autoimmunity and is used to encode the autoantibodies of autoimmune disease. It is also clear that no particular Ig V region genes are absolutely required for the production of autoantibodies (reviewed in reference 218). Immunoglobulin genes that are present in a nonautoimmune animal clearly are capable of forming pathogenic autoantibodies. The offspring of a nonautoimmune SWR mouse and an NZB mouse (SNF1 mice) spontaneously produce autoantibodies,[219] with a large percentage of the anti-DNA antibodies that are deposited in the kidneys of SNF1 mice having been encoded by Ig genes derived from the nonautoimmune SWR parent.[219] In fact, both idiotypic and molecular studies show that the V region genes used to produce autoantibodies in lupus are also used in a protective antibody response in nonautoimmune individuals.[220,221] Autoantibodies bear cross-reactive idiotypes that also are present on the antibodies that are made in response to foreign antigens, and V region genes used to encode autoantibodies also encode antibodies to foreign antigen.[222-225] Indeed, a number of autoantibodies cross-react with foreign antigens, demonstrating that the same V region gene segments can be used in both protective and potentially pathogenic responses.[226-228] These cross-reactive antibodies are capable of binding to bacterial antigen with high affinity, but they also possess specificity for a self-antigen. Patients with *Klebsiella* infections and individuals vaccinated with pneumococcal polysaccharide develop antibacterial antibodies expressing anti-DNA cross-reactive idiotypes.[220,229] In vivo, cross-reactive antibodies with specificity to both pneumococcus and dsDNA are protective in mice against an otherwise lethal bacterial infection, yet they also can deposit in the kidney and cause glomerular damage.[230] It appears that cross-reactive antibodies are routinely generated during the course of the normal immune response in the nonautoimmune individual. Ordinarily, however, autoreactive B cells expressing a self-specificity are actively downregulated and contribute little to the expressed antibody repertoire.[114]

Although there is no evidence that specific genes encode only autoantibodies, some data suggest that autoantibodies are encoded by a somewhat restricted number of immunoglobulin V region genes.[231-233] In murine lupus, extensive analyses of anti-DNA–producing B cells show that 15 to 20 heavy-chain V region genes encode most anti-DNA antibodies.[165,234-236] One study found a dramatic increase in the frequency of use of a particular *J558* heavy-chain gene in autoimmune than in normal mice, whereas nonautoimmune mice that were immunized with an immunogenic DNA/DNA-binding peptide complex displayed intermediate usage.[233] This finding supports the concept that differences in V gene usage that may be seen between autoimmune and nonautoimmune mice are quantitative rather than reflecting a true qualitative difference. Although molecular studies of human antibodies are more limited, idiotypic analyses also suggest restricted V gene usage. This observation is important because it suggests that antiidiotypes can play a role in therapeutic strategies. Furthermore, analysis of restriction fragment length polymorphisms, which is a tool used to identify the similarities and differences among particular genes in a population, has been used to examine whether distinct Ig gene polymorphisms are associated with SLE.[237-239] A deletion of a specific heavy-chain V gene, *hv-3,* was reported to be more frequent in individuals with SLE or rheumatoid arthritis.[240,241] A specific germline Vκ gene, *A30,* was found to increase the cationicity (and therefore the pathogenicity) of human anti-DNA antibodies. A defective A30 gene was found in eight of nine patients with lupus without nephritis, but this gene was normal in all nine patients with lupus with nephritis.[242] Polymorphism at the Vκ gene locus may then contribute to susceptibility to lupus nephritis. Although these studies look at only small numbers of patients, they suggest that polymorphisms in immunoglobulin genes may make some contribution to the generation of autoantibodies and expression of human lupus. Nevertheless, the anti-DNA response is no more restricted than are many responses to foreign antigen, and the restricted V region gene usage does not appear to be skewed toward particular gene families.

SHM is one mechanism by which protective, antiforeign antibodies may evolve into pathogenic autoantibodies (see Figure 8-4).[243,244] The characteristics and mechanics of SHM in SLE are, therefore, of interest. Examining ten human antibodies positive for a specific, lupus-associated idiotype (F4), Manheimer-Lory[245] found no change in the frequency of somatic mutations or the distributions of such mutations in CDRs. Although the normal process of somatic mutation is generally random, there is some bias for mutation at specific sequence motifs, termed mutational "hot spots." Surprisingly, F4-positive antibodies displayed abnormal somatic mutation, as shown by a decrease in hot-spot targeting. Mice transgenic for the antiapoptotic gene *bcl-2* also display this decreased targeting of mutations to hot spots,[246] so the decreased targeting in F4-positive antibodies derived from patients with lupus may reflect an abnormal process of B-cell selection rather than defective machinery for somatic mutation. Studies have been performed on the mutational process in the V gene repertoire in individual B cells from a small number of patients with lupus.[247] The frequency of mutations was increased in both productive and unproductive Vκ rearrangements, with evidence of increased targeting to mutational hot spots in framework regions, consistent with altered selection. A single study in mice found essentially no differences in somatic mutation between B cells of an autoreactive strain and those of a normal strain.[248] Conflicting data prevent drawing firm conclusions as yet.

AUTOANTIBODY INDUCTION

Autoantibodies that are present in SLE may be germline-encoded or may reflect the process of SHM,[95,249] suggesting exposure to antigen and T-cell help. For some autoantibodies, mutation of the germline sequences clearly is crucial in generating the autoantigenic specificity.[95] These antibodies have a high R:S ratio, primarily in CDRs; however, the pitfalls of R:S ratio calculations have been discussed and should be considered in the analysis of anti-DNA antibodies.[120,121] There also are lupus autoantibodies that have a high R:S ratio in framework regions.[250] Because these framework region mutations are less likely to alter antigenic specificity, it is tempting to speculate that they instead may facilitate escape from a putative regulatory mechanism.

There are various hypotheses regarding the nature of an eliciting antigen or antigens in SLE (Box 8-2). Several lines of evidence support the role of foreign microbial antigens in the generation of autoantibodies.[251] Lupus-prone strains of mice carrying the xid mutation, which impairs production of the antipolysaccharide antibodies that are required for antibacterial immunity, demonstrate much lower titers of anti-DNA antibodies and decreased renal disease.[252]

Box 8-2 Antigenic Triggers for Anti–Double-Stranded (ds) DNA Antibodies

Foreign antigen:
- Molecular mimics
- Bacterial DNA
- Complexes of DNA and DNA-binding proteins

Self-antigen:
- Ribonucleoprotein autoepitopes
- Histone peptides
- Peptides derived from anti-dsDNA antibodies
- Cryptic autoepitopes (sequestered autoantigens, altered processing/presentation)

Idiotypic network (antiidiotypic antibody-autoantigen)

Similarly, autoimmune-prone NZB mice raised in a germ-free environment produce reduced titers of anti-DNA antibodies and show delayed onset of autoimmune manifestations.[253] It has been shown that raising lupus-prone lymphoproliferative (MRL/lpr/lpr) mice in a germ-free environment and feeding them a filtered, antigen-free diet significantly decreases the severity of renal disease.[254] Evidence that an antipneumococcal antibody can spontaneously mutate to become an anti-DNA antibody in an in vitro system,[113] as well as in response to immunization with a pneumococcal antigen in vivo,[114] also supports a close structural relationship between the autoantibody response and a protective antibacterial response. Finally, to further demonstrate the close relationship between a protective antibacterial and autoantibody response in lupus, Kowal[255] generated a combinatorial immunoglobulin expression library in phage from splenocytes of a patient with lupus who was immunized with pneumococcal polysaccharide. Four of eight of the monovalent Fab fragments selected for expression of an SLE-associated idiotype bound both pneumococcal polysaccharide and dsDNA, indicating that a significant portion of the human antipneumococcal response in SLE is cross-reactive with self-antigen.[52]

Molecular mimicry and SHM might be important mechanisms by which exposure to foreign, bacterial antigen can elicit autoantibodies. *Molecular mimicry* refers to a sufficient structural homology between foreign antigen and self-antigen that both antigens are recognized by a single, cross-reactive B cell. The best-known example of this mechanism in autoimmunity is rheumatic fever, in which the antibodies arising in the antistreptococcal response cross-react with cardiac myosin, leading to antibody deposition in cardiac muscle and carditis. A molecular mimic induces an autoantibody response by activating cross-reactive B cells specific for both foreign antigen and self-antigen. These B cells receive T-cell help for autoantibody production from T cells activated by microbial proteins. In support of a possible role for molecular mimicry in induction of anti-DNA antibodies is the rise in autoantibodies seen even in nonautoimmune hosts following infection.[256] Furthermore, nonautoimmune individuals vaccinated with pneumococcal polysaccharide generate antipneumococcal antibodies idiotypically related to anti-DNA antibodies.[220] Infection does not usually lead to self-perpetuating autoimmunity, because the T-cell help available for cross-reactive B cells dissipates after the clearing of the infectious agent. Failure to resolve the autoimmune process induced by a molecular mimic may be due to a defect in re-induction of tolerance or to the persistence of the foreign antigen. Some possible causes for a lack of return to a tolerant state are activation of T cells specific for antigenic epitopes to which T-cell tolerance had never been established (cryptic epitopes),[257] upregulation of co-stimulatory molecules, the presence of immunomodulatory cytokines, and abnormally enhanced intracellular signaling. It is also possible that regulatory cells are critical in the maintenance of peripheral tolerance following antigen activation and may be dysfunctional in SLE.[258,259] Finally, it may be that lupus-specific immune complexes containing RNA or DNA activate dendritic cells to create an immunogenic environment.[260,261]

Peptide antigens that structurally mimic DNA can also elicit an autoantibody response.[262,263] Screening of a phage peptide display library with a pathogenic IgG2b anti-dsDNA antibody revealed the D/E WD/E Y S/G consensus motif that is recognized by both murine and human anti-DNA antibodies.[263] DWEYS inhibits the binding of a high percentage of anti-DNA antibodies to dsDNA in vitro and to glomeruli in vivo. Immunization of nonautoimmune BALB/c mice with a multimeric peptide containing the consensus motif induces significant serum titers of IgG anti-dsDNA antibodies as well as antihistone, anti-Sm/RNP, and anticardiolipin antibodies. Monoclonal antibodies from peptide-immunized BALB/c mice resemble anti-dsDNA antibodies present in spontaneous murine lupus, with similar V_H and V_L gene usage, and exhibiting arginines in heavy-chain CDR3 regions.[264]

Another possible model for induction of anti-DNA antibodies is by a hapten carrier–like mechanism, in which T cells recognize epitopes of a protein carrier associated with DNA and provide help for autoreactive B cells specific for hapten (DNA). Novel peptide determinants of the protein component of the complex may then be presented by DNA-specific B cells to recruit autoreactive T cells and further perpetuate an immune response. Immunization of nonautoimmune animals with DNA together with DNA-binding proteins such as DNase I,[265] Fus 1 (derived from *Trypanosoma cruzi*),[266] and the polyomavirus transcription factor T antigen[267] results in the generation of anti-dsDNA antibodies with structural similarity to anti-dsDNA antibodies present in spontaneous murine lupus.

There are several studies demonstrating autoreactive T cells in SLE. Investigators have identified T cells in SNF1 lupus-prone mice that are pathogenic in vivo and accelerate the development of an immune complex glomerulonephritis in mice.[268] Many of these pathogenic T-cell clones were found to respond to nucleosomal antigens, specifically histone peptides. Stimulating these T-cell clones with the histone peptides leads to increased anti-DNA antibody secretion in a B-T cell co-culture system, and peptide immunization in vivo induces severe glomerulonephritis.[269] Other investigators have focused on the immunogenicity of peptides derived from the V_H regions of anti-DNA antibodies themselves.[270,271] One of the studies reported that three V_H-derived 12-mer peptides induce a class II restricted proliferation of unprimed T cells from preautoimmune NZB X New Zealand white (NZW) F1 mice.[270] Immunization of NZBxNZW F1 mice with one peptide, or transfer of a T-cell line reactive with this peptide, increased the titer of anti-dsDNA antibodies and the severity of the nephritis. Further support for a possible role of self-peptide in induction of anti-dsDNA antibodies can be found in studies showing that tolerization with self-peptides can downregulate anti-dsDNA antibody production and nephritis in murine lupus.[271-273] This observation suggests a potential therapeutic strategy in SLE.

Because antiidiotypic antibodies can function like antigen to induce an antibody response, some investigators have emphasized a potential role for antiidiotype in activating autoantibody production. For example, the Ku antigen is a DNA-binding protein.[274] Studies of anti-DNA and anti-Ku antibodies suggest that the anti-Ku antibodies are antiidiotypic to anti-DNA antibodies.[275] Several studies have found that mice immunized with an anti-DNA antibody and mice immunized with an antiidiotypic antibody to an anti-DNA antibody each develop autoantibodies.[276,277] This development has also been shown for other autoantigen-autoantibody systems important in lupus, such as anticardiolipin antibodies.[278] Interestingly, immunization with antibodies recognizing a DNA-binding protein (anti-p53 antibodies) can generate anti-DNA antibodies.[279] Although such studies suggest that the idiotypic network may contribute to the production of autoantibodies, others have suggested that antiidiotypes may function to induce or maintain clinical remissions and that the failure to generate an antiidiotypic response may perpetuate autoantibody production.[280] There is some evidence to suggest that nucleic acids can induce anti-dsDNA antibodies (see later). Although investigators have long known that mammalian dsDNA is poorly immunogenic, later studies have focused on bacterial DNA as a potential trigger for induction of anti-dsDNA antibodies. Bacterial DNA contains unmethylated CpG motifs, which can bind to and activate TLR9 and may be an important adjuvant in the immune system.[281] Preautoimmune lupus-prone mice immunized with bacterial DNA produce antibodies that not only bind to the immunizing antigen, but also are cross-reactive with mammalian DNA.[282] However, the response of nonautoimmune mice to bacterial DNA is non–cross-reactive, indicating that bacterial DNA alone is not sufficient to induce anti-dsDNA antibodies in a non–lupus-prone host. Although mammalian DNA contains fewer CpG motifs, these motifs are present and can activate TLR9 and perhaps other TLRs or scavenger receptors that are involved in dendritic cell activation. Failure to clear DNA properly and degrade it to nonimmunogenic fragments may contribute to production of anti-DNA antibody. In the pristane-induced model of SLE, anti-DNA antibodies arise in a TLR-dependent fashion, but the initial impetus appears to be inflammation with enhancement of TLR signaling rather than enhanced presentation of self-antigen.

Autoantibody responses to DNA and other nuclear antigens are often simultaneously present in established SLE (Ro/La, Sm/RNP). Longitudinal studies begun early in the disease course demonstrate that a particular response may initially be limited to a particular peptide epitope and may be followed by intramolecular (other epitopes in the same polypeptide) and intermolecular (epitopes in distinct, but structurally linked molecules) spread of the response.[283] This process, termed *epitope spreading,* is the result of processing by antigen-presenting cells (including B cells) of the multimolecular complex and of presentation of novel epitopes to nontolerized T cells. The initial target for epitope spreading may be a molecular mimic derived from a microorganism or a self-antigen. Some data have suggested that apoptosis can generate novel nuclear autoantigen fragments[284] that may become accessible to interaction with antibody molecules by translocation to the cell surface.[214,285] Neoepitopes of particular antigens generated by specific forms of apoptosis, for example, granzyme induced rather than caspase involved, might also explain defined autoantibody profiles that are associated with SLE.

The potential role for epitope spreading in diversification of the autoantibody response in SLE has been clearly demonstrated for the anti-Sm response. James and Harley[286] identified two B/B′ octapeptides that were early targets of an anti-Sm response in patients with lupus. Over time, rabbits[287] and some inbred mouse strains[286] immunized with one of these octapeptides, PPPGMRPP, develop an immune response against other regions of Sm B/B′ and Sm D. Furthermore, in some animals antinuclear antibodies and anti-dsDNA antibodies also arise. B-cell epitope spreading has also been demonstrated in the Ro/La autoantigen system.[288]

B-CELL TOLERANCE

Several transgenic mouse models have been described in which immunoglobulin V regions encoding anti-DNA or other autoantibodies have been introduced into the germline. The importance of these models is multifold: (1) they afford perhaps the best direct evidence that certain anti-DNA antibodies are pathogenic, (2) they have contributed significantly to understanding the tolerizing mechanisms that regulate anti-DNA–producing B cells and the defects that allow the survival and activation of these cells, and (3) they provide models in which to test novel therapies designed to block tissue injury or inactivate pathogenic B cells.

B cells expressing autoreactive immunoglobulin arise in all hosts at times of B-cell receptor diversification, both during formation of the naïve B-cell repertoire and again during the germinal center response. Regulation of these autoreactive receptors occurs through inactivation or deletion (Box 8-3).[289] These mechanisms appear to operate when membrane immunoglobulins are cross-linked by antigen in the absence of T-cell help or co-stimulatory influences. Whether anergy or deletion occurs depends in part on the extent of membrane immunoglobulin cross-linking.[290] Normally, the serum of nonautoimmune mice does not contain high-affinity IgG autoantibodies, illustrating that the normal immune system can efficiently regulate autoantibody-producing B cells. Initial studies of anti-DNA transgenic nonautoimmune mice showed that anti-DNA antibodies are eliminated from the immune repertoire through functional inactivation (i.e., anergy) or deletion.[291,292] In lupus-prone mice, there appears to be a defect in some aspects of regulation, allowing the

autoreactive B cells to survive and contribute to the expressed antibody repertoire. A later study demonstrated that "ignorance" is an additional possible fate of DNA-binding B cells.[293] Bynoe[293] isolated low-affinity, DNA-binding B cells from a nonautoimmune mouse transgenic for an anti-DNA heavy chain. These B cells were in a resting state and produced unmutated, nonpathogenic antibodies. These cells may be a potential source of pathogenic autoantibodies; they may be recruited into an ongoing immune response and then become high-affinity (and pathogenic) antibodies through somatic mutation.

Studies have also now shown that an overabundance of molecules that rescue B cells from negative selection leads to the development of a lupus-like serology in mice. BAFF, a B-cell survival factor, is critical to the ability of transitional B cells to acquire a mature B cell phenotype and achieve immunocompetence. BAFF overexpression, however, leads to the survival of autoreactive B cells that would normally be deleted at an immature stage of development. Presumably, BAFF receptor activation impedes the apoptotic pathway triggered by BCR engagement.

Activation of TLR9 or TLR7 in B cells by DNA-IgG or RNA-IgG immune complexes, respectively, can also rescue B cells from negative selection and induce class-switched anti-DNA or anti-RNA (ribonucleoprotein) antibodies. Moreover, it has been shown that the engagement of the type I IFN receptor on B cells can also lead to B-cell activation by otherwise weak self-DNA and RNA stimulatory signals. Thus, immune complexes and increased IFN exposure that are characteristic of lupus probably contribute to sustaining the maturation and activation of DNA-reactive B cells that might otherwise undergo tolerance induction.[294] Patients with defective IRAK-4 (interleukin-1 receptor–associated kinase 4), MyD88 (myeloid differentiation factor 88), or the endoplasmic reticulum membrane protein UNC-93B—all of which are required for normal TLR signaling—exhibit increased numbers of circulating autoreactive B cells, further supporting the role of TLR in B-cell tolerance.[295]

In humans it has been suggested that B cells expressing antinuclear antibodies (ANAs) and polyreactive antibodies represent 55% to 75% of the repertoire expressed in the bone marrow. The majority of these autoreactive B cells are efficiently removed from the naïve repertoire at an immature stage before exiting the bone marrow.[296] Analysis of the B-cell repertoire from three patients newly diagnosed with SLE showed that autoreactive B cells accounted for 25% to 50% of the total mature naïve B cells, compared with a proportion of 5% to 20% observed in control subjects. Although the study showed a deficiency in removal of autoreactive B cells from the immature and transitional stages, implying a defect in negative selection, the autoantibodies that remained were mostly polyreactive against cytoplasmic antigens, insulin, or ssDNA and rarely against dsDNA. Hence, they may be precursors of lupus B cells, but they are not themselves pathogenic B cells.

Receptor editing (see previous discussion of antibody assembly) is another mechanism that can be used by B cells to maintain tolerance.[297] A second immunoglobulin rearrangement occurs, so that the transgenic heavy chain is paired with an endogenous light chain to generate a V_H-V_L combination that is no longer autoreactive.[298]

Transgenic studies have bred anti-DNA transgenes onto autoimmune genetic backgrounds to enable better understanding of the differential regulation of the anti-dsDNA specificity in lupus-prone mice.[299] An additional innovation has been the application of "knock-in" technology (in which the immunoglobulin transgene is inserted into its proper genetic locus), which provides a more physiologic system in that somatic mutation and isotype switching of the inserted V region may occur.[300-302] No single defect could be identified in tolerance mechanisms (deletion, anergy, receptor editing) to account for the selective expansion of anti-DNA–specific B cells in lupus mice. In fact, it has been reported that autoimmune MRL-lpr/lpr mice can efficiently delete B lymphocytes with a transgenic autoreactive receptor.[303]

Box 8-3 Mechanisms of B-Cell Tolerance

Clonal anergy
Clonal deletion
Clonal ignorance
Receptor editing

Box 8-4 Single Gene Defects Causing Autoimmunity

Molecules involved in apoptosis:
  lpr deficiency
  gld deficiency
  bcl-2 overexpression
Serum amyloid protein deficiency:
  DNAse I deficiency
  C1q deficiency
Signaling molecules:
  CD19 overexpression
  CD22 deficiency
  Lyn deficiency
  SHP-1 (Src homology phosphatase 1) deficiency

It is important to understand that the various thresholds for tolerance induction in autoreactive B cells (deletion, anergy, indifference) are not static but, rather, may be dynamically altered by immune modulators such as cytokines, hormones, and co-stimulatory molecules. Studies of transgenic and knockout mice, engineered to overexpress or be deficient in molecules of interest, have begun to unravel genes and pathways involved in B-cell regulation and B-cell tolerance.

The finding that expression of a lupus-like syndrome in MRL-lpr/lpr and C3H gld/gld mice is due to a single defect in the apoptosis gene *Fas* and Fas ligand, respectively,[304-306] has generated a large amount of interest in examining the role of dysregulated apoptosis in human autoimmunity (Box 8-4). Alterations in *Fas* and Fas ligand have been described in patients with systemic lupus, with some studies describing a correlation with manifestations of disease and clinical activity.[307-311] Interestingly, humans with a variety of defects in the Fas receptor have been described, some of which manifest as significant lymphadenopathy (Canale-Smith syndrome) reminiscent of the lymphoproliferative phenotype of lpr mice with defective *Fas*.[312] Although only a single patient with lupus has been described with a Fas defect, Fas mutations are clearly associated with dysregulated lymphocytes.[313]

Other apoptosis genes have also been implicated in the induction of autoimmunity. Transgenic mice overexpressing bcl-2 have long-lived lymphocytes and enhanced immune responses to immunization and, when the transgene is present on certain genetic backgrounds, spontaneously demonstrate antinuclear antigens and immune complex glomerulonephritis.[314] Enforced bcl-2 expression allows recovery of cross-reactive anti-dsDNA, antipneumococcal antibodies from the primary response of nonautoimmune hosts immunized with a pneumococcal cell wall antigen.[315] Furthermore, normally anergized or deleted autoreactive anti-DNA B cells could be recovered from mice transgenic both for bcl-2 and an anti-dsDNA heavy chain.[316] Hormones can also modify the expressed B-cell repertoire in mice transgenic for an anti-DNA heavy chain and facilitate the recovery of high-affinity B cells.[317] Estrogen upregulates bcl-2 and may be interfering with tolerance induction by this mechanism as well as by decreasing the strength of BCR signaling. Prolactin also permits the survival and activation of DNA-reactive B cells. It appears to act by increasing co-stimulatory pathways that can rescue B cells destined for apoptosis.

Another possible link between apoptosis and autoimmunity can be found in studies showing that altered clearance of apoptotic particles and, persistence of nuclear material in the circulation may induce anti-DNA antibodies. Immunizing nonautoimmune mice intravenously with syngeneic apoptotic cells induces antinuclear antibodies with specificity for cardiolipin and ssDNA.[318] Furthermore, these mice also demonstrate renal immunoglobulin deposition. Other studies demonstrate a role for complement receptors in clearing of apoptotic cells from the circulation, thus perhaps explaining the apparent paradox that humans with a deficiency in early complement components are more susceptible to SLE. Serum markedly enhances the uptake of apoptotic cells by phagocytes; components of both classical and alternative pathways of complement are responsible for the enhanced uptake.[319] Phosphatidylserine on the apoptotic cell surface may activate complement, coating apoptotic cells with C3bi, which facilitates apoptotic cell uptake by complement receptors on macrophages and leads to the degradation of apoptotic material.[319] Clearance of apoptotic cells by a complement receptor–mediated pathway may be important in maintaining self-tolerance to nuclear antigens. Deficiency in complement receptor CD21/CD35 or complement protein C4 in *Fas*-deficient mice[320] and C1q deficiency in normal mice[190] accelerates or induces lupus-like features. C1q binding to apoptotic cells or exposure of anionic proteins on the surfaces of cells undergoing apoptosis, like annexin V, can lead to a proinflammatory cytokine profile of phagocytic macrophages or induce a preferential uptake of these cells by dendritic cells, which can facilitate an autoimmune response.[321,322]

Serum amyloid P may also play a role in handling of chromatin from apoptotic cells. Serum amyloid P–deficient mice spontaneously demonstrate antinuclear antibodies and severe glomerulonephritis, and they display increased anti-DNA antibody levels in response to chromatin immunization.[323] A lupus phenotype occurs in mice with a targeted deletion in DNase 1, an enzyme that may be important in degrading DNA generated by apoptosis.[192] Interestingly, one study has suggested that patients with SLE have significantly lower serum levels of DNase 1 than controls with nephritis from other causes.[324] In mice, the complete phenotypic expression of autoimmunity caused by the lpr defect[325] or the bcl-2 transgene[326] is highly dependent on the genetic background. It seems reasonable to speculate that many of these same genes, bcl-2, and other genes and regulators of apoptosis, in combination with additional as yet unidentified genes, may be sufficient to induce many of the phenotypic features of systemic lupus in humans, although it is evident that defects in *Fas* expression lead to a different human disease.

The B-cell receptor is a complex of surface immunoglobulin with the accessory molecules Igα and Igβ. Following receptor cross-linking by binding of antigen to the BCR, a complex cascade of signaling molecules becomes involved in transducing the signal from the BCR to eventually result in B-cell activation and proliferation, or anergy and death. Abnormalities in signaling pathways can alter thresholds for induction of B-cell tolerance. The BCR is associated with several molecules that make up the B-cell co-receptor complex. CD19 is part of the co-receptor complex and plays a role in regulating signaling thresholds that modulate B-cell activation and autoimmunity.[327] CD19 overexpression leads to an increased strength of the BCR signal, resulting in B-cell hyperresponsiveness and breakdown of peripheral tolerance, as manifested by increased levels of anti-DNA antibodies and rheumatoid factor in mice.[328] CD22 is a B-cell surface glycoprotein that becomes rapidly phosphorylated following BCR cross-linking. CD22 is a negative regulator of BCR signaling, as shown by hyperresponsiveness to receptor signaling in mice deficient for the molecule.[329] CD22-deficient mice display a heightened immune response, increased numbers of B-1 B cells, and serum autoantibodies.[330] The structure of the antigen can determine the nature of the B-cell response. Highly immunogenic antigens can be transformed into tolerogenic antigens by the addition of sialosides, which bind the inhibitory molecules CD22 and Siglec-G.[331] Associated with CD22 are Lyn and SHP-1 (Src homology phosphatase-1). Targeted deletion of the genes encoding either of these molecules also leads to autoimmune manifestations.[332-334] The effects of alterations of these signaling molecules on regulation of tolerance and autoimmunity are evident in mice; however, a definite role for altered signaling in the autoimmune diathesis in patients with lupus remains speculative at this time. Another inhibitory co-receptor of the BCR is FcRIIb, the only Fc receptor expressed on B cells. Levels of expression of this receptor are low on B cells of lupus-prone strains and on memory B cells and plasmablasts of patients with lupus. In mice, increased expressions of FcRIIb in B cells restore immune tolerance.[335]

As mentioned previously, increased prolactin can potentiate autoimmunity by upregulating CD40 on B cells and CD40L on T cells. Engagement of CD40 is another mechanism for blocking the completion of an apoptotic program induced by BCR engagement of immature B cells. Not surprisingly, therefore, overexpression of CD40 in mice can also lead to autoantibody production. Several studies have suggested an increased expression of CD40L on both T and B cells in patients with SLE that may function to prevent B-cell tolerance induction and to enhance activation.[336]

Studies of autoimmune-prone mice and patients with lupus or rheumatoid arthritis have identified several susceptibility genes that appear to alter BCR signaling and modulate B cell tolerance (e.g., PTPN22, FCGR2B, LYN, CD40, CR2, TLR7).[331]

THERAPEUTIC INTERVENTIONS

Classic therapeutic interventions in SLE are characterized by their lack of specificity for B cells making particular pathogenic antibodies. Besides the desired decrease in autoantibody production by B cells, these therapies also cause a more generalized immune suppression, with potentially devastating consequences. There have been, however, several new and intriguing developments in the treatment of SLE (Box 8-5). Important advances in the molecular biology of B lymphocytes and their regulation have improved our understanding of the immunologic mechanisms that mediate B-cell tolerance and offer new opportunities and novel targets for therapeutic manipulation. Although many of these approaches are not selective for autoreactive B cells, they may have the advantage of causing fewer deleterious side effects than conventional cytotoxic therapy. Furthermore, antigen-specific therapies may increase the selectivity of the intervention, offering efficacy while potentially decreasing unwanted side effects.

NON–ANTIGEN-SPECIFIC THERAPIES
Depleting Autoreactive B Cells

BAFF, a member of the tumor necrosis factor family that plays an important role in B-cell survival, is often upregulated in patients with SLE. BAFF can be expressed on the cell surface or secreted mostly by immune cells, including activated T cells, monocytes, macrophages, and dendritic cells. BAFF mediates its signaling through three receptors, BAFF-R, TACI (transmembrane activator and calcium modulator interactor) and BCMA (B-cell maturation antigen). There have also been encouraging results with BAFF blockade in murine SLE. Clinical studies in human lupus with anti-BAFF (belimumab) have

shown significant clinical efficacy through large phase 3 studies,[345] and belimumab is now approved for treatment of active SLE in the United States. Mechanistic studies demonstrated that patients receiving belimumab had modest decreases in anti-dsDNA titers, total B cells, and plasmablasts.[346]

A vast clinical experience in the treatment of non-Hodgkin lymphoma has accumulated on the use of a humanized chimeric antibody specific for human CD20 (rituximab). This pan–B-cell surface marker is expressed on immature and mature B cells but is almost undetectable on plasma cells.[347] Rituximab depletes B cells from peripheral blood but does not eliminate plasma cells. Early open-label studies and case reports showed promise in patients with active lupus; however, the placebo-controlled studies in lupus (EXPLORER trial) and lupus nephritis (LUNAR trial) failed to meet primary and secondary end points. B-cell depletion increases serum BAFF levels, an effect that can rescue autoreactive B cells and may enhance the autoreactive repertoire in patients with lupus. Therefore, it has been proposed that the combination of B-cell depletion with BAFF inhibition might work synergistically in lupus.

Another cytokine that has been targeted as a therapeutic pathway in lupus is type I interferon. Antibodies to IFN-α are in randomized controlled phase 2 studies.

Interfering with T-Cell Help

Because the proliferation of autoreactive B cells and generation of IgG autoantibodies in SLE are T-cell–dependent, current therapeutic approaches include inhibition of lymphocyte proliferation, suppression of T-cell activation, and blockade of the accessory molecules important in B cell–T cell interaction.

Mycophenolate mofetil inhibits inosine monophosphate dehydrogenase, an enzyme important in the de novo synthesis of guanine nucleotides. Inhibition of this metabolic pathway inhibits B-cell and T-cell proliferation and results in immunosuppression.[348] Although mycophenolate mofetil acts as a cytotoxic agent by inhibiting cell division, this effect is relatively selective and limited to lymphocytes. In MRL-lpr/lpr[349] and NZB x NZW F1[350] murine lupus models, mycophenolate mofetil improves renal disease, decreases serum anti-dsDNA antibody levels, and significantly prolongs survival. In a study in human lupus, mycophenolate mofetil showed beneficial effects in the treatment of lupus nephritis.[351]

Rapamycin is an immunosuppressive macrolide drug that inhibits lymphocyte proliferation. Rapamycin binds to a protein kinase important in regulating cell cycle progression.[352] In MRL-lpr/lpr mice, treatment with rapamycin significantly reduces serologic manifestations of lupus as well as tissue damage.[353] Inhibition of co-stimulatory molecules important for T-cell activation was found to be beneficial in lupus. Selective inhibition of the interaction of co-stimulatory molecule B7-CD28 by cytotoxic T-lymphocyte antigen 4 (CTLA-4)–Ig (a recombinant fusion molecule between CTLA-4 and the Fc portion of an immunoglobulin molecule) blocks autoantibody production and prolongs life in NZB X NZW F1 mice, even when given late in the course of disease.[340,341] This intervention prevents T-cell activation, thereby preventing T-cell–dependent B-cell activation. In addition, blocking of CD28 signaling directly impairs survival of long-lived plasma cells.[354] Another member of the CD28 family of co-stimulatory molecules, ICOS, is expressed on activated T cells. Its ligand, ICOSL, is constitutively expressed by B cells. Increased ICOS expression on T cells causes a lupus-like syndrome in mice. Blockade of ICOS/ICOSL interaction impairs the development of follicular T-helper cells and germinal center reactions. In humans, ICOS expression is also elevated on T cells in patients with active SLE. Anti-ICOSL antibody is in clinical trials.

Among other important accessory molecules for B cell–T cell interaction, CD40L (gp39) is also expressed on activated T cells and binds to antigen-specific B cells to transduce a second signal for B-cell proliferation and differentiation (see Figure 8-3) and, as mentioned previously, rescues autoreactive B cells from deletion at an immature stage. A short treatment of young SNF1 lupus-prone mice with a monoclonal antibody to CD40L markedly delays and reduces the incidence of lupus nephritis for long after the antibody has been cleared.[337] Furthermore, treatment of older SNF1 mice with established nephritis reduces the severity of nephritis and prolongs survival.[338] Similarly, treating NZB X NZW F1 mice with anti-CD40L leads to decreased anti-dsDNA antibody titers, less renal disease, and, most importantly, improved survival in comparison with the control group.[339] Simultaneous blockade of B7/CD28 and CD40/CD40L with a short course of CTLA-4–Ig and anti-CD40L was significantly more effective than either intervention alone.[342] Clinical trials with anti-CD40L antibody in lupus were terminated because of a higher incidence of thromboembolic events.[343] Investigation into the possible mechanisms leading to increased thrombosis revealed that human platelets express CD40L, which interacts with integrins. This interaction apparently is important to maintain stability of a platelet thrombus; in the presence of anti-CD40L antibody, preformed platelet clots become unstable and release smaller thrombi. Mechanistic studies performed in a limited number of patients who received this antibody demonstrated, however, decreases in the number of peripheral anti-dsDNA B cells and in the titers of anti-dsDNA antibodies.[344] A clinical trial using CTLA-4–Ig in the treatment of human lupus did not meet the primary or secondary end point but did show evidence of a therapeutic effect. The use of CTLA-4–Ig in conjunction with cyclophosphamide for the treatment of lupus nephritis is being investigated.

Activation and proliferation of effector T cells can also be suppressed by regulatory T cells (Tregs). The peripheral Treg population is a mixture of natural Tregs developed in the thymus and induced Tregs converted extrathymically from peripheral $CD4^+$ T cells. The transcription factor Foxp3 is essential for Treg development and function. Mutations in Foxp3 in mice lead to a fatal autoimmune lymphoproliferative disorder, and those in humans cause a severe autoimmune disease known as immune dysregulation, polyendocrinopathy, enteropathy X-linked syndrome. The importance of Tregs in regulating the development of SLE has been underscored in mouse lupus models showing that a decrease in the number and function of Tregs has been linked to lupus susceptibility genes; depletion of Tregs results in an accelerated autoantibody production, and administration of Tregs could inhibit autoantibody responses. However, efforts to investigate Treg frequency and function in patients with SLE at different phases of disease has generated controversial data, mainly because the markers used to identify Tregs, such as CD25 and Foxp3, are transiently upregulated in activated T cells, which are numerous in patients with SLE. Nevertheless, mesenchymal stem cell transplantation in both mice and humans with active SLE significantly increases $CD4^+oxp3^+$ cells and reverses multiorgan dysfunction. Thus, adoptive Treg therapy may aid additional future strategies for SLE treatment.

ANTIGEN-BASED THERAPIES

There are two theoretical ways by which antigen conjugates might improve the course of disease in lupus. First, antigen conjugates may specifically block pathogenic autoantibodies from binding to their target antigens and initiating a tissue-destructive inflammatory cascade. Second, antigen conjugates may downregulate antigen-specific B cells and induce specific B-cell tolerance, which is ordinarily induced by BCR ligation in the absence of co-stimulation. One such conjugate, polyethylene-glycol with tetrameric oligonucleotides, was administered to BXSB male lupus-prone mice.[355] Treatment decreased the number of anti-dsDNA–producing cells, reduced proteinuria, and significantly increased survival. Early studies with abetimus (LJP-394), which contains four strands of dsDNA bound to a carrier, suggested a decrease in serum anti-dsDNA titers,[356-358] but subsequent randomized clinical trials of the agent failed to show any benefit in the treatment or prevention of renal flares.[359] A putative role for peptides in induction of anti-DNA antibodies has been discussed; these small antigens may also be suitable for therapeutic

use. Intravenous treatment of pre-autoimmune SNF1 mice with nucleosomal peptides postpones the onset of nephritis, whereas long-term treatment of older mice with established disease improves survival.[272] Immunization of mice with peptides derived from anti-dsDNA antibodies have been shown to activate autoreactive T cells that provide help for the production of autoantibodies (discussed previously). Treating NZB X NZW F1 mice with several T-cell peptide epitopes derived from an anti-dsDNA antibody induces T-cell tolerance to these peptides and results in significantly improved renal disease and prolonged mean survival.[273] Similarly, mice treated neonatally with CDR-based peptides acquire resistance to subsequent induction of autoimmunity through the generation of $CD8^+$ regulatory T cells.[271] These results suggest that tolerization to peptides may modulate the immune system and serve as adjunctive therapy in lupus.

The technology of displaying random peptides in phage permits the identification of peptides that function as surrogate antigens to autoantibodies. The selected peptide does not necessarily have to be the actual sequence that is recognized by pathogenic antibody (although it can be). Whether peptide dsDNA mimotopes will be useful in inhibiting polyclonal antibody deposition and/or directly tolerizing pathogenic B cells in lupus mouse models is currently under investigation.

SUMMARY

Sequences of many anti-dsDNA antibodies have been analyzed to see how they differ from the human and murine antibody responses to foreign antigens. As expected from idiotypic studies in SLE, certain V region genes or families are used preferentially in the anti-DNA response. However, observations of restricted gene usage do not differ in principle from those made in the response of nonautoimmune animals to foreign antigen, in which a small number of V regions dominate the response to any particular antigen. No particular gene family is absolutely necessary for the production of autoantibodies; nonetheless, investigation is continuing into genetic polymorphisms in the Ig locus that are associated with human lupus. It appears, however, that all individuals are capable of generating pathogenic autoantibodies; in autoimmune individuals, autoantibodies that have developed high affinity for autoantigen through somatic mutation are present in the expressed B-cell repertoire. This finding appears to primarily reflect a defect in the mechanisms of self-tolerance rather than an abnormality in V-gene repertoire, the process of gene rearrangement, or the process of somatic mutation. Although a defect in central tolerance permitting exodus of autoreactive B cells from the bone marrow (perhaps through lack of proper receptor editing or through aberrant signaling) seems to occur in lupus, it is equally possible that the defect is in peripheral tolerance (in the regulation of B cells maturing in the germinal centers), in which responsible mechanisms are not yet delineated.

The autoantibody response in SLE has the characteristics of an antigen-selected response. Cognate B- and T-cell interactions are crucial to the maturation of pathogenic anti-dsDNA antibodies, which are primarily IgG, are mono- or oligo-specific, and have high affinity for the antigen (dsDNA). Together with the higher than random R:S ratio in the CDRs of many anti-dsDNA antibodies, this finding suggests that the anti-DNA response is both driven and selected by an antigen. Pathogenic IgG anti-dsDNA antibodies in SLE seem to arise from the conventional B-cell lineage, possibly through somatic mutation of genes encoding protective antibodies. There is some speculation that natural autoantibodies, perhaps from the B-1 lineage, also could be precursors for anti-DNA antibodies.

It is clear that more than one constellation of immunologic defects can result in the clinical syndrome collectively known as SLE, and almost certainly there is heterogeneity in the patient population, but advances in understanding aspects of both B-cell biology and disease pathogenesis have led to the development of new potential therapeutic modalities. Integration of inhibition of co-stimulation or antigen-specific therapies into the routine management of patients with systemic lupus has just entered our armamentarium with the approval of anti-BAFF therapy. Other targeted pathways are likely to become available as well in the near future.

References

1. Tan EM. Autoantibodies to nuclear antigens (ANA): their immunobiology and medicine. *Adv Immunol* 33:167–240, 1982.
2. Gharavi AE, Harris EN, Lockshin MD, et al: IgG subclass and light chain distribution of anticardiolipin and anti-DNA antibodies in systemic lupus erythematosus. *Ann Rheum Dis* 47(4):286–290, 1988.
3. Bootsma H, Spronk PE, Ter Borg EJ, et al: The predictive value of fluctuations in IgM and IgG class anti-dsDNA antibodies for relapses in systemic lupus erythematosus. A prospective long-term observation. *Ann Rheum Dis* 56(11):661–666, 1997.
4. Koffler D: Immunopathogenesis of systemic lupus erythematosus. *Annu Rev Med* 25:149–164, 1974.
5. Tan EM, Chan EK, Sullivan KF, et al: Antinuclear antibodies (ANAs): diagnostically specific immune markers and clues toward the understanding of systemic autoimmunity. *Clin Immunol Immunopathol* 47(2):121–141, 1988.
6. Winfield JB, Faiferman I, Koffler D: Avidity of anti-DNA antibodies in serum and IgG glomerular eluates from patients with systemic lupus erythematosus. Association of high avidity antinative DNA antibody with glomerulonephritis. *J Clin Invest* 59(1):90–96, 1977.
7. Spiegelberg HL: Biological activities of immunoglobulins of different classes and subclasses. *Adv Immunol* 19:259–294, 1974.
8. Torres M, May R, Scharff MD, et al: Variable-region-identical antibodies differing in isotype demonstrate differences in fine specificity and idiotype. *J Immunol* 174(4):2132–4212, 2005.
9. Cooper LJ, Shikhman AR, Glass DD, et al: Role of heavy chain constant domains in antibody-antigen interaction. Apparent specificity differences among streptococcal IgG antibodies expressing identical variable domains. *J Immunol* 150(6):2231–2242, 1993.
10. Niles MJ, Matsuuchi L, Koshland ME: Polymer IgM assembly and secretion in lymphoid and nonlymphoid cell lines: evidence that J chain is required for pentamer IgM synthesis. *Proc Natl Acad Sci USA* 92(7):2884–2888, 1995.
11. Sorensen V, Rasmussen IB, Sundvold V, et al: Structural requirements for incorporation of J chain into human IgM and IgA. *Int Immunol* 12(1):19–27, 2000.
12. Maddison PJ: Autoantibodies in SLE. Disease associations. *Adv Exp Med Biol* 455:141–145, 1999.
13. Hendrickson BA, Conner DA, Ladd DJ, et al: Altered hepatic transport of immunoglobulin A in mice lacking the J chain. *J Exp Med* 182(6):1905–1911, 1995.
14. Kabat EA, Wu TT: Attempts to locate complementarity-determining residues in the variable positions of light and heavy chains. *Ann NY Acad Sci* 190:382–393, 1971.
15. Poljak RJ, Amzel LM, Avey HP, et al: Three-dimensional structure of the Fab′ fragment of a human immunoglobulin at 2,8-A resolution. *Proc Natl Acad Sci USA* 70(12):3305–3310, 1973.
16. Padlan EA: Anatomy of the antibody molecule. *Mol Immunol* 31(3):169–217, 1994.
17. Porter RR: The hydrolysis of rabbit gamma-globulin and antibodies with crystalline papain. *Biochem J* 73:119–126, 1959.
18. Nisonoff A, Wissler FC, Lipman LN, et al: Separation of univalent fragments from the bivalent rabbit antibody molecule by reduction of disulfide bonds. *Arch Biochem Biophys* 89:230–244, 1960.
19. Gerstein M, Lesk AM, Chothia C: Structural mechanisms for domain movements in proteins. *Biochemistry* 33(22):6739–6749, 1994.
20. Yamaguchi Y, Kim H, Kato K, et al: Proteolytic fragmentation with high specificity of mouse immunoglobulin G. Mapping of proteolytic cleavage sites in the hinge region. *J Immunol Methods* 181(2):259–267, 1995.
21. Capra JD, Kehoe JM, Winchester RJ, et al: Structure-function relationships among anti-gamma globulin antibodies. *Ann NY Acad Sci* 190:371–381, 1971.
22. Oudin J, Cazenave PA: Similar idiotypic specificities in immunoglobulin fractions with different antibody functions or even without detectable antibody function. *Proc Natl Acad Sci USA* 68(10):2616–2620, 1971.
23. Schiff C, Milili M, Hue I, et al: Genetic basis for expression of the idiotypic network. One unique Ig VH germline gene accounts for the major family of Ab1 and Ab3 (Ab1′) antibodies of the GAT system. *J Exp Med* 163(3):573–587, 1986.
24. Rajewsky K, Takemori T: Genetics, expression, and function of idiotypes. *Annu Rev Immunol* 1:569–607, 1983.
25. Bottomly K: All idiotypes are equal, but some are more equal than others. *Immunol Rev* 79:45–61, 1984.
26. Jerne NK: Towards a network theory of the immune system. *Ann Immunol (Paris)* 125C(1–2):373–389, 1974.
27. Urbain J, Wuilmart C, Cazenave PA: Idiotypic regulation in immune networks. *Contemp Top Mol Immunol* 8:113–148, 1981.
28. Tonegawa S: The Nobel Lectures in Immunology. The Nobel Prize for Physiology or Medicine, 1987. Somatic generation of immune diversity. *Scand J Immunol* 38(4):303–319, 1993.
29. Waldmann TA: The arrangement of immunoglobulin and T cell receptor genes in human lymphoproliferative disorders. *Adv Immunol* 40:247–321, 1987.
30. Early P, Huang H, Davis M, et al: An immunoglobulin heavy chain variable region gene is generated from three segments of DNA: VH, D and JH. *Cell* 19(4):981–992, 1980.
31. Kurosawa Y, Tonegawa S: Organization, structure, and assembly of immunoglobulin heavy chain diversity DNA segments. *J Exp Med* 155(1):201–218, 1982.
32. Sakano H, Maki R, Kurosawa Y, et al: Two types of somatic recombination are necessary for the generation of complete immunoglobulin heavy-chain genes. *Nature* 286(5774):676–683, 1980.
33. Kodaira M, Kinashi T, Umemura I, et al: Organization and evolution of variable region genes of the human immunoglobulin heavy chain. *J Mol Biol* 190(4):529–541, 1986.
34. Walter MA, Surti U, Hofker MH, et al: The physical organization of the human immunoglobulin heavy chain gene complex. *EMBO J* 9(10):3303–3313, 1990.
35. Cook GP, Tomlinson IM: The human immunoglobulin VH repertoire. *Immunol Today* 16(5):237–242, 1995.
36. Berman JE, Mellis SJ, Pollock R, et al: Content and organization of the human Ig VH locus: definition of three new VH families and linkage to the Ig CH locus. *EMBO J* 7(3):727–738, 1988.
37. Pascual V, Capra JD: Human immunoglobulin heavy-chain variable region genes: organization, polymorphism, and expression. *Adv Immunol* 49:1–74, 1991.
38. Honjo T, Habu S: Origin of immune diversity: genetic variation and selection. *Annu Rev Biochem* 54:803–830, 1985.
39. Lewis SM: The mechanism of V(D)J joining: lessons from molecular, immunological, and comparative analyses. *Adv Immunol* 56:27–150, 1994.
40. Schatz DG, Oettinger MA, Baltimore D: The V(D)J recombination activating gene, RAG-1. *Cell* 59(6):1035–1048, 1989.
41. Muraguchi A, Tagoh H, Kitagawa T, et al: Stromal cells and cytokines in the induction of recombination activating gene (RAG) expression in a human lymphoid progenitor cell. *Leuk Lymphoma* 30(1–2):73–85, 1998.
42. Paull TT, Gellert M: The 3′ to 5′ exonuclease activity of Mre 11 facilitates repair of DNA double-strand breaks. *Mol Cell* 1(7):969–979, 1998.
43. van Gent DC, Hiom K, Paull TT, et al: Stimulation of V(D)J cleavage by high mobility group proteins. *EMBO J* 16(10):2665–2670, 1997.
44. Jeggo PA, Taccioli GE, Jackson SP: Menage a trois: double strand break repair, V(D)J recombination and DNA-PK. *Bioessays* 17(11):949–957, 1995.
45. Weaver DT: What to do at an end: DNA double-strand-break repair. *Trends Genet* 11(10):388–392, 1995.
46. Desiderio SV, Yancopoulos GD, Paskind M, et al: Insertion of N regions into heavy-chain genes is correlated with expression of terminal deoxytransferase in B cells. *Nature* 311(5988):752–755, 1984.
47. Feeney AJ: Lack of N regions in fetal and neonatal mouse immunoglobulin V-D-J junctional sequences. *J Exp Med* 172(5):1377–1390, 1990.
48. Schable KF, Zachau HG: The variable genes of the human immunoglobulin kappa locus. *Biol Chem Hoppe Seyler* 374(11):1001–1022, 1993.
49. Jaenichen HR, Pech M, Lindenmaier W, et al: Composite human VK genes and a model of their evolution. *Nucleic Acids Res* 12(13):5249–5263, 1984.
50. Klobeck HG, Meindl A, Combriato G, et al: Human immunoglobulin kappa light chain genes of subgroups II and III. *Nucleic Acids Res* 13(18):6499–6513, 1985.
51. Klobeck HG, Bornkamm GW, Combriato G, et al: Subgroup IV of human immunoglobulin K light chains is encoded by a single germline gene. *Nucleic Acids Res* 13(18):6515–6529, 1985.
52. Meindl A, Klobeck HG, Ohnheiser R, et al: The V kappa gene repertoire in the human germ line. *Eur J Immunol* 20(8):1855–1863, 1990.
53. Frippiat JP, Lefranc MP: Genomic organisation of 34 kb of the human immunoglobulin lambda locus (IGLV): restriction map and sequences of new V lambda III genes. *Mol Immunol* 31(9):657–670, 1994.

54. Chuchana P, Blancher A, Brockly F, et al: Definition of the human immunoglobulin variable lambda (IGLV) gene subgroups. *Eur J Immunol* 20(6):1317–1325, 1990.

55. Solomon A, Weiss DT: Serologically defined V region subgroups of human lambda light chains. *J Immunol* 139(3):824–830, 1987.

56. Lai E, Wilson RK, Hood LE: Physical maps of the mouse and human immunoglobulin-like loci. *Adv Immunol* 46:1–59, 1989.

57. Ch'ang LY, Yen CP, Besl L, et al: Identification and characterization of a functional human Ig V lambda VI germline gene. *Mol Immunol* 31(7):531–536, 1994.

58. Heller M, Owens JD, Mushinski JF, et al: Amino acids at the site of V kappa-J kappa recombination not encoded by germline sequences. *J Exp Med* 166(3):637–646, 1987.

59. Chen J, Shinkai Y, Young F, et al: Probing immune functions in RAG-deficient mice. *Curr Opin Immunol* 6(2):313–319, 1994.

60. Schwarz K, Gauss GH, Ludwig L, et al: RAG mutations in human B cell-negative SCID. *Science* 274(5284):97–99, 1996.

61. Abe T, Tsuge I, Kamachi Y, et al: Evidence for defects in V(D)J rearrangements in patients with severe combined immunodeficiency. *J Immunol* 152(11):5504–5513, 1994.

62. Schwarz K, Hansen-Hagge TE, Knobloch C, et al: Severe combined immunodeficiency (SCID) in man: B cell-negative (B-) SCID patients exhibit an irregular recombination pattern at the JH locus. *J Exp Med* 174(5):1039–1048, 1991.

63. Villa A, Santagata S, Bozzi F, et al: Omenn syndrome: a disorder of Rag1 and Rag2 genes. *J Clin Immunol* 19(2):87–97, 1999.

64. Notarangelo LD, Villa A, Schwarz K: RAG and RAG defects. *Curr Opin Immunol* 11(4):435–442, 1999.

65. Gritzmacher CA: Molecular aspects of heavy-chain class switching. *Crit Rev Immunol* 9(3):173–200, 1989.

66. Matsuoka M, Yoshida K, Maeda T, et al: Switch circular DNA formed in cytokine-treated mouse splenocytes: evidence for intramolecular DNA deletion in immunoglobulin class switching. *Cell* 62(1):135–142, 1990.

67. Shimizu A, Honjo T: Immunoglobulin class switching. *Cell* 36(4):801–803, 1984.

68. Davis MM, Kim SK, Hood LE: DNA sequences mediating class switching in alpha-immunoglobulins. *Science* 209(4463):1360–1365, 1980.

69. Bergman Y, Cedar H: A stepwise epigenetic process controls immunoglobulin allelic exclusion. *Nat Rev Immunol* 4(10):753–761, 2004.

70. Singh N, Bergman Y, Cedar H, et al: Biallelic germline transcription at the kappa immunoglobulin locus. *J Exp Med* 197(6):743–750, 2003.

71. Mostoslavsky R, Singh N, Tenzen T, et al: Asynchronous replication and allelic exclusion in the immune system. *Nature* 414(6860):221–225, 2001.

72. Cherry SR, Baltimore D: Chromatin remodeling directly activates V(D)J recombination. *Proc Natl Acad Sci USA* 96(19):10788–10793, 1999.

73. Hieter PA, Korsmeyer SJ, Waldmann TA, et al: Human immunoglobulin kappa light-chain genes are deleted or rearranged in lambda-producing B cells. *Nature* 290(5805):368–372, 1981.

74. Korsmeyer SJ, Hieter PA, Ravetch JV, et al: Developmental hierarchy of immunoglobulin gene rearrangements in human leukemic pre-B-cells. *Proc Natl Acad Sci USA* 78(11):7096–7100, 1981.

75. Retter MW, Nemazee D: Receptor editing occurs frequently during normal B cell development. *J Exp Med* 188(7):1231–1238, 1998.

76. Melamed D, Benschop RJ, Cambier JC, et al: Developmental regulation of B lymphocyte immune tolerance compartmentalizes clonal selection from receptor selection. *Cell* 92(2):173–182, 1998.

77. Chen C, Prak EL, Weigert M, et al: Editing disease-associated autoantibodies. Immune receptor editing: revise and select. *Cell* 95(7):875–878, 1998.

78. Chen C, Prak EL, Weigert M: Editing disease-associated autoantibodies. *Immunity* 6(1):97–105, 1997.

79. Nemazee D: Receptor editing in B cells. *Adv Immunol* 74:89–126, 2000.

80. Ghia P, Gratwohl A, Signer E, et al: Immature B cells from human and mouse bone marrow can change their surface light chain expression. *Eur J Immunol* 25(11):3108–3114, 1995.

81. Hikida M, Mori M, Takai T, et al: Reexpression of RAG-1 and RAG-2 genes in activated mature mouse B cells. *Science* 274(5295):2092–2094, 1996.

82. Han S, Dillon SR, Zheng B, et al: V(D)J recombinase activity in a subset of germinal center B lymphocytes. *Science* 278(5336):301–305, 1997.

83. Papavasiliou F, Casellas R, Suh H, et al: V(D)J recombination in mature B cells: a mechanism for altering antibody responses. *Science* 278(5336):298–301, 1997.

84. Hikida M, Nakayama Y, Yamashita Y, et al: Expression of recombination activating genes in germinal center B cells: involvement of interleukin 7 (IL-7) and the IL-7 receptor. *J Exp Med* 188(2):365–372, 1998.

85. Rice JS, Newman J, Wang C, et al: Receptor editing in peripheral B cell tolerance. *Proc Natl Acad Sci USA* 102(5):1608–1613, 2005.

86. Berek C, Griffiths GM, Milstein C: Molecular events during maturation of the immune response to oxazolone. *Nature* 316(6027):412–418, 1985.

87. Noelle RJ, Ledbetter JA, Aruffo A: CD40 and its ligand, an essential ligand-receptor pair for thymus-dependent B-cell activation. *Immunol Today* 13(11):431–433, 1992.

88. Allen RC, Armitage RJ, Conley ME, et al: CD40 ligand gene defects responsible for X-linked hyper-IgM syndrome. *Science* 259(5097):990–993, 1993.

89. DiSanto JP, Bonnefoy JY, Gauchat JF, et al: CD40 ligand mutations in x-linked immunodeficiency with hyper-IgM. *Nature* 361(6412):541–543, 1993.

90. Ikematsu H, Harindranath N, Ueki Y, et al: Clonal analysis of a human antibody response. II. Sequences of the VH genes of human IgM, IgG, and IgA to rabies virus reveal preferential utilization of VHIII segments and somatic hypermutation. *J Immunol* 150(4):1325–1337, 1993.

91. Berek C, Milstein C: Mutation drift and repertoire shift in the maturation of the immune response. *Immunol Rev* 96:23–41, 1987.

92. Manser T, Wysocki LJ, Margolies MN, et al: Evolution of antibody variable region structure during the immune response. *Immunol Rev* 96:141–162, 1987.

93. Diamond B, Katz JB, Paul E, et al: The role of somatic mutation in the pathogenic anti-DNA response. *Annu Rev Immunol* 10:731–757, 1992.

94. Radic MZ, Weigert M: Genetic and structural evidence for antigen selection of anti-DNA antibodies. *Annu Rev Immunol* 12:487–520, 1994.

95. van Es JH, Gmelig Meyling FH, van de Akker WR, et al: Somatic mutations in the variable regions of a human IgG anti-double-stranded DNA autoantibody suggest a role for antigen in the induction of systemic lupus erythematosus. *J Exp Med* 173(2):461–470, 1991.

96. Marion TN, Tillman DM, Jou NT, et al: Selection of immunoglobulin variable regions in autoimmunity to DNA. *Immunol Rev* 128:123–149, 1992.

97. Clarke SH, Huppi K, Ruezinsky D, et al: Inter- and intraclonal diversity in the antibody response to influenza hemagglutinin. *J Exp Med* 161(4):687–704, 1985.

98. Clarke SH, Rudikoff S: Evidence for gene conversion among immunoglobulin heavy chain variable region genes. *J Exp Med* 159(3):773–782, 1984.

99. Reynaud CA, Anquez V, Dahan A, et al: A single rearrangement event generates most of the chicken immunoglobulin light chain diversity. *Cell* 40(2):283–291, 1985.

100. Wabl M, Steinberg C: Affinity maturation and class switching. *Curr Opin Immunol* 8(1):89–92, 1996.

101. Cascalho M, Wong J, Steinberg C, et al: Mismatch repair co-opted by hypermutation. *Science* 279(5354):1207–1210, 1998.

102. Wiesendanger M, Kneitz B, Edelmann W, et al: Somatic hypermutation in MutS homologue (MSH)3-, MSH6-, and MSH3/MSH6-deficient mice reveals a role for the MSH2-MSH6 heterodimer in modulating the base substitution pattern. *J Exp Med* 191(3):579–584, 2000.

103. Muramatsu M, Kinoshita K, Fagarasan S, et al: Class switch recombination and hypermutation require activation-induced cytidine deaminase (AID), a potential RNA editing enzyme. *Cell* 102(5):553–563, 2000.

104. Pham P, Bransteitter R, Goodman MF: Reward versus risk: DNA cytidine deaminases triggering immunity and disease. *Biochemistry* 44(8):2703–2715, 2005.

105. Revy P, Muto T, Levy Y, et al: Activation-induced cytidine deaminase (AID) deficiency causes the autosomal recessive form of the hyper-IgM syndrome (HIGM2). *Cell* 102(5):565–575, 2000.

106. Martin A, Bardwell PD, Woo CJ, et al: Activation-induced cytidine deaminase turns on somatic hypermutation in hybridomas. *Nature* 415(6873):802–806, 2002.

107. Okazaki IM, Kinoshita K, Muramatsu M, et al: The AID enzyme induces class switch recombination in fibroblasts. *Nature* 416(6878):340–345, 2002.

108. French DL, Laskov R, Scharff MD: The role of somatic hypermutation in the generation of antibody diversity. *Science* 244(4909):1152–1157, 1989.

109. Griffiths GM, Berek C, Kaartinen M, et al: Somatic mutation and the maturation of immune response to 2-phenyl oxazolone. *Nature* 312(5991):271–275, 1984.

110. Kim S, Davis M, Sinn E, et al: Antibody diversity: somatic hypermutation of rearranged VH genes. *Cell* 27(3 Pt 2):573–581, 1981.

111. Sablitzky F, Wildner G, Rajewsky K: Somatic mutation and clonal expansion of B cells in an antigen-driven immune response. *EMBO J* 4(2):345–350, 1985.

112. Levy Y, Gupta N, Le DF, et al: Defect in IgV gene somatic hypermutation in common variable immuno-deficiency syndrome. *Proc Natl Acad Sci USA* 95(22):13135–13140, 1998.

113. Diamond B, Scharff MD: Somatic mutation of the T15 heavy chain gives rise to an antibody with autoantibody specificity. *Proc Natl Acad Sci USA* 81(18):5841–5844, 1984.

114. Ray SK, Putterman C, Diamond B: Pathogenic autoantibodies are routinely generated during the response to foreign antigen: a paradigm for autoimmune disease. *Proc Natl Acad Sci USA* 93(5):2019–2024, 1996.

115. Hande S, Notidis E, Manser T: Bcl-2 obstructs negative selection of autoreactive, hypermutated antibody V regions during memory B cell development. *Immunity* 8(2):189–198, 1998.

116. Shlomchik MJ, Nemazee DA, Sato VL, et al: Variable region sequences of murine IgM anti-IgG monoclonal autoantibodies (rheumatoid factors). A structural explanation for the high frequency of IgM anti-IgG B cells. *J Exp Med* 164(2):407–427, 1986.

117. Jukes TH, King JL: Evolutionary nucleotide replacements in DNA. *Nature* 281(5732):605–606, 1979.

118. Chang B, Casali P: The CDR1 sequences of a major proportion of human germline Ig VH genes are inherently susceptible to amino acid replacement. *Immunol Today* 15(8):367–373, 1994.

119. Reynaud CA, Garcia C, Hein WR, et al: Hypermutation generating the sheep immunoglobulin repertoire is an antigen-independent process. *Cell* 80(1):115–125, 1995.

120. Betz AG, Neuberger MS, Milstein C: Discriminating intrinsic and antigen-selected mutational hotspots in immunoglobulin V genes. *Immunol Today* 14(8):405–411, 1993.

121. Berek C, Milstein C: The dynamic nature of the antibody repertoire. *Immunol Rev* 105:5–26, 1988.

122. Sharon J, Gefter ML, Wysocki LJ, et al: Recurrent somatic mutations in mouse antibodies to p-azophenylarsonate increase affinity for hapten. *J Immunol* 142(2):596–601, 1989.

123. Herzenberg LA, Stall AM, Lalor PA, et al: The Ly-1 B cell lineage. *Immunol Rev* 93:81–102, 1986.

124. Hardy RR, Carmack CE, Li YS, et al: Distinctive developmental origins and specificities of murine CD5+ B cells. *Immunol Rev* 137:91–118, 1994.

125. Baumgarth N: The double life of a B-1 cell: self-reactivity selects for protective effector functions. *Nat Rev Immunol* 11(1):34–46, 2011.

126. Hippen KL, Tze LE, Behrens TW: CD5 maintains tolerance in anergic B cells. *J Exp Med* 191(5):883–890, 2000.

127. Bikah G, Carey J, Ciallella JR, et al: CD5-mediated negative regulation of antigen receptor-induced growth signals in B-1 B cells. *Science* 274(5294):1906–1909, 1996.

128. Griffin DO, Holodick NE, Rothstein TL: Human B1 cells in umbilical cord and adult peripheral blood express the novel phenotype CD20+ CD27+ CD43+ CD70. *J Exp Med* 208(1):67–80, 2011.

129. Hardy RR, Hayakawa K: CD5 B cells, a fetal B cell lineage. *Adv Immunol* 55:297–339, 1994.

130. Kasaian MT, Casali P: Autoimmunity-prone B-1 (CD5 B) cells, natural antibodies and self recognition. *Autoimmunity* 15(4):315–329, 1993.

131. Hayakawa K, Hardy RR, Honda M, et al: Ly-1 B cells: functionally distinct lymphocytes that secrete IgM autoantibodies. *Proc Natl Acad Sci USA* 81(8):2494–2498, 1984.

132. Conger JD, Sage HJ, Corley RB: Correlation of antibody multireactivity with variable region primary structure among murine anti-erythrocyte autoantibodies. *Eur J Immunol* 22(3):783–790, 1992.

133. Murakami M, Yoshioka H, Shirai T, et al: Prevention of autoimmune symptoms in autoimmune-prone mice by elimination of B-1 cells. *Int Immunol* 7(5):877–882, 1995.

134. Casali P, Burastero SE, Balow JE, et al: High-affinity antibodies to ssDNA are produced by CD-B cells in systemic lupus erythematosus patients. *J Immunol* 143(11):3476–3483, 1989.

135. Casali P, Notkins AL: Probing the human B-cell repertoire with EBV: polyreactive antibodies and CD5+ B lymphocytes. *Annu Rev Immunol* 7:513–535, 1989.

136. Suzuki N, Sakane T, Engleman EG: Anti-DNA antibody production by CD5+ and CD5- B cells of patients with systemic lupus erythematosus. *J Clin Invest* 85(1):238–247, 1990.

137. Linton PJ, Lo D, Lai L, et al: Among naive precursor cell subpopulations only progenitors of memory B cells originate germinal centers. *Eur J Immunol* 22(5):1293–1297, 1992.

138. Mantovani L, Wilder RL, Casali P: Human rheumatoid B-1a (CD5+ B) cells make somatically hypermutated high affinity IgM rheumatoid factors. *J Immunol* 151(1):473–848, 1993.

139. Martin F, Kearney JF: Marginal-zone B cells. *Nat Rev Immunol* 2(5):323–335, 2002.

140. Hao Z, Rajewsky K: Homeostasis of peripheral B cells in the absence of B cell influx from the bone marrow. *J Exp Med* 194(8):1151–1164, 2001.

141. Martin F, Kearney JF: Positive selection from newly formed to marginal zone B cells depends on the rate of clonal production, CD19, and btk. *Immunity* 12(1):39–49, 2000.

142. Weller S, Braun MC, Tan BK, et al: Human blood IgM "memory" B cells are circulating splenic marginal zone B cells harboring a prediversified immunoglobulin repertoire. *Blood* 104(12):3647–3654, 2004.

143. Kruetzmann S, Rosado MM, Weber H, et al: Human immunoglobulin M memory B cells controlling *Streptococcus pneumoniae* infections are generated in the spleen. *J Exp Med* 197(7):939–945, 2003.

144. Viau M, Zouali M: B-lymphocytes, innate immunity, and autoimmunity. *Clin Immunol* 114(1):17–26, 2005.

145. Lacroix-Desmazes S, Kaveri SV, Mouthon L, et al: Self-reactive antibodies (natural autoantibodies) in healthy individuals. *J Immunol Methods* 216(1–2):117–137, 1998.

146. Dighiero G, Lymberi P, Holmberg D, et al: High frequency of natural autoantibodies in normal newborn mice. *J Immunol* 134(2):765–771, 1985.

147. Cairns E, Block J, Bell DA: Anti-DNA autoantibody-producing hybridomas of normal human lymphoid cell origin. *J Clin Invest* 74(3):880–887, 1984.

148. Guilbert B, Dighiero G, Avrameas S: Naturally occurring antibodies against nine common antigens in human sera. I. Detection, isolation and characterization. *J Immunol* 128(6):2779–2787, 1982.

149. Ternynck T, Avrameas S: Murine natural monoclonal autoantibodies: a study of their polyspecificities and their affinities. *Immunol Rev* 94:99–112, 1986.

150. Andrzejewski C, Jr, Rauch J, Lafer E, et al: Antigen-binding diversity and idiotypic cross-reactions among hybridoma autoantibodies to DNA. *J Immunol* 126(1):226–231, 1981.

151. Bell DA, Cairns E, Cikalo K, et al: Antinucleic acid autoantibody responses of normal human origin: antigen specificity and idiotypic characteristics compared to patients with systemic lupus erythematosus and patients with monoclonal IgM. *J Rheumatol Suppl* 14(Suppl 13): 127–131, 1987.

152. Peng Y, Kowalewski R, Kim S, et al: The role of IgM antibodies in the recognition and clearance of apoptotic cells. *Mol Immunol* 42(7):781–787, 2005.

153. Davidson A, Manheimer-Lory A, Aranow C, et al: Molecular characterization of a somatically mutated anti-DNA antibody bearing two systemic lupus erythematosus-related idiotypes. *J Clin Invest* 85(5): 1401–1409, 1990.

154. Baccala R, Quang TV, Gilbert M, et al: Two murine natural polyreactive autoantibodies are encoded by nonmutated germ-line genes. *Proc Natl Acad Sci USA* 86(12):4624–4628, 1989.

155. Hoch S, Schwaber J: Identification and sequence of the VH gene elements encoding a human anti-DNA antibody. *J Immunol* 139(5):1689–1693, 1987.

156. Manser T, Gefter ML: The molecular evolution of the immune response: idiotype-specific suppression indicates that B cells express germ-line-encoded V genes prior to antigenic stimulation. *Eur J Immunol* 16(11): 1439–1444, 1986.

157. Sanz I, Casali P, Thomas JW, et al: Nucleotide sequences of eight human natural autoantibody VH regions reveals apparent restricted use of VH families. *J Immunol* 142(11):4054–4061, 1989.

158. Avrameas S, Ternynck T: The natural autoantibodies system: between hypotheses and facts. *Mol Immunol* 30(12):1133–1142, 1993.

159. Halpern R, Davidson A, Lazo A, et al: Familial systemic lupus erythematosus. Presence of a cross-reactive idiotype in healthy family members. *J Clin Invest* 76(2):731–736, 1985.

160. Isenberg DA, Shoenfeld Y, Walport M, et al: Detection of cross-reactive anti-DNA antibody idiotypes in the serum of systemic lupus erythematosus patients and of their relatives. *Arthritis Rheum* 28(9):999–1007, 1985.

161. Dersimonian H, Schwartz RS, Barrett KJ, et al: Relationship of human variable region heavy chain germ-line genes to genes encoding anti-DNA autoantibodies. *J Immunol* 139(7):2496–2501, 1987.

162. Naparstek Y, Andre-Schwartz J, Manser T, et al: A single germline VH gene segment of normal A/J mice encodes autoantibodies characteristic of systemic lupus erythematosus. *J Exp Med* 164(2):614–626, 1986.

163. Shlomchik M, Mascelli M, Shan H, et al: Anti-DNA antibodies from autoimmune mice arise by clonal expansion and somatic mutation. *J Exp Med* 171(1):265–292, 1990.

164. Marion TN, Bothwell AL, Briles DE, et al: IgG anti-DNA autoantibodies within an individual autoimmune mouse are the products of clonal selection. *J Immunol* 142(12):4269–4274, 1989.

165. Marion TN, Tillman DM, Jou NT: Interclonal and intraclonal diversity among anti-DNA antibodies from an (NZB x NZW)F1 mouse. *J Immunol* 145(7):2322–2332, 1990.

166. O'Keefe TL, Bandyopadhyay S, Datta SK, et al: V region sequences of an idiotypically connected family of pathogenic anti-DNA autoantibodies. *J Immunol* 144(11):4275–4283, 1990.

167. Shlomchik MJ, Aucoin AH, Pisetsky DS, et al: Structure and function of anti-DNA autoantibodies derived from a single autoimmune mouse. *Proc Natl Acad Sci USA* 84(24):9150–9154, 1987.

168. Shlomchik MJ, Marshak-Rothstein A, Wolfowicz CB, et al: The role of clonal selection and somatic mutation in autoimmunity. *Nature* 328(6133):805–811, 1987.

169. Taki S, Schmitt M, Tarlinton D, et al: T cell-dependent antibody production by Ly-1 B cells. *Ann NY Acad Sci* 651:328–835, 1992.

170. Song H, Cerny J: Functional heterogeneity of marginal zone B cells revealed by their ability to generate both early antibody-forming cells and germinal centers with hypermutation and memory in response to a T-dependent antigen. *J Exp Med* 198(12):1923–1935, 2003.

171. Milner EC, Anolik J, Cappione A, et al: Human innate B cells: a link between host defense and autoimmunity? *Springer Semin Immunopathol* 26(4):433–452, 2005.

172. Liu Z, Bethunaickan R, Huang W, et al: Interferon-alpha accelerates murine systemic lupus erythematosus in a T cell-dependent manner. *Arthritis Rheum* 63(1):219–229, 2011.

173. Kim SJ, Caton M, Wang C, et al: Increased IL-12 inhibits B cells' differentiation to germinal center cells and promotes differentiation to short-lived plasmablasts. *J Exp Med* 205(10):2437–2448, 2008.

174. Yu D, Tan AH, Hu X, et al: Roquin represses autoimmunity by limiting inducible T-cell co-stimulator messenger RNA. *Nature* 450(7167):299–303, 2007.

175. Bernasconi NL, Onai N, Lanzavecchia A: A role for Toll-like receptors in acquired immunity: up-regulation of TLR9 by BCR triggering in naive B cells and constitutive expression in memory B cells. *Blood* 101(11):4500–4504, 2003.

176. Leadbetter EA, Rifkin IR, Hohlbaum AM, et al: Chromatin-IgG complexes activate B cells by dual engagement of IgM and Toll-like receptors. *Nature* 416(6881):603–607, 2002.

177. Viglianti GA, Lau CM, Hanley TM, et al: Activation of autoreactive B cells by CpG dsDNA. *Immunity* 19(6):837–847, 2003.

178. Vabulas RM, Wagner H, Schild H: Heat shock proteins as ligands of Toll-like receptors. *Curr Top Microbiol Immunol* 270:169–184, 2002.

179. Shlomchik MJ: Activating systemic autoimmunity: B's, T's, and tolls. *Curr Opin Immunol* 21(6):626–633, 2009.

180. Lenert P, Brummel R, Field EH, et al: TLR-9 activation of marginal zone B cells in lupus mice regulates immunity through increased IL-10 production. *J Clin Immunol* 25(1):29–40, 2005.

181. Houssiau FA, Lefebvre C, Vanden BM, et al: Serum interleukin 10 titers in systemic lupus erythematosus reflect disease activity. *Lupus* 4(5):393–395, 1995.

182. Park YB, Lee SK, Kim DS, et al: Elevated interleukin-10 levels correlated with disease activity in systemic lupus erythematosus. *Clin Exp Rheumatol* 16(3):283–288, 1998.

183. Llorente L, Richaud-Patin Y, Garcia-Padilla C, et al: Clinical and biologic effects of anti-interleukin-10 monoclonal antibody administration in systemic lupus erythematosus. *Arthritis Rheum* 43(8):1790–1800, 2000.

184. Ishida H, Muchamuel T, Sakaguchi S, et al: Continuous administration of anti-interleukin 10 antibodies delays onset of autoimmunity in NZB/W F1 mice. *J Exp Med* 179(1):305–310, 1994.

185. Yin Z, Bahtiyar G, Zhang N, et al: IL-10 regulates murine lupus. *J Immunol* 169(4):2148–2155, 2002.

186. Mauri C, Blair PA: Regulatory B cells in autoimmunity: developments and controversies. *Nat Rev Rheumatol* 6(11):636–643, 2010.

187. Evans JG, Chavez-Rueda KA, Eddaoudi A, et al: Novel suppressive function of transitional 2 B cells in experimental arthritis. *J Immunol* 178(12):7868–7878, 2007.

188. Tsao BP, Ohnishi K, Cheroutre H, et al: Failed self-tolerance and autoimmunity in IgG anti-DNA transgenic mice. *J Immunol* 149(1):350–358, 1992.

189. Mackay F, Woodcock SA, Lawton P, et al: Mice transgenic for BAFF develop lymphocytic disorders along with autoimmune manifestations. *J Exp Med* 190(11):1697–1710, 1999.

190. Botto M, Dell'Agnola C, Bygrave AE, et al: Homozygous C1q deficiency causes glomerulonephritis associated with multiple apoptotic bodies. *Nat Genet* 19(1):56–59, 1998.

191. Ehrenstein MR, Cook HT, Neuberger MS: Deficiency in serum immunoglobulin (Ig)M predisposes to development of IgG autoantibodies. *J Exp Med* 191(7):1253–1258, 2000.

192. Napirei M, Karsunky H, Zevnik B, et al: Features of systemic lupus erythematosus in Dnase1-deficient mice. *Nat Genet* 25(2):177–181, 2000.

193. Raz E, Brezis M, Rosenmann E, et al: Anti-DNA antibodies bind directly to renal antigens and induce kidney dysfunction in the isolated perfused rat kidney. *J Immunol* 142(9):3076–3082, 1989.

194. Bernstein K, Bolshoun D, Gilkeson G, et al: Detection of glomerular-binding immune elements in murine lupus using a tissue-based ELISA. *Clin Exp Immunol* 91(3):449–455, 1993.

195. Madaio MP, Carlson J, Cataldo J, et al: Murine monoclonal anti-DNA antibodies bind directly to glomerular antigens and form immune deposits. *J Immunol* 138(9):2883–2889, 1987.

196. Vlahakos DV, Foster MH, Adams S, et al: Anti-DNA antibodies form immune deposits at distinct glomerular and vascular sites. *Kidney Int* 41(6):1690–1700, 1992.

197. Ohnishi K, Ebling FM, Mitchell B, et al: Comparison of pathogenic and non-pathogenic murine antibodies to DNA: antigen binding and structural characteristics. *Int Immunol* 6(6):817–830, 1994.

198. Putterman C, Limpanasithikul W, Edelman M, et al: The double edged sword of the immune response: mutational analysis of a murine anti-pneumococcal, anti-DNA antibody. *J Clin Invest* 97(10):2251–2259, 1996.

199. Waters ST, McDuffie M, Bagavant H, et al: Breaking tolerance to double stranded DNA, nucleosome, and other nuclear antigens is not required for the pathogenesis of lupus glomerulonephritis. *J Exp Med* 199(2):255–264, 2004.

200. Boutjdir M, Chen L, Zhang ZH, et al: Arrhythmogenicity of IgG and anti-52-kD SSA/Ro affinity-purified antibodies from mothers of children with congenital heart block. *Circ Res* 80(3):354–362, 1997.

201. Miranda-Carus ME, Boutjdir M, Tseng CE, et al: Induction of antibodies reactive with SSA/Ro-SSB/La and development of congenital heart block in a murine model. *J Immunol* 161(11):5886–5892, 1998.

202. Mazel JA, el-Sherif N, Buyon J, et al: Electrocardiographic abnormalities in a murine model injected with IgG from mothers of children with congenital heart block. *Circulation* 99(14):1914–1918, 1999.

203. Pierangeli SS, Liu XW, Barker JH, et al: Induction of thrombosis in a mouse model by IgG, IgM and IgA immunoglobulins from patients with the antiphospholipid syndrome. *Thromb Haemost* 74(5):1361–1367, 1995.

204. Ikematsu W, Luan FL, La RL, et al: Human anticardiolipin monoclonal autoantibodies cause placental necrosis and fetal loss in BALB/c mice. *Arthritis Rheum* 41(6):1026–1039, 1998.

205. Piona A, La RL, Tincani A, et al: Placental thrombosis and fetal loss after passive transfer of mouse lupus monoclonal or human polyclonal anti-cardiolipin antibodies in pregnant naive BALB/c mice. *Scand J Immunol* 41(5):427–432, 1995.

206. Fossati-Jimack L, Ioan-Facsinay A, Reininger L, et al: Markedly different pathogenicity of four immunoglobulin G isotype-switch variants of an antierythrocyte autoantibody is based on their capacity to interact in vivo with the low-affinity Fcgamma receptor III. *J Exp Med* 191(8):1293–1302, 2000.

207. Papoian R, Pillarisetty R, Talal N: Immunological regulation of spontaneous antibodies to DNA and RNA. II. Sequential switch from IgM to IgG in NZB/NZW F1 mice. *Immunology* 32(1):75–79, 1977.

208. Neuwirth R, Singhal P, Diamond B, et al: Evidence for immunoglobulin Fc receptor-mediated prostaglandin2 and platelet-activating factor formation by cultured rat mesangial cells. *J Clin Invest* 82(3):936–944, 1988.

209. Lopez-Soto A, Cervera R, Font J, et al: Isotype distribution and clinical significance of antibodies to cardiolipin, phosphatidic acid, phosphatidylinositol and phosphatidylserine in systemic lupus erythematosus: prospective analysis of a series of 92 patients. *Clin Exp Rheumatol* 15(2):143–149, 1997.

210. Vlahakos D, Foster MH, Ucci AA, et al: Murine monoclonal anti-DNA antibodies penetrate cells, bind to nuclei, and induce glomerular proliferation and proteinuria in vivo. *J Am Soc Nephrol* 2(8):1345–1354, 1992.

211. Yanase K, Smith RM, Puccetti A, et al: Receptor-mediated cellular entry of nuclear localizing anti-DNA antibodies via myosin 1. *J Clin Invest* 100(1):25–31, 1997.

212. Koscec M, Koren E, Wolfson-Reichlin M, et al: Autoantibodies to ribosomal P proteins penetrate into live hepatocytes and cause cellular dysfunction in culture. *J Immunol* 159(4):2033–2041, 1997.

213. Miranda ME, Tseng CE, Rashbaum W, et al: Accessibility of SSA/Ro and SSB/La antigens to maternal autoantibodies in apoptotic human fetal cardiac myocytes. *J Immunol* 161(9):5061–5069, 1998.

214. Casciola-Rosen LA, Anhalt G, Rosen A: Autoantigens targeted in systemic lupus erythematosus are clustered in two populations of surface structures on apoptotic keratinocytes. *J Exp Med* 179(4):1317–1330, 1994.

215. Tadmor B, Putterman C, Naparstek Y: Embryonal germ-layer antigens: target for autoimmunity. *Lancet* 339(8799):975–978, 1992.

216. Liao L, Sindhwani R, Rojkind M, et al: Antibody-mediated autoimmune myocarditis depends on genetically determined target organ sensitivity. *J Exp Med* 181(3):1123–1131, 1995.

217. Crary GS, Katz A, Fish AJ, et al: Role of a basement membrane glycoprotein in anti-tubular basement membrane nephritis. *Kidney Int* 43(1):140–146, 1993.

218. Dorner T, Lipsky PE: Molecular basis of immunoglobulin variable region gene usage in systemic autoimmunity. *ClinExpMed* 4(4):159–169, 2005.

219. Gavalchin J, Nicklas JA, Eastcott JW, et al: Lupus prone (SWR x NZB) F1 mice produce potentially nephritogenic autoantibodies inherited from the normal SWR parent. *J Immunol* 134(2):885–894, 1985.

220. Grayzel A, Solomon A, Aranow C, et al: Antibodies elicited by pneumococcal antigens bear an anti-DNA–associated idiotype. *J Clin Invest* 87(3):842–846, 1991.

221. Shoenfeld Y, Vilner Y, Coates AR, et al: Monoclonal anti-tuberculosis antibodies react with DNA, and monoclonal anti-DNA autoantibodies react with *Mycobacterium tuberculosis*. *Clin Exp Immunol* 66(2):255–261, 1986.

222. Kofler R, Noonan DJ, Levy DE, et al: Genetic elements used for a murine lupus anti-DNA autoantibody are closely related to those for antibodies to exogenous antigens. *J Exp Med* 161(4):805–815, 1985.

223. Kworth-Young C, Sabbaga J, Schwartz RS: Idiotypic markers of polyclonal B cell activation. Public idiotypes shared by monoclonal antibodies derived from patients with systemic lupus erythematosus or leprosy. *J Clin Invest* 79(2):572–581, 1987.

224. Monestier M, Bonin B, Migliorini P, et al: Autoantibodies of various specificities encoded by genes from the VH J558 family bind to foreign antigens and share idiotopes of antibodies specific for self and foreign antigens. *J Exp Med* 166(4):1109–1124, 1987.

225. Naparstek Y, Duggan D, Schattner A, et al: Immunochemical similarities between monoclonal antibacterial Waldenstrom's macroglobulins and monoclonal anti-DNA lupus autoantibodies. *J Exp Med* 161(6):1525–1538, 1985.

226. Carroll P, Stafford D, Schwartz RS, et al: Murine monoclonal anti-DNA autoantibodies bind to endogenous bacteria. *J Immunol* 135(2):1086–1090, 1985.

227. Kabat EA, Nickerson KG, Liao J, et al: A human monoclonal macroglobulin with specificity for alpha(2–8)-linked poly-N-acetyl neuraminic acid, the capsular polysaccharide of group B meningococci and *Escherichia coli* K1, which crossreacts with polynucleotides and with denatured DNA. *J Exp Med* 164(2):642–654, 1986.

228. Query CC, Keene JD: A human autoimmune protein associated with U1 RNA contains a region of homology that is cross-reactive with retroviral p30gag antigen. *Cell* 51(2):211–220, 1987.

229. el-Roiey A, Sela O, Isenberg DA, et al: The sera of patients with *Klebsiella* infections contain a common anti-DNA idiotype (16/6) Id and anti-polynucleotide activity. *Clin Exp Immunol* 67(3):507–515, 1987.

230. Limpanasithikul W, Ray S, Diamond B: Cross-reactive antibodies have both protective and pathogenic potential. *J Immunol* 155(2):967–973, 1995.

231. Sanz I, Capra JD: The genetic origin of human autoantibodies. *J Immunol* 140(10):3283–3285, 1988.

232. Trepicchio W, Jr, Barrett KJ: Eleven MRL-lpr/lpr anti-DNA autoantibodies are encoded by genes from four VH gene families: a potentially biased usage of VH genes. *J Immunol* 138(7):2323–2331, 1987.

233. Ash-Lerner A, Ginsberg-Strauss M, Pewzner-Jung Y, et al: Expression of an anti-DNA-associated VH gene in immunized and autoimmune mice. *J Immunol* 159(3):1508–1519, 1997.

234. Radic MZ, Weigert M: Origins of anti-DNA antibodies and their implications for B-cell tolerance. *Ann NY Acad Sci* 764:384–396, 1995.

235. Eilat D, Webster DM, Rees AR: V region sequences of anti-DNA and anti-RNA autoantibodies from NZB/NZW F1 mice. *J Immunol* 141(5):1745–1753, 1988.

236. Yaoita Y, Takahashi M, Azuma C, et al: Biased expression of variable region gene families of the immunoglobulin heavy chain in autoimmune-prone mice. *J Biochem (Tokyo)* 104(3):337–343, 1988.

237. Sanz I, Kelly P, Williams C, et al: The smaller human VH gene families display remarkably little polymorphism. *EMBO J* 8(12):3741–3748, 1989.

238. Souroujon MC, Rubinstein DB, Schwartz RS, et al: Polymorphisms in human H chain V region genes from the VHIII gene family. *J Immunol* 143(2):706–711, 1989.

239. Zouali M, Madaio MP, Canoso RT, et al: Restriction fragment length polymorphism analysis of the V kappa locus in human lupus. *Eur J Immunol* 19(9):1757–1760, 1989.

240. Olee T, Yang PM, Siminovitch KA, et al: Molecular basis of an autoantibody-associated restriction fragment length polymorphism that confers susceptibility to autoimmune diseases. *J Clin Invest* 88(1):193–203, 1991.

241. Huang DF, Siminovitch KA, Liu XY, et al: Population and family studies of three disease-related polymorphic genes in systemic lupus erythematosus. *J Clin Invest* 95(4):1766–1772, 1995.

242. Suzuki N, Harada T, Mihara S, et al: Characterization of a germline Vk gene encoding cationic anti-DNA antibody and role of receptor editing for development of the autoantibody in patients with systemic lupus erythematosus. *J Clin Invest* 98(8):1843–1850, 1996.

243. Davidson A, Manheimer-Lory A, Aranow C, et al: Possible mechanisms of autoantibody production. *Biomed Pharmacother* 43(8):563–570, 1989.

244. Rahman MA, Isenberg DA: Autoantibodies in systemic lupus erythematosus. *Curr Opin Rheumatol* 6(5):468–473, 1994.

245. Manheimer-Lory AJ, Zandman-Goddard G, Davidson A, et al: Lupus-specific antibodies reveal an altered pattern of somatic mutation. *J Clin Invest* 100(10):2538–2546, 1997.

246. Kuo P, Alban A, Gebhard D, et al: Overexpression of bcl-2 alters usage of mutational hot spots in germinal center B cells. *Mol Immunol* 34(14):1011–1018, 1997.

247. Dorner T, Heimbacher C, Farner NL, et al: Enhanced mutational activity of Vkappa gene rearrangements in systemic lupus erythematosus. *Clin Immunol* 92(2):188–196, 1999.

248. Smith DS, Creadon G, Jena PK, et al: Di- and trinucleotide target preferences of somatic mutagenesis in normal and autoreactive B cells. *J Immunol* 156(7):2642–2652, 1996.

249. Shefner R, Kleiner G, Turken A, et al: A novel class of anti-DNA antibodies identified in BALB/c mice. *J Exp Med* 173(2):287–296, 1991.

250. Behar SM, Scharff MD: Somatic diversification of the S107 (T15) VH11 germ-line gene that encodes the heavy-chain variable region of antibodies to double-stranded DNA in (NZB x NZW)F1 mice. *Proc Natl Acad Sci USA* 85(11):3970–3974, 1988.

251. Kuo P, Kowal C, Tadmor B, et al: Microbial antigens can elicit autoantibody production. A potential pathway to autoimmune disease. *Ann NY Acad Sci* 815:230–236, 1997.

252. Steinberg BJ, Smathers PA, Frederiksen K, et al: Ability of the xid gene to prevent autoimmunity in (NZB X NZW)F1 mice during the course of their natural history, after polyclonal stimulation, or following immunization with DNA. *J Clin Invest* 70(3):587–597, 1982.

253. Unni KK, Holley KE, McDuffie FC, et al: Comparative study of NZB mice under germfree and conventional conditions. *J Rheumatol* 2(1):36–44, 1975.

254. Maldonado MA, Kakkanaiah V, MacDonald GC, et al: The role of environmental antigens in the spontaneous development of autoimmunity in MRL-lpr mice. *J Immunol* 162(11):6322–6330, 1999.

255. Kowal C, Weinstein A, Diamond B: Molecular mimicry between bacterial and self antigen in a patient with systemic lupus erythematosus. *Eur J Immunol* 29(6):1901–1911, 1999.

256. Argov S, Jaffe CL, Krupp M, et al: Autoantibody production by patients infected with *Leishmania*. *Clin Exp Immunol* 76(2):190–197, 1989.

257. Moudgil KD, Sercarz EE: The T cell repertoire against cryptic self determinants and its involvement in autoimmunity and cancer. *Clin Immunol Immunopathol* 73(3):283–289, 1994.

258. Monk CR, Spachidou M, Rovis F, et al: MRL/Mp CD4+,CD25− T cells show reduced sensitivity to suppression by CD4+,CD25+ regulatory T cells in vitro: a novel defect of T cell regulation in systemic lupus erythematosus. *Arthritis Rheum* 52(4):1180–1184, 2005.

259. Salaman MR: A two-step hypothesis for the appearance of autoimmune disease. *Autoimmunity* 36(2):57–61, 2003.

260. Means TK, Latz E, Hayashi F, et al: Human lupus autoantibody-DNA complexes activate DCs through cooperation of CD32 and TLR9. *J Clin Invest* 115(2):407–417, 2005.

261. Decker P, Singh-Jasuja H, Haager S, et al: Nucleosome, the main autoantigen in systemic lupus erythematosus, induces direct dendritic cell activation via a MyD88-independent pathway: consequences on inflammation. *J Immunol* 174(6):3326–3334, 2005.

262. Sibille P, Ternynck T, Nato F, et al: Mimotopes of polyreactive anti-DNA antibodies identified using phage-display peptide libraries. *Eur J Immunol* 27(5):1221–1228, 1997.

263. Gaynor B, Putterman C, Valadon P, et al: Peptide inhibition of glomerular deposition of an anti-DNA antibody. *Proc Natl Acad Sci USA* 94(5):1955–1960, 1997.

264. Putterman C, Deocharan B, Diamond B: Molecular analysis of the autoantibody response in peptide-induced autoimmunity. *J Immunol* 164(5):2542–2549, 2000.

265. Marchini B, Puccetti A, Dolcher MP, et al: Induction of anti-DNA antibodies in non autoimmune mice by immunization with a DNA-DNAase I complex. *Clin Exp Rheumatol* 13(1):7–10, 1995.

266. Desai DD, Krishnan MR, Swindle JT, et al: Antigen-specific induction of antibodies against native mammalian DNA in nonautoimmune mice. *J Immunol* 151(3):1614–1626, 1993.

267. Rekvig OP, Moens U, Sundsfjord A, et al: Experimental expression in mice and spontaneous expression in human SLE of polyomavirus T-antigen. A molecular basis for induction of antibodies to DNA and eukaryotic transcription factors. *J Clin Invest* 99(8):2045–2054, 1997.

268. Mohan C, Adams S, Stanik V, et al: Nucleosome: a major immunogen for pathogenic autoantibody-inducing T cells of lupus. *J Exp Med* 177(5):1367–1381, 1993.

269. Kaliyaperumal A, Mohan C, Wu W, et al: Nucleosomal peptide epitopes for nephritis-inducing T helper cells of murine lupus. *J Exp Med* 183(6):2459–2469, 1996.

270. Singh RR, Kumar V, Ebling FM, et al: T cell determinants from autoantibodies to DNA can upregulate autoimmunity in murine systemic lupus erythematosus. *J Exp Med* 181(6):2017–2027, 1995.

271. Waisman A, Ruiz PJ, Israeli E, et al: Modulation of murine systemic lupus erythematosus with peptides based on complementarity determining regions of a pathogenic anti-DNA monoclonal antibody. *Proc Natl Acad Sci USA* 94(9):4620–4625, 1997.

272. Kaliyaperumal A, Michaels MA, Datta SK: Antigen-specific therapy of murine lupus nephritis using nucleosomal peptides: tolerance spreading impairs pathogenic function of autoimmune T and B cells. *J Immunol* 162(10):5775–5783, 1999.

273. Singh RR, Ebling FM, Sercarz EE, et al: Immune tolerance to autoantibody-derived peptides delays development of autoimmunity in murine lupus. *J Clin Invest* 96(6):2990–2996, 1995.

274. Mimori T, Hardin JA: Mechanism of interaction between Ku protein and DNA. *J Biol Chem* 261(22):10375–10379, 1986.

275. Reeves WH, Chiorazzi N: Interaction between anti-DNA and anti-DNA-binding protein autoantibodies in cryoglobulins from sera of patients with systemic lupus erythematosus. *J Exp Med* 164(4):1029–1042, 1986.

276. Mendlovic S, Brocke S, Shoenfeld Y, et al: Induction of a systemic lupus erythematosus-like disease in mice by a common human anti-DNA idiotype. *Proc Natl Acad Sci USA* 85(7):2260–2264, 1988.

277. Mendlovic S, Fricke H, Shoenfeld Y, et al: The role of anti-idiotypic antibodies in the induction of experimental systemic lupus erythematosus in mice. *Eur J Immunol* 19(4):729–734, 1989.

278. Bakimer R, Fishman P, Blank M, et al: Induction of primary antiphospholipid syndrome in mice by immunization with a human monoclonal anticardiolipin antibody (H-3). *J Clin Invest* 89(5):1558–1563, 1992.

279. Erez-Alon N, Herkel J, Wolkowicz R, et al: Immunity to p53 induced by an idiotypic network of anti-p53 antibodies: generation of sequence-specific anti-DNA antibodies and protection from tumor metastasis. *Cancer Res* 58(23):5447–5452, 1998.

280. Abdou NI, Wall H, Lindsley HB, et al: Network theory in autoimmunity. In vitro suppression of serum anti-DNA antibody binding to DNA by anti-idiotypic antibody in systemic lupus erythematosus. *J Clin Invest* 67(5):1297–1304, 1981.

281. Pisetsky DS: The immunologic properties of DNA. *J Immunol* 156(2):421–423, 1996.

282. Gilkeson GS, Pippen AM, Pisetsky DS: Induction of cross-reactive anti-dsDNA antibodies in preautoimmune NZB/NZW mice by immunization with bacterial DNA. *J Clin Invest* 95(3):1398–1402, 1995.

283. Harley JB, James JA: Autoepitopes in lupus. *J Lab Clin Med* 126(6):509–516, 1995.

284. Casciola-Rosen L, Andrade F, Ulanet D, et al: Cleavage by granzyme B is strongly predictive of autoantigen status: implications for initiation of autoimmunity. *J Exp Med* 190(6):815–826, 1999.

285. Golan TD, Elkon KB, Gharavi AE, et al: Enhanced membrane binding of autoantibodies to cultured keratinocytes of systemic lupus erythematosus patients after ultraviolet B/ultraviolet A irradiation. *J Clin Invest* 90(3):1067–1076, 1992.

286. James JA, Harley JB: A model of peptide-induced lupus autoimmune B cell epitope spreading is strain specific and is not H-2 restricted in mice. *J Immunol* 160(1):502–508, 1998.

287. James JA, Gross T, Scofield RH, et al: Immunoglobulin epitope spreading and autoimmune disease after peptide immunization: Sm B/B'-derived PPPGMRPP and PPPGIRGP induce spliceosome autoimmunity. *J Exp Med* 181(2):453–461, 1995.

288. Reynolds P, Gordon TP, Purcell AW, et al: Hierarchical self-tolerance to T cell determinants within the ubiquitous nuclear self-antigen La (SS-B) permits induction of systemic autoimmunity in normal mice. *J Exp Med* 184(5):1857–1870, 1996.

289. Goodnow CC: Transgenic mice and analysis of B-cell tolerance. *Annu Rev Immunol* 10:489–518, 1992.

290. Hartley SB, Crosbie J, Brink R, et al: Elimination from peripheral lymphoid tissues of self-reactive B lymphocytes recognizing membrane-bound antigens. *Nature* 353(6346):765–769, 1991.

291. Offen D, Spatz L, Escowitz H, et al: Induction of tolerance to an IgG autoantibody. *Proc Natl Acad Sci USA* 89(17):8332–8336, 1992.

292. Tsao BP, Chow A, Cheroutre H, et al: B cells are anergic in transgenic mice that express IgM anti-DNA antibodies. *Eur J Immunol* 23(9):2332–2339, 1993.

293. Bynoe MS, Spatz L, Diamond B: Characterization of anti-DNA B cells that escape negative selection. *Eur J Immunol* 29(4):1304–1313, 1999.

294. Avalos AM, Busconi L, Marshak-Rothstein A: Regulation of autoreactive B cell responses to endogenous TLR ligands. *Autoimmunity* 43(1):76–83, 2010.

295. Isnardi I, Ng YS, Srdanovic I, et al: IRAK-4- and MyD88-dependent pathways are essential for the removal of developing autoreactive B cells in humans. *Immunity* 29(5):746–757, 2008.

296. Wardemann H, Nussenzweig MC: B-cell self-tolerance in humans. *Adv Immunol* 95:83–110, 2007.

297. Gay D, Saunders T, Camper S, et al: Receptor editing: an approach by autoreactive B cells to escape tolerance. *J Exp Med* 177(4):999–1008, 1993.

298. Radic MZ, Erikson J, Litwin S, et al: B lymphocytes may escape tolerance by revising their antigen receptors. *J Exp Med* 177(4):1165–1173, 1993.

299. Spatz L, Saenko V, Iliev A, et al: Light chain usage in anti-double-stranded DNA B cell subsets: role in cell fate determination. *J Exp Med* 185(7):1317–1326, 1997.

300. Pewzner-Jung Y, Friedmann D, Sonoda E, et al: B cell deletion, anergy, and receptor editing in "knock in" mice targeted with a germline-encoded or somatically mutated anti-DNA heavy chain. *J Immunol* 161(9):4634–4645, 1998.

301. Friedmann D, Yachimovich N, Mostoslavsky G, et al: Production of high affinity autoantibodies in autoimmune New Zealand Black/New Zealand white F1 mice targeted with an anti-DNA heavy chain. *J Immunol* 162(8):4406–4416, 1999.

302. Brard F, Shannon M, Prak EL, et al: Somatic mutation and light chain rearrangement generate autoimmunity in anti-single-stranded DNA transgenic MRL/lpr mice. *J Exp Med* 190(5):691–704, 1999.

303. Kench JA, Russell DM, Nemazee D: Efficient peripheral clonal elimination of B lymphocytes in MRL/lpr mice bearing autoantibody transgenes. *J Exp Med* 188(5):909–917, 1998.

304. Watanabe-Fukunaga R, Brannan CI, Copeland NG, et al: Lymphoproliferation disorder in mice explained by defects in Fas antigen that mediates apoptosis. *Nature* 356(6367):314–317, 1992.

305. Chu JL, Drappa J, Parnassa A, et al: The defect in Fas mRNA expression in MRL/lpr mice is associated with insertion of the retrotransposon, ETn. *J Exp Med* 178(2):723–730, 1993.

306. Takahashi T, Tanaka M, Brannan CI, et al: Generalized lymphoproliferative disease in mice, caused by a point mutation in the Fas ligand. *Cell* 76(6):969–976, 1994.

307. Suzuki N, Ichino M, Mihara S, et al: Inhibition of Fas/Fas ligand-mediated apoptotic cell death of lymphocytes in vitro by circulating anti-Fas ligand autoantibodies in patients with systemic lupus erythematosus. *Arthritis Rheum* 41(2):344–353, 1998.

308. Courtney PA, Crockard AD, Williamson K, et al: Lymphocyte apoptosis in systemic lupus erythematosus: relationships with Fas expression, serum soluble Fas and disease activity. *Lupus* 8(7):508–513, 1999.

309. van LT, Bijl M, Hart M, et al: Patients with systemic lupus erythematosus with high plasma levels of sFas risk relapse. *J Rheumatol* 26(1):60–67, 1999.

310. McNally J, Yoo DH, Drappa J, et al: Fas ligand expression and function in systemic lupus erythematosus. *J Immunol* 159(9):4628–4636, 1997.

311. Nozawa K, Kayagaki N, Tokano Y, et al: Soluble Fas (APO-1, CD95) and soluble Fas ligand in rheumatic diseases. *Arthritis Rheum* 40(6):1126–1129, 1997.

312. Vaishnaw AK, Toubi E, Ohsako S, et al: The spectrum of apoptotic defects and clinical manifestations, including systemic lupus erythematosus, in humans with CD95 (Fas/APO-1) mutations. *Arthritis Rheum* 42(9):1833–1842, 1999.

313. Drappa J, Vaishnaw AK, Sullivan KE, et al: Fas gene mutations in the Canale-Smith syndrome, an inherited lymphoproliferative disorder associated with autoimmunity. *N Engl J Med* 335(22):1643–1649, 1996.

314. Strasser A, Whittingham S, Vaux DL, et al: Enforced BCL2 expression in B-lymphoid cells prolongs antibody responses and elicits autoimmune disease. *Proc Natl Acad Sci USA* 88(19):8661–8665, 1991.

315. Kuo P, Bynoe M, Diamond B: Crossreactive B cells are present during a primary but not secondary response in BALB/c mice expressing a bcl-2 transgene. *Mol Immunol* 36(7):471–479, 1999.

316. Kuo P, Bynoe MS, Wang C, et al: Bcl-2 leads to expression of anti-DNA B cells but no nephritis: a model for a clinical subset. *Eur J Immunol* 29(10):3168–3178, 1999.

317. Bynoe MS, Grimaldi CM, Diamond B: Estrogen up-regulates Bcl-2 and blocks tolerance induction of naive B cells. *Proc Natl Acad Sci USA* 97(6):2703–2708, 2000.

318. Mevorach D, Zhou JL, Song X, et al: Systemic exposure to irradiated apoptotic cells induces autoantibody production. *J Exp Med* 188(2):387–392, 1998.

319. Mevorach D, Mascarenhas JO, Gershov D, et al: Complement-dependent clearance of apoptotic cells by human macrophages. *J Exp Med* 188(12):2313–2320, 1998.

320. Prodeus AP, Goerg S, Shen LM, et al: A critical role for complement in maintenance of self-tolerance. *Immunity* 9(5):721–731, 1998.

321. Nauta AJ, Castellano G, Xu W, et al: Opsonization with C1q and mannose-binding lectin targets apoptotic cells to dendritic cells. *J Immunol* 173(5):3044–3050, 2004.

322. Gaipl US, Beyer TD, Baumann I, et al: Exposure of anionic phospholipids serves as anti-inflammatory and immunosuppressive signal—implications for antiphospholipid syndrome and systemic lupus erythematosus. *Immunobiology* 207(1):73–81, 2003.

323. Bickerstaff MC, Botto M, Hutchinson WL, et al: Serum amyloid P component controls chromatin degradation and prevents antinuclear autoimmunity. *Nat Med* 5(6):694–697, 1999.

324. Yasutomo K, Horiuchi T, Kagami S, et al: Mutation of DNASE1 in people with systemic lupus erythematosus. *Nat Genet* 28(4):313–314, 2001.

325. Izui S, Kelley VE, Masuda K, et al: Induction of various autoantibodies by mutant gene lpr in several strains of mice. *J Immunol* 133(1):227–233, 1984.

326. Strasser A, Harris AW, Cory S: The role of bcl-2 in lymphoid differentiation and neoplastic transformation. *Curr Top Microbiol Immunol* 182:299–302, 1992.

327. Sato S, Ono N, Steeber DA, et al: CD19 regulates B lymphocyte signaling thresholds critical for the development of B-1 lineage cells and autoimmunity. *J Immunol* 157(10):4371–4378, 1996.

328. Inaoki M, Sato S, Weintraub BC, et al: CD19-regulated signaling thresholds control peripheral tolerance and autoantibody production in B lymphocytes. *J Exp Med* 186(11):1923–1931, 1997.

329. O'Keefe TL, Williams GT, Davies SL, et al: Hyperresponsive B cells in CD22-deficient mice. *Science* 274(5288):798–801, 1996.

330. O'Keefe TL, Williams GT, Batista FD, et al: Deficiency in CD22, a B cell-specific inhibitory receptor, is sufficient to predispose to development of high affinity autoantibodies. *J Exp Med* 189(8):1307–1313, 1999.

331. Basten A, Silveira PA: B-cell tolerance: mechanisms and implications. *Curr Opin Immunol* 22(5):566–574, 2010.

332. Chan VW, Meng F, Soriano P, et al: Characterization of the B lymphocyte populations in Lyn-deficient mice and the role of Lyn in signal initiation and down-regulation. *Immunity* 7(1):69–81, 1997.

333. Westhoff CM, Whittier A, Kathol S, et al: DNA-binding antibodies from viable motheaten mutant mice: implications for B cell tolerance. *J Immunol* 159(6):3024–3033, 1997.

334. Cornall RJ, Cyster JG, Hibbs ML, et al: Polygenic autoimmune traits: Lyn, CD22, and SHP-1 are limiting elements of a biochemical pathway regulating BCR signaling and selection. *Immunity* 8(4):497–508, 1998.

335. McGaha TL, Karlsson MC, Ravetch JV: FcgammaRIIB deficiency leads to autoimmunity and a defective response to apoptosis in Mrl-MpJ mice. *J Immunol* 180(8):5670–5679, 2008.

336. sai-Mehta A, Lu L, Ramsey-Goldman R, et al: Hyperexpression of CD40 ligand by B and T cells in human lupus and its role in pathogenic autoantibody production. *J Clin Invest* 97(9):2063–2073, 1996.

337. Mohan C, Shi Y, Laman JD, et al: Interaction between CD40 and its ligand gp39 in the development of murine lupus nephritis. *J Immunol* 154(3):1470–1480, 1995.

338. Kalled SL, Cutler AH, Datta SK, et al: Anti-CD40 ligand antibody treatment of SNF1 mice with established nephritis: preservation of kidney function. *J Immunol* 160(5):2158–2165, 1998.

339. Early GS, Zhao W, Burns CM: Anti-CD40 ligand antibody treatment prevents the development of lupus-like nephritis in a subset of New Zealand black x New Zealand white mice. Response correlates with the absence of an anti-antibody response. *J Immunol* 157(7):3159–3164, 1996.

340. Finck BK, Linsley PS, Wofsy D: Treatment of murine lupus with CTLA4Ig. *Science* 265(5176):1225–1227, 1994.

341. Mihara M, Tan I, Chuzhin Y, et al: CTLA4Ig inhibits T cell-dependent B-cell maturation in murine systemic lupus erythematosus. *J Clin Invest* 106(1):91–101, 2000.

342. Daikh DI, Finck BK, Linsley PS, et al: Long-term inhibition of murine lupus by brief simultaneous blockade of the B7/CD28 and CD40/gp39 costimulation pathways. *J Immunol* 159(7):3104–3108, 1997.

343. Boumpas DT, Furie R, Manzi S, et al: A short course of BG9588 (anti-CD40 ligand antibody) improves serologic activity and decreases hematuria in patients with proliferative lupus glomerulonephritis. *Arthritis Rheum* 48(3):719–727, 2003.

344. Huang W, Sinha J, Newman J, et al: The effect of anti-CD40 ligand antibody on B cells in human systemic lupus erythematosus. *Arthritis Rheum* 46(6):1554–1562, 2002.

345. Navarra SV, Guzman RM, Gallacher AE, et al: Efficacy and safety of belimumab in patients with active systemic lupus erythematosus: a randomised, placebo-controlled, phase 3 trial. *Lancet* 377(9767):721–731, 2011.

346. Jacobi AM, Huang W, Wang T, et al: Effect of long-term belimumab treatment on B cells in systemic lupus erythematosus: extension of a phase II, double-blind, placebo-controlled, dose-ranging study. *Arthritis Rheum* 62(1):201–210, 2010.

347. Silverman GJ: Anti-CD20 therapy in systemic lupus erythematosus: a step closer to the clinic. *Arthritis Rheum* 52(2):371–377, 2005.

348. Sievers TM, Rossi SJ, Ghobrial RM, et al: Mycophenolate mofetil. *Pharmacotherapy* 17(6):1178–1197, 1997.

349. Jonsson CA, Svensson L, Carlsten H: Beneficial effect of the inosine monophosphate dehydrogenase inhibitor mycophenolate mofetil on survival and severity of glomerulonephritis in systemic lupus erythematosus (SLE)-prone MRL lpr/lpr mice. *Clin Exp Immunol* 116(3):534–541, 1999.

350. McMurray RW, Elbourne KB, Lagoo A, et al: Mycophenolate mofetil suppresses autoimmunity and mortality in the female NZB x NZW F1 mouse model of systemic lupus erythematosus. *J Rheumatol* 25(12):2364–2370, 1998.

351. Gaubitz M, Schorat A, Schotte H, et al: Mycophenolate mofetil for the treatment of systemic lupus erythematosus: an open pilot trial. *Lupus* 8(9):731–736, 1999.

352. Abraham RT: Mammalian target of rapamycin: immunosuppressive drugs uncover a novel pathway of cytokine receptor signaling. *Curr Opin Immunol* 10(3):330–336, 1998.

353. Warner LM, Adams LM, Sehgal SN: Rapamycin prolongs survival and arrests pathophysiologic changes in murine systemic lupus erythematosus. *Arthritis Rheum* 37(2):289–297, 1994.

354. Rozanski CH, Arens R, Carlson LM, et al: Sustained antibody responses depend on CD28 function in bone marrow-resident plasma cells. *J Exp Med* 208(7):1435–1446, 2011.

355. Jones DS, Hachmann JP, Osgood SA, et al: Conjugates of double-stranded oligonucleotides with poly(ethylene glycol) and keyhole limpet hemocyanin: a model for treating systemic lupus erythematosus. *Bioconjug Chem* 5(5):390–399, 1994.

356. Arcon-Segovia D, Tumlin JA, Furie RA, et al: LJP 394 for the prevention of renal flare in patients with systemic lupus erythematosus: results from a randomized, double-blind, placebo-controlled study. *Arthritis Rheum* 48(2):442–454, 2003.

357. Linnik MD, Hu JZ, Heilbrunn KR, et al: Relationship between anti-double-stranded DNA antibodies and exacerbation of renal disease in patients with systemic lupus erythematosus. *Arthritis Rheum* 52(4):1129–1137, 2005.

358. Strand V, Aranow C, Cardiel MH, et al: Improvement in health-related quality of life in systemic lupus erythematosus patients enrolled in a randomized clinical trial comparing LJP 394 treatment with placebo. *Lupus* 12(9):677–686, 2003.

359. Cardiel MH, Tumlin JA, Furie RA, et al: Abetimus sodium for renal flare in systemic lupus erythematosus: results of a randomized, controlled phase III trial. *Arthritis Rheum* 58(8):2470–8240, 2008.

T Cells

José C. Crispín and George C. Tsokos

T cells are central regulators of the immune response through their actions on lymphoid and myeloid cells. By expressing membrane-bound molecules and secreting soluble mediators, they modulate antibody responses, activate innate immune cells, and lyse target cells. Certain T-cell subsets perform suppressive functions and limit the duration of immune responses. Therefore, inadequate T-cell function has widespread repercussions for the immune response.

Extensive evidence indicates that T cells are involved in the pathogenesis of systemic lupus erythematosus (SLE).[1] The phenotype of T cells isolated from patients with SLE is abnormal: SLE T cells partially resemble activated cells and partially behave like anergic (unresponsive) cells.[2] Their response to stimulation through the T-cell receptor (TCR) is exaggerated,[3] and their gene expression profile is altered in comparison with cells obtained from healthy individuals.[4] Moreover, the tolerance breach and self-directed response developed by patients with SLE have all the characteristics of a T-cell–driven immune response, including clonal expansion and somatic hypermutation,[5] and T-cell depletion prevents lupus in murine models.[6] Thus, even though SLE is a complex disease caused by multiple factors, evidence supports the role of T cells as promoters of the pathologic autoimmune response and as direct instigators of target organ damage. The aim of this chapter is to discuss the mechanisms by which T cells contribute to SLE and the intrinsic abnormalities that alter the behavior of the SLE T cells contributing to their pathogenicity.

ROLE OF T CELLS IN AUTOIMMUNITY AND INFLAMMATION

Help to B Cells

CD4+ T cells regulate production of antibodies in germinal centers (GCs), specialized lymphoid structures where B-cell proliferation and differentiation occur simultaneously with isotype switching and somatic hypermutation. In normal immune responses, these processes ensure the selection of high-affinity antibodies and memory B cells. In patients with SLE, the response to autoantigens and the development of high-affinity autoantibodies are poorly understood. However, the fact that the autoantibodies are mostly high-affinity immunoglobulin (Ig) G that have undergone somatic hypermutation suggests that they have developed in GCs or analogous structures.[7] Moreover, the presence of certain activated B-cell subsets in the peripheral blood of patients with SLE has been proposed to reflect increased GC activity,[8] probably related to increased CD40 ligand (CD40L) expression.[9]

Follicular T-helper cells (T_{FH} cells) represent the CD4+ helper subset specialized in providing help to B cells in GCs (Figure 9-1)[10] T_{FH} differentiate from naïve CD4+ T cells activated in the presence of interleukins IL-6 and IL-21 and co-stimulation through the co-stimulatory molecule ICOS. T_{FH} cells localize to lymph node B cell zones and induce isotype switching and somatic hypermutation through IL-21 and CD40L.[10] Their pathogenic capacity was shown in mice deficient in the ubiquitin ligase roquin. These mice demonstrated an expansion of T_{FH} cells and systemic lupus-like autoimmunity.[11] On the other hand, a mutation that disrupted the capacity of regulatory CD8+ T cells to suppress T_{FH} cells also triggered autoimmunity.[12] IL-21 and T_{FH} cells have been shown to play a role in disease development in murine models of lupus.[13-15] In lupus-prone B6-Yaa mice, defective CD8 regulatory function was associated with increased T_{FH} activity and systemic autoimmunity.[16] In MRL/*lpr* mice, deficiency of ICOS was protective because of the loss of extrafollicular T helper cells, an analogous CD4+ subset that promotes antibody production in extrafollicular compartments in autoimmune mice.[13] A subset of patients with SLE was shown to have increased numbers of T_{FH} cells in the peripheral blood, suggesting that indeed overactivation of this T-cell subset could be involved in human SLE.[17] The aforementioned studies, along with the presence of high titers of high-affinity IgG autoantibodies in most patients with lupus, indicate that T-cell–driven B-cell hyperactivity is an key event in the self-directed immune response that underlies pathology in patients with SLE.[18]

Production of IL-10, another cytokine able to promote B-cell function, is increased in patients with SLE.[19] In certain populations, high IL-10 production has been associated with polymorphisms of the *Il10* gene. IL-10 stimulates B cells and promotes immunoglobulin production by mononuclear cells of patients with SLE.[20] Interestingly, in patients with SLE most IL-10 derives from B cells and monocytes. Blockade of IL-10 delayed disease in NZB/NZW mice[21] and led to joint and skin disease improvement in a small group of patients with SLE,[22] suggesting that it may indeed play a role in disease pathogenesis.

Promotion of Inflammation

Inflammation is controlled locally by the regulation of vascular permeability and tissue access to immune cells. T cells from patients with SLE produce large amounts of proinflammatory cytokines and express high levels of adhesion molecules. A 2011 study highlighted the prognostic importance of kidney tubulointerstitial infiltrates in patients with SLE, emphasizing the relevance of target organ infiltration by immune cells.[23]

Th17 cells are a cell subset generated from naïve CD4+ T cells activated in the presence of transforming growth factor beta (TGF-β) and certain proinflammatory cytokines, including IL-1β, IL-6, and IL-21.[24] Th17 cells induce inflammation through the release of IL-17A, IL-17F, and IL-22. Abnormally high levels of IL-17 are found in the serum of patients with SLE.[25] Accordingly, abnormally high numbers of T cells produce IL-17 in patients with SLE.[26,27] In lupus, however, Th17 CD4+ cells are not the only relevant source of IL-17, because expansion of a normally rare IL-17–producing T-cell population that lacks CD4 and CD8 (hence called double-negative, DN) is common.[26] The heightened production of IL-17 in patients with SLE correlates with disease activity.[25] Further, IL-17–producing T cells have been found within kidney infiltrates from patients with lupus nephritis.[26]

IL-17 production is also increased in murine models of lupus. Spleen cells from SNF1 mice produce high amounts of IL-17 in the presence of nucleosomes.[28] As in patients, IL-17–producing T cells have been found in kidneys of mice with lupus-like nephritis.[28,29]

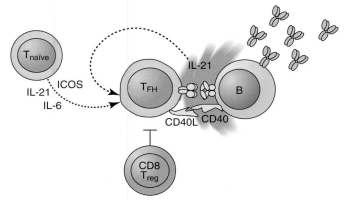

FIGURE 9-1 T follicular helper cells (T_{FH}) are the CD4 subset specialized in providing help to B cells. Naïve CD4$^+$ T cells become T_{FH} cells when they are primed in the presence of interleukin IL-6 and/or IL-21 and receive co-stimulation through the co-stimulatory molecule ICOS. T_{FH} cells migrate to the B-cell zone of lymph nodes thanks to their expression of CXCR5. They provide help to B cells by producing IL-21 and expressing CD40 ligand (CD40L). In mice, CD8$^+$ regulatory T cells limit T_{FH} cell numbers and function. Increased activity or decreased suppression of T_{FH} cells causes a lupus-like disease in mice. Indirect evidence suggests that in human SLE, activity of T_{FH} cells is augmented.

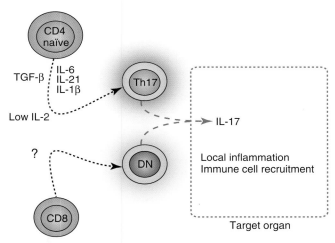

FIGURE 9-2 Generation of proinflammatory T-cell subsets able to produce interleukin 17 (IL-17) and infiltrate target organs contributes to SLE pathogenesis. Naïve CD4$^+$ T cells primed in the presence of transforming growth factor beta (TGF-β) and certain proinflammatory cytokines (i.e., interleukins IL-1β, IL-6, IL-21, and IL-23) become Th17 cells, an effector subset that produces IL-17A, IL-17F, and IL-22 and facilitates cell migration into target tissues through the induction of local chemokine production. Patients with SLE have increased amounts of Th17 cells. Probably the inflammatory milieu and the decreased production of IL-2 contribute to this phenomenon. CD8$^+$ T cells can lose CD8 and become DN (double-negative) T cells that also produce proinflammatory cytokines. This process is also increased in patients with SLE.

Interestingly, disease amelioration was accompanied by a reduction of IL-17 production in two murine studies.[28,30]

Different factors could account for the increased production of IL-17 in patients with SLE (Figure 9-2). Abundance of the Th17-promoting cytokines IL-6 and IL-21,[31] along with reduced levels of IL-2,[32] which promotes regulatory T-cell differentiation and inhibits Th17-cell generation,[33] could skew the CD4$^+$ T-cell priming. On the other hand, expansion of DN T cells increases the frequency of

IL-17–producing cells.[26] Thus, underlying inflammation, as well as lupus-specific factors (such as low IL-2 production), probably skews the effector differentiation of CD4$^+$ and CD8$^+$ T cells toward proinflammatory subsets that release cytokines that amplify the autoimmune response.

Interferon gamma (IFN-γ) is a proinflammatory cytokine produced by Th1, CD8$^+$, and natural killer (NK) cells. Although some reports argue that IFN-γ production is decreased in patients with SLE,[34,35] this decrease has not been uniformly documented.[27,36,37] Importantly, IFN-γ–positive cells and IFN-γ RNA transcripts have been found in glomeruli from kidneys affected by lupus nephritis.[38,39] In murine lupus models (e.g., NZB/NZW and MRL/*lpr*), IFN-γ plays a demonstrated pathogenic role.[40,41]

T cells are guided by adhesion molecules into lymphoid organs or peripheral tissues. CD44 is an adhesion molecule that binds to hyaluronic acid and other components of extracellular matrix. Its expression is increased on T cells from patients with SLE.[42] Moreover, the affinity of CD44 is enhanced in SLE T cells, allowing increased migration of T cells into inflamed organs.[42,43] The *CD44* gene can yield variant isoforms through alternative splicing. The expression of two variants, CD44v3 and CD44v6, is increased on T cells from patients with lupus and correlates with disease activity, renal disease, and anti–double-stranded DNA (anti-dsDNA) antibody production.[44] The relevance of this finding is exemplified by the fact that T cells that infiltrate kidneys in patients with lupus nephritis express CD44v3 and CD44v6.[45]

CD8$^+$ and Double-Negative T Cells

The phenotype and function of CD8$^+$ T cells has been scarcely studied in patients with SLE. Activity of peripheral blood CD8$^+$ T cells may be increased in patients with active SLE,[46] because a higher fraction of these cells express perforin and granzyme B.[47] Importantly, CD8$^+$ T cells are also found within cellular infiltrates in kidney biopsy specimens from patients with SLE, particularly in the interstitial and periglomerular areas,[48] suggesting that the cells may participate in target organ tissue injury. On the other hand, cytotoxic capacity of CD8$^+$ cells has been reported to be hampered in SLE.[49]

Although scarce in healthy individuals, DN T cells constitute a significant proportion of T cells in patients with SLE.[26,50] When expanded, DN T cells probably play a pathogenic role in patients with SLE. They can provide B-cell help,[50,51] produce proinflammatory cytokines (e.g., IL-1β, IL-17, and IFN-γ), and are found in cellular infiltrates in kidneys of patients with lupus.[26] At least a fraction of DN T cells is derived from activated CD8$^+$ T cells.[52] In SLE, DN T-cell expansion is probably explained by either increased conversion of CD8$^+$ T cells into DN T cells or abnormal survival of the latter.

Regulatory Function

T cells also suppress immune responses. This function allows the duration and intensity of the immune response to be controlled. Moreover, it protects the host tissues from immune-mediated damage.[53] Complete absence of regulatory T (Treg) cells causes a severe autoimmune disorder in mice and humans (immunodysregulation polyendocrinopathy enteropathy X-linked syndrome [IPEX]).[54] On the other hand, partial defects in numbers and function of Tregs have been linked to several autoimmune disorders, including SLE. Reduced Treg numbers are observed in the peripheral blood of patients with SLE, particularly during active disease periods.[55-57] The suppressive function of SLE-derived Tregs has also been studied, but the results are conflicting. Some reports claim they are unable to efficiently suppress proliferation and cytokine production.[58,59] However, others suggest that the function of Tregs is conserved and that the suboptimal T-cell suppression observed in in vitro assays is the consequence of SLE T cells being abnormally resistant to Treg-induced suppression.[60,61] One study has identified a CD8$^+$ FoxP3$^+$ regulatory cell subset present in patients with severe lupus subjected to autologous hematopoietic stem cell transplantation. Interestingly, the presence of these cells was associated with disease remission.[62]

INTRINSIC T-CELL DEFECTS
Assembly and Selection of the T-Cell Repertoire

Assembly of the T-cell receptor is complex and involves DNA recombination. In the thymus, gene segments that code for different sections of the TCR are combined in a stochastic process. This creates a diverse T-cell repertoire but entails the creation of a large number of flawed receptors. T-cell precursors are then selected to eliminate cells whose receptors cannot bind to self–major histocompatibility complex (MHC) molecules and those that bind self-antigens with high affinity. During these stages (known as positive and negative selection, respectively) most thymocytes are deleted. The remaining cells constitute the T-cell repertoire that exits the thymus and populates secondary lymphoid organs.

Deficient removal of autoreactive T cells can cause autoimmunity. In patients with autoimmune polyendocrinopathy (APECED), absence of *AIRE,* a gene that allows the thymic expression of tissue-restricted antigens, hampers negative selection, allowing autoreactive T cells to egress the thymus.[63] In patients with SLE, central tolerance has been studied indirectly through analysis of the frequency of peripheral blood autoreactive T cells.[64,65] Histone-reactive T cells have been identified with a similar frequency in healthy controls, suggesting that negative selection occurs normally.[64,65] In murine models of lupus, this process has also been evaluated on transgenic mice that express a specific preformed TCR.[66,67] In mice with lupus-like diseases, thymocyte deletion is unremarkable when the cognate antigen is expressed in the thymus.[66-68]

Taken together, studies performed in patients and mice with lupus indicate that no gross defect in central tolerance processes underlies SLE. However, because T-cell selection is based on the molecules of the MHC, the array of MHC molecules present in each person determines the T-cell repertoire and the peptides to be presented in the thymus and during immune responses. Thus, even if no defects have been found in the central tolerance processes of patients with SLE, the characteristics of the T-cell repertoire created in the thymus are likely involved in the proclivity of patients with lupus to mount self-aimed responses. This likelihood may explain why the MHC locus is the region most commonly linked to lupus in genetic association studies.[69]

T-Cell Activation and Signaling

T-cell activation is abnormal in patients with SLE. Defects in key molecules involved in modulating the T-cell response to antigen presentation alter the signaling pathways elicited through the TCR. This phenomenon skews the expression of genes that control T-cell function.[3,70]

Intracellular residues of proteins associated to the TCR (CD3 complex) deliver activation signals into the cell by becoming phosphorylated following antigen recognition. The expression of a central component of CD3, the ζ chain, is decreased in T cells from patients with SLE.[70] However, this decrease is paradoxically associated with an increased response to TCR stimulation. The reason is that CD3ζ is replaced by a closely related molecule, the common γ chain of the immunoglobulin receptor (FcRγ).[71] The substitution of CD3ζ by FcRγ affects the intensity of the TCR-derived signal. FcRγ couples with spleen tyrosine kinase (Syk) instead of with ZAP-70 (ζ-associated protein 70).[72] As a consequence, TCR engagement is followed by an abnormally high influx of calcium (Figure 9-3).[73]

Decreased expression and altered membrane localization of CD3ζ is thought to be a central defect in this process. Interestingly, multiple molecular mechanisms have been described in SLE T cells that contribute to the diminished expression of CD3ζ. They include decreased production,[74-76] decreased stability,[77,78] and increased degradation.[79]

A closely related phenomenon described in SLE T cells is the presence of preaggregated lipid rafts in the T-cell membrane. These cholesterol-rich membrane areas carry signaling molecules and fuse at the pole of the cell where antigen is being presented. In quiescent T cells, lipid rafts are distributed throughout the cellular surface and coalesce after activation. The clustering allows signal transduction to

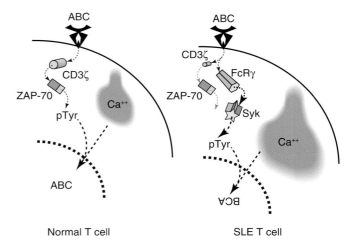

Figure 9-3 Structural differences alter the T-cell receptor (TCR) signaling process of the SLE T cell. Decreased levels of CD3ζ and a reciprocal increase in the expression of the Fc receptor FcRγ cause the TCR-initiated signal to relay on FcRγ and Syk, instead of on CD3ζ and ZAP-70. This "rewired" TCR signaling is associated with stronger phosphorylation of signaling molecules and a heightened calcium influx. Thus, in the presence of the same signal (e.g., ABC), a T cell from a patient with SLE receives a different, distorted message that affects its response.

occur effectively because all the necessary elements are rapidly drawn together. In T cells from patients with SLE, lipid rafts are clustered even in the absence of stimulation.[80,42] This phenomenon likely contributes to the increased signal transduction observed after TCR stimulation in SLE T cells.[81,82] Administration of a lipid raft–clustering agent accelerated disease onset in a murine model of lupus (MRL/*lpr*), whereas injection of a drug that disrupts lipid raft clustering had the opposite effect; these findings suggest that lipid raft clustering can indeed promote T-cell activation in vivo.[83]

The events that are initiated at the cell membrane when the TCR engages its cognate antigen are delivered through complex signaling pathways that cause immediate reactions in the cell and activate transcription factors. Activation of mitogen-activated protein (MAP) kinases mediates several cellular processes, such as proliferation, gene expression, and apoptosis induction. In T cells from patients with lupus, the MAP kinase activity is abnormal.[84,85] The abnormality could contribute to autoimmunity, because MAP kinase function has been linked to maintenance of tolerance.[86] In fact, mice deficient in RasGRP1 (RAS guanyl–releasing protein 1)[87] or in protein kinase C (PKC) δ (a MAP kinase activator)[88] demonstrate spontaneous autoimmune diseases.

Other signaling pathways are also affected in SLE T cells. Cyclic adenosine monophosphate (AMP)–dependent protein phosphorylation has been reported to be impaired,[89] probably because of reduced levels of the protein kinase A.[90] The activities of PKC and Lck (lymphocyte-specific protein tyrosine kinase) are also low in SLE T cells.[91,92] In contrast, activity of the protein kinase PKR (involved in the phosphorylation of translation initiation factors) is increased.[93] Likewise, activity of phosphatidylinositol-3 kinase (PI3K), the enzyme that produces the second messengers PIP_2 and PIP_3, is increased in mice with a lupus-like disease induced by alloreactivity.[94] The importance of this pathway was further supported by studies proving that pharmacologic inhibition of class IB PI3K can ameliorate disease in MRL/*lpr* mice.[95,96]

Regulation of Gene Expression

The activation process of SLE T cells has several alterations that probably contribute to T-cell overactivation. Clustered lipid rafts and the abnormally configured transduction system cause a disproportionally high calcium response unbalanced with other signals such as

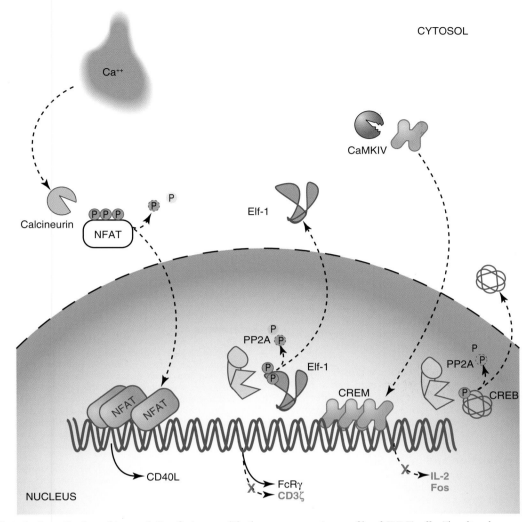

CYTOSOL

Ca⁺⁺

CaMKIV

Calcineurin

NFAT

Elf-1

NUCLEUS

PP2A

Elf-1

CREM

PP2A

CREB

NFAT NFAT

CD40L

X → FcRγ
X → CD3ζ

X → IL-2
Fos

FIGURE 9-4 Defects in the activation of transcription factors modify the gene expression profile of SLE T cells. The altered response to T-cell receptor (TCR)–initiated signals, along with changes in the levels and activity of certain kinases and phosphatases, modifies the transcription factor activity. Increased calcium signaling leads to a heightened activation of NFAT (nuclear factor of activated T cells), which is responsible for the overexpression of CD40 ligand (CD40L). On the other hand, increased levels and activity of the phosphatase PP2A inactivate (by dephosphorylating) the transcription factors Elf-1 and CREB (cyclic AMP response element [CRE]–binding protein). Reduced activity of Elf-1 is associated with decreased transcription of CD3ζ and increased production of FcRγ. Decreased activity of CREB, coupled with increased activity of CREM (CRE-modulator, an inhibitory transcription factor of the same family), decreases production of IL-2 and of yet another transcription factor, Fos. Together, these alterations severely distort gene expression in SLE T cells.

MAP kinases. These alterations lead to unbalanced activation of transcription factors and, thus, abnormal gene expression (Figure 9-4).[2] The altered gene transcription pattern produces a characteristic phenotype that in some aspects suggests overactivation but in others indicates failure of activation (anergy).

Nuclear factor of activated T cells (NFAT) is a transcription factor activated by calcium influx through the action of the phosphatase calcineurin. SLE T cells have increased activation of NFAT as consequence of their altered calcium response.[9] Thus, the expression of certain genes regulated by NFAT is altered. For example, expression of CD40L, an important co-stimulatory molecule used by T cells to stimulate antibody production and dendritic cell activation, is increased.[9,97]

A cyclic AMP response element (CRE)—a DNA sequence where the transcription factors CRE-binding protein (CREB) and CRE-modulator (CREM) bind—has been shown to be significant in the regulation of IL-2 in patients with SLE.[98] CREM and CREB compete for this site, where they exert antagonistic effects. CREB favors transcription, whereas CREM represses it. The balance between CREB

and CREM is altered in SLE T cells. Lower CREB and higher CREM levels contribute to an IL-2 production deficiency.[99] Other genes known to be affected by the disturbed CREB : CREM ratio in SLE T cells are *CD247* (CD3ζ),[76] *FOS*,[100] and *CD86*.[101] Because Fos is also a transcription factor, the transcriptional effects of decreased CREB and increased CREM levels extend to genes regulated by Fos.[100]

The altered CREB : CREM ratio of SLE T cells results from several factors. Anti–T-cell antibodies commonly present in the sera of patients with SLE induce the activation of CaMKIV (calcium/calmodulin-dependent kinase IV).[102] CaMKIV increases CREM activity, probably through phosphorylation.[102] On the other hand, levels of protein phosphatase 2A (PP2A) are increased in T cells from patients with lupus.[103] PP2A dephosphorylates and thus inactivates CREB (see Figure 9-4).[104]

By modulating their transcription, transcription factor Elf-1 promotes the production of CD3ζ and represses FcRγ.[75] Increased levels of PP2A promote dephosphorylation of Elf-1 to its inactive form, which lacks DNA-binding activity and is confined to the cytoplasm of the cell. Thus, in SLE T cells, increased PP2A activity leads to an inversion of the CD3ζ:FcRγ ratio. Transcriptional activity of CD3ζ is diminished and that of FcRγ is derepressed (see Figure 9-2).[75]

The accessibility of transcription factor binding sites can be regulated by modifications in DNA and histones (mainly acetylation and methylation). These changes, known as *epigenetic regulation,* represent an additional layer of control of gene expression. DNA methylation suppresses gene expression, and in comparison with T cells from healthy individuals, T cells from SLE patients have abnormally low levels of DNA methylation.[105] This relative lack of methylation causes overexpression of several genes and has been proposed as a mechanism underlying drug-induced lupus, because some of the "culprit" drugs inhibit DNA methylation (e.g., procainamide and hydralazine).[106,107]

Importantly, some of the signaling alterations mentioned previously have been associated with the reduced DNA methylation characteristic of SLE T cells. Hence, altered MAP kinase and PKCδ activities have been associated with deficient DNA methyltransferase 1 (DNMT1) function in SLE T cells.[88,108,109]

Histone acetylation, another epigenetic regulatory mechanism, has been proposed to alter gene expression in SLE T cells. Some of the effects of CREM, particularly its effect on the *IL2* promoter, depend on its capacity to recruit histone deacetylase (HDAC) 1.[110] PP2A also regulates the activity of HDAC, and some of its effects are known to be mediated through histone acetylation.[111] Treatment of SLE T cells with trichostatin A, an HDAC inhibitor, has been found to diminish the expression of CD40L and the production of IL-10, suggesting that histone acetylation plays a role in the overexpression of these molecules in lupus.[112]

In summary, T cells from SLE patients have a grossly distorted pattern of gene expression. This defect, which is in part a consequence of the alterations in cell activation and signaling, affects the phenotype and function of the cells, creating a vicious circle in which altered signaling skews gene expression that further alters cell signaling and activation.

Mitochondrial Dysfunction and mTOR Signaling

Several mitochondrial defects, including increased mass, ultrastructural damage, and elevated transmembrane potential ($\Delta\Psi_m$), have been described in T cells from patients with SLE.[113] Elevated $\Delta\Psi_m$ and increased levels of nitric oxide increase activity of the protein kinase mTOR in T cells from patients with SLE.[114] This situation contributes to the decreased expression of CD3ζ and thus to the increased calcium response upon TCR stimulation.[115] The importance of these alterations was suggested by the results of a small clinical trial in which patients with SLE received rapamycin, an inhibitor of mTOR. Clinical disease activity, as well as calcium response following T-cell activation, improved significantly.[115]

Apoptosis Induction

T-cell clones able to recognize an antigen expand exponentially during immune responses. When the stimulus has ceased, programmed cell death is triggered in most cells, and only a few survive as memory cells. This process allows the immune system to expand its useful clones temporarily and to select the cells with highest affinity to persist. In patients with SLE, T-cell apoptosis is faulty. The rate of spontaneous apoptosis of resting CD4[+] T cells is increased and has been linked to lymphopenia, a commonly observed phenomenon in lupus.[116] On the other hand, deletion of activated T cells is defective in patients with SLE.[113,117-119] T cells from patients with SLE exhibit an abnormal elevation of the $\Delta\Psi_m$, produce increased levels of reactive oxygen intermediates, and have decreased amounts of adenosine triphosphate (ATP).[113] These changes, proposed to be caused by repeated cellular activation, facilitate spontaneous apoptosis and decrease activation-induced apoptosis. Moreover, they sensitize T cells to undergo necrosis instead of apoptosis.[113] Decreased abundance of IL-2 is an important cue that triggers apoptosis at the end of immune responses. The Bβ regulatory subunit of PP2A is upregulated in T cells when IL-2 levels fall and initiates apoptosis. In a subset

of patients with SLE, resistance to apoptosis is associated with failed induction of Bβ upon low IL-2.[119] Taken together, these data indicate that several molecular defects alter the sensitivity of resting and activated SLE T cells to apoptosis. This altered sensitivity could contribute to the persistence of activated T cells. In murine models of lupus, absence of the molecule Fas or its ligand acts as a powerful accelerator of autoimmune disease in several backgrounds.[120] Interestingly, Fas signaling has been found to be normal in cells from patients with SLE.[117]

CONCLUSION

T cells, along with other components of the immune system, are profoundly affected in patients with SLE. Some T-cell defects are probably secondary to chronic inflammatory signals present in patients with SLE. Other defects are probably genetically determined and inherited as traits that in isolation are not severe enough to cause disease. It is probably the combination of several defects triggered by proinflammatory environmental stimulation that induces the T-cell functional defects that have been described in this chapter. A more thorough knowledge of these alterations will enable us to better understand the disease pathogenesis and also to determine which defects are primary, thus representing adequate therapeutic targets or potential biomarkers to predict disease outcomes.

References

1. Crispin JC, Kyttaris VC, Terhorst C, et al: T cells as therapeutic targets in systemic lupus erythematosus. *Nat Rev Rheumatol* 6:317–325, 2010.
2. Crispin JC, Kyttaris VC, Juang YT, et al: How signaling and gene transcription aberrations dictate the systemic lupus erythematosus T cell phenotype. *Trends Immunol* 29:110–115, 2008.
3. Vassilopoulos D, Kovacs B, Tsokos GC: TCR/CD3 complex-mediated signal transduction pathway in T cells and T cell lines from patients with systemic lupus erythematosus. *J Immunol* 155:2269–2281, 1995.
4. Juang YT, Peoples C, Kafri R, et al: A systemic lupus erythematosus gene expression array in disease diagnosis and classification: a preliminary report. *Lupus* 20:243–249, 2011.
5. Shlomchik M, Mascelli M, Shan H, et al: Anti-DNA antibodies from autoimmune mice arise by clonal expansion and somatic mutation. *J Exp Med* 171:265–292, 1990.
6. Hang L, Theofilopoulos AN, Balderas RS, et al: The effect of thymectomy on lupus-prone mice. *J Immunol* 132:1809–1813, 1984.
7. Ravirajan CT, Rahman MA, Papadaki L, et al: Genetic, structural and functional properties of an IgG DNA-binding monoclonal antibody from a lupus patient with nephritis. *Eur J Immunol* 28:339–350, 1998.
8. Grammer AC, Slota R, Fischer R, et al: Abnormal germinal center reactions in systemic lupus erythematosus demonstrated by blockade of CD154-CD40 interactions. *J Clin Invest* 112:1506–1520, 2003.
9. Kyttaris VC, Wang Y, Juang YT, et al: Increased levels of NF-ATc2 differentially regulate CD154 and IL-2 genes in T cells from patients with systemic lupus erythematosus. *J Immunol* 178:1960–1966, 2007.
10. Crotty S: Follicular helper CD4 T cells (TFH). *Annu Rev Immunol* 29:621–663, 2011.
11. Vinuesa CG, Cook MC, Angelucci C, et al: A RING-type ubiquitin ligase family member required to repress follicular helper T cells and autoimmunity. *Nature* 435:452–458, 2005.
12. Kim HJ, Verbinnen B, Tang X, et al: Inhibition of follicular T-helper cells by CD8[+] regulatory T cells is essential for self tolerance. *Nature* 467:328–332, 2010.
13. Odegard JM, Marks BR, DiPlacido LD, et al: ICOS-dependent extrafollicular helper T cells elicit IgG production via IL-21 in systemic autoimmunity. *J Exp Med* 205:2873–2886, 2008.
14. Bubier JA, Sproule TJ, Foreman O, et al: A critical role for IL-21 receptor signaling in the pathogenesis of systemic lupus erythematosus in BXSB-Yaa mice. *Proc Natl Acad Sci U S A* 106:1518–1523, 2009.
15. Foster AD, Haas M, Puliaeva I, et al: Donor CD8 T cell activation is critical for greater renal disease severity in female chronic graft-vs.-host mice and is associated with increased splenic ICOS(hi) host CD4 T cells and IL-21 expression. *Clin Immunol* 136:61–73, 2010.
16. Kim HJ, Wang X, Radfar S, et al: CD8+ T regulatory cells express the Ly49 Class I MHC receptor and are defective in autoimmune prone B6-Yaa mice. *Proc Natl Acad Sci U S A* 108:2010–2015, 2011.

17. Simpson N, Gatenby PA, Wilson A, et al: Expansion of circulating T cells resembling follicular helper T cells is a fixed phenotype that identifies a subset of severe systemic lupus erythematosus. *Arthritis Rheum* 62:234–244, 2010.

18. Shlomchik MJ, Craft JE, Mamula MJ: From T to B and back again: positive feedback in systemic autoimmune disease. *Nat Rev Immunol* 1:147–153, 2001.

19. Llorente L, Richaud-Patin Y, Couderc J, et al: Dysregulation of interleukin-10 production in relatives of patients with systemic lupus erythematosus. *Arthritis Rheum* 40:1429–1435, 1997.

20. Llorente L, Zou W, Levy Y, et al: Role of interleukin 10 in the B lymphocyte hyperactivity and autoantibody production of human systemic lupus erythematosus. *J Exp Med* 181:839–844, 1995.

21. Ishida H, Muchamuel T, Sakaguchi S, et al: Continuous administration of anti-interleukin 10 antibodies delays onset of autoimmunity in NZB/W F1 mice. *J Exp Med* 179:305–310, 1994.

22. Llorente L, Richaud-Patin Y, Garcia-Padilla C, et al: Clinical and biologic effects of anti-interleukin-10 monoclonal antibody administration in systemic lupus erythematosus. *Arthritis Rheum* 43:1790–1800, 2000.

23. Hsieh C, Chang A, Brandt D, et al: Predicting outcomes of lupus nephritis with tubulointerstitial inflammation and scarring. *Arthritis Care Res (Hoboken)* 63:865–874, 2011.

24. Korn T, Bettelli E, Oukka M, et al: IL-17 and Th17 Cells. *Annu Rev Immunol* 27:485–517, 2009.

25. Doreau A, Belot A, Bastid J, et al: Interleukin 17 acts in synergy with B cell-activating factor to influence B cell biology and the pathophysiology of systemic lupus erythematosus. *Nat Immunol* 10:778–785, 2009.

26. Crispin JC, Oukka M, Bayliss G, et al: Expanded double negative T cells in patients with systemic lupus erythematosus produce IL-17 and infiltrate the kidneys. *J Immunol* 181:8761–8766, 2008.

27. Shah K, Lee WW, Lee SH, et al: Dysregulated balance of Th17 and Th1 cells in systemic lupus erythematosus. *Arthritis Res Ther* 12:R53–R63, 2010.

28. Kang HK, Liu M, Datta SK: Low-dose peptide tolerance therapy of lupus generates plasmacytoid dendritic cells that cause expansion of autoantigen-specific regulatory T cells and contraction of inflammatory Th17 cells. *J Immunol* 178:7849–7858, 2007.

29. Zhang Z, Kyttaris VC, Tsokos GC: The role of IL-23/IL-17 axis in lupus nephritis. *J Immunol* 183:3160–3169, 2009.

30. Wu HY, Quintana FJ, Weiner HL: Nasal anti-CD3 antibody ameliorates lupus by inducing an IL-10-secreting CD4+. *J Immunol* 181:6038–6050, 2008.

31. Linker-Israeli M, Deans RJ, Wallace DJ, et al: Elevated levels of endogenous IL-6 in systemic lupus erythematosus. A putative role in pathogenesis. *J Immunol* 147:117–123, 1991.

32. Alcocer-Varela J, Alarcon-Segovia D: Decreased production of and response to interleukin-2 by cultured lymphocytes from patients with systemic lupus erythematosus. *J Clin Invest* 69:1388–1392, 1982.

33. Yang XP, Ghoreschi K, Steward-Tharp SM, et al: Opposing regulation of the locus encoding IL-17 through direct, reciprocal actions of STAT3 and STAT5. *Nat Immunol* 12:247–254, 2011.

34. Tsokos GC, Boumpas DT, Smith PL, et al: Deficient gamma-interferon production in patients with systemic lupus erythematosus. *Arthritis Rheum* 29:1210–1215, 1986.

35. Neighbour PA, Grayzel AI: Interferon production of vitro by leucocytes from patients with systemic lupus erythematosus and rheumatoid arthritis. *Clin Exp Immunol* 45:576–582, 1981.

36. Harigai M, Kawamoto M, Hara M, et al: Excessive production of IFN-gamma in patients with systemic lupus erythematosus and its contribution to induction of B lymphocyte stimulator/B cell-activating factor/TNF ligand superfamily-13B. *J Immunol* 181:2211–2219, 2008.

37. Basu D, Liu Y, Wu A, et al: Stimulatory and inhibitory killer Ig-like receptor molecules are expressed and functional on lupus T cells. *J Immunol* 183:3481–3487, 2009.

38. Uhm WS, Na K, Song GW, et al: Cytokine balance in kidney tissue from lupus nephritis patients. *Rheumatology (Oxford)* 42:935–938, 2003.

39. Chan RW, Lai FM, Li EK, et al: Intrarenal cytokine gene expression in lupus nephritis. *Ann Rheum Dis* 66:886–892, 2007.

40. Haas C, Ryffel B, Le HM: IFN-gamma receptor deletion prevents autoantibody production and glomerulonephritis in lupus-prone (NZB x NZW)F1 mice. *J Immunol* 160:3713–3718, 1998.

41. Balomenos D, Rumold R, Theofilopoulos AN: Interferon-gamma is required for lupus-like disease and lymphoaccumulation in MRL-lpr mice. *J Clin Invest* 101:364–371, 1998.

42. Li Y, Harada T, Juang YT, et al: Phosphorylated ERM is responsible for increased T cell polarization, adhesion, and migration in patients with systemic lupus erythematosus. *J Immunol* 178:1938–1947, 2007.

43. Estess P, DeGrendele HC, Pascual V, et al: Functional activation of lymphocyte CD44 in peripheral blood is a marker of autoimmune disease activity. *J Clin Invest* 102:1173–1182, 1998.

44. Crispin JC, Keenan BT, Finnell MD, et al: Expression of CD44 variant isoforms CD44v3 and CD44v6 is increased on T cells from patients with systemic lupus erythematosus and is correlated with disease activity. *Arthritis Rheum* 62:1431–1437, 2010.

45. Cohen RA, Bayliss G, Crispin JC, et al: T cells and in situ cryoglobulin deposition in the pathogenesis of lupus nephritis. *Clin Immunol* 128:1–7, 2008.

46. Viallard JF, Bloch-Michel C, Neau-Cransac M, et al: HLA-DR expression on lymphocyte subsets as a marker of disease activity in patients with systemic lupus erythematosus. *Clin Exp Immunol* 125:485–491, 2001.

47. Blanco P, Pitard V, Viallard JF, et al: Increase in activated CD8+ T lymphocytes expressing perforin and granzyme B correlates with disease activity in patients with systemic lupus erythematosus. *Arthritis Rheum* 52:201–211, 2005.

48. Couzi L, Merville P, Deminiere C, et al: Predominance of CD8+ T lymphocytes among periglomerular infiltrating cells and link to the prognosis of class III and class IV lupus nephritis. *Arthritis Rheum* 56:2362–2370, 2007.

49. Stohl W: Impaired polyclonal T cell cytolytic activity. A possible risk factor for systemic lupus erythematosus. *Arthritis Rheum* 38:506–516, 1995.

50. Shivakumar S, Tsokos GC, Datta SK: T cell receptor alpha/beta expressing double-negative (CD4−/CD8−) and CD4+ T helper cells in humans augment the production of pathogenic anti-DNA autoantibodies associated with lupus nephritis. *J Immunol* 143:103–112, 1989.

51. Sieling PA, Porcelli SA, Duong BT, et al: Human double-negative T cells in systemic lupus erythematosus provide help for IgG and are restricted by CD1c. *J Immunol* 165:5338–5344, 2000.

52. Crispin JC, Tsokos GC: Human TCR-αβ+ CD4- CD8- T cells can derive from CD8+ T cells and display an inflammatory effector phenotype. *J Immunol* 183:4675–4681, 2009.

53. Sakaguchi S, Yamaguchi T, Nomura T, et al: Regulatory T cells and immune tolerance. *Cell* 133:775–787, 2008.

54. Le BS, Geha RS: IPEX and the role of Foxp3 in the development and function of human Tregs. *J Clin Invest* 116:1473–1475, 2006.

55. Crispin JC, Martinez A, Alcocer-Varela J: Quantification of regulatory T cells in patients with systemic lupus erythematosus. *J Autoimmun* 21:273–276, 2003.

56. Miyara M, Amoura Z, Parizot C, et al: Global natural regulatory T cell depletion in active systemic lupus erythematosus. *J Immunol* 175:8392–8400, 2005.

57. Lee JH, Wang LC, Lin YT, et al: Inverse correlation between CD4+ regulatory T-cell population and autoantibody levels in paediatric patients with systemic lupus erythematosus. *Immunology* 117:280–286, 2006.

58. Valencia X, Yarboro C, Illei G, et al: Deficient CD4+CD25high T regulatory cell function in patients with active systemic lupus erythematosus. *J Immunol* 178:2579–2588, 2007.

59. Bonelli M, Savitskaya A, von DK, et al: Quantitative and qualitative deficiencies of regulatory T cells in patients with systemic lupus erythematosus (SLE). *Int Immunol* 20:861–868, 2008.

60. Vargas-Rojas MI, Crispin JC, Richaud-Patin Y, et al: Quantitative and qualitative normal regulatory T cells are not capable of inducing suppression in SLE patients due to T-cell resistance. *Lupus* 17:289–294, 2008.

61. Monk CR, Spachidou M, Rovis F, et al: MRL/Mp CD4+CD25- T cells show reduced sensitivity to suppression by CD4+CD25+ regulatory T cells in vitro: a novel defect of T cell regulation in systemic lupus erythematosus. *Arthritis Rheum* 52:1180–1184, 2005.

62. Zhang L, Bertucci AM, Ramsey-Goldman R, et al: Regulatory T cell (Treg) subsets return in patients with refractory lupus following stem cell transplantation, and TGF-beta-producing CD8+ Treg cells are associated with immunological remission of lupus. *J Immunol* 183:6346–6358, 2009.

63. Anderson MS, Su MA: Aire and T cell development. *Curr Opin Immunol* 23:198–206, 2011.

64. Andreassen K, Bendiksen S, Kjeldsen E, et al: T cell autoimmunity to histones and nucleosomes is a latent property of the normal immune system. *Arthritis Rheum* 46:1270–1281, 2002.

65. Voll RE, Roth EA, Girkontaite I, et al: Histone-specific Th0 and Th1 clones derived from systemic lupus erythematosus patients induce double-stranded DNA antibody production. *Arthritis Rheum* 40:2162–2171, 1997.

66. Kotzin BL, Kappler JW, Marrack PC, et al: T cell tolerance to self antigens in New Zealand hybrid mice with lupus-like disease. *J Immunol* 143:89–94, 1989.

67. Herron LR, Eisenberg RA, Roper E, et al: Selection of the T cell receptor repertoire in Lpr mice. *J Immunol* 151:3450–3459, 1993.

68. Fatenejad S, Peng SL, Disorbo O, et al: Central T cell tolerance in lupus-prone mice: influence of autoimmune background and the lpr mutation. *J Immunol* 161:6427–6432, 1998.

69. Harley IT, Kaufman KM, Langefeld CD, et al: Genetic susceptibility to SLE: new insights from fine mapping and genome-wide association studies. *Nat Rev Genet* 10:285–290, 2009.

70. Liossis SN, Ding XZ, Dennis GJ, et al: Altered pattern of TCR/CD3-mediated protein-tyrosyl phosphorylation in T cells from patients with systemic lupus erythematosus. Deficient expression of the T cell receptor zeta chain. *J Clin Invest* 101:1448–1457, 1998.

71. Enyedy EJ, Nambiar MP, Liossis SN, et al: Fc epsilon receptor type I gamma chain replaces the deficient T cell receptor zeta chain in T cells of patients with systemic lupus erythematosus. *Arthritis Rheum* 44:1114–1121, 2001.

72. Krishnan S, Juang YT, Chowdhury B, et al: Differential expression and molecular associations of Syk in systemic lupus erythematosus T cells. *J Immunol* 181:8145–8152, 2008.

73. Tsokos GC, Nambiar MP, Tenbrock K, et al: Rewiring the T-cell: signaling defects and novel prospects for the treatment of SLE. *Trends Immunol* 24:259–263, 2003.

74. Juang YT, Tenbrock K, Nambiar MP, et al: Defective production of functional 98-kDa form of Elf-1 is responsible for the decreased expression of TCR zeta-chain in patients with systemic lupus erythematosus. *J Immunol* 169:6048–6055, 2002.

75. Juang YT, Wang Y, Jiang G, et al: PP2A dephosphorylates Elf-1 and determines the expression of CD3zeta and FcRgamma in human systemic lupus erythematosus T cells. *J Immunol* 181:3658–3664, 2008.

76. Tenbrock K, Kyttaris VC, Ahlmann M, et al: The cyclic AMP response element modulator regulates transcription of the TCR zeta-chain. *J Immunol* 175:5975–5980, 2005.

77. Moulton VR, Kyttaris VC, Juang YT, et al: The RNA-stabilizing protein HuR regulates the expression of zeta chain of the human T cell receptor-associated CD3 complex. *J Biol Chem* 283:20037–20044, 2008.

78. Chowdhury B, Tsokos CG, Krishnan S, et al: Decreased stability and translation of T cell receptor zeta mRNA with an alternatively spliced 3'-untranslated region contribute to zeta chain down-regulation in patients with systemic lupus erythematosus. *J Biol Chem* 280:18959–18966, 2005.

79. Krishnan S, Kiang JG, Fisher CU, et al: Increased caspase-3 expression and activity contribute to reduced CD3zeta expression in systemic lupus erythematosus T cells. *J Immunol* 175:3417–3423, 2005.

80. Jury EC, Kabouridis PS, Flores-Borja F, et al: Altered lipid raft-associated signaling and ganglioside expression in T lymphocytes from patients with systemic lupus erythematosus. *J Clin Invest* 113:1176–1187, 2004.

81. Krishnan S, Nambiar MP, Warke VG, et al: Alterations in lipid raft composition and dynamics contribute to abnormal T cell responses in systemic lupus erythematosus. *J Immunol* 172:7821–7831, 2004.

82. Jury EC, Isenberg DA, Mauri C, et al: Atorvastatin restores Lck expression and lipid raft-associated signaling in T cells from patients with systemic lupus erythematosus. *J Immunol* 177:7416–7422, 2006.

83. Deng GM, Tsokos GC: Cholera toxin B accelerates disease progression in lupus-prone mice by promoting lipid raft aggregation. *J Immunol* 181:4019–4026, 2008.

84. Cedeno S, Cifarelli DF, Blasini AM, et al: Defective activity of ERK-1 and ERK-2 mitogen-activated protein kinases in peripheral blood T lymphocytes from patients with systemic lupus erythematosus: potential role of altered coupling of Ras guanine nucleotide exchange factor hSos to adapter protein Grb2 in lupus T cells. *Clin Immunol* 106:41–49, 2003.

85. Mor A, Philips MR, Pillinger MH: The role of Ras signaling in lupus T lymphocytes: biology and pathogenesis. *Clin Immunol* 125:215–223, 2007.

86. Rui L, Vinuesa CG, Blasioli J, et al: Resistance to CpG DNA-induced autoimmunity through tolerogenic B cell antigen receptor ERK signaling. *Nat Immunol* 4:594–600, 2003.

87. Layer K, Lin G, Nencioni A, et al: Autoimmunity as the consequence of a spontaneous mutation in Rasgrp1. *Immunity* 19:243–255, 2003.

88. Gorelik G, Fang JY, Wu A, et al: Impaired T cell protein kinase C delta activation decreases ERK pathway signaling in idiopathic and hydralazine-induced lupus. *J Immunol* 179:5553–5563, 2007.

89. Mandler R, Birch RE, Polmar SH, et al: Abnormal adenosine-induced immunosuppression and cAMP metabolism in T lymphocytes of patients with systemic lupus erythematosus. *Proc Natl Acad Sci U S A* 79:7542–7546, 1982.

90. Kammer GM, Khan IU, Malemud CJ: Deficient type I protein kinase A isozyme activity in systemic lupus erythematosus T lymphocytes. *J Clin Invest* 94:422–430, 1994.

91. Tada Y, Nagasawa K, Yamauchi Y, et al: A defect in the protein kinase C system in T cells from patients with systemic lupus erythematosus. *Clin Immunol Immunopathol* 60:220–231, 1991.

92. Matache C, Stefanescu M, Onu A, et al: p56lck activity and expression in peripheral blood lymphocytes from patients with systemic lupus erythematosus. *Autoimmunity* 29:111–120, 1999.

93. Grolleau A, Kaplan MJ, Hanash SM, et al: Impaired translational response and increased protein kinase PKR expression in T cells from lupus patients. *J Clin Invest* 106:1561–1568, 2000.

94. Niculescu F, Nguyen P, Niculescu T, et al: Pathogenic T cells in murine lupus exhibit spontaneous signaling activity through phosphatidylinositol 3-kinase and mitogen-activated protein kinase pathways. *Arthritis Rheum* 48:1071–1079, 2003.

95. Barber DF, Bartolome A, Hernandez C, et al: PI3Kgamma inhibition blocks glomerulonephritis and extends lifespan in a mouse model of systemic lupus. *Nat Med* 11:933–935, 2005.

96. Barber DF, Bartolome A, Hernandez C, et al: Class IB-phosphatidylinositol 3-kinase (PI3K) deficiency ameliorates IA-PI3K-induced systemic lupus but not T cell invasion. *J Immunol* 176:589–593, 2006.

97. Yi Y, McNerney M, Datta SK: Regulatory defects in Cbl and mitogen-activated protein kinase (extracellular signal-related kinase) pathways cause persistent hyperexpression of CD40 ligand in human lupus T cells. *J Immunol* 165:6627–6634, 2000.

98. Tenbrock K, Tsokos GC: Transcriptional regulation of interleukin 2 in SLE T cells. *Int Rev Immunol* 23:333–345, 2004.

99. Solomou EE, Juang YT, Gourley MF, et al: Molecular basis of deficient IL-2 production in T cells from patients with systemic lupus erythematosus. *J Immunol* 166:4216–4222, 2001.

100. Kyttaris VC, Juang YT, Tenbrock K, et al: Cyclic adenosine 5'-monophosphate response element modulator is responsible for the decreased expression of c-fos and activator protein-1 binding in T cells from patients with systemic lupus erythematosus. *J Immunol* 173:3557–3563, 2004.

101. Ahlmann M, Varga G, Sturm K, et al: The cyclic AMP response element modulator {alpha} suppresses CD86 expression and APC function. *J Immunol* 182:4167–4174, 2009.

102. Juang YT, Wang Y, Solomou EE, et al: Systemic lupus erythematosus serum IgG increases CREM binding to the IL-2 promoter and suppresses IL-2 production through CaMKIV. *J Clin Invest* 115:996–1005, 2005.

103. Katsiari CG, Kyttaris VC, Juang YT, et al: Protein phosphatase 2A is a negative regulator of IL-2 production in patients with systemic lupus erythematosus. *J Clin Invest* 115:3193–3204, 2005.

104. Wadzinski BE, Wheat WH, Jaspers S, et al: Nuclear protein phosphatase 2A dephosphorylates protein kinase A-phosphorylated CREB and regulates CREB transcriptional stimulation. *Mol Cell Biol* 13:2822–2834, 1993.

105. Richardson B, Scheinbart L, Strahler J, et al: Evidence for impaired T cell DNA methylation in systemic lupus erythematosus and rheumatoid arthritis. *Arthritis Rheum* 33:1665–1673, 1990.

106. Scheinbart LS, Johnson MA, Gross LA, et al: Procainamide inhibits DNA methyltransferase in a human T cell line. *J Rheumatol* 18:530–534, 1991.

107. Deng C, Lu Q, Zhang Z, et al: Hydralazine may induce autoimmunity by inhibiting extracellular signal-regulated kinase pathway signaling. *Arthritis Rheum* 48:746–756, 2003.

108. Deng C, Kaplan MJ, Yang J, et al: Decreased Ras-mitogen-activated protein kinase signaling may cause DNA hypomethylation in T lymphocytes from lupus patients. *Arthritis Rheum* 44:397–407, 2001.

109. Sawalha AH, Jeffries M, Webb R, et al: Defective T-cell ERK signaling induces interferon-regulated gene expression and overexpression of methylation-sensitive genes similar to lupus patients. *Genes Immun* 9:368–378, 2008.

110. Tenbrock K, Juang YT, Leukert N, et al: The transcriptional repressor cAMP response element modulator alpha interacts with histone deacetylase 1 to repress promoter activity. *J Immunol* 177:6159–6164, 2006.

111. Martin M, Potente M, Janssens V, et al: Protein phosphatase 2A controls the activity of histone deacetylase 7 during T cell apoptosis and angiogenesis. *Proc Natl Acad Sci U S A* 105:4727–4732, 2008.

112. Mishra N, Brown DR, Olorenshaw IM, et al: Trichostatin A reverses skewed expression of CD154, interleukin-10, and interferon-gamma gene and protein expression in lupus T cells. *Proc Natl Acad Sci U S A* 98:2628–2633, 2001.

113. Gergely P, Jr., Grossman C, Niland B, et al: Mitochondrial hyperpolarization and ATP depletion in patients with systemic lupus erythematosus. *Arthritis Rheum* 46:175–190, 2002.

114. Nagy G, Barcza M, Gonchoroff N, et al: Nitric oxide-dependent mitochondrial biogenesis generates Ca2+ signaling profile of lupus T cells. *J Immunol* 173:3676–3683, 2004.

115. Fernandez D, Bonilla E, Mirza N, et al: Rapamycin reduces disease activity and normalizes T cell activation-induced calcium fluxing in patients with systemic lupus erythematosus. *Arthritis Rheum* 54:2983–2988, 2006.

116. Emlen W, Niebur J, Kadera R: Accelerated in vitro apoptosis of lymphocytes from patients with systemic lupus erythematosus. *J Immunol* 152:3685–3692, 1994.

117. Kovacs B, Vassilopoulos D, Vogelgesang SA, et al: Defective CD3-mediated cell death in activated T cells from patients with systemic lupus erythematosus: role of decreased intracellular TNF-alpha. *Clin Immunol Immunopathol* 81:293–302, 1996.

118. Xu L, Zhang L, Yi Y, et al: Human lupus T cells resist inactivation and escape death by upregulating COX-2. *Nat Med* 10:411–415, 2004.

119. Crispin JC, Apostolidis SA, Finnell MI, et al: Induction of PP2A Bβ, a regulator of IL-2 deprivation-induced T-cell apoptosis, is deficient in systemic lupus erythematosus. *Proc Natl Acad Sci U S A* 108(30):12443–12448, 2011.

120. Cohen PL, Eisenberg RA: Lpr and gld: single gene models of systemic autoimmunity and lymphoproliferative disease. *Annu Rev Immunol* 9:243–269, 1991.

Regulatory Cells in SLE

Antonio La Cava

Several subsets of immune cells endowed with regulatory functions can significantly influence the onset and progression of SLE. As a disease in which many etiopathogenetic aspects and clinical manifestations depend on a dysfunctional immune system, SLE represents a prototypical systemic autoimmune disease in which the checkpoints that normally control immune tolerance to self-antigens become impaired. One of the checkpoints that ensure the prevention of autoimmunity is the peripheral tolerance to self-antigens; it involves the activity of immunoregulatory cells that suppress autoreactive and/or inflammatory responses. Suppressor cells are part of both the adaptive and innate immune systems and include different immune cell populations with defined characteristics that have been identified at the phenotypic and functional levels. This chapter describes what is currently known about the roles and activities of immunoregulatory cells in the control and/or modulation of SLE.

One evident consequence of the dysfunction of immunoregulatory cells in SLE is the inability to properly suppress the proinflammatory events that lead to tissue damage and subsequent loss of organ function. Once tolerance to self-components is progressively impaired in SLE, the immune homeostatic mechanisms become insufficient to control the development of autoreactive immune responses and chronic inflammation. Local factors and immune cells can then sustain and/or amplify the inhibition of the suppressive activity of immunoregulatory cells.

The effects of regulatory cells on SLE depend on their number and function in relation to the stage of the disease and on the anatomic location where the response takes place. Simplistically, immunoregulatory cells take part in the mechanisms that control immune responses against self-antigens, or immune tolerance, at both central and peripheral levels. Central tolerance occurs in the thymus and bone marrow and eliminates immune cells that have a high avidity for self-antigens. However, low-affinity self-reactive immune cells escape negative selection and have the potential to cause autoimmunity. To avoid that possibility, several peripheral mechanisms of immune tolerance keep autoreactive immune responses under control. In addition to immunoregulatory/suppressor cells, peripheral tolerance mechanisms include clonal deletion, anergy, ignorance, and downregulation or editing of cell surface receptors.

The suppressive activity of regulatory cells appears crucial in preventing autoimmunity, in reducing inflammatory responses caused by pathogens and environmental insults, and in maintaining immune homeostasis. Here we focus on this specific aspect of immune tolerance by discussing the individual subsets of immunoregulatory cells in relation to SLE (Table 10-1; Figure 10-1).

REGULATORY T CELLS

T cells that suppress immune effector cells and proinflammatory cytokines belong to both the $CD4^+$ and $CD8^+$ cell subsets.

CD4+ Regulatory T Cells

$CD4^+$ regulatory T cells (Tregs) are the most-studied subset of immunoregulatory/suppressor cells. These cells help control immune self-reactivity, allograft rejection, and allergy, and they inhibit effector cell functions in infections and tumors. The deficiency or reduction of Tregs in normal mice leads to the development of autoimmune responses because these cells actively suppress the activation and expansion of autoreactive immune cells, and a restoration of the number of Tregs associates with the reversal of autoimmune phenotypes in several experimental animal models.[1,2]

$CD4^+$ Tregs are generally classified into two main categories, the thymus-derived natural Tregs (nTregs), and the Tregs that can be induced peripherally from $CD25^-$ precursors in vivo[3]—called adaptive or induced Tregs (iTregs) or—in vitro with interleukin-2 (IL-2) and transforming growth factor (TGF)-β[4] or IL-10 (the IL-10–producing type 1 Tregs are generally called Tr1 cells).[5] Both Treg types suppress $CD4^+$ effector cell activation, proliferation, and cytokine production as well as $CD8^+$ effector cell activation, proliferation, and cytotoxic activity in vitro, and B lymphocytes.[6] At present, there are no reliable phenotypic or functional markers that make it possible to reliably distinguish between natural and induced Tregs.

Natural Tregs represent 5% to 10% of peripheral $CD4^+$ T cells in mice and are characterized by the constitutive expression of CD25 (IL-2 receptor α-chain). In humans, they make up 1% to 2% of the peripheral blood $CD4^+$ T cells, particularly the ones with the highest CD25 expression ($CD25^{high}$ or $CD25^{bright}$).[7] However, CD25 is not a unique marker for Tregs because it is also present on activated T cells—and is thus also expressed by effector T cells.[8] To discriminate Tregs from conventional (activated) $CD4^+$ T cells, particularly in humans, it may be useful to include additional markers such as a low expression of CD127 (the α chain of the IL-7 receptor)[9] and a modulated CD45RB expression, together with the expression of $CD25^{high}$ and the intracellular expression of FOXP3.[10] FOXP3 (forkhead box P3) is an X chromosome–encoded member of the forkhead/winged-helix family of transcription regulators whose discovery led to a significant advancement in the understanding of the biology of Tregs.[11] Mice and humans harboring a loss-of-function mutation in the *FOXP3* gene are affected by fatal lymphoproliferative immune-mediated disease, the IPEX (immune dysregulation, polyendocrinopathy, enteropathy, X-linked) syndrome in humans[12] and the scurfy phenotype in mice.[13,14] FOXP3 is required for the development, maintenance, and suppressor function of Tregs,[11,15] and the loss of FOXP3 in Tregs—or its reduced expression—leads to the acquisition of effector T-cell properties that include the production of non-Treg-specific cytokines.[16,17] However, the expression of FOXP3 per se may not be sufficient for a regulatory cell function, because human activated T cells can also express FOXP3 even without possessing a suppressive capacity.[18] Yet, FOXP3 remains at present the best marker for the identification of Tregs.

Another marker that discriminates two subsets of thymus-derived $FOXP3^+$ Tregs is the co-stimulatory molecule ICOS,[19] which distinguishes $ICOS^+$ Tregs with high IL-10–producing capacity from $ICOS^-$ Tregs that produce TGF-β.[19] Additional markers that also describe Tregs are the cytotoxic T lymphocyte–associated antigen 4 (CTLA-4), the glucocorticoid-induced TNF receptor (GITR), $CD45RB^{low}$ and $CD62L^{high}$ expression, neuropilin-1, CD103 (integrin $\alpha E\beta 7$), CD5, CD27, CD38, CD39, CD73, CD122, OX-40 (CD134),

TABLE 10-1 Schematic Summary of the Phenotypic Markers of the Main Subsets of Immunoregulatory Cells in SLE

CELL TYPE	MOUSE	HUMAN
Regulatory T cells:		
CD4+ Tregs	CD4+CD25+Foxp3+	CD4+CD25highFoxP3+CD127−
		CD4+CD25highFoxP3+ICOS+/−
	Additional markers: CTLA-4, GITR, CD45RBlow, CD62Lhigh, neuropilin-1, CD103, CD5, CD27, CD38, CD39, CD73, CD122, OX-40 (CD134), TNFR2, LAG-3, CCR4, CCR7, CCR8	
CD8+ Tregs	CD8+CD28−	CD8+CD28−
	CD8+CD25+Foxp3+	CD8+CD25+FoxP3+
	CD8+CD122+	CD8+CD122+
	CD8+CD103+Foxp3+	CD8+CXCR3+
		CD8+CD27+CD45RA+
	Additional markers: CTLA-4, GITR, CD44, Ly49	
Regulatory B cells	CD1dhighCD5+B220+	CD19+CD24highCD38high
	CD1dhighCD21highCD23+IgMhigh	
Myeloid-derived suppressor cells	CD11b+GR-1low	
Dendritic cells	CD11c+CD103+	
Natural killer cells	NKG2D+, CD56bright	
Invariant natural killer T cells	Vα14Jα18/Vβ8.2	Vα24JαQ/Vβ11

GITR, glucocorticoid-induced tumor necrosis factor receptor; LAG-3, lymphocyte activation gene 3; TNFR, tumor necrosis factor receptor.

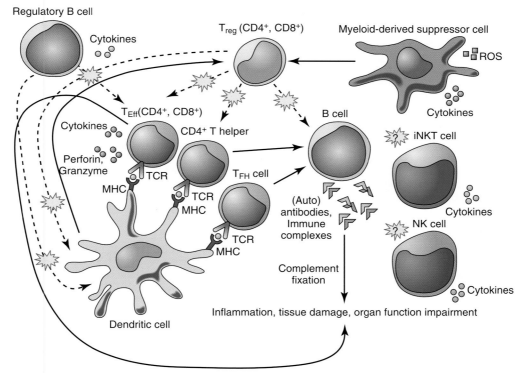

FIGURE 10-1 Immunoregulatory cells in SLE. Full lines indicate facilitating activities, dashed lines indicate suppressive effects. iNKT cell, invariant natural killer cell; MHC, major histocompatibility complex; NK, natural killer; ROS, reactive oxygen species; TCR, T-cell receptor; T$_{Eff}$, T effector cells; Treg, T-regulatory cell; T$_{FH}$ cell, T follicular helper cell.

tumor necrosis factor receptor 2 (TNFR2), lymphocyte activation gene 3 (LAG-3), C-C chemokine receptor type 4 (CCR4), CCR7, and CCR8.[20]

In regard to Treg development, nTregs originate in the thymus through high-avidity major histocompatibility complex (MHC) class II–dependent/T-cell receptor (TCR) interactions,[21-23] with the induction of FOXP3 upon TCR engagement in thymus,[24] whereas peripherally, FOXP3 expression appears influenced by factors such as intracellular signaling, cell proliferation, and the synergy with TGF-β

and IL-2.[25-26] In addition to the TCR, CD28 co-stimulation also seems to play an important role in the differentiation of Tregs, and a marked decrease in the frequency of Tregs is observed in CD28-deficient and CD80/CD86-deficient mice.[27,28] Of interest, the CD28/B7 signaling pathway is essential for the development of nTregs but it may not be needed for the development of iTregs (although it promotes their expansion).[27] Additionally, the development and function of both nTregs and iTregs appear negatively regulated by OX40, a member of the TNF–TNF receptor superfamily.[29,30]

IL-2 and TGF-β play an essential role in the differentiation and development of iTregs, and the combination of IL-2 and TGF-β can induce CD25⁻FOXP3⁻ precursors to express FOXP3 and acquire a suppressive phenotype.[3,4] Interestingly, iTregs generated in vivo and Tr1 cells may not express FOXP3, whereas iTregs induced ex vivo by IL-2 and TGF-β typically express FOXP3 and share many phenotypic and functional characteristics with nTregs.[25,31,32] In this context, it has been reported that the *foxp3* gene locus and its enhancer in nTregs could be structurally distinct from those in iTregs. DNA methylation can affect Tregs' stability and their suppressive capacity in vitro, and although demethylation of CpG motifs within the *foxp3* locus is observed in nTregs, only partial demethylation of CpG motifs is observed in iTregs.[33] Furthermore, a specific site within a unique and evolutionarily conserved CpG-rich island of *foxp3* upstream enhancer has been found unmethylated in nTregs but not in iTregs.[34] It is not known why methylation status in the TSDR (Tregs-specific demethylated region) of iTregs generated in vitro is different from that found in those generated in vivo, but it seems that iTregs induced in vivo have both stable FOXP3 expression and demethylated TSDR.[35]

The mechanisms of action of human and mouse Tregs have been studied mostly in vitro. Targets of the activity of Tregs include CD4⁺CD25⁻ T cells, CD8⁺ T cells, B cells, monocytes, and dendritic cells (DCs).[2,20,36,37] Tregs (particularly nTregs) operate through cell-to-cell contact mechanisms that involve the release of cytotoxic molecules, including perforin and granzymes A and B.[38] Gene expression arrays showed that granzyme B was upregulated in mouse Tregs,[39] and human Tregs expressed granzyme A and lysed activated CD4⁺ and CD8⁺ T cells in a perforin-dependent manner.[40,41] Tregs could also kill B cells in a granzyme B–dependent and partially perforin-dependent manner,[1,42] or could induce apoptosis of effector T cells upon the upregulation of the TRAIL-DR5 (tumor necrosis factor–related apoptosis inducing ligand-death receptor 5) pathway[43] or galectin-1.[44] Other means by which Tregs can suppress target cells is a metabolic disruption that includes cytokine deprivation–mediated apoptosis, cyclic AMP (cAMP)–mediated inhibition,[45] and the expression of the ectoenzymes CD39 and CD73 (which can generate pericellular adenosine, which inhibits activated T cells or inhibits DCs through the activation of the adenosine receptor 2A).[46-48]

Regarding the cytokines that influence Treg activity, TGF-β seems to play a key role. In vitro studies that used neutralizing antibodies to this cytokine—or that employed Tregs that lacked TGF-β indicated that TGF-β was dispensable for Tregs' suppressive functions.[49,50] However, other studies found a relevant role for cell membrane–tethered TGF-β on Tregs in their suppressive activity, both in vitro and in vivo.[51,52]

Another newly described inhibitory cytokine, IL-35, which can be expressed by Tregs, might also contribute to their suppressive capacity or could operate on targets.[53]

Lastly, other mechanisms employed by Tregs can involve direct effects on maturation and function of antigen-presenting cells (APCs) through the expression of CTLA-4[54,55] and the inhibitory lymphocyte activation gene 3 (LAG-3, or CD223, a CD4 homolog that binds MHC class II molecules with very high affinity).[56]

CD4⁺ Tregs and SLE
Lupus-prone mice have a lower frequency of Tregs than non-autoimmune mouse strains.[57] Although a deficit of Tregs in murine SLE was found to contribute to the development of the disease in mice,[58] adoptive transfer of in vitro–expanded CD4⁺CD25⁺CD62L^high Tregs slowed the progression of renal disease and decreased mortality in lupus mice.[57] However, the effect of adoptive transfer in mice in which proteinuria had already developed was modest.[57] The Tregs that could confer protection and increase the survival in mice with established SLE were the iTregs that could prevent the help of T cells to B cells for the production of anti-DNA antibodies, with a resulting inhibition of immune complex glomerulonephritis and proteinuria.[59,60]

In human SLE, the investigation of the role of Tregs in the disease has sometimes yielded controversial results. Most studies found a reduced frequency of Tregs in SLE, although other studies showed normal or even increased numbers.[60] Although a normal suppressive capacity of Tregs has been described in patients with both active and inactive SLE, it seems overall that the number of Tregs is lower in patients with active disease than in patients with inactive SLE and in normal controls, and this lower number would be associated with reduced levels of FOXP3 and a poor suppressive capacity in patients with active disease.[61-64] Another consideration is that the finding of a reduced inhibition of autoreactive immune responses in SLE could be associated with a resistance of effector target cells to an otherwise normal activity of Tregs.[65]

Nothwithstanding these aspects, it is interesting to note that a rise in the numbers of Tregs was observed after rituximab-induced B-cell depletion at the time of B-cell repopulation,[66] and that therapy with corticosteroids and/or immunosuppressive agents promoted an increase in the number of functional Tregs.[67]

CD8⁺ Tregs
Like CD4⁺ Tregs, CD8⁺ Tregs can be classified as either natural or induced. CD8⁺ nTregs develop in the thymus, whereas iTregs likely arise in the periphery from cells that initially do not express regulatory functions but acquire them after antigenic stimulation. The phenotype of CD8⁺ nTregs resembles that of CD4⁺ nTregs, and these cells generally express FOXP3 as well as CD25 in addition to surface CTLA-4 and GITR.[68] Other subsets of CD8⁺ Tregs are CD8⁺CD28⁻ T cells[69]; CD8⁺CD103⁺FOXP3⁺GITR⁺CTLA-4⁺ T cells induced by allostimulation and facilitated in culture by IL-10, IL-4, and TGF-β[70]; and CD8⁺CD122⁺[71] or CD8⁺ T cells that coexpress CD44 and Ly49 and directly suppress follicular T helper (T_FH) cells (and thus autoantibody production) by recognizing Qa-1/peptide complexes on T_FH cells and depend on IL-15 for development and function.[72]

As mechanisms of suppression, CD8⁺ Tregs employ the secretion of the cytokines IL-10 (used by human CD8⁺CXCR3⁺, CD8⁺CD122⁺, and CD8⁺CD27⁺CD45RA⁺ Tregs), TGF-β, IFN-γ, and IL-16,[73-79] cell-to-cell contact (e.g., in a membrane-bound TGF-β—and in a CTLA-4–mediated, contact-dependent manner),[68] and cytotoxicity (e.g., on activated CD4⁺ Th cells, which depends on the expression of the MHC class 1b molecule Qa-1 or HLA-E in humans).[80-82] CD8⁺ Tregs could also induce a tolerogenic phenotype in APCs that would in turn favor the induction of CD4⁺ Tregs.[68]

CD8⁺ Tregs and SLE
Murine models of tolerogenic vaccination with peptides have shown that the induction of Tregs (both CD4⁺ and CD8⁺ Tregs) protected mice from SLE manifestations.[59,77,83-85] Tolerization of (NZB × NZW) F₁ (BWF₁) mice with the anti-DNA Ig–based peptide pCons expanded CD8⁺ Tregs capable of suppressing (1) anti-DNA autoantibodies in vivo and in vitro, (2) CD4⁺ T-cell proliferation, and (3) IFN-γ production.[86] These CD8⁺ iTregs secreted TGF-β and required FOXP3 for their suppressive function.[86,87] Their induction was associated with a reduced expression of programmed death 1 (PD-1) molecules on those cells,[88] which influenced their immunoregulation capacity.[89] In the same BWF₁ lupus model, another tolerogenic peptide based on human anti-dsDNA antibodies also induced CD8⁺CD28⁻ Tregs that suppressed lymphocyte proliferation and autoantibody production, increased TGF-β production, and decreased IFN-γ and IL-10 production as well as lymphocyte apoptosis.[85,90,91] Similarly, a histone-derived tolerizing peptide (H4_71-94) in (SWR × NZB)F₁ (SNF₁) lupus-prone mice increased survival and decreased anti-dsDNA autoantibodies in lupus mice, expanding CD8⁺ Tregs that expressed GITR and TGF-β.[77] Finally, in a graft-versus-host disease (GVHD) murine model of lupus, both CD4⁺ and CD8⁺ Tregs that required IL-2 and TGF-β increased survival.[92]

In patients with SLE, some studies reported defective and/or reduced numbers of or no difference in CD8⁺ Tregs in comparison with healthy controls.[93-95] One study comparing CD8⁺ Tregs from

SLE patients and healthy controls generated by culture of CD8$^+$ T cells with IL-2 and granulocyte-monocyte colony-stimulating factor (GM-CSF) showed that CD8$^+$ Tregs from patients with active SLE could not suppress effector T cells, whereas CD8$^+$ Tregs from patients whose SLE was in remission had a suppressive capacity similar to that of cells from healthy controls.[93] In another study on the effects of autologous hematopoietic stem cell transplantation in patients with refractory lupus, patients who showed clinical improvement after transplantation had an increase in the number of CD4$^+$ and CD8$^+$ Tregs, including the CD8$^+$CD103$^+$ T-cell susbset.[96]

REGULATORY B CELLS

Certain autoantibodies can be found in healthy individuals, but in autoimmune settings these antibodies can cause tissue damage through local inflammation that ultimately leads to impaired organ function. B cells are key contributors to the pathogenesis of SLE, not only because they make autoantibodies but also because they can present self-antigens and because they secrete cytokines that can sustain or amplify the autoimmune response. On the other hand, it has become apparent that certain subsets of B cells can also exert immunoregulatory functions and contribute to the inhibition of autoimmune responses. In mice, the regulatory function of B cells is almost exclusively dependent on IL-10.[97] The cell surface phenotype of murine regulatory B cells is typically CD1d^{high}CD5$^+$ or CD1d^{high}CD21^{high}CD23$^+$IgM^{high}, and thus it overlaps with that of CD5$^+$ B-1a cells, CD1d^{high}CD21^{high}CD23^{low}IgM^{high} marginal zone (MZ) B cells, and CD1d^{high}CD21^{high}CD23^{high}IgM^{high} transitional type 2 (T2)–MZ precursor B cells.[98] As such, a regulatory function for B cells seems to be present in MZ B cells, T2-like B cells, and CD5$^+$ B cells.

In comparison with mouse regulatory B cells, less is known about human regulatory B cells: It seems that human CD19$^+$D24^{high}CD38^{high} B cells have regulatory capacity.[99]

The initial suggestion that B cells could exert immunoregulatory functions came from studies in mice in which the depletion of B cells abolished the inhibition of skin inflammation.[100] Subsequent studies showed that B cells could have immunoregulatory functions in humans and in several murine animal models, and some underlying mechanisms of action have been elucidated. The activation of regulatory B cells seems to require three signals: BCR, CD40, and Toll-like receptors (TLRs).[101] CD19 has also been found to be important in the development of regulatory B cells.[102-104] Genetic deficiency of CD19 resulted in an increased and prolonged inflammation in autoimmune-prone mice, whereas overexpression of CD19 associated with the expansion of regulatory B cells.[104] For CD40, signaling through this molecule expressed on B cells was required for regulatory B-cell development, and CD40 appeared to be involved in the regulatory mechanisms used by B cells.[105] In this context, B cells also express the ligand for CD40 (CD40L), which makes possible an autonomous B-cell control of IL-10 production (the production of IL-10 in CD40L$^+$ B cells correlates with CD40L expression levels in some autoimmune diseases).[104,106]

Currently the following two models are proposed for the B cell–mediated immunoregulation of effector CD4$^+$ T cells, Tregs, invariant natural killer T (iNKT) cells, and DCs: (1) a direct regulation due to cell interactions or the secretion of soluble factors and (2) an indirect regulation via effects on intermediate cells. For example, regulatory B cells could suppress APC function by producing IL-10 or C-X-C motif chemokine 13 (CXCL13) or could downregulate CD4$^+$ T-cell responses by engaging their TCRs.[107] Regulatory B cells could also activate iNKT cells through an increased CD1d expression.[108,109] The regulatory effects could involve CD40 or B7 co-stimulatory molecules for the mechanisms involving cell-to-cell contacts[98] or soluble factors (i.e., the B cell–derived IL-10, considering that B cells from IL-10–deficient mice cannot protect from autoimmunity[98] and that activated B cells in the presence of neutralizing anti-IL-10R fail to exert regulatory functions[110]).

B cells that produce IL-10 include peritoneal CD5$^+$ B-1a cells, CD5$^-$CD11c$^-$CD21$^+$ B cells in Peyer patches, and lupus CD21$^+$CD23$^-$ MZ cells (in response to CpG stimulation).[111-113] A B-2–like phenotype (CD5$^-$CD11b$^-$IgD$^+$) of IL-10–producing regulatory B cells detectable after IL-7 stimulation has also been identified.[114] Subsets of B regulatory cells that produce TGF-β have also been described, suggesting that certain B cells could use TGF-β to inhibit Th1 autoimmunity (by inducing apoptosis in Th1 cells) and/or by inhibiting antigen presentation[98,115] or inducing CD8$^+$ T-cell anergy.[116] Another suppressive mechanisms used by B cells could be the secretion of antibodies, because under certain circumstances, antibodies can contribute to the downregulation of inflammatory responses and participate in immunoregulation by binding the Fcγ receptor FcγRIIB on DCs to suppress APC function.[117,118] Incidentally, passive administration of antibodies associated with the reversal of inflammation in B cell–deficient mice[119] and beneficial effects in some patients with SLE.[120]

Regulatory B Cells and SLE

In one study, low-dose CD20 monoclonal antibody (mAb) treatment in BWF$_1$ mice at 12 to 28 weeks of age followed by administrations every 4 weeks delayed SLE, whereas B-cell depletion initiated in 4-week-old mice hastened the onset of disease concomitantly with the depletion of IL-10–producing regulatory B10 cells.[121] In another study, CD19-deficient BWF$_1$ mice had delayed development of antinuclear antibodies in comparison with wild-type BWF$_1$ mice, but showed pathologic signs of lupus nephritis much earlier and had reduced survival, indicating both disease-promoting and protective roles for B cells in the pathogenesis of SLE.[122] Also in the second study, IL-10–producing regulatory B cells (CD1d^{high}CD5$^+$B220$^+$) were increased in wild-type BWF$_1$ mice and were deficient in CD19-deficient BWF$_1$ mice, and the transfer of these cells from wild-type animals into the CD19-deficient ones prolonged the latters' survival.[122]

In humans, CD19$^+$CD24^{high}CD38^{high} regulatory B cells were found to suppress the differentiation of Th1 cells after CD40 stimulation in the presence of IL-10 but not TGF-β, and their suppressive capacity was reversed by blockade of CD80 and CD86.[123] Also, CD19$^+$D24^{high}CD38^{high} from patients with SLE were refractory to further CD40 stimulation, produced less IL-10, and lacked the suppressive capacity of their healthy counterparts.[123]

MYELOID-DERIVED SUPPRESSOR CELLS

Myeloid-derived suppressor cells (MDSCs) are a heterogeneous population of cells that expands during the course of inflammation, infection, and cancer.[124] MDSCs include immature granulocytes, monocytes/macrophages, certain DCs, and early myeloid progenitors, and in mice they express CD11b and GR-1.[125] The mechanisms of suppression used by these cells include the production of arginase-1 (which depletes the target cells of L-arginine), the formation of nitric oxide and reactive oxygen species (ROS),[126] and the induction of CD4$^+$ Tregs.[127] Certain macrophages also display similar suppressive capacities associated with the production of IL-10 and the capacity to influence tryptophan catabolism in target cells in addition to modulating levels of ROS and L-arginine. For example, macrophages stimulated with M-CSF (macrophage colony-stimulating factor) were found to express indoleamine 2,3-dioxygenase, which reduced tryptophan availability and inhibited T-cell proliferation.[128]

Myeloid-Derived Suppressor Cells and SLE

In MRL(lpr-lpr) lupus mice, CD11b$^+$GR-1^{low} cells were found to suppress CD4$^+$ T-cell proliferation, which was restored by the arginase-1 inhibitor nor-NOHA. These MDSCs regulated immunologic responses via signaling by chemokine (C-C motif) ligands CCL2/CCR2.[129]

In a chronic graft-versus-host disease model of lupus, *Csf3r* was identified as the causative gene of the lupus-susceptible Sle2c2 interval in NZM2410 lupus mice that was used by MDSCs in the suppression of T cells.[130]

DENDRITIC CELLS

Central and peripheral mechanisms act in parallel to inactivate, eliminate, or control autoreactive immune cells, and DCs play a key role in the development of both central and peripheral immune tolerance. Classically, when DCs are in an immature stage (characterized by elevated endocytic capacity and by low surface expression of MHC and co-stimulatory molecules), these professional APCs typically favor tolerogenic responses and promote T-cell tolerance by modulating the differentiation and the maintenance of Tregs. However, when DCs mature and become activated (e.g., in the presence of inflammation due to pathogens), they can promote immunogenic responses (aimed at the removal of the pathogen).

DCs are found in multiple tissues, including the gut, lung, skin, internal organs, blood, lymphoid tissues, and bone marrow and may display different functions that depend on the tissue microenvironment.[131] Schematically, DCs can be classified into conventional DCs and pre-DCs (which need further differentiation into DCs). Conventional DCs are further classified into migratory DCs (which move to draining lymph nodes) and lymphoid tissue–resident DCs, which capture the antigen in lymphoid organs. In addition to these conventional DC subtypes, a DC population that produces large amounts of type I IFNs is represented by the plasmacytoid DCs (pDCs). Migratory and lymphoid tissue–resident DCs can be classified into subtypes. For migratory DCs the classification is based on the tissue of origin, whereas for lymphoid tissue–resident mainly DCs it is based on specific markers.[132-134] For example, mouse skin contains two populations of langerin+ DCs: epidermal Langerhans cells (LCs) and dermal DCs (DDCs). The dermis also contains migratory LCs and langerin− DC. The skin draining lymph nodes contain different DC populations that express CD11c: CD8+DEC205+ resident DCs, CD8−DEC205− (both CD4− and CD4+ resident DCs), CD8lowCD205int DCs (migratory DDCs), and CD8lowDEC205high DCs (migratory LCs).[135] Under homeostatic conditions, DDCs and LCs continuously migrate to draining lymph nodes,[136] and the spontaneous migration of the DCs to lymph nodes in steady-state conditions contributes to the maintenance of immune tolerance to tissue antigens.[137,138] Other DCs are found in Peyer patches or in the lamina propria in the gut (where they produce IL-10 and perform local immunoregulatory functions).[139] DCs at these locations could be responsible for maintaining tolerance to commensal bacteria and food.[140,141]

The immunoregulatory function of DCs in the gut has been attributed to a CD103+ DC subpopulation that efficiently mediates the conversion of naïve T cells into iTregs. Studies in vitro have shown that CD103+ DCs isolated from the lamina propria of the small intestine and from mesenteric lymph nodes can induce iTregs' differentiation in the presence of TGF-β and retinoic acid, the active derivative of vitamin A.[142]

It is thought that conventional DCs can be tolerogenic if antigen presentation occurs in the absence of inflammation, through mechanisms that could involve apoptosis, anergy, and Treg activation and expansion.[143] In this regard, the conversion of naïve CD4+ T cells into iTregs has been attributed to migratory DCs reaching the skin-draining lymph nodes and displaying a semimature phenotype.[144] In one study, DC-mediated expansion of Tregs appeared to be contact-dependent and required IL-2 and the expression of B7 co-stimulatory molecules.[145] Studies with CD40-deficient mice also showed that DCs helped maintain Treg homeostasis through cell-cell contact, CD40-CD40L interaction, and IL-2 production.[146] Of interest, DCs could tolerize not only CD4+ T cells but also CD8+ T cells via the cross-presentation of exogenous antigens and the involvement of inhibitory molecules such as PD-1 and CTLA-4.[147]

Typically, DCs that have presented their antigens to T cells are eliminated by apoptosis,[148] so that in physiologic conditions DCs die by apoptosis 48 hours after activation.[149] Significant accumulation of DCs was observed in patients with autoimmune lymphoproliferative syndrome type II (who have a defect in apoptosis)[150] and in *lpr* mutant mice (DC apoptosis may be Fas-dependent or Fas-independent),[151] suggesting that defects in DC apoptosis might contribute to autoimmunity.

Dendritic Cells and SLE

Low-dose tolerance achieved with the histone-derived peptide H4$_{71-94}$ prolonged the lifespan of lupus mice and effectively induced CD4+ and CD8+ Tregs that suppressed autoreactive Th and B cells and renal inflammation.[77] In investigating these findings, it was found that the peptide H4$_{71-94}$ induced a tolerogenic phenotype in splenic DCs that captured the peptide, facilitated the production of local TGF-β, and allowed DC-mediated induction of Tregs together with the inhibition of Th17 cells that infiltrated the kidney of the lupus mice.[152] Tregs could also be induced in SLE by mature human monocyte-derived DCs that expressed indoleamine 2,3-dioxygenase (IDO).[153] Other DC-mediated effects on SLE were found to be secondary to immune complexes/Ig that inhibited DC maturation and enhanced tolerogenicity of DCs (through the engagement of FcγRIIb and the induction of prostaglandin E$_2$).[154]

NATURAL KILLER CELLS

Natural killer (NK) cells are large granular cells of the innate immune system that constitute about 5% to 10% of the circulating lymphocytes in humans and 1% to 3% in mice. These cells are cytotoxic to their targets without the need of MHC restriction, do not require APCs for activation, and can produce cytokines that can significantly influence the adaptive immune response, including IFN-γ, TNF-α, TGF-β, IL-5, IL-10, IL-13, IL-22, GM-CSF, and the chemokines macrophage inflammatory protein (MIP)-1α, MIP-1β, IL-8, and RANTES (regulated upon activation, normal T-cell expressed, and secreted). NK cells can be found in both lymphoid and non-lymphoid tissues and can rapidly mobilize to tissues in the course of inflammation or under pathologic conditions.[155]

The activity of NK cells is regulated by signaling through inhibitory and activating receptors that are expressed on the surfaces of these cells.[156] Inhibitory receptors include Ly49, which is a receptor for MHC I molecules in mice but not in humans, LIRs (leukocyte inhibitory receptors), and KIRs (killer-cell immunoglobulin-like receptors) for both classical MHC class I (HLA-A, HLA-B, HLA-C) and nonclassical MHC molecules like HLA-G. The activating receptors include FcγRIII, or CD16, which allows NK cells to bind the Fc part of antibodies and to lyse cells through antibody-dependent cellular cytotoxicity (ADCC). An increased expression of the activating receptor NKp46/CD335 has been observed on NK cells from patients with SLE.[157] The stimulatory NKG2D receptor on NK cells has been found to mediate tumor immunity but could also promote immune suppression when the NKG2D ligand was induced persistently, such as in certain tumors and autoimmune diseases.[158] In a genetic association study of SLE with one of the NKG2D gene variants, it was found that the *NKG2D* alanine/alanine (G/G) gene variant was significantly associated with SLE in a German cohort.[159]

Once activated, NK cells display two main activities, cytotoxicity and cytokine production. Cytotoxicity is typically directed against transformed or infected cells and appears to be controlled by the levels of self MHC class I expression on the target cells.[160] As such, reduced MHC class I molecule expression can be associated with NK cell activation, particularly when coupled with chronic infection and (increased) IFN production.[161] Human NK cells with elevated cytotoxic capacity express CD16highCD56dim, and cytokine-producing NK cells are typically CD16dim/−CD56bright. Cytotoxic NK cells usually have high levels of KIRs and low levels of NKG2A, whereas cytokine-producing NK cells express low levels of KIRs and high levels of NKG2A.[162]

The immunoregulatory function of NK cells is often ascribed to the cytokine-producing CD56bright NK cell subset, and an increased proportion of CD56bright NK cells has been observed in SLE regardless of disease activity.[157] Also, an inverse correlation between increased frequency of NKG2D+CD4+ T cells (which produce IL-10) and disease activity was described in juvenile-onset SLE, suggesting that these cells may have regulatory effects.[163]

It is generally thought that the promotion or inhibition of immune responses by NK cells may depend on the stage of the immune response and the organ where the response takes place. For example, NK cells and APCs can activate each other through cytokine release and/or co-stimulatory interactions, or kill APCs and/or T cells, or collaborate with CD4[+] Tregs and NKT cells.[164-166]

NK Cells and SLE

The role of NK cells in animal models of SLE has also been investigated. The administration of NK1.1-depleting antibodies was found to accelerate the disease, suggesting a possible protective role for NK cells.[167] Two weeks after being injected intravenously with spleen cells (SCs) from the parental DBA/2 mice that developed serum anti-dsDNA antibodies, (C57BL/6 × DBA/2) F_1 (BDF$_1$) mice had increased NK activity, but subsequently the activity dropped dramatically, suggesting that NK cells might have a protective role in lupus-like disease in the early stages of the disease.[168] The levels of serum autoantibodies were influenced by NK cells in these BDF$_1$ mice because NK cell depletion with anti-NK1.1 antibodies accelerated the development of anti-dsDNA antibodies, but the administration of polyinosine-polycytidylic acid, or poly(I:C), which expands NK cells, inhibited the production of autoantibodies.[168]

Studies of NK cells in human SLE have been mainly descriptive. In general, NK cells in patients with SLE are found numerically decreased in comparison with healthy matched controls.[169] A deficiency of NK cells, particularly CD226[+] NK cells, was reported to be prominent in patients with active SLE,[170] and a later study identified an association of CD226 polymorphism with SLE in 1163 patients with SLE and 1482 healthy controls of European ancestry.[171] Importantly, NK cells in SLE are reported to be defective in cytokine production and cytotoxic capacity.[169,172]

In human SLE, at the time of diagnosis of pediatric SLE, a significant decrease in CD16[+] or CD56[+] NK cells was observed concomitantly with a reduction of cytotoxic NK-cell activity.[173] Adult patients with lupus also exhibited a low NK killing ability in comparison with controls,[174,175] a feature that did not depend on the depressed IL-2 production that is typical of SLE.[176] Most studies found that patients with active SLE had the greatest impairment in NK-cell number and cytotoxicity,[177,178] but other studies could not link impairment of NK-cell activity in SLE with disease activity.[179] It has been speculated that the observed lower cytotoxic capacity of NK cells in patients with SLE might have a genetic component and that NK cells in those patients might produce insufficient levels of the cytokines required for the regulation of antibody production (the NK cytotoxic capacity was also found to be decreased in relatives of patients with SLE).[180]

INVARIANT NKT CELLS

NKT cells express NK cell markers together with the TCRs of T cells. Invariant NKT cells express a TCR containing an invariant (i) Vα chain (Vα14Jα18/Vβ8.2 in mice and Vα24JαQ/Vβ11 in humans).[181] The iNKT cells represent an important innate immunoregulatory cell subset that links signals of cellular distress with adaptive immune responses. These cells have anti-microbial and anti-tumor capacity and the ability to contribute to the maintenance of peripheral immune T-cell tolerance, mainly through the modulation of the activity of DCs via cell-cell interactions. In that sense, iNKT cells can favor immunogenic responses by facilitating the maturation of proinflammatory DCs or promote immune tolerance through the induction of tolerogenic DCs.

Unlike conventional T cells, which recognize antigenic peptides presented by MHC molecules, iNKT cells recognize lipid antigens presented by the non-polymorphic MHC class I–like molecule CD1d.[182] Several glycolipids and phospholipids that can activate iNKT cells have been identified,[183,184] but the natural ligands recognized by these cells remain elusive. To activate iNKT cells—both in vivo and in vitro—the glycosphingolipid α-galactosylceramide

(αGalCer), which was originally isolated from a marine sponge, has been used extensively.[185] Several microorganisms can also produce CD1d-restricted ligands that can activate iNKT cell subsets, for instance, during infection.[186-188] For example, during infection with *Salmonella typhimurium*, iNKT cells can be activated by the recognition of the endogenous glycosphingolipid isoglobotrihexosylceramide (iGb3) presented by DCs onto CD1d molecules.[189]

It was initially thought that most of the iNKT effects on the immune response, including the suppression of autoimmune reactivity, could be ascribed to the ability of these cells to release elevated amounts of cytokines. For example, it was believed that the release of type 2 cytokines such as IL-4 and IL-10 by iNKT cells could explain their protective effects in some autoimmune diseases.[190] This hypothesis was revisited upon the finding that the iNKT cell–mediated prevention of autoimmunity in Vα14Jα18 TCR transgenic mice did not require IL-4 or IL-10 (or IL-13 and TGF-β).[191,192] Additionally, iNKT cells did not promote immune tolerance in IL-10–deficient mice,[193] yet iNKT cell activation by αGalCer is associated with protection in IL-10–deficient mice.[194] It was then found that iNKT cells can anergize autoreactive CD4[+] T cells[195] and induce tolerogenic DCs.[196] Importantly, iNKT cells could also directly inhibit autoantibody-producing B cells in a contact- and CD1d-dependent manner. In vivo reconstitution of iNKT-deficient mice with iNKT cells reduced autoantibody production, and iNKT cells inhibited antibody production in SCID mice implanted with B cells.[197] Thus, different outcomes could depend on the timing, route, and frequency of administration of αGalCer (e.g., the interaction of iNKT cells with immature DCs would favor immune tolerance, whereas the interaction with mature DCs would promote immunogenic responses).

Invariant NKT Cells and SLE

Both disease-suppressive and -promoting roles of NKT cells have been reported for murine SLE. Some researchers found that NKT cells increased Ig production and anti-dsDNA antibodies in B-1 and MZ B cells.[198] In another study, the development of SLE in BWF$_1$ mice was associated with an expansion and activation of iNKT cells, and in aging mice, the immunoregulatory role of iNKT cells varied over time, with an increase in the production of IFN-γ with advancing age and progression of the disease.[199] Another study found that the activation of NKT cells exacerbated lupus in BWF$_1$ mice by increasing Th1 responses and anti-dsDNA autoantibody production and that anti-CD1d mAb was beneficial for lupus treatment.[200] Also, treatment with βGalCer, a glycolipid that reduces the cytokine secretion induced by αGalCer in NKT cells, ameliorated lupus and improved proteinuria, renal histopathology, IgG autoantibody formation, and survival in BWF$_1$ mice.[201] On the other hand, the deficiency or reduction of iNKT cells, as well as the deficiency of CD1d on B cells (which is required for the interaction between iNKT cells and B cells) was found to be associated with SLE manifestations and to increase B-cell autoreactivity.[202] In another study, CD1d deficiency, which eliminated iNKT cells, exacerbated lupus nephritis induced by the hydrocarbon oil pristane through the reduction of TNF-α and IL-4 production by T cells as well as through an expansion of MZ B cells.[203] Germline deletion of CD1d in lupus-prone BWF$_1$ mice also has been reported to exacerbate lupus-like disease.[204]

It is possible that NKT-cell activation by αGalCer could either suppress or promote lupus-like disease depending on the genetic background and other factors, including the dose of αGalCer, the number of injections, and the stage of the disease at which treatment was performed. Indeed, CD1d deficiency in BALB/c mice exacerbates lupus nephritis and autoantibody production induced by pristane, yet repeated in vivo treatment of pristane-injected BALB/c mice with αGalCer suppresses proteinuria in a CD1d- and IL-4–dependent manner.[205]

In BWF$_1$ mice, genome-wide quantitative trait locus analyses and association studies identified a locus linked to D11Mit14 on chromosome 11 in NZW mice (a parent of the hybrid BWF$_1$) as being involved in the regulation of cytokine production by NKT cells after αGalCer stimulation.[206] Another study that introgressed homozygous NZB chromosome 4 intervals onto the lupus-resistant C57BL/6 background identified a region that promotes CD1d-restricted NKT cell expansion on chromosome 4 of the other BWF$_1$ parent.[207]

The role of NKT cells in inflammatory dermatitis was also investigated in lupus-prone MRL(lpr/lpr) mice. NKT cells were found to be reduced in MRL(lpr/lpr) mice in comparison with control mice, and repeated administration of αGalCer in MRL(lpr/lpr) mice alleviated the inflammatory dermatitis but did not influence kidney disease. The mechanisms by which protection was exerted involved an expansion of iNKT cells and possibly a Th2 immune deviation (as suggested by the increased levels of serum IgE in treated animals).[208]

In one study of human SLE, the percentages and absolute numbers of NKT cells were lower in peripheral blood specimens from 128 patients as compared to 92 matched healthy controls, and so was the cytokine production after αGalCer stimulation. The NKT cell deficit correlated with the SLE Disease Activity Index (SLEDAI) score.[209] The reduction of iNKT cells also correlated with SLE progression.[210]

It is possible that as for NK cells, a genetically determined alteration of NKT cell numbers might predispose first-degree relatives of patients with lupus to an increased susceptibility to the disease, as indicated by a study that found a lower proportion of NKT cells in 367 first-degree relatives of patients with SLE than in 102 controls.[211] However, another study found not a lower frequency of NKT cells in the relatives of patients with SLE but only an inverse correlation between NKT frequency and IgG in the relatives.[212]

CONCLUSIONS

The study of immunoregulatory cells in SLE has received increasing interest that has been instrumental in a considerable advance of the field. Nonetheless, a better definitions of specific markers that can identify unique immunoregulatory cell subsets may still be required for immunotherapies aimed at modulating the activity of these cells in the disease.

In summary, it has become clear that multiple immunoregulatory cell populations play an important role in influencing the disease onset, progression, and complications of SLE. As in other autoimmune diseases in which pilot studies have been initiated, new immunotherapies using regulatory cells might be developed to possibly harness the beneficial potential of these cells in SLE.

References

1. Sakaguchi S, Sakaguchi N, Asano M, et al: Immunologic self-tolerance maintained by activated T cells expressing IL-2 receptor α-chains (CD25). Breakdown of a single mechanism of self-tolerance causes various autoimmune diseases. *J Immunol* 155:1151–1164, 1995.
2. Shevach EM: CD4$^+$CD25$^+$ suppressor T cells: more questions than answers. *Nat Rev Immunol* 2:389–400, 2002.
3. Chen W, Jin W, Hardegen N, et al: Conversion of peripheral CD4$^+$CD25$^-$ naïve T cells to CD4$^+$CD25$^+$ regulatory T cells by TGFβ induction of transcription factor Foxp3. *J Exp Med* 198:1875–1886, 2003.
4. Zheng SG, Wang JH, Gray JD, et al: Natural and induced CD4$^+$CD25$^+$ cells educate CD4$^+$CD25$^-$ cells to develop suppressive activity: the role of IL-2, TGFβ and IL-10. *J Immunol* 172:5213–5221, 2004.
5. Vieira PL, Christensen JR, Minaee S, et al: IL-10-secreting regulatory T cells do not express Foxp3 but have comparable regulatory function to naturally occurring CD4$^+$CD25$^+$ regulatory T cells. *J Immunol* 172:5986–5993, 2004.
6. Sakaguchi S: Regulatory T cells: key controllers of immunologic self-tolerance. *Cell* 101:455–458, 2000.
7. Baecher-Allan C, Brown JA, Freeman GJ, et al: CD4$^+$CD25^{high} regulatory cells in human peripheral blood. *J Immunol* 167:1245–1253, 2001.
8. Mills KH: Regulatory T cells: friend or foe in immunity to infection? *Nat Rev Immunol* 4:841–855, 2004.
9. Liu W, Putnam AL, Xu-Yu Z, et al: CD127 expression inversely correlates with FoxP3 and suppressive function of human CD4$^+$ Treg cells. *J Exp Med* 203:1701–1711, 2006.
10. Miyara M, Yoshioka Y, Kitoh A, et al: Functional delineation and differentiation dynamics of human CD4$^+$ T cells expressing the FoxP3 transcription factor. *Immunity* 19:899–911, 2009.
11. Hori S, Nomura T, Sakaguchi S: Control of regulatory T cell development by the transcription factor Foxp3. *Science* 299:1057–1061, 2003.
12. Bennett CL, Christie J, Ramsdell F, et al: The immune dysregulation, polyendocrinopathy, enteropathy, X-linked syndrome (IPEX) is caused by mutations of FOXP3. *Nat Genet* 27:20–21, 2001.
13. Brunkow ME, Jeffery EW, Hjerrild KA, et al: Disruption of a new forkhead/winged-helix protein, scurfin, results in the fatal lymphoproliferative disorder of the scurfy mouse. *Nat Genet* 27:68–73, 2001.
14. Wildin RS, Ramsdell F, Peake J, et al: X-linked neonatal diabetes mellitus, enteropathy and endocrinopathy syndrome is the human equivalent of mouse scurfy. *Nat Genet* 27:18–20, 2001.
15. Gavin M, Rudensky A: Control of immune homeostasis by naturally arising regulatory CD4$^+$ T cells. *Curr Opin Immunol* 15:690–696, 2003.
16. Wan YY, Flavell RA: Regulatory T-cell functions are subverted and converted owing to attenuated Foxp3 expression. *Nature* 445:766–770, 2007.
17. Williams LM, Rudensky AY: Maintenance of the Foxp3-dependent developmental program in mature regulatory T cells requires continued expression of Foxp3. *Nat Immunol* 8:277–284, 2007.
18. Bonelli M, von Dalwigk K, Savitskaya A, et al: FOXP3 expression in CD4$^+$ T cells of patients with systemic lupus erythematosus: a comparative phenotypic analysis. *Ann Rheum Dis* 67:664–671, 2008.
19. Ito T, Hanabuchi S, Wang YH, et al: Two functional subsets of FOXP3$^+$ regulatory T cells in human thymus and periphery. *Immunity* 28:870–880, 2008.
20. La Cava A: Natural Tregs and autoimmunity. *Front Biosci* 14:333–343, 2009.
21. Apostolou I, Sarukhan A, Klein L, et al: Origin of regulatory T cells with known specificity for antigen. *Nat Immunol* 3:756–763, 2002.
22. Bensinger SJ, Bandeira A, Jordan MS, et al: Major histocompatibility complex class II-positive cortical epithelium mediates the selection of CD4$^+$25$^+$ immunoregulatory T cells. *J Exp Med* 194:427–438, 2001.
23. Jordan MS, Boesteanu A, Reed AJ, et al: Thymic selection of CD4$^+$CD25$^+$ regulatory T cells induced by an agonist self-peptide. *Nat Immunol* 2:301–306, 2001.
24. Olivares-Villagomez D, Wang Y, Lafaille JJ: Regulatory CD4$^+$ T cells expressing endogenous T cell receptor chains protect myelin basic protein-specific transgenic mice from spontaneous autoimmune encephalomyelitis. *J Exp Med* 188:1883–1894, 1998.
25. Horwitz DA, Zheng SG, Gray JD: Natural and TGFβ-induced Foxp3$^+$CD4$^+$CD25$^+$ regulatory T cells are not mirror images of each other. *Trends Immunol* 29:429–435, 2008.
26. Bluestone JA, Abbas AK: Natural versus adaptive regulatory T cells. *Nat Rev Immunol* 3:253–257, 2003.
27. Salomon B, Lenschow DJ, Rhee L, et al: B7/CD28 costimulation is essential for the homeostasis of the CD4$^+$CD25$^+$ immunoregulatory T cells that control autoimmune diabetes. *Immunity* 12:431–440, 2000.
28. Tai X, Cowan M, Feigenbaum L, et al: CD28 costimulation of developing thymocytes induces Foxp3 expression and regulatory T cell differentiation independently of interleukin 2. *Nat Immunol* 6:152–162, 2005.
29. So T, Croft M: Cutting edge: OX40 inhibits TGFβ- and antigen-driven conversion of naïve CD4 T cells into CD25$^+$Foxp3$^+$ T cells. *J Immunol* 179:1427–1430, 2007.
30. Vu MD, Xiao X, Gao W, et al: OX40 costimulation turns off Foxp3$^+$ Tregs. *Blood* 110:2501–2510, 2007.
31. Battaglia M, Gregori S, Bacchetta R, et al: Tr1 cells: from discovery to their clinical application. *Semin Immunol* 18:120–127, 2006.
32. Zheng SG, Gray JD, Ohtsuka K, et al: Generation ex vivo of TGFβ-producing regulatory T cells from CD4$^+$CD25$^-$ precursors. *J Immunol* 169:4183–4189, 2002.
33. Floess S, Freyer J, Siewert C, et al: Epigenetic control of the Foxp3 locus in regulatory T cells. *PLoS Biol* 5:e38, 2007.
34. Lal G, Zhang N, van der Touw W, et al: Epigenetic regulation of Foxp3 expression in regulatory T cells by DNA methylation. *J Immunol* 182:259–273, 2009.
35. Polansky JK, Kretschmer K, Freyer J, et al: DNA methylation controls Foxp3 gene expression. *Eur J Immunol* 38:1654–1663, 2008.
36. Sakaguchi S: Naturally arising CD4$^+$ regulatory T cells for immunologic self-tolerance and negative control of immune responses. *Annu Rev Immunol* 22:531–562, 2004.
37. Iikuni N, Lourenco EV, Hahn BH, et al: Cutting edge: regulatory T cells directly suppress B cells in systemic lupus erythematosus. *J Immunol* 183:1518–1522, 2009.
38. Vignali DA, Collison LW, Workman CJ: How regulatory T cells work. *Nat Rev Immunol* 8:523–532, 2008.
39. McHugh RS, Whitters MJ, Piccirillo CA, et al: CD4$^+$CD25$^+$ immunoregulatory T cells: gene expression analysis reveals a functional role

for the glucocorticoid-induced TNF receptor. *Immunity* 16:311–323, 2002.

40. Grossman WJ, Verbsky JW, Tollefsen BL, et al: Differential expression of granzymes A and B in human cytotoxic lymphocyte subsets and T regulatory cells. *Blood* 104:2840–2848, 2004.

41. Gondek DC, Lu LF, Quezada SA, et al: Cutting edge: contact-mediated suppression by CD4⁺CD25⁺ regulatory cells involves a granzyme B-dependent, perforin-independent mechanism. *J Immunol* 174:1783–1786, 2005.

42. Zhao DM, Thornton AM, DiPaolo RJ, et al: Activated CD4⁺CD25⁺ T cells selectively kill B lymphocytes. *Blood* 107:3925–3932, 2006.

43. Ren X, Ye F, Jiang Z, et al: Involvement of cellular death in TRAIL/DR5-dependent suppression induced by CD4⁺CD25⁺ regulatory T cells. *Cell Death Differ* 14:2076–2084, 2007.

44. Garin MI, Chu CC, Golshayan D, et al: Galectin-1: a key effector of regulation mediated by CD4⁺CD25⁺ T cells. *Blood* 109:2058–2065, 2007.

45. Bopp T, Becker C, Klein M, et al: Cyclic adenosine monophosphate is a key component of regulatory T cell-mediated suppression. *J Exp Med* 204:1303–1310, 2007.

46. Deaglio S, Dwyer KM, Gao W, et al: Adenosine generation catalyzed by CD39 and CD73 expressed on regulatory T cells mediates immune suppression. *J Exp Med* 204:1257–1265, 2007.

47. Borsellino G, Kleinewietfeld M, Di Mitri D, et al: Expression of ecto-nucleotidase CD39 by Foxp3⁺ Treg cells: hydrolysis of extracellular ATP and immune suppression. *Blood* 110:1225–1232, 2007.

48. Kobie JJ, Shah PR, Yang L, et al: T regulatory and primed uncommitted CD4 T cells express CD73, which suppresses effector CD4 T cells by converting 5′-adenosine monophosphate to adenosine. *J Immunol* 177:6780–6786, 2006.

49. Takahashi T, Kuniyasu Y, Toda M, et al: Immunologic self-tolerance maintained by CD4⁺CD25⁺ naturally anergic and suppressive T cells: induction of autoimmune disease by breaking their anergic/suppressive state. *Int Immunol* 10:1969–1980, 1998.

50. Piccirillo CA, Letterio JJ, Thornton AM, et al: CD4⁺CD25⁺ regulatory T cells can mediate suppressor function in the absence of transforming growth factor b1 production and responsiveness. *J Exp Med* 196:237–246, 2002.

51. Nakamura K, Kitani A, Strober W: Cell contact-dependent immunosuppression by CD4⁺CD25⁺ regulatory T cells is mediated by cell surface-bound transforming growth factor β. *J Exp Med* 194:629–644, 2001.

52. Green EA, Gorelik L, McGregor CM, et al: CD4⁺CD25⁺ T regulatory cells control anti-islet CD8⁺ T cells through TGFβ-TGFβ receptor interactions in type 1 diabetes. *Proc Natl Acad Sci USA* 100:10878–10883, 2003.

53. La Cava A: Tregs are regulated by cytokines: implications for autoimmunity. *Autoimmun Rev* 8:83–87, 2008.

54. Misra N, Bayry J, Lacroix-Desmazes S, et al: Cutting edge: human CD4⁺CD25⁺ T cells restrain the maturation and antigen-presenting function of dendritic cells. *J Immunol* 172:4676–4680, 2004.

55. Read S, Greenwald R, Izcue A, et al: Blockade of CTLA-4 on CD4⁺CD25⁺ regulatory T cells abrogates their function in vivo. *J Immunol* 177:4376–4383, 2006.

56. Liang B, Workman C, Lee J, et al: Regulatory T cells inhibit dendritic cells by lymphocyte activation gene-3 engagement of MHC class II. *J Immunol* 180:5916–5926, 2008.

57. Scalapino KJ, Tang Q, Bluestone JA, et al: Suppression of disease in New Zealand Black/New Zealand White lupus-prone mice by adoptive transfer of ex vivo expanded regulatory T cells. *J Immunol* 177:1451–1459, 2006.

58. Wolf D, Hochegger K, Wolf AM, et al: CD4⁺CD25⁺ regulatory T cells inhibit experimental anti-glomerular basement membrane glomerulonephritis in mice. *J Am Soc Nephrol* 16:1360–1370, 2005.

59. La Cava A, Ebling FM, Hahn BH: Ig-Reactive CD4⁺CD25⁺ T cells from tolerized (New Zealand Black x New Zealand White)F₁ mice suppress in vitro production of antibodies to DNA. *J Immunol* 173:3542–3548, 2004.

60. La Cava A: T-regulatory cells in systemic lupus erythematosus. *Lupus* 17:421–425, 2008.

61. Mellor-Pita S, Citores MJ, Castejon R, et al: Decrease of regulatory T cells in patients with systemic lupus erythematosus. *Ann Rheum Dis* 65:553–554, 2006.

62. Miyara M, Amoura Z, Parizot C, et al: Global natural regulatory T cell depletion in active systemic lupus erythematosus. *J Immunol* 175:8392–8400, 2005.

63. Valencia X, Yarboro C, Illei G, et al: Deficient CD4⁺CD25ʰⁱᵍʰ T regulatory cell function in patients with active systemic lupus erythematosus. *J Immunol* 178:2579–2588, 2007.

64. Lyssuk EY, Torgashina AV, Soloviev SK, et al: Reduced number and function of CD4⁺CD25ʰⁱᵍʰFoxP3⁺ regulatory T cells in patients with systemic lupus erythematosus. *Adv Exp Med Biol* 601:113–119, 2007.

65. Vargas-Rojas MI, Crispín JC, Richaud-Patin Y, et al: Quantitative and qualitative normal regulatory T cells are not capable of inducing suppression in SLE patients due to T-cell resistance. *Lupus* 17:289–294, 2008.

66. Sfikakis PP, Souliotis VL, Fragiadaki KG, et al: Increased expression of the FoxP3 functional marker of regulatory T cells following B cell depletion with rituximab in patients with lupus nephritis. *Clin Immunol* 123:66–73, 2007.

67. Cepika AM, Marinic I, Morovic-Vergles J, et al: Effect of steroids on the frequency of regulatory T cells and expression of FOXP3 in a patient with systemic lupus erythematosus: a two-year follow-up. *Lupus* 16:374–377, 2007.

68. Dinesh RK, Skaggs BJ, La Cava A, et al: CD8⁺ Tregs in lupus, autoimmunity, and beyond. *Autoimmun Rev* 9:560–568, 2010.

69. Filaci G, Fravega M, Negrini S, et al: Nonantigen specific CD8+ T suppressor lymphocytes originate from CD8⁺CD28⁻ T cells and inhibits both T-cell proliferation and CTL function. *Hum Immunol* 65:142–156, 2004.

70. Uss E, Rowshani AT, Hooibrink B, et al: CD103 is a marker for alloantigen-induced regulatory CD8⁺ T cells. *J Immunol* 177:2775–2783, 2006.

71. Rifa'i M, Kawamoto Y, Nakashima I, et al: Essential roles of CD8⁺D122⁺ regulatory T cells in the maintenance of T cell homeostasis. *J Exp Med* 200:1123–1134, 2004.

72. Kim HJ, Wang X, Radfar S, et al: CD8⁺ T regulatory cells express the Ly49 class I MHC receptor and are defective in autoimmune prone B6-Yaa mice. *Proc Natl Acad Sci USA* 108:2010–2015, 2011.

73. Menager-Marcq I, Pomie C, Romagnoli P, et al: CD8⁺D28⁻ regulatory T lymphocytes prevent experimental inflammatory bowel disease in mice. *Gastroenterology* 131:1775–1785, 2006.

74. Endharti AT, Rifa IMS, Shi Z, et al: Cutting edge: CD8⁺D122⁺ regulatory T cells produce IL-10 to suppress IFNγ production and proliferation of CD8⁺ T cells. *J Immunol* 175:7093–7097, 2005.

75. Saitoh O, Abiru N, Nakahara M, et al: CD8⁺D122⁺ T cells, a newly identified regulatory T subset, negatively regulate Graves' hyperthyroidism in a murine model. *Endocrinology* 148:6040–6046, 2007.

76. Hahn BH, Singh RP, La Cava A, et al: Tolerogenic treatment of lupus mice with consensus peptide induces Foxp3-expressing, apoptosis-resistant, TGFβ-secreting CD8⁺ T cell suppressors. *J Immunol* 175:7728–7737, 2005.

77. Kang HK, Michaels MA, Berner BR, et al: Very low-dose tolerance with nucleosomal peptides controls lupus and induces potent regulatory T cell subsets. *J Immunol* 174:3247–3255, 2005.

78. Filaci G, Fenoglio D, Fravega M, et al: CD8⁺CD28⁻ T regulatory lymphocytes inhibiting T cell proliferative and cytotoxic functions infiltrate human cancers. *J Immunol* 179:4323–4334, 2007.

79. Klimiuk PA, Goronzy JJ, Weyand CM: IL-16 as an anti-inflammatory cytokine in rheumatoid synovitis. *J Immunol* 162:4293–4299, 1999.

80. Jiang H, Ware R, Stall A, et al: Murine CD8⁺ T cells that specifically delete autologous CD4⁺ T cells expressing Vβ8 TCR: a role of the Qa-1 molecule. *Immunity* 2:185–194, 1995.

81. Sarantopoulos S, Lu L, Cantor H: Qa-1 restriction of CD8⁺ suppressor T cells. *J Clin Invest* 114:1218–1221, 2004.

82. Hu D, Ikizawa K, Lu L, et al: Analysis of regulatory CD8 T cells in Qa-1-deficient mice. *Nat Immunol* 5:516–523, 2004.

83. Hahn BH, Singh RP, La Cava A, et al: Tolerogenic treatment of lupus mice with consensus peptide induces Foxp3-expressing, apoptosis-resistant, TGFβ secreting CD8⁺ T cell suppressors. *J Immunol* 175:7728–7737, 2005.

84. Ferrera F, Hahn BH, Rizzi M, et al: Protection against renal disease in (NZB x NZW)F₁ lupus-prone mice after somatic B cell gene vaccination with anti-DNA immunoglobulin consensus peptide. *Arthritis Rheum* 56:1945–1953, 2007.

85. Sharabi A, Zinger H, Zborowsky M, et al: A peptide based on the complementarity-determining region 1 of an autoantibody ameliorates lupus by up-regulating CD4⁺CD25⁺ cells and TGFβ. *Proc Natl Acad Sci USA* 103:8810–8815, 2006.

86. Singh RP, Hahn BH, Wong M, et al: CD8⁺ T cell-mediated suppression of autoimmunity in a murine lupus model of peptide-induced immune

tolerance depends on Foxp3 expression. *J Immunol* 178:7649–7657, 2007.

87. Hahn BH, Singh RP, La Cava A, et al: Tolerogenic treatment of lupus mice with consensus peptide induces Foxp3-expressing, apoptosis-resistant, TGFβ-secreting CD8+ T cell suppressors. *J Immunol* 175:7728–7737, 2005.

88. Singh RP, La Cava A, Hahn BH: pConsensus peptide induces tolerogenic CD8+ T cells in lupus-prone (NZB x NZW)F₁ mice by differentially regulating Foxp3 and PD1 molecules. *J Immunol* 180:2069–2080, 2008.

89. Wong M, La Cava A, Singh RP, et al: Blockade of programmed death-1 in young (New Zealand black x New Zealand white)F₁ mice promotes the activity of suppressive CD8+ T cells that protect from lupus-like disease. *J Immunol* 185:6563–6571, 2010.

90. Eilat E, Dayan M, Zinger H, et al: The mechanism by which a peptide based on complementarity determining region-1 of a pathogenic anti-DNA auto-Ab ameliorates experimental systemic lupus erythematosus. *Proc Natl Acad Sci USA* 98:1148–1153, 2001.

91. Sharabi A, Haviv A, Zinger H, et al: Amelioration of murine lupus by a peptide, based on the complementarity determining region-1 of an auto-antibody as compared to dexamethasone: different effects on cytokines and apoptosis. *Clin Immunol* 119:146–155, 2006.

92. Horwitz DA, Gray JD, Zheng SG: The potential of human regulatory T cells generated *ex vivo* as a treatment for lupus and other chronic inflammatory diseases. *Arthritis Res* 4:241–246, 2002.

93. Filaci G, Bacilieri S, Fravega M, et al: Impairment of CD8+ T suppressor cell function in patients with active systemic lupus erythematosus. *J Immunol* 166:6452–6457, 2001.

94. Tulunay A, Yavuz S, Direskeneli H, et al: CD8+D28−, suppressive T cells in systemic lupus erythematosus. *Lupus* 17:630–637, 2008.

95. Alvarado-Sanchez B, Hernandez-Castro B, Portales-Perez D, et al: Regulatory T cells in patients with systemic lupus erythematosus. *J Autoimmun* 27:110–118, 2006.

96. Zhang L, Bertucci AM, Ramsey-Goldman R, et al: Regulatory T cell (Treg) subsets return in patients with refractory lupus following stem cell transplantation, and TGFβ-producing CD8+ Treg cells are associated with immunological remission of lupus. *J Immunol* 183:6346–6358, 2009.

97. Fujimoto M: Regulatory B cells in skin and connective tissue diseases. *J Dermatol Sci* 2010 Oct;60:1–7.

98. Li X, Braun J, Wei B: Regulatory B cells in autoimmune diseases and mucosal immune homeostasis. *Autoimmunity* 44:58–68, 2011.

99. Mauri C: Regulation of immunity and autoimmunity by B cells. *Curr Opin Immunol* 22:761–767, 2010.

100. Katz SI, Parker D, Turk JL: B-cell suppression of delayed hypersensitivity reactions. *Nature* 251:550–551, 1974.

101. Yanaba K, Bouaziz JD, Matsushita T, et al: The development and function of regulatory B cells expressing IL-10 (B10 cells) requires antigen receptor diversity and TLR signals. *J Immunol* 182:7459–7472, 2009.

102. Matsushita T, Fujimoto M, Hasegawa M, et al: Inhibitory role of CD19 in the progression of experimental autoimmune encephalomyelitis by regulating cytokine response. *Am J Pathol* 168:812–821, 2006.

103. Watanabe R, Fujimoto M, Ishiura N, et al: CD19 expression in B cells is important for suppression of contact hypersensitivity. *Am J Pathol* 171:560–570, 2007.

104. Yanaba K, Bouaziz J-D, Haas KM, et al: A regulatory B cell subset with a unique CD1d^hiCD5+ phenotype controls T cell-dependent inflammatory responses. *Immunity* 28:639–650, 2008.

105. Richards S, Watanabe C, Santos L, et al: Regulation of B-cell entry into the cell cycle. *Immunol Rev* 224:183–200, 2008.

106. Desai-Mehta A, Lu L, Ramsey-Goldman R, et al: Hyperexpression of CD40 ligand by B and T cells in human lupus and its role in pathogenic autoantibody production. *J Clin Invest* 97:2063–2073, 1996.

107. Subramanian S, Yates M, Vandenbark AA, et al: Oestrogen-mediated protection of experimental autoimmune encephalomyelitis in the absence of Foxp3+ regulatory T cells implicates compensatory pathways including regulatory B cells. *Immunology* 132:340–347, 2011.

108. Mizoguchi A, Mizoguchi E, Takedatsu H, et al: Chronic intestinal inflammatory condition generates IL-10-producing regulatory B cell subset characterized by CD1d upregulation. *Immunity* 16:219–230, 2002.

109. Koh-Hei S, Joan SS: CD1d on antigen-transporting APC and splenic marginal zone B cells promotes NKT cell-dependent tolerance. *Eur J Immunol* 32:848–857, 2002.

110. Mauri C, Gray D, Mushtaq N, et al: Prevention of arthritis by interleukin-10-producing B cells. *J Exp Med* 197:489–501, 2003.

111. Madan R, Demircik F, Surianarayanan S, et al: Nonredundant roles for B cell-derived IL-10 in immune counter-regulation. *J Immunol* 183:2312–2320, 2009.

112. Spencer NF, Daynes RA: IL-12 directly stimulates expression of IL-10 by CD5+ B cells and IL-6 by both CD5+ and CD5− B cells: possible involvement in age-associated cytokine dysregulation. *Int Immunol* 9:745–754, 1997.

113. Brummel R, Lenert P: Activation of marginal zone B cells from lupus mice with type A(D) CpG-oligodeoxynucleotides. *J Immunol* 174:2429–2434, 2005.

114. Mizoguchi A, Bhan AK: A case for regulatory B cells. *J Immunol* 176:705–710, 2006.

115. Tian J, Zekzer D, Hanssen L, et al: Lipopolysaccharide-activated B cells down-regulate Th1 immunity and prevent autoimmune diabetes in non-obese diabetic mice. *J Immunol* 167:1081–1089, 2001.

116. Parekh VV, Prasad DVR, Banerjee PP, et al: B cells activated by lipopolysaccharide, but not by anti-Ig and anti-CD40 antibody, induce anergy in CD8+ T cells: role of TGFβ1. *J Immunol* 170:5897–5911, 2003.

117. Buendia AJ, Del Rio L, Ortega N, et al: B-cell-deficient mice show an exacerbated inflammatory response in a model of *Chlamydophila abortus* infection. *Infect Immun* 70:6911–6918, 2002.

118. Diamond MS, Shrestha B, Marri A, et al: B cells and antibody play critical roles in the immediate defense of disseminated infection by West Nile encephalitis virus. *J Virol* 77:2578–2586, 2003.

119. Mizoguchi A, Mizoguchi E, Smith RN, et al: Suppressive role of B cells in chronic colitis of T cell receptor α mutant mice. *J Exp Med* 186:1749–1756, 1997.

120. Siragam V, Brinc D, Crow AR, et al: Can antibodies with specificity for soluble antigens mimic the therapeutic effects of intravenous IgG in the treatment of autoimmune disease? *J Clin Invest* 115:155–160, 2005.

121. Haas KM, Watanabe R, Matsushita T, et al: Protective and pathogenic roles for B cells during systemic autoimmunity in NZB/W F₁ mice. *J Immunol* 184:4789–4800, 2010.

122. Watanabe R, Ishiura N, Nakashima H, et al: Regulatory B cells (B10 cells) have a suppressive role in murine lupus: CD19 and B10 cell deficiency exacerbates systemic autoimmunity. *J Immunol* 184:4801–4809, 2010.

123. Blair PA, Noreña LY, Flores-Borja F, et al: CD19+CD24^hiCD38^hi B cells exhibit regulatory capacity in healthy individuals but are functionally impaired in systemic lupus erythematosus patients. *Immunity* 32:129–140, 2010.

124. Frumento G, Piazza T, Di Carlo E, et al: Targeting tumor-related immunosuppression for cancer immunotherapy. *Endocr Metab Immune Disord Drug Targets* 6:233–237, 2006.

125. Mahnke K, Bedke T, Enk AH: Regulatory conversation between antigen presenting cells and regulatory T cells enhance immune suppression. *Cell Immunol* 250:1–13, 2007.

126. Gelderman KA, Hultqvist M, Pizzolla A, et al: Macrophages suppress T cell responses and arthritis development in mice by producing reactive oxygen species. *J Clin Invest* 117:3020–3028, 2007.

127. Hoves S, Krause SW, Schutz C, et al: Monocyte-derived human macrophages mediate anergy in allogeneic T cells and induce regulatory T cells. *J Immunol* 177:2691–2698, 2006.

128. Munn DH, Shafizadeh E, Attwood JT, et al: Inhibition of T cell proliferation by macrophage tryptophan catabolism. *J Exp Med* 189:1363–1372, 1999.

129. Iwata Y, Furuichi K, Kitagawa K, et al: Involvement of CD11b+GR-1^low cells in autoimmune disorder in MRL-Fas^lpr mouse. *Clin Exp Nephrol* 14:411–417, 2010.

130. Xu Z, Vallurupalli A, Fuhrman C, et al: A New Zealand black-derived locus suppresses chronic graft-versus-host disease and autoantibody production through nonlymphoid bone marrow-derived cells. *J Immunol* 186:4130–4139, 2011.

131. Everson MP, McDuffie DS, Lemak DG, et al: Dendritic cells from different tissues induce production of different T cell cytokine profiles. *J Leukoc Biol* 59:494–498, 1996.

132. Ardavin C: Origin, precursors and differentiation of mouse dendritic cells. *Nat Rev Immunol* 3:582–590, 2003.

133. Shortman K, Liu YJ: Mouse and human dendritic cell subtypes. *Nat Rev Immunol* 2:151–161, 2002.

134. Henri S, Vremec D, Kamath A, et al: The dendritic cell populations of mouse lymph nodes. *J Immunol* 167:741–748, 2001.

135. Zanoni I, Granucci F: The regulatory role of dendritic cells in the induction and maintenance of T-cell tolerance. *Autoimmunity* 44:23–32, 2011.

136. Steinman RM, Nussenzweig MC: Avoiding horror autotoxicus: the importance of dendritic cells in peripheral T cell tolerance. *Proc Natl Acad Sci USA* 99:351–358, 2002.

137. Kamath AT, Henri S, Battye F, et al: Developmental kinetics and lifespan of dendritic cells in mouse lymphoid organs. *Blood* 100:1734–1741, 2002.

138. Merad M, Manz MG, Karsunky H, et al: Langerhans cells renew in the skin throughout life under steady-state conditions. *Nat Immunol* 3:1135–1141, 2002.

139. Hart AL, Al-Hassi HO, Rigby RJ, et al: Characteristics of intestinal dendritic cells in inflammatory bowel diseases. *Gastroenterology* 129:50–65, 2005.

140. Iwasaki A, Kelsall BL: Mucosal immunity and inflammation. I. Mucosal dendritic cells: their specialized role in initiating T cell responses. *Am J Physiol* 276:G1074-G1078, 1999.

141. Worbs T, Bode U, Yan S, et al: Oral tolerance originates in the intestinal immune system and relies on antigen carriage by dendritic cells. *J Exp Med* 203:519–527, 2006.

142. Coombes JL, Siddiqui KR, Arancibia-Carcamo CV, et al: A functionally specialized population of mucosal CD103$^+$ DCs induces Foxp3$^+$ regulatory T cells via a TGFβ and retinoic acid-dependent mechanism. *J Exp Med* 204:1757–1764, 2007.

143. Steinbrink K, Mahnke K, Grabbe S, et al: Myeloid dendritic cell: from sentinel of immunity to key player of peripheral tolerance? *Hum Immunol* 70:289–293, 2009.

144. Lutz MB, Kurts C: Induction of peripheral CD4$^+$ T-cell tolerance and CD8$^+$ T-cell cross-tolerance by dendritic cells. *Eur J Immunol* 39:2325–2330, 2009.

145. Yamazaki S, Iyoda T, Tarbell K, et al: Direct expansion of functional CD25$^+$CD4$^+$ regulatory T cells by antigen-processing dendritic cells. *J Exp Med* 198:235–247, 2003.

146. Guiducci C, Valzasina B, Dislich H, et al: CD40/CD40L interaction regulates CD4$^+$CD25$^+$ Treg homeostasis through dendritic cell-produced IL-2. *Eur J Immunol* 35:557–567, 2005.

147. Probst HC, McCoy K, Okazaki T, et al: Resting dendritic cells induce peripheral CD8$^+$ T cell tolerance through PD-1 and CTLA-4. *Nat Immunol* 6:280–286, 2005.

148. Matsue H, Takashima A: Apoptosis in dendritic cell biology. *J Dermatol Sci* 20:159–171, 1999.

149. Kamath AT, Henri S, Battye F, et al: Developmental kinetics and lifespan of dendritic cells in mouse lymphoid organs. *Blood* 100:1734–1741, 2002.

150. Wang J, Zheng L, Lobito A, et al: Inherited human caspase 10 mutations underlie defective lymphocyte and dendritic cell apoptosis in autoimmune lymphoproliferative syndrome type II. *Cell* 98:47–58, 1999.

151. Fields ML, Sokol CL, Eaton-Bassiri A, et al: Fas/Fas ligand deficiency results in altered localization of anti-double-stranded DNA B cells and dendritic cells. *J Immunol* 167:2370–2378, 2001.

152. Kang HK, Liu M, Datta SK: Low-dose peptide tolerance therapy of lupus generates plasmacytoid dendritic cells that cause expansion of autoantigen-specific regulatory T cells and contraction of inflammatory Th17 cells. *J Immunol* 178:7849–7858, 2007.

153. Kast RE, Altschuler EL: Indoleamine 2,3-dioxygenase-expressing mature human monocyte-derived dendritic cells expand potent autologous regulatory T cells: consideration of triamterene to treat lupus. *Med Hypotheses* 74:957, 2010.

154. Zhang Y, Liu S, Yu Y, et al: Immune complex enhances tolerogenicity of immature dendritic cells via FcγRIIb and promotes FcγRIIb-overexpressing dendritic cells to attenuate lupus. *Eur J Immunol* 41:1154–1164, 2011.

155. Flodström-Tullberg M, Bryceson YT, Shi FD, et al: Natural killer cells in human autoimmunity. *Curr Opin Immunol* 21:634–640, 2009.

156. Shi FD, Van Kaer L: Reciprocal regulation between natural killer cells and autoreactive T cells. *Nat Rev Immunol* 6:751–760, 2006.

157. Schepis D, Gunnarsson I, Eloranta ML, et al: Increased proportion of CD56(bright) natural killer cells in active and inactive systemic lupus erythematosus. *Immunology* 126:140–146, 2009.

158. Champsaur M, Lanier LL: Effect of NKG2D ligand expression on host immune responses. *Immunol Rev* 235:267–285, 2010.

159. Kabalak G, Thomas RM, Martin J, et al: Association of an NKG2D gene variant with systemic lupus erythematosus in two populations. *Hum Immunol* 71:74–78, 2010.

160. Moins-Teisserenc HT, Gadola SD, Cella M, et al: Association of a syndrome resembling Wegener's granulomatosis with low surface expression of HLA class-I molecules. *Lancet* 354:1598–1603, 1999.

161. Zimmer J, Bausinger H, de la Salle H: Autoimmunity mediated by innate immune effector cells. *Trends Immunol* 22:300–301, 2001.

162. Galiani MD, Aguado E, Tarazona R, et al: Expression of killer inhibitory receptors on cytotoxic cells from HIV-1-infected individuals. *Clin Exp Immunol* 115:472–476, 1999.

163. Dai Z, Turtle CJ, Booth GC, et al: Normally occurring NKG2D$^+$CD4$^+$ T cells are immunosuppressive and inversely correlated with disease activity in juvenile-onset lupus. *J Exp Med* 206:793–805, 2009.

164. O'Garra A: Cytokines induce the development of functionally heterogeneous T helper cell subsets. *Immunity* 8:275–283, 1998.

165. Chung Y, Chang SH, Martinez GJ, et al: Critical regulation of early Th17 cell differentiation by interleukin-1 signaling. *Immunity* 30:576–587, 2009.

166. Xu W, Fazekas G, Hara H, et al: Mechanism of natural killer (NK) cell regulatory role in experimental autoimmune encephalomyelitis. *J Neuroimmunol* 163:24–30, 2005.

167. Nilsson N, Bremell T, Tarkowski A, et al: Protective role of NK1.1$^+$ cells in experimental *Staphylococcus aureus* arthritis. *Clin Exp Immunol* 117:63–69, 1999.

168. Harada M, Lin T, Kurosawa S, et al: Natural killer cells inhibit the development of autoantibody production in (C57BL/6 x DBA/2) F$_1$ hybrid mice injected with DBA/2 spleen cells. *Cell Immunol* 161:42–49, 1995.

169. Park YW, Kee SJ, Cho YN, et al: Impaired differentiation and cytotoxicity of natural killer cells in systemic lupus erythematosus. *Arthritis Rheum* 60:1753–1763, 2009.

170. Huang Z, Fu B, Zheng SG, et al: Involvement of CD226$^+$ NK cells in immunopathogenesis of systemic lupus erythematosus. *J Immunol* 186:3421–3431, 2011.

171. Löfgren SE, Delgado-Vega AM, Gallant CJ, et al: A 3′-untranslated region variant is associated with impaired expression of CD226 in T and natural killer T cells and is associated with susceptibility to systemic lupus erythematosus. *Arthritis Rheum* 62:3404–3414, 2010.

172. Green MR, Kennell AS, Larche MJ, et al: Natural killer cell activity in families of patients with systemic lupus erythematosus: demonstration of a killing defect in patients. *Clin Exp Immunol* 141:165–173, 2005.

173. Yabuhara A, Yang FC, Nakazawa T, et al: A killing defect of natural killer cells as an underlying immunologic abnormality in childhood systemic lupus erythematosus. *J Rheumatol* 23:171–177, 1996.

174. Egan ML, Mendelsohn SL, Abo T, et al: Natural killer cells in systemic lupus erythematosus. Abnormal numbers and functional immaturity of HNK-1$^+$ cells. *Arthritis Rheum* 26:623–629, 1983.

175. Ytterberg SR, Schnitzer TJ: Inhibition of natural killer cell activity by serum from patients with systemic lupus erythematosus: roles of disease activity and serum interferon. *Ann Rheum Dis* 43:457–461, 1984.

176. Sibbitt WL Jr, Likar L, Spellman CW, et al: Impaired natural killer cell function in systemic lupus erythematosus. Relationship to interleukin-2 production. *Arthritis Rheum* 26:1316–1320, 1983.

177. Hervier B, Beziat V, Haroche J, et al: Phenotype and function of natural killer cells in systemic lupus erythematosus: over IFNγ production in active patients. *Arthritis Rheum* 63:1698–1706, 2011.

178. Katz P, Zaytoun AM, Lee JH Jr, et al: Abnormal natural killer cell activity in systemic lupus erythematosus: an intrinsic defect in the lytic event. *J Immunol* 129:1966–1971, 1982.

179. Ewan PW, Barrett HM, Pusey CD: Defective natural killer (NK) and killer (K) cell function in systemic lupus erythematosus. *J Clin Lab Immunol* 10:71–76, 1983.

180. Green MR, Kennell AS, Larche MJ, et al: Natural killer cell activity in families of patients with systemic lupus erythematosus: demonstration of a killing defect in patients. *Clin Exp Immunol* 141:165–173, 2005.

181. Van Kaer L: NKT cells: T lymphocytes with innate effector functions. *Curr Opin Immunol* 19:354–364, 2007.

182. Brigl M, Brenner MB: CD1: antigen presentation and T cell function. *Annu Rev Immunol* 22:817–890, 2004.

183. Gumperz JE, Roy C, Makowska A, et al: Murine CD1d-restricted T cell recognition of cellular lipids. *Immunity* 12:211–221, 2000.

184. Kawano T, Cui J, Koezuka Y, et al: CD1d-restricted and TCR-mediated activation of Vα14 NKT cells by glycosylceramides. *Science* 278:1626–1629, 1997.

185. Kobayashi E, Motoki K, Uchida T, et al: KRN7000, a novel immunomodulator, and its antitumor activities. *Oncol Res* 7:529–534, 1995.

186. Mattner J, Debord KL, Ismail N, et al: Exogenous and endogenous glycolipid antigens activate NKT cells during microbial infections. *Nature* 434:525–529, 2005.

187. Kinjo Y, Wu D, Kim G, et al: Recognition of bacterial glycosphingolipids by natural killer T cells. *Nature* 434:520–525, 2005.

188. Amprey JL, Im JS, Turco SJ, et al: A subset of liver NK T cells is activated during *Leishmania donovani* infection by CD1d-bound lipophosphoglycan. *J Exp Med* 200:895–904, 2004.

189. Zajonc DM, Cantu C 3rd, Mattner J, et al: Structure and function of a potent agonist for the semi-invariant natural killer T cell receptor. *Nat Immunol* 6:810–818, 2005.

190. Miyamoto K, Miyake S, Yamamura T: A synthetic glycolipid prevents autoimmune encephalomyelitis by inducing Th2 bias of natural killer T cells. *Nature* 413:531–534, 2001.

191. Hugues S, Mougneau E, Ferlin W, et al: Tolerance to islet antigens and prevention from diabetes induced by limited apoptosis of pancreatic β cells. *Immunity* 16:169–181, 2002.

192. Beaudoin L, Laloux V, Novak J, et al: NKT cells inhibit the onset of diabetes by impairing the development of pathogenic T cells specific for pancreatic b cells. *Immunity* 17:725–736, 2002.

193. Sonoda KH, Faunce DE, Taniguchi M, et al: NK T cell-derived IL-10 is essential for the differentiation of antigen-specific T regulatory cells in systemic tolerance. *J Immunol* 166:42–50, 2001.

194. Mi QS, Ly D, Zucker P, et al: Interleukin-4 but not interleukin-10 protects against spontaneous and recurrent type 1 diabetes by activated CD1d-restricted invariant natural killer T-cells. *Diabetes* 53:1303–1310, 2004.

195. Novak J, Beaudoin L, Griseri T, et al: Inhibition of T cell differentiation into effectors by NKT cells requires cell contacts. *J Immunol* 174:1954–1961, 2005.

196. Naumov YN, Bahjat KS, Gausling R, et al: Activation of CD1d-restricted T cells protects NOD mice from developing diabetes by regulating dendritic cell subsets. *Proc Natl Acad Sci USA* 98:13838–13843, 2001.

197. Yang JQ, Wen X, Kim PJ, et al: Invariant NKT cells inhibit autoreactive B cells in a contact- and CD1d-dependent manner. *J Immunol* 186:1512–1520, 2011.

198. Takahashi T, Strober S: Natural killer T cells and innate immune B cells from lupus-prone NZB/W mice interact to generate IgM and IgG autoantibodies. *Eur J Immunol* 38:156–165, 2008.

199. Forestier C, Molano A, Im JS, et al: Expansion and hyperactivity of CD1d-restricted NKT cells during the progression of systemic lupus erythematosus in (New Zealand Black x New Zealand White)F₁ mice. *J Immunol* 175:763–770, 2005.

200. Zeng D, Liu Y, Sidobre S, et al: Activation of natural killer T cells in NZB/W mice induces Th1-type immune responses exacerbating lupus. *J Clin Invest* 112:1211–1222, 2003.

201. Morshed SR, Takahashi T, Savage PB, et al: β-galactosylceramide alters invariant natural killer T cell function and is effective treatment for lupus. *Clin Immunol* 132:321–333, 2009.

202. Wermeling F, Lind SM, Jordö ED, et al: Invariant NKT cells limit activation of autoreactive CD1d⁺ B cells. *J Exp Med* 207:943–952, 2010.

203. Yang JQ, Singh AK, Wilson MT, et al: Immunoregulatory role of CD1d in the hydrocarbon oil-induced model of lupus nephritis. *J Immunol* 171:2142–2153, 2003.

204. Yang JQ, Wen X, Liu H, et al: Examining the role of CD1d and natural killer T cells in the development of nephritis in a genetically susceptible lupus model. *Arthritis Rheum* 56:1219–1233, 2007.

205. Singh AK, Yang JQ, Parekh VV, et al: The natural killer T cell ligand α-galactosylceramide prevents or promotes pristane-induced lupus in mice. *Eur J Immunol* 35:1143–1154, 2005.

206. Tsukamoto K, Ohtsuji M, Shiroiwa W, et al: Aberrant genetic control of invariant TCR-bearing NKT cell function in New Zealand mouse strains: possible involvement in systemic lupus erythematosus pathogenesis. *J Immunol* 180:4530–4539, 2008.

207. Loh C, Cai YC, Bonventi G, et al: Dissociation of the genetic loci leading to b1a and NKT cell expansions from autoantibody production and renal disease in B6 mice with an introgressed New Zealand Black chromosome 4 interval. *J Immunol* 178:1608–1617, 2007.

208. Yang JQ, Saxena V, Xu H, et al: Repeated α-galactosylceramide administration results in expansion of NK T cells and alleviates inflammatory dermatitis in MRL-lpr/lpr mice. *J Immunol* 171:4439–4446, 2003.

209. Cho YN, Kee SJ, Lee SJ, et al: Numerical and functional deficiencies of natural killer T cells in systemic lupus erythematosus: their deficiency related to disease activity. *Rheumatology (Oxford)* 50:1054–1063, 2011.

210. Oishi Y, Sumida T, Sakamoto A, et al: Selective reduction and recovery of invariant Vα24JαQ T cell receptor T cells in correlation with disease activity in patients with systemic lupus erythematosus. *J Rheumatol* 28:275–283, 2001.

211. Wither J, Cai YC, Lim S, et al; CaNIOS Investigators, Fortin PR: Reduced proportions of natural killer T cells are present in the relatives of lupus patients and are associated with autoimmunity. *Arthritis Res Ther* 10:R108, 2008.

212. Green MR, Kennell AS, Larche MJ, et al: Natural killer T cells in families of patients with systemic lupus erythematosus: their possible role in regulation of IgG production. *Arthritis Rheum* 56:303–310, 2007.

Apoptosis, Necrosis, and Autophagy

Keith B. Elkon

DEFINITIONS

Apoptosis

The modern understanding of apoptosis began with the electron-microscopic descriptions of morphologic changes characterized by shrinkage of hepatocytes (i.e., shrinkage necrosis) after ischemic or toxic injury to the liver. The name *apoptosis* was coined by Kerr in 1972 to describe the form of death that was "consistent with an active, inherently controlled phenomenon" characterized by cell shrinkage, nuclear condensation, and cell blebbing (Figure 11-1).[1] This term also conveyed the concept of cell death that was similar to leaves falling from a tree (*apo* means "from" and *ptosis* "a fall" in Greek), implying a regulated "mechanism of cell deletion, which is complementary to mitosis."[1]

Further developments in our understanding of apoptosis paralleled advances in molecular biology, genetics, and biochemistry. The detection of a nucleosomal ladder[2] was of considerable importance, because it defined a biochemical event (i.e., nucleosomal cleavage) and provided a simple electrophoretic test for detection of apoptotic cell death that remains a standard in the field. Studies in the 1980s demonstrated that the death of cells during nematode development was under strict genetic control. Remarkably, the death of these cells could be perturbed by mutation of a small number of genes called *ced* (for cell death abnormal) genes.[3] Horvitz determined that two ced genes, *ced3* and *ced4*, encoded death effectors, whereas *ced9* was an antiapoptotic gene. Most of the remaining ced genes were responsible for engulfment and removal of the "corpses." This simple model, in which CED-3 is the main death protease that is activated by CED-4 and inhibited by CED-9, has served as a paradigm for defining apoptotic pathways in mammalian cells. Mammalian cells are more complex and, as discussed here in detail, have multiple defined pathways that follow the basic *Caenorhabditis elegans* model. The molecules within these pathways, the downstream effectors of apoptosis, the caspases (cysteine aspartate proteases), and the proteins implicated in the clearance of apoptotic cells are discussed in detail. The control of cell death is of seminal importance in a number of diseases, including cancers, autoimmune diseases, and degenerative disorders.[4] Regulation of apoptosis and handling of dying cells are especially relevant to SLE, as also discussed here.

Necrosis

Necrosis has traditionally been viewed as a passive form of cell death resulting from toxic or physical insults leading to adenosine triphosphate (ATP) depletion, although later studies indicate that some changes can be biochemically mediated. Morphologically, necrosis is notable for plasma cell membrane disruption leading to cellular swelling and cytoplasmic vacuolation (see Figure 11-1). In contradistinction to apoptosis, necrotic death induces inflammation around the dying cell as a result of the release of various intracellular components (see Figure 11-1). Although chromatin degradation is evident in necrotic cells, the condensation and organized DNA fragmentation seen in apoptotic cells are usually absent. Notably, the same inducers (e.g., ischemia, hydrogen peroxide) may produce apoptosis or necrosis, depending on the severity of the injury and the

rapidity of cell death. The cell's fate is determined in part by cellular energy reserves such as ATP. When removal of the apoptotic cells is delayed, some inducers initially cause apoptosis followed by necrosis (postapoptotic necrosis). This transition from apoptotic to necrotic cells is likely to be important in the context of autoimmunity (see later).

Autophagy

Autophagy, which means to eat oneself, occurs during nutrient stress when cells switch to a catabolic program and degrade cytoplasmic constituents as a survival mechanism.[5] It does not necessarily lead to cell death. During autophagy, more than 20 members of the ATG family of proteins orchestrate the initiation, elongation, and closure of the characteristic double-membrane vesicle called the *autophagosome*. The autophagosome then fuses with lysosomes (see Figure 11-1), the contents are degraded, and the products recycled for energy utilization. Autophagy has been implicated in a wide spectrum of diseases ranging from degenerative neurologic diseases associated with polyglutamine repeats to cancer and immunologic diseases such as Crohn disease.[5]

Autophagy is important in immune functions, such as the intracellular host response to pathogens, survival of lymphocytes following growth factor withdrawal, Toll-like receptor (TLR) stimulation in plasmacytoid dendritic cells (pDCs), and major histocompatibility complex (MHC) class II presentation of antigen.[5,6] The association between a genetic variant of ATG16L1 as well as IRGM (immunity-related guanosine triphosphatase gene), another protein that regulates autophagy, and Crohn disease is unclear but could potentially involve thymic selection, macrophage function, or intestinal immunity.[5] Of relevance to SLE is the identification in patients with the disease of an increased frequency of single-nucleotide polymorphisms) (SNPs) in *ATG5* that could potentially predispose to disease through alterations in T-cell selection, clearance of apoptotic cells, or regulation of type I interferon (IFN).[5]

Other Forms of Cell Death

Pyroptosis (from the Greek, "pyro" meaning fire) is distinguished from the other forms of cell death by the activation of caspase 1 (interleukin-1beta [IL-1β]–converting enzyme) and secretion of the inflammatory cytokine IL-1β. Pyroptosis is most strongly associated with infections by intracellular bacteria such as *Salmonella, Yersinia,* and *Legionella,* although it may also be seen following tissue infarction.[7] Cells undergoing pyroptosis demonstrate nuclear condensation associated with DNA damage, cell swelling, and, ultimately, cell lysis associated with release of IL-1β. The mechanisms responsible for this process involve intracellular sensors of bacterial products and formation of the inflammasome.

Necroptosis is a programmed form of necrosis that has so far mainly been described in response to certain death ligands such as Fas ligand and tumor necrosis factor alpha (TNF-α; see Biochemistry of Apoptosis). It has long been known that in addition, a stimulation of inflammation through activation of nuclear factor kappa B (NF-κb), TNF-α can induce necrosis (tumor *necrosis* factor). Only recently

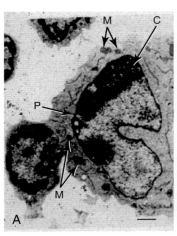
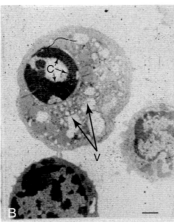
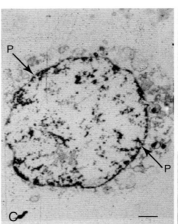
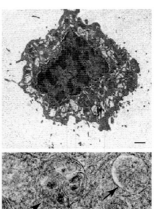

FIGURE 11-1 **Electron-microscopic morphology of cell death. A,** A cytotoxic T cell (*lower left*) conjugated to its target, P815, a murine mast cell before the initiation of cell death. **B,** Induction of apoptotic changes in P815. Note the reduction in target cell size, nuclear condensation, and vacuoles with the relative preservation of organelles. **C,** Osmotic lysis and necrosis in P815 induced by antibody and complement. Note the increased size of the nucleus and apparently random fragmentation of the chromatin. Organelles are severely disrupted. **D,** Autophagic cell death of L929 cells treated for 12 hours with caspase inhibitor (zVAD). *Arrows* show membrane-bound vacuoles characteristic of autophagosomes. C, dense chromatin; M, mitochondria; P, nuclear pore; V, vacuoles. *(Autophagy image courtesy of Dr. Mike Lenardo. Adapted from Russell JH, Masakowski V, Rucinsky T, et al: Mechanisms of immune lysis III: Characterization of the nature and kinetics of the cytotoxic T lymphocyte induced nuclear lesion in the target. J Immunol 128:2087, 1982.)*

has the pathway become clear, and it is described in the section Initiation and Pathways of Apoptosis.

BIOCHEMISTRY OF APOPTOSIS

Figures 11-2 and 11-3 show schematic overviews of the cell death program. A brief outline of each major functional component within the program, from the signals for death to removal of the apoptotic cells, is discussed here, but space limitations preclude a detailed analysis of the layers of regulation at each step of the pathway. For a more comprehensive discussion of the biochemical pathways controlling apoptosis, the reader is referred to excellent reviews.[8,9]

Numerous proteins involved in apoptosis, including receptors, adaptors, effectors, and inhibitors, contain modules/domains that are structurally similar and evolutionarily conserved. Interestingly, these motifs are predominantly involved in promoting homotypic protein-protein interactions (see Figure 11-3). Furthermore, as discussed later, these domains occur in proteins involved in apoptosis as well as inflammation. It has been suggested that death domain (DD), death effector domain (DED), caspase recruitment domain (CARD), and pyrin domains all evolved from the prototypic DD-fold corresponding to an antiparallel six-helix bundle.[10] Because of the central role for caspases, deoxyribonucleases (DNases), and the bcl-2 family of proteins, each is briefly described in greater detail later, before the discussion of how these families of proteins interact.

The cell death process can be divided into a number of stages, as follows: inductive stimulus, signal transduction, activation of caspases, activation of nuclease(s) with nuclear condensation, redistribution of the cellular contents into apoptotic bodies, and removal of the dying cells (see Figures 11-2 and 11-3). Because the nature of the inductive stimulus dictates the initial biochemical pathways engaged, extrinsic ("death receptor") and intrinsic (damage- and stress-induced) pathways are discussed separately.

Caspases

The cysteine protease family of caspases plays a central role in apoptosis, and the orthologs in *C. elegans* and *Drosophila* demonstrate evolutionary conservation. Caspases are produced as catalytically inactive zymogens and function as homodimers, with each monomer composed of a large subunit and a small subunit. Caspases can be divided into two categories reflecting both structural and functional

differences; "initiator" and "effector" caspases (Table 11-1; for a comprehensive review, see reference 11).

The "initiator" caspases, which in mammals include caspases 2, 8, 9, and 10, have extended *N*-terminal prodomains that allow for clustering and autoactivation of the zymogens. The clustering of the initiator caspases depends on adaptor proteins that utilize homophilic interactions between conserved nonenzymatic domains present on both the adaptor and the caspase. These adaptors include Fas-associating protein with death domain (FADD), which recruits caspase 8 via homophilic interactions between DEDs in both proteins (see later and Figures 11-2 and 11-3), and apoptotic protease activating factor 1 (Apaf-1), which recruits caspase 9 through a homophilic interaction in CARD (caspase recruitment domain). The recruitment and activation of various initiator caspases occur in response to unique sets of stimuli and in separate cellular compartments. Autoactivation of initiator caspases likely occurs through oligomerization, ultimately leading to the activation of downstream effector caspases (caspases 3, 6, and 7). As discussed later, caspase 8, considered a pro-apoptotic protease, functions both in Fas-induced apoptosis and in lymphocyte activation and protective immunity.

The "effector" caspases are necessary for the execution of apoptosis. They cleave specific substrates, such as the structural proteins fodrin, gelsolin, and lamins, key intracellular enzymes involved in DNA repair (e.g., poly[ADP]ribose polymerase, DNA-dependent protein kinase [DNA-PK]). These changes facilitate inactivation of synthetic functions of the cell, dissolution of the nuclear membrane, and packaging of cellular proteins into apoptotic blebs on the cell surface. Caspases also cleave regulatory proteins such as Bcl family members and the inhibitor of caspase-activated DNase (ICAD). Cleavage of ICAD leads to the release of active CAD, which enters the nucleus and cleaves nucleosomes at the linker region, yielding the characteristic "DNA ladder."

Not all caspases are involved in the execution of apoptosis. Human caspases 1, 4, and 5 are most likely involved in inflammation. Caspase 1 was originally defined as the enzyme that cleaves IL-1 (interleukin-1–converting enzyme [ICE]) into its active form. It has been shown that caspases 1 and 5 interact to form a multiprotein complex that has been called the *inflammasome* (analogous to the apoptosome).[12] Caspases 1 and 5 bind to the adaptor proteins ASC (pyrin CARD

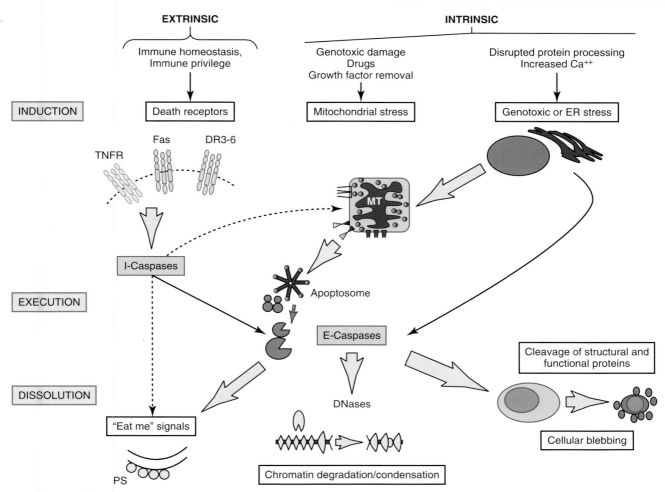

FIGURE 11-2 Mammalian apoptotic pathways. Cell death can be initiated by multiple pathways, including extrinsic (*left panel*) and intrinsic pathways (*middle and right panels*). Apoptosis occurs in discrete stages, with induction stimuli leading to further execution and dissolution steps. Examples of stimuli that can induce each of these pathways are shown and discussed in further detail in the text. These various death pathways differ in the upstream initiator caspases (I-Caspases) that are activated but converge to cleave the effector caspases (E-Caspases), such as caspase 3, during execution of apoptosis. Central to the apoptotic program is the formation of the apoptosome, which functions to amplify the death signal and leads to activation of effector caspases 3, 5, and 7. The alterations that occur during dissolution of the cell are too numerous to mention, but a few are highlighted in view of their potential relevance to autoimmunity (see text). Exposure of phosphatidylserine (PS) on the cell surface (*lower left*) may be relevant to the generation of antiphospholipid autoantibodies and coagulation disorders in vivo. Cleavage products of chromatin by various DNases (*lower middle*) as well as proteins, such as lamins and DNA-dependent protein kinase (DNA-PK), may be antigenic.

[PYCARD]) and NALP1 (DECAP), respectively, by their CARD domains. The protein, pyrin, which is mutated in familial Mediterranean fever (FMF), binds to ASC. Mutation of pyrin therefore most likely leads to inflammation through uncontrolled activation of caspase 1, generating active IL-1 and IL-18.

Inhibition of Caspases—Intracellular Inhibitors of Apoptosis

Intracellular inhibitors of apoptosis (IAPs) are a family of antiapoptotic proteins that are highly conserved through evolution. Members of the family (cellular IAPs c-IAP-1 and c-IAP-2, X-linked IAP [X-IAP], survivin, IAP-like protein 2 [ILP2], ML-IAP (melanoma IAP), Bruce, and neuronal apoptosis inhibitory protein [NAIP]) share a baculovirus IAP repeat (BIR) domain and most contain a RING domain that functions as an E3 ligase. IAPs such as X-IAP directly inhibit effector caspases, especially caspase 9, whereas c-IAPs modulate cell survival by ubiquitylation of substrates such as ribosome-inactivating protein (RIP) and proteins in the NF-κB pathway. IAPs block apoptosis induced by a variety of stimuli, including Fas, TNF-α, ultraviolet (UV) irradiation, and serum withdrawal. IAPs themselves are inhibited by two mitochondrial proteins named Smac/Diablo and HtrA2/Omi, which are released into the cytosol during the intrinsic and some extrinsic apoptotic programs (see Figure 11-3).

Nucleases and the Degradation of Cellular DNA and RNA

Nucleic acids are of high relevance to SLE as they are prominent targets of autoantibodies in this disease and can potently stimulate the production of type I IFN. RNase 1 and DNase I are the predominant serum nucleases thought to be crucial for the degradation of nucleic acids released from dead and dying cells into blood or tissue. Mice deficient in DNase I, at least on some strain backgrounds, demonstrate a lupus-like phenotype,[13] but whether altered DNase activity represents a genetic susceptibility factor in human lupus remains controversial.

A hallmark of programmed cell death is internucleosomal cleavage of DNA, which results in nuclear condensation and a nucleosomal

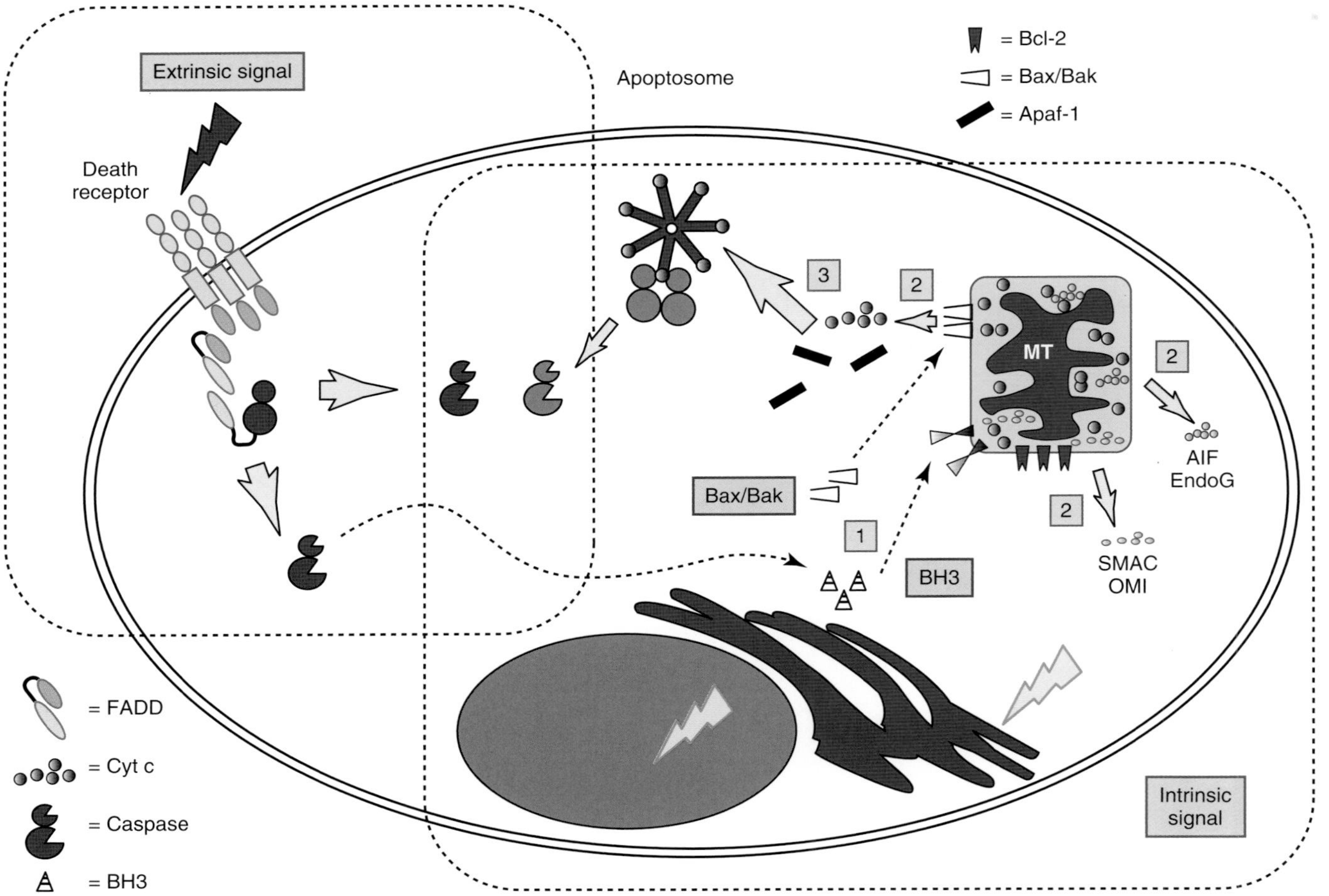

FIGURE 11-3 Overview of extrinsic and intrinsic apoptotic pathways. Death receptor extrinsic signaling is shown on the left, as modeled by Fas-induced apoptosis. Fas aggregation leads to formation of the death-inducing signaling complex (DISC), which contains the bifunctional adaptor FADD (Fas-associated protein with death domain) and the initiator caspase 8. High local caspase concentrations lead to the dimerization, activation, and subsequent release of caspase 8 from the cell membrane. The intrinsic apoptotic signaling pathway is schematized on the *right* (see text for specifics of various proapoptotic and antiapoptotic proteins). Signals from cellular stress lead to the translocation of the proapoptotic Bax/Bak and BH3-only proteins to the mitochondria (shown as 1). BH3-only proteins antagonize the protective effects of Bcl-2 on cellular viability. Bax/Bak in turn aggregates and forms large oligomers in the mitochondrial membrane leading to the release of cytochrome *c* into the cytosol (shown as 2). Apaf-1 (apoptotic protease activating factor 1) forms a large scaffold for caspase activation, known as the *apoptosome,* in the presence of cytochrome-*c* (shown as 3). Both pathways lead to the activation of effector caspases and subsequent cleavage of a multiplicity of cellular substrates.

"ladder." Numerous DNases have been implicated in this process, including caspase-activated DNase (CAD/DFF40) and apoptosis-inducing factor (AIF)/endonuclease G (Endo G) (located in mitochondria) (see Table 11-1). Initially, degradation of chromatin into large DNA fragments to produce large (50-200 kb) fragments occurs through cooperative interaction between endo G and AIF. Subsequently, while the cell membrane remains intact, CAD/DFF40 cleaves DNA into internucleosomal units, producing a characteristic 180-bp ladder. Following phagocytic ingestion of apoptotic cells with partially processed DNA, DNase II, another DNase located in lysosomes, completes DNA digestion. Mice deficient in both CAD/DFF40 and DNase II have defects in thymic development associated with production of inflammatory cytokines, supporting a model in which DNA degradation during apoptosis is a sequential process that requires initiation in a cell-autonomous way and is then fully executed by the phagocyte. Of interest, mice doubly deficient in DNAseII and IFN receptors demonstrate a disease similar to rheumatoid arthritis.[14]

A third category of nucleases are those involved in processing of normal or abnormal (e.g., virus) nucleic acids. TREX1 (three prime repair enxonuclease 1) is a 3-5′ exonuclease that appears to be necessary for degradation of cytoplasmic single-stranded DNA.[15] Loss of

TREX1 function stimulates the production of type I IFN through an unknown DNA sensor.

The Bcl-2 Family: Central Regulators of Apoptosis

There are at least 20 known Bcl-2 family members in mammals that have diverse cellular localization and function and are broadly divided into three interacting groups (see Table 11-1; and reviewed in reference 16). All Bcl-2 family members possess one or more BH (Bcl-2 homology) domains, which allow for interaction with a variety of proapoptotic or antiapoptotic proteins. Multidomain prosurvival members Bcl-2, and closely related Bcl-xL, Mcl-1, and A1, can protect cells from a wide range of potentially death-inducing stimuli, including irradiation (UV and gamma), growth factor withdrawal, and chemotherapy. The proapoptotic multidomain group that includes Bax, Bak, and Bok likely functions by altering the permeability or conductance of mitochondrial and other membranes, resulting in the release of additional proapoptotic mediators (see later). Finally, the "BH3-only" group of proapoptotic proteins contains at least eight members and functions primarily by antagonizing the protective effects of the Bcl-2 family. Some BH3-only proteins may sensitize cells for apoptosis, whereas others likely function more directly in activating apoptosis.[8] The BH3-only members act as sentinels in various organelles, integrating proximal death or survival signals and ultimately facilitating Bax/Bak-induced apoptosis.

The cellular localization of the Bcl-2 family members is diverse and likely reflects the complexity of networks that sense cellular damage and govern life or death. The antiapoptotic Bcl-2 subfamily is associated with membranes, including the cytoplasmic face of the mitochondrial membrane. Although Bcl-2 itself inserts into membranes in healthy cells, other related proteins must undergo allosteric changes prior to membrane association, allowing for the unique response to cytotoxic stressors. Similarly, the proapoptotic Bax family has both cytosolic (e.g., Bax) and membrane-associated (e.g., Bak) members in healthy cells that translocate to the outer mitochondrial membrane after appropriate stimuli. The BH3-only family adds to the complexity of apoptosis regulation because individual members are expressed in a cell-type specific manner and may allow for the response to organelle-specific signals. Constitutively expressed BH3-only members remain latent until released by a variety of stimuli. Examples are Bad (sequestered to 14-3-3 scaffold proteins) and Bid (undergoes cleavage). Finally, some BH3-only members are transcriptionally regulated so that certain forms of apoptosis resulting from cellular stress increase the expression of proapoptotic proteins.

Abnormalities in the Expression of Bcl-2 Family Members Cause Lupus-Like Autoimmunity in Mice

Mice that overexpress the antiapoptotic protein Bcl-2 or are deficient in the proapoptotic protein Bim demonstrate a lupus-like disease on certain strain backgrounds.[17] Bcl-2 is not a critical player in positive or negative thymic selection but may promote autoimmunity by enhancing cell survival in peripheral lymphocytes. In contrast, loss of Bim does affect thymic selection, as evidenced in a Bim-deficient T-cell receptor transgenic model in which T cells targeted against the male antigen HY have impaired deletion of autoreactive $CD4^+8^+$ thymocytes in male mice.[18] Bim may also regulate B-cell survival.

INITIATION AND PATHWAYS OF APOPTOSIS
Extrinsic Signaling Through Death Receptors

Our understanding of the molecular basis for apoptosis has been guided by the dissection of the signal transduction pathways downstream of Fas and TNF. The "death receptor" family has six members, all of which contain an 80–amino acid cytoplasmic tail known as the "death domain" that is required for apoptosis (Table 11-2; Figure 11-4). In addition to receptors for signaling apoptosis, there are a number of "decoy receptors" (DcRs) that also bind the same ligands

TABLE 11-1 Families of Intracellular Proteins Involved in Apoptosis

Caspases		
Initiator	Pro-Domain	Function
Caspase 8, 10	Long, with DED	Extrinsic (death receptor) pathway
Caspase 9	Long, with CARD	Intrinsic pathway
Caspase 2	Long, with CARD	Both extrinsic (death receptor) and intrinsic (chemotherapy) pathways
Executioner		
Caspase 3/6/7	Short	Cleavage of apoptotic substrates
Caspase Inhibitors		
IAPs	—	Active-site blockage of caspases
p35, CrmA	—	Pan-caspase inhibitors
cFLIP	DED	Cell inhibitor of DISC formation
Bcl-2 Members		
	Prototype	Others
Anti-apoptosis: Bcl-2 sub-family	Bcl-2	Bcl-xL, Bcl-w, Mcl-1
Pro-apoptosis: Bax sub-family BH3-only sub-family	Bax Bid	Bak, Bok Bim, Bad, Puma, Noxa, Bik
DNases		
DNase	Activation	DNA substrates
CAD	Caspase	Cell autonomous, generates nucleosomes
AIF + Endo G	Mitochondrial	Cell autonomous, cleaves chromatin
DNase II	Low pH	Ingested DNA in phagocytes
DNase I	—	Extracellular DNA
TREX1	—	Intracellular single-stranded DNA

AIF, apoptosis-inducing factor; CAD,; CARD, caspase recruitment domain; cFLIP, cellular FLICE (FADD [Fas-associated protein with death domain]–like interleukin-1β–converting enzyme)–inhibitory protein; DED, death effector domain; DISC, death-inducing signaling complex; Endo G, endonuclease G; IAP, inhibitor of apoptosis; TREX1, three prime repair exonuclease 1.

TABLE 11-2 Death Receptor Family Members

RECEPTOR	LIGAND	MAIN FUNCTIONS
Fas/ CD95 (TNFRSF6)	FasL	Activation-induced cell death, T-cell proliferation
TNF-R1 (TNFRSF1A)	TNF	Immune activation and cell survival, apoptosis
TNF-R2 (TNFRSF1B)	TNF	Immune activation and cell survival
DR3 (TNFRSF12)	TL1a (TWEAK)	T-cell co-stimulation
*DcR3 (TNFRSF6B)	TL1a, FasL	Suppress T-cell responses
DR4/TRAIL-R1(TNFRSF10A)	TRAIL	For DR4 and 5, cell death of certain tumor cells
DR5/TRAIL-R2 (TNFRSF10B)	TRAIL	death or activation of NF-κB
*DcR1/TRAIL-R3 (TNFRSF10C)	TRAIL	Competes for ligand
*DcR2/TRAIL-R4 (TNFRSF10D)	TRAIL	Competes for ligand
*Osteoprotegerin (OPG) (TNFRSF11b)	TRAIL, receptor activator of NF-κB ligand (RANKL)	Competes for ligands
DR6 (TNFRSF21)	†N-APP	Suppresses T- and B-cell responses

*Decoy receptors.
†N-APP, the extracellular fragment of the β-amyloid precursor protein that binds DR6 and triggers neuronal degeneration through activation of caspase 6 in Alzheimer' disease. The ligand in the immune system is unknown.
DcR, decoy receptor; DR, death receptor; L, ligand; NF-κB, nuclear factor kappa B; R, receptor; TNF, tumor necrosis factor; TRAIL, TNF-related apoptosis–inducing ligand; TWEAK, TNF-like weak inducer of apoptosis.

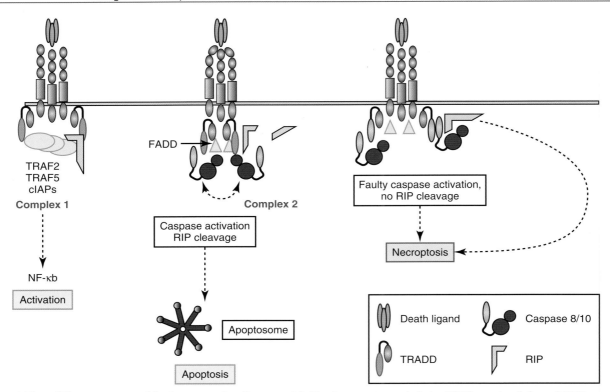

TRAF2
TRAF5
cIAPs
Complex 1

FADD

Complex 2

NF-κb

Activation

Caspase activation
RIP cleavage

Faulty caspase activation,
no RIP cleavage

Necroptosis

Apoptosome

Death ligand

Caspase 8/10

TRADD

RIP

Apoptosis

FIGURE 11-4 Three different outcomes of death receptor signaling as modeled by the tumor necrosis factor (TNF) receptor. *Left panel,* TNF-α recruits the death domain–containing adaptor TRADD (tumor necrosis factor receptor type 1–associated death domain) as well as a number of additional proteins to form complex 1. In this complex, the cellular inhibitors of apoptosis (c-IAPs) ubiquitinate the RIP (ribosome-inactivating protein) kinases, leading to downstream activation of nuclear factor kappa B (NF-κB). *Middle panel,* In the absence of c-IAP ubiquitinition of RIP, internalization of the ligand/receptor/TRADD complex recruits FADD (Fas-associated protein with death domain), RIP1, and RIP3. These kinases are cleaved by caspase 8, resulting in apoptosis by mechanisms similar to that shown in previous figures. *Right panel,* If caspase 8 is defective or inhibited, the RIP kinases are not cleaved and remain constitutively active, inducing necroptosis through reactive oxygen intermediates (ROIs) and activation of JNK (c-Jun *N*-terminal kinase) and calpains. In addition, the process involves lipid peroxidation and disintegration of lipid membranes. In contrast to apoptosis, NFkB activation and necroptosis are inflammatory.

of the TNF superfamily. These receptors either lack functional intracellular death domains (e.g., DcR3) or exist as soluble receptors (e.g., OPG) and are therefore unable to transmit an intracellular signal. By sequestration of death ligands, decoy receptors may prevent signal transduction from death receptors.

Fas/CD95 is a member of the TNF receptor (TNFR) superfamily and plays a central role in T-cell homeostasis.[19] Restimulation of activated human T cells through the TCR results in Fas translocation into lipid raft microdomains and renders the cells sensitive to apoptosis by un-crosslinked Fas ligand (FasL), most likely as a result of increased proximity and preassociation of receptor subunits (see Figure 11-4).

Upon binding by FasL, Fas further oligomerizes, and a number of apoptosis-related proteins are recruited via homotypic interactions and collectively form the death-inducing signaling complex (DISC). Fas itself binds to the adaptor protein FADD via death-domain interactions, and FADD binds to caspase 8 through DEDs (see Figure 11-4). The recruitment and activation of caspase 8 requires "induced proximity" and likely proceeds through dimerization of monomeric zymogens. Signaling through other death receptors, including TNF, and death receptor 3 (DR3), depends on the FADD as well as other adapter-induced recruitment of caspases. Activation of initiator caspases by death receptors leads to initiation of the "effector" caspase cascade, as described in greater detail later (*intrinsic death pathways*).

Although the six DD-containing receptors initiate cell death in certain contexts, all may signal cell survival/proliferation in different cell types and/or in different contexts. The ability to signal an opposite cell fate seems to depend on the recruitment of proteins such as the TNFR-associated factors (TRAFs) that activate NF-κB, thereby

promoting cell survival (see later). The increasingly complex roles of "death" receptors and caspase 8 are illustrated by impaired T-cell activation coupled with lymphocyte accumulation in patients with caspase 8 deficiency.

Like Fas, TNFR1 signals through FADD and caspase 8, and this signaling depends on the adaptor molecule TRADD (tumor necrosis factor receptor type 1–associated death domain), which has a region homologous to the FADD death domain. TNFR1 signaling involves assembly of two molecularly and spatially distinct signaling complexes that sequentially activate NF-κB and caspases (see Figure 11-4). Early after TNF binding, RIP1, TRADD, TRAF2, and c-IAP-1 are recruited to TNFR1 to form complex I, leading to NF-κB translocation, which protects cells from apoptosis. At later time points, RIP1, TRADD, and TRAF2 dissociate from TNFR1 and recruit FADD and caspase 8 to form complex II. In the absence of NF-κB activity from complex I, complex II can initiate caspase 8 activation and cell death. If caspase 8 is defective, persistent activation of the Ser/Thr protein kinases 1 (RIPK1) and RIPK3 (see Figure 11-4) results in necroptosis—inflammatory cell death.[20]

Regulation of Death Receptors

In most resting cell types that express Fas on their cell surfaces, the receptor does not appear to signal apoptosis, and in lymphocytes it may actually promote proliferation.[21] Resistance to death is explained by low levels of expression of the receptor, by physical separation of Fas from lipid rafts,[22] and by active inhibition by a protein called FLIP—FLICE (FADD-like interleukin-1β–converting enzyme)–inhibitory protein). FLIP resembles the adaptor protein FADD in structure, binds to Fas, and prevents FADD from initiating apoptosis. When lymphocytes become activated, FLIP is usually degraded, allowing Fas signal transduction to occur unimpeded. FLIP can affect sensitivity to both Fas and TNFR signaling by competing with caspase 8 for FADD.

Function in Immune Regulation

Fas and TNFR play little or no role in thymic selection. In contrast, Fas is involved in the maintenance of immune privilege in the eye and the testis, in the pathogenesis of graft-versus-host disease, and in immune evasion by tumors.[23] The major physiologic function of Fas and FasL in the immune system is the preservation of peripheral tolerance. This is achieved by the phenomenon of activation-induced cell death (AICD), whereby CD8+ T cells, T-helper 1 (Th1) cells, CD4+ T cells, and possibly natural killer (NK) cells induce apoptosis of activated T cells, B cells, and macrophages. The deletion of activated immune cells removes the source of proinflammatory molecules, prevents the continued presentation of self-peptides by primed (high levels of co-stimulatory molecules) antigen-presenting cells, and eliminates B cells that have mutated to self-specificity in the germinal centers.[24] Neutrophil homeostasis is also maintained by the Fas/FasL system. The Foxo3a forkhead transcription factor maintains neutrophil viability during inflammation by suppressing FasL, whereas TRAIL (TNF-related apoptosis–inducing ligand) signals apoptosis through DR4 and DR5 predominantly in tumor cells; TRAIL may play a role in negative selection of thymocytes.[25] Similarly, DR3 (the receptor for TWEAK [TNF-like weak inducer of apoptosis]) has also been implicated in negative selection.[26] Finally, DR6 plays a role in immunologic homeostasis, as evidenced by enhanced T- and B-cell proliferation in DR6-deficient mice.[27]

Deficiencies in Death Receptor Signaling Lead to Systemic Autoimmunity

Death receptors have been clearly implicated in both murine and human autoimmune diseases.[28] Mutations in Fas and FasL were first identified in the lpr and gld mouse models of lupus. Since that time numerous spontaneous and induced genetic alterations that affect apoptosis have been shown to predispose to systemic autoimmunity.[29] The autoimmune lymphoproliferative syndrome (ALPS) is an extremely rare disease usually detected during childhood.[30,31] Patients with ALPS present clinically with a nonmalignant accumulation of lymphocytes in lymphoid organs, hypergammaglobulinemia, cytopenias, autoantibodies, and, occasionally, glomerulonephritis or arthritis. The diagnosis of ALPS is made in patients with chronic (>6 months) nonmalignant and noninfectious lymphadenopathy and/or splenomegaly and the presence of increased circulating CD3+/TCRαβ+/CD4−/CD8− ("double-negative") T-cells (≥1.5% of total lymphocytes or 2.5% of CD3+ lymphocytes) with normal or elevated lymphocyte counts. It is confirmed by demonstrating defective lymphocyte apoptosis in two separate assays or the detection of somatic or germline pathogenic mutation in Fas, FasL, or caspase 10.[32] Either environmental and/or other genetic modifiers are necessary for disease onset, because not all humans or mice (lpr) with Fas mutations have the disease.

Mutations in the p55/TNFR1/CD120a receptor in humans results in a periodic autoinflammatory syndrome called TNFR-associated periodic syndrome (TRAPS). Mutations occur predominantly in the first two CRDs (cysteine rich domains) of the receptor, which may in some cases result in reduced shedding of the extracellular domain of the receptor and reduced neutralization of circulating TNF-α. Other hypotheses include abnormal intracellular stress resulting in NF-κB and mitogen-activated protein kinase (MAPK) activation or reduced apoptosis of activated cells.[33]

Intrinsic Death Pathways from Cellular Damage or Stress

Cells depend on a variety of signals for active maintenance of survival, including those relating to overall nutritional and bioenergetic status. Loss of signals from neighboring cells or withdrawal of growth factors or cytokines results in initiation of a cell death program.

Damage or stress to intracellular organelles may be induced from outside or within the cell, and these pathways depend on the dynamic interplay of the Bcl-2 family of proteins and other regulators.

The Mitochondria as an Integrator of Cell Metabolism and Apoptosis

Mitochondria are cytoplasmic organelles that contain their own 16-kb genome encased by inner and outer membranes with a number of proteins, including cytochrome-*c*, situated between these membranes. Mitochondria help to maintain redox potential and are the energy powerhouse of the cell through the generation of ATP by oxidative phosphorylation. The discovery that many bcl-2 family members constitutively or inducibly localize to the mitochondrion illuminated a central role for this organelle in orchestrating apoptosis.

The mitochondrion contains numerous proteins that are crucial to the apoptotic machinery. Cytochrome-*c* and Apaf-1 are cofactors for the activation of caspase 9. Additionally, the inner mitochondrial membrane contains inhibitors of antiapoptotic proteins Smac/Diablo and HtrA2/Omi as well as inactive endonucleases (Endo G, AIF), which become active following their release from the mitochondria (see Figure 11-3). The proapoptotic BAX and BAK proteins are essential for mitochondrial permeabilization, and mice doubly deficient in BAX and BAK are resistant to multiple forms of apoptosis.[34] These proteins undergo changes, allowing oligomerization and permeabilization of the mitochondrial outer membrane. The permeabilization in turn promotes release of proapoptotic proteins and formation of a complex including Apaf-1, cytochrome-*c* (Apaf-2), and caspase 9 (Apaf-3). This multiprotein complex, aptly termed the *apoptosome*, amplifies the death signal and leads to activation of the effector caspases 3, 5, and 7 (see Figure 11-3). The mechanism whereby BAX/BAK promotes release of these proteins is controversial and may involve the formation of pores or may occur by alteration of intrinsic mitochondrial proteins triggering permeability transition. Once the mitochondrial membrane has been disrupted, multiple proapoptotic molecules are released, including cytochrome-*c*, the IAP inhibitors Smac/Diablo and HtrA2/Omi, and the proteins involved in chromatin degradation (Endo G, AIF).

Metabolic Stress

Withdrawal of either growth factors or nutritional sources leads to metabolic changes including lower oxygen consumption and a reduction in both ATP levels and protein production. In many cell types, these conditions lead to a form of apoptosis that can be blocked by overexpression of either Bcl-2 or Bcl-xL.[9] A link has been identified between proteins involved in sensing bioenergetic status of a cell and those controlling apoptosis. The proapoptotic BH3-only protein BAD forms part of a multiprotein holoenzyme complex that includes glucokinase and that regulates glucose-driven mitochondrial respiration.[35] In response to withdrawal of survival factors, BAD is phosphorylated and orchestrates cell death. BAD additionally serves to help regulate blood glucose levels, and mice deficient in BAD have defective glucokinase activity that manifests as diabetes.

Another example of the connection between the apoptotic machinery and mitochondrial function is the interaction between a mitochondrial voltage–dependent anion channel (VDAC) and Bcl-2 family members. The Akt kinase, which promotes cell growth and inhibits apoptosis, also facilitates localization of hexokinase to the mitochondrial membrane. Hexokinase, in turn, associates with VDAC and prevents Bax toxicity.[36] Interestingly, Akt requires glucose to regulate hexokinase (and hence to protect against apoptosis), demonstrating a connection between the protein machinery regulating energy stores and the promotion of survival with the interface at the mitochondrial membrane.

Genotoxic Stress

Mutations occur frequently in mammalian DNA and are usually promptly repaired. However, if repair fails or DNA is severely damaged by radiation or drugs, the transcription factor p53 is upregulated and phosphorylated by DNA damage sensors such as ATM (ataxia telangiectasia mutated). Activated p53 induces a cell cycle arrest through induction of the cyclin-dependent kinase inhibitor, p21. If the DNA damage is repaired, cell cycle arrest is abrogated, whereas if the injury cannot be repaired, the cell undergoes apoptosis. The critical importance of p53 as a tumor suppressor is illustrated by the high frequency of p53 mutations in cancers.[37] The transcription factor induces apoptosis, in part, by transcription of death effectors such as Bax that cause mitochondrial stress as well as two BH3-only bcl-2 family members, Puma and Noxa.[38] This example illustrates how apoptotic signals that originate in the nucleus are transmitted to the mitochondria.

Endoplasmic Reticulum Stress

The endoplasmic reticulum (ER) is now recognized as an important organelle that regulates the intrinsic apoptotic pathway. The ER is the major intracellular store of calcium, and in addition, functions to ensure proper protein folding. Disruptions in protein folding can lead to the *unfolded protein response* (UPR) and trigger cell death.[39] One ER-stress response in mice has been shown to depend on caspase 12. Both Huntington disease and Alzheimer disease have been implicated in ER stress–induced apoptosis due to misfolded or mutant proteins. The signal for apoptosis due to ER stress may depend on calcium release, although the mechanism remains uncertain.

Bcl-2 and Bax/Bak also function in ER stress–induced apoptosis in opposing ways. Bcl-2 blocks transmission of a stress signal from the ER to the mitochondria. Mice doubly deficient in Bax and Bak have markedly reduced ER calcium concentrations and defects in ER stress–induced apoptosis that could be corrected with overexpression of calcium pumps [sarcoplasmic/endoplasmic reticulum calcium ATPases (SERCA)].[40] These studies highlight the role of calcium dynamics in apoptosis and the functional interaction between the ER and mitochondria.

REMOVAL OF APOPTOTIC CELLS
Receptors and Ligands

Within the immune system alone, more than 10^{12} apoptotic cells are removed from the body each day. These apoptotic cells are generated in vast numbers in the central lymphoid organs, such as the thymus and bone marrow, by out-of-frame rearrangements of antigen receptors, negative selection, or simple "neglect." A significant load of apoptotic cells is produced in the peripheral immune system because of both the relatively short lifespan of lymphocytes and myeloid cells and the secondary selection of high-affinity B cells in germinal centers. The specialized sites of selection (e.g., thymus, bone marrow, lymphoid follicles) have remarkably efficient phagocytes that rapidly remove the dying cells (a process also called *efferocytosis*). At other sites, "find me" signals (sphingosine-1-phosphate and the nucleotides ATP and UTP [uridine 5′-triphosphate], which are released by dying cells—especially as the plasma membrane becomes damaged) may be necessary for phagocytes to remove apoptotic cells.

An early event in apoptosis is the appearance of phosphatidylserine (PS) on the cell surface membrane (Figure 11-5). This membrane asymmetry (PS is usually located on the inner surface of the membrane) is caused by the reduced function of a translocase and by activation of a lipid scramblase. PS is an important ligand for phagocytosis of apoptotic cells.[41] Despite the detection of only limited chemical alterations in lipids and sugars on the apoptotic cell membrane, blockade of a large and diverse number of receptors on

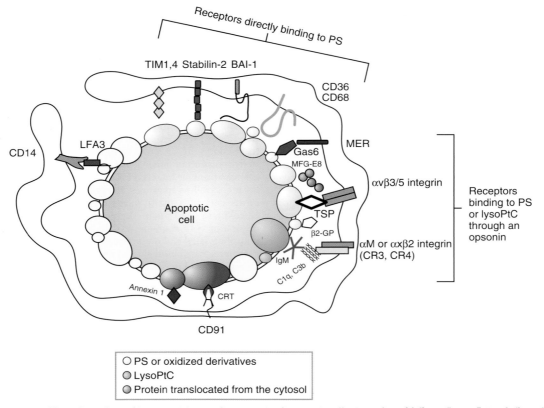

FIGURE 11-5 Receptors and ligands implicated in recognition or phagocytosis of apoptotic cells. A number of different "eat me" signals (ligands) are expressed on apoptotic, but not live, cells. In fact, live cells may express repulsive signals, such as CD47, that prevent them from being engulfed. The multiplicity of signals reflects different contexts and kinetics and the fact that certain ligands promote ("tethering") and others engulfment ("tickling"). Many ligands are serum proteins that coat exposed cell surface molecules and serve as opsonins for phagocytosis (*right* side of figure). C, complement; CRT, calreticulin; LyPtC, lysophosphatidylcholine; PS, phosphatidylserine; TSP, thrombospondin.

phagocytes can impair the uptake of apoptotic cells (reviewed in reference 42) (see Figure 11-5). This diversity likely reflects redundancy, the fact that some receptors tether the dying cell but others trigger the engulfment, and in vivo variables such as the location and homeostatic versus inflammatory clearance. All of the receptors identified have other functions, perhaps reflecting an evolution from receptors designed to remove apoptotic cells during development to pattern recognition receptors useful for host defense.[43] Many of the receptors are integrins, such as the vitronectin receptor $\alpha_v\beta_3$, $\alpha_v\beta_5$, complement receptors 3 (CD11b/CD18) and 4 (CD11c/CD18), and class A and B scavenger receptors. Nonintegrin receptors include CD14, CD91, and members of the TIM (T-cell immunoglobulin and mucin domain–containing molecule) and TAM (Tyro, Axl, and Mer) families.

Some receptors (Bal-1, TIM1, 4) recognize PS directly on the dying cell, whereas in most cases, efficient phagocytosis requires a bridging protein (opsonin). Opsonins include serum factors such as thrombospondin that bridge the $\alpha_v\beta_3$ and CD36 receptors, classical complement components that are amplified on apoptotic cell membranes by natural immunoglobulin M (IgM) antibodies,[44,45] mannose-binding protein, and acute-phase proteins such as C-reactive protein (CRP) (see Figure 11-5). Other opsonins (calreticulin, annexin 1) are translocated from the dying cell itself or are secreted by the phagocyte (MFG-E8 [milk fat globule factor E8]). A special class of receptors belong to a closely related family of TAM receptor tyrosine kinases, which link to PS on apoptotic cells through the serum opsonins Gas6 and protein S (see Figure 11-5).[46]

Function in Immune Regulation
Apoptotic cell death is an integral part of development as well as of normal tissue homeostasis, so it is crucial that the immune consequence of removal of these cells is absence of inflammation and failure to stimulate adaptive immune responses to self-antigens. Most dead and dying cells are removed by professional phagocytes (macrophages and dendritic cells); but the release of lactoferrin from apoptotic cells prevents ingestion by neutrophils, minimizing the risk of neutrophil activation. Activation of macrophages is suppressed by the release of inhibitory cytokines including IL-10 and TGF-β. Although DCs are less abundant, they are potent activators of T cells and are also pivotal to the maintenance of T-cell tolerance via the presentation of self-antigen derived from apoptotic cells in the absence of co-stimulation ("steady state" condition).[47] Apoptotic cells suppress myeloid DC activation of T cells, in part, through suppression of IL-12[48,49] and attenuation of type I IFN signaling by engagement of TAM receptors.[46]

In contrast, DCs exposed to necrotic or tumor cells undergo maturation and activate both CD4+ and CD8+ T cells.[50] Necrotic cells release proinflammatory constituents, including heat shock proteins (HSPs), HMGB-1 (high-mobility group protein B1), and nucleoproteins themselves.[51] Maturation of DCs has clearly emerged as a critical switch to stimulate effector T-cell development. Maturation may be effected by engagement of either PAMPS (pathogen-associated molecular patterns) or DAMPS (damage-associated molecular patterns).[51] Especially potent are nucleic acids that, whether derived from the host or microbes, stimulate intracellular sensors belonging to the TLR family (TLRs 3, 7, 8, and 9), the RIG-I (retinoic acid inducible gene I) family (RIG-I and MDA-5 [melanoma differentiation–associated protein 5]), and the PYHIN family.[52]

Defective Clearance of Apoptotic Cells Predisposes to Lupus-Like Disease in Mice
Deficiencies of a number of proteins implicated in the removal of apoptotic cells have been reported to cause lupus-like diseases in mice. They include deficiencies of receptors such as mer as well as serum opsonins such as natural IgM antibodies, C1q, SAP (serum amyloid P component), and MFG-E8 (reviewed in reference 53). The mechanisms involved differ; in mer deficiency, antigen-presenting cells (APCs) receive a proinflammatory rather than antiinflammatory

signal upon ingestion of apoptotic cells. Defective clearance of apoptotic cells in mice deficient (knockout) in serum IgM, C1q, SAP, and MFG-E8 may predispose to lupus through slow clearance of apoptotic cells,[54,55] leading to postapoptotic necrosis, and/or through lack of engagement with specific inhibitory receptors on the phagocyte. Interestingly, the sites at which defective apoptosis manifests differ—in C1q-deficient, mice apoptotic cells accumulate in the kidney, whereas in MFG-E8 knockout mice, apoptotic cells accumulate in germinal centers. Lack of MFG-E8 also results in abnormal processing of apoptotic cell debris by dendritic cells, leading to enhanced—cell responses against self.[56]

APOPTOSIS ABNORMALITIES IN HUMAN SLE
Evidence implicating the products of dying cells in the immunization of patients with SLE includes the strong focus of the autoimmune response on nucleosomes. Autoantibodies to nucleosomes precede those to DNA and histones,[57] and nucleosomes, but not isolated DNA or histones, deposit in the glomeruli, suggesting that it is the in situ fixation of nucleosomes, rather than DNA/anti-DNA immune complexes (ICs), that causes lupus nephritis.[58] Another prominent feature of SLE is lymphopenia, indicating either that cell death is excessive or that lymphocyte homeostasis is abnormal. An increase in apoptosis of SLE peripheral blood mononuclear cells has been observed in vitro[59] and ex vivo.[60] This increase may result from the higher number of activated lymphocytes (activation-induced cell death) in SLE or may be an effect of elevations of cytokines such as IL-10 and IFN-α (see later). A brief outline of apoptosis abnormalities that are relevant to SLE or have been observed in SLE patients is offered here (Figure 11-6).

Is the Process of Cell Death Normal in SLE?
As discussed previously, although mutations in Fas and FasL predispose to the ALPS syndrome in children, Fas/FasL mutations are exceptionally rare in SLE. However, both the generation of autoimmunity to blood cells in ALPS and the presence of antinuclear antibodies (ANA) in patients with caspase 10 mutations indicate that the extrinsic cell death pathway remains informative with regard to understanding loss of tolerance to cellular antigens. Although alterations in FasL or Bcl-2 have been reported, there is currently no compelling evidence to implicate intrinsic defects in apoptosis regulators in SLE. Whether other death processes, such as autophagy, pyroptosis, and necroptosis, are relevant to disease pathogenesis remains to be determined.

Is the Response to Dying Cells Abnormal?
Why the immune system targets a select subset of self-antigens in each disease has never been satisfactorily explained, although illegitimate stimulation of one of the nucleic acid sensors previously mentioned may well play a role. An important early discovery was the observation that autoantigens, including those normally found in the nucleus, cluster and concentrate in surface blebs.[61] Either these antigens, or autoantigen-coated microparticles released from apoptotic cells,[62] have the potential to engage and therefore tolerize or activate B cells (see Figure 11-6).

As noted previously, apoptosis leads to the controlled activation of multiple intracellular nucleases and proteases, which in turn leads to the cleavage of numerous cellular molecules; one consequence of this autodigestion is the generation of "neoepitopes."[63] Some of these antigens undergo modification, including cleavage, phosphorylation, and oxidation. However, it is expected that under normal conditions, these neoepitopes are also generated in the thymus and bone marrow, leading to deletion of potentially self-reactive cells. In addition, the oxidation of lipids such as PS and lysophosphatidyl choline (LPC) are recognized by IgM natural antibodies, which protect against inflammation and response to self.[64,65] In contrast, inflammatory changes in the peripheral immune system, as might occur secondary to UV light, oxidation, or cleavage by granzyme B delivered by cytotoxic T cells, could qualitatively alter self-antigens released by dying cells and thereby stimulate immune responses.

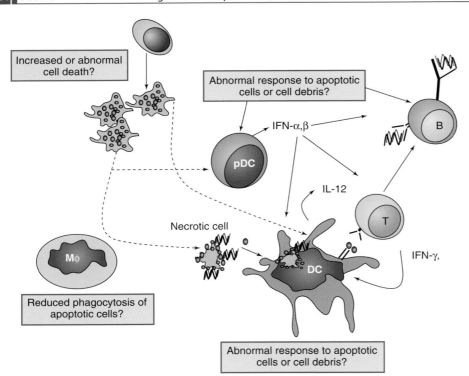

FIGURE 11-6 Role of apoptotic cells in the generation of autoantibodies to self-antigen in SLE. Autoantibodies to cellular antigens in SLE may be generated by abnormalities in one or more of the pathways shown. See text for details.

Type I IFNs have emerged as critical cytokines in SLE.[66] Studies of both patients with SLE and lupus-prone mice suggest that activation of type I IFNs likely plays an important role in disease pathogenesis. It has long been known that serum values of IFN-α are elevated in many patients with SLE, and gene expression profiling revealed that peripheral blood mononuclear cells (PBMCs) of such patients demonstrate upregulation of IFN-responsive genes.[67,68] Apoptotic cells have not been shown to directly induce type I IFN, but when engaged by antinuclear autoantibodies to form immune complexes (ICs), they are internalized by pDCs and activate intracellular TLRs.[69] A similar mechanism has been shown to activate B cells in a model of murine lupus.[70] Together, these results strongly implicate endogenous DNA or nucleoproteins from dead or dying cells as immunostimulants for pDCs, B cells, and, possibly, myeloid dendritic cells. Although these very important experiments support a process whereby IFN production can by amplified by circulating ICs to perpetuate disease, the stimulus driving the original loss of tolerance remains unclear (see Figure 11-6). Because about 1% of patients with SLE have mutations in the DNA exonuclease TREX1,[71] cell-intrinsic stimulation of type I IFN could be important in the initiation of inflammation. Furthermore, patients with SLE have an increased frequency of single-nucleotide polymorphisms in genes encoding proteins in the type I IFN pathway, such as IRF5 (interferon regulatory factor 5) and STAT4 (signal transducer and activator of transcription 4) (see Chapter 4), with the consequence that such patients may show a more vigorous response to nucleic acid stimuli.

Do Patients with SLE Have Reduced Clearance of Apoptotic Cells?

Like several spontaneous lupus strains of mice, some patients with lupus may have reduced clearance of apoptotic cells, as exemplified by an increased number of apoptotic cells in the germinal centers of patients with SLE.[72] Both in vitro and in vivo experiments strongly support the idea that the early complement components are required for the clearance of apoptotic cells.[44,73] The high frequency of SLE in patients with C1q, C4, and C2 deficiencies (reviewed in reference 74) could therefore be explained by impaired clearance of dying cells,

although it has also been shown that C1q protects against IFN-α stimulation by ICs by promoting IC removal by monocytes.[75] Because serum CRP levels are inappropriately low in SLE and CRP is a potent scavenger of intact apoptotic cells[76] as well as small nuclear ribonucleoproteins (snRNPs) and chromatin, reduced levels of CRP are likely to impair efficient removal of apoptotic cells and their debris.

CONCLUSIONS

Our understanding of the apoptotic program has grown exponentially over the past two decades. Numerous human diseases have been directly linked to genetic defects in the apoptotic pathways, including cancer, neurodegenerative disorders, and autoimmune diseases. Caspases initiate and amplify a variety of death signals, allowing for selective and ordered cellular demolition. The fine balance between proapoptotic and antiapoptotic Bcl-2 family members regulates the cell fate in response to many (but not all) stress or signaling pathways. New discoveries highlight the complex integration of signals from various organelles that determine cell fate, and the multiple functions of central players in the apoptotic process. It is likely that the knowledge obtained in a relatively short time will translate into better diagnostics and therapies to enhance or retard cell death or to facilitate the removal of cell debris in the appropriate clinical circumstances.

ACKNOWLEDGMENTS

The author appreciates the prior contributions of David Martin, helpful discussions from past and present laboratory members, and permission from Drs. Li Yu, Eric Baehrecke, and Mike Lenardo for the use of published electron micrographs.

References

1. Kerr JF, Wyllie AH, Currie AR: Apoptosis: a basic biological phenomenon with wide-ranging implications in tissue kinetics. *Br J Cancer* 26:239–257, 1972.
2. Wyllie AH, Morris RG, Smith AL, et al: Chromatin cleavage in apoptosis: association with condensed chromatin morphology and dependence on macromolecular synthesis. *J Pathol* 142:67–77, 1984.

3. Ellis H, Horvitz H: Genetic control of programmed cell death in the nematode *C. elegans*. *Cell* 44:817–829, 1986.

4. Hotchkiss RS, Strasser A, McDunn JE, et al: Cell death. *N Engl J Med* 361:1570–1583, 2009.

5. Levine B, Mizushima N, Virgin HW: Autophagy in immunity and inflammation. *Nature* 469:323–335, 2011.

6. Deretic V: Autophagy in immunity and cell-autonomous defense against intracellular microbes. *Immunol Rev* 240:92–104, 2011.

7. Bergsbaken T, Fink SL, Cookson BT: Pyroptosis: host cell death and inflammation. *Nat Rev Microbiol* 7:99–109, 2009.

8. Danial NN, Korsmeyer SJ: Cell death: critical control points. *Cell* 116:205–219, 2004.

9. Adams JM: Ways of dying: multiple pathways to apoptosis. *Genes Dev* 17:2481–2495, 2003.

10. Aravind L, Dixit VM, Koonin EV: The domains of death: evolution of the apoptosis machinery. *Trends Biochem Sci* 24:47–53, 1999.

11. Li J, Yuan J: Caspases in apoptosis and beyond. *Oncogene* 27:6194–6206, 2008.

12. Schroder K, Tschopp J: The inflammasomes. *Cell* 140:821–832, 2010.

13. Napirei M, Karsunky H, Zevnik B, et al: Features of systemic lupus erythematosus in Dnase1-deficient mice [see comments]. *Nat Genet* 25:177–181, 2000.

14. Kawane K, Ohtani M, Miwa K, et al: Chronic polyarthritis caused by mammalian DNA that escapes from degradation in macrophages. *Nature* 443:998–1002, 2006.

15. Stetson DB, Ko JS, Heidmann T, et al: Trex1 prevents cell-intrinsic initiation of autoimmunity. *Cell* 134:587–598, 2008.

16. Youle RJ, Strasser A: The BCL-2 protein family: opposing activities that mediate cell death. *Nat Rev Mol Cell Biol* 9:47–59, 2008.

17. Strasser A, Whittingham S, Vaux DL, et al: Enforced Bcl-2 expression in B-lymphoid cells prolongs antibody responses and elicits autoimmune disease. *Proc Natl Acad Sci U S A* 88:8661–8665, 1991.

18. Bouillet P, Purton JF, Godfrey DI, et al: BH3-only Bcl-2 family member Bim is required for apoptosis of autoreactive thymocytes. *Nature* 415:922–926, 2002.

19. Peter ME, Budd RC, Desbarats J, et al: The CD95 receptor: apoptosis revisited. *Cell* 129:447–450, 2007.

20. Vandenabeele P, Galluzzi L, Vanden Berghe T, et al: Molecular mechanisms of necroptosis: an ordered cellular explosion. *Nat Rev Mol Cell Biol* 11:700–714, 2010.

21. Elkon KB: Caspases: multifunctional proteases. *J Exp Med* 190:1725–1728, 1999.

22. Muppidi JR, Siegel RM: Ligand-independent redistribution of Fas (CD95) into lipid rafts mediates clonotypic T cell death. *Nat Immunol* 5:182–189, 2004.

23. Strasser A, Jost PJ, Nagata S: The many roles of FAS receptor signaling in the immune system. *Immunity* 30:180–192, 2009.

24. Elkon KB, Marshak-Rothstein A: B cells in systemic autoimmune disease: recent insights from Fas-deficient mice and men. *Curr Opin Immunol* 8:852–859, 1996.

25. Gonzalvez F, Ashkenazi A: New insights into apoptosis signaling by Apo2L/TRAIL. *Oncogene* 29:4752–4765, 2010.

26. Wang EC, Thern A, Denzel A, et al: DR3 regulates negative selection during thymocyte development. *Mol Cell Biol* 21:3451–3461, 2001.

27. Schmidt CS, Liu J, Zhang T, et al: Enhanced B cell expansion, survival, and humoral responses by targeting death receptor 6. *J Exp Med* 197:51–62, 2003.

28. Siegel RM, Muppidi J, Roberts M, et al: Death receptor signaling and autoimmunity. *Immunol Res* 27:499–512, 2003.

29. Kim SJ, Gershov D, Ma X, et al: Opsonization of apoptotic cells and its effect on macrophage and T cell immune responses. *Ann N Y Acad Sci* 987:68–78, 2003.

30. Martin DA, Zheng L, Siegel RM, et al: Defective CD95/APO-1/Fas signal complex formation in the human autoimmune lymphoproliferative syndrome, type Ia [in process citation]. *Proc Natl Acad Sci U S A* 96:4552–4557, 1999.

31. Vaishnaw AK, Orlinick JR, Chu JL, et al: Molecular basis for the apoptotic defects in patients with CD95 (Fas/Apo-1) mutations. *J Clin Invest* 103:355–363, 1999.

32. Oliveira JB, Bleesing JJ, Dianzani U, et al: Revised diagnostic criteria and classification for the autoimmune lymphoproliferative syndrome (ALPS): report from the 2009 NIH International Workshop. *Blood* 116:e35–e40, 2010.

33. Lobito AA, Gabriel TL, Medema JP, et al: Disease causing mutations in the TNF and TNFR superfamilies: focus on molecular mechanisms driving disease. *Trends Mol Med* 17:494–505, 2011.

34. Ruiz-Vela A, Opferman JT, Cheng EH, et al: Proapoptotic BAX and BAK control multiple initiator caspases. *EMBO Rep* 6:379–385, 2005.

35. Danial NN, Gramm CF, Scorrano L, et al: BAD and glucokinase reside in a mitochondrial complex that integrates glycolysis and apoptosis. *Nature* 424:952–956, 2003.

36. Pastorino JG, Shulga N, Hoek JB: Mitochondrial binding of hexokinase II inhibits Bax-induced cytochrome c release and apoptosis. *J Biol Chem* 277:7610–7618, 2002.

37. Levine AJ, Hu W, Feng Z: The P53 pathway: what questions remain to be explored? *Cell Death Differ* 13:1027–1036, 2006.

38. Villunger A, Michalak EM, Coultas L, et al: p53- and drug-induced apoptotic responses mediated by BH3-only proteins puma and noxa. *Science* 302:1036–1038, 2003.

39. Kaufman RJ: Orchestrating the unfolded protein response in health and disease. *J Clin Invest* 110:1389–1398, 2002.

40. Scorrano L, Oakes SA, Opferman JT, et al: BAX and BAK regulation of endoplasmic reticulum Ca2+: a control point for apoptosis. *Science* 300:135–139, 2003.

41. Fadok VA, Voelker DR, Campbell PA, et al: Exposure of phosphatidyl serine on the surface of apoptotic lymphocytes triggers specific recognition and removal by macrophages. *J Immunol* 148:2207–2216, 1992.

42. Gregory CD, Pound JD: Microenvironmental influences of apoptosis in vivo and in vitro. *Apoptosis* 15:1029–1049, 2010.

43. Franc NC, Dimarcq J-L, Lagueux M, et al: Croquemort, a novel drosophila hemocyte/macrophage receptor that recognizes apoptotic cells. *Immunity* 4:431–443, 1996.

44. Mevorach D, Mascarenhas J, Gershov DA, et al: Complement-dependent clearance of apoptotic cells by human macrophages. *J Exp Med* 188:2313–2320, 1998.

45. Kim G, Jun JB, Elkon KB: Necessary role of phosphatidylinositol 3-kinase in transforming growth factor beta-mediated activation of Akt in normal and rheumatoid arthritis synovial fibroblasts. *Arthritis Rheum* 46:1504–1511, 2002.

46. Lemke G, Rothlin CV: Immunobiology of the TAM receptors. *Nat Rev Immunol* 8:327–336, 2008.

47. Steinman RM, Hawiger D, Nussenzweig MC: Tolerogenic dendritic cells. *Annu Rev Immunol* 21:685–711, 2003.

48. Stuart LM, Lucas M, Simpson C, et al: Inhibitory effects of apoptotic cell ingestion upon endotoxin-driven myeloid dendritic cell maturation. *J Immunol* 168:1627–1635, 2002.

49. Kim SJ, Elkon KB, Ma X: Transcriptional suppression of interleukin-12 gene expression following phagocytosis of apoptotic cells. *Immunity* 21:643–653, 2004.

50. Sauter B, Albert ML, Francisco L, et al: Consequences of cell death: exposure to necrotic tumor cells, but not primary tissue cells or apoptotic cells, induces the maturation of immunostimulatory dendritic cells. *J Exp Med* 191:423–434, 2000.

51. Rock KL, Kono H: The inflammatory response to cell death. *Annu Rev Pathol* 3:99–126, 2008.

52. Theofilopoulos AN, Gonzalez-Quintial R, Lawson BR, et al: Sensors of the innate immune system: their link to rheumatic diseases. *Nat Rev Rheumatol* 6:146–156, 2010.

53. Nagata S, Hanayama R, Kawane K: Autoimmunity and the clearance of dead cells. *Cell* 140:619–630, 2010.

54. Quartier P, Potter PK, Ehrenstein MR, et al: Predominant role of IgM-dependent activation of the classical pathway in the clearance of dying cells by murine bone marrow-derived macrophages in vitro. *Eur J Immunol* 35:252–260, 2005.

55. Ogden CA, Kowalewski R, Peng YF, et al: IgM is required for efficient complement mediated phagocytosis of apoptotic cells in vivo. *Autoimmunity* 38:259–264, 2005.

56. Peng Y-F, Elkon KB: Autoimmunity in MFG-E8 deficient mice is associated with altered trafficking of apoptotic cell antigens and enhanced cross presentation. *J Clin Invest* 121:2221–2241, 2011.

57. Burlingame RW, Rubin RL, Balderas RS, et al: Genesis and evolution of anti-chromatin autoantibodies in murine lupus implicates T-dependent immunization and self antigen. *J Clin Invest* 91:1687–1696, 1993.

58. Kalaaji M, Fenton KA, Mortensen ES, et al: Glomerular apoptotic nucleosomes are central target structures for nephritogenic antibodies in human SLE nephritis. *Kidney Int* 71:664–672, 2007.

59. Emlen W, Niebur J-A, Kadera R: Accelerated in vitro apoptosis of lymphocytes from patients with systemic lupus erythematosus. *J Immunol* 152:3685–3692, 1994.

60. Perniok A, Wedekind F, Herrmann M, et al: High levels of circulating early apoptotic peripheral blood mononuclear cells in systemic lupus erythematosus. *Lupus* 7:113–118, 1998.

61. Casciola-Rosen LA, Anhalt G, Rosen A: Autoantigens targeted in systemic lupus erythematosus are clustered in two populations of surface structures on apoptotic keratinocytes. *J Exp Med* 179:1317–1330, 1994.

62. Pisetsky DS, Lipsky PE: Microparticles as autoadjuvants in the pathogenesis of SLE. *Nat Rev Rheumatol* 6:368–372, 2010.

63. Hall JC, Casciola-Rosen L, Rosen A: Altered structure of autoantigens during apoptosis. *Rheum Dis Clin North Am* 30:455–471, vii, 2004.

64. Kim SJ, Gershov D, Ma X, et al: I-PLA^2 activation during apoptosis promotes the exposure of membrane lysophosphatidylcholine leading to binding by natural immunoglobulin M antibodies and complement activation. *J Exp Med* 196:655–665, 2002.

65. Chen Y, Park YB, Patel E, et al: IgM antibodies to apoptosis-associated determinants recruit C1q and enhance dendritic cell phagocytosis of apoptotic cells. *J Immunol* 182:6031–6043, 2009.

66. Dall'era MC, Cardarelli PM, Preston BT, et al: Type I interferon correlates with clinical and serologic manifestations of systemic lupus erythematosus. *Ann Rheum Dis* 2005.

67. Baechler EC, Batliwalla FM, Karypis G, et al: Interferon-inducible gene expression signature in peripheral blood cells of patients with severe lupus. *Proc Natl Acad Sci U S A* 100:2610–2615, 2003.

68. Bennett L, Palucka AK, Arce E, et al: Interferon and granulopoiesis signatures in systemic lupus erythematosus blood. *J Exp Med* 197:711–723, 2003.

69. Ronnblom L, Eloranta ML, Alm GV: The type I interferon system in systemic lupus erythematosus. *Arthritis Rheum* 54:408–420, 2006.

70. Leadbetter EA, Rifkin IR, Hohlbaum AM, et al: Chromatin-IgG complexes activate B cells by dual engagement of IgM and Toll-like receptors. *Nature* 416:603–607, 2002.

71. Namjou B, Kothari PH, Kelly JA, et al: Evaluation of the TREX1 gene in a large multi-ancestral lupus cohort. *Genes Immun* 12:270–279, 2011.

72. Baumann I, Kolowos W, Voll RE, et al: Impaired uptake of apoptotic cells into tingible body macrophages in germinal centers of patients with systemic lupus erythematosus. *Arthritis Rheum* 46:191–201, 2002.

73. Botto M, Dell'Agnola C, Bygrave AE, et al: Homozygous C1q deficiency causes glomerulonephritis associated with multiple apoptotic bodies. *Nat Genet* 19:56–59, 1998.

74. Manderson AP, Botto M, Walport MJ: The role of complement in the development of systemic lupus erythematosus. *Annu Rev Immunol* 22:431–456, 2004.

75. Santer D, Hall BE, George TC, et al: C1q deficiency leads to the defective suppression of IFN-alpha in response to nucleoprotein containing immune complexes. *J Immunol* 185:4738–4749, 2010.

76. Gershov D, Kim S, Brot N, et al: C-reactive protein binds to apoptotic cells, protects the cells from assembly of the terminal complement components, and sustains an antiinflammatory innate immune response. Implications for systemic autoimmunity. *J Exp Med* 192:1353–1364, 2000.

Chapter 12

Abnormalities in Immune Complex Clearance and Fcγ Receptor Function

Jane E. Salmon and Robert P. Kimberly

Systemic lupus erythematosus (SLE), the prototype human disease mediated by immune complexes, is characterized by circulating antigen/antibody complexes that may be removed by the mononuclear phagocyte system or deposited in tissues. The fate of circulating immune complexes depends on the lattice of the immune complexes (i.e., number of antigens and antibody molecules in a given complex), the nature of the antigen and antibodies composing the immune complexes, and the status of the mononuclear phagocyte system. The efficiency of mononuclear phagocyte system immune complex clearance depends on the function of Fc gamma receptors (FcγR)—receptors recognizing the Fc region of immunoglobulin—and the complement receptors. In SLE, inadequate clearance results in tissue immune complex deposition, detected by immunofluorescence and electron microscopy, that initiates release of inflammatory mediators and influx of inflammatory cells. If sustained, this situation leads to tissue damage with resultant, clinically apparent disease, such as glomerulonephritis. Through in vivo and in vitro studies of patients with SLE, there clearly is both FcγR-dependent and complement-dependent mononuclear phagocyte dysfunctions in SLE that have inherited genetic variation and acquired components. This chapter reviews the role of the mononuclear phagocyte system in immune complex clearance, describes abnormalities in the mononuclear phagocyte function in SLE, and discusses mononuclear phagocyte system FcγR dysfunction as a mechanism for abnormal immune complex clearance in SLE.

THE ROLE OF THE MONONUCLEAR PHAGOCYTE SYSTEM IN THE CLEARANCE OF IMMUNE COMPLEXES

Early studies of the blood clearance of bacteria in mice, rabbits, and guinea pigs demonstrated that the mononuclear phagocyte system performed this function for opsonized particles. Infused bacteria were internalized by hepatic and splenic phagocytes.[1] The rate of clearance of bacteria from the blood and the site of their clearance depended on the level of antibodies to the bacteria in the serum of the animal. Rapidly cleared, well-opsonized bacteria were principally phagocytosed in the liver, whereas the more slowly cleared, less efficiently internalized (and presumably less opsonized) bacteria were removed by splenic phagocytes. These observations are remarkable for their similarity to the models of immune complex clearance in animals and humans that are described later.

Animal models have shown that the mononuclear phagocyte system serves an important role as a site for removal of soluble immune complexes.[2,3] This system may be saturated with increasing amounts of infused immune complexes, resulting in glomerular deposition of complexes, as seen in SLE.[4] Although impairment of immune complex clearance leads to increased deposition in tissues, the absence of activating FcγR on phagocytes prevents an inflammatory response to the localized immune complexes. Mice with targeted

deletions of activating FcγR are protected from fatal antigen-antibody Arthus reactions and immune complex–mediated glomerulonephritis. In contrast, mice lacking inhibitory FcγRs have exaggerated responses to immune complexes.[5-7]

Animal models of endogenous immune complex deposition also support the relationship between depressed mononuclear phagocyte system clearance and the genesis of glomerulonephritis. In chronic serum sickness, there is decreased clearance of aggregated albumin[8] and aggregated human immunoglobulin G (IgG).[9] Decreased clearance of heat-aggregated IgG in murine nephritis[10] and of polyvinyl pyrrolidine in New Zealand black/white (NZB/W) mice[11] has been observed, although some studies of endogenous immune complex–mediated disease have not found dysfunction of the mononuclear phagocyte system. The principle to be derived from these animal models of immune complex disease, whether from infused immune complexes or endogenous disease, is that immune complex deposition is influenced by the efficiency of mononuclear phagocyte system clearance. Specifically, impairment of mononuclear phagocyte system clearance is associated with tissue deposition of immune complexes and the potential for local organ damage.

MECHANISMS OF IMMUNE COMPLEX CLEARANCE

A number of factors govern the physical characteristics of immune complexes and, hence, their biologic properties (Box 12-1). These include the nature of the antibody in the complex, the nature of the antigen, and the antigen-antibody interaction. Antigen and antibodies in the circulation may rapidly form immune complexes, but the immunochemical properties of these circulating immune complexes determine their ultimate fate, either removal by the mononuclear phagocyte system or deposition in tissues. The potential of immune complexes to interact with FcγRs, to fix complement, and to react with complement receptors influences their rate of clearance. Immune complexes without complement are cleared primarily by FcγRs on fixed-tissue macrophages. Complexes that are opsonized with sufficient complement may bind to the receptor for C3b on circulating erythrocytes and subsequently may be removed by FcγRs and complement receptors. Thus, two classes of receptors, the FcγRs on phagocytes and the complement receptors on both erythrocytes and phagocytes, participate in the clearance of immune complexes (Figure 12-1).

Complement Mechanisms: Immune Adherence and the Erythrocyte CR1 System

Complement component 3 and the receptor for C3b on erythrocytes are important in processing and transporting large immune complexes[12] (see Chapter 13). Incorporation of complement components, C3b in particular, modifies the solubility of large immune complexes[13,14] and mediates the binding of immune complexes to human and other primate erythrocytes. Although both the liver and spleen are the major sites of immune complex uptake, erythrocytes in primates[12,15] and platelets in rodents[16,17] are important in clearing/processing immune complexes from the circulation. It has long been known that large complement-opsonized immune complexes bind to human erythrocytes.[18] Termed *immune adherence*, this reaction has been shown to participate in the handling of nascent circulating immune complexes in primates.[19]

Human erythrocytes express complement receptor type 1 (CR1), which permits binding of complement-fixing immune complexes. CR1 on erythrocytes can be conceptualized as having three main functions, which are not mutually exclusive: buffering, transporting, and processing (see Figure 12-1). The role of immune complex buffer has been suggested for erythrocytes because erythrocyte-bound immune complexes are unavailable for tissue deposition but non-bound complexes can deposit in the tissues. Bound immune complexes are transported to the liver or spleen, where fixed-tissue phagocyte FcγRs and complement receptors strip the immune complexes from the erythrocytes, which then return to the circulation to continue this process, thus performing the transporting function. Finally, CR1 promotes degradation of captured C3b on immune complexes, thereby modifying their subsequent handling.

The human CR1 (the complement receptor for C3b/C4b and, to a lesser degree, iC3b) is a single-chain, intrinsic membrane glycoprotein expressed on several different cells, including erythrocytes, granulocytes, monocytes, and macrophages (see Chapter 13). There are four codominantly expressed alleles of CR1, with molecular weights of 220,000, 250,000, 190,000, and 280,000 daltons (Da).[20-23] Inherited and acquired differences in the numeric expression of CR1 on erythrocytes have been described and associated with SLE.[24-28] Two alleles with codominant expression determine erythrocyte CR1 number in healthy individuals.[27,29] Although the CR1 number

---

Box 12-1 Factors Influencing the Characteristics of Immune Complexes

Antigen	**Antibody**
Availability	Quantity
Valence, size	Class, subclass
Epitope density and distribution	Capacity to fix complement
Tissue tropism/charge	Binding avidity
	Charge and distribution
	Antigen-Antibody Interaction
	Molar ratio

---

expressed on erythrocytes is low compared with that on leukocytes, approximately 90% of total circulating CR1 is on erythrocytes, because there are far more erythrocytes than leukocytes in the circulation.[30,31]

The binding of immune complexes to CR1 occurs rapidly in vivo, and it represents multivalent binding between multiple C3b molecules on the complex and clusters of CR1 on erythrocytes.[19,32-35] In vivo studies have demonstrated that immune complexes preferentially bind to circulating erythrocytes that express multiple CR1 clusters and that the capacity of each erythrocyte for binding correlates with the density of cell surface CR1. Because CR1 on erythrocytes tends to cluster more than that on resting neutrophils, most immune complexes that are bound to circulating cells are bound to erythrocytes.[13,15,30,31,36-40] A reduction in the number of functional CR1s limits the capacity of erythrocytes to transport and buffer immune complexes, and in vivo studies have demonstrated that repeated administration of antigens in immunized humans and primates with immune complex formation results in a decrease in erythrocyte CR1 levels.[36,41] Studies with primates have suggested that circulating immune complexes that are not bound to erythrocytes are more easily trapped in the microvasculature and can be recovered in the lungs and kidneys.[40,42] Taken together, these findings have obvious implications for immune complex–mediated diseases.

The erythrocyte CR1 system may also have a second physiologic function: providing a processing mechanism for immune complexes.[43] In addition to being a carrier for opsonized immune complexes, CR1 has a potent inhibitory function in the complement cascade, a function that may enhance clearance. It participates in the inactivation of C3b and may alter the size of complexes, thus affecting their subsequent handling. Specifically, CR1 is a cofactor for factor I in the cleavage of C3b to iC3b and then to C3dg.[44,45] Therefore, the binding of immune complexes containing C3b to erythrocyte CR1 facilitates proteolytic cleavage of the C3b to iC3b and C3dg, which do not bind to CR1. This reaction is the basis for the degradation of complement on immune complexes with their subsequent release from the receptor,[46] and its rate varies with the physicochemical properties of the individual complexes.[47] If the immune complex can again activate complement and bind C3b, it can rebind to CR1.[48] The fraction of immune complexes in whole blood that is erythrocyte bound depends on several dynamic processes: complement fixation and C3b capture, erythrocyte binding, and C3b degradation and immune complex release.

Fcγ Receptor Mechanisms

Immune complexes are removed from the circulation by the mononuclear phagocyte system of the liver and spleen through engagement of FcγRs and complement receptors. The interaction of immune complexes with the phagocyte involves a qualitatively different

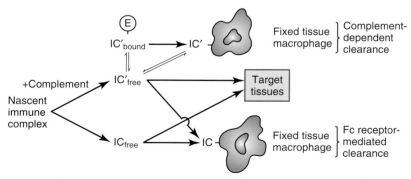

FIGURE 12-1 Framework for immune complex handling. Nascent immune complexes (ICs) that fix complement efficiently are rapidly bound by erythrocytes (E). ICs containing complement may cycle between E-bound and unbound (free); they usually are rapidly taken up in the liver. Unbound complexes also may deposit in the tissues, and with impaired complement-dependent uptake, they may be taken up by Fc receptor–dependent mechanisms. ICs that do not bind complement are either taken up by Fc receptor–dependent mechanisms or deposited in tissues. (*Redrawn from Kimberly RP: Immune complexes in rheumatic diseases.* Rheum Dis Clin North Am *13:583–596, 1987.*)

ABNORMALITIES IN IMMUNE COMPLEX CLEARANCE
AND Fc RECEPTOR FUNCTION

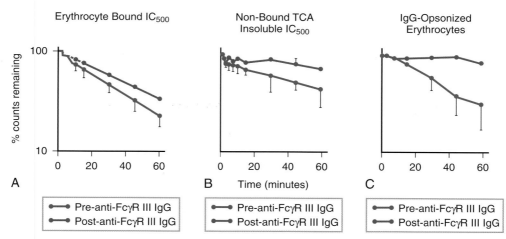

FIGURE 12-2 Effect of monoclonal antibody against Fcγ receptor III (anti-FcγRIII MAb) on the handling of soluble immune complex (IC). The effects of anti-FcγRIII MAb infusions on the handling of several different radiolabeled model IC probes in chimpanzees are presented, with data expressed as the percentage counts remaining relative to the counts infused. **A,** Following intravenous infusion of soluble radiolabeled IC, clearance of erythrocyte (E)–bound IC was measured and found to be slowed by treatment with anti-FcγRIII MAb immunoglobulin (Ig) G. **B,** After intravenous infusion of soluble IC, clearance of non–E-bound IC was slowed more by anti-FcγRIII MAb IgG. **C,** Clearance of IgG-opsonized E was most markedly slowed by anti-FcγRIII infusions. *(From Kimberly RP, Edberg JC, Merriam LT, et al: In vivo handling of soluble complement fixing Ab/dsDNA immune complexes in chimpanzees.* J Clin Invest 84:962–970, 1989.)

process from that with erythrocytes.[37] The relative contribution of each receptor system depends on the immunochemical properties of the complex. The liver, which is much larger than the spleen, is the principal site for the uptake of immune complexes[42,49,50]; however, immune complexes that escape clearance by hepatic macrophages, which may be smaller and of lower valence, are taken up by the spleen.[49] The role of FcγRs in clearance of both soluble and particulate immune complexes is shown by studies wherein blockade of FcγRs by an infusion of aggregated IgG into the portal venous system[30] or of antibodies against FcγRs[37] suppresses uptake of these immune complexes (Figure 12-2). Supporting the pivotal role of FcγRs in handling certain immune complexes, studies of complement depletion show no effect on the efficiency of uptake of immune complexes by the liver or spleen and actually show an acceleration in the rate of removal of complexes from the circulation, presumably resulting from their being trapped in the microvasculature.[40]

FcγRs appear to play a key role in the transfer and retention of immune complexes by mononuclear phagocytes. Studies of DNA/anti-DNA complexes that are bound to radiolabeled erythrocytes and injected into chimpanzees show that whereas immune complexes are removed by the mononuclear phagocyte system, the erythrocytes are not sequestered; rather, they are stripped of immune complexes and promptly recirculated.[15] Although the mechanism of this stripping is not well defined, the involvement of complement proteases has been implicated.[51] In this model of immune complex clearance, infusion of erythrocyte-bound DNA/anti-DNA complexes after treatment with anti-FcγR monoclonal antibody results in a significant amount of non–erythrocyte-bound circulating immune complexes, documenting the participation of FcγRs in the retention of immune complexes by phagocytes (see Figure 12-2B).[37]

In addition to stripping erythrocyte-bound complexes, FcγRs as well as CR3/CR4 are responsible for the clearance of those complexes that are unable to bind to erythrocyte CR1 because of inadequate C3b capture or degradation of C3b. This interpretation is supported by experiments in which primates treated with anti-FcγR monoclonal antibodies showed impaired clearance of infused immune complexes, which was most pronounced in the fraction of complexes that did not bind to erythrocytes.[37] It has been shown that immune adherence is not a prerequisite for the efficient handling of immune complexes

by the mononuclear phagocyte system,[41] but immune complexes that do not fix complement or that fix complement poorly cannot be cleared if FcγR function is impaired (see Figure 12-1).

ABNORMAL IMMUNE COMPLEX CLEARANCE IN SLE
Human Models of Immune Complex Clearance
Probes that have been used to assess the efficiency of immune complex clearance in humans are (1) autologous erythrocytes sensitized with IgG antibodies that are directed against the D antigen of the Rh system, (2) preformed immune complexes or aggregated IgG, and (3) antigen infused into passively immunized subjects. Because each of these probes has distinct immunochemical properties, they interact differently with the complement and FcγR systems, as expected. Thus, the results of in vivo studies comparing immune clearance in patients with SLE and in healthy individuals vary with the probe used.

Analysis of the Clearance of IgG-Sensitized Autologous Erythrocytes
The technique introduced by Frank[52] to measure mononuclear phagocyte system function employs autologous chromium Cr 51–labeled erythrocytes that are sensitized with IgG anti-(Rh)D antibodies and injected into study subjects, and clearance or removal of these cells from the circulation is determined by serial bleeding. External surface counting of sensitized radiolabeled erythrocytes shows initial rapid sequestration in the liver, followed by splenic accumulation of most of the injected cells. The semilogarithmic plot of mean data for the clearance of sensitized cells in normal control subjects is curvilinear, with a rapid initial loss of radiolabeled cells followed by a slower, sustained loss of radioactivity (Figure 12-3).[53-55]

Although originally conceptualized as a measure of FcγR capacity, kinetic analysis of in vivo clearance studies and in vitro studies with IgG anti-(Rh)D–coated erythrocytes suggests that complement also plays a role in clearance of this probe.[56] A proposed model to describe the series of steps in handling of IgG anti-(Rh)D–sensitized erythrocytes is as follows: Circulating cells initially sequestered by a complement-dependent process are deactivated and released back into the circulation or are phagocytosed. Released cells are

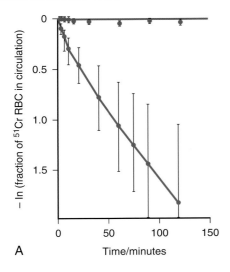

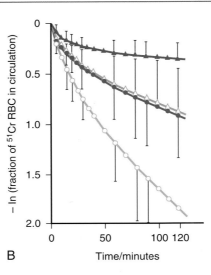

FIGURE 12-3 A, Survival of chromium Cr 51–labeled autologous erythrocytes in normal controls. Data are shown for unsensitized erythrocytes in six normal controls (*pink curve*) and that of anti-Rh(D)–sensitized erythrocytes in 49 normal controls (*green curve*). **B,** Survival of Cr 51–labeled autologous anti-Rh(D)–sensitized erythrocytes in 32 patients with SLE; comparison between disease active subgroups: ○–○, inactive/nonrenal disease (n = 5); •–• active/nonrenal disease (n = 7); △–△, active/nonrenal disease (n = 12); ▲–▲, active/renal (n = 8). *(From Kimberly RP, Meryhew NL, Runquist OA: Mononuclear phagocyte function in SLE. I: Bipartite Fc- and complement-dependent dysfunction. J Immunol 137:91–96, 1986. Copyright 1986. The American Association of Immunologists, Inc.)*

sequestered and phagocytosed by an FcγR-mediated process. Circulating cells may also be directly sequestered and phagocytosed by FcγRs.[54-56]

Abnormal mononuclear phagocyte system function in patients with SLE has been demonstrated in several studies performed with IgG anti-(Rh)D–sensitized erythrocytes.[52,57-60] Clearance half-times for radiolabeled autologous IgG-sensitized erythrocytes were longer in these patients than in normal individuals and longer in patients with renal disease than in those without renal disease (Figures 12-3 and 12-4). When clinical activity in patients with SLE was assessed, there was a significant but independent association between impaired FcγR clearance and the level of both renal and nonrenal disease activity.[59] Increased activity along either parameter was associated with more impaired clearance (see Figure 12-4). Longitudinal studies in patients with SLE showed that mononuclear phagocyte system function changed concordantly with changes in clinical status, indicating that clearance dysfunction is dynamic and closely related to disease activity.[57,58]

Although partly acquired and related to disease activity, the FcγR mononuclear phagocyte dysfunction has a genetic component. Allelic polymorphisms of FcγR are potential inherited factors influencing immune complex clearance (discussed later). Thus, basal genetically determined mononuclear phagocyte clearance in normal individuals may contribute to the predisposition and pathogenesis of SLE.

Analysis of Clearance of Infused Soluble Immune Complexes

As another measure of mononuclear phagocyte system function, the clearance of preformed, large, soluble, complement-fixing immune complexes has been studied in humans. Radiolabeled tetanus toxoid/antitetanus toxoid, hepatitis B surface antigen/antibody, or aggregated human IgG is infused, and then sequential blood samples are obtained and analyzed for whole blood and erythrocyte-bound radioactivity to monitor clearance.[38,61,62] Clearance of these preformed immune complexes (free or erythrocyte bound) from the circulation of humans has been shown to involve the activation of complement with capture of C3b, binding to erythrocyte CR1 receptors, uptake by complement, and FcγR tissue mononuclear phagocytes, as described earlier. Factors that cause the erythrocyte transport system to fail, such as hypocomplementemia and CR1 deficiency, are associated with an initially more rapid disappearance of immune complexes, presumably caused by trapping in capillary beds outside the mononuclear phagocyte system. Given the different kinds of information obtained from each of these in vivo probes, examination of multiple models of immune complex clearance is necessary to define the mechanisms of immune complex deposition in SLE.

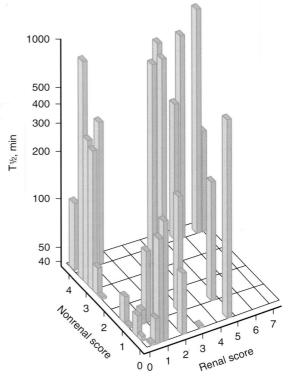

FIGURE 12-4 Relationship of clinical activity and Fc gamma receptor (FcγR)–mediated mononuclear phagocyte system dysfunction. Clinical activity was assessed in terms of both renal and nonrenal manifestations. Longer (taller) clearance half-time values represent greater degrees of dysfunction. Patients with active renal and nonrenal disease showed the greatest degree of FcγR-mediated clearance impairment. *(From Kimberly RP, Salmon JE, Edberg JC, et al: The role of Fc receptors in mononuclear phagocyte system function. Clin Exp Rheum 7(Suppl):S130–S138, 1989.)*

In vivo studies of infused soluble immune complexes complement the sensitized erythrocyte model of clearance and demonstrate multifactorial mononuclear phagocyte dysfunction. Abnormalities in the erythrocyte CR1 system, the early buffer for circulating immune complexes, are described in patients with SLE, and for these models it is important to recognize that such patients tend to have an acquired, decreased numeric expression of CR1 on erythrocytes that correlates with disease activity[63,64] and may result from repeated

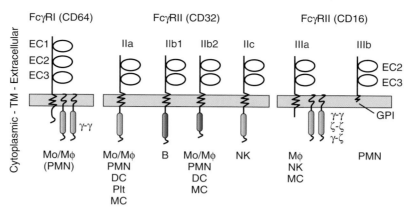

FIGURE 12-5 Schematic representation of the human Fc gamma receptor (FcγR) family members. FcγR α chains contain two or three disulfide-linked immunoglobulin (Ig)–like extracellular domains (*ellipses*) that mediate binding to IgG. All FcγRs, except the glycosyl phosphatidylinositol (GPI)–anchored FcγRIIIb, have transmembrane regions (TMs), some of which can interact with accessory chains to yield a multichain signaling complex. The cytoplasmic domains of FcγRs or their associated subunits are responsible for signal transduction. FcγRIIIb is the only FcγR that lacks a cytoplasmic tail. FcγRI and FcγRIIIa are multichain receptors that associate with immunoreceptor tyrosine activation motif (ITAM)–containing γ- or ζ-chain dimers (*green cylinders*) to mediate positive signaling. FcγRIIa and FcγRIIc are single-chain stimulatory receptors containing ITAM motifs in their cytoplasmic tails. FcγRIIb (isoforms FcγRIIb1 and FcγRIIb2) are single-chain inhibitory receptors containing immunoreceptor tyrosine inhibitory motif (ITIM) in their cytoplasmic tails (*pink cylinders*). The cellular distribution of each FcγR is listed below it. B, B lymphocyte; DC, dendritic cell; MC, mast cell; B, Mφ, macrophage; Mo, monocyte; NK, natural killer cell; Plt, platelet; PNM, polymorphonuclear leukocyte (PMN). (*Adapted from Salmon JE, Pricop L: Human receptors for immunoglobulin G: Key elements in the pathogenesis of rheumatic disease. Arthritis Rheum 44:739–750, 2001.*)

immune complex/erythrocyte CR1 interactions.[38,41] There also is evidence of an inherited deficiency of CR1 in some patients.[26,28] With these model immune complexes, a rapid first phase of elimination was noted in patients with low complement, low CR1, and low immune adherence, which was ascribed to inappropriate tissue deposition of complexes.[39] The second, slower elimination phase of infused aggregated IgG is also abnormal in SLE, presumably because of impaired splenic uptake as well as generalized mononuclear phagocyte dysfunction. Regardless of the mechanism, abnormalities in both splenic and hepatic clearance functions allow for a spillover of complexes beyond the mononuclear phagocyte system in SLE.

Blockade of FcγRs by elevations of IgG interferes with this key mechanism for the elimination of soluble circulating immune complexes.[65,66] That serum concentrations of IgG are an important factor predicting the rate of aggregated IgG clearance in SLE[67] emphasizes the importance of FcγR mechanisms in this model and supports the conclusions derived from the sensitized erythrocyte model of immune complex clearance. Specifically, FcγR-mediated clearance efficiency is crucial in SLE because of the defects in complement-dependent function.

BIOLOGY OF HUMAN Fcγ RECEPTORS

With evidence for both the genetic and acquired components of FcγR-mediated clearance defects, further information about FcγR structure and function should enhance our understanding of immune complex handling and provide insight into novel therapeutic options. More than simply one type of receptor for IgG, as assumed in many of the early studies cited in this chapter, human FcγR structures are quite varied in terms of ligand binding and signaling properties. With their expression dynamically regulated by cytokines and other inflammatory stimuli and with their having cell type–specific patterns of expression, our knowledge of FcγRs has revealed extreme diversity accompanied by great complexity.

Structure and Distribution

FcγRs are an essential receptor system that is engaged by immune complexes as they trigger internalization, release of inflammatory mediators, cytokines, and degranulation. In contrast to complement receptors, FcγRs recognize ligand in its native form. In humans, there are three distinct but closely related families of FcγRs—FcγRI (CD64), FcγRII (CD32), and FcγRIII (CD16)—that share many

immunochemical and physicochemical properties and cellular distribution, and have highly homologous DNA sequences.[68-72] Each of the eight FcγR genes leads to protein products with some unique features, including differences in binding capacity, distinct signal transduction elements, and cell-specific expression patterns (Figure 12-5). The structure-function relationships of each receptor family provide a framework for understanding how FcγRs may contribute to disease susceptibility, pathogenesis, and therapeutic intervention in SLE.

Both stimulatory and inhibitory FcγRs are often coexpressed on surfaces of hematopoietic cells, providing a mechanism to modulate cell activation initiated by stimulatory FcγRs. Studies have suggested that inhibitory FcγRs, which modulate thresholds for activation and can terminate activation signals, are a key element in the regulation of effector function.[6,7] Inhibitory FcγRs play a central role in afferent and efferent immune responses as negative regulators of both antibody production and immune complex–triggered activation.

FcγRs belong to the immunoglobulin supergene family and are encoded by multiple genes on the long arm of chromosome 1q21-23.[73-75] The presence of multiple distinct genes (arising from gene reduplication) and alternative splicing variants leads to a variety of receptor isoforms that are most strikingly different in transmembrane and intracellular regions, whereas they share similar but not precisely identical extracellular domains (see Figure 12-5).

FcγRs capable of triggering cellular activation possess intracellular activation motifs, termed immunoreceptor tyrosine-based activation motifs (ITAMs), similar to those of B-cell receptors and T-cell receptors.[76,77] Inhibitory FcγRs have extracellular domains that are homologous to their activating counterparts, but their cytoplasmic domains contain an immunoreceptor tyrosine-based inhibitory motif (ITIM). The stimulatory FcγRI, a high-affinity receptor for IgG that binds monomeric IgG, and FcγRIIIa, an intermediate-affinity receptor that binds only multivalent IgG, are multichain receptors composed of a ligand-binding α-subunit, which confers ligand specificity and affinity, and associated signaling subunits with ITAMs in their respective cytoplasmic domains (Figure 12-5). FcγR α-chains are transmembrane molecules that share the structural motif of two or three extracellular immunoglobulin-like domains but vary in their affinity for IgG and in their preferences for binding different IgG subclasses (IgG1, IgG2, IgG3, and IgG4). Allelic variations in the ligand-binding regions of specific FcγRs influence the ability to bind certain IgG subclasses and alter the responses of phagocytes to IgG-opsonized antigens.[78-80] The transmembrane domains of the α subunits contain a basic residue, which mediates the physical interaction with associated signal transducing chains required for efficient expression and signal transduction. Homodimeric γ-chains are transducing modules for FcγRI and FcγRIIIa (see Figure 12-5). Heterodimers of γ-ζ chains or homodimers of ζ chains can also transduce signals through FcγRIIIa in human natural killer (NK) cells. Another isoform, FcγRIIb, has neither an ITAM nor a transmembrane domain, but is maintained in the plasma membrane outer leaflet by a glycosyl phosphatidylinositol (GPI) anchor (see Figure 12-5). In addition to multichain receptors, there are two other types of activating FcγRs and one inhibitory receptor with two different splice variants. FcγRIIa and FcγRIIc are single-chain receptors that include an extracellular ligand-binding domain and an ITAM in the cytoplasmic domain. Inhibitory FcγRs, FcγRIIb1 and FcγRIIb2, are single-chain receptors with extracellular domains highly homologous to their activating counterparts and cytoplasmic domains with ITIMs (see Figure 12-5).[81]

FcγRI (CD64) is distinguished by three extracellular immunoglobulin-like domains, a relatively high affinity for IgG,[82] and the capacity for binding monomeric IgG (see Figure 12-5).[83-85] FcγRIa, a heavily glycosylated 72-kDa protein, associates with homodimers of the Fc common γ-chain, which also can associate with the high-affinity receptor for IgE (see Figure 12-5).[86] FcγRIa is present on monocytes, macrophages, and myeloid-derived dendritic cells.[87] Monocyte expression of FcγRI is markedly enhanced by interferon-γ (IFN-γ),[88,89] and neutrophils that do not constitutively express FcγRI can be induced to express this receptor by IFN-γ and granulocyte colony-stimulating factor (G-CSF).[90,91]

The FcγRII (CD32) family contains three genes encoding receptors that have low affinity for IgG and interact only with multimeric IgG in complexes. CD32 family gene products are the most widely expressed FcγRs and are found on most leukocytes and platelets.[92-94] Density of expression varies with cell type but generally is higher than that for FcγRI.[95] The structural heterogeneity of FcγRII family reflects three genes, *FCGR2A, FCGR2B,* and *FCGR2C,* which encode FcγRIIa, FcγRIIb, and FcγRIIc proteins, respectively, as well as several splice variants (see Figure 12-5).[69-72,96] With near identity in their extracellular and transmembrane domains, the gene products show divergence in cytoplasmic tails, which determines the effector functions that are mediated by each isoform (see Figure 12-5). Among the FcγRII family members, there are activating and inhibiting receptors that differ mainly in the signaling motif in the cytoplasmic domain. FcγRIIa and FcγRIIc contain ITAMs and they are preferentially expressed on cells of myeloid lineage, monocytes, neutrophils, certain dendritic cells, platelets, and NK cells. In addition to different isoforms, there are two allelic forms of FcγRIIa (R131 and H131), which are expressed codominantly and have differing IgG subclass–binding specificities and functional capacities (discussed later).[70,78,79]

Although ITAMs can assume an inhibitory function is some special circumstances, *FCGR2B* is the only FCGR gene encoding an ITIM, the canonical motif for an inhibitory receptor (see Figure 12-5).[81] A single-chain low-affinity receptor with extracellular domains highly homologous to FcγRIIa and FcγRIIc, FcγRIIb has two alternative splice isoforms, FcγRIIb1 and FcγRIIb2, which differ only in their intracytoplasmic regions.[96] FcγRIIb1 contains an insertion of 19 amino acids that alters intracellular targeting pathways. Neither isoform can trigger cell activation. Instead, both isoforms of FcγRIIb, when coaggregated with ITAM-bearing receptors, are negative regulators of activation. In addition, FcγRIIb2 participates in endocytosis of multivalent ligands by phagocytes and antigen-presenting cells, and the intracytoplasmic insertion in FcγRIIb1 inhibits internalization.[97] FcγRIIb can modulate tyrosine phosphorylation–based cell activation by stimulatory FcγR, B-cell receptor (BCR), T-cell receptor (TCR), Fc receptors for IgE,[98] Toll-like receptors (TLRs), and others. However, to inhibit cell activation, FcγRIIbs are typically coclustered with the other activating receptors.[99] For example, FcγRIIb coaggregation with FcγRIIa by

IgG-opsonized particles blocks phagocytosis, and FcγRIIb coligation to BCRs by antibody-antigen complexes inhibits B-cell proliferation and antibody production.[100,101] Thus, FcγRIIb-mediated negative regulation of ITAM-dependent cell activation endows IgG-containing immune complexes with the capacity to regulate B cells and inflammatory cells. Because activating and inhibitory FcγRs are often coexpressed, the balance between stimulatory and inhibitory inputs determines cellular response. Allelic polymorphisms have been described in FcγRIIb; those in the transmembrane domain alter inhibitory function in B cells, and those in the promoter region alter receptor expression.[102-104]

The low-affinity FcγRIII (CD16) family contains two proteins, each with cell type–specific expression and each encoded by distinct, yet highly homologous genes (*FCGR3A* and *FCGR3B*).[70,71,105] FcγRIIIa is the most abundant FcγR on tissue-specific macrophages and thus is a key receptor of the mononuclear phagocyte system. It is present at high density on Kupffer cells in the liver and on macrophages in the spleen, both important areas for immune complex clearance binding and internalization. In addition, it is expressed on dendritic cells, NK cells, γ/δ T cells, and mesangial cells.[106] Different glycoforms of FcγRIIIa, with different affinities for IgG, are expressed on NK cells and macrophages.[107] The FcγRIIIa α-chain is most typically associated with the Fc common γ-chain, a member of the family of signal transduction molecules that bear ITAMs within their cytoplasmic domains (see Figure 12-5).[108] These signal transduction partners also are used by FcγRI, the high-affinity receptor for IgE and the T-cell receptor/CD3 complex. These accessory molecules form disulfide-linked dimeric complexes (homodimers or heterodimers) that noncovalently associate with the transmembrane region of FcγRIIIa to enable cell surface expression and signal transduction. FcγRIIIa also has the capacity to associate with the β-subunit of the high-affinity IgE receptor.[109]

FcγRIIIb is expressed at high levels on neutrophils and is the most abundant FcγR in the circulation. As a GPI-anchored receptor, it differs from FcγRIIIa, which is expressed on macrophages and NK cells as a conventional transmembrane protein (see Figure 12-5).[110,111] FcγRIIIb on the surfaces of neutrophils interacts with β integrin CD11b/CD18, a finding of interest because of the strong genetic association of CD11b/ITGAM (integrin alpha M) locus and SLE. Further diversity in FcγRIII structure is provided by an allotypic variation in FcγRIIIb. The two most commonly recognized allelic forms of the GPI-anchored neutrophil isoform of FcγRIIIb, termed NA1 and NA2, differ by several amino acids and N-linked glycosylation sites.[112,113] The alleles are inherited in a classic mendelian manner and are expressed in a codominant fashion. In addition to different isoforms, there are two allelic forms of FcγRIIIa (F176 and V176), which differ (1) in one amino acid at position 176 in the extracellular domain (phenylalanine and valine, respectively)[80,114,115] and (2) in binding capacity for IgG1 and IgG3 (discussed later).

Ligands

Ligand specificity for FcγRs is relative rather than absolute, and it depends on the valency or degree of opsonization of the study probe.[116] Table 12-1 shows the binding specificity of human FcγRs for human IgG subclasses. A multivalent immune complex may bind simultaneously to different classes of FcγR. FcγRI, the high-affinity receptor and the only FcγR capable of univalent binding of IgG,[69,70] and FcγRII and FcγRIIIb, which are lower-affinity FcγRs, preferentially bind IgG1 and IgG3. There is differential binding affinity for allelic variants of FcγRIIIa[80] and for different glycoforms. Although the affinity of FcγRIIIa expressed on macrophages and NK cells is higher than that of FcγRIIIb on neutrophils, the pattern of specificity for subclasses is similar for all FcγRs.[107] For all three classes of FcγR, IgG2 is the ligand with lowest affinity (see Table 12-1), although studies have shown efficient binding to IgG2 by the H131 allele of FcγRIIa (discussed later).[78,79,117]

In addition to classic IgG-FcγR interactions, FcγRI and FcγRIIa function as receptors for innate immune opsonins, including

TABLE 12-1 Fcγ Receptor (FcγR) Affinity and Immunoglobulin (Ig) G Subclass Specificity

RECEPTOR FAMILY	MOLECULAR WEIGHT (kDa)	RECEPTOR(S)	AFFINITY FOR IgG (kA)	IgG SPECIFICITY
FcγRI	72	FcγRI	10^8-10^9 M^{-1}	1, 3 > 4 >> 2
FcγRII	40-50	FcγRIIA-R131	$<10^7$ M^{-1}	1, 3 >> 2, 4
		FcγRIIA-H131	$<10^7$ M^{-1}	1, 3, 2 >>> 4
		FcγRIIB, C	$<10^7$ M^{-1}	1, 3 >> 2, 4
FcγRIII	60-70	FcγRIIIA	10^7 M^{-1}	1, 3 >>> 2, 4
	50-80	FcγRIIIB	$<10^7$ M^{-1}	1, 3 >> 2, 4

C-reactive protein (CRP) and serum amyloid protein. FcγRIIa, the main receptor on human phagocytes for CRP, may contribute to the uptake and clearance of nucleosomes bound to CRP, which may be influenced by allelic polymorphisms[118-120] and could provide one mechanism responsible for the association of FcγRIIa polymorphisms with SLE in genome-wide association studies.

FcγR Signal Transduction

Clustering of FcγRs at the cell surface by multivalent antigen-antibody complexes initiates signal transduction and involves tyrosine phosphorylation as a critical early signaling event.[76,77] Typically, membrane-anchored src family kinases mediate phosphorylation of the YxxL tyrosines within the ITAM motifs, which enables docking of the protein tyrosine kinase *syk*. Subsequent tyrosine phosphorylation targets many intracellular substrates, including phospholipid kinases, phospholipases, adapter molecules, and cytoskeletal proteins.[121] Activation of the ras pathway can lead to phosphorylation of mitogen-activated protein (MAP) kinases, activation of transcription factors, and induction of gene expression.[122]

FcγRIIb isoforms are important negative regulators of ITAM-dependent activation and establish the threshold for effector cell activation. The ITIM motif (V/IxYxxL), contained in a 13–amino-acid sequence present in the intracytoplasmic domain of both FcγRIIb1 and FcγRIIb2, is essential for the negative regulatory properties of FcγRIIbs and other inhibitory receptors (reviewed in references 123-125). Like ITAMs, ITIMs are phosphorylated by protein src family kinases, and they then recruit SH2 (Src homology region 2 domain)–containing protein tyrosine phosphatases such as SHP-1 (SH2-containing phosphatases-1) and SHP-2. The inositol polyphosphate 5′-phosphatase SHIP is preferentially recruited to FcγRIIb and appears to play the predominant role in FcγRIIb-mediated inhibition by preventing Ca^{2+} influx.[126-128]

In cells that express both stimulatory and inhibitory receptors for IgG, the relative levels of these two types of receptors determine the state of cell activation after interaction with immune complexes. Cross-talk among different receptor systems, the role of the α-chain cytoplasmic domain, and the capacity of ITAM-associated receptors, such as the IgA receptor FcαRI, to have paradoxically inhibitory effects in certain circumstances add further nuance to the regulation of inflammatory responses.[129]

FcγR-Mediated Effector Functions

The multivalent interaction of phagocytes with immune complexes leads to internalization of the complex, generation of reactive oxygen intermediates, and release of inflammatory mediators, including prostaglandins, leukotrienes, hydrolytic enzymes, and cytokines.[130-134] Although there may be significant overlap among the biologic activities mediated by each family of FcγRs, there is also specialization among the receptors, and the relative contribution of each receptor family depends on the nature of the ligand, the state of phagocyte activation, and the effector function being assessed. Through binding via FcγRs, antibodies modulate immune responses, triggering an array of activities (reviewed in reference 135).

Binding and internalization are the most important effector functions for immune complex clearance. Experiments using erythrocytes coated with Fab fragments of anti-FcγR monoclonal antibodies show that in cultured human monocytes (a model system for fixed-tissue macrophages), FcγRI, FcγRIIa, and FcγRIIIa mediate phagocytosis.[136] A key role for FcγRIIIa is evident from studies showing that blockade of FcγRIII by infusion of anti-FcγRIII monoclonal antibody in humans and nonhuman primates inhibits clearance of IgG anti-D–sensitized erythrocytes (see Figure 12-2).[37,137,138] The intermediate affinity of this receptor on fixed-tissue macrophages is ideal for capture and clearance of soluble immune complexes with contributions from other FcγRs and complement receptors.

On neutrophils, FcγRIIIb, the GPI-anchored molecule that is abundantly expressed, serves to capture circulating immune complexes and focuses IgG ligand for more efficient recognition and phagocytosis by other FcγR species.[71,136,139] FcγRIIIb can generate some intracellular signals and is a potentiator of other receptors on the cell. Crosslinking of FcγRIIIb enhances the amount of FcγRIIa-specific internalization, and coligation of FcγRII and FcγRIIIb results in a synergistic phagocytic response: internalization that is greater than the sum of the FcγRII and FcγRIIIb responses.[139-141] This synergistic capacity of FcγRIIIb also enables complement receptor-mediated phagocytosis.

Cytokines elaborated during an immune response alter FcγR expression and functional capacity. For example, IFN-γ and G-CSF upregulate FcγRI on monocytes and induce its expression on polymorphonuclear cells (PMNs), whereas interleukin-4 (IL-4) inhibits the expression of all ITAM-bearing FcγRs.[142-144] Granulocyte-macrophage CSF (GM-CSF) specifically increases FcγRIIa, and transforming growth factor beta (TGF-β) increases FcγRIIIa.[144] In contrast to their effects on stimulatory receptors, IFN-γ decreases and IL-4 increases the expression of the inhibitory receptor FcγRIIb2 on human monocytes.[145] That IFN-γ (a prototypic T-helper-1 [Th1] cytokine) and IL-4 (a prototypic Th2 cytokine) differentially regulate the expression of FcγR isoforms with opposite functions provides a mechanism for regulation of activating and inhibitory signals delivered by FcγRs on phagocytes.[146] Cytokines released with in an inflammatory milieu thus act in an autocrine and paracrine manner to modulate effector cell function.

Inherited Differences in FcγRs

Germline differences in FcγR structure, expression, or function provide the basis for differences in FcγR function among individuals, and these differences may contribute to disease susceptibility and pathogenesis. Heritable differences include sequence polymorphisms in regulatory and coding regions and gene copy number polymorphisms with duplications and deletions. Individuals with the rare deficiency of FcγRIa1 are free of clinical disease and circulating immune complexes, and they do not show greater susceptibility to infection.[147] Duplications and deletions of *FCGR3B* have been implicated in a number of autoimmune conditions,[148] supporting the proposed role for neutrophil extracellular trap (NET) formation in SLE pathogenesis.[149-154]

The concept that the balance of stimulatory and inhibitory FcγRs is a determinant of the susceptibility to and severity of immune complex–induced inflammatory disease is supported by murine models.[5-7] Reduced expression of FcγRIIb on macrophages and activated B cells, whether naturally occurring or engineered, predisposes mice to the development of autoantibodies and autoimmune

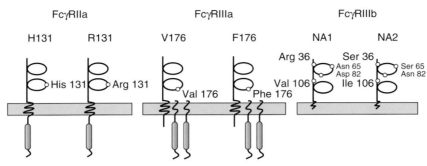

FIGURE 12-6 Allelic variants of activating human Fc gamma receptors (FcγRs). *Left,* The FcγRIIa polymorphism is a consequence of an arginine (R131)–to-histidine (H131) substitution at amino acid position 131 in the extracellular domain, which causes differences in binding affinity for human immunoglobulin (Ig) G2 and C-reactive protein (CRP). *Middle,* The FcγRIIIa polymorphism is the consequence of a valine (V176)–to–phenylalanine (F176) substitution at position 176, leading to changes in binding affinity for human IgG1 and IgG3. *Right,* The neutrophil antigen 1 (NA1) and NA2 polymorphism of FcγRIIIb reflects four amino acid substitutions with consequent differences in *N*-linked glycosylation sites and quantitative differences in phagocytic function. Arg, arginine; Asn, asparagine; Asp, aspartic acid; His, histine; Ile, isoleucine; Phe, phenylalanine; Ser, serine; Val, valine. *(Adapted from Salmon JE, Pricop L: Human receptors for immunoglobulin G: Key elements in the pathogenesis of rheumatic disease.* Arthritis Rheum *44:739–750, 2001.)*

glomerulonephritis in a strain-dependent fashion.[155-158] Conversely, increases in FcγRIIb expression in these mice restores tolerance and ameliorates the autoimmune phenotype.[159] In humans, single-nucleotide polymorphisms in regulatory regions of the promoter alter receptor expression and are associated with both alterations in cell function and antibody-mediated autoimmunity.[102,160] A nonsynonymous T-to-C single-nucleotide polymorphism in the *FCR2B* gene that results in a change from isoleucine to threonine at position 187 (187T allele) in the transmembrane domain of the FcγRIIb protein excludes the receptor from lipid rafts, decreases the inhibitory potential for BCR signaling, and alters the inhibitory function in B cells.[104,161] In addition, homozygosity of the hypofunctional allele associated with SLE (the minor allele) is protective against severe malaria.[162,163] Metaanalysis of association studies of this variant of *FCGR2B* in SLE demonstrated and association of I87T allele in Asian and perhaps Caucasian populations.[103,162]

Germline polymorphisms in coding regions, leading to subtle variations in FcγR structure, provide a basis for inherited predisposition to disease. Single amino acid substitutions within the extracellular domain can alter the capacity to bind different IgG subclasses. Substitutions in the transmembrane domain affect lateral mobility in the plane of the membrane and partitioning to lipid domains. These allelic variants of human FcγRs profoundly influence phagocyte biologic activity and have been associated with both autoimmune and infectious disease (Figure 12-6).

FcγRIIa, expressed on mononuclear phagocytes, neutrophils, and platelets, has two codominantly expressed alleles, which differ at amino acid position 131 in the ligand-binding contact region of the extracellular domain (see Figure 12-6). Unlike the arginine allele (R131), the histidine allele (H131) is able to bind human IgG2.[78,79,97,164] Because IgG2 is a poor activator of the classical complement pathway, FcγRIIa-H131 is essential for handling IgG2 immune complexes. Even with model immune complexes containing IgG2 in combination with other IgG subclasses, there is differential handling by PMNs from homozygous individuals in relation to host FcγRIIa genotype.[165] The allele frequency of H131 in Caucasian and African-American populations is approximately 0.50. Among Asians the frequency of the R131 allele is much lower, and less than 10% of the population is homozygous for R131 (reviewed in reference 166).

FcγRIIa alleles have important clinical implications for host defense against infection with encapsulated bacteria known to elicit IgG2 responses, such as *Neisseria meningitidis, Haemophilus influenzae,* and *Streptococcus pneumoniae.*[167-169] The increased frequency of homozygosity for FcγRIIa-R131 among otherwise healthy children who suffer from recurrent respiratory tract infections or fulminant meningococcal sepsis and the risk for invasive pneumococcal infection in patients with SLE is predictable and underscores the importance of these allelic polymorphisms to disease susceptibility.[170]

Partially offsetting this risk for infectious disease may be the reciprocal relationship between the binding affinities of IgG2 and of CRP for FcγRIIa alleles.[119] Because FcγRIIa is the main receptor for CRP, the handling of nucleosomes/CRP may also be influenced by allelic polymorphisms.[120]

FcγRIIIa, expressed on mononuclear phagocytes and NK cells, also has two codominantly expressed allelic variants, F176 and V176, which differ in one amino acid at position 176 within the ligand-binding contact point of the extracellular domain (phenylalanine and valine, respectively) (see Figure 12-6).[80,114,115] The higher binding affinity of the V176 allele for IgG1 and IgG3 has important implications for antibody-mediated immune surveillance (antibody-dependent cell-mediated toxicity [ADCC]), antibody-mediated host defense against pathogens, and autoimmune disease. The distribution of genotypes of *FCGR3A* in disease-free Caucasian and African-American populations has been reported to be 40% to 50% homozygous F176, 40% to 50% heterozygous, and 8% to 18% homozygous V176.[166]

The two most common allelic variants of FcγRIIIb, neutrophil antigen (NA) 1 and NA2, differ by five nucleotides, resulting in a substitution of four amino acids in the membrane-distal first extracellular domain (see Figure 12-6).[113] Although binding of IgG does not seem to be affected, the NA1 and NA2 allelic forms do have different quantitative levels of function,[79,141,171,172] with NA1 neutrophils having a more robust FcγR-mediated phagocytic response than NA2 neutrophils, despite equivalent density of receptor expression.[171,172] Correspondingly, homozygous NA1 individuals may be more resistant to bacterial infection, especially when FcγRIIa cannot be effectively engaged, as suggested by the finding of increased *Neisseria meningitidis* infection among hosts with complement component 6 or 8 deficiency who are homozygous for FcγRIIIb-NA2 and FcγRIIa-R131.[173]

ABNORMALITIES IN Fcγ RECEPTORS IN SLE

Studies of mononuclear phagocyte system clearance function in SLE have indicated a profound impairment of clearance as measured by immunospecific techniques in many patients despite the apparently normal clearance assessed by nonimmunologic techniques. Demonstration of specific FcγR-mediated dysfunction raised the possibility of saturation by circulating immune complexes with decreased receptor availability as a potential mechanism for defective FcγR-mediated clearance.[52] Despite the in vitro induction of loss of surface FcγRs in monocytes by culture with immune complexes[174,175] and the in vivo production of mononuclear phagocyte blockade by infusion of immune complexes,[4] studies of blood monocytes from patients with SLE demonstrated an increase rather than the anticipated decrease in FcγR-mediated binding.[176-178] Despite such an increase, which might result from exposure to cytokines and cellular activation,[179-181] an in vitro study found FcγR-mediated phagocytosis of IgG-sensitized erythrocytes to be markedly impaired in monocytes derived from patients with SLE.[177] The defect in phagocytosis in vitro was most profound in those patients with the most significantly impaired in vivo mononuclear phagocyte system clearance, thus supporting the role of defective phagocytosis as an important component of altered FcγR-mediated clearance.[66,182]

The net FcγR-mediated phagocytic capacity in SLE is a result of at least two factors. The first is inherited and associated with allelic polymorphisms of FcγR, and the second is disease acquired with a relationship to disease activity. Association studies indicate that the low-binding FcγRIIa-R131 and FcγRIIIa-F176 alleles are enriched in some groups of patients with SLE,[183-188] suggesting that patients with the potential for less efficient immune complex clearance are at a greater risk for immune complex deposition. Indeed, genome-wide association studies confirm the association of FcγR alleles with SLE.[80,183,189-192] Metaanalyses have shown that FcγRIIa-R131 is associated with SLE, especially in African Americans, and that FcγRIIIa-F176 is associated with SLE in Caucasians and in other groups.[158,193] The association for FcγRIIIa low-binding alleles may be most important for risk for lupus nephritis.[194]

The qualitative nature of the immune response is an important principle in all association studies. Differences in the IgG subclass of pathogenic autoantibodies may influence the relative importance of FcγR alleles in disease. For example, in the presence of anti-C1q antibodies, which correlate with severe renal disease and are largely of the IgG2 subclass, *FCGR2A* genes appear to play a crucial role in determining disease severity.[195,196] Two studies have found that FcγRIIa-R131 alleles were associated with renal disease among Caucasian patients with lupus who had anti-C1q antibodies, whereas analysis of the population as a whole revealed no significant difference in the frequencies of FcγRIIa-R131 and -H131 alleles in comparison with controls.[195,196] Indeed, IgG2 is a predominant IgG subclass found in glomeruli of patients with proliferative nephritis. In one study, the frequency of genotypes containing the low-binding IgG2 allele FcγRIIa-R131 was significantly greater than expected in patients with class III or class IV nephritis and in patients with intense IgG2 deposition. CRP, a ligand with particular affinity for FcγRIIa-R131, was consistently present in the renal immune deposits of lupus nephritis specimens.[197] Thus, with precisely defined phenotypes, FcγRIIa variants have been identified as disease modifiers, in this example conferring inherited risk for nephritis.

The finding that other autoantibodies associated with nephritis, specifically anti–double-stranded DNA (anti-dsDNA) and antinucleosome antibodies, are predominantly IgG1 and IgG3 supports the importance of *FCGR3A* variants as disease-modifying genes.[198,199] For both FcγRIIa and FcγRIIIa, optimal handling of pathogenic immune complexes is provided by homozygous high-binding alleles. The low affinity of FcγRIIa-R131 for IgG2-containing immune complexes, and that of FcγRIIIa-F176 for IgG1 and IgG3, results in impaired removal of circulating immune complexes, increased tissue deposition, and accelerated organ damage. The combination of low-affinity alleles may be particularly important, as demonstrated in a cohort of Hispanic patients with a high prevalence of lupus nephritis in patients with haplotypes containing both FcγRIIa-R131 and FcγRIIIa-F176.[200] Thus, the physiology of FcγR alleles provides a new framework within which the interplay between humoral immune response and host genotype may be defined and heritable risk factors for disease susceptibility and disease severity may be identified.[201-204]

In addition to FcγR dysfunction, there is impaired phagocytosis of other probes in SLE monocytes. As predicted by the in vivo clearance studies,[55,56] bipartite defects in internalization by SLE monocytes include complement-mediated mechanisms.[177,205] Reduced internalization of apoptotic cells in SLE may also promote autoimmunity.[206]

Collectively, in vivo clearance data and in vitro monocyte data indicate that FcγRs play a central role in immune complex handling. Decreased complement-dependent immune complex uptake by fixed-tissue macrophages may also contribute and may be influenced

---

Box 12-2 Strategies for Modulating FcγR-Mediated IC Clearance and Receptor Function*

1. Direct receptor engagement (agonist or antagonist):
   a. Agonists: Monoclonal antibodies that engage FcγR with high affinity[217]
   b. Antagonists: Blocking peptides[218] and soluble FcγR[219]
2. Alter receptor expression (ratio of activating/inhibitory receptors):
   a. Cytokines[88,144-146,207,208,210]
   b. Complement products—C5a[220]
3. Inhibit receptor signaling:
   a. Syk inhibitors[212,213]
   b. Btk inhibitors[221]
4. Modulate cooperative signaling:
   a. TLR inhibitors[215,216]
   b. Adenosine receptors[222,223]
   c. Cross-talk among ITAM-receptors[129]
5. Multiple mechanisms/unknown:
   a. Glucocorticoids[224,225]
   b. Intravenous pulse methylprednisolone[181,226]
   c. Intravenous gammaglobulin:
      i. Increase FcγRIIb expression[220]
      ii. Scavenge complement activation fragments
      iii. Anti-inflammatory properties of sialylated IgG[146]
      iv. Increase catabolism of autoantibodies by blocking FcRn[224]

*Superscript numbers indicate chapter references.

by hypocomplementemia, deficiency in erythrocyte CR1 receptors, or perhaps polymorphisms in CR3 (CD11/18). Even in the face of intact complement mechanisms, immune complexes that do not fix complement, or that fix complement poorly (e.g., such as IgG2 containing complexes), are cleared less efficiently if FcγR-mediated function is abnormal (see Figure 12-1).

STRATEGIES FOR MODULATING FcγR-MEDIATED IMMUNE COMPLEX CLEARANCE AND RECEPTOR FUNCTION

The emerging picture of the extensive structural diversity of human FcγRs, the importance of FcγRs in immune complex clearance, and the evidence for FcγR dysfunction in SLE presents the opportunity for novel treatment strategies. A broad range of approaches to target FcγRs is presented in Box 12-2, and specific aspects are highlighted here.

Blockade of activating FcγRs or co-stimulation of FcγRIIb with monoclonal antibodies alters the threshold of inflammatory effector responses. Cytokines regulate total receptor expression, modulate relative isoform predominance, and modulate receptor function.[95] In vivo and in vitro studies have shown that IFN-γ and G-CSF upregulate expression of different stimulatory FcγRs on monocytes,[89,95,144,207-209] whereas IL-4 and IL-13 downregulate expression of all three classes of stimulatory FcγRs.[170,210] In contrast, IL-4 and IL-33 increase the expression of FcγRIIb2 on monocytes.[145,146] The complement split product C5a generated at sites of immune complex–triggered inflammation also alters the balance of FcγRs, upregulating stimulatory FcγRIIIa expression and downregulating inhibitory FcγRIIb expression on macrophages, thereby lowering the threshold of activation for effector cells and augmenting immune-mediated tissue damage.[211]

Responses to immune complexes may also be modulated by targeted pharmacologic manipulation of protein kinases or phosphatases. *Syk* inhibitors, which block activating FcγR signaling, are in clinical trials for rheumatoid arthritis and have been found to suppress skin and kidney disease in lupus-prone mice.[212,213] ITAM signaling is influenced by cross-talk with other signal transduction pathways, such as β2 integrins and TLRs, and these pathways may be targeted to regulate inflammatory responses.[129,214] Immune complexes containing nucleosomes engage TLRs and FcγRs; blockade of cooperative signaling by TLRs on dendritic cells and B cells may alter autoimmune and inflammatory responses.[215,216] In addition, ITAM-bearing receptors, such as FcαRI, may have paradoxical inhibitory effects, raise the threshold required for immune complexes to trigger activation, and attenuate autoantibody-triggered inflammatory diseases.[129] The mechanisms by which glucocorticoids and intravenous gammaglobulin modulate responses of immune complexes are multifactorial and are summarized in Box 12-2.

With our increasing recognition of the role of FcγRs in the pathophysiology of SLE and such a range of receptor-modulating agents, successful therapeutic intervention will be feasible and will form the basis for further advances in the treatment of SLE.

ACKNOWLEDGMENTS

We are grateful for support from the Mary Kirkland Center for Lupus Research at the Hospital for Special Surgery and from the National Institute of Arthritis and Musculoskeletal and Skin Diseases (NIAMS).

References

1. Benacerraf B, Sebestyen MM, Schlossman S: A quantitative study of the kinetics of blood clearance of P32-labelled *Escherichia coli* and *Staphylococci* by the reticuloendothelial system. *J Exp Med* 110:27–48, 1959.
2. Arend WP, Mannik M: Studies on antigen-antibody complexes. II. Quantification of tissue uptake of soluble complexes in normal and complement-depleted rabbits. *J Immunol* 107:63–75, 1971.
3. Mannik M, Arend MP, Hall AP, et al: Studies on antigen-antibody complexes. I. Elimination of soluble complexes from rabbit circulation. *J Exp Med* 133:713–739, 1971.
4. Haakenstad AO, Mannik M: Saturation of the reticuloendothelial system with soluble immune complexes. *J Immunol* 112:1939–1948, 1974.
5. Ravetch JV, Clynes RA: Divergent roles for Fc receptors and complement in vivo. *Annu Rev Immunol* 16:421–432, 1998.
6. Takai T, Ono M, Hikida M, et al: Augmented humoral and anaphylactic responses in Fc gamma RII-deficient mice. *Nature* 379:346–349, 1996.
7. Clynes R, Maizes JS, Guinamard R, et al: Modulation of immune complex-induced inflammation in vivo by the coordinate expression of activation and inhibitory Fc receptors. *J Exp Med* 189:179–185, 1999.
8. Wilson CB, Dixon FJ: Quantitation of acute and chronic serum sickness in the rabbit. *J Exp Med* 134(Suppl):7s–8s, 1971.
9. Wardle EN: Reticuloendothelial clearance studies in the course of horse serum induced nephritis. *Br J Exp Pathol* 55:149–152, 1974.
10. Hoffsten PE, Swerdlin A, Bartell M, et al: Reticuloendothelial and mesangial function in murine immune complex glomerulonephritis. *Kidney Int* 15:144–159, 1979.
11. Morgan AG, Steward MW: Macrophage clearance function and immune complex disease in New Zealand Black/White F1 hybrid mice. *Clin Exp Immunol* 26:133–136, 1976.
12. Hebert LA: The clearance of immune complexes from the circulation of man and other primates. *Am J Kidney Dis* 17:352–361, 1991.
13. Schifferli JA, Bartolotti SR, Peters DK: Inhibition of immune precipitation by complement. *Clin Exp Immunol* 42:387–394, 1980.
14. Schifferli JA, Steiger G, Hauptmann G, et al: Formation of soluble immune complexes by complement in sera of patients with various hypocomplementemic states. Difference between inhibition of immune precipitation and solubilization. *J Clin Invest* 76:2127–2133, 1985.
15. Cornacoff JB, Hebert LA, Smead WL, et al: Primate erythrocyte-immune complex-clearing mechanism. *J Clin Invest* 71:236–247, 1983.
16. Manthei U, Nickells MW, Barnes SH, et al: Identification of a C3b/iC3 binding protein of rabbit platelets and leukocytes. A CR1-like candidate for the immune adherence receptor. *J Immunol* 140:1228–1235, 1988.
17. Taylor RP, Kujala G, Wilson K, et al: In vivo and in vitro studies of the binding of antibody/dsDNA immune complexes to rabbit and guinea pig platelets. *J Immunol* 134:2550–2558, 1985.
18. Nelson D: Immune adherence. *Adv Immunol* 3:131–180, 1963.
19. Edberg JC, Kujala GA, Taylor RP: Rapid immune adherence reactivity of nascent, soluble antibody/DNA immune complexes in the circulation. *J Immunol* 139:1240–1244, 1987.
20. Dykman TR, Cole JL, Iida K, et al: Polymorphism of human erythrocyte C3b/C4b receptor. *Proc Natl Acad Sci U S A* 80:1698–1702, 1983.
21. Dykman TR, Hatch JA, Atkinson JP: Polymorphism of the human C3b/C4b receptor. Identification of a third allele and analysis of receptor phenotypes in families and patients with systemic lupus erythematosus. *J Exp Med* 159:691–703, 1984.
22. Holers VM, Seya T, Brown E, et al: Structural and functional studies on the human C3b/C4b receptor (CR1) purified by affinity chromatography using a monoclonal antibody. *Complement* 3:63–78, 1986.
23. Wong WW, Wilson JG, Fearon DT: Genetic regulation of a structural polymorphism of human C3b receptor. *J Clin Invest* 72:685–693, 1983.
24. Walport MJ, Ross GD, Mackworth-Young C, et al: Family studies of erythrocyte complement receptor type 1 levels: reduced levels in patients with SLE are acquired, not inherited. *Clin Exp Immunol* 59:547–554, 1985.
25. Wilson JG, Fearon DT: Altered expression of complement receptors as a pathogenetic factor in systemic lupus erythematosus. *Arthritis Rheum* 27:1321–1328, 1984.
26. Wilson JG, Murphy EE, Wong WW, et al: Identification of a restriction fragment length polymorphism by a CR1 cDNA that correlates with the number of CR1 on erythrocytes. *J Exp Med* 164:50–59, 1986.
27. Wilson JG, Wong WW, Murphy EE, 3rd, et al: Deficiency of the C3b/C4b receptor (CR1) of erythrocytes in systemic lupus erythematosus: analysis of the stability of the defect and of a restriction fragment length polymorphism of the CR1 gene. *J Immunol* 138:2708–2710, 1987.
28. Wilson JG, Wong WW, Schur PH, et al: Mode of inheritance of decreased C3b receptors on erythrocytes of patients with systemic lupus erythematosus. *N Engl J Med* 307:981–986, 1982.
29. Moldenhauer F, David J, Fielder AH, et al: Inherited deficiency of erythrocyte complement receptor type 1 does not cause susceptibility to systemic lupus erythematosus. *Arthritis Rheum* 30:961–966, 1987.
30. Hebert LA, Cosio G: The erythrocyte-immune complex-glomerulonephritis connection in man. *Kidney Int* 31:877–885, 1987.
31. Schifferli JA, Ng YC, Peters DK: The role of complement and its receptor in the elimination of immune complexes. *N Engl J Med* 315:488–495, 1986.
32. Chevalier J, Kazatchkine MD: Distribution in clusters of complement receptor type one (CR1) on human erythrocytes. *J Immunol* 142:2031–2036, 1989.
33. Edberg JC, Wright E, Taylor RP: Quantitative analyses of the binding of soluble complement-fixing antibody/dsDNA immune complexes to CR1 on human red blood cells. *J Immunol* 139:3739–3747, 1987.
34. Horgan C, Taylor RP: Studies on the kinetics of binding of complement-fixing dsDNA/anti-dsDNA immune complexes to the red blood cells of normal individuals and patients with systemic lupus erythematosus. *Arthritis Rheum* 27:320–329, 1984.
35. Paccaud JP, Carpentier JL, Schifferli JA: Direct evidence for the clustered nature of complement receptors type 1 on the erythrocyte membrane. *J Immunol* 141:3889–3894, 1988.
36. Davies KA, Hird V, Stewart S, et al: A study of in vivo immune complex formation and clearance in man. *J Immunol* 144:4613–4620, 1990.
37. Kimberly RP, Edberg JC, Merriam LT, et al: In vivo handling of soluble complement fixing Ab/dsDNA immune complexes in chimpanzees. *J Clin Invest* 84:962–970, 1989.
38. Schifferli JA, Ng YC, Estreicher J, et al: The clearance of tetanus toxoid/anti-tetanus toxoid immune complexes from the circulation of humans. Complement- and erythrocyte complement receptor 1-dependent mechanisms. *J Immunol* 140:899–904, 1988.
39. Schifferli JA, Ng YC, Paccaud JP, et al: The role of hypocomplementaemia and low erythrocyte complement receptor type 1 numbers in determining abnormal immune complex clearance in humans. *Clin Exp Immunol* 75:329–335, 1989.
40. Waxman FJ, Hebert LA, Cornacoff JB, et al: Complement depletion accelerates the clearance of immune complexes from the circulation of primates. *J Clin Invest* 74:1329–1340, 1984.
41. Hebert LA, Cosio FG, Birmingham DJ, et al: Experimental immune complex-mediated glomerulonephritis in the nonhuman primate. *Kidney Int* 39:44–56, 1991.
42. Waxman FJ, Hebert LA, Cosio FG, et al: Differential binding of immunoglobulin A and immunoglobulin G1 immune complexes to primate erythrocytes in vivo. Immunoglobulin A immune complexes bind less well to erythrocytes and are preferentially deposited in glomeruli. *J Clin Invest* 77:82–89, 1986.
43. Medof ME: Complement-dependent maintenance of immune complex solubility. In Rother K, Till GO, editors: *The complement system*, Berlin, 1988, Springer-Verlag, pp 418–443.

44. Medof ME, Iida K, Mold C, et al: Unique role of the complement receptor CR1 in the degradation of C3b associated with immune complexes. *J Exp Med* 156:1739–1754, 1982.

45. Ross GD, Lambris JD, Cain JA, et al: Generation of three different fragments of bound C3 with purified factor I or serum. I. Requirements for factor H vs CR1 cofactor activity. *J Immunol* 129:2051–2060, 1982.

46. Davis AE, 3rd, Harrison RA, Lachmann PJ: Physiologic inactivation of fluid phase C3b: isolation and structural analysis of C3c, C3d,g (alpha 2D), and C3g. *J Immunol* 132:1960–1966, 1984.

47. Horgan C, Burge J, Crawford L, et al: The kinetics of [3H]-dsDNA/anti-DNA immune complex formation, binding by red blood cells, and release into serum: effect of DNA molecular weight and conditions of antibody excess. *J Immunol* 133:2079–2084, 1984.

48. Medof ME, Lam T, Prince GM, et al: Requirement for human red blood cells in inactivation of C3b in immune complexes and enhancement of binding to spleen cells. *J Immunol* 130:1336–1340, 1983.

49. Hosea SW, Brown EJ, Hamburger MI, et al: Opsonic requirements for intravascular clearance after splenectomy. *N Engl J Med* 304:245–250, 1981.

50. Lobatto S, Daha MR, Breedveld FC, et al: Abnormal clearance of soluble aggregates of human immunoglobulin G in patients with systemic lupus erythematosus. *Clin Exp Immunol* 72:55–59, 1988.

51. Medof ME, Prince GM, Mold C: Release of soluble immune complexes from immune adherence receptors on human erythrocytes is mediated by C3b inactivator independently of Beta 1H and is accompanied by generation of C3c. *Proc Natl Acad Sci U S A* 79:5047–5051, 1982.

52. Frank MM, Hamburger MI, Lawley TJ, et al: Defective reticuloendothelial system Fc-receptor function in systemic lupus erythematosus. *N Engl J Med* 300:518–523, 1979.

53. Schreiber AD, Frank MM: Role of antibody and complement in the immune clearance and destruction of erythrocytes. I. In vivo effects of IgG and IgM complement-fixing sites. *J Clin Invest* 51:575–582, 1972.

54. Meryhew NL, Runquist OA: A kinetic analysis of immune-mediated clearance of erythrocytes. *J Immunol* 126:2443–2449, 1981.

55. Kimberly RP, Meryhew NL, Runquist OA: Mononuclear phagocyte function in SLE. I. Bipartite Fc- and complement-dependent dysfunction. *J Immunol* 137:91–96, 1986.

56. Meryhew NL, Kimberly RP, Messner RP, et al: Mononuclear phagocyte system in SLE. II. A kinetic model of immune complex handling in systemic lupus erythematosus. *J Immunol* 137:97–102, 1986.

57. Kimberly RP, Parris TM, Inman RD, et al: Dynamics of mononuclear phagocyte system Fc receptor function in systemic lupus erythematosus. Relation to disease activity and circulating immune complexes. *Clin Exp Immunol* 51:261–268, 1983.

58. Hamburger MI, Lawley TJ, Kimberly RP, et al: A serial study of splenic reticuloendothelial system Fc receptor functional activity in systemic lupus erythematosus. *Arthritis Rheum* 25:48–54, 1982.

59. Parris TM, Kimberly RP, Inman RD, et al: Defective Fc receptor-mediated function of the mononuclear phagocyte system in lupus nephritis. *Ann Intern Med* 97:526–532, 1982.

60. van der Woude FJ, van der Giessen M, Kallenberg CG, et al: Reticuloendothelial Fc receptor function in SLE patients. I. Primary HLA linked defect or acquired dysfunction secondary to disease activity? *Clin Exp Immunol* 55:473–480, 1984.

61. Madi N, Steiger G, Estreicher J, et al: Defective immune adherence and elimination of hepatitis B surface antigen/antibody complexes in patients with mixed essential cryoglobulinemia type II. *J Immunol* 147:495–502, 1991.

62. Halma C, Breedveld FC, Daha MR, et al: Elimination of soluble 123I-labeled aggregates of IgG in patients with systemic lupus erythematosus. Effect of serum IgG and numbers of erythrocyte complement receptor type 1. *Arthritis Rheum* 34:442–452, 1991.

63. Ross GD, Yount WJ, Walport MJ, et al: Disease-associated loss of erythrocyte complement receptors (CR1, C3b receptors) in patients with systemic lupus erythematosus and other diseases involving autoantibodies and/or complement activation. *J Immunol* 135:2005–2014, 1985.

64. Walport MJ, Lachmann PJ: Erythrocyte complement receptor type 1, immune complexes, and the rheumatic diseases. *Arthritis Rheum* 31:153–158, 1988.

65. Kelton JG, Singer J, Rodger C, et al: The concentration of IgG in the serum is a major determinant of Fc-dependent reticuloendothelial function. *Blood* 66:490–495, 1985.

66. Kimberly RP, Salmon JE, Bussel JB, et al: Modulation of mononuclear phagocyte function by intravenous gamma-globulin. *J Immunol* 132:745–750, 1984.

67. Lawley TJ: Immune complexes and reticuloendothelial system function in human disease. *J Invest Dermatol* 74:339–343, 1980.

68. Heijnen IA, van de Winkel JG: Human IgG Fc receptors. *Int Rev Immunol* 16:29–55, 1997.

69. Hulett MD, Hogarth PM: Molecular basis of Fc receptor function. *Adv Immunol* 57:1–127, 1994.

70. Salmon JE, Pricop L: Human receptors for immunoglobulin G: key elements in the pathogenesis of rheumatic disease. *Arthritis Rheum* 44:739–750, 2001.

71. Kimberly RP, Salmon JE, Edberg JC: Receptors for immunoglobulin G. Molecular diversity and implications for disease. *Arthritis Rheum* 38:306–314, 1995.

72. Daeron M: Fc receptor biology. *Annu Rev Immunol* 15:203–234, 1997.

73. Grundy HO, Peltz G, Moore KW, et al: The polymorphic Fc gamma receptor II gene maps to human chromosome 1q. *Immunogenetics* 29:331–339, 1989.

74. Qiu WQ, de Bruin D, Brownstein BH, et al: Organization of the human and mouse low-affinity Fc gamma R genes: duplication and recombination. *Science* 248:732–735, 1990.

75. Peltz GA, Grundy HO, Lebo RV, et al: Human Fc gamma RIII: cloning, expression, and identification of the chromosomal locus of two Fc receptors for IgG. *Proc Natl Acad Sci U S A* 86:1013–1017, 1989.

76. Reth M: Antigen receptor tail clue. *Nature* 338:383–384, 1989.

77. Cambier JC: Antigen and Fc receptor signaling. The awesome power of the immunoreceptor tyrosine-based activation motif (ITAM). *J Immunol* 155:3281–3285, 1995.

78. Warmerdam PA, van de Winkel JG, Vlug A, et al: A single amino acid in the second Ig-like domain of the human Fc gamma receptor II is critical for human IgG2 binding. *J Immunol* 147:1338–1343, 1991.

79. Salmon JE, Edberg JC, Brogle NL, et al: Allelic polymorphisms of human Fc gamma receptor IIA and Fc gamma receptor IIIB. Independent mechanisms for differences in human phagocyte function. *J Clin Invest* 89:1274–1281, 1992.

80. Wu J, Edberg JC, Redecha PB, et al: A novel polymorphism of FcgammaRIIIa (CD16) alters receptor function and predisposes to autoimmune disease. *J Clin Invest* 100:1059–1070, 1997.

81. Muta T, Kurosaki T, Misulovin Z, et al: A 13-amino-acid motif in the cytoplasmic domain of Fc gamma RIIB modulates B-cell receptor signalling. *Nature* 368:70–73, 1994.

82. Anderson CL: Isolation of the receptor for IgG from a human monocyte cell line (U937) and from human peripheral blood monocytes. *J Exp Med* 156:1794–1806, 1982.

83. Allen JM, Seed B: Isolation and expression of functional high-affinity Fc receptor complementary DNAs. *Science* 243:378–381, 1989.

84. van de Winkel JG, Ernst LK, Anderson CL, et al: Gene organization of the human high affinity receptor for IgG, Fc gamma RI (CD64). Characterization and evidence for a second gene. *J Biol Chem* 266:13449–13455, 1991.

85. Ernst LK, van de Winkel JG, Chiu IM, et al: Three genes for the human high affinity Fc receptor for IgG (Fc gamma RI) encode four distinct transcription products. *J Biol Chem* 267:15692–15700, 1992.

86. Ernst LK, Duchemin AM, Anderson CL: Association of the high-affinity receptor for IgG (Fc gamma RI) with the gamma subunit of the IgE receptor. *Proc Natl Acad Sci U S A* 90:6023–6027, 1993.

87. Fanger NA, Voigtlaender D, Liu C, et al: Characterization of expression, cytokine regulation, and effector function of the high affinity IgG receptor Fc gamma RI (CD64) expressed on human blood dendritic cells. *J Immunol* 158:3090–3098, 1997.

88. Guyre PM, Morganelli PM, Miller R: Recombinant immune interferon increases immunoglobulin G Fc receptors on cultured human mononuclear phagocytes. *J Clin Invest* 72:393–397, 1983.

89. Perussia B, Dayton ET, Lazarus R, et al: Immune interferon induces the receptor for monomeric IgG1 on human monocytic and myeloid cells. *J Exp Med* 158:1092–1113, 1983.

90. Shen L, Guyre PM, Fanger MW: Polymorphonuclear leukocyte function triggered through the high affinity Fc receptor for monomeric IgG. *J Immunol* 139:534–538, 1987.

91. Buckle AM, Hogg N: The effect of IFN-gamma and colony-stimulating factors on the expression of neutrophil cell membrane receptors. *J Immunol* 143:2295–2301, 1989.

92. Looney RJ, Abraham GN, Anderson CL: Human monocytes and U937 cells bear two distinct Fc receptors for IgG. *J Immunol* 136:1641–1647, 1986.

93. Looney RJ, Anderson CL, Ryan DH, et al: Structural polymorphism of the human platelet Fc gamma receptor. *J Immunol* 141:2680–2683, 1988.

94. Looney RJ, Ryan DH, Takahashi K, et al: Identification of a second class of IgG Fc receptors on human neutrophils. A 40 kilodalton molecule also found on eosinophils. *J Exp Med* 163:826–836, 1986.

95. Fanger MW, Shen L, Graziano RF, et al: Cytotoxicity mediated by human Fc receptors for IgG. *Immunol Today* 10:92–99, 1989.

96. Brooks DG, Qiu WQ, Luster AD, et al: Structure and expression of human IgG FcRII (CD32). Functional heterogeneity is encoded by the alternatively spliced products of multiple genes. *J Exp Med* 170:1369–1385, 1989.

97. Van Den Herik-Oudijk IE, Westerdaal NA, Henriquez NV, et al: Functional analysis of human Fc gamma RII (CD32) isoforms expressed in B lymphocytes. *J Immunol* 152:574–585, 1994.

98. Daeron M, Latour S, Malbec O, et al: The same tyrosine-based inhibition motif, in the intracytoplasmic domain of Fc gamma RIIB, regulates negatively BCR-, TCR-, and FcR-dependent cell activation. *Immunity* 3:635–646, 1995.

99. Daeron M, Malbec O, Latour S, et al: Regulation of high-affinity IgE receptor-mediated mast cell activation by murine low-affinity IgG receptors. *J Clin Invest* 95:577–585, 1995.

100. Hunter S, Indik ZK, Kim MK, et al: Inhibition of Fcgamma receptor-mediated phagocytosis by a nonphagocytic Fcgamma receptor. *Blood* 91:1762–1768, 1998.

101. Phillips NE, Parker DC: Cross-linking of B lymphocyte Fc gamma receptors and membrane immunoglobulin inhibits anti-immunoglobulin-induced blastogenesis. *J Immunol* 132:627–632, 1984.

102. Su K, Wu J, Edberg JC, et al: A promoter haplotype of the immunoreceptor tyrosine-based inhibitory motif-bearing FcgammaRIIb alters receptor expression and associates with autoimmunity. I. Regulatory FCGR2B polymorphisms and their association with systemic lupus erythematosus. *J Immunol* 172:7186–7191, 2004.

103. Kono H, Kyogoku C, Suzuki T, et al: FcgammaRIIB Ile232Thr transmembrane polymorphism associated with human systemic lupus erythematosus decreases affinity to lipid rafts and attenuates inhibitory effects on B cell receptor signaling. *Hum Mol Genet* 14:2881–2892, 2005.

104. Floto RA, Clatworthy MR, Heilbronn KR, et al: Loss of function of a lupus-associated FcgammaRIIb polymorphism through exclusion from lipid rafts. *Nat Med* 11:1056–1058, 2005.

105. Kurosaki T, Ravetch JV: A single amino acid in the glycosyl phosphatidylinositol attachment domain determines the membrane topology of Fc gamma RIII. *Nature* 342:805–807, 1989.

106. Santiago A, Satriano J, DeCandido S, et al: A specific Fc gamma receptor on cultured rat mesangial cells. *J Immunol* 143:2575–2582, 1989.

107. Edberg JC, Barinsky M, Redecha PB, et al: Fc gamma RIII expressed on cultured monocytes is a N-glycosylated transmembrane protein distinct from Fc gamma RIII expressed on natural killer cells. *J Immunol* 144:4729–4734, 1990.

108. Anderson P, Caligiuri M, O'Brien C, et al: Fc gamma receptor type III (CD16) is included in the zeta NK receptor complex expressed by human natural killer cells. *Proc Natl Acad Sci U S A* 87:2274–2278, 1990.

109. Kurosaki T, Gander I, Wirthmueller U, et al: The beta subunit of the Fc epsilon RI is associated with the Fc gamma RIII on mast cells. *J Exp Med* 175:447–451, 1992.

110. Ravetch JV, Perussia B: Alternative membrane forms of Fc gamma RIII(CD16) on human natural killer cells and neutrophils. Cell type-specific expression of two genes that differ in single nucleotide substitutions. *J Exp Med* 170:481–497, 1989.

111. Selvaraj P, Rosse WF, Silber R, et al: The major Fc receptor in blood has a phosphatidylinositol anchor and is deficient in paroxysmal nocturnal haemoglobinuria. *Nature* 333:565–567, 1988.

112. Huizinga TW, Kleijer M, Tetteroo PA, et al: Biallelic neutrophil Na-antigen system is associated with a polymorphism on the phospho-inositol-linked Fc gamma receptor III (CD16). *Blood* 75:213–217, 1990.

113. Ory PA, Goldstein IM, Kwoh EE, et al: Characterization of polymorphic forms of Fc receptor III on human neutrophils. *J Clin Invest* 83:1676–1681, 1989.

114. de Haas M, Koene HR, Kleijer M, et al: A triallelic Fc gamma receptor type IIIA polymorphism influences the binding of human IgG by NK cell Fc gamma RIIIa. *J Immunol* 156:3948–3955, 1996.

115. Koene HR, Kleijer M, Algra J, et al: Fc gammaRIIIa-158 V/F polymorphism influences the binding of IgG by natural killer cell Fc gammaRIIIa, independently of the Fc gammaRIIIa-48 L/R/H phenotype. *Blood* 90:1109–1114, 1997.

116. Jeffries R: Structure/function relationships of IgG subclasses. In Shakib F, editor: *The human IgG subclasses: molecular analysis of structure, function and regulation*, Oxford, 1990, Pergamon Press, pp 93–108.

117. Parren PW, Warmerdam PA, Boeije LC, et al: On the interaction of IgG subclasses with the low affinity Fc gamma RIIa (CD32) on human monocytes, neutrophils, and platelets. Analysis of a functional polymorphism to human IgG2. *J Clin Invest* 90:1537–1546, 1992.

118. Marnell LL, Mold C, Volzer MA, et al: C-reactive protein binds to Fc gamma RI in transfected COS cells. *J Immunol* 155:2185–2193, 1995.

119. Bharadwaj D, Stein MP, Volzer M, et al: The major receptor for C-reactive protein on leukocytes is fcgamma receptor II. *J Exp Med* 190:585–590, 1999.

120. Stein MP, Edberg JC, Kimberly RP, et al: C-reactive protein binding to FcgammaRIIa on human monocytes and neutrophils is allele-specific. *J Clin Invest* 105:369–376, 2000.

121. Lowry MB, Duchemin AM, Coggeshall KM, et al: Chimeric receptors composed of phosphoinositide 3-kinase domains and FCgamma receptor ligand-binding domains mediate phagocytosis in COS fibroblasts. *J Biol Chem* 273:24513–24520, 1998.

122. Karimi K, Lennartz MR: Mitogen-activated protein kinase is activated during IgG-mediated phagocytosis, but is not required for target ingestion. *Inflammation* 22:67–82, 1998.

123. Bolland S, Ravetch JV: Inhibitory pathways triggered by ITIM-containing receptors. *Adv Immunol* 72:149–177, 1999.

124. Malbec O, Fridman WH, Daeron M: Negative regulation of hematopoietic cell activation and proliferation by Fc gamma RIIB. *Curr Top Microbiol Immunol* 244:13–27, 1999.

125. Coggeshall KM: Negative signaling in health and disease. *Immunol Res* 19:47–64, 1999.

126. Ono M, Bolland S, Tempst P, et al: Role of the inositol phosphatase SHIP in negative regulation of the immune system by the receptor Fc(gamma) RIIB. *Nature* 383:263–266, 1996.

127. Bolland S, Pearse RN, Kurosaki T, et al: SHIP modulates immune receptor responses by regulating membrane association of Btk. *Immunity* 8:509–516, 1998.

128. Chacko GW, Tridandapani S, Damen JE, et al: Negative signaling in B lymphocytes induces tyrosine phosphorylation of the 145-kDa inositol polyphosphate 5-phosphatase, SHIP. *J Immunol* 157:2234–2238, 1996.

129. Ivashkiv LB: How ITAMs inhibit signaling. *Sci Signal* 4:pe20, 2011.

130. Anegon I, Cuturi MC, Trinchieri G, et al: Interaction of Fc receptor (CD16) ligands induces transcription of interleukin 2 receptor (CD25) and lymphokine genes and expression of their products in human natural killer cells. *J Exp Med* 167:452–472, 1988.

131. Cardella CJ, Davies P, Allison AC: Immune complexes induce selective release of lysosomal hydrolases from macrophages. *Nature* 247:46–48, 1974.

132. Debets JM, Van de Winkel JG, Ceuppens JL, et al: Cross-linking of both Fc gamma RI and Fc gamma RII induces secretion of tumor necrosis factor by human monocytes, requiring high affinity Fc-Fc gamma R interactions. Functional activation of Fc gamma RII by treatment with proteases or neuraminidase. *J Immunol* 144:1304–1310, 1990.

133. Krutmann J, Kirnbauer R, Kock A, et al: Cross-linking Fc receptors on monocytes triggers IL-6 production. Role in anti-CD3-induced T cell activation. *J Immunol* 145:1337–1342, 1990.

134. Rouzer CA, Scott WA, Kempe J, et al: Prostaglandin synthesis by macrophages requires a specific receptor-ligand interaction. *Proc Natl Acad Sci U S A* 77:4279–4282, 1980.

135. Nimmerjahn F, Ravetch JV: Antibody-mediated modulation of immune responses. *Immunol Rev* 236:265–275, 2010.

136. Anderson CL, Shen L, Eicher DM, et al: Phagocytosis mediated by three distinct Fc gamma receptor classes on human leukocytes. *J Exp Med* 171:1333–1345, 1990.

137. Clarkson SB, Bussel JB, Kimberly RP, et al: Treatment of refractory immune thrombocytopenic purpura with an anti-Fc gamma-receptor antibody. *N Engl J Med* 314:1236–1239, 1986.

138. Clarkson SB, Kimberly RP, Valinsky JE, et al: Blockade of clearance of immune complexes by an anti-Fc gamma receptor monoclonal antibody. *J Exp Med* 164:474–489, 1986.

139. Salmon JE, Brogle NL, Edberg JC, et al: Fc gamma receptor III induces actin polymerization in human neutrophils and primes phagocytosis mediated by Fc gamma receptor II. *J Immunol* 146:997–1004, 1991.

140. Edberg JC, Kimberly RP: Modulation of Fc gamma and complement receptor function by the glycosyl-phosphatidylinositol-anchored form of Fc gamma RIII. *J Immunol* 152:5826–5835, 1994.

141. Salmon JE, Millard SS, Brogle NL, et al: Fc gamma receptor IIIb enhances Fc gamma receptor IIa function in an oxidant-dependent and allele-sensitive manner. *J Clin Invest* 95:2877–2885, 1995.

142. Pan LY, Mendel DB, Zurlo J, et al: Regulation of the steady state level of Fc gamma RI mRNA by IFN-gamma and dexamethasone in human monocytes, neutrophils, and U-937 cells. *J Immunol* 145:267–275, 1990.

143. te Velde AA, Huijbens RJ, de Vries JE, et al: IL-4 decreases Fc gamma R membrane expression and Fc gamma R-mediated cytotoxic activity of human monocytes. *J Immunol* 144:3046–3051, 1990.

144. Welch GR, Wong HL, Wahl SM: Selective induction of Fc gamma RIII on human monocytes by transforming growth factor-beta. *J Immunol* 144:3444–3448, 1990.

145. Pricop L, Redecha P, Teillaud JL, et al: Differential modulation of stimulatory and inhibitory Fc gamma receptors on human monocytes by Th1 and Th2 cytokines. *J Immunol* 166:531–537, 2001.

146. Anthony RM, Kobayashi T, Wermeling F, et al: Intravenous gammaglobulin suppresses inflammation through a novel T(H)2 pathway. *Nature* 475:110–113, 2011.

147. Ceuppens JL, Baroja ML, Van Vaeck F, et al: Defect in the membrane expression of high affinity 72-kD Fc gamma receptors on phagocytic cells in four healthy subjects. *J Clin Invest* 82:571–578, 1988.

148. Morris DL, Roberts AL, Witherden AS, et al: Evidence for both copy number and allelic (NA1/NA2) risk at the FCGR3B locus in systemic lupus erythematosus. *Eur J Hum Genet* 18:1027–1031, 2010.

149. Clark MR, Liu L, Clarkson SB, et al: An abnormality of the gene that encodes neutrophil Fc receptor III in a patient with systemic lupus erythematosus. *J Clin Invest* 86:341–346, 1990.

150. Huizinga TW, Kuijpers RW, Kleijer M, et al: Maternal genomic neutrophil FcRIII deficiency leading to neonatal isoimmune neutropenia. *Blood* 76:1927–1932, 1990.

151. Stroncek DF, Skubitz KM, Plachta LB, et al: Alloimmune neonatal neutropenia due to an antibody to the neutrophil Fc-gamma receptor III with maternal deficiency of CD16 antigen. *Blood* 77:1572–1580, 1991.

152. Fromont P, Bettaieb A, Skouri H, et al: Frequency of the polymorphonuclear neutrophil Fc gamma receptor III deficiency in the French population and its involvement in the development of neonatal alloimmune neutropenia. *Blood* 79:2131–2134, 1992.

153. Cartron J, Celton JL, Gane P, et al: Iso-immune neonatal neutropenia due to an anti-Fc receptor III (CD16) antibody. *Eur J Pediatr* 151:438–441, 1992.

154. Lande R, Ganguly D, Facchinetti V, et al: Neutrophils activate plasmacytoid dendritic cells by releasing self-DNA-peptide complexes in systemic lupus erythematosus. *Sci Transl Med* 3:73ra19, 2011.

155. Luan JJ, Monteiro RC, Sautes C, et al: Defective Fc gamma RII gene expression in macrophages of NOD mice: genetic linkage with up-regulation of IgG1 and IgG2b in serum. *J Immunol* 157:4707–4716, 1996.

156. Pritchard NR, Cutler AJ, Uribe S, et al: Autoimmune-prone mice share a promoter haplotype associated with reduced expression and function of the Fc receptor FcgammaRII. *Curr Biol* 10:227–230, 2000.

157. Jiang Y, Hirose S, Abe M, et al: Polymorphisms in IgG Fc receptor IIB regulatory regions associated with autoimmune susceptibility. *Immunogenetics* 51:429–435, 2000.

158. Bolland S, Ravetch JV: Spontaneous autoimmune disease in Fc(gamma) RIIB-deficient mice results from strain-specific epistasis. *Immunity* 13:277–285, 2000.

159. McGaha TL, Sorrentino B, Ravetch JV: Restoration of tolerance in lupus by targeted inhibitory receptor expression. *Science* 307:590–593, 2005.

160. Su K, Li X, Edberg JC, et al: A promoter haplotype of the immunoreceptor tyrosine-based inhibitory motif-bearing FcgammaRIIb alters receptor expression and associates with autoimmunity. II. Differential binding of GATA4 and Yin-Yang1 transcription factors and correlated receptor expression and function. *J Immunol* 172:7192–7199, 2004.

161. Li X, Wu J, Carter RH, et al: A novel polymorphism in the Fcgamma receptor IIB (CD32B) transmembrane region alters receptor signaling. *Arthritis Rheum* 48:3242–3252, 2003.

162. Willcocks LC, Carr EJ, Niederer HA, et al: A defunctioning polymorphism in FCGR2B is associated with protection against malaria but susceptibility to systemic lupus erythematosus. *Proc Natl Acad Sci U S A* 107:7881–7885, 2010.

163. Waisberg M, Tarasenko T, Vickers BK, et al: Genetic susceptibility to systemic lupus erythematosus protects against cerebral malaria in mice. *Proc Natl Acad Sci U S A* 108:1122–1127, 2011.

164. Clark MR, Stuart SG, Kimberly RP, et al: A single amino acid distinguishes the high-responder from the low-responder form of Fc receptor II on human monocytes. *Eur J Immunol* 21:1911–1916, 1991.

165. Raij L, Sibley RK, Keane WF: Mononuclear phagocytic system stimulation. Protective role from glomerular immune complex deposition. *J Lab Clin Med* 98:558–567, 1981.

166. Lehrnbecher T, Foster CB, Zhu S, et al: Variant genotypes of the low-affinity Fcgamma receptors in two control populations and a review of low-affinity Fcgamma receptor polymorphisms in control and disease populations. *Blood* 94:4220–4232, 1999.

167. Sanders LA, van de Winkel JG, Rijkers GT, et al: Fc gamma receptor IIa (CD32) heterogeneity in patients with recurrent bacterial respiratory tract infections. *J Infect Dis* 170:854–861, 1994.

168. Bredius RG, Derkx BH, Fijen CA, et al: Fc gamma receptor IIa (CD32) polymorphism in fulminant meningococcal septic shock in children. *J Infect Dis* 170:848–853, 1994.

169. Platonov AE, Shipulin GA, Vershinina IV, et al: Association of human Fc gamma RIIa (CD32) polymorphism with susceptibility to and severity of meningococcal disease. *Clin Infect Dis* 27:746–750, 1998.

170. Yee AM, Ng SC, Sobel RE, et al: Fc gammaRIIA polymorphism as a risk factor for invasive pneumococcal infections in systemic lupus erythematosus. *Arthritis Rheum* 40:1180–1182, 1997.

171. Salmon JE, Edberg JC, Kimberly RP: Fc gamma receptor III on human neutrophils. Allelic variants have functionally distinct capacities. *J Clin Invest* 85:1287–1295, 1990.

172. Bredius RG, Fijen CA, De Haas M, et al: Role of neutrophil Fc gamma RIIa (CD32) and Fc gamma RIIIb (CD16) polymorphic forms in phagocytosis of human IgG1- and IgG3-opsonized bacteria and erythrocytes. *Immunology* 83:624–630, 1994.

173. Platonov AE, Kuijper EJ, Vershinina IV, et al: Meningococcal disease and polymorphism of FcgammaRIIa (CD32) in late complement component-deficient individuals. *Clin Exp Immunol* 111:97–101, 1998.

174. Mellman IS, Plutner H, Steinman RM, et al: Internalization and degradation of macrophage Fc receptors during receptor-mediated phagocytosis. *J Cell Biol* 96:887–895, 1983.

175. Michl J, Unkeless JC, Pieczonka MM, et al: Modulation of Fc receptors of mononuclear phagocytes by immobilized antigen-antibody complexes. Quantitative analysis of the relationship between ligand number and Fc receptor response. *J Exp Med* 157:1746–1757, 1983.

176. Fries LF, Mullins WW, Cho KR, et al: Monocyte receptors for the Fc portion of IgG are increased in systemic lupus erythematosus. *J Immunol* 132:695–700, 1984.

177. Kavai M, Lukacs K, Sonkoly I, et al: Circulating immune complexes and monocyte Fc function in autoimmune diseases. *Ann Rheum Dis* 38:79–83, 1979.

178. Salmon JE, Kimberly RP, Gibofsky A, et al: Defective mononuclear phagocyte function in systemic lupus erythematosus: dissociation of Fc receptor-ligand binding and internalization. *J Immunol* 133:2525–2531, 1984.

179. Salmon JE, Kimberly RP: Phagocytosis of concanavalin A-treated erythrocytes is mediated by the Fc gamma receptor. *J Immunol* 137:456–462, 1986.

180. Kavai M, Zsindely A, Sonkoly I, et al: Signals of monocyte activation in patients with SLE. *Clin Exp Immunol* 51:255–260, 1983.

181. Salmon JE, Kapur S, Meryhew NL, et al: High-dose, pulse intravenous methylprednisolone enhances Fc gamma receptor-mediated mononuclear phagocyte function in systemic lupus erythematosus. *Arthritis Rheum* 32:717–725, 1989.

182. Kimberly RP, Gibofsky A, Salmon JE, et al: Impaired fc-mediated mononuclear phagocyte system clearance in HLA-DR2 and MT1-positive healthy young adults. *J Exp Med* 157:1698–1703, 1983.

183. Salmon JE, Millard S, Schachter LA, et al: Fc gamma RIIA alleles are heritable risk factors for lupus nephritis in African Americans. *J Clin Invest* 97:1348–1354, 1996.

184. Duits AJ, Bootsma H, Derksen RH, et al: Skewed distribution of IgG Fc receptor IIa (CD32) polymorphism is associated with renal disease in systemic lupus erythematosus patients. *Arthritis Rheum* 38:1832–1836, 1995.

185. Salmon JE, Ng S, Yoo DH, et al: Altered distribution of Fcgamma receptor IIIA alleles in a cohort of Korean patients with lupus nephritis. *Arthritis Rheum* 42:818–819, 1999.

186. Koene HR, Kleijer M, Swaak AJ, et al: The Fc gammaRIIIA-158F allele is a risk factor for systemic lupus erythematosus. *Arthritis Rheum* 41:1813–1818, 1998.

187. Manger K, Repp R, Spriewald BM, et al: Fcgamma receptor IIa polymorphism in Caucasian patients with systemic lupus erythematosus: association with clinical symptoms. *Arthritis Rheum* 41:1181–1189, 1998.

188. Song YW, Han CW, Kang SW, et al: Abnormal distribution of Fc gamma receptor type IIa polymorphisms in Korean patients with systemic lupus erythematosus. *Arthritis Rheum* 41:421–426, 1998.

189. Moser KL, Neas BR, Salmon JE, et al: Genome scan of human systemic lupus erythematosus: evidence for linkage on chromosome 1q in

African-American pedigrees. *Proc Natl Acad Sci U S A* 95:14869–14874, 1998.

190. Botto M, Theodoridis E, Thompson EM, et al: Fc gamma RIIa polymorphism in systemic lupus erythematosus (SLE): no association with disease. *Clin Exp Immunol* 104:264–268, 1996.

191. Smyth LJ, Snowden N, Carthy D, et al: Fc gamma RIIa polymorphism in systemic lupus erythematosus. *Ann Rheum Dis* 56:744–746, 1997.

192. Oh M, Petri MA, Kim NA, et al: Frequency of the Fc gamma RIIIA-158F allele in African American patients with systemic lupus erythematosus. *J Rheumatol* 26:1486–1489, 1999.

193. Karassa FB, Trikalinos TA, Ioannidis JP: Role of the Fcgamma receptor IIa polymorphism in susceptibility to systemic lupus erythematosus and lupus nephritis: a meta-analysis. *Arthritis Rheum* 46:1563–1571, 2002.

194. Karassa FB, Trikalinos TA, Ioannidis JP: The Fc gamma RIIIA-F158 allele is a risk factor for the development of lupus nephritis: a meta-analysis. *Kidney Int* 63:1475–1482, 2003.

195. Haseley LA, Wisnieski JJ, Denburg MR, et al: Antibodies to C1q in systemic lupus erythematosus: characteristics and relation to Fc gamma RIIA alleles. *Kidney Int* 52:1375–1380, 1997.

196. Norsworthy P, Theodoridis E, Botto M, et al: Overrepresentation of the Fcgamma receptor type IIA R131/R131 genotype in caucasoid systemic lupus erythematosus patients with autoantibodies to C1q and glomerulonephritis. *Arthritis Rheum* 42:1828–1832, 1999.

197. Zuniga R, Markowitz GS, Arkachaisri T, et al: Identification of IgG subclasses and C-reactive protein in lupus nephritis: the relationship between the composition of immune deposits and Fcgamma receptor type IIA alleles. *Arthritis Rheum* 48:460–470, 2003.

198. Amoura Z, Koutouzov S, Chabre H, et al: Presence of antinucleosome autoantibodies in a restricted set of connective tissue diseases: antinucleosome antibodies of the IgG3 subclass are markers of renal pathogenicity in systemic lupus erythematosus. *Arthritis Rheum* 43:76–84, 2000.

199. Zouali M, Jefferis R, Eyquem A: IgG subclass distribution of autoantibodies to DNA and to nuclear ribonucleoproteins in autoimmune diseases. *Immunology* 51:595–600, 1984.

200. Zuniga R, Ng S, Peterson MG, et al: Low-binding alleles of Fcgamma receptor types IIA and IIIA are inherited independently and are associated with systemic lupus erythematosus in Hispanic patients. *Arthritis Rheum* 44:361–367, 2001.

201. Lewis EJ, Busch GJ, Schur PH: Gamma G globulin subgroup composition of the glomerular deposits in human renal diseases. *J Clin Invest* 49:1103–1113, 1970.

202. Imai H, Hamai K, Komatsuda A, et al: IgG subclasses in patients with membranoproliferative glomerulonephritis, membranous nephropathy, and lupus nephritis. *Kidney Int* 51:270–276, 1997.

203. Zuniga R, Markowitz G, D'Agati V, et al: IgG subclass glomerular deposition and its relationship to FcgammaRIIA alleles in lupus. *Arthritis Rheum* 42:S174, 1999.

204. Edberg JC, Langefeld CD, Wu J, et al: Genetic linkage and association of Fcgamma receptor IIIA (CD16A) on chromosome 1q23 with human systemic lupus erythematosus. *Arthritis Rheum* 46:2132–2140, 2002.

205. Hurst NP, Nuki G, Wallington T: Evidence for intrinsic cellular defects of "complement" receptor-mediated phagocytosis in patients with systemic lupus erythematosus (SLE). *Clin Exp Immunol* 55:303–312, 1984.

206. Herrmann M, Voll RE, Zoller OM, et al: Impaired phagocytosis of apoptotic cell material by monocyte-derived macrophages from patients with systemic lupus erythematosus. *Arthritis Rheum* 41:1241–1250, 1998.

207. Guyre PM, Campbell AS, Kniffin WD, et al: Monocytes and polymorphonuclear neutrophils of patients with streptococcal pharyngitis express increased numbers of type I IgG Fc receptors. *J Clin Invest* 86:1892–1896, 1990.

208. Valerius T, Repp R, de Wit TP, et al: Involvement of the high-affinity receptor for IgG (Fc gamma RI; CD64) in enhanced tumor cell cytotoxicity of neutrophils during granulocyte colony-stimulating factor therapy. *Blood* 82:931–939, 1993.

209. Allen JB, Wong HL, Guyre PM, et al: Association of circulating receptor Fc gamma RIII-positive monocytes in AIDS patients with elevated levels of transforming growth factor-beta. *J Clin Invest* 87:1773–1779, 1991.

210. de Waal Malefyt R, Figdor CG, de Vries JE: Effects of interleukin 4 on monocyte functions: comparison to interleukin 13. *Res Immunol* 144:629–633, 1993.

211. Shushakova N, Skokowa J, Schulman J, et al: C5a anaphylatoxin is a major regulator of activating versus inhibitory FcgammaRs in immune complex-induced lung disease. *J Clin Invest* 110:1823–1830, 2002.

212. Genovese MC, Kavanaugh A, Weinblatt ME, et al: An oral syk kinase inhibitor in the treatment of rheumatoid arthritis: a 3 month randomized placebo controlled phase 2 study in patients with active RA who had failed biologic agents. *Arthritis Rheum* 2011.

213. Deng GM, Liu L, Bahjat FR, et al: Suppression of skin and kidney disease by inhibition of spleen tyrosine kinase in lupus-prone mice. *Arthritis Rheum* 62:2086–2092, 2010.

214. Ivashkiv LB: Cross-regulation of signaling by ITAM-associated receptors. *Nat Immunol* 10:340–347, 2009.

215. Craft JE: Dissecting the immune cell mayhem that drives lupus pathogenesis. *Sci Transl Med* 3:73–79, 2011.

216. Green NM, Marshak-Rothstein A: Toll-like receptor driven B cell activation in the induction of systemic autoimmunity. *Semin Immunol* 23:106–112, 2011.

217. Horton HM, Chu SY, Ortiz EC, et al: Antibody-mediated coengagement of FcgammaRIIb and B cell receptor complex suppresses humoral immunity in systemic lupus erythematosus. *J Immunol* 186:4223–4233, 2011.

218. Marino M, Ruvo M, De Falco S, et al: Prevention of systemic lupus erythematosus in MRL/lpr mice by administration of an immunoglobulin-binding peptide. *Nat Biotechnol* 18:735–739, 2000.

219. Ierino FL, Powell MS, McKenzie IF, et al: Recombinant soluble human Fc gamma RII: production, characterization, and inhibition of the Arthus reaction. *J Exp Med* 178:1617–1628, 1993.

220. Samuelsson A, Towers TL, Ravetch JV: Anti-inflammatory activity of IVIG mediated through the inhibitory Fc receptor. *Science* 291:484–486, 2001.

221. Honigberg LA, Smith AM, Sirisawad M, et al: The Bruton tyrosine kinase inhibitor PCI-32765 blocks B-cell activation and is efficacious in models of autoimmune disease and B-cell malignancy. *Proc Natl Acad Sci U S A* 107:13075–13080, 2010.

222. Girard MT, Hjaltadottir S, Fejes-Toth AN, et al: Glucocorticoids enhance the gamma-interferon augmentation of human monocyte immunoglobulin G Fc receptor expression. *J Immunol* 138:3235–3241, 1987.

223. Salmon JE, Cronstein BN: Fc gamma receptor-mediated functions in neutrophils are modulated by adenosine receptor occupancy. A1 receptors are stimulatory and A2 receptors are inhibitory. *J Immunol* 145:2235–2240, 1990.

224. Roopenian DC, Akilesh S: FcRn: the neonatal Fc receptor comes of age. *Nat Rev Immuno* 7:715–725, 2007.

225. Hoyoux C, Foidart J, Rigo P, et al: Effects of methylprednisolone on the Fc-receptor function of human reticuloendothelial system in vivo. *Eur J Clin Invest* 14:60–66, 1984.

226. Guiducci C, Gong M, Xu Z, et al: TLR recognition of self nucleic acids hampers glucocorticoid activity in lupus. *Nature* 465:937–941, 2010.

Chapter 13

Neural-Immune Interactions: Principles and Relevance to SLE

Cherie L. Butts and Esther M. Sternberg

The immune and central nervous systems are the body's primary tools for interfacing with constant environmental perturbations that threaten homeostasis. Chemical, antigenic, or infectious agents recognized by the immune system and psychological or physical stimuli recognized by the central nervous system (CNS) often activate similar transducing pathways to translate perturbing signals into stabilizing responses. Numerous studies (human and animal model) also provide evidence for bidirectional communication between the CNS and the immune system. Cytokines produced by cells of the immune system stimulate the CNS, leading to "sickness behavior" following an infection—characterized by loss of appetite, decreased mobility, loss of libido, withdrawal from social interaction, depressed mood, increased somnolence, and fever—whereas hormones and proteins generated by the CNS modulate immunity to influence the course of immune-related disease (Figure 13-1).[1] Disruptions in communication between these systems can increase susceptibility to and severity of a variety of diseases, including autoimmune and inflammatory conditions such as systemic lupus erythematosus (SLE).[2] This chapter outlines the general principles of communication between the CNS and immune system and how this interaction could play a significant role in SLE disease outcome. In addition, it defines the afferent and efferent limbs of CNS regulation of immunity, the contribution of specific immune cell populations and their actions in initiating autoimmune/inflammatory conditions, and evidence from studies with humans and using animal models that demonstrate how this interaction operates in SLE.

Communication between the CNS and the immune system impacts physiologic processes at multiple levels (local, regional, systemic), and interruptions at any point in this dialogue could disrupt homeostasis and lead to disease. The strength of an immune response and of inflammation when a foreign stimulus is encountered depends not only on the nature, potency, dose, route, and duration of exposure but also on the contribution of CNS influences—including under conditions of stress.[3] This fact has important implications with the use of pharmacologic agents because drugs aimed at ameliorating autoimmune/inflammatory disease could alter the course of disease if they modify activity of the CNS or be ineffective when administered while the individual is stressed, because hormones generated during the stress response have a profound effect on immune responses and are likely to affect disease outcome.

THE IMMUNE SYSTEM

Activation of the immune system is important for preventing disease when a pathogen is introduced; however, if uncontrolled, immunopathology can result in autoimmune/inflammatory conditions. Responses generated by the immune system are generally divided into two groups: innate and adaptive. Innate immunity provides early—minutes to hours—immunologic events and an initial defense against pathogens and also supplies signals (cytokines, chemokines, costimulatory molecules, etc.) necessary to stimulate adaptive immunity.[4,5] Several different cell types are involved in innate immunity, including granulocytes, monocytes, dendritic cells (DCs), and natural killer (NK) cells. Granulocytes (basophils, eosinophils, and neutrophils) are found throughout the body and are among the first immune cells recruited after an injury.[6,7] Monocytes originate in the bone marrow and are a population of antigen-presenting cells (APCs) with phagocytic properties that can produce cytokines and chemokines to attract other immune cells to initiate an inflammatory response.[8,9] DCs are a more potent APC population that recognizes pathogens using receptors for pattern-associated molecular patterns (PAMPs) to drive strong immune responses by producing cytokines and expressing molecules on their cell surfaces that stimulates other immune cells.[10,11] NK cells have cytotoxic function and kill by producing perforin and granzyme, which break up the plasma membrane of a target cell or induce apoptosis using death receptors, such as Fas ligand (FasL) and tumor necrosis factor (TNF)–related apoptosis–inducing ligand (TRAIL).[7,12]

Adaptive immunity provides long-term protection against such pathogens as viruses, parasites, and tumor cells. Although the time required to initiate adaptive immune responses is more extensive (days to weeks), a second exposure to the pathogen is eliminated much more rapidly.[13,14] The majority of autoimmune/inflammatory conditions, such as SLE, are mediated by overactive or uncontrolled adaptive immune responses; therefore, controlling adaptive immunity is critical. Cells of adaptive immune responses consist primarily of B and T lymphocytes but require the efforts of innate immune cells to drive their responses. B cells are antibody-producing cells that develop in bone marrow and form germinal centers—sites of B-cell proliferation—upon activation to generate humoral immune responses, and these cells' lack of controlled activity is a key component in development of SLE.[15,16] Antibodies are important for neutralizing pathogens but can also stimulate other immune cell activity, including complement-mediated immune responses. T cells, also an important population in adaptive immunity, generate cellular immunity, including CD8+ T cells, which are cytotoxic to target cells (similar to NK cells) and assist in the promotion of other immune responses. The various immune cell populations work together to provide the host with an efficient system for eliminating pathogens and ameliorating disease, and additional information on the involvement of specific populations of innate and adaptive immune cells in SLE is discussed elsewhere in this text.

CENTRAL NERVOUS SYSTEM REGULATION OF IMMUNITY

The CNS regulates immunity primarily through three outflow pathways: neuroendocrine responses (hypothalamic-pituitary-adrenal [HPA] and hypothalamic-pituitary-gonadal [HPG] axes), the autonomic nervous system (sympathetic and parasympathetic), and the peripheral nervous system. The HPA and HPG axes regulate immunity systemically through the effects of glucocorticoids released from the adrenal glands and sex steroids from the gonads, respectively. The

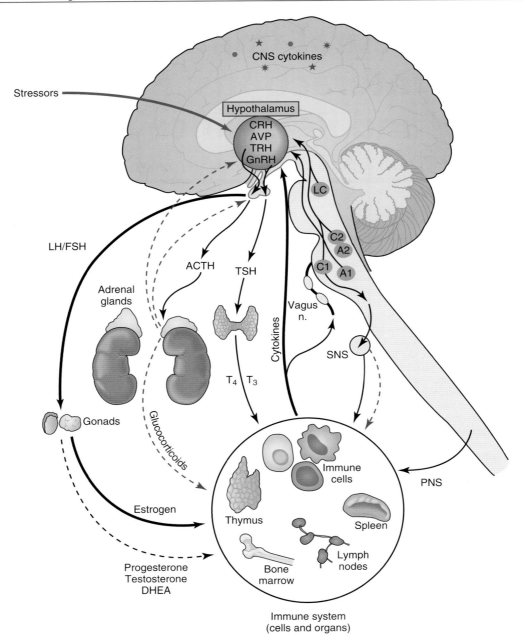

FIGURE 13-1 Schematic illustration of neural immune connections, including immune signaling of central nervous system (CNS) via systemic routes and the vagus nerve (Vagus n.) and CNS regulation of immunity via the hypothalamic-pituitary-adrenal (HPA) axis, sympathetic nervous system (SNS) and parasympathetic nervous system, and peripheral nervous system (PNS). Cytokine expression within the CNS is represented by *asterisks* within the brain. *Dotted lines* represent negative regulatory pathways, and *solid lines* represent positive regulatory pathways. CRH, corticotropin releasing hormone; AVP, arginine vasopressin; A1, C1, A2, C2, brainstem adrenergic nuclei; ACTH, adrenocorticotropin hormone; LC, locus ceruleus; PNS, peripheral nervous system; SNS, sympathetic nervous system. *(From Marques-Deak A, Cizza G, Sternberg E: Brain-immune interactions and disease susceptibility.* Mol Psychiatry 10:239–250, 2005.)

autonomic nervous system tends to regulate immunity regionally, at the level of immune organs such as the spleen, lymph nodes, and thymus, and the peripheral nervous system regulates immunity at local sites of inflammation. The various neurotransmitters and hormones generated by the CNS impact function of immune cells and strength of immune responses. Dysregulation of these pathways can, therefore, contribute to susceptibility to and the severity and course of autoimmune-inflammatory diseases, such as SLE.

The Neuroendocrine System

The neuroendocrine system comprises the hypothalamus, the pituitary, and glands involved in release of their respective hormones,

that is, the adrenal glands and the gonads. The HPA axis exerts its effects primarily through release of glucocorticoids and mineralocorticoids[17,18] by the cortex of the adrenal glands. The neuroendocrine stress response generated through the HPA axis is activated by stressful stimuli and is a powerful regulator of immune responses. The HPG axis exerts its effects on immunity through the sex hormones estrogen, progesterone, and testosterone.[19,20] These hormones bind to a family of related nuclear hormone receptors. Activity of the HPG axis fluctuates throughout the life cycle, whereas activity of the HPA axis tends to be more consistent. Together these systems can affect immunity to, susceptibility to, and the course of autoimmune/inflammatory diseases. Temporal and quantitative changes in these systems and their effects on immunity are discussed in detail later.

The Stress Response

The *stress response* can be defined as the brain's physiologic and behavioral reaction to psychological or physical stressors. The hypothalamus responds to internal and external stimuli by synthesizing the neuropeptide corticotropin-releasing hormone (CRH) from cells of the paraventricular nucleus (PVN)—neurons in the hypothalamus that project to the sympathetic brainstem nuclei, parasympathetic brainstem preganglionic neurons, and spinal cord.[21] CRH secreted into the rich hypophyseal portal blood supply stimulates the anterior pituitary gland to secrete adrenocorticotropin hormone (ACTH), which in turn stimulates the adrenal glands to synthesize and secrete glucocorticoids.[22] Hypothalamic CRH secretion is held under tight regulatory control by several positive and negative neurotransmitter systems to regulate glucocorticoid release from the adrenal glands. The noradrenergic, serotonergic, and dopaminergic systems upregulate CRH via α_1-adrenergic receptors,[23] serotonin (5-hydroxytryptamine [5-HT]) receptors,[24] and dopamine (D1) receptors,[25] respectively, whereas opiates, gamma-aminobutyric acid (GABA)/benzodiazepine, and glucocorticoid feedback suppress CRH production via opiate receptors,[26] GABAergic receptors,[27] and glucocorticoid receptors,[28] respectively.[29,30]

In addition to its neuroendocrine effects via the pituitary gland, CRH also acts centrally within the brain as a neuropeptide to induce a set of behaviors that are characterized by cautious avoidance, vigilance, enhanced attention, and suppression of vegetative functions, such as feeding and reproduction,[31,32] which make up the classic "fight or flight" pattern of behavior.[23,33] Many of these effects are mediated through the hypothalamus and neurotransmitter systems, such as the brainstem-noradrenergic system and sympathetic nervous system.[34,35] The hypothalamic CRH system also communicates with noradrenergic pathways during the stress response via anatomic connections between the hypothalamus and noradrenergic centers in the brainstem.[36] In turn, the brainstem-noradrenergic system sends signals to the periphery via the sympathetic nerves. Through such connections, the physiologic components of the stress response (i.e., increased heart rate, muscle tone, and sweating) are coordinated with behavioral responses to form the generalized stress response. Many studies suggest that modulation of immune responses by both the sympathetic and neuroendocrine systems are an important physiologic component of the stress response.[37-42]

Sex Hormones

Another group of steroid hormones whose production is controlled by the neuroendocrine system and that are shown to be important in autoimmune/inflammatory conditions are sex hormones, and their involvement in SLE is discussed in more detail elsewhere in this text. Both males and females produce the different sex hormones—estrogen, progesterone, testosterone—but with varying concentrations. These hormones are critical in the development of secondary sexual characteristics and during pregnancy but also play a role in modifying immune responses. The hypothalamus responds to rhythmic signals to produce gonadotropin-releasing hormone (GnRH).[43,44] GnRH acts to stimulate pituitary gland cells to produce luteinizing hormone (LH) and follicle-stimulating hormone (FSH), which enter the bloodstream and interact with gonadal cells (testes, ovaries) that activate gametogenesis and produce sex hormones, such as testosterone by interstitial cells and estrogen and progesterone by granulosa cells.[45] Production of sex hormones in females is especially sensitive to rhythmic changes throughout the reproductive cycle.[46]

Interactions between the HPA and HPG Axes

There is an important interplay between the HPA and HPG axes. In addition to regulating its own activity, the HPA axis is able to modify activity of the HPG axis, and vice versa. Psychological or physical stressors that generate elevations of glucocorticoids for extended periods or other events leading to overactivity of the HPA axis can initiate a negative feedback loop by acting on the hypothalamus and limit further production of glucocorticoids. Stressors that cause classic "sickness behavior" can also reduce the libido and limit production of sex hormones by suppressing HPG axis activity.[47] Conversely, the HPG axis is able to regulate activities of the HPA axis, such as elevated concentrations of sex hormones limiting glucocorticoid release by adrenal glands.[48] Co-regulation between the HPA and HPG axes could, therefore, impact activation of the immune system and potency of immune responses following a trigger.

Molecular Mechanisms of Steroid Hormone Actions

Receptors for glucocorticoids and other steroid hormones are members of the nuclear receptor superfamily and are structurally related. They include glucocorticoid receptor (GR), which that binds corticosterone and dexamethasone; mineralocorticoid receptor (MR), which binds corticosterone and aldosterone; androgen receptor (AR), which binds testosterone and its derivatives; estrogen receptor, which binds estradiol (ER); progesterone receptor (PR), which binds progestins; thyroid hormone receptor, which binds thyroxine; and retinoic acid receptors, which bind all-*trans* retinoic acid. Structurally, these receptors are made up of three functional regions: (1) a C-terminal hormone–binding region, (2) a DNA-binding region, and (3) an N-terminal immunogenic region involved in transactivation.[49,50] The unbound receptor located in the cytosol is folded and inactive, bound to a 90-kilodalton (kDa) heat shock protein[51] (HSP90) and immunophilins (Figure 13-2). When the ligand (hormone) binds to its receptor, hsp90 is displaced, resulting in a conformational change in the receptor that allows the active ligand-receptor complex to displace to the nucleus and bind to hormone receptor–binding elements (HREs) on DNA as either a homodimer or heterodimer. For example, although GR generally binds to GR DNA-binding elements[52] as homodimers, it is also possible for GRs and MRs to form heterodimers.[53,54] These different mechanisms of binding to DNA response elements confer additional specificity of action to the steroid hormone receptors. The hormone receptor complex then translocates to the nucleus and acts as a transcription factor, either suppressing or stimulating DNA gene transcription. In addition, the GRs and other steroid hormone receptors interact with more than 200 nuclear cofactors. The recruitment of either coactivators or co-repressor complexes is involved in transcriptional regulation and can determine whether or not a gene is transcribed.[55] Other accessory proteins, such as (histone deacetylase 6) HDAC6, also contribute to transcriptional regulation,[56] and steroid hormone receptors can interact with other transcription factors, such as NF-κB and (activator protein 1) AP-1, to inhibit their activity in immune and other cells.[57,58]

Further specificity of action of these receptors is conferred by tissue distribution within tissues. This process is well-documented for the relationship between GRs and MRs. The primary glucocorticoid receptor in immune cells is GR, which is consistent with the physiologic role of glucocorticoid regulation of the immune system by stress levels of these hormones[1,59,60]; however, an additional level of specificity is conferred by tissue distribution of the corticosterone-metabolizing enzyme 11β-hydroxysteroid, which metabolizes corticosterone but not aldosterone. Thus, where 11β-hydroxysteroid is present (e.g., kidney), the primary ligand that is available for binding to MRs is aldosterone rather than corticosterone,[52] whereas where the enzyme is not present (e.g., brain), the primary ligand for MRs is corticosterone. MRs in the brain play a role in regulation of basal HPA function, such as circadian rhythm.

Impact of Neuroendocrine Factors on Immunity

Several neuroendocrine factors, including steroid hormones, have been shown to alter immunity and impact immune-related disease outcome. This effect was demonstrated dramatically when it was shown that hormonal fluctuations could influence the size of lymphoid organs, such as experiments using restraint and psychological

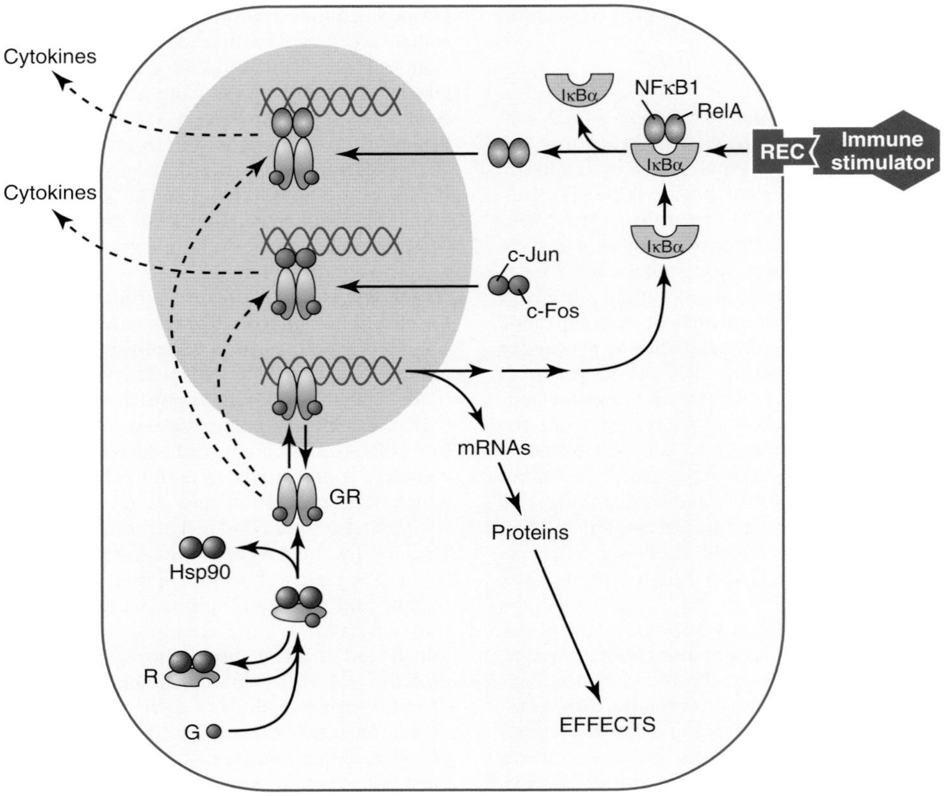

FIGURE 13-2 Schematic diagram of the molecular mechanism of glucocorticoid receptor regulation of cytokine production. Glucocorticoid hormone (G) binds to the cytosolic glucocorticoid receptor (GR), displacing heat shock protein 90 (HSP90). This allows dimerization, movement into the nucleus, and binding of the G-GR complex to DNA, with resultant transcription and translation of proteins, including the IκB protein. IκB indirectly suppresses cytokine production by sequestration of nuclear factor kappa B (NF-κB). In addition, the G-GR complex can interact with NF-κB directly to suppress cytokine production.

stressors that activate the HPA axis and led to shrinkage of the thymus and other lymphoid tissues.[61] In addition, many of the autoimmune/inflammatory conditions exhibit differences in incidences in males and females (being up to tenfold higher in women), suggesting a role for sex hormones in immune-mediated disease.

Glucocorticoid Modulation of the Immune System

Glucocorticoids are able to modulate immune cell function by acting through intracellular GRs in immune cells. The overall functional effect of glucocorticoids on the immune response depends on the preparation, dose (whether pharmacologic or physiologic), and temporal sequence of glucocorticoid exposure in relation to antigenic or proinflammatory challenge and has profound effects at molecular, cellular, and whole-organ levels.[62-64] Exposure to stress levels of glucocorticoids results in rapid involution of the thymus as a result of glucocorticoid-induced thymocyte apoptosis, and glucocorticoids can regulate immune responses by inducing apoptosis in proliferating lymphocytes.[49] There is evidence to suggest that such glucocorticoid-regulated apoptosis could take place within the thymus through induction of an intrathymic glucocorticoid system because the enzymatic machinery for glucocorticoid synthesis is present within the thymus.[65] Glucocorticoids also orchestrate redistribution of circulating white blood cells with neutrophilic leukocytosis, eosinopenia, monocytopenia, and altered ratios of T-lymphocyte subtypes—resulting in decreased peripheral blood CD4+ cells and increased CD8+ cells—as well as decreased infiltration of neutrophils and monocytes into tissues.[66]

Glucocorticoids have effects on both innate and adaptive immune cell populations, including granulocytes, NK cells, monocytes, DCs, and B and T lymphocytes.[67] Mice treated with glucocorticoids show

a reduction in the number of splenic NK cells, and remaining NK cells exhibit reduced cytolytic activity.[68] Glucocorticoids inhibit cytokine release and other activity of eosinophils in asthma[69,70] and of neutrophils in chronic obstructive pulmonary disease (COPD),[71,72] and inhaled glucocorticoids prevent histamine release by basophils in allergic disease.[73] Monocytes and neutrophils are thought to be primary targets of glucocorticoid actions in diminishing contact hypersensitivity reactions, as evidenced by repression of monocyte production of cytokines and chemokines.[74] Glucocorticoids have also been shown to reduce DC production of interleukin-12 (IL-12), limit upregulation of co-stimulatory molecules expressed by mature DCs to reduce recognition of antigen, and strongly reduce allostimulatory capacity.[74,75] However, the suppressive effect was not observed with DCs previously activated by lipopolysaccharide (LPS), indicating that the influence of glucocorticoids depends on stage of DC maturation.[76] In a study of children with asthma, glucocorticoids were shown to decrease expression of intracellular adhesion molecule 1 (ICAM-1) and L-selectin, leading to an inhibition of the ability of immune cells to migrate to inflammatory sites.[77]

In addition to effects on innate immune cells, extensive studies have shown immunomodulatory consequences of glucocorticoids on adaptive immunity. Glucocorticoids suppress differentiation and maturation of T cells as well as altering the function of T-cell subtypes, such as cytolytic (CD8+) and helper (CD4+) T cells. In addition, several studies have reported that glucocorticoids suppress mitogen- and antigen-stimulated T-cell proliferation.[78] This is thought to be most critical in T-helper (Th) cell populations, which are skewed from a Th1 toward a Th2 or other T-helper cell responses in the presence of glucocorticoids, with inhibition of TNF-α, IL-2, IL-6, IL-12, and interferon gamma (IFN-γ) production and increases in IL-10,

IL-4, and IL-13 production.[79-81] The impact of glucocorticoids on B-cell proliferation is variable, depending on the stimulus and dose of glucocorticoids used and age-dependent expression of GRs.[82,83] In general, B-cell proliferation is suppressed by glucocorticoids to a lesser extent than T-cell proliferation, but suppression of Th2 subsets that assist in antibody production could inhibit B-cell activity. Although the overall effects of glucocorticoids on immune responses at the cellular level are immunosuppressive, this effect is attained through suppression of many stimulatory components of the immune cascade and stimulation of some immunosuppressive or antiinflammatory elements. The relatively greater sensitivity to glucocorticoid suppression of components of cellular versus humoral immunity tends to shift immune responses from a cellular to a humoral pattern,[1] which is important in SLE.

Effects of Sex Hormones on Immunity

Immune suppression or modulation of immunity by sex hormones has been reported in many diseases.[84-87] In female mice, surgical removal of ovaries (oophorectomy, essentially eliminating available estrogen and progesterone) followed by hormone treatment, such as estrogen, has been used to show their effects on immune responses. In male mice that have undergone castration (orchidectomy) and been given estrogen, increases in susceptibility to autoimmune/inflammatory disease to levels that are similar to those in females have been reported. Sex hormones can have direct effects on immune cells because they express receptors for estrogen (ERs), progesterone (PRs), and testosterone (ARs) but may also modify immunity through indirect effects on the HPA or HPG axis.[88,89] In the female genital tract, the number of uterine NK cells changes during the reproductive cycle and with pregnancy,[90] and progesterone receptor (PR)$^{-/-}$ mice do not have uterine NK cells.[91] In addition, women are more susceptible to a variety of infections during pregnancy, including the bacterium *Listeria monocytogenes*, which poses a significant health problem.[92] Taken together, these findings indicate a role of sex hormones in the regulation of immunity.

Although the impact is not as dramatic as has been shown with glucocorticoids, sex hormones are able to modify both innate and adaptive immune cell populations. Estrogens can prevent production of free radicals[93] and adhesion to endothelial cells by neutrophils[94]; in ovariectomy experiments using mice, an infiltration of neutrophils was found in the endometrium[95,96]; and monocyte populations are also responsive to sex hormones. Bacterial lipopolysaccharide–activated splenic macrophages treated with estrogen have reduced production of proinflammatory cytokines.[97] Testosterone induces Fas ligand (FasL)–dependent apoptosis in bone marrow–derived macrophages,[98] and progesterone increases expression of FasL, inhibits TNF-α production in uterine macrophages,[99] and decreases cytokine (IL-12, IL-1β) production by monocytes from varicella-zoster virus (VZV)–stimulated peripheral blood mononuclear cells (PBMCs) from healthy subjects.[100] Progesterone has also been reported to inhibit DC phagocytosis of *Candida albicans*,[101] to contribute to susceptibility to human immunodeficiency virus (HIV) in women by increasing the number of Langerhans cells available for HIV infection,[102] and to increase susceptibility to *Chlamydia* infection in rats as a result of increased bacterial infiltrates in the uterine epithelium and vaginal secretions of these animals.[103] In addition, estrogen has been shown to affect DC function in the development of experimental autoimmune encephalomyelitis (EAE)—the mouse model for the autoimmune disease multiple sclerosis.[104,105]

Sex hormones also have a profound influence on adaptive immune responses. The two forms of estrogen receptor, ERα and ERβ,[106] have been identified in lymphocytes,[107] and the presence of estrogen increases the severity of autoimmune diseases driven by B and T cells in mice and humans. Progesterone inhibits T-cell proliferation,[108] whereas estrogen at elevated concentrations (achieved during pregnancy) is thought to be important in immune suppression during pregnancy, possibly by increasing T-regulatory cell (Treg) populations to prevent fetal rejection.[109,110] In addition, estradiol has been shown to increase antibody production by B cells and has been implicated in the improper regulation of B-cell development.[15,114] The ability of estrogen to aggravate SLE symptoms is related at least in part to dose. In one study, administration of hormone replacement therapy (Premarin 0.625 mg (CLB) conjugated estrogen) to women with SLE increased their risk for mild-to-moderate flares of disease.[111] In another study, however, administration of lower doses of estradiol-containing oral contraceptives (30 to 35 μg (CLB) estradiol, plus methindrone), compared to placebo, to women with stable SLE (and no history of clotting) was not associated with increased flare rates.[112]

Autonomic and Peripheral Nervous System Regulation of Immunity

The CNS can also utilize the autonomic and peripheral nervous systems to regulate immune responses and influence development of autoimmune/inflammatory conditions.[3] The sympathetic nervous system releases neurotransmitters, such as norepinephrine, and connects CNS adrenergic brainstem regions to lymphoid organs.[113,114] The parasympathetic nervous system modulates immune responses through efferent and afferent fibers of the vagus nerve. The peripheral nervous system regulates immunity through release of neuropeptides from sensory peripheral nerves involved in pain, touch, and temperature perception. Interplay between these systems provide the feedback loop that optimizes immune responses by amplifying immunity to clear a pathogen and then dampening the response to prevent overactivation of the immune response that would lead to autoimmune/inflammatory conditions, such as SLE.

Sympathetic Nervous System Effects on Inflammation and the Immune System

The sympathetic nervous system serves an important role in regional regulation of immunity.[115,116] Many lymphoid organs—including spleen, thymus, and lymph nodes—are richly innervated by sympathetic nerves.[117] A number of studies, including denervation and ablation studies, indicate that these anatomic connections as well as the neurotransmitters of the sympathetic nervous system play an important physiologic role in inflammatory responses.[115] The sympathetic nervous system mediates its effects through release of norepinephrine from sympathetic nerve fibers and epinephrine released from the adrenal medulla. Both norepinephrine and epinephrine exert their actions through adrenergic receptors. The beta-2 adrenergic receptor (β$_2$AR), a G-protein–coupled receptor, is the main receptor found on lymphocytes.[118,119] Adrenergic influences on immune cells potently inhibit Th1 cytokine production and thereby suppress cell-mediated immune responses. Norepinephrine and epinephrine also stimulate production of Th2 cytokines, such as IL-10, that could drive immune cell activity in SLE.[120]

Evidence that the sympathetic nervous system affects the exudation component of peripheral inflammation is provided by sympathetic ablation studies using 6-OH dopamine (6-OHDA)[121] or sympathetic ganglionic blockers such as chlorisondamine,[122] or noradrenergic antagonists and agonists.[123] Noradrenergic denervation studies using rodent models have shown differential effects on inflammation depending on the location of denervation. Thus, denervation of the noradrenergic fibers of lymph nodes[124] is associated with exacerbation of inflammation, but systemic sympathectomy or denervation of joints is associated with decreased severity of inflammation.[125,126] Treatment of neonatal rats with 6-OHDA, which interrupts both central and peripheral noradrenergic systems, is associated with exacerbation of experimental allergic encephalomyelitis.[127] Pharmacologic studies show decreased inflammation in experimental arthritis with beta-blockade[128] and decreased severity of experimental allergic encephalomyelitis with β-adrenergic agonists.[127]

Parasympathetic Nervous System and Immunity

The parasympathetic nervous system both sends immune signals to the CNS through the afferent fibers of the vagus nerve and modulates immune responses regionally through efferent fibers of the vagus nerve. Ganglia outside the spinal cord receive projections from the brainstem and further innervate visceral organs, such as the heart, lungs, gut, liver, and spleen. IL-1 receptors on paraganglia cells located adjacent to parasympathetic ganglia bind IL-1 and activate the vagus nerve, thus signaling the presence of peripheral inflammation to the brain.[129-131] Inflammation in the gut or peritoneum leads to the *inflammatory reflex,* which results in the release of acetylcholine from efferent vagus nerve fibers and negative feedback control of inflammation.[40] Cutting the vagus nerve prevents immune signaling to the brain and therefore prevents further activation of cholinergic brainstem regions.[40,132,133] Acetylcholine is the primary parasympathetic neurotransmitter, which binds to two receptor subtypes, nicotinic and muscarinic cholinergic receptors, each of which consist of several different subunits that heterodimerize to provide cell and tissue specificity of cholinergic effects. Immune cells contain both receptors, but the α7 subunit of the nicotinic receptors specifically mediates cholinergic antiinflammatory effects in macrophages.

Peripheral Nervous System Effects on Inflammation and the Immune System

Peripheral nerves that release neuropeptides, such as substance P (SP), calcitonin gene–related protein (CGRP), and vasoactive intestinal peptide (VIP) that play a role in peripheral inflammation, innervating immune organs and local sites of inflammation.[134-136] CRH is also released from peripheral nerves and, in this context, induces inflammation.

Substance P has also been shown to be a key mediator of severity in arthritis[125,137] and in the cellular component of inflammation.[138] Substance P, which can be released in retrograde fashion from sensory nerve endings at sites of inflammation, acts as a chemoattractant and stimulator of cellular proliferation and cytokine production. It also plays a role in the early arteriolar changes associated with inflammation.[139] Both denervation of substance P nerve fibers with local capsaicin denervation of lymph nodes and systemic capsaicin treatment are associated with diminished peripheral inflammation.[124,125,137] The peripheral neuropeptides VIP and CGRP are generally thought to suppress inflammatory responses.[140-144]

PHYSIOLOGIC IMPACT OF MISCOMMUNICATIONS BETWEEN THE CNS AND IMMUNE SYSTEM

A multilevel infrastructure exists to allow anatomic, molecular, and functional communications between the CNS and the immune system.[145-147] Animal studies in which these communications are interrupted on a genetic, pharmacologic, or surgical basis provide evidence that this interaction plays an important role in regulating susceptibility to and severity of autoimmune/inflammatory diseases. Human studies also provide evidence that dysregulation of neural-immune interactions are associated with autoimmune/inflammatory disease, which has been shown in Sjögren syndrome, rheumatoid arthritis, asthma, dermatitis, irritable bowel syndrome, and SLE.[148,149] Some genetically inbred animal strains show a simple association between a relatively blunted HPA axis and autoimmune disease. The obese-strain chicken, in which thyroiditis develops spontaneously, and its thyroiditis-resistant counterpart also exhibit relative HPA-axis hyporesponsiveness and hyperresponsiveness.[146] Some, but not all, lupus-prone mouse strains (MRL but not NZB) have a relatively blunted HPA axis response.[150] The concept that an intact HPA axis response protects against autoimmune/inflammatory disease has also been shown through intervention studies in disease models, including streptococcal cell wall–induced arthritis,[151] experimental autoimmune encephalomyelitis induced by myelin basic protein,[152] and the lethal effects of salmonella.[153] Interruptions of the HPA axis in these models by surgical means, through adrenalectomy or hypophysectomy (i.e., pituitary excision), or by pharmacologic means, through the glucocorticoid-receptor antagonist RU486, results in enhanced

inflammatory disease mortality. Conversely, surgical or pharmacologic reconstitution of the HPA axis reverses inflammatory disease susceptibility in inflammation-susceptible strains.[151,152,154]

Glucocorticoid Resistance

Impaired glucocorticoid control of inflammation may also result from a lack of responsiveness, in cells and tissues that normally respond to circulating glucocorticoids, due to impaired receptor function. Glucocorticoid resistance may result from polymorphisms of the receptor or associated cofactors that are necessary for it to function or from overexpression of glucocorticoid receptor β (GR-β), an inactive form of GR that binds hormone but not DNA.[1,155,156] Chronic inflammation can itself result in enhanced expression of GR-β and associated glucocorticoid resistance. Glucocorticoid resistance has been associated with several autoimmune, inflammatory, and allergic diseases (reviewed in references 3 and 149). Patients with severe SLE often require large doses of glucocorticoids before a therapeutic effect is seen, and some have Cushingoid features following glucocorticoid therapy.[157] The contribution of the glucocorticoid receptor to potential glucocorticoid resistance has been explored in some studies examining the binding number and affinity characteristics of GR in lupus. Patients who exhibit hormone resistance have been found to have abnormally high levels of GRβ[158] or defective, mutated GR.[159,160] A decrease in GR number in mononuclear cells has also been found in patient s with lupus patients,[159] and such patients have been reported to have a higher percentage of lymphocytes with high activity of P-glycoprotein—a molecule responsible for transporting steroids outside the cell that would limit glucocorticoid's effects.[161] In a study of patients with SLE who had not received steroid treatment within the previous 6 months, glucocorticoid receptor numbers in PBMCs were significantly higher than in PBMCs of controls.[162] There was no correlation with disease activity, nor was there a difference in affinity of the GR in these patients. In another study, no difference in GR number was found between patients and controls; however, patients who were undergoing low-dose glucocorticoid treatment were not excluded from this study.[163] Because exogenous treatment with glucocorticoids suppresses the responsiveness of the HPA axis, the GR numbers measured in glucocorticoid-treated patients may reflect treatment rather than intrinsic factors. Thus, the discrepancy between these studies could be related to differences in exogenous glucocorticoid exposure in these patients, underscoring the inherent difficulty in studying GR binding and number in such patients. Later studies have examined GRs in SLE and show that not only is GR expression reduced in patients with the disease but also its binding affinity for glucocorticoids is lower in such patients.[164]

Effects of Stress in SLE

Until recently, studies of the effects of stress on physical illness, including autoimmune diseases such as SLE, were viewed with skepticism. This reaction is related in part to the inherent difficulty in accurately defining and quantifying stressful stimuli and response outcomes. However, advances in defining and quantifying not only stressors but also neuroendocrine transducing signals, disease outcomes, and molecular components of the immune/inflammatory response in animals and humans have allowed more accurate assessment of the effects of stress on autoimmune/inflammatory disease and of the mechanisms by which such effects are transduced. Although most of these studies have been carried out in models of infectious disease,[165,166] it is clear from such studies that activation of both the HPA axis and the sympathetic system play an important role in modulating immunity during stress. The evidence from animal models that these systems interact provides direction for the future design of human studies to substantiate old or anecdotal claims that stress is associated with exacerbation or precipitation of disease in SLE.

A number of studies have suggested that emotional stress might trigger the onset of SLE or worsen its course, and some studies have shown an association between flares of disease and emotional stress or number and severity of daily stressors.[167-169] Chronic stress can also lead to burnout—a state of emotional and physical exhaustion in which the stress hormone cortisol is initially elevated and in later stages depleted.[170,171] This condition could contribute to triggering of autoimmune diseases, such as SLE, through impairment of negative feedback with inflammation. Similarly, there have been some reports of the onset of glucocorticoid resistance in burnout, which could further contribute to exacerbation of inflammatory disease tendencies.[172-175]

Chronic inflammation itself can be viewed as a stressor that can alter HPA axis responses. Rodent models have been used to demonstrate the effects of chronic inflammation, which include hypercortisolism and a shift from primarily CRH control of the stress response to primarily vasopressin (AVP) control.[176,177] The latter shift results from a switch from CRH to AVP expression in hypothalamic neurons[178] and occurs in response to cytokines such as IL-1.[179] Human studies in multiple sclerosis (MS) have shown both a shift toward an AVP-driven stress response[176] as well as glucocorticoid resistance in PBMCs in some subsets of patients with MS (relapsing remitting),[180] indicating that an impairment of HPA and glucocorticoid responses in addition to glucocorticoid resistance may contribute to the pathogenesis of the disease in different subpopulations of patients.

Neuroendocrine Mechanisms in SLE

Neuroendocrine immune interactions could play a role in the pathogenesis of SLE in several ways. As in susceptibility or resistance to other inflammatory illnesses, premorbid neuroendocrine responsiveness might predispose to an increased susceptibility to the development of SLE. Once SLE develops, and if the CNS is involved, the local effects of cytokines on neuronal tissue could contribute to some of the specific neuropathologic or neuropsychiatric features of SLE. At the effector end point of the HPA axis, differences in GR number or sensitivity could play a role in the pathogenesis of SLE as well as in clinical response to treatment with steroids. In addition, regardless of the premorbid reactivity of the HPA axis, chronic inflammation itself could alter HPA axis responses. Studies supporting these possibilities in both animal models and humans suggest that a variety of neuroimmune mechanisms may be relevant to many features in the pathogenesis of SLE. Several studies have shown a blunted HPA axis response to a variety of stimuli in human autoimmune/inflammatory and allergic diseases, including SLE (Box 13-1). In these studies, there is no difference between basal cortisol responses in patients and controls, but patients with SLE show significantly lower cortisol rises in response to stimuli than did controls. Specifically, patients with SLE showed lower cortisol responses to ovine CRH than controls.[181] Studies of HPA axis responsiveness in mouse models of SLE have shown relatively blunted corticosterone responses in MRL, but not NZB/NZW F, mice.[182]

Together, these studies underline the biologic principle that neuroendocrine responsiveness plays an important modulating role in susceptibility and resistance to autoimmune/inflammatory disease.

Box 13-1 Inflammatory/Autoimmune Diseases Correlated with a Dysfunctional Hypothalamic-Pituitary-Adrenal Axis in Humans*

Rheumatoid arthritis[191,192]
  SLE[181]
  Sjögren syndrome[193]
  Dermatitis[194]
  Multiple sclerosis[176,195]

*Superscript numbers are chapter references.
Adapted from Marques-Deak A, Cizza G, Sternberg E: Brain-immune interactions and disease susceptibility. *Mol Psychiatry* 10:239–250, 2005.

When feedback suppression of the immune system by antiinflammatory/immunosuppressive glucocorticoids is interrupted—either by blocking production of glucocorticoids, preventing their action using receptor antagonists, or in the presence of impaired receptor function—overactive inflammatory responses lead to autoimmune susceptibility. It is likely that in human autoimmune/inflammatory diseases the HPA axis could be impaired or interrupted at different points in different diseases or in the same disease in different individuals. Neuroendocrine responsiveness also varies with time on a circadian basis, in females in relation to the reproductive cycle, and throughout life with aging—emphasizing the influence of sex hormones on autoimmune/inflammatory conditions. Thus, the degree to which neuroendocrine responses modulate inflammatory disease also may vary over time, and this variation may account for some of the temporal waxing and waning of these illnesses. Understanding the degree to which such hormonal and neuronal inputs control inflammatory disease will provide new insights for future therapeutic approaches in these diseases.

Autonomic and Peripheral Nervous System Activity in SLE

In addition to changes in neuroendocrine function in SLE, other neuronal regulatory systems, such as the sympathetic, parasympathetic, and peripheral nervous systems, may be dysregulated in SLE. Norepinephrine and epinephrine production is reported to be dysregulated in SLE and suspected to contribute to disease activity.[183-185] Sympathetic nervous system outflow has been shown to be increased in patients with SLE, as demonstrated by increased levels of serum neuropeptide Y (NPY),[186,187] and a mouse model of SLE also showed elevated NPY levels.[188,189] The peripheral nervous system can also contribute to disease development in SLE but clinically is considered to be less frequently affected. In addition, peripheral neuropeptides such as VIP, substance P, and CGRP are increased in SLE[189,190]; therefore, further investigation of the connection between these systems and symptoms exhibited by SLE patients or predisposition to other conditions is needed.

SUMMARY

It is apparent that neural-immune interactions play an important role in the pathogenesis of many features of SLE at multiple levels, within and outside the CNS and at the molecular and whole-organ level. This chapter has mainly focused on how the CNS influences immunity to impact SLE, but it is also possible that cytokines and other factors produced by the immune system can influence CNS activity to further exacerbate conditions that promote SLE. Many additional neural factors play important roles in modulating immune function and could be important in the development of SLE.

References

1. Webster JI, Tonelli L, Sternberg EM: Neuroendocrine regulation of immunity. *Annu Rev Immunol* 20:125–163, 2002.
2. Butts C, Sternberg E: Different approaches to understanding autoimmune rheumatic diseases: the neuroimmunoendocrine system. *Best Pract Res Clin Rheumatol* 18:125–139, 2004.
3. Sternberg EM: Neural regulation of innate immunity: a coordinated nonspecific host response to pathogens. *Nat Rev Immunol* 6:318–328, 2006.
4. Trinchieri G, Sher A: Cooperation of Toll-like receptor signals in innate immune defence. *Nat Rev Immunol* 7:179–190, 2007.
5. Coffman RL, Sher A, Seder RA: Vaccine adjuvants: putting innate immunity to work. *Immunity* 33:492–503, 2010.
6. Fahey TJ, 3rd, Sherry B, Tracey KJ, et al: Cytokine production in a model of wound healing: the appearance of MIP-1, MIP-2, cachectin/TNF and IL-1. *Cytokine* 2:92–99, 1990.
7. Cooper MA, Fehniger TA, Caligiuri MA: The biology of human natural killer-cell subsets. *Trends Immunol* 22:633–640, 2001.
8. Weber C, Belge KU, von Hundelshausen P, et al: Differential chemokine receptor expression and function in human monocyte subpopulations. *J Leukoc Biol* 67:699–704, 2000.

9. Gordon S, Taylor PR: Monocyte and macrophage heterogeneity. *Nat Rev Immunol* 5:953–964, 2005.

10. Mellman I, Steinman RM: Dendritic cells: specialized and regulated antigen processing machines. *Cell* 106:255–258, 2001.

11. Colonna M, Pulendran B, Iwasaki A: Dendritic cells at the host-pathogen interface. *Nat Immunol* 7:117–120, 2006.

12. Tiemessen CT, Shalekoff S, Meddows-Taylor S, et al: Cutting edge: unusual NK cell responses to HIV-1 peptides are associated with protection against maternal-infant transmission of HIV-1. *J Immunol* 182:5914–5918, 2009.

13. Pasare C, Medzhitov R: Toll-like receptors: linking innate and adaptive immunity. *Microbes Infect* 6:1382–1387, 2004.

14. Verdeil G, Marquardt K, Surh CD, et al: Adjuvants targeting innate and adaptive immunity synergize to enhance tumor immunotherapy. *Proc Natl Acad Sci U S A* 105:16683–16688, 2008.

15. Grimaldi CM, Hill L, Xu X, et al: Hormonal modulation of B cell development and repertoire selection. *Mol Immunol* 42:811–820, 2005.

16. Lipsky PE: Systemic lupus erythematosus: an autoimmune disease of B cell hyperactivity. *Nat Immunol* 2:764–766, 2001.

17. Smith CC, Omeljaniuk RJ, Whitfield HJ, Jr, et al: Differential mineralocorticoid (type 1) and glucocorticoid (type 2) receptor expression in Lewis and Fischer rats. *Neuroimmunomodulation* 1:66–73, 1994.

18. Tsugita M, Iwasaki Y, Nishiyama M, et al: Glucocorticoid receptor plays an indispensable role in mineralocorticoid receptor-dependent transcription in GR-deficient BE(2)C and T84 cells in vitro. *Mol Cell Endocrinol* 302:18–25, 2009.

19. Lahita RG: The role of sex hormones in systemic lupus erythematosus. *Curr Opin Rheumatol* 11:352–356, 1999.

20. Cutolo M, Sulli A, Capellino S, et al: Sex hormones influence on the immune system: basic and clinical aspects in autoimmunity. *Lupus* 13:635–638, 2004.

21. Vale W, Spiess J, Rivier C, et al: Characterization of a 41-residue ovine hypothalamic peptide that stimulates secretion of corticotropin and beta-endorphin. *Science* 213:1394–1397, 1981.

22. Williams RH, Larsen PR: *Williams textbook of endocrinology*, Philadelphia, 2003, Saunders.

23. Forray MI, Gysling K: Role of noradrenergic projections to the bed nucleus of the stria terminalis in the regulation of the hypothalamic-pituitary-adrenal axis. *Brain Res Brain Res Rev* 47:145–160, 2004.

24. Mikkelsen JD, Hay-Schmidt A, Kiss A: Serotonergic stimulation of the rat hypothalamo-pituitary-adrenal axis: interaction between 5-HT1A and 5-HT2A receptors. *Ann N Y Acad Sci* 1018:65–70, 2004.

25. Zhou Y, Spangler R, Ho A, et al: Hypothalamic CRH mRNA levels are differentially modulated by repeated "binge" cocaine with or without D(1) dopamine receptor blockade. *Brain Res Mol Brain Res* 94:112–118, 2001.

26. McNally GP, Akil H: Role of corticotropin-releasing hormone in the amygdala and bed nucleus of the stria terminalis in the behavioral, pain modulatory, endocrine consequences of opiate withdrawal. *Neuroscience* 112:605–617, 2002.

27. Grottoli S, Giordano R, Maccagno B, et al: The stimulatory effect of canrenoate, a mineralocorticoid antagonist, on the activity of the hypothalamus-pituitary-adrenal axis is abolished by alprazolam, a benzodiazepine, in humans. *J Clin Endocrinol Metab* 87:4616–4620, 2002.

28. Kovacs KJ, Foldes A, Sawchenko PE: Glucocorticoid negative feedback selectively targets vasopressin transcription in parvocellular neurosecretory neurons. *J Neurosci* 20:3843–3852, 2000.

29. Calogero AE, Gallucci WT, Gold PW, et al: Multiple feedback regulatory loops upon rat hypothalamic corticotropin-releasing hormone secretion. Potential clinical implications. *J Clin Invest* 82:767–774, 1988.

30. Imaki T, Nahan JL, Rivier C, et al: Differential regulation of corticotropin-releasing factor mRNA in rat brain regions by glucocorticoids and stress. *J Neurosci* 11:585–599, 1991.

31. Sutton RE, Koob GF, Le Moal M, et al: Corticotropin releasing factor produces behavioural activation in rats. *Nature* 297:331–333, 1982.

32. Servatius RJ, Beck KD, Moldow RL, et al: A stress-induced anxious state in male rats: corticotropin-releasing hormone induces persistent changes in associative learning and startle reactivity. *Biol Psychiatry* 57:865–872, 2005.

33. Hsu SY, Hsueh AJ: Human stresscopin and stresscopin-related peptide are selective ligands for the type 2 corticotropin-releasing hormone receptor. *Nat Med* 7:605–611, 2001.

34. Valentino RJ, Foote SL, Aston-Jones G: Corticotropin-releasing factor activates noradrenergic neurons of the locus coeruleus. *Brain Res* 270:363–367, 1983.

35. Jansen AS, Nguyen XV, Karpitskiy V, et al: Central command neurons of the sympathetic nervous system: basis of the fight-or-flight response. *Science* 270:644–646, 1995.

36. Cunningham ET, Jr, Bohn MC, et al: Organization of adrenergic inputs to the paraventricular and supraoptic nuclei of the hypothalamus in the rat. *J Comp Neurol* 292:651–667, 1990.

37. Madden KS, Moynihan JA, Brenner GJ, et al: Sympathetic nervous system modulation of the immune system. III: Alterations in T and B cell proliferation and differentiation in vitro following chemical sympathectomy. *J Neuroimmunol* 49:77–87, 1994.

38. Harle P, Mobius D, Carr DJ, et al: An opposing time-dependent immune-modulating effect of the sympathetic nervous system conferred by altering the cytokine profile in the local lymph nodes and spleen of mice with type II collagen-induced arthritis. *Arthritis Rheum* 52:1305–1313, 2005.

39. Li X, Taylor S, Zegarelli B, et al: The induction of splenic suppressor T cells through an immune-privileged site requires an intact sympathetic nervous system. *J Neuroimmunol* 153:40–49, 2004.

40. Tracey KJ: The inflammatory reflex. *Nature* 420:853–859, 2002.

41. Sanders VM, Kasprowicz DJ, Kohm AP, et al: *Neurotransmitter receptors on lymphocytes and other lymphoid cells*, New York, 2001, New York.

42. Fleshner M, Laudenslager ML: Psychoneuroimmunology: then and now. *Behav Cogn Neurosci Rev* 3:114–130, 2004.

43. Christian CA, Moenter SM: The neurobiology of preovulatory and estradiol-induced gonadotropin-releasing hormone surges. *Endocr Rev* 31:544–577, 2010.

44. Christian CA, Glidewell-Kenney C, Jameson JL, et al: Classical estrogen receptor alpha signaling mediates negative and positive feedback on gonadotropin-releasing hormone neuron firing. *Endocrinology* 149:5328–5334, 2008.

45. Szoltys M, Galas J, Jablonka A, et al: Some morphological and hormonal aspects of ovulation and superovulation in the rat. *J Endocrinol* 141:91–100, 1994.

46. Galas J, Slomczynska M, Knapczyk-Stwora K, et al: Steroid levels and the spatiotemporal expression of steroidogenic enzymes and androgen receptor in developing ovaries of immature rats. *Acta Histochem* 114:207–214, 2012.

47. Szeto A, Gonzales JA, Spitzer SB, et al: Circulating levels of glucocorticoid hormones in WHHL and NZW rabbits: circadian cycle and response to repeated social encounter. *Psychoneuroendocrinology* 29:861–866, 2004.

48. Lee TJ, Chang HH, Lee HC, et al: Axo-axonal interaction in autonomic regulation of the cerebral circulation. *Acta Physiol (Oxf)* 203:25–35, 2011.

49. Evans RM: The nuclear receptor superfamily: a Rosetta stone for physiology. *Mol Endocrinol* 19:1429–1438, 2005.

50. Adcock IM: Molecular mechanisms of glucocorticosteroid actions. *Pulm Pharmacol Ther* 13:115–126, 2000.

51. Schaaf MJ, Cidlowski JA: Molecular mechanisms of glucocorticoid action and resistance. *J Steroid Biochem Mol Biol* 83:37–48, 2002.

52. Funder JW: Mineralocorticoids, glucocorticoids, receptors and response elements. *Science* 259:1132–1133, 1993.

53. Ou XM, Storring JM, Kushwaha N, et al: Heterodimerization of mineralocorticoid and glucocorticoid receptors at a novel negative response element of the 5-HT1A receptor gene. *J Biol Chem* 276:14299–14307, 2001.

54. Savory JG, Prefontaine GG, Lamprecht C, et al: Glucocorticoid receptor homodimers and glucocorticoid-mineralocorticoid receptor heterodimers form in the cytoplasm through alternative dimerization interfaces. *Mol Cell Biol* 21:781–793, 2001.

55. Shi Y, Downes M, Xie W, et al: Sharp, an inducible cofactor that integrates nuclear receptor repression and activation. *Genes Dev* 15:1140–1151, 2001.

56. Kovacs JJ, Murphy PJ, Gaillard S, et al: HDAC6 regulates Hsp90 acetylation and chaperone-dependent activation of glucocorticoid receptor. *Mol Cell* 18:601–607, 2005.

57. Tao Y, Williams-Skipp C, Scheinman RI: Mapping of glucocorticoid receptor DNA binding domain surfaces contributing to transrepression of NF-kappa B and induction of apoptosis. *J Biol Chem* 276:2329–2332, 2001.

58. De Bosscher K, Vanden Berghe W, Haegeman G: The interplay between the glucocorticoid receptor and nuclear factor-kappaB or activator protein-1: molecular mechanisms for gene repression. *Endocr Rev* 24:488–522, 2003.

59. Moldow RL, Beck KD, Weaver S, et al: Blockage of glucocorticoid, but not mineralocorticoid receptors prevents the persistent increase in

circulating basal corticosterone concentrations following stress in the rat. *Neurosci Lett* 374:25–28, 2005.

60. Dhabhar FS, McEwen BS: Enhancing versus suppressive effects of stress hormones on skin immune function. *Proc Natl Acad Sci U S A* 96:1059–1064, 1999.

61. Selye H: Variations in organ size caused by chronic treatment with adrenal cortical compounds: an example of a dissociated adaptation to a hormone. *J Anat* 76:94–99, 1941.

62. Franchimont D, Galon J, Gadina M, et al: Inhibition of Th1 immune response by glucocorticoids: dexamethasone selectively inhibits IL-12-induced Stat4 phosphorylation in T lymphocytes. *J Immunol* 164:1768–1774, 2000.

63. Hara Y, Shiraishi A, Kobayashi T, et al: Alteration of TLR3 pathways by glucocorticoids may be responsible for immunosusceptibility of human corneal epithelial cells to viral infections. *Mol Vis* 15:937–948, 2009.

64. Papasian CJ, Qureshi N, Morrison DC: Endogenous and exogenous glucocorticoids in experimental enterococcal infection. *Clin Vaccine Immunol* 13:349–355, 2006.

65. Vacchio MS, Ashwell JD: Glucocorticoids and thymocyte development. *Semin Immunol* 12:475–485, 2000.

66. Tuckermann JP, Kleiman A, Moriggl R, et al: Macrophages and neutrophils are the targets for immune suppression by glucocorticoids in contact allergy. *J Clin Invest* 117:1381–1390, 2007.

67. Tait AS, Butts CL, Sternberg EM: The role of glucocorticoids and progestins in inflammatory, autoimmune, infectious disease. *J Leukoc Biol* 84:924–931, 2008.

68. Raja Gabaglia C, Diaz de Durana Y, Graham FL, et al: Attenuation of the glucocorticoid response during Ad5IL-12 adenovirus vector treatment enhances natural killer cell-mediated killing of MHC class I-negative LNCaP prostate tumors. *Cancer Res* 67:2290–2297, 2007.

69. Adcock IM, Caramori G, Ito K: New insights into the molecular mechanisms of corticosteroids actions. *Curr Drug Targets* 7:649–660, 2006.

70. Kay AB: The role of eosinophils in the pathogenesis of asthma. *Trends Mol Med* 11:148–152, 2005.

71. Adcock IM, Marwick J, Casolari P, et al: Mechanisms of corticosteroid resistance in severe asthma and chronic obstructive pulmonary disease (COPD). *Curr Pharm Des* 16:3554–3573, 2010.

72. Jeffery P: Anti-inflammatory effects of inhaled corticosteroids in chronic obstructive pulmonary disease: similarities and differences to asthma. *Expert Opin Investig Drugs* 14:619–632, 2005.

73. Schroeder JT, MacGlashan DW, Jr, MacDonald SM, et al: Regulation of IgE-dependent IL-4 generation by human basophils treated with glucocorticoids. *J Immunol* 158:5448–5454, 1997.

74. Woltman AM, Massacrier C, de Fijter JW, et al: Corticosteroids prevent generation of CD34+-derived dermal dendritic cells but do not inhibit Langerhans cell development. *J Immunol* 168:6181–6188, 2002.

75. Yawalkar N, Karlen S, Egli F, et al: Down-regulation of IL-12 by topical corticosteroids in chronic atopic dermatitis. *J Allergy Clin Immunol* 106:941–947, 2000.

76. de Jong EC, Vieira PL, Kalinski P, et al: Corticosteroids inhibit the production of inflammatory mediators in immature monocyte-derived DC and induce the development of tolerogenic DC3. *J Leukoc Biol* 66:201–204, 1999.

77. Lin SJ, Chang LY, Yan DC, et al: Decreased intercellular adhesion molecule-1 (CD54) and L-selectin (CD62L) expression on peripheral blood natural killer cells in asthmatic children with acute exacerbation. *Allergy* 58:67–71, 2003.

78. Cupps TR, Fauci AS: Corticosteroid-mediated immunoregulation in man. *Immunol Rev* 65:133–155, 1982.

79. Elenkov IJ, Chrousos GP: Stress hormones, proinflammatory and anti-inflammatory cytokines, and autoimmunity. *Ann N Y Acad Sci* 966:290–303, 2002.

80. Munck A, Guyre PM: Glucocorticoid physiology, pharmacology and stress. *Adv Exp Med Biol* 196:81–96, 1986.

81. Snijdewint FG, Kapsenberg ML, Wauben-Penris PJ, et al: Corticosteroids class-dependently inhibit in vitro Th1- and Th2-type cytokine production. *Immunopharmacology* 29:93–101, 1995.

82. Igarashi H, Kouro T, Yokota T, et al: Age and stage dependency of estrogen receptor expression by lymphocyte precursors. *Proc Natl Acad Sci U S A* 98:15131–15136, 2001.

83. Medina KL, Garrett KP, Thompson LF, et al: Identification of very early lymphoid precursors in bone marrow and their regulation by estrogen. *Nat Immunol* 2:718–724, 2001.

84. Nalbandian G, Kovats S: Understanding sex biases in immunity: effects of estrogen on the differentiation and function of antigen-presenting cells. *Immunol Res* 31:91–106, 2005.

85. Medina KL, Kincade PW: Pregnancy-related steroids are potential negative regulators of B lymphopoiesis. *Proc Natl Acad Sci U S A* 91:5382–5386, 1994.

86. Fukuzuka K, Edwards CK, 3rd, Clare-Salzer M, et al: Glucocorticoid and Fas ligand induced mucosal lymphocyte apoptosis after burn injury. *J Trauma* 49:710–716, 2000.

87. Fukuzuka K, Edwards CK, 3rd, Clare-Salzler M, et al: Glucocorticoid-induced, caspase-dependent organ apoptosis early after burn injury. *Am J Physiol Regul Integr Comp Physiol* 278:R1005–R1018, 2000.

88. Cutolo M, Seriolo B, Villaggio B, et al: Androgens and estrogens modulate the immune and inflammatory responses in rheumatoid arthritis. *Ann N Y Acad Sci* 966:131–142, 2002.

89. Isgor C, Cecchi M, Kabbaj M, et al: Estrogen receptor beta in the paraventricular nucleus of hypothalamus regulates the neuroendocrine response to stress and is regulated by corticosterone. *Neuroscience* 121:837–845, 2003.

90. Tayade C, Black GP, Fang Y, et al: Differential gene expression in endometrium, endometrial lymphocytes, trophoblasts during successful and abortive embryo implantation. *J Immunol* 176:148–156, 2006.

91. Mulac-Jericevic B, Mullinax RA, DeMayo FJ, et al: Subgroup of reproductive functions of progesterone mediated by progesterone receptor-B isoform. *Science* 289:1751–1754, 2000.

92. Bakardjiev AI, Theriot JA, Portnoy DA: *Listeria monocytogenes* traffics from maternal organs to the placenta and back. *PLoS Pathog* 2:e66, 2006.

93. Buyon JP, Korchak HM, Rutherford LE, et al: Female hormones reduce neutrophil responsiveness in vitro. *Arthritis Rheum* 27:623–630, 1984.

94. Geraldes P, Gagnon S, Hadjadj S, et al: Estradiol blocks the induction of CD40 and CD40L expression on endothelial cells and prevents neutrophil adhesion: an ERalpha-mediated pathway. *Cardiovasc Res* 71:566–573, 2006.

95. Staples LD, Heap RB, Wooding FB, et al: Migration of leucocytes into the uterus after acute removal of ovarian progesterone during early pregnancy in the sheep. *Placenta* 4:339–349, 1983.

96. Gottshall SL, Hansen PJ: Regulation of leucocyte subpopulations in the sheep endometrium by progesterone. *Immunology* 76:636–641, 1992.

97. Deshpande R, Khalili H, Pergolizzi RG, et al: Estradiol down-regulates LPS-induced cytokine production and NFκB activation in murine macrophages. *Am J Reprod Immunol* 38:46–54, 1997.

98. Jin L, Ai X, Liu L, et al: Testosterone induces apoptosis via Fas/FasL-dependent pathway in bone marrow-derived macrophages. *Methods Find Exp Clin Pharmacol* 28:283–293, 2006.

99. Tibbetts TA, Conneely OM, O'Malley BW: Progesterone via its receptor antagonizes the pro-inflammatory activity of estrogen in the mouse uterus. *Biol Reprod* 60:1158–1165, 1999.

100. Enomoto LM, Kloberdanz KJ, Mack DG, et al: Ex vivo effect of estrogen and progesterone compared with dexamethasone on cell-mediated immunity of HIV-infected and uninfected subjects. *J Acquir Immune Defic Syndr* 45:137–143, 2007.

101. Pepe M, Jirillo E, Covelli V: In vitro infection of human monocyte-derived dendritic cells with *Candida albicans*: receptorial involvement and therapeutic implications. *Curr Pharm Des* 12:4263–4269, 2006.

102. Mingjia L, Short R: How oestrogen or progesterone might change a woman's susceptibility to HIV-1 infection. *Aust N Z J Obstet Gynaecol* 42:472–475, 2002.

103. Kaushic C, Zhou F, Murdin AD, et al: Effects of estradiol and progesterone on susceptibility and early immune responses to *Chlamydia trachomatis* infection in the female reproductive tract. *Infect Immun* 68:4207–4216, 2000.

104. Elloso MM, Phiel K, Henderson RA, et al: Suppression of experimental autoimmune encephalomyelitis using estrogen receptor-selective ligands. *J Endocrinol* 185:243–252, 2005.

105. van den Broek HH, Damoiseaux JG, De Baets MH, et al: The influence of sex hormones on cytokines in multiple sclerosis and experimental autoimmune encephalomyelitis: a review. *Mult Scler* 11:349–359, 2005.

106. Nilsson M, Dahlman-Wright K, Gustafsson JA: Nuclear receptors in disease: the oestrogen receptors. *Essays Biochem* 40:157–167, 2004.

107. Danel L, Souweine G, Monier JC, et al: Specific estrogen binding sites in human lymphoid cells and thymic cells. *J Steroid Biochem* 18:559–563, 1983.

108. Butts CL, Shukair SA, Duncan KM, et al: Progesterone inhibits mature rat dendritic cells in a receptor-mediated fashion. *Int Immunol* 19:287–296, 2007.

109. Piccinni MP: Role of immune cells in pregnancy. *Autoimmunity* 36:1–4, 2003.

110. Polanczyk MJ, Hopke C, Huan J, et al: Enhanced FoxP3 expression and Treg cell function in pregnant and estrogen-treated mice. *J Neuroimmunol* 170:85–92, 2005.

111. Buyon JP, Petri MA, Kim MY, et al: The effect of combined estrogen and progesterone hormone replacement therapy on disease activity in systemic lupus erythematosus: a randomized trial. *Ann Intern Med* 142:953–962, 2005.

112. Petri M, Kim MY, Kalunian KC, et al: Combined oral contraceptives in women with systemic lupus erythematosus. *N Engl J Med* 353:2550–2558, 2005.

113. Perez SD, Silva D, Millar AB, et al: Sympathetic innervation of the spleen in male Brown Norway rats: a longitudinal aging study. *Brain Res* 1302:106–117, 2009.

114. Di Comite G, Grazia Sabbadini M, Corti A, et al: Conversation galante: how the immune and the neuroendocrine systems talk to each other. *Autoimmun Rev* 7:23–29, 2007.

115. Sanders VM, Straub RH: Norepinephrine, the beta-adrenergic receptor, immunity. *Brain Behav Immun* 16:290–332, 2002.

116. Madden KS, Sanders VM, Felten DL: Catecholamine influences and sympathetic neural modulation of immune responsiveness. *Annu Rev Pharmacol Toxicol* 35:417–448, 1995.

117. Felten DL: Neurotransmitter signaling of cells of the immune system: important progress, major gaps. *Brain Behav Immun* 5:2–8, 1991.

118. Sanders JD, Happe HK, Bylund DB, et al: Differential effects of neonatal norepinephrine lesions on immediate early gene expression in developing and adult rat brain. *Neuroscience* 157:821–832, 2008.

119. Sanders RD, Brian D, Maze M: G-protein-coupled receptors. *Handb Exp Pharmacol* (182):93–117, 2008.

120. Elenkov IJ, Chrousos GP: Stress hormones, Th1/Th2 patterns, pro/anti-inflammatory cytokines and susceptibility to disease. *Trends Endocrinol Metab* 10:359–368, 1999.

121. Green PG, Luo J, Heller PH, et al: Further substantiation of a significant role for the sympathetic nervous system in inflammation. *Neuroscience* 55:1037–1043, 1993.

122. Sundar SK, Cierpial MA, Kilts C, et al: Brain IL-1-induced immunosuppression occurs through activation of both pituitary-adrenal axis and sympathetic nervous system by corticotropin-releasing factor. *J Neurosci* 10:3701–3706, 1990.

123. Green PG, Luo J, Heller P, et al: Modulation of bradykinin-induced plasma extravasation in the rat knee joint by sympathetic co-transmitters. *Neuroscience* 52:451–458, 1993.

124. Felten DL, Felten SY, Bellinger DL, et al: Noradrenergic and peptidergic innervation of secondary lymphoid organs: role in experimental rheumatoid arthritis. *Eur J Clin Invest* 22(Suppl 1):37–41, 1992.

125. Helme RD, Andrews PV: The effect of nerve lesions on the inflammatory response to injury. *J Neurosci Res* 13:453–459, 1985.

126. Levine JD, Dardick SJ, Roizen MF, et al: Contribution of sensory afferents and sympathetic efferents to joint injury in experimental arthritis. *J Neurosci* 6:3423–3429, 1986.

127. Chelmicka-Schorr E, Kwasniewski MN, Thomas BE, et al: The beta-adrenergic agonist isoproterenol suppresses experimental allergic encephalomyelitis in Lewis rats. *J Neuroimmunol* 25:203–207, 1989.

128. Levine JD, Coderre TJ, Helms C, et al: Beta 2-adrenergic mechanisms in experimental arthritis. *Proc Natl Acad Sci U S A* 85:4553–4556, 1988.

129. Thayer JF, Loerbroks A, Sternberg EM: Inflammation and cardiorespiratory control: the role of the vagus nerve. *Respir Physiol Neurobiol* 178:387–394, 2011.

130. Tracey KJ: Understanding immunity requires more than immunology. *Nat Immunol* 11:561–564, 2010.

131. Rosas-Ballina M, Tracey KJ: Cholinergic control of inflammation. *J Intern Med* 265:663–676, 2009.

132. Watkins LR, Maier SF: Implications of immune-to-brain communication for sickness and pain. *Proc Natl Acad Sci U S A* 96:7710–7713, 1999.

133. Laye S, Bluthe RM, Kent S, et al: Subdiaphragmatic vagotomy blocks induction of IL-1 beta mRNA in mice brain in response to peripheral LPS. *Am J Physiol* 268:R1327–1331, 1995.

134. Bulloch K, Sadamatsu M, Patel A, et al: Calcitonin gene-related peptide immunoreactivity in the hippocampus and its relationship to cellular changes following exposure to trimethylin. *J Neurosci Res* 55:441–457, 1999.

135. Tan YR, Yang T, Liu SP, et al: Pulmonary peptidergic innervation remodeling and development of airway hyperresponsiveness induced by RSV persistent infection. *Peptides* 29:47–56, 2008.

136. Kulka M, Sheen CH, Tancowny BP, et al: Neuropeptides activate human mast cell degranulation and chemokine production. *Immunology* 123:398–410, 2008.

137. Levine JD, Clark R, Devor M, et al: Intraneuronal substance P contributes to the severity of experimental arthritis. *Science* 226:547–549, 1984.

138. Weinstock JV: Neuropeptides and the regulation of granulomatous inflammation. *Clin Immunol Immunopathol* 64:17–22, 1992.

139. Pothoulakis C, Castagliuolo I, LaMont JT, et al: CP-96,345, a substance P antagonist, inhibits rat intestinal responses to *Clostridium difficile* toxin A but not cholera toxin. *Proc Natl Acad Sci U S A* 91:947–951, 1994.

140. Bulloch K, Milner TA, Prasad A, et al: Induction of calcitonin gene-related peptide-like immunoreactivity in hippocampal neurons following ischemia: a putative regional modulator of the CNS injury/immune response. *Exp Neurol* 150:195–205, 1998.

141. Carucci JA, Ignatius R, Wei Y, et al: Calcitonin gene-related peptide decreases expression of HLA-DR and CD86 by human dendritic cells and dampens dendritic cell-driven T cell-proliferative responses via the type I calcitonin gene-related peptide receptor. *J Immunol* 164:3494–3499, 2000.

142. Delgado M, Munoz-Elias EJ, Gomariz RP, et al: Vasoactive intestinal peptide and pituitary adenylate cyclase-activating polypeptide enhance IL-10 production by murine macrophages: in vitro and in vivo studies. *J Immunol* 162:1707–1716, 1999.

143. Hernanz A, Tato E, De la Fuente M, et al: Differential effects of gastrin-releasing peptide, neuropeptide Y, somatostatin and vasoactive intestinal peptide on interleukin-1 beta, interleukin-6 and tumor necrosis factor-alpha production by whole blood cells from healthy young and old subjects. *J Neuroimmunol* 71:25–30, 1996.

144. Martinez C, Delgado M, Pozo D, et al: Vasoactive intestinal peptide and pituitary adenylate cyclase-activating polypeptide modulate endotoxin-induced IL-6 production by murine peritoneal macrophages. *J Leukoc Biol* 63:591–601, 1998.

145. Sternberg EM, Chrousos GP, Wilder RL, et al: The stress response and the regulation of inflammatory disease. *Ann Intern Med* 117:854–866, 1992.

146. Wick G, Hu Y, Schwarz S, et al: Immunoendocrine communication via the hypothalamo-pituitary-adrenal axis in autoimmune diseases. *Endocr Rev* 14:539–563, 1993.

147. Reichlin S: Neuroendocrine-immune interactions. *N Engl J Med* 329:1246–1253, 1993.

148. Eskandari F, Webster JI, Sternberg EM: Neural immune pathways and their connection to inflammatory diseases. *Arthritis Res Ther* 5:251–265, 2003.

149. Marques-Deak A, Cizza G, Sternberg E: Brain-immune interactions and disease susceptibility. *Mol Psychiatry* 10:239–250, 2005.

150. Wick G, Sgonc R, Lechner O: Neuroendocrine-immune disturbances in animal models with spontaneous autoimmune diseases. *Ann N Y Acad Sci* 840:591–598, 1998.

151. Sternberg EM, Hill JM, Chrousos GP, et al: Inflammatory mediator-induced hypothalamic-pituitary-adrenal axis activation is defective in streptococcal cell wall arthritis-susceptible Lewis rats. *Proc Natl Acad Sci U S A* 86:2374–2378, 1989.

152. Mason D, MacPhee I, Antoni F: The role of the neuroendocrine system in determining genetic susceptibility to experimental allergic encephalomyelitis in the rat. *Immunology* 70:1–5, 1990.

153. Edwards CK, 3rd, Yunger LM, et al: The pituitary gland is required for protection against lethal effects of *Salmonella typhimurium*. *Proc Natl Acad Sci U S A* 88:2274–2277, 1991.

154. Misiewicz B, Poltorak M, Raybourne RB, et al: Intracerebroventricular transplantation of embryonic neuronal tissue from inflammatory resistant into inflammatory susceptible rats suppresses specific components of inflammation. *Exp Neurol* 146:305–314, 1997.

155. Gross KL, Oakley RH, Scoltock AB, et al: Glucocorticoid receptor α isoform-selective regulation of antiapoptotic genes in osteosarcoma cells: a new mechanism for glucocorticoid resistance. *Mol Endocrinol* 25:1087–1099, 2011.

156. DeRijk RH, Schaaf M, de Kloet ER: Glucocorticoid receptor variants: clinical implications. *J Steroid Biochem Mol Biol* 81:103–122, 2002.

157. Greenstein B: Steroid resistance: implications for lupus. *Lupus* 3:143, 1994.

158. Rai T, Ohira H, Tojo J, et al: Expression of human glucocorticoid receptor in lymphocytes of patients with autoimmune hepatitis. *Hepatol Res* 29:148–152, 2004.

159. Jiang T, Liu S, Tan M, et al: The phase-shift mutation in the glucocorticoid receptor gene: potential etiologic significance of neuroendocrine mechanisms in lupus nephritis. *Clin Chim Acta* 313:113–117, 2001.

160. Lee YM, Fujiwara J, Munakata Y, et al: A mutation of the glucocorticoid receptor gene in patients with systemic lupus erythematosus. *Tohoku J Exp Med* 203:69–76, 2004.

161. Diaz-Borjon A, Richaud-Patin Y, Alvarado de la Barrera C, et al: Multi-drug resistance-1 (MDR-1) in rheumatic autoimmune disorders. Part II: increased P-glycoprotein activity in lymphocytes from systemic lupus erythematosus patients might affect steroid requirements for disease control. *Joint Bone Spine* 67:40–48, 2000.

162. Gladman DD, Urowitz MB, Doris F, et al: Glucocorticoid receptors in systemic lupus erythematosus. *J Rheumatol* 18:681–684, 1991.

163. Tanaka H, Akama H, Ichikawa Y, et al: Glucocorticoid receptor in patients with lupus nephritis: relationship between receptor levels in mononuclear leukocytes and effect of glucocorticoid therapy. *J Rheumatol* 19:878–883, 1992.

164. Du J, Li M, Zhang D, et al: Flow cytometry analysis of glucocorticoid receptor expression and binding in steroid-sensitive and steroid-resistant patients with systemic lupus erythematosus. *Arthritis Res Ther* 11:R108, 2009.

165. Hermann G, Tovar CA, Beck FM, et al: Restraint stress differentially affects the pathogenesis of an experimental influenza viral infection in three inbred strains of mice. *J Neuroimmunol* 47:83–94, 1993.

166. Brown DH, Sheridan J, Pearl D, et al: Regulation of mycobacterial growth by the hypothalamus-pituitary-adrenal axis: differential responses of *Mycobacterium bovis* BCG-resistant and -susceptible mice. *Infect Immun* 61:4793–4800, 1993.

167. Peralta-Ramirez MI, Jimenez-Alonso J, Godoy-Garcia JF, et al: The effects of daily stress and stressful life events on the clinical symptomatology of patients with lupus erythematosus. *Psychosom Med* 66:788–794, 2004.

168. Pawlak CR, Witte T, Heiken H, et al: Flares in patients with systemic lupus erythematosus are associated with daily psychological stress. *Psychother Psychosom* 72:159–165, 2003.

169. Da Costa D, Dobkin PL, Pinard L, et al: The role of stress in functional disability among women with systemic lupus erythematosus: a prospective study. *Arthritis Care Res* 12:112–119, 1999.

170. Ayala AR, Pushkas J, Higley JD, et al: Behavioral, adrenal, sympathetic responses to long-term administration of an oral corticotropin-releasing hormone receptor antagonist in a primate stress paradigm. *J Clin Endocrinol Metab* 89:5729–5737, 2004.

171. Dhabhar FS: Stress-induced augmentation of immune function—the role of stress hormones, leukocyte trafficking, and cytokines. *Brain Behav Immun* 16:785–798, 2002.

172. Unterbrink T, Hack A, Pfeifer R, et al: Burnout and effort-reward-imbalance in a sample of 949 German teachers. *Int Arch Occup Environ Health* 80:433–441, 2007.

173. Bauer J, Stamm A, Virnich K, et al: Correlation between burnout syndrome and psychological and psychosomatic symptoms among teachers. *Int Arch Occup Environ Health* 79:199–204, 2006.

174. Bella GP, Garcia MC, Spadari-Bratfisch RC: Salivary cortisol, stress, and health in primary caregivers (mothers) of children with cerebral palsy. *Psychoneuroendocrinology* 36:834–842, 2011.

175. Pruessner JC, Hellhammer DH, Kirschbaum C: Burnout, perceived stress, and cortisol responses to awakening. *Psychosom Med* 61:197–204, 1999.

176. Michelson D, Stone L, Galliven E, et al: Multiple sclerosis is associated with alterations in hypothalamic-pituitary-adrenal axis function. *J Clin Endocrinol Metab* 79:848–853, 1994.

177. Ma XM, Lightman SL: The arginine vasopressin and corticotrophin-releasing hormone gene transcription responses to varied frequencies of repeated stress in rats. *J Physiol* 510(Pt 2):605–614, 1998.

178. Whitnall MH, Anderson KA, Lane CA, et al: Decreased vasopressin content in parvocellular CRH neurosecretory system of Lewis rats. *Neuroreport* 5:1635–1637, 1994.

179. Schmidt ED, Janszen AW, Wouterlood FG, et al: Interleukin-1-induced long-lasting changes in hypothalamic corticotropin-releasing hormone (CRH)—neurons and hyperresponsiveness of the hypothalamus-pituitary-adrenal axis. *J Neurosci* 15:7417–7426, 1995.

180. DeRijk RH, Eskandari F, Sternberg EM: Corticosteroid resistance in a subpopulation of multiple sclerosis patients as measured by ex vivo dexamethasone inhibition of LPS induced IL-6 production. *J Neuroimmunol* 151:180–188, 2004.

181. Gutierrez MA, Garcia ME, Rodriguez JA, et al: Hypothalamic-pituitary-adrenal axis function and prolactin secretion in systemic lupus erythematosus. *Lupus* 7:404–408, 1998.

182. Tehrani MJ, Hu Y, Marquette C, et al: Interleukin-1 receptor deficiency in brains from NZB and (NZB/NZW)F1 autoimmune mice. *J Neuroimmunol* 53:91–99, 1994.

183. Hinrichsen H, Barth J, Ruckemann M, et al: Influence of prolonged neuropsychological testing on immunoregulatory cells and hormonal parameters in patients with systemic lupus erythematosus. *Rheumatol Int* 12:47–51, 1992.

184. Huang ST, Chen GY, Wu CH, et al: Effect of disease activity and position on autonomic nervous modulation in patients with systemic lupus erythematosus. *Clin Rheumatol* 27:295–300, 2008.

185. Harle P, Straub RH, Wiest R, et al: Increase of sympathetic outflow measured by neuropeptide Y and decrease of the hypothalamic-pituitary-adrenal axis tone in patients with systemic lupus erythematosus and rheumatoid arthritis: another example of uncoupling of response systems. *Ann Rheum Dis* 65:51–56, 2006.

186. Handa SR, Deepak KK, et al: Autonomic dysfunction in systemic lupus erythematosus. *Rheumatol Int* 26:837–840, 2006.

187. Harle P, Straub RH, Wiest R, et al: Increase of sympathetic outflow measured by NPY and decrease of the hypothalamic-pituitary-adrenal axis tone in patients with SLE and RA—another example of uncoupling of response systems. *Ann Rheum Dis* 65:51–56, 2006.

188. Bracci-Laudiero L, Aloe L, Lundeberg T, et al: Altered levels of neuropeptides characterize the brain of lupus prone mice. *Neurosci Lett* 275:57–60, 1999.

189. Bracci-Laudiero L, Aloe L, Stenfors C, et al: Development of systemic lupus erythematosus in mice is associated with alteration of neuropeptide concentrations in inflamed kidneys and immunoregulatory organs. *Neurosci Lett* 248:97–100, 1998.

190. Bangale Y, Cavill D, Gordon T, et al: Vasoactive intestinal peptide binding autoantibodies in autoimmune humans and mice. *Peptides* 23:2251–2257, 2002.

191. Cash JM, Crofford LJ, Gallucci WT, et al: Pituitary-adrenal axis responsiveness to ovine corticotropin releasing hormone in patients with rheumatoid arthritis treated with low dose prednisone. *J Rheumatol* 19:1692–1696, 1992.

192. Chikanza IC: Mechanisms of corticosteroid resistance in rheumatoid arthritis: a putative role for the corticosteroid receptor beta isoform. *Ann N Y Acad Sci* 966:39–48, 2002.

193. Johnson EO, Vlachoyiannopoulos PG, Skopouli FN, et al: Hypofunction of the stress axis in Sjögren's syndrome. *J Rheumatol* 25:1508–1514, 1998.

194. Buske-Kirschbaum A, Geiben A, Hollig H, et al: Altered responsiveness of the hypothalamus-pituitary-adrenal axis and the sympathetic adrenomedullary system to stress in patients with atopic dermatitis. *J Clin Endocrinol Metab* 87:4245–4251, 2002.

195. Wei T, Lightman SL: The neuroendocrine axis in patients with multiple sclerosis. *Brain* 120(Pt 6):1067–1076, 1997.

Chapter 14

Complement and SLE

Chau-Ching Liu, Susan Manzi, and Joseph M. Ahearn

HISTORICAL OVERVIEW

The complement system is arguably linked more intimately to systemic lupus erythematosus (SLE) than to any other human disease. This association has been recognized for decades and, until recently, was viewed as inexplicably paradoxical. Two seemingly irreconcilable early observations formed the foundation for this conundrum. First, in 1951 Vaughan was the first to assay serum complement in cases of SLE.[1] His team determined from four cases that a diminished total complement activity (CH_{50}) value correlated with disease activity. Elliott confirmed this finding and noted complement depression to be particularly associated with "albuminuria."[2] Lange discovered that complement was diminished in virtually all cases of acute, but not in chronic, glomerulonephritis, and that low complement was characteristic of SLE whether or not there was renal involvement.[3] Schur, in the largest study to that time, found CH_{50} to be below 50% of normal in 24% of patients with active SLE and in 46% of those with renal involvement, but in only 4% with inactive disease.[4] Schur suggested that complement levels were of particular value in following and evaluating patients with SLE, especially those with nephritis. These seminal observations were followed by a large body of work from many laboratories demonstrating that complement activation, reflected by diminished serum levels of C3, C4, and diminished CH_{50}, plays a major role in the tissue inflammation and organ damage that result from lupus pathogenesis.

Seemingly paradoxical to these findings was a second set of observations that demonstrated a strong association between hereditary homozygous deficiency of the classical pathway components and development of SLE.[5] In fact, inherited complement deficiency is still recognized as conferring the greatest known risk for development of SLE. Thus, for decades this paradox has been pondered. How is it that complement deficiency may be causative in SLE yet activation of this same inflammatory cascade is detrimental in patients who already have the disease?

Discoveries made during the past several years have begun to explain this perplexing link between complement and SLE and have concomitantly identified potential strategies and opportunities for mining the complement system for lupus genes, biomarkers, and therapeutics. In this chapter we review the biology of the complement system in relation to SLE, summarize common methods for measurement of complement, revisit the utility of complement assays in clinical management of SLE, and consider the potential for targeting the complement system for therapeutic intervention.

BIOLOGY OF THE COMPLEMENT SYSTEM

Investigation of complement originated in the late 19th century, when a heat-labile serum component with nonspecific activity (now known to be complement) was found capable of facilitating the killing of bacteria by a heat-stable serum component with antigen specificity (now known to be antibodies).[6] Subsequently, similar heat-labile and heat-stable factors were demonstrated to mediate lysis of erythrocytes sensitized by immune sera. In 1899, the term *complement* was introduced by Paul Ehrlich to emphasize that the heat-labile factors present in fresh serum "complemented" the heat-stable

specific factors mediating immune bacteriolysis and hemolysis.[7] Although its name may imply an ancillary role in immunity, later studies have demonstrated that the complement system is not only a vital component of host defense, through participation in innate immune response and adaptive immunity, but also an "accidental" culprit in the pathogenesis of SLE and other immune-inflammatory diseases.

Protein biochemistry studies conducted in the late 1960s and throughout the 1970s and 1980s have greatly advanced our understanding of the biochemical nature of the complement system.[8] The complement system comprises more than 30 plasma and membrane-bound proteins that form three distinct pathways (classical, alternative, and lectin) designed to protect against invading pathogens (Table 14-1 and Figure 14-1).[9-11] Many of the complement proteins exist in plasma as functionally inactive zymogens until appropriate events trigger their activation. Once activated, the proteins within each pathway undergo a cascade of sequential serine protease–mediated cleavage events, release biologically active fragments, and self-assemble into multimolecular complexes. In general, activation of the complement system can be viewed as a two-stage process. The first stage, unique to each of the three activation pathways, involves the early complement components that lead to the formation of the C3 convertases. The second stage, common to all three pathways once they converge, results in the formation of activation products (such as C3a and C5a) and a lytic complex consisting of the terminal complement components (see Figure 14-1).

Complement Activation Pathways

The classical pathway of complement activation is thought to play an important role in SLE pathogenesis. There are five proteins specific to activation of the classical pathway: C1q, C1r, C1s, C4, and C2 (see Figure 14-1). Activation of this pathway begins when C1q binds to the Fc portion of immunoglobulin G (IgG) (particularly IgG1 and IgG3) or IgM molecules that are bound to an antigen. The binding of C1q to an antigen-antibody complex (immune complex) leads to activation of C1r (a serine protease), which, in turn, leads to activation of C1s (also a serine protease). C1s enzymatically cleaves the other two classical pathway proteins, C4 and C2, generating and releasing two small soluble polypeptides, C4a and C2b. At the same time, this proteolytic cleavage leads to the formation of a surface-bound bimolecular complex, C4b2a, which functions as an enzyme and is referred to as the *classical pathway C3 convertase*. Studies have now shown that in addition to immune complexes, molecules of the "pentraxin" family (such as C-reactive protein and serum amyloid P) and DNA have also been shown capable of directly interacting with C1q and thus initiating the classical pathway.[11]

Unlike activation of the classical pathway, activation of the alternative pathway does not depend on antibodies but can be triggered by carbohydrates, lipid, and proteins found on surfaces of microbial pathogens. Three plasma proteins are unique to the alternative pathway: factor B, factor D, and properdin (see Figure 14-1). Normally, native C3 molecules undergo a so-called C3 tickover process, a continuous, low-rate hydrolysis of the thioester group that

TABLE 14-1 Components of the Human Complement System

Effector Protein	Function /Pathway Involved	M_r (kd)
C1q	Recognition, binding/classical	450 (a six-subunit bundle)
C1r	Serine protease/classical	85
C1s	Serine protease/classical	85
C4*	Serine protease (C4b); anaphylatoxin (C4a)/classical	205 (a 3-chain, αβγ, complex)
C2	Serine protease (C2a); small fragment with kinin activity (C2b)/classical	102
C3†	Membrane binding, opsonization (C3b); anaphylatoxin (C3a)/terminal	190 (a 2-chain, αβ, complex)
C5	MAC component (C5b), anaphylatoxin (C5a)/terminal	190 (a 2-chain, αβ, complex)
C6	MAC component/terminal	110
C7	MAC component/terminal	100
C8	MAC component/terminal	150 (a 3-chain, αβγ, complex)
C9	MAC component/terminal	70
Factor B	Serine protease/alternative	90
Factor D	Serine protease/alternative	24
Properdin	Stabilizing of C3bBb complexes/alternative	55 (monomers); 110, 165, 220, or higher (oligomers)
MBL	Recognition, binding/lectin	200-400 (2-4 subunits with three 32 KD chains each)
MASP-1	Serine protease/lectin	100
MASP-2	Serine protease/lectin	76

Soluble Regulatory Protein	Function	M_r (kd)
C1 inhibitor (C1-INH)	Removal of activated C1r and C1s from the C1 complex	105
C4-binding protein (C4bp)	Binding to C4b and displacing C2a in the C4bC2a complex; accelerating decay of C3 convertase; cofactor for factor I	570 (an 8-subunit complex)
Factor H	Displacing Bb in the C3bBb complex; cofactor for factor I	160
Factor I	Serine protease cleaving C3b and C4b	88
Clusterin	Preventing insertion of soluble C_{5b-9} complexes into cell membranes	70
S protein (vitronectin)	Preventing insertion of soluble C_{5b-9} complexes into cell membranes	84
Carboxypeptidase N	Inactivating anaphylatoxins	280 (a multi-subunit complex)

Membrane-Bound Regulatory Protein	Function	M_r (kd)
CD35 (CR1)	Binding C3b and C4b; cofactor for factor I	190-280 (four isoforms)
CD46 (MCP)	Promoting C3b and C4b inactivation by factor I	45-70 (different glycosylation forms)
CD55 (DAF)	Accelerating decay of the C3bBb and C4b2a complexes	70
CD59 (protectin; H19)	Preventing C9 incorporation into the MAC in a homologous restriction manner	18-20

Complement Receptor	Structure/M_r (kd)	Complement Ligand(s)‡
CR1 (CD35)	Single chain/190-280§	C3b; C4b; iC3b; C1q
CR2 (CD21)	Single chain/140-145	C3dg/C3d; iC3b;
CR3 (CD11b/CD18)	Two-chain, α/β/ 170/95	iC3b
CR4 (CD11c/CD18)	Two-chain, α/β/150/95	iC3b
cC1qR (calreticulin)	Single chain/60	C1q (collagenous tail); MBL
gC1qR	Tetramer/33 per subunit	C1q (globular head)
C1qRP	Single chain/126	C1q (collagenous tail)
C3a receptor	Single chain/50?	C3a
C5a receptor (CD88)	Single chain/50	C5a

DAF, decay-accelerating factor; kd, kilodalton; MAC, membrane attack complex; MASP, mannose-binding protein–associated serine protease; MBL, mannose-binding lectin; MCP, membrane cofactor protein; M_r, molecular mass (molecular weight); r, receptor.

*Serum concentration range considered normal: 20-50 mg/dL.

†Serum concentration range considered normal: 55-120 mg/dL.

‡Noncomplement ligands (e.g., Epstein-Barr virus for CR2 and fibrinogen for CR3 and CR4) not listed.

§Four allotypes with different numbers of SCR and displaying distinct M_r under reducing condition: CR1-A (220 kd), CR1-B (250 kd), CR1-C (190 d), and CR1-D (280 kd).

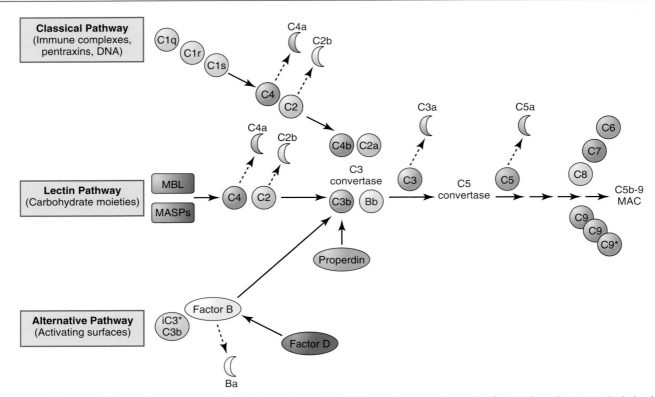

FIGURE 14-1 Overview of the complement system and activation pathways. C_{5b-9} MAC, membrane attack complex for C5b through C9; iC3*, hydrolized C3; MASP, mannose-binding protein–associated serine protease; MBL, mannose-binding lectin.

generates iC3* (hydrolyzed C3) and, subsequently, C3b fragments.[12] A fraction of these spontaneously generated C3b fragments may covalently attach to the surface of microbial pathogens and host cells via thioester bonds. The bound C3b molecules are capable of binding factor B. Once bound, factor B is cleaved into Ba and Bb fragments by factor D (a serine protease). While the small, soluble Ba fragment diffuses away from the activation site, the Bb fragment remains associated with C3b. Like the C4b2a complex in the classical pathway, the surface-bound C3bBb complex serves as the alternative pathway C3 convertase. The C3bBb complexes, if bound to host cells, are rapidly degraded by several regulatory proteins, thereby preventing self-damage. However, the C3bBb complexes associated with microbial pathogens are stabilized by the binding of properdin and prevented from being degraded by factor H and factor I. It has been suggested that properdin can also function as pattern-recognition molecules and initiate complement activation on apoptotic and necrotic cells.[13]

The lectin pathway shares several components with the classical pathway (see Figure 14-1). Initiation of the lectin pathway is mediated through the binding of mannose-binding lectin (MBL; also known as mannose-binding protein [MBP]) or ficolin to a variety of repetitive carbohydrate moieties such as mannose, *N*-acetyl-D-glucosamine, and *N*-acetyl-mannosamine, which are abundantly present on a variety of microorganisms.[14] MBL, a plasma protein composed of a collagen-like region and a carbohydrate-binding domain, is structurally similar to C1q. As in the case of the C1qC1rC1s complex, MBL forms complexes in the plasma with other proteins, such as mannose-binding protein–associated serine proteases (MASPs).[15] Under physiologic conditions, MBL does not bind to mammalian cells, probably because these cells lack mannose residues on their surfaces. Once bound to microbial pathogens, MASPs undergo conformational changes and become active enzymes that are capable of cleaving C4 into C4a and C4b fragments. At this point, the lectin pathway intersects with the classical pathway, and a C3 convertase, that is, the C4b2a complex, is eventually generated. One

study, however, has shown that MBL, in the absence of C4 or C2, is still capable of activating the complement system by engaging the alternative pathway.[16] This finding suggests that this unconventional lectin-initiated complement activation process may serve as a "backup" protective mechanism in individuals deficient in C4 or C2.

C3 convertases generated during the first stage of complement activation cleave C3, the central and most abundant component of the complement system. This proteolytic cleavage gives rise to a smaller C3a fragment and a larger C3b fragment. The C3b molecules associate with C4bC2a or with C3bBb complexes to form the classical and alternative C5 convertases, respectively. The C5 convertases cleave C5 to form C5a and C5b. C5b then recruits C6, C7, C8, and multiple molecules of C9, which together form the C_{5b-9} membrane attack complex (MAC; also called terminal complement complex [TCC]) on the surfaces of foreign pathogens (see Figure 14-1).

Regulators of Complement Activation

In humans and other mammals, complement activation is controlled by a multitude of regulatory proteins to ensure that this effective machinery is not inappropriately activated on host cells and tissues (see references 17 and 18 for reviews; see Table 14-1). To control the potentially harmful consequence of complement activation, soluble or cell-surface regulatory molecules need to act at multiple steps of the activation pathways using different mechanisms, functioning as proteolytic enzymes (carboxypeptidases, factor I), cofactors for proteolytic enzymes (factor H, complement receptor 1, membrane cofactor protein), protease inhibitors (C1 inhibitor), physical dissociators or competitive inhibitors of multimolecular convertases (C4-binding protein, decay-accelerating factor, factor H), or inhibitors of MAC formation and membrane insertion (CD59, homologous restriction factor). For example, C1 inhibitor (C1-INH) is capable of inactivating C1r, C1s, and MASPs, preventing the activation of the classical pathway and the lectin pathway. Further downstream, plasma carboxypeptidases can quickly remove an arginine residue from the

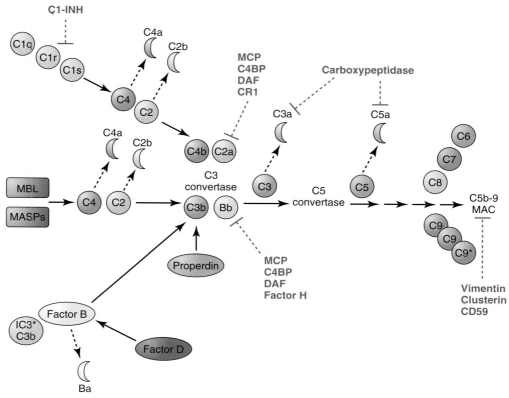

FIGURE 14-2 Overview of the regulation of complement activation. C1-INH, C1 inhibitor; C_{5b-9} MAC, membrane attack complex for C5b through C9; Cr1, complement receptor 1; DAF, decay-accelerating factor; iC3*, hydrolyzed C3; MASP, mannose-binding protein–associated serine protease; MBL, mannose-binding lectin.

C-terminus of C3a and C5a and generate C3a desArg and C5a desArg, which lose more than 90% of their original biological activities. C3b and C4b are also converted into proteolytic fragments such as iC3b, C3c, C3dg, C4c, and C4d by the serine protease factor I in the presence of cofactors such as factor H and membrane cofactor protein (MCP), thereby preventing the formation of C3 convertases. C3 convertases, once formed on cell surfaces, can be dissembled by the action of decay-accelerating factor (DAF; CD55), C4-binding protein (C4BP), and factor H. Finally, if all these gatekeepers fail, a membrane protein CD59 (also known as "protectin") will take action to prevent the formation of the MACs, the lytic "terminator" of cells, within the plasma membrane (Figure 14-2).

Receptors for Complement Proteins
Receptors for proteolytic fragments of complement proteins (e.g., C3b, C4b, iC3b, C3d) and, in some circumstances, for complement proteins with altered conformation (e.g., C1q) are expressed by a wide spectrum of cells and serve pivotal roles in executing many of the effector functions of complement previously described (see references 19 and 20 for reviews). Studies have now led to the identification of at least four receptors for C1q, cC1qR (calreticulin; a collectin receptor), gC1qR, C1qRp, and complement receptor 1 (CR1; also know as CD35). Binding of C1q-opsonized immune complexes to endothelial cells via C1q receptors has been reported to induce expression of adhesion molecules on endothelial cells and thus to enhance leukocyte binding/extravasation. On other cell types, C1q binding, presumably via distinct receptors, has been shown to enhance phagocytosis, increase generation of reactive oxygen intermediates, and activate platelets.

Receptors for C3a and C5a have been identified and cloned. The C3a receptor (C3aR) and C5a receptor (C5aR; CD88), which belong to the rhodopsin family of the G protein–coupled 7 transmembrane–domain receptors, are expressed on leukocytes, endothelial cells, podocytes, and proximal tubular epithelial cells in the kidney.[21] Interactions of C3aR and C5aR with their respective ligands (C3a and C3a desArg, and C5a and C5a desArg) are essential for the intracellular signaling processes that lead to leukocyte degranulation, production of cytokines, release of vasoactive substances, and other anaphylaxis and inflammatory responses.[22]

CR1 (CD35) and CR2 (CD21), two major receptors for C3- and C4-derived fragments, belong to the *regulators of complement activation* (RCA) family.[23] CR1 is widely expressed by erythrocytes, neutrophils, monocytes/macrophages, B lymphocytes, some T lymphocytes, and glomerular podocytes. CR1 primarily binds C3b and C4b. One important function of CR1 expressed on erythrocytes is to bind and clear immune complexes. CR1 also plays a role in regulation of complement activation by serving as a cofactor for factor I, which is responsible for cleaving C3b and C4b to iC3b and iC4b, respectively. CR2 is expressed mainly on B lymphocytes, activated T lymphocytes, and follicular dendritic cells, and binds primarily iC3b, C3dg, and C3d. CR2, together with its cognate complement ligands, is a critical link between the innate and adaptive immune systems. For example, coligation of CR2 (as part of the CD19/CD21/CD81 B-cell co-receptor complex) and B-cell receptors on the surfaces of B lymphocytes via the binding of C3d-decorated immune complexes or antigens enhances B-cell activation, proliferation, and antibody production. Antigens and immune complexes opsonized by C3-derived fragments can be retained in the germinal centers of secondary lymphoid follicles via binding to CR2 expressed on follicular dendritic cells; the retained antigens provide essential signals for survival and affinity maturation of B cells as well as for generation of memory B cells.[24]

CR3 and CR4 belong to the β_2 integrin family and are composed of two subunits, a common β chain (CD18) and a specific α chain (CD11b in CR3 and CD11c in CR4). These receptors are expressed on phagocytic cells (e.g., neutrophils, monocytes, and macrophages), antigen-presenting cells (e.g., dendritic cells), and follicular dendritic cells. CR3 and CR4 not only play important roles in phagocytic removal of C3-opsonized pathogens but also participate in mediating adhesion of mononuclear phagocytes to endothelial cells.

Effector Functions of Complement

The complement system is traditionally thought to have the following four biological functions in protecting against invasion by pathogens: (1) initiation of the inflammatory response, (2) opsonization and clearance of pathogens, (3) opsonization and clearance of immune complexes, and (4) osmotic lysis of invading microorganisms.[20,25] During SLE pathogenesis, complement activation and its inflammatory consequences are generated by self-antigens and autoimmune complexes rather than by foreign microbes.

The soluble proteolytic fragments, C3a, C4a, and C5a, are highly potent proinflammatory molecules. These *anaphylatoxins* act as potent chemoattractants to recruit leukocytes into sites of infection or injury and activate these cells by binding to specific receptors (e.g., C3aR and C5aR).[22] The larger fragments, C3b, C4b, and their derivatives (e.g., iC3b and iC4b), can remain bound to the surfaces of microbial pathogens (or autoantigens) and facilitate recognition and uptake of the opsonized particles by phagocytic cells. This function is mediated through the binding of these complement-derived fragments to CR1 (for C3b and C4b), CR3 (for iC3b), and CR4 (for iC3b) expressed on phagocytes.

The binding of C4b and C3b to immune complexes also prevents their aggregation into insoluble complexes and enhances their clearance. The clearance of C3b/C4b-opsonized immune complexes is mediated by erythrocytes that express CR1 and are capable of transporting immune complexes to macrophages of the reticuloendothelial system in the spleen and liver. In addition, C3b/C4b-opsonized immune complexes may bind to B lymphocytes, monocytes, and neutrophils. Phagocytosis of opsonized pathogens or immune complexes by neutrophils and monocytes is often accompanied by release of lysosomal enzymes. Finally, the C_{5b-9} MACs may perturb the osmotic equilibrium and/or disrupt the integrity of the surface membranes of target cells, thereby causing lysis of these cells.

Complement: An Important Bridge between Innate Immunity and Adaptive Immunity

For several decades, the role of the complement system was thought to be limited to the four effector functions already discussed. However, there has been an explosion in discovery of additional roles for complement. A growing number of studies have shown that innate immunity and adaptive immunity, the two arms of the immune system, collaborate in an intricate way to elicit efficient immune responses against infectious agents (see references 24, 26, and 27 for reviews).

The complement system—particularly C3, its derivative fragments, and their cognate receptors—plays an important role in this collaboration. First, C3 plays important roles in B-cell biology. Antigens (and immune complexes) decorated with C3d, the end cleavage product of C3 and a major ligand for CR2, are capable of cross-linking the B-cell receptors to the CR2/CD19/TAPA-1 co-receptor complexes and thus facilitating B-cell activation and enhancing humoral immune responses.[24] Second, antigens (and immune complexes) opsonized by C3 can be retained in the germinal centers of secondary lymphoid follicles via binding to CR2-expressing follicular dendritic cells; the retained antigens provide essential signals for survival and affinity maturation of B cells as well as for generation of memory B cells.[24] Third, complement is also involved in regulating T-cell activities.[26] For example, decay-accelerating factor appears to negatively regulate T cells and prevents T-cell overproliferation during an immune response[28]; C3a and C5a, via binding to their respective receptors expressed on T cells and antigen-presenting cells, may participate in maintaining T-cell viability, proliferation, and differentiation.[29] Fourth, opsonization of pathogens by complement components facilitates their uptake by phagocytes and antigen-presenting cells and thus may enhance presentation of antigens and initiation of specific immune responses. Fifth, complement activation products generated at sites of infection can recruit inflammatory cells and immune effector cells to help eliminate pathogenic antigens. In addition, complement appears to play an important role in opsonizing apoptotic cells and facilitating their clearance (see further discussion later).

COMPLEMENT AND SLE

The involvement of complement in the etiopathogenesis of SLE has been scrutinized over the past several decades. Suffice it to say that the role of complement in SLE is both complex and paradoxically intriguing. On the one hand, activation of the complement system is thought to play an important role in tissue inflammation/damage in SLE as a consequence of tissue deposition of immune complexes formed by autoantigens and autoantibodies.[30,31] On the other hand, a hereditary deficiency of a component of the classical pathway (C1, C2, or C4) has been associated with the development of SLE.[5] These seemingly discordant roles for complement may be reconciled by studies performed during the past several years. Those studies have demonstrated that, although the complement system plays a role in maintaining immune tolerance to prevent the development of SLE, it also participates in tissue-destructive inflammatory processes once SLE is established in a patient.

Immune Complex Abnormalities, Complement Activation, and Tissue Injury

Considerable evidence has indicated that many of the clinical manifestations and pathology in patients with SLE can be attributed to immune complex abnormalities (e.g., decreased solubility and impaired disposal of immune complexes) and consequent complement activation. In patients with SLE, decreased serum levels of C3 and C4 (due to genetic and/or acquired factors) may not permit sufficient binding of C3 and C4 fragments to the antigen-antibody lattice, thereby preventing the formation of small, soluble immune complexes.[32] Furthermore, reduced levels of CR1 on erythrocytes, frequently detected in patients with SLE, may lead to impaired binding, processing, and transporting of immune complexes to phagocytes of the reticuloendothelial system. Consequently, abnormally large quantities of immune complexes are likely to circulate for prolonged periods and form insoluble aggregates that may deposit in various tissues. Alternatively, insoluble immune complexes may form in situ as a result of the "planting" of autoantigens and subsequent binding of autoantibodies at specific loci. Deposited immune complexes do not seem to cause tissue damage directly but provide ample binding sites for complement components. The ensuing activation of the complement system causes the release of various mediators, promotes cellular infiltration and interaction, and culminates in tissue damage. The vascular endothelium and glomerular basement membrane appear to be highly susceptible to this mode of inflammatory damage. This pathogenic sequence provides a molecular basis underlying vasculitis and glomerulonephritis, two hallmark manifestations of SLE.

Complement Deficiency and SLE

Hereditary complement deficiency in humans has been reported for almost every component of the complement system.[33,34] Although the overall incidence of hereditary complement deficiency is low in the general population, a deficiency of any complement component is significantly associated with specific human diseases (Table 14-2). The clinical manifestations associated with the hereditary deficiency of individual complement components vary widely and depend on the position of the deficient component within the complement activation cascade.[34] Patients with homozygous deficiency of the early

TABLE 14-2 Complement Component Deficiencies and Associated Diseases

DEFICIENT COMPONENT	FUNCTIONAL DEFECT(S)	ASSOCIATED DISEASES
C1	Impaired clearance of immune complexes and apoptotic cells	Systemic lupus erythematosus (SLE)[*,†] Glomerulonephritis Bacterial infections
C2	Impaired clearance of immune complexes?	SLE[*,†] Glomerulonephritis Bacterial infections
C4	Impaired clearance of immune complexes	SLE[*,†] Glomerulonephritis Scleroderma Sjögren syndrome Bacterial infections
C3	Impaired opsonization; impaired clearance of apoptotic cells?	Bacterial infections[*,‡] SLE[§]
C5	Impaired chemotaxis; absence of lytic activity	Bacterial infections[c]
C6	Absence of lytic activity	Bacterial infections[§]
C7	Absence of lytic activity	Bacterial infections[§]
C8	Absence of lytic activity	Bacterial infections[§]
C9	Impaired lytic activity	Bacterial infections[§]
Properdin	Impaired alternative pathway activation	Bacterial infections[§]
Mannose-binding lectin (MBL)	Impaired lectin pathway activation	Bacterial and viral infections[*] SLE?
C1-inhibitor	Excessive C2 and kininogen activation	Hereditary angioedema[*] SLE?
Factor H	Excessive alternative pathway activation	Atypical hemolytic uremic syndrome (aHUS) Age-related macular degeneration (AMD) Bacterial infections
Factor I	Excessive alternative pathway activation	Bacterial infections
Membrane cofactor protein (MCP)	Excessive alternative pathway activity	aHUS AMD
CD55/CD59	Excessive MAC formation and cytolysis	Paroxysmal nocturnal hematuria

[*]Predominant phenotype.
[†]Risk hierarchy for development of SLE: C1 deficiency (~90%) > C4 deficiency (~80%) > C2 deficiency (~30%).
[‡]Most frequently infections with encapsulated bacteria, especially *Neisseria meningitidis.*
[§]SLE occasionally reported for patients with homozygous deficiency.

components of the classical pathway, C1, C4, and C2, are particularly at risk for development of SLE.[5]

In humans, there are two isotypes of C4, C4A and C4B.[35] Complete C4 deficiency (homozygous deficiency of both C4A and C4B) is extremely rare. It was first reported in 1974 in a patient who manifested an acute SLE-like disease,[36] and a total of 24 cases have since been reported.[5] However, homozygous deficiency of C4A alone and heterozygous deficiency of C4A and/or C4B is relatively frequent. Increased incidences of deficiency of C4A and, less commonly, of

C4B, have been reported in patients with SLE.[37] A review of clinical cases of SLE associated with complement deficiency revealed a hierarchical correlation between the position of the deficient component within the classical pathway and the prevalence of SLE. It has been estimated that SLE occurs in approximately 90%, 80%, and 30% of patients deficient in C1q, C4, and C2, respectively.[5] This risk for SLE in complement-deficient individuals is greater than concordance of this disease in monozygotic twins. This observation indicates that the classical complement pathway loci encode "lupus genes."

Clinically, patients with SLE associated with homozygous C1q or C1r/s deficiency usually present with symptomatic disease at an early age (before 20 years), have severe disease with prominent cutaneous manifestations, and do not exhibit the usual female predilection.[5,34] Similarly, SLE associated with homozygous C4 deficiency often occurs at an early age and manifests cutaneous lesions more frequently than renal disease. Patients with SLE and homozygous C2 deficiency also have less renal involvement but have more cutaneous involvement (especially photosensitivity) and arthralgia. Serologically, the prevalence of antinuclear antibodies (ANAs) and anti–double-stranded DNA (anti-dsDNA) antibodies is often lower in patients with complement deficiency–associated SLE than in patients with idiopathic SLE, but the presence of anti-Ro antibodies appears to be common in SLE associated with C2 or C4 deficiency.

In contrast to the high incidence of SLE and SLE-like disease in patients with homozygous deficiency of the classical pathway components, patients with homozygous C3 deficiency seldom have SLE. Of the reported 24 cases of C3 deficiency, only four patients were described to have SLE-like disease and all tested negative for ANA.[5] As for terminal complement components, there have been occasional case reports of patients with SLE and C6 deficiency, C7 deficiency, C8 deficiency, and C9 deficiency. However, the predominant phenotype of homozygous deficiencies of terminal complement components is the recurrence of infection (see Table 14-2).

MBL, the initiating component of the lectin pathway, is structurally homologous and functionally analogous to C1q. Polymorphisms in the promoter and coding regions of the MBL gene that lead to altered serum levels of MBL or encode defective MBL proteins incapable of activating the complement system have been reported. Like C1q deficiency, MBL deficiency has been associated with increased susceptibility to SLE.[38] Higher frequencies of an MBL gene variant that encodes a defective MBL protein (due to changes in amino acid residues 54 and 57) have been found in patients with SLE of different ethnic origins. Associations between low serum levels of MBL and SLE have also been reported. Clinically, MBL deficiency in patients with SLE appears to increase their susceptibility to infections.

In patients with SLE, autoantibodies against complement components have also been found to cause acquired complement deficiency. For example, C3 nephritic factor, an autoantibody capable of stabilizing the alternative pathway C3 convertase BbC3b, can cause consumption of complement proteins via unregulated activation of the alternative and terminal pathways.[39] Another autoantibody reactive with the first complement component, C1q, has been detected at increased frequencies in patients with SLE. A significant portion of patients with SLE also demonstrate functional C1q deficiency secondary to the presence of anti-C1q antibodies.[5] Although the pathophysiologic role of anti-C1q in SLE is largely unknown, its presence in patients with SLE has been associated with lupus nephritis.[40]

Possible Mechanisms Underlying the Complement Deficiency–SLE Association

Currently, there are three non–mutually exclusive hypotheses explaining the intriguing clinical association between complement deficiency and SLE. The first hypothetical mechanism envisions that impaired clearance of immune complexes in the absence of early complement components may trigger/augment the development of SLE. It is interesting to note that of the two isotypes of human C4, C4A has predominantly been implicated in the binding and solubilization of immune complexes.[41] Consequently, it is not unexpected that the prevalence of C4A deficiency is reportedly higher in patients with SLE than in the general population.[37] Several studies have demonstrated abnormal processing of immune complexes in such patients.[42] These studies showed that the initial clearance of immune complexes was impaired in the spleen, supporting the concept that impaired clearance of immune complexes may contribute to the development of SLE in the context of complement deficiency.

The second hypothetical mechanism, "impaired waste disposal," originated from the discovery that C1q can bind directly to apoptotic keratinocytes.[43] Subsequent observations in support of this hypothesis demonstrated that endothelial cells and monocytes that are undergoing apoptosis also bind C1q,[44] and this binding can subsequently trigger activation and deposition of C4 and C3 on these apoptotic cells.[45] Thus, apoptotic cells and blebs become opsonized and can be effectively taken up by phagocytic cells via a complement receptor–mediated mechanism.[45] During apoptosis, normally hidden intracellular constituents are often biochemically modified and redistributed/segregated into surface blebs of dying cells.[46] Impaired clearance of apoptotic cells due to complement deficiency may lead to persistence of such "altered-self" constituents, which may be recognized by the immune system, breach immune tolerance, and trigger autoimmune responses.[47] Indeed, it has been reported that immunization of mice with apoptotic cells can lead to the generation of anti-DNA antibodies in those mice.[48] Taken together, these studies suggest that complement is involved in facilitating the clearance of autoantigen-containing apoptotic bodies and therefore plays a pivotal role in maintaining immune tolerance.

Using a mouse model, Botto was the first to report accumulation of apoptotic cells in the kidneys and spontaneous development of autoimmune responses to nuclear autoantigens and glomerulonephritis in the absence of C1q.[49] Subsequently, Taylor reported similar, but less severe, defects in the clearance of apoptotic cells and spontaneous autoantibody production in C4-deficient mice.[50] Likewise, the persistence of apoptotic cells may lead to the development of autoimmunity and tissue damage in humans. Reduced phagocytic activity of neutrophils, monocytes, and macrophages of patients with SLE has been observed previously. Specifically, a reduced capacity of SLE-derived macrophages to phagocytose apoptotic cells was reported by Hermann.[51] Moreover, impaired clearance of iC3b-opsonized apoptotic cells in vitro through the use of monocyte-derived macrophages prepared from SLE patients has been reported. Evidence has also been generated in vivo to support impaired clearance of apoptotic cells in human SLE. Bermann reported an abnormal accumulation of apoptotic cells, accompanied by a significantly decreased number of tangible body macrophages (cells responsible for removing apoptotic nuclei), in the germinal centers of lymph nodes in a small subset of patients with SLE.[52] Collectively, data from both animal and human studies not only substantiate the observed hierarchical correlations between the deficiency of C1, C4, or C2 and the risks for development of SLE but also provide a strong mechanistic basis linking complement deficiency and SLE.

The third hypothetical mechanism relates to the capacity of complement to determine activation thresholds of B and T lymphocytes, suggesting that complement deficiency may alter the normal mechanism of negative selection of self-reactive lymphocytes (see reference 53 for a review). Because coligation of CR2 and BCR augments B-cell activation by decreasing the threshold for antigenic stimulation, it has been postulated that self-antigens not opsonized by C4b or C3b are unlikely to trigger sufficient activation of self-reactive B cells and that, as a result, these cells may escape negative selection. The escaped cells may become activated once they encounter relevant autoantigens in the periphery and thus may breach self-tolerance to autoantigens.

ANALYSES OF COMPLEMENT

During clinical inflammatory states in which complement activation occurs, for example, in flares of SLE, complement proteins would presumably be consumed at a rate proportional to activity of the disease. Thus, measuring complement activation may be useful for diagnosing disease, assessing disease activity, and determining response to therapy. Measuring complement activity and individual component levels is also essential for detecting and diagnosing complement deficiency. Conventionally, the complement system is measured by one of two types of assays. Functional assays assess the integrity of individual activation pathways, CH_{50} (indicative of the activity of the classical pathway) and AH_{50} (indicative of the activity of the alternative pathway). Immunochemical assays measure serum concentrations of individual complement components and their proteolytic fragments (hereafter referred to as "complement activation products"). Although complement analyses associated with measurement of serum C3 and C4 have been used in the clinic for decades, novel assays for detecting complement activation products and genetic analysis of complement genes have been utilized increasingly.[54]

Measurement of Complement Functional Activity

Assays that measure complement-mediated hemolysis, such as the CH_{50} and AH_{50} assays, are simple quantitative tests for functional complement components in serum or other fluid samples. These assays are useful not only in detecting complement deficiencies but also in guiding subsequent specific complement analyses. Because complement activation in SLE is triggered predominantly by immune complexes that active the classical pathway, it is common to perform the CH_{50} assay in patients with SLE. Complement activity is quantified by determining the dilution of a serum (or other fluid sample) required to lyse 50% of a fixed amount of sheep erythrocytes sensitized with anti-sheep IgM (for CH_{50} assays) or unsensitized rabbit erythrocytes (for AH_{50} assays) under standard conditions. The reciprocal of this dilution represents complement activity in units per milliliter of serum. For example, if a 1:160 dilution of a serum sample lyses 50% of erythrocytes, complement activity in that sample is reported as 160 CH_{50} U/mL.

A complement functional assay employing the enzyme-linked immunosorbent assay (ELISA) methodology has become available for general use.[55] This assay was developed on the basis of findings first reported by Zwirner that various complement components in the serum could deposit on a suitable surface during activation in vitro.[56] In principle, individual wells of a microtiter plate are coated with IgM, lipopolysaccharide, and mannan for activating the classical, alternative, and lectin pathways, respectively. Diluted serum is added to the plate to allow activation of the complement system. After incubation, complement activation is detected with the use of a monoclonal antibody reactive to a C9 neoepitope that is exposed upon incorporation of C9 into the MAC. The use of specific buffer (e.g., Ca^{++}/Mg^{++}–containing buffer for the classical pathway; Mg^{++}/ethylene glycol tetraacetic acid (EGTA)–containing buffer for the alternative pathway) and the addition of an anti-C1q antibody that inhibits the classical pathway (to allow activation of the lectin pathway only) grant the specificity for assessing each individual pathway and the feasibility of screening all three pathways in the same assay.

A general precaution should be taken during the collection and storing of samples for complement analysis. Because some complement components are heat-labile, serum samples, if not used immediately, should be stored at −70°C to optimize the preservation of complement proteins in functionally active forms.

Measurement of Complement Proteins

Measurement of serum levels of individual complement components is commonly used to diagnose and assess disease activity in SLE. These tests also help identify deficiencies of specific complement proteins.

Traditionally, serum is used for complement measurements. As cautioned previously for the functional assays, serum samples should be handled promptly and carefully to minimize possible degradation of complement proteins. A number of immunochemical methods, such as radial immunodiffusion and nephelometry, which are generally based on the antigen-antibody reactivity between complement components in the test sample and added anticomplement antibodies, are available for such measurement. The selection of a proper method depends on several factors, such as the level of sensitivity required, the availability of specific antibody, the number of samples, and the types of samples. In most clinical immunology laboratories, nephelometry is routinely used to measure complement components that are present at relatively high concentrations in the serum (e.g., C3 and C4). Other components that are usually present at low concentrations (e.g., C1, C2, C5 through C9, factor B, factor D, properdin) can be measured with the use of radial immunodiffusion (RID) or ELISA. When C3 and C4 concentrations are too low to be measured accurately by nephelometry—less than 20 mg/dL and less than 10 mg/dL, respectively—RID is the alternative method of choice. For other body fluids or cell culture supernatants, in which the levels of complement components may be very low, ELISA is the most practical method to use.

It should be pointed out that the commonly used methods employ polyclonal antibodies that recognize multiple protein variants. For example, the polyclonal antibodies used in assays quantifying C3 and C4 react with not only the native molecules but also their proteolytic fragments C3c and C4c, which are formed during activation (occurring in vivo or in vitro). Therefore, the results must be interpreted with caution.

Measurement of Complement Activation Products

Measurement of serum concentrations of complement components is essentially a static appraisal of an extremely dynamic process that includes activation, consumption, catabolism, and synthesis of these components. Because most complement components are acute-phase proteins and complement activation in vivo is often inevitably associated with inflammation (an acute-phase reaction), levels of complement components may remain within the normal range as a consequence of the counterbalance between ongoing consumption and increased production.[57] Unlike the native molecules, complement activation products (CAPs) are generated only when complement activation occurs, and thus acute-phase responses alone do not increase their concentrations. Therefore, direct determination of CAPs is thought to reflect more precisely the activation process of complement in vivo and hence the disease activity. Measures of CAPs in the plasma, yielded from activation of the classical pathway (C1rs–C1 inhibitor complex, C4a, C4b/c, and C4d), the alternative pathway (Ba, Bb, and C3bBbP), the lectin pathway (C4a, C4b/c, and C4d), and the terminal pathway (C3a, C3b/c, iC3b, C3d, C5a, and soluble c5b-9 [sC_{5b-9}]), are currently performed in many clinical immunology laboratories.

When CAPs are to be measured, plasma, instead of serum, should be used. Plasma (EDTA-anticoagulated) is used to avoid generating CAPs in vitro. Because only low levels of CAPs may be present in the circulation, even after significantly increased complement activation, ELISA and enzyme immunoassay (EIA) are the most practical methods for their measurement. Currently, many CAP assays are commercially available and utilize monoclonal antibodies that react specifically with neoepitopes that are triggered to be exposed on complement proteins upon activation. Because various CAPs have widely different half-life in vivo, it is important to carefully choose the molecules to be measured. Some CAPs, such as C3a, C4a, and C5a, are quickly converted to more stable, less active forms, such as C3a desArg, C4a desArg, and C5a desArg, respectively. The measurement of C5a is further compounded by its rapid receptor binding and therefore is difficult to measure in samples obtained in vivo. Moreover, in measurement of a CAP derived from a single complement protein (e.g., C3a or C4d), the fact that the amount of CAP generated during activation in vivo is proportional to the level of the parental molecule should be taken into consideration. Therefore, the ratio between the amounts of the CAP and the parental molecule is considered to be a more sensitive indicator of complement activation

than the CAP level alone. In comparison with single-molecule CAPs, CAPs that form multimolecular complexes usually have relatively long half-lives in the circulation. Examples of the latter include C1rs–C1 inhibitor complexes (products of classical pathway activation), C3bBbP complexes (products of alternative pathway activation), and sC_{5b-9} (the ultimate product of complement activation). The half-life of sC_{5b-9}, the soluble form of MAC that consists of C5b, C6, C7, C8, poly-C9, and the solubilizing protein, protein S, is 50 to 60 minutes. The MAC reflects the final activation step of all three pathways, so sC_{5b-9} is a particularly good candidate for general assessment of complement activation.

Proteomics Approaches for Complement Analyses

Proteomics technology has also been adopted for developing novel assays aimed at high-throughput analyses of various complement components in the serum. Although most novel assays, such as antibody-based microarrays, are still investigational, they have already shown great promise in multiplexed protein profiling. The antibody-based microarray technology has made significant advance over the past several years largely because of the availability of phage display libraries of recombinant single-chain variable region (scFv) of human antibodies that cover virtually any antigenic specificity. Through incubation of a small volume (as little as 1 μL) of serum on a microarray slide that has been spotted with scFv antibodies specific for the native form, the activation products, and the genetic polymorphic variants of various complement components, the presence of those molecules present can be simultaneously profiled and (semi-) quantified with use of a single serum sample.[58]

Conversely, a large number of serum samples can be screened for a specific complement protein or CAP of interest in a single microarray assay with use of a reverse format. In such a "reverse phase" microarray, multiple tested samples are spotted on a microarray slide and the slide is then incubated with an antibody recognizing a given protein. This format allows a large number of serum (or plasma) samples to be analyzed simultaneously under identical conditions. This method has been used for analysis of serum C3 and IgA,[59] suggesting its potential in high-throughput screening of sera from patients with SLE for specific proteins of clinical relevance.

In addition to profiling of protein expression, microarray technology may also be used for analysis of protein functional activity. A unique application of this approach, although not directly pertinent to complement measurement, is worth mentioning. Antigen microarrays in which various antigens are spotted on the slide are commonly used for profiling antibodies in serum samples. Prechl reported a novel "on-chip complement activation" feature of antigen microarrays, whereby antigen microarray slides were incubated with serum under conditions that favor complement activation, and the complement components deposited on antigen spots were detected with use of fluorescently labeled anticomplement antibodies.[60] Using two-color detection, this investigator found that antigens on the array slides either could bind and initiate complement activation directly or were recognized by antibodies that in turn activated the complement system. This method, if performed with an appropriate array of antigens, can be applied to detecting autoantibodies, particularly those that are capable of activating the complement cascade, present in the sera of patients with SLE (or other immune/inflammatory diseases).[61] Results obtained from this type of assay may help uncover the autoantibody profile that is relevant to the pathogenesis and clinical disease in a given patient.

SOLUBLE COMPLEMENT COMPONENTS AS BIOMARKERS FOR SLE
Soluble Complement Components and SLE Activity

Since Vaughan first reported an association between decreased complement proteins and active SLE five decades ago,[1] most patients with SLE are commonly monitored by measures of serum C3 levels, serum C4 levels, and CH_{50}. Numerous studies have been conducted to evaluate the potential utility of these assays in the diagnosis and monitoring of SLE. A succinct review of noteworthy data and precautions is offered here.

First, although it has generally been thought that decreased levels of complement components reflect activation of the classical and/or alternative pathway and correlate with clinical disease activity, there is still no consensus regarding the actual value of complement measures in SLE monitoring (see references 62 and 63 for reviews). Evidence in support of the usefulness of CH_{50}, C3, and C4 measurements include the following observations: (1) significantly decreased values of CH_{50} and serum C3 and C4 have been associated with increased SLE disease activity manifested by active nephritis and extrarenal involvement; (2) an increase/decrease in serum C3 levels has coincided significantly with remission/relapse of lupus nephritis; (3) a decrease in serum C4 levels has been noted to precede clinical exacerbation; (4) progressive fall of serum C3 or C4 levels may indicate an impending flare of SLE; and (5) serum C3 and C4 levels have frequently normalized on resolution of disease flares. On the contrary, the following observations argue against the usefulness of conventional complement measurement: (1) serum C4 and C3 levels have been found to remain normal in some patients during disease flares; (2) persistently low C4 levels have been detected in patients with inactive SLE; (3) decreases in C3 and C4 have not always been accompanied by increases in their split products (e.g., C3a, C3d, and C4d); and (4) the extent of changes in serum C3 and C4 levels do not correlate quantitatively with disease severity.

Second, although direct determination of complement activation products, in comparison with conventional complement measurement, should theoretically reflect more precisely the activation process of complement in vivo and thus, more specifically, clinically active disease, controversy regarding utility of these assays remains. Studies arguing in favor of the value of these assays have generally shown that plasma concentrations of complement split products, including C1–C1 inhibitor complex, C3a, C4a, C5a, C3d, C4d, C_{5b-9}, Ba, and Bb, increased before or during clinical exacerbation, and in some cases, the plasma levels correlated strongly with SLE disease activity scores. However, elevated C1-C1 inhibitor complex and C3d levels have been reported not only in almost all clinically ill patients but also in a significant fraction of patients with quiescent disease, suggesting that plasma levels of C1-C1 inhibitor complex and C3d bear little relationship to clinical activity. Moreover, inconsistent results have been reported for the utility of plasma levels of a given complement split product in differentiating patients with different disease activity or severity.

Complement Measurement in Lupus Nephritis

Lupus nephritis is one of the most serious clinical manifestations of SLE. Nephritic flare has been shown to be a predictor of a poor long-term outcome in patients with SLE. Measurements of complement components and activation products in the plasma or in the urine may be a useful tool for evaluating the extent of active inflammation in the kidneys. Patients with SLE who had renal involvement were found to more frequently have markedly reduced serum levels of C3 and C4 than patients with extrarenal involvement only. Patients with SLE with normal C3 and C4 levels were rarely found to have active nephritis. Therefore, the absence of a low C3 or C4 level in a patient with SLE may help exclude the possibility of ongoing renal disease. Low C3 and C4 levels may also be helpful in predicting long-term outcome in SLE, because low C3 levels have been reported to be predictive of persistently active glomerular disease and to be associated with end-stage renal disease. In addition to low C3 and C4 levels, very low levels of serum C1q were detected in patients with SLE who had, but not in those who did not have, active renal disease. In patients who had lupus nephritis requiring intense treatment, persistently low C1q levels before and after treatment have been shown to be indicative of continuously progressive damages in the kidneys and hence a poor outcome.

Because it seems likely that C3d generated in the kidney at sites of immune complex deposition would pass into the urine, measurement

of C3d in the urine has been pursued as a test for specific and accurate estimation of inflammation in the kidney. Kelly[64] and Manzi[65] have reported the detection of C3d in the urine in patients with SLE who had acute nephritis and in patients without evidence of renal involvement. These results suggest that urinary C3d may also come from nonrenal origins and thus may not be viewed as a specific marker of acute nephritis or a prognostic indicator of renal disease. Nevertheless, in the study by Manzi , urinary C3d was shown to be better than serum C3, plasma C4d, Bb, and C_{5b-9} in distinguishing patients with acute lupus nephritis from those without such disease activity.[65] Negi reported that C3d levels were elevated in the urine of patients with active disease, more so in patients with active lupus nephritis (0.87 arbitrary units [AU]/mL) than in patients with active extrarenal disease (0.31 AU/mL) or in patients with inactive lupus nephritis (0.06 AU/mL).[66] Taken together, these results suggest that increased levels of urinary C3d may reflect active SLE, particularly active lupus nephritis.

Problems Associated with Measurement of Soluble Complement Components

The discrepant reports on the value of measuring serum C4 and C3 to monitor disease activity of chronic inflammatory diseases such as SLE may originate from several factors that particularly confound measurement of C3 and C4 in disease. First, there is a wide range of variation in serum C3 and C4 levels among healthy individuals, and this range overlaps with that observed in patients with different diseases. Second, traditional concentration measurements reflect the presence of C3 and C4 protein entities irrespective of their functional integrity. Third, acute-phase responses during inflammation may lead to an increase in C4 and C3 synthesis,[57] which can counterbalance the consumption of these proteins during activation. Fourth, enhanced catabolism and altered synthesis of C3 and C4 have been reported to occur in patients with SLE, which clearly can interfere with static measures of serum C3 and C4 levels. Fifth, genetic variations such as partial deficiency of C4, which is commonly present in the general population and in patients with autoimmune diseases, may result in lower than normal serum C4 levels in some patients because of decreased synthesis rather than increased complement consumption during disease flares. Sixth, tissue deposition of immune complexes may result in complement activation at local sites in patients with certain diseases; such activity may not be faithfully reflected by the levels of complement products in the systemic circulation. Additional concerns should be raised about the measurements of complement activation products. As mentioned previously, many of the activation products have an undefined, most likely short, half-life both in vivo and in vitro. Moreover, complement activation can easily occur in vitro after blood sampling. In combination, these factors may hamper accurate measures of activation products that are derived solely from complement activation occurring in patients.

Given the numerous confounding factors summarized here, it is not surprising that irreconcilable results have prevailed in the research arena of complement and SLE disease activity. However, it should be kept in mind that complement measures may still be informative if they are performed chronologically in the same patient and interpretation is based on the specific genetic and clinical characteristics of the patient.

CELL-BOUND COMPLEMENT AS A BIOMARKER FOR SLE

The historical value yet inadequate performance of soluble complement components as lupus biomarkers provides strong incentive for developing the next generation of complement-based biomarkers for lupus diagnosis, monitoring, and/or stratification.

Rationale for Cell-Bound Complement Biomarkers

Complement proteins are abundant in the circulation and in tissues. Besides floating freely as soluble proteins, both the parental molecules and their activation derivatives can readily interact with cells circulating in the blood (e.g., erythrocytes and lymphocytes) or tissues (e.g., endothelial cells). Conceivably, complement activation products generated during SLE flares may bind to various circulating and tissue cells and alter physiologic functions of those cells. Studies have explored the hypothesis that cell-bound CAPs (CB-CAPs) may serve as biomarkers for SLE diagnosis and monitoring. This hypothesis was based on the following rationale. First, most soluble complement activation products are easily subjected to hydrolysis in circulation or in tissue fluids and thus are short-lived. Second, activation products derived from C3 and C4 contain thioester bonds capable of covalently attaching to circulating cells and may decorate the surfaces for the lifespans of those cells.[67] Third, many circulating cells express receptors for proteolytic fragments generated upon complement activation. Fourth, products of C4 activation are known to be present on surfaces of erythrocytes of healthy individuals.[68] Fifth, CB-CAPs on specific cell types might provide additional disease information by reflecting unique cellular properties such as the lifespans of erythrocytes and reticulocytes. Therefore, cell-bound complement components have the potential to be long-lived and may perform more reliably than soluble complement proteins as biomarkers for SLE.

Investigational Studies of Cell-Bound Complement Activation Products

Several studies have focused on the discovery and validation of CB-CAPs as potential lupus biomarkers. With the use of flow cytometry assays, a unique CB-CAP phenotype of circulating blood cells that is highly specific for SLE has been identified.[69-72]

In consideration of the physiologic abundance and localization of erythrocytes, it was hypothesized that erythrocytes, circulating throughout the body and hence having easy assess to products derived from systemic as well as local activation of the complement system, may serve as biological beacons of the inflammatory condition in vivo (and hence the disease activity) in patients with SLE or other inflammatory diseases. To verify this hypothesis, the first CB-CAP study was a cross-sectional investigation examining erythrocyte-bound C4d (E-C4d) levels in patients with SLE (n = 100), patients with other inflammatory and immune-mediated diseases (n = 133), and healthy controls (n = 84).[69] In light of the previous reported association of low E-CR1 levels with SLE, erythrocyte-CR1 (E-CR1) was determined simultaneously. This study demonstrated unambiguously for the first time that patients with SLE have significantly higher levels of E-C4d) than patients with other diseases and healthy individuals.

A subsequent study took advantage of the knowledge that erythrocytes develop from hematopoietic stem cells in the bone marrow and emerge as reticulocytes, which then maintain distinct phenotypic features for 1 or 2 days before fully maturing into erythrocytes. Reticulocytes, if released into the peripheral circulation during an active disease state, may immediately be exposed to and bind C4-derived fragments generated from activation of the complement system. Therefore, it was hypothesized that the levels of C4d bound on reticulocytes (R-C4d) may effectively and precisely reflect the current disease activity in a given SLE patient at a specific point in time. The results of a cross-sectional study involving 156 patients with SLE, 140 patients with other autoimmune and inflammatory diseases, and 159 healthy controls showed that (1) R-C4d levels of patients with SLE were significantly higher than those of patients with other diseases or healthy controls) and (2) R-C4d levels fluctuated over time in patients with SLE.[70]

Additional studies explored the possibility that CAPs may also bind to nonerythroid lineages of circulating cells, such as platelets and lymphocytes. A cross-sectional comparison of platelet-bound C4d (P-C4d) in patients with SLE (n = 105), patients with other inflammatory and immune-mediated diseases (n = 115), and healthy controls (n = 100) showed that abnormal levels of C4d were present on platelets in 18% of patients with SLE, 1.7% of patients with other diseases, and 0% of healthy controls.[71] In a later study, flow

TABLE 14-3 Potential Clinical Applications of Cell-Bound Complement Activation Products (CB-CAPs) as Lupus Biomarkers

CELL TYPE	CB-CAP	CLINICAL APPLICATION(S)
Erythrocyte	E-C4d, E-C3d	Diagnosis; monitoring
Reticulocyte	R-C4d (R-C3d)	Monitoring
Platelet	P-C4d (P-C3d)	Diagnosis; stratification
T lymphocyte	T-C4d, T-C3d	Diagnosis; others (under investigation)
B lymphocyte	B-C4d, B-C3d	Diagnosis; others (under investigation)

cytometric analysis was performed to detect C4d on T and B lymphocytes (referred to as T-C4d and B-C4d, respectively) from patients with SLE (n = 224), patients with other diseases (n = 179), and healthy controls (n = 114). Both T-C4d and B-C4d values were significantly and specifically elevated in patients with SLE in comparison with healthy controls and patients with other diseases.[72]

Collectively, these studies strongly suggest a CB-CAP phenotype that is highly specific for patients with SLE. Moreover, it has been noted that high levels of C4d are not necessarily concurrently present on erythrocytes, reticulocytes, platelets, and lymphocytes of a given patient with SLE at a particular time (Liu, unpublished data, 2010). These findings suggest that binding of CAP to circulating blood cells does not merely reflect complement activation occurring during SLE disease flares but may also reflect specific cellular and molecular mechanisms in lupus pathogenesis.

Clinical Applications of Cell-Bound Complement Activation Products as Lupus Biomarkers

Despite extensive research and numerous trials of potential new therapeutics, SLE remains one of the greatest challenges for physicians. It is of importance to develop accurate and easy-to-use biomarkers to improve daily management of patients with SLE and to facilitate the development of new SLE therapeutics. CB-CAPs appear to have the potential to serve as clinically practical biomarkers for SLE (Table 14-3).

Cell-Bound Complement Activation Products as Diagnostic Biomarkers for SLE

The diagnostic utility of CB-CAPs has been demonstrated for E-C4d, P-C4d, T-C4d, and B-C4d. In the inaugural CB-CAP study, an abnormally high level of E-C4d in combination with an abnormally low level of E-CR1 was shown to be 72% sensitive and 79% specific in differentiating SLE from other inflammatory or immune-mediated diseases, and 81% sensitive and 91% specific in differentiating SLE from healthy conditions, with an overall negative predictive value of 92%.[69] Similarly, T-C4d and B-C4d levels, as diagnostic tools, were 56% sensitive/80% specific and 60% sensitive/82% specific in differentiating SLE from other diseases and healthy conditions, respectively.[72] Despite being present in only a subset of patients with SLE evaluated in a cross-sectional study, an abnormal P-C4d test result has high diagnostic specificity, being 100% specific for a diagnosis of SLE in comparison with healthy controls and 98% specific for SLE in comparison with other diseases.[71]

Until recently, the single most useful laboratory test for confirming a diagnosis of SLE has been determination of anti-dsDNA antibodies. This test is highly specific for SLE, being detected in less than 5% of patients with other diseases. However, the mean sensitivity of anti-dsDNA testing for SLE among published studies is only 57%.[73] In contrast, the commonly used ANA test is sensitive (>95%) but highly nonspecific for a diagnosis of SLE, with a positive predictive value as low as 11% in some studies.[74] Therefore, the reported diagnostic specificities and sensitivities of E-C4d, P-C4d, T-C4d, and B-C4d tests indicate that a single CB-CAP assay in general may be more sensitive than the anti-dsDNA test and more specific than the ANA test. Whether combinations of CB-CAP assays of different cell types will provide greater diagnostic utility than individual CB-CAP assays of a particular cell type remains to be determined.

Cell-Bound Complement Activation Products as Biomarkers for SLE Disease Activity

Initial studies demonstrated that E-C4d levels in the same SLE patient examined on different days varied considerably, suggesting that changes in E-C4d levels in patients with SLE might reflect fluctuations in disease activity.[69] The utility of E-C4d as a biomarker for monitoring SLE disease activity was subsequently investigated through a longitudinal study.[75] This study was conducted in 157 patients with SLE, 290 patients with other diseases, and 256 healthy individuals who were followed prospectively over a 5-year period (2001-2005), encompassing 1005 patient-visits in patients with SLE, 660 patient-visits in patients with other diseases, and 395 subject-visits in healthy individuals. The disease activity in patients with SLE was measured using the Systemic Lupus Activity Measure (SLAM) and the Safety of Estrogen in Lupus Erythematosus—National Assessment version of the Systemic Lupus Erythematosus Disease Activity Index (SELENA-SLEDAI). Consistent with the initial cross-sectional study, the results showed that patients with SLE had higher levels of E-C4d and E-C3d than did the healthy controls and patients with other diseases. The variances of E-C4d and E-C3d were high, not only within the same SLE patient but also between different patients with SLE, suggesting again the possibility that levels of these biomarkers may track with changes in disease activity over time. This possibility was verified by a regression formulation in which each patient's evolving clinical status was regressed on each of the biomarkers, with the use of both univariate and multivariate analyses. Although the univariate analysis demonstrated that E-C4d and E-C3d, as well as the gold standard anti-dsDNA and serum C3 levels, were significantly associated with disease activity in patients with SLE, the multivariate analysis showed that only E-C4d and E-C3d remained significant predictors of SLE disease activity measured by SELENA-SLEDAI (E-C4d) and/or SLAM (E-C4d and E-C3d), even after data were adjusted for serum C3, C4, and anti-dsDNA antibody. These observations suggest that erythrocyte-bound CAPs can serve as informative measures of SLE disease activity as compared with anti-dsDNA and serum complement levels and should be considered for monitoring disease activity in patients with SLE.

To devise a laboratory test that can differentiate ongoing active disease from cumulative past disease activity in a patient with SLE, a series of studies has focused on analyzing C4d levels on reticulocytes. The rationale underlying these studies is that the level of CAPs bound to reticulocytes (e.g., R-C4d), which are short-lived (0-2 days) intermediates transiting into mature erythrocytes, should reflect precisely and promptly the extent of complement activation (and disease activity) at the time of blood sample procurement. During longitudinal follow-up of 156 patients with SLE, it was noted that the R-C4d levels in a significant fraction of patients with SLE varied considerably over time,[70] suggesting that fluctuations in R-C4d levels coincide with changes in disease activity. Indeed, initial studies showed that, within the SLE patient population, the level of R-C4d appeared proportionate to the clinical disease activity in a given SLE patient—that is, patients with higher R-C4d levels have higher disease activity as measured using the SLAM and SELENA-SLEDAI.[70] In cross-sectional comparison, patients with R-C4d levels in the highest quartile, in comparison with those in the lowest quartile, had significantly higher SELENA-SLEDAI ($P < 0.001$) and SLAM ($P = 0.02$) scores. Moreover, longitudinal observations showed that the R-C4d levels appeared to change promptly in relation to the clinical course in individual patients with SLE.[70] Taken together, these results suggest that R-C4d levels, compared with C4d levels on the 120 day-lived erythrocytes, may more precisely reflect ongoing disease activity in a patient with SLE, supporting a potential role for CAP-bearing reticulocytes as "instant messengers" of SLE disease activity.

Cell-Bound Complement Activation Products as Biomarkers for Stratifying Clinical Subsets of SLE Patients

The various studies previously outlined indicate that the paradigm of CB-CAPs as lupus biomarkers is not limited to a particular lineage of circulating cells. Observations to date also suggest that CB-CAPs associated with a particular cell type may provide clues to clinical stratification or establishing subsets of patients with SLE. In view of the biological role of platelets in hemostasis and coagulation, the presence of abnormal levels of CAPs on platelets may serve as a useful biomarker for patients with SLE who are at increased risk of cardiovascular and cerebrovascular events. Indeed, the previous cross-sectional study of 100 patients with SLE showed that P-C4d values correlated with a history of neurologic events (seizure and psychosis; $P = 0.006$) and positive antiphospholipid antibody test results ($P = 0.013$), a clinical manifestation and a known risk factor for thrombotic complications of SLE, respectively.[71] A later longitudinal study of 341 patients with SLE who had at least three consecutive office visits identified 57 patients (17%) with abnormal P-C4d levels in general screening tests (unpublished data, 2011). Moreover, the P-C4d–positive patients with SLE, in comparison with the P-C4d–negative patients, were found to be more likely to have a history of seizure disorder and positive antiphospholipid antibody test result. Furthermore, P-C4d–positive patients had a significantly higher frequency of cardiovascular events associated with acute thrombosis than P-C4d–negative patients (unpublished data, 2011). The results of the cross-sectional and longitudinal studies together suggest that patients with SLE who have abnormal P-C4d levels may represent a subset of patients with increased thrombotic tendency and higher risk of cardiovascular and cerebrovascular complications.

ANTICOMPLEMENT THERAPEUTICS FOR SLE

The fundamental role of complement activation in SLE pathogenesis has led naturally to exploration of the complement system as a target for therapeutic intervention. A controlled, localized regulation of the complement cascade is considered to be the most desired approach. To date, a variety of reagents that inhibit or modulate complement activation at different steps of the cascade have been developed (see references 76 and 77 for reviews). Although various factors such as short half-lives and lack of specificity have so far limited the clinical success of many of these reagents, the potential of anticomplement therapeutics is undeniable and warrants continuing investigation.

The complement-targeted reagents can be classified into two broad categories: (1) inhibitors of the early steps of complement activation and (2) inhibitors of the terminal pathway that do not interfere with early activation events (Figure 14-3). Examples of the first group include soluble CR1 (sCR1; capable of regulating the generation of C3/C4 fragments and C3 convertases), heparin (a polyanionic glycosamine capable of binding/inhibiting C1, inhibiting C1q binding to immune complexes, blocking C3 convertase formation, and interfering with MAC assembly), compstatin (a cyclic tridecapeptide capable of binding C3 and preventing its proteolytic cleavage), and protease inhibitors. Prominent among the second group are anti-C5 monoclonal antibodies (mAbs) that can bind C5, block its cleavage and formation of C5a, and abrogate MAC assembly. Synthetic antagonists of C5a receptors also belong to the second group and have been exploited to block the anaphylactic and chemotactic effects of C5a.

Considering that C3b opsonization of pathogens and immune complexes is crucial for host defense and for prevention of immune complex–associated adverse reactions, it is reasonable to postulate that inhibitors of complement activation at a downstream step, such as C5 cleavage, would have therapeutic effects for patients with inflammatory diseases but would be less likely to increase the risk for infection in these patients. Eculizumab, a humanized anti-C5 mAb approved by the U.S. Food and Drug Administration for treating paroxysmal nocturnal hematuria, has been shown to significantly improve renal disease and increase survival in the NZB/W F1 mouse model of SLE. A phase 1 clinical trial of eculizumab in patients with SLE concluded that the agent was safe and well tolerated without

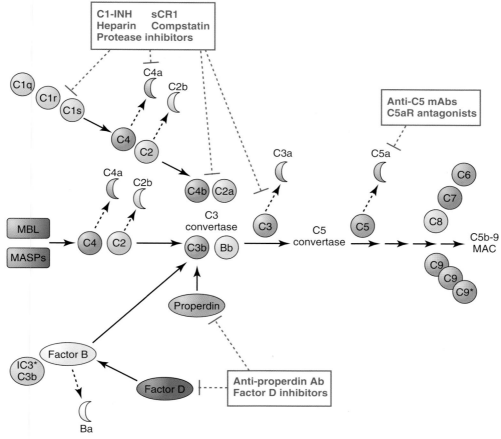

FIGURE 14-3 Anticomplement therapeutics and potential target molecules. Ab, antibody; Ba, Bb, fragments of factor B; C1-INH, C1 inhibitor; C5aR, complement 5a receptor; C_{5b-9} MAC, membrane attack complex for C5b through C9; Cr1, complement receptor 1; iC3*, hydrolyzed C3; mAb, monoclonal antibody; MASP, mannose-binding protein–associated serine protease; MBL, mannose-binding lectin; s, soluble.

significant adverse effects. Heparin, traditionally used as an anticoagulant and known to inhibit complement activation, has been demonstrated to prevent antiphospholipid antibody/complement–induced fetal loss in a murine model.[78] This seminal observation suggests that heparin at "subtherapeutic" (non-anticoagulating) doses may be beneficial in pathologic situations in which excess complement activation is unfavorable, such as ischemia/reperfusion injury, antiphospholipid antibody syndrome, and lupus nephritis.

CONCLUSION

In 1948, Hargraves reported discovery of the LE cell,[79] although the origin and significance of the structure were unknown at the time. Shortly after that discovery, it was determined that in vitro generation of LE cells depends on complement activation.[80] More than 60 years later, the LE cell is recognized as a neutrophil that has engulfed the remnants of apoptosis, thus linking complement, apoptosis, and SLE. So the LE cell can be considered a lupus biomarker relic and an early icon of the disease. Perhaps this cell's history should instruct us to forge ahead with microarrays, proteomics, molecular signatures, and genome-wide explorations, but also to carry with us and occasionally revisit simpler observations of the past. The complement system holds at least one important clue to the mystery of SLE, and recent progress is cause for optimism that a solution to the puzzle may be within reach.

References

1. Vaughan JH, Bayles TB, Favour CB: The response of serum gamma globulin level and complement titer to adrenocorticotropic hormone (ACTH) therapy in lupus erythematosus disseminatus. *J Lab Clin Med* 37:698–702, 1951.
2. Elliott JA, Mathieson DR: Complement in disseminated (systemic) lupus erythematosus. *AMA Arch Dermat Syphilol* 68:119–128, 1953.
3. Lange K, Wasserman E, Slobody LB: The significance of serum complement levels for the diagnosis and prognosis of acute and subacute glomerulonephritis and lupus erythematosus disseminatus. *Ann Intern Med* 53:636–646, 1960.
4. Schur PH, Sandson J: Immunological factors and clinical activity in systemic lupus erythematosus. *N Engl J Med* 278:533–538, 1968.
5. Pickering MC, Botto M, Taylor PR, et al: Systemic lupus erythematosus, complement deficiency, and apoptosis. *Adv Immunol* 76:227–324, 2000.
6. Bordet J, Gengou O: Sur l'existences de substance sensibiliatrices dans la plupart des serum antimicrobiens. *Ann Inst Pasteur* 15:289–302, 1901.
7. Ehrlich P, Morgenroth J: Uber Hamolysine. Berlin Klin. *Wochenschr* 36:481–486, 1899.
8. Muller-Eberhard HJ: Molecular organization and function of the complement system. *Annu Rev Biochem* 57:321–347, 1988.
9. Walport MJ: Complement. First of two parts. *N Engl J Med* 344:1058–1066, 2001.
10. Sarma JV, Ward PA: The complement system. *Cell Tissue Res* 343:227–235, 2011.
11. Sjoberg AP, Trouw LA, Blom AM: Complement activation and inhibition: a delicate balance. *Trends Immunol* 30:83–90, 2009.
12. Pangburn MK, Muller-Eberhard HJ: Relation of putative thioester bond in C3 to activation of the alternative pathway and the binding of C3b to biological targets of complement. *J Exp Med* 152:1102–1114, 1980.
13. Kemper C, Atkinson JP, Hourcade DE: Properdin: emerging roles of a pattern-recognition molecule. *Annu Rev Immunol* 28:131–155, 2010.
14. Thiel S, Gadjeva M: Humoral pattern recognition molecules: mannan-binding lectin and ficolins. *Adv Exp Med Biol* 653:58–73, 2009.

15. Takahashi M, Mori S, Shigeta S, et al: Role of MBL-associated serine protease (MASP) on activation of the lectin complement pathway. *Adv Exp Med Biol* 598:93–104, 2007.

16. Selander B, Martensson U, Weintraub A, et al: Mannan-binding lectin activates C3 and the alternative complement pathway without involvement of C2. *J Clin Invest* 116:1425–1434, 2006.

17. Song WC: Complement regulatory proteins and autoimmunity. *Autoimmunity* 39:403–410, 2006.

18. Zipfel PF, Skerka C: Complement regulators and inhibitory proteins. *Nat Rev Immunol* 9:729–740, 2009.

19. Carroll MC: The role of complement and complement receptors in induction and regulation of immunity. *Annu Rev Immunol* 16:545–568, 1998.

20. Prodinger WM, Wurzner R, Stoiber H, et al: Complement. In Paul WE, editor: *Fundamental Immunology*, ed 5, Philadelphia, 2003, Lippincott Williams & Wilkins, pp 1077–1103.

21. Wetsel RA: Structure, function and cellular expression of complement anaphylatoxin receptors. *Curr Opin Immunol* 7:48–53, 1995.

22. Klos A, Tenner AJ, Johswich KO, et al: The role of the anaphylatoxins in health and disease. *Mol Immunol* 46:2753–2766, 2009.

23. Hourcade D, Holers VM, Atkinson JP: The regulators of complement activation (RCA) gene cluster. *Adv Immunol* 45:381–416, 1989.

24. Carroll MC: Complement and humoral immunity. *Vaccine* 26(Suppl 8):I28–I33, 2008.

25. Walport MJ: Complement. Second of two parts. *N Engl J Med* 344:1140–1144, 2001.

26. Kemper C, Atkinson JP: T-cell regulation: with complements from innate immunity. *Nat Rev Immunol* 7:9–18, 2007.

27. Dunkelberger JR, Song WC: Complement and its role in innate and adaptive immune responses. *Cell Res* 20:34–50, 2010.

28. Heeger PS, Lalli PN, Lin F, et al: Decay-accelerating factor modulates induction of T cell immunity. *J Exp Med* 201:1523–1530, 2005.

29. Strainic MG, Liu J, Huang D, et al: Locally produced complement fragments C5a and C3a provide both costimulatory and survival signals to naive CD4+ T cells. *Immunity* 28:425–435, 2008.

30. Cook HT, Botto M: Mechanisms of disease: the complement system and the pathogenesis of systemic lupus erythematosus. *Nat Clin Pract Rheumatol* 2:330–337, 2006.

31. Manderson AP, Botto M, Walport MJ: The role of complement in the development of systemic lupus erythematosus. *Annu Rev Immunol* 22:431–456, 2004.

32. Schifferli JA, Steiger G, Hauptmann G, et al: Formation of soluble immune complexes by complement in sera of patients with various hypocomplementemic states. Difference between inhibition of immune precipitation and solubilization. *J Clin Invest* 76:2127–2133, 1985.

33. Colten HR, Rosen FS: Complement deficiencies. *Annu Rev Immunol* 10:809–834, 1992.

34. Botto M, Kirschfink M, Macor P, et al: Complement in human diseases: lessons from complement deficiencies. *Mol Immunol* 46:2774–2783, 2009.

35. Yu CY, Belt KT, Giles CM, et al: Structural basis of the polymorphism of human complement component C4A and C4B: gene size, reactivity and antigenicity. *EMBO J* 5:2873–2881, 1986.

36. Hauptmann G, Grosshans E, Heid E: Systemic lupus erythematosus and hereditary complement deficiency: a case with total C4 defect. *Ann Dermatol Syphil Paris* 101:479–496, 1974.

37. Yang Y, Chung EK, Zhou B, et al: The intricate role of complement component C4 in human systemic lupus erythematosus. *Curr Dir Autoimmun* 7:98–132, 2004.

38. Monticielo OA, Mucenic T, Xavier RM, et al: The role of mannose-binding lectin in systemic lupus erythematosus. *Clin Rheumatol* 27:413–419, 2008.

39. Walport MJ, Davies KA, Botto M, et al: C3 nephritic factor and SLE: report of four cases and review of the literature. *QJM* 87:609–615, 1994.

40. Kallenberg CG: Anti-C1q autoantibodies. *Autoimmun Rev* 7:612–615, 2008.

41. Schifferli JA, Steiger G, Paccaud JP, et al: Difference in the biological properties of the two forms of the fourth component of human complement (C4). *Clin Exp Immunol* 63:473–477, 1986.

42. Davies KA, Peters AM, Beynon HL, et al: Immune complex processing in patients with systemic lupus erythematosus. In vivo imaging and clearance studies. *J Clin Invest* 90:2075–2083, 1992.

43. Korb LC, Ahearn JM: C1q binds directly and specifically to surface blebs of apoptotic human keratinocytes: complement deficiency and systemic lupus erythematosus revisited. *J Immunol* 158:4525–4528, 1997.

44. Navratil JS, Watkins SC, Wisnieski JJ, et al: The globular heads of C1q specifically recognize surface blebs of apoptotic vascular endothelial cells. *J Immunol* 166:3231–3239, 2001.

45. Nauta AJ, Trouw LA, Daha MR, et al: Direct binding of C1q to apoptotic cells and cell blebs induces complement activation. *Eur J Immunol* 32:1726–1736, 2002.

46. Rosen A, Casciola-Rosen L, Ahearn J: Novel packages of viral and self-antigens are generated during apoptosis. *J Exp Med* 181:1557–1561, 1995.

47. Liu CC, Navratil JS, Sabatine JM, et al: Apoptosis, complement and systemic lupus erythematosus: a mechanistic view. *Curr Dir Autoimmun* 7:49–86, 2004.

48. Mevorach D, Zhou JL, Song X, et al: Systemic exposure to irradiated apoptotic cells induces autoantibody production. *J Exp Med* 188:387–392, 1998.

49. Botto M, Dell'Agnola C, Bygrave AE, et al: Homozygous C1q deficiency causes glomerulonephritis associated with multiple apoptotic bodies [see comment]. *Nature Genetics* 19:56–59, 1998.

50. Taylor PR, Carugati A, Fadok VA, et al: A hierarchical role for classical pathway complement proteins in the clearance of apoptotic cells in vivo. *J Exp Med* 192:359–366, 2000.

51. Herrmann M, Voll RE, Zoller OM, et al: Impaired phagocytosis of apoptotic cell material by monocyte-derived macrophages from patients with systemic lupus erythematosus. *Arthritis Rheum* 41:1241–1250, 1998.

52. Baumann I, Kolowos W, Voll RE, et al: Impaired uptake of apoptotic cells into tingible body macrophages in germinal centers of patients with systemic lupus erythematosus. *Arthritis Rheum* 46:191–201, 2002.

53. Carroll MC: The role of complement in B cell activation and tolerance. *Adv Immunol* 74:61–88, 2000.

54. Mollnes TE, Jokiranta TS, Truedsson L, et al: Complement analysis in the 21st century. *Mol Immunol* 44:3838–3849, 2007.

55. Seelen MA, Roos A, Wieslander J, et al: Functional analysis of the classical, alternative, and MBL pathways of the complement system: standardization and validation of a simple ELISA. *J Immunol Methods* 296:187–198, 2005.

56. Zwirner J, Felber E, Reiter C, et al: Deposition of complement activation products on plastic-adsorbed immunoglobulins. A simple ELISA technique for the detection of defined complement deficiencies. *J Immunol Methods* 124:121–129, 1989.

57. Sturfelt G, Sjoholm AG: Complement components, complement activation, and acute phase response in systemic lupus erythematosus. *Int Arch Allergy Appl Immunol* 75:75–83, 1984.

58. Ingvarsson J, Larsson A, Sjoholm AG, et al: Design of recombinant antibody microarrays for serum protein profiling: targeting of complement proteins. *J Proteome Res* 6:3527–3536, 2007.

59. Janzi M, Odling J, Pan-Hammarstrom Q, et al: Serum microarrays for large scale screening of protein levels. *Mol Cell Proteomics* 4:1942–1947, 2005.

60. Papp K, Szekeres Z, Terenyi N, et al: On-chip complement activation adds an extra dimension to antigen microarrays. *Mol Cell Proteomics* 6:133–140, 2007.

61. Papp K, Vegh P, Miklos K, et al: Detection of complement activation on antigen microarrays generates functional antibody profiles and helps characterization of disease-associated changes of the antibody repertoire. *J Immunol* 181:8162–8169, 2008.

62. Esdaile JM, Abrahamowicz M, Joseph L, et al: Laboratory tests as predictors of disease exacerbations in systemic lupus erythematosus. Why some tests fail. *Arthritis Rheum* 39:370–378, 1996.

63. Liu CC, Ahearn JM, Manzi S: Complement as a source of biomarkers in systemic lupus erythematosus: past, present, and future. *Curr Rheumatol Rep* 6:85–88, 2004.

64. Kelly RH, Carpenter AB, Sudol KS, et al: Complement C3 fragments in urine detection in systemic lupus erythematosus patients by Western blotting. *Appl Theor Electroph* 3:265–269, 1993.

65. Manzi S, Rairie JE, Carpenter AB, et al: Sensitivity and specificity of plasma and urine complement split products as indicators of lupus disease activity. *Arthritis Rheum* 39:1178–1188, 1996.

66. Negi VS, Aggarwal A, Dayal R, et al: Complement degradation product C3d in urine: marker of lupus nephritis. *J Rheumatol* 27:380–383, 2000.

67. Law SKA: The covalent binding reaction of C3 and C4. *Ann NY Acad Sci* 246–258, 1983.

68. Atkinson JP, Chan AC, Karp DR, et al: Origin of the fourth component of complement related Chido and Rodgers blood group antigens. *Complement* 5:65–76, 1988.

69. Manzi S, Navratil JS, Ruffing MJ, et al: Measurement of erythrocyte C4d and complement receptor 1 in systemic lupus erythematosus. *Arthritis Rheum* 50:3596–3604, 2004.

70. Liu CC, Manzi S, Kao AH, et al: Reticulocytes bearing C4d as biomarkers of disease activity for systemic lupus erythematosus. *Arthritis Rheum* 52:3087–3099, 2005.
71. Navratil JS, Manzi S, Kao AH, et al: Platelet C4d is highly specific for systemic lupus erythematosus. *Arthritis Rheum* 54:670–674, 2006.
72. Liu CC, Kao AH, Hawkins DM, et al: Lymphocyte-bound complement activation products as biomarkers for diagnosis of systemic lupus erythematosus. *Clin Transl Sci* 2:300–308, 2009.
73. Solomon DH, Kavanaugh AJ, Schur PH: Evidence-based guidelines for the use of immunologic tests: antinuclear antibody testing. *Arthritis Rheum* 47:434–444, 2002.
74. Slater CA, Davis RB, Shmerling RH: Antinuclear antibody testing. A study of clinical utility. *Arch Intern Med* 156:1421–1425, 1996.
75. Kao AH, Navratil JS, Ruffing MJ, et al: Erythrocyte C3d and C4d for monitoring disease activity in systemic lupus erythematosus. *Arthritis Rheum* 62:837–844, 2010.
76. Ricklin D, Lambris JD: Complement-targeted therapeutics. *Nat Biotechnol* 25:1265–1275, 2007.
77. Wagner E, Frank MM: Therapeutic potential of complement modulation. *Nat Rev Drug Discov* 9:43–56, 2010.
78. Girardi G, Redecha P, Salmon JE: Heparin prevents antiphospholipid antibody-induced fetal loss by inhibiting complement activation. *Nature Medicine* 10:1222–1226, 2004.
79. Hargraves MM, Richmond H, Morton R: Presentation of two bone marrow elements: the "tart" cell and the "LE" cell. *Proc Staff Meetings Mayo Clinic* 23:25–28, 1948.
80. McDuffie FC, Drexler E, Golden HE: Immunologic factors in lupus erythematosus cell formation. *Mayo Clin Proc* 44:620–629, 1969.

Chapter 15

Mechanisms of Acute Inflammation and Vascular Injury in SLE

J. Michelle Kahlenberg and Mariana J. Kaplan

Inflammation and injury of blood vessels in systemic lupus erythematosus (SLE) has been a topic of study for the past several decades. Although inflammatory, necrotizing damage to blood vessel walls can rarely be seen in various organs in SLE, chronic vasculopathy that promotes endothelial dysfunction and premature atherosclerosis is prevalent in this disease and causes significant morbidity and mortality.

EPIDEMIOLOGY OF PREMATURE VASCULAR DAMAGE IN SLE

Accelerated atherosclerosis is an important problem in patients with SLE (see Chapter 26 for more detail). Enhanced atherosclerotic risk increases with each year of disease duration. This is especially the case in young females with SLE, in whom the cardiovascular risk can be up to 50-fold higher than in age-matched controls (Figure 15-1).[1,2] Clinically evident coronary artery disease affects approximately 6% to 10% of patients with SLE.[1] There is also evidence that SLE, like diabetes mellitus, increases risk of poor outcomes after acute myocardial infarction.[3]

Traditional Framingham Study risk factors likely contribute to CVD in SLE, but they cannot fully account for the increased risk. Therefore, the pathogenesis of premature CVD in SLE may also rely on factors unique to the disease itself.[4] Many investigators agree with the hypothesis that long-term exposure to lupus immune dysregulation promotes CVD.

The type of cardiovascular lesion may provide clues to its etiology. The pathology of SLE-related CVD can involve atherosclerotic lesions[5] and also fibrointimal hyperplasia, which may reflect chronic endothelial injury (Figure 15-2).[6] Noncalcified coronary plaque is more common in patients with currently active or recently active SLE, suggesting that disease-specific factors directly contribute to development of new plaque.[7] Contrarily, calcified plaque correlates with traditional cardiovascular risk factors in patients with lupus, suggesting that factors such as age and obesity may advance calcified disease.[8]

Systemic inflammation has been linked to atherosclerosis development in the general population and in specific conditions. Interestingly, patients with SLE typically display a lower "classical inflammatory burden" than the burden that would be seen in patients with inflammatory arthritis, including rheumatoid arthritis and spondyloarthropathies; yet lupus is associated with a higher cardiovascular risk than these other diseases. This observation indicates that the triggers of accelerated atherosclerosis in lupus differ from the typical proinflammatory factors (i.e., high C-reactive protein [CRP]) linked to "idiopathic" atherosclerosis.

SUBCLINICAL AND CLINICAL VASCULAR DAMAGE IN SLE

Premature damage in SLE has been described in both the macrovasculature and microvasculature. Vascular functional abnormalities in lupus appear to develop early during the course of the disease,[9]

although it is unclear whether they precede SLE diagnosis. Subclinical vascular dysfunction can be quantified with a variety of invasive and noninvasive tests (see Chapter 26); patients with SLE have significantly decreased flow-mediated dilation (FMD) of the brachial artery—a function of endothelial cells—and this decrease correlates with increased carotid intima media thickness (IMT) in such patients.[10] Additionally, carotid plaque can be detected in 21% of patients with SLE younger than 35 years and in up to 100% of those older than 65.[11] Aortic atherosclerosis is also increased in SLE.[12] Subclinical macrovascular disease in SLE correlates with disease activity and disease duration.[10-12] Damage to the coronary circulation is also common in patients with SLE; in one study, more than half of the tested patients displayed noncalcified coronary plaque.[7] There is also evidence of impairment of the coronary microvasculature flow reserve and altered coronary vasomotor function, even in those patients with lupus who have grossly normal coronary arteries.[13] This dysfunction correlates with disease duration and severity, suggesting that microvascular damage and dysfunction are also part of SLE-related cardiovascular pathology.[14]

MECHANISMS OF ATHEROSCLEROSIS DEVELOPMENT IN THE GENERAL POPULATION

The vascular endothelium is a barrier between the blood which regulates vascular tone, cell migration into the vasculature, and localized inflammatory responses. Various groups have proposed that CVD, endothelial dysfunction, and atherosclerosis arise from chronic injury to the endothelium, which allows for invasion of inflammatory cells and lipid deposition. This endothelial injury can occur via shear stress or through toxic or inflammatory factors that result in endothelial cell apoptosis.

Inflammation is considered to play a crucial role in the pathogenesis of atherosclerosis and is present throughout the various stages of the vascular damage process. In early lesions of atherosclerosis, the fatty streak and infiltration by macrophages and T cells are prominent. Indeed, factors such as oxidized LDL (ox-LDL) activate the endothelium to secrete chemokines that recruit inflammatory cells, including T lymphocytes, dendritic cells (DCs), and monocytes. The monocytes differentiate into macrophages and foam cells under the influence of locally secreted factors and further stimulation by ox-LDL.[15,16] Cholesterol crystals and other stimuli activate macrophages and foam cells to secrete inflammatory cytokines, reactive oxygen and nitrogen species, and proteases. All these factors can contribute to the atherogenic phenotype in the blood vessel.[17] Invasion of the atherosclerotic plaque by CD4+ T cells also contributes to vascular pathology, through these cells' recognition of epitopes of various molecules, such as ox-LDL, and secretion of interferon gamma (IFN-γ), which then leads to increased inflammatory cytokine production. Chronic and unabated synthesis of proteases and inflammatory cytokines promotes thinning of the atherosclerotic plaque wall and eventual rupture. Rupture leads to exposure of the blood to phospholipids, tissue factor, and platelet-adhesive matrix

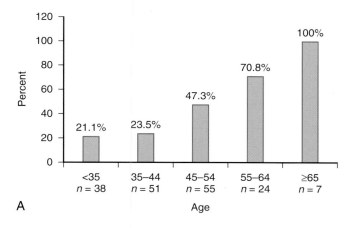

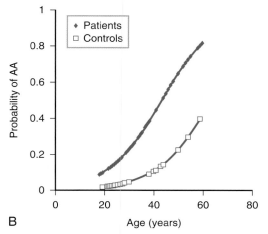

FIGURE 15-1 Cardiovascular disease is increased in SLE. A, Prevalence of focal carotid plaque by age in 175 women evaluated by carotid ultrasound. **B,** Probability of aortic atherosclerosis (AA) as a function of age in patients with SLE versus healthy controls. (*A from Manzi S, et al: Prevalence and risk factors of carotid plaque in women with systemic lupus erythematosus.* Arthritis Rheum *42:51–60, 1999; **B** from Roldan C, et al: Premature aortic atherosclerosis in systemic lupus erythematosus: a controlled transesophageal echocardiographic study.* J Rheumatol *37:71–78, 2010.)

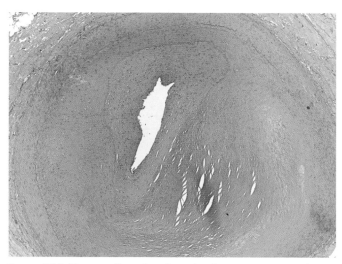

FIGURE 15-2 Hematoxylin and eosin stain of a coronary artery from a 35-year-old woman with lupus. Her disease manifested as cardiovascular disease, which consisted of three myocardial infarctions, cerebritis, myocarditis, mesenteric vasculitis, and antiphospholipid syndrome. The lesion is characterized by a dense fibrous infiltrate without significant calcium or lipid deposition. (*Photomicrograph courtesy of Dr. Gerald Abrams.*)

Box 15-1 Mechanisms of Vascular injury in SLE

1. Increased endothelial damage:
   a. Complement- and immune complex–mediated damage.
   b. Oxidative stress.
2. Decreased vascular repair:
   a. Interferon alpha (IFN-α) mediates dysfunction of endothelial progenitor cells (EPCs)/circulating angiogenic cells (CACs).
   b. Low-density granulocytes are toxic to the endothelium.
3. Enhanced plaque formation by IFN-α.
4. Neutrophil extracellular traps induce endothelial cell death.
5. IFN-α–activated platelets promote vascular inflammation.
6. Dysregulated cytokine production:
   a. Tumor necrosis factor alpha (TNF-α, interleukin–17, adiponectin.
7. CD154-CD40 interactions and CD137 co-stimulation lead to vascular damage by T cells.
8. Aberrant lipid processing:
   a. Increased oxidized low-density lipoprotein cholesterol.
   b. Decreased high-density lipoprotein (HDL) cholesterol and increased proinflammatory HDL cholesterol.
   c. Elevated very-low-density lipoprotein cholesterol and triglycerides.
9. Autoantibodies with various targets affecting many steps in the atherogenic cycle.

---

molecules, eventually promoting thrombosis and acute cardiovascular events.[15]

Under normal conditions, vascular damage triggers a response that leads to an attempt to repair the endothelium. If this repair fails or is incomplete, the vessel may be at a higher risk for atherosclerotic disease. Repair of the damaged endothelium has been proposed to occur primarily by circulating bone marrow–derived endothelial progenitor cells (EPCs) and by myelomonocytic circulating angiogenic cells (CACs).[18] Decreased numbers or dysfunction of these cell types may contribute to CVD in persons with various diseases as well as in the general population, because EPC numbers inversely correlate with CVD risk, time to first cardiovascular event, and in-stent re-stenosis risk.[19,20] Additionally, functional impairment of EPCs correlates with coronary artery disease risk.[21]

MECHANISMS OF ENDOTHELIAL INFLAMMATION, INJURY, AND ATHEROSCLEROSIS IN SLE

Because of the profound immune dysregulation present in SLE, the increased risk of CVD is likely secondary to a combination of many factors that alter the endothelium and inflammatory response. Indeed, variables that enhance traditional mechanisms of atherosclerosis and create novel injury pathways are present in this disease

(Box 15-1). As such, understanding the putative mechanisms that promote accelerated vascular damage in SLE may also provide novel information about the pathways by which the immune system may promote atherosclerosis in the general population.

Endothelial damage is increased in SLE. Patients with SLE have increased numbers of circulating apoptotic endothelial cells, which correlate with endothelial dysfunction (as assessed by brachial artery FMD) and circulating levels of tissue factor (Figure 15-3A).[9] Various soluble adhesion molecules, such as vascular cell adhesion molecule (VCAM), intercellular adhesion molecule (ICAM), and E-selectin, which are released after endothelial cell damage, are increased in SLE and correlate with higher coronary calcium scores.[22] Additionally,

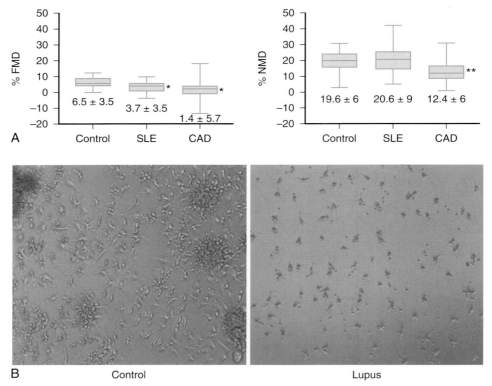

FIGURE 15-3 A, Endothelial dysfunction is characteristic of SLE-mediated cardiovascular disease. Box-and-whisker plots representing flow-mediated vaso-dilation (FMD), which depends on endothelial function, and nitroglycerin-mediated vasodilation (NMD), which is present on intact smooth muscle function, in control subjects and cohorts of patients with SLE and coronary artery disease (CAD) and patients with CAD but not SLE. Numbers below the box plots are means ± SEM. *$P < 0.01$ versus controls and †$P < 0.001$ versus controls and SLE. **B,** Vascular repair is dysfunctional in SLE. Endothelial progenitor cells (EPCs)/circulating angiogenic cells (CACs) from patients with SLE are unable to differentiate into mature endothelial cells in culture. Photomicrographs of primary blood mononuclear cells from a healthy control subject (*left*) and a patient with SLE (*right*) after 2 weeks of culture in proangiogenic media on fibronectin-coated plates. Cells were imaged via inverted-phase microscopy at a total magnification of 100×. (*A from Rajagopalan S, et al: Endothelial cell apoptosis in systemic lupus erythematosus: a common pathway for abnormal vascular function and thrombosis propensity. Blood 103:3677-3683, 2004.*)

soluble levels of the antithrombotic endothelial protein C receptor, which is typically released secondary to inflammatory activation of metalloproteinases, are increased in SLE and correlate with the presence of carotid plaque.[23] These findings indicate that the endothelium is under chronic assault in SLE, a phenomenon that could lead to atherosclerotic pathology if the damage is not adequately repaired.

However, despite evidence that accelerated endothelial cell death occurs in lupus, a phenomenon that should trigger enhanced vascular repair, the latter is significantly impaired in SLE. Patients with lupus, even those with very stable disease, have decreased circulating EPCs. Further, EPCs/CACs in SLE exhibit enhanced apoptosis and demonstrate decreased capacity to synthesize proangiogenic molecules, to be incorporated into vascular structures, and to differentiate into mature endothelial cells (Figure 15-3B).[24-26] Thus, patients with SLE have compromised repair of the damaged endothelium, and we can hypothesize that this phenomenon may contribute to the establishment of a milieu that promotes the development of vascular plaque.

Type I Interferons and SLE-Related Cardiovascular Disease

One mechanism by which vascular repair is impaired in SLE is through increased levels and enhanced effects of type I IFNs, cytokines known to play important roles in innate immunity and antiviral responses. Human and murine studies from various groups indicate that IFN-α may be crucial in the pathogenesis of SLE. Approximately 60% of patients with SLE have elevations of serum IFN-α and carry an "IFN signature" in peripheral blood mononuclear cells, kidneys, and other tissues, in correlation with disease activity.[27,28] Further,

lupus cells appear to be more sensitive to the effects of type I IFNs.[29] Because of the role of type I IFNs in SLE pathology, these cytokines have been investigated as a contributing factor to the development of lupus-related CVD. A summary of the mechanisms by which IFN-α insults the vasculature is shown in Figure 15-4.

Over the past few years, evidence has surfaced that type I IFNs correlate with atherosclerosis and endothelial dysfunction. Patients with lupus and a high type I IFN signature have decreased endothelial function, as assessed by peripheral arterial tone measurements.[30] Additionally, type I IFN serum activity in SLE was found to be positively associated with increased carotid IMT, coronary calcification, and decreased brachial artery FMD in a cohort of patients with lupus who had low traditional cardiovascular risk factors, stable disease, and no previous cardiovascular events.[31] Importantly, in this cohort, factors such as high-sensitivity CRP, serum levels of adhesion molecules, and lupus disease activity were not associated with functional or anatomic evidence of vascular damage in SLE. Thus, enhanced type I IFN effects may be one of the unique factors in SLE that results in increased cardiovascular risk.

Induction of an Imbalance of Vascular Damage and Repair by Type I Interferons

Type I IFNs promote decreased vascular repair. In SLE, dysfunction of EPC/CAC differentiation is mediated by IFN-α, because neutralization of this cytokine restores a normal phenotype of these cells.[26] This theory is further reinforced by the observation of abrogated EPC/CAC numbers and function in lupus-prone New Zealand Black/New Zealand White F_1 mice, a strain that depends on type I IFNs for disease development and severity. Additionally, non–lupus-prone

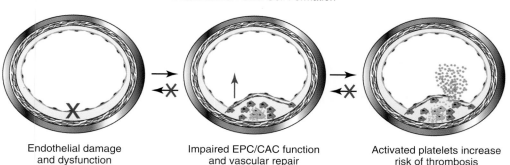

FIGURE 15-4 Interferon-α (IFN-α) contributes to SLE-mediated vascular disease in a variety of ways. IFN-α contributes to endothelial dysfunction and decreased repair of endothelial damage by decreasing numbers and function of endothelial progenitor cells (EPCs) (*orange symbols*) and circulating angiogenic cells (CACs (*pink symbols*). In addition to synthesizing type I IFNs, low-density granulocytes (LDGs) present in patients with SLE are directly toxic to the endothelium. Locally produced IFN-α contributes to plaque inflammation, and modulation of macrophages by IFN-α increases oxidized low-density lipoprotein (ox-LDL) uptake and foam cell formation. Additionally, activation of platelets by IFN-α results in upregulation of adhesion molecules and further platelet-mediated IFN-α production, which promotes vascular inflammation and thrombus formation. (*Artwork partially contributed by Seth G Thacker.*)

mouse EPCs are unable to properly differentiate into mature endothelial cells in the presence of IFN-α.[32,33] The pathways by which IFN-α mediates aberrant vascular repair may depend on repression of the proangiogenic factors interleukin-1β (IL-1β) and vascular endothelial growth factor (VEGF) and on upregulation of the cytokine IL-18 and the antiangiogenic IL-1 receptor antagonist. Indeed, addition of recombinant human IL-1β to SLE EPC/CAC cultures restores normal endothelial differentiation.[32,34] Further, blockade of IL-18 signaling improves endothelial differentiation, suggesting that the balance between IL-1β and IL-18, which is modulated by IFN-α, may be important in vascular health.[34] There is evidence that an antiangiogenic phenotype is operational in vivo in patients with SLE, as manifested by decreased vascular density and increased vascular rarefaction in renal blood vessels, in association with upregulation of the IL-1 receptor antagonist and decreased vascular endothelial growth factor in the kidney and serum.[26,32]

The cellular source of type I IFNs leading to abnormal vascular repair has been examined. Depletion of plasmacytoid DCs (pDCs; the major in vivo producers of IFN-α) does not lead to abrogation of abnormal lupus EPC/CAC differentiation in culture.[35] Therefore, other cellular sources for this cytokine in the context of interactions with the endothelium have been sought. Neutrophil-specific genes are abundant in peripheral blood mononuclear cell microarrays from patients with lupus because of the presence of low-density granulocytes (LDGs) in mononuclear cell fractions.[18,36] These LDGs have the capacity to secrete sufficient amounts of IFN-α to interfere with vascular repair. Indeed, LDG depletion from lupus peripheral blood mononuclear cells restores the ability of EPC/CACs to differentiate in vitro into endothelial monolayers.[35]

IFN-α and Plaque Formation

In addition to the role type I IFNs play in modulating endothelial cell death and repair, they may also contribute to plaque development through other mechanisms. For example, IFN-α–producing plasmacytoid DCs have been identified in areas of atheromatous plaque from patients without SLE. IFN-α then activates plaque-residing CD4⁺ T cells to increase expression of tumor necrosis factor (TNF)–related apoptosis-inducing ligand (TRAIL), which results in killing of plaque-stabilizing cells and a potential increase in the risk of plaque rupture. Additionally, IFN-α sensitizes plaque-residing myeloid DCs, potentially promoting further inflammation and plaque destabilization. This cytokine can act in conjunction with bacterial products (such as lipopolysaccharide [LPS]) to increase the

synthesis of various proinflammatory cytokines and metalloproteinases.[32,37,38] Importantly, IFN-α has also been shown to upregulate the macrophage scavenger receptor A (SRA), which allows for ox-LDL uptake and foam cell formation. Indeed, SRA and CD36 have been implicated in foam cell formation and in the regulation of inflammatory signaling pathways leading to lesional macrophage apoptosis and plaque necrosis in other conditions. The presence of a strong interferon gene signature correlates with higher levels of macrophage SRA messenger RNA (mRNA) in patients with SLE, indicating an additional mechanism by which type I IFNs may modulate deleterious vascular responses in SLE.[39] These findings indicate that type I IFNs could potentially be involved in atherosclerosis development not only in persons with autoimmune disorders but also in the general population in the context of idiopathic atherosclerosis and microbial infections.

Platelet Abnormalities Induced by IFN-α

Platelets are crucial players in the development of acute cardiovascular events, including acute coronary syndrome (ACS). It has now been found that platelets from SLE patients have a more activated phenotype that correlates with the presence of both vascular disease and an interferon signature.[40] Indeed, the platelet transcriptome in SLE shows evidence of an interferogenic signature. Additionally, platelets from patients with SLE can activate pDCs in a CD154 (CD 40 ligand)–dependent manner, resulting in greater IFN-α production.[41] IFN-α is also able to increase platelet adhesion to endothelial cells in a P-selectin–dependent manner. This greater adhesion results in increased monocyte rolling and invasion of the vasculature, suggesting that IFN-α positively affects vascular inflammation.[42] Additionally, SLE-prone mice have decreased renal involvement and immune complex formation after platelet depletion or platelet inhibition with clopidogrel, suggesting that activation of platelets, possibly via IFN-α, plays an important role in SLE pathogenesis and possibly CVD.[41] Thus, the development of a feed-forward loop, wherein type I IFNs induce platelet activation leading to the induction of IFN-α synthesis by platelets and enhancing thrombotic risk, could be a mechanism by which type I IFNs enhance cardiovascular events.

Neutrophil Extracellular Traps

One mechanism of antimicrobial defense by neutrophils is the formation of neutrophil extracellular traps (NETs), which are composed of DNA and antimicrobial proteins. Research has demonstrated

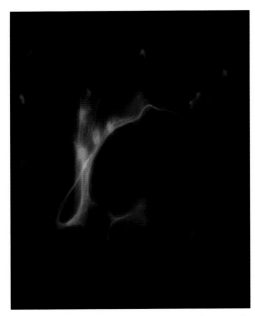

FIGURE 15-5 **Lupus low-density granulocytes (LDGs) externalize double-stranded DNA (dsDNA) through NETosis.** Representative image of lupus LDGs after isolation from peripheral blood. Cells were stained for detection of neutrophil elastase (*green*), DNA (Hoechst 33342, *blue*), and dsDNA (*red*). Photograph is a merged image of dsDNA, elastase, and Hoechst. Magnification is 40×. (*Picture obtained by Eneida Villanueva.*)

that these NETs may also contribute to endothelial injury. In SLE, neutrophils (and particularly LDGs) are primed to make NETs (Figure 15-5).[43,44] Autoantibodies, including anti-ribonucleoprotein and antibodies directed against antimicrobial proteins like LL37 and human neutrophil peptide, are increased in patients with lupus and are able to stimulate NET production in neutrophils in patients with SLE with greater frequency than in healthy controls.[43,45] When in contact with the endothelium, NETs provide cytotoxic signals that result in endothelial damage.[46] Indeed, spontaneous NET formation by LDGs induces enhanced endothelial apoptosis, which may further hamper the balance between vascular damage and repair in lupus.[44] Further enhancement of endothelial cytotoxicity may be induced by stimulation of NET formation by activated platelets, which are enhanced in SLE.[40] Intravascular NETs are also able to trap and activate platelets, possibly predisposing to thrombosis at sites of vascular injury.[47] In addition, lupus neutrophils induced to make NETs have enhanced capacity to stimulate pDCs to synthesize IFN-α,[43-45] potentially contributing to the perpetuation of the cycle of aberrant vascular damage and repair in this disease. Thus, interplay among endothelial activation, NET formation, endothelial cytotoxicity secondary to enhanced NET exposure, and thrombosis may contribute to enhanced cardiovascular events in SLE.

Other Cytokines

Cytokines in addition to type I IFNs play a role in cardiovascular disease development. TNF-α has been proposed to play a prominent role in the initiation and perpetuation of atherosclerotic lesions in the general population. This cytokine achieves its effect in part by enhancing the levels of adhesion molecules on the surface of vascular endothelium and by inducing chemotactic proteins, allowing for recruitment of monocytes and T cells into the endothelial wall.[16] In SLE, serum TNF-α values have been reported to be elevated and to correlate with coronary calcium scores.[22] TNF-α levels are also higher in patients with SLE and CVD than in those without CVD, and the higher levels correlate with altered lipid profiles.[48] Additionally, elevations of TNF-α may increase soluble vascular cell adhesion

molecule 1 in SLE.[49] To date, however, the exact role that TNF-α plays in the development of vascular damage in SLE remains unclear.

IL-17 stimulates synthesis of other proinflammatory cytokines and upregulation of chemokines and adhesion molecules. IL-17 has also been linked to atherosclerotic plaque development in non–lupus-prone mouse models. Indeed, atherosclerosis-prone mice have reduced plaque burden when transplanted with bone marrow deficient in the IL-17 receptor (IL-17R).[50] Additionally, IL-17 and IFN-γ dual-producing T cells are increased in CVD, have been localized to atherosclerotic plaque, and have been shown to be increased during ACS.[51,52] A link has been proposed between circulating levels of IL-17A and vascular dysfunction in rheumatoid arthritis.[53] Patients with SLE have increased levels of circulating IL-17, and T-helper 17 (Th17) cells are expanded in SLE and can induce upregulation of endothelial adhesion molecules.[54,55] Thus, there is a theoretical role for Th17 and IL-17 in the induction of cardiovascular damage in SLE, but this possibility needs to be further investigated.

The adipocytokine adiponectin inhibits monocyte adhesion to endothelial cells and migration and proliferation of vascular smooth muscle cells. Adiponectin is increased in lupus serum,[23,56] and this increase is associated with heightened severity of carotid plaque in this disease.[23] This discrepancy could be explained by long-term lupus vascular damage leading to positive feedback on adiponectin-secreting cells. Although this process could lead to increases in levels of adiponectin, its effects may be blunted at the site of endothelial damage because of the lupus inflammatory milieu.[57] Indeed, a protective role for adiponectin in lupus is supported by the observations of its absolute requirement for the protective effects against lupus cardiovascular disease by the drug rosiglitazone in murine models.[58]

T Cells

In addition to circulating and locally produced cytokines that contribute to the increased risk of CVD in SLE, SLE T cells may also play a pathogenic role. The differentiation of Th1 CD4⁺ T cells is promoted in atherosclerotic lesions by the greater expression of IFN-γ and IL-12.[16] These cells may also play a role in SLE-related CVD, because atherosclerosis-prone mice deficient in LDL receptors have increased vascular inflammation and CD4⁺ T-cell infiltration in their plaques after bone marrow transplantation with lupus-susceptible cells.[59] CD4⁺ T cells also increase (TNF)–related apoptosis-inducing ligand (TRAIL) expression when exposed to IFN-α, possibly leading to plaque destabilization and the development of ACS.[38]

CD154 (CD40 ligand) plays a crucial role in T-cell activation and is aberrantly upregulated on SLE T cells.[60] CD154-CD40 interactions between T cells and CD40-expressing endothelial cells can lead to upregulation of tissue factor and adhesion molecules by the endothelium.[61] These changes may promote a procoagulant state and initiation and perpetuation of vascular damage. In fact, atherosclerosis-prone mice that are treated with an antibody to disrupt CD40-CD154 interactions show lower plaque burden and less vessel inflammation.[62] These observations suggest a putative link between aberrant CD154 regulation in SLE and CVD.

CD137, an inducible T-cell co-stimulatory receptor present on both activated CD4⁺ and CD8⁺ T cells has previously been shown to be involved in the development of murine SLE.[63] A link between CD137 and vascular damage has also been demonstrated, as atherosclerosis-prone mice deficient in CD137 had lower plaque burden and less IFN-γ production by T cells.[64] The same study found that CD137 signaling activation in endothelial cells promotes enhanced synthesis of proinflammatory cytokines and adhesion molecules.[64]

Autoreactive CD4⁺ T cells present in patients with SLE could play a role in the induction of endothelial damage. This possibility is supported by the observation that SLE-autoreactive T cells can kill antigen-presenting cells (APCs).[65] Endothelial cells have the ability to act as APCs upon activation, and studies focused on transplant rejection indicate that graft endothelial cells are activated and killed by host T cells during antigen presentation.[66] Further research focused on the potentially deleterious interactions between endothelial cells and SLE-autoreactive T cells should be considered.

Other T-cell subsets may contribute to the increased risk of CVD in SLE. Invariant natural killer T (iNKT) cells, which recognize glycolipids and increase with the duration of lupus, may be proatherogenic.[67] The role of the abnormalities observed in T-regulatory cells in cardiovascular damage also warrants further investigation.[68] Indeed, regulatory T-cell function is compromised in mouse models of atherosclerosis.[23]

Complement and Immune Complexes

Characteristic of SLE is the formation of complement-containing immune complexes (ICs) that promote organ damage and may contribute to vascular disease. Indeed, inhibition of complement regulatory proteins exacerbates atherosclerosis in mice, whereas abrogation of the membrane attack complex attenuates atherosclerotic plaque formation.[69] Complement-IC interactions can lead to upregulation of endothelial adhesion molecules, leading to enhancement of neutrophil recruitment and vascular damage.[70] Increases in ox-LDL/beta-2 glycoprotein I (ox-LDL/β_2-GPI) complexes and anti-ox-LDL/β_2-GPI complex immunoglobulin (Ig) G or IgM have been reported in SLE. Because the titers of these complexes correlate with a number of cardiovascular risk factors,[71] it is possible that the complexes could be proatherogenic. In addition, the C1q complex has antiatherogenic effects, at least in part, in that it promotes macrophage clearance of oxidized and acetylated LDL. These observations indicate that C1q deficiency or antibodies that inactivate C1q could play a role in the vascular damage observed in SLE.[72] ICs may also play a role in vascular damage and atherosclerosis development. In rabbit models, ICs can accelerate diet-induced atherosclerosis; in addition, mice deficient in IC receptors have decreases in vascular damage.[73]

Oxidative Stress

Damage to the endothelium and the initiation and perpetuation of the atherogenic cycle may be influenced by the redox environment. Patients with SLE have increased levels of reactive oxygen and nitrogen species as well as antibodies to resultant protein adducts. These abnormalities correlate with disease activity and provide an environment for oxidation of lipoproteins and promotion of atherosclerosis.[74] Homocysteine, which has the capacity to increase reactive oxygen species in the bloodstream, is also increased in patients with SLE. Higher levels of homocysteine have been found to correlate with carotid IMT and with coronary calcification.[75-77] In addition, defense mechanisms against an altered redox environment appear to be downregulated in SLE. For example, paraoxonase, an enzyme with antioxidant activity that circulates attached to HDL and prevents LDL oxidation, is decreased in this disease. This finding correlates with the presence of antibodies to HDL and β_2-glycoprotein and with enhanced atherosclerosis risk.[78]

Ox-LDL, which is produced when LDL is exposed to reactive oxygen species, promotes cytokine secretion by endothelial cells, resulting in monocyte recruitment and differentiation into macrophages. Ox-LDL is increased in patients with SLE and the increase correlates with cardiovascular disease and renal involvement.[79] As mentioned previously, IFN-α upregulates SRA and may modulate foam cell formation in the presence of ox-LDL.[39] However, variations in uptake of ox-LDL may not necessarily explain the increased risk of atherosclerosis in SLE. Indeed, no differences have been found between the ability of monocytes from patients with lupus to bind and endocytose ox-LDL and that of monocytes from matched healthy controls.[80]

Oxidized LDL may also be proatherogenic via its associated molecules. Platelet-activating factor–acetylhydrolase (PAF-AH), also known as lipoprotein-associated phospholipase-A$_2$, binds to ox-LDL and may increase atherosclerotic plaque inflammation via the production of lysophosphatidylcholine. This molecule is increased in patients with SLE and established CVD.[81] Annexin V can bind to PAF-AH and prevent lysophosphatidylcholine generation. Because annexin V has been found to decrease endothelial binding capacity in patients with SLE and CVD, it is possible that this abnormality could play a role in cardiovascular risk in SLE.[82]

Lupus-Related Dyslipidemias

Dysfunctional cholesterol processing and elevated LDL are well-established risk factors for CVD in the general population (see Chapter 26 for additional information). In patients with SLE, the disturbances in lipoprotein levels and their processing in the bloodstream are well documented and result in higher cardiovascular risk profiles than in the general population. In clinically active lupus, HDL is decreased, whereas LDL, very-low-density lipoprotein (VLDL), and triglyceride levels are increased. As a result, ratios of total cholesterol to HDL-cholesterol and of LDL to HDL-cholesterol are increased. The triglyceride levels may be influenced by abnormal chylomicron processing secondary to low levels of lipoprotein lipase.[83] In addition, increased levels of proinflammatory HDL (piHDL) have been described in SLE and occur in approximately half of patients. Pro-inflammatory HDL is unable to protect LDL from oxidation and promotes endothelial injury. Indeed, increased piHDL levels in SLE have been associated with increases in carotid IMT.[84]

There is also evidence that the lipid profiles in lupus mice are more susceptible to environmental effects. Lupus-prone mice exposed to high-fat chow exhibit higher piHDL and greater lipid deposition in vessels than nonlupus mice.[85] A high-fat diet administered to LDL receptor–deficient mice that had been made susceptible to SLE via bone marrow transplantation promoted enhanced lipid levels and significant increases in mortality in comparison with similar mice fed regular chow.[59] These observations suggest that SLE may increase sensitivity to the lipid perturbations induced by diet and other environmental stimuli.

Antiphospholipid Antibodies

The role of antiphospholipid (APL) antibodies in premature CVD remains a matter of debate. It has been hypothesized that β_2-GPI, a molecule that is abundant in vascular plaques, may be atheroprotective. On the other hand, some groups have proposed that β_2-GPI may induce a cellular immune response in a subpopulation of patients with carotid atherosclerosis, thus contributing to the inflammatory responses involved in atherosclerotic disease. Previous studies have shown in vitro cross-reactivity of APL antibodies with ox-LDL as well as an interaction between ox-LDL and β_2-glycoprotein. These results may indicate a pro-atherogenic role for β_2-GPI and APL antibodies.[86,87] Antibodies against β_2-GPI could, in theory, be detrimental to the vessel wall and promote activation of inflammatory cascades by IC formation.[88] APL antibodies may increase the likelihood of abnormal ankle-brachial index, and anticardiolipin antibody titers correlate with carotid IMT.[75,89] A study examining FMD and EPC numbers in patients with primary APL syndrome (APS), however, did not detect any difference in their levels of these early markers of cardiovascular risk and levels in age- and gender-matched healthy controls.[90] This observation is supported by previous work in which the presence of APL antibodies did not correlate with endothelial dysfunction or carotid IMT in SLE.[7,87] In one study using cardiac magnetic resonance imaging (MRI) to find evidence of subclinical ischemic disease, 26% of patients with APS had occult myocardial scarring, compared with 11% of controls. In this study, however, 22% of the enrolled patients had APS in association with SLE (and it is unclear whether a significant number of the patients with myocardial damage also had lupus).[91] Thus, the role of APL antibodies in the development of atherosclerosis in SLE remains unclear and requires further investigation. Nevertheless, because APS is clearly linked to the development of arterial thrombosis, a putative role for APL antibodies in triggering unstable angina and acute coronary syndromes should be considered (see Chapter 42 for more information on antiphospholipid antibodies).

Other Autoantibodies

Autoantibodies against regulatory proteins in the atherogenic cycle in SLE may potentially contribute to CVD. Antibodies to the antiatherogenic HDL and one of its components, apolipoprotein (apo) A-1, are increased in SLE and rise with disease flares.[92] Apo A-1 IgG correlates with an increased risk of a major cardiovascular event and may have positive chronotropic effects, further contributing to an enhanced risk of cardiac death.[93] Although these antibodies have also been shown to be independent predictors of major cardiovascular events in rheumatoid arthritis,[94] their role in promoting damage to the vasculature in SLE remains to be determined.

Patients with SLE have increased levels of anti–lipoprotein lipase antibodies, which rise with disease activity. These antibodies may contribute to hypertriglyceridemia and may be proatherogenic.[95] Anti–endothelial cell antibodies (AECAs) represent a heterogeneous family of autoantibodies directed against structural endothelial proteins. These antibodies can be detected in a heterogeneous group of autoimmune and inflammatory conditions, including SLE. AECAs can induce a proinflammatory and proadhesive endothelial cell phenotype leading to increased monocyte adhesion. AECAs have also been implicated in mediating enhanced endothelial apoptosis.[96] However, the precise contribution of AECAs to atherosclerosis-related chronic endothelial activation in SLE is unclear.[97] Additionally, antibodies to ox-LDL, lipoprotein lipase, CRP, and annexin V have may have a putative role in CVD in SLE.[98,99]

Naturally occurring IgM antibodies against phosphorylcholine, which plays a role in platelet-activating factor (PAF) receptor signaling, are inversely correlated with atherosclerosis.[100] Additionally, both IgG and IgM antiphosphorylcholine antibodies, which are able to inhibit expression of endothelial cell adhesion molecules in response to platelet-activating factor, are decreased in patients with SLE in proportion to disease activity.[101] Evidence now indicates that low levels of antiphosphorylcholine IgM are independently associated with the prevalence of carotid atherosclerotic plaque in patients with SLE.[102]

CONCLUSION

The cardiovascular risk in patients with SLE stems from a combination of traditional risk factors and SLE-specific mechanisms that incorporate chronic inflammation, endothelial dysfunction, decreased vascular repair through a type I IFN effect, antibody formation, enhanced NETosis and aberrant neutrophil function, and a perturbed lipid homeostasis and redox environment. It is hoped that continued research into the mechanisms of lupus-related CVD will provide effective tools and targets to improve patient survival and overall quality of life.

References

1. Manzi S, Meilahn EN, Rairie JE, et al: Age-specific incidence rates of myocardial infarction and angina in women with systemic lupus erythematosus: comparison with the Framingham Study. *American Journal of Epidemiology* 145:408–415, 1997.
2. Hak AE, Karlson EW, Feskanich D, et al: Systemic lupus erythematosus and the risk of cardiovascular disease: results from the nurses' health study. *Arthritis Care & Research* 61:1396–1402, doi:10.1002/art.24537, 2009.
3. Shah MA, Shah AM, Krishnan E: Poor outcomes after acute myocardial infarction in systemic lupus erythematosus. *The Journal of rheumatology* 36:570–575, 2009.
4. Esdaile JM, Abrahamowicz M, Grodzicky T, et al: Traditional Framingham risk factors fail to fully account for accelerated atherosclerosis in systemic lupus erythematosus. *Arthritis and rheumatism* 44:2331–2337, 2001.
5. Haider YS, Roberts WC: Coronary arterial disease in systemic lupus erythematosus; quantification of degrees of narrowing in 22 necropsy patients (21 women) aged 16 to 37 years. *Am J Med* 70:775–781, 1981.
6. Sipek-Dolnicar A, Hojnik M, Bozic B, et al: Clinical presentations and vascular histopathology in autopsied patients with systemic lupus erythematosus and anticardiolipin antibodies. *Clinical and experimental rheumatology* 20:335–342, 2002.
7. Kiani AN, Vogel-Claussen J, Magder LS, et al: Noncalcified coronary plaque in systemic lupus erythematosus. *J Rheumatol* 37:579–584, 2010.
8. Kiani AN, Magder L, Petri M: Coronary calcium in systemic lupus erythematosus is associated with traditional cardiovascular risk factors, but not with disease activity. *J Rheumatol* 35:1300–1306, 2008.
9. Rajagopalan S, Somers EC, Brook RD, et al: Endothelial cell apoptosis in systemic lupus erythematosus: a common pathway for abnormal vascular function and thrombosis propensity. *Blood* 103:3677–3683, 2004.
10. El-Magadmi M, Bodill H, Ahmad Y, et al: Systemic lupus erythematosus: an independent risk factor for endothelial dysfunction in women. *Circulation* 110:399–404, 2004.
11. Manzi S, Selzer F, Sutton-Tyrrell K, et al: Prevalence and risk factors of carotid plaque in women with systemic lupus erythematosus. *Arthritis and rheumatism* 42:51–60, 1999.
12. Roldan C, Joson J, Sharrar J, et al: Premature aortic atherosclerosis in systemic lupus erythematosus: a controlled transesophageal echocardiographic study. *The Journal of rheumatology* 37:71–78, 2010.
13. Hirata K, Kadirvelu A, Kinjo M, et al: Altered coronary vasomotor function in young patients with systemic lupus erythematosus. *Arthritis & Rheumatism* 56:1904–1909, 2007.
14. Recio-Mayoral A, Mason J, Kaski J, et al: Chronic inflammation and coronary microvascular dysfunction in patients without risk factors for coronary artery disease. *European Heart Journal* 30:1837–1843, 2009.
15. Hansson GK: Inflammation, atherosclerosis, and coronary artery disease. *New England Journal of Medicine* 352:1685–1695, 2005.
16. McMahon M, Hahn BH: Atherosclerosis and systemic lupus erythematosus—mechanistic basis of the association. *Current Opinion in Immunology* 19:633–639, 2007.
17. Duewell P, Kono H, Rayner KJ, et al: NLRP3 inflammasomes are required for atherogenesis and activated by cholesterol crystals. *Nature* 464:1357–1361, 2010.
18. Briasoulis A, Tousoulis D, Antoniades C, et al: The role of endothelial progenitor cells in vascular repair after arterial injury and atherosclerotic plaque development. *Cardiovascular Therapeutics* 29:125–139, 2011.
19. Schmidt-Lucke C, Rssig L, Fichtlscherer S, et al: Reduced number of circulating endothelial progenitor cells predicts future cardiovascular events: proof of concept for the clinical importance of endogenous vascular repair. *Circulation* 111:2981–2987, 2005.
20. George J, Herz I, Goldstein E, et al: Number and adhesive properties of circulating endothelial progenitor cells in patients with in-stent restenosis. *Arterioscler Thromb Vasc Biol* 23:e57–e60, doi:10.1161/01. ATV.0000017029.65274.db, 2003.
21. Vasa M, Fichtlscherer S, Aicher A, et al: Number and migratory activity of circulating endothelial progenitor cells inversely correlate with risk factors for coronary artery disease. *Circulation research* 89:E1–E7, 2001.
22. Rho Y, Chung C, Oeser A, et al: Novel cardiovascular risk factors in premature coronary atherosclerosis associated with systemic lupus erythematosus. *The Journal of rheumatology* 35:1789–1794, 2008.
23. Reynolds HR, Buyon J, Kim M, et al: Association of plasma soluble E-selectin and adiponectin with carotid plaque in patients with systemic lupus erythematosus. *Atherosclerosis* 210:569–574, 2010.
24. Baker JF, Zhang L, Imadojemu S, et al: Circulating endothelial progenitor cells are reduced in SLE in the absence of coronary artery calcification. *Rheumatology international* 32:997–1002, 2012.
25. Westerweel P, Luijten RKMAC, Hoefer I, et al: Haematopoietic and endothelial progenitor cells are deficient in quiescent systemic lupus erythematosus. *Annals of the Rheumatic Diseases* 66:865–870, 2007.
26. Denny MF, Thacker S, Mehta H, et al: Interferon-alpha promotes abnormal vasculogenesis in lupus: a potential pathway for premature atherosclerosis. *Blood* 110:2907–2915, 2007.
27. Baechler E, Batliwalla F, Karypis G, et al: Interferon-inducible gene expression signature in peripheral blood cells of patients with severe lupus. *Proceedings of the National Academy of Sciences of the United States of America* 100:2610–2615, 2003.
28. Kim T, Kanayama Y, Negoro N, et al: Serum levels of interferons in patients with systemic lupus erythematosus. *Clinical and experimental immunology* 70:562–569, 1987.
29. Mallat Z, Benamer H, Hugel B, et al: Elevated levels of shed membrane microparticles with procoagulant potential in the peripheral circulating blood of patients with acute coronary syndromes. *Circulation* 101:841–843, 2000.
30. Lee P, Li Y, Richards H, et al: Type I interferon as a novel risk factor for endothelial progenitor cell depletion and endothelial dysfunction in systemic lupus erythematosus. *Arthritis and rheumatism* 56:3759–3769, 2007.

31. Somers EC, Zhao W, Lewis EE, et al: *Type I Interferon signatures are associated with vascular risk and atherosclerosis in systemic lupus erythematosus. Abstract# 10223. Presented at the annual meeting of the American College of Rheumatology and the Association of Rheumatology Health Professionals, Philadelphia.* October 16–21, 2009.

32. Thacker S, Berthier C, Mattinzoli D, et al: The detrimental effects of IFN-α on vasculogenesis in lupus are mediated by repression of IL-1 pathways: potential role in atherogenesis and renal vascular rarefaction. *The journal of immunology* 185:4457–4469, 2010.

33. Thacker SG, Duquaine D, Park J, et al: Lupus-prone New Zealand Black/New Zealand White F1 mice display endothelial dysfunction and abnormal phenotype and function of endothelial progenitor cells. *Lupus* 19:288–299, 2010.

34. Kahlenberg JM, Thacker SG, Berthier CC, et al: Inflammasome activation of IL-18 results in endothelial progenitor cell dysfunction in systemic lupus erythematosus. *J Immunol* 187(11):6143–6156, doi:jimmunol.1101284 [pii]10.4049/jimmunol.1101284, 2011.

35. Denny M, Yalavarthi S, Zhao W, et al: A distinct subset of proinflammatory neutrophils isolated from patients with systemic lupus erythematosus induces vascular damage and synthesizes type I IFNs. *The journal of immunology* 184:3284–3297, 2010.

36. Bonelli M, Smolen JS, Scheinecker C: Treg and lupus. *Annals of the Rheumatic Diseases* 69:i65–i66, 2010.

37. Niessner A, Shin M, Pryshchep O, et al: Synergistic proinflammatory effects of the antiviral cytokine interferon-alpha and Toll-like receptor 4 ligands in the atherosclerotic plaque. *Circulation* 116:2043–2052, 2007.

38. Niessner A, Weyand CM: Dendritic cells in atherosclerotic disease. *Clinical Immunology* 134:25–32, 2010.

39. Li J, Fu Q, Cui H, et al: Interferon-α priming promotes lipid uptake and macrophage-derived foam cell formation: a novel link between interferon-α and atherosclerosis in lupus. *Arthritis & Rheumatism* 63:492–502, 2011.

40. Lood C, Amisten S, Gullstrand B, et al: Platelet transcriptional profile and protein expression in patients with systemic lupus erythematosus: up-regulation of the type I interferon system is strongly associated with vascular disease. *Blood* 116:1951–1957, 2010.

41. Duffau P, Seneschal J, Nicco C, et al: Platelet CD154 potentiates interferon-alpha secretion by plasmacytoid dendritic cells in systemic lupus erythematosus. *Science translational medicine* 2:47ra63–47ra63, 2010.

42. Higashiyama M, Hokari R, Kurihara C, et al: Interferon-α increases monocyte migration via platelet-monocyte interaction in murine intestinal microvessels. *Clinical & Experimental Immunology* 162:156–162, 2010.

43. Garcia-Romo GS, Caielli S, Vega B, et al: Netting neutrophils are major inducers of type I IFN production in pediatric systemic lupus erythematosus. *Sci Transl Med* 3:73ra20, 2011.

44. Villanueva E, Yalavarthi S, Berthier CC, et al: Netting neutrophils induce endothelial damage, infiltrate tissues, and expose immunostimulatory molecules in systemic lupus erythematosus. *J Immunol* 187:538–552, 2011.

45. Lande R, Ganguly D, Facchinetti V, et al: Neutrophils activate plasmacytoid dendritic cells by releasing self-DNA-peptide complexes in systemic lupus erythematosus. *Sci Transl Med* 3:73ra19, 2011.

46. Gupta AK, Joshi MB, Philippova M, et al: Activated endothelial cells induce neutrophil extracellular traps and are susceptible to NETosis-mediated cell death. *FEBS Letters* 584:3193–3197, 2010.

47. Fuchs TA, Brill A, Duerschmied D, et al: Extracellular DNA traps promote thrombosis. *Proceedings of the National Academy of Sciences* 107:15880–15885, 2010.

48. Svenungsson E, Fei GZ, Jensen-Urstad K, et al: TNF-alpha: a link between hypertriglyceridaemia and inflammation in SLE patients with cardiovascular disease. *Lupus* 12:454–461, 2003.

49. Svenungsson E, Cederholm A, Jensen-Urstad K, et al: Endothelial function and markers of endothelial activation in relation to cardiovascular disease in systemic lupus erythematosus. *Scandinavian Journal of Rheumatology* 37:352–359, 2008.

50. van Es T, van Puijvelde GHM, Ramos OH, et al: Attenuated atherosclerosis upon IL-17R signaling disruption in LDLr deficient mice. *Biochemical and Biophysical Research Communications* 388:261–265, 2009.

51. Wang Z, Lee J, Zhang Y, et al: Increased Th17 cells in coronary artery disease are associated with neutrophilic inflammation. Scandinavian Cardiovascular Journal 45:54–61, 2011.

52. Chen S, Crother T, Arditi M: Emerging role of IL-17 in atherosclerosis. Journal of innate *immunity* 2:325–333, 2010.

53. Marder W, Myles KS, Yalavarthi J, et al: Interleukin-17 as a novel predictor of vascular function in rheumatoid arthritis. *Annals of Rheumatic Diseases* 70:1550–1555, 2011.

54. Mok MY, Wu HJ, Lo Y, et al: The relation of interleukin 17 (IL-17) and IL-23 to Th1/Th2 cytokines and disease activity in systemic lupus erythematosus. *The Journal of rheumatology*, 37(10):2046–2052, doi:10.3899/jrheum.100293, 2010.

55. Yang J, Chu Y, Yang X, et al: Th17 and natural Treg cell population dynamics in systemic lupus erythematosus. *Arthritis and rheumatism* 60:1472–1483, 2009.

56. Chung CP, Long AG, Solus JF, et al: Adipocytokines in systemic lupus erythematosus: relationship to inflammation, insulin resistance and coronary atherosclerosis. *Lupus* 18:799–806, 2009.

57. Clancy R, Ginzler E: Endothelial function and its implications for cardiovascular and renal disease in systemic lupus erythematosus. *Rheumatic diseases clinics of North America* 36:145–160, ix, 2010.

58. Aprahamian T, Bonegio RG, Richez C, et al: The peroxisome proliferator-activated receptor γ agonist rosiglitazone ameliorates murine lupus by induction of adiponectin. *J Immunol* 182:340–346, 2009.

59. Braun N, Wade N, Wakeland E, et al: Accelerated atherosclerosis is independent of feeding high fat diet in systemic lupus erythematosus-susceptible LDLr−/− mice. *Lupus* 17:1070–1078, 2008.

60. Koshy M, Berger D, Crow MK: Increased expression of CD40 ligand on systemic lupus erythematosus lymphocytes. *The Journal of clinical investigation* 98:826–837, 1996.

61. Yellin MJ, Thienel U: T cells in the pathogenesis of systemic lupus erythematosus: potential roles of CD154-CD40 interactions and costimulatory molecules. *Curr Rheumatol Rep* 2:24–31, 2000.

62. Mach F, Schnbeck U, Sukhova GK, et al: Reduction of atherosclerosis in mice by inhibition of CD40 signalling. *Nature* 394:200–203, 1998.

63. Foell J, Strahotin S, O'Neil S, et al: CD137 costimulatory T cell receptor engagement reverses acute disease in lupus-prone NZB × NZW F1 mice. *The Journal of clinical investigation* 111:1505–1518, 2003.

64. Jeon H, Choi J-H, Jung I-H, et al: CD137 (4-1BB) deficiency reduces atherosclerosis in hyperlipidemic mice. *Circulation* 121:1124–1133, 2010.

65. Kaplan M, Lewis E, Shelden E, et al: The apoptotic ligands TRAIL, TWEAK, and Fas ligand mediate monocyte death induced by autologous lupus T cells. *The journal of immunology* 169:6020–6029, 2002.

66. Al-Lamki R, Bradley J, Pober J: Endothelial cells in allograft rejection. *Transplantation* 86:1340–1348, 2008.

67. Major AS, Singh RR, Joyce S, et al: The role of invariant natural killer T cells in lupus and atherogenesis. *Immunol Res* 34:49–66, 2006.

68. Urowitz MB, Gladman DD, Tom BDM, et al: Changing patterns in mortality and disease outcomes for patients with systemic lupus erythematosus. *The Journal of rheumatology* 35:2152–2158, 2008.

69. Wu G, Hu W, Shahsafaei A, et al: Complement regulator CD59 protects against atherosclerosis by restricting the formation of complement membrane attack complex. *Circ Res* 104:550–558, 2009.

70. Clancy RM: Circulating endothelial cells and vascular injury in systemic lupus erythematosus. *Current Rheumatology Reports* 2:39–43, 2000.

71. Bassi N, Zampieri S, Ghirardello A, et al: Oxldl/2gpI complex and anti-oxldl/2gpi in SLE: prevalence and correlates. *Autoimmunity* 42:289–291, 2009.

72. Fraser DA, Tenner AJ: Innate immune proteins C1q and mannan-binding lectin enhance clearance of atherogenic lipoproteins by human monocytes and macrophages. *J Immunol* 185:3932–3939, 2010.

73. Mayadas TN, Tsokos GC, Tsuboi N: Mechanisms of immune complex-mediated neutrophil recruitment and tissue injury. *Circulation* 120: 2012–2024, 2009.

74. Wang G, Pierangeli SS, Papalardo E, et al: Markers of oxidative and nitrosative stress in systemic lupus erythematosus: correlation with disease activity. *Arthritis Rheum* 62:2064–2072, 2010.

75. Ames PRJ, Margarita A, Alves JD, et al: Anticardiolipin antibody titre and plasma homocysteine level independently predict intima media thickness of carotid arteries in subjects with idiopathic antiphospholipid antibodies. *Lupus* 11:208–214, 2002.

76. Roman MJ, Crow MK, Lockshin MD, et al: Rate and determinants of progression of atherosclerosis in systemic lupus erythematosus. *Arthritis & Rheumatism* 56:3412–3419, 2007.

77. Kiani AN, Magder L, Petri M: Coronary calcium in systemic lupus erythematosus is associated with traditional cardiovascular risk factors, but not with disease activity. *J Rheumatology* 35:1300–1306, 2008.

78. Alves JD, Ames PRJ, Donohue S, et al: Antibodies to high-density lipoprotein and beta2-glycoprotein I are inversely correlated with paraoxonase

activity in systemic lupus erythematosus and primary antiphospholipid syndrome. *Arthritis and rheumatism* 46:2686–2694, 2002.

79. Frostegård J, Svenungsson E, Wu R, et al: Lipid peroxidation is enhanced in patients with systemic lupus erythematosus and is associated with arterial and renal disease manifestations. *Arthritis & Rheumatism* 52:192–200, 2005.

80. Yassin LM, Londoño J, Montoya G, et al: Atherosclerosis development in SLE patients is not determined by monocytes ability to bind/endocytose Ox-LDL. *Autoimmunity* 44:201–210, 2011.

81. Cederholm A, Svenungsson E, Stengel D, et al: Platelet-activating factor-acetylhydrolase and other novel risk and protective factors for cardiovascular disease in systemic lupus erythematosus. *Arthritis & Rheumatism* 50:2869–2876, 2004.

82. Cederholm A, Frostegard J: Frostegard, J Annexin A5 as a novel player in prevention of atherothrombosis in SLE and in the general population. *Ann N Y Acad Sci* 1108:96–103, 2007.

83. Borba EF, Bonf E, Vinagre CG, et al: Chylomicron metabolism is markedly altered in systemic lupus erythematosus. *Arthritis and rheumatism* 43:1033–1040, 2000.

84. McMahon M, Grossman J, Skaggs B, et al: Dysfunctional proinflammatory high-density lipoproteins confer increased risk of atherosclerosis in women with systemic lupus erythematosus. *Arthritis and rheumatism* 60:2428–2437, 2009.

85. Hahn B, Lourencço E, McMahon M, et al: Pro-inflammatory high-density lipoproteins and atherosclerosis are induced in lupus-prone mice by a high-fat diet and leptin. *Lupus* 19:913–917, 2010.

86. Kobayashi K, Kishi M, Atsumi T, et al: Circulating oxidized LDL forms complexes with beta2-glycoprotein I: implication as an atherogenic autoantigen. *J Lipid Res* 44:716–726, 2003.

87. Profumo E, Buttari B, Alessandri C, et al: Beta2-glycoprotein I is a target of T cell reactivity in patients with advanced carotid atherosclerotic plaques. *Int J Immunopathol Pharmacol* 23:73–80, 2010.

88. George J, Harats D, Gilburd B, et al: Immunolocalization of beta2-glycoprotein I (apolipoprotein H) to human atherosclerotic plaques: potential implications for lesion progression. *Circulation* 99:2227–2230, 1999.

89. Baron MA, Khamashta MA, Hughes GRV, et al: Prevalence of an abnormal ankle-brachial index in patients with primary antiphospholipid syndrome: preliminary data. *Annals of the Rheumatic Diseases* 64:144–146, 2005.

90. Gresele P, Migliacci R, Vedovati MC, et al: Patients with primary antiphospholipid antibody syndrome and without associated vascular risk factors present a normal endothelial function. *Thrombosis Research* 123:444–451, 2009.

91. Sacre K, Brihaye B, Hyafil F, et al: Asymptomatic myocardial ischemic disease in antiphospholipid syndrome: a controlled cardiac magnetic resonance imaging study. *Arthritis and rheumatism* 62:2093–2100, 2010.

92. O'Neill S, Giles I, Lambrianides A, et al: Antibodies to apolipoprotein A-I, high-density lipoprotein, and C-reactive protein are associated with disease activity in patients with systemic lupus erythematosus. *Arthritis and rheumatism* 62:845–854, 2010.

93. Vuilleumier N, Rossier M, Pagano S, et al: Anti-apolipoprotein A-1 IgG as an independent cardiovascular prognostic marker affecting basal heart rate in myocardial infarction. *European Heart Journal* 31:815–823, 2010.

94. Vuilleumier N, Bas S, Pagano S, et al: Anti-apolipoprotein A-1 IgG predicts major cardiovascular events in patients with rheumatoid arthritis. *Arthritis Rheum* 62:2640–2650, 2010.

95. Rodrigues CEM, Bonfá E, Carvalho JF: Review on anti-lipoprotein lipase antibodies. *Clinica Chimica Acta* 411:1603–1605, 2011.

96. Domiciano D, Carvalho J, Shoenfeld Y: Pathogenic role of anti-endothelial cell antibodies in autoimmune rheumatic diseases. *Lupus* 18:1233–1238, 2009.

97. Duval A, Helley D, Capron L, et al: Endothelial dysfunction in systemic lupus patients with low disease activity: evaluation by quantification and characterization of circulating endothelial microparticles, role of anti-endothelial cell antibodies. *Rheumatology* 49:1049–1055, 2010.

98. Elliott J, Manzi S: Cardiovascular risk assessment and treatment in systemic lupus erythematosus. Best Practice & Research *Clinical Rheumatology* 23:481–494, 2009.

99. Meyer O: Anti-CRP antibodies in systemic lupus erythematosus. *Joint bone spine* 77:384–389, 2010.

100. Su J, Georgiades A, Wu R, et al: Antibodies of IgM subclass to phosphorylcholine and oxidized LDL are protective factors for atherosclerosis in patients with hypertension. *Atherosclerosis* 188:160–166, 2006.

101. Su J, Hua X, Concha H, et al: Natural antibodies against phosphorylcholine as potential protective factors in SLE. *Rheumatology* 47:1144–1150, 2008.

102. Anania C, Gustafsson T, Hua X, et al: Increased prevalence of vulnerable atherosclerotic plaques and low levels of natural IgM antibodies against phosphorylcholine in patients with systemic lupus erythematosus. *Arthritis research & therapy* 12:R214–R214, 2010.

Mechanisms of Tissue Damage—Free Radicals and Fibrosis

Biji T. Kurien, Chandra Mohan, and R. Hal Scofield

Systemic lupus erythematosus (SLE) is a chronic, complex inflammatory autoimmune disease involving multisystem manifestations. Diverse autoantibody response, directed against a multitude of self-antigens, is a characteristic of the disease. The targets of these antibodies are localized in the nucleus, cytoplasm, or cell membranes. SLE it thought to arise as a consequence of genetic and environmental factors.[1] To date, multiple mechanisms of tissue damage have been implicated in SLE, including oxidative stress and free radicals, fibrosis, complement-mediated pathways, and a panoply of enzymatic cascades including matrix metalloproteinases, the renin-angiotensin system, plasmin, and kallikreins. This review focuses on two of these mechanisms: free radicals and oxidative stress and fibrosis.

FREE RADICALS AND OXIDATIVE STRESS

Free radicals (reactive oxygen species, oxygen-based free radicals, reactive nitrogen species, and nitrogen-based free radicals), free radical–mediated oxidative damage, and its natural corollary—namely, oxidative modification of proteins—are seen in SLE.[2-10] That oxidative stress, through the process of lipid peroxidation and resulting products of oxidative damage, may be implicated in the pathogenesis of SLE is evidenced by (1) an enhanced urinary excretion of isoprostanes, a well-established index of lipid peroxidation, in patients with SLE; (2) the fact that lipid peroxidation–derived short-chain aldehyde levels are significantly elevated in children with high SLE disease activity; and (3) the finding of oxidized LDL elevations along with increased levels of autoantibodies against oxidized LDL in women with SLE. The involvement of free radical–mediated lipid peroxidation is also suggested by the observation that lipid peroxidation–specific epitopes are detected in tissues from the patients.[11]

Free Radicals, Antioxidant Enzymes, and Lipid Peroxidation

Compared with most anaerobic organisms, aerobes have an efficient metabolism owing to the high reduction potential of molecular oxygen, which acts as the terminal electron acceptor for respiration. However, because both chemical reduction and metabolic reduction of oxygen result in the production of highly toxic free radicals, this advantage comes with a price.[12]

Free radicals are chemical species that contain atoms with one or more unpaired electrons occupying an outer orbital. This arrangement of electrons means that free radicals readily engage in chemical reactions by donating the unpaired, outer-orbit electron to another molecule. Thus, free radicals are highly reactive and generally have an extremely short lifespan.

Detection of Radicals

Free radicals possess unique physical properties that permit their detection and analysis. These properties derive from the fact that any charged particle that is spinning generates a magnetic field. Therefore, electrons and protons create a weak magnetic field. Paired electrons occupying an orbital, owing to their opposing spins, cancel each other's magnetic fields. On the other hand, a free radical can be detected and analyzed by means of electron paramagnetic resonance spectroscopy because free radicals have a weak magnetic field as a result of the unopposed electron.[13]

Radical Chemistry—A Brief Outline

A free radical state can be induced by physical means such as irradiation with x rays or ultraviolet (UV) light or by chemical means such as with compounds known as *initiators*. Most importantly, substances attain an unusual chemistry and molecular configurational changes once they become free radicals. Substances change their physical-chemical properties and shapes considerably as free radicals. Free radicals blaze their own patterns of chemical reactions. In order to distinguish them from the normal organic reactions, such chemical reactions are sometimes referred to as anti-Markownikoff or Kharasch mechanisms. The important aspect regarding radical chemistry is the altered function of molecules involved consequent to the altered size and shape.[13]

Free radicals are generally known as reactive oxygen species (ROS) when oxygen-based and reactive nitrogen species (RNS) when nitrogen-based.

Reactive Oxygen Species

ROS are highly reactive and are produced even at basal conditions in living organisms by a number of ways. The superoxide anion radical O_2^- is formed consequent to the one-electron reduction of oxygen. The two-electron reduction product of oxygen in the fully protonated form is hydrogen peroxide (H_2O_2), and the hydroxyl radical ($OH\cdot$) results from the three-electron reduction of oxygen.[2,3,8,9]

Oxygen is reduced to the more reactive superoxide radical by a variety of enzymic and nonenzymic reactions.[14] The divalent reduction of oxygen by the enzymes urate oxidase, D-amino-acid oxidase, and glycolate oxidase leads to formation of superoxide. The univalent reduction of oxygen to superoxide followed by the action of superoxide dismutase leads to the formation of hydrogen peroxide. Hydrogen peroxide, though not a free radical itself, can lead to the formation of the more dangerous hydroxyl radical through the Fenton reaction. Autoxidation of dehydrogenases, catechols, thiols, flavins, and oxidases, as well as UV radiation, can also generate superoxide anion and hydrogen peroxide.[3,14]

Aerobic organisms have developed protective mechanisms to escape from the hazards of oxygen toxicity, which is the result of ROS. Superoxide dismutase, catalase, and the peroxidases form the enzymatic free radical defense system. Ascorbic acid, vitamin E, and reduced glutathione serve as the nonenzymatic antioxidant sentinels that guard against oxidative damage. Superoxide dismutase (SOD) catalyzes the conversion of superoxide to hydrogen peroxide, which is then converted to water by catalase/glutathione peroxidase.

Superoxide dismutases are virtually ubiquitous among living organisms. However, there are three SOD metalloisoenzymes, and these isoenzymes display different intracellular and species distributions. Copper-zinc–containing SOD (SOD1) is found in the cytoplasm of virtually all eukaryotic cells. Manganese-containing SOD

(SOD2) is located in the mitochondrial matrix of all aerobes. Mammals have extracellular copper-zinc (Cu-Zn) SOD (SOD3) in extracellular fluids or associated with membrane.[15] Bacteria possess an iron SOD (FeSOD), a manganese SOD (MnSOD), or both in the cytosol. In addition, higher plants generally contain a Cu-Zn SOD isozyme in the chloroplast. Some plants also have chloroplast FeSOD, chloroplast MnSOD, and leaf peroxisomal MnSOD.[15]

Anaerobes generally do not have the Cu-Zn SOD or catalase genes. This lack of such genes is shown by their absence from the complete genome sequences now available for the anaerobic *Methanococcus jannaschii*, *Archaeoglobus fulgidus*, *Pyrococcus horikoshii*, *Pyrococcus abyssi*, and *Thermotoga maritima* as well as the incomplete genome of *Clostridium acetobutylicum*.[12] However, *Photobacterium leiognathi*, *Caulobacter crescentus*,[15] as well as the opportunistic pathogen *Bacteroides fragilis* (the most aerotolerant species among anaerobic bacteria), do have Cu-Zn SOD in addition to Fe SOD.[12]

Interaction of Reactive Oxygen Species with Lipids

Compromise of the activity of SOD, catalase, or peroxidases by stress or any other factor could result in the triggering of a potentially dangerous pathway of lipoperoxidative damage. *Lipid peroxidation* has been defined as oxidative degeneration of polyunsaturated fatty acids, set into motion by free radicals. Oxidative damage brought about by ROS is involved in the pathogenesis of several diseases.[2-10]

The unsaturated acyl chains in membrane phospholipids and cholesterol in membranes, among biomolecules, are highly susceptible to pathologic free radical damage for the following reasons[16]: First, the inherent structure of polyunsaturated fatty acid chains (polyunsaturated acyl chains are normally unconjugated, and the alpha-methylenic carbons between carbons with double bonds have allylic hydrogen that can readily enter into free radical reaction.[13,16] Second, the solubility of molecular oxygen is 700% higher within nonpolar than aqueous milieus (the hydrophobic regions of the membrane are generally the most nonpolar regions of the cell). Third, molecular oxygen has unpaired electrons in the outer orbitals. This feature confers upon oxygen certain properties of free radicals, such as magnetic susceptibility (owing to the magnetic moment of an unpaired electron in orbit) and the propensity to initiate free radical chain reactions among susceptible molecules that lack enough neighboring antioxidant molecules.[13,16,17]

Oxidation of any polyunsaturated fatty acid results in a number of deleterious end products and is a chain reaction involving initiation, propagation, and termination (Figure 16-1A).[17] In the initiation phase, a primary reactive radical molecule (x•) containing an unpaired electron interacts with polyunsaturated fatty acid to initiate the peroxidation process. The reactive radical molecule has enough reactivity to abstract a hydrogen atom from a methylene group (—CH$_2$—). An unpaired electron is left on the carbon (—CH—), because a hydrogen atom has only one electron. The carbon radical tends to stabilize itself by molecular rearrangement to form a conjugated diene. The carbon-centered fatty acid radicals combine with molecular oxygen in the propagation phase, yielding highly reactive peroxyl radicals that react with other lipid molecules to form hydroperoxides. Peroxyl radicals are capable of producing new fatty acid radicals, resulting in a radical chain reaction. The peroxyl radicals themselves, in this reaction, are converted to stable termination products (lipid hydroperoxides) (see Figure 16-1A). Thus, the lipid peroxidation process can result in a variety of harmful end products. Markers of oxidative damage include conjugated dienes, isoprostanes, 4-hydroxy-2-nonenal (HNE), HNE-modified proteins, malondialdehyde (MDA), MDA-modified proteins, protein-bound acrolein, ROS-modified DNA, and protein carbonylation.[3,4,13,17-19]

Interaction of Reactive Oxygen Species with Proteins

Enzymes and other proteins, when subjected to lipid peroxidation in aqueous solutions, undergo polymerization, polypeptide chain scission, and chemical changes in individual amino acids. In spite of the fact that all these chemical reactions are important to the sequence of damage that occurs, current interest focuses on the polymerization or cross-linking of proteins. Pure enzymes undergo cross-linking when exposed to lipid peroxidation, resulting in a several-fold increase in molecular weight in comparison with their original molecular weights. Thus, the biological activities of enzymes and other proteins and their precise arrangement in organelles and subcellular membranes can be lost or impaired by this process. Methionine, histidine, cystine, and lysine are among the most labile amino acids in a variety of proteins.[3,17,19]

Aldehydic lipid peroxidation products (α,β-unsaturated aldehydes), chiefly the 4-hydroxy-2-alkenals, form adducts with the free amino groups of lysine and other amino acids. Aldehyde-modified proteins are highly immunogenic.[3,20,21]

Among the 4-hydroxy-2-alkenals the most studied molecule is HNE. This molecule, and related compounds, possesses two very reactive electrophilic sites: the aldehyde group and the alkene bond. The free aldehyde in the open-chain form of the alkenal adduct can react with a second lysine, histidine, or cysteine and then can act as a heterobifunctional cross-linking reagent. The alkene bond reacts via Michael-type addition with the three nucleophilic amino acids cysteine, histidine, and lysine. HNE also reacts avidly with certain antioxidants and enzyme cofactors, including glutathione and lipoic acid (the cofactor for α-ketoglutarate dehydrogenase).[3,20,21]

Reactive Nitrogen Species

RNS are free radicals that possess biological activity in vivo and are capable of carrying out targeted modification of proteins and lipids. RNS include all nitrogen-based reactive species, such as nitric oxide (•NO) and its nitrogen oxide derivatives, including higher-nitrogen oxide (N$_2$O$_3$) and peroxynitrite (ONOO$^-$).[22]

The most studied RNS, NO, is a membrane-soluble free radical that is synthesized by nitric oxide synthase (NOS). NOS utilizes oxygen and L-arginine as substrates and converts them to NO and L-citrulline (Figure 16-1B). There are three isoforms of NOS, each transcribed by separate genes. Endothelial NOS (eNOS) and neuronal NOS (nNOS) are the two constitutively expressed isoforms, and inducible NOS (iNOS) is transcriptionally regulated.[22-24]

The pathogenic potential of NO depends on its concentration and whether its production occurs near ROS such as superoxide. NO interacts through a first-order, diffusion-limited reaction with superoxide to form peroxynitrite. Because NO freely diffuses across cell membranes and superoxide cannot, the reaction occurs within cells/organelles (activated leukocytes, endothelial cells, and mitochondria) that produce superoxide in close proximity to diffusible NO exuding from the target cell or a neighboring cell.

NO possesses an apparently contradictory ability—that is, the capacity to bring about both physiologic and pathologic effects. NO effects in vivo largely depend on its concentration and whether it is produced in proximity to other free radicals like superoxide. NO has a direct effect on processes such as proliferation and cell survival at lower concentrations. At higher concentrations, NO has an indirect effect through oxidative stress, leading to nitrosative modification of both proteins and lipids.[22-24]

Nitrosative modifications refers to selective processes that target precise molecular sites in lipids or proteins for loss or gain of function, in a manner somewhat similar to the well-known phosphorylation or acetylation signal transduction mechanisms. These modifications manifest in proteins, with the exception of heme iron binding, either as *S*-nitros(yl)ation—the general attachment of NO to nucleophilic centers is defined as *nitrosation*, and the covalent attachment of the diatomic NO group to reactive thiol sulfhydryl residues in proteins in a redox-dependent fashion is referred to as *S-nitrosylation*—of cysteine thiols or as nitration of tyrosine residues. Tyrosine nitration occurs through the covalent addition of a triatomic nitro group (NO$_2$) to the phenolic ring of tyrosine residues. Interaction of proteins with NO or other reactive nitrogen intermediates may lead to both *S*-nitrosylation and tyrosine nitration. N$_2$O$_3$,

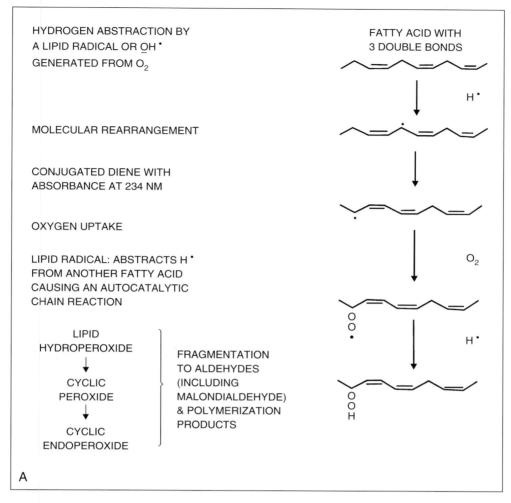

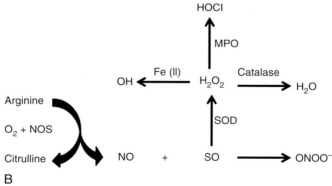

Figure 16-1 **A, Phases of lipid peroxidation.** The various phases of lipid peroxidation occurring in a polyunsaturated fatty acid, shown on the *right,* is described on the *left,* along the same line. **B,** Formation of reactive nitrogen species and reactive oxygen species. MPO, myeloperoxidase; SOD, superoxide dismutase; NOS, nitric oxide synthase; OH, hydroxyl radical; NO, nitric oxide; SO, superoxide; H_2O_2, hydrogen peroxide; ONOO$^-$, peroxynitrite; HOCl, hypochlorous acid.

resulting from reaction of NO with O_2, is thought to be a major *S*-nitrosylating species.[22-25]

Peroxynitrite, derived from the reaction of NO with superoxide anion (see Figure 16-1B), is also regarded as a major cellular nitrating agent. Myeloperoxidase-catalyzed nitrosonium cation ($\cdot NO_2$), formed from the reaction of nitrite (NO_2^-) with hydrogen peroxide (H_2O_2), and nitroso-peroxocarbonate ($ONOOCO_2^-$) produced through the reaction of carbon dioxide (CO_2) with peroxynitrite are some of the other notable nitrating agents. Data show that lipid peroxyl radicals (LOO·) promote tyrosine nitration by inducing tyrosine oxidation and also by reacting with NO_2^- to produce $\cdot NO_2$.[22-28]

Oxidation and Immune Response

Autoantibodies targeting epitopes in MDA- and HNE-modified low-density lipoprotein (LDL) particles are present in plasma of rabbits and mice immunized with oxidized LDL (ox-LDL). Several

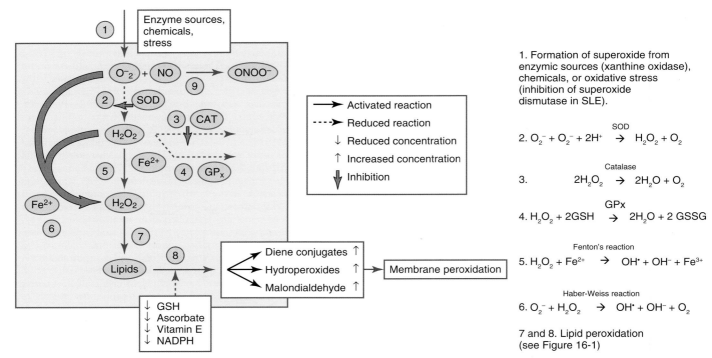

Figure 16-2 Mechanism of free radical mediated oxidative damage. SOD, superoxide dismutase; CAT, catalase; GP_x, glutathione peroxidase; O_2^-, superoxide; H_2O_2, hydrogen peroxide; NO, nitric oxide; $ONOO^-$, peroxynitrite; GSH, reduced glutathione; GSSG, oxidized glutathione; NADPH, Nicotinamide adenine dinucleotide phosphate (reduced form). Steps 2 to 8 describe the reactions given in Figure 16-2.

investigators have demonstrated the presence of antibodies directed against ox-LDL or MDA-LDL in atherosclerotic plaques and oxidation-specific antigens on the surfaces of apoptotic cells. The presence of antibodies to ox-LDL is associated with more rapid progression of atherosclerosis. Antigens modified by oxidative by-products induce immune responses in alcoholic liver disease.

Oxidative processes enhance the reaction of the adaptive response. Oxidation of carbohydrates has been shown to the antibody response to co-administered co-antigens. Moreover, the use of the Schiff base-forming agent tucaresol during immunization with protein antigen increases T cell–dependent immune response. Direct modification of protein antigen has been shown to enhance the immune response.[3,29,30]

Oxidative Damage and Oxidative Modification of Proteins in Autoimmune Disease

Autoimmunity results from the abrogation of self-tolerance and is involved in several human diseases. Autoimmune diseases fall into two categories, organ-specific and systemic. Organ-specific disorders include type 1 diabetes mellitus, thyroiditis, myasthenia gravis, primary biliary cirrhosis, and Goodpasture syndrome, to name only a few. Systemic diseases include rheumatoid arthritis, progressive systemic sclerosis, and SLE. Nearly all these diseases have autoantibodies. Autoantibodies are typically present several years prior to diagnosis of SLE and serve as markers for future disease. Inflammation, infection, drugs, and environmental factors induce formation of neoantigens with involvement of ROS. Thus, oxidative damage is involved in several autoimmune disorders, including SLE.[3,4,10,31,32]

Free Radical Damage in SLE

The disruption of the homeostasis of reactive intermediates (ROS and RNS) in SLE may lead to a loss of self-tolerance, greater tissue damage, and altered enzyme functions.[23]

ROS-mediated oxidative damage occurs in SLE.[3-10] The greater oxidative damage observed in SLE is mediated by free radicals and is the direct result of a change in the delicate balance between the oxidants and antioxidants and an imbalance in the pro- and anti-inflammatory molecules (Figure 16-2). Oxidative damage in SLE is reviewed in the following sections to show how aberrant generation of superoxide and hydrogen peroxide aided by decreased levels of antioxidant enzymes and antioxidants can lead to the increased production of lipid peroxides (see Figure 16-2), altered fatty acid metabolism, and free radical–induced anti-DNA antibodies.

Increased Oxygen Free Radical Production in SLE

Normal cellular metabolism produces ROS, especially in the physiologic role of defense against infectious agents and to maintain cellular redox homeostasis.[33] Overproduction of ROS, however, results in oxidative stress, which can lead to oxidatively modified neo-autoantigens that can promote loss of tolerance to self and induction of autoantibodies in a variety of diseases, including SLE (Table 16-1).[3]

In one study, neutrophils of patients with SLE who had clinical manifestations associated with autoantibodies (leukopenia, thrombocytopenia, and hemolytic anemia) were found to have decreased superoxide anion production mediated by the immunoglobulin (Ig) G receptor (Fc gamma receptor [FcγR]) with the cooperation of complement receptors. Neutrophils from patients with SLE who have manifestations associated with the immune complex (nephritis, arthritis, skin symptoms, serositis, and neuropsychiatric disorders), excluding cytopenia, were also found to behave similarly. However, neutrophils from patients with SLE sharing clinical manifestations related to autoantibodies and immune complexes were found to produce significantly more superoxide anion than those from controls. The study concluded that differences in oxidative metabolism of neutrophils brought about by FcγR/complement receptors may reflect an acquired characteristic of SLE linked to specific clinical manifestations.[34]

Suryaprabha, investigating free radical production, lipid peroxidation, and the levels of essential fatty acids and their metabolites in SLE, found increased levels of superoxide and hydrogen peroxide production by peripheral leukocytes in patients with SLE without any elevations of MDA (as measured by the thiobarbituric acid assay). Furthermore, fatty acid analysis of human plasma showed that both

TABLE 16-1 Free Radicals and Antioxidants in SLE

STUDY	SUPEROXIDE	HYDROGEN PEROXIDE	REDUCED GLUTATHIONE	NITRIC OXIDE	TISSUES/CELLS STUDIED
Alves et al, 2008[34]	↓ and ↑				Neutrophils
Suryaprabha et al, 1991[34a]	↑	↑			Peripheral leukocytes
Casellas et al, 199[36]	↑				Neutrophils
Turi et al, 1997[8]	↑	↑	↓		Leukocytes, RBCs
Furusu et al, 1998[89]				↑	Kidney
Das, 1998[90]	↑			↓	Plasma
Shah et al, 2010[39]			↓		RBCs
Serban et al, 1994[6]			↓		RBCs
Oates & Gilkeson, 2006[91]				↑	Serum
Belmont et al, 1997[53]				↑	Kidney
Oates et al, 2008[92]				↑	Kidney
Ghiran et al, 2011[54]				↑	RBCs

RBC, red blood cell; ↑, significantly raised levels; ↓, significantly diminished levels.

linoleic acid (omega-6 series) and alpha-linolenic acid (omega-3 series) metabolites were significantly lower in the plasma phospholipid fraction of patients with SLE than in controls, suggesting altered essential fatty acid metabolism in these patients.[34a,35]

Casellas showed in vitro production of superoxide was enhanced in normal and lupus polymorphonuclear neutrophils stimulated with lupus serum. When stimulated by N-formyl-methionyl-leucyl-phenylalanine, lupus polymorphonuclear neutrophils exhibited a 5.2-fold increase in superoxide production over the response of normal polymorphonuclear neutrophils so stimulated.[36] The results of this study demonstrate the existence of serum factors in patients with SLE that stimulate O_2^- production by polymorphonuclear neutrophils. Casellas proposes that increased superoxide production by polymorphonuclear neutrophils in patients with SLE could be important in the development of vasculitis and tissue damage in the disease.[36]

In addition, several studies show that patients with SLE exhibit increased superoxide and hydrogen peroxide contents in peripheral leukocytes (Table 16-1).[8,35] Higher production of ROS can also contribute to oxidative modification of DNA, which becomes more immunogenic and induces antibody production directed against native DNA.[37] Studies by Jiang and Chen suggest that excessive free radical production is responsible for the higher lipid peroxide levels in patients with SLE (especially in the active phase of disease) than in controls.[10] Gallelli showed significantly higher levels of ROS in patients with lupus nephritis who had carotid plaques than in those nephritis patients without plaques.[38] Yet another study observed an increase in superoxide generation during the active phase of SLE with a concomitant decrease in NO levels.[4]

Altered Antioxidant Enzyme and Antioxidant Levels in SLE

Several studies of SLE have found significantly reduced activities of the antioxidant enzymes SOD, catalase, and glutathione peroxidase as well as reduced levels of antioxidants such as reduced glutathione (Table 16-2), including the study of Shah, who examined North Indian patients with SLE compared to controls.[39] Turi found that red blood cell (RBC) SOD and catalase activities as well as activity of reduced glutathione were significantly decreased in pediatric patients with lupus nephropathy.[8] A decrease in reduced glutathione and glutathione peroxidase activities was reported in 66 patients with SLE and systemic vasculitides treated with glucocorticoids.[6]

Disease activity has been correlated with antioxidant enzymes and their metabolites. Zhang found significantly lower protein thiol and SOD levels in patients with SLE who tested positive for anti–double-stranded DNA (anti-dsDNA) antibodies than in patients with SLE who tested negative.[40] Anti-dsDNA is a frequent correlate of active disease. Others have studied active disease directly. Zhang showed that the disease activity index correlated negatively with superoxide dismutase, glutathione peroxidase, and catalase activities in patients with SLE.[41] Vipartene reported that decreased SOD and glutathione peroxidase in patients with SLE may promote oxidative stress.[42] When the activities of SOD and glutathione peroxidase were studied during the active and inactive phases of the disease, activity of each was found to be decreased during active disease.[35] Agisheva and Salikhov have studied the antioxidant system in 30 patients with SLE by measuring the concentration of alpha-tocopherol and free fatty acids. Shifts in the levels of these antioxidants and lipid peroxidation correlated with the clinical appearance of SLE.[35] Kurien and Scofield[4] as well as Jiang and Chen[10] have also shown decreased SOD1 activity in SLE.

However, some studies have found increased SOD and catalase levels in SLE, suggesting that this protective mechanism could be an adaptation to the greater oxidative stress seen in human SLE. Higher glomerular SOD has been observed in human lupus nephritis, especially diffuse proliferative lupus nephritis.[43] Similarly, Taysi showed higher superoxide dismutase activity in the serum of patients with SLE compared to healthy controls.[43a] Interestingly, in this study, disease activity index in the patients correlated negatively with serum SOD, suggesting that superoxide dismutase is protective. Catalase and SOD activities were also found to be significantly elevated in the sera of patients with SLE in another study.[44] Significantly higher glutathione peroxidase activity has been reported in a group of patients with SLE who tested positive for anticardiolipin and in patients with SLE whose Systemic Lupus Erythematosus Disease Activity Index (SLEDAI) scores were higher than 3, compared to patients with SLEDAI less than 3.[45]

Antibodies to Catalase, Superoxide Dismutase, and Oxidized Low-Density Lipoprotein

Kurien and Scofield[4] as well as Mansour[44] have demonstrated antibodies to SOD1 in the sera of patients with SLE. Mansour's group have, in addition, shown that antibodies to catalase are present in patients with SLE.[44] These investigators also found a positive correlation between anticatalase antibodies and antisuperoxide antibodies in patients with SLE. Significantly higher titers of autoantibodies against ox-LDL were found in a group of patients with SLE who

TABLE 16-2 Antioxidant Enzymes, Inducible Nitric Oxide Synthase (iNOS) and Lipid Peroxidation in SLE

STUDY	SUPEROXIDE DISMUTASE	CATALASE	GLUTATHIONE PEROXIDASE	INOS	LIPID PEROXIDATION	TISSUES/CELLS STUDIED
Shah et al, 2010[39]					↑	RBCs
Agisheva & Salikhov, 1990[93]					↑	Plasma
Serban & Negru, 1998[94]			↓		↑	Serum
Jiang & Chen, 1992[10]	↓				↑	Serum
Das, 1998[90]	↓		↓		↑	Plasma
Turi et al, 1997[8]	↓	↓			↑	RBCs
Kurien & Scofield, 2003[4]	↓				↑	Serum
Nuttall et al, 2003[46]					↑	Plasma
Taysi et al, 2002[43a]	↑	↓	↓		↑	Serum
Zhang et al, 2008[40]	↓				↑	Plasma
Zhang et al, 2010[41]	↑	↓	↓		↑	Serum
Vipartene et al, 2006[42]	↓		↓		↑	Blood
Mansour et al, 2008[44]	↑	↑			↑	Serum
Wang et al, 2010[50]	↓			↑		Serum
Belmont et al, 1997[53]				↑		Endothelial cells, keratinocytes

RBC, red blood cell; ↑, significantly elevated levels; ↓, significantly diminished levels.

TABLE 16-3 Antibodies against Antioxidant Enzymes and Oxidatively Modified Proteins as well as Levels of Oxidatively Modified Proteins in SLE

STUDY	ANTI-SOD ANTIBODY	ANTI-CATALASE ANTIBODY	ANTI-OXIDIZED LDL	ANTI-MDA-SOD OR CATALASE	ANTI-MDA OR HNE ADDUCT	HNE-MODIFIED PROTEINS	MDA-MODIFIED PROTEINS	TISSUES/CELLS STUDIED
Kurien & Scofield, 2003[4]	↑							Serum
Mansour et al, 2008[44]	↑	↑						Serum
Mansour et al, 2010[49]				↑			↑	Serum
Huang et al, 2007[45]			↑					Serum
Toyoda et al, 2007[47]					↑	↑		Serum, epidermal cells
Grune et al, 1997[7]						↑		Plasma
Wang et al, 2010[50]					↑	↑	↑	Serum
Fesmire et al, 2010[51]			↑					Serum
Vaarala et al, 1993[95]			↑					Serum
Matsuura et al, 2004[96]			↑					Serum

HNE, 4-hydroxy-2-nonenal; LDL, low-density lipoprotein; MDA, malondialdehyde; SOD, superoxide dismutase; ↑, significantly elevated levels.

tested positive for antibodies against cardiolipin and in patients with an SLEDAI score higher than 3 (Table 16-3).[45]

Lipid Peroxidation

Numerous studies have found increased lipid peroxidation in patients with SLE. Shah showed a significant increase in the level of lipid peroxidation, measured as MDA, in the erythrocyte hemolysate of patients with SLE.[39] The level of MDA correlated positively with SLEDAI score.[35,39] Several other studies demonstrated increased lipid peroxidation in erythrocytes and blood plasma of patients with SLE.[35,36] Mansour[44] reported that MDA and conjugated dienes were significantly higher in the sera of patients with SLE than in healthy controls. Patients with SLE who tested positive for anticardiolipin

antibodies as well as patients with an SLEDAI score higher than 3 also had significantly higher thiobarbituric acid–reactive substance levels than healthy controls.[44]

In a study of oxidative stress in pediatric patients with lupus nephropathy, Turi found an increase in lipid peroxidation in the peripheral RBCs and also a correlation between the presence of active glomerular disease and evidence of oxidative changes in the various parameters measured in peripheral RBCs.[8] Serban also found increased lipid peroxidation in patients with SLE who had systemic vasculitides that were treated with glucocorticoid, an increase caused by the dyslipidemias induced by the use of glucocorticoid.[6] MDA levels and conjugate dienes have been found to be elevated in patients with SLE.[4,10,35]

Isoprostanes, products of lipid peroxidation, are thought to be particularly important in the context of vascular disease, and the measure of this parameter has been projected as a reliable, sensitive, and noninvasive marker of oxidative stress in vivo as well as having relevance to vascular disease.[35] 8-Isoprostaglandin F_{2alpha} (8-iso-$PGF_{2\alpha}$) has been measured in the serum of 60 patients with SLE and 20 age- and sex-matched controls. The serum concentration of 8-iso-$PGF_{2\alpha}$ was found to be significantly higher in the patients with SLE than in controls. Lipid peroxides were also found to be increased in patients with SLE. Peroxidation of the LDL subfraction may contribute to severe and premature cardiovascular diseases in patients with SLE.[46]

Protein Modification and Antibodies against Modified Proteins
Specific immunohistochemical studies have clearly shown accumulation of HNE-modified proteins in the dermis of patients with SLE. The observation of intracellular accumulation of HNE-specific epitopes in human SLE for the first time raised the possibility that the higher lipid peroxidation may be directly involved in the pathogenesis of autoimmune disorders.[47] Significantly higher HNE-modified protein levels occur in children with SLE.[7]

Protein-bound carbonyls were found to be elevated in SLE and to correlate with disease activity. Oxidation of proteins is thought to play a role in the pathogenesis of chronic organ damage in SLE.[40] For example, MDA, an end product of lipid peroxidation (see Figure 16-2), can be covalently linked to proteins generating intramolecular and intermolecular adducts.[48] Elevations of MDA-modified proteins and a significant decrease in the concentration of thiol groups in the sera were observed among 65 patients with SLE ($P < 0.05$) in comparison with levels found in 60 healthy controls. In addition, the patients with SLE exhibited significantly enhanced levels of IgG antibodies against catalase and SOD-modified proteins (MDA-modified SOD and catalase). Such antibodies are potentially responsible for the increased oxidative damage seen in SLE.[49]

An analysis of 72 sera from patients with SLE showed significantly higher levels of both anti-MDA/anti-HNE protein adduct antibodies and MDA/HNE protein adducts than sera from 36 age- and sex-matched healthy controls. Interestingly, a higher number of patients were positive for anti-MDA as well as anti-HNE antibodies, and the levels of both of these antibodies were statistically significantly higher among patients with SLE with SLEDAI scores of 6 or more than among patients with SLEDAI scores lower than 6. This study also found a significant correlation between the levels of anti-MDA or anti-HNE antibodies with SLEDAI score ($r = 0.734$ and $r = 0.647$, respectively). This observation suggested a possible causal relationship between these antibodies and SLE.[50]

Antibodies against Oxidatively Modified Proteins
Oxidant stress has been attributed to the development of anti-phospholipid antibodies, and oxidatively modified LDL particles have been shown to elicit autoantibodies. Elevations of anti–ox-LDL autoantibodies occur in patients with SLE, and studies show that anti–ox-LDL positively correlates with antiphospholipid antibodies and anti–beta 2-glycoprotein (β_2-GP). Antibodies to ox-LDL that are cross-reactive with phospholipids are thought to be due to binding to oxidized phospholipids. Circulating ox-LDL/β_2-GP complexes and IgG immune complexes containing ox-LDL/β_2-GP occur in SLE and/or antiphospholipid syndrome.[3] Fesmire, et al. observed significantly higher levels of antibodies directed against ox-LDL in patients with SLE than in controls matched for age and sex.[51]

Oxidative Modification of DNA
DNA damage induced by superoxide anion radicals has been implicated in several inflammatory disorders. DNA damaged in this manner has been reported to display hyperchromicity, decrease in melting temperatures, single-stranded breaks, and modifications of bases. Rabbits immunized with superoxide-modified DNA demonstrated high-titer antibodies against different antigens, including native DNA and other nucleic acid polymers. Superoxide anion–modified DNA preferentially bound anti-DNA IgG from SLE sera (purified on a Protein-A-Sepharose column) compared to native DNA.[35]

Hydroxyl radicals mediate damage to guanine residues of polyguanylic acid. Native and oxidatively modified polyG DNA sequences were found to be highly immunogenic and induced high-titer antibodies in rabbits. The antigen-binding characteristics of these antibodies resembled those of the anti-dsDNA antibodies found in patients with SLE. The antibodies from patients with SLE preferentially bound oxidatively modified poly-guanine rather than native polyguanine.[35]

Lymphocytes from patients with SLE have higher levels of 8-oxo-deoxyguanine (8-oxodG).[3] An investigation of blood monocytes from patients with SLE showed an impairment in the removal of 8-oxodG consequent to a deficient repair system.[3]

Reactive Nitrogen Species in SLE
Nitration and NO in SLE
Disease activity index has been found to correlate positively with erythrocyte sedimentation rate and levels of serum protein carbonyl and 3-nitrotyrosine.[41] Wang, studying 72 sera from patients with SLE and 36 matched controls, found that the SLE sera had lower levels of SOD and higher levels of iNOS and nitrotyrosine.[50] In one study, the autoantigen Ro52 was found by immunohistochemistry to undergo nuclear localization in inflamed tissue that expressed iNOS (this tissue was obtained from patients with cutaneous lupus).[52] The investigators verified this observation in NO-treated cultures of patient-derived primary keratinocytes. NO was identified as the extrinsic factor that induced nuclear translocation of Ro52, expression of iNOS and nuclear Ro52 in biopsies of cutaneous lupus lesions.[52]

Many independent studies show a significant correlation between global lupus disease activity and markers of systemic NO production. One investigation showed significant elevation in NO production markers among African-Americans with SLE disease activity. Because two NOS2 polymorphisms were significantly more common among African-American women with SLE than among matched controls, this predisposition to generate elevated NO associated with disease activity is likely to be inherited. Studies demonstrating improved malaria survival associated with elevated markers of systemic NO production in some African populations with these polymorphisms lends support to the functional role for the polymorphisms.[24]

Expression of iNOS in skin appears to reflect SLE disease activity (the skin reflects SLE disease activity usually). iNOS protein and messenger RNA (mRNA) were shown, by immunostaining methods, to be increased in 33% of epidermal tissue samples obtained from subjects with cutaneous lupus prior to UV B irradiation exposure. However, the expression was elevated in all samples after UV B exposure. Skin biopsy specimens obtained from the buttocks of subjects with systemic disease showed higher iNOS expression in endothelial cells (the endothelial expression correlated with lupus disease activity) and keratinocytes than specimens obtained from controls.[24,53]

Patients with SLE have decreased endothelium-dependent vasodilation and often possess a phenotype of defective eNOS function. The reason is not known. However, patients with lupus have higher levels of circulating endothelial cells, which may be a marker of endothelial damage. The level of endothelial cells in circulation in such patients has been found to correlate inversely with levels of complement, and the endothelial cells stained positively for nitrotyrosine. This finding, along with the fact that eNOS cells stain for iNOS even in nonlesional skin, implies an immune complex–mediated formation of peroxynitrite by iNOS in endothelial cells.[24,53]

Higher levels of systemic NO production markers have been shown in later longitudinal observational studies in subjects with proliferative lupus nephritis than in those with nonproliferative renal disease or those with lupus but without nephritis. In the same subjects with nephritis, those who showed no renal response to therapy had significantly higher levels of systemic NO production markers in the first 3 months of therapy than those who showed a renal response. This finding supports the hypothesis that continuous RNS production leads to renal damage in lupus nephritis.[24]

In one study, incubation of RBCs derived from healthy universal donors (type O, Rh negative) with sera from subjects with SLE brought about NO production by the RBCs. However, the RBCs did not release NO when they were incubated with control sera.[54]

Several investigators have reported elevated iNOS expression in the glomeruli of patients with proliferative lupus nephritis. In biopsy specimens from those with class IV disease, citrulline staining increased with iNOS staining, suggesting that the iNOS was functionally active.[24]

Glomerular iNOS staining colocalized with apoptosis markers and p53 (a proapoptotic signaling molecule) in one study. This result is in agreement with the reported effect of increased levels of NO on p53 phosphorylation. In another study, iNOS expression was elevated in subjects with class IV lupus nephritis in glomerular, tubular, and interstitial cells. Expression of iNOS in the tubulointerstitium correlated significantly with total lesion index on biopsy as well as the degree of proteinuria and creatinine clearance at the time of biopsy. Nuclear factor–kappa B (NF-κB) and iNOS colocalized with apoptotic cells in the glomerulus. These data suggest that signaling for apoptosis via increased p53 activity and through activation of nuclear factor–kappa are the two mechanisms for iNOS-mediated glomerular damage in proliferative nephritis.[24,55]

The creation of neoepitopes by peroxynitrite-mediated nitration of nucleophilic domains on self-antigens is one mechanism through which NO can be pathogenic in SLE. Sera from patients with SLE were shown in one study to bind more avidly to peroxynitrite nitrated poly-L-tyrosine than to nonnitrated molecules. Binding of anti-dsDNA sera to nitrated poly-L-tyrosine was inhibited by nitrated poly-L-tyrosine, nitrated BSA, nitrated DNA, and nitrated chromatin significantly more than by the nonnitrated forms of these antigens. Nitrated DNA serves as a better immunogen for inducing anti-dsDNA antibody production in experimental animals. Peroxynitrite-treated DNA, similarly, is more immunogenic than native DNA as the antigen for dsDNA antibody screening of serum from patients with SLE. These studies point to the possibility that peroxynitrite modifications of self-antigens can create neoepitopes that possess higher binding affinity than native antigens. However, it has not been determined whether the enhanced immunogenicity of nitrated DNA originates from cross-reactivity of these epitopes with native DNA or from epitope spreading to unmodified epitopes.[24,56]

Normal T cells do not express iNOS but do express eNOS and nNOS. Co-stimulation with CD3/CD28 increases T-cell expression of these NOS isoforms. In addition, NO induces an increase of mitochondrial hyperpolarization in normal human T cells. On the other hand, T lymphocytes of subjects with SLE in one study showed persistent mitochondrial hyperpolarization and mitochondrial mass, accounting for elevated formation of ROS. This raises the possibility that depletion of adenosine triphosphate (ATP) resulting from mitochondrial dysfunction is finally the cause for reduced activation-induced apoptosis and sensitizes lupus T cells to necrosis. Activation of mTOR, a mitochondrial potential sensor and target of the drug rapamycin, was shown by later studies to be caused by NO-induced mitochondrial hyperpolarization in SLE T cells.[24,57]

Animal Models of SLE and Oxidative Damage
Animal Models of SLE and Reactive Oxygen Species
Serum SOD is elevated in the MRL.lpr strain of mice, a model of spontaneous lupus. However, this effect is not seen in other strains of mice (e.g., B6.*Sle1.Sle3*). In the B6.*Sle1.Sle3* strain, urinary SOD, predominantly renal in origin, correlates well with glomerular nephritis score and renal disease activity indices.[58]

In a passive animal model of anti–glomerular basement membrane (GBM)–induced experimental nephritis, urinary protease,

prostaglandin D synthase, serum amyloid P, and SOD were found to be novel biomarkers of anti-GBM disease and lupus nephritis, having stronger correlation to renal disease.[58]

Because our (BTK and RHS) laboratory observed greater oxidative damage and HNE modification of proteins in SLE patients than in normal controls, we immunized rabbits with HNE-modified Ro60 and unmodified Ro60 to test the hypothesis that immunization of animals with HNE-modified Ro60 would result in accelerated epitope spreading. Ro60 ribonucleoprotein (RNP) is a common target of autoantibodies in both SLE and Sjögren syndrome. Ro60 RNP is made up of a 60,000-molecular-weight (MW) protein noncovalently associated with at least one of four short uridine-rich RNAs (the hY RNAs). These hY RNAs are also associated with the 48,000-MW La (or SSB) autoantigen. Anti-Ro60 is found in up to 50% of patients with SLE, and anti-La is found in substantially fewer patients. As hypothesized, we found a rapid autoimmune response and development of lupus-like disease in the HNE-Ro–immunized group. Thus, immunization with an oxidatively modified autoantigen accelerates the disease process in this animal model of SLE.[3]

Oxidative modification of Ro60 might result in the formation of chemical adducts that could serve as neoantigens to which the immune system has probably not been exposed. The Ro60 modified in this fashion might be more readily internalized, on account of its neoconformation, than the unmodified Ro, by antigen-presenting cells, such as dendritic cells and macrophages. These cells in turn present novel self-peptides to T cells, which can provide help to autoreactive B cells to elicit intramolecular spreading. B cells specific for either the modified or unmodified Ro could internalize the antigen, along with associated antigens, by means of their cell surface Ig receptor. Epitopes from each of these proteins could be then presented to naïve T cells, in the context of major histocompatibility complex class II, resulting in a diversification of autoreactive T cells, which assist a diversified B-cell response that can recognize separate B-cell antigenic determinants from the different antigens, resulting in autoreactivity to numerous antigens (Figure 16-3).

The fact that human Ro60 was found to be oxidatively modified in human liver lends credibility to the possibility that Ro60 in patients with SLE may be subject to modification, especially because increased oxidative damage and HNE-modified proteins, including HNE-modified catalase, have been found to occur in SLE.[3,5-9,59] Such a scenario proposes development of antibodies to Ro60 and thus autoimmunity to the entire Ro RNP particle after an initial immune response to oxidized Ro60. This effect was seen under experimental conditions when we immunized rabbits with HNE-modified Ro60. Distinct intramolecular and intermolecular epitope spreading effects were seen in these animals.

Toyoda demonstrated the occurrence of molecular mimicry between anti-dsDNA autoantibodies and antibodies raised against HNE-modified protein.[47] The anti-HNE monoclonal antibodies (mAbs) raised by the Toyoda group, in an earlier work, were found to bind the (R)-HNE-histidine Michael adducts. These investigators also found that the anti-HNE monoclonal antibody sequence was highly homologous to anti-dsDNA autoantibodies. In addition, they characterized the binding site of the monoclonal antibody to dsDNA as the 4-Oxo-2-nonenal (ONE)–modified 2″-deoxynucleoside (7-(2-oxo-heptyl)-substituted 1,N-etheno-type 4-oxo-2-nonenal-2″-deoxynucleoside). On the basis of these results, the Toyoda group hypothesized that HNE-modified protein could trigger the production of anti-dsDNA autoantibodies in autoimmune diseases. The investigators immunized BALB/c mice with HNE-modified keyhole limpet hemocyanin (KLH) and observed a progressive increase in the anti-dsDNA titer. All the mice immunized with HNE-modified KLH developed an IgG anti-dsDNA response that was comparable to the anti-HNE response. Immunization with KLH alone did not induce any significant anti-DNA response in the control mice.[47]

These data suggest that oxidatively modified autoantigens can serve as neoantigens and promote loss of tolerance to self, thus leading to autoimmune diseases such as SLE.

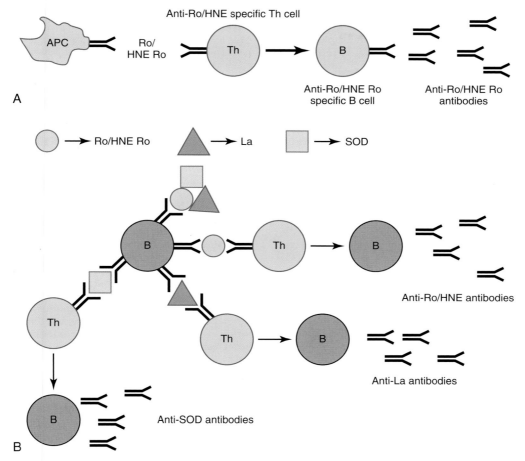

Figure 16-3 Model showing mechanisms of B- and T-cell epitope spreading. A, Antigen presenting cells (APCs) (macrophages or dendritic cells) present novel self peptides from 60-kD Ro or the 60-kD HNE-Ro neoantigen to T cells, which in turn provide help to autoreactive B cells. Clonal expansion of B cells capable of binding to 60-kD Ro or 60-kD HNE Ro occurs. **B,** B cells internalize multiple proteins such as 60-kD Ro, HNE-modified 60-kD Ro or SOD1, present epitopes from each protein to naïve T cells resulting in diversification of autoreactive T cells. Finally, T cells assist a diversified B-cell response. The cascade continues, with T cells activating additional autoreactive B cells and B cells presenting additional self-epitopes, until there is autoreactivity to numerous autoantigens.

Animal Models of SLE and Reactive Nitrogen Species

Weinberg observed increasing urinary NO metabolites in MRL/lpr mice side by side with the development of glomerulonephritis.[60] This elevation in NO production was linked to the production of 3-nitrotyrosine, a product of NO_2 or $ONOO^-$ and tyrosine. MRL/lpr kidney catalase activity decreased as a result of tyrosine nitration. Owing to its role in eliminating hydrogen peroxide, inactivation of catalase may have exposed the kidney cells to enhanced oxidative stress. The formation of immune complex and its deposition in tissues appear to be independent of iNOS activity in MRL/lpr mice, because iNOS inhibitor therapy did not have any effect on glomerular immune complex deposition in MRL/lpr mice even though it improved renal histopathology. iNOS expression, instead, may be triggered by downstream innate immune responses consequent to immune complex generation with autoantigens. For example, 3-nitrotyrosine/iNOS generation has been seen in models of passive transfer of anti-GBM and myeloperoxidase antibody glomerulonephritis.[23,24,60]

There is evidence to show that interferon regulatory factor 1 (IRF1) may play a role in expression of iNOS. With inactivation of the *IRF1* gene, the expression of iNOS induced by lipopolysaccharide/interferon gamma (LPS/IFN-γ) can be abrogated in MRL/lpr mesangial cells. Expression of iNOS is reduced in MRL/lpr mice lacking the functional IRF1 gene. Because this also reduces the anti-dsDNA

formation as well as glomerular immune complex deposition in these mice, it is difficult to conclude that the genetic manipulation is directly responsible for the decreased iNOS expression.[61] Certain interventions decrease the expression of iNOS without directly inhibiting the enzyme. Oral administration of mycophenolate mofetil as well as chemical induction of heme oxygenase 1, for example, were found to effectively reduce iNOS expression in the kidney and to treat glomerulitis in MRL/lpr mice.[24,61]

The use of NG-monomethyl-L-arginine (nonspecific arginine analog) to inhibit iNOS activity in MRL/lpr mice prior to disease onset lowers 3-nitrotyrosine production in the kidney, inhibits cellular proliferation and necrosis in the glomerulus, and partially restores kidney catalase activity.[60] This effect happens without the occurrence of altered complement or immunoglobulin deposition in the glomerulus and thus suggests that elevated expression of iNOS occurs downstream of complement activation and immune complex deposition.[60] A similar effect was observed when the same strain of mice were treated with L-N6-(1-iminoethyl)lysine, a partially selective iNOS inhibitor, before onset of disease. Mice treated with this inhibitor showed significantly better glomerular pathology scores than controls. Compared with NG-monomethyl-L-arginine given prior to disease onset in NZB/W mice, NG-monomethyl-L-arginine given to NZB/W mice with nephritis had a similar but less profound effect on renal histopathology and proteinuria. For treating the rapidly progressive nephritis observed in MRL/lpr mice, stand-alone therapy with NG-monomethyl-L-arginine was less effective.[24,60]

Even though iNOS−/− MRL/lpr mice showed ameliorated signs of vasculitis and IgG rheumatoid factor production, these mice had glomerular pathology that was similar to that in their MRL/lpr wild-type littermates. This result is in contrast to the effectiveness of pharmacologic iNOS inhibition in murine lupus. In order to see whether the beneficial effect of NG-monomethyl-L-arginine in SLE was related to iNOS, researchers gave MRL/lpr NOS−/− mice an iNOS-selective inhibitor before disease onset and during disease progression. NOS2−/− mice did not have a significant decrease in glomerular pathology or proteinuria and had elevations of anti-dsDNA antibody. iNOS inhibitor therapy, however, significantly lowered the level of proteinuria and podocyte flattening/eNOS cell swelling, as observed by electron microscopy. These observations suggest that iNOS inhibitor therapy reduces pathologic changes in podocyte and endothelial cell pathology in an iNOS-independent and possibly eNOS-dependent manner in this model.[24,62]

The pathogenic mechanisms of iNOS activity in SLE have been studied in animal models. As mentioned earlier, peroxynitrite formed as a result of iNOS activity can nitrate amino acid residues and alter catalytic activity of enzymes such as the antioxidant enzyme catalase. The inactivation of prostacyclin synthase and eNOS in the vascular tissue by peroxynitrite brings about vasoconstriction. The results of these studies suggest that deactivation of tissue protective enzymes is one mechanism through which iNOS activity is pathogenic.[24]

Regulation of apoptosis and clearance of apoptotic cells is an important area of investigation because SLE-related nuclear antigens are presented in late apoptotic blebs. NO and peroxynitrite are both essential in regulating non–receptor-mediated apoptosis in several cellular systems. MRL/lpr mice with active disease were treated with the iNOS inhibitor NG-monomethyl-L-arginine in order to investigate the role of iNOS activity in apoptosis. The treated mice showed lower levels of splenocyte apoptosis than controls. Elevations of apoptosis were seen when cultured splenocytes isolated from mice with active disease were treated with a NO donor. Even though MRL/lpr mice have the well-described defect in receptor-mediated apoptosis, non–receptor-mediated apoptosis appears to be increased by NO or other RNS.[24,63]

As mentioned previously, $ONOO_2$ can be produced by iNOS only if iNOS activity is present in close proximity to a cell with equimolar superoxide levels. Parallel production of superoxide by the reductase domain of iNOS itself is one mechanism for simultaneous production of superoxide and NO. Studies involving pharmacologic inhibition of iNOS in MRL/lpr and NZB/W mouse models lend support for this mechanism in lupus. Significantly lower levels of urinary F_2 isoprostanes were seen in mice administered iNOS2-specific or nonspecific inhibitors than in control mice given only distilled water. Thus, the ability of iNOS activity to form ROS close to NO could be a possible means by which iNOS exerts pathogenic effects in SLE.[24,64]

Therapy in SLE

The effect of prednisolone therapy on the levels of plasma 8-epi-$PGF_{2\alpha}$(8-iso-$PGF_{2\alpha}$) has been studied in a group of 36 patients with SLE and in 23 healthy controls, as a part of a larger study group, with the use of gas chromatography-mass spectrometry. SLE patients with SLE not undergoing prednisolone therapy displayed higher 8-epi-$PGF_{2\alpha}$ levels than patients with SLE undergoing prednisolone treatment.[65]

Mohan and Das determined the plasma concentrations of lipid peroxides, NO, and antioxidants such as catalase, SOD, glutathione peroxidase, and vitamin E in patients with SLE both prior to and following administration of eicosapentaenoic acid/docosahexaenoic acid. The investigators showed elevated values of lipid peroxides and decreased values of NO, SOD, and glutathione peroxidase in SLE prior to supplementation with eicosapentaenoic acid and docosahexaenoic acid supplementation. Following eicosapentaenoic acid/docosahexaenoic acid administration, they found that lipid

peroxides, NO, superoxide dismutase, and glutathione peroxidase reverted to near normal levels. These data suggest that oxidant stress, NO, and antioxidants play a significant role in SLE and that eicosapentaenoic acid/docosahexaenoic acid can modulate oxidant stress and NO synthesis. This interaction may have a regulatory role in the synthesis of antioxidant enzymes such as SOD and glutathione peroxidase. Pottathil showed that serum arachidonic acid content is significantly lower in patients with SLE sera than in controls.[65a]

Jiang and Chen[10] showed that there is a gradual decline in lipid peroxidation levels and an increase in SOD activity from the active phase to the inactive phase of SLE. In addition, as the patients with SLE improved in health, these researchers found that there was an increase in SOD activity with a concomitant decrease in lipid peroxidation.[10]

FIBROSIS IN SLE
Renal Fibrosis in Lupus Nephritis

Lupus nephritis is a major cause of morbidity and mortality in SLE. To progress to lupus nephritis, the subject must break immune tolerance and form autoantibodies that deposit in the kidney. The subject must have a number of predisposing factors for this event to produce renal pathology and finally lead to end-stage renal fibrosis or glomerular sclerosis.[66]

To date, histologic parameters of nephritis remain the best predictor of renal survival and patient mortality in SLE.[67-73] Class III or higher nephritis, a high renal activity index (>7; the presence of cellular crescents and extensive fibrinoid necrosis, in particular), a high renal chronicity index (>4), and the presence of subepithelial and subendothelial deposits on electron microscopy are all associated with worse prognosis, that is, poorer renal survival over time due to end-stage renal disease.[67-73] The renal pathology chronicity index is computed by summing the individual scores of four histologic features—glomerular sclerosis, fibrous crescents, tubular atrophy, and interstitial fibrosis. In particular, interstitial fibrosis and glomerular crescents have repeatedly been identified as having the highest predictive value for poor renal and patient survival in lupus nephritis.

The amount of extracellular matrix within the kidneys hinges upon the balance between its deposition and its degradation, as illustrated in Figure 16-4. Extracellular matrix degradation depends on two key interrelated enzyme systems, matrix metalloproteinases (MMPs) and plasmin, that break down collagen as well as other components of the matrix. The activation of MMPs can be initiated by urokinase-type (uPA) and tissue-type (tPA) plasminogen activators, both of which cleave plasminogen into active plasmin. Active plasmin not only activates MMPs and cleaves matrix but also cleaves fibrin. Finally, proinflammatory cytokines can augment MMP generation and activity.

MMP9, in particular, has the potential to upregulate several biologically active proteins, such as the profibrotic growth factor transforming growth factor–beta (TGF-β). The latter plays a critical role in promoting fibrosis, as indicated in Figure 16-4. In addition, two other key systems play a key role in keeping matrix breakdown in check, tissue inhibitor of metalloproteinases (TIMPs) and plasminogen activator inhibitor 1 (PAI-1). TIMPs and PAI-1 block matrix degradation at successive stages of the cascade portrayed in Figure 16-4 and are associated with an influx of macrophages, which are important for the repair process. The balance between deposition and degradation is changed in favor of progressive fibrosis, in most instances, among patients with lupus nephritis.[74] Indeed, several molecules portrayed in Figure 16-4, including PIA-1, MMPs, and TGF-β, have been shown to be upregulated in lupus nephritis.[75-79]

TGF-β is a major mediator of renal fibrosis, as in most forms of fibrosis. In the mid- to late stages of an animal model of lupus nephritis, the levels of TGF-β and other profibrotic mediators increase. Indeed, in mouse models, TGF-β has been shown to have a pathogenic role in lupus nephritis.[79] Consistent with this observation, renal and urinary (but not serum) levels of TGF-β have been reported to

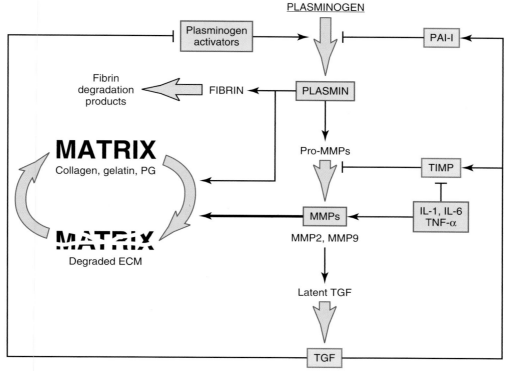

Figure 16-4 Enzymes and factors that dictate extracellular matrix balance. ECM, extracellular matrix; IL, interleukin; MMP, matrix metalloproteinases; PAI-1, plasminogen activator inhibitor 1; TGF, transforming growth factor; TIMPs, tissue inhibitor of metalloproteinases.

be increased in isolated studies. In addition to TGF-β, a large number of related growth factors, including connective tissue growth factor (CTGF), fibroblast growth factor (FGF), vascular endothelial growth factor (VEGF), platelet-derived growth factor (PDGF), and bone morphogenetic proteins (BMPs), are now known to be equally important in dictating the degree of renal fibrosis. However, the roles of these molecules in lupus nephritis are poorly understood, with the exception of isolated studies with BMP-7.[80]

Glomerular sclerosis and interstitial fibrosis is reversible in animal models. With regard to MMPs and their inhibitors, a single injection of puromycin aminonucleoside (PAN) led to fibrosis early on in a PAN-induced nephrosis model in one study. Although MMPs stayed relatively constant, the fibrosis was accompanied by upregulation of TIMP-1 and followed by resolution of the fibrosis over several weeks with a decrease in TIMP-1 as fibrosis resolved. Patients with lupus have also been studied in this regard. Hill carried out initial renal biopsies on 71 patients with lupus nephritis and systematic control biopsies 6 months following therapy.[74] The investigating group found that renal interstitial fibrosis was partially reversible in 17 patients and that glomerular segmental scarring was partially reversible in 11 patients, both of which were accompanied by an excellent outcome. Reversal of glomerular and interstitial fibrotic lesions in humans has been formally demonstrated in diabetic nephropathy,[74] and similar studies in other chronic nephritis are awaited.

Pulmonary Fibrosis in SLE
Pulmonary disease has the potential to complicate SLE and is a major cause of morbidity and mortality. Pleuritis (other pleural involvement is also seen), pulmonary vascular disease, parenchymal disease, diaphragmatic dysfunction, and upper airway dysfunction are some of the most common pulmonary problems seen in SLE.[81] In an autopsy study of 120 subjects with SLE, after exclusions of abnormalities not thought to be "directly related" to SLE, 18% of subjects were found to have significant lung pathology, including 22 with

pleuritis, 11 with cellular interstitial pneumonia, and 5 with mixed inflammatory/fibrotic interstitial disease.[82]

Fibrotic Lupus Pneumonitis (Chronic Interstitial Lung Disease)
Chronic interstitial lung disease, also known as fibrotic lupus pneumonitis, is observed in 3% to 13% of patients with SLE. Interstitial lung disease occurs mainly in patients with long-standing disease. Anti-Ro60 (or anti-SSA) antibodies are associated with interstitial lung disease. Anti-Ro60 antibodies were found in 81% of patients with lupus pneumonitis, compared with 38% of all patients with SLE. Controversy remains regarding the prevalence of chronic interstitial lung disease in SLE, because interstitial lung disease can manifest in primary Sjögren syndrome or with other lupus overlap syndromes. Interstitial lung disease often develops gradually and stealthily. A worsening nonproductive cough, exertion-related dyspnea, and recurrent pleurisy are seen in interstitial lung disease. This disorder can also develop after an episode of acute lupus pneumonitis. Bibasilar inspiratory pulmonary crackles, which are evident upon physical examination, are similar to idiopathic pulmonary fibrosis. A restrictive pattern with reduced lung volumes is observed during lung function tests, along with diminished diffusing capacity of the lung for carbon monoxide.[81]

Chest radiographs may appear normal or may show bibasilar irregular linear opacities early in the course of the disease. Later in the disease course, more diffuse infiltrates, pleural disease, or honeycombing appears. In order to evaluate for the ground-glass appearance found with cellular infiltration or fibrosis and for the reticular pattern found with fibrotic disease, high-resolution computed tomography (HRCT) is useful. A biopsy is occasionally employed to exclude other causes of interstitial lung disease, including infections, even though HRCT results are predictive of the pathologic pattern of interstitial lung disease observed on lung biopsy. Alveolar septal thickening, lymphocytic infiltrates, interstitial fibrosis, alveolar septal immune deposits, and type II pneumocyte hyperplasia are the major histopathologic findings in chronic interstitial lung disease in SLE. Nonspecific interstitial pneumonia, normal interstitial pneumonia, and the rarer lymphocytic interstitial pneumonia are the most common pathologic patterns that occur in interstitial lung disease.[81]

There have been no controlled treatment trials for chronic interstitial lung disease in SLE as there have been for acute lupus pneumonitis. For symptomatic patients, oral corticosteroids form a reasonable first-line therapy. Respiratory symptoms were found to improve in all 14 patients with SLE-related interstitial lung disease in an open-label trial of prednisone (60 mg/day for at least 4 weeks). Three of the patients died, 2 from lung fibrosis and 1 from bacterial pneumonia. However, diffusing capacity of the lung for carbon monoxide was found to be improved in the majority of the survivors during the follow-up period.[81a] Beyond corticosteroids, our guidance on the choice of immunosuppressant treatment parallels the treatment guidelines for scleroderma interstitial lung disease, supported by a similar histopathologic appearance between the two diseases. For medications other than corticosteroids, the optimal choice for SLE-related interstitial lung disease is not certain. However, azathioprine, cyclophosphamide, and mycophenolate have all been attempted in patients who showed an inadequate response to corticosteroids.[81]

Pulmonary Arterial Hypertension

The prevalence of pulmonary arterial hypertension in patients with SLE is unknown but is lower than that seen in scleroderma. Pulmonary arterial hypertension has been identified, with use of transthoracic echocardiography, in approximately 6% to 14% of patients with SLE. One half of these, approximately, do not have an identifiable cause other than the presence of SLE. The prevalence of pulmonary arterial hypertension (as determined by transthoracic echocardiography) was found to increase from 14% to 43% after 5 years in a small longitudinal study (n = 36). Raynaud phenomenon is found in 75% of subjects with SLE and pulmonary arterial hypertension, versus only 20% to 35% of those without clinically evident pulmonary arterial hypertension. Fibrocollagenous intimal thickening, medial thickening, changes in the elastic lamina, and luminal narrowing of muscular arteries are identified pathologically. Histologic vasculitis was reported in one study in approximately 50% of cases. Immune deposits are thought to be involved in the pathogenesis of SLE-related pulmonary arterial hypertension, considering the fact that granular IgG deposits and the C1q complement protein (and to a lesser extent IgM and C3) have been observed in vessel walls.[82]

Immunomodulatory therapy appears to be of help to patients with SLE and pulmonary arterial hypertension. After 6 months of a randomized study comparing monthly intravenous cyclophosphamide with oral enalapril, transthoracic echocardiography–derived pulmonary artery systolic pressure was found to decline in both groups. However, the effect was found to be significantly higher in patients who received intravenous cyclophosphamide (decrease of 15 mm Hg vs. 7 mm Hg; $P = 0.04$). Glucocorticoids given orally (usually combined with an immunomodulatory agent) lower pulmonary artery systolic pressure, improve 6-minute walk distance, and possibly prolong 5-year survival. Epoprostenol, bosentan, sitaxsentan, and sildenafil have also been shown to be effective in later studies.

Drug-Induced Pulmonary Fibrosis

Pulmonary complications from drugs used to treat SLE manifestations have not been studied systematically. Azathioprine and mycophenolate mofetil have been reported in some studies to cause cellular interstitial pneumonia. Nonsteroidal antiinflammatory drugs have a penchant to cause chronic eosinophilic pneumonia.[82]

Cyclophosphamide causes two types of lung injuries, early-onset pneumonitis and late-onset lung injury (reported up to 13 years after cyclophosphamide exposure). Early-onset pneumonitis develops within the first 6 months of cyclophosphamide exposure and responds to drug withdrawal and treatment with glucocorticoids. Late-onset lung injury manifests as upper lobe–predominant fibrosis and bilateral pleural thickening, which respond poorly to glucocorticoid therapy.

Lung injury brought about by methotrexate is seen in 2% to 12% of recipients and is not related to total or current dose, underlying disease, or duration of therapy. There are varying degrees of inflammation and/or fibrosis, and the histologic findings are variable and nonspecific. Elevated tissue eosinophils have been observed, and peripheral eosinophilia is found in up to 40% of patients. The lung injury brought about by methotrexate is responsive to glucocorticoid treatment and methotrexate withdrawal.[82]

Cirrhosis or Periportal Hepatitis in SLE

Advanced liver disease with cirrhosis and liver failure is rare in patients with SLE, even though clinical and biochemical evidence of associated liver abnormalities is common. Coincident viral hepatitis or earlier treatment with potentially hepatotoxic drugs has been normally implicated as the main reason for liver disease in subjects with SLE. The important question, even after careful exclusion of these causes, is whether to consider the subject as having a primary liver disease with related autoimmune, clinical, and laboratory features or as displaying liver disease due to SLE. A good example of this pathogenetic conundrum is that of autoimmune hepatitis and SLE-associated hepatitis. They have been considered different entities even though they have features in common. However, numerous clinical and histologic features aid in discriminating autoimmune hepatitis from SLE. In autoimmune hepatitis, periportal piecemeal necrosis variably linked with lobular activity, rosetting of liver cells, and dense lymphoid infiltrates are prominent. In SLE, however, the inflammation is normally lobular and occasionally periportal in association with a paucity of lymphoid infiltrates. A differential diagnosis between the two disorders poses a major challenge only in the 2% of SLE cases associated with periportal hepatitis and in cases of autoimmune hepatitis with extrahepatic manifestations, particularly those associated with arthralgia and presence of antinuclear antibodies (ANAs). The occurrence of cirrhosis or periportal (interface hepatitis) would be indicative of autoimmune hepatitis. However, this does not exclude SLE, even though only the occurrence of lobular hepatitis is more compatible with SLE.

One study reviewed more than 200 patients meeting diagnostic criteria for SLE. From the liver biopsy specimens available for 33 of these patients, a variety of hepatic lesions were found. The lesions included nonspecific portal inflammation, chronic active hepatitis, and established cirrhosis. Hepatic steatosis, observed in more than one third of patients who underwent biopsy, was the most common finding. Granulomatous hepatitis, nodular hyperplasia, idiopathic portal hypertension, and features of primary biliary cirrhosis have been documented by other reports.[83]

Retroperitoneal Fibrosis

Retroperitoneal fibrosis is a rare disorder characterized by the development of widespread fibrosis throughout the retroperitoneum, often leading to entrapment and obstruction of retroperitoneal structures, notably the ureters. Retroperitoneal fibrosis is not associated with a specific disease. Only five patents with retroperitoneal fibrosis and SLE have been reported thus far. Because animal models of retroperitoneal fibrosis are unavailable, the pathogenic origin of this disease is not clear, although association with elevated IgG4 has been reported. All the reported patients with SLE with retroperitoneal fibrosis, except one, have shown response to treatment with glucocorticoids (especially in the active inflammatory stage of retroperitoneal fibrosis).[84]

Mechanisms of Fibrosis in SLE

Deposition of immune complexes (containing autoantibodies) in target organs such as kidneys or T-cell infiltration of these target organs in autoimmune diseases induces early inflammatory lesions.

This injury is thought to trigger several events, such as complement activation, production of chemokines, more inflammatory cell infiltration, and release of inflammatory cytokines. These mediators play a role in triggering the breakdown of extracellular matrix through MMP- and plasmin-mediated pathways, as discussed previously, and described in Figure 16-4. In the chronic phases of the disease, these events culminate in excessive deposition of extracellular matrix and progressive fibrosis within the inflamed organs, including the kidneys, lungs, and other sites. As shown in Figure 16-4, TGF-β is believed to play a major role in the development of tissue fibrosis. Indeed, mice transgenic for TGF-β1 show fibrogenesis in multiple organs.[79,85]

TGF-β plays two conflicting roles during the induction and progression of immune-mediated organ damage. Diminished TGF-β production by immune cells induces immune dysregulation that results in the development of autoimmunity in early life. TGF-β1 or T cells that produce TGF-β1 suppress production of antibodies. Saxena demonstrated diminished expression of TGF-β1 in T cells in lupus-prone New Zealand Black and White F1 mice.[79] The reduced expression predisposes to increases in T-cell activation and autoantibody production. These increases cause inflammation in tissues, which leads to the production of antiinflammatory cytokines like TGF-β as well as its signaling molecules and type II TGF-β receptor (TβRII), the protein SMAD3, and phospho-SMAD3 in target organs to regulate inflammation. The continuous and/or increased production of these cytokines initially helps in tissue repair and remodeling. However, it eventually brings about local fibrogenesis that culminates in end-stage organ disease. Consistent with these results, in vivo blockade of TGF-β by monoclonal antibody treatment selectively inhibits the development of chronic fibrotic lesions but does not appear to affect local inflammation or autoantibody production.[79]

The key role played by TGF-β in fibrosis can be further seen in autoimmune congenital heart block (CHB), a model of acquired passive immunity. The characteristic lesion seen in this condition is fibrosis of the heart conducting tissue (specifically fibrosis of the atrioventricular node) and sometimes the surrounding myocardium. Anti-Ro60 and anti-La (or SSB) are present in more than 85% of mothers of fetuses with abnormalities in conduction (even though the fetuses have structurally normal hearts). However, there is only a 2% risk for a woman with these autoantibodies to have a baby with CHB. The exact mechanism by which these antibodies induce atrioventricular scarring is unclear. It is well known, though, that these candidate antibodies alone are insufficient to bring about disease, and fetal factors are thought to have a contributory role. One pathologic cascade has been suggested, on the basis of in vitro and in vivo studies, that is initiated through apoptosis. Maternal autoantibodies have been shown to bind to Ro60 and La antigens that translocate to the cell surface consequent to apoptosis. Following this event, the Fc regions of bound immunoglobulins bind to Fc receptors on tissue macrophages. Ingestion of such opsonized apoptosed cardiocytes by macrophages induces an inflammatory response. This response results in the increased release of TGF-β that brings about a profibrotic environment and leads to irreversible tissue scarring. This pathway also activates tissue-specific TGF-β, which induces the conversion of fibroblasts into myofibroblasts, leading to scarring.[86] Clancy delineated a model for fibrosis injury in CHB, linking Ro60-associated, single-stranded RNA–mediated macrophage activation through Toll-like receptor (TLR) engagement to fibrosis.[87] This model proposes the engagement of Toll-like receptor 7 following FcγR-mediated phagocytosis of immune complexes. The immune complexes result from the binding of anti-Ro60 antibodies to the apoptosis-released Ro60-bound single-stranded RNA on apoptotic cardiocytes.

Finally, as noted earlier, connective tissue growth factor (CTGF), fibroblast growth factor (FGF), vascular endothelial growth factor (VEGF), platelet-derived growth factor (PDGF), and bone morphogenetic proteins (BMPs) constitute additional molecules that shape the evolution of tissue fibrosis, but our understanding of how these molecules affect fibrosis in SLE remains incomplete. Whether fibrosis is a consequence of both matrix breakdown products leading to matrix and fibrin deposition or just the deposition of fibrin alone is unknown. Alternatively, both of these processes could occur independently, leading to organ damage.

CONCLUSION

The involvement of ROS and RNS in the pathogenesis and development of diseases is well known. Formation of these reactive intermediates along with enzymatic and nonenzymatic control of these harmful molecules is an ongoing process. Antibodies to antioxidant enzymes could result in the disruption in this balance resulting in oxidative stress, which in turn leads to pathologic changes. This process could lead to oxidatively modified autoantigens that serve as neoantigens in promoting loss of tolerance to self and thus lead to autoimmune diseases such as SLE. Immunization with modified autoantigens has been shown to accelerate epitope spreading and to induce disease. Administration of antioxidants or related dietary modulations has not been systematically studied in autoimmune diseases but could be helpful in preventing or ameliorating disease, although results in cardiovascular disease have not been encouraging.[88] Fibrosis constitutes a second major determinant of tissue damage in SLE, affecting the kidneys and lungs primarily. The balance set by plasmin and MMPs on the one hand, and TIMPs, PAI-I, and TGF-β on the other, dictate the degree of extracellular matrix breakdown versus fibrotic buildup. The latter bodes poorly for end-organ and patient survival in SLE. Currently, TGF-β is emerging as a major final determinant and potential therapeutic target in this complex network of pathogenic cascades, but future research is sure to clarify the respective roles of related growth factors. Thus, effective regulation of free radical–induced damage and end-organ fibrosis can have a profound impact not only in SLE but also in a myriad of other chronic diseases.

References

1. Boyd GW: An evolution-based hypothesis on the origin and mechanisms of autoimmune disease. *Immunol Cell Biol* 75:503–507, 1997.
2. Wang G, Pierangeli SS, Papalardo E, et al: Markers of oxidative and nitrosative stress in systemic lupus erythematosus: correlation with disease activity. *Arthritis Rheum* 62:2064–2072, 2010.
3. Kurien BT, Hensley K, Bachmann M, et al: Oxidatively modified autoantigens in autoimmune diseases. *Free Radic Biol Med* 41:549–556, 2006.
4. Kurien BT, Scofield RH: Free radical mediated peroxidative damage in systemic lupus erythematosus. *Life Sci* 73:1655–1666, 2003.
5. Michel P, Eggert W, Albrecht-Nebe H, et al: Increased lipid peroxidation in children with autoimmune diseases. *Acta Paediatr* 86:609–612, 1997.
6. Serban MG, Balanescu E, Nita V: Lipid peroxidase and erythrocyte redox system in systemic vasculitides treated with corticoids. Effect of vitamin E administration. *Rom J Intern Med* 32:283, 1994.
7. Grune T, Michel P, Sitte N, et al: Increased levels of 4-hydroxynonenal modified proteins in plasma of children with autoimmune diseases. *Free Radic Biol Med* 23:357–360, 1997.
8. Turi S, Nemeth I, Torkos A, et al: Oxidative stress and antioxidant defense mechanism in glomerular diseases. *Free Radic Biol Med* 22:161–168, 1997.
9. Serban MG, Tanaseanu S, Bara C: Oxidant stress and antioxidant protection in lupus nephropathy. *Rom J Intern Med* 34:105–109, 1996.
10. Jiang X, Chen F: The effect of lipid peroxides and superoxide dismutase on systemic lupus erythematosus: a preliminary study. *Clin Immunol Immunopathol* 63:39–44, 1992.
11. Otaki N, Chikazawa M, Nagae R, et al: Identification of a lipid peroxidation product as the source of oxidation-specific epitopes recognized by anti-DNA autoantibodies. *J Biol Chem* 285:33834–33842, 2010.
12. Jenney FE, Jr, Verhagen MF, Cui X, et al: Anaerobic microbes: oxygen detoxification without superoxide dismutase. *Science* 286:306–309, 1999 Oct 8.
13. Demopoulos HB: The basis of free radical pathology. *Fed Proc* 32:1859–1861, 1973.

14. Fridovich I: In Hayaishi O, editor: *Molecular mechanism of oxygen activation*. New York, 1974, Academic Press, p 453.

15. Steinman HM, Ely B: Copper-zinc superoxide dismutase of *Caulobacter crescentus*: cloning, sequencing and mapping of the gene and periplasmic location of the enzyme. *J Bacteriol* 172:2901–2910, 1990.

16. Seligman ML, Mitamura J, Shera N, et al: Corticosteroid (methylprednisolone) modulation of photoperoxidation by ultraviolet light in liposomes. *Photochemistry and Photobiology* 29:549–558, March 1979.

17. Gutteridge JMC, Westermarck T, Halliwell B: Oxygen radical damage in biological systems. In Johnson JE, Walford R, Harman D, Miquel J, editors: *Free radicals, aging, and degenerative diseases*, New York, 1985, A. R. Liss, pp 99–139.

18. Rimbach G, Hohler D, Fischer A, et al: Methods to assess free radicals and oxidative stress in biological systems. *Arch Tierernahr* 52:203–222, 1999.

19. Tappel AL: Lipid peroxidation damage to cell components. *Fed Proc* 32:1870–1874, 1973.

20. Esterbauer H, Schaur RJ, Zollner H: Chemistry and biochemistry of 4-hydroxynonenal, malonaldehyde and related aldehydes. *Free Radic Biol Med* 11:81–128, 1991.

21. Humphries KM, Szweda LI: Selective inactivation of alpha-ketoglutarate dehydrogenase and pyruvate dehydrogenase: reaction of lipoic acid with 4-hydroxy-2-nonenal. *Biochemistry* 37:15835–15841, 1998.

22. White PJ, Charbonneau A, Cooney GJ, et al: Nitrosative modifications of protein and lipid signaling molecules by reactive nitrogen species. *Am J Physiol Endocrinol Metab* 299:E868–E878, 2010, Review.

23. Mashmoushi AK, Gilkeson GS, Oates JC: Role of reactive nitrogen and oxygen-intermediates in systemic lupus erythematosus. Dubois' systemic lupus erythematosus. I. Basis of disease pathogenesis. 199–211.

24. Oates JC. The biology of reactive intermediates in systemic lupus erythematosus. *Autoimmunity* 43:56–63, 2010.

25. Stamler JS, Lamas S, Fang Nitrosylation FC: The prototypic redox-based signaling mechanism. *Cell* 106:675–683, 2001.

26. Hogg N: The biochemistry and physiology of S-nitrosothiols. *Annu Rev Pharmacol Toxicol* 42:585–600, 2002.

27. Eiserich JP, Hristova M, Cross CE, et al: Formation of nitric oxide-derived inflammatory oxidants by myeloperoxidase in neutrophils. *Nature* 391:393–397, 1998.

28. Bartesaghi S, Wenzel J, Trujillo M, et al: Lipid peroxyl radicals mediate tyrosine dimerization and nitration in membranes. *Chem Res Toxicol* 23:821–835, 2010.

29. Zheng B, Brett SJ, Tite JP, et al: Galactose oxidation in the design of immunogenic vaccines. *Science* 256:1560–1563, 1992.

30. Rhodes J, Chen H, Hall SR, et al: Therapeutic potentiation of the immune system by costimulatory Schiff-base-forming drugs. *Nature* 377:71–75, 1995.

31. Arbuckle MR, McClain MT, Rubertone MV, et al: Development of autoantibodies before the clinical onset of systemic lupus erythematosus. *N Engl J Med* 349:1526–1533, 2003.

32. Scofield RH: Autoantibodies as predictors of disease. *Lancet* 363:1544–1546, 2004.

33. Valko M, Leibfritz D, Moncol J, et al: Free radicals and antioxidants in normal physiological functions and human disease. *Int J Biochem Cell Biol* 39:44–84, 2007.

34. Alves CM, Marzocchi-Machado CM, Louzada-Junior P, et al: Superoxide anion production by neutrophils is associated with prevalent clinical manifestations in systemic lupus erythematosus. *Clin Rheumatol* 27:701–708, 2008.

34a. Suryaprabha P, Das UN, Ramesh G, et al: Reactive oxygen species, lipid peroxides and essential fatty acids in patients with arthritis and systemic lupus erythematosus. *Prostaglandins Leukot Essent Fatty Acids* 43:251–255, 1991.

35. Kurien BT, Scofield RH: Lipid peroxidation in systemic lupus erythematosus. *Ind J Exp Biol* 44:349–356, 2006.

36. Casellas AM, Prat A, Llera A, et al: Increased superoxide production by polymorphonuclear leukocytes in systemic lupus erythematosus. *Clin Exp Rheumatol* 9:511–514, 1991.

37. Ahmad R, Alam K, Ali R: Antigen binding characteristics of antibodies against hydroxyl radical modified thymidine monophosphate. *Immunol Lett* 71:111–115, 2000.

38. Gallelli B, Burdick L, Quaglini S, et al: Carotid plaques in patients with long-term lupus nephritis. *Clin Exp Rheumatol* 28:386–392, 2010, May–Jun.

39. Shah D, Kiran R, Wanchu A, et al: Oxidative stress in systemic lupus erythematosus: relationship to Th1 cytokine and disease activity. *Immunol Lett* 129:7–12, 2010.

40. Zhang Q, Ye DQ, Chen GP: (Study on the relationship between protein oxidation and disease activity in systemic lupus erythematosus). (Article in Chinese). Zhonghua Liu Xing Bing Xue Za Zhi 29:181–184, 2008.

41. Zhang Q, Ye DQ, Chen GP, et al: Oxidative protein damage and antioxidant status in systemic lupus erythematosus. *Clin Exp Dermatol* 35:287–294, 2010.

42. Vipartene D, Iasiulevichute L, Butkene B, et al: (Pro- and antioxidant blood system in patients with rheumatoid arthritis and systemic lupus erythematosus). *Ter Arkh* 78(6):10–14, 2006 (Article in Russian).

43. Wang JS, Ger LP, Tseng HH: Expression of glomerular antioxidant enzymes in human glomerulonephritis. *Nephron* 76:32–38, 1997.

43a. Taysi S, Gul M, Sari RA, et al: Serum oxidant/antioxidant status of patients with systemic lupus erythematosus. *Clin Chem Lab Med* 40:684–688, 2002.

44. Mansour RB, Lassoued S, Gargouri B, et al: Increased levels of autoantibodies against catalase and superoxide dismutase associated with oxidative stress in patients with rheumatoid arthritis and systemic lupus erythematosus. *Scand J Rheumatol* 37:103–108, 2008.

45. Huang WN, Tso TK, Huang HY: Enhanced oxidative status but not corresponding elevated antioxidative status by anticardiolipin antibody and disease activity in patients with systemic lupus erythematosus. *Rheumatol Int* 27:453–458, 2007.

46. Nuttall SL, Heaton S, Piper MK, et al: Gordon Cardiovascular risk in systemic lupus erythematosus—evidence of increased oxidative stress and dyslipidaemia. *Rheumatology* 42:758–762, 2003.

47. Toyoda K, Nagae R, Akagawa M, et al: Protein-bound 4-hydroxy-2-nonenal: an endogenous triggering antigen of anti-DNA response. *J Biol Chem* 282:25769–25778, 2007.

48. Haberland ME, Olch C, Folgeman AM: Role of lysine in mediating interaction of modified low density lipoproteins with the scavenger receptor of human monocyte macrophages. *J Biol Chem* 259:11305–11311, 1984.

49. Ben Mansour R, Lassoued S, Elgaied A, et al: Enhanced reactivity to malondialdehyde-modified proteins by systemic lupus erythematosus autoantibodies. *Scand J Rheumatol* 39:247–253, 2010.

50. Wang G, Pierangeli SS, Papalardo E, et al: Markers of oxidative and nitrosative stress in systemic lupus erythematosus: correlation with disease activity. *Arthritis Rheum* 62:2064–2072, 2010.

51. Fesmire J, Wolfson-Reichlin M, Reichlin M: Effects of autoimmune antibodies anti-lipoprotein lipase, anti-low density lipoprotein, and anti-oxidized low density lipoprotein on lipid metabolism and atherosclerosis in systemic lupus erythematosus. *Rev Bras Reumatol* 50:539–551, 2010 Oct (Article in English, Portuguese).

52. Espinosa A, Oke V, Elfving A, et al: The autoantigen Ro52 is an E3 ligase resident in the cytoplasm but enters the nucleus upon cellular exposure to nitric oxide. *Exp Cell Res* 314:3605–3613, 2008.

53. Belmont HM, Levartovsky D, Goel A, et al: Increased nitric oxide production accompanied by the up-regulation of inducible nitric oxide synthase in vascular endothelium from patients with systemic lupus erythematosus. *Arthritis Rheum* 40:1810–1816, 1997.

54. Ghiran IC, Zeidel ML, Shevkoplyas SS, et al: Systemic lupus erythematosus serum deposits C4d on red blood cells, decreases red blood cell membrane deformability, and promotes nitric oxide production. *Arthritis Rheum* 63:503–512, 2011.

55. Thomas DD, Ridnour LA, Isenberg JS, et al: The chemical biology of nitric oxide: implications in cellular signaling. *Free Radic Biol Med* 45:18–31, 2008.

56. Habib S, Moinuddin Ali R: Peroxynitrite-modified DNA: a better antigen for systemic lupus erythematosus anti-DNA autoantibodies. *Biotechnol Appl Biochem* 43(Pt 2):65–70, 2006.

57. Nagy G, Koncz A, Perl A: T cell activation-induced mitochondrial hyperpolarization is mediated by Ca2þ- and redox-dependent production of nitric oxide. *J Immunol* 171:5188–5197, 2003.

58. Wu T, Fu Y, Brekken D, et al: Urine proteome scans uncover total urinary protease, prostaglandin D synthase, serum amyloid P, and superoxide dismutase as potential markers of lupus nephritis. *J Immunol* 184:2183–2193, 2010.

59. D'souza A, Kurien BT, Rodgers R, et al: Detection of catalase as a major protein target of the lipid peroxidation product 4-HNE and the lack of its genetic association as a risk factor in SLE. *BMC Med Genet* 9:62, 2008.

60. Weinberg JB, Granger DL, Pisetsky DS, et al: The role of nitric oxide in the pathogenesis of spontaneous murine autoimmune disease: increased nitric oxide production and nitric oxide synthase expression in MRL-lpr/lpr mice, and reduction of spontaneous glomerulonephritis and arthritis

by orally administered NG-monomethyl-L-arginine. *J Exp Med* 179:651–660, 1994.

61. Reilly CM, Olgun S, Goodwin D, et al: Interferon regulatory factor-1 gene deletion decreases glomerulonephritis in MRL/lpr mice. *Eur J Immunol* 36:1296–1308, 2006.

62. Gilkeson GS, Mudgett JS, Seldin MF, et al: Clinical and serologic manifestations of autoimmune disease in MRL-lpr/lpr mice lacking nitric oxide synthase type 2. *J Exp Med* 186:365–373, 1997.

63. Boyd CS, Cadenas E: Nitric oxide and cell signaling pathways in mitochondrial-dependent apoptosis. *Biol Chem* 383:411–423, 2002.

64. Njoku CJ, Patrick KS, Ruiz P, Jr, et al: Inducible nitric oxide synthase inhibitors reduce urinary markers of systemic oxidant stress in murine proliferative lupus nephritis. *J Investig Med* 53:347–352, 2005.

65. Ames PR, Alves J, Murat I, et al: Oxidative stress in systemic lupus erythematosus and allied conditions with vascular involvement. *Rheumatology (Oxford)* 38:529, 1999.

65a. Pottathil R, Huang SW, Chandrabose KA, et al: Essential fatty acids in diabetes and systemic lupus erythematosus (SLE) patients. *Biochem Biophys Res Commun* 128:803–808, 1985.

66. Oates JC, Gilkeson GS: Mediators of injury in lupus nephritis. *Curr Opin Rheumatol* 14:498–503, 2002, Review.

67. Austin HA 3rd, Muenz LR, Joyce KM, et al: Diffuse proliferative lupus nephritis: identification of specific pathologic features affecting renal outcome. *Kidney Int* 25:689–695, 1984.

68. Austin HA III, Boumpas DT, Vaughan EM, et al. High-risk features of lupus nephritis: importance of race and clinical and histological factors in 166 patients. *Nephrol Dial Transplant* 10:1620–1628, 1995.

69. Nossent HC, Henzen-Logmans SC, Vroom TM, et al: Contribution of renal biopsy data in predicting outcome in lupus nephritis. Analysis of 116 patients. *Arthritis Rheum* 33:970–977, 1990.

70. Esdaile JM, Federgreen W, Quintal H, et al: Predictors of one year outcome in lupus nephritis: the importance of renal biopsy. *Q J Med* 81:879–881, 1991.

71. Schwartz MM, Lan SP, Bernstein J, et al: Role of pathology indices in the management of severe lupus glomerulonephritis. *Kidney Int* 42:743–748, 1992.

72. Moroni G, Pasquali S, Quaglini S, et al: Clinical and prognostic value of serial renal biopsies in lupus nephritis. *Amer J Kidney Dis* 34:530–539, 1999.

73. Contreras G, Pardo V, Cely C, et al: Factors associated with poor outcomes in patients with lupus nephritis. *Lupus* 14:890–895, 2005.

74. Hill GS, Delahousse M, Nochy D, et al: Outcome of relapse in lupus nephritis: roles of reversal of renal fibrosis and response of inflammation to therapy. *Kidney Int* 61:2176–2186, 2002.

75. Triantafyllopoulou A, Franzke CW, Seshan SV, et al: Proliferative lesions and metalloproteinase activity in murine lupus nephritis mediated by type I interferons and macrophages. *PNAS* 107:3012–3017, 2010, February 16.

76. Tveita A, Rekvig OP, Zykova SN: Glomerular matrix metalloproteinases and their regulators in the pathogenesis of lupus nephritis. *Arthritis Res Ther* 10:229, 2008.

77. Moll S, Menoud PA, Fulpius T, et al: Induction of plasminogen activator inhibitor type 1 in murine lupus-like glomerulonephritis. *Kidney Int* 48(5):1459–1468, 1995 Nov.

78. Yamamoto K, Loskutoff DJ: Expression of transforming growth factor-beta and tumor necrosis factor-alpha in the plasma and tissues of mice with lupus nephritis. *Lab Invest* 80:1561–1570, 2000 Oct.

79. Saxena V, Lienesch DW, Zhou M, et al: Dual roles of immunoregulatory cytokine TGF-beta in the pathogenesis of autoimmunity-mediated organ damage. *J Immunol* 180:1903–1912, 2008.

80. Zeisberg M, Bottiglio C, Kumar N, et al: Müller and Raghu Kalluri. Bone morphogenic protein-7 inhibits progression of chronic renal fibrosis associated with two genetic mouse models. *Am J Physiol Renal Physiol* 285:F1060–F1067, 2003.

81. Kamen DL, Strange C: Pulmonary manifestations of systemic lupus erythematosus. *Clin Chest Med* 31:479–488, 2010.

81a. Weinrib L, Sharma OP, Quismorio FP Jr: A long-term study of interstitial lung disease in systemic lupus erythematosus. *Semin Arthritis Rheum* 20:48–56, 1990.

82. Swigris JJ, Fischer A, Gillis J, et al: Pulmonary and thrombotic manifestations of systemic lupus erythematosus. *Chest* 133:271–280, 2008.

83. Youssef WI, Tavill AS: Connective tissue diseases and the liver. *J Clin Gastroenterol* 35:345–349, 2002.

84. Okada H, Takahira S, Sugahara S, et al: Retroperitoneal fibrosis and systemic lupus erythematosus. *Nephrol Dial Transplant* 14:1300–1302, 1999.

85. Kopp JB, Factor VM, Mozes M, et al: Transgenic mice with increased plasma levels of TGF-beta 1 develop progressive renal disease. *Lab Invest* 74:991–1003, 1996.

86. Clancy RM, Buyon JP: Autoimmune-associated congenital heart block: dissecting the cascade from immunologic insult to relentless fibrosis. *Anat Rec A Discov Mol Cell Evol Biol* 280:1027–1035, 2004.

87. Clancy RM, Alvarez D, Komissarova E, et al: Ro60-associated single-stranded RNA links inflammation with fetal cardiac fibrosis via ligation of TLRs: a novel pathway to autoimmune-associated heart block. *J Immunol* 184:2148–2155, 2010.

88. Shekelle PG, Morton SC, Jungvig LK, et al: Effect of supplemental vitamin E for the prevention and treatment of cardiovascular disease. *J Gen Intern Med* 19:380–389, 2004.

89. Furusu A, Miyazaki M, Abe K, et al: Expression of endothelial and inducible nitric oxide synthase in human glomerulonephritis. *Kidney Int* 53:1760–1768, 1998.

90. Das UN: Oxidants, antioxidants, essential fatty acids, eicosanoids, cytokines, gene/oncogene expression and apoptosis in systemic lupus erythematosus. *J Assoc Physic India* 46:630–634, 1998.

91. Oates JC, Gilkeson GS: The biology of nitric oxide and other reactive intermediates in systemic lupus erythematosus. *Clin Immunol* 121:243–250, 2006.

92. Oates JC, Shaftman SR, Self SE, et al: Association of serum nitrate and nitrite levels with longitudinal assessments of disease activity and damage in systemic lupus erythematosus and lupus nephritis. *Arthritis Rheum* 58:263–272, 2008.

93. Agisheva KN, Salikhov IG: [Lipid peroxidation and state of antioxidant system in patients with systemic lupus erythematosus] *Klin Med (Mosk)* 68:99–102, 1990. Russian.

94. Serban MG, Negru T: Antioxidant protection in collagen-vascular diseases. *Rom J Intern Med* 36:245–250, 1998.

95. Vaarala O, Alfthan G, Jauhiainen M, et al: Crossreaction between antibodies to oxidised low-density lipoprotein and to cardiolipin in systemic lupus erythematosus. *Lancet* 341:923–925, 1993.

96. Matsuura E, Lopez LR: Are oxidized LDL/beta2-glycoprotein I complexes pathogenic antigens in autoimmune-mediated atherosclerosis? *Clin Dev Immunol* 11:103–111, 2004.

Animal Models of SLE

Bevra Hannahs Hahn and Dwight Kono

Animal models of SLE have provided an invaluable resource for defining disease pathophysiology, genetics, and therapeutic approaches. Furthermore, in human SLE, heterogeneity in disease expression is an obstacle to devising targeted interventions that apply to all patients. Consequently, many investigators have turned to murine lupus models, both spontaneous and induced, that develop relatively homogeneous disease recapitulating some of the serologic and histopathologic features of SLE. Murine SLE is characterized by the presence of autoantibodies against nuclear and a variety of other ubiquitous and cell type–specific self-antigens, and end-organ injury, most commonly immune-mediated glomerulonephritis (GN).[1] Another noteworthy finding is that virtually all cases of spontaneous and induced murine lupus require a susceptible genetic background. There are informative differences in disease in different strains. For example, BALB/c mice injected with a DNA surrogate peptide demonstrate extensive glomerular immune deposition but no renal inflammation,[2] whereas in BALB/c mice injected with hydrocarbon oil pristane immune deposition and limited kidney inflammation (focal GN) develop, but no kidney failure.[3,4] In contrast, many multigenic lupus-prone mouse strains spontaneously develop immune deposition–mediated renal disease that is lethal, with strain-dependent variation in disease patterns and severity.[5] Numerous single-gene knockout and transgenic strains also develop autoimmune features[6,7] that recapitulate some aspects of SLE-like disease.

A few lupus-like murine strains develop coronary occlusions and myocardial infarction as a result of immune complex deposition, but the relevance of this mechanism to the increased cardiovascular disease in human SLE is unclear. Some strains develop dermatitis, autoimmune hemolytic anemia, arthritis, and vasculitis, but the incidence of these disorders is generally variable and may depend at least in part on environment. Mouse models have not recapitulated the waxing and waning nature or the full spectrum of human SLE. Spontaneous SLE also develops in dogs. Tables 17-1 to 17-3 provide an overview of major characteristics of mice and dogs with lupus-like disease.

CLINICAL DISEASE, AUTOANTIBODIES, IMMUNOLOGIC ABNORMALITIES, AND GENETICS IN SPONTANEOUS MULTIGENIC MURINE SLE

This section reviews the principal characteristics of the most extensively studied mouse strains that spontaneously develop lupus-like disease.

New Zealand Mice

NZB/BL (NZB) Mice

The New Zealand Bielschowsky black (NZB/Bl) mouse was bred by Bielschowsky, who was mating mice by coat color to derive cancer-susceptible strains. In 1959, she reported that NZB mice died early from autoimmune hemolytic anemia.[8] Shortly thereafter, her colleagues described a hybrid between NZB and unrelated strains including the New Zealand white (NZW) that was characterized by

early death in females from nephritis associated with lupus erythematosus (LE) cells, thus providing the first animal models of lupus nephritis.[9]

The characteristics of NZB mice are shown in Tables 17-1 to 17-3 and Box 17-1. They also are discussed in several review articles.[10,11]

Clinical Characteristics and Autoantibodies

NZB mice are characterized by hyperactive B cells, present in fetal life, that produce primarily immunoglobulin M (IgM) antibodies to thymocytes, erythrocytes, single-stranded DNA (ssDNA), and the gp70 glycoprotein of murine leukemia virus.[10-12] The first antibody to appear in serum is natural thymocytotoxic antibody (NTA)[13,14]; by 3 months of age, 100% of mice have this antibody. NTAs are cytotoxic for all thymocytes, 50% to 60% of thoracic duct and peripheral blood lymphocytes (both CD4[+] and CD8[+] populations), 50% of lymph node cells, 33% of spleen cells, and 5% of bone marrow cells. These figures are similar to the reactivity of anti–Thy-l sera. Some NTAs react with cell surface molecules on B lymphocytes, granulocytes, and bone marrow myeloid cells; others react with a 55-kd molecule on most T cells. Other reported reactivities include an 88-kd glycoprotein, which is thought to be a T-cell differentiation antigen, and surface molecules of 33 and 30 kd.[11,15-17]

The primary clinical problem in NZB mice is hemolytic anemia, which is fatal in most (60%-90%) between 15 and 18 months of age.[8,10,11] There is mild disease acceleration in females, with death 1 month earlier than in males. IgM and IgG antibodies to erythrocytes (red blood cells [RBCs]) cause hemolysis,[18,19] appear by 3 months of age, and are found in 100% by 9 to 10 months of age. Antibodies to RBCs are directed against (1) RBC surface antigens exposed by bromelain, (2) anion exchanger membrane protein band 3,[20-22] or (3) spectrin.[23] Early in life, the RBC antibodies are polyreactive; later, they become more specific for band 3 or spectrin, suggesting antigenic stimulation.[23] However, genetic deletion of the band 3 antigen does not protect NZB mice against anti-RBC: they simply make autoantibodies to antigens other than B and 3.[21] Polyclonal B-cell activation, B-cell proliferation, high IgM production, and class-switching in response to activation by Toll-like receptors (TLRs) are largely independent of T-cell help and may be influenced by elevations of B cell–activating factor (BAFF) in this strain.[24] However, hemolysis is primarily mediated by IgG anti-RBC, and the characteristic mild clinical GN[25,26] depends on deposition of IgG autoantibodies (particularly to nucleosome and dsDNA), especially of the T helper–1 cell (Th1)–driven, IgG2a complement–fixing subclass. Knockout of CD40L (which mediates 2nd signal B-T interactions that result in Ig class switch) abrogates most IgG autoantibody production, and largely prevents glomerular disease, but does not affect abnormalities in B220[+] cells and in IgM production.[24] In NZB mice, antinuclear antibodies (ANAs) are not regularly present in high titers as in other lupus-prone strains, although approximately 80% of mice test ANA positive by 9 months of age.[10] Some NZB mice exhibit learning disabilities,[27] probably related both to the cortical ectopias that occur in 40% and to the autoimmune process. Autoantibodies to Purkinje cells of the cerebellum have been found,[28] and the

TABLE 17-1 Major Characteristics of Animal Strains Developing Systemic Lupus Erythematosus (SLE): Disease Manifestations in Lupus-Prone Animals

STRAIN/ MODEL	Nephritis	Dermatitis	Arthritis	Neuropsychiatric	Hematologic	Vascular	Other
			Manifestation				
NZB/Bl	Mild, late life				Hemolytic anemia		Peptic ulcer 50%
(NZB/NZW) F1 (BWF1)	Proliferative, progressive			Yes	Mild leukopenia		Choroiditis 60%-90%, oophoritis 35%
NZM.2410	Early glomerulosclerosis			Yes			
NZM.2328	Proliferative, progressive						Sialoadenitis, dacryoadenitis
(NZB/SWR) F1 (SNF1)	Proliferative, progressive						
MRL/Mp-lpr/lpr (MRL-1)	Diffuse proliferative; severe interstitial inflammation	50% by 5 mo of age Epidermal hyperplasia, ulceration, chronic on back, neck, face	75%, pannus and infiltrate	Yes		Vasculitis in 56% Myocardial infarct in small percent	Sialoadenitis 100%, conjunctivitis 85%, band keratopathy 90%, choroiditis 100%, oophoritis 72%
MRL/Mp-+/+	Mild, late life	Mild, late life	75%, pannus and infiltrate			Vasculitis in 8%	Milder/later than in MRL-1; sialoadenitis 95%, conjunctivitis 50%, band keratopathy 90%, choroiditis 100%, oophoritis 72%
BXSB	Diffuse proliferative						Neutrophilic infiltrate in joints
BXD2	Diffuse proliferative		Erosive				Splenomegaly, large germinal centers in spleen, lymph nodes
NZW/BXSB (WBF1)						Atherosclerosis	Myocardial, myocardial infarcts, high-titer antiphospholipid
Hydrocarbon oil-induced	Focal proliferative		Yes				Hepatitis
Anti-DNA idiotype induced	Yes				Leukopenia	Thrombosis	Elevated erythrocyte sedimentation rate
Dog	65%	60%	90%		Thrombocytopenia, hemolytic anemia	Clotting	Relapsing/remitting disease, fever, lymphadenopathy, splenomegaly
Heparan sulfate–induced in dog	100%	100%	40%		Anemia		Interstitial pneumonitis

numbers of interleukin-1 receptors (IL-1Rs) expressed in the dentate gyrus are lower than in normal mice.[29]

Abnormalities of Stem Cells and B Cells

NZB mice are remarkable for inherent abnormalities in their B cells that probably originate in bone marrow stem cells, because hyperactivation of B cells is detectable in fetal liver. In comparison with normal mice, there are higher numbers of IgM-secreting cells and greater synthesis of IgM by individual B cells—characteristics that may be controlled by different genes.[30-32] Splenic $CD21^{hi}CD23^-$ (marginal zone [MZ] B cells) and $CD21^{lo}CD23^-$ (immature B, memory B, and preplasma cells) subsets are particularly expanded, as are spleen and bone marrow plasma cells.[24] Putative bone marrow pre-B cells exhibit increased growth both in vitro and in vivo[33]; this property is lost after 10 months of age.[34] Mature B cells are resistant to normal control mechanisms involving engagement of the B-cell receptor (BCR).[35] Another B-cell abnormality highly characteristic of NZB mice is the appearance of aneuploidy in B cells, primarily in B-1 B

TABLE 17-2 Major Characteristics of Animal Strains Developing Systemic Lupus Erythematosus (SLE): Autoantibodies in Lupus-Prone Animals*

STRAIN/MODEL	Double-Stranded DNA	Anticardiolipin	Rheumatoid Factors	Erythrocyte	Small Nuclear Ribonucleoprotein	Cryoglobulin	Others
			Autoantibody				
NZB/Bl				+			gp70, natural thymocytotoxic antibody, ANA late life
NZB/NZW F1 (BWF1)	100% (4-5 mo), IgG	+	+ (rare)	20%-40%	0	+	gp70, RNA polymerase I, RNA, ubiquitin, helicase ANAs in 100%
NZM.2410	IgG						
NZM.2328	IgG						
NZB/SWR F1 (SNF1)	IgG in 100% of females, IgG2b cationic						ANA in all females
MRL/Mp-+/+	100%		+	10%	83% (9 mo)	+	gp70, albumin, transferrin, La, Ro, ribosome P, S10 RNA polymerase I
MRL/Mp-lpr/lpr (MRL-1)	100% (4-5 mo), IgG	+	+	10%	37% (5 mo)	+	gp70, albumin, transferrin, La, Ro, Su, ribosome P, S10 RNA polymerase I, laminin, collagen, ubiquitin, mitochondria, circulating immune complexes
BXSB	IgG, 100% (4-5 mo)			20%-40%		+	gp70, albumin, transferrin
BXD2	+		+				
NZW/BXSB (WBF1)		+					
Hydrocarbon oil–induced	+	+	+		+		Su, ribosomal P, tRNA synthetase, helicase
Anti-DNA idiotype induced	+						
Dog	<30				<30		ANA (90%), histones (90%), <30% Ro, lymphocytes, and platelets
Heparan sulfate–induced in dog	0						ANA titer > 1:128 (100%), heparan sulfate

ANA, antinuclear antibody; gp, glycoprotein; Ig, immunoglobulin.
*Numbers indicate frequency of specific autoantibody (at tested age, if known). All strains have ANA positivity.

cells (also designated Ly-1 or CD5+), as the mice age. Hyperdiploid B-1 B cells with additional chromosomes 10, 15, 17, and X are common.[36] Lymphoid malignancies are more common in NZB than in other murine lupus strains, prevalence varying in different colonies between 1% and 20%; they may be a model of B-cell chronic lymphocytic leukemia. Malignant B-1 B cells secrete large quantities of IL-10, which can skew T-cell repertoires away from T-helper 1 (Th1) and toward Th2 phenotypes.[37] In young NZB mice, numbers of nonmalignant B-1 B cells are increased in the spleen and peritoneum[38]; these cells make IgM autoantibodies to RBCs, thymocytes, and ssDNA. B-1 cells are also present among MZ B cells in lymphoid tissues.[39] B-2 (CD5−) B cells, however, are more likely to be the source

TABLE 17-3 Major Characteristics of Animal Strains Developing Systemic Lupus Erythematosus (SLE): Genetic and Other Features of Lupus-Prone Animals

STRAIN/MODEL	Coat Color	Sex Dominance	Life Span (days)	Age for 50% Mortality (mo)	H-2 Locus	Mls-1 Locus	Vα	Vβ	IgH-C	IgH-V
(NZB/NZW) F1 (BWF1)	Brown	F	245 F, 406 M	8.5	d/z (d/u)	a/b				
NZB/Bl	Black	M/	430 F 469 M	16	d	a	c	b	n	d
NZW	White	F			z (u)		d	*a*	n	d
NZM.2410	Agouti	F/M								
NZM.2328	Agouti	F	~9.5							
(NZB/SWR) F1 (SNF1)	Brown	F		6	d/q	a/a	c	a/b	n/p	
SWR					q		c	a	p	
MRL/Mp-+/+	White		476 F, 546 M		k			a	b	j	j
75% LG/J					d/f		a	b	d	j
12.6% AKR					k		a	b	j	d
12.1% C3H/Di					k		a	b	b	k
0.3% C57BL/6					b		b			b
MRL/Mp-lpr/lpr (MRL-1)	White	M/F	143 F, 154 M	6	k	b	a	b	J	h
BXSB	Brown	M	574 F, 161 M	5	b	b	b	b		b
50% C57BL/6										
50% SB/Le										
BXD2			14 mo							

F, female; Ig, immunoglobulin; M, male.

Box 17-1 Characteristics of NZB/Bl Mice

Clinical
1. Females live a mean of 431 days, males 467 days.
2. Death usually is caused by autoimmune hemolytic anemia.
3. 50% mortality by 15 to 17 months of age.

Histologic
1. Glomerulonephritis with Ig and C3 deposits.
2. Marked thymic atrophy.
3. Mild lymphoid hyperplasia.

Autoantibodies
1. IgM natural thymocytotoxic antibody.
2. IgM and IgG antierythrocyte.
3. IgM anti-ssDNA.
4. Anti–glycoprotein 70.
5. Antinuclear antibodies by late life.
6. Modest elevations of circulating immune complexes.

Immune Abnormalities
1. B cells are unusually mature and hyperactivated, and they secrete Ig spontaneously from a very early age (in fetus and in newborn mice); this abnormality is required for autoimmune disease in NZB mice and in hybrids mated with NZB mice.
2. Numbers of B-1 (CD5+) B cells in spleen and peritoneum are increased; these cells make primarily IgM autoantibodies; their elimination protects from SLE.

3. B cells resist tolerance to T cell–independent antigens.
4. Older mice develop aneuploidy in B-1 B cells.
5. Thymic epithelium is strikingly atrophic by 1 month of age.
6. Antithymocyte antibodies react with immune T cells and may inactivate/delete precursors of suppressor T-cell populations.
7. T cells are required for maximal autoantibody formation.
8. High quantities of a unique form of retroviral gp70 antigen in serum.
9. Clearance of immune complexes by Fc-mediated mechanisms is defective.

Genetics
1. Multiple dominant, codominant, and recessive genes participate in the immune abnormalities.
2. One set of genes controls the constellation of polyclonal B-cell activation, expression of gp70, and antithymocyte antibodies; another set of genes controls B-cell tolerance defects, antibodies to gp70, anti-ssDNA, and anti–red blood cells; the gene sets segregate independently; neither of these sets is dependent on H-2.
3. The disease is linked to major histocompatibility class.
4. NZB has two to five susceptibility genes located on different chromosomes, some transmitted in a dominant and others in a recessive fashion. *Nba2* region on chromosome 1 plays a major role in susceptibility to lupus in mice with NZ backgrounds.

gp, glycoprotein; Ig, immunoglobulin; ssDNA, single-stranded DNA.

for IgG autoantibodies.[40] Nevertheless, elimination of B-1 B cells by lysing of the cells with water in the peritoneal cavity (where these cells are renewed) reduces antibodies to RBC and hemolytic anemia,[41] thus demonstrating the importance of B-1 cells to NZB disease. Finally, splenic B cells in NZB mice are probably resistant to apoptosis because of the influence of the *Ifi202* gene (in the Nba2 region),

which is upregulated in this strain and plays a major role in sustained autoantibody production in NZB hybrids.[42,43]

Abnormalities of Dendritic Cells

Since the recognition of the connections between innate and acquired immunity, there has been great interest in the role of dendritic cells

(DCs) as mediators of immune tolerance, as a source of antigen-presenting cells (APCs) that activate T cells, and as a source of interferon alpha (IFN-α). Notably, pDCs express TLR9 and TLR7, which can bind immune complexes containing, respectively, DNA and ssRNA, thus becoming activated pDCs that enhance autoimmune responses to nucleic acids or material containing nucleic acids. In fact, NZB mice, compared with normal strains, respond to injections of CpG oligodeoxynucleotide (CpG ODN), a synthetic DNA, with increased release of IFN-α. Furthermore, cell numbers of DCs and messenger RNA (mRNA) for TLR9 are increased in NZB mice. On the other hand, other features of DCs that promote inflammation are abnormally low in NZB DCs, including production of IL-12 and expression of the homing chemokine CCR7 and the activation surface marker CD62L.[44] Whether these DC abnormalities represent primary defects contributing to autoimmunity or secondary activation stages remains to be determined.

Abnormalities of Thymus and T Cells

NZB mice characteristically exhibit a dramatic involution of thymic tissue; thymic epithelium is atrophied and immunologically defective by 1 month of age (before the appearance of NTA), with epithelial cell degeneration, accumulation of terminal deoxynucleotidyl transferase-positive (TdT$^+$) large immature T cells in the subcapsular region of the cortex, cortical atrophy, and increased lymphoid and plasma cell infiltrates in the medulla.[10,17,45-47] NZB thymic epithelial cells are functionally defective compared with cells from normal mice, having low expression of Aire and RelB proteins, low numbers of surface Ia molecules and major histocompatibility complex (MHC) class II molecules, low secretion of IL-1, high secretion of prostaglandin E$_2$ (PGE$_2$) and PGE$_3$, and diminished ability to educate nonthymic cells to express Thy-l.[46-49] NZB bone marrow contains greater prothymocyte activity, and the prothymocytes have an increased growth advantage when they are transferred to histocompatible recipients.[50] Thymic DCs are also abnormal; they are defective in mediating negative T-cell selection, possibly because they express less E-cadherin than thymic DCs from nonautoimmune mice.[51]

CD4$^+$ T cells play an essential role in NZB disease. Accordingly, the MHC class II (also called H-2 in mice) is an important predisposing factor for autoimmunity. The hybrid combination of NZB (H-2d/d haplotype) and NZW (z/z) or SWR (q/q) to make d/z or d/q MHC haplotypes enhances susceptibility to GN mediated by IgG anti-dsDNA,[52-62] which are antibodies that NZB mice do not make. NZB mice that are congenic for H-2b (NZB.H-2b) have less disease than the wild-type NZB.H-2d. However, introduction of a mutated I-A chain (bm12) converts this animal (i.e., NZB.H-2bm12) to a phenotype that is similar to the BWF1 hybrid, with high-titer IgG anti-dsDNA and severe clinical GN.[63,64] MHC class II likely plays a role in disease by shaping the repertoires of CD4$^+$ T cells. In fact, CD4$^+$ cells that proliferate in response to the RBC membrane protein band 3 and to spectrin have been isolated from NZB spleens.[22] The importance of T cells to autoantibody formation is also indicated by experiments in which anti-CD4 nondepleting antibody was administered to NZB mice; antierythrocyte antibodies were significantly decreased, although anemia was not prevented.[65]

Genetics

Genetic susceptibility in NZB mice is polygenically inherited, with genes having a partial and additive effect similar to that in most human SLE. With use of crosses of NZB to lupus-prone and non-lupus strains, loci linked to one or more lupus traits have been mapped to ten chromosomes.[52-62] The underlying genetic variants for most loci are not yet defined. For the most prominent disease manifestation, anti-RBC antibodies, loci on chromosomes 1 (called Nba2), 4 (Aia1, Aem1), 7 (Aem2), and 10 (Aem3) have been confirmed by more than one study or in congenic mice.[57,63-67] Among these, the distal chromosome 4 locus (also called Lbw2) was further dissected with subcongenic mice and shown to consist of at least three loci.[66]

This locus also increased susceptibility to GN and B-cell hyperactivity on the BWF1 background.[68] IgM hypergammaglobulinemia and increased peritoneal B-1 cells also map to the same interval.[36,60,69,70] Within this interval, a promoter variant of Cdkn2c (encodes the cyclin-dependent kinase inhibitor p18INK4c) associated with reduced expression in a B6-Sle2c1 congenic strain containing a small NZB chromosome 4 genome on the B6 background, was identified as a likely candidate for the increase in B-1 cells.[70] The lower expression of Cdkn2c was postulated to impair normal cell cycle arrest in B-1 but not B-2 cells because of inherent differences in their cell cycle regulation.

Two other loci already mentioned, Aem2 and Nba2, on chromosomes 7 and 1, respectively, were also confirmed in B6 congenic mice carrying the corresponding NZB locus.[26,66] However, only low levels of anti-RBC and incomplete penetrance were observed in the Aem2 congenic mice, and for the Nba2 congenic mice, detection of anti-RBC required the addition of the lupus-enhancing Yaa (Y-linked accelerated autoimmunity) mutation (see section on BXSB mice for information about Yaa). Nba2 can also promote other lupus traits, such as IgG ANAs and severe GN in F1 hybrids of B6.Nba2 crosses with other lupus strains, such as the NZW.[47] Further dissection of the Nba2 interval on chromosome 1 with a panel of subcongenic mice indicated at least two loci, one containing the SLAM (signaling lymphocyte activation molecule) family (see NZW genetics) and the other Fcγ receptors (FcγRs), that evidence now suggests additively contribute to autoimmunity.[71,72] The subcongenic containing Ifi202, a candidate for Nba2, however, was not associated with lupus traits.[43] Within the Fcγ interval, regulatory region variants of FcγRIIB that were associated with reduced expression were found in all major lupus-prone strains.[73,74] This finding is supported by studies showing that deficiency of FcγRIIB promotes autoimmune susceptibility[75] and further that the deficiency is related to the deficiency may result in failure to adequately block IgG anti-DNA plasma cell generation.[76]

NZB mice are among the inbred strains of mice deficient in C5 owing to deletion of two base pairs (TA, positions 62-63) that lack terminal complement activity.[77] Autoantibody-coated RBCs are therefore removed primarily by sequestration of agglutinated RBCs in the spleen and liver, through the use of Fc receptor–dependent phagocytosis, but not by complement-mediated hemolysis.[78]

Summary

In NZB mice, the combination of inherent B-cell hyperactivity, IgM hypergammaglobulinemia, high levels of BAFF, and thymic loss, in addition to expansion and activation of DCs in bone marrow, probably results in the abnormal shaping of T- and B-cell repertoires. NZB mice are characterized by a fatal hemolytic anemia that is induced by antierythrocyte antibodies. Other autoantibodies in their repertoire are predominantly IgM NTA, anti-ssDNA, and anti-gp70. Their dominant immunologic abnormalities are hyperactivated B cells from fetal life onward, early degeneration of thymic epithelium, and increased numbers of B-1 B cells that develop aneuploidy with age. These manifestations are controlled by multiple different genes. Sex differences are present but not marked.

New Zealand White Mice

The New Zealand white (NZW) mouse strain is of great interest because although it is clinically healthy, its genes can synergize with those of other lupus-prone and even normal strains to produce highly susceptible F1 hybrids or congenics.[11,53,59,61,79-94] Therefore, the NZW genome likely contains controlling, repressor, or epistatic genes that protect from SLE, and such controlling genes must be powerful enough to allow the animal to effectively resist disease.

Clinical Characteristics and Autoantibodies

The NZW mouse has a slightly shortened life span and develops largely nonpathogenic autoantibodies, some of which are only intermittently detectable. The autoantibody pattern is characterized primarily by IgG antibodies to ssDNA and histones.[86,95]

Genetics

Lupus-affecting loci have been mapped to 12 chromosomes using crosses of NZW to lupus-predisposed and normal strains or by interval congenic mice containing introgressed NZW loci.[53,86,96-101] Only a few have been further characterized, but they have provided significant insights. Of substantial interest because of its strong effect in human SLE is the MHC class II region, where NZW is H-2z and NZB is H-2d. Notably, BWF1 background mice expressing H-2d/z have a 30-fold greater risk of nephritis than H-2d/d mice.[100] This increased susceptibility has been linked to class switching of various autoantibodies from IgM to IgG[94] as well as antibodies to ssDNA, dsDNA, chromatin, and histones, but not to gp70.[81-83] Also, within the MHC region is a variant NZW tumor necrosis factor alpha (TNF-α) gene with a polymorphism in the 3′UT region associated with lower TNF levels.[84] Because of linkage disequilibrium within the MHC region, it has been difficult to separate the roles of class II and TNF; however, Fujimura and colleagues made three H-2 congenic BWF1 mice bearing distinct haplotypes at class II and TNF-α regions and showed that nephritis was affected by both the NZW MHC class II and the unique TNF-α allele.[102] Also, within the MHC region is another recessive locus, Sles1 (Sle suppressor 1), which reduced the incidence of severe nephritis in B6-Sle1/Sle3 bicongenic and B6-Sle1/Yaa+ lupus-susceptible mice by about 50%.[79,87,103] Thus, the MHC region of the NZW mice is rather complex with at least two lupus-promoting and one lupus-suppressing genetic variants.

Three other major NZW loci, Sle1, Sle2, and Sle3/5, on chromosomes 1, 4, and 7, respectively, have been studied in detail.[103] They were derived from the mixed NZW/NZB background NZM2410 strain but are entirely NZW in origin except for an NZB region covering the telomeric half of Sle2. Sle1 is situated on the distal half of chromosome 1,[85] overlapping with the NZB Nba2 locus, and contains many similar genetic variants. On the basis of panels of B6 subcongenic lines, Sle1 was subdivided into Sle1a, 1b, and 1c, and later these were further subdivided.[103] Sle1a consists of two subloci, Sle1a.1 and Sle1a.2, with hyperactivity in B cells, ANA, and antichromatin tracking with Sle1a.1, whereas both Sle1a.1 and Sle1a.2 are required for hyperproliferation in CD4+ T cells and defects in CD4+ regulatory T (Treg) cells.[86] Remarkably, the B6-Sle1a.1 subcongenic interval contains a single gene, Pbx1, a transcription factor in the TALE (three amino acid loop extension) family that participates in embryonic development and retinoic acid function.[104] SPbx1 has no coding region variation; however, a higher level of a Pbx1-d isoform has been detected, which studies suggest promotes T-cell activation and inhibits retinoic acid–mediated apoptosis. Increased Pbx1 was also detected in T cells from patients with SLE.

Sle1b, which has the strongest effect on autoimmunity, promotes breaking of tolerance to chromatin.[79,81] When NZW mice were compared with B6 mice, polymorphisms in the NZW (or NZM2410) involving at least 10 genes within the SLAM/CD2 gene cluster were identified,[105] including expansion of 2B4 from one to four copies; coding changes in LY9, CD48, and CD84; transcription level variation in Ly108, CS1, CD84, and CD48; and differences in the predominant isoform of Ly108.[106] Although dissecting the role of individual genes is difficult because of their close proximity, studies suggest that Ly108 is a major candidate that affects B- and T-cell tolerance and germinal center selection.[107,108] The SLAM/CD2 family participates in a wide range of immune activities that encompass humoral immunity, cell survival, lymphocyte development, and cell adhesion,[106,109] and it is likely that genetic variations promote autoimmunity by multiple mechanisms. The NZW Sle1b haplotype (haplotype 2) is present in most inbred and some wild strains, whereas the B6 haplotype 1 is found mainly in the C57BL-derived strains.[106] Accordingly, B6 mice congenic for the Sle1b interval from normal haplotype 2 mice also develop lupus-like disease, further confirming the significance of this haplotype and providing evidence for susceptibility genes in the B6 strain.[110]

The most distal Sle1c is also associated with three subloci, two of which enhance autoimmunity in a chronic graft-versus-host disease

(GVHD) model, and the third, which contains a variant complement receptor 2 (Cr2) gene, impairs humoral immune response and germinal center (GC) formation.[111,112]

The Sle2 locus on chromosome 4 promotes B-cell hyperactivity and B-1–cell expansion in B6.Sle2 congenic mice.[69] It consists of at least three subloci, Sle2a and 2b of NZW origin and the aforementioned Sle2c from the NZB. The NZW-derived loci increase lymphocyte expansion and renal disease, whereas Sle2c, as mentioned previously, is associated with the increase in B-1 B cells.[85] Sle2a also has been found to promote the loss of tolerance to DNA and alter splenic B-cell populations.[113] Another locus, Sle3/5, is associated with generalized T-cell activation—elevated CD4:CD8 ratios, expansion of CD4+ T cells, and reduced apoptosis—caused by defective DCs and an intrinsic T-cell abnormality.[114,115] Sle3/5, as its name implies, consists of two subloci, Sle3 and Sle5, that map to mid- and proximal chromosome 7, respectively.[115] Single congenic B6.Sle3 or B6.Sle5 mice do not develop systemic autoimmunity, but double congenic mice that combine either of these with Sle1 develop splenomegaly, activated lymphocytes, ANAs, and glomerular immune complex deposits. The additive contribution of these lupus-predisposing loci to overall disease development has been further illustrated by the finding that single–Sle locus congenic mice had no to minimal autoimmunity, but those with two Sle loci had intermediate severity that depended on the specific combination of loci, and triple congenic mice exhibited severe nephritis similar to that in the original NZM2410.[80,87]

In addition to the candidate genes associated with Sle loci, several other NZW variants that might modulate autoimmune susceptibility have been identified. The P2RX7 gene, within the Lbw3 region on chromosome 5, encodes the purinergic receptor P2X7, which initiates programmed cell death by aponecrosis, and NZW mice express the P2X-P allele associated with greater sensitivity to stimulation by adenosine triphosphate (ATP).[62,89] It has been postulated that this variant might promote lupus by enhancing programmed cell death and increasing the release of cellular autoantigens such as nucleosomes. NZW mice also have a unique deletion of the T-cell receptor (TCR) α/β-chain gene, encompassing the Db2-Jb2 region on chromosome 6, which in one study was shown to segregate with lupus; however, this finding was not confirmed.[57,58,92] In NZW mice, one of two murine Rt6 genes, Art2a-ps, on chromosome 7 is deleted.[91] Rt6, a member of the family of mono–adenosine diphosphate (ADP)–ribosyl transferases, is a T cell-restricted, glycoprotein I (GPI)–anchored membrane protein that is activated by apoptosis and participates in DNA repair. It was suggested that the lack of Rt6 might increase susceptibility to lupus; however, no immune defects are associated with this variant, and an association with autoimmunity has yet to be established. Another NZW candidate susceptibility gene is CD22, a B-cell adhesion molecule that modulates BCR-mediated signal transduction, located between the Sle3/5 loci on chromosome 7.[116] The NZW CD22a allele contains a 794-bp insertion in the second intron that causes altered splicing, the production of aberrant mRNA species, and reduced surface expression of the CD22 protein. Although it was not directly shown that this variant promotes lupus, heterozygous deficiency of CD22 was documented to markedly enhance the production of anti-DNA in Yaa+ mice.

(NZB/NZW) F1 Mice (BWF1)

The disease in BWF1 hybrid cross between NZB and NZW mice resembles human SLE in that disease is more severe and earlier in females, with high titers of IgG anti-dsDNA, antichromatin, ANAs, and LE cells occurring in virtually all; Treg- and B-cell networks fail, and death results from immune GN with tissue damage (Tables 17-1 to 17-3 and Box 17-2).[10,26] Involvement of the innate immune system, elevation of BAFF, and increased type-1 IFN–induced gene expression are similar to features in human lupus.[117-133] Both NZB and NZW parents contribute genetically to the immune abnormalities that cause disease, as discussed in the preceding sections. The B-cell hyperactivity characteristic of the NZB is inherited by the BWF1,

Characteristics of (NZB/NZW) F1 Mice

Clinical

1. Females live a mean of 280 days, males 439 days.
2. Death usually is caused by immune glomerulonephritis.
3. 50% mortality by 8 months in females and 15 months in males.

Histologic

1. Glomerulonephritis with proliferative changes in mesangial and endothelial cells of glomeruli, capillary basement membrane thickening, and chronic obliterative changes; mononuclear cell infiltrates in interstitium.
2. Glomerular immune deposits of IgG (predominantly IgG2a) and C3; similar deposits in tubular basement membrane and interstitium.
3. Thymic cortical atrophy by 6 months of age, including epithelial cell atrophy.
4. Myocardial infarcts with hyaline thickening of small arteries.
5. Mild lymph node hyperplasia and splenomegaly.

Autoantibodies

1. IgG anti-dsDNA (also binds single-stranded DNA), enriched in IgG2a and 2b.
2. Antinuclear antibody (ANA) and lupus erythematosus (LE) cells in all.
3. IgG antibodies bind chromatin, nucleosomes, and phospholipids.
4. Antithymocyte in most females and some males.
5. Renal eluates contain IgG anti-dsDNA concentrated 25 to 30 times greater than in serum; IgG2a isotype is dominant.
6. Modest elevations of circulating immune complexes; these include glycoprotein (gp) 70–anti-gp70.
7. Low serum complement levels by 6 months of age in females.

Immune Abnormalities

1. Polyclonal B-cell activation.
2. B cells are resistant to tolerance to some antigens.
3. Strict dependence on T-cell help for formation of pathogenic IgG anti-DNA, CD4+CD8−, and CD4−CD8− α/β TCR cells, as well as CD4−CD8− γ/δ TCR cells, can provide help.
4. IgG repertoire becomes restricted with age to certain public idiotypes; there is some restriction of B-cell clonality in the IgG anti-DNA response.
5. Clearance of immune complexes by Fc- and complement-mediated mechanisms is defective.
6. Disease and autoantibody production are sensitive to sex hormone influences.

Genetics

1. The expression of high-titer IgG anti-dsDNA requires heterozygosity at the major histocompatibility complex, namely, H-2(d/z).
2. Additional complementary non–H-2-linked genes are required from both NZB and NZW parents to permit full expression of the IgG anti-DNA response. By microsatellite analysis of DNA, there are approximately 10 genes on as many chromosomes, with multiple genes required for early mortality, glomerulonephritis, antichromatin, and splenomegaly; this suggests a multigenic inheritance, with certain groupings predisposing more strongly than others to disease, rather than a simple additive model. NZW also provides a resistance gene.
3. The large deletion in the β chain of the TCR of the NZW parent probably does not predispose to disease.

dsDNA, double-stranded DNA; Ig, immunoglobulin; TCR, T-cell receptor.

with abnormally high secretion of Ig being detectable by 1 month of age.[11] However, the T-cell dependence of the response is more striking than in the NZB parent and is responsible for the isotype shift from IgM anti-DNA to IgG anti-DNA that precedes clinical disease.[134]

Clinical Characteristics and Autoantibodies

Large quantities of IgG antibodies that bind nucleosomes, chromatin, dsDNA, and ssDNA in BWF1 mice are striking and can be abrogated by removal or inactivation of CD4+ T cells.[94,135] IgG antibodies to dsDNA contain subsets that cause nephritis. Transfer of selected monoclonal BWF1 IgG2 anti-dsDNA antibodies to normal BALB/c mice induces nephritis.[136,137] Infusion of anti-DNA into rodent kidneys induces proteinuria,[138] and normal mice secreting BWF1 IgG anti-dsDNA (encoded by transgenes) develop GN.[139] Anti-DNA, antinucleosome antibody, and immune complexes containing gp70 and anti-gp70s all contribute to nephritis.[140,141] ANAs are detectable in most 3-month-old females; they include antibodies that bind subnucleosomes, nucleosomes, chromatin, dsDNA, ssDNA, dsRNA, transfer RNA (tRNA), polynucleotides, and histones.[134-141] IgM anti-DNAs arise first; by 6 months of age, IgG anti-DNAs appear.[10,134] The IgG 2a and 2b subclasses are most common; these subclasses fix complement and bind FcγRs. Antibodies to erythrocytes are found in 35% to 78% of BWF1 females but rarely cause hemolytic anemia. Approximately 50% of females develop NTAs by 6 months of age. Because the genes governing NTA, anti-DNA, and antierythrocyte antibodies probably segregate separately,* New Zealand mouse strains have been bred that have high-titer NTAs but no autoimmune disease. However, NTAs, by altering T cell functions, may serve as accelerators of the disease process that occurs in mice with IgG anti-DNA. Both IgM and IgG antiphospholipid antibodies have been detected and obtained as monoclonal antibodies from BWF1 mice.[150] Some have anticardiolipin (aCL) activity, and others lupus anticoagulant properties. However, clotting disorders are not characteristic of BWF1 mice. Antibodies to ubiquitin and fibrillarin have been reported, as have cryoglobulins.[151-153]

Nephritis in BWF1 Females: the Autoantibodies, the Infiltrating Cells, and the Predisposing Glomerular Structures

Shortly after the switch from IgM to IgG, IgG and complement deposit in the mesangia of BWF1 glomeruli, spreading later to capillary loops and interstitial tubular regions.[10] Proteinuria appears between 5 and 7 months of age; azotemia followed by death occurs in females at 6 to 12 months of age. Approximately half of females are dead by 8.5 months and 90% at 12 months.[10,136]

Antibodies eluted from BWF1 glomeruli are composed predominantly of IgG anti-DNA/antinucleosome antibody (anti-NUC); 50% of the total IgG is anti-DNA according to some reports.[154,155] In our laboratory, anti-DNA accounts for as much as 85% of the total glomerular IgG.[156] IgG2a is the dominant isotype in glomerular deposits, suggesting a role for Th1 cells, because production of IgG2a depends on IFN-γ. Immune complexes containing gp70/anti-gp70 are also found in glomeruli of BWF1 mice. Gp70 is an endogenous retroviral glycoprotein produced by hepatic cells that is found in all mouse strains but is quantitatively higher in some, including the main lupus-prone strains.[157] Among the IgG anti-dsDNA antibodies made by BWF1 mice are subsets that cause nephritis by (1) passive trapping of immune complexes containing them, (2) direct attachment to planted (e.g., chromatin/nucleosomes/DNA) or cross-reactive (e.g., laminin) glomerular and tubular antigens, and (3) cationic charge, which binds to anionic glomerular areas.[141,156] For gp70/anti-gp70 immune complexes, passive trapping is probably the major mechanism. NZB chromosome regions Nba2 (on chromosome 1; contains the *Ifi202* gene) and H2 (on chromosome 17) are linked both to high levels of gp70/anti-gp70 immune complex production and to high titers of IgG anti-DNA.[142] Plasma cells making antibodies to dsDNA and to histone 2B are found in renal tissue of BWF1 mice as well as

*References 11, 52, 54, 79-88, 100, 142-149.

in their bone marrow and spleens,[158,159] so local synthesis of nephritogenic antibodies occurs. Regarding the role of anti-dsDNA/NUC in BWF1 nephritis, the availability of apoptotic chromatin planted in glomerular membrane is important in pathogenicity.[160] Furthermore, BWF1 mice have lower levels of renal DNAse1 after the development of nephritis; thus nucleosomal DNA fragmentation during apoptosis is decreased in kidney tissue, and partial fragmentation may induce more production and binding of anti-DNA/NUC.[161] In support of this idea, one study has reported that administration of heparin to BWF1 mice increased enzymatic degradation of nucleosomes, inhibited their binding to laminin and collagen, reduced glomerular deposition of IgG, and delayed development of nephritis.[162] Various epitopes in chromatin can be targeted by autoantibodies: some antibodies against apoptotic chromatin recognize acetylated epitopes.[163] Epigenetic changes in DNA, including acetylation and methylation, are controlled in part by microRNA; at least three dysregulated miRNAs have been found in splenocytes of BWF1 mice at the onset of nephritis.[164] Finally, some BWF1 antibodies to DNA/NUC can bind to and/or penetrate living cells; some induce proliferation of glomerular cells and impair intracellular production of protein.[165-167]

Other antigens and antibodies have been reported in glomerular eluates, including antihistones, anti-C1q, and anti-RNA polymerase.[168,169] Hypocomplementemia occurs concomitantly with high serum levels of IgG anti-DNA.[10]

Histologic changes in kidneys include chronic obliterative changes in glomeruli, mesangial and peripheral proliferative changes, capillary membrane thickening, glomerular sclerosis, tubular atrophy, infiltration by mononuclear lymphocytes and monocyte/macrophages, and vasculopathy (primarily degenerative, occasionally inflammatory) (Figure 17-1).[10,26] Some studies suggest that after deposition of complement-fixing IgG in glomeruli, the next local

abnormality is upregulation of genes associated with macrophage activation,[120,170] followed later by upregulation of genes characteristic of T and B cells. Successful treatment of nephritis is associated with downregulation of the initial macrophage signature.[118,120] These tissue macrophages derive from peripheral blood GR1^{lo} monocytes.[117] At the beginning of nephritis, the renal F4/80^{hi}Cd11c^{int} macrophages upregulate cell surface CD11b, acquire cathepsin and matrix metalloproteinase activity, accumulate autophagocytic vacuoles, and upregulate expression of proinflammatory and tissue repair/degradation genes.[171] In contrast, dendritic cells (F4/80^{lo}CD11c^{hi}) appear in kidneys later, after proteinuria onset, and disappear more rapidly after treatment.[117] Renal infiltration of T and B lymphocytes that follows glomerular/tubular innate cell infiltration is associated with upregulation of MHC class II on T cells and secretion of IFN-γ.[120] Inhibition of macrophage migration inhibitory factor (which promotes retention of monocytes in tissue via the CD74 receptor) reduces leukocyte accumulation and expression of proinflammatory cytokines and chemokines in renal tissue of BWF1 mice.[172] Additional evidence for the crucial role of monocytes/macrophages in BWF1 nephritis are the observations that renal inflammation after Ig deposition is abrogated by knocking out activating gamma globulin FcRs in infiltrating monocytes/macrophages but not by impairing FcRs on mesangial cells.[170] Apart from infiltrating inflammatory cells, glomeruli in BWF1 mice differ from nonautoimmune mice in ways that may promote glomerular disease. Embryonic forms of collagen IVα chains are more abundant than in normal strains,[173] and IL-20 (in the IL-10 family) and C-IVα receptors are upregulated in mesangial cells. Activation of these receptors upregulates expression of the chemokines/receptors monocyte chemoattractant protein-1 (MCP-1) and RANTES (regulated upon activation, normal T-cell expressed, and secreted) as well as mediators of oxidative damage inducible

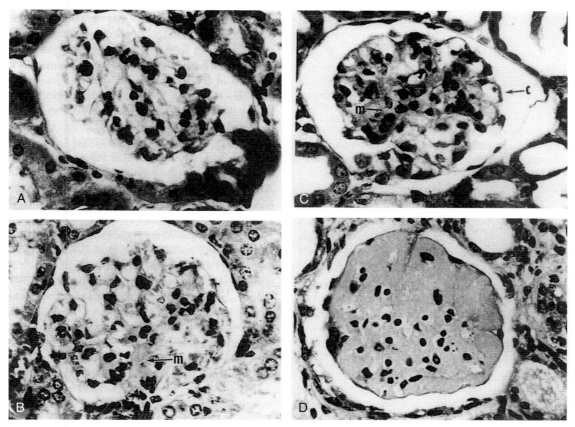

FIGURE 17-1 Glomerulonephritis in New Zealand mice. Panel A is a sample from a NZW mouse. Other panels are from BWF1 mice. **A,** Normal mouse glomerulus. **B,** Mesangial proliferation and thickening (m). **C,** Proliferative glomerulonephritis with thickened glomerular capillaries (c). **D,** End-stage glomerulopathy; the glomerulus is obliterated.

nitric oxide synthase (iNOS) and reactive oxygen species (ROS).[174] BWF1 mice are also prone to chronic nephritis because their renal tissue expresses high levels of the inflammatory chemokine CXCL13/ BCL, which attracts leukocytes into interstitial areas.[172] Upregulation of the canonical Wnt/beta-catenin pathway is also a characteristic in BWF1 renal tissue as nephritis develops, paralleled in renal tissue and serum by increase in the Wnt inhibitor Dkk-1.[175] Dkk-1 at these high levels can induce apoptosis in mesangial and renal tubular cells—an additional factor contributing to tissue damage. In summary, a combination of multiple hematopoietic cells attracted into renal tissue after deposition of autoreactive Ig and activation of complement mediate acute and chronic renal disease in BWF1 mice, and the renal tissue itself differs from that of non-lupus strains in ways that make the tissue more susceptible to damage.

Neurologic Tissue

IgG1 antibodies have been eluted from the neurons of BWF1 mice[176]; it is not known whether they cross-react extensively with lymphocytes, as do some human lupus antineuronal antibodies. BWF1 mice exhibit anxiety-like behavior and have inflammatory infiltrates and deposition of IgG and C3 in hippocampi.[177]

Lymphoproliferation

The lymphoproliferative features of NZB mice occur in BWF1 hybrids, which exhibit mild lymphadenopathy and splenomegaly.[10] Lymphoid neoplasia is far less common in BWF1 than in NZB mice. Some investigators have reported a relatively high incidence of thymoma, from 1% to 5%,[178] but that has been rare in our colonies unless mice are treated with cytotoxic agents.[179] Extrarenal lesions occur in BWF1 mice, including lymphocytic infiltration of salivary glands, mild inflammation around bile ducts in the liver, pancarditis, vasculitis (less common than in MRL-Fas[lpr] and BXSB mice), myocardial infarcts, and deposits of DNA and anti-DNA in the dermo-epidermal junction of skin and in the choroid plexus.[10,180]

Sex Hormone Influences on Lupus in BWF1 Mice

Female BWF1 mice have earlier and more severe autoimmune disease than males. Most BWF1 males develop ANAs, including antibodies to DNA, but the switch from IgM to IgG occurs late in life, usually after 12 months. Histologic evidence of nephritis can be found in males, and most die of slowly progressive chronic nephritis by 15 to 20 months of age.[10]

The BWF1 mouse is particularly sensitive to the effects of sex hormones on disease. In general, androgens are protective and suppress the expression of autoantibodies and disease, and estrogens are permissive.[181-186] Males that are castrated and/or treated with estrogens or testosterone antagonists assume a female pattern: early IgM-to-IgG switch of anti-DNA antibodies and early, fatal nephritis. Females that are treated with castration and androgens, or antiestrogens, have prolonged survival, with suppression of IgG anti-DNA and nephritis.[181,185,187] Administration of ethinylestradiol to BWF1 mice accelerates disease.[182] In old females, androgens can suppress disease without altering the elevations of IgG anti-DNA.[181] Female and male BWF1 mice deficient for estrogen receptor alpha (ERα) have lower blood levels of IgG anti-dsDNA and IFN-γ than ERα-intact controls, and increased survival.[185] In addition, expression of several sex hormone–regulated genes in antigen-presenting splenocytes is different in female and male BWF1 mice.[188] Prolactin also influences BWF1 disease: administration of prolactin accelerates disease, whereas bromocriptine suppresses it.[189-191] Continuous treatment of premorbid BWF1 females with high doses of depot medroxyprogesterone acetate reduces IgG2a deposition in glomeruli, histologic glomerular damage, proteinuria, and mortality.[192] These benefits may relate to the ability of progesterone to suppress activation of plasmacytoid DCs (pDCs) and their production of IFN-α, whereas 7beta-estradiol (E2) can increase pDC activation and cytokine production, depending on the age of the BWF1 mouse at the time of treatment.[193]

There are receptors for estrogens, progestogens, and prolactin on lymphocytes and natural killer (NK) cells.[191,194] The administration of estradiol in vivo dramatically suppresses NK cell function, and NK cells downregulate activated B cells.[194] In addition, normal mice transgenic for a murine IgG antibody to DNA show defective B-cell tolerance if they are treated with exogenous estradiol.[195] Such mice fail to delete B cells that are producing anti-DNA from unmutated germline genes; this failure of negative selection is particularly marked at the transitional cell type 1/type 2 selection checkpoint.[196] Data now suggest that estradiol is linked to SLE in part via effects on type 1 IFN pathways. For example, female BWF1 mice have higher expression of Irf5 mRNA (Irf5 is a molecule in the pathway of plasmacytoid dendritic cell activation that results in type 1 IFN production) than both BWF1 males and normal mice; and those levels are reduced in ERα$^{-/-}$ mice.[131] Activation of spleen cells by IFN (either α or γ) upregulates expression of ERα, and both IFN-α– and ERα–responsive genes are upregulated in BWF1 females.[128,197] In vivo treatment of castrated BWF1 males with 17β-estradiol increases steady-state levels of *Ifi202* mRNA in splenic cells (*Ifi202* is an interferon-inducible gene); dihydrotestosterone decreases those levels. In contrast, *Ifi202* mRNA levels are not detectable in female BWF1 mice that were Esrα$^{-/-}$. Thus, female and male hormones differentially regulate the expression of some IFN-inducible genes, including *Ifi202*, which has been suggested to be a susceptibility gene for murine lupus.[198]

Interferons and SLE in BWF1 Mice

High levels of IFN-γ in plasma and lymphoid tissues are characteristic of BWF1 mice. IFN-γ is a major cytokine produced by Th1 cells, which provide help to B cells. The high IFN-γ levels may relate to low levels of the negative regulator suppressor of cytokine signaling 1 (SOCS-1).[199] Elevated genetic signatures associated with type 1 IFN (e.g., IFN-α) are also characteristic of BWF1 mice, similar to those in human SLE.[133] Enhanced expression of IFN-α (by infection of their cells with DNA encoding IFN-α) increases short-lived plasma cells in healthy and BWF1 mice, but only the BWF1 mice make autoantibodies and develop accelerated lupus[129]; this acceleration requires CD4+ T-cell help.[130] Conversely, inhibition of IFN-α by inhibitory antibodies induced by vaccination with an IFN-α kinoid protect mice from severe nephritis.[132]

Abnormalities of Hematopoietic Cells in BWF1 Mice

BWF1 mice exhibit the hyperactivated B-cell phenotype of their NZB parent, except that defects appear later with abnormally elevated IgM occurring by 1 month of age. Pre-B lineage cells can partially transfer disease: severe combined immunodeficiency disease (SCID) mice (a mutant strain that lacks most T cells) inoculated with BWF1 bone marrow pre-B cells develop autoantibodies (including IgG anti-dsDNA) and, in approximately 25%, clinical nephritis.[200] Thus, BWF1 B cells alone can induce lupus-like disease, albeit less globally than in the presence of T-cell help; the B-cell repertoire that expresses anti-DNA is also somewhat restricted. In this regard, public idiotypes (Ids) that are expressed on total serum IgG become increasingly restricted as the mice age.[201] Although many different V genes can be used to assemble antibodies that bind DNA,[202] most BWF1 anti-DNA monoclonal antibodies belong to one of approximately 12 families.[203-205] This type of restriction is seen in normal, antigen-driven antibody responses. In BWF1 mice, B-1 B cells and MZ B cells are increased in number. Depleting some of these cells by administering a B-cell superantigen (protein A from *Staphylococcus aureus*) delays appearance of serum IgG anti-DNA and reduces proteinuria, further suggesting participation of these cells in autoimmunity in this strain.[206] Depleting mature B2 cells (MZ) plus peritoneal B1 cells can be achieved by repeated doses of anti-mouse CD20 plus a BR3-Fc fusion protein (which blocks BAFF): These treatments delay disease in young mice and prolong life in old nephritic mice without reducing autoantibody levels.[207] Murine B cells from spleen, bone marrow, and peritoneum can express BAFF when activated via innate immune pathways; in BWF1 mice, splenic MZ and germinal center B-cell populations express high levels of BAFF,[127] indicating their continued activation.

Abnormalities of Thymus and T Cells

The characteristic degeneration of thymic epithelial cells seen in NZB mice at 1 month of age also occurs in BWF1 mice, but at 6 months.[11] Responses to thymectomy have been variable; there are reports of thymectomy failing to alter disease or even accelerating it.[46] Full-blown BWF1 lupus depends on the presence of CD4+ Th cells; T-cell lines from nephritic mice can accelerate disease in naive young syngeneic mice.[208,209] Elimination or inactivation of CD4+ T cells prevents the onset of disease and can even partially reverse established nephritis.[135,210] As BWF1 mice age, the numbers of CD4+ T cells increase fivefold, and these cells are polyclonal.[211,212] T cells from nephritic BWF1 mice can drive B cells from young normal mice to make pathogenic autoantibodies,[208,209] but T cells from young mice do not have this property. Several T-cell subsets influence BWF1 disease. These include Th1 cells (require IL-12 for development; secrete IFN-γ; mediate cell-mediated immunity; express Tbet transcription factor), Th2 cells (require IL-4 for development; support B-cell production of autoantibodies; express transcription factor GATA3), Th17 cells (require transforming growth factor beta [TGF-β] plus IL-6 plus IL-2 for development; secrete proinflammatory IL-17, which attracts neutrophils; require IL-21 for maintenance; help B cells make autoantibodies; express the protein RORγT), and Treg cells (CD4+CD25+; require TGF-β plus IL-2 for development; may secrete TGF-β or IL-10; downregulate CD4+ Th cells and autoreactive B cells by contact; express the protein FoxP3). Another major Th cell promoting IgG autoantibody formation is located in lymphoid follicles: these follicular CD4+ Th (T$_{FH}$) cells stimulate GC B cells to produce autoantibodies via interactions between inducible T-cell co-stimulator) ICOS and its ligand, B7-related protein 1 (B7RP-1). Interrupting second signals between these T cells and B cells alters BWF1 disease.[212,213] In addition, blockade of the CD28/cytotoxic T-lymphocyte antigen 4 (CTLA-4) T-cell surface molecule's interactions with CD80/CD86 (also called B7-1/B7-2) on APCs prevents disease. Experiments showing this include the administration of CTLA-4–Ig, which binds to CD80 and CD86, thus preventing interaction with CD28,[214] and the administration of antibodies to CD80 and CD86.[215] In addition, blocking second signals that activate B cells (CD40 interacting with CD40 ligand [CD40L]) by administration of antibody to CD40L prolongs survival in BWF1 and other New Zealand–background lupus mice.[216,217] Blocking both CD28/B7 and CD40/CD40L interactions is probably more effective than blocking either one alone.[218] This multiple-blockade strategy was used in one study to reverse nephritis in BWF1 mice, along with doses of cyclophosphamide, but disease recurred when the therapies were stopped.[120] Enhancing proinflammatory T-cell function by administration of IL-6 accelerates disease, and antibodies to IL-6 delay it.[219] Administration of anti–IL-10, which also suppresses IL-6, delays disease in BWF1 mice.[220]

TGF-β is essential for the suppression by some CD4+CD25+ Treg cells[221] and by CD8+ T cells,[222] which delay autoimmunity in BWF1 mice tolerized with histone or Ig peptides; a similar process protects healthy mice from autoimmunity.[223] However, late in disease TGF-β contributes to glomerular scarring and thus to shortened survival.[1] IL-1 and TNF-α are both proinflammatory and may be abnormally elevated in BWF1 lupus.[224] The role of TNF-α in murine and human lupus has been debated for several years. In support of its role, NZW mice have a variant gene that encodes lower levels of TNF-α, and short-term administration of TNF-α to BWF1 mice delays disease.[225] However, long-term administration of the cytokine worsens disease.[226]

Abnormalities of Monocytes/Macrophages

Monocytes/macrophages are primary sources of IL-1, production of which is reduced in BWF1 and other murine lupus strains.[227] Macrophages also produce IL-12, the major cytokine stimulating Th1

responses. The ability of C-reactive protein (CRP) treatment to delay disease onset in BWF1 mice may relate to the fact that CRP reduces IL-12 production by macrophages following ingestion of apoptotic materials; those macrophages have reduced ability to activate T cells.[228-231] Monocytes that differentiate into macrophages in renal tissue (and possibly others that express activating FcR) seem to govern the inflammatory response to Ig deposition and complement activation in BWF1 kidneys; those cells are discussed in the previous section on nephritis.[120,170] BWF1 monocytes and dendritic cells exposed to apoptotic cells can activate Th cells in BWF1 mice, consistent with the presentation of autoantigens by APCs, but the T-cell responses are more vigorous in lupus-prone mice than in normal mice.[232]

The Role of Defective Regulatory Cells in BWF1 Lupus (CD4+CD25+, CD8+, NK T Cells, B-1 B Cells)

Finally, there is strong evidence that numbers and functions of regulatory cells that ordinarily suppress activated T and/or B cells are defective in BWF1 F1 mice. As the mice age, CD8+ cytotoxic/suppressive T cells fail to expand, whereas CD4+ T and B cells are increasing greatly in numbers, and very few CD8+ cells express surface markers of activation and memory. Furthermore, stimulation of CD8+ T cells from old BWF1 mice results in apoptosis rather than activation.[212] Tolerizing regimens with autoantibody- or histone-derived peptides induce both suppressive CD8+ T cells and classic CD4+CD25+ Treg cells, each of which can prolong survival in BWF1 or (NZB/SWR) F1 mice, indicating that Treg-cell defects can be "repaired" in vivo.[221-233] The regulatory capacity of CD8+ T cells depends on their expression of Foxp3 and of programmed death 1 (PD-1), a member of the CTLA-4 family that helps determine whether a CD8+ T cell has suppressive capabilities.[234] Regulatory B cells have also been described; these cells (called B-10 cells) in mice are CD1d^{hi}CD5+ B cells (B-1 cells) that secrete IL-10. B-10 B cells expand as disease develops in BWF1 but are not able to overcome the effects of hyperactivated autoantibody-producing plasma cells.[235] CD1-restricted NK T cells prevent the development of autoimmune manifestations if activated in early stages of disease in BWF1 (nephritis), pristane-injected BALB/c (nephritis), and MRL-lpr (dermatitis) mice,[1,4] but not in late stages of disease in BWF1 or pristane-injected SJL mice.[236,237] As BWF1 mice age, NK T cells expand in number and become hyperactive; they can actually increase production of IFN-γ—a major cytokine that, as noted previously, enhances SLE in this strain.[238]

Abnormalities of Dendritic Cells in BWF1 Mice

DCs, which connect innate and acquired immunity, can be activated by RNA and/or DNA produced by viruses and bacteria and by patients with SLE, in complex with antibodies to nucleoproteins. As BWF1 mice age, DCs expand in number and acquire the ability to attract B cells and to present antigen.[239] This activity is particularly brisk in the spleen, where DCs stimulate nucleosome-reactive T cells to a much greater extent than normal,[240] promoting induction of autoantibodies to apoptotic materials.[241] Furthermore, pDCs are a major source of type 1 IFNs. High production of these IFNs is characteristic of BWF1 mice and of humans with SLE.[6] Deficiency of the type I IFN receptor protects NZB mice from disease,[242] and administration of IFN-α accelerates it.[243] Therefore, abnormal DCs and their production of IFN-α play a critical role in promoting lupus-like disease in BWF1 mice.

Genetic Predisposition

Genetic predisposition is reviewed in the preceding sections on NZB and NZW mice. In BWF1 mice, genetic contributions to disease are provided by both NZB and NZW parents. Although in F1 hybrids these must be dominantly transmitted, most loci identified in mapping and congenic studies of NZB and NZW loci exhibit additive inheritance. The most important contributors are the MHC genes (heterozygosity for H-2 d/z) and loci on chromosome 4 (Lbw2, Nba1) that were shown to directly affect autoimmunity in BWF1 mice.[6,43]

Likely of major importance are genes on chromosome 1 from the NZB (Nba2) and NZW (Sle1) and chromosome 7 from the NZW (Sle3/5). In addition, multiple non-MHC genes on at least eight different chromosomes contribute to disease susceptibility.[56-72,74-81,83-88]

Summary

BWF1 mice develop fatal GN, mediated primarily by IgG antibodies to dsDNA, chromatin, and nucleosomes, with participation of immune complexes of gp70 and anti-gp70. Disease occurs earlier and is more severe in females and can be modulated by sex hormones. Nephritis is mediated initially by deposition of autoantibodies and complement activation products in glomeruli. Monocytes/macrophages that infiltrate renal tissue are probably crucial in establishing acute and chronic injury, although DCs and T, B, and plasma cells that follow also participate in the disease. Multiple genes inherited from both NZB and NZW parents, both MHC and non-MHC, are required for the development of high-titer IgG anti-dsDNA and clinical nephritis. Abnormalities in B-1 and MZ B cells, in CD4$^+$ Th cells and CD4$^+$CD25$^+$ Treg cells, in CD8$^+$ and NK T suppressor cells, and in DCs are all required for the disease to be fully manifest.

(SWR × NZB) F1 (SNF1) Mice

The SNF1 mouse is a model of lupus nephritis that is produced by mating the normal Swiss Webster (SWR) mouse with the autoimmune NZB mouse (Box 17-3).[244-246] In contrast to NZW mice that mated with NZB to produce the BWF1 strain, SWR mice are completely healthy, with normal life spans, low levels of serum gp70, and no evidence of autoimmune disease.[244] Their B cells can produce Igs bearing the same public Ids that dominate serum Ig in MRL-Fas(lpr) mice.[247,248]

Clinical Characteristics and Autoantibodies

SNF1 mice are similar to BWF1 mice. Females typically succumb by 10 to 12 months of age (50% mortality at 6 months) from an immune GN mediated primarily by IgG2b complement-fixing antibodies to

---

Box 17-3 Characteristics of NZB X SWR F1 (SNF1) Mice

Clinical
1. Mean survival in females is 297 days; mean survival in males is 531 days.
2. Females die from immune glomerulonephritis between 5 and 13 months of age.

Histologic
1. Glomerulonephritis with proliferative and obliterative lesions.

Autoantibodies
1. IgG anti-dsDNA is made by all females.
2. Anti-dsDNA is dominated by IgG2b cationic populations with restricted idiotypes.
3. ANAs in all females.

Immune Abnormalities
1. B cells are hyperactivated.
2. The development of nephritis depends on the presence of T-cell help for production of IgG anti-DNA.
3. Cationic IgG anti-dsDNA may use the allotype of either the NZB or healthy SWR parent.
4. Anti-dsDNA deposited in glomeruli cluster into two main groups defined by their idiotypes.
5. CD4$^+$D8$^-$ and CD4$^-$CD8$^-$ T cells can provide help for the synthesis of cationic IgG anti-dsDNA.

Genetics
1. Probably similar to genetics of BWF1 mice.

dsDNA, double-stranded DNA; Ig, immunoglobulin.

---

dsDNA.[245,249] Activated B cells of NZB mice make anti-DNAs that are predominantly IgM, bind ssDNA rather than dsDNA, and are anionic in charge.[249] In contrast, B cells of SNF1 mice make predominantly cationic IgG2b anti-dsDNA. Such positively charged antibodies (or antigens or immune complexes), also found in BWF1 mice, probably contribute to the initiation of nephritis by binding to polyanions in glomerular basement membranes.[141,156] The presumed pathogenic IgG2b cationic anti-dsDNAs are also restricted in Id expression. The IgG in the glomeruli of SNF1 mice can be grouped into two families of Ids.[249] The first, Id564, is composed entirely of cationic IgG, and most members bear the Igh allotype of the SWR parent. The second Id cluster, Id512, contains Ig of anionic, neutral, and cationic charges; the allotypes expressed are both SWR and NZB derived. Id564 is unique to SNF1 mice and absent in either parent. Sequence data show that the expression of Id564 depends on the heavy chain variable (V$_H$) region of the Ig molecule; Id564$^+$ monoclonal antibodies are closely related structurally and probably derive from a germline gene unique to the SNF1 mouse.[247] SNF1 mice also make antibodies to histones, with some clonal restriction and somatic mutation, like most autoantibodies in the mouse models.[250]

Abnormalities in Stem Cells and B Cells

The interesting features of this model include the demonstration that a nephritogenic anti-DNA subset can be constructed from the allotype of a normal parent given the appropriate additional genetic background. Idiotypic connectivity between B and T cells has also been particularly well described.[246-251] IdLNF$^+$ Ig does not contain much antibody to DNA, but nephritis and early death correlate with high serum levels of IdLNF$^+$ Ig and glomerular deposits of the Id, thus illustrating the role of non–DNA-binding Ig in the glomerular disease. Suppression of IdLNF$^+$ Ig by the administration of a specific anti-Id does not downregulate serum levels of IgG anti-DNA, but nephritis is delayed and survival prolonged.[252]

Abnormalities in T Cells

Studies suggest that the T-cell abnormalities of BWF1 mice are reiterated in the SNF1 model. B cells from SNF1 spleens (or BWF1 spleens) secrete IgG anti-dsDNA only when they are stimulated by T cells in culture.[253] Those T cells may bear the classic CD4$^+$D8$^-$ phenotype of Th cells, or they may be CD4$^-$CD8$^-$.

As mice age, their CD4$^+$, IdLNF$^+$-specific repertoire expands greatly. There is little TCR restriction in the expanding CD4$^+$ cells. Transfer of a few T-cell clones that are specific for the Id increase the Id$^+$ Ig production in young SNF1 mice.[251] Some of the T cells that help anti-DNA production recognize peptides in the histones found in nucleosomes[254]; autoantibody production and disease can be dramatically delayed by administration of some of those peptides in very small quantities.[221] Another example of the critical importance of T cells in this model are studies inducing immune tolerance by oral administration of anti-CD3.[255] As with other tolerance strategies in lupus mice, this treatment induces Treg cells; in this case the Tregs can suppress IL17$^+$CD4$^+$ICOS$^-$CXCR5$^+$ T$_{FH}$ cells, along with memory B cells and plasma cells. Pathogenic T cells can also be suppressed in SNF1 mice by administration of a flavonoid (apigenin), which increases apoptosis in APCs and T and B cells by inhibiting the antiapoptotic molecules COX-1 and c-FLIP.[256]

Genetics

As in the BWF1 mouse, genes contributed from both parents are necessary for disease in the SNF1 with genes from loci on chromosomes 1, 14, and 18 from the SWR identified in a (SWR×NZB) F2 mapping study.[61] Some genes clearly are linked to H-2. In fact, heterozygosity at H-2 correlates strongly with GN; the MHC alleles seemed to confer susceptibility independently and are additive.

Summary

The SNF1 mouse is another example of female-dominant, T cell–dependent lupus nephritis in a hybrid mouse with an NZB background. The nature of the antibodies that deposit in glomeruli has been particularly well studied and is somewhat oligoclonal, thus providing important information about the characteristics and genetic control of pathogenic subsets of autoantibodies.

Additional NZB hybrids that show female predominance of disease that can be influenced by treatment with sex hormones include (NZB×SJL) F1 (NS) mice.[257-259]

New Zealand Mixed Mice

In 1993, Rudofsky and colleagues performed selective inbreeding of the progeny of one cross between NZB and NZW mice, selecting for severity of nephritis and coat colors.[260] They reported 27 new strains and studied 12 for extent of NZB and NZW genes and lupus-like disease. Most New Zealand mixed (NZM) strains had IgG anti-dsDNA antibodies. However, the incidence of nephritis was variable, ranging from severe to absent. Females were more susceptible in some strains, whereas in others males were also affected. These initial studies showed that there is not a strict requirement for H-2d/z (MHC) heterozygosity (as in BWF1 mice) to develop nephritis, but such heterozygosity increases susceptibility. The best characterized of the NZM strains is the NZM/Aeg2410 (NZM2410), for which studies have revealed additive and epistatic polygenic inheritance of lupus, multiple subloci within initially mapped regions, and identification of several candidate genes (reviewed in reference 261). This model is similar to the BWF1, with anti-DNA and nephritis, but exhibits equal nephritis severity in males and females.

Another NZM strain, NZM2328, develops autoantibodies and severe GN that occurs in two phases—acute and chronic with glomerular sclerosis and tubular atrophy, and has female predominance similar to BWF1 and human SLE.[98] Genome-wide mapping of (NZM2328×C57L/J) F1×NZM2328 backcrosses identified loci on chromosome 1 (Cgnz1 linked to chronic and Agnz1 to acute GN) and suggestive loci on chromosomes 4 (Adnz1) and 17.[98] Cgnz1 and Adnz1 were verified with replacement of the corresponding NZM2328 chromosome 1 and 4 regions with normal C57L genome. The congenic NZM.C57Lc1 mice with the substituted C57L chromosome 1 had reduced autoantibodies and GN; interestingly, NZM.C57Lc4 had no ANAs but yet developed severe chronic GN. The latter finding clearly documented the presence of independent genetic influences on ANAs and chronic GN. It suggests that development of chronic renal changes has genetic controls that determine whether initial glomerular injury either heals or progresses to end-stage renal disease.

Further, in NZM2328 mice, adoptive transfer of CD4+CD25+ Treg cells suppresses anti-DNA antibody production but does not influence the development of chronic GN.[98] Treg cells may be important in acute nephritis; male NZM2328 mice that normally do not develop GN experience an acute GN after day 3 thymectomy but the disease does not progress to chronic GN.

Compared with MRL-lpr and BWF1 mice, NZM2410 mice develop an accelerated onset of chronic glomerulosclerosis that can be suppressed by in vivo blockade of IL-4 by monoclonal antibody treatment or by genetic deletion of Stat6, a transcription factor that mediates response to type 2 cytokines such as IL-4.[262] In fact, levels of IL-4 are markedly elevated in NZM.2410 mice. Germline deletion of Stat6 in NZM2328 mice has a similar ameliorating effect on glomerulosclerosis.[263] Strikingly, antibody blockade or Stat6 deletion has no effect on IgG anti-dsDNA antibody levels and on renal IgG deposition in NZM2410 and NZM2328 strains. Thus, IL-4 effects on lupus nephritis in NZM2410 and NZM2328 models appear to be independent of IL-4 effects on autoantibody production. On the other hand, the germline deletion of signal transducer and activator of transcription 4 (STAT4), a transcription factor for type 1 cytokines, suppresses anti-dsDNA antibody production but does not reduce the incidence of GN in these models.[262,263]

These observations suggest that anti-DNA autoantibody production and development of acute or chronic GN are all uncoupled in some models, raising the question of the direct cause-and-effect

relationships between the presence of autoantibodies and lupus nephritis in at least some of the NZM strains.

See previous discussion of genetics in NZB and NZW mice for more details on genetic information obtained from NZM mice.

MRL/MP (Mrl+/+) and MRL-Fas(lpr) Mice

The Murphy Roths Large/lymphoproliferation MRL-Fas(lpr) strain and the congenic MRL/Mp (MRL/+/+) (also called MRL/n) were developed by Murphy and Roths in 1976.[264] They were derived from LG/J mice crossed with AKR/J, C3H/HeDi, and C57BL/6. By the 12th generation of inbreeding, the MRL-Fas(lpr), which is characterized by marked lymphadenopathy and splenomegaly, large quantities of antibodies to DNA, antibodies to Sm, and lethal immune nephritis, was derived. Lacking the lpr mutation, MRL/+/+ mice share more than 95% of the genetic material of the MRL-Fas(lpr). The lpr (i.e., lymphoproliferation) trait occurred as a spontaneous mutation in a single autosomal recessive gene and results in a defective Fas molecule.[265-269] Interactions of Fas and Fas ligand (FasL) are required for the initiation of apoptosis in activated B and T lymphocytes under normal immunoregulatory conditions.[270] Therefore, mice homozygous for the lpr mutation (i.e., Fas [lpr]) develop massive lymphoproliferation and large quantities of IgG autoantibodies but varying degrees of autoimmune disease, depending on the strain.[271-273] Features of the MRL-lpr strain are listed in Box 17-4.

Clinical Characteristics and Autoantibodies

MRL/+/+ mice develop late-life lupus. They make anti-DNA, anti-Sm, and rheumatoid factors, but serum levels are lower than those in MRL-Fas(lpr) mice. Male and female MRL/+/+ are similarly affected; most develop clinical nephritis with advancing age and are dead by 24 months.[10,264,274]

In MRL-Fas(lpr) mice, the quantities of antibodies that are provided by the MRL/+/+ background are greatly amplified by T-cell help delivered by the CD4+ cells expanded by lymphoproliferation.[275-285] In normal immune responses, activated, expanded CD4+ T cells are reduced in numbers by apoptosis, which is mediated by Fas/FasL interactions and Fas-independent pathways such as those involving Bcl2 family members.[286] In MRL-Fas(lpr) mice, the defective apoptosis is associated with expansions of CD4+, CD8+, and B cells, but the most numerous cells that pack lymph nodes and spleen are the so-called double-negative (DN) T cells that express on their surface α/β TCRs, CD3+, CD4−, CD8−, and B220+. These mice die at 3 to 7 months of age.

Both male and female MRL-Fas(lpr) mice develop high serum levels of Igs, monoclonal paraproteins, ANAs, and immune complexes (the highest of all murine lupus strains).[10,274] They make IgM and IgG anti-ssDNA and anti-dsDNA, and they die from immune nephritis at a young age (90% dead by 9 months of age). Other autoantibodies in their repertoire are IgG antibodies that bind chromatin, histone, nucleosomes, nucleobindin (i.e., a DNA-binding protein), cardiolipin, erythrocyte surfaces, thyroglobulin, lymphocyte surfaces, Sm, U1 small nuclear ribonucleoprotein (U1-snRNP), Ro (SSA [Sjögren syndrome antigen A]), La (SSB [Sjögren syndrome antigen B]), Ku, Su, proteoglycans on endothelial cell membranes, neurons, ribosomal P, RNA polymerase I, C1q, and heat-shock proteins.[283-304] In addition, they have gp70/anti-gp70 immune complexes.[140] A substantial portion of MRL-Fas(lpr) mice develop IgG3 cryoglobulins, some containing rheumatoid factor activity.[151,305,306] Many antibodies are cross-reactive: antibodies to Sm, La, C1q, and nucleobindin also bind DNA. Anti-DNA, anti-Sm, and anti-La frequently use highly similar V_H genes. The following features are found in MRL-Fas(lpr) and never, or rarely, in NZB mice and their hybrids: (1) massive lymphoproliferation, (2) inflammatory erosive polyarthritis (usually detected microscopically rather than grossly), (3) IgM rheumatoid factors, (4) severe necrotizing arteritis, and (5) antibodies to snRNP particles.* In addition to fatal nephritis, most MRL-Fas(lpr) mice

---

*References 10, 264, 274, 284, 297-301, 307-309.

Box 17-4 Characteristics of MRL/*lpr* Mice

Clinical

1. Massive lymphadenopathy with expansion of CD3$^+$, Thy-1$^+$, B220$^+$, CD4$^-$, CD8$^-$, TCR $\alpha\beta^+$ (TCR double-negative or DN T) cells.
2. Early death in males and females (50% mortality at 6 months).
3. Congenic strain MRL/$^{++}$ lacks *lpr*; 50% mortality at 17 months.
4. Deaths usually result from immune glomerulonephritis.
5. Approximately one half develop acute necrotizing polyarteritis.
6. In some colonies, approximately 25% develop destructive polyarthritis.
7. Approximately one half develop dermatitis over dorsal region and face.

Histologic

1. Subacute proliferation of mesangial and endothelial cells, occasional glomerular crescents, basement membrane thickening; deposits of Ig and C3 in glomeruli, especially in capillary walls; marked mononuclear cell infiltrate in interstitium.
2. Acute polyarteritis of coronary and renal arteries.
3. Proliferative synovitis, pannus formation, and destruction of articular cartilage—usually detected microscopically, not grossly.
4. Thymic atrophy.
5. Massive hyperplasia of all lymphoid organs, sometimes with hemorrhage and cystic necrosis.

Autoantibodies

1. Monoclonal paraproteins in approximately 40%; IgG3 cryoglobulins are common.
2. Most marked elevations of serum IgG, IgM, and immune complexes of all murine SLE models.
3. Antinuclear antibodies at highest levels of all murine SLE models.
4. IgG and IgM anti–double-stranded DNA and anti–single-stranded DNA.
5. Anti-Sm in 10% of females and 35% of males.
6. IgM and IgG rheumatoid factors in 65%; some IgG-IgG complexes.
7. gp70–anti-gp70 complexes.
8. IgM and IgG antibodies to DNA, small nuclear ribonucleoprotein (snRNP) particles, and phospholipid often are cross-reactive, suggesting that any of the antigens can activate the entire repertoire.
9. Hypocomplementemia.

Immune Abnormalities

1. Lymphoid hyperplasia primarily results from expansion of unusual CD3,$^+$ CD4$^-$, CD8$^-$, B220$^+$, TCR α/β^+ T cells; they probably derive from activated CD8$^+$ cells that failed to undergo apoptosis.
2. Appearance of these T cells and of early disease is strictly dependent on the *lpr* gene and also is thymus dependent; thymectomy prevents disease.
3. High numbers of hyperactivated B cells appear just before onset of clinical disease.
4. Autoantibodies, nephritis, arthritis, and central nervous system disease are prevented by elimination of CD4$^+$ cells; lymphoproliferation is not.
5. Lymphoproliferation is prevented by elimination of CD8$^+$ cells; autoantibodies, nephritis, and arthritis are not affected.
6. Defective Fc-mediated phagocytosis and clearance of immune complexes.
7. Monocytes/macrophages are abnormal, with low expression of interleukin-1β and defective function.

Genetics

1. Accelerated disease is produced by a single autosomal recessive gene, *lpr*; this mutation encodes a defective Fas molecule, so that very low levels of Fas are expressed on cell surfaces; engagement between Fas and Fas ligand (FasL) is infrequent, making Fas-mediated apoptosis defective; Fas-FasL interaction delivers a major signal for deleting activated T cells by apoptosis; mice homozygous for *lpr* develop lymphoproliferation on most backgrounds, but clinical autoimmune disease primarily appears in permissive backgrounds, such as MRL/$^{++}$ and NZB.
2. The congenic MRL/$^{++}$ has a B-cell repertoire that makes anti-DNA, anti-Sm, and rheumatoid factors; these autoantibodies are probably controlled by multiple genes, as in the NZB.

gp, glycoprotein; Ig, immunoglobulin; TCR, T-cell receptor.

develop lymphocytic infiltration of salivary glands, pancreas, peripheral muscles and nerves, uvea, and thyroid.[310-314] In fact, they develop clinical thyroiditis with hypothyroidism, abnormal electrical transmission in muscles and nerves (suggesting clinical polymyositis and polyneuritis), learning disabilities, sensorineural hearing loss, and band keratopathy.[312-316]

In females, anti-DNA is detectable in the circulation by 6 to 8 weeks of age, proteinuria begins at 1 to 3 months, and death associated with azotemia occurs at 3 to 6 months.[10,274] Males lag behind females by approximately 1 month. IgG2a antibodies to DNA deposit in glomeruli, as do IgG1 and IgG3. The IgG3 cryoglobulins may be associated with either wire-loop, membranous-type lesions or focal proliferative glomerular disease.[151,305,306] The IgG anti-DNA repertoire is dominated by a public Id, H130.[248] Such dominance is reminiscent of the nephritis of BWF1 and SNF1 mice. As for BWF1 mice, there is some evidence that the first stimulating autoantigen is DNA linked to protein, such as chromatin or nucleosomes.[302,303] After these antibodies mutate, specificities for other autoantigens could develop (e.g., ssDNA, dsDNA, phospholipid, Sm, La, and so on).[294,297,298] Antibodies to snRNP antigens, such as Sm, Ro (SSA), and La(SSB), occur in the MRL-*Fas(lpr)* and MRL/$^{+/+}$ lupus-prone strains,[10,274,295-298,304] but not in New Zealand strains. However, antibodies to snRNP have been found in the Palmerston North, a less commonly studied lupus-prone strain.[317] Antibodies to snRNP antigens are found in approximately 25% of MRL mice. The reason that some MRL-Fas(*lpr*) mice express anti-Sm and others do not is unclear; no demonstrable genetic or environmental factors account for these differences.[318] There may be a role for antibody specificities, however. The D epitope of Sm may contain helper epitopes that induce antibody production, and the B epitope may contain suppressor epitopes.[295] Antigen specificity for components of the polypeptides/nRNP complex is similar to the specificities of human anti-Sm. The anti-Sm response is dominated by public Ids (e.g., Y2), which can be found on human anti-Sm and on other human and murine autoantibodies.[319,320] The ability to make anti-Sm does not correlate with clinical nephritis.

Histologic examination of the kidneys shows proliferation of mesangial and endothelial cells in glomeruli, occasional crescent formation, and basement membrane thickening, as well as interstitial infiltration by lymphocytes. IgG, C3, and anti-DNA are deposited in glomeruli; the presence of gp70 is variable and less constant than in NZB and related strains.[321] Antibodies to RNA polymerase I may also contribute to nephritis.[287] Renal failure is the primary cause of death.

Polyarthritis occurs in some MRL-*Fas(lpr)* mice with a prevalence between 15% and 25%,[10,274,307,308] usually observed histologically rather than clinically.[308] By 14 weeks of age, there is synovial cell proliferation with early subchondral bone destruction and marginal erosions. Cartilage is intact in this early lesion, and the synovial stroma is devoid of inflammatory cells. By 19 weeks of age, there is destruction of cartilage and subchondral bone, which is associated with proliferating synovial lining cells and pannus formation. Mild inflammation occurs in synovial stroma but is remote from areas of cartilage damage. Focal arteriolitis can occur. By 25 weeks of age, the inflammatory response in synovium is more marked, but proliferating synovial lining cells continue to be present. In addition, joint destruction has progressed to the development of periarticular fibrous scar tissue and new bone formation. The animals have rheumatoid factors and antibodies to collagen type II.[10,274,307] There also is a correlation between the presence of IgM rheumatoid factor and arthritis. The rheumatoid factors in MRL-Fas(lpr) mice differ from those in MRL[/+/+] and C57BL/6-lpr/lpr in that the former are more likely to bind IgG2a than to bind other IgG isotypes.[306,309] All of these features raise the possibility that MRL-Fas(lpr) mice are a model of spontaneous, genetically controlled arthritis, albeit arthritis that is relatively subtle. It is particularly fascinating that the initial destructive lesions are formed by proliferating synovium without inflammatory cells.

Acute necrotizing arteritis, primarily of coronary and renal arteries, is found in more than half of MRL-Fas(lpr) males and females.[10,274] Many have myocardial infarctions, but these seem to be related histologically more to small vessel vasculopathy than to inflammation of medium-sized arteries. The degenerative vascular disease consists of periodic acid–Schiff–positive eosinophilic deposits in the intima and media of small vessels without inflammation. Ig, C3, and occasionally gp70 can be found in the walls of medium and small arteries, venules, and arterioles.

T Cells, B Cells, Stem Cells, and the Thymus

Lymphoproliferation is the hallmark of MRL-Fas(lpr) mice. In both males and females, lymphadenopathy begins by 3 months of age.[10,274] Nodes can reach 100 times their normal size and may develop hemorrhage and necrosis. Lymphoid malignancies are rare. Normal mouse strains onto which the Fas(lpr) gene is engrafted yield homozygotes with lymphoproliferation. Most of these develop anti-DNA, and varying proportions develop nephritis—not as universal or severe as in MRL-Fas(lpr) mice.[272,274] Therefore, the lpr gene encoding a defective Fas molecule with resultant diminished apoptosis creates a T-lymphocyte population in which highly autoreactive cells are not eliminated in a normal fashion. Other T cells, and probably B cells as well, also proliferate in the absence of some of the usual control mechanisms.

The development of lymphoproliferation may depend on CD8[+] cells, which are precursors of the DN T cells, or some DN T cells may arise from a separate autoreactive lineage usually deleted in mice with normal tolerance mechanisms. MRL-Fas(lpr) mice that are treated with antibodies to CD8 or genetically engineered to fail to express CD8 or MHC class I molecules do not develop lymphoproliferation[322-325] or the expansion of DN T cells. Further studies have identified CD3[+] DN T cells that secrete IL-17; such cells are proinflammatory and particularly rich among infiltrating cells in kidney; they may also express IL-23 receptors, which support survival of IL-17–secreting cells.[326,327] Some T cells cloned from kidney infiltrates have the DN surface phenotype and are autoreactive and kidney-specific, proliferating to renal tubular epithelial and mesangial cells.[328,329] When activated in vitro, they induce MHC class II and intracellular adhesion molecule 1 (ICAM-1) on cultured tubular epithelial cells, which can process antigen and act as APCs.[330] The cytokines encoded by mRNA in the DN T-cell clones include IL-4, TNF-α, and IFN-γ. The chemokine CXCR3 mediates tissue infiltration by both Th1 and Th17 cells.[326] Some DN cells may be an independent lineage,[331] and some can express perforin and become cytolytic.[332] The autoantibodies, vasculitis, arthritis, and Ig-induced nephritis of MRL-Fas(lpr) mice depend largely on CD4[+] cells. Studies of mice (1) after the administration of antibodies to CD4, (2) in which MHC class II is knocked out (thus preventing development of CD4[+] T cells), or (3) that lack CD4 molecules show that these disease features do not develop.[278,322,323,333,334] The presence of the lpr gene

causes marked expansion of CD4[+] cells at the same time that the DN population is increasing. In fact, T-cell help for syngeneic B cells is more marked in MRL-Fas(lpr) than in NZB or BXSB mice.[274] T cells probably are not entirely incapable of undergoing apoptosis; the protein kinase C–dependent pathway for apoptosis is intact.[335] The genes that are used to assemble the TCRs on MRL-Fas(lpr) cells are diverse.[279] There may be some restriction in clonality at the onset of disease; TCR-BV8 families were abundant in lymphoid or salivary glands in some studies.[336] As disease progresses, however, multiple different clones are involved.[279,337] T cells in the periphery have other abnormal features. The ability of MRL-Fas(lpr) T cells to cap, proliferate, and express IL-2 surface receptors and to secrete IL-2 after antigenic or mitogenic stimulation is impaired.[281,338] This impairment may result from deficient signaling via the phosphoinositide pathway.[339] There is increased tyrosine phosphorylation of p561ck in splenic T cells of MRL-Fas(lpr) mice, with increased levels of intracellular polyamines.[340] In lymph nodes, quantities of mRNA encoding IL-6, IL-10, and IFN-γ are increased,[341] suggesting the participation of both Th1 and Th2 cells in disease. Cytokine gene therapy has been studied,[342] and monthly intramuscular injection of complementary DNA (cDNA) expression vectors encoding for TGF-β or IL-2 altered MRL-Fas(lpr) disease. TGF-β prolonged survival, decreased autoantibodies and total IgG, and suppressed histologic damage to kidneys. IL-2 decreased survival and increased autoantibody and IgG production. Inhibition of the Jak/STAT signaling pathway (stimulated by IFN-γ from Th1 cells and by TNF-α, IL-6, platelet-derived growth factor [PDGF], and MCP-1, all of which are increased in MRL-Fas/lpr nephritic tissue) reduced infiltration of T cells and macrophages, expression of cytokines, and proteinuria.[343] Similarly, inhibition of spleen tyrosine kinase (Syk) which is involved in transmitting signals from several cell-surface receptors, including the B-cell antigen receptor, reduced nephritis and dermatitis.[344]

The Fas-defective T cells of MRL-Fas(lpr) mice can be destructive in non-lpr backgrounds. When bone marrow or such T cells are transferred to MRL[/+/+] or SCID mice, a severe GVHD–like wasting disease occurs.[345] This has been attributed to a marked elevation of FasL expression in donor T cells, particularly the DN subset, that induces apoptosis of Fas-expressing recipient cells, resulting in a syndrome that resembles GVHD.[346-348]

There is debate regarding the role of B cells in the pathogenesis of MRL-Fas(lpr) lupus. The hyperactivation of B cells and abnormalities of pre-B stem cells that clearly are present in NZB mice, their hybrids, and BXSB mice are far less dramatic in the MRL background. However, MRL-Fas(lpr) B cells that are isolated from T cells are hyperactivated.[349] They hyperrespond to stimulation with lipopolysaccharide (LPS) or IL-1,[350-352] display increased quantities of IL-6 receptors on their surfaces,[353] and do not undergo anergy or receptor editing (two mechanisms of B-cell tolerance) as efficiently as B cells in normal mice.[354] Perhaps all of these qualities reflect the importance of normal Fas/FasL interactions in B cells, or the influence of the large populations of Th cells to which the B cells are exposed. There is restricted B-cell clonality to several autoantigens, such as rheumatoid factor that binds IgG2a, but this is similar to the situation in both BWF1 and normal mice making antibody responses after stimulation by specific antigens.[355] In MRL-Fas(lpr) mice, the contribution of the MRL background apparently provides B cells with appropriate antibody repertoires to cause autoimmunity.

Stem cells in these mice may be less abnormal than stem cells in other SLE mouse models. One group has reported significant delay in disease onset after syngeneic bone marrow transplantation.[356] MRL-Fas(lpr) mice underwent immunoablation with high-dose cyclophosphamide and then received syngeneic bone marrow that was depleted of Thy1.2 cells. Mean survival was 350 days, compared with 197 days in untreated controls, and lymphadenopathy did not develop. This is a curious finding, because all background genes, as well as the lpr gene, would be transferred with the marrow. It suggests that removing T cells can reset the thermostat for autoimmunity, and many weeks are required for disease to begin again.

The thymus is structurally abnormal in MRL-*Fas*(*lpr*) mice, as it is in all strains that develop spontaneous SLE.[357] Thymic cortical atrophy is severe and medullary hyperplasia common, as in NZB and BWF1 mice.[45,46] The numbers of epithelial cells in the subcapsular and medullary regions are decreased, and there are cortical holes in which no epithelial cells can be seen. Total cortical thymocytes are decreased in number. Levels of DN cells are high, whereas levels of single-positive cells are low, thus suggesting the inability of activated DN cells to undergo apoptosis. Studies with superantigens have suggested that intrathymic deletion of autoreactive T cells is normal early in the lives of MRL-*Fas*(*lpr*) mice[358,359] but that it may be impaired in older mice.[360,361] Both thymic and peripheral deletion mechanisms for T cells likely are affected profoundly by the defect in apoptosis, which eliminates highly autoreactive activated T cells from the repertoire.[270-273,360,361] In fact, SLE in MRL-*Fas*(*lpr*) mice may be more thymus dependent than in other strains. Thymectomy of newborn MRL-*Fas*(*lpr*) mice prevents development of lymphoproliferation and autoimmune disease,[274,362,363] and MRL-*Fas*(*lpr*) thymus engrafted into MRL/+/+ mice causes lymphoproliferation and early death from autoimmune nephritis.[274]

Abnormal cell functions also extend to populations other than lymphocytes. Neutrophils from MRL-*Fas*(*lpr*) (but not MRL/+/+) mice have a marked defect in Fc receptor–mediated phagocytosis, which develops at the time of onset of autoimmune disease; this may result from elevations of TGF-β in the serum. The ability of such neutrophils to access areas of inflammation also may be impaired.[364] Macrophages make abnormally small quantities of IL-1,[227,365] and immune complexes are not cleared as efficiently as in normal mice.[366]

Genetics

The lpr allele on chromosome 19 is the major disease accelerator in the MRL-lpr mice. Deficiency of Fas is caused by an early retroviral transposon insertion in the second intron that results in abnormal RNA splicing, a frame shift, premature termination of the mRNA product, and markedly reduced Fas surface expression in mice homozygous for lpr.[265-270] Normal mice express high levels of Fas on activated T and B lymphocytes and on CD4+CD8+ thymocytes, and lower levels on proliferating cells in the thymus, gut, skin, heart, liver, and ovary. Engagement of Fas by Fas ligand leads to trimerization and formation of the death-inducing signaling complex (DISC), which activates caspase 8.[367,368] Depending on the strength of the signal, this activation can initiate apoptosis directly by activating caspase 3 and 7 (extrinsic apoptosis pathway) or indirectly by activating the proapoptotic Bcl-2 member, Bid, which then induces the release of cytochrome *c* from the mitochondria, which in turn induces the formation of the apoptosome and its activation of caspase 3 (intrinsic apoptosis pathway). Stimulation of Fas can also trigger other nonapoptotic pathways, but these pathways and their role in autoimmunity are less well defined.[369]

Deficiency of Fas or Fas ligand leads to massive lymphoproliferation with particularly prominent accumulation of a normally rare B220+CD4−CD8− DN T-cell population that are mostly derived from CD8+ T cells.[370,371] DN T cells, however, do not appear to play a significant role in the development of autoimmunity. Expansion of DN T cells is not observed with specific deletion of Fas in B cells, DCs, or myeloid cells through the use of conditional knockout mice, a finding consistent with accumulation due to resistance of certain T cells to Fas-mediated apoptosis.[372,373] Notably, Fas is not required for the elimination of expanded T cells following activation (activation-induced cell death), which is mediated by the proapoptotic Bcl-2 family member Bim,[374] but has been suggested to play a role in eliminating T cells exposed to long-term activation with weak signals, such as autoreactivity.[373] Studies using conditional knockouts of Fas to define the specific immune cell population mediating autoimmunity somewhat unexpectedly found that elimination of Fas in all populations tested, including T cells, B cells, DCs, and myeloid cells, resulted in lupus-like disease.[372,373,375] Thus, Fas deficiency leads not only to failure to eliminate autoreactive T and B lymphocytes but also

directly (DCs) or indirectly (myeloid cells) to enhanced autoantigen presentation.

The introduction of the lpr mutation into any mouse strain results in lymphadenopathy of various degrees and production of autoantibodies, but only strains that are genetically susceptible to SLE develop high-titer autoantibodies and severe clinical autoimmune disease. For example, MRL+/+ background genes are essential for the development of full-blown SLE, whereas B6 background genes result in only late-onset autoantibodies (mostly rheumatoid factor [RF] and anti-ssDNA) and minimal end-organ disease. To define these genetic variants, initial genome-wide mapping studies have identified at least 8 loci on chromosomes 1, 2, 4, 5, 7, 10, 11, 12, and 16 in MRL mice in association with one or more lupus traits, including lymphoproliferation, autoantibody production, GN, and vasculitis.[266,376-380] Several have been confirmed in congenics. Four loci from a genome scanning of MRL-lpr and B6-lpr mice[380] showed that lymphadenopathy and splenomegaly are linked to regions on chromosomes 4, 5, 7, and 10, designated Lmb l-4. Lmbs l, 2, and 3 were also linked to anti-DNA but not to nephritis; in contrast, Lmb4 was linked to nephritis. Lmb 1 was derived from the B6 background; Lmbs 2, 3, and 4 were from MRL. Reciprocal congenic mice were generated, confirming a modest effect of each locus on autoimmune traits except for Lmb3 on chromosome 7.[381,382] Lmb3 contained a centromeric MRL locus that promoted lupus,[382] and more distally there was a spontaneously arising nonsense Q262X mutation in the *Coro1a* gene from a B6-lpr colony that suppressed autoimmunity.[383] The function-impairing mutation in the actin cytoskeleton regulatory protein coronin-1A resulted in impairment of T-cell migration, activation, and survival, leading to defective T cell–dependent humoral responses and marked reduction in lymphoproliferation, autoantibody production, and GN. Thus, the *Coro1a* variant Lmb3 locus was an example of an autoimmune disease modifier that illustrated the complexity of autoimmune disease susceptibility.[384] In an additional study, B6 congenic mice (not lpr), containing the MRL chromosome 1 (82-100 centimorgans [cM]) region corresponding to Sle1, Nba2, and Bxs3, have been shown to develop autoantibodies and immune complex–mediated GN.[376] This finding is consistent with MRL's having the same Sle1 haplotype 2 genotype as most inbred strains.

Summary

MRL-*Fas*(*lpr*) mice are particularly interesting as a model of the accelerating factor for autoimmunity that can be provided by the addition of a single gene to a susceptible host. The massive lymphoproliferation that is associated with the autosomal recessive *lpr* gene almost surely results from defective apoptosis. The resultant expansion in CD4+ T cells and inability to delete autoreactive B cells after somatic hypermutation/class switch recombination drives predisposed MRL B cells to make the largest array of autoantibodies seen in murine lupus. The production of pathogenic autoantibodies and the presence of cytolytic DN cells and of CD4+ T cells in target organs such as kidneys and salivary glands result in accelerated autoimmunity and early death from lupus-like nephritis. Some MRL-*Fas*(*lpr*) mice develop destructive polyarthritis, which often is associated with IgM rheumatoid factors. MRL mice are the only strains that spontaneously make anti-Sm. They also develop vasculitis, which can be severe.

BXSB Mice

The BXSB strain was developed by Murphy and Roths.[385] BXSB is a recombinant inbred (RI) strain; RI mice are derived through brother/sister matings within each generation, usually extending for 20 generations. The RI technique is used to produce strains with high frequencies of homozygosity at many loci to observe the expression of recessive genes. The initial mating was between a C57BL/6 (B6) female and a satin beige (SB/Le male)—hence the designation BXSB. BXSB develops severe lupus-like disease with hypergammaglobulinemia, high titers of anti-DNA, marked lymphoproliferation and monocytosis, acute severe GN, and early mortality.[386]

A unique feature of BXSB mice is the disease predominance in males, which is due to a major disease-accelerating gene on the Y chromosome, *Yaa* (Y-linked accelerated autoimmunity and lympho-proliferation transposition). *Yaa* is a duplication of a telomeric segment of the X chromosome (containing TLR7) on the Y chromosome.[387,388] *Yaa* males express two *Tlr7* genes, compared with one in XX females that have one X inactivated. Upon exposure to ssRNA in immune complexes or through direct binding to self-reactive B-cell antigen receptors, the additional TLR7 copy enhances activation of pDCs and conventional DCs, which generate IFN-α, and B cells, including those that make autoantibodies.[389] In comparison with female B cells, male B cells respond more vigorously to TLR7 ligands and even more to the combination of TLR7 plus BCR ligation.[390] Introduction of *Tlr7*-null mutation to mice expressing *Yaa* reduces autoantibodies and disease, but not to zero, indicating that other genes within the *Yaa* interval also participate.[391] Female BXSB mice develop late-life lupus, and B6.Yaa males exhibit only minor lupus-like manifestations, consistent with background genes outside the Y chromosome contributing significantly to lupus-like disease (Box 17-5).

Clinical Manifestations and Autoantibodies

BXSB mice make an autoantibody repertoire that includes IgG antibodies to ssDNA and dsDNA, chromatin, C1q, ANAs, and antibodies that are directed against brain cells.[10,274,392,393] In addition, a small proportion make antierythrocyte, NTAs, monoclonal paraproteins, and gp70anti-gp70 immune complexes.[10,274] By an early age (3 months), they have elevations of circulating immune complexes and hypocomplementemia.[10] Serum levels of C4 diminish as clinical disease appears.[394]

Death is caused by immune GN.[10,274,393] Histologically, the disease is more exudative than in other mouse models—that is, there are neutrophils invading glomeruli along with IgG and C3 deposition, proliferative changes in mesangia and endothelial cells, and basement membrane thickening.[10] The progression from nephritis to death is rapid, with 50% of males dead by 5 months of age.[10,274,393,394]

T Cells, B Cells, Stem Cells, and the Thymus

Lymphoproliferation occurs in BXSB mice; it is more marked than in BWF1 but less dramatic than in MRL-*Fas*(lpr) mice.[10,274] Unlike in MRL-*Fas*(lpr) mice, the hyperplastic nodes in BXSB mice contain predominantly B cells,[274,362] and for some time it was thought that B-cell defects were the primary abnormality in this strain. As in the other models, B cells are hyperactivated, higher portions are mature (expressing IgD and IgM on their surfaces), higher proportions display CD40L on their surfaces, and secretion of IgG and IgM is increased.[274,362,395] A rather unique property of BXSB is that MZ B cells are depleted (unrelated to the *Yaa* gene[391]). The B cells are resistant to tolerance with human gamma globulin; resistance is a property of the B cell itself and does not reflect abnormalities in APCs or T cells.[396] Studies in *Yaa*+*Yaa*− double–bone marrow chimeric mice show that *Yaa*− T cells can activate *Yaa*+ B cells to make autoantibodies but *Yaa*+ T cells cannot drive *Yaa*− B cells to do so.[397] This finding probably indicates that *Yaa*+ B cells present antigen to T cells and the two cells cross-activate each other. However, BXSB T cells play an important role in disease by providing help for autoantibody formation.[398,399] As mice age, they develop the typical T-cell defects of SLE mice (i.e., abnormally low proliferative responses to antigens/mitogens, reduced production of IL-2). Elimination of CD4+ (but not CD8+) T cells suppresses autoantibodies, monocytosis, and nephritis.[399] In sum, it is clear that BXSB B cells are intrinsically abnormal but that T cells are required for development of full-blown disease. Disease is delayed by the prevention of second signal–mediated T-cell activation after administration of CTLA-4–Ig.[400] Although some authorities consider BXSB disease to be primarily related to Th cells, there is evidence for involvement of a unique type of CD4+ T cell. As BXSB males age, their T cells acquire a memory phenotype and secrete lymphokines that are characteristic of both Th1 and Th2

cells.[1,401,402] Th2 are probably not disease-promoting, as BXSB disease is not altered in mice deficient in IL-4.[403] In contrast, deficiency of the IL-21 receptor (usually expressed by Th17 cells and T$_{FH}$ cells) prevents hypergammaglobulinemia, autoantibody production, depletion of MZ B cells, monocytosis, and renal disease. IL-21 was derived from ICOS+CD4+ splenic T cells, an unusual source of this cytokine, in addition to the usual T$_{FH}$ and Th17 cells. This

---

Box 17-5 Characteristics of BXSB Mice

Clinical
1. Males die early of lupus (50% mortality at 5 months; 90% at 8 months).
2. Females have late-onset lupus (50% mortality at 15 months; 90% at 24 months).
3. Major cause of death is immune glomerulonephritis.

Histologic
1. Males show severe acute to subacute glomerulonephritis, with proliferation and exudation of neutrophils into glomeruli.
2. In males, IgG and C3 deposit in mesangium and glomerular capillary walls by 3 months of age; deposits in tubular basement membranes and interstitium also occur.
3. Lymph node hyperplasia (10-20 times normal size) in males.
4. Myocardial infarcts in 25%, without arteritis.
5. Thymic cortical atrophy with medullary hyperplasia; thymic epithelial cells contain crystalline inclusions.

Autoantibodies
1. All males develop antinuclear antibodies and IgG anti–double-stranded DNA and anti–single-stranded DNA.
2. Less than half of males develop monoclonal paraproteins, antierythrocyte antibodies, gp70–anti-gp70, and thymocytotoxic antibodies.
3. Hypocomplementemia in males by 3 months of age; low C4 levels.
4. Elevations of circulating immune complexes.
5. Defective monocyte/macrophages.

Immune Abnormalities
1. B cell is the most common cell in hyperplastic lymph nodes.
2. B-cell hyperactivation and advanced maturity.
3. B cells are resistant to tolerance with some antigens.
4. Male bone marrow transferred to female BXSB mice produces accelerated disease; female bone marrow confers late lupus when transferred to males; mature male B cells do not accelerate disease; abnormality is contained in marrow stem cells.
5. Monocytosis occurs.
6. Elimination of CD4+ T cells diminishes anti-DNA, monocytosis, nephritis, and mortality.
7. Disease is not influenced substantially by thymectomy.
8. Disease is not influenced substantially by sex hormone therapies and/or castration.
9. Defective Fc-mediated immune complex clearance.

Genetics
1. A single gene that accelerates disease (formerly called *Yaa*, now known to be *Tlr7*, is present on the Y chromosome. It has translocated from X (its usual location), producing increased copy numbers of TLR7 and therefore increased innate immune activation by RNA/protein containing antigens that trigger TLR7 receptors in dendritic cells and B cells.
2. Additional genes that behave like X-linked recessives confer susceptibility to disease; they may account for late-life SLE in females.

gp, glycoprotein; Ig, immunoglobulin; TLR, Toll-like receptor.

IL-21–producing T-cell population may be a unique feature of BXSB mice.[404] The thymus shows cortical atrophy and defects in thymic epithelial cells and dendritic cells similar to those in other SLE strains.[51,357,405] Crystalline structures have been described in the thymic epithelial cells of BXSB males; they are thought to represent abnormal storage of thymic hormones.[406] Apoptosis of thymic cells is delayed in all SLE strains studied, including BXSB. Thymectomy has accelerated disease in some studies and has not altered it in others.[362,407] The effects are not as consistent and dramatic as the protection from disease that is conferred by thymectomy in MRL-Fas(lpr) mice.[274,362,363]

An additional feature of BXSB mice is monocytosis. By 2 weeks of age, BXSB males have increased numbers of monocyte colony-forming units in spleen and lymph nodes.[408] Further, the monocytes/macrophages are abnormal; they make unusually large quantities of procoagulants, which might contribute to the rapid damage to glomeruli that characterizes lupus in this strain.[409] Monocytes, neutrophils, and B cells all have increased expression of CXCR4; its ligand, CXCL12, is increased in kidneys, so inflammatory and autoantibody-producing cells can home to their target organ.[410] The monocytosis is related to the *Yaa* gene,[411] probably as a result of an epistatic interaction between *Yaa* and the telomeric region of chromosome 1 that contains the Bxs3 susceptibility locus.[411] Studies of lymph nodes show dramatic increases in mRNA for IL-1, with some increase in IL-10 and TGF-β, all of which probably come from monocytes. IFN-γ is also increased, suggesting simultaneous increase in Th1 activity.[341]

There is good evidence that a stem cell abnormality may underlie all of these cellular abnormalities in BXSB mice,[274,412] because male BXSB bone marrow can transfer disease, and normal marrow grafted into male BXSB mice can prevent disease.[274,412-414] Production of mixed chimerics in BXSB mice created by lethal irradiation followed by transfer of bone marrow from nonautoimmune BALB/c mice plus congenic marrow depleted of T cells prolongs survival, prevents nephritis, and restores normal primary immune responses. Depletion of BXSB T cells is essential for the success of this approach.[415] This stem-cell defect may lead to a single abnormality that affects both B and T cells, or there may be multiple genes influencing multiple responses leading to hyperactivity in each type of lymphocyte, and perhaps in monocytes.

Sex Hormones and Disease

Manipulations such as castration and androgen therapy do not dramatically alter outcome in BXSB mice,[274,416] in contrast to mice with New Zealand backgrounds.

Genetics

Multiple genes predispose to SLE in BXSB mice, as in the other models. There is an inherent tendency toward autoimmune disease in BXSB mice of both sexes; that tendency is dramatically accelerated by a higher number of copies of the *Yaa* gene, created by translocation of TLR7 from the X to the Y chromosome. It accounts for the earlier, more severe disease in males. If normal mice are generated that bear the Sle1 gene from NZW mice (a gene associated with the ability to break tolerance to nucleosomes) and the *Yaa* gene, fatal autoimmune nephritis occurs.[88] However, the *Yaa* gene alone is not sufficient to permit the development of autoimmunity: MHC and other genes play important roles.[417-419] The *Yaa* gene encodes TLR7, a molecule in endosomes of pDCs and B cells that binds RNA-containing nucleotides and can activate these cells. See the preceding section for more discussion of the Y chromosome and BXSB disease. Mice of the H-2b haplotype (BXSB is H-2b) do not express MHC class II I-E molecules; introduction of the I-E α chain into BXSB males permits the mice to display I-E on cell surfaces and prevents disease.[420-422] This effect occurs only in mouse strains with "permissive" MHC such as H-2b.[423] The I-A molecule in the transgenic mice contains peptides from I-E, and it is possible that those peptides prevent the presentation of other peptides that induce and sustain pathogenic autoantibody production.[423] Susceptibility to autoimmunity is transmitted as an autosomal

dominant trait in some F1 hybrids that are derived from BXSB,[417-419] and in others, susceptibility behaves as if it were controlled by autosomal recessive genes.[274]

Results of genome scans of back-crosses between BXSB and other strains have identified eight loci linked to autoantibodies, lymphoproliferation, GN, autoimmune thrombocytopenia, and/or myocardial infarction.[424-426] Among the loci associated with traits in parental BXSB males, three or four regions on chromosome 1 and one region on chromosome 3 are linked to nephritis. There are at least six non-MHC loci (*Yaa, Bsx1-4,* and *Bxs6*) linked to disease susceptibility, with another locus, *Bsx5*, as a possible suppressor. Loci on chromosome 1 contribute the most to overall variance, and examination of congenic mice has confirmed several chromosome 1 loci and tentatively identified candidate genes.[427,428] It should be noted that the BXSB chromosome 1 contains the *Sle1* haplotype 2, like the NZW and NZB strains, and it is likely that the same predisposing genetic variants are contributing significantly to susceptibility in BXSB mice. Another interesting related observation is that BXSB/long-lived mice, thought originally to be a subline, were actually a closely related recombinant inbred strain derived from a common BXSB stock before the line was fixed and this strain was resistant to lupus despite having major susceptibility loci such as *Bxs3*.[426] It was postulated that this observation supports the presence of one or more potent suppressor genes in the parental B6 and SB/Le strains that have not yet been defined.

Summary

In summary, BXSB mice are unique in that lupus nephritis is more severe and occurs earlier in males than in females. This feature results largely from the accelerating effect of a single gene, *Yaa*, which encodes *Tlr7*. Ordinarily on the X chromosome, *Tlr7* is translocated from the X to the Y chromosome, resulting in males that have gene duplication for TLR7 and thus are hyperresponsive to RNA nucleotide–containing ligands of TLR7. Disease develops rapidly in BXSB males, with 50% dead of immune GN by 5 months of age.

B cells, T cells, and monocytes are all abnormal in BXSB, with good evidence for hematopoietic stem cell defects. There is a somewhat unique peripheral CD4+ T cell that produces IL-21, which helps promote the synthesis of anti-DNA by a subpopulation of B-1 cells. The autoantibody repertoire is directed primarily against nucleosomal and DNA antigens. Multiple genes participate in disease susceptibility.

The BXD2 (C57BL/6J×DBA2J) Model of Spontaneous Erosive Arthritis and Glomerulonephritis ("Rhupus")

The BXD2 strain of mice is one of approximately 80 BXD RI mouse strains that were generated originally by Dr. Benjamin A. Taylor at the Jackson Laboratory (Bar Harbor, ME, USA) by inbreeding the intercross progeny of a cross between C57BL/6J and DBA/2J strains for more than 20 generations.[429] During the course of a survey to discover genetic loci that influence T-cell senescence, Mountz and colleagues observed the development of not only GN that is less severe than BWF1 mice but also erosive arthritis in the BXD2 strain in specific pathogen–free conditions.[430] Increased serum titers of RF and anti-DNA antibody appear in females, and their arthritis is characterized histologically by mononuclear cell infiltration, synovial hyperplasia, and bone and cartilage erosion. The arthritis affects 50% of female mice by 8 months and 90% after 12 months. Splenomegaly is characterized by increased numbers and sizes of GCs; this feature of BXD2 mice has been the subject of studies providing novel information regarding the role of GCs in autoimmunity. In mammals, GCs occur not only in spleens but in all secondary lymphoid tissues, including tonsils, Peyer patches of mucosa-associated lymphoid tissue, and lymph nodes. Autoantibody specificities are to a large extent produced in GCs through a series of interactions between B cells, T_{FH} cells, and follicular dendritic cells—interactions that may be facilitated by migration of B-cell subsets between the follicle and MZs.[430] With exposure to immune complexes, GC pDCs are activated via their activating FcγR and complement receptors; they express the chemokine ligand CXCL13, release IFN-α, and present antigens. These features attract premarginal B cells into areas of GCs where they interact with pDCs and come into contact with CD4$^+$ T cells. At the same time, the CD4$^+$ follicular T cells produce IL-17, which keeps the B cells in the follicular DC network by upregulating intracellular regulators of G-protein signals, which modify CSCL12/CSCL13 receptors. Thus, the B cells stay in contact with DCs and T cells for longer-than-usual periods, providing greater opportunity to generate pathogenic autoantibodies. Activation-induced cytidine deaminase (AID), which is required for somatic hypermutation and class switch recombination in B cells, is also elevated in BXD2 mice.[431,432] The increased formation of GCs with B-cell activation and retention is largely prevented in BXD2 mice with the inactivation of AID in B cells.[433] The features of lupus and arthritis developed by BXD2 mice segregate in F2 recombinant inbred mice, generated by crossing BXD2 mice with the parental B6 and D2 strains. Using the available BXD recombinant inbred strains, genetic mapping analysis of anti-DNA and RF showed linkage to loci on mouse chromosome 2 near the marker D2Mit412 (78 cM, 163 Mb) and on chromosome 4 near D4Mit146 (53.6 cM, 109 Mb), respectively. Both loci are close to the B-cell hyperactivity, lupus, or GN susceptibility loci that have been identified previously in other lupus-prone strains. Thus, the BXD2 strain of mice is a novel polygenic model for complex autoimmune disease that spontaneously develops generalized autoimmune disease that includes expanded GCs, autoantibody production, nephritis, and chronic erosive arthritis.[430]

The (NZW×BXSB) F1 Model of Antiphospholipid Syndrome and Coronary Artery Disease
Disease Characteristics and Autoantibodies
Male hybrid (NZW×BXSB) F1 mice have been particularly interesting as models of autoimmunity linked to antiphospholipid antibodies and accelerated degenerative coronary artery disease, a combination seen in some patients with SLE. Apparently the combination of NZW lupus susceptibility genes and the Yaa plus other background genes in BXSB is enough to produce high titers of aCL. In these mice, 50% of the males are dead by 24 weeks of age, usually with extensive myocardial infarction, with occlusive disease and intimal thickening in small coronary arteries but not extramyocardial coronary arteries. These mice also develop high serum levels of anti-DNA and immune complexes, with antibodies against both platelets (causing thrombocytopenia) and phospholipids. Most of the antiphospholipids bind β$_2$ GPI; such subsets may be more likely to be associated with clotting than subsets without that characteristic.[434] The males also develop GN, hypertension, leukocytosis, and gastrointestinal vasculitis.[434,435] Females develop nephritis late in life but generally do not generate antibodies to cardiolipin.

Abnormalities in Hematopoietic Stem Cells, T Cells, and B Cells
Hematopoietic stem cell, T cells, and B cells are abnormal, as in BXSB parents. Numbers of DCs are increased in multiple organs, probably increasing B-cell activation.[436] Serum levels of IFN-γ and IL-10 rise as mice age. Treatment with antibodies to CD4 delays disease, whereas treatment with antibodies to CD8 accelerates it.[437] Lethal irradiation of (NZW×BXSB) F1 mice followed by transfer of bone marrow from normal C57BL/6 mice prevents nephritis, coronary artery disease, and thrombocytopenia, suggesting that hybrid stem cells are abnormal.[438] Treatment with the calcium channel blocker ticlopidine prolongs survival and lowers the prevalence of myocardial infarction without affecting nephritis.[431] Similarly, treatment with nifedipine lowers blood pressure and prolongs survival, protects partially from coronary artery stenosis and myocardial infarction, and reduces the amount of histologic nephritis.[439] Administration of IFN-α (which is stimulated by ligation of Tlr7) to female (NZW×BXSB) F1 mice does not completely recapitulate the male disease: It accelerates nephritis but cannot induce high titer

antiphospholipids or thrombocytopenia,[440] suggesting that these properties require abnormalities on the Y chromosome (Yaa mutation with Tlr7 duplication) and/or male hormones. In fact, the inhibitory IgG Fc (fcrg2b) receptor polymorphism associated with low production of the FcrγIIB inhibitory protein on monocyte/macrophages and B cells in many of the SLE models, including this one, has an epistatic interaction with Yaa that enhances disease.[441] Administration of BAFF receptor Ig (BAFF-R–Ig) and TACI (transmembrane activator and calcium-modulator and cyclophilin ligand interactor)–Ig both prevented disease, with fewer B cells, fewer activated and memory T cells, and substantially less nephritis.[442] Interestingly, BAFF blockade did not prevent the appearance of aCL, and mice developed thrombocytopenia, but fewer myocardial infarcts than controls. This finding suggests that aCL is generated in the GCs (relatively independent of BAFF) and that the myocardial infarcts not only depend on presence of the antibodies but also require immune/inflammatory responses.

Genetics
A single genome scan has shown linkage between various disease features and different chromosomal regions. Antibodies to cardiolipin, platelet-binding antibodies, thrombocytopenia, and myocardial infarction were each controlled by independently segregating dominant loci. Anticardiolipin was linked to regions on chromosomes 4 and 17, antiplatelet antibodies and thrombocytopenia to chromosomes 8 and 17, and myocardial infarction to chromosomes 7 and 14.[443] Taken together, these findings suggest there is not a simple direct association between antiphospholipid and myocardial infarct or thrombocytopenia, and overall that antibodies and disease expression have complex genetic requirements.

Gld/Gld Mice with Absence of Functional Fas Ligand
In 1984, Roths and associates[444] reported a spontaneous autosomal recessive mutation that occurred in the inbred mouse strain C3H/HeJ, which they called gld (for generalized lymphoproliferative disorder). It now is known that the mutation is a single base change in the C-terminal extracellular domain of the FasL molecule, which is encoded on mouse chromosome 6[445-447]; functional membrane-bound FasL molecules are not generated.[448] FasL is expressed on cell surfaces, but the mutation interferes with its ability to bind Fas. Therefore, apoptosis does not proceed normally, highly autoreactive T and B cells persist instead of dying, and SLE results.

FasL plays a major role in apoptosis. Clinically, C3H/gld/gld mice of both sexes develop lymphadenopathy and splenomegaly by 13 weeks of age. Lymphoid organs contain increased numbers of B, T, and DN lymphocytes. The B220$^+$, CD4$^-$, CD8$^-$, TCR$^+$ T cell that expands so dramatically in MRL-Fas(lpr) mice is identical to the major expanded population in gld/gld mice, consistent with major defects in both strains of apoptosis mediated by Fas/FasL interactions. These DN cells require MHC class I expression for expansion and contain populations with high avidity for self-antigens such as endogenous retroviral superantigens; such a dangerous population is deleted in normal mice.[449] C3H/gld/gld mice have shorter life spans than wild-type C3H/HeJ mice; male C3H/gld/gld mice live a mean of 396 days and females 368 days, compared with 688 days in females that are not homozygous for gld. Lymphoid cells and macrophages infiltrate the interstitium of lungs extensively, but other organs are rarely involved. Vasculitis does not occur. Most of these mice do not develop histologic lupus nephritis, although all mice older than 22 weeks have Ig deposits in glomeruli (primarily confined to the mesangium). By that age, serum levels of gamma globulin are approximately five times normal; this increase occurs in all isotypes but is most dramatic in IgA and IgG2b. ANAs begin to appear at 8 weeks of age, and all C3H/gld/gld mice are ANA-positive by 16 weeks. By 20 weeks, all have antibodies to thymocytes and dsDNA.[444,450] The primary cause of early mortality probably is the pulmonary disease. In C3H/gld/gld and BALB/gld/gld mice that live to 1 year of age, B-cell malignancies are common (usually CD5$^+$

malignant plasmacytoid lymphomas).[451] As in other lupus models, genetic backgrounds in addition to the single-point mutation determine the extent of disease: B6/gld/gld mice have milder disease than C3H/gld/gld, but develop autoantibodies. T-cell studies in gld/gld mice show expansion of Th17 cells that does not require IFN-γ (in contrast to other types of T cells), and resistance of Th1 cells (responsible for helping synthesis of IgG2a) to CD4+ Treg cells.[449]

Examination of the gld mutation has greatly improved our understanding of the importance of Fas/FasL interactions and of apoptosis in maintaining normal immune homeostasis. For example, lethally irradiated mice reconstituted with stem cells from Fas-deficient MRL/lpr mice develop chronic GVHD, but stem cells deficient in both Fas and FasL do not produce GVHD, showing that FasL is an important effector in this syndrome. Interestingly, these double-deficient T cells can induce normal B cells to produce autoantibodies.[452] In pristane-induced murine lupus, lpr and gld mutations affect some autoantibody production but not others, suggesting that autoantibodies differ in their dependence on Fas and FasL expression.[453] B6/gld/gld mice can clear cytomegalovirus after infection, but they cannot downregulate the resultant inflammatory responses.[454] Non-obese diabetic (NOD) mice spontaneously develop autoimmune diabetes, resulting from immune destruction of pancreatic beta cells. NOD/gld/gld mice are protected from disease, showing the dependence of the process on FasL-mediated apoptosis.[455] Interestingly, lupus-like disease in C3H/gld/gld mice also requires TNF-α: Mice deficient in that cytokine or treated with antibodies to it have milder disease.[456] C3H/gld/gld disease can be prevented by lethal irradiation followed by reconstitution with a mixture of normal and gld bone marrow, as long as the normal marrow is not depleted of Thy1+ cells, suggesting that T cells expressing FasL can correct the gld defect; CD8+ FasL+ cells are primarily responsible for suppression of lymphoproliferation.[457]

In summary, autoimmune-permissive strains with defective production of FasL develop lymphoproliferation, autoantibodies, and infiltration of organs with lymphocytes that cannot be deleted normally. Their disease has similarities to human SLE, as does disease associated with production of a defective Fas molecule in lpr-bearing strains.

INDUCTION OF LUPUS IN NORMAL MOUSE STRAINS

In the previously discussed models of spontaneous SLE, multiple genetic factors likely provide the major if not the only important risk factors. Mutations in Fas (Fas-lpr) and FasL (gld) accelerate autoimmunity in these susceptible strains. However, there are several examples of the induction of SLE-like disease in mice that are otherwise healthy, with genetic backgrounds that do not predispose to autoimmunity. These include (1) induction of chronic GVHD; (2) alteration of expression of single molecules (either upregulation via transgene insertion or deletion in knockout mice); (3) transfer of pathogenic autoantibodies or the B cells that secrete them; (4) forced expression of pathogenic autoantibodies via the introduction of transgenes; (5) activation of idiotypic networks that result in the production of pathogenic autoantibodies; (6) inoculations of DNA, DNA/protein, other autoreactive proteins or oligopeptides; and (7) injections of hydrocarbon oils such as pristane or heavy metals such as mercury. In most of these models, some strains of mice are more susceptible than others, again suggesting that most if not all murine genetic backgrounds contain genes that permit autoimmunity.

Chronic GVHD

GVHD is produced in mice by injection of lymphocytes from a parent into an F1 hybrid differing at one MHC locus from that parent. Disease is caused by CD4+ T cells recognizing certain foreign MHC class II antigens.[458-464] A struggle ensues between graft-versus-host and host-versus-graft reactions, with host and donor cytolytic CD8+ T cells, stimulated by IFN-γ, attacking the donor CD4+ T cells. If after 2 to 12 weeks the CD4+ donor T cells persist and expand,

mice develop chronic GVHD.[458,459,465] Chronic GVHD resembles SLE.[458,459,461-464] Several IgG autoantibodies are made, including anti-dsDNA, anti-ssDNA, and antihistone.[458,461,464] In some combinations, fatal lupus-like nephritis mediated by IgG anti-DNA occurs. One MHC interaction that results in fatal nephritis of chronic GVHD is between H-2d donor lymphocytes and an H-2b recipient.[463,464] In contrast, most recipient H2k haplotypes are resistant. A common model is parental DBA/2 (H2d) splenocytes transferred into B6xD2 (H2b/d) F1 mice. The development of clinical nephritis and of autoantibodies can be separated. Many parental hybrid combinations result in the ability of the recipient to make high-titer IgG anti-DNA, but class II genes I-A and I-E (equivalent to human HLA class II DR and DQ) must contain a susceptible haplotype, such as b, for severe nephritis to result.[464] In animals without nephritis renal deposits of IgG are confined to mesangial regions of glomeruli; in animals with nephritis, IgG deposits occur along the capillary loops. Renal damage can be reduced by blockade of TWEAK (TNF-like weak inducer of apoptosis). TWEAK induces proinflammatory cytokines upon interaction with its Fn14 receptor, which is expressed in kidney cells.[466]

Disease is initiated by donor CD4+ cells activated by host APCs to secrete IL-4, which promotes B-cell stimulation with autoantibody production.[467] The "pathogenic" T cells include CD44hiCD62lo peripheral CD4+ T cells and ICOShi CD4+ TFH cells, which secrete IL-21.[468] These CD4+ effector cells require expression of TRAIL (TNF-related apoptosis–inducing ligand) to sustain their numbers, help to B cells, and resultant severe nephritis.[469] Ability of the host to mount CD8+ cells that kill the B cells determines whether acute (wasting disease) or chronic (lupus-like) GVHD will occur. Both the acute and chronic forms of GVHD begin as IL-4–mediated B-cell stimulation; transition to acute GVHD depends on the education in the host thymus of donor-derived pro-T and pre-T cells to develop into CD8+ T cells that eliminate activated B cells (both perforin-mediated cytotoxicity and Fas/FasL killing occur). These donor-derived CD8+ cytolytic T cells mediate acute GVHD. If generation of the CD8+ T cells does not occur, IL-4 secretion continues, and T cell–activated B cells survive; sustained autoantibody production and lupus-like chronic GVHD result.[470-472] The tyrosine kinase associated with the Mer receptor on B cells is required for activation of B cells by CD4+ T in chronic GVHD.[473] The major source of autoantibodies among B-cell subsets is mature B cells, especially those with MZ phenotype.[474] Mice with severe chronic GVHD usually have high levels of IgE and IgG1 in their sera, confirming the important role of Th2 cells (which secrete IL-4) in disease. Antibodies to IL-4 or infusion of soluble IL-4 receptor prevents or suppresses disease.[475]

Genetic Alteration of the Expression of Single Molecules
Deletions and Increased Expression
Studies in which single genes are overexpressed in transgenic mice, or single genes are deleted in knockout mice, have all suggested that strategies that permit extended lifetimes for autoreactive lymphocytes or for autoantigens promote the development of SLE-like disease in normal mice. For example, overexpression of bcl-2 (which protects cells from apoptotic death) in normal mice transgenic for that molecule causes them to develop mild autoimmunity.[476] Bcl-2 transgenic C57BL/6-lpr mice have lymphadenopathy but no abnormal autoantibodies.[477] In C57BL/6-lpr mice transgenic for Pim-l (a cytoplasmic serine/threonine protein kinase that also inhibits apoptosis), lymphoproliferation resulting from the accumulation of B220+ T cells also occurs.[478] BAFF, also known as BLyS (B-lymphocyte stimulator) promotes B-cell survival and differentiation by production of antiapoptotic proteins.[479] BAFF is made by monocytes, DCs, activated T and B lymphocytes, and some epithelial cells. Naïve B cells require BAFF for survival and selection. Autoantigen-stimulated B cells maturing from transitional phases 1 to 2 are usually deleted; in the presence of high quantities of BAFF they may survive. BAFF is also important in the switch to IgG and the maturation of memory B cells into plasma cells. BAFF enhances humoral responses to T

cell–independent and T cell–dependent antigens by protecting antigen-activated B cells from apoptosis.[479-482] Thus, overexpression of BAFF in transgeneic mice can induce autoimmunity that includes autoantibodies to DNA.

Deleted Molecules in Knockout Mice

Two general categories of single-gene deletions have led to generation of lupus-like disease in otherwise healthy mice: (1) removal of genes that downregulate accumulation and/or activation of B or T lymphocytes and (2) deletion of genes that regulate normal degradation and clearing of DNA, immune complexes, or apoptotic cells and bodies. In the first category, normal mice with deletion of *Lyn* have a marked increase in IgM-secreting B cells and develop high levels of immune complexes and anti-DNA along with a GN similar to SLE.[483,484] *Lyn* is an Src protein tyrosine kinase associated with the BCR that participates in an inhibitory signal after BCR activation; *Lyn* phosphorylates the BCR co-receptor CD22, a process that recruits the tyrosine phosphatase SHP-1 to the BCR/CD22 complex and controls B-cell activation. In the absence of *Lyn,* B cells exhibit spontaneous hyperreactivity, doubtless contributing to their lupus-like phenotype.[485] Moth-eaten mice (so called because of patchy alopecia) have spontaneous deletion of a single residue in the *N*-terminal SH2 domain of the protein tyrosine phosphatase 1C gene (PTP1c). PTP1c activity is absent, removing an inhibitory signal for the activation of *Lyn* and *Syk*, with resultant B-cell hyperactivation. IgM levels are high, B-1 B cells are abnormally activated, and high-titer ANAs develop, with immune complex deposition in many tissues.[486,487] Deletion of IRAK1 (IL-1 receptor–associated kinase-1), which is on the X chromosome, has been reported to abrogate autoantibody production and nephritis in normal mice congenic for the *Sle1* or *Sle3* susceptibility genes.[488] IRAK1 is recruited to IL-1β (predominantly in monocytes/ macrophages and DCs) and enables subsequent activation of nuclear factor kappa B (NF-κB) and JNK pathways, leading to immune responses and inflammation. On the T-cell side, deletion of PD-1, an Ig superfamily member bearing an immunoreceptor tyrosine–based inhibitory motif (ITIM) that affects primarily CD4⁻CD8⁻ thymocytes and CD8+ Treg cells, also results in lupus-like disease.[234,489] Similarly, expression of the cell-cycle regulator p21 prevents accumulation of CD4⁺ memory cells; deletion of that molecule in normal mice results in loss of tolerance for nuclear antigens. Interestingly, female mice with a p21 deletion are particularly prone to development of SLE; they develop IgG antibodies to dsDNA, lymphadenopathy, Ig-mediated GN, and shortened survival.[490] In the sanroque mouse strain, a novel gene, *Roquin,* associates with failure to tolerize self-reactive germinal center T cells; anti-dsDNA and a lupus phenotype result.[491]

In the second category—gene deletions that influence clearing of DNA, nucleosomes, apoptotic cells, and apoptotic bodies—several single-gene deletions have produced lupus-like phenotypes in normal mice. Humans with homozygous deletions of C1q have a very high prevalence of SLE. Similarly, among mice in which the C1q gene has been deleted, approximately half develop high-titer ANAs and 25% have clinical nephritis by the age of 8 months; glomeruli show unusually abundant deposits of apoptotic bodies.[492] C1q probably plays a role in clearance of immune complexes, of apoptotic cells, and of apoptotic bodies.[493] Mice deficient in DNAse1 also develop ANAs, Ig deposition in glomeruli, and clinical nephritis.[494]

In summary, these single-gene knockout mice show that one alteration that either permits B- or T-cell hyperactivation, or interferes with the elimination of DNA/nucleosomes or of apoptotic and necrotic cells that provide stimulatory nucleosomes and other self-antigens, is powerful enough to produce lupus-like phenotypes in mice that otherwise are resistant to clinical autoimmunity.

Lupus Induced by Direct Transfer of Pathogenic Autoantibodies or B Cells That Secrete Those Antibodies

Our laboratory has demonstrated that transfer of B-cell hybridomas secreting pathogenic IgG anti-dsDNA to normal BALB/c mice results in the development of SLE, with circulating IgG anti-dsDNA, immune complex deposition in glomeruli, and severe Ig-mediated GN.[136,137] Injections of the Ig into C57BL/6 mice does not produce any disease, suggesting that background susceptibility genes, perhaps influencing the composition of the kidney, must be present for this approach to induce disease. In another study, SCID mice that were populated with BWF1 pre-B cells developed SLE with the expected secretion of autoantibodies by their adopted B cells.[200] Similarly, another group has reported that some human monoclonal antibody anti-DNA inoculated into SCID mice deposited in glomeruli and induced proteinuria.[495]

Lupus in Mice Transgenic for Pathogenic Autoantibodies

Transient lupus nephritis has been reported to develop in normal mice that were transgenic for an IgG2b anti-dsDNA derived from a nephritic BWF1 female.[139] The gene construct permitted only small quantities of the transgenic IgG2b to be expressed on B-cell surfaces, thus bypassing early tolerance mechanisms. Therefore, the transgenic mice secreted IgG2b anti-dsDNA for several weeks and, during that time, developed proteinuria. Later, B-cell receptor editing occurred, with resultant elimination of the ability of the Ig to bind DNA; the proteinuria disappeared, and the mice lived a normal life span. Mice carrying transgenes encoding anti-DNA from MRL-*Fas(lpr)* mice have also been generated and studied for B-cell tolerance. In MRL-*Fas(lpr)* mice, anti-dsDNA B cells undergo receptor editing, but anti-ssDNA B cells are functionally silenced.[496] Unlike in normal BALB/c mice, developmental arrest of autoreactive B cells does not occur in the lupus mice; in the presence of the *Fas/lpr* mutation anti-dsDNA, B cells find their way to lymphoid follicles, along with CD4⁺ T cells, so that T cell–B cell interactions continue to drive clinical autoimmunity.[497] To summarize, if normal mice express the transgene-encoded Ig on B-cell surfaces, the cells are developmentally arrested, deleted, anergized, or receptor-edited; cells do not reach T cell–B cell interaction sites in lymphoid organs, and secretion of the anti-DNA is short-lived if it occurs at all. If the transgenic mouse has an *lpr* background, these mechanisms of tolerance degrade over time, pathogenic B cells reach follicles where they can interact with T cells, and ANAs encoded by the transgene are secreted with steadily increasing titers. Another model uses normal BALB/c mice transgenic for the R4A-γ 2b heavy chain of a BALB/c anti-DNA monoclonal antibody. This heavy chain can combine with multiple light chains to make a dsDNA-binding Ig. In the BALB/c mouse, B cells with high affinity for dsDNA are either deleted or anergic, whereas a third population that produces germline-encoded antibodies with low affinity for dsDNA reaches maturity and survives without producing SLE. Several manipulations of R4A transgenic mice can permit high-affinity DNA-binding B cells to escape tolerance and cause disease. For example, after administration of estradiol, high-affinity DNA-reactive B cells mature to a MZ phenotype, and the mice make high tiers of anti-DNA. This outcome requires DNA antigen and is accompanied by high levels of BAFF and induction of an IFN signature.[498] Overexpression of BAFF also permits maturation of pathogenic R4A B cells in the MZ and follicular splenic compartments, with anti-dsDNA B cells escaping a regulatory checkpoint in the transitional stage of B-cell development.[499]

Lupus Following Activation of Idiotype/Anti-Idiotype Networks

Idiotypes are immunogenic amino acid sequences in the variable regions of Ig molecules. Manipulation of the idiotypic network can induce or suppress SLE in mice and has been used to develop tolerizing peptides, some of which have reached clinical trials in patients with SLE. Immunization with an Id induces anti-Id; immunization with an anti-Id induces anti–anti-Id and/or Id. This principle has been used to study murine models of SLE and of antiphospholipid syndrome. After immunization of BALB/c or other susceptible strains with Id 16/6 (a frequently occurring Id on Ig in patients with SLE) or anti-Id 16/6, a full Id/anti-Id network appeared in the mice along with autoantibodies to DNA, to phospholipids, and to snRNP particles. The mice developed leukopenia, elevated erythrocyte sedimentation rates, and Ig deposits in glomeruli.[500-502] Normal mice that were immunized with a monoclonal antiphospholipid IgM with lupus anticoagulant activity also developed an Id/anti-Id network, along with thrombocytopenia, lupus anticoagulant, and fetal loss.[503,504] These models have also been used to test multiple therapeutic interventions.[505-510] Both CD4+ and CD8+ cells may be necessary for the development of full-blown disease.[509,511]

Lupus Induced by Immunization with DNA, DNA/Proteins, RNA/Proteins, or Oligopeptides

There has been great debate regarding the nature of the inciting antigens in SLE. Most investigators agree that DNA/protein and RNA/protein molecules and particles are likely the true immunogens in mice or humans who are predisposed to SLE. In general, naked mammalian DNA is a weak immunogen and does not induce SLE in normal mice unless it is bound to a protein.[512-514] In contrast, bacterial DNA used to immunize normal mice can induce IgG antibodies to DNA (almost exclusively to ssDNA rather than dsDNA), and some animals develop immune complex nephritis.[515] Whether this DNA acquires protein after immunization is unknown. Mammalian DNA used as an immunogen also can induce IgG anti-DNA and nephritis in normal mice if it is bound to protein. Thus, immunization with nucleobindin, which probably combines with nucleosomes that are released from the thymus and other tissues, can induce anti-DNA in normal subjects,[289] as can DNA that is combined with a fusion protein.[513] Nucleosomes are particles in which DNA is wrapped around histones; they likely are direct immunogens that induce many of the autoantibodies characteristic of SLE.

Immunization of rabbits, mice, and baboons with protein or oligopeptide autoantigens (from Sm B/51, Ro 60-kd peptides, and La/SSB) have induced epitope spreading, ANAs, and proteinuria in a proportion of animals.[516-519] However, one group of investigators found more limited epitope spreading in rabbits and mice after immunization with a peptide of Sm B/B8, less ANA production, and no clinical disease.[520] These findings may reflect differences in environmental stimuli to which animals are exposed in different laboratories.

Lupus Induced by Injection of Hydrocarbon Oil

Chronic peritoneal inflammation caused by injections of hydrocarbon oils induces autoantibodies and lupus-like disease in susceptible normal mice. Activation of autoimmunity over a period of several months depends on apoptosis of peritoneal mesothelial cells providing antigens, uptake of the antigens by phagocytic cells in the peritoneum, and production of type 1 IFNs by immature monocytes and pDCs responding to TLR7 activation.[521,522] Ectopic lymphoid tissue (lipogranulomas) develops, in which B cells undergo GC-like reactions, including class switch that produces IgG autoantibodies.[523] Pristane is 2,6,10,14-tetramethylpentadecane, a terpenoid alkane usually obtained from shark liver oil and contained in mineral oil.[524] Approximately half of BALB/c mice injected once with pristane develop hypergammaglobulinemia, IgM anti-ssDNA, IgM antihistone, IgG anti-Sm, and IgG anti-Su.[525] IgG anti-RNP and anti-dsDNA can also be induced.[526] The antibodies to RNA/protein (anti-RNP and anti-Sm) depend on the expression of TLR7, but anti-dsDNA does not (it is probably mediated by TLR9).[526,527] A single injection of pristane in SJL/J mice induces anti–ribosomal P autoantibodies. SJL mice are also susceptible to experimental autoimmune encephalomyelitis, so the prominence of immune response in neurologic tissue is interesting. Furthermore, transgenic SJL mice (gonadally similar in females and males) with XX sex chromosome have greater susceptibility to pristane-induced lupus than mice with XY chromosome.[528] In association with these autoimmune responses, mice of susceptible strains develop immune complex–mediated GN.[4,525] IgM, IgG, and C3 are found in glomeruli, predominantly in mesangial areas, but proliferative GN can occur. Disease in wild-type mice (deficient for

either TLR9 or TLR4) injected with pristane shows that both TLR molecules participate. Absence of TLR9 associated with decreased glomerular Ig deposition and renal injury in the setting of reduced Th1 cytokine production and reduced titers of anti-RNP but sustained IgG anti-dsDNA. TLR4 deficiency associated with decreased renal injury in the setting of reduced Th1- and Th17-cell activation as well as reduction of both anti-RNP and anti-dsDNA.[526] Thus, activation of TLRs 4, 7, and 9 plays a role in pristane-induced lupus.

The finding that BALB/c, CBA, and DBA mice develop an inflammatory joint disease similar to rheumatoid arthritis after two intraperitoneal injections of pristane further increases interest in this animal model.[529] A variety of autoantibodies, including RF, autoantibodies to collagen type II, and antibodies to stress proteins, are detected in the serum of affected mice. Pristane-induced arthritis does not develop in specific pathogen–free mice, indicating a role for environmental infectious agents.

Because pristane selectively induces lupus-specific autoantibodies in virtually any strain of mouse regardless of its genetic background,[530] this model is increasingly being used in testing the role of various genes on lupus manifestations in transgenic and knockout mice that are generated in normal mouse backgrounds. The use of the hydrocarbon model in these experiments saves time and resources that would be required to back-cross the null mutation from the stock (usually C57BL/6-Sv129) onto genetically lupus-prone strains. Furthermore, pristane injection broadens the spectrum of lupus-like autoantibodies produced in genetically lupus-prone mice. For example, it induces anti-nRNP/Sm and Su antibodies, which are not generally detected in genetically lupus-prone NZB/NZW F1 mice. Injection with adjuvant mineral oils, such as Bayol F (incomplete Freund's adjuvant [IFA]) and squalene (MF59), also induces lupus-like autoantibody production in otherwise normal BALB/c mice.[531]

A Brief Overview of the Pathogenesis of Murine Lupus

Chapter 3 summarizes current concepts regarding the pathogenesis of SLE. Spontaneous SLE in genetically predisposed mice is associated with stem-cell abnormalities that affect both B and T lymphocytes; thymic atrophy and epithelial cell dysfunction, which diminish tolerance of autoreactive T cells; abnormalities in B-cell checkpoints that delete or anergize autoreactive cells; increases in type 1 IFN and in BAFF that result at least in part from activation of TLRs in pDCs and B cells; enhanced activation of monocytes and tissue macrophages, DCs, T and B cells; and sometimes, changes in the ability of the animal to clear apoptotic materials or immune complexes—permitting sustained antigenic stimulation and monocyte/macrophage/DC activation. Ultimately, autoantibodies that contain pathogenic subsets or form pathogenic immune complexes arise and are even synthesized locally in renal tissue. These autoantibodies/immune complexes deposit in target tissues, particularly glomeruli, where they fix complement, initiate tissue macrophage activation, attract activated monocytes, DCs, and T and B cells. Pathways leading to injury of endothelial, mesangial, and renal tubular endothelial cells are initiated, as are pathways leading to production of damaging reactive oxidative species and those leading to glomerular sclerosis and fibrosis. In different mouse strains with different genetic backgrounds, various of these processes dominate. For example, some strains develop autoantibodies with glomerular deposition and complement fixation, but little tissue damage, whereas in others the renal damage is rapid and lethal. See Box 17-6 for a summary of these processes. In otherwise healthy mice, animals can be induced to develop various manifestations and severity of lupus by manipulation of one of these several pathways to autoimmune disease (see Box 17-6). For almost all of these manipulations, susceptibility varies among mouse strains, indicating the strong role of genetics. In some cases, manipulation of the environment (including the intrinsic environment of sex hormones and the extrinsic environment of bacteria) can influence disease, but the genetics are always crucial. Addition

Box 17-6 Pathogenesis of Autoimmunity in Murine Models of SLE

- Genetic susceptibility:
  - MHC genes (NZ and BXSB)
  - Multiple genes on different chromosomes, not linked to MHC; *Nba2* from NZB, and *Sle 1, 2, 3* in New Zealand Black/White mixtures
  - Single accelerating genes: *lpr, Yaa, me* on susceptible backgrounds
- Immune abnormalities:
  - Excessive T-cell help by $CD4^+$ and $CD4^-$, $CD8^-$ cells, particularly Th1 (IFN-γ–producing), and by Th17 and by follicular T-helper (T_{FH}) cells
  - Promotion of tissue inflammation by infiltrating Th17 cells
  - Excessive B-cell activation, both T cell–dependent (in follicles) and T cell–independent (including B-1 B cells)
  - Defective generation of regulatory/inhibitory T cells, including $CD4^+CD25^+Foxp3^+$ and $CD8^+Foxp3^+$
  - Defects in bone marrow stem cells (NZ and BXSB mice)
  - Abnormal architecture and function of the thymus, with marked cortical atrophy
  - Defective clearance of apoptotic materials and immune complexes
- Production of autoantibodies:
  - Antibodies against DNA/protein and RNA/protein antigens
  - Antibodies against cell surface molecules, including erythrocytes, lymphocytes, and neurons
  - Antibodies against phospholipids
- Infiltration of target organs by T cells capable of damaging the organ
- Activation of DCs by oligonucleotides from bacteria, viruses, and DNA/anti-DNA complexes: DCs then activate various subsets of Th cells; plasmacytoid DCs release IFN-α
- Elevation of B-cell activating factor (BAFF,) which promotes survival of naïve B cells, maturation/survival to memory B cells, and plasma cells, both long- and short-lived
- Environmental factors influencing disease:
  - Diet
  - Sex hormone status
  - Infections
  - Neuroendocrine system

DC, dendritic cell; IFN, interferon; MHC, major histocompatibility complex; Th, T-helper (cell).

TABLE 17-4 Gene Targeted Strains with Lupus-Like Phenotypes

POTENTIAL MECHANISM	TARGETED GENE(S)*
Impaired apoptosis and cell cycle	Bcl-2^{Tg}, Bim, CD95^{DIT}, CDK, E2F2, Fas, Fas ligand, GADD45, IEX-1^{Tg}, Pten^{Het}, Pten$^{T cell-CKO}$
Defective clearance of DNA, apoptotic cells, and immune complexes	C1q, C4, DNase, IgM (secreted), Mer, MFG-E8, SAP
Dysregulated lymphocyte activation caused by mutations in cell receptors and their ligands	BAFF^{Tg}, CD22, CD21/CD35, CD45^{PMt}, CD152, FcγRIIB, G2A, IL-2Rβ, PD-1, Roquin, TACI, TCR-α, TGF-βRII$^{DNT or T cell-CKO}$
Dysregulated lymphocyte activation caused by intracellular signaling molecule mutations	Aiolos, Cbl-b/Vav-1, E2F2, Fli-1^{Tg}, Gadd45a, LIGHT^{Tg}, Lyn, PKC-d, P21, Rasgrp1, SHP-1, SOCS-1, Stra13, TSAd, IRAK-1 (reduces SLE)
Cytokine production abnormalities	IFN-γ^{Tg}, IL-4^{Tg}, IL-10, TGF-β
Defective hormone signaling	ER-α

*Gene-targeted mice are conventional knockout mutations unless marked as Tg (transgenic overexpression), DIT (dominant interfering transgene that causes deficiency of the targeted molecule), Het (heterozygous for the targeted gene), CKO (conditional knockout), PMT (a point mutation in CD45 prevents dimerization and negative regulation of phosphatase activity), or DNT (dominant negative transgene).

All successful interventions are most effective when they are introduced before the development of full-blown clinical lupus. The most interesting ones also are effective in mice with established disease.

Strategies That Are Widely Immunosuppressive

Cytotoxic and immunosuppressive drugs that are currently used in the management of SLE in patients have been studied in murine models of lupus. These include glucocorticoids, azathioprine, cyclophosphamide, methotrexate, cyclosporine, mycophenolate mofetil, rapamycin, and inhibition of BLyS/BAFF. Glucocorticoids suppress hemolysis and prolong life in NZB mice.[532] In BWF1 mice, murine chronic GVHD mice, and MRL-*Fas*(lpr) mice, immunosuppressive agents suppress IgG anti-dsDNA, proteinuria, glomerular Ig deposits, and nephritis, with resultant prolonged survival.[393,532-560] These agents are effective even in animals with established nephritis, although better when introduced before clinical disease appears. The effects on survival of strategies from comparable studies are shown in Figure 17-2.

Azathioprine as a single agent does not prolong survival in NZB, BWF1, or chronic GVHD mice. When it is added to glucocorticoids and/or cyclophosphamide, however, the combination is more effective than any single drug alone.[536,537]

As a single-drug intervention, cyclophosphamide is superior to glucocorticoids and azathioprine in suppressing nephritis and IgG autoantibodies, and it prolongs life in NZB, BWF1, and chronic GVHD mice.[179,536,540-544,546] It is equally effective when given daily and intermittently (Figure 17-3). In combination with glucocorticoid, it suppresses disease in MRL-*Fas*(lpr) mice[540]; combinations of cyclophosphamide and another immunosuppressive drug, such as glucocorticoid or FK506, are more effective than either drug alone.[540,548] Administration of cyclophosphamide in any regimen is associated with substantial increases in malignancies, and in some colonies azathioprine also has this effect.[179,539,545] Any combination therapy that includes cyclophosphamide suppresses lupus nephritis effectively.[540] Cyclophosphamide combined with CTLA-4–Ig (which blocks T-cell/B-cell signaling through CD80/86) is more effective than cyclophosphamide alone in suppressing nephritis, particularly in BWF1 mice that already have established disease.[561] A combination that has been used to suppress established murine lupus nephritis, then withdrawn to permit flare in order to study the biologies of

of accelerator genes to otherwise mildly susceptible genetic environments makes the disease appear earlier and progress faster, such as *Fas/1pr, gld,* and *Yaa/Tlr7,* each of which has already been discussed. In most if not all strains, MHC class II genes are critical, probably because they shape the CD4$^+$ T-cell responses that drive abnormal B cells, which are already prone to secrete large quantities of IgM and autoantibodies. Microsatellite analysis of DNA in the mouse genome has shown that multiple genes on different chromosomes are required for development of all SLE manifestations that are known to develop in susceptible strains (Table 17-4).

MURINE LUPUS MODELS USED TO TEST THERAPEUTIC INTERVENTIONS

A major advantage of each mouse model of SLE is its availability for studies of therapeutic interventions. These interventions include strategies to (1) provide general immunosuppression, (2) eliminate or inactivate Th cells, (3) inactivate/eliminate pathogenic B cells, (4) activate suppressor networks, (5) alter cytokines, (6) replace stem cells, (7) alter generation of eicosanoids, (8) alter immunoregulation via sex hormones, and (9) alter tissue damage in target organs. Interventions are summarized in Table 17-5.

TABLE 17-5 Therapeutic Interventions in Murine Lupus

INTERVENTION	STRAINS STUDIED	EFFECTS
Immunosuppressive Regimens		
1. Glucocorticoids	NZB, BWF1, MRL/*lpr*, BXSB, chronic GVHD	Prolong survival Suppress GN Suppress autoAbs Suppress T-cell abnormalities
2. Cyclophosphamide	Same as 1	Same as 1
3. Azathioprine	BWF1, chronic GVHD	Not effective as single drug; effective in combination
4. Combinations of 1-3	BWF1	More effective than one drug alone
5. Mycophenolate mofetil	BWF1, MRL/lpr	Decreases autoAb and nephritis, including sclerosis
6. Cyclosporin A	MRL/*lpr*, BXSB, BWF1	Suppresses lymphoproliferation No suppression of anti-DNA, circulating immune complexes Suppresses GN, arthritis Prolongs survival
7. FK506	MRL/*lpr*	Prolongs survival Suppresses lymphoproliferation Suppresses anti-DNA Suppresses nephritis
8. Total nodal irradiation	BWF1, MRL/lpr	Prolongs survival No suppression of anti-DNA Suppresses GN Reduction of T-cell help for months, suppression for weeks
Inhibition of T Cells		
1. Anti-CD4 (L3T4)	BWF1, MRL/*lpr*, BXSB	Prolongs life survival in pre-dz and post- Depletes or inactivates CD4$^+$ T cells, suppresses accumulation of CD8$^+$ T cells, B cells, and monocytes in lymphoid organs and kidneys Suppresses anti-DNA Suppresses GN
2. CTLA-4–Ig	BWF1	Suppresses autoAb and GN if given before disease begins Effective after nephritis onset if combined with cyclophosphamide or anti-CD40L
3. Anti-CD40L	BWF1	Suppresses autoAb and GN with reduced expression of TGF-β, interleukin-10, and TNF-α in kidneys, better effects combined with CTLA-4–Ig
4. Anti-CD137	BWF1	Suppresses autoAb and nephritis

5. Anti-Ia	BWF1	Anti-IAz:
		  Prolongs survival
		  Suppresses anti-DNA
		  Suppresses GN
		Anti-IAd less effective

6. Rapamycin	BWF1, MRL/lpr	Suppresses nephritis, suppresses innate immunity
7. Inhibition of CaMKIV	BWF1, MRL/lpr	Suppresses GN, dermatitis
Inhibition of B Cells		
1. Anti-CD20	BWF1	Suppresses GN, improved results if BAFF blockade added
2. Blockade of BAFF or BAFF/APRIL	BWF1, NZM2410, BXSB	Decreases renal damage, better results if combined with CTLA-4–Ig
3. Antiidiotypes	BWF1, MRL/*lpr*	Prolong survival Suppress anti-DNA Suppress GN
4. Deplete/diminish B-1 B cells (introduce Xid gene, give B cell superantigen)	BWF1	Suppress anti-DNA and GN
5. TACI-Ig (or ad-encoded TACI)	BWF1, MRL/lpr	Suppresses anti-DNA and GN
6. Ig peptide minigenes	BWF1	CD8$^+$ T cells that ablate anti-DNA B cells and suppress GN
7. Inhibition of Btk, Syk kinases	MRL/lpr, BWF1	Suppresses GN, dermatitis, lymphoproliferation

TABLE 17-5 Therapeutic Interventions in Murine Lupus—cont'd

INTERVENTION	STRAINS STUDIED	EFFECTS
Induction of Immune Tolerance in T and/or B Cells		
1. LJP394 (abetimus sodium; Riquent)	BXSB	Suppresses anti-DNA and GN
2. Peptides from Ig	BWF1, idiotype-induced lupus	Suppress autoAb and GN: Induce CD4$^+$CD25$^+$ and CD8$^+$ regulatory/inhibitory T cells
3. Peptides from histones	SNF1	Suppress autoAb and GN: Induce CD4$^+$CD25$^+$ and CD8$^+$ regulatory/inhibitory T cells
4. Peptide from D1 protein of Sm antigen	BWF1	Suppresses anti-DNA, induces CD4$^+$ IL-10–secreting regulatory T cells
Manipulation of Cytokines		
1. Inhibit IFN-γ	BWF1, MRL/lpr	Suppresses autoAb and GN
2. Inhibit IL-4	BWF1, NZM.2410, NZM.2328	Decreases glomerulosclerosis
3. Inhibit IL-10 (including with C-reactive protein)	BWF1, MRL/lpr	Decreases autoAb and GN
4. Inhibit IFN-α	NZB	Decreases autoAb and GN
5. Inhibit TNF-α	BWF1	Mixed results—see text
6. Inhibit TGF-β	BWF1	Supresses chronic renal lesions
7. Inhibit STAT4	MRL/lpr, C6.Sle123	Decreases autoantibodies and GN
8. Inhibit STAT6	MRL/lpr	Decreases glomerulosclerosis
9. Inhibit IL21	MRL/lpr	Decreases anti-DNA, glomerular Ig deposits
Inhibition of Innate Immunity		
1. Inhibition of Toll-like receptor 7	MRL/lpr	Decreases GN and renal damage
2. Replace bone marrow stem cells with allogeneic or T cell–depleted syngeneic cells	MRL/lpr, BWF1, BXSB	Diminishes disease
3. Reduce eicosanoids (low-calorie/fat diet, prostaglandin E, omega-3 fatty acid enriched)	NZB, BWF1, MRL/lpr, BXSB	Delays and diminishes disease
Sex Hormone Therapies		
1. Estrogens, castration	BWF1, MRL/*lpr*, BXSB	Accelerate male dz Increase IgG anti-DNA Increase nephritis Decrease survival Dramatic in BWF1, modest effects in MRL/*lpr*, no effect in BXSB males
2. Androgens plus castration or antiestrogens	BWF1, MRL/*lpr*	Suppress female dz Prolong survival Delay IgG anti-DNA Delay nephritis Dramatic in BWF1, modest effects in MRL/*lpr* females
3. Antisense nucleotides for G proteins	BWF1	Diminish anti-DNA and GN
4. Indole-3-carbinol	BWF1	Antiestrogen effect, prolongs survival

Ab, antibody; BAFF, B-cell activating factor; CTLA, cytotoxic T-lymphocyte antigen; GN, glomerulonephritis; GVHD, graft-versus-host disease; IFN, interferon; Ig, immunoglobulin; IL, interleukin; STAT, signal transducer and activator of transcription; TACI, transmembrane activator and calcium modulator and cyclophilin ligand interactor; TGF, transforming growth factor; TNF, tumor necrosis factor.

disease onset and flare, is cyclophosphamide, CTLA-4I–g and anti-CD40L.[120]

In one study, methotrexate delayed the appearance of proteinuria and prolonged survival (without decreasing anti-DNA) in BWF1 and MRL-*Fas(lpr)* mice, but it did not affect disease in (NZW×BXSB) F1 males.[547]

The effects of cyclosporine A in MRL-*Fas(lpr)*, BXSB, and NZB mice also have been studied. This drug is highly effective in suppressing lymphoproliferation; the DN T cells that are associated with *Fas/lpr* do not expand.[550-553] Cyclosporine in high doses can suppress the synthesis of anti-DNA in vitro.[553] However, B-cell hyperactivation with production of high levels of Ig, circulating immune complexes, RFs, and anti-DNA was not suppressed when the drug was given in vivo.[551,552] The effects on nephritis were variable. One group reported

no suppression of nephritis and no improvement in survival for either MRL-*Fas(lpr)* or BXSB mice,[551] whereas another reported reduction of nephritis and prolonged survival.[552] Apparently, renal damage can be suppressed without diminishing B-cell activation and autoantibody synthesis, suggesting that autoantibodies alone may be necessary, but not sufficient, for the development of lethal lupus nephritis. In one study, FK506 when given to young MRL-*Fas(lpr)* mice prevented lymphoproliferation and nephritis and also reduced titers of anti-dsDNA[554]; in another study, FK506 was more effective in combination with cyclophosphamide.[548]

Mycophenolate mofetil has been studied in BWF1 and MRL-*Fas(lpr)* mice. Mycophenolate is an inhibitor of inosine monophosphate dehydrogenase, thus inhibiting guanosine nucleotide synthesis. T and B lymphocytes depend on this pathway for their purine synthesis, whereas other types of cells have alternate pathways. Therefore, mycophenolate is relatively specific for suppression of lymphocytes, in contrast to the other drugs already discussed. In both murine lupus strains, development of nephritis was suppressed, along with autoantibodies and total numbers of lymphocytes. In comparison with cyclophosphamide, the numbers of cells infiltrating renal tissue were less with cyclophosphamide.[558-560] Mycophenolate has benefits other than reducing autoantibody levels (it is particularly effective at reducing IgG2a).[562] In particular, administration of mycophenolate (or its active metabolite, mycophenolic acid) suppresses oxidative

damage in kidneys: It decreases renal cortical expression of iNOS and urinary nitrite production, along with reducing glomerular fibronectin synthesis and glomerular sclerosis.[563,564] In support of combination therapy, a study in which mycophenolate was combined with a cyclooxygenase-2 inhibitor to reduce production of thromboxane A_2 (an eicosanoid that promotes ischemia), survival of lupus mice was better than with mycophenolate alone.[565]

Several Asian herbal preparations act as general immunosuppressants. Some of these have been effective in suppressing various manifestations of lupus in MRL-*Fas*(*lpr*) mice.[566,567]

Therapeutic irradiation has been studied in murine as well as human SLE.[546,568-572] Irradiation of BWF1 or MRL-*Fas*(*lpr*) mice, even after clinical disease is established, results in prolonged survival and markedly diminished nephritis with decreased serum levels of anti-DNA and reduced lymphoproliferation. Repeated gamma irradiation of MRL/lpr is associated with suppression of CD3+CD4−CD8− B220+ T cells that are unique to this model, upregulation of CD4+ CD25+Foxp3+ Treg cells, reduction of autoantibodies and IL-6, and suppression of nephritis.[573] In summary, immunosuppressive regimens that include glucocorticoids and/or immunosuppressive drugs, or irradiation, are impressive in their ability to reverse established nephritis, at least partially.

Strategies That Deplete, Inactivate, or Interfere with Activation Pathways in T Cells

Because CD4+ Th cells amplify autoantibody production and are required for the development of full-blown SLE in all SLE mouse models that have been studied to date, elimination or inactivation of those cells is effective in preventing disease, and even in partially reversing it once clinical nephritis is manifest. Administration of antibodies to CD4 prolongs survival, suppresses IgG anti-dsDNA and other autoantibodies, and suppresses nephritis and lymphoproliferation in NZ-derived, MRL-*Fas*(*lpr*), and BXSB mice and in normal mice that have been induced to express antiphospholipid antibodies.*
Long-term benefits require repeated treatments throughout the lifetime of the mouse. Apparently, CD4+ cells are not entirely eliminated,

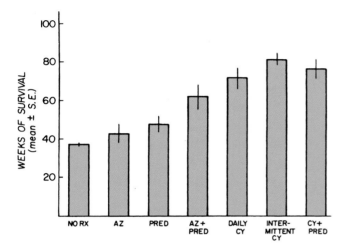

FIGURE 17-2 Survival in (NZB×N2W) F1 female mice treated from 6 weeks of age with daily oral doses of azathioprine (AZ), prednisolone (Pred), cyclophosphamide (Cy), combination therapies, or nothing (No Rx). *Bars* indicate mean weeks of survival; each *vertical line* is 1 SEM. Survival was significantly better in Pred vs. No Rx and in AZ plus Pred vs. AZ alone, Pred alone, and no RX, and was best in all groups receiving Cy, whether daily or intermittently. (*See* Hahn et al.[179])

*References 135, 210, 278, 322, 334, 399, 509, 574, 575.

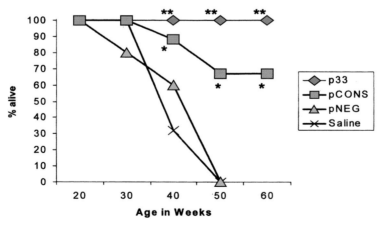

** p<.01-.05 compared to saline and APLneg, chi square test

* p<.05 compared to saline, chi square test

FIGURE 17-3 Effect of immune tolerance to peptides from autoantibody molecules on survival in (NZB/NZW) F1 mice. BWF1 females were treated from the age of 12 weeks with saline (-×-), a negative control peptide that binds major histocompatibility complex (MHC) class II I-Ed but does not cause T-cell activation (pNEG: -Δ-), a wild immunoglobulin (Ig) peptide stimulatory for BWF1 T cells, (p33: -◇-), or a synthetic peptide based on T-cell stimulatory Ig sequences (pCONSENSUS or pCONS: -□-) until 60 weeks of age. Peptides were administered as tolerogens, high doses intravenously once a month. Each group contained 5 to 15 mice. Note that all mice in the saline and pNEG groups were dead by 50 weeks of age, whereas 70% to 100% of mice tolerized with peptides that are stimulatory for T cells were still alive. Survival was significantly longer in the effectively treated groups, *P* < .01 to .05 in the p33 group compared to the saline group and pNEG by chi square test, *P* < .05 in the pCONS group compared to the saline group. Autoantibodies and cytokine increases in interferon-γ (IFN-γ) and interleukin-4 (IL-4) were all significantly delayed in the tolerized groups. These mice mounted normal T- and B-cell responses to immunization with HEL, an external foreign antigen.

or their numbers are repopulated, so that autoantibodies and disease eventually appear if the treatment is stopped.[576]

The monoclonal antibody used in all of these studies is a rat anti-mouse L3T4 (CD4); it has the advantage of inducing tolerance to itself in the recipient by preventing antibody responses that require T-cell help.[135,577,578] In earlier studies using antibodies against lymphocytes or thymocytes or Thy-1[+] cells (CD2[+] in humans), results were often obscured by the development of inactivating antibodies and of serum sickness nephritis caused by the immune response to the antilymphocyte globulin.[579-582] The rat anti-L3T4 monoclonal antibody is cytotoxic to Th cells and deletes them from the repertoire. The F(ab)₂ fragment of the monoclonal antibody is not cytotoxic because it cannot fix complement, but it inactivates L3T4[+] T cells and is as effective as the whole antibody molecule in preventing the development of anti-DNA and nephritis in BWF1 mice.[577] In addition to the predictable effects of anti-L3T4 on diminishing T-cell help and autoantibody formation, CD8[+] T cells and B220[+] B cells that infiltrate tissues, as well as CD4[+] T cells, are all diminished.[578] This finding confirms a central role for CD4[+] T cells in the evolution of activated CD8[+] and activated mature B cells, which evolve from the follicles of lymphoid tissue where they interact with T cells. In contrast to the benefit of anti-CD4 in (NZW × BXSB) F1 mice, administration of anti-CD8 worsened disease.[437]

Anti-CD4 therapy of MRL-*Fas(lpr)* mice is particularly interesting, because the lymphoproliferative component of their disease is dominated by CD3[+]CD4[−]CD8[−] B200[+] TCR α/β T cells. However, the autoantibodies, arthritis, nephritis, and central nervous system disease depend on CD4[+] T cells.[322] Treatment of MRL-*Fas(lpr)* mice with a combination of anti-CD4 and anti-CD8 abrogates most disease manifestations. However, treatment with anti-CD4 alone suppresses autoantibodies, proteinuria, histologic nephritis, arthritis, and central nervous system disease but does not affect lymphocytic proliferation and actually worsens lacrimal gland destruction.[310,322,334] The BWF1 mouse has a predictable response, because its disease depends primarily on CD4[+] cells: Administration of anti-CD8 to tolerized BWF1 mice has been found to deplete CD8[+] cells but not to influence autoantibody titers, nephritis, or survival.[583] Although anti-CD4 therapy is remarkably effective in murine lupus, its use in human disease has had disappointing results. Perhaps by the time a patient is diagnosed, desirable immune regulation has developed and depends in part on CD4[+] Treg cells, so eliminating T-cell help also eliminates T-cell regulation.

BWF1 mice have also been bred with nude mice to produce BWF1.nu/nu offspring. Nu/nu homozygotes are athymic and develop T-cell repertoires that are small in number and uneducated in the thymus. BWF1-nu/nu mice have prolonged survival associated with decreased levels of IgG anti-DNA and little development of nephritis or lymphoproliferation.[584,585] There has also been interest in interfering with second signals to disable activated CD4[+] T cells rather than all CD4[+] cells. T cells receiving only one signal (binding of their TCRs by peptides or anti-CD3) usually undergo activation only if they receive second signals via CD28/CTLA-4 interacting with CD80 and CD86 (B7-1 and B7-2) on APCs, or via CD40 interacting with CD40L (gp39, CD154) on B cells. Several groups have investigated the effect of disabling CD80 or CD86. Antibodies to CD80 plus CD86 interrupt signaling, as does soluble CTLA-4–Ig, which binds CD80 and CD86 so they cannot interact with CD28 and deliver a second signal. Such treatments are effective in delaying disease in BWF1 and BXSB mice.[214,215,400] In a study using BWF1 mice, one dose of adenovirus containing CTLA-4–Ig reduced numbers of activated T cells and affected disease as long as the protein was present. B cells requiring T-cell help were impaired, although there was no effect on intrinsic B-cell abnormalities.[586] In other studies, CTLA-4–Ig administered to lupus mice delayed autoantibody production if given prior to disease onset but was less effective in established disease. However, when it was combined with anti-CD40L (anti-CD154), TACI-Ig, or cyclophosphamide, there was dramatic suppression of autoantibodies and healing of renal lesions. Induction therapy with the combination of

CTLA-4–Ig and cyclophosphamide arrested the progression of murine lupus nephritis and precluded the need for additional therapy—a finding very exciting for its potential implications in the therapy of human lupus nephritis.[218,561,587,588]

Impairment of CD40/CD40L interactions has also been studied in murine lupus. BWF1 mice treated with anti-CD40L had reduced anti-DNA levels, diminished proteinuria, and prolonged survival.[216] Treatment with anti-CD40L also prolonged survival in SNF1 mice even if started after nephritis was clinically evident.[217] Anti-CD40L is effective in a higher proportion of mice if administered before nephritis begins, but it can suppress established renal disease in subsets of older mice, which respond with rapid reductions in renal mRNA for TGF-β, IL-10, and TNF-α.[589] One group reported that better clinical results are obtained in BWF1 mice by blocking of both CD28/B7 interactions with CTLA-4–Ig, and of CD40/CD40L interactions with anti-CD40L. In fact, 10 months after a 2-week course of both therapies, 70% of mice were alive compared with 0% to 18% of mice treated with only one of the agents.[218] It is likely that combination therapy will be more useful in human disease as well, because there are several routes to B-cell production of autoantibodies.

Inhibition of MHC class II (thus blocking the first signal to CD4[+] T cells) has been effective in treating murine lupus. One group studied the efficacy of antibodies to I-A in murine lupus.[590] (NZB/NZW) F1 mice express I-A and I-E MHC class II molecules with two alleles, d and z. Administration of antibodies directed against I-Az suppressed production of anti-DNA and development of nephritis in BWF1 mice. Anti–I-Ad was somewhat immunosuppressive, but less effective than anti–I-Az. Knockout of MHC class II in MRL-*Fas(lpr)* mice prevented the development of autoantibodies and nephritis but not of lymphoproliferation.[333] A safer strategy to block MHC-peptide activation of TCR is to provide tolerizing peptides in MHC class II molecules, discussed later. Other strategies that block T-cell function have been assessed in murine lupus. Rapamycin, which binds to mTOR (mammalian target of rapamycin) receptors in T cells, suppresses both activation in CD4[+] Th cells, including phosphorylation of proteins in the P13K and Akt pathways, and disease in BWF1 mice.[591] T cells cannot activate in the absence of formation of lipid rafts that bring mediators of activation into close physical proximity; administration of galectin, which impairs lipid raft formation, has been reported to protect young BWF1 mice from developing disease.[592] Once T cells are activated via their TCR, intracellular calcium release occurs; this process is significantly higher in T cells from humans and mice with lupus. Dipyridamole decreases activation of nuclear factor of activated T cells (NFAT), required for calcium release, and upon administration to MRL/lpr mice, suppresses production of pro-inflammatory cytokines such as IFN-γ, IL-17, and IL-6, with subsequent downregulation of Ig production.[593] High levels of calcium/calmodulin-dependent protein kinase type IV (CaMKIV) translocates to the nucleus after engagement of the TCR; inhibition of CaMKIV suppressed both nephritis and dermatitis in MRL/lpr mice as well as reducing co-stimulatory molecules on B cells and suppressing IFN-γ production.[594] Another small molecule, 4SC-101, inhibits dihydroorotate dehydrogenase, suppressing numbers of T, B, and plasma cells; it is effective in MRL/lpr lupus.[595]

Strategies That Deplete B cells or Prevent B-Cell Activation

Many interventions that deplete or interrupt B-cell development or activation also suppress murine SLE. In BWF1 females, depletion of follicular and kidney-infiltrating B cells with murine anti-CD20 in multiple doses (to also deplete relatively resistant peritoneal and MZ B cells) delayed disease onset in young mice and prolonged survival when started in mice with clinical nephritis. Addition of BAFF blockade improved results.[207]

BAFF (also called BLyS) is secreted by monocytes and other APCs and binds receptors TACI, B-cell maturation antigen (BCMA), and BAFF-R on B cells[482,596-598]; it is essential for survival of mature naïve B cells, IgG switch, and generation/survival of Ig-secreting plasma cells. BAFF also stimulates innate immunity, specifically by increasing type 1 IFN synthesis by pDCs. Blockade of BAFF with BAFF-R–Ig suppresses BWF1 lupus.[596] In one study in NZM2410 mice, blocking BAFF with soluble BAFF-R or blocking both BAFF and APRIL with TACI-Ig did not prevent autoantibody formation but depleted some B cells and memory CD4+ T cells, and decreased lymphoproliferation and activation of monocytes. Although Ig deposited in glomeruli, activation of tissue endothelial and dendritic cells was decreased, as was renal damage.[599] This work supports observations that activated B cells contribute to lupus via activation of other non-B cells, independent of their production of Ig. BAFF blockade was also found to be effective in prolonging survival in BXSB mice.[600] Administration of TACI-Ig fusion protein delayed onset of autoimmunity in BWF1 mice.[598] Administration of adenovirus-encoded soluble TACI for the purpose of inhibiting BAFF pathways reduced GN and proteinuria in MRL/lpr mice but was ineffective in BWF1 mice because of the appearance of antibodies to TACI.[601] In contrast, in the presence of T-cell blockade with CTLA-4-Ig, TACI-Ig was highly effective in BWF1 mice: It depleted B cells matured past the T1 stage, decreased numbers of activated and memory CD4+ T cells, and delayed proteinuria in spite of high titers of autoantibodies that appeared after therapy was stopped.[602] This last study suggests that treatment of SLE might require sequential or combined cytotoxics and biologics, with different times of administration or duration of therapies to optimize disease suppression. Antibody to BAFF (belimumab) has been approved for treatment of patients with SLE,[603] and TACI-Ig is currently in clinical trials in human SLE.

Specific blockade of several pathways of B-cell activation also suppresses clinical lupus in mice. *Xid* is a mutated nonreceptor, Bruton's tyrosine kinase (BTK); unmutated BTK promotes activation of nuclear factor kappa B following activation of the BCR, resulting in IgM production.[604,605] Introduction of the *Xid* gene into NZB or BWF1 mice in one study resulted in near-deletion of B-1 B cells with reduced levels of IgM. NZB.*xid* and BWF1.*xid* mice did not develop their characteristic early-life, severe lupus.[31,606,607] Inhibiting BTK with the small molecule PCI-32765 also inhibited autoantibody production and nephritis in MRL/lpr mice.[608] Stimulation of the BCR (or Fc receptors) activates pathways that include spleen tyrosine kinase. The R788 Syk kinase inhibitor prevented dermatitis and suppressed nephritis and lymphoproliferation in MRL/lpr mice[344] and in BWF1 mice, in which numbers of activated CD4+ T cells were also reduced, indicating the known interactions of T and B cells in activating each other during murine and human SLE.[609]

Cyclin-dependent kinases are involved in both T- and B-cell proliferation. Administration of a cyclin-dependent kinase inhibitor (seliciclib) to BWF1 mice has been found to delay nephritis and histologic renal damage and, in combination with methylprednisolone, to be effective in prolonging life in mice with established nephritis.[610] Another characteristic of SLE T cells is that in comparison with normal cells, the DNA is hypomethylated and the histones are hypoacetylated.[611] These epigenetic changes generally result in inability to transcribe DNA into protein. MRL/lpr mice infected with the histone deacetylase sirtuin 1 (silent mating type information regulation 2 homolog)–small interfering RNA (SIRT1-siRNA) had suppression of SIRT1 expression, elevations of acetylation on histones H3 and H4 in CD4+ T cells, and reductions of serum anti-dsDNA, glomerular IgG deposition, and histologic renal inflammation.[612] MRL/lpr mice treated with trichostatin A (an inhibitor of histone deacetylases) had reduction in nephritis.[613] DNAse treatment of BWF1 mice designed to remove DNA antigen so it could not trigger BCRs reduced numbers of anti-DNA–secreting B cells for 1 month but did not alter cytokine production, GN, or survival.[614]

Manipulation of the idiotypic network by administration of Id or anti-Id can have profound effects on the immune system, and those effects can result in either upregulation or downregulation of autoantibodies. Administration of carefully chosen Ids or anti-Ids in proper doses at the correct time can suppress Id+ anti-dsDNA and delay the onset of nephritis in BWF1 mice,[615-619] as well as

MRL-*Fas(lpr)* and SNF1 mice.[252,620] Treatment with anti-Ids conjugated to cytotoxic compounds such as neocarzinostatin is also effective in suppressing autoantibodies and nephritis in BWF1 mice, particularly if multiple anti-Ids are included in the regimen.[618,619] Anti-Ids also can suppress in vitro synthesis of autoantibodies by human B cells.[621] There are limitations to Id/anti-Id therapies, however. Some anti-Ids upregulate autoantibodies and induce lupus in mice,[622] and variations in dose and time of administration to lupus mice can profoundly influence whether immune responses are enhanced or suppressed. Beneficial responses can be short-lived, abrogated either by the escape of pathogen-enriched Ids from suppression or by emergence of autoantibodies with different Ids.

Induction of Tolerance in T and B Cells

There are several mechanisms of immune tolerance: ignorance, anergy, deletion, receptor editing (in B cells), and active suppression. One can induce tolerance in T or B lymphocytes in lupus mice by inhibiting the first activating signal (i.e., binding the TCR or BCR with the peptide or antigen it recognizes), without a second signal (via CD28, CD40, or CD137), thus inducing anergy. Alternatively tolerance results from induction of apoptosis in autoreactive cells (deletion). Finally, one can induce regulatory cells to control autoimmunity. Induction of tolerance to autoantigens in either helper T or B cells in individuals with SLE could abrogate production of pathogenic antibodies. Several laboratories have developed strategies to tolerize mice with lupus to DNA and related antigens.[623-628] Mice so treated have significant delays in the appearance of autoantibodies and nephritis. For example, intrathymic inoculation of H1-stripped chromatin into BXSB males significantly reduced T-cell proliferation to nucleosomal antigens, as well as production of IgG antichromatin, anti-dsDNA, and anti-ssDNA, for 8 to 10 weeks.[627]

Success was achieved in BXSB murine lupus by tolerizing B cells to a molecule containing short nucleotides displayed on a tetrameric scaffold (LJP294; abetimus sodium [Riquent]).[628,629] The mice had delayed appearance of IgG anti-dsDNA and nephritis and significantly prolonged survival. Administration of this agent to patients with lupus nephritis reduced antibodies to DNA (although not usually to zero) but did not prolong time to flare.[630] Another strategy for cross-linking B cells to inactivate them is to administer DNA/anti-DNA soluble immune complexes. That has been effective in improving survival of MRL-*Fas(lpr)* mice.[631]

In BWF1 mice, repeated tolerization with monthly intravenous doses of a synthetic peptide based on Th determinants in the V_H region of murine antibodies to DNA, or of combined wild Ig-derived peptides, produced dramatic delays in nephritis and prolonged survival.[632-634] Results of one series of experiments are shown in Figure 17-3. Similarly, tolerization to Th cell–activating peptides from the histone moieties of nucleosomes reduces autoantibody formation and delays Ig deposition in glomeruli in (SWR×NZB) F1 mice.[635] In all these studies, peptides that are both T-cell and B-cell epitopes and that induce tolerance to first signals in both T and B cells, were the most effective in delaying clinical disease. One group has reported that repeated oral administration of low doses of whole kidney extract reduced IgG1 and IgG3 anti-dsDNA antibody levels, diminished numbers of inflammatory cells and expression of IL-4 and IL-10 in kidney tissue (while increasing expression of IL-1, IFN-γ, and TNF-α), and prolonged survival.[636] This effect is interesting and may depend on timing of the oral preparation, because aged BWF1 mice have low intestinal IgA levels and are quite resistant to oral tolerance, which usually depends on the production of regulatory and inhibitory T cells in the mucosa-associated lymphoid tissue.[637] Our group has been successful in delaying lupus in young BWF1 mice with oral administration of a tolerogen.[638]

Strategies That Activate Suppressor Networks

Most experts suspect that one of the defects in murine and human SLE is an absence of normal suppressive immunoregulatory networks. In normal mice, Treg cells develop in both thymus and periphery; they can be CD4,[+] CD8,[+] or DN; some secrete TGF-β, others secrete IL-10, and still others suppress effector cells by contact.[639] It is also clear that regulatory B cells exist (which secrete IL-10) and there is growing evidence for regulatory monocytes/macrophages and regulatory hematopoietic cells. These cells have the capacity to prevent autoimmunity and probably function to do so in most normal individuals. Vaccination of mice with disease-inducing T cells or with certain peptides can activate suppressive networks, with at least some of the regulatory cells (CD4[+]) recognizing the TCR of the disease-upregulating T cells. De Alboran and colleagues[640] inoculated young MRL-*Fas(lpr)* mice with irradiated cells from the diseased lymph nodes of older MRL-*Fas(lpr)* mice; peripheral T cells were obtained that protected against disease in adoptive transfer experiments. Normal B cells may also serve a regulatory function; transfer of MHC-matched normal B cells into nonirradiated BWF1 mice decreased serum IgG autoantibody levels, delayed proteinuria, and prolonged life.[641] It is likely that attempts to induce regulatory networks in SLE will be successful in the near future.

Given these observations, there is currently great interest in devising strategies to induce regulatory/inhibitory T cells to prevent autoimmunity. In the tolerance therapies previously discussed, multiple simultaneous processes suppress autoimmunity. For example, in the tolerance induced in BWF1 mice by administration of a soluble 15-mer artificial peptide based on T-cell epitopes in anti-DNA, CD4[+] T-cell help is anergized, but at least two subsets of regulatory/inhibitory T cells are induced—CD4[+]CD25[+]CTLA-4[+] antigen-specific cells that suppress B cells making anti-DNA by direct contact, and CD8[+] suppressors that prevent proliferation of CD4[+] helper T cells via secretion of TGF-β.[222,233] Similarly, administration of nanomolar quantities of histone peptides that contain T-cell epitopes suppress disease in SNF1 mice, at least in part by inducing CD4[+]CD25[+] regulatory and CD8[+] inhibitory cells—each of which depends on secretion of TGF-β for activity.[221] Administration of human Ig CDR1-derived peptide (also containing T-cell epitope) to BWF1 mice also suppresses autoantibodies and nephritis and induces regulatory CD4[+]CD25[+] T cells.[642] One group reported induction of different Treg cells in BWF1 mice by intravenous injection of the D1 protein from Sm antigen; those cells were CD4[+] and secreted IFN-γ and IL-10 (but not TGF-β); the cells suppressed Th-cell proliferation and B-cell synthesis of anti-DNA.[643] The classic CD4[+]CD25[+] Treg cells are characterized by expression of Foxp3, a DNA-binding protein that may contribute to protection of the regulatory/inhibitory cells from apoptosis.[222,233] SLE can be suppressed in BWF1 mice by administration of peptide tolerogen, or by blocking of PD-1, a molecule on T cells, particularly CD8[+] T cells, that seems to control whether that cell is anergic and nonfunctional (exhausted) or can express Foxp3 and downregulate effector T and B cells.[234] Strategies to induce such cells are in progress for control of many autoimmune diseases. For example, human Treg cells with stable expression of Foxp3 can be induced in vitro by incubation with IL-2, TGF-β, and the vitamin A metabolite all-*trans* retinoic acid; these cells can protect mice from human-antimouse GVHD.[644]

Fan and Singh used a minigene vaccination approach to elicit cytotoxic/regulatory CD8[+] T cells.[645] They showed that impairment in the activation of CD8[+] Treg cells can be overcome in BWF1 mice by administering plasmid DNA vectors that encode MHC class I–binding peptides. These minigenes encoding single or multiple peptides preferentially induced CD8[+] T cells that could kill anti-DNA B cells and suppress GN in BWF1 mice. In another study, cytotoxic/regulatory CD8[+] T cells that suppressed nephritis were also induced in BWF1 mice by gene vaccination with an Ig construct encoding the immunoregulatory peptide pConsensus.[646]

Therapeutic Strategies Targeting Cytokines and Chemokines

Manipulation of cytokines/chemokines that affect T cells, B cells, or target tissue alters murine lupus. A therapy that inhibits multiple cytokines and chemokines central to SLE has been shown to be effective in MRL/lpr mice even when started after proteinuria appeared.[647] Activated protein C is a serine protease, known to be an anticoagulant and to minimize gaps between endothelial cells; when administered to the mice for 5 weeks, it reduced Th1 and Th17 cytokines, numbers of short-lived and long-lived plasma cells, numbers of total and activated DCs, inflammatory infiltrates including macrophages in glomeruli, dermis, and lungs, autoantibody levels, and serum levels of IL-12p40, IL-6, and MCP-1 (but not TNF-α). There was protection from damage in kidneys and skin. Thus the treatment served as a multitarget inhibitor of cytokines/chemokines, expansion of proinflammatory cells, and access of those cells to target organs. This might be a more effective approach than treatments targeted to single cytokines.

T cells from virtually all SLE mice develop defects in the production of IL-2 and the presentation of IL-2 receptors on their surfaces. IL-2 is required for generation of Treg cells and other suppressors, and inability of such cells to survive probably increases susceptibility to the hyperactivated T cells, B cells, monocytes, and pDCs that mediate SLE.[648] However, manipulation of IL-2 to treat murine lupus has had variable effects. Treatment of MRL-lpr mice with the human *IL2* gene delivered via live vaccinia recombinant viruses or with the murine *Il2* delivered via *Salmonella typhimurium* suppressed GN, autoantibody production, and lymph node enlargement.[649,650] However, intramuscular injections with complementary DNA expression vectors encoding the *Il2* gene increased autoantibody production in MRL-*Fas(lpr)* mice.[342] Furthermore, treatment with immunosuppressives that inhibit IL-2, such as cyclosporine and FK506, are beneficial (as discussed earlier). Rapamycin has some effects similar to those of cyclosporine and FK506—it prolongs life and reduces lymphoproliferation and nephritis in MRL-*Fas(lpr)* mice[651] and BWF1 mice.[652] Rapamycin inhibits production of many cytokines and chemokines, including renal expression of MCP-1, a feature that may account for some of its effectiveness in suppressing ingress of inflammatory cells that mediate renal damage.

IL-4 is another multifunctional cytokine. Among its antiinflammatory effects, such as promoting Th2-cell differentiation, IL-4 may directly promote damage by increasing extracellular matrix deposition in the glomeruli. Consistent with this idea, blockade of IL-4 by antibody or drug treatment, or of its signaling by inactivation of the *Stat6* gene, ameliorates glomerulosclerosis and delays or even prevents the development of end-stage renal disease, despite the presence of high levels of IgG anti-dsDNA antibodies.[262,653]

IL-6 is generally considered proinflammatory because of its promotion of Th17-cell differentiation and of B-cell activation. In BWF1 mice, administration of anti–IL-6 (with anti-CD4 to prevent T-cell responses to the Ig of the antibody) improved disease.[219] In MRL-lpr mice, IL-10 deficiency exacerbates lupus manifestations, whereas administration of recombinant IL-10 reduces IgG2a anti-dsDNA autoantibody production, presumably through inhibition of pathogenic Th1 cytokine responses, probably by Treg and B cells.[654]

In addition to increases in Th1 and Th2 cytokines in lupus mice, proinflammatory cytokines and chemokines, including IL-1, IL12, TNF-α, and MCP-—derived primarily from monocytes/macrophages—and IFN-α—derived primarily from pDCs—are increased in most strains.[341] Inhibitors of *Stat4*, through which IL-1 and IL12 signal, ameliorated nephritis in MRL/lpr mice[655]; knockout of *Stat 4* suppressed disease in B6 Sle1,Sle2,Sle3 mice.[656] Other strategies that decrease production of IL-12/IL-12 p40 and suppress murine lupus are induction of tolerance by administration of the Ig peptide hCDR1,[657] knockout of *MyD88*,[658] which mediates signaling from many TLRs, and administration of inhibitory oligodeoxynucleotides.[659] BWF1 mice, in contrast to other murine lupus strains, produce abnormally low quantities of TNF-α, which is a defect that correlates with an unusual restriction fragment–length polymorphism in the TNF-α gene.[225,660] Administration of normal recombinant TNF-α delayed the development of nephritis and prolonged survival.[225] The benefit was lost after a few months. Another study reported that low doses of TNF-α accelerated nephritis.[661]

IFN-γ, made by Th1 cells, is a cytokine of central importance in several strains of murine lupus. Administration of this cytokine worsens murine SLE in BWF1 mice; administration of antibodies to IFN-γ or of soluble IFN-γ receptors to BWF1 mice before disease begins significantly prolongs survival and diminishes Ig deposition and lymphocytic infiltration of kidneys.[171] In MRL-*Fas(lpr)* mice, antibodies to IFN-γ do not alter disease,[662] but lowering serum levels of IFN-γ with IFN-γ R/Fc molecules was effective.[663] Gene therapy of MRL-*Fas(lpr)* mice with intramuscular injections of plasmids containing complementary DNA (cDNA) encoding IFN-γ R/Fc molecules resulted in reduced serum levels of IFN-γ and diminished levels of autoantibodies, lymphoid hyperplasia, and GN, with prolonged survival. Treatment after mice had established nephritis was also effective.[663] Genetic deletion of the IFN-γ receptor significantly delayed nephritis in BWF1 mice, although the mice developed lethal lymphomas at 1 year of age.[664]

Th17 cells are proinflammatory and are found in abundance in renal lesions of BWF1 mice. Generating and sustaining Th17 depends in part on presence of IL-21. An antibody to IL-21R was effective in reducing anti-dsDNA and IgG glomerular deposits in MRL/lpr mice.[665] Th17 secretion is also characteristic of T_{FH} cells; an oral anti-CD3 preparation induced CD4$^+$ Treg cells that prevented expansion of T_{FH} in SNF1 mice.[255] Other cytokines have been studied as therapeutic agents in murine lupus. The response of MRL-*Fas(lpr)* mice to granulocyte colony–stimulating factor (G-CSF) was complex: Long-term administration of low doses accelerated nephritis, whereas high doses prolonged survival and prevented inflammation in glomeruli even in the presence of Ig deposits.[666] Another strategy for changing regulation is to provide large quantities of cytokines. Gene therapy in which cytokines in vectors were injected intramuscularly into MRL-*Fas(lpr)* mice once a month showed that IL-2 accelerated disease whereas TGF-β suppressed it.[342] TGF-β, a cytokine required for the generation of regulatory/suppressive T cells early in immune responses that is also involved in promoting glomerular sclerosis in later disease, was inhibited by administration of the angiotensin-converting enzyme inhibitor captopril to BWF1 or MRL/lpr mice either before or after proteinuria appeared. Treatment delayed proteinuria in premorbid mice and reduced chronic renal lesions in older mice, without affecting autoantibody production. Expression of both TGF-β$_1$ and TGF-β$_2$ isoforms was reduced in the kidneys, and IL-4 and IL-10 were reduced in spleen cells.[653] It is likely that timing and quantities of TGF-β are critical in obtaining either immunosuppression or suppression of sclerosis. There has also been great interest in the role of type I IFNs, particularly IFN-α, in promoting SLE. Evidence that IFN-α is important was discussed previously. Increased expression of IFN-α accelerates disease in BWF1 mice.[667] Reduction of IFN-α occurs when innate immune responses are interrupted, as discussed in the next section.

Strategies that impair chemokines that play a major role in attracting monocytes and other inflammatory cells into target tissues in SLE are effective in mouse models. For example, rapamycin suppresses MCP-1 and is clinically effective in MRL/lpr and BWF1 mice.[652,668] An RNA ODN that inhibits CCL2 prolongs survival with suppression of nephritis, dermatitis, and pulmonitis in MRL/lpr mice.[669] Administration of a CCR1 antagonist suppresses nephritis in MRL/lpr mice, with reduction of renal expression of CCL2, CCL3, CCL4, and CCL5 chemokines and of the receptors CCR1, CCR2, and CCR5.[670]

In summary, cytokines and chemokines appear to have multiple effects on the development of lupus disease. Some cytokines, such as IL-10, TGF-β, and IL-4, appear to have suppressor effects in early stages of disease through modulation of immune responses, whereas they may exacerbate late stages of disease by promoting local tissue repair and remodeling. This effect is clearly represented in many examples in which autoantibody production persists but renal damage is diminished. Doses, timing, and duration of cytokine manipulation are critical to outcome and may be achieved by many different mechanisms. In the next section we discuss inhibition of cytokine/chemokine pathways by interference with receptors that trigger innate immunity.

Strategies That Target Innate Immunity

Strategies that alter interactions among the host, innate immune responses (mediated by DCs, monocytes/macrophages, neutrophils, NK cells, and MZ B cells), and acquired immune responses (mediated by T cells, APCs, and B cells) result in reduced inflammatory responses and therefore might benefit lupus. CRP interaction with apoptotic materials facilitates their phagocytosis and clearance.[228] It is likely that this process must be intact to reduce the quantitative level of autoantigen presentation by apoptotic cells and bodies that stimulate autoantibody production. Suppressive oligonucleotides expressing TTAGGG motifs impair the activation of DCs and macrophages and therefore their release of IFNs, TNF-α, and IL-12. In one study, administration of CRP to BWF1 mice delayed nephritis but not anti-DNA formation; the benefit depended on IL-10.[230] In another, BWF1 mice transgenic for human CRP expressed primarily in renal tissue showed reduced deposition of IgM and IgG and glomerular damage.[231]

DCs, the source of many proinflammatory cytokines, recognize "dangerous" protein/lipopolysaccharide/nucleotide sequences in foreign organisms that invade the host. One of the receptor sets involved in such recognition is TLRs. Several TLRs are important in SLE. Infections may worsen SLE in part via TLR activation. For example, TLR2 is expressed on renal podocytes and endothelial cells, and TLR3 on renal mesangial cells. Triggering TLR2 with bacterial lipopeptide or TLR3 with viral dsRNA worsened murine lupus nephritis.[671,672] Inhibiting the TLRs that promote SLE (particularly endosomal TLR7, which recognizes RNA/protein, and TLR9, which recognizes DNA/protein and is upregulated by type 1 IFNs) protects from or downregulates SLE in mouse models. Blocking CpG-induced inflammation with an inhibitory ODN has been reported to protect MRL/lpr mice that already had glomerular deposits of IgG and C3 from developing renal damage.[673] Synthetic ODNs that inhibit TLR7 and/or TLR7-plus-TLR9 reduced inflammation and damage in MRL/lpr kidneys and lung.[674] (For a review, see reference 675.)

Strategies to Replace Stem Cells

An important question in SLE is whether replacement of bone marrow stem cells with allogeneic cells from MHC-compatible normal mice, or syngeneic cells that have been depleted of T cells,[356] or stem cells from humans, will prevent, delay, or heal disease. Immunoablated MRL-*Fas(lpr)* mice receiving bone marrow from MRL$^{+/+}$ or other H-2–matched strains have been found to have prolonged survival.[676] Immunoablation with radiation or high-dose cyclophosphamide followed by transfer of T cell–depleted syngeneic bone marrow also prolonged survival.[356] In BWF1 mice, transfer of bone marrow–derived pre-B cells from normal donors also suppressed autoantibody production.[677] Such stem cells can even be provided from human cord blood.[678] Mesenchymal stem cells from human bone marrow transferred to a small number of MRL/lpr mice reduced anti-DNA, proteinuria, and renal inflammation.[679] Bone marrow stem cell transfer also has benefited BXSB mice.[680] The idea behind these strategies is that stem cells inhibit host T- and - cell proliferation and autoantibody production, possibly through a paracrine effect independent of how the stem cells differentiate in vivo.

Strategies to Alter Generation of Eicosanoids: The Role of Diet

Because inflammation in murine SLE is mediated by multiple molecules, including products of arachidonic acid (AA) metabolism, there has been interest in deviating the products of AA toward less proinflammatory metabolites than the leukotrienes and thromboxanes. This can be done by giving PGE or its analogues or by altering diets. Repeated injections of PGE$_1$ suppress nephritis and prolong survival.[681-683] Two days of treating MRL-*Fas(lpr)* mice with a PGE analogue, misoprostol, reduced renal cortical IL-1 mRNA levels but not leukotrienes.[684]

Dietary factors have a major influence on murine lupus. Calorie reduction alone, to approximately 40% of the usual laboratory mouse dietary intake, significantly prolongs survival and suppresses lymphoproliferation, autoantibody production, increases in Th1 and Th2 cytokine production, and nephritis in NZB, BWF1, MRL-*Fas(lpr)*, and BXSB mice.[685-690] Restriction of dietary fat seems to be more important than restriction of protein. Diets that are rich in unsaturated fats and in omega-3 fatty acids, such as fish oil, flaxseed, menhaden oil, and eicosapentaenoic acid, are associated with better survival and markedly less lymphoproliferation, autoantibody production, nephritis, and vasculitis in NZB, BWF1, and MRL-*Fas(lpr)* mice.[686,687,691-701] In contrast, diets that are enriched in saturated fats and in omega-9 and omega-6 fatty acids are associated with reduced survival and more severe lymphoproliferation.[686,687,696,698,702]

Presumably, the omega-3 fatty acids are precursors of molecules that are less inflammatory and/or immunostimulatory than the products of omega-9 and omega-6 fatty acids. Omega-3–rich diets reduce production of leukotriene B$_4$ and tetraene peptidoleukotrienes by peritoneal macrophages, presumably reducing inflammation.[701] In addition, they increase antioxidant enzyme gene expression and decrease tissue levels of proinflammatory cytokines such as IL-6 and TNF-α.[689,702] T cells from SNF1 mice express increased levels of cyclooxygenase-2. Blockade of prostaglandin production by administration of a cyclooxygenase 2 enzyme inhibitor (celecoxib) to SNF1 mice decreased autoantibodies and T-cell responses to nucleosomes, and prolonged survival when doses were low and intermittent.[703]

Dietary factors that are unrelated to lipids also influence murine lupus. BWF1 mice raised on a casein-free diet had diminished anti-DNA and nephritis and improved survival.[704] Alfalfa seeds fed to cynomolgus macaque monkeys were associated with the development of autoimmune hemolytic anemia and ANAs.[705] When the seeds were autoclaved before administration, however, the disease did not occur.[706] Several investigators have attributed this phenomenon to the presence of L-canavanine, which is a nonprotein amino acid, in alfalfa. L-Canavanine is immunostimulatory and increases the proliferation of lymphocytes to mitogens and antigens.[707,708] The importance of this finding in human SLE, however, is unknown. Supplementation of diet with soy isoflavones reduced disease severity and improved survival in MRL/lpr mice; anti-DNA and IFN-γ production was lower than in controls, but levels of ERβ were higher.[709]

Strategies That Manipulate Sex Hormones

The influence of sex hormones on murine lupus is highly variable, depending on the strain. Hybrid mice that are derived from NZ backgrounds, especially BWF1 mice, are exquisitely sensitive to the effects of sex hormones. Females are protected from severe early-life lupus by castration plus androgenic hormone or by antiestrogens.* Estrogens worsen their disease, probably through toxic effects as well as immunostimulation.[183] Males develop early-onset severe SLE rather than their usual late-onset disease if they are castrated and treated with estrogenic hormones or antiandrogens.[185,187,710] Whether this development relates to the modification of immune responses by sex hormone receptors in immune cells or to modification of gene expression is unclear. In contrast, male BXSB mice develop rapid-onset, early-life lupus whether or not they are castrated or receive sex hormones.[710] The effects in MRL-*Fas(lpr)* mice are intermediate; that is, estrogenic hormones tend to worsen and androgenic hormones to suppress disease manifestations, but the effects are less dramatic than in BWF1 mice.[710] In fact, the effects of estrogen in MRL-*Fas(lpr)* mice are to worsen renal disease but to lessen vasculitis and sialadenitis.[712] This could result from the simultaneous stimulation of antibody responses and suppression of T cell– and NK cell–mediated

immunity,[194] but the effects of sex hormones are doubtless more complicated than that. Studies in normal mice transgenic for Ig genes that encode anti-DNA show that estrogen affects B-cell tolerance and permits survival of autoreactive B cells.[195] Administration of tamoxifen to MRL-*Fas(lpr)* mice and to BWF1 mice reduces renal damage and prolongs survival.[713] Prolactin worsens lupus in BWF1 mice, whereas bromocriptine suppresses it.[189-191,714] Strategies that reduce sex hormone levels include administration of antisense oligonucleotides to Galpha(Q/11), which inhibits the G proteins required to transmit the effect of gonadotropin-releasing hormone. BWF1 mice receiving the antisense oligonucleotides had reduced levels of autoantibodies and proteinuria, with inhibition of IL-6 production.[715] A diet enriched in indole-3-carbinol, an anti-estrogen abundant in cruciferous vegetables, when given to BWF1 mice resulted in lower levels of anti-DNA, less severe nephritis, and dramatic improvement in survival.[716] Studies in this interesting area are likely to expand in the next few years.

Strategies That Protect Target Organs from Damage after Immunoglobulin Deposition

Protecting tissue from damage induced by deposition of Igs, rather than altering Ig production, is another strategy for treating lupus. For example, administration of NG-monomethyl-L-arginine, which suppresses nitric oxide production, reduces the severity of arthritis and nephritis in MRL-*Fas(lpr)* mice.[717] High quantities of iNOS are expressed in kidneys of MRL-*Fas(lpr)* mice after nephritis begins; administration of linomide significantly decreases iNOS mRNA levels and prevents development of nephritis.[718] Similarly, administration of aminoguanidine reduced glomerular expression of both iNOS and TGF-β mRNA in BWF1 mice: This effect was associated with less glomerulosclerosis.[719] Rapamycin administration to BWF1 mice inhibits monocyte/macrophage and lymphocytic infiltration into kidneys, even though deposition of Ig and complement fixation have occurred, with resultant improvement in survival.[652] Combined treatment with antibodies to LFA-1A and ICAM-1 reduced Ig and C3 deposition in glomeruli and prolonged survival in mice treated after induction of chronic GVHD.[720] Inhibition of thromboxane A and endothelin receptors reduced histologic renal damage, hypertension, and proteinuria in BWF1 mice.[721] Administration of heparin or a heparinoid prevented binding of nucleosome/antinucleosome immune complexes to glomerular basement membrane of BALB/c mice and delayed proteinuria and histologic glomerular damage in MRL-*Fas(lpr)* mice for several weeks.[722] Another method to prevent damage is to inhibit development of activated terminal components of complement proteins. Administration of a monoclonal antibody specific for the C5 component of complement blocked cleavage of C5 and generation of C5a and C5b-9. Continuous therapy with anti-C5 for 6 months reduced nephritis and increased survival in BWF1 mice.[723] Finally, deposition of immune complexes in glomeruli can be prevented by administration of a soluble peptide selected from a peptide display library for reaction with a mouse monoclonal pathogenic anti-DNA antibody (but not with nonpathogenic monoclonal antibodies).[724]

Miscellaneous Interventions

A review by Perl highlights several additional strategies that might suppress SLE.[725] Exposure of BWF1 mice to ultraviolet (UV) A light was associated with prolonged survival, reduced lymphoproliferation, and suppression of anti-DNA antibodies.[726] In contrast, exposure of BXSB mice to ultraviolet B light exacerbated disease.[727]

Disease in MRL-*Fas(lpr)* mice has been successfully suppressed by the administration of cholera toxin[728] and of a platelet-activating factor receptor antagonist.[729] Administration of a single dose of thalidomide to NZB, MRL/++, and MRL-*Fas(lpr)* mice diminished the production of IgM and/or IgG, probably by reducing the numbers of CD5+ B cells.[730] The value of these strategies (and of others not mentioned here) depends on whether these findings can be confirmed and the role of these compounds in altering disease elucidated.

*References 181, 184, 185, 187, 710, 711.

LUPUS IN DOMESTIC ANIMALS

Spontaneous lupus-like disease has been reported in several animal species other than mice, including dogs, cats, rats, rabbits, guinea pigs, pigs, monkeys, hamsters, and Aleutian minks.[731-744] The largest body of literature addresses SLE in dogs.

Spontaneous Canine SLE

The canine lupus model is particularly interesting because of its clinical similarity to human SLE. Like human SLE, canine lupus is a chronic disease with alternating periods of remission and relapse. In contrast, such a cyclic evolution is not observed in mice with lupus, in which the disease steadily progresses to its terminal stage. Frequent manifestations in canine lupus include fever, polyarthritis (91%), GN (65%), mucocutaneous lesions (60%), ulcerating dermatitis, lymphadenopathy, and splenomegaly.[742] Other less common manifestations include hemolytic anemia, thrombocytopenia, and clotting.[738,740-742,744-747] Bullous, discoid, and systemic type skin lesions can occur. The predominant autoantibodies, occurring in more than 90% of dogs with SLE, are ANAs and antibodies directed against individual histones. ANAs are induced commonly in dogs with various infections.[748] Homogeneous patterns in Hep2 cells are characteristic of SLE.[749] Antibodies against ssDNA, dsDNA, Ro/SSA, Sm, RNP, lymphocytes, and platelets are found, but in less than 30%.[737,741,746,747,750-752] The H130 Id that is characteristic of anti-DNA from MRL-*Fas(lpr)* mice has been found on anti-DNA in dogs.[753] Effective interventions include glucocorticoids, levamisole, apheresis, and tetracyclines. Most dogs show responses.

In dogs, the disease can be sporadic or familial. A colony of dogs particularly susceptible to SLE was created by breeding a male and female German shepherd, each of which had SLE. As healthy sires were introduced to mate with F1 and F2 generations, the disease prevalence declined.[732,738] There is a genetic association with MHC, particularly DR (class II) as in mice and in humans.[754] A genome-wide association mapping in Nova Scotia duck-trolling retrievers (a breed with a high prevalence of SLE) showed that HLA and four additional gene regions increased risk for canine SLE. Most of the gene regions are associated with T-cell activation, particularly via the NFAT pathway that controls calcium influx.[755]

Because of concern that SLE may be transmitted by viruses, studies have been done to determine whether SLE in humans is more common among owners of dogs with SLE. A study of 83 members of 23 households with 19 dogs that had high-titer ANAs showed no excess in the number of cases of human SLE.[756]

Induced Model of Canine SLE

Normal dogs immunized with heparan sulfate, the major glycosaminoglycan of the glomerular basement membrane, have been reported to develop ANAs, proteinuria, and skin disease as well as marked deposition of IgM and C3 in the dermoepidermal junctions of the skin.[757] Cutaneous signs associated with SLE included alopecia, erythema, crusting, scaling, and seborrhea. Three of eight dogs showed lameness. Therefore, the heparan sulfate–immunized dog can be useful as a canine SLE model for studying immune-mediated skin disease and autoimmunity.

SLE in Cats, Monkeys, and Horses

SLE in cats usually is a spontaneous disease.[758] Analyses of clinical features in 22 cases showed that GN (in 10 cases), neurologic signs (in 9 cases), arthritis (in 9), anemia (in 8), and dermatologic signs (in 7) were frequent manifestations.[759] Other manifestations were fever, lymphadenopathy, mucocutaneous ulcers, and thrombocytopenia. In addition to spontaneous diseases, there has been interest in a series of experiments in which the administration of propylthiouracil to cats induces autoantibodies and autoimmune hemolytic anemia.[760]

SLE in monkeys can be induced by feeding macaques alfalfa seeds, probably because of the immunostimulatory properties of the L-canavanine nonprotein amino acid that the seeds contain.[705-708]

SLE is rarely reported in horses. In these cases, the horses were reported to demonstrate polyarthritis, proteinuria, thrombocytopenia, and presence of ANAs in one case[761] and weight loss, Coombs-positive anemia, alopecia, ulcerative glossitis, generalized lymphadenopathy, and skin inflammation with dermoepidermal Ig deposits on biopsy in another case.[762]

Attempts have been made to induce SLE in animals by transferring plasma from patients with SLE. Histologic evidence of GN was produced by repeated infusions of human plasma containing LE factors into healthy dogs in one set of experiments[763] but not in another.[764] Similar experiments were unsuccessful in guinea pigs.

Efforts to induce lupus-like disease in various animals by administering lupus-inducing drugs have been largely unsuccessful. Hydralazine and procainamide have been given to dogs, guinea pigs, swine, and rats, but with little evidence of autoimmune responses.[765] On the other hand, immunization of rabbits, mice, and baboons with protein or oligopeptide autoantigens (from Sm B/B8, Ro 60-kd peptides, and La/SSB) have induced epitope spreading, ANAs, and proteinuria in a proportion of animals.[516-519] Differences in proportions of animals that develop autoantibodies in different experiments may reflect differences in environmental stimuli to which animals are exposed in different laboratories.

Finally, dogs have been studied for evidence of vertical transmission of infectious agents that cause SLE. In breeding studies performed by Lewis and Schwartz, the incidence of positive LE cell test results in inbred back-crosses and out-cross matings was not consistent with any conventional mechanisms of inheritance.[733] The investigators concluded that the results could be explained by vertical transmission of an infectious agent in a genetically susceptible individual. Cell-free filtrates of tissues from seropositive dogs also have been injected into newborn mice,[733] and these mice developed ANAs and, in some cases, lymphomas. Passage of cells or filtrates from the tumors to normal newborn puppies resulted in ANA production or positive LE cell test results. C-type RNA viruses were identified in the tumors. In cats, autoimmunity is highly associated with the feline leukemia virus.[735] It may be that autoimmune disease similar to human SLE is more closely linked to viral infections in dogs and cats than in humans.

USE AND ANALYSIS OF ANIMAL STRAINS FOR LUPUS RESEARCH

A variety of animal strains develop lupus-like disease, each with particular clinical manifestations and pathogenesis, representing different stages or subsets of SLE. Although selection of the model that truly represents human SLE remains debated, investigators have chosen models based on the clinical manifestation or phenomena of interest within the lupus autoimmune spectrum. For example, NZB/Bl mice may be most suitable to study autoimmune hemolytic anemia; BWF1 and NZM strains have been extensively studied for anti-dsDNA antibody production, T-cell autoreactivity, and typical progressive lupus nephritis. MRL-lpr/lpr mice, on the other hand, can serve as a model for a more multisystem disease, such as lupus dermatitis, arthritis, fulminant interstitial nephritis, or lymphadenopathy as well as for autoantibodies against multiple antigens. Although not extensively investigated, canine SLE may serve as a model for relapsing-remitting disease with clinical manifestations that more closely mimic those of human SLE. Induced SLE models such as hydrocarbon oil–induced lupus in otherwise normal mouse strains may be particularly useful in investigating the role of various genes in the pathogenesis of lupus using gene-targeted strains that are not normally lupus-prone, because it may save the 2 years or more that is required to back-cross the null genotype from the stock strains (usually C57BL6/Sv129) onto the lupus-prone backgrounds.

References

1. Singh RR: SLE: translating lessons from model systems to human disease. *Trends Immunol* 26:572–579, 2005.

2. Deocharan B, Marambio P, Edelman M, et al: Differential effects of interleukin-4 in peptide induced autoimmunity. *Clin Immunol* 108:80–88, 2003.
3. Richards HB, Satoh M, Jennette JC, et al: Interferon-gamma is required for lupus nephritis in mice treated with the hydrocarbon oil pristane. *Kidney Int* 60:2173–2180, 2001.
4. Yang JQ, Singh AK, Wilson MT, et al: Immunoregulatory role of CD1d in the hydrocarbon oil-induced model of lupus nephritis. *J Immunol* 171:2142–2153, 2003.
5. Peng SL: Experimental use of murine lupus models. *Methods Mol Med* 102:227–272, 2004.
6. Jorgensen TN, Gubbels MR, Kotzin BL: Links between type I interferons and the genetic basis of disease in mouse lupus. *Autoimmunity* 36:491–502, 2003.
7. Wakeland EK, Liu K, Graham RR, et al: Delineating the genetic basis of systemic lupus erythematosus. *Immunity* 15:397–408, 2001.
8. Bielschowsky M, Helyer BJ, Howie JB: Spontaneous haemolytic anaemia in mice of the NZB/B1 strain. *Proc Univ Otago Med Sch (NZ)* 37:9–11, 1959.
9. Helyer BJ, Howie JB: The thymus and autoimmune disease. *Lancet* 2(7316):1026–1029, 1963.
10. Andrews BS, Eisenberg RA, Theofilopoulos AN, et al: Spontaneous murine lupus-like syndromes. Clinical and immunopathological manifestations in several strains. *J Exp Med* 148:1198–1215, 1978.
11. Yoshida S, Castles JJ, Gershwin ME: The pathogenesis of autoimmunity in New Zealand mice. *Semin Arthritis Rheum* 19:224–242, 1990.
12. DeHeer DH, Edgington TS: Evidence for a B lymphocyte defect underlying the anti-X anti-erythrocyte autoantibody response of NZB mice. *J Immunol* 118:1858–1863, 1977.
13. Milich DR, Gershwin ME: The pathogenesis of autoimmunity in New Zealand mice. *Semin Arthritis Rheum* 10:111–147, 1980.
14. Shirai T, Mellors RC: Natural thymocytotoxic autoantibody and reactive antigen in New Zealand black and other mice. *Proc Natl Acad Sci U S A* 68:1412–1415, 1971.
15. Bray KR, Gershwin ME, Ahmed A, et al: Tissue localization and biochemical characteristics of a new thymic antigen recognized by a monoclonal thymocytotoxic autoantibody from New Zealand black mice. *J Immunol* 134:4001–4008, 1985.
16. Bray KR, Gershwin ME, Chused T, et al: Characteristics of a spontaneous monoclonal thymocytotoxic antibody from New Zealand Black mice: recognition of a specific NTA determinant. *J Immunol* 133:1318–1324, 1984.
17. Ohgaki M, Ueda G, Shiota J, et al: Two distinct monoclonal natural thymocytotoxic autoantibodies from New Zealand black mouse. *Clin Immunol Immunopathol* 53:475–487, 1989.
18. De Heer DH, Edgington TS: Clonal heterogeneity of the anti-erythrocyte autoantibody responses of NZB mice. *J Immunol* 113:1184–1189, 1974.
19. Meryhew NL, Handwerger BS, Messner RP: Monoclonal antibody-induced murine hemolytic anemia. *J Lab Clin Med* 104:591–601, 1984.
20. Barker RN, de Sa Oliveira GG, Elson CJ, et al: Pathogenic autoantibodies in the NZB mouse are specific for erythrocyte band 3 protein. *Eur J Immunol* 23:1723–1726, 1993.
21. Hall AM, Ward FJ, Shen CR, et al: Deletion of the dominant autoantigen in NZB mice with autoimmune hemolytic anemia: effects on autoantibody and T-helper responses. *Blood* 110:4511–4517, 2007.
22. Perry FE, Barker RN, Mazza G, et al: Autoreactive T cell specificity in autoimmune hemolytic anemia of the NZB mouse. *Eur J Immunol* 26:136–141, 1996.
23. Hentati B, Payelle-Brogard B, Jouanne C, et al: Natural autoantibodies are involved in the haemolytic anaemia of NZB mice. *J Autoimmun* 7:425–439, 1994.
24. Pau E, Chang NH, Loh C, et al: Abrogation of pathogenic IgG autoantibody production in CD40L gene-deleted lupus-prone New Zealand Black mice. *Clin Immunol* 139:215–227, 2011.
25. Bielschowsky M, D'Ath EF: The kidneys of NZB-B1, NZO-B1, NZC-B1 and NZY-B1 mice. *J Pathol* 103:97–105, 1971.
26. Hicks JD, Burnet FM: Renal lesions in the "auto-immune" mouse strains NZB and F1 NZB × NZW. *J Pathol Bacteriol* 91:467–476, 1966.
27. Schrott LM, Denenberg VH, Sherman GF, et al: Environmental enrichment, neocortical ectopias, and behavior in the autoimmune NZB mouse. *Brain Res Dev Brain Res* 67:85–93, 1992.
28. Harbeck RJ, Hoffman AA, Hoffman SA, et al: A naturally occurring antibody in New Zealand mice cytotoxic to dissociated cerebellar cells. *Clin Exp Immunol* 31:313–320, 1978.
29. Tehrani MJ, Hu Y, Marquette C, et al: Interleukin-1 receptor deficiency in brains from NZB and (NZB/NZW)F1 autoimmune mice. *J Neuroimmunol* 53:91–99, 1994.
30. Moutsopoulos HM, Boehm-Truitt M, Kassan SS, et al: Demonstration of activation of B lymphocytes in New Zealand black mice at birth by an immunoradiometric assay for murine IgM. *J Immunol* 119:1639–1644, 1977.
31. Taurog JD, Moutsopoulos HM, Rosenberg YJ, et al: CBA/N X-linked B-cell defect prevents NZB B-cell hyperactivity in F1 mice. *J Exp Med* 150:31–43, 1979.
32. Theofilopoulos AN, Shawler DL, Eisenberg RA, et al: Splenic immunoglobulin-secreting cells and their regulation in autoimmune mice. *J Exp Med* 151:446–466, 1980.
33. Schwieterman WD, Manoussakis M, Klinman DM, et al: Studies of marrow progenitor abnormalities in lupus-prone mice. II. Further studies of NZB Thy 1(neg)Lin(neg) bone marrow cells. *Clin Immunol Immunopathol* 72:114–120, 1994.
34. Merchant MS, Garvy BA, Riley RL: B220-bone marrow progenitor cells from New Zealand black autoimmune mice exhibit an age-associated decline in pre-B and B-cell generation. *Blood* 85:1850–1857, 1995.
35. Anderson CC, Cairns E, Rudofsky UH, et al: Defective antigen-receptor-mediated regulation of immunoglobulin production in B cells from autoimmune strains of mice. *Cell Immunol* 164:141–149, 1995.
36. Marti GE, Metcalf RA, Raveche E: The natural history of a lymphoproliferative disorder in aged NZB mice. *Curr Top Microbiol Immunol* 194:117–126, 1995.
37. Raveche ES, Phillips J, Mahboudi F, et al: Regulatory aspects of clonally expanded B-1 (CD5+ B) cells. *Int J Clin Lab Res* 22:220–234, 1992.
38. Hayakawa K, Hardy RR, Herzenberg LA: Peritoneal Ly-1 B cells: genetic control, autoantibody production, increased lambda light chain expression. *Eur J Immunol* 16:450–456, 1986.
39. Brummel R, Lenert P: Activation of marginal zone B cells from lupus mice with type A(D) CpG-oligodeoxynucleotides. *J Immunol* 174:2429–2434, 2005.
40. Conger JD, Pike BL, Nossal GJ: Clonal analysis of the anti-DNA repertoire of murine B lymphocytes. *Proc Natl Acad Sci U S A* 84:2931–2935, 1987.
41. Murakami M, Yoshioka H, Shirai T, et al: Prevention of autoimmune symptoms in autoimmune-prone mice by elimination of B-1 cells. *Int Immunol* 7:877–882, 1995.
42. Dinesh R, Hahn BH, La Cava A, et al: Interferon-inducible gene 202b controls CD8(+) T cell-mediated suppression in anti-DNA Ig peptide-treated (NZB×NZW) F1 lupus mice. *Genes Immun* 12:360–369, 2011.
43. Rozzo SJ, Allard JD, Choubey D, et al: Evidence for an interferon-inducible gene, Ifi202, in the susceptibility to systemic lupus. *Immunity* 15:435–443, 2001.
44. Lian ZX, Kikuchi K, Yang GX, et al: Expansion of bone marrow IFN-alpha-producing dendritic cells in New Zealand Black (NZB) mice: high level expression of TLR9 and secretion of IFN-alpha in NZB bone marrow. *J Immunol* 173:5283–5289, 2004.
45. de Vries MJ, Hijmans W: Pathological changes of thymic epithelial cells and autoimmune disease in NZB, NZW and (NZB×NZW)F1 mice. *Immunology* 12:179–196, 1967.
46. Gershwin ME, Ikeda RM, Kruse WL, et al: Age-dependent loss in New Zealand mice of morphological and functional characteristics of thymic epithelial cells. *J Immunol* 120:971–979, 1978.
47. Whittum J, Goldschneider I, Greiner D, et al: Developmental abnormalities of terminal deoxynucleotidyl transferase positive bone marrow cells and thymocytes in New Zealand mice: effects of prostaglandin E1. *J Immunol* 135:272–280, 1985.
48. Fletcher AL, Seach N, Reiseger JJ, et al: Reduced thymic Aire expression and abnormal NF-kappa B2 signaling in a model of systemic autoimmunity. *J Immunol* 182:2690–2699, 2009.
49. Minoda M, Senda S, Horiuchi A: The relationship between the defect in the syngeneic mixed lymphocyte reaction and thymic abnormality in New Zealand mice. *J Clin Lab Immunol* 23:101–108, 1987.
50. Hayes SM, Greiner DL: Evidence for elevated prothymocyte activity in the bone marrow of New Zealand Black (NZB) mice. Elevated prothymocyte activity in NZB mice. *Thymus* 19:157–172, 1992.
51. Okada T, Inaba M, Naiki M, et al: Comparative immunobiology of thymic DC mRNA in autoimmune-prone mice. *J Autoimmun* 28:41–45, 2007.
52. Drake CG, Babcock SK, Palmer E, et al: Genetic analysis of the NZB contribution to lupus-like autoimmune disease in (NZB×NZW)F1 mice. *Proc Natl Acad Sci U S A* 91:4062–4066, 1994.

53. Kono DH, Burlingame RW, Owens DG, et al: Lupus susceptibility loci in New Zealand mice. *Proc Natl Acad Sci U S A* 91(21):10168–10172, 1994.

54. Vyse TJ, Rozzo SJ, Drake CG, et al: Control of multiple autoantibodies linked with a lupus nephritis susceptibility locus in New Zealand black mice. *J Immunol* 158:5566–5574, 1997.

55. Rozzo SJ, Vyse TJ, Drake CG, et al: Effect of genetic background on the contribution of New Zealand black loci to autoimmune lupus nephritis. *Proc Natl Acad Sci U S A* 93(26):15164–15168, 1996.

56. Rigby RJ, Rozzo SJ, Boyle JJ, et al: New loci from New Zealand Black and New Zealand White mice on chromosomes 4 and 12 contribute to lupus-like disease in the context of BALB/c. *J Immunol* 172:4609–4617, 2004.

57. Ochiai K, Ozaki S, Tanino A, et al: Genetic regulation of anti-erythrocyte autoantibodies and splenomegaly in autoimmune hemolytic anemia-prone New Zealand black mice. *Int Immunol* 12:1–8, 2000.

58. Drake CG, Rozzo SJ, Hirschfeld HF, et al: Analysis of the New Zealand Black contribution to lupus-like renal disease. Multiple genes that operate in a threshold manner. *J Immunol* 154:2441–2447, 1995.

59. Hirose S, Tsurui H, Nishimura H, et al: Mapping of a gene for hypergammaglobulinemia to the distal region on chromosome 4 in NZB mice and its contribution to systemic lupus erythematosus in (NZB×NZW)F1 mice. *Int Immunol* 6:1857–1864, 1994.

60. Jiang Y, Hirose S, Hamano Y, et al: Mapping of a gene for the increased susceptibility of B1 cells to Mott cell formation in murine autoimmune disease. *J Immunol* 158:992–997, 1997.

61. Xie S, Li L, Chang S, et al: Genetic origin of lupus in NZB/SWR hybrids: lessons from an intercross study. *Arthritis Rheum* 52:659–667, 2005.

62. Vyse TJ, Drake CG, Rozzo SJ, et al: Genetic linkage of IgG autoantibody production in relation to lupus nephritis in New Zealand hybrid mice. *J Clin Invest* 98:1762–1772, 1996.

63. Lee NJ, Rigby RJ, Gill H, et al: Multiple loci are linked with anti-red blood cell antibody production in NZB mice—comparison with other phenotypes implies complex modes of action. *Clin Exp Immunol* 138:39–46, 2004.

64. Kikuchi S, Amano H, Amano E, et al: Identification of 2 major loci linked to autoimmune hemolytic anemia in NZB mice. *Blood* 106:1323–1329, 2005.

65. Ozaki S, Honda H, Maruyama N, et al: Genetic regulation of erythrocyte autoantibody production in New Zealand black mice. *Immunogenetics* 18:241–254, 1983.

66. Scatizzi JC, Haraldsson KM, Pollard KM, et al: The *Lbw2* locus promotes autoimmune hemolytic anemia. *J Immunol* 188:3307–3314, 2012.

67. Knight JG, Adams DD: Genes determining autoimmune disease in New Zealand mice. *J Clin Lab Immunol* 5:165–170, 1981.

68. Haraldsson MK, dela Paz NG, Kuan JG, et al: Autoimmune alterations induced by the New Zealand Black Lbw2 locus in BWF1 mice. *J Immunol* 174:5065–5073, 2005.

69. Xu Z, Duan B, Croker BP, et al: Genetic dissection of the murine lupus susceptibility locus Sle2: contributions to increased peritoneal B-1a cells and lupus nephritis map to different loci. *J Immunol* 175:936–943, 2005.

70. Xu Z, Potula HH, Vallurupalli A, et al: Cyclin-dependent kinase inhibitor Cdkn2c regulates B cell homeostasis and function in the NZM2410-derived murine lupus susceptibility locus Sle2c1. *J Immunol* 186:6673–6682, 2011.

71. Jorgensen TN, Alfaro J, Enriquez HL, et al: Development of murine lupus involves the combined genetic contribution of the SLAM and FcgammaR intervals within the Nba2 autoimmune susceptibility locus. *J Immunol* 184:775–786, 2010.

72. Fujii T, Hou R, Sato-Hayashizaki A, et al: Susceptibility loci for the defective foreign protein-induced tolerance in New Zealand Black mice: implication of epistatic effects of Fcgr2b and Slam family genes. *Eur J Immunol* 41:2333–2340, 2011.

73. Jiang Y, Hirose S, Abe M, et al: Polymorphisms in IgG Fc receptor IIB regulatory regions associated with autoimmune susceptibility. *Immunogenetics* 51:429–435, 2000.

74. Xiu Y, Nakamura K, Abe M, et al: Transcriptional regulation of Fcgr2b gene by polymorphic promoter region and its contribution to humoral immune responses. *J Immunol* 169:4340–4346, 2002.

75. Boross P, Arandhara VL, Martin-Ramirez J, et al: The inhibiting Fc receptor for IgG, FcgammaRIIB, is a modifier of autoimmune susceptibility. *J Immunol* 187:1304–1313, 2011.

76. Fukuyama H, Nimmerjahn F, Ravetch JV: The inhibitory Fcgamma receptor modulates autoimmunity by limiting the accumulation of immunoglobulin G+ anti-DNA plasma cells. *Nat Immunol* 6:99–106, 2005.

77. Wetsel RA, Fleischer DT, Haviland DL: Deficiency of the murine fifth complement component (C5). A 2-base pair gene deletion in a 5′-exon. *J Biol Chem* 265:2435–2440, 1990.

78. Shibata T, Berney T, Reininger L, et al: Monoclonal anti-erythrocyte autoantibodies derived from NZB mice cause autoimmune hemolytic anemia by two distinct pathogenic mechanisms. *Int Immunol* 2:1133–1141, 1990.

79. Mohan C, Morel L, Yang P, et al: Genetic dissection of lupus pathogenesis: a recipe for nephrophilic autoantibodies. *J Clin Invest* 103:1685–1695, 1999.

80. Mohan C, Yu Y, Morel L, et al: Genetic dissection of SLE pathogenesis: Sle3 on murine chromosome 7 impacts T cell activation, differentiation, and cell death. *J Immunol* 162:6492–6502, 1999.

81. Sobel ES, Mohan C, Morel L, et al: Genetic dissection of SLE pathogenesis: adoptive transfer of Sle1 mediates the loss of tolerance by bone marrow-derived B cells. *J Immunol* 162:2415–2421, 1999.

82. Mohan C, Morel L, Yang P, et al: Accumulation of splenic B1a cells with potent antigen-presenting capability in NZM2410 lupus-prone mice. *Arthritis Rheum* 41:1652–1662, 1998.

83. Mohan C, Alas E, Morel L, et al: Genetic dissection of SLE pathogenesis. Sle1 on murine chromosome 1 leads to a selective loss of tolerance to H2A/H2B/DNA subnucleosomes. *J Clin Invest* 101:1362–1372, 1998.

84. Mohan C, Morel L, Yang P, et al: Genetic dissection of systemic lupus erythematosus pathogenesis: Sle2 on murine chromosome 4 leads to B cell hyperactivity. *J Immunol* 159:454–465, 1997.

85. Morel L, Mohan C, Yu Y, et al: Functional dissection of systemic lupus erythematosus using congenic mouse strains. *J Immunol* 158:6019–6028, 1997.

86. Vyse TJ, Morel L, Tanner FJ, et al: Backcross analysis of genes linked to autoantibody production in New Zealand White mice. *J Immunol* 157:2719–2727, 1996.

87. Morel L, Yu Y, Blenman KR, et al: Production of congenic mouse strains carrying genomic intervals containing SLE-susceptibility genes derived from the SLE-prone NZM2410 strain. *Mamm Genome* 7:335–339, 1996.

88. Morel L, Croker BP, Blenman KR, et al: Genetic reconstitution of systemic lupus erythematosus immunopathology with polycongenic murine strains. *Proc Natl Acad Sci U S A* 97:6670–6675, 2000.

89. Schiffenbauer J, McCarthy DM, Nygard NR, et al: A unique sequence of the NZW I-E beta chain and its possible contribution to autoimmunity in the (NZB×NZW)F1 mouse. *J Exp Med* 170:971–984, 1989.

90. Kotzin BL, Palmer E: The contribution of NZW genes to lupus-like disease in (NZB×NZW)F1 mice. *J Exp Med* 165:1237–1251, 1987.

91. Hirose S, Kinoshita K, Nozawa S, et al: Effects of major histocompatibility complex on autoimmune disease of H-2-congenic New Zealand mice. *Int Immunol* 2:1091–1095, 1990.

92. Nygard NR, McCarthy DM, Schiffenbauer J, et al: Mixed haplotypes and autoimmunity. *Immunol Today* 14:53–56, 1993.

93. Song YW, Tsao BP, Hahn BH: Contribution of major histocompatibility complex (MHC) to upregulation of anti-DNA antibody in transgenic mice. *J Autoimmun* 6:1–9, 1993.

94. Tokushima M, Koarada S, Hirose S, et al: In vivo induction of IgG anti-DNA antibody by autoreactive mixed haplotype A beta z/A alpha d MHC class II molecule-specific CD4+ T-cell clones. *Immunology* 83:221–226, 1994.

95. Hahn BH, Shulman LE: Autoantibodies and nephritis in the white strain (NZW) of New Zealand mice. *Arthritis Rheum* 12:355–364, 1969.

96. Morel L, Mohan C, Yu Y, et al: Multiplex inheritance of component phenotypes in a murine model of lupus. *Mamm Genome* 10:176–181, 1999.

97. Morel L, Rudofsky UH, Longmate JA, et al: Polygenic control of susceptibility to murine systemic lupus erythematosus. *Immunity* 1:219–229, 1994.

98. Waters ST, Fu SM, Gaskin F, et al: NZM2328: a new mouse model of systemic lupus erythematosus with unique genetic susceptibility loci. *Clin Immunol* 100:372–383, 2001.

99. Rahman ZS, Tin SK, Buenaventura PN, et al: A novel susceptibility locus on chromosome 2 in the (New Zealand Black×New Zealand White)F1 hybrid mouse model of systemic lupus erythematosus. *J Immunol* 168:3042–3049, 2002.

100. Morel L, Tian XH, Croker BP, et al: Epistatic modifiers of autoimmunity in a murine model of lupus nephritis. *Immunity* 11:131–139, 1999.

101. Santiago ML, Mary C, Parzy D, et al: Linkage of a major quantitative trait locus to Yaa gene-induced lupus-like nephritis in (NZW × C57BL/6) F1 mice. *Eur J Immunol* 28:4257–4267, 1998.

102. Fujimura T, Hirose S, Jiang Y, et al: Dissection of the effects of tumor necrosis factor-alpha and class II gene polymorphisms within the MHC on murine systemic lupus erythematosus (SLE). *Int Immunol* 10:1467–1472, 1998.

103. Subramanian S, Yim YS, Liu K, et al: Epistatic suppression of systemic lupus erythematosus: fine mapping of Sle1 to less than 1 mb. *J Immunol* 175:1062–1072, 2005.

104. Cuda CM, Li S, Liang S, et al: Pre-B cell leukemia homeobox 1 is associated with lupus susceptibility in mice and humans. *J Immunol* 188:604–614, 2012.

105. Wandstrat AE, Nguyen C, Limaye N, et al: Association of extensive polymorphisms in the SLAM/CD2 gene cluster with murine lupus. *Immunity* 21:769–780, 2004.

106. Wang A, Batteux F, Wakeland EK: The role of SLAM/CD2 polymorphisms in systemic autoimmunity. *Curr Opin Immunol* 22:706–714, 2010.

107. Kumar KR, Li L, Yan M, et al: Regulation of B cell tolerance by the lupus susceptibility gene Ly108. *Science* 312:1665–1669, 2006.

108. Vuyyuru R, Mohan C, Manser T, et al: The lupus susceptibility locus Sle1 breaches peripheral B cell tolerance at the antibody-forming cell and germinal center checkpoints. *J Immunol* 183:5716–5727, 2009.

109. Cannons JL, Tangye SG, Schwartzberg PL: SLAM family receptors and SAP adaptors in immunity. *Annu Rev Immunol* 29:665–705, 2011.

110. Heidari Y, Fossati-Jimack L, Carlucci F, et al: A lupus-susceptibility C57BL/6 locus on chromosome 3 (Sle18) contributes to autoantibody production in 129 mice. *Genes Immun* 10:47–55, 2009.

111. Boackle SA, Holers VM, Chen X, et al: Cr2, a candidate gene in the murine Sle1c lupus susceptibility locus, encodes a dysfunctional protein. *Immunity* 15:775–785, 2001.

112. Chen Y, Perry D, Boackle SA, et al: Several genes contribute to the production of autoreactive B and T cells in the murine lupus susceptibility locus Sle1c. *J Immunol* 175:1080–1089, 2005.

113. Zeumer L, Sang A, Niu H, et al: Murine lupus susceptibility locus Sle2 activates DNA-reactive B cells through two sub-loci with distinct phenotypes. *Genes Immun* 12:199–207, 2011.

114. Sobel ES, Morel L, Baert R, et al: Genetic dissection of systemic lupus erythematosus pathogenesis: evidence for functional expression of Sle3/5 by non-T cells. *J Immunol* 169:4025–4032, 2002.

115. Liu K, Li QZ, Yu Y, et al: Sle3 and Sle5 can independently couple with Sle1 to mediate severe lupus nephritis. *Genes Immun* 8:634–645, 2007.

116. Mary C, Laporte C, Parzy D, et al: Dysregulated expression of the Cd22 gene as a result of a short interspersed nucleotide element insertion in Cd22a lupus-prone mice. *J Immunol* 165:2987–2996, 2000.

117. Bethunaickan R, Berthier CC, Ramanujam M, et al: A unique hybrid renal mononuclear phagocyte activation phenotype in murine systemic lupus erythematosus nephritis. *J Immunol* 186:4994–5003, 2011.

118. Leng L, Chen L, Fan J, et al: A small-molecule macrophage migration inhibitory factor antagonist protects against glomerulonephritis in lupus-prone NZB/NZW F1 and MRL/lpr mice. *J Immunol* 186:527–538, 2011.

119. Okamoto A, Fujio K, van Rooijen N, et al: Splenic phagocytes promote responses to nucleosomes in (NZB × NZW) F1 mice. *J Immunol* 181:5264–5271, 2008.

120. Schiffer L, Bethunaickan R, Ramanujam M, et al: Activated renal macrophages are markers of disease onset and disease remission in lupus nephritis. *J Immunol* 180:1938–1947, 2008.

121. Santiago-Raber ML, Dunand-Sauthier I, Wu T, et al: Critical role of TLR7 in the acceleration of systemic lupus erythematosus in TLR9-deficient mice. *J Autoimmun* 34:339–348, 2010.

122. Takahashi T, Strober S: Natural killer T cells and innate immune B cells from lupus-prone NZB/W mice interact to generate IgM and IgG autoantibodies. *Eur J Immunol* 38:156–165, 2008.

123. Benigni A, Caroli C, Longaretti L, et al: Involvement of renal tubular Toll-like receptor 9 in the development of tubulointerstitial injury in systemic lupus. *Arthritis Rheum* 56:1569–1578, 2007.

124. Yang JQ, Wen X, Liu H, et al: Examining the role of CD1d and natural killer T cells in the development of nephritis in a genetically susceptible lupus model. *Arthritis Rheum* 56:1219–1233, 2007.

125. Barrat FJ, Meeker T, Chan JH, et al: Treatment of lupus-prone mice with a dual inhibitor of TLR7 and TLR9 leads to reduction of autoantibody production and amelioration of disease symptoms. *Eur J Immunol* 37:3582–3586, 2007.

126. Martin DA, Zhang K, Kenkel J, et al: Autoimmunity stimulated by adoptively transferred dendritic cells is initiated by both alphabeta and gammadelta T cells but does not require MyD88 signaling. *J Immunol* 179:5819–5828, 2007.

127. Chu VT, Enghard P, Riemekasten G, et al: In vitro and in vivo activation induces BAFF and APRIL expression in B cells. *J Immunol* 179:5947–5957, 2007.

128. Panchanathan R, Shen H, Bupp MG, et al: Female and male sex hormones differentially regulate expression of Ifi202, an interferon-inducible lupus susceptibility gene within the Nba2 interval. *J Immunol* 183:7031–7038, 2009.

129. Mathian A, Gallegos M, Pascual V, et al: Interferon-alpha induces unabated production of short-lived plasma cells in pre-autoimmune lupus-prone (NZB × NZW)F1 mice but not in BALB/c mice. *Eur J Immunol* 41:863–872, 2011.

130. Liu Z, Bethunaickan R, Huang W, et al: Interferon-alpha accelerates murine systemic lupus erythematosus in a T cell-dependent manner. *Arthritis Rheum* 63:219–229, 2011.

131. Shen H, Panchanathan R, Rajavelu P, et al: Gender-dependent expression of murine Irf5 gene: implications for sex bias in autoimmunity. *J Mol Cell Biol* 2:284–290, 2010.

132. Zagury D, Le Buanec H, Mathian A, et al: IFNalpha kinoid vaccine-induced neutralizing antibodies prevent clinical manifestations in a lupus flare murine model. *Proc Natl Acad Sci U S A* 106:5294–5299, 2009.

133. Lu Q, Shen N, Li XM, et al: Genomic view of IFN-alpha response in pre-autoimmune NZB/W and MRL/lpr mice. *Genes Immun* 8:590–603, 2007.

134. Papoian R, Pillarisetty R, Talal N: Immunological regulation of spontaneous antibodies to DNA and RNA. II. Sequential switch from IgM to IgG in NZB/NZW F1 mice. *Immunology* 32:75–79, 1977.

135. Wofsy D, Seaman WE: Successful treatment of autoimmunity in NZB/NZW F1 mice with monoclonal antibody to L3T4. *J Exp Med* 161:378–391, 1985.

136. Ohnishi K, Ebling FM, Mitchell B, et al: Comparison of pathogenic and non-pathogenic murine antibodies to DNA: antigen binding and structural characteristics. *Int Immunol* 6:817–830, 1994.

137. Tsao BP, Ebling FM, Roman C, et al: Structural characteristics of the variable regions of immunoglobulin genes encoding a pathogenic autoantibody in murine lupus. *J Clin Invest* 85:530–540, 1990.

138. Raz E, Brezis M, Rosenmann E, et al: Anti-DNA antibodies bind directly to renal antigens and induce kidney dysfunction in the isolated perfused rat kidney. *J Immunol* 142:3076–3082, 1989.

139. Tsao BP, Ohnishi K, Cheroutre H, et al: Failed self-tolerance and autoimmunity in IgG anti-DNA transgenic mice. *J Immunol* 149:350–358, 1992.

140. Tucker RM, Vyse TJ, Rozzo S, et al: Genetic control of glycoprotein 70 autoantigen production and its influence on immune complex levels and nephritis in murine lupus. *J Immunol* 165:1665–1672, 2000.

141. Ebling FM, Hahn BH: Pathogenic subsets of antibodies to DNA. *Int Rev Immunol* 5:79–95, 1989.

142. Raveche ES, Novotny EA, Hansen CT, et al: Genetic studies in NZB mice. V. Recombinant inbred lines demonstrate that separate genes control autoimmune phenotype. *J Exp Med* 153:1187–1197, 1981.

143. Datta SK, Owen FL, Womack JE, et al: Analysis of recombinant inbred lines derived from "autoimmune" (NZB) and "high leukemia" (C58) strains: independent multigenic systems control B cell hyperactivity, retrovirus expression, and autoimmunity. *J Immunol* 129:1539–1544, 1982.

144. Maruyama N, Furukawa F, Nakai Y, et al: Genetic studies of autoimmunity in New Zealand mice. IV. Contribution of NZB and NZW genes to the spontaneous occurrence of retroviral gp70 immune complexes in (NZB × NZW)F1 hybrid and the correlation to renal disease. *J Immunol* 130:740–746, 1983.

145. Koch-Nolte F, Klein J, Hollmann C, et al: Defects in the structure and expression of the genes for the T cell marker Rt6 in NZW and (NZB × NZW)F1 mice. *Int Immunol* 7:883–890, 1995.

146. Maeda T, Webb DR, Chen J, et al: Deletion of signaling molecule genes resembling the cytoplasmic domain of Igbeta in autoimmune-prone mice. *Int Immunol* 10:815–821, 1998.

147. Babcock SK, Appel VB, Schiff M, et al: Genetic analysis of the imperfect association of H-2 haplotype with lupus-like autoimmune disease. *Proc Natl Acad Sci U S A* 86(19):7552–7555, 1989.

148. Cuda CM, Zeumer L, Sobel ES, et al: Murine lupus susceptibility locus Sle1a requires the expression of two sub-loci to induce inflammatory T cells. *Genes Immun* 11:542–553, 2010.

149. Jacob CO, Lee SK, Strassmann G: Mutational analysis of TNF-alpha gene reveals a regulatory role for the 3′-untranslated region in the genetic predisposition to lupus-like autoimmune disease. *J Immunol* 156:3043–3050, 1996;

150. Adachi Y, Inaba M, Amoh Y, et al: Effect of bone marrow transplantation on antiphospholipid antibody syndrome in murine lupus mice. *Immunobiology* 192:218–2130, 1995.

151. Lemoine R, Berney T, Shibata T, et al: Induction of "wire-loop" lesions by murine monoclonal IgG3 cryoglobulins. *Kidney Int* 41:65–72, 1992.

152. Elouaai F, Lule J, Benoist H, et al: Autoimmunity to histones, ubiquitin, and ubiquitinated histone H2A in NZB×NZW and MRL-lpr/lpr mice. Anti-histone antibodies are concentrated in glomerular eluates of lupus mice. *Nephrol Dial Transplant* 9:362–366, 1994.

153. Takeuchi K, Turley SJ, Tan EM, et al: Analysis of the autoantibody response to fibrillarin in human disease and murine models of autoimmunity. *J Immunol* 154:961–971, 1995.

154. Lambert PH, Dixon FJ: Pathogenesis of the glomerulonephritis of NZB/W mice. *J Exp Med* 127:507–522, 1968.

155. Dixon FJ, Oldstone MB, Tonietti G: Pathogenesis of immune complex glomerulonephritis of New Zealand mice. *J Exp Med* 134:65–71, 1971.

156. Ebling F, Hahn BH: Restricted subpopulations of DNA antibodies in kidneys of mice with systemic lupus. Comparison of antibodies in serum and renal eluates. *Arthritis Rheum* 23:392–403, 1980.

157. Tucker RM, Roark CL, Santiago-Raber ML, et al: Association between nuclear antigens and endogenous retrovirus in the generation of autoantibody responses in murine lupus. *Arthritis Rheum* 50:3626–3636, 2004.

158. Espeli M, Bokers S, Giannico G, et al: Local renal autoantibody production in lupus nephritis. *J Am Soc Nephrol* 22:296–305, 2011.

159. Lacotte S, Dumortier H, Decossas M, et al: Identification of new pathogenic players in lupus: autoantibody-secreting cells are present in nephritic kidneys of (NZB×NZW)F1 mice. *J Immunol* 184:3937–3945, 2010.

160. Mjelle JE, Kalaaji M, Rekvig OP: Exposure of chromatin and not high affinity for dsDNA determines the nephritogenic impact of anti-dsDNA antibodies in (NZB×NZW)F1 mice. *Autoimmunity* 42:104–111, 2009.

161. Zykova SN, Seredkina N, Benjaminsen J, et al: Reduced fragmentation of apoptotic chromatin is associated with nephritis in lupus-prone (NZB×NZW)F mice. *Arthritis Rheum* 58:813–825, 2008.

162. Hedberg A, Fismen S, Fenton KA, et al: Heparin exerts a dual effect on murine lupus nephritis by enhancing enzymatic chromatin degradation and preventing chromatin binding in glomerular membranes. *Arthritis Rheum* 63:1065–1075, 2011.

163. van Bavel CC, Dieker JW, Tamboer WP, et al: Lupus-derived monoclonal autoantibodies against apoptotic chromatin recognize acetylated conformational epitopes. *Mol Immunol* 48:248–256, 2010.

164. Dai R, Zhang Y, Khan D, et al: Identification of a common lupus disease-associated microRNA expression pattern in three different murine models of lupus. *PLoS One* 5:e14302, 2010.

165. Reichlin M: Cellular dysfunction induced by penetration of autoantibodies into living cells: cellular damage and dysfunction mediated by antibodies to dsDNA and ribosomal P proteins. *J Autoimmun* 11:557–561, 1998.

166. Koren E, Koscec M, Wolfson-Reichlin M, et al: Murine and human antibodies to native DNA that cross-react with the A and D SnRNP polypeptides cause direct injury of cultured kidney cells. *J Immunol* 154:4857–4864, 1995.

167. Vlahakos D, Foster MH, Ucci AA, et al: Murine monoclonal anti-DNA antibodies penetrate cells, bind to nuclei, and induce glomerular proliferation and proteinuria in vivo. *J Am Soc Nephrol* 2:1345–1354, 1992.

168. Stetler DA, Cavallo T: Anti-RNA polymerase I antibodies: potential role in the induction and progression of murine lupus nephritis. *J Immunol* 138:2119–2123, 1987.

169. Schmiedeke T, Stoeckl F, Muller S, et al: Glomerular immune deposits in murine lupus models may contain histones. *Clin Exp Immunol* 90:453–458, 1992.

170. Bergtold A, Gavhane A, D'Agati V, et al: FcR-bearing myeloid cells are responsible for triggering murine lupus nephritis. *J Immunol* 177:7287–7295, 2006.

171. Ozmen L, Roman D, Fountoulakis M, et al: Experimental therapy of systemic lupus erythematosus: the treatment of NZB/W mice with mouse soluble interferon-gamma receptor inhibits the onset of glomerulonephritis. *Eur J Immunol* 25:6–12, 1995.

172. Adalid-Peralta L, Mathian A, Tran T, et al: Leukocytes and the kidney contribute to interstitial inflammation in lupus nephritis. *Kidney Int* 73:172–180, 2008.

173. Tveita AA, Ninomiya Y, Sado Y, et al: Development of lupus nephritis is associated with qualitative changes in the glomerular collagen IV matrix composition. *Lupus* 18:355–360, 2009.

174. Li HH, Cheng HH, Sun KH, et al: Interleukin-20 targets renal mesangial cells and is associated with lupus nephritis. *Clin Immunol* 129:277–385, 2008.

175. Tveita AA, Rekvig OP: Alterations in Wnt pathway activity in mouse serum and kidneys during lupus development. *Arthritis Rheum* 63:513–522, 2011.

176. Moore PM: Evidence for bound antineuronal antibodies in brains of NZB/W mice. *J Neuroimmunol* 38(1–2):147–154, 1992.

177. Lapter S, Marom A, Meshorer A, et al: Amelioration of brain pathology and behavioral dysfunction in mice with lupus following treatment with a tolerogenic peptide. *Arthritis Rheum* 60:3744–3754, 2009.

178. Talal N, Steinberg AD: The pathogenesis of autoimmunity in New Zealand black mice. *Curr Top Microbiol Immunol* 64:79–103, 1974.

179. Hahn BH, Knotts L, Ng M, et al: Influence of cyclophosphamide and other immunosuppressive drugs on immune disorders and neoplasia in NZB/NZW mice. *Arthritis Rheum* 18:145–152, 1975.

180. Jabs DA, Prendergast RA: Murine models of Sjögren's syndrome. *Adv Exp Med Biol* 350:623–630, 1994.

181. Roubinian JR, Talal N, Greenspan JS, et al: Delayed androgen treatment prolongs survival in murine lupus. *J Clin Invest* 63:902–911, 1979.

182. Verheul HA, Verveld M, Hoefakker S, et al: Effects of ethinylestradiol on the course of spontaneous autoimmune disease in NZB/W and NOD mice. *Immunopharmacol Immunotoxicol* 7:163–180, 1995.

183. Walker SE, Besch-Williford CL, Keisler DH: Accelerated deaths from systemic lupus erythematosus in NZB×NZW F1 mice treated with the testosterone-blocking drug flutamide. *J Lab Clin Med* 124:401–407, 1994.

184. Duvic M, Steinberg AD, Klassen LW: Effect of the anti-estrogen, Nafoxidine, on NZB/W autoimmune disease. *Arthritis Rheum* 21:414–417, 1978.

185. Roubinian JR, Talal N, Greenspan JS, et al: Effect of castration and sex hormone treatment on survival, anti-nucleic acid antibodies, and glomerulonephritis in NZB/NZW F1 mice. *J Exp Med* 147:1568–1583, 1978.

186. Bynote KK, Hackenberg JM, Korach KS, et al: Estrogen receptor-alpha deficiency attenuates autoimmune disease in (NZB×NZW)F1 mice. *Genes Immun* 9:137–152, 2008.

187. Roubinian J, Talal N, Siiteri PK, et al: Sex hormone modulation of autoimmunity in NZB/NZW mice. *Arthritis Rheum* 22:1162–1169, 1979.

188. Gubbels Bupp MR, Jorgensen TN, Kotzin BL: Identification of candidate genes that influence sex hormone-dependent disease phenotypes in mouse lupus. *Genes Immun* 9:47–56, 2008.

189. Elbourne KB, Keisler D, McMurray RW: Differential effects of estrogen and prolactin on autoimmune disease in the NZB/NZW F1 mouse model of systemic lupus erythematosus. *Lupus* 7:420–427, 1998.

190. McMurray R, Keisler D, Izui S, et al: Hyperprolactinemia in male NZB/NZW (B/W) F1 mice: accelerated autoimmune disease with normal circulating testosterone. *Clin Immunol Immunopathol* 71:338–343, 1994.

191. Walker SE, Allen SH, Hoffman RW, et al: Prolactin: a stimulator of disease activity in systemic lupus erythematosus. *Lupus* 4:3–9, 1995.

192. Hughes GC, Martin D, Zhang K, et al: Decrease in glomerulonephritis and Th1-associated autoantibody production after progesterone treatment in NZB/NZW mice. *Arthritis Rheum* 60:1775–1784, 2009.

193. Jiang B, Sun L, Hao S, et al: Estrogen distinctively modulates spleen DC from (NZB×NZW) F1 female mice in various disease development stages. *Cell Immunol* 248:95–102, 2007.

194. Nilsson N, Carlsten H: Estrogen induces suppression of natural killer cell cytotoxicity and augmentation of polyclonal B cell activation. *Cell Immunol* 158:131–139, 1994.

195. Bynoe MS, Grimaldi CM, Diamond B: Estrogen up-regulates Bcl-2 and blocks tolerance induction of naive B cells. *Proc Natl Acad Sci U S A* 97:2703–2708, 2000.

196. Zhang Y, Saha S, Rosenfeld G, et al: Raloxifene modulates estrogen-mediated B cell autoreactivity in NZB/W F1 mice. *J Rheumatol* 37:1646–1657, 2010.

197. Panchanathan R, Shen H, Zhang X, et al: Mutually positive regulatory feedback loop between interferons and estrogen receptor-alpha in mice: implications for sex bias in autoimmunity. *PLoS One* 5:e10868, 2010.

198. Singh RP, Dinesh R, Elashoff D, et al: Distinct gene signature revealed in white blood cells, CD4(+) and CD8(+) T cells in (NZB × NZW) F1 lupus mice after tolerization with anti-DNA Ig peptide. *Genes Immun* 11:294–309, 2010.

199. Sharabi A, Sthoeger ZM, Mahlab K, et al: A tolerogenic peptide that induces suppressor of cytokine signaling (SOCS)-1 restores the aberrant control of IFN-gamma signaling in lupus-affected (NZB × NZW)F1 mice. *Clin Immunol* 133:61–68, 2009.

200. Reininger L, Radaszkiewicz T, Kosco M, et al: Development of autoimmune disease in SCID mice populated with long-term "in vitro" proliferating (NZB × NZW)F1 pre-B cells. *J Exp Med* 176:1343–1353, 1992.

201. Hahn BH, Ebling FM: Idiotype restriction in murine lupus; high frequency of three public idiotypes on serum IgG in nephritic NZB/NZW F1 mice. *J Immunol* 138:2110–2118, 1987.

202. Panosian-Sahakian N, Klotz JL, Ebling F, et al: Diversity of Ig V gene segments found in anti-DNA autoantibodies from a single (NZB × NZW) F1 mouse. *J Immunol* 142:4500–4506, 1989.

203. Marion TN, Bothwell AL, Briles DE, et al: IgG anti-DNA autoantibodies within an individual autoimmune mouse are the products of clonal selection. *J Immunol* 142:4269–4274, 1989.

204. Shlomchik M, Mascelli M, Shan H, et al: Anti-DNA antibodies from autoimmune mice arise by clonal expansion and somatic mutation. *J Exp Med* 171:265–292, 1990.

205. Tillman DM, Jou NT, Hill RJ, et al: Both IgM and IgG anti-DNA antibodies are the products of clonally selective B cell stimulation in (NZB × NZW)F1 mice. *J Exp Med* 176:761–779, 1992.

206. Viau M, Zouali M: Effect of the B cell superantigen protein A from *S. aureus* on the early lupus disease of (NZB × NZW) F1 mice. *Mol Immunol* 42:849–855, 2005.

207. Bekar KW, Owen T, Dunn R, et al: Prolonged effects of short-term anti-CD20 B cell depletion therapy in murine systemic lupus erythematosus. *Arthritis Rheum* 62:2443–2457, 2010.

208. Ando DG, Sercarz EE, Hahn BH: Mechanisms of T and B cell collaboration in the in vitro production of anti-DNA antibodies in the NZB/NZW F1 murine SLE model. *J Immunol* 138:3185–3190, 1987.

209. Singh RR, Kumar V, Ebling FM, et al: T cell determinants from autoantibodies to DNA can upregulate autoimmunity in murine systemic lupus erythematosus. *J Exp Med* 181:2017–2027, 1995.

210. Wofsy D, Seaman WE: Reversal of advanced murine lupus in NZB/NZW F1 mice by treatment with monoclonal antibody to L3T4. *J Immunol* 138:3247–3253, 1987.

211. Rozzo SJ, Drake CG, Chiang BL, et al: Evidence for polyclonal T cell activation in murine models of systemic lupus erythematosus. *J Immunol* 153:1340–1351, 1994.

212. Karpouzas GA, La Cava A, Ebling FM, et al: Differences between CD8+ T cells in lupus-prone (NZB × NZW) F1 mice and healthy (BALB/c × NZW) F1 mice may influence autoimmunity in the lupus model. *Eur J Immunol* 34:2489–2499, 2004.

213. Hu YL, Metz DP, Chung J, et al: B7RP-1 blockade ameliorates autoimmunity through regulation of follicular helper T cells. *J Immunol* 182:1421–1428, 2009.

214. Finck BK, Linsley PS, Wofsy D: Treatment of murine lupus with CTLA4Ig. *Science* 265:1225–1227, 1994.

215. Nakajima A, Azuma M, Kodera S, et al: Preferential dependence of autoantibody production in murine lupus on CD86 costimulatory molecule. *Eur J Immunol* 25:3060–3069, 1995.

216. Early GS, Zhao W, Burns CM: Anti-CD40 ligand antibody treatment prevents the development of lupus-like nephritis in a subset of New Zealand black × New Zealand white mice. Response correlates with the absence of an anti-antibody response. *J Immunol* 157:3159–3164, 1996.

217. Kalled SL, Cutler AH, Datta SK, et al: Anti-CD40 ligand antibody treatment of SNF1 mice with established nephritis: preservation of kidney function. *J Immunol* 160:2158–2165, 1998;

218. Daikh DI, Finck BK, Linsley PS, et al: Long-term inhibition of murine lupus by brief simultaneous blockade of the B7/CD28 and CD40/gp39 costimulation pathways. *J Immunol* 159:3104–3108, 1997.

219. Finck BK, Chan B, Wofsy D: Interleukin 6 promotes murine lupus in NZB/NZW F1 mice. *J Clin Invest* 94:585–591, 1994.

220. Ishida H, Muchamuel T, Sakaguchi S, et al: Continuous administration of anti-interleukin 10 antibodies delays onset of autoimmunity in NZB/W F1 mice. *J Exp Med* 179:305–310, 1994.

221. Kang HK, Michaels MA, Berner BR, et al: Very low-dose tolerance with nucleosomal peptides controls lupus and induces potent regulatory T cell subsets. *J Immunol* 174:3247–3255, 2005.

222. Hahn BH, Singh RP, La Cava A, et al: Tolerogenic treatment of lupus mice with consensus peptide induces Foxp3-expressing, apoptosis-resistant, TGFbeta-secreting CD8+ T cell suppressors. *J Immunol* 175:7728–7737, 2005.

223. Singh RR, Ebling FM, Albuquerque DA, et al: Induction of autoantibody production is limited in nonautoimmune mice. *J Immunol* 169:587–594, 2002.

224. Brennan DC, Yui MA, Wuthrich RP, et al: Tumor necrosis factor and IL-1 in New Zealand Black/White mice. Enhanced gene expression and acceleration of renal injury. *J Immunol* 143:3470–3475, 1989.

225. Jacob CO, McDevitt HO: Tumour necrosis factor-alpha in murine autoimmune "lupus" nephritis. *Nature* 331(6154):356–358, 1988.

226. Gordon C, Wofsy D: Effects of recombinant murine tumor necrosis factor-alpha on immune function. *J Immunol* 144:1753–1758, 1990.

227. Hartwell DW, Fenton MJ, Levine JS, et al: Aberrant cytokine regulation in macrophages from young autoimmune-prone mice: evidence that the intrinsic defect in MRL macrophage IL-1 expression is transcriptionally controlled. *Mol Immunol* 32:743–751, 1995.

228. Du Clos TW, Zlock LT, Hicks PS, et al: Decreased autoantibody levels and enhanced survival of (NZB × NZW) F1 mice treated with C-reactive protein. *Clin Immunol Immunopathol* 70:22–27, 1994.

229. Kim SJ, Gershov D, Ma X, et al: Opsonization of apoptotic cells and its effect on macrophage and T cell immune responses. *Ann N Y Acad Sci* 987:68–78, 2003.

230. Rodriguez W, Mold C, Kataranovski M, et al: Reversal of ongoing proteinuria in autoimmune mice by treatment with C-reactive protein. *Arthritis Rheum* 52:642–650, 2005.

231. Szalai AJ, Weaver CT, McCrory MA, et al: Delayed lupus onset in (NZB × NZW)F1 mice expressing a human C-reactive protein transgene. *Arthritis Rheum* 48:1602–1611, 2003.

232. Tzeng TC, Suen JL, Chiang BL: Dendritic cells pulsed with apoptotic cells activate self-reactive T-cells of lupus mice both in vitro and in vivo. *Rheumatology (Oxford)* 45:1230–1237, 2006.

233. La Cava A, Ebling FM, Hahn BH: Ig-reactive CD4+CD25+ T cells from tolerized (New Zealand Black × New Zealand White)F1 mice suppress in vitro production of antibodies to DNA. *J Immunol* 173:3542–3548, 2004.

234. Wong M, La Cava A, Singh RP, et al: Blockade of programmed death-1 in young (New Zealand black × New Zealand white)F1 mice promotes the activity of suppressive CD8+ T cells that protect from lupus-like disease. *J Immunol* 185:6563–6571, 2010.

235. Watanabe R, Ishiura N, Nakashima H, et al: Regulatory B cells (B10 cells) have a suppressive role in murine lupus: CD19 and B10 cell deficiency exacerbates systemic autoimmunity. *J Immunol* 184:4801–4809, 2010.

236. Singh AK, Yang JQ, Parekh VV, et al: The natural killer T cell ligand alpha-galactosylceramide prevents or promotes pristane-induced lupus in mice. *Eur J Immunol* 35:1143–1154, 2005.

237. Zeng D, Liu Y, Sidobre S, et al: Activation of natural killer T cells in NZB/W mice induces Th1-type immune responses exacerbating lupus. *J Clin Invest* 112:1211–1222, 2003.

238. Forestier C, Molano A, Im JS, et al: Expansion and hyperactivity of CD1d-restricted NKT cells during the progression of systemic lupus erythematosus in (New Zealand Black × New Zealand White)F1 mice. *J Immunol* 175:763–770, 2005.

239. Ishikawa S, Nagai S, Sato T, et al: Increased circulating CD11b+CD11c+ dendritic cells (DC) in aged BWF1 mice which can be matured by TNF-alpha into BLC/CXCL13-producing DC. *Eur J Immunol* 32:1881–1887, 2002.

240. Fujio K, Okamoto A, Tahara H, et al: Nucleosome-specific regulatory T cells engineered by triple gene transfer suppress a systemic autoimmune disease. *J Immunol* 173:2118–2125, 2004.

241. Bondanza A, Zimmermann VS, Dell'Antonio G, et al: Requirement of dying cells and environmental adjuvants for the induction of autoimmunity. *Arthritis Rheum* 50:1549–1560, 2004.

242. Santiago-Raber ML, Baccala R, Haraldsson KM, et al: Type-I interferon receptor deficiency reduces lupus-like disease in NZB mice. *J Exp Med* 197:777–788, 2003.

243. Mathian A, Weinberg A, Gallegos M, et al: IFN-alpha induces early lethal lupus in preautoimmune (New Zealand Black × New Zealand White) F1 but not in BALB/c mice. *J Immunol* 174:2499–2506, 2005.

244. Datta SK, Manny N, Andrzejewski C, et al: Genetic studies of autoimmunity and retrovirus expression in crosses of New Zealand black mice I. Xenotropic virus. *J Exp Med* 147:854–871, 1978.

245. Eastcott JW, Schwartz RS, Datta SK: Genetic analysis of the inheritance of B cell hyperactivity in relation to the development of autoantibodies and glomerulonephritis in NZB×SWR crosses. *J Immunol* 131:2232–2329, 1983.

246. Gavalchin J, Datta SK: The NZB×SWR model of lupus nephritis. II. Autoantibodies deposited in renal lesions show a distinctive and restricted idiotypic diversity. *J Immunol* 138:138–148, 1987.

247. O'Keefe TL, Bandyopadhyay S, Datta SK, et al: V region sequences of an idiotypically connected family of pathogenic anti-DNA autoantibodies. *J Immunol* 144:4275–4283, 1990.

248. Rauch J, Murphy E, Roths JB, et al: A high frequency idiotypic marker of anti-DNA autoantibodies in MRL-lpr/lpr mice. *J Immunol* 129:236–241, 1982.

249. Gavalchin J, Nicklas JA, Eastcott JW, et al: Lupus prone (SWR×NZB)F1 mice produce potentially nephritogenic autoantibodies inherited from the normal SWR parent. *J Immunol* 134:885–894, 1985.

250. Portanova JP, Creadon G, Zhang X, et al: An early post-mutational selection event directs expansion of autoreactive B cells in murine lupus. *Mol Immunol* 32:117–135, 1995.

251. Knupp CJ, Uner AH, Tatum AH, et al: IdLNF1-specific T cell clones accelerate the production of IdLNF1 + IgG and nephritis in SNF1 mice. *J Autoimmun* 8:367–380, 1995.

252. Uner AH, Knupp CJ, Tatum AH, et al: Treatment with antibody reactive with the nephritogenic idiotype, IdLNF1, suppresses its production and leads to prolonged survival of (NZB×SWR)F1 mice. *J Autoimmun* 7:27–44, 1994.

253. Datta SK, Patel H, Berry D: Induction of a cationic shift in IgG anti-DNA autoantibodies. Role of T helper cells with classical and novel phenotypes in three murine models of lupus nephritis. *J Exp Med* 165:1252–1268, 1987.

254. Mohan C, Adams S, Stanik V, et al: Nucleosome: a major immunogen for pathogenic autoantibody-inducing T cells of lupus. *J Exp Med* 177:1367–1381, 1993.

255. Wu HY, Center EM, Tsokos GC, et al: Suppression of murine SLE by oral anti-CD3: inducible CD4+CD25-LAP+ regulatory T cells control the expansion of IL-17+ follicular helper T cells. *Lupus* 18:586–596, 2009.

256. Kang HK, Ecklund D, Liu M, et al: Apigenin, a non-mutagenic dietary flavonoid, suppresses lupus by inhibiting autoantigen presentation for expansion of autoreactive Th1 and Th17 cells. *Arthritis Res Ther* 11:R59, 2009.

257. Dumont F, Monier JC: Sex-dependent systemic lupus erythematosus-like syndrome in (NZB×SJL)F1 mice. *Clin Immunol Immunopathol* 29:306–317, 1983.

258. Dumont F, Robert F: Age- and sex-dependent thymic abnormalities in NZB×SJL F1 hybrid mice. *Clin Exp Immunol* 41:63–72, 1980.

259. Dumont F: Effects of ovariectomy and androgen treatment on the thymic pathology of NZB×SJL mice. *Thymus* 7:37–48, 1985.

260. Rudofsky UH, Evans BD, Balaban SL, et al: Differences in expression of lupus nephritis in New Zealand mixed H-2z homozygous inbred strains of mice derived from New Zealand black and New Zealand white mice. Origins and initial characterization. *Lab Invest* 68:419–426, 1993.

261. Perry D, Sang A, Yin Y, et al: Murine models of systemic lupus erythematosus. *J Biomed Biotechnol* 2011:271694, 2011.

262. Singh RR, Saxena V, Zang S, et al: Differential contribution of IL-4 and STAT6 vs STAT4 to the development of lupus nephritis. *J Immunol* 170:4818–4825, 2003.

263. Jacob CO, Zang S, Li L, et al: Pivotal role of Stat4 and Stat6 in the pathogenesis of the lupus-like disease in the New Zealand mixed 2328 mice. *J Immunol* 171:1564–1571, 2003.

264. Murphy ED, Roths JB: A single gene for massive lymphoproliferation with immune complex disease in a new mouse strain MRL. In: Seno S, Takaku F, Irino S, eds. Topics in Hematology: Proceedings of the 16th International Congress in Hematology, Kyoto, September 5–11, 1976. *Excerpta Medica* 69–72, 1977.

265. Watanabe-Fukunaga R, Brannan CI, Copeland NG, et al: Lymphoproliferation disorder in mice explained by defects in Fas antigen that mediates apoptosis. *Nature* 356:314–317, 1992.

266. Watson ML, Rao JK, Gilkeson GS, et al: Genetic analysis of MRL-lpr mice: relationship of the Fas apoptosis gene to disease manifestations and renal disease-modifying loci. *J Exp Med* 176:1645–1656, 1992.

267. Wu J, Zhou T, He J, et al: Autoimmune disease in mice due to integration of an endogenous retrovirus in an apoptosis gene. *J Exp Med* 178:461–468, 1993.

268. Chu JL, Drappa J, Parnassa A, et al: The defect in Fas mRNA expression in MRL/lpr mice is associated with insertion of the retrotransposon, ETn. *J Exp Med* 178:723–730, 1993.

269. Adachi M, Watanabe-Fukunaga R, Nagata S: Aberrant transcription caused by the insertion of an early transposable element in an intron of the Fas antigen gene of lpr mice. *Proc Natl Acad Sci U S A* 90:1756–1760, 1993.

270. Nagata S, Golstein P: The Fas death factor. *Science* 267:1449–1456, 1995.

271. Drappa J, Brot N, Elkon KB: The Fas protein is expressed at high levels on CD4+CD8+ thymocytes and activated mature lymphocytes in normal mice but not in the lupus-prone strain, MRL lpr/lpr. *Proc Natl Acad Sci U S A* 90:10340–10344, 1993.

272. Lynch DH, Ramsdell F, Alderson MR: Fas and FasL in the homeostatic regulation of immune responses. *Immunol Today* 16:569–574, 1995.

273. Mountz JD, Bluethmann H, Zhou T, et al: Defective clonal deletion and anergy induction in TCR transgenic lpr/lpr mice. *Semin Immunol* 6:27–37, 1994.

274. Theofilopoulos AN, Dixon FJ: Etiopathogenesis of murine SLE. *Immunol Rev* 55:179–216, 1981.

275. Morse HC, 3rd, Davidson WF, Yetter RA, et al: Abnormalities induced by the mutant gene lpr: expansion of a unique lymphocyte subset. *J Immunol* 129:2612–2615, 1982.

276. Izui S, Kelley VE, Masuda K, et al: Induction of various autoantibodies by mutant gene lpr in several strains of mice. *J Immunol* 133:227–233, 1984.

277. Katagiri T, Cohen PL, Eisenberg RA: The lpr gene causes an intrinsic T cell abnormality that is required for hyperproliferation. *J Exp Med* 167:741–751, 1988.

278. Jabs DA, Burek CL, Hu Q, et al: Anti-CD4 monoclonal antibody therapy suppresses autoimmune disease in MRL/Mp-lpr/lpr mice. *Cell Immunol* 141:496–507, 1992.

279. Singer PA, McEvilly RJ, Noonan DJ, et al: Clonal diversity and T-cell receptor beta-chain variable gene expression in enlarged lymph nodes of MRL-lpr/lpr lupus mice. *Proc Natl Acad Sci U S A* 83:7018–7022, 1986.

280. Singer PA, Theofilopoulos AN: Novel origin of lpr and gld cells and possible implications in autoimmunity. *J Autoimmun* 3:123–135, 1990.

281. Altman A, Theofilopoulos AN, Weiner R, et al: Analysis of T cell function in autoimmune murine strains. Defects in production and responsiveness to interleukin 2. *J Exp Med* 154:791–808, 1981.

282. Cohen PL, Rapoport R, Eisenberg RA: Characterization of functional T-cell lines derived from MRL mice. *Clin Immunol Immunopathol* 40:485–496, 1986.

283. Fisher CL, Shores EW, Eisenberg RA, et al: Cellular interactions for the in vitro production of anti-chromatin autoantibodies in MRL/Mp-lpr/lpr mice. *Clin Immunol Immunopathol* 50:231–240, 1989.

284. Shores EW, Eisenberg RA, Cohen PL: T-B collaboration in the in vitro anti-Sm autoantibody response of MRL/Mp-lpr/lpr mice. *J Immunol* 140:2977–2982, 1988.

285. Santoro TJ, Portanova JP, Kotzin BL: The contribution of L3T4+ T cells to lymphoproliferation and autoantibody production in MRL-lpr/lpr mice. *J Exp Med* 167:1713–1718, 1988.

286. Puliaeva I, Puliaev R, Shustov A, et al: Fas expression on antigen-specific T cells has costimulatory, helper, and down-regulatory functions in vivo for cytotoxic T cell responses but not for T cell-dependent B cell responses. *J Immunol* 181:5912–5929, 2008.

287. Stetler DA, Sipes DE, Jacob ST: Anti-RNA polymerase I antibodies in sera of MRL lpr/lpr and MRL +/+ autoimmune mice. Correlation of antibody production with delayed onset of lupus-like disease in MRL +/+ mice. *J Exp Med* 162:1760–1770, 1985.

288. Kanai Y, Miura K, Uehara T, et al: Natural occurrence of Nuc in the sera of autoimmune-prone MRL/lpr mice. *Biochem Biophys Res Commun* 196:729–736, 1993.

289. Kanai Y, Takeda O, Miura K, et al: Novel autoimmune phenomena induced in vivo by a new DNA binding protein Nuc: a study on MRL/n mice. *Immunol Lett* 39:83–89, 1993.

290. Kita Y, Sumida T, Ichikawa K, et al: V gene analysis of anticardiolipin antibodies from MRL-lpr/lpr mice. *J Immunol* 151:849–856, 1993.

291. Treadwell EL, Cohen P, Williams D, et al: MRL mice produce anti-Su autoantibody, a specificity associated with systemic lupus erythematosus. *J Immunol* 150:695–699, 1993.

292. Wang J, Chou CH, Blankson J, et al: Murine monoclonal antibodies specific for conserved and non-conserved antigenic determinants of the human and murine Ku autoantigens. *Mol Biol Rep* 18:15–28, 1993.

293. Uwatoko S, Mannik M, Oppliger IR, et al: C1q-binding immunoglobulin G in MRL/l mice consists of immune complexes containing antibodies to DNA. *Clin Immunol Immunopathol* 75:140–146, 1995.

294. Bloom DD, St Clair EW, Pisetsky DS, et al: The anti-La response of a single MRL/Mp-lpr/lpr mouse: specificity for DNA and VH gene usage. *Eur J Immunol* 24:1332–1338, 1994.

295. James JA, Mamula MJ, Harley JB: Sequential autoantigenic determinants of the small nuclear ribonucleoprotein Sm D shared by human lupus autoantibodies and MRL lpr/lpr antibodies. *Clin Exp Immunol* 98:419–426, 1994.

296. Fatenejad S, Brooks W, Schwartz A, et al: Pattern of anti-small nuclear ribonucleoprotein antibodies in MRL/Mp-lpr/lpr mice suggests that the intact U1 snRNP particle is their autoimmunogenic target. *J Immunol* 152:5523–5531, 1994.

297. Bloom DD, Davignon JL, Cohen PL, et al: Overlap of the anti-Sm and anti-DNA responses of MRL/Mp-lpr/lpr mice. *J Immunol* 150:1579–1590, 1993.

298. Retter MW, Eisenberg RA, Cohen PL, et al: Sm and DNA binding by dual reactive B cells requires distinct VH, V kappa, and VH CDR3 structures. *J Immunol* 155:2248–2257, 1995.

299. Bernstein KA, Valerio RD, Lefkowith JB: Glomerular binding activity in MRL lpr serum consists of antibodies that bind to a DNA/histone/type IV collagen complex. *J Immunol* 154:2424–2433, 1995.

300. Faulds G, Conroy S, Madaio M, et al: Increased levels of antibodies to heat shock proteins with increasing age in Mrl/Mp-lpr/lpr mice. *Br J Rheumatol* 34:610–615, 1995.

301. Dimitriu-Bona A, Matic M, Ding W, et al: Cytotoxicity to endothelial cells by sera from aged MRL/lpr/lpr mice is associated with autoimmunity to cell surface heparan sulfate. *Clin Immunol Immunopathol* 76:234–240, 1995.

302. Amoura Z, Chabre H, Koutouzov S, et al: Nucleosome-restricted antibodies are detected before anti-dsDNA and/or antihistone antibodies in serum of MRL-Mp lpr/lpr and +/+ mice, and are present in kidney eluates of lupus mice with proteinuria. *Arthritis Rheum* 37:1684–1688, 1994.

303. Burlingame RW, Rubin RL, Balderas RS, et al: Genesis and evolution of antichromatin autoantibodies in murine lupus implicates T-dependent immunization with self antigen. *J Clin Invest* 91:1687–1696, 1993.

304. Wahren M, Skarstein K, Blange I, et al: MRL/lpr mice produce anti-Ro 52,000 MW antibodies: detection, analysis of specificity and site of production. *Immunology* 83:9–15, 1994.

305. Panka DJ, Salant DJ, Jacobson BA, et al: The effect of VH residues 6 and 23 on IgG3 cryoprecipitation and glomerular deposition. *Eur J Immunol* 25:279–284, 1995.

306. Berney T, Fulpius T, Shibata T, et al: Selective pathogenicity of murine rheumatoid factors of the cryoprecipitable IgG3 subclass. *Int Immunol* 4:93–99, 1992.

307. Hang L, Theofilopoulos AN, Dixon FJ: A spontaneous rheumatoid arthritis-like disease in MRL/l mice. *J Exp Med* 155:1690–1701, 1982.

308. O'Sullivan FX, Fassbender HG, Gay S, et al: Etiopathogenesis of the rheumatoid arthritis-like disease in MRL/l mice. I. The histomorphologic basis of joint destruction. *Arthritis Rheum* 28:529–536, 1985.

309. Aguado MT, Balderas RS, Rubin RL, et al: Specificity and molecular characteristics of monoclonal IgM rheumatoid factors from arthritic and non-arthritic mice. *J Immunol* 139:1080–1087, 1987.

310. O'Sullivan FX, Vogelweid CM, Besch-Williford CL, et al: Differential effects of CD4+ T cell depletion on inflammatory central nervous system disease, arthritis and sialadenitis in MRL/lpr mice. *J Autoimmun* 8:163–175, 1995.

311. Kanno H, Nose M, Itoh J, et al: Spontaneous development of pancreatitis in the MRL/Mp strain of mice in autoimmune mechanism. *Clin Exp Immunol* 89:68–73, 1992.

312. Green LM, LaBue M, Lazarus JP, et al: Characterization of autoimmune thyroiditis in MRL-lpr/lpr mice. *Lupus* 4:187–196, 1995.

313. Brey RL, Cote S, Barohn R, et al: Model for the neuromuscular complications of systemic lupus erythematosus. *Lupus* 4:209–212, 1995.

314. Hoffman RW, Yang HK, Waggie KS, et al: Band keratopathy in MRL/l and MRL/n mice. *Arthritis Rheum* 26:645–652, 1983.

315. Hess DC, Taormina M, Thompson J, et al: Cognitive and neurologic deficits in the MRL/lpr mouse: a clinicopathologic study. *J Rheumatol* 20:610–617, 1993.

316. Kusakari C, Hozawa K, Koike S, et al: MRL/MP-lpr/lpr mouse as a model of immune-induced sensorineural hearing loss. *Ann Otol Rhinol Laryngol Suppl* 157:82–86, 1992.

317. Handwerger BS, Storrer CE, Wasson CS, et al: Further characterization of the autoantibody response of Palmerston North mice. *J Clin Immunol* 19:45–57, 1999.

318. Eisenberg RA, Craven SY, Fisher CL, et al: The genetics of autoantibody production in MRL/lpr lupus mice. *Clin Exp Rheumatol* 7(Suppl 3):S35-S40, 1989.

319. Pisetsky DS, Semper KF, Eisenberg RA: Idiotypic analysis of a monoclonal anti-Sm antibody. II. Strain distribution of a common idiotypic determinant and its relationship to anti-Sm expression. *J Immunol* 133:2085–2089, 1984.

320. Dang H, Takei M, Isenberg D, et al: Expression of an interspecies idiotype in sera of SLE patients and their first-degree relatives. *Clin Exp Immunol* 71:445–450, 1988.

321. Andrews J, Hang L, Theofilopoulos AN, et al: Lack of relationship between serum gp70 levels and the severity of systemic lupus erythematosus in MRL/l mice. *J Exp Med* 163:458–462, 1986.

322. Merino R, Fossati L, Iwamoto M, et al: Effect of long-term anti-CD4 or anti-CD8 treatment on the development of lpr CD4- CD8- double negative T cells and of the autoimmune syndrome in MRL-lpr/lpr mice. *J Autoimmun* 8:33–45, 1995.

323. Koh DR, Ho A, Rahemtulla A, et al: Murine lupus in MRL/lpr mice lacking CD4 or CD8 T cells. *Eur J Immunol* 25:2558–2562, 1995.

324. Ohteki T, Iwamoto M, Izui S, et al: Reduced development of CD4-8-B220+ T cells but normal autoantibody production in lpr/lpr mice lacking major histocompatibility complex class I molecules. *Eur J Immunol* 25:37–41, 1995.

325. Mixter PF, Russell JQ, Budd RC: Delayed kinetics of T lymphocyte anergy and deletion in lpr mice. *J Autoimmun* 7:697–710, 1994.

326. Steinmetz OM, Turner JE, Paust HJ, et al: CXCR3 mediates renal Th1 and Th17 immune response in murine lupus nephritis. *J Immunol* 183:4693–4704, 2009.

327. Zhang Z, Kyttaris VC, Tsokos GC: The role of IL-23/IL-17 axis in lupus nephritis. *J Immunol* 183:3160–3169, 2009.

328. Diaz Gallo C, Jevnikar AM, Brennan DC, et al: Autoreactive kidney-infiltrating T-cell clones in murine lupus nephritis. *Kidney Int* 42:851–859, 1992.

329. Diaz-Gallo C, Kelley VR: Self-regulation of autoreactive kidney-infiltrating T cells in MRL-lpr nephritis. *Kidney Int* 44:692–699, 1993.

330. Kelley VR, Singer GG: The antigen presentation function of renal tubular epithelial cells. *Exp Nephrol* 1:102–111, 1993.

331. Sobel ES, Kakkanaiah VN, Rapoport RG, et al: The abnormal lpr double-negative T cell fails to proliferate in vivo. *Clin Immunol Immunopathol* 74:177–184, 1995.

332. Hammond DM, Nagarkatti PS, Gote LR, et al: Double-negative T cells from MRL-lpr/lpr mice mediate cytolytic activity when triggered through adhesion molecules and constitutively express perforin gene. *J Exp Med* 178:2225–2230, 1993.

333. Jevnikar AM, Grusby MJ, Glimcher LH: Prevention of nephritis in major histocompatibility complex class II-deficient MRL-lpr mice. *J Exp Med* 179:1137–1143, 1994.

334. Gilkeson GS, Spurney R, Coffman TM, et al: Effect of anti-CD4 antibody treatment on inflammatory arthritis in MRL-lpr/lpr mice. *Clin Immunol Immunopathol* 64:166–172, 1992.

335. Ohkusu K, Isobe K, Hidaka H, et al: Elucidation of the protein kinase C-dependent apoptosis pathway in distinct subsets of T lymphocytes in MRL-lpr/lpr mice. *Eur J Immunol* 25:3180–3186, 1995.

336. Hayashi Y, Hamano H, Haneji N, et al: Biased T cell receptor V beta gene usage during specific stages of the development of autoimmune sialadenitis in the MRL/lpr mouse model of Sjögren's syndrome. *Arthritis Rheum* 38:1077–1084, 1995.

337. de Alboran IM, Gonzalo JA, Kroemer G, et al: Attenuation of autoimmune disease and lymphocyte accumulation in MRL/lpr mice by treatment with anti-V beta 8 antibodies. *Eur J Immunol* 22:2153–2158, 1992.

338. Davignon JL, Cohen PL, Eisenberg RA: Rapid T cell receptor modulation accompanies lack of in vitro mitogenic responsiveness of double negative T cells to anti-CD3 monoclonal antibody in MRL/Mp-lpr mice. *J Immunol* 141:1848–1854, 1988.

339. Scholz W, Isakov N, Mally MI, et al: Lpr T cell hyporesponsiveness to mitogens linked to deficient receptor-stimulated phosphoinositide hydrolysis. *J Biol Chem* 263:3626–3631, 1988.

340. Thomas TJ, Gunnia UB, Seibold JR, et al: Defective signal-transduction pathways in T-cells from autoimmune MRL-lpr/lpr mice are associated with increased polyamine concentrations. *Biochem J* 311:175–182, 1995.

341. Prud'homme GJ, Kono DH, Theofilopoulos AN: Quantitative polymerase chain reaction analysis reveals marked overexpression of

interleukin-1 beta, interleukin-1 and interferon-gamma mRNA in the lymph nodes of lupus-prone mice. *Mol Immunol* 32:495–503, 1995.

342. Raz E, Dudler J, Lotz M, et al: Modulation of disease activity in murine systemic lupus erythematosus by cytokine gene delivery. *Lupus* 4:286–292, 1995.

343. Wang S, Yang N, Zhang L, et al: Jak/STAT signaling is involved in the inflammatory infiltration of the kidneys in MRL/lpr mice. *Lupus* 19:1171–1180, 2010.

344. Deng GM, Liu L, Bahjat FR, et al: Suppression of skin and kidney disease by inhibition of spleen tyrosine kinase in lupus-prone mice. *Arthritis Rheum* 62:2086–2092, 2010.

345. Theofilopoulos AN, Balderas RS, Gozes Y, et al: Association of lpr gene with graft-vs.-host disease-like syndrome. *J Exp Med* 162:1–18, 1985.

346. Hosaka N, Nagata N, Nakagawa T, et al: Analyses of lpr-GVHD by adoptive transfer experiments using MRL/lpr-Thy-1.1 congenic mice. *Autoimmunity* 17:217–224, 1994.

347. Hosaka N, Nagata N, Miyashima S, et al: Attenuation of lpr-graft-versus-host disease (GVHD) in MRL/lpr spleen cell-injected SCID mice by in vivo treatment with anti-V beta 8.1,2 monoclonal antibody. *Clin Exp Immunol* 96:500–507, 1994.

348. Ashany D, Hines JJ, Gharavi AE, et al: MRL/lpr−>severe combined immunodeficiency mouse allografts produce autoantibodies, acute graft-versus-host disease or a wasting syndrome depending on the source of cells. *Clin Exp Immunol* 90:466–475, 1992.

349. Sobel ES, Katagiri T, Katagiri K, et al: An intrinsic B cell defect is required for the production of autoantibodies in the lpr model of murine systemic autoimmunity. *J Exp Med* 173:1441–1449, 1991.

350. Cavallo T, Granholm NA: Lipopolysaccharide from gram-negative bacteria enhances polyclonal B cell activation and exacerbates nephritis in MRL/lpr mice. *Clin Exp Immunol* 82:515–521, 1990.

351. Klinman DM, Eisenberg RA, Steinberg AD: Development of the autoimmune B cell repertoire in MRL-lpr/lpr mice. *J Immunol* 144:506–511, 1990.

352. Lebedeva TV, Singh AK: Increased responsiveness of B cells in the murine MRL/lpr model of lupus nephritis to interleukin-1 beta. *J Am Soc Nephrol* 5:1530–1534, 1995.

353. Kobayashi I, Matsuda T, Saito T, et al: Abnormal distribution of IL-6 receptor in aged MRL/lpr mice: elevated expression on B cells and absence on CD4+ cells. *Int Immunol* 4:1407–1412, 1992.

354. Roark JH, Kuntz CL, Nguyen KA, et al: Breakdown of B cell tolerance in a mouse model of systemic lupus erythematosus. *J Exp Med* 181:1157–1167, 1995.

355. Shan H, Shlomchik MJ, Marshak-Rothstein A, et al: The mechanism of autoantibody production in an autoimmune MRL/lpr mouse. *J Immunol* 153:5104–5120, 1994.

356. Karussis DM, Vourka-Karussis U, Lehmann D, et al: Immunomodulation of autoimmunity in MRL/lpr mice with syngeneic bone marrow transplantation (SBMT). *Clin Exp Immunol* 100:111–117, 1995.

357. Takeoka Y, Yoshida SH, Van de Water J, et al: Thymic microenvironmental abnormalities in MRL/MP-lpr/lpr, BXSB/MpJ Yaa and C3H HeJ/gld/gld mice. *J Autoimmun* 8:145–161, 1995.

358. Kotzin BL, Herron LR, Babcock SK, et al: Self-reactive T cells in murine lupus: analysis of genetic contributions and development of self-tolerance. *Clin Immunol Immunopathol* 53:S35–S46, 1989.

359. Singer PA, Balderas RS, McEvilly RJ, et al: Tolerance-related V beta clonal deletions in normal CD4-8-, TCR-alpha/beta + and abnormal lpr and gld cell populations. *J Exp Med* 170:1869–1877, 1989.

360. Papiernik M, Pontoux C, Golstein P: Non-exclusive Fas control and age dependence of viral superantigen-induced clonal deletion in lupus-prone mice. *Eur J Immunol* 25:1517–1523, 1995.

361. Zhou T, Bluethmann H, Zhang J, et al: Defective maintenance of T cell tolerance to a superantigen in MRL-lpr/lpr mice. *J Exp Med* 176:1063–1072, 1992.

362. Steinberg AD, Huston DP, Taurog JD, et al: The cellular and genetic basis of murine lupus. *Immunol Rev* 55:121–154, 1981.

363. Steinberg AD, Roths JB, Murphy ED, et al: Effects of thymectomy or androgen administration upon the autoimmune disease of MRL/Mp-lpr/lpr mice. *J Immunol* 125:871–873, 1980.

364. Gresham HD, Ray CJ, O'Sullivan FX: Defective neutrophil function in the autoimmune mouse strain MRL/lpr. Potential role of transforming growth factor-beta. *J Immunol* 146:3911–3921, 1991.

365. Levine JS, Pugh BJ, Hartwell D, et al: Interleukin-1 dysregulation is an intrinsic defect in macrophages from MRL autoimmune-prone mice. *Eur J Immunol* 23:2951–2958, 1993.

366. Field M, Brennan FM, Melsom RD, et al: MRL mice show an age-related impairment of IgG aggregate removal from the circulation. *Clin Exp Immunol* 61:195–202, 1985.

367. Kaufmann T, Strasser A, Jost PJ: Fas death receptor signalling: roles of Bid and XIAP. *Cell Death Differ* 19:42–50, 2012.

368. Lavrik IN, Krammer PH: Regulation of CD95/Fas signaling at the DISC. *Cell Death Differ* 19:36–41, 2012.

369. Peter ME, Budd RC, Desbarats J, et al: The CD95 receptor: apoptosis revisited. *Cell* 129:447–450, 2007.

370. Strasser A, Jost PJ, Nagata S: The many roles of FAS receptor signaling in the immune system. *Immunity* 30:180–192, 2009.

371. Nagata S: Fas ligand-induced apoptosis. *Annu Rev Genet* 33:29–55, 1999.

372. Cuda CM, Agrawal H, Misharin AV, et al: Requirement of myeloid cell-specific Fas expression for prevention of systemic autoimmunity in mice. *Arthritis Rheum* 64:808–820, 2012.

373. Stranges PB, Watson J, Cooper CJ, et al: Elimination of antigen-presenting cells and autoreactive T cells by Fas contributes to prevention of autoimmunity. *Immunity* 26:629–641, 2007.

374. Hildeman DA, Zhu Y, Mitchell TC, et al: Molecular mechanisms of activated T cell death in vivo. *Curr Opin Immunol* 14:354–359, 2002.

375. Hao Z, Hampel B, Yagita H, et al: T cell-specific ablation of Fas leads to Fas ligand-mediated lymphocyte depletion and inflammatory pulmonary fibrosis. *J Exp Med* 199:1355–1365, 2004.

376. Ichii O, Konno A, Sasaki N, et al: Autoimmune glomerulonephritis induced in congenic mouse strain carrying telomeric region of chromosome 1 derived from MRL/MpJ. *Histol Histopathol* 23:411–422, 2008.

377. Gu L, Weinreb A, Wang XP, et al: Genetic determinants of autoimmune disease and coronary vasculitis in the MRL-lpr/lpr mouse model of systemic lupus erythematosus. *J Immunol* 161:6999–7006, 1998.

378. Miyazaki T, Ono M, Qu WM, et al: Implication of allelic polymorphism of osteopontin in the development of lupus nephritis in MRL/lpr mice. *Eur J Immunol* 35:1510–1520, 2005.

379. Wang Y, Nose M, Kamoto T, et al: Host modifier genes affect mouse autoimmunity induced by the lpr gene. *Am J Pathol* 151:1791–1798, 1997.

380. Vidal S, Kono DH, Theofilopoulos AN: Loci predisposing to autoimmunity in MRL-Fas lpr and C57BL/6-Faslpr mice. *J Clin Invest* 101:696–702, 1998.

381. Santiago-Raber M-L, Haraldsson MK, Theofilopoulos AN, et al: Characterization of reciprocal Lmb1–4 interval MRL-Fas[lpr] and B6-Fas[lpr] congenic mice reveals significant effects from Lmb3. *J Immunol* 178: 8195–8202, 2007.

382. Kong PL, Morel L, Croker BP, et al: The centromeric region of chromosome 7 from MRL mice (Lmb3) is an epistatic modifier of Fas for autoimmune disease expression. *J Immunol* 172:2785–2794, 2004.

383. Haraldsson MK, Louis-Dit-Sully CA, Lawson BR, et al: The lupus-related Lmb3 locus contains a disease-suppressing Coronin-1A gene mutation. *Immunity* 28:40–51, 2008.

384. Vyse TJ: Understanding lupus: fishing genes out of mice and men. *Immunity* 28:8–10, 2008.

385. Murphy ED, Roths JB: A Y chromosome associated factor in strain BXSB producing accelerated autoimmunity and lymphoproliferation. *Arthritis Rheum* 22:1188–1194, 1979.

386. Theofilopoulos AN, Dixon FJ: Murine models of systemic lupus erythematosus. *Adv Immunol* 37:269–390, 1985.

387. Subramanian S, Tus K, Li QZ, et al: A Tlr7 translocation accelerates systemic autoimmunity in murine lupus. *Proc Natl Acad Sci U S A* 103: 9970–9975, 2006.

388. Pisitkun P, Deane JA, Difilippantonio MJ, et al: Autoreactive B cell responses to RNA-related antigens due to TLR7 gene duplication. *Science* 312:1669–1672, 2006.

389. Deane JA, Pisitkun P, Barrett RS, et al: Control of toll-like receptor 7 expression is essential to restrict autoimmunity and dendritic cell proliferation. *Immunity* 27:801–810, 2007.

390. Layer T, Steele A, Goeken JA, et al: Engagement of the B cell receptor for antigen differentially affects B cell responses to Toll-like receptor-7 agonists and antagonists in BXSB mice. *Clin Exp Immunol* 163:392–403, 2011.

391. Santiago-Raber ML, Kikuchi S, Borel P, et al: Evidence for genes in addition to Tlr7 in the Yaa translocation linked with acceleration of systemic lupus erythematosus. *J Immunol* 181:1556–1562, 2008.

392. Hoffman SA, Arbogast DN, Ford PM, et al: Brain-reactive autoantibody levels in the sera of ageing autoimmune mice. *Clin Exp Immunol* 70:74–83, 1987.

393. Makino M, Fujiwara M, Aoyagi T, et al: Immunosuppressive activities of deoxyspergualin. I. Effect of the long-term administration of the drug on the development of murine lupus. *Immunopharmacology* 14:107–113, 1987.

394. Garlepp MJ, Hart DA, Fritzler MJ: Regulation of plasma complement C4 and factor b levels in murine systemic lupus erythematosus. *J Clin Lab Immunol* 28:137–141, 1989.

395. Blossom S, Chu EB, Weigle WO, et al: CD40 ligand expressed on B cells in the BXSB mouse model of systemic lupus erythematosus. *J Immunol* 159:4580–4586, 1997.

396. Fossati L, Iwamoto M, Merino R, et al: Selective enhancing effect of the Yaa gene on immune responses against self and foreign antigens. *Eur J Immunol* 25:166–173, 1995.

397. Fossati L, Sobel ES, Iwamoto M, et al: The Yaa gene-mediated acceleration of murine lupus: Yaa- T cells from non-autoimmune mice collaborate with Yaa+ B cells to produce lupus autoantibodies in vivo. *Eur J Immunol* 25:3412–3417, 1995.

398. Dumont FJ, Habbersett RC: Alterations of the T-cell population in BXSB mice: early imbalance of 9F3-defined Lyt-2+ subsets occurs in the males with rapid onset lupic syndrome. *Cell Immunol* 101:39–50, 1986.

399. Wofsy D: Administration of monoclonal anti-T cell antibodies retards murine lupus in BXSB mice. *J Immunol* 136:4554–4560, 1986.

400. Chu EB, Hobbs MV, Wilson CB, et al: Intervention of CD4+ cell subset shifts and autoimmunity in the BXSB mouse by murine CTLA4Ig. *J Immunol* 156:1262–1268, 1996.

401. Chu EB, Ernst DN, Hobbs MV, et al: Maturational changes in CD4+ cell subsets and lymphokine production in BXSB mice. *J Immunol* 152:4129–4138, 1994.

402. Chu EB, Hobbs MV, Ernst DN, et al: In vivo tolerance induction and associated cytokine production by subsets of murine CD4+ T cells. *J Immunol* 154:4909–4914, 1995.

403. Kono DH, Balomenos D, Park MS, et al: Development of lupus in BXSB mice is independent of IL-4. *J Immunol* 164:38–42, 2000.

404. Bubier JA, Sproule TJ, Foreman O, et al: A critical role for IL-21 receptor signaling in the pathogenesis of systemic lupus erythematosus in BXSB-Yaa mice. *Proc Natl Acad Sci U S A* 106:1518–1523, 2009.

405. Takeoka Y, Taguchi N, Shultz L, et al: Apoptosis and the thymic microenvironment in murine lupus. *J Autoimmun* 13:325–334, 1999.

406. Dardenne M, Savino W, Nabarra B, et al: Male BXSB mice develop a thymic hormonal dysfunction with presence of intraepithelial crystalline inclusions. *Clin Immunol Immunopathol* 52:392–405, 1989.

407. Smith HR, Chused TM, Smathers PA, et al: Evidence for thymic regulation of autoimmunity in BXSB mice: acceleration of disease by neonatal thymectomy. *J Immunol* 130:1200–1204, 1983.

408. Vieten G, Grams B, Muller M, et al: Examination of the mononuclear phagocyte system in lupus-prone male BXSB mice. *J Leukoc Biol* 59:325–332, 1996.

409. Cole EH, Sweet J, Levy GA: Expression of macrophage procoagulant activity in murine systemic lupus erythematosus. *J Clin Invest* 78:887–893, 1986.

410. Wang A, Fairhurst AM, Tus K, et al: CXCR4/CXCL12 hyperexpression plays a pivotal role in the pathogenesis of lupus. *J Immunol* 182:4448–4458, 2009.

411. Rogers NJ, Gabriel L, Nunes CT, et al: Monocytosis in BXSB mice is due to epistasis between Yaa and the telomeric region of chromosome 1 but does not drive the disease process. *Genes Immun* 8:619–627, 2007.

412. Scribner CL, Steinberg AD: The role of splenic colony-forming units in autoimmune disease. *Clin Immunol Immunopathol* 49:133–142, 1988.

413. Eisenberg RA, Izui S, McConahey PJ, et al: Male determined accelerated autoimmune disease in BXSB mice: transfer by bone marrow and spleen cells. *J Immunol* 125:1032–1036, 1980.

414. Ikehara S, Nakamura T, Sekita K, et al: Treatment of systemic and organ-specific autoimmune disease in mice by allogeneic bone marrow transplantation. *Prog Clin Biol Res* 229:131–146, 1987.

415. Wang B, Yamamoto Y, El-Badri NS, et al: Effective treatment of autoimmune disease and progressive renal disease by mixed bone-marrow transplantation that establishes a stable mixed chimerism in BXSB recipient mice. *Proc Natl Acad Sci U S A* 96:3012–3016, 1999.

416. Eisenberg RA, Dixon FJ: Effect of castration on male-determined acceleration of autoimmune disease in BXSB mice. *J Immunol* 125:1959–1961, 1980.

417. Merino R, Fossati L, Lacour M, et al: H-2-linked control of the Yaa gene-induced acceleration of lupus-like autoimmune disease in BXSB mice. *Eur J Immunol* 22:295–299, 1992.

418. Kawano H, Abe M, Zhang D, et al: Heterozygosity of the major histocompatibility complex controls the autoimmune disease in (NZW x BXSB) F1 mice. *Clin Immunol Immunopathol* 65:308–314, 1992.

419. Izui S, Iwamoto M, Fossati L, et al: The Yaa gene model of systemic lupus erythematosus. *Immunol Rev* 144:137–156, 1995.

420. Merino R, Iwamoto M, Fossati L, et al: Prevention of systemic lupus erythematosus in autoimmune BXSB mice by a transgene encoding I-E alpha chain. *J Exp Med* 178:1189–1197, 1993.

421. Iwamoto M, Ibnou-Zekri N, Araki K, et al: Prevention of murine lupus by an I-E alpha chain transgene: protective role of I-E alpha chain-derived peptides with a high affinity to I-Ab molecules. *Eur J Immunol* 26:307–314, 1996.

422. Ibnou-Zekri N, Iwamoto M, Fossati L, et al: Role of the major histocompatibility complex class II Ea gene in lupus susceptibility in mice. *Proc Natl Acad Sci U S A* 94(26):14654–14659, 1997.

423. Ibnou-Zekri N, Iwamoto M, Gershwin ME, et al: Protection of murine lupus by the Ead transgene is MHC haplotype-dependent. *J Immunol* 164:505–511, 2000.

424. Hogarth MB, Slingsby JH, Allen PJ, et al: Multiple lupus susceptibility loci map to chromosome 1 in BXSB mice. *J Immunol* 161:2753–2761, 1998.

425. Haywood ME, Hogarth MB, Slingsby JH, et al: Identification of intervals on chromosomes 1, 3, and 13 linked to the development of lupus in BXSB mice. *Arthritis Rheum* 43:349–355, 2000.

426. Haywood ME, Gabriel L, Rose SJ, et al: BXSB/long-lived is a recombinant inbred strain containing powerful disease suppressor loci. *J Immunol* 179:2428–2434, 2007.

427. Haywood ME, Rose SJ, Horswell S, et al: Overlapping BXSB congenic intervals, in combination with microarray gene expression, reveal novel lupus candidate genes. *Genes Immun* 7:250–263, 2006.

428. Haywood ME, Rogers NJ, Rose SJ, et al: Dissection of BXSB lupus phenotype using mice congenic for chromosome 1 demonstrates that separate intervals direct different aspects of disease. *J Immunol* 173:4277–4285, 2004.

429. Morse HC, 3rd, Chused TM, Hartley JW, et al: Expression of xenotropic murine leukemia viruses as cell-surface gp70 in genetic crosses between strains DBA/2 and C57BL/6. *J Exp Med* 149:1183–1196, 1979.

430. Mountz JD, Wang JH, Xie S, et al: Cytokine regulation of B-cell migratory behavior favors formation of germinal centers in autoimmune disease. *Discov Med* 11:76–85, 2011.

431. Suzuka H, Fujiwara H, Tanaka M, et al: Antithrombotic effect of ticlopidine on occlusive thrombi of small coronary arteries in (NZW × BXSB) F1 male mice with myocardial infarction and systemic lupus erythematosus. *J Cardiovasc Pharmacol* 25:9–13, 1995.

432. Hsu HC, Wu Y, Yang P, et al: Overexpression of activation-induced cytidine deaminase in B cells is associated with production of highly pathogenic autoantibodies. *J Immunol* 178:5357–5365, 2007.

433. Hsu HC, Yang P, Wu Q, et al: Inhibition of the catalytic function of activation-induced cytidine deaminase promotes apoptosis of germinal center B cells in BXD2 mice. *Arthritis Rheum* 63:2038–2048, 2011.

434. Hashimoto Y, Kawamura M, Ichikawa K, et al: Anticardiolipin antibodies in NZW × BXSB F1 mice. A model of antiphospholipid syndrome. *J Immunol* 149:1063–1068, 1992.

435. Mizutani H, Engelman RW, Kinjoh K, et al: Gastrointestinal vasculitis in autoimmune-prone (NZW × BXSB)F1 mice: association with anticardiolipin autoantibodies. *Proc Soc Exp Biol Med* 209:279–285, 1995.

436. Tokuyama Y, Adachi Y, Minamino K, et al: Abnormal distribution of dendritic cells in (NZW x BXSB)F1 mice. *Autoimmunity* 42:399–405, 2009.

437. Adachi Y, Inaba M, Sugihara A, et al: Effects of administration of monoclonal antibodies (anti-CD4 or anti-CD8) on the development of autoimmune diseases in (NZW × BXSB)F1 mice. *Immunobiology* 198:451–464, 1998.

438. Mizutani H, Engelman RW, Kurata Y, et al: Development and characterization of monoclonal antiplatelet autoantibodies from autoimmune thrombocytopenic purpura-prone (NZW × BXSB)F1 mice. *Blood* 82:837–844, 1993.

439. Tanaka M, Fujiwara H, Shibata Y, et al: Effects of chronic oral administration of nifedipine and diltiazem on occlusive thrombus of small coronary arteries in (NZW × BXSB)F1 male mice. *Cardiovasc Res* 26:586–592, 1992.

440. Ramanujam M, Kahn P, Huang W, et al: Interferon-alpha treatment of female (NZW × BXSB)F mice mimics some but not all features associated with the Yaa mutation. *Arthritis Rheum* 60:1096–1101, 2009.

441. Lin Q, Hou R, Sato A, et al: Inhibitory IgG Fc receptor promoter region polymorphism is a key genetic element for murine systemic lupus erythematosus. *J Autoimmun* 34:356–363, 2010.

442. Kahn P, Ramanujam M, Bethunaickan R, et al: Prevention of murine antiphospholipid syndrome by BAFF blockade. *Arthritis Rheum* 58:2824–2834, 2008.

443. Ida A, Hirose S, Hamano Y, et al: Multigenic control of lupus-associated antiphospholipid syndrome in a model of (NZW × BXSB) F1 mice. *Eur J Immunol* 28:2694–2703, 1998.

444. Roths JB, Murphy ED, Eicher EM: A new mutation, gld, that produces lymphoproliferation and autoimmunity in C3H/HeJ mice. *J Exp Med* 159:1–20, 1984.

445. Takahashi T, Tanaka M, Brannan CI, et al: Generalized lymphoproliferative disease in mice, caused by a point mutation in the Fas ligand. *Cell* 76:969–976, 1994.

446. Lynch DH, Watson ML, Alderson MR, et al: The mouse Fas-ligand gene is mutated in gld mice and is part of a TNF family gene cluster. *Immunity* 1:131–136, 1994.

447. Hahne M, Peitsch MC, Irmler M, et al: Characterization of the non-functional Fas ligand of gld mice. *Int Immunol* 7:1381–1386, 1995.

448. O'Reilly LA, Tai L, Lee L, et al: Membrane-bound Fas ligand only is essential for Fas-induced apoptosis. *Nature* 461:659–663, 2009.

449. Mixter PF, Russell JQ, Morrissette GJ, et al: A model for the origin of TCR-alphabeta+ CD4-CD8- B220+ cells based on high affinity TCR signals. *J Immunol* 162:5747–5756, 1999.

450. Bhandoola A, Yui K, Siegel RM, et al: Gld and lpr mice: single gene mutant models for failed self tolerance. *Int Rev Immunol* 11:231–244, 1994.

451. Davidson WF, Giese T, Fredrickson TN: Spontaneous development of plasmacytoid tumors in mice with defective Fas-Fas ligand interactions. *J Exp Med* 187:1825–1838, 1998.

452. Zhu B, Beaudette BC, Rifkin IR, et al: Double mutant MRL-lpr/lpr-gld/gld cells fail to trigger lpr-graft-versus-host disease in syngeneic wild-type recipient mice, but can induce wild-type B cells to make autoantibody. *Eur J Immunol* 2000;30:1778–1784.

453. Satoh M, Weintraub JP, Yoshida H, et al: Fas and Fas ligand mutations inhibit autoantibody production in pristane-induced lupus. *J Immunol* 165:1036–1043, 2000.

454. Zhang HG, Fleck M, Kern ER, et al: Antigen presenting cells expressing Fas ligand down-modulate chronic inflammatory disease in Fas ligand-deficient mice. *J Clin Invest* 105:813–821, 2000.

455. Su X, Hu Q, Kristan JM, et al: Significant role for Fas in the pathogenesis of autoimmune diabetes. *J Immunol* 164:2523–2532, 2000.

456. Korner H, Cretney E, Wilhelm P, et al: Tumor necrosis factor sustains the generalized lymphoproliferative disorder (gld) phenotype. *J Exp Med* 191:89–96, 2000.

457. Maldonado MA, MacDonald GC, Kakkanaiah VN, et al: Differential control of autoantibodies and lymphoproliferation by Fas ligand expression on CD4+ and CD8+ T cells in vivo. *J Immunol* 163:3138–3142, 1999.

458. van Elven EH, van der Veen FM, Rolink AG, et al: Diseases caused by reactions of T lymphocytes to incompatible structures of the major histocompatibility complex. V. High titers of IgG autoantibodies to double-stranded DNA. *J Immunol* 127:2435–2438, 1981.

459. Rolink AG, Pals ST, Gleichmann E: Allosuppressor and allohelper T cells in acute and chronic graft-vs.-host disease. II. F1 recipients carrying mutations at H-2K and/or I-A. *J Exp Med* 157:755–771, 1983.

460. Chu JL, Ramos P, Rosendorff A, et al: Massive upregulation of the Fas ligand in lpr and gld mice: implications for Fas regulation and the graft-versus-host disease-like wasting syndrome. *J Exp Med* 181:393–398, 1995.

461. Gleichmann E, Van Elven EH, Van der Veen JP: A systemic lupus erythematosus (SLE)-like disease in mice induced by abnormal T-B cell cooperation. Preferential formation of autoantibodies characteristic of SLE. *Eur J Immunol* 12:152–159, 1982.

462. Gleichmann H, Gleichmann E, Andre-Schwartz J, et al: Chronic allogeneic disease. 3. Genetic requirements for the induction of glomerulonephritis. *J Exp Med* 135:516–532, 1972.

463. Kimura M, van Rappard-van der Veen FM, Gleichmann E: Requirement of H-2-subregion differences for graft-versus-host autoimmunity in mice: superiority of the differences at class-II H-2 antigens (I-A/I-E). *Clin Exp Immunol* 65:542–552, 1986.

464. Portanova JP, Ebling FM, Hammond WS, et al: Allogeneic MHC antigen requirements for lupus-like autoantibody production and nephritis in murine graft-vs-host disease. *J Immunol* 141:3370–3376, 1988.

465. Foster AD, Soloviova K, Puliaeva I, et al: Donor CD8 T cells and IFN-gamma are critical for sex-based differences in donor CD4 T cell engraftment and lupus-like phenotype in short-term chronic graft-versus-host disease mice. *J Immunol* 186:6238–6254, 2011.

466. Zhao Z, Burkly LC, Campbell S, et al: TWEAK/Fn14 interactions are instrumental in the pathogenesis of nephritis in the chronic graft-versus-host model of systemic lupus erythematosus. *J Immunol* 179:7949–7958, 2007.

467. Choudhury A, Cohen PL, Eisenberg RA: B cells require "nurturing" by CD4 T cells during development in order to respond in chronic graft-versus-host model of systemic lupus erythematosus. *Clin Immunol* 136:105–115, 2010.

468. Foster AD, Haas M, Puliaeva I, et al: Donor CD8 T cell activation is critical for greater renal disease severity in female chronic graft-vs.-host mice and is associated with increased splenic ICOS(hi) host CD4 T cells and IL-21 expression. *Clin Immunol* 136:61–73, 2010.

469. Rus V, Nguyen V, Puliaev R, et al: T cell TRAIL promotes murine lupus by sustaining effector CD4 Th cell numbers and by inhibiting CD8 CTL activity. *J Immunol* 178:3962–3972, 2007.

470. Rus V, Svetic A, Nguyen P, et al: Kinetics of Th1 and Th2 cytokine production during the early course of acute and chronic murine graft-versus-host disease. Regulatory role of donor CD8+ T cells. *J Immunol* 155:2396–2406, 1995.

471. Shustov A, Nguyen P, Finkelman F, et al: Differential expression of Fas and Fas ligand in acute and chronic graft-versus-host disease: up-regulation of Fas and Fas ligand requires CD8+ T cell activation and IFN-gamma production. *J Immunol* 161:2848–2855, 1998.

472. Shustov A, Luzina I, Nguyen P, et al: Role of perforin in controlling B-cell hyperactivity and humoral autoimmunity. *J Clin Invest* 106:R39–R47, 2000.

473. Shao WH, Eisenberg RA, Cohen PL: The Mer receptor tyrosine kinase is required for the loss of B cell tolerance in the chronic graft-versus-host disease model of systemic lupus erythematosus. *J Immunol* 180:7728–7735, 2008.

474. Choudhury A, Cohen PL, Eisenberg RA: Mature B cells preferentially lose tolerance in the chronic graft-versus-host disease model of systemic lupus erythematosus. *J Immunol* 179:5564–5570, 2007.

475. Schorlemmer HU, Dickneite G, Kanzy EJ, et al: Modulation of the immunoglobulin dysregulation in GvH- and SLE-like diseases by the murine IL-4 receptor (IL-4-R). *Inflamm Res* 44(Suppl 2):S194–S196, 1995.

476. Strasser A, Whittingham S, Vaux DL, et al: Enforced BCL2 expression in B-lymphoid cells prolongs antibody responses and elicits autoimmune disease. *Proc Natl Acad Sci U S A* 88:8661–8665, 1991.

477. Reap EA, Felix NJ, Wolthusen PA, et al: bcl-2 transgenic Lpr mice show profound enhancement of lymphadenopathy. *J Immunol* 155:5455–5462, 1995.

478. Moroy T, Grzeschiczek A, Petzold S, et al: Expression of a Pim-1 transgene accelerates lymphoproliferation and inhibits apoptosis in lpr/lpr mice. *Proc Natl Acad Sci U S A* 90:10734–10738, 1993.

479. Liu Z, Davidson A: BAFF inhibition: a new class of drugs for the treatment of autoimmunity. *Exp Cell Res* 317:1270–1277, 2011.

480. Marsters SA, Yan M, Pitti RM, et al: Interaction of the TNF homologues BLyS and APRIL with the TNF receptor homologues BCMA and TACI. *Curr Biol* 10:785–788, 2000.

481. Laabi Y, Strasser A: Immunology. Lymphocyte survival—ignorance is BLys. *Science* 289:883–884, 2000.

482. Khare SD, Sarosi I, Xia XZ, et al: Severe B cell hyperplasia and autoimmune disease in TALL-1 transgenic mice. *Proc Natl Acad Sci U S A* 97:3370–3375, 2000.

483. Hibbs ML, Tarlinton DM, Armes J, et al: Multiple defects in the immune system of Lyn-deficient mice, culminating in autoimmune disease. *Cell* 83:301–311, 1995.

484. Nishizumi H, Taniuchi I, Yamanashi Y, et al: Impaired proliferation of peripheral B cells and indication of autoimmune disease in lyn-deficient mice. *Immunity* 3:549–560, 1995.

485. Cornall RJ, Cyster JG, Hibbs ML, et al: Polygenic autoimmune traits: Lyn, CD22, and SHP-1 are limiting elements of a biochemical pathway regulating BCR signaling and selection. *Immunity* 8:497–508, 1998.

486. Shultz LD, Schweitzer PA, Rajan TV, et al: Mutations at the murine motheaten locus are within the hematopoietic cell protein-tyrosine phosphatase (Hcph) gene. *Cell* 73:1445–1454, 1993.

487. Tsui HW, Siminovitch KA, de Souza L, et al: Motheaten and viable motheaten mice have mutations in the haematopoietic cell phosphatase gene. *Nat Genet* 4:124–129, 1993.

488. Jacob CO, Zhu J, Armstrong DL, et al: Identification of IRAK1 as a risk gene with critical role in the pathogenesis of systemic lupus erythematosus. *Proc Natl Acad Sci U S A* 106:6256–6261, 2009.
489. Nishimura H, Honjo T, Minato N: Facilitation of beta selection and modification of positive selection in the thymus of PD-1-deficient mice. *J Exp Med* 191:891–898, 2000.
490. Balomenos D, Martin-Caballero J, Garcia MI, et al: The cell cycle inhibitor p21 controls T-cell proliferation and sex-linked lupus development. *Nat Med* 6:171–176, 2000.
491. Vinuesa CG, Cook MC: Genetic analysis of systemic autoimmunity. *Novartis Found Symp* 281:103–120, 2007; discussion 20–28, 208–209.
492. Walport MJ, Davies KA, Botto M: C1q and systemic lupus erythematosus. *Immunobiology* 199:265–285, 1998.
493. Taylor PR, Carugati A, Fadok VA, et al: A hierarchical role for classical pathway complement proteins in the clearance of apoptotic cells in vivo. *J Exp Med* 192:359–366, 2000.
494. Napirei M, Karsunky H, Zevnik B, et al: Features of systemic lupus erythematosus in Dnase1-deficient mice. *Nat Genet* 25:177–181, 2000.
495. Ehrenstein MR, Katz DR, Griffiths MH, et al: Human IgG anti-DNA antibodies deposit in kidneys and induce proteinuria in SCID mice. *Kidney Int* 48:705–711, 1995.
496. Xu H, Li H, Suri-Payer E, et al: Regulation of anti-DNA B cells in recombination-activating gene-deficient mice. *J Exp Med* 188:1247–1254, 1998.
497. Mandik-Nayak L, Seo SJ, Sokol C, et al: MRL-lpr/lpr mice exhibit a defect in maintaining developmental arrest and follicular exclusion of anti-double-stranded DNA B cells. *J Exp Med* 189:1799–1814, 1999.
498. Venkatesh J, Yoshifuji H, Kawabata D, et al: Antigen is required for maturation and activation of pathogenic anti-DNA antibodies and systemic inflammation. *J Immunol* 186:5304–5312, 2011.
499. Thorn M, Lewis RH, Mumbey-Wafula A, et al: BAFF overexpression promotes anti-dsDNA B-cell maturation and antibody secretion. *Cell Immunol* 261:9–22, 2010.
500. Mendlovic S, Brocke S, Shoenfeld Y, et al: Induction of a systemic lupus erythematosus-like disease in mice by a common human anti-DNA idiotype. *Proc Natl Acad Sci U S A* 85:2260–2264, 1988.
501. Mendlovic S, Fricke H, Shoenfeld Y, et al: The role of anti-idiotypic antibodies in the induction of experimental systemic lupus erythematosus in mice. *Eur J Immunol* 19:729–734, 1989.
502. Shoenfeld Y: Idiotypic induction of autoimmunity: a new aspect of the idiotypic network. *FASEB J* 8:1296–1301, 1994.
503. Bakimer R, Fishman P, Blank M, et al: Induction of primary antiphospholipid syndrome in mice by immunization with a human monoclonal anticardiolipin antibody (H-3). *J Clin Invest* 89:1558–1563, 1992.
504. Sthoeger ZM, Tartakovsky B, Bentwich Z, et al: Monoclonal anticardiolipin antibodies derived from mice with experimental lupus erythematosus: characterization and the induction of a secondary antiphospholipid syndrome. *J Clin Immunol* 13:127–138, 1993.
505. Krause I, Blank M, Kopolovic J, et al: Abrogation of experimental systemic lupus erythematosus and primary antiphospholipid syndrome with intravenous gamma globulin. *J Rheumatol* 22:1068–1074, 1995.
506. Blank M, Tomer Y, Slavin S, et al: Induction of tolerance to experimental anti-phospholipid syndrome (APS) by syngeneic bone marrow cell transplantation. *Scand J Immunol* 42:226–234, 1995.
507. Blank M, Krause I, Buskila D, et al: Bromocriptine immunomodulation of experimental SLE and primary antiphospholipid syndrome via induction of nonspecific T suppressor cells. *Cell Immunol* 162:114–122, 1995.
508. Shoenfeld Y, Blank M: Effect of long-acting thromboxane receptor antagonist (BMS 180,291) on experimental antiphospholipid syndrome. *Lupus* 3:397–400, 1994.
509. Tomer Y, Blank M, Shoenfeld Y: Suppression of experimental antiphospholipid syndrome and systemic lupus erythematosus in mice by anti-CD4 monoclonal antibodies. *Arthritis Rheum* 37:1236–1244, 1994.
510. Levite M, Zinger H, Zisman E, et al: Beneficial effects of bone marrow transplantation on the serological manifestations and kidney pathology of experimental systemic lupus erythematosus. *Cell Immunol* 162:138–145, 1995.
511. Mozes E, Kohn LD, Hakim F, et al: Resistance of MHC class I-deficient mice to experimental systemic lupus erythematosus. *Science* 261:91–93, 1993.
512. Hardin JA: The lupus autoantigens and the pathogenesis of systemic lupus erythematosus. *Arthritis Rheum* 29:457–460, 1986.
513. Desai DD, Krishnan MR, Swindle JT, et al: Antigen-specific induction of antibodies against native mammalian DNA in nonautoimmune mice. *J Immunol* 151:1614–1626, 1993.
514. Reeves WH, Satoh M, Wang J, et al: Systemic lupus erythematosus. Antibodies to DNA, DNA-binding proteins, and histones. *Rheum Dis Clin North Am* 20:1–28, 1994.
515. Gilkeson GS, Grudier JP, Karounos DG, et al: Induction of anti-double stranded DNA antibodies in normal mice by immunization with bacterial DNA. *J Immunol* 142:1482–1486, 1989.
516. Scofield RH, Henry WE, Kurien BT, et al: Immunization with short peptides from the sequence of the systemic lupus erythematosus-associated 60-kDa Ro autoantigen results in anti-Ro ribonucleoprotein autoimmunity. *J Immunol* 156:4059–4066, 1996.
517. Arbuckle MR, Gross T, Scofield RH, et al: Lupus humoral autoimmunity induced in a primate model by short peptide immunization. *J Investig Med* 46:58–65, 1998.
518. Scofield RH, Kaufman KM, Baber U, et al: Immunization of mice with human 60-kd Ro peptides results in epitope spreading if the peptides are highly homologous between human and mouse. *Arthritis Rheum* 42:1017–1024, 1999.
519. Farris AD, Brown L, Reynolds P, et al: Induction of autoimmunity by multivalent immunodominant and subdominant T cell determinants of La (SS-B). *J Immunol* 1999;162:3079–3087.
520. Mason LJ, Timothy LM, Isenberg DA, et al: Immunization with a peptide of Sm B/B' results in limited epitope spreading but not autoimmune disease. *J Immunol* 162:5099–5105, 1999.
521. Reeves WH, Lee PY, Weinstein JS, et al: Induction of autoimmunity by pristane and other naturally occurring hydrocarbons. *Trends Immunol* 30:455–464, 2009.
522. Lech M, Skuginna V, Kulkarni OP, et al: Lack of SIGIRR/TIR8 aggravates hydrocarbon oil-induced lupus nephritis. *J Pathol* 220:596–607, 2010.
523. Nacionales DC, Weinstein JS, Yan XJ, et al: B cell proliferation, somatic hypermutation, class switch recombination, and autoantibody production in ectopic lymphoid tissue in murine lupus. *J Immunol* 182:4226–4236, 2009.
524. Pristane Available at en.wikipedia.org/Pristane.
525. Satoh M, Kumar A, Kanwar YS, et al: Anti-nuclear antibody production and immune-complex glomerulonephritis in BALB/c mice treated with pristane. *Proc Natl Acad Sci U S A* 92:10934–10938, 1995.
526. Summers SA, Hoi A, Steinmetz OM, et al: TLR9 and TLR4 are required for the development of autoimmunity and lupus nephritis in pristane nephropathy. *J Autoimmun* 35:291–298, 2010.
527. Savarese E, Steinberg C, Pawar RD, et al: Requirement of Toll-like receptor 7 for pristane-induced production of autoantibodies and development of murine lupus nephritis. *Arthritis Rheum* 58:1107–1115, 2008.
528. Smith-Bouvier DL, Divekar AA, Sasidhar M, et al: A role for sex chromosome complement in the female bias in autoimmune disease. *J Exp Med* 205:1099–1108, 2008.
529. Lu S, Holmdahl R: Different therapeutic and bystander effects by intranasal administration of homologous type II and type IX collagens on the collagen-induced arthritis and pristane-induced arthritis in rats. *Clin Immunol* 90:119–127, 1999.
530. Satoh M, Richards HB, Shaheen VM, et al: Widespread susceptibility among inbred mouse strains to the induction of lupus autoantibodies by pristane. *Clin Exp Immunol* 121:399–405, 2000.
531. Kuroda Y, Nacionales DC, Akaogi J, et al: Autoimmunity induced by adjuvant hydrocarbon oil components of vaccine. *Biomed Pharmacother* 58:325–337, 2004.
532. Casey TP, Howie JB: Autoimmune hemolytic anemia in NZB/B1 mice treated with the corticosteroid drug betamethasone. *Blood* 25:423–431, 1965.
533. Nakamura T, Ebihara I, Nagaoka I, et al: Effect of methylprednisolone on transforming growth factor-beta, insulin-like growth factor-I, and basic fibroblast growth factor gene expression in the kidneys of NZB/W F1 mice. *Ren Physiol Biochem* 16:105–116, 1993.
534. Appleby P, Webber DG, Bowen JG: Murine chronic graft-versus-host disease as a model of systemic lupus erythematosus: effect of immunosuppressive drugs on disease development. *Clin Exp Immunol* 78:449–453, 1989.
535. Casey TP: Systemic lupus erythematosus in NZB x NZW hybrid mice treated with the corticosteroid drug betamethasone. *J Lab Clin Med* 71:390–399, 1968.
536. Gelfand MC, Steinberg AD: Therapeutic studies in NZB-W mice. II. Relative efficacy of azathioprine, cyclophosphamide and methylprednisolone. *Arthritis Rheum* 15:247–252, 1972.
537. Hahn BH, Bagby MK, Hamilton TR, et al: Comparison of therapeutic and immunosuppressive effects of azathioprine, prednisolone and combined therapy in NZP-NZW mice. *Arthritis Rheum* 16:163–170, 1973.

538. Jevnikar AM, Singer GG, Brennan DC, et al: Dexamethasone prevents autoimmune nephritis and reduces renal expression of Ia but not costimulatory signals. *Am J Pathol* 141:743–751, 1992.

539. Casey TP: Azathioprine (Imuran) administration and the development of malignant lymphomas in NZB mice. *Clin Exp Immunol* 3:305–312, 1968.

540. Kiberd BA, Young ID: Modulation of glomerular structure and function in murine lupus nephritis by methylprednisolone and cyclophosphamide. *J Lab Clin Med* 124:496–506, 1994.

541. Archer RL, Cunningham AC, Moore PF, et al: Effects of dazmegrel, piroxicam and cyclophosphamide on the NZB/W model of SLE. *Agents Actions* 27:369–374, 1989.

542. Casey TP: Immunosuppression by cyclophosphamide in NZB × NZW mice with lupus nephritis. *Blood* 32:436–444, 1968.

543. Horowitz RE, Dubois EL, Weiner J, et al: Cyclophosphamide treatment of mouse systemic lupus erythematosus. *Lab Invest* 21:199–206, 1969.

544. Russell PJ, Hicks JD, Burnet FM: Cyclophosphamide treatment of kidney disease in (NZB × NZW) F1 mice. *Lancet* 1(7450):1280–1284, 1966.

545. Walker SE, Bole GG: Augmented incidence of neoplasia in female New Zealand black-New Zealand white (NZB-NZW) mice treated with long-term cyclophosphamide. *J Lab Clin Med* 78:978–979, 1971.

546. Waer M, Van Damme B, Leenaerts P, et al: Treatment of murine lupus nephritis with cyclophosphamide or total lymphoid irradiation. *Kidney Int* 34:678–682, 1988.

547. Mihara M, Katsume A, Takeda Y: Effect of methotrexate treatment on the onset of autoimmune kidney disease in lupus mice. *Chem Pharm Bull (Tokyo)* 40:2177–2181, 1992.

548. Woo J, Wright TM, Lemster B, et al: Combined effects of FK506 (tacrolimus) and cyclophosphamide on atypical B220+ T cells, cytokine gene expression and disease activity in MRL/MpJ-lpr/lpr mice. *Clin Exp Immunol* 100:118–125, 1995.

549. Mihara M, Takagi N, Urakawa K, et al: A novel antifolate, MX-68, inhibits the development of autoimmune disease in MRL/lpr mice. *Int Arch Allergy Immunol* 113:454–459, 1997.

550. Halloran PF, Urmson J, Ramassar V, et al: Increased class I and class II MHC products and mRNA in kidneys of MRL-lpr/lpr mice during autoimmune nephritis and inhibition by cyclosporine. *J Immunol* 141:2303–2312, 1988.

551. Berden JH, Faaber P, Assmann KJ, et al: Effects of cyclosporin A on autoimmune disease in MRL/1 and BXSB mice. *Scand J Immunol* 24:405–411, 1986.

552. Mountz JD, Smith HR, Wilder RL, et al: CS-A therapy in MRL-lpr/lpr mice: amelioration of immunopathology despite autoantibody production. *J Immunol* 138:157–163, 1987.

553. Pisetsky DS: Inhibition of in vitro NZB antibody responses by cyclosporine. *Clin Exp Immunol* 71:155–158, 1988.

554. Yamamoto K, Mori A, Nakahama T, et al: Experimental treatment of autoimmune MRL-lpr/lpr mice with immunosuppressive compound FK506. *Immunology* 69:222–227, 1990.

555. Ito S, Ueno M, Arakawa M, et al: Therapeutic effect of 15-deoxyspergualin on the progression of lupus nephritis in MRL mice. I. Immunopathological analyses. *Clin Exp Immunol* 81:446–453, 1990.

556. Nemoto K, Mae T, Saiga K, et al: Autoimmune-prone (NZW × BXSB) F1 (W/BF1) mice escape severe thrombocytopenia after treatment with deoxyspergualin, an immunosuppressant. *Br J Haematol* 91:691–696, 1995.

557. Hayashi T, Kameyama Y, Shirachi T: Long-term treatment with dimethylthiourea inhibits the development of autoimmune disease in NZB x NZWF1 mice. *J Comp Pathol* 112:423–428, 1995.

558. Van Bruggen MC, Walgreen B, Rijke TP, et al: Attenuation of murine lupus nephritis by mycophenolate mofetil. *J Am Soc Nephrol* 9:1407–1415, 1998.

559. Jonsson CA, Erlandsson M, Svensson L, et al: Mycophenolate mofetil ameliorates perivascular T lymphocyte inflammation and reduces the double-negative T cell population in SLE-prone MRLlpr/lpr mice. *Cell Immunol* 197:136–144, 1999.

560. Jonsson CA, Svensson L, Carlsten H: Beneficial effect of the inosine monophosphate dehydrogenase inhibitor mycophenolate mofetil on survival and severity of glomerulonephritis in systemic lupus erythematosus (SLE)-prone MRLlpr/lpr mice. *Clin Exp Immunol* 116:534–541, 1999.

561. Daikh DI, Wofsy D: Cutting edge: reversal of murine lupus nephritis with CTLA4Ig and cyclophosphamide. *J Immunol* 166:2913–2916, 2001.

562. Ramos MA, Pinera C, Cibrian E, et al: Effects of mycophenolate mofetil in the development of systemic lupus erythematosus in (NZB × NZW) F1 mice. *Transplant Proc* 33:3316–3317, 2001.

563. Yu CC, Yang CW, Wu MS, et al: Mycophenolate mofetil reduces renal cortical inducible nitric oxide synthase mRNA expression and diminishes glomerulosclerosis in MRL/lpr mice. *J Lab Clin Med* 138:69–77, 2001.

564. Yung S, Zhang Q, Zhang CZ, et al: Anti-DNA antibody induction of protein kinase C phosphorylation and fibronectin synthesis in human and murine lupus and the effect of mycophenolic acid. *Arthritis Rheum* 60:2071–2082, 2009.

565. Zoja C, Benigni A, Noris M, et al: Mycophenolate mofetil combined with a cyclooxygenase-2 inhibitor ameliorates murine lupus nephritis. *Kidney Int* 60:653–663, 2001.

566. Kanauchi H, Imamura S, Takigawa M, et al: Evaluation of the Japanese-Chinese herbal medicine, kampo, for the treatment of lupus dermatoses in autoimmune prone MRL/Mp-lpr/lpr mice. *J Dermatol* 21:935–939, 1994.

567. Zhou NN, Nakai S, Kawakita T, et al: Combined treatment of autoimmune MRL/MP-lpr/lpr mice with a herbal medicine, Ren-shen-yang-rong-tang (Japanese name: Ninjin-youei-to) plus suboptimal dosage of prednisolone. *Int J Immunopharmacol* 16:845–854, 1994.

568. Slavin S: Successful treatment of autoimmune disease in (NZB/NZW) F1 female mice by using fractionated total lymphoid irradiation. *Proc Natl Acad Sci U S A* 76:5274–5276, 1979.

569. Kotzin BL, Strober S: Reversal of nzb/nzw disease with total lymphoid irradiation. *J Exp Med* 150:371–377, 1979.

570. Theofilopoulos AN, Balderas R, Shawler DL, et al: Inhibition of T cells proliferation and SLE-like syndrome of MRL/1 mice by whole body or total lymphoid irradiation. *J Immunol* 125:2137–2142, 1980.

571. Kotzin BL, Arndt R, Okada S, et al: Treatment of NZB/NZW mice with total lymphoid irradiation: long-lasting suppression of disease without generalized immune suppression. *J Immunol* 136:3259–3265, 1986.

572. Moscovitch M, Rosenmann E, Neeman Z, et al: Successful treatment of autoimmune manifestations in MRL/l and MRL/n mice using total lymphoid irradiation (TLI). *Exp Mol Pathol* 38:33–47, 1983.

573. Tago F, Tsukimoto M, Nakatsukasa H, et al: Repeated 0.5-Gy gamma irradiation attenuates autoimmune disease in MRL-lpr/lpr mice with suppression of CD3+CD4-CD8-B220+ T-cell proliferation and with up-regulation of CD4+CD25+Foxp3+ regulatory T cells. *Radiat Res* 169:59–66, 2008.

574. Oliveira GG, Hutchings PR, Lydyard PM: Anti-CD4 treatment of NZB mice prevents the development of erythrocyte autoantibodies but hastens the appearance of anaemia. *Immunol Lett* 39:153–156, 1994.

575. Oliveira GG, Hutchings PR, Roitt IM, et al: Production of erythrocyte autoantibodies in NZB mice is inhibited by CD4 antibodies. *Clin Exp Immunol* 96:297–302, 1994.

576. Connolly K, Roubinian JR, Wofsy D: Development of murine lupus in CD4-depleted NZB/NZW mice. Sustained inhibition of residual CD4+ T cells is required to suppress autoimmunity. *J Immunol* 149:3083–3088, 1992.

577. Carteron NL, Schimenti CL, Wofsy D: Treatment of murine lupus with F(ab′)2 fragments of monoclonal antibody to L3T4. Suppression of autoimmunity does not depend on T helper cell depletion. *J Immunol* 142:1470–1475, 1989.

578. Carteron NL, Wofsy D, Schimenti C, et al: F(ab′)2 anti-CD4 and intact anti-CD4 monoclonal antibodies inhibit the accumulation of CD4+ T cells, CD8+ T cells, and B cells in the kidneys of lupus-prone NZB/NZW mice. *Clin Immunol Immunopathol* 56:373–383, 1990.

579. Denman AM, Russell AS, Denman EJ: Renal disease in (NZB × NZW) F1 hybrid mice treated with anti-lymphocytic antibody. *Clin Exp Immunol* 6:325–335, 1970.

580. Denman AM, Russell AS, Loewi G, et al: Immunopathology of New Zealand Black mice treated with antilymphocyte globulin. *Immunology* 20:973–1000, 1971.

581. Hahn BH, Mehta J, Knotts LL, et al: The effect of altered lymphocyte function on the immunologic disorders of NZB/NZW mice. Response to anti-thymocyte globulin. *Clin Immunol Immunopathol* 8:225–237, 1977.

582. Wofsy D, Ledbetter JA, Hendler PL, et al: Treatment of murine lupus with monoclonal anti-T cell antibody. *J Immunol* 134:852–857, 1985.

583. Wofsy D: The role of Lyt-2+ T cells in the regulation of autoimmunity in murine lupus. *J Autoimmun* 1:207–217, 1988.

584. Gershwin ME, Castles JJ, Saito W, et al: Studies of congenitally immunologically mutant New Zealand mice. VII: the ontogeny of thymic

abnormalities and reconstitution of nude NZB/W mice. *J Immunol* 129:2150–2155, 1982.

585. Mihara M, Ohsugi Y, Saito K, et al: Immunologic abnormality in NZB/NZW F1 mice. Thymus-independent occurrence of B cell abnormality and requirement for T cells in the development of autoimmune disease, as evidenced by an analysis of the athymic nude individuals. *J Immunol* 141:85–90, 1988.

586. Mihara M, Tan I, Chuzhin Y, et al: CTLA4Ig inhibits T cell-dependent B-cell maturation in murine systemic lupus erythematosus. *J Clin Invest* 106:91–101, 2000.

587. Cunnane G, Chan OT, Cassafer G, et al: Prevention of renal damage in murine lupus nephritis by CTLA-4Ig and cyclophosphamide. *Arthritis Rheum* 50:1539–1548, 2004.

588. Ramanujam M, Wang X, Huang W, et al: Mechanism of action of transmembrane activator and calcium modulator ligand interactor-Ig in murine systemic lupus erythematosus. *J Immunol* 173:3524–3534, 2004.

589. Quezada SA, Eckert M, Adeyi OA, et al: Distinct mechanisms of action of anti-CD154 in early versus late treatment of murine lupus nephritis. *Arthritis Rheum* 48:2541–2554, 2003.

590. Adelman NE, Watling DL, McDevitt HO: Treatment of (NZB × NZW) F1 disease with anti-I-A monoclonal antibodies. *J Exp Med* 158:1350–1355, 1983.

591. Stylianou K, Petrakis I, Mavroeidi V, et al: The PI3K/Akt/mTOR pathway is activated in murine lupus nephritis and downregulated by rapamycin. *Nephrol Dial Transplant* 26:498–508, 2011.

592. Liu SD, Lee S, La Cava A, et al: Galectin-1-induced down-regulation of T lymphocyte activation protects (NZB × NZW) F1 mice from lupus-like disease. *Lupus* 20:473–484, 2011.

593. Kyttaris VC, Zhang Z, Kampagianni O, et al: Calcium signaling in systemic lupus erythematosus T cells: a treatment target. *Arthritis Rheum* 63:2058–2066, 2011.

594. Ichinose K, Juang YT, Crispin JC, et al: Suppression of autoimmunity and organ pathology in lupus-prone mice upon inhibition of calcium/calmodulin-dependent protein kinase type IV. *Arthritis Rheum* 63:523–529, 2011.

595. Kulkarni OP, Sayyed SG, Kantner C, et al: 4SC-101, a novel small molecule dihydroorotate dehydrogenase inhibitor, suppresses systemic lupus erythematosus in MRL-(Fas)lpr mice. *Am J Pathol* 176:2840–2847, 2010.

596. Mackay F, Woodcock SA, Lawton P, et al: Mice transgenic for BAFF develop lymphocytic disorders along with autoimmune manifestations. *J Exp Med* 190:1697–1710, 1999.

597. Do RK, Hatada E, Lee H, et al: Attenuation of apoptosis underlies B lymphocyte stimulator enhancement of humoral immune response. *J Exp Med* 192:953–964, 2000.

598. Gross JA, Johnston J, Mudri S, et al: TACI and BCMA are receptors for a TNF homologue implicated in B-cell autoimmune disease. *Nature* 404(6781):995–999, 2000.

599. Ramanujam M, Bethunaickan R, Huang W, et al: Selective blockade of BAFF for the prevention and treatment of systemic lupus erythematosus nephritis in NZM2410 mice. *Arthritis Rheum* 62:1457–1468, 2010.

600. Ding H, Wang L, Wu X, et al: Blockade of B-cell-activating factor suppresses lupus-like syndrome in autoimmune BXSB mice. *J Cell Mol Med* 14:1717–1725, 2010.

601. Liu W, Szalai A, Zhao L, et al: Control of spontaneous B lymphocyte autoimmunity with adenovirus-encoded soluble TACI. *Arthritis Rheum* 50:1884–1896, 2004.

602. Davidson A, Aranow C: Lupus nephritis: lessons from murine models. *Nat Rev Rheumatol* 6:13–20, 2010.

603. Navarra SV, Guzman RM, Gallacher AE, et al: Efficacy and safety of belimumab in patients with active systemic lupus erythematosus: a randomised, placebo-controlled, phase 3 trial. *Lancet* 377:721–731, 2011.

604. Li T, Tsukada S, Satterthwaite A, Havlik MH, et al: Activation of Bruton's tyrosine kinase (BTK) by a point mutation in its pleckstrin homology (PH) domain. *Immunity* 2:451–460, 1995.

605. Bajpai UD, Zhang K, Teutsch M, et al: Bruton's tyrosine kinase links the B cell receptor to nuclear factor kappaB activation. *J Exp Med* 191:1735–1744, 2000.

606. Ohsugi Y, Gershwin ME, Ahmed A, et al: Studies of congenitally immunologic mutant New Zealand mice. VI. Spontaneous and induced autoantibodies to red cells and DNA occur in New Zealand X-linked immunodeficient (Xid) mice without phenotypic alternations of the Xid gene or generalized polyclonal B cell activation. *J Immunol* 128:2220–2227, 1982.

607. Klinman DM, Steinberg AD: Similar in vivo expansion of B cells from normal DBA/2 and autoimmune NZB mice in xid recipients. *J Immunol* 139:2284–2289, 1987.

608. Honigberg LA, Smith AM, Sirisawad M, et al: The Bruton tyrosine kinase inhibitor PCI-32765 blocks B-cell activation and is efficacious in models of autoimmune disease and B-cell malignancy. *Proc Natl Acad Sci U S A* 107:13075–13080, 2010.

609. Bahjat FR, Pine PR, Reitsma A, et al: An orally bioavailable spleen tyrosine kinase inhibitor delays disease progression and prolongs survival in murine lupus. *Arthritis Rheum* 58:1433–1444, 2008.

610. Zoja C, Casiraghi F, Conti S, et al: Cyclin-dependent kinase inhibition limits glomerulonephritis and extends lifespan of mice with systemic lupus. *Arthritis Rheum* 56:1629–1637, 2007.

611. Javierre BM, Richardson B: A new epigenetic challenge: systemic lupus erythematosus. *Adv Exp Med Biol* 711:117–136, 2011.

612. Hu N, Long H, Zhao M, et al: Aberrant expression pattern of histone acetylation modifiers and mitigation of lupus by SIRT1-siRNA in MRL/lpr mice. *Scand J Rheumatol* 38:464–471, 2009.

613. Mishra N, Reilly CM, Brown DR, et al: Histone deacetylase inhibitors modulate renal disease in the MRL-lpr/lpr mouse. *J Clin Invest* 111:539–552, 2003.

614. Verthelyi D, Dybdal N, Elias KA, et al: DNAse treatment does not improve the survival of lupus prone (NZB × NZW)F1 mice. *Lupus* 7:223–230, 1998.

615. Hahn BH, Ebling FM: Suppression of NZB/NZW murine nephritis by administration of a syngeneic monoclonal antibody to DNA. Possible role of anti-idiotypic antibodies. *J Clin Invest* 71:1728–1736, 1983.

616. Hahn BH, Ebling FM: Suppression of murine lupus nephritis by administration of an anti-idiotypic antibody to anti-DNA. *J Immunol* 132:187–190, 1984.

617. Ebling FM, Ando DG, Panosian-Sahakian N, et al: Idiotypic spreading promotes the production of pathogenic autoantibodies. *J Autoimmun* 1:47–61, 1988.

618. Sasaki T, Muryoi T, Takai O, et al: Selective elimination of anti-DNA antibody-producing cells by antiidiotypic antibody conjugated with neocarzinostatin. *J Clin Invest* 77:1382–1386, 1986.

619. Harata N, Sasaki T, Osaki H, et al: Therapeutic treatment of New Zealand mouse disease by a limited number of anti-idiotypic antibodies conjugated with neocarzinostatin. *J Clin Invest* 86:769–776, 1990.

620. Mahana W, Guilbert B, Avrameas S: Suppression of anti-DNA antibody production in MRL mice by treatment with anti-idiotypic antibodies. *Clin Exp Immunol* 70:538–545, 1987.

621. Sasaki T, Tamate E, Muryoi T, et al: In vitro manipulation of human anti-DNA antibody production by anti-idiotypic antibodies conjugated with neocarzinostatin. *J Immunol* 142:1159–1165, 1989.

622. Teitelbaum D, Rauch J, Stollar BD, et al: In vivo effects of antibodies against a high frequency idiotype of anti-DNA antibodies in MRL mice. *J Immunol* 132:1282–1285, 1984.

623. Borel Y, Lewis RM, Stollar BD: revention of murine lupus nephritis by carrier-dependent induction of immunologic tolerance to denatured DNA. *Science* 182:76–78, 1973.

624. Parker LP, Hahn BH, Osterland CK: Modification of NZB-NZW F1 autoimmune disease by development of tolerance to DNA. *J Immunol* 113:292–297, 1974.

625. Eshhar Z, Benacerraf B, Katz DH: Induction of tolerance to nucleic acid determinants by administration of a complex of nucleoside D-glutamic acid and D-lysine (D-GL). *J Immunol* 114:872–876, 1975.

626. Borel Y, Lewis RM, Andre-Schwartz J, et al: Treatment of lupus nephritis in adult (NZB + NZW)F1 mice by cortisone-facilitated tolerance to nucleic acid antigens. *J Clin Invest* 61:276–286, 1978.

627. Duncan SR, Rubin RL, Burlingame RW, et al: Intrathymic injection of polynucleosomes delays autoantibody production in BXSB mice. *Clin Immunol Immunopathol* 79:171–181, 1996.

628. Weisman MH, Bluestein HG, Berner CM, et al: Reduction in circulating dsDNA antibody titer after administration of LJP 394. *J Rheumatol* 24:314–318, 1997.

629. Coutts SM, Plunkett ML, Iverson GM, et al: Pharmacological intervention in antibody mediated disease. *Lupus* 5:158–159, 1996.

630. Alarcon-Segovia D, Tumlin JA, Furie RA, et al: LJP 394 for the prevention of renal flare in patients with systemic lupus erythematosus: results from a randomized, double-blind, placebo-controlled study. *Arthritis Rheum* 48:442–454, 2003.

631. Burny W, Lebrun P, Cosyns JP, et al: Treatment with dsDNA-anti-dsDNA antibody complexes extends survival, decreases anti-dsDNA

antibody production and reduces severity of nephritis in MRLlpr mice. *Lupus* 6:4–17, 1997.

632. Singh RR, Ebling FM, Sercarz EE, et al: Immune tolerance to autoantibody-derived peptides delays development of autoimmunity in murine lupus. *J Clin Invest* 96:2990–2996, 1995.

633. Hahn BH, Ebling FM: Immune tolerance to the artificial peptide pCONSENSUS (pCONS) delays murine lupus by multiple mechanisms, including induction of regulatory cells. *Arthritis Rheum* 43:S93, 2000 (abstract).

634. Hahn BH, Singh RR, Wong WK, et al: Treatment with a consensus peptide based on amino acid sequences in autoantibodies prevents T cell activation by autoantigens and delays disease onset in murine lupus. *Arthritis Rheum* 44:432–441, 2001.

635. Kaliyaperumal A, Michaels MA, Datta SK: Antigen-specific therapy of murine lupus nephritis using nucleosomal peptides: tolerance spreading impairs pathogenic function of autoimmune T and B cells. *J Immunol* 162:5775–5783, 1999.

636. Ofosu-Appiah W, Sfeir G, Viti D, et al: Suppression of systemic lupus erythematosus disease in mice by oral administration of kidney extract. *J Autoimmun* 13:405–414, 1999.

637. Akadegawa K, Ishikawa S, Sato T, et al: Breakdown of mucosal immunity in the gut and resultant systemic sensitization by oral antigens in a murine model for systemic lupus erythematosus. *J Immunol* 174:5499–5506, 2005.

638. Skaggs BJ, Lourenco EV, Hahn BH: Oral administration of different forms of a tolerogenic peptide to define the preparations and doses that delay anti-DNA antibody production and nephritis and prolong survival in SLE-prone mice. *Lupus* 20:912–920, 2011.

639. La Cava A: Regulatory immune cell subsets in autoimmunity. *Autoimmunity* 44:1–2, 2011.

640. De Alboran IM, Gutierrez JC, Gonzalo JA, et al: Lpr T cells vaccinate against lupus in MRL/lpr mice. *Eur J Immunol* 22:1089–1093, 1992.

641. Ono S, Shao D, Yamada S, et al: A novel function of B lymphocytes from normal mice to suppress autoimmunity in (NZB×NZW)F1 mice. *Immunology* 100:99–109, 2000.

642. Luger D, Dayan M, Zinger H, et al: A peptide based on the complementarity determining region 1 of a human monoclonal autoantibody ameliorates spontaneous and induced lupus manifestations in correlation with cytokine immunomodulation. *J Clin Immunol* 24:579–590, 2004.

643. Riemekasten G, Langnickel D, Enghard P, et al: Intravenous injection of a D1 protein of the Smith proteins postpones murine lupus and induces type 1 regulatory T cells. *J Immunol* 173:5835–5842, 2004.

644. Lu L, Zhou X, Wang J, et al: Characterization of protective human CD4CD25 FOXP3 regulatory T cells generated with IL-2, TGF-beta and retinoic acid. *PLoS One* 5:e15150, 2010.

645. Fan GC, Singh RR: Vaccination with minigenes encoding V(H)-derived major histocompatibility complex class I-binding epitopes activates cytotoxic T cells that ablate autoantibody-producing B cells and inhibit lupus. *J Exp Med* 196:731–741, 2002.

646. Ferrera F, Hahn BH, Rizzi M, et al: Protection against renal disease in (NZB x NZW)F lupus-prone mice after somatic B cell gene vaccination with anti-DNA immunoglobulin consensus peptide. *Arthritis Rheum* 56:1945–1953, 2007.

647. Lichtnekert J, Rupanagudi KV, Kulkarni OP, et al: Activated protein C attenuates systemic lupus erythematosus and lupus nephritis in MRL-Fas(lpr) mice. *J Immunol* 187:3413–3421, 2011.

648. Humrich JY, Morbach H, Undeutsch R, et al: Homeostatic imbalance of regulatory and effector T cells due to IL-2 deprivation amplifies murine lupus. *Proc Natl Acad Sci U S A* 107:204–209, 2010.

649. Gutierrez-Ramos JC, Andreu JL, Revilla Y, et al: Recovery from autoimmunity of MRL/lpr mice after infection with an interleukin-2/vaccinia recombinant virus. *Nature* 346:271–274, 1990.

650. Huggins ML, Huang FP, Xu D, et al: Modulation of autoimmune disease in the MRL-lpr/lpr mouse by IL-2 and TGF-beta1 gene therapy using attenuated *Salmonella typhimurium* as gene carrier. *Lupus* 8:29–38, 1999.

651. Warner LM, Adams LM, Sehgal SN: Rapamycin prolongs survival and arrests pathophysiologic changes in murine systemic lupus erythematosus. *Arthritis Rheum* 37:289–297, 1994.

652. Lui SL, Yung S, Tsang R, et al: Rapamycin prevents the development of nephritis in lupus-prone NZB/W F1 mice. *Lupus* 17:305–313, 2008.

653. De Albuquerque DA, Saxena V, Adams DE, et al: An ACE inhibitor reduces Th2 cytokines and TGF-beta1 and TGF-beta2 isoforms in murine lupus nephritis. *Kidney Int* 65:846–859, 2004.

654. Yin Z, Bahtiyar G, Zhang N, et al: IL-10 regulates murine lupus. *J Immunol* 169:2148–2155, 2002.

655. Menke J, Bork T, Kutska B, et al: Targeting transcription factor Stat4 uncovers a role for interleukin-18 in the pathogenesis of severe lupus nephritis in mice. *Kidney Int* 79:452–463, 2011.

656. Xu Z, Duan B, Croker BP, et al: STAT4 deficiency reduces autoantibody production and glomerulonephritis in a mouse model of lupus. *Clin Immunol* 120:189–198, 2006.

657. Sela U, Sharabi A, Dayan M, et al: The role of dendritic cells in the mechanism of action of a peptide that ameliorates lupus in murine models. *Immunology* 128(Suppl):e395–e405, 2009.

658. Sadanaga A, Nakashima H, Akahoshi M, et al: Protection against autoimmune nephritis in MyD88-deficient MRL/lpr mice. *Arthritis Rheum* 56:1618–1628, 2007.

659. Dong L, Ito S, Ishii KJ, et al: Suppressive oligodeoxynucleotides delay the onset of glomerulonephritis and prolong survival in lupus-prone NZB×NZW mice. *Arthritis Rheum* 52:651–658, 2005.

660. Bazzoni F, Beutler B: Comparative expression of TNF-alpha alleles from normal and autoimmune-prone MHC haplotypes. *J Inflamm* 45:106–114, 1995.

661. Gordon C, Ranges GE, Greenspan JS, et al: Chronic therapy with recombinant tumor necrosis factor-alpha in autoimmune NZB/NZW F1 mice. *Clin Immunol Immunopathol* 52:421–434, 1989.

662. Nicoletti F, Meroni P, Di Marco R, et al: In vivo treatment with a monoclonal antibody to interferon-gamma neither affects the survival nor the incidence of lupus-nephritis in the MRL/lpr-lpr mouse. *Immunopharmacology* 24:11–16, 1992.

663. Lawson BR, Prud'homme GJ, Chang Y, et al: Treatment of murine lupus with cDNA encoding IFN-gammaR/Fc. *J Clin Invest* 106:207–215, 2000.

664. Haas C, Ryffel B, Le Hir M: IFN-gamma receptor deletion prevents autoantibody production and glomerulonephritis in lupus-prone (NZB x NZW)F1 mice. *J Immunol* 160:3713–3718, 1998.

665. Vugmeyster Y, Guay H, Szklut P, et al: In vitro potency, pharmacokinetic profiles, and pharmacological activity of optimized anti-IL-21R antibodies in a mouse model of lupus. *MAbs* 2:335–346, 2010.

666. Zavala F, Masson A, Hadaya K, et al: Granulocyte-colony stimulating factor treatment of lupus autoimmune disease in MRL-lpr/lpr mice. *J Immunol* 163:5125–5132, 1999.

667. Liu Z, Bethunaickan R, Huang W, et al: IFN-alpha confers resistance of systemic lupus erythematosus nephritis to therapy in NZB/W F1 mice. *J Immunol* 187:1506–1513, 2011.

668. Sironi M, Guglielmotti A, Polentarutti N, et al: A small synthetic molecule capable of preferentially inhibiting the production of the CC chemokine monocyte chemotactic protein-1. *Eur Cytokine Netw* 10:437–442, 1999.

669. Kulkarni O, Pawar RD, Purschke W, et al: Spiegelmer inhibition of CCL2/MCP-1 ameliorates lupus nephritis in MRL-(Fas)lpr mice. *J Am Soc Nephrol* 18:2350–2358, 2007.

670. Anders HJ, Belemezova E, Eis V, et al: Late onset of treatment with a chemokine receptor CCR1 antagonist prevents progression of lupus nephritis in MRL-Fas(lpr) mice. *J Am Soc Nephrol* 15:1504–1513, 2004.

671. Patole PS, Grone HJ, Segerer S, et al: Viral double-stranded RNA aggravates lupus nephritis through Toll-like receptor 3 on glomerular mesangial cells and antigen-presenting cells. *J Am Soc Nephrol* 16:1326–1338, 2005.

672. Pawar RD, Castrezana-Lopez L, Allam R, et al: Bacterial lipopeptide triggers massive albuminuria in murine lupus nephritis by activating Toll-like receptor 2 at the glomerular filtration barrier. *Immunology* 128(Suppl):e206–e221, 2009.

673. Hoshi N, Watanabe H, Kobayashi H, et al: Inhibitory oligodeoxynucleotide improves glomerulonephritis and prolongs survival in MRL-lpr/lpr mice. *Fukushima J Med Sci* 53:70–84, 2007.

674. Pawar RD, Ramanjaneyulu A, Kulkarni OP, et al: Inhibition of Toll-like receptor-7 (TLR-7) or TLR-7 plus TLR-9 attenuates glomerulonephritis and lung injury in experimental lupus. *J Am Soc Nephrol* 18:1721–1731, 2007.

675. Hennessy EJ, Parker AE, O'Neill LA: Targeting Toll-like receptors: emerging therapeutics? *Nat Rev Drug Discov* 9:293–307, 2010.

676. Ishida T, Inaba M, Hisha H, et al: Requirement of donor-derived stromal cells in the bone marrow for successful allogeneic bone marrow transplantation. Complete prevention of recurrence of autoimmune diseases in MRL/MP-lpr/lpr mice by transplantation of bone marrow plus bones (stromal cells) from the same donor. *J Immunol* 152:3119–3127, 1994.

677. Shao DZ, Yamada S, Hirayama K, et al: Modulation of B-cell abnormalities in lupus-prone (NZB×NZW)F1 mice by normal bone marrow-derived B-lineage cells. *Immunology* 85:16–25, 1995.

678. Ende N, Czarneski J, Raveche E: Effect of human cord blood transfer on survival and disease activity in MRL-lpr/lpr mice. *Clin Immunol Immunopathol* 75:190–195, 1995.

679. Zhou K, Zhang H, Jin O, et al: Transplantation of human bone marrow mesenchymal stem cell ameliorates the autoimmune pathogenesis in MRL/lpr mice. *Cell Mol Immunol* 5:417–424, 2008.

680. Himeno K, Good RA: Marrow transplantation from tolerant donors to treat and prevent autoimmune diseases in BXSB mice. *Proc Natl Acad Sci U S A* 85:2235–2239, 1988.

681. Zurier RB, Sayadoff DM, Torrey AB, et al: Prostaglandin E treatment of NZB/NZW mice. *Arthritis Rheum* 20:723–728, 1977.

682. Zurier RB, Damjanov I, Sayadoff DM, et al: Prostaglandin E1 treatment of NZB/NZW F1 hybrid mice. II. Prevention of glomerulonephritis. *Arthritis Rheum* 20:1449–1456, 1977.

683. Yoshikawa T, Suzuki H, Sugiyama E, et al: Effects of prostaglandin E1 on the production of IgM and IgG class anti-dsDNA antibodies in NZB/W F1 mice. *J Rheumatol* 20:1701–1706, 1993.

684. Fan PY, Ruiz P, Pisetsky DS, et al: The effects of short-term treatment with the prostaglandin E1 (PGE1) analog misoprostol on inflammatory mediator production in murine lupus nephritis. *Clin Immunol Immunopathol* 75:125–130, 1995.

685. Hurd ER, Johnston JM, Okita JR, et al: Prevention of glomerulonephritis and prolonged survival in New Zealand Black/New Zealand White F1 hybrid mice fed an essential fatty acid-deficient diet. *J Clin Invest* 67:476–485, 1981.

686. Johnson BC, Gajjar A, Kubo C, et al: Calories versus protein in onset of renal disease in NZB x NZW mice. *Proc Natl Acad Sci U S A* 83:5659–5662, 1986.

687. Fernandes G, Venkatraman J, Khare A, et al: Modulation of gene expression in autoimmune disease and aging by food restriction and dietary lipids. *Proc Soc Exp Biol Med* 193:16–22, 1990.

688. Kubo C, Johnson BC, Day NK, et al: Effects of calorie restriction on immunologic functions and development of autoimmune disease in NZB mice. *Proc Soc Exp Biol Med* 201:192–199, 1992.

689. Chandrasekar B, McGuff HS, Aufdermorte TB, et al: Effects of calorie restriction on transforming growth factor beta 1 and proinflammatory cytokines in murine Sjögren's syndrome. *Clin Immunol Immunopathol* 76:291–296, 1995.

690. Jolly CA, Fernandes G: Diet modulates Th-1 and Th-2 cytokine production in the peripheral blood of lupus-prone mice. *J Clin Immunol* 19:172–178, 1999.

691. Prickett JD, Robinson DR, Steinberg AD: Dietary enrichment with the polyunsaturated fatty acid eicosapentaenoic acid prevents proteinuria and prolongs survival in NZB x NZW F1 mice. *J Clin Invest* 68:556–559, 1981.

692. Morrow WJ, Ohashi Y, Hall J, et al: Dietary fat and immune function. I. Antibody responses, lymphocyte and accessory cell function in (NZB×NZW)F1 mice. *J Immunol* 135:3857–3863, 1985.

693. Yumura W, Hattori S, Morrow WJ, et al: Dietary fat and immune function. II. Effects on immune complex nephritis in (NZB×NZW)F1 mice. *J Immunol* 135:3864–3868, 1985.

694. Robinson DR, Prickett JD, Polisson R, et al: The protective effect of dietary fish oil on murine lupus. *Prostaglandins* 30:51–75, 1985.

695. Godfrey DG, Stimson WH, Watson J, et al: Effects of dietary supplementation on autoimmunity in the MRL/lpr mouse: a preliminary investigation. *Ann Rheum Dis* 45:1019–1024, 1986.

696. Alexander NJ, Smythe NL, Jokinen MP: The type of dietary fat affects the severity of autoimmune disease in NZB/NZW mice. *Am J Pathol* 127:106–121, 1987.

697. Watson J, Godfrey D, Stimson WH, et al: The therapeutic effects of dietary fatty acid supplementation in the autoimmune disease of the MRL-mp-lpr/lpr mouse. *Int J Immunopharmacol* 10:467–471, 1988.

698. Westberg G, Tarkowski A, Svalander C: Effect of eicosapentaenoic acid rich menhaden oil and MaxEPA on the autoimmune disease of Mrl/l mice. *Int Arch Allergy Appl Immunol* 88:454–461, 1989.

699. Hall AV, Parbtani A, Clark WF, et al: Abrogation of MRL/lpr lupus nephritis by dietary flaxseed. *Am J Kidney Dis* 22:326–332, 1993.

700. Clark WF, Parbtani A: Omega-3 fatty acid supplementation in clinical and experimental lupus nephritis. *Am J Kidney Dis* 23:644–647, 1994.

701. Spurney RF, Ruiz P, Albrightson CR, et al: Fish oil feeding modulates leukotriene production in murine lupus nephritis. *Prostaglandins* 48:331–348, 1994.

702. Chandrasekar B, Fernandes G: Decreased pro-inflammatory cytokines and increased antioxidant enzyme gene expression by omega-3 lipids in murine lupus nephritis. *Biochem Biophys Res Commun* 200:893–898, 1994.

703. Zhang L, Bertucci AM, Smith KA, et al: Hyperexpression of cyclooxygenase 2 in the lupus immune system and effect of cyclooxygenase 2 inhibitor diet therapy in a murine model of systemic lupus erythematosus. *Arthritis Rheum* 56:4132–4141, 2007.

704. Carr R, Forsyth S, Sadi D: Abnormal responses to ingested substances in murine systemic lupus erythematosus: apparent effect of a casein-free diet on the development of systemic lupus erythematosus in NZB/W mice. *J Rheumatol Suppl* 14(Suppl 13):158–165, 1987.

705. Malinow MR, Bardana EJ, Jr, Pirofsky B, et al: Systemic lupus erythematosus-like syndrome in monkeys fed alfalfa sprouts: role of a nonprotein amino acid. *Science* 216:415–417, 1982.

706. Malinow MR, McLaughlin P, Bardana EJ, Jr, et al: Elimination of toxicity from diets containing alfalfa seeds. *Food Chem Toxicol* 22:583–587, 1984.

707. Alcocer-Varela J, Iglesias A, Llorente L, et al: Effects of L-canavanine on T cells may explain the induction of systemic lupus erythematosus by alfalfa. *Arthritis Rheum* 28:52–57, 1985.

708. Prete PE: Effects of L-canavanine on immune function in normal and autoimmune mice: disordered B-cell function by a dietary amino acid in the immunoregulation of autoimmune disease. *Can J Physiol Pharmacol* 63:843–854, 1985.

709. Hong Y, Wang T, Huang C, et al: Soy isoflavones supplementation alleviates disease severity in autoimmune-prone MRL-lpr/lpr mice. *Lupus* 17:814–821, 2008.

710. Steinberg AD, Melez KA, Raveche ES, et al: Approach to the study of the role of sex hormones in autoimmunity. *Arthritis Rheum* 22:1170–1176, 1979.

711. Matsunaga A, Miller BC, Cottam GL: Dehydroisoandrosterone prevention of autoimmune disease in NZB/W F1 mice: lack of an effect on associated immunological abnormalities. *Biochim Biophys Acta* 992:265–271, 1989.

712. Carlsten H, Nilsson N, Jonsson R, et al: Estrogen accelerates immune complex glomerulonephritis but ameliorates T cell-mediated vasculitis and sialadenitis in autoimmune MRL lpr/lpr mice. *Cell Immunol* 144:190–202, 1992.

713. Wu WM, Lin BF, Su YC, et al: Tamoxifen decreases renal inflammation and alleviates disease severity in autoimmune NZB/W F1 mice. *Scand J Immunol* 52:393–400, 2000.

714. Walker SE, McMurray RW, Houri JM, et al: Effects of prolactin in stimulating disease activity in systemic lupus erythematosus. *Ann N Y Acad Sci* 840:762–772, 1998.

715. Ansari MA, Dhar M, Muthukrishnan V, et al: Administration of antisense oligonucleotides to Galpha(Q/11) reduces the severity of murine lupus. *Biochimie* 85:627–632, 2003.

716. Auborn KJ, Qi M, Yan XJ, et al: Lifespan is prolonged in autoimmune-prone (NZB/NZW) F1 mice fed a diet supplemented with indole-3-carbinol. *J Nutr* 133:3610–3613, 2003.

717. Weinberg JB, Granger DL, Pisetsky DS, et al: The role of nitric oxide in the pathogenesis of spontaneous murine autoimmune disease: increased nitric oxide production and nitric oxide synthase expression in MRL-lpr/lpr mice, and reduction of spontaneous glomerulonephritis and arthritis by orally administered NG-monomethyl-L-arginine. *J Exp Med* 179:651–660, 1994.

718. Hortelano S, Diaz-Guerra MJ, Gonzalez-Garcia A, et al: Linomide administration to mice attenuates the induction of nitric oxide synthase elicited by lipopolysaccharide-activated macrophages and prevents nephritis in MRL/Mp-lpr/lpr mice. *J Immunol* 158:1402–1408, 1997.

719. Yang CW, Yu CC, Ko YC, et al: Aminoguanidine reduces glomerular inducible nitric oxide synthase (iNOS) and transforming growth factor-beta 1 (TGF-beta1) mRNA expression and diminishes glomerulosclerosis in NZB/W F1 mice. *Clin Exp Immunol* 113:258–264, 1998.

720. Kootstra CJ, Van Der Giezen DM, Van Krieken JH, et al: Effective treatment of experimental lupus nephritis by combined administration of anti-CD11a and anti-CD54 antibodies. *Clin Exp Immunol* 108:324–332, 1997.

721. Matsuo Y, Takagawa I, Koshida H, et al: Antiproteinuric effect of a thromboxane receptor antagonist, S-1452, on rat diabetic nephropathy and murine lupus nephritis. *Pharmacology* 50:1–8, 1995.

722. van Bruggen MC, Walgreen B, Rijke TP, et al: Heparin and heparinoids prevent the binding of immune complexes containing nucleosomal antigens to the GBM and delay nephritis in MRL/lpr mice. *Kidney Int* 50:1555–1564, 1996.

723. Wang Y, Hu Q, Madri JA, et al: Amelioration of lupus-like autoimmune disease in NZB/WF1 mice after treatment with a blocking monoclonal

antibody specific for complement component C5. *Proc Natl Acad Sci U S A* 93:8563–8568, 1996.

724. Gaynor B, Putterman C, Valadon P, et al: Peptide inhibition of glomerular deposition of an anti-DNA antibody. *Proc Natl Acad Sci U S A* 94:1955–1960, 1997.

725. Perl A: Pathogenic mechanisms in systemic lupus erythematosus. *Autoimmunity* 43:1–6, 2010.

726. McGrath H, Jr, Bak E, Michalski JP: Ultraviolet-A light prolongs survival and improves immune function in (New Zealand black x New Zealand white)F1 hybrid mice. *Arthritis Rheum* 30:557–561, 1987.

727. Ansel JC, Mountz J, Steinberg AD, et al: Effects of UV radiation on autoimmune strains of mice: increased mortality and accelerated autoimmunity in BXSB male mice. *J Invest Dermatol* 85:181–186, 1985.

728. Fan JL, Himeno K, Tsuru S, et al: Treatment of autoimmune MRL/Mp-lpr/lpr mice with cholera toxin. *Clin Exp Immunol* 70:94–101, 1987.

729. Baldi E, Emancipator SN, Hassan MO, et al: Platelet activating factor receptor blockade ameliorates murine systemic lupus erythematosus. *Kidney Int* 38:1030–1038, 1990.

730. Vilanova M, Ribeiro A, Carneiro J, et al: The effects of thalidomide treatment on autoimmune-prone NZB and MRL mice are consistent with stimulation of the central immune system. *Scand J Immunol* 40:543–548, 1994.

731. Lewis RM, Schwartz R, Henry WB, Jr: Canine systemic lupus erythematosus. *Blood* 25:143–160, 1965.

732. Lewis RM, Schwartz RS: Canine systemic lupus erythematosus. Genetic analysis of an established breeding colony. *J Exp Med* 134:417–438, 1971.

733. Lewis RM, Schwartz RS: The transmissibility of canine systemic lupus erythematosus (SLE). *J Clin Invest* 51, 1974.

734. Monier JC, Dardenne M, Rigal D, et al: Clinical and laboratory features of canine lupus syndromes. *Arthritis Rheum* 23:294–301, 1980.

735. Halliwell RE: Autoimmune diseases in domestic animals. *J Am Vet Med Assoc* 181:1088–1096, 1982.

736. Shanley KJ: Lupus erythematosus in small animals. *Clin Dermatol* 3:131–138, 1985.

737. Welin Henriksson E, Hansson H, Karlsson-Parra A, et al: Autoantibody profiles in canine ANA-positive sera investigated by immunoblot and ELISA. *Vet Immunol Immunopathol* 61(2-4):157–170, 1998.

738. Monier JC, Fournel C, Lapras M, et al: Systemic lupus erythematosus in a colony of dogs. *Am J Vet Res* 49:46–51, 1988.

739. Teichner M, Krumbacher K, Doxiadis I, et al: Systemic lupus erythematosus in dogs: association to the major histocompatibility complex class I antigen DLA-A7. *Clin Immunol Immunopathol* 55:255–262, 1990.

740. Center SA, Smith CA, Wilkinson E, et al: Clinicopathologic, renal immunofluorescent, and light microscopic features of glomerulonephritis in the dog: 41 cases (1975-1985). *J Am Vet Med Assoc* 190:81–90, 1987.

741. Costa O, Fournel C, Lotchouang E, et al: Specificities of antinuclear antibodies detected in dogs with systemic lupus erythematosus. *Vet Immunol Immunopathol* 7:369–382, 1984.

742. Fournel C, Chabanne L, Caux C, et al: Canine systemic lupus erythematosus. I: A study of 75 cases. *Lupus* 1:133–139, 1992.

743. Jones DR: Canine systemic lupus erythematosus: new insights and their implications. *J Comp Pathol* 108:215–228, 1993.

744. Stone MS, Johnstone IB, Brooks M, et al: Lupus-type "anticoagulant" in a dog with hemolysis and thrombosis. *J Vet Intern Med* 8:57–61, 1994.

745. Halla JT, Volanakis JE, Schrohenloher RE: Circulating immune complexes in mixed connective tissue disease. *Arthritis Rheum* 22:484–489, 1979.

746. Taylor RP, Kujala G, Wilson K, et al: In vivo and in vitro studies of the binding of antibody/dsDNA immune complexes to rabbit and guinea pig platelets. *J Immunol* 134:2550–2558, 1985.

747. Brinet A, Fournel C, Faure JR, et al: Anti-histone antibodies (ELISA and immunoblot) in canine lupus erythematosus. *Clin Exp Immunol* 74:105–109, 1988.

748. Smee NM, Harkin KR, Wilkerson MJ: Measurement of serum antinuclear antibody titer in dogs with and without systemic lupus erythematosus: 120 cases (1997-2005). *J Am Vet Med Assoc* 230:1180–1183, 2007.

749. Hansson-Hamlin H, Lilliehook I, Trowald-Wigh G: Subgroups of canine antinuclear antibodies in relation to laboratory and clinical findings in immune-mediated disease. *Vet Clin Pathol* 35:397–404, 2006.

750. Kristensen AT, Weiss DJ, Klausner JS, et al: Detection of antiplatelet antibody with a platelet immunofluorescence assay. *J Vet Intern Med* 8:36–39, 1994.

751. Monestier M, Novick KE, Karam ET, et al: Autoantibodies to histone, DNA and nucleosome antigens in canine systemic lupus erythematosus. *Clin Exp Immunol* 99:37–41, 1995.

752. White SD, Rosychuk RA, Schur PH: Investigation of antibodies to extractable nuclear antigens in dogs. *Am J Vet Res* 53:1019–1021, 1992.

753. Zouali M, Migliorini P, Mackworth-Young CG, et al: Nucleic acid-binding specificity and idiotypic expression of canine anti-DNA antibodies. *Eur J Immunol* 18:923–927, 1988.

754. Wilbe M, Jokinen P, Hermanrud C, et al: MHC class II polymorphism is associated with a canine SLE-related disease complex. *Immunogenetics* 61:557–564, 2009.

755. Wilbe M, Jokinen P, Truve K, et al: Genome-wide association mapping identifies multiple loci for a canine SLE-related disease complex. *Nat Genet* 42:250–254, 2010.

756. Reinertsen JL, Kaslow RA, Klippel JH, et al: An epidemiologic study of households exposed to canine systemic lupus erythematosus. *Arthritis Rheum* 23:564–568, 1980.

757. Choi E, Shin I, Youn H, et al: Development of canine systemic lupus erythematosus model. *J Vet Med A Physiol Pathol Clin Med* 51:375–383, 2004.

758. Lusson D, Billiemaz B, Chabanne JL: Circulating lupus anticoagulant and probable systemic lupus erythematosus in a cat. *J Feline Med Surg* 1:193–196, 1999.

759. Halliwell REW: Systemic lupus erythematosus in domestic animals. In: Lahita RG, editor: *Systemic Lupus Erythematosus*, ed 3, San Diego, 1999, Academic Press, pp 183–195.

760. Aucoin DP, Rubin RL, Peterson ME, et al: Dose-dependent induction of anti-native DNA antibodies in cats by propylthiouracil. *Arthritis Rheum* 31:688–692, 1988.

761. Vrins A, Feldman B: Lupus erythematosus-like syndrome in a horse. *Equine Pract* 5:18, 1983.

762. Geor RJ, Clark EG, Haines DM, et al: Systemic lupus erythematosus in a filly. *J Am Vet Med Assoc* 197:1489–1492, 1990.

763. Clifford GO, McClure J, Conway M: Renal lesions in dogs produced by plasma from patients with systemic lupus erythematosus. *J Lab Clin Med* 58:807–814, 1961.

764. Bencze G, Tiboldi T, Lakatos L. Experiments on the pathogenetic role of the L.E. factor in dogs and guinea-pigs. *Acta Rheumatol Scand* 9:209–211, 1963.

765. Dubois EL, Katz YJ, Freeman V, et al: Chronic toxicity studies of hydralazine (apresoline) in dogs with particular reference to the production of the hydralazine syndrome. *J Lab Clin Med* 50:119–126, 1957.

Chapter 18

Pathogenetic Mechanisms in Lupus Nephritis

Anne Davidson, Celine Berthier, and Matthias Kretzler

The kidneys maintain homeostasis of water, minerals, electrolytes, and hydrogen ions and eliminate toxic substances produced by the body. Each kidney contains more than 1 million nephrons, each consisting of a glomerulus and tubule. The glomerulus is a capillary filter under arteriolar pressure that filters out cells and large molecules to produce an ultrafiltrate that empties into the tubule of the nephron. The final urine is produced in the tubule as a result of both reabsorption of substances and secretion of substances into the tubular fluid. The other critical function of the kidney is the secretion of hormones that regulate blood pressure, calcium metabolism, and red blood cell production. Thus any process that threatens kidney viability has a major impact on patient health.

SLE nephritis is characterized by glomerular and tubulointerstitial inflammation most often initiated by the renal deposition of immune complexes[1-4] that trigger a cascade of inflammatory events including complement activation,[5] engagement of activating Fc receptors on mononuclear cells,[6] activation of intrinsic renal cells, and recruitment of inflammatory cells. Renal deposition of autoantibodies and complement is not, however, sufficient to cause renal damage. Signals from the innate immune system and cellular immunity also contribute to renal disease. Immune complexes directly activate resident renal cells through Toll-like receptors (TLRs) to produce inflammatory mediators.[7] Chemokines produced by intrinsic renal cells attract multiple subsets of inflammatory cells.[8] Cytokines induce endothelial cells to express adhesion molecules, increasing the probability that they will recruit inflammatory cells after contact with immune complexes. In one animal model of nephritis, T cell–mediated interstitial renal disease and vasculitis together with mild glomerular changes occur even in the complete absence of circulating immunoglobulins.[9] Similarly, in human SLE some pauci-immune forms of nephritis have been observed. Microvascular damage and thromboses also occur in the setting of SLE nephritis and may be more common in patients with antiphospholipid antibodies.[10] Inadequately treated disease or repeated disease flares can lead to chronic changes, including glomerulosclerosis, tubular atrophy, and tissue fibrosis, that may ultimately lead to the death of the organ.

RENAL ANATOMY AND PHYSIOLOGY
Glomerular Structure and Function
The glomerulus is an intricately organized structure that is highly permeable to water while at the same time acting as a filtration barrier for larger molecules (Figure 18-1).[10a] Each glomerulus consists of a spherical tuft of capillaries under arteriolar pressure that is held together by the mesangium, a supporting tissue consisting of mesangial cells and their matrix. The highly negatively charged glomerular filtration barrier consists of endothelial cells, the glomerular basement membrane, and a series of foot processes that emanate from podocytes, specialized epithelial cells located within the urinary space. Maintenance of the structural integrity of the glomerular capillary loops and of the glomerular filtration barrier depends on intricate "cross talk" between podocytes, endothelial cells, and mesangial cells; injury of any of the three cell types may lead to proteinuria. The urinary space of each glomerulus is located between and outside the

podocytes and is surrounded by a single layer of parietal epithelial cells that is continuous with the podocyte layer. Importantly, the effluent blood flow from the glomerulus provides the sole blood supply for peritubular capillaries, so any decrease in glomerular blood flow will threaten the viability of the tubules.

Glomerular Filtration Barrier
The glomerular filtration barrier has several layers.[11] The first is a glycocalyx made up of proteoglycans and an adsorbed layer of plasma proteins that is located between the endothelial cells and the capillary lumen. Fenestrated endothelial cells form the next layer. Next is the thick glomerular basement membrane (GBM), which is synthesized by podocytes and endothelial cells and has an inner layer composed of collagen type IV and laminin sandwiched between layers of heparin sulfate. Podocyte foot processes line the epithelial side of the GBM; the intercellular junctions between adjacent foot processes are closed by the slit diaphragm, a specialized intercellular junction that acts as a molecular sieve and the final component of the filtration barrier. The slit diaphragm comprises several proteins, including nephrin, CD-associated protein (CD2AP), podocin, the tight junction protein ZO-1 (zonula occludens 1), P-cadherin, catenins, and the calcium channel TRPC6 (transient receptor potential cation channel, subfamily C, member 6), each of which is required for slit diaphragm integrity. Slit diaphragm proteins are supported by the highly dynamic podocyte actin cytoskeleton that in turn is anchored to an integrin complex that fastens each podocyte foot process to the GBM.

Podocytes
Podocytes play a crucial role in maintaining glomerular integrity and function. Apart from synthesizing the GBM, podocytes secret angiopoietin 1 and vascular endothelial growth factor 1 (VEGF-1), which help maintain the endothelial cells; loss of podocyte-derived VEGF results in renal thrombotic microangiopathy. Podocytes also express the immunoglobulin (Ig) receptor FcRn (neonatal Fc receptor), which helps clear trapped immunoglobulin, and express angiotensin receptors and angiotensin-converting enzyme (ACE).[12] Inhibition of the latter pathway can improve proteinuria via systemic hemodynamic and local metabolic effects. During inflammatory states, including SLE nephritis, podocytes can be induced by TLR engagement to express B7-1, which binds to the integrin complex and displaces the foot process from the GBM, thus inducing proteinuria.[13] Loss of podocytes into the urine is a feature of active SLE nephritis. Although some forms of podocyte injury are reversible, chronic injury leading to excessive podocyte loss eventually results in glomerulosclerosis and loss of renal function.[13]

Mesangium
The mesangium consists of mesangial cells and the mesangial matrix that contains collagens, laminin, proteoglycans, heparin sulfate, fibronectin, entactin, and nidogen. Mesangial cells are smooth muscle–like cells that contain actin and myosin; they connect to each other via gap junctions and to the GBM via cell processes.

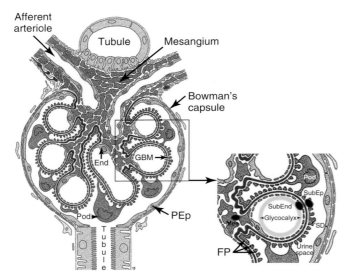

FIGURE 18-1 Anatomy of the glomerulus, consisting of a tuft of capillary loops fed by the afferent arteriole. The tuft is held together by the mesangium. The enlarged capillary loop shows the components of the glomerular filtration barrier. The barrier is formed by the glycocalyx, fenestrated endothelial cells (End), glomerular basement membrane (GBM), podocyte foot processes (Pod and FP), and slit diaphragm (SD). The podocyte layer is contiguous with the parietal epithelial layer (PEp), which is surrounded by the Bowman capsule. Immune deposits may be found on either side of the GBM (SubEnd or SubEp) or in the mesangium (Mes).

Contraction of mesangial cells regulates the size of the capillary lumen and thus the amount of glomerular blood flow. Mesangial cells are in direct contact with the vascular system via the fenestrations in the endothelial capillary cells, and their survival depends on platelet-derived growth factor (PDGF) secreted by endothelial cells. Mesangial cells produce growth factors, cytokines, adhesion molecules, chemokines, and vasoactive factors, and they express Fc receptors, C-type lectins, and some TLRs including TLR3.[14,15] Mesangial deposition of immune complexes occurs in most forms of SLE nephritis, and both mesangial cell proliferation and mesangiolysis (loss of matrix) have been observed. Nevertheless, deposits restricted to the mesangium are usually associated with mild disease.

Glomerular Endothelial Cells
To facilitate maximal selective solute flux, the renal glomerular vascular bed is lined by specialized endothelial cells. The negatively charged glycocalyx serves to reflect cellular elements and negatively charged molecules, whereas a dense network of endothelial transcellular fenestrae facilitate solute exposure to the next layers of the filtration barrier; in mature kidneys the fenestrae occupy 20-50% of the glomerular capillary wall surface area. Capillary endothelial cells deliver signals to circulating cells and are themselves targets of intraglomerular "cross talk" and soluble mediators.

The Renal Tubules and the Kidney Interstitium
Renal Tubular Epithelial Cells
Proximal tubular epithelial cells can assume a proinflammatory and profibrotic role during chronic renal disease in which they express inflammatory mediators including complement proteins, tumor necrosis factor alpha (TNF-α), chemokines, and growth factors. Sensitive markers of renal tubular injury include kidney injury molecule 1 (KIM-1) and lipocalin 2 (LCN-2), which are both produced by proximal tubular cells and appear in the urine promptly after ischemic damage.[16]

Epithelial-to-mesenchymal transition is a process by which epithelial cells transform into mesenchymal cells that contribute to chronic renal fibrosis. This transition is posited to occur in response to cell

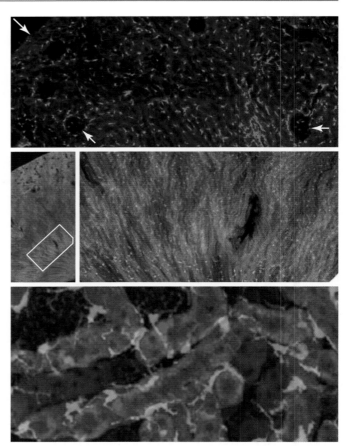

FIGURE 18-2 A resident renal mononuclear phagocyte network. A network of CXC3CR1⁺ (*green*) interstitial dendritic cells is found throughout the interstitium of normal mouse kidneys. This network of cells surrounds glomeruli in the cortex (*arrows*) and is intricately associated with renal tubules (*red*) in the medulla. (*From Soos TJ, Sims TN, Barisoni L, et al: CX3CR1⁺ interstitial dendritic cells form a contiguous network throughout the entire kidney.* Kidney Int *70:591–596, 2006.*)

injury and exposure to transforming growth factor–beta (TGF-β) and is followed by secretion of collagen and extracellular matrix. Definitive cell-tracing experiments have now shown that despite the acquisition of some mesenchymal markers, renal tubular cells do not transform into cells that cause fibrosis, calling into question the existence of this process.[17]

Renal Interstitial Fibroblasts
Renal fibroblasts form a structural network that helps maintain kidney architecture; they are also the source of erythropoietin. These cells form focal contacts with each other as well as capillaries and tubules. The current consensus is that renal interstitial fibroblasts are the origin of myofibroblasts that cause renal fibrosis during chronic injury.[16,17] Fibroblast proliferation is enhanced by basic fibroblast growth factor (FGF-2), which is induced by TGF-β1.[18]

Resident Renal Mononuclear Phagocytes
Resident renal mononuclear phagocytes have variably been called resident macrophages and resident renal dendritic cells.[19] In mice, the major population of phagocytes express F4/80, CD11b, and intermediate levels of CD11c, and they are positive for major histocompatibility complex (MHC) class II molecules but express low levels of co-stimulatory molecules. The generation of CX3CR1-GFP–labeled mice has allowed visualization of these cells in a network surrounding glomerular tubules (Figure 18-2).[20] These cells are capable of phagocytosis and constantly retract and extend dendritic processes

into the interstitium.[20,21] Their role is probably a sentinel one under physiologic circumstances, but they can contribute to renal injury once activated. In addition to these cells, other small populations of renal mononuclear phagocytes can be detected. Lymphocytes are rare in normal kidneys, with the exception of a small population of CD4[+] T cells whose function is not known.

MECHANISMS FOR IMMUNE COMPLEX DEPOSITION IN THE KIDNEYS
Site of Immune Complex Deposition in SLE

Immune deposits may deposit on either side of the GBM (Figure 18-1), and both the amount and location of deposits correlate with the severity of the disease. Deposits limited to the mesangium and sparing the capillary loops are associated with International Society of Nephrology (ISN) class I and class II disease. Subendothelial deposits, located between the endothelium and the GBM, are found in ISN class III and class IV disease. These have access to the vascular space and can therefore mediate recruitment of inflammatory cells and subsequent endothelial damage. Subepithelial deposits located at the base of the podocyte foot processes outside the GBM are found in class V disease. In this type of disease, complement-mediated injury of podocytes induces them to lay down excessive matrix material that alters the structure of the basement membrane, leading to proteinuria. Inflammatory mediators recruited by subepithelial deposits are diluted into the urinary space and are excreted, limiting recruitment of inflammatory cells and local damage. Mesangial deposits are found in most classes of lupus nephritis and can induce mesangial cells to overproduce inflammatory mediators, growth factors, and extracellular matrix. Deposits of immune complexes have also been reported in the tubulointerstitium and in the vasculature.

The Characteristics of Pathogenic Autoantibodies

The precise properties of pathogenic antibodies that deposit in the kidneys and elicit an inflammatory response have still not been completely defined. Antibodies eluted from kidneys of both mice and humans with SLE are predominantly class switched, are enriched for anti-DNA activity, and are cross-reactive with multiple autoantigens, including GBM components, whereas lupus serum anti-DNA antibodies are less cross-reactive and "natural" anti-DNA antibodies derived from normal serum have no cross-reactivity.[22,23] Some of this polyreactivity may be artifactual, resulting from tight binding of nuclear material to the anti-DNA antibodies, thereby forming a "bridge" to other antigens such as collagen, histones, and glomerular material.[24,25] Antibodies eluted from the kidneys also have higher avidity for DNA than those antibodies in the circulation, although there is considerable variability in both compartments.[22] Binding to nucleosomal components may be more important than binding to DNA because nucleosomes may become trapped in the kidneys.[22] However, binding to chromatin is not the only mechanism for renal deposition, because antibodies without specificity for any nuclear components may also deposit in the kidneys and cause renal damage in murine lupus models.[3] Similarly, only a variable proportion of the antibodies eluted from kidneys of patients with SLE are specific for DNA or other known nuclear antigens.[23] Another characteristic of pathogenic antibodies is cationic charge, which may confer binding specificity for negatively charged DNA or heparan sulfate (HS) in the GBM. In mice, charged residues such as arginine, lysine, and asparagine in the complementarity-determining regions, particularly of the heavy chain, are associated with anti-DNA–binding activity and pathogenicity.[25,26] A number of investigators have reported that anti-DNA antibodies penetrate into live cells, including resident renal cells, via a mechanism dependent on the antigen-binding region of the antibody.[27] Although localization of antibodies in nuclei could cause alterations in protein synthesis or impair other nuclear functions, it remains to be shown whether this phenomenon is actually associated with pathogenicity. Studies in vitro have shown that anti-DNA antibodies directly induce proinflammatory cytokine release in

Box 18-1 Factors That May Contribute to Pathogenicity of Anti–Double-Stranded DNA Antibodies

1. Functional features associated with antibody deposition:
   a. Cross-reactivity with target organ antigens.
   b. Avidity for DNA.
   c. Ability to bind glomerular basement membranes in vitro.
   d. Binding to C1q.
   e. Ability to penetrate cells or activate cell surface molecules—thereby influencing cellular functions.
2. Structural features of the Ig component that influence antigen binding or recruitment of downstream effector pathways:
   a. Charge—positively charged antibodies are more likely to bind to negatively charged DNA or to the negatively charged glomerular basement membrane.
   b. Use of particular amino acids in V region genes that confer charge differences.
   c. Isotype—determines antibody effector functions such as complement fixation and binding to Fc receptors.
3. Features of the complexes themselves that affect the amount of renal damage:
   a. Size of immune complexes.
   b. Site of deposition.
   c. Amount of deposit.
   d. Composition of the deposits.

mesangial and tubular cells as well as increased proliferation and changes in viability. The mechanisms for these effects are not yet fully elucidated. Finally the isotype of the antibody dictates its effector properties, particularly the ability to bind to Fc receptors and to activate complement (Box 18-1).

Not all anti-DNA antibodies are pathogenic. In one study, infusion of 24 different monoclonal anti-DNA antibodies into mice in vivo resulted in variable patterns of deposition and only some induced pathologic renal changes and proteinuria, indicating heterogeneity in renal specificity.[28] Furthermore, the ability to bind to glomeruli in vitro or to induce renal pathology in vivo was found in a second study to be independent of relative avidity for DNA.[29] Another comprehensive study of a large panel of monoclonal antibodies derived from SLE-prone mice showed that antibodies to double-stranded DNA (dsDNA) were more pathogenic than antibodies to histones or non-nuclear antigens and that anti-DNA antibodies with glomerular binding specificity were more pathogenic than those that did not bind to glomeruli.[25] The abrogation of glomerular binding by DNAse treatment of either the antibodies or the glomerular substrate, with the restoration of binding activity by the addition of chromatin, suggests that much of the glomerular binding of these in vitro glomerular binding monoclonal antibodies is mediated via antigenic bridges.[1]

To determine whether there are any serum autoantibody specificities that correlate with or predict renal disease in human SLE, clinical studies have compared the specificity of antibodies in the sera of patients with and without nephritis. On a proteome array consisting of multiple autoantigens and renal antigens, serologic reactivity of IgG antibodies with an antigenic cluster that included nuclear antigens and whole glomerular lysates correlated with current renal activity and with overall disease activity as indicated by Systemic Lupus Erythematosus Disease Activity Index (SLEDAI) score.[2] As shown for mouse monoclonal antibodies, pretreatment of lupus sera with DNAse reduced binding to glomerular lysates on the proteome array but not to all of the individual glomerular antigens. Another study used the glomerular binding assay to test sera from a well-characterized cohort of patients with SLE with and without nephritis. In this study glomerular binding activity was present in 92% of sera from those individuals with both renal disease and anti-dsDNA antibodies, compared with 25% of sera from individuals with anti-dsDNA antibodies but without nephritis. However, glomerular

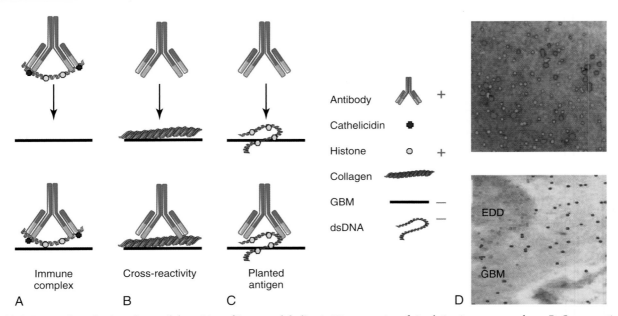

FIGURE 18-3 Proposed mechanisms for renal deposition of immunoglobulin. A, Direct trapping of circulating immune complexes. **B,** Cross-reactivity with renal antigen. **C,** Indirect binding to nuclear material planted on the glomerular basement membrane. **D,** *Top,* An electron-dense deposit (EDD) in the glomerular basement membrane (GBM) of a BWF1 lupus mouse stained with TUNEL (*red*) for chromatin and anti-immunoglobulin (anti-Ig) (*green*). *Bottom,* The GBM from a BWF1 mouse stains for laminin (*red*) but the deposited Ig (*green*) is localized to the EDD. *(D adapted from van Bavel CC, Fenton KA, Rekvig OP, et al: Glomerular targets of nephritogenic autoantibodies in systemic lupus erythematosus. Arthritis Rheum 58:1892–1899, 2008.)*

binding activity did not correlate with either the type or the severity of the renal lesion and was only rarely present in nephritic individuals who did not have anti-dsDNA antibodies in their serum.[30] Although these studies in sum show that glomerular binding antibodies are detected more commonly in the sera of patients with nephritis than in those without it and correlate with the presence of anti-DNA antibodies, they also reflect the heterogeneous characteristics of the circulating autoantibodies. Importantly, circulating autoantibodies may not fully reflect the characteristics of those antibodies that actually deposit in the kidneys.

Mechanisms of Tissue Deposition of Immune Complexes

Several overlapping hypotheses have been proposed to explain how autoantibodies deposit in the kidneys (Figure 18-3, *A* to *C*).

Trapping of Preformed Immune Complexes

The kidney is particularly susceptible to immune complex trapping because it receives a large amount of the cardiac output and has a large glomerular capillary bed. On the basis of findings in mouse lupus models, it was initially thought that circulating immune complexes of antibodies with nucleic acids formed in the blood of patients with SLE become trapped in the mesangium or in the subendothelial space; these are too large to cross into the subepithelial space unless they dissociate. Because small complexes are soluble and do not bind complement efficiently and large complexes are rapidly removed from the circulation by phagocytosis, it has been hypothesized that medium-sized complexes are the most likely to deposit.[31] The charge of the complexes may also be important because the GBM is highly negatively charged. Although circulating immune complexes have been detected in animal models of SLE nephritis and have been reported by some investigators in humans with active nephritis, they have been difficult to detect by standard methods.[32-33] On the basis of these data and the inability to show that preformed antibody/free DNA complexes deposit in the kidneys, the immune complex–trapping hypothesis was subsequently discredited. However, this hypothesis has now been revisited because it has become clear that a major cause of SLE is a failure to adequately clear apoptotic cell debris and nucleosomes that are rich sources of nucleic acids. Circulating autoantibodies can bind to autoantigens that are exposed in this debris. In fact, nucleosome-complexed antibodies bind more avidly to the GBM than antibodies that have been highly purified and no longer contain nucleosomal material.[4] One hypothesis is that binding of positively charged anti-DNA antibodies to the negatively charged DNA of the nucleosome leaves the positively charged nucleosomal histones available to bind to the negatively charged GBM (see Figure 18-3A). This idea is supported by the observation that binding of autoantibodies to the GBM can be blocked by heparin, which acts as an inhibitor of HS binding. In contrast, antihistone antibodies that mask the nucleosomal positive charges prevent binding to the GBM and thus are less pathogenic.[24]

It has also been shown that circulating microparticles that are released from a variety of cell types are coated with IgG more frequently in plasma from patients with lupus than in plasma from normal controls.[34] Patients with SLE also have abnormal neutrophils that are activated in patients with active disease and more prone to cell death via a process called NETosis, in which neutrophils extrude weblike structures, called neutrophil extracellular traps (NETs), that contain large amounts of nuclear DNA. This DNA is complexed with neutrophil-derived antimicrobial proteins such as LL37 (cathelicidin) and human neutrophil peptides belonging to the α-defensin family. Immune complexes containing DNA complexed to these neutrophil peptides have been detected in SLE sera. Not only are these complexes strong inducers of type I interferons (IFNs) but they are also prone to form particulates that are resistant to DNAse treatment.[35] Resistance to DNAse can be due to circulating inhibitors or to antibodies that cover the NETs and protect them from the enzyme. Importantly, preliminary studies have suggested that failure to degrade NETs is associated with a higher incidence of nephritis.[36]

These studies all suggest that nuclear material tightly complexed to antibodies can be found circulating in the peripheral blood of patients with SLE and help explain the results of glomerular binding assays in which binding is not always abrogated by DNAse treatment.

Cross-Reactive Renal Antigens

The second proposed mechanism for tissue deposition is in situ immune complex deposition by direct cross-reactivity with renal antigens other than nucleic acids. The glomerular antigen that is the target in most cases of idiopathic membranous nephritis in humans, phospholipase A_2 receptor, has now been identified. However, antibodies to this antigen are only rarely found in cases of membranous SLE nephritis. Nevertheless, many studies have shown that antinuclear antibodies (ANAs) may cross-react with a variety of renal antigens, including laminin, fibronectin, collagen IV, HS, and α-actinin.[1] Furthermore, anti-DNA antibodies from patients with SLE nephritis deposit directly in rat glomeruli when perfused into the renal artery, whereas anti-DNA antibodies from patients without nephritis do not.[37] Studies of monoclonal antibodies from lupus-prone mice showed that antibodies with cross-reactivities to different glomerular proteins can bind to different types of glomerular cells and may elicit different types of renal diseases.[28] One of the problems with using serum antibodies or even monoclonal antibodies for these studies is that they have a strong tendency to bind to circulating nuclear material or to nucleosomes released into the culture supernatants of the hybridoma cells, and it can be very difficult to remove all the nuclear antigens even with DNAse. Thus some of these findings may be explained by the presence of nuclear material bridges. It is also clear that immune complex–mediated renal disease can occur both in SLE-prone mice and in patients without anti-DNA antibodies in their sera; the relevant antigens and mechanisms in the latter remain to be determined.

In Situ Immune Complex Formation

The third major hypothesized mechanism for tissue deposition of autoantibodies is the entrapment of circulating autoantibodies by nucleosomal material ("planted antigen") that has already bound to renal antigens. Deposition of nuclear material is mediated by binding of positively charged histones to the negatively charged GBM. Relevant GBM antigens include heparan sulfate, collagen type IV, and anionic phospholipids. The source of this material could include circulating chromatin,[24] microparticles,[34] neutrophil-derived NETs,[36] or debris released from locally damaged cells. Further evidence for the planted antigen theory has come from elegant immunohistochemical studies in NZB/W mice showing that in vivo–bound autoantibodies fail to colocalize with the putative cross-reactive antigens, α-actinin, laminin, and collagen IV, but rather colocalize with electron-dense deposits containing chromatin (see Figure 18-3, *D*).[24] Deposition may then be amplified by circulating rheumatoid factors that bind to the Fc region of the antibodies or by antibodies to C1q that bind to fixed complement. Antibodies to C1q may also bind directly to apoptotic material, perhaps through binding to exposed phosphatidyl serine.[38] A better understanding of the sources of renal chromatin may lead to new interventions directed at preventing its renal deposition or enhancing its clearance. For example, it has been shown by one group of investigators that SLE nephritic kidneys downregulate their production of DNAse and therefore may be less able to clear planted nuclear antigens.[4]

PAUCI-IMMUNE GLOMERULONEPHRITIS

Some cases of lupus nephritis are associated with only small amounts of immune deposits. This pauci-immune nephritis may be associated with thrombotic microangiopathy, with vasculitis, or with a podocytopathy that is presumably due to circulating immune mediators that induce activation and damage of intrinsic renal cells.[39] In the MRL/lpr mouse model, mild to moderate renal disease can occur even when circulating immunoglobulins are absent, suggesting that innate and T cell–mediated mechanisms may be sufficient to cause tissue damage.[9] Several new studies have investigated the role of cell-mediated immunity in the induction of renal damage. There is evidence that interstitial renal dendritic cells, when activated by renal injury, can capture renal antigens that have been degraded and transported from the tubular lumen by tubular epithelial cells. Because self-antigens constitute the majority of peptides expressed in the peptide-binding groove of MHC class I molecules, renal cells may then become targets of activated cytotoxic T cells.[40]

MOUSE MODELS OF LUPUS NEPHRITIS

The study of the effector phase of SLE nephritis in humans is hampered by the small amount of biopsy material available, by the cost and invasive nature of repeated biopsy, and by the therapeutic interventions that are already in place before the biopsy is performed. Murine models of nephritis have therefore been invaluable for studying the mechanisms of renal inflammation in SLE.

Two main categories of mouse models exist, namely, spontaneous models[41] and induced models. Not surprisingly, striking differences in both pathogenic mechanisms and responses to immunologic interventions have been observed in the different mouse models, suggesting that multiple animal models will be needed to dissect the pathogenetic mechanisms of SLE nephritis and to study responses to new therapies. These differences among the mouse models parallel the emerging appreciation of heterogeneity in human SLE nephritis.[42] Apart from the limited heterogeneity of the mouse models, a further limitation of the mouse in comparison with human and other species such as rat is the relative resistance to the development of end-stage kidney disease, most likely as a consequence of a higher nephron endowment relative to body mass than in other species. However, given the vast literature on mouse models of SLE on which potential new therapies are often based, this chapter contains a brief description of several murine models in which the renal disease has been well characterized.

Diffuse Proliferative Glomerulonephritis with Anti-DNA Antibodies

The NZB/W F1 hybrid, the oldest classic SLE model, has a phenotype comparable to that of patients with lupus, with the production of IgG2a anti-dsDNA antibodies and some genetic similarities to human SLE. Nephritic kidneys are characterized by proliferative glomerulonephritis with glomerular enlargement and hypercellularity, extensive infiltration with activated renal macrophages in the tubulointerstitial region, and accumulation of T and B cells along with dendritic cells in disorganized perivascular and periglomerular aggregates,[43] similar to those reported in SLE biopsy specimens. These mice can also be used to study disease remission and relapse because complete remission of established nephritis is achieved in more than 80% of mice by combination therapy either with a short course of cyclophosphamide (Cytoxan) together with co-stimulatory blockade or with a short course of cytotoxic T-lymphocyte antigen 4 (CTLA-4) Ig together with B-cell activating factor (BAFF) blockade.[44] A similar hybrid is the SNF1 mouse, a hybrid of SWR with NZB. This mouse demonstrates proliferative disease with glomerular hypercellularity with crescents, thickening of capillary loops and basement membrane as well as mesangial thickening, large perivascular infiltrates of lymphoid cells, and eventually, glomerulosclerosis and fibrosis.[45]

Sclerotic Glomerulonephritis with Antinucleosome and Anti-DNA Antibodies

The NZM2410 strain of mice was derived from a back-cross between NZB/W F1 and NZW mice followed by brother-sister mating. Twenty-seven different recombinant inbred strains of New Zealand Mixed (NZM) mice were obtained; among them, NZM2410 and NZM2328 have been used most commonly as lupus models. NZM2410 mice are dominated by an interleukin-4 (IL-4) response, and they produce IgG1 and IgE antichromatin antibodies. They demonstrate sclerotic glomerulonephritis with early loss of podocytes, and they accumulate activated interstitial macrophages but have little lymphocytic or dendritic cell infiltration.[46] These mice are very responsive to treatment, and BAFF blockade alone induces long-term survival and may even induce remission of established nephritis.[47] A congenic strain of C57BL/6 mice named Sle1,2,3 has been generated with the use of three genetic loci from the NZM2410 mouse.

NZM2328 Mice and Congenic Strains—Proliferative Disease without Antinuclear Antibodies

NZM2328 are phenotypically similar to NZB/W and have been used extensively to study the effects of single-gene deletions on the immune system. An important finding in this system is that deficiency of signal transducer and activator of transcription 4 (STAT4), which decreases T-helper 1 cell (Th1) cytokine responses, results in accelerated nephritis despite a marked decrease in serum IgG2a autoantibodies, whereas deficiency of STAT6, which decreases Th2 cytokine responses, ameliorates nephritis despite the presence of high-titer serum IgG2a autoantibodies.[48] Both STAT4- and STAT6-deficient mice have less renal immune complex deposition than wt NZM2328 mice, indicating the complex relationships between autoantibody specificity, autoantibody deposition, and renal pathology. NZM2328 congenic mice have been derived by back-crossing to C57L. One of these strains demonstrates immune complex–mediated glomerulonephritis but has no ANAs or rheumatoid factor activity in either the serum or renal eluates.[3] The relevant renal antigens have not yet been identified.

Proliferative Disease Associated with Anti-RNA and Antiphospholipid Antibodies

BXSB.Yaa mice exhibit monocytosis and lymphoid hyperplasia, circulating immune complexes, and proliferative immune complex glomerulonephritis. Male BXSB mice carry the Yaa (Y chromosome–linked autoimmunity accelerator) locus, consisting of a reduplication of at least 17 genes from the X chromosome, including TLR7; the resulting dysregulation of the innate immune response induces the development of antibodies to RNA antigens and accelerates disease onset.[49] NZW/BXSB F1 (W/B) mice produce anti-Sm/RNP (ribonucleoprotein) antibodies and antiphospholipid antibodies, which cause clots within the myocardial small vessels. These mice have severe proliferative glomerulonephritis, with disorganized large lymphoid infiltrates, scattered interstitial T cells, sheets of macrophages in the interstitium and periglomerular regions, renal vasculitis, and the accumulation of dendritic cells within the glomeruli.[50] Serologically active W/B mice are resistant to therapy with cyclophosphamide and co-stimulatory blockade but have a partial response to treatment with BAFF blockade.[50] The discovery of the TLR7 gene within the Yaa locus has led to the development of a TLR7 transgenic mouse that is on a nonautoimmune genetic background; even females carrying more than four copies of TLR7 spontaneously demonstrate SLE with features similar to those in the BXSB mouse.

Proliferative and Interstitial Disease Associated with Anti-DNA, Anti-RNA, and Rheumatoid Factor Autoantibodies

MRL/lpr mice have a permissive genetic background and are also deficient in the proapoptotic molecule Fas, resulting in accumulation of double-negative (CD4−/CD8−) T cells and B220+ cells[51] as well as massive lymphoproliferation. These mice have elevations of multiple autoantibodies, including ANA, anti–single-stranded DNA, anti-Sm, and rheumatoid factors, and make large quantities of IFN-γ and IgG2a autoantibodies.[46] They demonstrate diffuse proliferative glomerulonephritis with mesangial cell proliferation and crescent formation as well as significant interstitial nephritis; mild glomerular disease and progressive interstitial disease can occur even in the total absence of circulating autoantibodies.[9] Macrophage infiltration is an essential feature of nephritis in this model and is driven by renal expression of colony-stimulating factor 1 (CSF-1).[52] The infiltrating cells have not as yet been well characterized in this model, although recruitment of F4/80lo/Ly6Chi inflammatory macrophages into the kidneys is observed 1 or 2 days after adoptive transfer of bone marrow–derived monocytes.[52] When MRL/lpr mice are rendered

deficient in the IL-27 receptor, their autoantibody response is skewed to a Th2 phenotype, they express high levels of IL-4, IgG1, and IgE,[53] and membranous nephropathy develops; these mice have longer renal survival than their IL-27R–sufficient counterparts. These findings indicate that even in mice with the same genetic susceptibility to SLE, the cytokine milieu can have a major impact on the type of nephritis that develops.

Nephrotoxic Nephritis

Acute immune complex–mediated glomerulonephritis is induced in rats and in certain strains of mice by infusion of sheep or rabbit antibodies specific for glomerular type IV collagen followed by disease induction with an innate immune trigger such as lipopolysaccharide (LPS).[54] The disease is characterized by acute neutrophil and inflammatory Gr1hi macrophage infiltration and T-cell infiltration occurring over days to weeks. The acute phase is followed by a period of renal repair and recovery. Much information is available about the mechanisms of tissue damage in this acute model, which has been invaluable in defining the cells and mediators necessary for acute renal inflammation. Both Fc receptors and complement activation are required, as are the acute-phase cytokines TNF-α, IL-1, and IL-6. The T cells involved appear to be skewed to a Th1 phenotype, and PDGF, a molecule that enhances mesangial cell proliferation and matrix formation, is also required. In addition, the observation that only some strains of mice are susceptible to disease induction led to elegant genetic studies in which polymorphisms of the kallikrein genes were identified as major determinants of disease susceptibility.[55] The nephrotoxic nephritis model has also been useful for identifying both the pathogenic role of inflammatory Gr1hi macrophages during the early phases of disease and the protective role of reparative macrophages during disease resolution. However, this disease has many differences from spontaneous SLE models, in which neutrophils and inflammatory Gr1hi macrophages are infrequent. Thus, although it is a useful model for studying the effector phase of acute inflammation, it is not adequate for the study of chronic SLE nephritis.

Pristane-Induced Nephritis

The hydrocarbon pristane can induce a lupus-like disease in several strains of mice with the induction of autoantibodies against DNA, chromatin, Sm, ribonucleoprotein, and ribosomal P. These mice demonstrate immune complex–mediated proliferative glomerulonephritis with mesangial and subendothelial deposits. Interestingly, although the absence of type I IFN signaling prevents the formation of antibodies to DNA and RNA, antinuclear and anticytoplasmic antibodies are still found in the serum, and IgG and complement deposition in the kidneys still occurs. Nevertheless the immune complexes do not induce renal damage, indicating that type I IFN signaling is required for the subsequent effector stage of disease.[56]

KIDNEY EFFECTOR MECHANISMS

Although immune complex deposition in the kidneys is a critical pathogenic component in most cases of SLE nephritis, it is not sufficient to cause inflammatory renal disease that injures the kidney. Multiple studies in mice have identified key pathways that are required for renal damage to occur. Immune complex deposition without renal damage has been reported in SLE-prone mice deficient in FcR γ-chain,[57] IFN-α/β receptor (IFNAR),[56] or monocyte chemotactic protein 1 (MCP-1),[58] and in mice treated with caspase inhibitors, total lymphoid irradiation, combination cyclophosphamide/co-stimulatory blockade,[43] or very high doses of anti-CD154 antibodies. These findings are consistent with a disease model in which immune complex deposition in the kidney triggers a cascade of inflammatory events mediated by activation of complement or engagement of FcRs on renal cells or circulating monocytes, followed by upregulation of renal and monocyte-derived inflammatory chemokines; transmigration of inflammatory cells into the renal parenchyma; release of damaged tissue, inflammatory cytokines, and

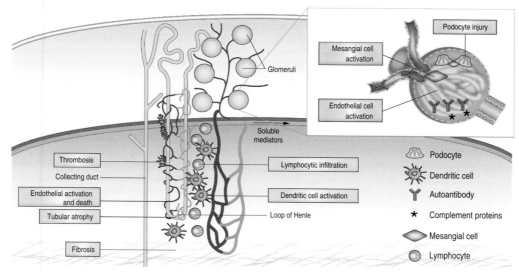

FIGURE 18-4 Mechanisms for renal injury. Disease starts in the glomerulus with the deposition of immunoglobulin and complement, activation of intrinsic renal cells, and engagement of Fc receptors on circulating myeloid cells. Upregulation of chemokines results in recruitment of inflammatory cells, which produce cytokines, more chemokines, and other inflammatory mediators that activate the endothelium and attract and activate resident renal mononuclear cells. Damage to the glomerular filtration barrier causes proteinuria. The inflammatory ultrafiltrate activates renal tubular cells and amplifies recruitment of interstitial infiltrates. Unabated inflammation causes tissue hypoxia and tubular atrophy. Dysregulated tissue repair mechanisms cause glomerulosclerosis and interstitial fibrosis. *(From Davidson A, Aranow C: Lupus nephritis: lessons from murine models. Nat Rev Rheumatol 6:13–20, 2010.)*

mediators that amplify the process; and, finally, irreversible renal damage. This model suggests many avenues for therapeutic intervention that are not necessarily based on systemic immune suppression (Figure 18-4).

Complement

Renal deposition of autoantibodies of the appropriate isotype is followed by recruitment of complement components.[5] The complement system comprises more than 30 proteins, some of which are activating and some of which are regulatory. Complement plays an important role in clearance of apoptotic material and immune complexes, and therefore, early component complement deficiencies that cause an overload of circulating nuclear material are highly associated with susceptibility to SLE in humans. In contrast, excessive activation of later complement components may be associated with failure to control inflammation or thrombosis; several renal diseases have been associated with loss-of-function mutations in complement regulatory proteins.

Activation of complement may occur through the classical pathway, which is activated by the binding of C1 to immunoglobulins in immune complexes, or the lectin pathway, which is activated by the binding of mannose-binding lectin to terminal carbohydrates on microbes. A third, "alternative" pathway is an amplification pathway that is activated by binding of hydrolyzed complement factors 3b and 3d, generated via the other two pathways, to factor B, resulting in formation of an alternative C3 convertase (Figure 18-5). An increase in synthesis of various complement components may occur at sites of inflammation or hypoxia; for example, IL-1, IL-6, IFN-γ, and TNF-α all upregulate C3 production. Studies in MRL/lpr SLE-prone mice have demonstrated that deficiency of factor B, an essential component of the alternative pathway, protects from renal disease, whereas deficiency of C3, which is required both for complement activation and for clearance of unwanted material, does not confer protection.[59,60]

Cleavage of complement components C3 and C5 by the complement convertases that are generated via the three complement activation pathways amplifies complement activation (C3b), releases proinflammatory products (C3a and C5a) that cause tissue damage through anaphylotoxin activity, and activates the terminal

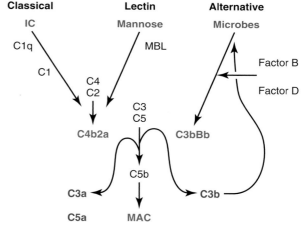

FIGURE 18-5 A simplified outline of the complement cascade. The three pathways have different activators (*blue*) and converge on two different convertases (*green*) to release inflammatory effectors (*purple*) or the terminal complex (*red*).

complement membrane attack complex (MAC C5b,C6-9). The MAC has both cytolytic and noncytolytic effects. Activation of the MAC in membranous disease results in podocyte injury, which disrupts the actin cytoskeleton and releases oxidants and proteases that damage the GBM. The MAC also induces proliferation of mesangial cells and stimulates their release of profibrotic mediators TGF-β and PDGF. Finally the terminal complement products can activate endothelial cells, inducing the expression of adhesion molecules and other inflammatory mediators and acting as procoagulants.[61]

Targeting of the effector molecules of the complement pathways, including C5 and the various regulatory proteins, may be therapeutic in renal inflammation. For example, a therapeutic agent that targets the soluble complement regulatory protein factor H to renal tubular sites of C3 binding has shown some efficacy in mouse models of renal ischemia.[62] Eculizumab, the only currently approved complement inhibitor, is a humanized monoclonal antibody that prevents the cleavage of human complement component C5 into its proinflammatory components. This agent is therapeutic in diseases associated with deficiency of complement regulatory proteins, such as hemolytic uremic syndrome, and is currently in clinical trials for several chronic inflammatory diseases, including nephritis.[61]

Another complement-based amplification mechanism is mediated by antibodies to tissue-bound C1q, which is the first component of the classical pathway and binds directly to apoptotic cells and to aggregated immunoglobulin, particularly IgG3. C1q binding causes a conformational change in the molecule that may render it immunogenic; thus, defective clearance mechanisms in SLE may predispose to the generation of anti-C1q autoantibodies in a fashion analogous to the generation of antibodies directed to nucleic acids. High titers of anti-C1q antibodies, particularly of the IgG2 isotype, have been associated with lupus nephritis in multiple studies of patients with SLE. When anti-C1q antibodies are infused into the kidneys of normal mice, they recruit C1q but do not cause renal injury. However when anti-C1q is infused into the kidneys of mice with low levels of immune complex deposition, they can trigger renal inflammation; this finding suggests that the antibodies bind to or recruit C1q onto immune complexes, thereby activating the classical complement pathway. C1q may also be recruited to damaged cells in the kidney that then act as targets for anti-C1q antibodies.[38,63] Alternatively, the antibodies may interfere with complement-mediated clearance of immune complexes and apoptotic material.

A final complement abnormality reported in SLE is the presence of autoantibodies that prevent the breakdown of the complement convertase C4b2a, thus increasing the formation of the MAC.

Fc Receptors

The crucial role of FcRs in renal injury was first shown in the NZBW F1 mouse model, in which absence of the FcR γ-chain, which is common to the activating FcRI and FcRIII, abrogated renal injury despite unabated immune complex deposition and an intact complement system. Although FcRs are present on intrinsic renal cells, experiments using bone marrow chimeras subsequently showed definitively that the FcRs need to be expressed on cells of hematopoietic origin, most likely myeloid cells.[57] Upregulation of FcRI on circulating monocytes has been detected in patients with active SLE and particularly in active SLE nephritis; this appears to be associated with monocyte activation and enhanced chemotactic ability.[64] IL-12, IFN-γ, and IFN-α are potential inducers of FcγRI/CD64 expression in SLE and thus may promote lupus nephritis by enhancing the renal recruitment of proinflammatory monocytes/macrophages. The dependence of renal damage on FcRs does not, however, hold true in all murine models, indicating that there is heterogeneity in the renal mechanisms for inflammatory cell recruitment to the kidneys.

Although FcR polymorphisms have been associated with SLE nephritis, they appear to confer a decrease rather than an increase in IgG binding, suggesting that their pathogenetic mechanism is to adversely influence clearance rather than augment FcR-mediated inflammatory cell recruitment by immune complexes. The FcγRIIa-R131 polymorphism that has been associated with nephritis in African Americans confers an increased affinity for C-reactive protein (CRP) and therefore may contribute to disease pathogenesis by triggering phagocyte activation and the release of inflammatory mediators at sites of immune complex deposition.[65]

Toll-Like Receptors and Other Innate Immune Receptors

TLRs are members of a large family of innate immune receptors that detect and respond to infection and to sterile tissue injury. TLRs on the cell surface recognize substances released during tissue injury, such as heat-shock proteins and high-mobility group protein B1 (HMGB1), whereas intracellular TLRs are specialized to recognize DNA and RNA. Recognition of innate stimuli by TLRs occurs within renal tissues. Renal immune complexes containing DNA may

stimulate intrarenal dendritic cells, which take up this material through their FcRs, resulting in release of inflammatory cytokines and type I IFNs that accelerate tissue damage. Antibody-mediated inflammatory kidney disease is markedly exacerbated by the coadministration of TLR agonists in mouse models. Comprehensive analysis of renal TLR expression and the effects of TLR agonists on renal disease have been performed in the MRL/lpr model.[7] These studies have demonstrated ubiquitous expression of TLRs 2, 3, and 4 in most renal cell types, whereas TLRs 7 and 9 are mostly restricted to resident and infiltrating antigen-presenting cells. Activation of TLRs induces the secretion of proinflammatory cytokines including type I IFNs. However, most of the TLR agonists used in these studies did not induce tissue injury in prediseased mice; thus transient exposure of healthy mouse kidneys to TLR agonists during infections does not cause renal damage. The one exception was the TLR9 agonist CpG DNA, which induced SLE onset even in young mice and induced a severe crescentic glomerulonephritis. Once proinflammatory cytokines were present, continuous administration of most TLR agonists increased renal immune complex deposition and infiltration by macrophages and inflammatory cells with variable effects on proteinuria. Interestingly, the TLR3 agonist accelerated renal disease without increasing immune complex deposition, suggesting that the pathologic effect was due to local renal cell activation. Similar findings were reported in NZB/W mice treated with the TLR3 agonist polyI:C. These studies, in sum, show that TLR activation can aggravate SLE nephritis but that each agonist induces a different pattern of renal damage. This observation suggests that environmental insults may induce different patterns of renal disease even in genetically similar individuals. Oligonucleotide antagonists of TLRs 7 and 9 have shown some efficacy in murine models of SLE nephritis and are being developed for human use.

Tissue injury may further amplify renal damage by releasing molecules known as danger-associated molecular pattern molecules (DAMPs), which activate innate immune receptors, including TLR2 and TLR4. Inciting molecules could include heat-shock proteins, HMGB1, fibrinogen, biglycans, or hyaluronic acid. HMGB proteins can also act as cofactors for the recognition of nucleic acids through TLRs 7 and 9. Viral infections could trigger flares of SLE nephritis through similar mechanisms.[66]

Cell Influx

One of the cardinal characteristics of proliferative lupus nephritis is the infiltration of the periglomerular regions and interstitium with inflammatory infiltrates. The role of these infiltrates is still not clear. Infiltrating cells may mediate pathogenesis by direct cytotoxicity, by the secretion of soluble factors such as cytokines and proteases, or by the amplification of immune responses. Extensive cellular infiltrates were first noted in early pathologic studies of lupus kidneys in patients who had not received immunosuppressive treatment. Later studies show that the extent of these infiltrates correlates with the clinical severity of the disease and with the serum level of creatinine[67] but not with the severity of glomerular disease. Most importantly, tubulointerstitial disease correlates with prognosis and the risk of eventual renal failure. A correlation of renal outcome with extensive morphologic characterization of the kidneys demonstrated that tubuloepithelial cell activation and infiltration of the interstitium with inflammatory cells and macrophages both correlated better than glomerular lesions with interstitial fibrosis and with deterioration of renal function (doubling of serum creatinine concentration) in lupus nephritis as well as in most other glomerular diseases.[67,68]

Several studies have determined the cell types present in the tubulointerstitial infiltrates of lupus renal biopsy specimens and have shown that they include B cells, plasma cells, T cells, macrophages, and dendritic cells. In approximately half of patients with SLE, tubulointerstitial infiltrates are scattered throughout the interstitium, whereas in the other half they are organized into aggregates that sometimes contain germinal centers and actively dividing cells (Figure 18-6).[69] These cells elaborate numerous inflammatory

CD3   CD20

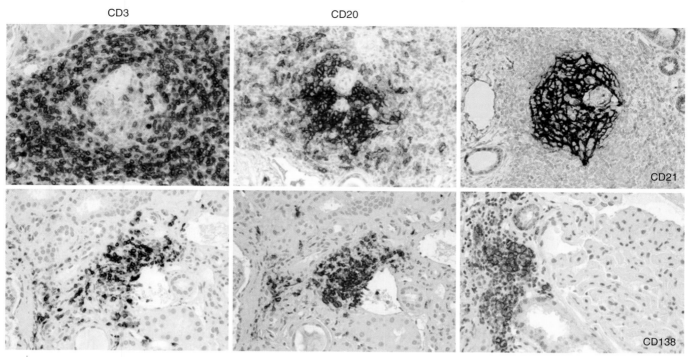

FIGURE 18-6 Inflammatory cell infiltrates in human SLE nephritis kidneys. Infiltrates may be organized and contain follicular structures with germinal centers (*upper three panels*) or may be diffuse (*lower three panels*). CD138+ plasma cells are prominent in the infiltrates (*lower right*). *Far left upper and lower panels* show cells staining for CD3 (T lymphocytes); *upper and lower middle panels* show cells staining for CD20 (B lymphocytes); *upper right panel* shows germinal center (GC)-like structure staining for follicular dendritic cells; lower right panel shows cells staining for CD138 (plasma cells). *(Adapted from Chang A, Henderson SG, Brandt D, et al: In situ B cell-mediated immune responses and tubulointerstitial inflammation in human lupus nephritis. J Immunol 186:1849–1860, 2011.)*

mediators and co-stimulatory molecules that could amplify inflammation.

T Cells

T cells are more common than B cells in renal infiltrates and include both CD4+ and CD8+ cells. Studying these cells has been difficult because of their small numbers and the limited numbers of biopsy specimens available. A few studies have suggested that CD4+ T cells in lupus kidneys are skewed toward a Th1 phenotype, particularly in patients with proliferative disease, but these findings have not been universally replicated. Th17 cells can be found within infiltrates in the kidneys in some but not all murine models, and a small study of human renal biopsies found IL-17–producing CD4−/CD8− T cells within tubulointerstitial infiltrates.[70] As in many other inflammatory tissues, Foxp3+ T-regulatory cells (Tregs) are also found in renal infiltrates, but their function is unknown.

CD8+ cells are located in periglomerular sites, where they often exceed the number of CD4+ T cells, and are associated with poor responses to induction therapy. Apart from their ability to secrete cytokines, it has been suggested from experiments in which model antigens were expressed in the glomerular podocytes that cytotoxic T cells with specificity for renal antigens are recruited by tubulointerstitial dendritic cells that have ingested antigens from damaged cells. Activation of these CD8+ T cells requires CD4+ T cells to provide help. Further cell death mediated by the cytotoxic T cells then releases more antigens and amplifies recruitment of T cells and dendritic cells, thus sustaining tubulointerstitial inflammation.[40] Analysis of T-cell receptor (TCR) repertoires of intrarenal T cells from a small number of biopsy specimens has shown oligoclonality, suggesting that T-cell clonal expansion may occur in situ.

B Cells

Both B cells and plasma cells are found in lupus kidneys, and studies in mice suggest that the inflamed tissue becomes an ectopic plasma

cell niche. Analysis of the Ig repertoires of B cells isolated from the aggregates of a small number of lupus renal biopsy specimens showed evidence of clonal expansion, indicating that immune responses occur in situ[69]; these findings, together with evidence of T-cell oligoclonal expansions, further support the hypothesis that renal antigens drive a local immune response that could amplify tissue damage.

Mononuclear Phagocytes

Macrophages and dendritic cells have long been known to be key players in acute renal inflammation,[19,71] and both cell types infiltrate the kidneys in SLE nephritis, where they may function to present local renal antigens to infiltrating T cells. As mentioned earlier, macrophage infiltration is correlated with poor renal outcome. Therefore, macrophages have become the subject of considerable interest in the past few years. These cells have a high degree of plasticity and have complex responses to inflammatory stimuli with distinct activation patterns and functions, depending on the stimuli to which they are exposed.[72] Inflammatory or classically activated (M1) macrophages are induced during cell-mediated immune responses in response to IFN-γ (or IFN-β) and TNF-α, and they produce large amounts of proinflammatory cytokines, including interleukins 1, 6, 12, and 23 and inflammatory mediators including iNOS and ROS. These inflammatory macrophages derive from peripheral Gr1hi/CCR2+ monocytes that egress from the blood during acute inflammation or infection.[73] M1 macrophages help recruit neutrophils to sites of inflammation and induce the differentiation of Th1 and Th17 cells. Depletion of these cells in the early stages of nephrotoxic nephritis results in attenuation of renal damage. Alternatively activated (M2) macrophages, which are induced by IL-4, secrete protective cytokines and promote wound healing. They derive from Gr1lo/CX3CR1+ monocytes that patrol the endothelium and extravasate very rapidly upon tissue damage.[74] Depletion of these cells during the late stages of nephrotoxic nephritis can exacerbate tissue injury. Finally, regulatory macrophages that are induced by immune complexes or by corticosteroids produce high levels of IL-10 and are antiinflammatory.[74] Other macrophage activation patterns represent a mixed phenotype likely resulting from simultaneous exposure to inflammatory and homeostatic/suppressive factors in vivo during chronic disease states.[75] Of relevance to SLE, macrophages exposed to immune complexes and TLR agonists are characterized by an IL-10hi/IL-12lo phenotype termed M2b.

Dendritic cells (DCs) belong to three main subgroups, plasmacytoid DCs that produce large amounts of type I IFNs, conventional DCs that have a major antigen presentation role, and migratory DCs that reside in peripheral tissue and capture antigen that they then deliver to T cells in lymphoid organs.[72] Conventional DCs are very heterogeneous; within tissues, the microenvironment can greatly influence their function and longevity.

Normal mouse kidneys have a heterogeneous resident population of mononuclear cells. The dominant population is high for F4/80, CX3CR1, and MHC class II, low for Gr1, and intermediate for CD86, CD11b, and CD11c. This cell population forms a network that is dense in the renal interstitium but less common in the renal cortex.[20] Studies in human kidneys from normal and diseased individuals have similarly found a network of CD68+ cells throughout the interstitium.[76] Functional studies in mice have confirmed that these cells have an antigen-presenting function, use dendrites to sample their local environment, and are poor NO producers, suggesting that they are dendritic cells.[20-21] Because these cells express F4/80, they have also often been referred to as a "resident macrophage population."[19]

A minor population of monocytic cells in normal kidneys test high for CD11b, CD62L, and Gr-1, and low for F4/80, CD11c MHCII and CD86; this population expresses CCR2, secretes inflammatory cytokines, and most resembles classic inflammatory M1 macrophages. During acute ischemic injury this inflammatory macrophage population increases markedly in the kidneys.[73] Small DC populations have also been found in the kidneys, including CD103+ DCs and plasmacytoid DCs.

Macrophage/DC populations have been characterized in the kidneys of several mouse SLE models. In NZB/W, NZW/BXSB, and NZM2410 mice, the onset of proteinuria was associated with expansion and activation of the F4/80hi resident population along with an increase in expression of the adhesion molecule CD11b and upregulation of CD86. Microarray analysis of this population from prediseased and diseased NZB/W mice identified a hybrid nephritis-associated profile of proinflammatory and antiinflammatory and tissue repair genes that was regulated upon remission. These findings suggest that mononuclear phagocytes with an aberrant activation profile contribute to tissue damage in lupus nephritis by mediating both local inflammation and excessive tissue remodeling.[77] In NZB/W and NZW/BXSB mice, proteinuria is also associated with the influx of a large number of CD11chi DCs into the kidneys. These cells localize within lymphoid aggregates, separate from the F4/80hi population. Studies in humans have similarly shown that there may be more than one population of mononuclear phagocytes in the kidneys during inflammatory disease with different phenotypic features of glomerular/periglomerular from those of interstitial cells.[76]

Soluble Mediators of Tissue Injury
Chemokines
Chemokines are a major class of chemoattractants that mediate migration of infiltrating cells expressing the corresponding chemokine receptors. Approximately 50 chemokines and 20 receptors have so far been identified. Secreted chemokines become immobilized by binding to glycosaminoglycans on cell surfaces or in the extracellular matrix. Upon binding to the relevant receptors on leukocytes, chemokines trigger an increase in integrin binding that leads to firm adhesion of the cell to the endothelium, followed by transmigration. Normal kidneys produce very low levels of chemokines, but chemokine production is induced by a variety of inflammatory stimuli, including IL-1, TNF-α, IFN-γ, TLR stimulation, immune complexes, ROS, and renal vasoactive hormones. Because chemokine expression is mostly regulated by transcription, molecular analyses of renal tissue from mouse SLE models have been informative.[8,78] Such studies have demonstrated that a limited number of inflammatory chemokines is expressed in the glomeruli shortly after immune complex deposition. In both MRL/lpr and NZB/W, mice CCL2 (MCP-1) and CCL5 (RANTES [regulated upon activation, normal T-cell expressed, and secreted]) are expressed early in the disease process; CCL2 (MCP-1) and CX3CL1 (fractalkine) have been identified by gene deletion or protein inhibitor studies as essential mediators of renal disease in the MRL/lpr model. IFN-induced chemokines CXCL9 (MIG [monokine induced by gamma interferon]) and CXCL10 (IP-10 [IFN-γ–induced protein 10]) are also expressed in the MRL/lpr model together with their T cell–expressed receptor CXCR3. CXCR3+ T cells have been found in human lupus renal biopsy specimens.[79] In the NZB/W model, CXCL13 and CCL20 are prominently expressed early in the disease together with parallel expression of the relevant chemokine receptors CXCR5 and CCR6.[43] CCR6 is also found in human renal inflammatory diseases. Finally CXCR4+ leukocytes of various types can be found in human SLE biopsy specimens along with their corresponding chemoattractant, CXCL12.[80]

Mesangial cells are an important source of chemokines initially, but as disease progresses, activated endothelial cells, infiltrating immune cells, activated resident macrophages and tubular epithelial cells may also express diverse chemokines, which recruit more circulating cells that express a range of chemokine receptors, including lymphocytes, polymorphonuclear leukocytes, and macrophages/DCs. Accordingly, more and more chemokines and their receptors are expressed as disease progresses, consistent with increasing cell infiltration.[43]

It is increasingly recognized that the kidney inflammatory environment may consist of more than one subenvironment in which different chemokines recruit different cell types. For example, in MRL/lpr mice, CCR1 is expressed by infiltrating T cells and macrophages in the interstitium, and a CCR1 inhibitor decreases interstitial inflammation and fibrosis without altering immune complex deposition or glomerular hypercellularity. In the same model, CCL2 deficiency results in a decrease in glomerular and interstitial macrophage infiltration with less proteinuria and less glomerular and tubulointerstitial injury without affecting perivascular T-cell infiltrates, consistent with the minimal expression of CCL2 in the perivascular zone. In contrast, CCL2 deficiency exacerbates nephrotoxic nephritis, pointing to different roles for cells expressing the relevant receptors in different disease phenotypes.[8,81]

In patients with SLE nephritis, chemokine ligands CCL2, CCL5, CCL3, and CCL4 are expressed in the glomeruli and recruit CCR2- and CCR5-expressing macrophages and T cells; CCL2 is also found in the urine during renal flares. Interstitial T cells express CCR5 and CXCR3, receptors that are expressed on polarized Th1 cells, whereas interstitial macrophages express CCR5 and CCR1. CX3CL1 colocalizes with infiltrates of T cells and mononuclear cells. These findings have led to the development and preclinical testing of chemokine inhibitors. A CCL2 inhibitor synergized with low-dose cyclophosphamide in the treatment of established nephritis in MRL/lpr mice. A CX3CL1 inhibitor similarly prevented glomerular and interstitial damage but did not alter pathology in the lungs or salivary glands, suggesting that chemokine expression may vary in different inflamed organs. CXCR4 inhibition has also been successful in murine models. Despite these encouraging findings, the complexity and redundancy of chemokine and chemokine receptor expression in the kidneys as well as the role of chemokines in systemic immunity and the possible protective role of some chemokines make chemokine targeting very challenging in human SLE nephritis.[8]

Cytokines
Sequential studies of kidneys from MRL/lpr mice have shown that an increase in renal proinflammatory cytokine expression occurs after the rise in chemokine expression and correlates with infiltration

by inflammatory cells. Polarized patterns of T-cell cytokine secretion have been observed in human crescentic glomerulonephritis (Th1) and membranous nephritis (Th2). IL-17–producing T cells have been detected in renal tissue of some mouse lupus models and some patients with SLE. In the MRL/lpr and NZB/W mouse models, antagonism of the Th1 cytokine IFN-γ is therapeutic during established disease and IL-4 is protective; however, in NZM2410 mice, IL-4 antagonism ameliorates nephritis. These differences illustrate the complexity of SLE, in that various effector cytokines may mediate different types of inflammation. For example, both Th1 and Th17 polarized CD4⁺ T cells can induce renal damage when ovalbumin-specific cells are transferred into mice infused with ovalbumin/antiovalbumin immune complexes. However, there are differences both in the pattern of chemokine expression and in the types of infiltrating cells, with more acute disease and more neutrophils in the mice given the Th17 polarized cells.[82] Similarly, IL-4 may exert reparative effects in the kidneys in some models but may increase collagen production and promote glomerulosclerosis in others.

Innate cytokines—IL-1β, type I IFNs, IL-18, TNF-α, and IL-6—are expressed in the kidneys during the effector phase of SLE nephritis, and antagonism of some of these cytokines is therapeutic in mouse models of inflammatory nephritis. The sources of these cytokines include infiltrating mononuclear cells and injured intrinsic renal cells. Studies in nephrotoxic nephritis using bone marrow chimeric mice have shown that TNF-α appears to be predominantly elaborated by intrinsic renal cells, whereas IL-1β is made predominantly by infiltrating cells. Furthermore, these studies have shown that IL-1β expression is required for TNF-α to be expressed, suggesting that IL-1β from infiltrating cells stimulates IL-1 receptor (IL-1R)–bearing intrinsic renal cells to produce TNF-α.[83]

Although TNF-α protects against the initiation of SLE in some murine models, it is highly expressed in glomeruli in mice and humans with SLE nephritis and correlates with disease activity. Antagonism of TNF-α with infliximab has been reported to significantly ameliorate proteinuria in a small number of patients with SLE with refractory nephritis, but toxicity, especially when this agent is used with other immunosuppressive medications, has so far precluded larger clinical trials.[84] In addition, TNF-α has pleiotropic roles in the immune response, raising concerns about the long-term safety of this approach in patients with SLE. For example, TNF-α deficiency causes an increase in SLE-related autoantibodies and in activation of Th17 cells that could potentially cause renal damage. There has been some interest in determining which renal TNF receptor is responsible for the pathogenic effects of excess TNF-α; these studies have yielded variable results depending on the model used. In the nephrotoxic nephritis model, disease depended on renal expression of TNF receptor 2 (TNFR2), but in the NZM2328 model, deficiency of TNFR2 was not protective.[85] A histologic study in humans showed that TNFR1 is expressed at high levels in proliferative SLE glomerulonephritis with little expression of TNFR2. Soluble receptors that may have a protective role are also released into the urine.[86]

Type I IFNs are secreted by mesangial cells via mechanisms that involve both TLRs and intracytoplasmic sensors for RNA and DNA; type I IFN–dependent genes, including IFN-induced chemokines, are upregulated in the nephritic kidneys of several mouse SLE models. IFN-α can also activate endothelial cells and thus may contribute to inflammatory cell recruitment. Importantly, lack of the IFN-α receptor IFNAR protects against ischemic renal damage in mice, suggesting a local proinflammatory role for IFN-α in the kidneys. The presence of a subset of IFN-inducible chemokines in the serum has been identified as a biomarker for risk of renal flare.[87] IFN-γ, induced by IL-12 and IL-18, is a pathogenic cytokine in the MRL/lpr and NZB/W models and can induce expression of adhesion molecules and chemokines in the kidneys. Macrophage production of IFN-γ is required for renal macrophage migration in the MRL/lpr model. Not surprisingly, therefore, therapies directed at IFN-γ or IL-18 are effective in the MRL/lpr and NZB/W models. As discussed previously, a Th1 profile is found in several models of SLE, and a predominance of renal Th1 cells is associated with proliferative forms of nephritis in humans.[88]

Lipid Mediators

Small lipids play an important role in normal kidney function and may also be involved in the pathogenesis of kidney diseases. The main precursor of bioactive lipids is arachidonic acid, which is metabolized to prostanoids by cyclooxygenase enzymes COX1 and COX2, both of which are expressed in the kidneys. Prostanoids interact with specific cell surface G-protein–coupled receptors or with nuclear receptors, such as peroxisome proliferator–activated receptor gamma (PPARγ) and PPARδ, and induce cell signaling via Ca²⁺ mobilization or cyclic adenosine monophosphate (cAMP) pathways. Production of some prostanoids is sensitive to inflammatory mediators. In the kidneys, prostanoids can be expressed by intrinsic renal cells or by inflammatory cells. Glomeruli of patients with SLE nephritis express increased levels of COX2, and COX2 inhibitors synergize with immunosuppressive agents in reducing renal damage in NZB/W mice. Arachidonic acid is also oxidized by lipooxygenases to leukotrienes, some of which have inflammatory, chemoattractant, or vasoconstrictive properties. Several leukotrienes are produced by injured glomeruli and may thus amplify renal injury. Arachidonic acid can also be metabolized by cytochrome P-450 monooxygenase to produce derivatives that are involved in regulating the renin-angiotensin syndrome and in maintaining the glomerular filtration barrier.[89]

Hypoxia and Reactive Oxygen and Nitrate Species

Hypoxia with the generation of free radicals is a characteristic feature of tissue inflammation and induces several factors that exaggerate tissue injury. Hypoxia also activates the renin-angiotensin system and enhances migration, recruitment, and retention of monocytes in inflammatory sites by altering the expression of adhesion molecules and chemoattractants. Despite its large blood supply, the kidney is particularly susceptible to hypoxia because of the architecture of the renal vascular system, in which the tubular capillary perfusion is downstream of glomerular capillary bed and thus sensitive to glomerular hemodynamic changes. In chronic kidney disease, loss of peritubular capillaries may exacerbate hypoxia. Hypoxia-inducible transcription factors (HIFs) fail to be normally degraded under hypoxic conditions and bind to hypoxic response elements in the promoter regions of a large number of target genes, whose role is to optimize cell functions and metabolism in the hypoxic environment.[90] HIFα expression is increased in patients with chronic kidney disease and in mouse models of SLE nephritis. Although HIFα has some protective functions, including increased production of erythropoietin and VEGF, there is also evidence that it can exacerbate tissue damage. Mice whose myeloid cells are deficient in HIFα have impaired innate inflammatory responses as a result of defects in activation of neutrophils, macrophages, and dendritic cells, including decreases in cytokine release and upregulation of co-stimulatory molecules; such mice have less inflammation in induced models of autoimmunity but are more susceptible to infections. HIFα also enhances podocyte expression of CXCR4, induces molecules involved in tissue remodeling, and exacerbates scar formation.[91]

Reactive nitrogen species (RNS) have also been detected in the serum of patients with lupus nephritis[92] and may be induced locally by complement split products that upregulate expression of *NOS2* and production of iNOS. Like ROS, RNS potentiate ongoing inflammation by altering multiple cellular functions; pharmacologic inhibition of iNOS decreases renal damage in the MRL/lpr model.

The Renin-Angiotensin System

Renin and ACE are required for the production of angiotensin II, which is a potent vasoconstrictor. ACE also degrades the vasodilator bradykinin. Angiotensin II binds to specific receptors on many tissue types to regulate vascular smooth muscle tone, aldosterone secretion, thirst, sympathetic nervous system stimulation, renal tubular Na⁺ reabsorption, and cardiac function. Several other receptors and mediators in this pathway have been described. Blockade of angiotensin II and of angiotensin receptors not only lowers blood pressure but has other salutary effects on kidney function, including improvement in renal blood flow and reductions in oxidative stress, podocyte loss, and proteinuria. Consistent with these data, ACE inhibition has been found to induce downmodulation of glomerular inflammation, reduction of mesangial cell proliferation, and decrease in chemokine expression in MRL/lpr mice; these beneficial effects were much more significant than those of treating hypertension alone. Benefits of ACE inhibitors and angiotensin receptor blocking agents have also been observed in small studies of patients with lupus.[93]

Matrix Metalloproteinases and Tissue Repair

Changes in the glomerular extracellular matrix, either expansion or mesangiolysis, may occur in lupus nephritis, and chronic breakdown of matrix components may release protein fragments that can act as antigens for local immune responses. Turnover of extracellular matrix proteins is regulated by the activity of matrix metalloproteinases (MMPs), Zn^{2+}-dependent proteinases that break down collagen, laminin, elastin, fibronectin, and the core proteins of proteoglycans. The gelatinases MMP-2 and MM-P9 are induced in the glomeruli in inflammatory glomerulonephritis. Regulators of MMP, especially tissue inhibitor of metalloproteinase 1 (TIMP-1), are also increased in the kidneys during inflammation, so that the overall physiologic effect may depend on the balance achieved in particular sites as well as on the rate of synthesis of matrix components.[94-95] In addition, MMPs have pleiomorphic functions, some of which, such as breakdown of cytokines and chemokines and antihypertensive effects, may be protective. This complexity is illustrated by the unexpected outcomes of MMP deficiencies in mice, in which fibrosis does not occur, and by the opposite effects of pharmacologic ablation of MMPs at early (protective) and late (pathogenic) disease stages in a model of renal fibrosis. For example, in the nephrotoxic nephritis model MMP-9–deficient mice manifest more severe disease owing to the decreased breakdown of fibrinogen.

Blood Vessels and Endothelium

Vascular damage occurs during active SLE as a result of excessive endothelial cell apoptosis with an imbalance between damage and repair. Circulating endothelial cells are a marker of endothelial damage and are increased in active SLE. Increased serum levels of endothelial cell–derived surface receptors are found in the serum, and aberrant circulating endothelial cell progenitors are found in the peripheral blood. Vascular abnormalities found in the SLE kidney include vascular immune complex deposition, glomerular necrosis, intracapillary thrombi, and noninflammatory vasculopathy. True renal vasculitis is rare in SLE. A decrease of expression of transcripts involved in endothelial proliferation and angiogenesis, including VEGF, has been noted in both mouse and human lupus nephritis kidneys. In addition, both the renal endothelium and renal cells can be induced by a variety of inflammatory mediators to elaborate members of the endothelin family that are potent vasoconstrictors. Excessive endothelin decreases renal blood flow and causes hypertension and also acts directly on renal parenchymal and inflammatory cells to enhance mesangial cell proliferation and inflammatory cell activation.[96] Activation of and damage to the endothelium may also be mediated by circulating cytokines including TN-Fα and type I IFNs, and by exposure to neutrophil NETs.[97] Increased renal expression of endothelial membrane protein C receptor, which helps protect against local thrombosis, has also been observed in SLE nephritis.[98] The contribution of antiphospholipid–mediated thrombotic microangiopathy and thrombotic thrombocytopenic purpura–hemolytic uremic syndrome (TTP-HUS) to the spectrum of SLE nephritis has not been well studied.

Integrin Ligands

Integrins are a family of adhesion molecules expressed on leukocytes and have been successfully targeted in several autoimmune diseases. Integrins have an external ligand-binding domain and a cytoplasmic signaling domain and function as both adhesion and activation molecules. Endothelial ligands for integrins include vascular cell adhesion molecule 1 (VCAM-1) and intercellular adhesion molecule (ICAM), both of which are upregulated in nephritic kidneys. Both are cleaved to soluble forms that can be detected in the serum and urine in patients with active SLE and SLE nephritis.[86] In murine models these ligands are upregulated in the kidney at or after the onset of proteinuria, and similarly, in humans they are expressed in patients with advanced histologic lesions and low levels of complement.[99] A polymorphism of the VCAM and ICAM binding integrin ITGAM (α-chain of CD11b) is associated with lupus and lupus nephritis in humans.

Heparan Sulfate

HS plays an important role in the recruitment, rolling, and firm adhesion of leukocytes to activated endothelium and is modified during endothelial activation. Glycosaminoglycans, including HS, bind chemokines, establishing a local concentration gradient that recruits leukocytes. N-sulfated and 6-O-sulfated HS domains on activated endothelial cells may also directly serve as ligands for L-selectin and CD11b, which are expressed on leukocytes. In addition, by virtue of its negative charge, HS can bind to positively charged autoantibodies. Heparins or heparinoid compounds without anticoagulant activity can block Ig deposition in the kidneys in murine SLE models and may have antiinflammatory effects as a result of a decrease in cellular recruitment.[100]

A decrease in HS in the GBM is associated with proteinuria in many glomerular diseases, and this is associated with an increase in expression of the HS-degrading enzyme heparanase, which is secreted by endothelial cells and podocytes. Proinflammatory cytokines increase heparanase production, and heparanase expression is increased in NZB/W kidneys.[77] The enzyme is active at acid pH, such as in inflammatory or hypoxic environments, and at the surface of the GBM. Heparanase digests HS and releases HS-bound factors that can enhance inflammation. The precise role of heparanase in disease pathogenesis is not fully defined, but heparanase inhibitors decrease proteinuria in a variety of kidney injury models.[100,101]

PROGRESSION TO FIBROSIS AND SCLEROSIS

Studies in both mouse and human lupus nephritis have shown that glomerular disease precedes tubulointerstitial disease. Mechanisms for renal injury are beginning to be better defined, allowing a unified set of mechanisms for organ loss to be proposed.[81,102] Activation of the mesangium by immune complexes induces release of chemokines, and activation of the glomerular endothelium allows migration of inflammatory cells in response to these chemokines. As inflammation proceeds within the glomerulus, proliferation and crescents may obstruct the urinary pole, leading to diminished ultrafiltrate flow; similarly, occlusion of glomerular capillaries leads to diminished peritubular capillary flow. In addition, damage to podocytes results in a decrease in production of VEGF, thus causing endothelial cell apoptosis and a further decrease in glomerular blood flow. Similarly, a decrease in endothelial cells results in a reduction in PDGF and less support for the mesangium. As the function of the nephrons declines, the workload for the remaining nephrons increases, leading to glomerular hypertension and hyperfiltration as well as hypertrophy of the remaining glomeruli. Further podocyte injury and loss occur, along with the development of progressive glomerulosclerosis of the denuded glomeruli. A decrease in glomerular blood flow now further jeopardizes the downstream peritubular blood flow, which has no collateral source of blood supply, causing oxidative stress. Inflammatory mediators released into glomerular vasculature by infiltrating cells, including lipid mediators, growth factors, cytokines, and chemokines, spill into the peritubular vasculature; this event activates the peritubular endothelium and induces inflammatory cell influx into the tubulointerstitium.

As disease progresses, the renal tubules may also be damaged by the glomerular ultrafiltrate, which now contains multiple inflammatory mediators and toxins that can activate tubular epithelial cells. Although high protein load alone has previously been postulated to cause tubular damage, this hypothesis has now been questioned because several clinical studies in humans failed to show a toxic effect of heavy proteinuria alone on renal function. Failure of removal of apoptotic material that accumulates as a result of hypoxia causes local endoplasmic reticulum stress, mitochondrial stress, activation of danger-associated molecular pattern molecules (DAMPs) and TLRs, and accumulation of reactive ROS, thus perpetuating apoptosis and aggravating the inflammation. Presentation of glomerular and tubular antigens derived from apoptotic cells to CD8[+] cells may result in cytotoxicity directed to glomerular antigens and more cell death. Tubules atrophy, and the tubular epithelial cells detach from their basement membrane and die. Activation of TGF-β by angiotensin II induces an increase in extracellular matrix formation, tissue remodeling, and replacement of apoptotic parenchyma by fibrous tissue. Activated intrinsic renal mononuclear phagocytes and infiltrating tubulointerstitial cells further contribute to tubular damage. If the inciting injury remains active and sites of tissue repair continue to be hypoxic, normal reparative processes become chronic, leading to amplification of inflammation and fibrosis (see Figure 18-4).[103] Importantly, nephron loss beyond the compensatory capacity of the kidney leads to glomerular hyperfiltration, hyperperfusion, and structural damage of the remaining nephrons, resulting in progressive loss of kidney function even if the initiating inflammatory process has been adequately contained.

Pathways That Contribute to or Protect from Fibrosis

Transforming Growth Factor–Beta 1

TGF-β1 is involved in both glomerulosclerosis and fibrosis of the kidneys in many chronic kidney diseases, including SLE. TGF-β1 is released from podocytes in latent form and is activated by a variety of mechanisms, including an increase in angiotensin II and advanced glycation end products. Together with its downstream mediator CTGF (connective tissue growth factor), TGF-β1 stimulates production of collagen and extracellular matrix and causes thickening of the GBM, resulting in podocyte detachment and apoptosis. This epithelial injury causes activation of mesenchymal cells and the differentiation of fibroblasts. Eventually glomerulosclerosis and interstitial fibrosis accompanied by inflammatory cell accumulation in the tubulointerstitum ensue.[95] Studies in laboratory models of fibrosis have suggested that blockade of epithelial cell injury and apoptosis might prevent tissue fibrosis, so TGF-β1 antagonists are now in clinical trials for several renal diseases. Because CTGF synergizes with TGF-β1 in mediating fibrosis, antibodies to CTGF have been generated and have been used successfully in mouse fibrosis models.[94] A human anti-CTGF antibody decreased microalbuminuria in a phase 1 study conducted in diabetic patients. Local renal antagonists of TGF-β1 include ACE inhibitors, bone morphogenetic protein 7 (BMP-7), and hepatocyte growth factor (HGF). High levels of HGF together with low levels of TGF-β1 correlate with a favorable outcome of SLE nephritis with immunosuppressive therapy, a finding consistent with studies showing that a finding of tubulointerstitial injury on biopsy is a bad prognostic marker.[104] Low levels of BMP-7 are found in models of renal fibrosis, and administration of BMP-7 was found to reverse renal fibrosis both in the nephrotoxic nephritis model and in MRL/lpr mice.[94]

Hepatocyte Growth Factor

HGF is a dimeric protein with a single receptor (c-met) that plays an essential role in cell growth and differentiation. The kidney is the highest producer of this protein in the body, and HGF is expressed by several renal cell types; c-met expression is ubiquitous. The exact function of HGF in the kidneys is unknown, but its expression is markedly upregulated upon acute renal injury, and it appears in the

urine as a biomarker. HGF helps degrade extracellular matrix, decreases TGF-β and collagen production, prevents hypoxia-induced cell injury, and has potent antifibrotic activity in a number of models of renal injury.[105]

Peroxisome Proliferator–Activated Receptor Gamma and Obesity

The role of obesity in renal dysfunction has now been explored. Adipocytes are increasingly recognized as an endocrine cell type that secretes a variety of hormones (leptin, adiponectin, and resistin) as well as proinflammatory cytokines. Adiponectin, a hormone that is decreased in obese individuals, has a protective effect on the endothelium and on podocytes. Adiponectin-deficient mice have albuminuria with podocyte foot process effacement, and MRL/lpr mice deficient in adiponectin have significantly worse renal disease than their wt counterparts.[106] Adiponectin levels can be elevated by the administration of PPARγ agonists. PPARγ is a nuclear hormone receptor that heterodimerizes with the retinoid X receptor and binds a specific response element on DNA. Agonists of PPARγ are currently in clinical use for diabetes, but the receptor has other important effects that may confer protection in the kidneys. PPARγ negatively regulates the renin-angiotensin system and thus lowers blood pressure. It also negatively regulates the thromboxane A_2 system and protects the endothelium and may therefore have an antiatherogenic effect. In the kidneys, PPARγ agonists prevent podocyte injury, decrease proteinuria and extracellular matrix accumulation, antagonize the effects of TGF-β1, and prevent renal macrophage accumulation in response to injury. PPARγ-deficient macrophages also fail to acquire an antiinflammatory phenotype upon engulfment of apoptotic cells, suggesting a role for PPARγ in immune clearance.[107] Two studies have shown remarkably beneficial effects of PPARγ agonists in murine models of SLE nephritis, suggesting that these drugs could be appropriate therapies for preventing chronic renal damage in SLE.

Lipocalin 2 and Kidney Injury Molecule 1

A search for biomarkers in the urine of mice and humans with kidney disease led to the identification of LCN-2 as a sensitive biomarker of tubular damage in many models of renal injury, including SLE nephritis. Analysis of the renal expression of this molecule using a reporter mouse line has shown that it is expressed primarily in proximal renal tubules. In a model of chronic kidney fibrosis and progressive glomerulosclerosis, LCN-2 deficiency markedly attenuated the development of renal tubular lesions, and fibrosis was prevented.[108] LCN-2 is regulated via the epidermal growth factor (EGF) receptor signaling pathway, which controls cell proliferation, differentiation, and apoptosis; the proliferative effect of EGF on renal tubular cells is abolished when LCN-2 is absent. Dysregulated EGF receptor (EGFR) signaling has been implicated in the development of fibrotic renal injury. LCN-2 also downregulates PPARγ expression and enhances adiposity; LCN-2 deficiency protects mice from the development of aging- and obesity-induced insulin resistance. Thus, several mechanisms may account for the protective effects of LCN-2 deficiency in the kidney. Importantly, however, LCN-2 is a potent bacteriostatic agent through its iron chelating properties. Thus, therapeutic targeting of LCN-2 could be associated with infectious toxicity.

KIM-1 (also called T cell–immunoglobulin-mucin 1 [TIM-1]), like LCN-2, is elaborated by the injured proximal renal tubule; it is a receptor for IgA and for TIM-4, which is present on antigen-presenting cells. The role of KIM-1 in renal damage is not known, but KIM-1–expressing atrophic tubules have been reported to be surrounded by fibrosis and inflammation; increased tubular KIM-1 expression is associated with tubulointerstitial inflammation and a decrease in renal function in humans. There is also some evidence that KIM-1 may function as a phagocytic receptor for apoptotic cells.[109] In mouse SLE models, KIM-1 expression in the kidneys, like LCN-2 expression, occurs after the onset of proteinuria, consistent with the later onset of tubulointerstitial disease relative to glomerular disease. Both LCN-2 and KIM-1 are potential biomarkers for renal flare in SLE. Two longitudinal studies involving approximately 100 patients each have shown some predictive capability of urinary LCN-2 levels for renal flare in children and adults with SLE.[110,111]

SYSTEMS BIOLOGY OF LUPUS NEPHRITIS: HARNESSING MOLECULAR MEDICINE TO DEFINE REGULATORY NETWORKS IN LUPUS NEPHRITIS

As previously described, lupus nephritis is a heterogeneous disease characterized by a complex inflammatory and fibrotic tissue response to local immune complex deposition and systemic inflammation. The current diagnosis and treatment of lupus nephritis is mainly based on clinical symptoms and histologic classification, which do not necessarily reflect the underlying pathophysiology. As a result, our ability to provide information about prognosis or expected response to therapy for each patient is quite limited. The ability to define specific disease mechanisms active in a given patient at a specific disease stage would provide prognostic information and form the basis for individualized therapeutic strategies. To reach this goal, an integrative analysis of regulatory events triggering and maintaining lupus nephritis is essential.

The emerging field of systems biology aims to integrate constantly growing complex biological information to provide a comprehensive description of regulatory events.[112] This approach has been greatly facilitated by the rapid development of molecular medicine, allowing the generation of large-scale datasets from minute patient samples. There are two aims of an integrative systems biology strategy. The first is to define molecular characteristics/features in the circulation or kidney and associate them with known disease phenotypes so as to obtain a better understanding of the pathophysiology of lupus nephritis. Hypotheses generated from these associative studies in humans can then be tested experimentally, either in vitro or in the murine disease models presented earlier in this chapter. For example, preclinical pharmacologic or genetic approaches in mice can validate novel treatment targets or pathways identified from the human studies and form the basis for subsequent clinical trials in patients with demonstrated activation of these molecules or pathways. The second goal of an integrated systems approach is to identify markers of disease progression and treatment response (referred to as *biomarkers*). Results from both aims are essential to identification of individualized therapeutic targets.

To obtain this comprehensive picture of regulatory cascades in lupus nephritis, several levels of clinical and molecular information from diverse sources need to be integrated (Box 18-2). However, our current ability to obtain each of these parameters in large enough patient cohorts varies widely, as does the ability to define clinically relevant associations between specific sets of molecular parameters in SLE. Strategies to integrate these large-scale datasets are still in their infancy. Here we delineate the current status of the field with a focus on gene expression studies, which are currently the sources of most published molecular information. We do not discuss the significant advances in the genetics of SLE, which are addressed in a separate chapter.

Defining Regulatory Networks in Lupus Nephritis

Gene expression profiles are currently the most comprehensive datasets to be integrated with known and predicted molecular regulatory mechanisms, clinical phenotypes and genetic information.[113,114] Gene expression in a specific compartment (single cell or whole tissue) can be measured by quantifying messenger RNA (mRNA) using a variety of technologies, including oligonucleotide microarrays, real-time quantitative reverse transcription–polymerase chain reaction (RT-PCR), or direct sequencing of transcripts. Steady-state mRNA levels are a consequence of a complex regulatory machinery ranging from regulation of mRNA transcription via transcription factors, modulation of mRNA accessibility, and stability by the translational machinery or by micro-RNAs, to selective mRNA degradation. The net effect is a tightly controlled transcriptional network that can be defined in a tissue- and disease-specific manner. Alternatively, protein levels can be measured in tissues using immunohistochemistry, proteomic arrays, two-dimensional gel electrophoresis, or mass spectrometry.

From Microarray Gene Expression Profiling to Pathway Mapping

As gene expression of cells is modified during disease, comprehensive mRNA profiling allows the evaluation of cell activity at a specific time point (e.g., time of biopsy) in a specific context (e.g., lupus nephritis) and comparison of it with another time point or context (e.g., previous biopsy or normal control cases). Our current knowledge of molecular regulatory cascades has been assembled into biological concepts (e.g. "antigen presentation" or "response to hypoxia") and maps of canonical pathways (e.g., "nuclear factor kappa B pathway") that are accessed via sophisticated software. This approach allows the integration of differentially regulated RNAs in their biological context. Biological concepts showing a significant enrichment in regulated transcripts in the cells or tissues of interest can be defined, and the significantly enriched signal transduction pathways and transcriptional programs associated with the regulated pathways can then be selected for further study and validation. In addition, current bioinformatics tools are able to identify regulatory transcriptional cascades by displaying interactions of transcription factors and their transcriptional targets.[115]

One of the first studies describing the human lupus nephritis renal transcriptome illustrates the opportunities and complexities of expression profiling in human lupus nephritis.[42] The kidney is a highly complex organ with tubulointerstitial and glomerular compartments containing multiple cell types. In addition, infiltrating cells (T cells, B cells, macrophages, etc.) add their own specific mRNAs to the transcriptional dataset. This challenge can be partially addressed by microdissecting renal tissue prior to RNA extraction. Peterson addressed this complexity by extracting glomeruli from renal biopsy specimens using a laser microdissection approach.[42] Because lupus nephritis is considered a disease primarily driven by intraglomerular immune complex deposition, an initial focus on the glomerular compartment was well justified. Gene expression profiles were used to group (cluster) patients according to their mRNA profiles into distinct subgroups. There was considerable kidney-to-kidney heterogeneity in increased transcript expression, resulting in four main gene clusters that identified the expression of type I IFN–inducible genes, presence of myelomonocytic lineages, B cells, and extracellular matrix formation. In addition, a large cluster of genes that were

---

Box 18-2 Examples of Systems Biology Analyses of Lupus Nephritis

Identify genetic variations to define genetic risk and protective alleles of the individual.

Analysis of epigenetic modulation in leukocytes and tissue to capture the effect of earlier live events on genetic information.

Transcriptional analysis of tissue and leukocytes to define currently activated disease processes.

Protein expression and function in plasma, tissue, and urine to capture the cellular machinery currently at work.

Metabolite levels in plasma, tissue, and urine to measure the metabolic status of the disease.

Histologic examination of tissue obtained by biopsy to define the net effect of the preceding regulatory cascade on structural composition of the diseased end organ.

Demographic and clinical characteristics to capture environmental exposures and mitigating factors, including treatment effects.

uniformly downregulated in all samples included genes involved in cellular growth and differentiation, such as transcription factors and ion channels and genes involved in endothelial cell proliferation and angiogenesis. Macrophage and myeloid DC transcripts were widely distributed in all biopsy samples. Interestingly the biopsy samples could be divided into two distinct groups, with one group expressing IFN-regulated genes and the other group expressing the fibrosis cluster. Importantly, the gene expression results did not correlate well with overall clinical phenotype or histologic features of the biopsy samples, although there was a tendency for those samples with IFN response elements to be associated with less crescent formation and those with fibrosis-related transcripts and B-cell infiltration to have more crescents. Whether this kind of analysis will be able to predict subsequent long-term outcomes remains to be determined.

Other investigators have focused their analyses on specific subsets of genes, such as cytokines. In one such study of laser-microdissected glomerular and tubulointerstitial compartments,[116] Th1 (e.g., T-bet, I-12, IFN-γ) and Th2 (e.g., transcription factor GATA-3) responses correlated with the degree of glomerular scarring and with chronic tubulointerstitial alterations, respectively.

The human studies previously cited define only the association of transcriptional signatures with lupus nephritis. Animal models can go beyond these associations to define a causal dependency by targeting the relevant pathways. A larger body of transcriptional data is available from murine models of lupus nephritis because they allow well-defined experimental conditions to be analyzed by comprehensive gene expression profiling. As an example of this approach, a genome-wide expression profile was generated from whole kidneys of prediseased and diseased NZB/W mice and from diseased mice that had been treated with the mTOR (mammalian target of rapamycin) inhibitor sirolimus.[117] These studies identified a set of 387 genes that were regulated during disease and a number of pathways associated with disease activity, including the antigen presentation pathway, complement pathway, IL-1 and IL-10 signaling pathways, and JAK-STAT and MAP (mitogen-activated protein) kinase signaling pathways. Many of these abnormalities reversed after treatment with sirolimus. Approximately 15% of the identified genes were found to directly or indirectly interact with the mTOR pathway, an important cellular pathway that regulates cell and organ size. Nevertheless, caution must be used in extrapolation of the results of these types of studies to the treatment of disease, because ubiquitous pathways such as mTOR are expressed in many cell types and may have heterogeneous effects. Indeed, although mTOR inhibitors are therapeutic in the lupus model, they are detrimental during the repair phase of acute renal injury and can exacerbate ischemic renal injury in humans.

Transcriptomic profiles generated from whole kidneys and laser-microdissected glomeruli from MRL/lpr mice confirmed the role of IFN-γ regulatory cascades in the development of lupus nephritis in this mouse model. Glomerular upregulated genes could be separated into major functional groups: the complement and coagulation cascades, chemokines/chemokine receptors, extracellular matrix and adhesion, MHC class II and antigen presentation/processing molecules, and IFN-regulated genes. Genes implicated in the inflammatory pathways in this model overlapped with those defined in the human study (e.g., antigen presentation, cytokines), confirming the recapitulation of a significant part of human lupus nephritis pathophysiology in this model system.[118,119] Importantly, glucocorticoid treatment by prednisolone significantly reduced the expression of inflammatory genes as well as the number of infiltrating cells and glomerular injury. This result implies that analysis of human data must be integrated with the known effects of therapeutic agents on gene expression.

As mentioned previously, a significant limitation of renal genome-wide gene expression profiling is the difficulty in evaluating the relative contributions of the accumulated infiltrating inflammatory cells (such as lymphocytes, macrophages, and neutrophils) and of intrinsic renal cell lineages (glomerular cells, tubular cell types, and renal fibroblasts). Therefore, another approach has been to isolate specific cell types from lupus nephritis kidneys via their specific surface markers. With use of this approach in NZB/W mice, a time sequence of resident macrophage–specific transcriptional profiles has been generated.[77] At nephritis onset, these cells upregulate cell surface CD11b, acquire cathepsin and MMP activity, and accumulate large numbers of autophagocytic vacuoles; these changes reverse after induction of remission. Gene expression profiling revealed that the levels of transcripts related to proinflammatory, regulatory, and tissue repair/degradation processes were increased; these transcripts were downregulated to basal levels after induction of remission by immunosuppressive therapy, supporting the conclusion that activated renal macrophages contribute to renal damage in lupus nephritis by mediating both local inflammation and excessive tissue remodeling. Importantly, many of the regulated genes overlap with the myeloid cluster defined by Petersen[42] in humans.

Integrating Genetic Predisposition with Transcriptional Regulation

A unique opportunity for systems biology is the integration of multidimensional genome-wide datasets. For example, it is possible to define the interdependence among the stable "genomic risk profile," the transcriptional status during disease, the dynamic disease phenotype, and the impact of environmental factors and treatment interventions. Linking these complex datasets can use established modes of interaction, that is, allelic variances alter transcript levels with subsequent alterations in cellular function, leading to more severe disease phenotypes. An elegant proof-of-concept study in the anti-GBM model of lupus nephritis identified an association of a decrease in renal expression of kallikrein genes with disease susceptibility in particular mouse strains. Kallikreins act through the generation of bradykinins; selective receptor blockade using pharmacologic inhibitors indicated that the biological effects of decreased kallikreins were mediated by the bradykinin B2 receptor such that blocking this receptor aggravated glomerulonephritis. Conversely, administration of bradykinins improved disease in susceptible mice. This result motivated the analysis of the orthologous locus in patients with lupus nephritis, leading to identification of single-nucleotide polymorphisms in the sequence of kallikrein 1 and 3 promoters that are strongly associated with lupus nephritis.[55]

Linking genome-wide mRNA expression with genome-wide association studies (GWASs) might therefore be a promising approach to integrate genes identified in GWASs into their functional disease context and prioritize genes for fine mapping and further functional studies. Using such an approach, one study has identified three microRNAs that together are predicted to target more than 50% of 72 lupus susceptibility genes.[120] MicroRNAs are small noncoding RNAs that interact with specific mRNAs using a partially complementary sequence; the bound mRNAs are blocked from translation and are targeted for degradation. Early studies of microRNA expression profiles in patients with lupus nephritis are starting to appear in the literature[121,122]; such studies will require confirmation but have potential functional and therapeutic implications.

Urinary Biomarkers of Lupus Nephritis: Defining the Disease State in Molecular Terms

The term *biomarker* characterizes a specific molecular feature (mRNA, micro-RNA, protein, metabolite, etc.) that can be measured and provides information about the biological status of the individual. The most specific source of a biomarker is the tissue manifesting the damage, that is, the kidney in lupus nephritis. However, renal biopsy is an invasive and costly procedure that cannot be repeated frequently. Therefore defining noninvasive modes to identify or predict disease flares, evaluate prognosis, determine appropriate therapy, and monitor treatment responses would be advantageous. The noninvasive compartments that are potentially informative for lupus nephritis include plasma, leukocytes, and urine. In SLE, however, the levels of noninvasive biomarkers in urine and plasma reflect not only alterations in the kidney but also a myriad of confounding factors not associated with nephritis. In the context of renal disease, urine might offer the best compromise of disease specificity and accessibility. A valid urinary biomarker needs to be shed into the urine at a constant rate, to be stable for variable periods in the bladder under variations of pH, and to be relatively easy to measure.

Several approaches have been applied to urine biomarker development. The first has been to test for candidate markers known to be expressed in the kidneys or that reflect general inflammatory processes. For example, inflammatory proteome arrays have identified VCAM-1 and CXCL16 as markers that distinguish subjects with active renal disease from other patients with lupus.[86] Other soluble markers identified this way that appear in the urine in lupus nephritis patients include MCP-1 and TWEAK (TNF-like weak inducer of apoptosis). A second approach is to analyze the protein content of the urine using various unbiased methods (e.g., two-dimensional gel electrophoresis, mass spectrometry) and correlate these results with the clinical or histologic activity of lupus nephritis.[123-125] With this approach, several associations of urinary proteins or peptide fingerprints with nephritis activity have been obtained. Of these, LCNn-2, hepcidin, and urinary protease have been the most rigorously studied. A third approach is to analyze the gene expression patterns in pellets of urinary cells. This analysis captures several steps of the inflammatory process, because these cells have undergone transendothelial migration, activation in the interstitium, and transepithelial migration into the renal ultrafiltrate. Unexpectedly, one such study showed an association between urinary Foxp3 and active lupus nephritis; a high urinary Foxp3 level was associated with a poor response to therapy. All of the markers identified by these exploratory studies must be rigorously validated in longitudinal studies of serum and urine from several independent cohorts to determine how they compare with simple measurements of proteinuria and to define their clinical utility for the individual patient. Extrapolation from biomarker efforts in other fields suggest that a significant attrition in the candidate markers is likely, but the unique capability of urine to reflect intrarenal events might allow the definition of robust, clinically useful biomarkers in the not too distant future. Several comprehensive critical appraisals of the literature have been published.[126-128]

Outlook and Clinical Applicability

Although lupus nephritis is currently defined in histologic terms, new technology is starting to allow a molecular definition based on profiling of renal tissue, urine, and inflammatory cells using multiple approaches. These early studies have provided new information about lupus nephritis pathogenesis in terms of which genes/pathways are activated during the different stages of lupus nephritis and can be used for defining biomarkers and therapeutic targets. Specific gene expression patterns from renal subcompartments are starting to provide further insight into the intrarenal pathophysiology of lupus nephritis in humans. Current efforts aim to define the exact contributions of various resident and infiltrating cell types and of kidney-specific response patterns to the inflammatory challenge and to identify reliable noninvasive markers that reflect the intrarenal molecular pathophysiology. Validations of these regulatory mechanisms[129] using independent methods and cohorts are still ongoing. Defining the functional status of lupus nephritis in patients with SLE should enable early detection of disease and relapses as well as guide the use of targeted therapies.

Importantly, human studies showed a poor correlation of the renal molecular expression pattern with histologically derived disease activity characteristics in lupus nephritis biopsy specimens, mirroring the relatively poor correlation of histologic scoring with clinical outcomes. Whether the gene expression profiles and emerging sets of biomarkers will have better prognostic power remains to be determined.

To improve the understanding of the renal molecular events that may eventually help define clinical outcomes, all publically available renal gene expression data, including several lupus nephritis datasets, have been deposited into a free available resource called Nephromine (*http://www.nephromine.org*). Nephromine is an example of how

systems biology is multidisciplinary, providing a huge amount of data to all interested investigators.

FUTURE DIRECTIONS IN SLE NEPHRITIS

Despite the disappointing results of a number of clinical trials in SLE nephritis that were directed at controlling systemic autoimmunity, many therapeutic targets have now been identified that provide a rich source of ideas for both prevention and treatment of this devastating SLE manifestation. There is still much room for uncovering the mechanisms that lead to chromatin and antibody deposition in the kidneys and the initiation of lupus nephritis. In addition, a consideration of pathogenetic mechanisms for chronic kidney disease and progression indicates a wide range of local processes that could be targeted. Therapies could be directed not only to local immunologically based mechanisms, such as complement activation, local T- and B-cell expansion, and activated renal mononuclear phagocytes, but also to broad nonimmunologic processes, such as epithelial cell death, tissue hypoxia, and fibrosis. Harnessing of normal renoprotective mechanisms may prevent damage without conferring systemic immune suppression. Simple interventions such as blood pressure control, appropriate nutrition, and avoidance of environmental insults all provide long-term patient benefits. Finally, identification of useful biomarkers may improve the ability to diagnose and treat disease flares and evaluate therapeutic responses. All of these new advances could translate into a decrease in rates of chronic renal failure in the coming decades.

References

1. Lefkowith JB, Kiehl M, Rubenstein J, et al: Heterogeneity and clinical significance of glomerular-binding antibodies in systemic lupus erythematosus. *J Clin Invest* 98:1373–1380, 1996.
2. Li QZ, Xie C, Wu T, et al: Identification of autoantibody clusters that best predict lupus disease activity using glomerular proteome arrays. *J Clin Invest* 115:3428–3439, 2005.
3. Bagavant H, Fu SM: Pathogenesis of kidney disease in systemic lupus erythematosus. *Curr Opin Rheumatol* 21:489–494, 2009.
4. Hedberg A, Mortensen ES, Rekvig OP: Chromatin as a target antigen in human and murine lupus nephritis. *Arthritis Res Ther* 13:214, 2011.
5. Turnberg D, Cook HT: Complement and glomerulonephritis: new insights. *Curr Opin Nephrol Hypertens* 14:223–228, 2005.
6. Clynes R, Dumitru C, Ravetch JV: Uncoupling of immune complex formation and kidney damage in autoimmune glomerulonephritis. *Science* 279:1052–1054, 1998.
7. Anders HJ, Schlondorff D: Toll-like receptors: emerging concepts in kidney disease. *Curr Opin Nephrol Hypertens* 16:177–183, 2007.
8. Vielhauer V, Anders HJ: Chemokines and chemokine receptors as therapeutic targets in chronic kidney disease. *Front Biosci (Schol Ed)* 1:1–12, 2009.
9. Chan OT, Hannum LG, Haberman AM, et al: A novel mouse with B cells but lacking serum antibody reveals an antibody-independent role for B cells in murine lupus. *J Exp Med* 189:1639–1648, 1999.
10. Lewis EJ, Schwartz MM: Pathology of lupus nephritis. *Lupus* 14:31–38, 2005.
10a. The Nephron by Dr. Fabian. Available at *http://www.youtube.com/watch?v=vEXx5YLcGmQ/*.
11. Salmon AH, Neal CR, Harper SJ: New aspects of glomerular filtration barrier structure and function: five layers (at least) not three. *Curr Opin Nephrol Hypertens* 18:197–205, 2009.
12. Mathieson PW: Update on the podocyte. *Curr Opin Nephrol Hypertens* 18:206–211, 2009.
13. Mundel P, Reiser J: Proteinuria: an enzymatic disease of the podocyte? *Kidney Int* 77:571–580, 2010.
14. Scindia YM, Deshmukh US, Bagavant H: Mesangial pathology in glomerular disease: targets for therapeutic intervention. *Adv Drug Deliv Rev* 62:1337–1343, 2010.
15. Schlondorff D, Banas B: The mesangial cell revisited: no cell is an island. *J Am Soc Nephrol* 20:1179–1187, 2009.
16. Kaissling B, Le Hir M: The renal cortical interstitium: morphological and functional aspects. *Histochem Cell Biol* 130:247–262, 2008.
17. Kriz W, Kaissling B, Le Hir M: Epithelial-mesenchymal transition (EMT) in kidney fibrosis: fact or fantasy? *J Clin Invest* 121:468–474, 2011.

18. Strutz F: The role of FGF-2 in renal fibrogenesis. *Front Biosci (Schol Ed)* 1:125–131, 2009.

19. Ferenbach D, Hughes J: Macrophages and dendritic cells: what is the difference? *Kidney Int* 74:5–7, 2008.

20. Soos TJ, Sims TN, Barisoni L, et al: CX3CR1+ interstitial dendritic cells form a contiguous network throughout the entire kidney. *Kidney Int* 70:591–596, 2006.

21. Kruger T, Benke D, Eitner F, et al: Identification and functional characterization of dendritic cells in the healthy murine kidney and in experimental glomerulonephritis. *J Am Soc Nephrol* 15:613–621, 2004.

22. Mjelle JE, Rekvig OP, Van Der Vlag J, et al: Nephritogenic antibodies bind in glomeruli through interaction with exposed chromatin fragments and not with renal cross-reactive antigens. *Autoimmunity* 42:104–111, 2011.

23. Mannik M, Merrill CE, Stamps LD, et al: Multiple autoantibodies form the glomerular immune deposits in patients with systemic lupus erythematosus. *J Rheumatol* 30:1495–1504, 2003.

24. van Bavel CC, Fenton KA, Rekvig OP, et al: Glomerular targets of nephritogenic autoantibodies in systemic lupus erythematosus. *Arthritis Rheum* 58:1892–1899, 2008.

25. Liang Z, Xie C, Chen C, et al: Pathogenic profiles and molecular signatures of antinuclear autoantibodies rescued from NZM2410 lupus mice. *J Exp Med* 199:381–398, 2004.

26. Radic MZ, Mackle J, Erikson J, et al: Residues that mediate DNA binding of autoimmune antibodies. *J Immunol* 150:4966–4977, 1993.

27. Vlahakos D, Foster MH, Ucci AA, et al: Murine monoclonal anti-DNA antibodies penetrate cells, bind to nuclei, and induce glomerular proliferation and proteinuria in vivo. *J Am Soc Nephrol* 2:1345–1354, 1992.

28. Vlahakos DV, Foster MH, Adams S, et al: Anti-DNA antibodies form immune deposits at distinct glomerular and vascular sites. *Kidney Int* 41:1690–1700, 1992.

29. Gilkeson GS, Bernstein K, Pippen AM, et al: The influence of variable-region somatic mutations on the specificity and pathogenicity of murine monoclonal anti-DNA antibodies. *Clin Immunol Immunopathol* 76:59–67, 1995.

30. Budhai L, Oh K, Davidson A: An in vitro assay for detection of glomerular binding IgG autoantibodies in patients with systemic lupus erythematosus. *J Clin Invest* 98:1585–1593, 1996.

31. Madaio MP: The role of autoantibodies in the pathogenesis of lupus nephritis. *Semin Nephrol* 19:48–56, 1999.

32. Fournie GJ: Circulating DNA and lupus nephritis. *Kidney Int* 33:487–497, 1988.

33. Izui S, Lambert PH, Miescher PA: Failure to detect circulating DNA–anti-DNA complexes by four radioimmunological methods in patients with systemic lupus erythematosus. *Clin Exp Immunol* 30:384–392, 1977.

34. Pisetsky DS, Gauley J, Ullal AJ: Microparticles as a source of extracellular DNA. *Immunol Res* 49:227–234, 2011.

35. Lande R, Ganguly D, Facchinetti V, et al: Neutrophils activate plasmacytoid dendritic cells by releasing self-DNA-peptide complexes in systemic lupus erythematosus. *Sci Transl Med* 3:73ra19, 2011.

36. Hakkim A, Furnrohr BG, Amann K, et al: Impairment of neutrophil extracellular trap degradation is associated with lupus nephritis. *Proc Natl Acad Sci U S A* 107:9813–9818, 2010.

37. Raz E, Brezis M, Rosenmann E, et al: Anti-DNA antibodies bind directly to renal antigens and induce kidney dysfunction in the isolated perfused rat kidney. *J Immunol* 142:3076–3082, 1989.

38. Tsirogianni A, Pipi E, Soufleros K: Relevance of anti-C1q autoantibodies to lupus nephritis. *Ann N Y Acad Sci* 1173:243–251, 2009.

39. Kraft SW, Schwartz MM, Korbet SM, et al: Glomerular podocytopathy in patients with systemic lupus erythematosus. *J Am Soc Nephrol* 16:175–179, 2005.

40. Heymann F, Meyer-Schwesinger C, Hamilton-Williams EE, et al: Kidney dendritic cell activation is required for progression of renal disease in a mouse model of glomerular injury. *J Clin Invest* 119:1286–1297, 2009.

41. Theofilopoulos AN, Dixon FJ: Murine models of systemic lupus erythematosus. *Adv Immunol* 37:269–390, 1985.

42. Peterson KS, Huang JF, Zhu J, et al: Characterization of heterogeneity in the molecular pathogenesis of lupus nephritis from transcriptional profiles of laser-captured glomeruli. *J Clin Invest* 113:1722–1733, 2004.

43. Schiffer L, Bethunaickan R, Ramanujam M, et al: Activated renal macrophages are markers of disease onset and disease remission in lupus nephritis. *J Immunol* 180:1938–1947, 2008.

44. Ramanujam M, Davidson A: Targeting of the immune system in systemic lupus erythematosus. *Expert Rev Mol Med* 10:e2, 2008.

45. Kalled SL, Cutler AH, Datta SK, et al: Anti-CD40 ligand antibody treatment of SNF1 mice with established nephritis: preservation of kidney function. *J Immunol* 160:2158–2165, 1998.

46. Singh RR, Saxena V, Zang S, et al: Differential contribution of IL-4 and STAT6 vs STAT4 to the development of lupus nephritis. *J Immunol* 170:4818–4825, 2003.

47. Ramanujam M, Davidson A: BAFF blockade for systemic lupus erythematosus: will the promise be fulfilled? *Immunol Rev* 223:156–174, 2008.

48. Jacob CO, Zang S, Li L, et al: Pivotal role of Stat4 and Stat6 in the pathogenesis of the lupus-like disease in the New Zealand mixed 2328 mice. *J Immunol* 171:1564–1571, 2003.

49. Subramanian S, Tus K, Li QZ, et al: A Tlr7 translocation accelerates systemic autoimmunity in murine lupus. *Proc Natl Acad Sci U S A* 103:9970–9975, 2006.

50. Kahn P, Ramanujam M, Bethunaickan R, et al: Prevention of murine antiphospholipid syndrome by BAFF blockade. *Arthritis Rheum* 58:2824–2834, 2008.

51. Watanabe-Fukunaga R, Brannan CI, Copeland NG, et al: Lymphoproliferation disorder in mice explained by defects in Fas antigen that mediates apoptosis. *Nature* 356:314–317, 1992.

52. Menke J, Rabacal WA, Byrne KT, et al: Circulating CSF-1 promotes monocyte and macrophage phenotypes that enhance lupus nephritis. *J Am Soc Nephrol* 20:2581–2592, 2009.

53. Shimizu S, Sugiyama N, Masutani K, et al: Membranous glomerulonephritis development with Th2-type immune deviations in MRL/lpr mice deficient for IL-27 receptor (WSX-1). *J Immunol* 175:7185–7192, 2005.

54. Fu Y, Du Y, Mohan C: Experimental anti-GBM disease as a tool for studying spontaneous lupus nephritis. *Clin Immunol* 124:109–118, 2007.

55. Liu K, Li QZ, Delgado-Vega AM, et al: Kallikrein genes are associated with lupus and glomerular basement membrane-specific antibody-induced nephritis in mice and humans. *J Clin Invest* 119:911–923, 2009.

56. Reeves WH, Lee PY, Weinstein JS, et al: Induction of autoimmunity by pristane and other naturally occurring hydrocarbons. *Trends Immunol* 30:455–464, 2009.

57. Bergtold A, Gavhane A, D'Agati V, et al: FcR-bearing myeloid cells are responsible for triggering murine lupus nephritis. *J Immunol* 177:7287–7295, 2006.

58. Tesch GH, Maifert S, Schwarting A, et al: Monocyte chemoattractant protein 1-dependent leukocytic infiltrates are responsible for autoimmune disease in MRL-Fas(lpr) mice. *J Exp Med* 190:1813–1824, 1999.

59. Lewis MJ, Botto M: Complement deficiencies in humans and animals: links to autoimmunity. *Autoimmunity* 39:367–378, 2006.

60. Watanabe H, Garnier G, Circolo A, et al: Modulation of renal disease in MRL/lpr mice genetically deficient in the alternative complement pathway factor B. *J Immunol* 164:786–794, 2000.

61. Woodruff TM, Nandakumar KS, Tedesco F: Inhibiting the C5-C5a receptor axis. *Mol Immunol* 48(14):1631–1642, 2011.

62. Renner B, Ferreira VP, Cortes C, et al: Binding of factor H to tubular epithelial cells limits interstitial complement activation in ischemic injury. *Kidney Int* 80(2):165–173, 2011.

63. Pickering MC, Botto M: Are anti-C1q antibodies different from other SLE autoantibodies? *Nat Rev Rheumatol* 6:490–493, 2010.

64. Li Y, Lee PY, Sobel ES, et al: Increased expression of FcgammaRI/CD64 on circulating monocytes parallels ongoing inflammation and nephritis in lupus. *Arthritis Res Ther* 11:R6, 2009.

65. Zuniga R, Markowitz GS, Arkachaisri T, et al: Identification of IgG subclasses and C-reactive protein in lupus nephritis: the relationship between the composition of immune deposits and FCgamma receptor type IIA alleles. *Arthritis Rheum* 48:460–470, 2003.

66. Anders HJ, Schlondorff DO: Innate immune receptors and autophagy: implications for autoimmune kidney injury. *Kidney Int* 78:29–37, 2010.

67. Hsieh C, Chang A, Brandt D, et al: Predicting outcomes of lupus nephritis with tubulointerstitial inflammation and scarring. *Arthritis Care Res (Hoboken)* 63:865–874, 2011.

68. Hill GS, Delahousse M, Nochy D, et al: Proteinuria and tubulointerstitial lesions in lupus nephritis. *Kidney Int* 60:1893–1903, 2001.

69. Chang A, Henderson SG, Brandt D, et al: In situ B cell-mediated immune responses and tubulointerstitial inflammation in human lupus nephritis. *J Immunol* 186:1849–1860, 2011.

70. Crispin JC, Oukka M, Bayliss G, et al: Expanded double negative T cells in patients with systemic lupus erythematosus produce IL-17 and infiltrate the kidneys. *J Immunol* 181:8761–8766, 2008.

71. Holdsworth SR, Tipping PG: Leukocytes in glomerular injury. *Semin Immunopathol* 29:355–374, 2007.

72. Geissmann F, Manz MG, Jung S, et al: Development of monocytes, macrophages, and dendritic cells. *Science* 327:656–661, 2010.

73. Li L, Huang L, Sung SS, et al: The chemokine receptors CCR2 and CX3CR1 mediate monocyte/macrophage trafficking in kidney ischemia-reperfusion injury. *Kidney Int* 74:1526–1537, 2008.

74. Hume DA: Differentiation and heterogeneity in the mononuclear phagocyte system. *Mucosal Immunol* 1:432–441, 2008.

75. Mosser DM, Edwards JP: Exploring the full spectrum of macrophage activation. *Nat Rev Immunol* 8:958–969, 2008.

76. Segerer S, Heller F, Lindenmeyer MT, et al: Compartment specific expression of dendritic cell markers in human glomerulonephritis. *Kidney Int* 74:37–46, 2008.

77. Bethunaickan R, Berthier CC, Ramanujam M, et al: A unique hybrid renal mononuclear phagocyte activation phenotype in murine systemic lupus erythematosus nephritis. *J Immunol* 186:4994–5003, 2011.

78. Panzer U, Steinmetz OM, Stahl RA, et al: Kidney diseases and chemokines. *Curr Drug Targets* 7:65–80, 2006.

79. Enghard P, Humrich JY, Rudolph B, et al: CXCR3+CD4+ T cells are enriched in inflamed kidneys and urine and provide a new biomarker for acute nephritis flares in systemic lupus erythematosus patients. *Arthritis Rheum* 60:199–206, 2009.

80. Wang A, Guilpain P, Chong BF, et al: Dysregulated expression of CXCR4/CXCL12 in subsets of patients with systemic lupus erythematosus. *Arthritis Rheum* 62:3436–3446, 2010.

81. Schlondorff DO: Overview of factors contributing to the pathophysiology of progressive renal disease. *Kidney Int* 74:860–866, 2008.

82. Kitching AR, Holdsworth SR: The emergence of TH17 cells as effectors of renal injury. *J Am Soc Nephrol* 22:235–238, 2011.

83. Timoshanko JR, Kitching AR, Iwakura Y, et al: Leukocyte-derived interleukin-1beta interacts with renal interleukin-1 receptor I to promote renal tumor necrosis factor and glomerular injury in murine crescentic glomerulonephritis. *Am J Pathol* 164:1967–1977, 2004.

84. Ernandez T, Mayadas TN: Immunoregulatory role of TNFalpha in inflammatory kidney diseases. *Kidney Int* 76:262–276, 2009.

85. Jacob N, Yang H, Pricop L, et al: Accelerated pathological and clinical nephritis in systemic lupus erythematosus-prone New Zealand Mixed 2328 mice doubly deficient in TNF receptor 1 and TNF receptor 2 via a Th17-associated pathway. *J Immunol* 182:2532–2541, 2009.

86. Wu T, Xie C, Wang HW, et al: Elevated urinary VCAM-1, P-selectin, soluble TNF receptor-1, and CXC chemokine ligand 16 in multiple murine lupus strains and human lupus nephritis. *J Immunol* 179:7166–7175, 2007.

87. Bauer JW, Baechler EC, Petri M, et al: Elevated serum levels of interferon-regulated chemokines are biomarkers for active human systemic lupus erythematosus. *PLoS Med* 3:e491, 2006.

88. Aringer M, Smolen JS: Cytokine expression in lupus kidneys. *Lupus* 14:13–18, 2005.

89. Hao CM, Breyer MD: Roles of lipid mediators in kidney injury. *Semin Nephrol* 27:338–351, 2007.

90. Eckardt KU, Bernhardt W, Willam C, et al: Hypoxia-inducible transcription factors and their role in renal disease. *Semin Nephrol* 27:363–372, 2007.

91. Nizet V, Johnson RS: Interdependence of hypoxic and innate immune responses. *Nat Rev Immunol* 9:609–617, 2009.

92. Oates JC, Shaftman SR, Self SE, et al: Association of serum nitrate and nitrite levels with longitudinal assessments of disease activity and damage in systemic lupus erythematosus and lupus nephritis. *Arthritis Rheum* 58:263–272, 2008.

93. Tse KC, Li FK, Tang S, et al: Angiotensin inhibition or blockade for the treatment of patients with quiescent lupus nephritis and persistent proteinuria. *Lupus* 14:947–952, 2005.

94. Nguyen TQ, Goldschmeding R: Bone morphogenetic protein-7 and connective tissue growth factor: novel targets for treatment of renal fibrosis? *Pharm Res* 25:2416–2426, 2008.

95. Bottinger EP: TGF-beta in renal injury and disease. *Semin Nephrol* 27:309–320, 2007.

96. Kohan DE: Endothelin, hypertension and chronic kidney disease: new insights. *Curr Opin Nephrol Hypertens* 19:134–139, 2010.

97. Thacker SG, Berthier CC, Mattinzoli D, et al: The detrimental effects of IFN-alpha on vasculogenesis in lupus are mediated by repression of IL-1 pathways: potential role in atherogenesis and renal vascular rarefaction. *J Immunol* 185:4457–4469, 2010.

98. Izmirly PM, Barisoni L, Buyon JP, et al: Expression of endothelial protein C receptor in cortical peritubular capillaries associates with a poor clinical response in lupus nephritis. *Rheumatology (Oxford)* 48:513–519, 2009.

99. Abd-Elkareem MI, Tamimy HMAl, Khamis OA, et al: Increased urinary levels of the leukocyte adhesion molecules ICAM-1 and VCAM-1 in human lupus nephritis with advanced renal histological changes: preliminary findings. *Clin Exp Nephrol* 14:548–557, 2010.

100. Gambaro G, Kong NC: Glycosaminoglycan treatment in glomerulonephritis? An interesting option to investigate. *J Nephrol* 23:244–252, 2010.

101. van den Hoven MJ, Rops AL, Vlodavsky I, et al: Heparanase in glomerular diseases. *Kidney Int* 72:543–548, 2007.

102. Wiggins RC: The spectrum of podocytopathies: a unifying view of glomerular diseases. *Kidney Int* 71:1205–1214, 2007.

103. Deelman L, Sharma K: Mechanisms of kidney fibrosis and the role of antifibrotic therapies. *Curr Opin Nephrol Hypertens* 18:85–90, 2009.

104. Capuano A, Costanzi S, Peluso G, et al: Hepatocyte growth factor and transforming growth factor beta1 ratio at baseline can predict early response to cyclophosphamide in systemic lupus erythematosus nephritis. *Arthritis Rheum* 54:3633–3639, 2006.

105. Liu Y: Hepatocyte growth factor and the kidney. *Curr Opin Nephrol Hypertens* 11:23–30, 2002.

106. Sharma K: The link between obesity and albuminuria: adiponectin and podocyte dysfunction. *Kidney Int* 76:145–148, 2009.

107. Fogo AB: PPARgamma and chronic kidney disease. *Pediatr Nephrol* 26:347–351, 2011.

108. Viau A, Karoui KEl, Laouari D, et al: Lipocalin 2 is essential for chronic kidney disease progression in mice and humans. *J Clin Invest* 120:4065–4076, 2010.

109. Waanders F, van Timmeren MM, Stegeman CA, et al: Kidney injury molecule-1 in renal disease. *J Pathol* 220:7–16, 2010.

110. Rubinstein T, Pitashny M, Levine B, et al: Urinary neutrophil gelatinase-associated lipocalin as a novel biomarker for disease activity in lupus nephritis. *Rheumatology (Oxford)* 49:960–971, 2010.

111. Hinze CH, Suzuki M, Klein-Gitelman M, et al: Neutrophil gelatinase-associated lipocalin is a predictor of the course of global and renal childhood-onset systemic lupus erythematosus disease activity. *Arthritis Rheum* 60:2772–2781, 2009.

112. Kretzler M, Cohen CD: Integrative biology of renal disease: toward a holistic understanding of the kidney's function and failure. *Semin Nephrol* 30:439–442, 2010.

113. Grant SF, Hakonarson H: Microarray technology and applications in the arena of genome-wide association. *Clin Chem* 54:1116–1124, 2008.

114. Stegall MD, Park W: What can be learned using microarrays? *Kidney Int* 72:783–784, 2007.

115. Werner T, Fessele S, Maier H, et al: Computer modeling of promoter organization as a tool to study transcriptional coregulation. *FASEB J* 17:1228–1237, 2003.

116. Chan RW, Lai FM, Li EK, et al: Intra-renal cytokine gene expression in lupus nephritis. *Ann Rheum Dis* 26:26, 2007.

117. Reddy PS, Legault HM, Sypek JP, et al: Mapping similarities in mTOR pathway perturbations in mouse lupus nephritis models and human lupus nephritis. *Arthritis Res Ther* 10:R127, 2008.

118. Teramoto K, Negoro N, Kitamoto K, et al: Microarray analysis of glomerular gene expression in murine lupus nephritis. *J Pharmacol Sci* 106:56–67, 2008.

119. Liu J, Karypis G, Hippen KL, et al: Genomic view of systemic autoimmunity in MRLlpr mice. *Genes Immun* 7:156–168, 2006.

120. Vinuesa CG, Rigby RJ, Yu D: Logic and extent of miRNA-mediated control of autoimmune gene expression. *Int Rev Immunol* 28:112–138, 2009.

121. Dai Y, Sui W, Lan H, et al: Comprehensive analysis of microRNA expression patterns in renal biopsies of lupus nephritis patients. *Rheumatol Int* 29:749–754, 2009.

122. Te JL, Dozmorov IM, Guthridge JM, et al: Identification of unique microRNA signature associated with lupus nephritis. *PLoS One* 5:e10344, 2010.

123. Oates JC, Varghese S, Bland AM, et al: Prediction of urinary protein markers in lupus nephritis. *Kidney Int* 68:2588–2592, 2005.

124. Zhang X, Jin M, Wu H, et al: Biomarkers of lupus nephritis determined by serial urine proteomics. *Kidney Int* 74:799–807, 2008.

125. Wu T, Fu Y, Brekken D, et al: Urine proteome scans uncover total urinary protease, prostaglandin D synthase, serum amyloid P, and superoxide

dismutase as potential markers of lupus nephritis. *J Immunol* 184:2183–2193, 2010.

126. Manoharan A, Madaio MP: Biomarkers in lupus nephritis. *Rheum Dis Clin North Am* 36:131–143, ix, 2010.

127. Mok CC: Biomarkers for lupus nephritis: a critical appraisal. *J Biomed Biotechnol* 2010:638413, 2010.

128. Rovin BH, Zhang X: Biomarkers for lupus nephritis: the quest continues. *Clin J Am Soc Nephrol* 4:1858–1865, 2009.

129. Chuaqui RF, Bonner RF, Best CJ, et al: Post-analysis follow-up and validation of microarray experiments. *Nat Genet* 32(Suppl):509–514, 2002.

130. Aprahamian T, Bonegio RG, Richez C, et al: The peroxisome proliferator-activated receptor gamma agonist rosiglitazone ameliorates murine lupus by induction of adiponectin. *J Immunol* 182:340–346, 2009.

131. Zhao W, Thacker SG, Hodgin JB, et al: The peroxisome proliferator-activated receptor gamma agonist pioglitazone improves cardiometabolic risk and renal inflammation in murine lupus. *J Immunol* 183:2729–2740, 2009.

SECTION III
AUTOANTIBODIES

Chapter 19
Immune Tolerance Defects in Lupus

Ram Raj Singh, Shweta Dubey, and Julia Pinkhasov

The presence of autoantibodies against a variety of ubiquitous self-antigens is a hallmark of systemic lupus erythematosus (SLE). Although primary impairments in B cells that produce autoantibodies have been described in lupus, T-cell help is paramount for the production of pathogenic autoantibodies. Thus, delineation of mechanisms of autoantibody production would require a thorough understanding of the loss of self-tolerance in both T and B cells.

Lack of central tolerance by negative selection in the thymus or bone marrow is an initial step in the development of autoreactive T or B cells, respectively.[1] Negative selection to ubiquitous self-antigens occurs in the cortex of the thymus, whereas negative selection to tissue-restricted self-antigens that are targeted in organ-specific autoimmune diseases occurs in the medulla of the thymus.[2,3] The loss of central T-cell tolerance, however, might be of little pathologic consequence, as robust peripheral tolerance mechanisms provide major control against pathologic autoimmunity.[2,4] Similarly, B cells that encounter self-antigens in the periphery face several tolerance checkpoints.[5,6] Patients with SLE have defects in B-cell tolerance at several of these checkpoints, including one at the transition from the early immature to the immature stage, another at the transitional to mature stage, a germinal center (GC) entry checkpoint, and a checkpoint between naïve and antigen-experienced B cells.[7,8] Belimumab, the only drug approved by the U.S. Food and Drug Administration (FDA) for SLE in more than 50 years, is assumed to act at one of these peripheral B-cell tolerance checkpoints via deletion of autoreactive transitional and naïve B cells.[8,9] It remains to be determined, however, whether treatment with belimumab also depletes a subset of transitional and naïve B cells that act as regulatory B (Breg) cells.[10-12] Depletion of such protective B cells can potentially tamper the therapeutic efficacy of belimumab.

In this chapter, we introduce concepts of normal immunologic tolerance, review potential mechanisms that lead to breakdown of tolerance in lupus, and discuss ways to reestablish immune tolerance in lupus.

IMMUNE TOLERANCE
Lymphocyte Homeostasis and Immune Tolerance
The immune system is unique in its ability to maintain a state of equilibrium despite its continuous exposure to self-antigens as well as its requirement to mount an adequate response to a variety of foreign antigens. After responding to an antigen, the immune system returns to its original state, so that the numbers and functional status of lymphocytes are reset at roughly the original state. This process, known as *lymphoid homeostasis*, allows the immune system to respond

to new antigenic challenges. The size and content of the preimmune lymphocyte repertoire are tightly regulated, as new emigrants from the lymphoid organs compete for "space" with resident cells.[13] Several groups have tried to define factors that control naïve and memory T-cell homeostasis under lymphoproliferative or lymphopenic conditions.[14] There has been a renewed interest in the hypothesis that in lymphopenic conditions, T cells expand to reestablish homeostasis by a process dependent on self–major histocompatibility complex (MHC)–peptide recognition and on the availability of cytokines that can promote the proliferation and survival of lymphocytes. Such lymphocyte expansion is believed to be a normal physiologic process. The constant recurrence of this process, however, might lead to the selection and accumulation of high-affinity self-reactive T-cell clones and ensuing autoimmune disease.[15] Experimental support for this hypothesis was reported in a study that showed that autoimmune nonobese diabetic (NOD) mice have reduced numbers of CD4+ T and B cells in comparison with control mouse strains.[16] Increasing T-cell numbers, such as by immunization with complete Freund's adjuvant (CFA), increases B-cell numbers as well and protects these mice from autoimmune diabetes. Interestingly, self-reactive T-cell receptor (TCR) transgenic T cells expand in the lymphopenic NOD mice, but not in NOD mice "filled" (reconstituted) with syngeneic T cells, in CFA-immunized NOD mice, and in congenic B6.idd3.NOD mice that have normal T- and B-cell numbers. Thus, lymphopenia and the resulting compensatory homeostatic expansion of effector lymphocytes reactive with self-antigens may precipitate autoimmunity.[16] Another example of lymphopenia-induced autoimmunity in rodents is the development of autoimmunity after neonatal thymectomy, discontinuation of cyclosporine treatment, or total lymphoid irradiation. Lymphopenia also accompanies human autoimmune diseases, such as SLE and Sjögren syndrome.[17]

Lymphocytes with receptors specific for self-antigens are generated continuously in the body, yet most individuals maintain a state of unresponsiveness to their own antigens, a process referred to as self–immune tolerance. Thus, immune *tolerance* can be broadly defined as a physiologic state in which the immune system does not react harmfully against the components of an organism that harbors it or against antigens that are introduced to it.[18] Harmful responses are prevented by a variety of mechanisms that operate during development of the immune system and during the generation of each immune response. These mechanisms can be broadly classified into four major groups: *Central tolerance*—which implies induction of tolerance in developing lymphocytes when they encounter self-antigens in the thymus or bone marrow—ensures tolerance to self-antigens that are present in high concentrations in the bone marrow and thymus. This process occurs by induction of apoptosis of self-reactive lymphocytes also known as *clonal deletion*. *Peripheral tolerance* is maintained by mechanisms that operate on mature lymphocytes once they exit the primary lymphoid organs. *Ignorance* may be the mechanism of tolerance for these self-antigens, which is believed to operate when the self-antigen is sequestered in anatomic sites, which are inaccessible to lymphocytes. *Clonal anergy* is another mechanism of lymphocyte tolerance in which the lymphocyte is functionally unresponsive following antigen encounter but remains alive for extended periods in a hyporesponsive state.[19] Self-antigen recognition without co-stimulatory signals is widely believed to induce lymphocyte anergy. However, the conditions or factors that determine whether a self-antigen can be functionally ignored or induces anergy remain to be fully understood. More importantly, so far we do not know which self-antigens can induce which form of self-tolerance or what is the relative contribution of each of these mechanisms in shaping the normal immune repertoire. There is also no proper understanding of which characteristics of a self-antigen can lead it to undergo central tolerance, peripheral tolerance, clonal ignorance, or clonal anergy. Nevertheless, substantial progress has been made in unraveling these basic tolerance mechanisms that are common to both B and T lymphocytes. Because current knowledge supports loss of tolerance in both B and T cells in eliciting pathologic autoimmunity, we discuss them separately (Table 19-1).

Mechanisms Underlying T-Cell Tolerance

Tolerance of self-reactive T cells occurs in both a central tolerance mode, occurring in the thymus, and in peripheral tolerance mode, occurring in the peripheral lymphoid organs. The sites of tolerance and potential mechanisms are depicted in Figure 19-1, *A*.

Thymic Selection

The recognition of self-peptides, in association with self-MHC molecules, presented to differentiating T cells by antigen-presenting cells (APCs) present in the thymus results in thymic selection of T cells.[1] This thymic selection process ensures that mature T cells are both self-MHC–restricted and self-tolerant. When the TCRs on a pre–T cell thymocyte are engaged, the thymocyte can be either positively or negatively selected, depending on the balancing effects of several other factors regulating this process. Thymic selection begins at the double-positive (DP; CD4$^+$CD8$^+$) stage in the thymus (when the α and β chain genes are expressed) and beyond. This process has two important outcomes: MHC restriction (positive selection) and central tolerance (negative selection). Thymic cortical epithelial cells function as the effector cells in a process known as *positive selection*. In positive selection, T cells that bear a TCR that can bind self-MHC are selected to survive and proliferate. T cells that are not positively selected are triggered to undergo apoptosis. Positively selected thymocytes must go through a second phase of selection known as *negative selection*. During negative selection, any T cell that is presented with antigenic peptide bound to MHC within the thymus is triggered to undergo apoptosis if the avidity between the TCR and the MHC/self-peptide is too strong.

TABLE 19-1 Mechanisms of Self-Tolerance in T and B Cells

MECHANISM	PRESENT IN T CELLS?	PRESENT IN B CELLS?
Clonal deletion	Yes	Yes
Ignorance	Yes	Yes
Anergy	Yes	Yes
Immune deviation	Yes	No
Regulatory T/B cells	Yes	Yes
Receptor editing	No	Yes

The self-peptides encountered in the thymus are derived from proteins expressed in the thymus as well as other proteins brought to the thymus via the bloodstream. Moreover, medullary thymic epithelial cells (mTECs) express the autoimmune regulator (Aire) transcription factor that allows promiscuous gene expression.[20] Aire allows mTECs to express not only antigens that are ubiquitously expressed but also antigens that are exclusively restricted in organ-specific cells. The Aire-controlled expression of tissue-restricted self-antigens provides a dynamic mechanism by which organ-specific self-tolerance is achieved. Mutations in the gene encoding Aire have been recognized as the molecular cause of the autoimmune polyendocrine syndrome type 1 (APS-1). In addition, dendritic cells (DCs) can functionally remove autoreactive T cells and express tissue-restricted self-antigens released from mTECs.[21,22] Surviving T cells continue to migrate to the medulla, where they undergo full maturation and finally leave the thymus through the postcapillary venules or efferent lymphatics. Data now suggest that negative selection to ubiquitous self-antigens occurs in the cortex of thymus without medullary involvement, whereas positive selection and migration to the medulla are required for negative selection to tissue-restricted self-antigens.[2,3]

Although thymic selection should enable the deletion of all self-reactive T cells, this process is not perfect because not all peptides that an organism may encounter in the lifetime are presented in the thymus. Other variables, such as peptide concentrations, affinity of TCRs, and state of APCs in the thymus, may all determine whether the threshold for receptor occupancy is reached for the positive or negative selection to occur. Potentially self-reactive T cells that escape central tolerance can still be tamed through several backup mechanisms for maintenance of self-tolerance.[2,4] These *peripheral tolerance* mechanisms include antigen-specific unresponsiveness or anergy, immune deviation, and elimination after repeated activation.[23] Variables that determine whether peripheral deletion proceeds efficiently include extent of TCR occupancy, affinity of antigenic peptide for the MHC, and affinity of TCR for the antigen peptide complex. High antigenic dose and chronic stimulation favor elimination both in CD4$^+$ and CD8$^+$ T cells. The silencing of T cells upon persistent activation in the periphery may thus represent a continuous process, ranging from the activation to unresponsiveness to deletion, with T-cell signal strength and exposure time together determining the outcome. A major mechanism for peripheral deletion of activated T cells involves activation-induced cell death (AICD) via the Fas-FasL pathway, as suggested by studies in mouse models, in which mutations in these molecules are associated with the development of autoimmunity. In mice deficient in Fas (MRL/Fas*lpr/lpr* [MRL/lpr]) or the Fas ligand (FasL) (gld mice), severe lymphoproliferative autoimmune disease develops as a result of accumulation of activated T cells. Mutations in *Fas* are associated with autoimmune disease in humans as well.[24] Some mouse strains carrying gld or lpr mutations demonstrate inflammatory disease, whereas the same mutations on other genetic backgrounds cause only excessive lymphoproliferation.[25] In humans, not all subjects carrying mutations in Fas or FasL experience autoimmune disease.[24,26] Thus, additional mechanisms must contribute to peripheral tolerance of autoreactive T cells.

Inhibitory co-stimulatory molecules like cytotoxic T-lymphocyte antigen 4 (CTLA-4) and programmed death 1 (PD-1) have been implicated in peripheral tolerance. These two molecules play distinct regulatory roles. Although CTLA-4 is involved in regulating initiation of immune response in the lymph node, PD-1 pathways act late at the tissue site to limit T-cell activation.[27]

Induction of Anergy

Anergy induction is another mechanism of lymphocyte tolerance, in which the lymphocyte is functionally unresponsive after antigen encounter but remains alive for extended periods in a hyporesponsive state.[19] The basic types of T-cell anergy fall in two groups. One is the principally growth arrest state clonal anergy, and the other is adaptive tolerance or in vivo anergy, a generalized inhibition of proliferation and effector functions.[28] According to the two-signal model

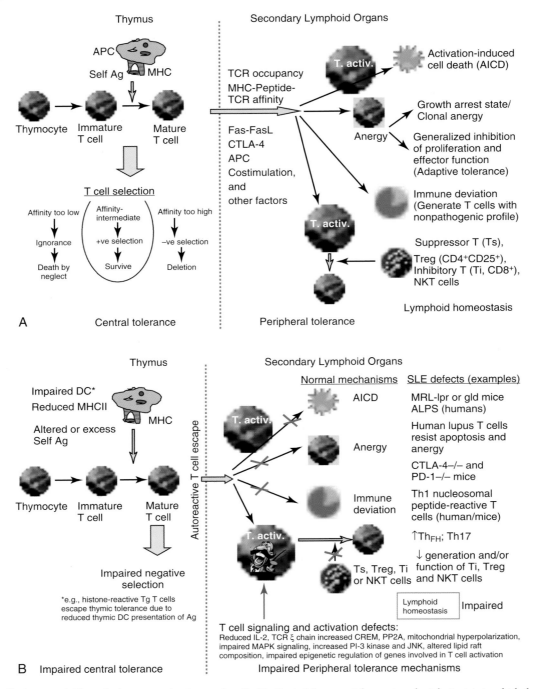

FIGURE 19-1 **T-cell tolerance. A,** Normal tolerance mechanisms as described in the text. Immune *tolerance* is a physiologic state in which the immune system does not react harmfully against the components of an organism that harbors it or against antigens that are introduced to it. Self-reactive T cells undergo negative selection in the thymus; those that escape thymic tolerance are subjected to multiple peripheral tolerance mechanisms at many levels. Normal mechanisms of tolerance induction and maintenance are indicated in *red*. **B,** Breakdown of T-cell tolerance in SLE as described in the text. T cells may escape negative selection in the thymus by impaired presentation of self-antigen (Ag) by thymic antigen-presenting cells (APC). The affinity of self-epitopes can also prevent them from undergoing negative selection. Self-reactive T cells exit the thymus and are activated by self Ag presented on APCs, inducing a hyperresponsive phenotype coupled with resistance to induction of anergy and/or apoptosis. Immune deviation and activation of T regulatory cells (Tregs) and T inhibitory (Ti) cells, which are additional mechanisms to control autoreactive T cells, fail to suppress them, thereby leading to the expansion and survival of autoreactive T cells. SLE T cells also exhibit an overexcitable phenotype, which further contributes to increased T-cell activation and T-cell receptor (TCR)–mediated signaling. Examples of impaired tolerance in SLE are indicated in *brown*.

of T-cell activation versus anergy, the APCs having the ability to offer T cells the prerequisite triggering of TCRs (signal 1) and co-stimulation (CD28/B7; signal 2) induce T-cell activation. However, not all APCs have the ability to offer T cells both of these signals, and signaling through the TCR alone induces a state of functional unresponsiveness, or clonal anergy. This could happen via two pathways: One is the direct inhibition of CD28 signaling by "anergy factors," and the other involves an indirect effect on cell cycle progression through growth factors such as interleukin-1 (IL-2).[29,30] Some studies have led to a better understanding of the cell-intrinsic program that establishes T-cell anergy. During the induction phase of anergy, "incomplete" stimulation of T cells (TCR triggering without co-stimulation) leads via calcium influx to an altered gene expression program that includes upregulation of several E3 ubiquitin ligases. When the anergic T cells contact APCs, intracellular signaling proteins are monoubiquitinated and targeted for lysosomal degradation, thus decreasing intracellular signaling and also resulting in decreased stability of the T cell–APC contact.[31] Ubiquitin ligases that have been implicated in T-cell anergy are c-Cbl, Cbl-b, GRAIL, ITCH, and Nedd4.[32] Interplay of these ubiquitin ligases has been shown to regulate T-cell anergy.

Immune Deviation

The immune system has also evolved to have a functional mechanism of tolerance in the face of persistent T-cell activation. Skewing of a T-cell response into a lineage that does not mediate disease and that prevents development of harmful T-cell responses is called *immune deviation*. In NOD mice, in which diabetes spontaneously develops, the presence of T-helper 1 (Th1) cells in islets was found to be associated with the clinical disease, whereas resistance to disease is associated with predominance of cells producing Th2-like cytokines.[33] Similarly, in experimental autoimmune encephalomyelitis (EAE) models, the Th1 responses are generally pathogenic, whereas Th2 responses are protective. Paradoxically, the blockade of Th1 differentiation in IL-12 receptor 2–deficient mice results in more severe EAE.[34] This led to the discovery of another T-helper cell type, known as Th17 cells because of their production of the proinflammatory cytokine IL-17.[35] It was quickly recognized that Th17 cells mediate major pathogenic functions in many autoimmune diseases, such as multiple sclerosis (MS), rheumatoid arthritis (RA), inflammatory bowel disease (IBD), diabetes, Sjögren syndrome, and psoriasis, and even Th2-mediated inflammatory diseases such as asthma.[36] Specific mechanisms, which allow skewing of T-cell immune deviation into Th1, Th2, Th17, and T-regulatory (Treg) cells, are not fully understood. Several explanations for the apparent dichotomy have been proposed, including the role of the types of APCs participating in the immune response, modulation of the co-stimulatory molecules, cytokine secretion, and signal transduction pathways. Interestingly, both Th17 and Treg cells can develop from naïve CD4+ T-cell precursors under the influence of transforming growth factor β1 (TGF-β1), depending on the other cytokines in the milieu. Therefore autoimmunity may result when the differentiation of CD4+ T cells is favored toward differentiation of Th17 cells instead of Treg cells.

Regulatory, Suppressor, or Inhibitory T cells

A number of T-cell subsets have been shown to regulate or suppress autoimmunity. The most studied of these subsets, Tregs, which are identified as CD4+CD25+Foxp3+ cells, are described in another chapter ('Regulatory Cells'). We have also described CD8+ inhibitory T cells that, by producing TGF-β, prevent or suppress autoimmunity,[37] and CD8+ cytotoxic T cells, which can ablate autoreactive B cells.[38] Natural killer T (NKT) cells, especially those that express invariant TCR, can induce self-tolerance in the periphery via multiple mechanisms, including the regulation of autoreactive B cells.[39-42]

Mechanism of B-Cell Tolerance

As with T cells, tolerance of self-reactive B cells occurs in both a central tolerance mode occurring in the bone marrow and in peripheral tolerance mode occurring at different stages of maturation of B cells as well as at the level of mature B cells, as depicted in Figure 19-2A.

More than half of all newly generated immature B cells in the bone marrow of healthy individuals appear to be polyautoreactive and capable of binding self-antigen, including nuclear antigens.[43,44] Elaborate control mechanisms must therefore exist to remove such potentially autoreactive B cells, ensuring self-tolerance. In fact, extensive studies in mouse models and some in humans with regard to B-cell selection suggest that there are a number of *distinct tolerance checkpoints* during B-cell development and maturation,[43,45] which can be broadly categorized into three stages. First, there is an initial checkpoint during the maturation of B cells in the bone marrow; second, there are many checkpoints during B-cell development in the periphery; and finally, there are checkpoints involving mature B-cell subsets (see Figure 19-2A).

The majority of polyreactive and antinuclear antibody B cells are removed at the immature B-cell stage in the bone marrow,[43] which essentially involves three mechanisms: deletion, anergy, and receptor editing.[5,44,46,47] B-cell receptor (BCR) signaling strength and the physical nature of the self-antigen (soluble versus membrane-bound) play major regulatory roles in the selection process.[5,48] Stronger signals result in apoptosis of B cells, called *clonal deletion*. Weaker signals render the B cell unresponsive to antigen stimulation, a state known as *anergy*. Anergic cells are susceptible to early death. In some B cells, re-expression of recombinant activating gene (RAG) proteins allows replacement of self-reactive receptors with non–self-reactive ones, a process known as *receptor editing*.

In the periphery, most remaining potentially autoreactive B cells are removed when newly emigrant B cells transition into naïve immunocompetent lymphocytes.[43] To develop from the immature state in the bone marrow to the mature naïve state in the peripheral lymphoid organs, a B cell must survive several checkpoints.[45] The first checkpoint is between the immature cell in the bone marrow and the transitional T1 cell in the spleen. The second is between the T1 and more mature T2/3 state, and the third is between the T2/T3 stage and mature B cells. This process depends not only on the strength of the BCR signal the B cells receive if and when they encounter a self-antigen but also on competition with non–self-reactive B cells for B cell–activating factor of the tumor necrosis factor family (BAFF).[8,49] The transitional B cells can be rescued from negative selection by co-stimulatory signals. For example, CD40 engagement by CD40 ligand (CD40L) can rescue B cells destined to undergo BCR-mediated apoptosis. Apoptotic cells, a source of endogenous TLR ligands, can activate Toll-like receptors (TLRs), which also promote T-independent class switching and differentiation of B cells. Apoptotic cells are normally removed from circulation by macrophages, thus preventing any autoreactivity via this mechanism.

B cells that escape tolerance mature into immunocompetent B cells having the phenotype of one of the following B-cell subsets: B-1 cells, marginal zone (MZ) B cells, short-lived plasma cells, and GC-matured long-lived plasma cells. The B1 cells express CD5, are restricted in diversity, and fail to generate a memory population. Self-reactive B-1 cells bearing low-affinity BCRs normally home to the peritoneal cavity (in mice) and produce autoantibodies that are thought to help avoid pathogenic autoreactivity by clearing apoptotic cells.[50] The human equivalent of B-1 cells, which express CD5, are normally present in the naïve repertoire, but they are usually excluded from the GC reactions.[51] The MZ B cells that mature rapidly into plasmablasts can produce autoantibodies.[52] How tolerance is regulated in the MZ B cell subset is unclear. Our group has recently shown that invariant NKT cells that normally activate MZ B cells control MZ B–cell homeostasis by promoting their activation-induced cell death and inhibiting their proliferation,[41] and thus reducing autoantibody production.[42] The follicular B cells, after they encounter antigen and receive T-cell help, generate GCs to mount an affinity-matured antibody response and generate memory B cells.

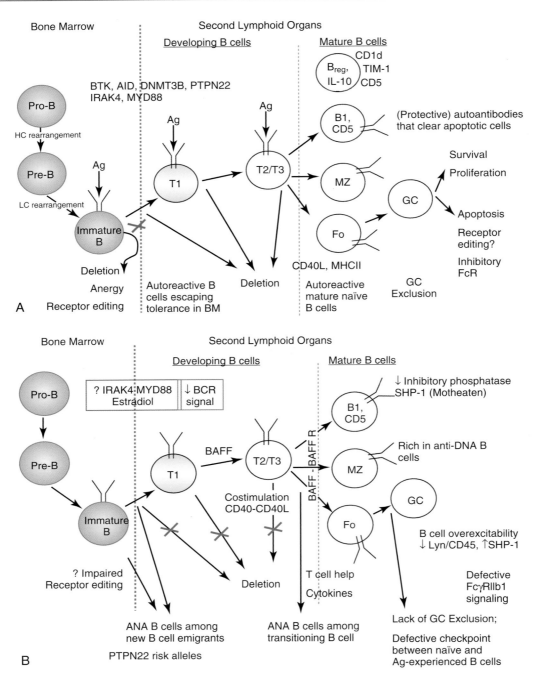

FIGURE 19-2 B-cell tolerance. A, Normal B cell tolerance checkpoints. There are three distinct tolerance checkpoints in B cells. First, there is a checkpoint during the maturation of B cells in the bone marrow; second, there are many checkpoints during B-cell development in the periphery; and finally, there are checkpoints involving mature B-cell subsets. Fo, follicular; GC, germinal center; HC, heavy chain; LC, light chain; MZ, marginal zone; T, transitional. Mechanisms of tolerance induction and maintenance are indicated in *red*. Details on the mechanisms involved at each of these stages can found in the text. **B,** Breakdown of B-cell tolerance in SLE, as described in the text. Defects found in humans and/or mice with SLE are indicated in *brown*.

Germinal center exclusion of potentially autoreactive B cells is an important checkpoint in mature B cells to preclude class switching and somatic hypermutation. In GCs, a stringent balance of proliferative and apoptotic signals is required to prevent the survival of self-reactive B cells while ensuring expansion of the normal B-cell repertoire. Mechanisms of positive and negative selection at the level of GC are not well understood. Receptor editing might contribute to negative selection at this stage,[53] and inhibitory Fc receptor FcγRIIB may regulate B-cell survival in the GC,[54] whereas T cells may serve

to mediate positive selection of GC B cells. Finally, autoreactive CD138+ preplasma cells can be prevented from differentiating into antibody-secreting plasma cells by long-term BCR engagement by self-antigen.

Studies of B-cell tolerance in patients with primary immune deficiency diseases can be instructive for tolerance breakdown in SLE.[6] Indeed, risk alleles encoding variants altering BCR signaling, such as PTPN22 alleles associated with the development of SLE, interfere with the removal of developing autoreactive B cells. Patients with deficiencies of IRAK4, MYD88, and UNC-93B, which are involved in TLR signaling, also have a defective central B-cell tolerance. Defective central B-cell tolerance is also seen in patients with activation-induced cytidine deaminase (AID) deficiency and X-linked agammaglobulinemia who carry mutations in the *BTK* gene, which encodes an essential BCR signaling component. In contrast, CD40L⁻ and MHC class II–deficient patients displayed only peripheral B-cell tolerance defects. Thus, central B-cell tolerance is mostly controlled by intrinsic B-cell factors that regulate BCR and TLR signaling, whereas peripheral B-cell tolerance seems to involve extrinsic B-cell factors, such as Treg cells and serum BAFF concentrations in humans. Furthermore, defects in peripheral B cell tolerance mechanisms are also detected in patients who have defects in central B-cell tolerance.

Studies have now demonstrated the existence of a subset of IL-10–producing splenic B cells that can serve as *regulatory B cells*. Bregs promote tolerance in a number of autoimmune models, including collagen-induced arthritis.[10] Lacking specific markers, such Breg activity appears to reside within uncommon IL-10–expressing B cells scattered within various B-cell subpopulations. One study characterized Bregs as CD1d^hiCD5+ B cells expressing T-cell Ig domain and mucin domain protein 1 (TIM-1) molecule.[12]

In summary, elaborate mechanisms of T- and B-cell tolerance act in concert to maintain normal lymphocyte homeostasis and avoid pathologic autoimmunity. Elucidating the nature of these mechanisms may lead to better approaches for sustaining a balanced response to self and promoting reactivity to nonself at the same time. How tolerance mechanisms fail, resulting in pathologic autoimmunity, is discussed in the next section.

IMMUNE TOLERANCE DEFECTS IN LUPUS

Although substantial progress has been made in understanding fundamental mechanisms of self-tolerance, how impairment in this process causes autoimmune disease remains largely unclear. A number of mechanisms have been proposed, and a few have been demonstrated in animal models of autoimmunity. As summarized in Table 19-2, some of these mechanisms depend on alterations in autoantigen itself,[55-57] some on changes in the processing and presentation of autoantigen at the level of APCs, some on changes in the T and B cells, and some on aberrant immune regulation. On the basis of our current understanding, alterations at different levels may account for loss of self-tolerance in different animal models and probably in different subsets of SLE, and multiple impairments could well account for the loss of self-tolerance in a single model or patient.[55]

Abnormalities at the Level of Autoantigens in Causing Tolerance Breakdown

Impaired removal of apoptotic cells could contribute to an overload of autoantigens, which can cause prolonged activation of immune cells. There are also several examples of autoimmunity being triggered by responses to foreign antigens via molecular mimicry. That only certain self-proteins frequently elicit an autoimmune response has intrigued many investigators to speculate that autoimmunity might occur because altered self or modified self serves as a potential source of autoantigen. Several mechanisms, including somatic mutations, genetic polymorphisms, alternative splicing, and posttranslational modifications, could generate epitopes for which the immune system is not tolerized.[58] Defective apoptosis and altered antigen processing can also result in the generation of neoepitopes. The modified antigens can be taken up, processed, and presented by APCs and recognized by existing potentially self-reactive B and T cells, resulting in breakdown of tolerance and induction of autoimmunity. These mechanisms are described in Chapter 21 'Autoantigenesis and Antigen-based Therapy and Vaccination in SLE'.

Impairment of Antigen-Presenting Cell Function in Tolerance Breakdown

Using nucleosome-specific TCR transgenic mice, Michaels demonstrated that thymic DCs from lupus-prone mice are less efficient than

TABLE 19-2 Mechanisms of Tolerance Breakdown in Lupus

SITE OF ALTERATION	ALTERATIONS

Autoantigen	Altered self:
	  Mutations in autoantigens
	  Excessive polymorphisms of autoantigens
	  Noncanonical alternative messenger RNA splicing at high frequency
	  Posttranslational modifications of autoantigens
	  Direct modification of host proteins by viruses
	Molecular mimicry
	Excess:
	  Altered proteolytic cleavage of autoantigens
	  Inducible autoantigen expression by cytokines such as interferon alpha
	  Reduced clearance
	Activation of Toll-like receptor ligands (e.g., high-mobility group protein B1 [HMGB1] acting as an alarmin and universal sentinel for nucleic acids)
	Altered recognition in endomembrane traffic

Antigen-presenting cells (APCs)	Altered antigen processing Altered major histocompatibility complex class II expression and presentation Altered migration of APCs to sites of tolerance induction
T cells	Disturbed homeostasis Reduced apoptosis Loss of anergy Enhanced constitutive signaling Immune deviation
B cells	Impaired tolerance at the early immature stage in bone marrow Impaired tolerance during transition to mature stages in the periphery Impaired regulation at the level of mature B cells Defective follicular exclusion Impaired receptor editing Apoptosis Enhanced constitutive signaling Presentation of autoantigens by B cells
Regulatory T cells and cytokines	Reduced induction or activation of CD8+ T inhibitory cells Reduced function of CD4+CD25+ T regulatory cells Insufficiency of natural killer T cells Reduced production of immunoregulatory cytokines such as transforming growth factor beta Expansion of follicular T helper cells

those from normal mice in presenting naturally processed nucleosomal peptides in the steady state.[4] Thus, insufficient presentation of self-antigens in the thymus may account for positive selection and/or lack of negative selection of autoreactive T cells in an autoimmune-prone background.

Specialized DC subsets that reside in peripheral tissues carry antigens from the tissue to draining lymph nodes to maintain tolerance to respective tissue antigens in steady state, thus avoiding autoimmunity. This process of peripheral tolerance is impaired in lupus, because Langerhans DCs in the skin of lupus-prone MRL/lpr mice display impaired capacity to migrate to draining lymph nodes in comparison with cells in normal strains.[59] Thus, impaired capacity of DCs to present self-antigens in the thymus[4] or reduced ability of tissue-resident DCs to migrate and carry self-antigens to draining lymph nodes[59] may contribute to a breakdown in central or peripheral tolerance, respectively.

Molecular mechanisms underlying DC defects in SLE are not defined. One study demonstrated a critical role for B-lymphocyte-induced maturation protein 1 (BLIMP-1), a key regulator of plasma-cell differentiation in B cells and of effector/memory function in T cells, in the tolerogenic function of DCs.[60] The investigators showed that a diminished expression of BLIMP-1 in DCs results in increased production of IL-6, preferential differentiation of follicular T-helper (T_{FH}) cells, and development of a lupus-like serology in female but not male mice. Of particular relevance to human SLE, a polymorphism of BLIMP-1 is associated with SLE.

B cells may also serve as important APCs in breaking T-cell tolerance. Using anti–small nuclear ribonucleoprotein immunoglobulin (anti-snRNP Ig) transgenic mice, Yan and Mamula showed that whereas both normal and autoimmune (MRL/lpr) mice harbor autoreactive T cells, transgenic B cells can tolerize autoreactive T cells in the periphery of normal mice only.[61] Thus, B cells (anti-snRNP transgenic B cells in this case) served as important APCs for T cell tolerance in normal mice and for T-cell activation in MRL mice. The study further suggested that anti-snRNP B-cell anergy in normal mice could be reversed by autoreactive T cells from autoimmune mice in a cognate manner, indicating an important role of T cells in the development of lupus (as described later).

T-Cell Abnormalities Contributing to Tolerance Breakdown

Studies of T-cell tolerance using animal models or human T cells have revealed a plethora of impairments at almost every level of central or peripheral tolerance mechanisms in SLE (see Figure 19-1, *B*).

Impaired Clonal Deletion of Lupus Autoreactive T-Helper Cells

To determine whether lupus T cells arise as a consequence of failed negative selection, Datta used transgenic mice expressing TCR of a pathogenic autoantibody-inducing Th cell that was specific for nucleosomes and its histone peptide H4$_{71-94}$. The investigators found that whereas thymocytes carrying lupus TCR were deleted in normal mice, such negative selection did not occur in the thymus of lupus-prone (SWR × NZB)F1 (SNF1) mice.[4] Thus, impaired central tolerance may contribute to the positive selection of autoreactive pathogenic Th cells in lupus (see Figure 19-1, *B*). This idea is further supported by a study in which procainamide-hydroxylamine (PAHA), a drug that induces lupus in humans, has been found to interfere with central tolerance mechanisms in the thymus, resulting in the emergence of chromatin-reactive T cells followed by humoral autoimmunity in C57BL/6xDBA/2 F1 mice.[62] To address this issue in humans, T cells from patients with SLE were cultured with thymic stromal cells. In these experiments, T cells from patients with SLE are more resistant to induction of apoptosis by thymic stromal cells than normal T cells. Thus, SLE T cells have intrinsically acquired a mechanism to evade central tolerance mechanisms in SLE, whereby interactions between thymic stromal and lymphoid cells lead to subsequent survival of autoimmune T cells.[63]

Neonatal and Adult Tolerance to Exogenously Administered Peptide Antigens in Lupus

To understand mechanisms and outcome of tolerance induction in lupus, our group administered MHC class II–binding foreign or self peptides, namely, hen egg lysozyme (HEL) 106-116 or self immunoglobulin A6.1 V_H58-69, to newborn lupus (NZB/NZW F1) or normal (BALB/c) mice.[64] A comparable level of tolerance, as measured by peptide-specific T-cell proliferation and IL-2 production in response to subsequent peptide challenge, was induced in both lupus-prone and normal mice. Lupus-prone mice, however, had increased anti-DNA antibody production in response to a neonatally administered self-V_H peptide. Comparable levels of tolerance were also induced in adult lupus-prone and normal control mice, when peptide antigens

were administered intravenously in high doses of soluble form or intraperitoneally in high doses of emulsified form.[65-67] The older lupus-prone animals, however, tended to have relatively more leakiness in tolerance, particularly in Th functions and peptide-specific antibody responses (RR Singh, unpublished data, 1999). These studies demonstrate lack of a major tolerance defect in the induction of experimental tolerance in lupus-prone mice.

Intact Central Tolerance but Impaired Peripheral T-Cell Control Mechanisms

Several groups have studied mechanisms and outcome of tolerance induction in lupus using transgenic mice expressing TCR of a T cell specific for a conventional peptide antigen (e.g., pigeon cytochrome C [PCC]). In the pigeon cytochrome C peptide TCR transgenic model, the relevant antigen exposure results in intrathymic deletion of immature CD4$^+$D8$^+$ double-positive thymocytes, TCR downregulation, and thymocyte apoptosis, which are comparable in a nonautoimmune mouse strain (B10.BR) and an autoimmune-prone MRL/MpJ strain.[68] Thus, central tolerance to a conventional antigen is intact in lupus-prone MRL mice. Using the NZB model, another study inferred that there is no generalized T-cell tolerance defect in lupus-prone mice.[69] Thus, lupus-autoreactive T cells may arise in the setting of incomplete but qualitatively normal tolerance or as a result of defects in peripheral control mechanisms.

Using gene microarray profiling and functional and biochemical studies, one study showed that activated T cells of patients with SLE resist anergy and apoptosis (see Figure 19-1, *B*) by upregulating and sustaining cyclooxygenase-2 (COX-2) expression, along with the antiapoptotic or survival molecule c-FLIP (cellular homolog of viral FLICE inhibitory protein).[70] Inhibition of COX-2 causes apoptosis of the anergy-resistant lupus T cells by augmenting Fas signaling and reducing c-FLIP. Studies with COX-2 inhibitors and Cox-2–deficient mice confirmed that anergy-resistant lupus T cells, and not cancer cells or other autoimmune T cells, selectively use this COX-2/FLIP antiapoptosis program. Thus, an imbalance in the proapoptotic and antiapoptotic mechanisms may contribute to the persistence of autoreactive clones.[70]

Studies in animals also show that CD4$^+$ T cells from lupus mice are more resistant than those in nonautoimmune mice to anergy induction (see Figure 19-1, *B*). Anergy avoidance in the periphery may be one of the causes for abnormal T-cell activation in response to self-antigen in SLE.[71] Indeed, T cells from patients with SLE and lupus-prone mice display phenotypes of in vivo activation, as defined by expression of CD25, HLA-DR, and CD40L.[72,73] Additionally, increased expression of perforin and granzyme on CD8$^+$ T cells correlates with disease activity in patients with SLE.[74] Thus, T-cell activation appears to be a hallmark of disease development in SLE. However, the mechanisms that cause T cells to become hyperactivated or overexcitable have not been well defined, except for those described in the following section on T cell–signaling defects.

Studies in lupus mice show that heightened response to peptide antigens, particularly those with low affinity for TCR, appears to drive the polyclonal T-cell activation.[75] Many studies have also demonstrated the presence of intrinsic T-cell abnormalities, such as diminished activation thresholds, in patients and mice with SLE. The following sections narrate efforts of several laboratories to define such intrinsic T-cell abnormalities in lupus.

T Cell–Signaling Defects in SLE

T cells use a cell surface multi-subunit structure, the TCR/CD3 complex, as an antigen-specific recognition site. The TCR α/β or γ/δ chains are the antigen-binding sites but, because of having very short cytoplasmic domains, they are not capable of any signal transduction, which is carried out by the CD3 complex. Human and murine SLE T cells, when stimulated through the TCR/CD3 complex, exhibit several abnormalities in T-cell signaling (see Figure 19-1, *B*). These include aberrant tyrosine phosphorylation, altered calcium flux, and heightened mitochondrial potential. A major and well-studied outcome of this aberrant signal transduction in SLE T cells is reduced IL-2 production, a phenotype of lupus T cells observed 30 years ago.[76,77] Reduced response to IL-2 by T cells accompanied reduced IL-2 production in some patients with SLE.[76] One study found a severe defect in IL-2 production by mononuclear cells from all 19 subjects, who were patients with SLE, regardless of the stimulant used and irrespective of the patients' disease activity.[78] Defective IL-2 production has also been reported in mouse models of lupus, including MRL/lpr, BXSB, and BWF1 mice.[77,79] In MRL/lpr mice, reduced IL-2 production precedes the onset of clinical illness and becomes increasingly severe with age[79] (S Dubey and RR Singh, unpublished data, 2005). Spleen cells from MRL/lpr mice also fail to respond normally to IL-2.[79] It is therefore important to focus on the IL-2 defect in SLE T cells, because it acts as an essential regulator of immune response by promoting activation of the immune system and terminating it when required by inducing activation-induced cell death of autoreactive T cells. In fact, treatment of MRL/lpr mice with the *Il-2* gene delivered via Vaccinia virus or attenuated Salmonella vectors results in significant improvement in lupus disease.[80] Consistent with reduced IL-2 production, proliferative responses of T cells from patients with SLE, when the cells are cultured with thymic stromal cells, are lower than those of their normal counterparts.[63] In addition to being a potent T-cell growth factor, IL-2 is essential for immune tolerance. Accordingly, mice deficient in IL-2 succumb to a rapidly progressing autoimmune disease that is caused by an uncontrolled activation of T and B cells.[81] It was thereafter discovered that IL-2 was critically required for the development, homeostatic maintenance, and suppressive function of Treg cells.[82] A number of reports have found a low prevalence and/or function of Treg cells in patients with SLE and murine SLE models.[83-85]

Several mechanisms have been proposed to explain defective IL-2 production in SLE. Reduced phosphorylation and expression of the TCR/CD3 ζ chain[86] is one such mechanism. Two patients with SLE have been reported to have a 36-bp exon 7 deletion in the TCR ζ messenger RNA (mRNA), and many other mutations found in patients with SLE have been mapped to the third immunoreceptor tyrosine–based activation motif (ITAM) or the guanosine triphosphate/guanosine diphosphate (GTP/GDP)–binding site in the TCR ζ molecule. These mutations have been implicated in the downregulation of the TCR ζ chain.[87] Transfection of SLE T cells with TCR ζ chain has been shown to normalize TCR/CD3-induced free intracytoplasmic calcium.[86,88]

Under physiologic conditions, the signal generated by the CD3 complex triggers phosphorylation of phospholipase C (PLC-γ) on Tyr and Ser residues, hydrolysis of phosphatidylinositol 4,5-biphosphate to phosphatidylinositol 1,4,5-biphosphate, and a rapid rise in intracellular Ca^{2+}. The rise in intracellular calcium upon activation has been reported to be higher in SLE T cells than in control T cells.[89] This increase in calcium flux in T cells, however, did not correlate with disease activity. The aberrant calcium flux is probably due to an IgG anti–TCR/CD3 complex antibody in human SLE serum.[90] Tsokos has shown that this anti–TCR/CD3 complex antibody stimulates translocation of Ca^{2+} calmodulin kinase from the cytosol to the nucleus.[86] This event induces upregulation of CREM (cyclic adenosine monophosphate [cAMP] response element [CRE] modulator) transcript and protein, phosphorylation of CREM and binding of pCREM homodimers to the −180 site of the IL-2 promoter, thus leading to decreased IL-2 production. Further studies suggest that protein phosphatase 2A (PP2A), the primary enzyme that dephosphorylates CREB (CRE binding) in T lymphocytes, is involved in the suppression of IL-2 production. Thus, PP2A represents a negative regulator of IL-2 promoter activity. Consistent with this idea, the mRNA, protein, and catalytic activity of PP2A are increased in patients with SLE regardless of disease activity and treatment.[90]

In contrast to the preceding studies showing increased calcium flux in SLE T cells, a study by Sierakowski found lower calcium flux upon anti-CD3 stimulation in patients with SLE than in controls.[91] Ionomycin-induced calcium flux, however, is similar in patients with

SLE and controls. The reduced calcium flux upon TCR stimulation in T cells was also seen in patients with mild disease and in those whose T cells produced normal amounts of IL-2.[91] We have observed reduced calcium flux upon TCR signaling in T cells from autoimmune MRL/lpr mice at an age (≥8 weeks) when they begin to develop disease. Interestingly, T cells from these mice display a split activation phenotype—that is, although these T cells show evidence of in vivo activation as exhibited by increased expression of activation markers and IFN-γ production, they have reduced IL-2 production and calcium flux upon TCR stimulation (S Dubey and RR Singh, unpublished data, 2005).

Two cytoplasmic intracellular signaling pathways important in T-cell activation, differentiation, and effector function are the mitogen-activated protein kinase (MAPK) and phosphatidylinositol 3-kinase (PI3K). There are three major groups of MAP kinases in mammalian cells[92]: extracellular signal regulated kinases (ERKs), p38 MAP kinases, and c-Jun *N*-terminal kinases (JNKs). Defects in the MAPK signaling pathway in T cells have been shown to account for reduced IL-2 production by SLE T cells. For example, the activity of ERK-1 and ERK-2 is diminished in resting as well as TCR-stimulated peripheral blood T cells from patients with SLE; such a diminution can lead to reduced translocation of nuclear factor AP-1 (activator protein 1), resulting in altered coordination of signals needed for normal IL-2 production and maintenance of tolerance in T cells.[93] Studies using the graft-versus-host disease (GVHD) model of murine lupus have found increased activity for PI3K and JNK but not for raf-1, p38 MAPK, or ERK-1. Increased PI-3 kinase activity in the chronic GVHD model is consistent with a role for persistent T-cell activation in lupus-like disease, as evidenced by increased phosphorylation of TCR-associated Src-family kinases (Lck and Fyn).[94] Consistent with these data, treatment with a PI3 kinase inhibitor improves disease in MRL/lpr lupus mice.[95] The PI3K pathway is also activated in peripheral blood mononuclear cells (PBMCs) and T cells from about 70% of patients with SLE, especially in patients with active disease. The magnitude of PI3K pathway activation in patients with SLE correlated with accumulation of activated/memory T cells. The study suggests that increased PI3K activity causes defective activation-induced cell death in patients with SLE. Moreover, defective activation-induced cell death in SLE T cells was found to be corrected after reduction of PI3Kδ activity, suggesting that PI3Kδ contributes to induction of enhanced memory T-cell survival in SLE.[96]

The mammalian target of rapamycin (mTOR), a key regulator of metabolic activity, and its major upstream activator, PI3K/AKT pathway, have been implicated in SLE pathogenesis.[97] mTOR affects many immune cells, including monocytes and dendritic cells, and influences the cytokine milieu during an immune response. The PI3K/AKT/mTOR pathway is upregulated in lupus B cells and T cells. Importantly, the mTOR inhibitor, rapamycin, has been found to ameliorate disease in lupus mice and reduce disease activity in patients with SLE who had been treated unsuccessfully with other immunosuppressive medications.[98,99] In T cells, rapamycin treatment alters the signaling through the TCR, which attenuates the inappropriate activation of autoreactive T cells in SLE. It has been shown that the TCR complex in SLE is different from normal T cells.[100] In SLE T cells, CD3ζ is replaced by the FcR γ chain, and instead of recruiting Lck, these cells recruit Syk. Rapamycin-treated T cells are reported to exhibit increased levels of CD3ζ and Lck, thereby normalizing calcium flux and IL-2 production.[101] Moreover, Syk is a downstream target of mTOR, and a Syk inhibitor, R788, ameliorates lupus nephritis.[102] Additionally, stimulating T cells through the TCR in the presence of rapamycin in vitro promotes the generation of Treg cells.[103] Thus, the spontaneous PI3K/AKT/mTOR signaling activity in pathogenic T cells might contribute to reduced Treg cell number and/or suppressive activity in patients with SLE and mouse models.[84,85,104]

T-cell abnormalities in lupus can also be explained by the alterations in lipid raft composition and dynamics. The organization of signaling molecules into discrete membrane-associated microdomains, called *lipid rafts,* is vital for regulation of T-lymphocyte activation pathways.[105,106] Lipid rafts play a central role in signal transduction, in the immune response, and in many pathologic conditions on the basis of two important raft properties, their capacity to incorporate or exclude proteins selectively and their ability to coalesce into small domains. As has been reported, SLE T cells contain larger pools of lipid rafts than normal T cells and produce lipid rafts more robustly upon anti-CD3 treatment than normal T cells. These changes are accompanied by a qualitative alteration in the composition of lipid rafts in SLE. Whereas CD3ζ and LAT (linker of activated T cells) are uniformly distributed on the surface of normal T-cell membranes, these molecules are organized in discrete clusters on membranes of SLE T cells. Unlike lipid rafts from normal T cells, those from SLE T cells contain FcRγ and activate Syk kinase.[107]

The localization of Lck to lipid rafts is essential for normal TCR-mediated signaling. The Lck is significantly reduced in both lipid rafts and nonraft portions of T lymphocytes from patients with SLE. Reduced expression of Lck in lupus T cells occurs because of increased ubiquitination and subsequent degradation of Lck, so that T cells become unresponsive to TCR-mediated signals.[108] These findings imply chronic in vivo activation of T cells in SLE. However, the direct pathogenetic implications of the reductions in Lck in lupus T cells as well as factors that regulate Lck homeostasis in lipid raft domains and cause degradation of Lck in lupus T cells remain to be clarified. Further studies have shown greater expression of raft-associated ganglioside GM1 in SLE T cells. CD45, a tyrosine phosphatase that regulates Lck activity, is also differentially expressed and its localization into lipid rafts is increased in SLE T cells. Such altered association of CD45 with lipid raft domains may regulate Lck expression in SLE T cells. The altered lipid raft occupancy is not induced by serum factors from patients with SLE, but cell-to-cell contact is required to activate proximal signaling pathways.[109]

Although most studies have focused on identifying genes associated with altered T-cell functions in SLE, epigenetic regulation of gene expression, such as histone acetylation and methylation, may also contribute to impaired SLE T cell function.[110] In fact, treatment with histone deacetylase inhibitors, such as trichostatin A, which corrects these impairments and suppresses lupus in mice,[111] holds promise for humans.

Expansion of Follicular Helper T Cells in Lupus

T_{FH}, which are known to help the formation of GCs and induce T cell–dependent B-cell responses, are increased in a subset of patients with severe SLE.[112] These cells may play a role in the breakdown of tolerance in SLE. Indeed, an abundance of T_{FH} has been linked to the excessive GC formation, increased autoantibody production, and end-organ damage in animal models.[113] T_{FH} produces high levels of IL-21, which promotes T_{FH} survival as well as B-cell proliferation, affinity maturation, and terminal differentiation into plasma cells.[114] Blockade of IL-21 with a receptor fusion protein in MRL/lpr mice was found to downregulate the production of pathogenic autoantibodies, leading to reduced skin lesions, lowered lymphadenopathy, and decreased renal damage.[115] Increase in IL-21–producing T cells is also reported in patients with SLE.[116]

T_{FH} express high levels of inducible co-stimulatory molecule (ICOS), which interacts with its ligand (ICOSL). The ICOS-ICOSL interaction stimulates the PI3-kinase pathway, which plays an essential role in T_{FH} development and GC formation.[117,118] ICOS-ICOSL interaction can also promote GC B-cell survival, maturation, and terminal differentiation into plasma cells, as well as CD40-CD154 pathway–mediated Ig class switching.[119] Importantly, the blockade of the ICOS-ICOSL pathway in NZB/W F1 lupus mice was found to result in diminished levels of T_{FH} and GC B cells, a decrease in IgG autoantibodies, and reduced inflammatory damage.[120]

The ICOS-ICOSL pathway and IL-21 have also been implicated in the development of Th17 cells.[121] IL-17 can promote the formation of GCs and drive B cells to undergo class switching to the IgG subtypes.[122] The increased expression of IL-17 in serum and tissues of patients with active SLE has been linked to the production of

autoantibodies and disease severity.[123,124] Interestingly, some work has demonstrated that the increased IL-17 levels in patients with SLE are produced by Th17 cells as well as TCRαβ+ double-negative (DN; CD4−CD8−) expanded T cells. IL-17–producing T cells have been detected in the kidneys of patients with lupus nephritis and in the SNF1 lupus mouse model. Taken together, these findings show that a cellular and molecular pathway linking T_{FH}, IL-21, and Th17, and ICOS-ICOSL appears to cause breakdown of tolerance in GC B cells and IgG autoantibody production.

B-Cell Abnormalities Contributing to Tolerance Breakdown
Breaking the B-Cell Tolerance Checkpoints

Appearance of self-reactive antibodies precedes the onset of clinical manifestations in humans and animals with SLE.[125] Where in the B-cell pathway tolerance is first broken and which mechanisms account for such breakdown remain to be fully elucidated (see Figure 19-2, B). As described previously, many B-cell tolerance checkpoints can be located at three broad steps of the B-cell pathway—the immature state in the bone marrow, then in the periphery from the immature state to the mature naïve state, and finally at the level of mature B-cell subsets (see Figure 19-2, A). At the immature B-cell stage in the bone marrow, most polyautoreactive and antinuclear B cells in healthy individuals are silenced through clonal deletion, anergy, or receptor editing.[43]

Analysis of the human B-cell repertoire in the peripheral blood of newly diagnosed, untreated patients with SLE has identified two early tolerance checkpoints that are defective in SLE, one at the transition from the early immature to the immature stage, and the other at the transitional to the mature naïve stage.[126] Because B cells at transitional stages T2 and T3 can be rescued from negative selection by co-stimulatory signals, increased expression of co-stimulatory molecules in patients with SLE[127] can rescue transitional B cells destined to undergo BCR-mediated apoptosis. BAFF, which can also enhance the survival of autoreactive transitional B cells,[128] is increased in the circulation of some patients with SLE.[129] Beyond the transitional stages, one study identified a defect at a GC entry checkpoint in patients with SLE. The investigators reported that VH4-34 antibody–expressing CD5+ B cells that produce pathogenic IgM antilymphocyte antibodies are normally excluded from GC reactions, but these cells enter GCs in patients with SLE and contribute to the memory B-cell pool.[51] Analysis of autoreactive B cells in tonsil biopsy specimens revealed that autoreactive B cells exist in normal individuals but they do not secrete IgG, whereas these cells in patients with SLE expand and secrete IgG.[130] In SLE, but not in RA, autoreactive B cells (9G4 B cells) escape normal censoring and actively participate in productive GC reactions, leading to the generation of increased levels of IgG memory and plasma cells.[130] The specific peripheral tolerance checkpoint that is broken occurs early in the GC reaction, during the transition from the pre-GC to the centroblast stage, thus implicating faulty GC exclusion of autoreactive B cells in the pathogenesis of SLE (see Figure 19-2, B). Using a synthetic peptide to track anti-DNA B cells, one study identified a tolerance checkpoint between naïve and antigen-experienced B cells that is compromised in active SLE.[131] Thus, B-cell tolerance is compromised at several checkpoints in patients with SLE; the site and type of defect appear to vary among patients.[8]

Studies in mouse models suggest that negative selection mediated by BCR signaling confers B-cell tolerance at the transitional stages in the periphery. In fact, evidence shows that clonal deletion of B cells at their T1 stage of development is defective in murine lupus.[132] In NZB mice, IgM cross-linking in resting or isolated T1 B cells prevents mitochondrial membrane damage and apoptosis induction.[132,133] Extrinsic factors such as the sex hormone estradiol can also diminish the BCR signal and thereby potentially diminishes the negative selection of autoreactive B cells (see Figure 19-2, B),[134] which likely occurs through estradiol-induced upregulation of the inhibitory phosphatase SHP-1 and of CD22. This might be one explanation for the predominance of SLE and several other autoimmune diseases in women.

Self-reactive B cells that escape tolerance processes throughout their transitional stages may mature to be autoantibody-secreting B cells. These mature autoantibody-secreting cells may assume the phenotypic characteristics of any B-cell subset: B-1 cells, marginal zone (MZ) B cells, and follicular B cells[45] (see Figure 19-2, B). However, it is unclear which of these B-cell subsets contributes to disease pathogenesis in mice and which is responsible for autoantibody production in humans with SLE. In mouse models, all three subsets can produce pathogenic autoantibodies. For example, B-1 cells produce high-affinity IgM anti–double stranded DNA (anti-dsDNA) autoantibodies in the moth-eaten mutant mouse strain that is deficient in SHP-1.[135] The human equivalent of murine B-1 cells, CD5-expressing B cells, generally produce polyreactive, low-affinity IgM autoantibodies using germline-encoded V genes. However, somatic mutation has been described in human autoreactive CD5+ B cells,[136] which can sometimes differentiate into cells with features of GC cells.[137] Thus, impaired generation or regulation of B-1 cells may be involved in the pathogenesis of SLE.

The MZ B cells have several features required to break T-cell tolerance. For example, they can act as APCs as they express co-stimulatory molecules and can activate T cells.[138] These cells are easily activated by dendritic cells and mature rapidly into plasmablasts.[52] MZ B cells can also generate T cell–independent autoimmune responses and undergo heavy-chain class switching and somatic mutation in extrafollicular regions of the spleen in lupus-prone mice.[139] MZ B cells can also initiate GC formation.[52] In humans these cells, which are present in circulation as IgD^low^IgM+CD27+, can populate all secondary lymphoid organs. The factors that regulate differentiation and entry of MZ B cells to GC or extrafollicular foci of antibody production are not known. MZ B-cell development depends on BAFF, which is upregulated in SLE. In fact, MZ B cells can produce pathogenic autoantibodies in lupus-prone (NZB/NZW)F1 mice.[134]

After antigen encounter and T-cell help, follicular B cells normally generate GCs, where they mount an affinity-matured antibody response and generate memory B cells. Because lupus autoantibodies are mostly somatically mutated and class-switched IgGs, they are likely to be produced by antigen-experienced B cells, implicating abnormalities in tolerance in late-stage, GC-matured B cells. Mechanisms of negative and positive selection in GCs are not well understood. The presence of autoreactive T cells and lack of inhibitory mechanisms such as inhibitory Fc receptor FcγRIIB on the B cells may contribute to positive selection and differentiation of autoreactive B cells at this stage.

Patients with SLE have high numbers of naïve B cells, which can secrete polyreactive antibodies that react with single-stranded DNA (ssDNA), dsDNA, insulin, and lipopolysaccharide (LPS).[126] It is not clear whether the polyreactive autoreactive B cells reflect a defect in negative selection that correlates with development of disease or represent precursors of the B cells that produce pathogenic autoantibodies.[45] Although patients with lupus have cross-reactive antibodies, the polyreactivity is usually restricted to a set of nuclear and nucleoprotein antigens. Thus, it will be important to know when the generalized polyreactivity is converted to restricted cross-reactivity in patients with SLE.

B-Cell Receptor Signaling Defects, Hyperactivation, and Loss of Tolerance in SLE

The strength and the duration of the B-cell response largely depend on the integrity of BCRs and availability of co-stimulatory (CD19, CD21) or inhibitory receptors. Patients with SLE manifest B-cell abnormalities that include B-cell proliferation, increased calcium flux, hyperresponsiveness to physiologic stimuli, and altered production of and response to cytokines.[140,141] One cause of the B-cell overexcitability in lupus is supposed to be increased signaling through the BCR. In this context, expression of Lyn protein, a key negative regulator of B-cell signaling, is reduced in B cells in a majority of

patients with SLE. SLE B cells also have altered translocation of Lyn to lipid rafts. This altered Lyn expression is associated with heightened spontaneous proliferation, anti-dsDNA autoantibodies, and elevated IL-10 production.[142] Another study has reported persistently reduced tyrosine phosphatase CD45 and elevated protein tyrosine phosphatase SHP-1 in the BCRs from patients with SLE. Because Lyn and SHP-1 act in concert within a negative signaling pathway in which CD45 counteracts SHP-1–mediated regulation, altered expression of these molecules may contribute to defective feedback regulation in SLE B cells.

B cells preferentially express the FcγRIIB isoform, cross-linking of which in normal B cells suppresses the B-cell signal transduction. Memory cells in patients with SLE do not upregulate FcγRIIB, increasing the chance for survival of autoreactive B cells.[143] In mice, the germline deficiency of FcγRIIB causes an accumulation of plasma cells secreting anti-DNA antibodies,[54] suggesting a role for this Fc receptor in regulating B-cell differentiation at the GC stage. In fact, FcγRIIB polymorphisms have been associated with autoimmunity in mice and humans. For example, a polymorphism in the FcγRIIb1 gene, FCGR2B c.695T>C, which results in the nonconservative replacement of 232Ile at the transmembrane helix to Thr, is associated with susceptibility to SLE in Asians. This polymorphism (FcγRIIB 232Thr) is less potent than the wild-type molecule (FcγRIIB 232Ile) in inhibiting BCR-mediated accumulation of phosphatidylinositol-3,4,5-trisphosphate, activation of Akt and PLCγ2, and calcium mobilization after IgG Fc–mediated coligation with BCR. Further, the FcγRIIB 232Thr is less effective than wild-type FcγRIIB 232Ile in its localization to detergent-insoluble lipid rafts.[144] Thus, altered balance between positive and negative signaling molecules may modify the BCR signaling thresholds and contribute to disruption of B-cell tolerance.[145]

BAFF and BAFF receptors appear to affect many stages of B-cell differentiation, ranging from the development, selection, and homeostasis of naïve B cells to antibody-producing plasma cells. Excessive BAFF rescues self-reactive B cells from anergy, thereby breaking B-cell tolerance.[146] Mice overexpressing BAFF exhibit increased B-cell numbers in spleen and lymph node and an autoimmune phenotype similar to that observed in patients with SLE.[128,147] Furthermore, self-reactive B cells that are destined for deletion during later stages of maturation are rescued by BAFF from undergoing apoptosis.[128] Inhibition of BAFF by transmembrane activator and calcium modulator and cyclophilin ligand interactor (TACI)-Ig and BAFF receptor Ig (BAFF-R-Ig) has been proven to be beneficial in murine models of SLE.[148] Elevated serum concentrations of BAFF have also been detected in some patients with SLE,[149] and BAFF-R is consistently occupied on blood B cells in patients with SLE. Thus, increased BAFF expression in SLE-prone individuals may precipitate autoimmunity through positive selection of B cells at their late stages of maturation.

There is evidence that diminished BCR signaling can also lead to loss of B-cell tolerance, likely by allowing self-reactive B cells to escape negative selection.[150,151] A polymorphism in the gene that encodes PTPN22 (protein tyrosine phosphatase, nonreceptor type 22), which acts as a phosphatase that inhibits BCR signal, leads to a gain-of-function mutation that attenuates BCR signaling during selection.[152] Intriguingly, the PTPN22 risk allele has been associated with a number of autoimmune diseases, including SLE, RA, type 1 diabetes, and autoimmune thyroid disease. BCR signal strength has been shown to affect B-cell fate after antigen activation. B cells with low affinity to antigen, therefore low BCR signal, participated in GC reactions and produced both memory and long-lived plasma cells. On the contrary, B cells with high affinity to antigen, therefore high BCR signal, were found to be excluded from GC reactions and differentiated into short-lived plasma cells.[153] As mentioned previously, estradiol was found to allow B cells to escape negative selection by attenuating BCR signal strength. Estrogen causes an expansion of the marginal zone populations, which may be due to its effect in diminishing BCR signal strength. Future studies to elucidate the role of BCR signal strength in germinal centers are of interest because of the high proportion of class-switched and affinity-matured antibodies in patients with lupus.

Role of B Cells in Breaking T-Cell Tolerance

The role of B cells beyond their traditional function of autoantibody production has been explored. B cells process and present self-antigens to naïve T cells.[154] Mamula and Janeway reported that mice are normally unresponsive to immunization with native mouse snRNP (a lupus autoantigen), suggesting that the tolerance to this self-antigen is intact in these animals. Such tolerance can be broken, however, if the animals are immunized with foreign (human) snRNPs. When mice are immunized with human and mouse snRNPs together in complete Freund's adjuvant, T cells specific for mouse snRNPs can be elicited. Furthermore, B cells purified from mice immunized with foreign antigen (human A protein), when transferred into naïve mice, can present self-antigen (mouse snRNP) and activate self-reactive $CD4^+$ T cells specific for mouse antigen.[155] Similarly, B cells induced to make autoantibody by immunization of mice with the non–self-protein human cytochrome c can present self-antigen mouse cytochrome c to activate autoreactive T cells. Taken together, these observations indicate that the foreign cross-reactive determinants can induce and activate self antigen specific B cells that in turn elicit autoreactive T cell response. This mechanism of breaking T-cell self-tolerance can account for the role of foreign antigens in breaking not only B-cell but also T-cell self-tolerance, leading to sustained auto-antibody production in the absence of the foreign antigen. In consonance with these observations, B cell–deficient MRL/lpr mice have fewer numbers of $CD4^+$ and $CD8^+$ memory cells than their B cell–intact counterparts,[156] whereas secreted Ig–deficient but B cell–intact MRL/lpr mice continue to have spontaneous T-cell activation and expansion.[157] Thus, B cells serve as an important APC role in inducing spontaneous activation of T cells in autoimmunity.

Impairments of Regulatory T Cells and Factors as Mechanisms of Loss of Tolerance

T and B cells are normally self-tolerant. Our group has reported that this tolerant state can be broken in otherwise healthy, nonautoim-mune mice by in vivo stimulation of the Th cells that are capable of promoting autoantibody production, for example, by immunization with autoantigenic peptides (such as anti-DNA V_H peptides). This state of loss of tolerance (or autoimmunity) is short-lived, however. Recovery from autoimmunity in these mice correlates temporally with the appearance of certain $CD8^+$ and $CD4^+$ T cells that are capable of suppressing autoantibody production.[37,158,159] In fact, $CD8^+$ regulatory T-cell lines derived from nonautoimmune mice can suppress in vivo autoantibody production and nephritis when implanted into lupus-prone (NZB/NZW)F1 mice.[160] $CD8^+$ regulatory T cells might confer this role via their suppressive effect on Qa-1$^+$ T_{FH} cells,[161] which are known to induce autoreactive B cells, as described previously. Thus, self-reactive B and Th cells exist in the normal immune repertoire but are kept in control to avoid pathologic autoimmunity. These control mechanisms are defective in lupus mice, which have impaired activation of such inhibitory, suppressor, and Treg cells.[37] Impairments in $CD8^+$ T-cell suppressor functions have also been described in human SLE.[162] These observations might have therapeutic implications, because this impairment in lupus mice can be corrected through modification of the delivery of peptide antigens, for example, by DNA vaccination with minigenes that encode T-cell epitopes from anti-DNA–variable regions.[38] Vaccination with nucleosome-derived peptides or administration of an Ig-derived peptide can also induce suppressor $CD8^+$ and $CD4^+D25^+$ T cells, which suppress disease in lupus mice.[163] Because similar T-cell epitopes exist in humans, strategies described here might be useful in therapy of the human disease.

The V_H peptide–reactive $CD8^+$ inhibitory T (Ti) cells described previously produce TGF-β,[37,38,164] which plays a critical role in maintaining self-tolerance.[165] In fact, TGF-β1 knockout mice demonstrate lethal systemic inflammation and autoantibodies.[166] This

TGF-β–mediated self-tolerance appears to act via controlling T-cell activation, as the deletion of the TGF-β receptor type II gene in T cells alone can cause severe autoinflammatory disease (D Adams and RR Singh, 2003, unpublished). TGF-β is also required for the normal functioning of Treg and Ti cells. The regulatory role of TGF-β in the development of lupus-like autoimmunity is further supported in studies that have shown reduced production of TGF-β by immune cells from patients with SLE; addition of TGF-β to the lupus PBMC cultures reduces production of autoantibodies.[167] However, TGF-β production is increased in patients with SLE who have advanced disease with tissue fibrosis. For example, patients with SLE who have congenital complete heart block that is believed to occur as a result of fibrosis of the cardiac conduction system have a TGF-β1 genotype that is associated with increased fibrosis. Further, their PBMCs secrete greater amounts of spontaneous and mitogen-stimulated TGF-β1.[168] Thus, TGF-β may play dual, seemingly paradoxic, roles during the development and progression of lupus disease[169]: In early stages of disease development, TGF-β deficiency may predispose to immune dysregulation, breakdown of immune tolerance, and development of autoimmunity, whereas in late stages of disease, increased TGF-β production in local tissues may predispose to impairment of tissue repair and remodeling and development of tissue fibrosis.[170]

The V_H peptide–reactive $CD4^+D25^+$ Treg cells can also inhibit autoantibody production in vitro in (NZB/NZW)F1 mice.[171] To test the role of such Treg cells on lupus disease in vivo, one study performed thymectomy on day 3 of life, a procedure known to cause deficiency of $CD4^+D25^+$ Treg cells and generalized autoimmune disease in normal background, in the NZM2328 model of lupus.[172] Indeed, the thymectomy on day 3 accelerated anti-dsDNA antibody production and proliferative glomerulonephritis and sialoadenitis and induced severe prostatitis, thyroiditis, and dacryoadenitis. To test whether "refilling" these thymectomized mice with Treg cells would obviate lupus exacerbation, the researchers transferred $CD25^+$ T cells from young, healthy NZM2328 mice into syngeneic mice 4 to 7 days after thymectomy. Such transfer prevented the development of prostatitis, thyroiditis, and dacryoadenitis, abolished the accelerated dsDNA antibody response, but had little or no influence on the accelerated development of lupus nephritis and sialoadenitis.[172] Thus, a deficiency of $CD4^+D25^+$ Treg cells may contribute to abnormal immunoregulation in NZM2328 mice, but it may not be sufficient to cause lupus nephritis.

Studies in patients with SLE demonstrate that $CD4^+CD25^{hi}$ T cells in peripheral blood are reduced in patients with active disease in comparison with patients with inactive SLE or healthy individuals.[173] Foxp3$^+$ Tregs are also reduced in the lymph nodes from patients with active SLE.[85] Despite a large number of studies on Tregs and SLE, their role in disease initiation and development remains unexplained. Qualitative and functional studies of Tregs in patients with SLE have produced conflicting results.

That regulatory mechanisms constitute an important checkpoint against the development of pathologic autoimmunity was also demonstrated in a study in which introduction of a transgenic TCR specific for a pathogenic nucleosome–specific T cell in a lupus-prone strain caused suppression of autoimmune disease despite positive selection of autoreactive Th cells. The autoimmune disease suppression in TCR transgenic lupus mice was associated with a marked downregulation of the transgenic TCR, upregulation of endogenous TCRs in the periphery, and induction of potent Treg cells. Thus, the presence of autoreactive Th cells in large numbers since birth may elicit regulatory mechanisms to preempt pathologic autoimmunity.[4]

Contrary to many reports on Treg cells in lupus, Divekar has found higher numbers of $CD4^+D25^+Foxp3^+$ cells in the spleen of MRL/lpr and MRL/Fas$^{+/+}$ mouse models of SLE than in nonautoimmune C3H/HeOuj mice. However, these cells have an altered phenotype ($CD62L^{low}CD69^+$) and a lower suppressive capacity in MRL strains than in control mice. This feature was associated with a profound reduction in the expression of Dicer, which is involved in the generation of microRNAs (miRNAsmiRs), small RNA fragments that act as posttranscriptional repressors. Consistently, MRL/lpr Treg cells were found to have an altered miRNA profile. Intriguingly, however, despite having a reduced level of Dicer, MRL/lpr Treg cells overexpressed several miRNAs, including let-7a, let-7f, miR-16, miR-23a, miR-23b, miR-27a, and miR-155, in comparison with control mice. Using computational and functional approaches, this study identified a new role for miR-155 in conferring the altered Treg cell phenotype defined by reduced CD62L expression in MRL/lpr mice. In fact, the induced overexpression of miR-155 in otherwise normal (C3H/HeOuj) Treg cells reduced their CD62L expression, mimicking the altered Treg-cell phenotype in MRL/lpr mice.[84]

STRATEGIES TO REESTABLISH TOLERANCE IN LUPUS

Tolerizing DNA-Specific B Cells

Because many pathogenic autoantibodies bind DNA, there have been attempts to tolerize DNA-specific B cells. Almost 40 years ago, Borel showed that it was possible to prevent lupus in an animal model by inducing tolerance to denatured DNA.[174] This finding was translated into human disease 15 years later by the demonstration that a DNA-IgG conjugate inhibits the formation of anti-dsDNA antibodies in vitro by lymphoid cells from patients with SLE.[175] These observations eventually led to a clinical trial to evaluate a dsDNA-directed B-cell tolerogen, a synthetic molecule with the ability to bind dsDNA antibodies, that is believed to induce anergy or apoptosis of B cells. It has been shown to delay renal flares and reduce anti-dsDNA antibodies in a subgroup of patients.[176] However, its phase 3 trial was terminated after an interim analysis failed to show clinical benefit overall in patients with SLE.

In another study, the tolerance to native DNA in human B cells was reestablished by a chimeric molecule consisting of a complement receptor type 1 (CR1)–specific monoclonal antibody coupled to the decapeptide DWEYSVWLSN, which mimics dsDNA. The CR1-dsDNA mimic chimera co–cross-linked selectively native DNA–specific BCR with the B-cell inhibitory receptor CR1 and caused the targeted inhibition of DNA-specific B cells in immune-deficient SCID mice transferred with PBMCs from patients with SLE.[177]

Tolerizing Lupus Th Cells

The DNA-based tolerogen just described, however, has had a limited success in human SLE to date. Because strong evidence favors the role of T-cell help for pathogenic autoantibody production,[178,179] several groups have attempted various strategies to induce tolerance to peptides that specifically target autoreactive T and B cells in lupus. Intravenous administration of high doses of these peptides induces high-zone tolerance in most T-cell functions, presumably through induction of apoptosis.[65,180,181] Mucosal delivery of histone peptides in lupus-prone mice can also induce peptide-specific tolerance, presumably via increased IL-10 production.[182] In another study, repeated subcutaneous injections of low doses of histone peptides were found to induce tolerance in pathogenic lupus T cells through the generation of CD8+ and CD4+CD25+ Treg cells.[163] Such peptide-specific tolerance achieved by diverse approaches results in suppressed autoantibody production and reduced lupus manifestations in murine models.[65,163,178,183] Studies using peptides to modulate lupus are described in Chapter 21.

Non–Antigen-Specific Approaches to Reestablishing Immune Tolerance in SLE

Belimumab, a fully human monoclonal antibody against B lymphocyte stimulator (Blys, also known as BAFF), plus standard therapy was shown to significantly improve SLE response index rate and to reduce SLE disease activity and severe flares in a phase 3, randomized, placebo-controlled trial.[184] Activated (CD20+CD69+) and naive (CD20+CD27−) B cells, CD19+CD27bright CD38bright plasma cells, and short-lived CD20−CD27bright plasma cells were reduced in belimumab-treated patients. No changes in CD4+ or CD8+ T cells or memory B cells (CD20+CD27+) occurred in belimumab-treated patients at week 52 or 76. Serum anti-dsDNA antibody levels were disproportionately reduced in comparison with total IgG level, suggesting a preferential inhibition of autoreactive B-cell survival and differentiation.[9] Although this effect needs to be demonstrated in patients, the main benefit of BAFF blockade is assumed to be the deletion of autoreactive transitional and naive B cells at a main peripheral checkpoint known to be defective in SLE.[8] Interestingly, transitional and naïve B-cell populations have been reported to contain IL-10–producing B cells with regulatory potential and to be functionally defective in SLE.[7] Although anti-dsDNA B cells in animals express higher levels of IL-10 than nonautoreactive B cells,[42] a subset of IL-10–producing cells also serves as regulatory B cells.[11] Hence, it will be important to determine whether inhibition of these potentially regulatory B cells underlies the relatively modest effect of belimumab treatment in SLE as well as its lack of effect in other autoimmune diseases.

Studies of B cells from patients with SLE undergoing B-cell depletion therapy using rituximab suggest that apparently nonspecific therapies may repair the specific tolerance defects at least in some patients with SLE.[185] Thus, CD20-targeted B-cell depletion effectively normalizes the disturbances in peripheral B-cell homeostasis that typically occur in SLE[186] and is accompanied by reduced activated peripheral T-cell populations of Treg cells.[187] In patients with prolonged remission after rituximab treatment, the memory B cells remain depleted but naïve B cells recover within 3 to 9 months, and the expression levels of CD40 and CD80 remain downregulated for 2 years. There is also a decrease of memory T cells relative to naïve T cells, and the expression of CD40L and ICOS on CD4+ T cells rapidly decreases and remains downregulated for 2 years.[188] In some patients, the number of memory B cells rises with upregulation of CD40 and CD80 expression just before relapse. In other patients with relapse, CD4+ memory T cells recover with upregulation of ICOS expression, without any change in the number of memory B cells. Thus, depletion of B cells appears to restore, albeit for a few months, tolerance in T cells at least in some patients.

Our group has reported that treatment with α-galactosylceramide, which activates iNKT cells, selectively inhibits the production of autoantibodies while leaving normal Ig production intact.[42] This effect occurs via selective targeting of autoreactive B cells that express high levels of CD1d and IL-10.

T cells from patients with SLE avoid peripheral tolerance by selectively using the COX-2/FLIP antiapoptosis program to resist anergy.[70] Interestingly, such a defect in lupus T cells can be reversed in vitro by some, but not all, COX-2 inhibitors, which cause apoptosis of the anergy-resistant T cells and suppress the production of pathogenic autoantibodies to DNA. Targeting such peripheral T-cell tolerance mechanisms in patients with SLE may open new avenues of treatment that reestablish immune tolerance but do not require the identification of specific antigens.

Until antigen-specific therapies are further developed, the preceding and several other approaches, such as CTLA-4-Ig and transmembrane activator and calcium modulator and cyclophilin ligand interactor (TACI)–Ig, which are at various stages of therapeutic testing, hold promise for SLE.[189] Available data suggest that these antigen "non-specific" treatment approaches may preferentially correct the impairments in immune phenotype and responses. Further studies are needed to develop treatments that equip the immune system to selectively target autoimmune diseases and to not compromise the ability to counteract infectious agents and cancers.

Stem Cell Transplantation to Reset Immune Tolerance in SLE

Autologous hematopoietic stem cell transplantation (HSCT) has been used as a therapy for severe and treatment-refractory autoimmune diseases. The premise for HSCT is the de novo generation of naïve B and T cells, which thereby resets the immunologic clock and reestablishes immune tolerance. Before HSCT, immunoablative chemotherapy is utilized to eliminate pathogenic cells from the host. A pertinent study clearly elucidated the ability of HSCT to establish reconstitution of T and B cells for up to 8 years after immunoablation and autologous HSCT therapy in patients with SLE.[190] This study clearly demonstrated the reactivation of the thymus and recovery of naïve T cell subsets to numbers comparable to those in healthy controls. Furthermore, the frequency of Treg cells reached normal levels for 2 to 7 years after HSCT. Importantly, T cells reacting to nucleosomes or SmD1 were not detected early after HSCT, autoreactive B cells were extinguished, and long-lived plasma cells were depleted from the bone marrow after HSCT. The majority of repopulating B cells showed a naïve (IgD$^+$) phenotype, with memory B cells (IgD$^-$) appearing later on. Remarkably, many patients have long-lasting clinical and serologic remission after HSCT and are no longer reliant on immunosuppressive therapy.

Looking Beyond Immune Tolerance in Lupus

Most studies on the pathogenesis of SLE have focused on the prevailing notion that pathogenic T cells help B cells to produce autoantibodies that deposit in tissues and cause tissue damage. Challenging this notion are many later studies, in which lupus-associated organ damage can be "uncoupled" from the production of antinuclear autoantibodies.[169,191-193] Consistent with this idea, some individuals have high levels of antinuclear autoantibodies but no SLE-associated organ damage, whereas many patients with SLE with end-organ damage have no antinuclear autoantibodies. In some cases, autoantibodies are deposited in tissues but do not cause any local inflammation and damage. Studies in other autoimmune diseases also provide credence to this idea. For example, the presence of autoantibodies to beta-cell antigens is not always related to the clinical onset of hyperglycemia and diabetes.[194] These studies, however, do not exclude the possibility that the more relevant pathogenic autoantibodies may differ in antigen specificity, binding affinity, and Ig isotype and/or subclass, making their detection more difficult. It is also possible that autoantibodies may contribute to tissue lesions in some individuals but not in others. Additionally, autoimmunity may play a role in the initiation, but not the perpetuation, of tissue lesions.

SYNTHESIS

Many different animal models and human tissues, including peripheral blood cells, tonsils, and spleen, and diverse methodologies are being used to uncover tolerance defects in SLE. These studies reveal that whereas breakdown of central tolerance involving positive and negative selection in bone marrow or thymus can explain lupus-like autoimmunity in some instances, impaired peripheral tolerance appears to confer self-reactivity in most cases. In the periphery, these impairments in SLE involve breakdown of anergy or deletion of autoreactive cells or loss of normal censoring at different checkpoints during the development of immune responses. Although impairments at the level of APCs, adhesion, co-stimulation and interactions between different immune cells, and lymphoid organization such as faulty GC exclusion of autoreactive B cells might explain the loss of normal censoring in some cases, the intrinsic ability of lupus T and B cells to become easily overexcitable contributes to lupus autoimmunity in other cases. Full understanding of these mechanisms will allow the development of new therapeutic approaches designed to repair specific immune alterations. Finally, some patients with SLE may come to clinic at a late stage, when their disease cannot be tackled by repairing faults in immune tolerance. Studies have also begun to show that faulty immune tolerance might not be the cause of lupus disease development in some cases. For such cases, we must understand the mechanisms of end-organ damage.

References

1. Stritesky GL, Jameson SC, Hogquist KA: Selection of self-reactive T cells in the thymus. *Annu Rev Immunol* 30:95–114, 2011.
2. Suen AY, Baldwin TA: Proapoptotic protein Bim is differentially required during thymic clonal deletion to ubiquitous versus tissue-restricted antigens. *Proc Natl Acad Sci U S A* 109:893–898, 2012.
3. McCaughtry TM, Hogquist KA: Central tolerance: what have we learned from mice? *Semin Immunopathol* 30:399–409, 2008.
4. Michaels MA, Kang HK, Kaliyaperumal A, et al: A defect in deletion of nucleosome-specific autoimmune T cells in lupus-prone thymus: role of thymic dendritic cells. *J Immunol* 175:5857–5865, 2005.
5. Goodnow CC, Vinuesa CG, Randall KL, et al: Control systems and decision making for antibody production. *Nat Immunol* 11:681688, 2010.
6. Meffre E: The establishment of early B cell tolerance in humans: lessons from primary immunodeficiency diseases. *Ann N Y Acad Sci* 1246:1–10, 2011.
7. Blair PA, Norena LY, Flores-Borja F, et al: CD19(+)CD24(hi)CD38(hi) B cells exhibit regulatory capacity in healthy individuals but are functionally impaired in systemic lupus erythematosus patients. *Immunity* 32:129–140, 2010.
8. Liu Z, Davidson A: BAFF and selection of autoreactive B cells. *Trends Immunol* 32:388–394, 2011.
9. Sanz I: Connective tissue diseases: targeting B cells in SLE: good news at last! *Nat Rev Rheumatol* 7:255–256, 2011.
10. Mauri C, Blair PA: Regulatory B cells in autoimmunity: developments and controversies. *Nat Rev Rheumatol* 6:636–643, 2010.
11. Yang M, Sun L, Wang S, et al: Novel function of B cell-activating factor in the induction of IL-10-producing regulatory B cells. *J Immunol* 184:3321–3325, 2010.
12. Ding Q, Yeung M, Camirand G, et al: Regulatory B cells are identified by expression of TIM-1 and can be induced through TIM-1 ligation to promote tolerance in mice. *J Clin Invest* 121:3645–3656, 2011.
13. Van Parijs L, Abbas AK: Homeostasis and self-tolerance in the immune system: turning lymphocytes off. *Science* 280(5361):243–248, 1998.
14. Surh CD, Sprent J: Homeostatic T cell proliferation: how far can T cells be activated to self-ligands? *J Exp Med* 192:F9–F14, 2000.
15. Baccala R, Theofilopoulos AN: The new paradigm of T-cell homeostatic proliferation-induced autoimmunity. *Trends Immunol* 26:5–8, 2005.
16. King C, Ilic A, Koelsch K, et al: Homeostatic expansion of T cells during immune insufficiency generates autoimmunity. *Cell* 117:265–277, 2004.
17. Theofilopoulos AN, Dummer W, Kono DH: T cell homeostasis and systemic autoimmunity. *J Clin Invest* 108:335–340, 2001.
18. Schwartz RH, Mueller DL: Immunological tolerance. In Paul WE, editor: *Fundamental immunology*, ed 5, Philadelphia, 2003, Lippincott Williams and Wilkins, pp 901–934.
19. Schwartz RH: T cell anergy. *Annu Rev Immunol* 21:305–334, 2003.
20. Mathis D, Benoist C: A decade of AIRE. *Nat Rev Immunol* 7:645–650, 2007.
21. Gallegos AM, Bevan MJ: Central tolerance: good but imperfect. *Immunological reviews* 209:290–296, 2006.
22. Brocker T, Riedinger M, Karjalainen K: Targeted expression of major histocompatibility complex (MHC) class II molecules demonstrates that dendritic cells can induce negative but not positive selection of thymocytes in vivo. *J Exp Med* 185:541–550, 1997.
23. Kruisbeek AM, Amsen D: Mechanisms underlying T-cell tolerance. *Curr Opin Immunol* 8:233–244, 1996.
24. Rieux-Laucat F, Le Deist F, Hivroz C, et al: Mutations in Fas associated with human lymphoproliferative syndrome and autoimmunity. *Science* 268(5215):1347–1349, 1995.
25. Nagata S, Suda T: Fas and Fas ligand: lpr and gld mutations. *Immunol Today* 16:39–43, 1995.
26. Fisher GH, Rosenberg FJ, Straus SE, et al: Dominant interfering Fas gene mutations impair apoptosis in a human autoimmune lymphoproliferative syndrome. *Cell* 81:935–946, 1995.
27. Fife BT, Bluestone JA: Control of peripheral T-cell tolerance and autoimmunity via the CTLA-4 and PD-1 pathways. *Immunol Rev* 224:166–182, 2008.
28. Perez VL, Van Parijs L, Biuckians A, et al: Induction of peripheral T cell tolerance in vivo requires CTLA-4 engagement. *Immunity* 6:411–417, 1997.
29. Becker JC, Brabletz T, Kirchner T, et al: Negative transcriptional regulation in anergic T cells. *Proc Natl Acad Sci U S A* 92:2375–2378, 1995.
30. Jenkins MK: The role of cell division in the induction of clonal anergy. *Immunol Today* 13:69–73, 1992.
31. Heissmeyer V, Macian F, Varma R, et al: A molecular dissection of lymphocyte unresponsiveness induced by sustained calcium signalling. *Novartis Found Symp* 267:165–174, 2005; discussion 174–179.
32. Mueller DL: E3 ubiquitin ligases as T cell anergy factors. *Nat Immunol* 5:883–890, 2004.

33. Liblau RS, Singer SM, McDevitt HO: Th1 and Th2 CD4+ T cells in the pathogenesis of organ-specific autoimmune diseases. *Immunol Today* 16:34–38, 1995.

34. Zhang GX, Gran B, Yu S, et al: Induction of experimental autoimmune encephalomyelitis in IL-12 receptor-beta 2-deficient mice: IL-12 responsiveness is not required in the pathogenesis of inflammatory demyelination in the central nervous system. *J Immunol* 170:2153–2160, 2003.

35. Harrington LE, Hatton RD, Mangan PR, et al: Interleukin 17-producing CD4+ effector T cells develop via a lineage distinct from the T helper type 1 and 2 lineages. *Nat Immunol* 6:1123–1132, 2005.

36. Hu Y, Shen F, Crellin NK, et al: The IL-17 pathway as a major therapeutic target in autoimmune diseases. *Ann N Y Acad Sci* 1217:60–76, 2011.

37. Singh RR, Ebling FM, Albuquerque DA, et al: Induction of autoantibody production is limited in nonautoimmune mice. *J Immunol* 169:587–594, 2002.

38. Fan GC, Singh RR: Vaccination with minigenes encoding V(H)-derived major histocompatibility complex class I-binding epitopes activates cytotoxic T cells that ablate autoantibody-producing B cells and inhibit lupus. *J Exp Med* 196:731–741, 2002.

39. Sonoda KH, Exley M, Snapper S, et al: CD1-reactive natural killer T cells are required for development of systemic tolerance through an immune-privileged site. *J Exp Med* 190:1215–1226, 1999.

40. Wermeling F, Lind SM, Jordo ED, et al: Invariant NKT cells limit activation of autoreactive CD1d-positive B cells. *J Exp Med* 207:943–952, 2010.

41. Wen X, Yang JQ, Kim PJ, et al: Homeostatic regulation of marginal zone B cells by invariant natural killer T cells. *PLoS One* 6:e26536, 2011.

42. Yang JQ, Wen X, Kim PJ, et al: Invariant NKT cells inhibit autoreactive B cells in a contact- and CD1d-dependent manner. *J Immunol* 186:1512–1520, 2011.

43. Wardemann H, Yurasov S, Schaefer A, et al: Predominant autoantibody production by early human B cell precursors. *Science* 301(5638):1374–1377, 2003.

44. Verkoczy LK, Martensson AS, Nemazee D: The scope of receptor editing and its association with autoimmunity. *Curr Opin Immunol* 16:808–814, 2004.

45. Jacobi AM, Diamond B: Balancing diversity and tolerance: lessons from patients with systemic lupus erythematosus. *J Exp Med* 202:341–344, 2005.

46. Gay D, Saunders T, Camper S, et al: Receptor editing: an approach by autoreactive B cells to escape tolerance. *J Exp Med* 177:999–1008, 1993.

47. Jankovic M, Casellas R, Yannoutsos N, et al: RAGs and regulation of autoantibodies. *Annu Rev Immunol* 22:485–501, 2004.

48. Rajewsky K: Clonal selection and learning in the antibody system. *Nature* 381(6585):751–758, 1996.

49. Loder F, Mutschler B, Ray RJ, et al: B cell development in the spleen takes place in discrete steps and is determined by the quality of B cell receptor-derived signals. *J Exp Med* 190:75–89, 1999.

50. Kim SJ, Gershov D, Ma X, et al: I-PLA activation during apoptosis promotes the exposure of membrane lysophosphatidylcholine leading to binding by natural immunoglobulin M antibodies and complement activation. *J Exp Med* 196:655–665, 2002.

51. Pugh-Bernard AE, Silverman GJ, Cappione AJ, et al: Regulation of inherently autoreactive VH4–34 B cells in the maintenance of human B cell tolerance. *J Clin Invest* 108:1061–1070, 2001.

52. Song H, Cerny J: Functional heterogeneity of marginal zone B cells revealed by their ability to generate both early antibody-forming cells and germinal centers with hypermutation and memory in response to a T-dependent antigen. *J Exp Med* 198:1923–1935, 2003.

53. Rice JS, Newman J, Wang C, et al: Receptor editing in peripheral B cell tolerance. *Proc Natl Acad Sci U S A* 102:1608–1613, 2005.

54. Fukuyama H, Nimmerjahn F, Ravetch JV: The inhibitory Fcgamma receptor modulates autoimmunity by limiting the accumulation of immunoglobulin G+ anti-DNA plasma cells. *Nat Immunol* 6:99–106, 2005.

55. Eisenberg R: Do autoantigens define autoimmunity or vice versa? *Eur J Immunol* 35:367–370, 2005.

56. Graham KL, Utz PJ: Sources of autoantigens in systemic lupus erythematosus. *Curr Opin Rheumatol* 17:513–517, 2005.

57. Wu CT, Gershwin ME, Davis PA: What makes an autoantigen an autoantigen? *Ann N Y Acad Sci* 1050:134–145, 2005.

58. Ng B, Yang F, Huston DP, et al: Increased noncanonical splicing of autoantigen transcripts provides the structural basis for expression of untolerized epitopes. *J Allergy Clin Immunol* 114:1463–1470, 2004.

59. Eriksson AU, Singh RR: Cutting edge: migration of Langerhans dendritic cells is impaired in autoimmune dermatitis. *J Immunol* 181:7468–7472, 2008.

60. Kim SJ, Zou YR, Goldstein J, et al: Tolerogenic function of Blimp-1 in dendritic cells. *J Exp Med* 208:2193–2199, 2011.

61. Yan J, Mamula MJ: Autoreactive T cells revealed in the normal repertoire: escape from negative selection and peripheral tolerance. *J Immunol* 168:3188–3194, 2002.

62. Kretz-Rommel A, Duncan SR, Rubin RL: Autoimmunity caused by disruption of central T cell tolerance. A murine model of drug-induced lupus. *J Clin Invest* 99:1888–1896, 1997.

63. Budagyan VM, Bulanova EG, Sharova NI, et al: The resistance of activated T-cells from SLE patients to apoptosis induced by human thymic stromal cells. *Immunol Lett* 60:1–5, 1998.

64. Singh RR, Hahn BH, Sercarz EE: Neonatal peptide exposure can prime T cells and, upon subsequent immunization, induce their immune deviation: implications for antibody vs. T cell-mediated autoimmunity. *J Exp Med* 183:1613–1621, 1996.

65. Singh RR, Ebling FM, Sercarz EE, et al: Immune tolerance to autoantibody-derived peptides delays development of autoimmunity in murine lupus. *J Clin Invest* 96:2990–2996, 1995.

66. Singh RR, Jacinto J, Sercarz EE, Hahn BH: Experimental split T cell tolerance to peptides in murine SLE: lack of a defect. *Lupus* 4(Suppl 2):83, 1995.

67. Singh RR, Ebling F, Jacinto J, Sercarz E, et al: Functional split tolerance in autoimmune mice: implications for Ab-mediated autoimmunity. *FASEB J* 8:A205, 1994.

68. Fatenejad S, Peng SL, Disorbo O, et al: Central T cell tolerance in lupus-prone mice: influence of autoimmune background and the lpr mutation. *J Immunol* 161:6427–6432, 1998.

69. Wither J, Vukusic B: Autoimmunity develops in lupus-prone NZB mice despite normal T cell tolerance. *J Immunol* 161:4555–4562, 1998.

70. Xu L, Zhang L, Yi Y, et al: Human lupus T cells resist inactivation and escape death by upregulating COX-2. *Nat Med* 10:411–415, 2004.

71. Bouzahzah F, Jung S, Craft J: CD4+ T cells from lupus-prone mice avoid antigen-specific tolerance induction in vivo. *J Immunol* 170:741–748, 2003.

72. Rozzo SJ, Drake CG, Chiang BL, et al: Evidence for polyclonal T cell activation in murine models of systemic lupus erythematosus. *J Immunol* 153:1340–13451, 1994.

73. Ishikawa S, Akakura S, Abe M, et al: A subset of CD4+ T cells expressing early activation antigen CD69 in murine lupus: possible abnormal regulatory role for cytokine imbalance. *J Immunol* 161:1267–1273, 1998.

74. Blanco P, Pitard V, Viallard JF, et al: Increase in activated CD8+ T lymphocytes expressing perforin and granzyme B correlates with disease activity in patients with systemic lupus erythematosus. *Arthritis Rheum* 52:201–211, 2005.

75. Vratsanos GS, Jung S, Park YM, et al: CD4(+) T cells from lupus-prone mice are hyperresponsive to T cell receptor engagement with low and high affinity peptide antigens: a model to explain spontaneous T cell activation in lupus. *J Exp Med* 193:329–337, 2001.

76. Alcocer-Varela J, Alarcon-Segovia D: Decreased production of and response to interleukin-2 by cultured lymphocytes from patients with systemic lupus erythematosus. *J Clin Invest* 69:1388–1392, 1982.

77. Altman A, Theofilopoulos AN, Weiner R, et al: Analysis of T cell function in autoimmune murine strains. Defects in production and responsiveness to interleukin 2. *J Exp Med* 154:791–808, 1981.

78. Linker-Israeli M, Bakke AC, Kitridou RC, et al: Defective production of interleukin 1 and interleukin 2 in patients with systemic lupus erythematosus (SLE). *J Immunol* 130:2651–2655, 1983.

79. Wofsy D, Murphy ED, Roths JB, et al: Deficient interleukin 2 activity in MRL/Mp and C57BL/6J mice bearing the lpr gene. *J Exp Med* 154:1671–1680, 1981.

80. Gutierrez-Ramos JC, Andreu JL, Revilla Y, et al: Recovery from autoimmunity of MRL/lpr mice after infection with an interleukin-2/vaccinia recombinant virus. *Nature* 346(6281):271–274, 1990.

81. Sadlack B, Lohler J, Schorle H, et al: Generalized autoimmune disease in interleukin-2-deficient mice is triggered by an uncontrolled activation and proliferation of CD4+ T cells. *Eur J Immunol* 25:3053–3059, 1995.

82. Fontenot JD, Rasmussen JP, Gavin MA, et al: A function for interleukin 2 in Foxp3-expressing regulatory T cells. *Nat Immunol* 6:1142–1151, 2005.

83. Scalapino KJ, Tang Q, Bluestone JA, et al: Suppression of disease in New Zealand Black/New Zealand White lupus-prone mice by adoptive transfer of ex vivo expanded regulatory T cells. *J Immunol* 177:1451–1459, 2006.

84. Divekar AA, Dubey S, Gangalum PR, et al: Dicer insufficiency and microRNA-155 overexpression in lupus regulatory T cells: an apparent paradox in the setting of an inflammatory milieu. *J Immunol* 186:924–930, 2011.

85. Miyara M, Amoura Z, Parizot C, et al: Global natural regulatory T cell depletion in active systemic lupus erythematosus. *J Immunol* 175:8392–8400, 2005.

86. Tsokos GC, Nambiar MP, Tenbrock K, et al: Rewiring the T-cell: signaling defects and novel prospects for the treatment of SLE. *Trends Immunol* 24:259–263, 2003.

87. Tsuzaka K, Fukuhara I, Setoyama Y, et al: TCR zeta mRNA with an alternatively spliced 3'-untranslated region detected in systemic lupus erythematosus patients leads to the down-regulation of TCR zeta and TCR/CD3 complex. *J Immunol* 171:2496–2503, 2003.

88. Nambiar MP, Juang YT, Krishnan S, et al: Dissecting the molecular mechanisms of TCR zeta chain downregulation and T cell signaling abnormalities in human systemic lupus erythematosus. *Int Rev Immunol* 23:245–263, 2004.

89. Vassilopoulos D, Kovacs B, Tsokos GC: TCR/CD3 complex-mediated signal transduction pathway in T cells and T cell lines from patients with systemic lupus erythematosus. *J Immunol* 155:2269–2281, 1995.

90. Juang YT, Wang Y, Solomou EE, et al: Systemic lupus erythematosus serum IgG increases CREM binding to the IL-2 promoter and suppresses IL-2 production through CaMKIV. *J Clin Invest* 115:996–1005, 2005.

91. Sierakowski S, Kucharz EJ, Lightfoot RW, et al: Impaired T-cell activation in patients with systemic lupus erythematosus. *J Clin Immunol* 9:469–476, 1989.

92. Dong C, Davis RJ, Flavell RA: MAP kinases in the immune response. *Annu Rev Immunol* 20:55–72, 2002.

93. Cedeno S, Cifarelli DF, Blasini AM, et al: Defective activity of ERK-1 and ERK-2 mitogen-activated protein kinases in peripheral blood T lymphocytes from patients with systemic lupus erythematosus: potential role of altered coupling of Ras guanine nucleotide exchange factor hSos to adapter protein Grb2 in lupus T cells. *Clin Immunol* 106:41–49, 2003.

94. Niculescu F, Nguyen P, Niculescu T, et al: Pathogenic T cells in murine lupus exhibit spontaneous signaling activity through phosphatidylinositol 3-kinase and mitogen-activated protein kinase pathways. *Arthritis Rheum* 48:1071–1079, 2003.

95. Barber DF, Bartolome A, Hernandez C, et al: PI3Kgamma inhibition blocks glomerulonephritis and extends lifespan in a mouse model of systemic lupus. *Nat Med* 11:933–935, 2005.

96. Suarez-Fueyo A, Barber DF, Martinez-Ara J, et al: Enhanced phosphoinositide 3-kinase delta activity is a frequent event in systemic lupus erythematosus that confers resistance to activation-induced T cell death. *J Immunol* 187:2376–2385, 2011.

97. Fernandez D, Perl A: mTOR signaling: a central pathway to pathogenesis in systemic lupus erythematosus? *Discovery Medicine* 9:173–178, 2010.

98. Warner LM, Adams LM, Sehgal SN: Rapamycin prolongs survival and arrests pathophysiologic changes in murine systemic lupus erythematosus. *Arthritis Rheum* 37:289–297, 1994.

99. Fernandez D, Bonilla E, Mirza N, et al: Rapamycin reduces disease activity and normalizes T cell activation-induced calcium fluxing in patients with systemic lupus erythematosus. *Arthritis Rheum* 54:2983–2988, 2006.

100. Enyedy EJ, Nambiar MP, Liossis SN, et al: Fc epsilon receptor type I gamma chain replaces the deficient T cell receptor zeta chain in T cells of patients with systemic lupus erythematosus. *Arthritis Rheum* 44:1114–1121, 2001.

101. Nambiar MP, Fisher CU, Warke VG, et al: Reconstitution of deficient T cell receptor zeta chain restores T cell signaling and augments T cell receptor/CD3-induced interleukin-2 production in patients with systemic lupus erythematosus. *Arthritis Rheum* 48:1948–1955, 2003.

102. Bahjat FR, Pine PR, Reitsma A, et al: An orally bioavailable spleen tyrosine kinase inhibitor delays disease progression and prolongs survival in murine lupus. *Arthritis and rheumatism* 58:1433–1444, 2008.

103. Sauer S, Bruno L, Hertweck A, et al: T cell receptor signaling controls Foxp3 expression via PI3K, Akt, and mTOR. *Proc Natl Acad Sci U S A* 105:7797–7802, 2008.

104. Valencia X, Yarboro C, Illei G, et al: Deficient CD4+CD25high T regulatory cell function in patients with active systemic lupus erythematosus. *J Immunol* 178:2579–2588, 2007.

105. Simons K, Ikonen E: Functional rafts in cell membranes. *Nature* 387:569–572, 1997.

106. Simons K, Toomre D: Lipid rafts and signal transduction. *Nat Rev Mol Cell Biol* 1:31–39, 2000.

107. Krishnan S, Nambiar MP, Warke VG, et al: Alterations in lipid raft composition and dynamics contribute to abnormal T cell responses in systemic lupus erythematosus. *J Immunol* 172:7821–7831, 2004.

108. Jury EC, Kabouridis PS, Abba A, et al: Increased ubiquitination and reduced expression of LCK in T lymphocytes from patients with systemic lupus erythematosus. *Arthritis Rheum* 48:1343–1354, 2003.

109. Jury EC, Kabouridis PS, Flores-Borja F, et al: Altered lipid raft-associated signaling and ganglioside expression in T lymphocytes from patients with systemic lupus erythematosus. *J Clin Invest* 113:1176–1187, 2004.

110. Garcia BA, Busby SA, Shabanowitz J, et al: Resetting the epigenetic histone code in the MRL-lpr/lpr mouse model of lupus by histone deacetylase inhibition. *J Proteome Res* 4:2032–2042, 2005.

111. Mishra N, Reilly CM, Brown DR, et al: Histone deacetylase inhibitors modulate renal disease in the MRL-lpr/lpr mouse. *J Clin Invest* 111:539–552, 2003.

112. Simpson N, Gatenby PA, Wilson A, et al: Expansion of circulating T cells resembling follicular helper T cells is a fixed phenotype that identifies a subset of severe systemic lupus erythematosus. *Arthritis Rheum* 62:234–244, 2010.

113. Linterman MA, Rigby RJ, Wong RK, et al: Follicular helper T cells are required for systemic autoimmunity. *J Exp Med* 206:561–576, 2009.

114. Bryant VL, Ma CS, Avery DT, et al: Cytokine-mediated regulation of human B cell differentiation into Ig-secreting cells: predominant role of IL-21 produced by CXCR5+ T follicular helper cells. *J Immunol* 179:8180–8190, 2007.

115. Herber D, Brown TP, Liang S, et al: IL-21 has a pathogenic role in a lupus-prone mouse model and its blockade with IL-21R.Fc reduces disease progression. *J Immunol* 178:3822–3830, 2007.

116. Dolff S, Abdulahad WH, Westra J, et al: Increase in IL-21 producing T-cells in patients with systemic lupus erythematosus. *Arthritis Res Ther* 13:R157, 2011.

117. Gigoux M, Shang J, Pak Y, et al: Inducible costimulator promotes helper T-cell differentiation through phosphoinositide 3-kinase. *Proc Natl Acad Sci U S A* 106:20371–20376, 2009.

118. Rolf J, Bell SE, Kovesdi D, et al: Phosphoinositide 3-kinase activity in T cells regulates the magnitude of the germinal center reaction. *J Immunol* 185:4042–4052, 2010.

119. McAdam AJ, Greenwald RJ, Levin MA, et al: ICOS is critical for CD40-mediated antibody class switching. *Nature* 409:102–105, 2001.

120. Hu YL, Metz DP, Chung J, et al: B7RP-1 blockade ameliorates autoimmunity through regulation of follicular helper T cells. *J Immunol* 182:1421–1428, 2009.

121. Bauquet AT, Jin H, Paterson AM, et al: The costimulatory molecule ICOS regulates the expression of c-Maf and IL-21 in the development of follicular T helper cells and TH-17 cells. *Nat Immunol* 10:167–175, 2009.

122. Mitsdoerffer M, Lee Y, Jager A, et al: Proinflammatory T helper type 17 cells are effective B-cell helpers. *Proc Natl Acad Sci U S A* 107:14292–14297, 2010.

123. Wong CK, Lit LC, Tam LS, et al: Hyperproduction of IL-23 and IL-17 in patients with systemic lupus erythematosus: implications for Th17-mediated inflammation in auto-immunity. *Clin Immunol* 127:385–393, 2008.

124. Zhang Z, Kyttaris VC, Tsokos GC: The role of IL-23/IL-17 axis in lupus nephritis. *J Immunol* 183:3160–3169, 2009.

125. Arbuckle MR, McClain MT, Rubertone MV, et al: Development of autoantibodies before the clinical onset of systemic lupus erythematosus. *N Engl J Med* 349:1526–1533, 2003.

126. Yurasov S, Wardemann H, Hammersen J, et al: Defective B cell tolerance checkpoints in systemic lupus erythematosus. *J Exp Med* 201:703–711, 2005.

127. Bijl M, Horst G, Limburg PC, et al: Expression of costimulatory molecules on peripheral blood lymphocytes of patients with systemic lupus erythematosus. *Ann Rheum Dis* 60:523–526, 2001.

128. Thien M, Phan TG, Gardam S, et al: Excess BAFF rescues self-reactive B cells from peripheral deletion and allows them to enter forbidden follicular and marginal zone niches. *Immunity* 20:785–798, 2004.

129. Zhang J, Roschke V, Baker KP, et al: Cutting edge: a role for B lymphocyte stimulator in systemic lupus erythematosus. *J Immunol* 166:6–10, 2001.

130. Cappione A, Anolik JH, Pugh-Bernard A, et al: Germinal center exclusion of autoreactive B cells is defective in human systemic lupus erythematosus. *J Clin Invest* 115:3205–3216, 2005.

131. Jacobi AM, Zhang J, Mackay M, et al: Phenotypic characterization of autoreactive B cells–checkpoints of B cell tolerance in patients with systemic lupus erythematosus. *PLoS One* 4:e5776, 2009.

132. Roy V, Chang NH, Cai Y, et al: Aberrant IgM signaling promotes survival of transitional T1 B cells and prevents tolerance induction in lupus-prone New Zealand black mice. *J Immunol* 175:7363–7371, 2005.

133. Kozono Y, Kotzin BL, Holers VM: Resting B cells from New Zealand Black mice demonstrate a defect in apoptosis induction following surface IgM ligation. *J Immunol* 156:4498–4503, 1996.

134. Grimaldi CM, Michael DJ, Diamond B: Cutting edge: expansion and activation of a population of autoreactive marginal zone B cells in a model of estrogen-induced lupus. *J Immunol* 167:1886–1890, 2001.

135. Westhoff CM, Whittier A, Kathol S, et al: DNA-binding antibodies from viable motheaten mutant mice: implications for B cell tolerance. *J Immunol* 159:3024–3033, 1997.

136. Mantovani L, Wilder RL, Casali P: Human rheumatoid B-1a (CD5+ B) cells make somatically hypermutated high affinity IgM rheumatoid factors. *J Immunol* 151:473–488, 1993.

137. Caligaris-Cappio F, Riva M, Tesio L, et al: Human normal CD5+ B lymphocytes can be induced to differentiate to CD5- B lymphocytes with germinal center cell features. *Blood* 73:1259–1263, 1989.

138. Attanavanich K, Kearney JF: Marginal zone, but not follicular B cells, are potent activators of naive CD4 T cells. *J Immunol* 172:803–811, 2004.

139. William J, Euler C, Christensen S, et al: Evolution of autoantibody responses via somatic hypermutation outside of germinal centers. *Science* 297:2066–2070, 2002.

140. Tsokos GC, Liossis SN: Immune cell signaling defects in lupus: activation, anergy and death. *Immunol Today* 20:119–124, 1999.

141. Tanaka Y, Shirakawa F, Ota T, et al: Mechanism of spontaneous activation of B cells in patients with systemic lupus erythematosus. Analysis with anti-class II antibody. *J Immunol* 140:761–767, 1988.

142. Flores-Borja F, Kabouridis PS, Jury EC, et al: Decreased Lyn expression and translocation to lipid raft signaling domains in B lymphocytes from patients with systemic lupus erythematosus. *Arthritis Rheum* 52:3955–3965, 2005.

143. Mackay M, Stanevsky A, Wang T, et al: Selective dysregulation of the FcgammaIIB receptor on memory B cells in SLE. *J Exp Med* 203:2157–2164, 2006.

144. Kono H, Kyogoku C, Suzuki T, et al: FcgammaRIIB Ile232Thr transmembrane polymorphism associated with human systemic lupus erythematosus decreases affinity to lipid rafts and attenuates inhibitory effects on B cell receptor signaling. *Hum Mol Genet* 14:2881–2892, 2005.

145. Huck S, Le Corre R, Youinou P, et al: Expression of B cell receptor-associated signaling molecules in human lupus. *Autoimmunity* 33:213–224, 2001.

146. Craxton A, Draves KE, Gruppi A, et al: BAFF regulates B cell survival by downregulating the BH3-only family member Bim via the ERK pathway. *J Exp Med* 202:1363–1374, 2005.

147. Carter RH, Zhao H, Liu X, et al: Expression and occupancy of BAFF-R on B cells in systemic lupus erythematosus. *Arthritis Rheum* 52:3943–3954, 2005.

148. Gross JA, Dillon SR, Mudri S, et al: TACI-Ig neutralizes molecules critical for B cell development and autoimmune disease impaired B cell maturation in mice lacking BLyS. *Immunity* 15:289–302, 2001.

149. Pers JO, Daridon C, Devauchelle V, et al: BAFF overexpression is associated with autoantibody production in autoimmune diseases. *Ann N Y Acad Sci* 1050:34–39, 2005.

150. Ng YS, Wardemann H, Chelnis J, et al: Bruton's tyrosine kinase is essential for human B cell tolerance. *J Exp Med* 200:927–934, 2004.

151. Wang C, Khalil M, Ravetch J, et al: The naive B cell repertoire predisposes to antigen-induced systemic lupus erythematosus. *J Immunol* 170:4826–4832, 2003.

152. Arechiga AF, Habib T, He Y, et al: Cutting edge: the PTPN22 allelic variant associated with autoimmunity impairs B cell signaling. *J Immunol* 182:3343–3347, 2009.

153. Benson MJ, Erickson LD, Gleeson MW, et al: Affinity of antigen encounter and other early B-cell signals determine B-cell fate. *Curr Opin Immunol* 19:275–280, 2007.

154. Mamula MJ, Janeway CA, Jr: Do B cells drive the diversification of immune responses? *Immunol Today* 14:151–152; discussion 3–4, 1993.

155. Mamula MJ, Fatenejad S, Craft J: B cells process and present lupus autoantigens that initiate autoimmune T cell responses. *J Immunol* 152:1453–1461, 1994.

156. Chan OT, Madaio MP, Shlomchik MJ: B cells are required for lupus nephritis in the polygenic, Fas-intact MRL model of systemic autoimmunity. *J Immunol* 163:3592–3596, 1999.

157. Chan OT, Hannum LG, Haberman AM, et al: A novel mouse with B cells but lacking serum antibody reveals an antibody-independent role for B cells in murine lupus. *J Exp Med* 189:1639–1648, 1999.

158. Singh RR, Ebling F, Kumar V, Hahn BH: Involvement of regulatory T cells in limiting induction of anti-DNA antibodies in non-autoimmune mice. *Arthritis Rheum* 42:S362, 1999.

159. Singh RR: Prevention and control of reciprocal T-B cell diversification: implications for lupus-like autoimmunity. *Mol Immunol* 40:1137–1145, 2004.

160. Karpouzas GA, La Cava A, Ebling FM, et al: Differences between CD8+ T cells in lupus-prone (NZB × NZW) F1 mice and healthy (BALB/c × NZW) F1 mice may influence autoimmunity in the lupus model. *Eur J Immunol* 34:2489–2499, 2004.

161. Kim HJ, Verbinnen B, Tang X, et al: Inhibition of follicular T-helper cells by CD8(+) regulatory T cells is essential for self tolerance. *Nature* 467:328–332, 2010.

162. Filaci G, Bacilieri S, Fravega M, et al: Impairment of CD8+ T suppressor cell function in patients with active systemic lupus erythematosus. *J Immunol* 166:6452–6457, 2001.

163. Kang HK, Michaels MA, Berner BR, et al: Very low-dose tolerance with nucleosomal peptides controls lupus and induces potent regulatory T cell subsets. *J Immunol* 174:3247–3255, 2005.

164. Hahn BH, Singh RP, La Cava A, et al: Tolerogenic treatment of lupus mice with consensus peptide induces Foxp3-expressing, apoptosis-resistant, TGFbeta-secreting CD8+ T cell suppressors. *J Immunol* 175:7728–7737, 2005.

165. Bommireddy R, Saxena V, Ormsby I, et al: TGF-beta 1 regulates lymphocyte homeostasis by preventing activation and subsequent apoptosis of peripheral lymphocytes. *J Immunol* 170:4612–4622, 2003.

166. Shull MM, Ormsby I, Kier AB, et al: Targeted disruption of the mouse transforming growth factor-beta 1 gene results in multifocal inflammatory disease. *Nature* 359(6397):693–699, 1992.

167. Ohtsuka K, Gray JD, Stimmler MM, et al: Decreased production of TGF-beta by lymphocytes from patients with systemic lupus erythematosus. *J Immunol* 160:2539–2545, 1998.

168. Cimaz R, Borghi MO, Gerosa M, et al: Transforming growth factor beta1 in the pathogenesis of autoimmune congenital complete heart block: lesson from twins and triplets discordant for the disease. *Arthritis Rheum* 54:356–359, 2006.

169. Singh RR: SLE: translating lessons from model systems to human disease. *Trends Immunol* 26:572–579, 2005.

170. Saxena V, Lienesch DW, Zhou M, et al: Dual roles of immunoregulatory cytokine TGF-beta in the pathogenesis of autoimmunity-mediated organ damage. *J Immunol* 180:1903–1912, 2008.

171. La Cava A, Ebling FM, Hahn BH: Ig-reactive CD4+CD25+ T cells from tolerized (New Zealand Black x New Zealand White)F1 mice suppress in vitro production of antibodies to DNA. *J Immunol* 173:3542–3548, 2004.

172. Waters ST, McDuffie M, Bagavant H, et al: Breaking tolerance to double stranded DNA, nucleosome, and other nuclear antigens is not required for the pathogenesis of lupus glomerulonephritis. *J Exp Med* 199:255–264, 2004.

173. Xing Q, Wang B, Su H, et al: Elevated Th17 cells are accompanied by FoxP3+ Treg cells decrease in patients with lupus nephritis. *Rheumatol Int* 32:949–958, 2011.

174. Borel Y, Lewis RM, Stollar BD: Prevention of murine lupus nephritis by carrier-dependent induction of immunologic tolerance to denatured DNA. *Science* 182:76–78, 1973.

175. Borel Y, Borel H: Oligonucleotide linked to human gammaglobulin specifically diminishes anti-DNA antibody formation in cultured lymphoid cells from patients with systemic lupus erythematosus. *J Clin Invest* 82:1901–1907, 1988.

176. Alarcon-Segovia D, Tumlin JA, Furie RA, et al: LJP 394 for the prevention of renal flare in patients with systemic lupus erythematosus: results from a randomized, double-blind, placebo-controlled study. *Arthritis Rheum* 48:442–454, 2003.

177. Kerekov NS, Mihaylova NM, Grozdev I, et al: Elimination of autoreactive B cells in humanized SCID mouse model of SLE. *Eur J Immunol* 41:3301–3311, 2011.

178. Datta SK: Major peptide autoepitopes for nucleosome-centered T and B cell interaction in human and murine lupus. *Ann N Y Acad Sci* 987:79–90, 2003.

179. Ando DG, Sercarz EE, Hahn BH: Mechanisms of T and B cell collaboration in the in vitro production of anti-DNA antibodies in the NZB/NZW F1 murine SLE model. *J Immunol* 138:3185–3190, 1987.

180. Liblau RS, Tisch R, Shokat K, et al: Intravenous injection of soluble antigen induces thymic and peripheral T-cells apoptosis. *Proc Natl Acad Sci U S A* 93:3031–3036, 1996.

181. Barron L, Knoechel B, Lohr J, et al: Cutting edge: contributions of apoptosis and anergy to systemic T cell tolerance. *J Immunol* 180:2762–2766, 2008.

182. Wu HY, Ward FJ, Staines NA: Histone peptide-induced nasal tolerance: suppression of murine lupus. *J Immunol* 169:1126–1134, 2002.

183. Wu HY, Staines NA: A deficiency of CD4+CD25+ T cells permits the development of spontaneous lupus-like disease in mice, and can be reversed by induction of mucosal tolerance to histone peptide autoantigen. *Lupus* 13:192–200, 2004.

184. Furie R, Petri M, Zamani O, et al: A phase III, randomized, placebo-controlled study of belimumab, a monoclonal antibody that inhibits B lymphocyte stimulator, in patients with systemic lupus erythematosus. *Arthritis Rheum* 63:3918–3930, 2011.

185. Anolik JH, Aringer M: New treatments for SLE: cell-depleting and anti-cytokine therapies. *Best Pract Res Clin Rheumatol* 19:859–878, 2005.

186. Anolik JH, Barnard J, Cappione A, et al: Rituximab improves peripheral B cell abnormalities in human systemic lupus erythematosus. *Arthritis Rheum* 50:3580–3590, 2004.

187. Sfikakis PP, Souliotis VL, Fragiadaki KG, et al: Increased expression of the FoxP3 functional marker of regulatory T cells following B cell depletion with rituximab in patients with lupus nephritis. *Clin Immunol* 123:66–73, 2007.

188. Iwata S, Saito K, Tokunaga M, et al: Phenotypic changes of lymphocytes in patients with systemic lupus erythematosus who are in longterm remission after B cell depletion therapy with rituximab. *J Rheumatol* 38:633–641, 2011.

189. Ramanujam M, Davidson A: Targeting of the immune system in systemic lupus erythematosus. *Expert Rev Mol Med* 10:e2, 2008.

190. Alexander T, Thiel A, Rosen O, et al: Depletion of autoreactive immunologic memory followed by autologous hematopoietic stem cell transplantation in patients with refractory SLE induces long-term remission through de novo generation of a juvenile and tolerant immune system. *Blood* 113:214–223, 2009.

191. De Albuquerque DA, Saxena V, Adams DE, et al: An ACE inhibitor reduces Th2 cytokines and TGF-beta1 and TGF-beta2 isoforms in murine lupus nephritis. *Kidney Int* 65:846–859, 2004.

192. Singh RR, Saxena V, Zang S, et al: Differential contribution of IL-4 and STAT6 vs STAT4 to the development of lupus nephritis. *J Immunol* 170:4818–4825, 2003.

193. Ramanujam M, Bethunaickan R, Huang W, et al: Selective blockade of BAFF for the prevention and treatment of systemic lupus erythematosus nephritis in NZM2410 mice. *Arthritis Rheum* 62:1457–1468, 2010.

194. Lernmark A, Agardh CD: Immunomodulation with human recombinant autoantigens. *Trends Immunol* 26:608–612, 2005.

Chapter 20

Autoantibodies

PART A Antibody Structure, Function, and Production

Jessica Manson

Under normal circumstances, the immune system is involved in host defense. A loss of self-tolerance leads to the development of autoimmunity. Some autoimmune diseases are mediated directly by autoreactive T cells, such as β islet cell destruction by CD8+ T cells in type 1 diabetes mellitus. The immunologic hallmark of SLE is the generation of autoantibodies, which are predominantly directed toward nuclear antigens. This section describes the normal structure and function of antibodies.

ANTIBODY STRUCTURE AND FUNCTION

All antibody molecules have a common core structure of two identical light chains and two identical heavy chains. The four chains are connected by disulfide bonds—each heavy chain to a light chain, and the heavy chains to each other. These four chains fold to form a globular motif, hence the term *immunoglobulin* (Figure 20-1).

Human antibody molecules are divided into five classes, or isotypes, IgA, IgD, IgE, IgG, and IgM, on the basis of their heavy chains. IgA and IgG molecules are further divided into subclasses. It is the heavy chain isotype of each antibody molecule that determines its effector mechanisms. There are two light chain isotypes, κ and λ, although no differences in function have been identified. In humans, usage of κ and λ light chains is approximately equal, but in mice the ratio is more like 10:1.[1] The structure and function of the different antibody isotypes are described in Table 20-1.

The specificity of an antibody is determined by the amino acid sequence of its antigen-binding site. The variability in sequence that accounts for the enormous diversity of the antibody repertoire is confined, as the name would suggest, to the variable regions of the heavy and light chains. Within these chains, there are three hypervariable regions, surrounded by relatively constant areas known as *framework regions*. The three heavy chain and three light chain hypervariable regions combine to form the antigen-binding site or complementarity-determining regions (CDRs).

Early investigation of immunoglobulin structure utilized the proteolytic enzyme papain.[2] Treatment with papain leads to disruption of the hinge region of the immunoglobulin molecule (see Figure 20-1) and the production of three fragments. Two of the fragments are identical, each consisting of a light chain plus the variable and first constant regions of a heavy chain, and were thus termed the antigen-binding fragments (Fab). The remaining fragment was noted to crystallize easily into diamond-shaped plates, and accordingly was called the Fc fragment.

ANTIBODY PRODUCTION AND THE GENERATION OF DIVERSITY

Cells of the B-cell lineage, which arise from the bone marrow, are the sole producers of antibody. B cells are capable of producing different isotypes of antibody at different stages of their maturation. Fully formed immunoglobulin molecules first appear at the immature B-cell stage, with the expression of surface IgM. At the mature B-cell stage, surface IgD can also be expressed. It is not until antigen is encountered and a B cell becomes activated that it can undergo isotype switching, which enables the expression of the other Ig isotypes and the increasing production of the secretory forms of antibody (which lack the transmembrane sequence).

Once a B cell has expressed an antibody molecule, affinity for its antigen can be increased by subtle changes in DNA encoding the variable regions, in an antigen-driven mechanism known as *affinity maturation*.

Loci for the different immunoglobulin chains are found on separate chromosomes.[1] In humans, the κ light (L) chain locus is on chromosome 2, the λ light chain locus on chromosome 22, and the heavy (H) chain locus on chromosome 14. Each locus contains multiple genes encoding the variable (V) and constant (C) regions. At the 5′ end of the locus are the V genes, and in humans, each heavy and light chain locus contains 100- to 200-V genes. However, many of these are nonfunctioning pseudogenes, and the actual number of genes that can be used is more like 50 V_H, 40 V_κ, and 30 V_λ. There is 1 gene in the human κ C region locus, and 3 to 6 genes in the λ locus. The heavy chain locus contains all the genes necessary to produce the different immunoglobulin isotypes. Between the V and C regions, there are additional genes named the joining (J) and diversity (D) segments. The latter are found only in the heavy chain locus. The third CDR of the variable chain is encoded by genes from the V region and the J/D segments. The structure of the human immunoglobulin chain loci are shown in Figure 20-2.

It is only in the developing B cell that the immunoglobulin genes rearrange, to allow the eventual production of functioning antibody. This mechanism is highly controlled. The heavy chains rearrange first, with one D and one J segment combining, before being joined by a V gene. RNA splicing leads to the combination of the VDJ with a constant region gene, most frequently μ in the first instance. The light chain genes are then combined in a similar manner, and the light and heavy chains assemble in the endoplasmic reticulum.

The enormous diversity in antibody specificity is achieved by a number of mechanisms. As discussed, there are multiple possible V, D, and J germline genes, and variability is further increased by different VDJ and different heavy and light chain combinations. In addition, small changes in the nucleotide sequences of junctional regions (i.e., between V, D, and J genes) occur from either imprecisions in the rearrangement mechanism or the addition of new nucleotides. Finally, after antigen is encountered, further diversity is

TABLE 20-1 Human Antibody Isotypes

ISOTYPE (FUNCTION)	SUBCLASS	HEAVY CHAIN	SERUM CONCENTRATION (MG/ML)	SECRETORY FORM	MOLECULAR WEIGHT* (KD)
IgA (mucosal immunity, ADCC)	IgA1	$\alpha 1$	3	Mono/di/trimer	150
	IgA2	$\alpha 2$	0.5	Mono/di/trimer	
IgD (BCR)	No	δ	Trace	n/a	180
IgE (Hypersensitivity, ADCC)	No	ε	Trace	Monomer	190
IgG (complement activation, opsonization, ADCC, neonatal immunity)	IgG1	$\gamma 1$	9	Monomer	150
	IgG2	$\gamma 2$	3	Monomer	150
	IgG3	$\gamma 3$	1	Monomer	150
	IgG4	$\gamma 4$	0.5	Monomer	150
IgM (complement activation, BCR)	No	μ	1.5	Pentamer	950

ADCC, antibody-dependent cell-mediated cytotoxicity; BCR, B-cell receptor; Ig, immunoglobulin.
*Molecular weight of the monomer.

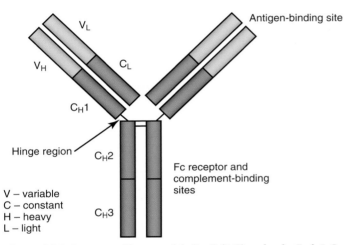

FIGURE 20-1 **Structure of immunoglobulin G (IgG) molecule.** Each IgG molecule is made up of two heavy and two light chains. The antigen-binding site is formed by the juxtaposition of the heavy and light chain variable domains.

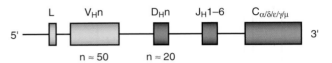

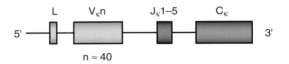

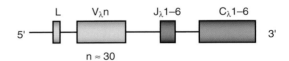

L leader
V variable
D diversity
J joining
C constant

FIGURE 20-2 **Human immunoglobulin chain loci.** The human immunoglobulin genes are arranged as shown. The number (n) relates to functional genes only. Leader peptides are involved in guiding protein synthesis. $C_{a/d/e/g/m}$; H, heavy; L, light.

achieved by somatic mutation, which accounts for affinity maturation of antibody, as described previously.[1,3]

References

1. Abbas AK, Lichtman AH, Pober JS: *Cellular and molecular immunology,* ed 2, Philadelphia, 1994, WB Saunders.
2. Porter RR: Structural studies of immunoglobulins. *Science* 180:713–716, 1973.
3. Janeway CA, Travers P, Walport M, et al: *Immunobiology: the immune system in health and disease,* ed 5, New York, 2001, Garland Science.

PART B Antibodies to DNA, Histones, and Nucleosomes

Anisur Rahman, Jessica Manson, and David Isenberg

ANTI-DNA ANTIBODIES IN LUPUS: HISTORICAL OVERVIEW

Anti-DNA antibodies were the first autoantibodies described in patients with systemic lupus erythematosus (SLE), having been reported by four separate research groups in 1957 (reviewed in reference 1). Over the next 50 years, evidence obtained through a variety of approaches suggested that these antibodies were important in the pathogenesis of the disease, that is, that they had direct and damaging effects on tissues. This suggestion is particularly true of antibodies to double-stranded DNA (anti-dsDNA) as opposed to single stranded DNA (anti-ssDNA).

Some of this evidence was derived from serologic studies in cohorts of patients with SLE. These studies showed that whereas anti-dsDNA antibodies can be found in up to 70% to 80% of patients with SLE at some time during the course of their disease, these antibodies are very rarely found in patients with other autoimmune conditions and in healthy controls. Using stored samples taken from American military recruits in whom SLE later developed, Arbuckle showed that in some cases anti-dsDNA antibodies are present several years before the onset of clinical disease.[2]

Furthermore, in many cases there is a relationship between disease activity and the serum titer of anti-dsDNA. For example, in an early study Schur and Sandson looked at serum samples taken from 96 patients with SLE (44 with nephritis) over a 2-year period.[2a] Anti-dsDNA and anti-ssDNA were found in more than 60% of patients with active nephritis but in only 10% to 15% of those with inactive disease. Characteristically, exacerbations of nephritis in these patients were preceded by the appearance of anti-DNA antibodies and a drop in serum complement. In a larger study, Swaak showed that a rise in levels of anti-dsDNA antibodies preceded renal flares in SLE,[3] and subsequent independent studies also showed that rises in anti-dsDNA antibody level were associated with flares of activity, either in the kidney or in other organs. In fact, one of the main disease activity indices in SLE—the Systemic Lupus Erythematosus Disease Activity Index (SLEDAI) actually includes raised anti-dsDNA antibodies as a scorable element of disease activity. Both isotype and binding properties of anti-DNA antibodies affect association with disease activity. Immunoglobulin (Ig) G anti-dsDNA antibodies are particularly important. Perhaps the clearest evidence for their importance came from a Japanese study in which renal biopsies were carried out in 40 patients with untreated lupus nephritis and the histologic degree of nephritis was compared with levels of IgG and IgM antibodies to dsDNA and ssDNA.[4] Levels of IgG anti-dsDNA were more closely correlated with nephritis than IgM anti-dsDNA or anti-ssDNA of either isotype.

In parallel with these serologic studies, other investigators showed that anti-DNA antibodies are present in inflamed organs of patients with SLE, with the clearest evidence relating to lupus nephritis. In a seminal experiment in 1967, Koffler showed deposition of IgG and complement in glomeruli of patients who had died from lupus nephritis.[5] Eluates from these kidneys bound nuclei, and this binding could be partially inhibited by the addition of dsDNA.[5] Winfield showed that glomerular eluates from autopsy specimens of patients who had died from lupus nephritis contained higher-avidity anti-dsDNA antibodies than serum from the same patients.[6] It is important to note, however, that other autopsy studies have shown that antibodies with different specificities (e.g., Ro, La, Sm, and C1q) can also be eluted from glomeruli of patients with lupus nephritis.

MEASUREMENT OF ANTI-dsDNA ANTIBODIES

The initial screen for anti-dsDNA antibodies usually involves testing for the presence of an antinuclear antibody (ANA), either by immunofluorescence (IF), or in an enzyme-linked immunosorbent assay (ELISA). Diffuse or homogeneous staining noted on IF testing is suggestive of binding to the DNA/histone complex, chromatin.

Anti-dsDNA antibody titer is most commonly measured by ELISA. The *Crithidia luciliae* IF assay is also widely used. This test detects antibodies that bind to the dsDNA in the kinetoplast of the *Crithidia*. It is relatively specific for anti-dsDNA antibodies. In particular, because the kinetoplast consists solely of dsDNA, anti-ssDNA antibodies do not bind. In contrast, ELISAs supposedly for detecting anti-dsDNA often show cross-reacts with anti-ssDNA and capture low-affinity antibodies of little pathologic consequence.

Historically, anti-dsDNA antibodies were measured in the Farr radioimmunoassay. The advantages of this assay are its accuracy and the fact that it detects antibodies with high avidity, which are considered to be more important clinically. The disadvantage, and the reason that the Farr assay is now rarely used routinely, is that the method involves the use of radioisotopes.

New forms of ELISA in which the source of dsDNA and the reaction conditions have been optimized are reported to give specificity for high-avidity antibodies as good as that of the Farr assay and are likely to come into more widespread use in the future. In a longitudinal study of 16 patients with newly diagnosed lupus nephritis, Manson found that one of these assays showed the same degree of association with measures of renal disease (such as urine protein/creatinine ratio) as measurement of antinucleosome level.[7] In fact

there is no strong evidence that replacing the currently available anti-dsDNA ELISAs with antinucleosome assays would be beneficial in the management of the majority of patients with SLE. There is a subgroup of patients with persistently high anti-dsDNA despite having no disease activity (serologically active, clinically quiescent [SACQ]). In these patients with SACQ disease, Ng reported that high antinucleosome levels were associated with a higher number of disease flares and reduced time to first flare over the next 5 years.[8] Thus, measuring antinucleosome levels might be worthwhile in patients with SACQ disease.

WORK FROM EXPERIMENTAL MODELS EMPHASING THE POTENTIAL IMPORTANCE OF ANTI-dsDNA ANTIBODIES

Although it is important to study patients to ensure clinical relevance, strong evidence for a directly pathogenic role of anti-dsDNA antibodies comes from work using animal models. The major studies have been reviewed in detail elsewhere.[1] Various groups have observed the effect of monoclonal anti-dsDNA antibodies in nonautoimmune mice strains. Ravirajan generated a human panel of anti-dsDNA antibody–producing hybridoma cells from the lymphocytes of patients with SLE.[9] Following intraperitoneal implantation of hybridoma cells producing one such antibody, RH14, severe combined immunodeficient (SCID) mice went on to demonstrate significant proteinuria with human immunoglobulin deposition within the kidney. Furthermore, electron microscopy findings were very suggestive of lupus nephritis–like disease, with mesangial cell hypertrophy, mesangial and endothelial cell deposits, and podocyte foot process effacement. It is important to note, however, that these pathogenic effects are not always observed. A second DNA-binding antibody, generated from a different patient, and noted to have much less diverse antigen binding in vitro, produced only minimal proteinuria and did not deposit in the mouse kidney or engender the pathologic changes observed with RH14.

Raz, using an isolation rat kidney perfusion system, showed that some murine monoclonal anti-dsDNA antibodies (and affinity-purified human anti-dsDNA antibodies) were able to increase proteinuria significantly.[10]

There is a significant body of work that examines the effect that small changes in the antigen-binding site have on antibody-binding properties in vitro and in vivo. By studying panels of murine[11] and human[12] monoclonal anti-dsDNA antibodies, it has been shown that there is a high prevalence of arginine, asparagine, and lysine residues in the complementarity-determining regions (CDRs) of anti-dsDNA antibodies. It is proposed that the presence and position of these amino acids facilitate the antibody-DNA interaction. The accumulation of these particular amino acids is driven by *somatic hypermutation*—the accumulation of beneficial mutations, which increase antigen affinity and promote survival of the B-cell clone.

HOW PATHOGENIC ANTI-dsDNA ANTIBODIES BIND TO TISSUES: THE IMPORTANCE OF BINDING TO NUCLEOSOMES

The previous section summarized evidence that circulating anti-dsDNA antibodies are deposited in tissues such as the kidney and cause inflammation. The mechanism whereby this process occurs has been studied intensively, and there are a number of theories that are not mutually exclusive. Within a single patient, these antibodies may be deposited by different mechanisms in different tissues or even within a single tissue. Though initial theories proposed that immune complexes of anti-dsDNA with dsDNA would be deposited in tissues, this now seems unlikely because there is very little circulating free dsDNA in human serum. Analysis of the molecular weight of DNA found in the circulation of patients with SLE showed that it occurred in fragments of 200 bp (or multiples thereof). The explanation is that this dsDNA is in the form of oligonucleosomes formed as debris from the breakdown of apoptotic cells. Nucleosomes are the base units of nuclear chromatin and consist of approximately 200 bp of dsDNA wrapped round a histone core. The identification of nucleosomes,[13] rather than free dsDNA, as the key antigen recognized by "anti-dsDNA" antibodies in SLE resolves a number of questions, as follows.

First, because dsDNA is present inside the nuclei of cells, it had been difficult to understand how anti-dsDNA antibodies could access their antigen. However, apoptotic cells release blebs in which previously intracellular antigens, such as nucleosomes, are exposed on the surface. The removal of this apoptotic debris is known to be slower in patients with SLE than in healthy controls,[14] so that such patients possess larger amounts of circulating nucleosome material, which could interact with antinucleosome antibodies.

Second, the concept that the pathogenic antibodies in SLE circulate in the form of nucleosome/antinucleosome complexes provided a possible mechanism for deposition of these complexes in the kidney and skin. This mechanism has been described and investigated by a Dutch group, who propose that positively charged histones in the nucleosomes of the nucleosome/antinucleosome complex interact with negatively charged heparan sulfate in the renal basement membrane.[15] In a series of elegant experiments in a perfused rat kidney model these investigators showed that deposition of IgG could be achieved by adding histones, then DNA, then antinucleosome antibody or by adding nucleosome/antinucleosome complexes generated in vitro. Deposition was reduced by prior perfusion with heparatinase, which removed heparan sulfate. The group has also shown deposition of antinucleosome antibodies in the skin of patients with lupus nephritis. Kalaaji has used electron microscopy to show that IgG in the kidneys of both patients with lupus nephritis and murine models of lupus colocalize with electron-dense extracellular deposits of chromatin, a finding consistent with the model that antibody-nucleosome interactions are important in the pathogenesis of lupus nephritis.[16]

Supporting these histologic findings are serologic studies showing that antinucleosome antibodies are present at a high prevalence in patients with SLE and may be related to disease activity. Studies by various groups have shown raised levels of antinucleosome antibodies in between 56% and 86% of patients with SLE.[17] The specificity of this test depends on the purity of the nucleosomes used.

CROSS-REACTION OF ANTI-DNA ANTIBODIES WITH INTRACELLULAR ANTIGENS

An alternative to the nucleosome-dependent mechanism just described is direct cross-reaction of anti-dsDNA antibodies with protein antigens within tissues. The major antigens implicated in this theory are laminin and α-actinin. In a murine model of lupus, treatment with peptides derived from laminin reduced renal antibody deposition and produced some amelioration in renal disease.

The antigen α-actinin-4 is produced by renal podocytes in glomeruli and plays an important role in the function of these cells. Point mutations in the α-actinin-4 gene cause a form of focal segmental glomerulosclerosis with nephrotic syndrome—although unlike lupus nephritis, this glomerulosclerosis is not characterized by deposition of antibodies and complement. Two groups working independently in mouse models of lupus showed that the ability of some murine monoclonal ANAs to cause glomerulonephritis after passive transfer depended on the ability to bind α-actinin rather than dsDNA. Subsequent clinical studies showed that anti–α-actinin antibodies are present in patients with SLE (though not specific for that disease) and that in some cohorts positivity for these antibodies might distinguish patients with and without renal involvement. However, most patients with lupus nephritis do not have anti–α-actinin antibodies, and a longitudinal study in 16 patients with newly diagnosed lupus nephritis showed that levels of anti-dsDNA and antinucleosome antibodies were much more closely associated with the presence of lupus nephritis and with clinical markers of renal function during the follow-up period than were levels of anti–α-actinin.[7] Currently, therefore, interaction with nucleosomes seems likely to be the predominant mechanism for renal deposition of pathogenic antibodies in lupus nephritis.

Antihistone Antibodies

Though the antinucleosome antibodies just described can bind to histones, the term *antihistone antibodies* is generally used to refer to a different type of antibody detected by ELISA using histones as the test antigen. Antihistone positivity is particularly characteristic of patients with drug-induced lupus caused by exposure to drugs such as hydralazine and procainamide. In general these patients have mild disease with a low frequency of nephritis that remits when the drug is stopped. However, patients with spontaneous (non–drug-induced) SLE can also test positive for antihistone antibodies, as shown by Gioud in 32 of 63 patients with SLE but only 1 of 70 patients with other rheumatic diseases.[18]

STRUCTURE AND ORIGIN OF PATHOGENIC ANTI-dsDNA AND ANTINUCLEOSOME ANTIBODIES

The fact that serologic studies showed that IgG anti-dsDNA antibodies were particularly closely related to disease activity in patients with SLE was supported by studies in which passive transfer of monoclonal human or murine anti-dsDNA antibodies caused glomerulonephritis in mice. In these studies, a consistent finding was that only some antibodies would cause nephritis. As previously described, in experiments in which six different hybridomas secreting monoclonal human IgG anti-dsDNA antibodies were introduced into severe combined immunodeficiency (SCID) mice, only two caused deposition similar to that seen in lupus nephritis.[9] A number of groups carried out sequence analysis of monoclonal human[12] and murine[11] anti-DNA antibodies, some of which were pathogenic in mouse models. The conclusion was that pathogenicity was more likely to be a property of antibodies that had gone through the processes of class switching and somatic mutation. The somatic mutations in these antibodies were clustered in the CDRs, implying that they had been accumulated nonrandomly as a result of antigen drive. This process typically occurs in germinal centers.

A B-lymphocyte clone, in the presence of T-helper cells, is stimulated to divide by antigen interacting with its surface immunoglobulin. The greater the affinity of the surface antibody for antigen, the more powerful the stimulus to divide and the faster the clone grows. As the cells divide, some incorporate somatic mutations owing to a specific hypermutation mechanism that operates only in B lymphocytes at this stage of their development and acts only upon the rearranged immunoglobulin sequences. Thus the different B cells in the clone contain a range of expressed antibody sequences that differ only at sites of somatic mutation. Any B cell that picks up a mutation that enhances binding to the driving antigen is stimulated to divide more strongly than its neighbors and has more descendants. Thus over time, the clone becomes dominated by cells containing mutations at positions in the sequence that improve binding to antigen. These positions are usually in or around the CDRs, because the CDRs encode the antigen-binding site. The accumulation of these mutations leads to a gradual increase in the antigen-binding affinity of the antibody secreted by the clone (affinity maturation). Within anti-DNA antibodies, it appears that mutations to the residues arginine, asparagine, and lysine within CDRs are particularly important to facilitate binding to dsDNA,[11,12] although this is not a universal rule and there are several examples of antibodies in which increased numbers of such residues are not associated with greater binding to dsDNA.

Which antigen drives the production of these high-affinity, somatically mutated IgG antibodies? The ideal antigen for this purpose would be one that is present in larger quantities in patients with SLE and that carries epitopes for both B cells and T-helper cells. Nucleosomes fit the bill. As noted previously, they are present on the surface of apoptotic blebs, which are not cleared quickly in patients with SLE.[14] This material can therefore be carried to lymphoid tissues, where it can stimulate both T-helper cells (via histone epitopes) and B cells that can then secrete antinucleosome antibodies.

If the nucleosome or apoptotic material really do provide the antigenic stimulus for development of somatically mutated autoantibodies in SLE, one would expect reversal of the mutations to reduce affinity for those antigens. Evidence supporting this expectation was produced by experiments in which antibodies were expressed from cloned cDNA in vitro and the cloned DNA was then altered to allow expression of antibodies in which one or more somatic mutations had been reverted to the germline sequence. The properties of the expressed antibodies containing different numbers of somatic mutations were then compared, and several researchers reported that mutations at single sites could alter binding to apoptotic cells, dsDNA, and other antigens typically found on apoptotic blebs. Thus, Cocca, who reverted a single mutation from arginine to serine at position 53 in CDR3 of the heavy chain of the pathogenic murine anti-dsDNA antibody 3H9, found that this change simultaneously reduced strength of binding to DNA, phospholipids, beta 2-glycoprotein I, and apoptotic cells.[19] Similarly, Wellman showed that three somatic mutations in CDRs of the pathogenic human anti-dsDNA antibody 33C9 were critical for binding to dsDNA, nucleosomes, and apoptotic cells.[20]

CAN MEASURING ANTI-dsDNA LEVELS HELP US MANAGE PATIENTS WITH SLE?

If levels of anti-dsDNA antibodies rise during periods of high disease activity, could we improve our management of patients with SLE by treating patients when these levels rise but before a clinical flare becomes apparent? The first trial to investigate this possibility was carried out by the Bootsma group in the mid-1990s.[21] They followed a cohort of 156 patients with SLE and identified 46 who experienced a rise in dsDNA. These 46 patients were randomly allocated to receive either conventional treatment (i.e., the dose of steroids was increased only if clinical symptoms of a flare developed) or increased prednisolone dose right away (the increase was 30 mg/day, followed by tapering over 18 weeks). The group in whom prednisolone dose was increased straightaway whenever anti-dsDNA level rose did have significantly fewer flares of disease but also experienced more adverse effects of steroids, and more than one quarter of this group discontinued the trial. A later study using a shorter course of higher steroid dose suggested that patients in whom both anti-dsDNA and C3a levels rose experienced significantly fewer flares when treated with prednisolone than when treated with placebo.[22]

Could we treat patients with SLE by targeting the production of anti-dsDNA antibodies? Because antibodies are produced by B lymphocytes, anti–B cell therapies would be expected to reduce anti-dsDNA levels. Both the anti-CD20 agent rituximab[23] and the anti–B lymphocyte stimulator agent belimumab[24] have been studied in randomized placebo-controlled clinical trials. The belimumab trial did show a benefit of drug over placebo, whereas the rituximab trial did not, although there is still much discussion about possible reasons for this difference, including the different trial designs and outcome measures used in the two trials. A number of previous open studies had suggested that treatment with rituximab is effective in many patients with SLE and leads to a fall in anti-dsDNA levels.[25] We await conclusive information about whether levels of anti-dsDNA antibodies can be used to guide selection of patients for treatment with either rituximab or belimumab.

In contrast, an ambitious attempt to treat SLE by specific deletion of B cells producing anti-dsDNA antibodies appears to have ended in failure. The therapeutic agent, called abetimus sodium, consisted of four oligonucleotide chains bound to an inert carrier. The theory was that the oligonucleotides would engage anti-dsDNA antibodies on the surface of B cells (and would thus not interact with any cells not producing anti-dsDNA antibodies). The lack of a T-cell epitope on the drug would mean that the engaged B cells could not recruit T-cell help and so would die. Treatment with abetimus sodium led to reduction of anti-dsDNA antibody levels and clinical improvements in a mouse model of SLE. In human trials, anti-dsDNA levels fell,[26] but it was not possible to demonstrate any significant difference between drug and placebo in the ability to delay the onset of renal flare.

SUMMARY

Anti-dsDNA antibodies were first reported in the blood of patients with SLE more than 50 years ago. Since then, a large body of evidence has been amassed to show that these antibodies play a critical role in pathogenesis of the disease, though it seems that this effect occurs via binding to nucleosomes rather than to free dsDNA. Thus the pathogenic antibodies should more accurately be called antinucleosome antibodies, which develop because the immune system is triggered by nucleosomes on apoptotic cell debris. This debris is not cleared efficiently in patients with SLE. Measurement of anti-dsDNA antibodies in clinical serum samples is routine in patients with SLE and helps clinicians assess disease activity. Therapies directed at the B cells that make anti-dsDNA antibodies show great promise for the treatment of SLE.

References

1. Isenberg DA, Manson JJ, Ehrenstein MR, et al: Fifty years of anti-ds DNA antibodies: are we approaching journey's end? *Rheumatology (Oxford)* 46:1052–1056, 2007.
2. Arbuckle MR, McClain MT, Rubertone MV, et al: Development of autoantibodies before the clinical onset of systemic lupus erythematosus. *N Engl J Med* 349:1526–1533, 2003.
2a. Schur PH, Sandson J: Immunologic factors and clinical activity in systemic lupus erythematosus. *N Engl J Med* 278:533–538, 1968.
3. Swaak AJ, Aarden LA, Statius van Eps LW, et al: Anti-dsDNA and complement profiles as prognostic guides in systemic lupus erythematosus. *Arthritis Rheum* 22:226–235, 1979.
4. Okamura M, Kanayama Y, Amastu K, et al: Significance of enzyme linked immunosorbent assay (ELISA) for antibodies to double stranded and single stranded DNA in patients with lupus nephritis: correlation with severity of renal histology. *Ann Rheum Dis* 52:14–20, 1993.
5. Koffler D, Schur PH, Kunkel HG: Immunological studies concerning the nephritis of systemic lupus erythematosus. *J Exp Med* 126:607–624, 1967.
6. Winifred JB, Faiferman I, Hoffler D: Avidity of anti-DNA antibodies in several IgG glomerular eluates from patients with systemic lupus erythematosus. Association of high avidity anti-native DNA antibody with glomerulonephritis. *J Clin Invest* 59:90–96, 1977.
7. Manson JJ, Ma A, Rogers P, et al: Relationship between anti-dsDNA, anti-nucleosome and anti-alpha-actinin antibodies and markers of renal disease in patients with lupus nephritis: a prospective longitudinal study. *Arthritis Res Ther* 11:R154, 2009.
8. Ng KP, Manson JJ, Rahman A, et al: Association of antinucleosome antibodies with disease flare in serologically active clinically quiescent patients with systemic lupus erythematosus. *Arthritis Rheum* 55:900–904, 2006.
9. Ravirajan CT, Rahman MA, Papadaki L, et al: Genetic, structural and functional properties of an IgG DNA-binding monoclonal antibody from a lupus patient with nephritis. *Eur J Immunol* 28:339–350, 1998.
10. Raz E, Brezis M, Rosenmann E, et al: Anti dsDNA antibodies bind directly to renal antigens and induce kidney dysfunction in the isolated perforated kidney. *J Immunol* 142:3076–3082, 1989.
11. Radic MZ, Weigert M: Genetic and structural evidence for antigen selection of anti-DNA antibodies. *Annu Rev Immunol* 12:487–520, 1994.
12. Rahman A, Giles I, Haley J, et al: Systematic analysis of sequences of anti-DNA antibodies—relevance to theories of origin and pathogenicity. *Lupus* 11:807–823, 2002.
13. Martensen ES, Fenton KA, Rekring OP: Lupus nephritis—the control role of nucleosomes revisited. *Am J Pathol* 172:275–283, 2008.
14. Munoz LE, Gaipl US, Franz S, et al: SLE—a disease of clearance deficiency? *Rheumatology (Oxford)* 44:1101–1107, 2005.
15. van Bavel CC, Fenton KA, Rekvig OP, et al: Glomerular targets of nephritogenic autoantibodies in systemic lupus erythematosus. *Arthritis Rheum* 58:1892–1899, 2008.
16. Kalaaji M, Sturfelt G, Mjelle JE, et al: Critical comparative analyses of anti-alpha-actinin and glomerulus-bound antibodies in human and murine lupus nephritis. *Arthritis Rheum* 54:914–926, 2006.
17. Amoura Z, Koutouzov S, Chabre H, et al: Presence of antinucleosome autoantibodies in a restricted set of connective tissue diseases: antinucleosome antibodies of the IgG3 subclass are markers of renal pathogenicity in systemic lupus erythematosus. *Arthritis Rheum* 43:76–84, 2000.

18. Gioud M, Kaci MA, Monier JC: Histone antibodies in systemic lupus erythematosus. A possible diagnostic tool. *Arthritis Rheum* 25:407–413, 1982.

19. Cocca BA, Seal SN, D'Agnillo P, et al: Structural basis for autoantibody recognition of phosphatidylserine-beta 2 glycoprotein I and apoptotic cells. *Proc Natl Acad Sci U S A* 98:13826–13831, 2001.

20. Wellmann U, Letz M, Herrmann M, et al: The evolution of human anti–double-stranded DNA autoantibodies. *Proc Natl Acad Sci U S A* 102:9258–9263, 2005.

21. Bootsma H, Spronk P, Derksen R, et al: Prevention of relapses in systemic lupus erythematosus. *Lancet* 345:1595–1599, 1995.

22. Tseng C, Buyon JP, Kim M, et al: The effect of moderate-dose corticosteroids in preventing severe flares in patients with serologically active, but clinically stable, systemic lupus erythematosus. *Arthritis Rheum* 54:3623–3632, 2006.

23. Merrill JT, Neuwelt CM, Wallace DJ, et al: Efficacy and safety of rituximab in moderately-to-severely active systemic lupus erythematosus: the randomized, double-blind, phase II/III systemic lupus erythematosus evaluation of rituximab trial. *Arthritis Rheum* 62:222–233, 2010.

24. Navarra SV, Guzman RM, Gallacher AE, et al: Efficacy and safety of belimumab in patients with active systemic lupus erythematosus: a randomised, placebo-controlled, phase 3 trial. *Lancet* 377:721–731, 2011.

25. Fava C, Isenberg D: B cell depletion therapy in SLE—what are the current prospects for its acceptance. *Nat Rev Rheum* 5:711–716, 2009.

26. Alarcon-Segovia D, Tumlin JA, Furie RA, et al: LJP 394 for the prevention of renal flare in patients with systemic lupus erythematosus: results from a randomized, double-blind, placebo-controlled study. *Arthritis Rheum* 48:442–454, 2003.

PART C Anti-lipoprotein and Anti–Endothelial Cell Antibodies

Anisur Rahman

The study of anti-lipoprotein antibodies in SLE has been motivated particularly by their possible involvement in the observed higher risk of development of cardiovascular disease in patients with SLE. The particular antigenic specificities studied have been antibodies to high-density lipoprotein (HDL) and its major component, apolipoprotein A1 (apo A-1).

HDL can protect against cardiovascular disease by several mechanisms.[1] These include reverse cholesterol transport (removing cholesterol from atherosclerotic plaques to the liver) and the presence of antioxidants, such as paraoxonase, attached to HDL. These antioxidants can inhibit oxidation of low-density lipoprotein, which is protective because oxidized low-density lipoprotein (ox-LDL) is a major promoter of atherosclerosis.

Delgado Alves, in a study of 32 patients with SLE, showed that they had higher IgG anti-HDL antibody levels and lower serum paraoxonase activity than 20 age- and sex-matched healthy controls.[2] A further study confirmed that IgG anti-HDL antibodies were higher in patients with SLE than in healthy controls and showed that the same was true for IgG anti–apo A-1 antibodies.[3] Anti–apo A-1 antibodies are of particular interest because of studies (in patients without SLE) showing that high levels of such antibodies are associated with increased risk of coronary disease. Batuca suggested that anti–apo A-1 and anti-HDL levels were higher in patients with disease flare at the time of sampling than in those with inactive disease.[3] However, one might argue that disease activity over a prolonged period prior to the date of sampling would be more relevant to the production of antibodies than the activity on the date of the sample. Therefore O'Neill carried out a retrospective study of samples from 37 patients with lupus with persistently high activity, 40 with persistently low activity, and 32 healthy controls.[4] Activity was defined using the British Isles Lupus Assessment Group (BILAG) index, which rates each of eight organs/systems between A (highly active) and E (never active). Persistently high activity was defined as BILAG A or B scores on at least three occasions and in at least two

separate systems over the previous 2 years. Persistently low activity was defined as no A or B scores in any system over the previous 2 years. The mean IgG anti-apo A-1 antibody levels were higher in the high activity group than in either the low activity group ($P < 0.01$) or the healthy control group ($P < 0.001$) and higher in the low activity group than in the healthy control group ($P < 0.05$).[4] Like the Batuca group,[3] O'Neill and I found raised levels of these antibodies at the time of a flare.[4] They did not demonstrate higher levels in patients with previous cardiovascular disease than in those without cardiovascular disease.

In a Finnish study, Vaarala showed raised levels of anti–ox-LDL antibodies in 80% of 61 patients with SLE. In many cases these antibodies cross-reacted with phospholipids.[5] Subsequently a Spanish group measured levels of anti–ox-LDL antibodies in 49 patients with SLE at two time points 3 to 4 months apart.[6] Though the majority of the patients tested positive for anti-ox-LDL antibodies at each time point, the level of anti–ox-LDL changed significantly in 15 of the 49 patients between the two measurements. Higher anti–ox-LDL antibody levels were associated with higher anti-dsDNA antibodies, higher disease activity, and lower complement levels.[6]

ANTI–ENDOTHELIAL CELL ANTIBODIES

Anti–endothelial cell antibodies (AECAs) in patients with SLE were first described by Cines in 1984 using a solid phase radioimmunoassay.[7] Comparing sera from 27 patients with SLE and 86 healthy control subjects, this group found significantly higher levels of AECAs in the patients with SLE.[7]

D'Cruz in 1991 measured AECAs by ELISA, in which live human umbilical vein endothelial cells (HUVECs) were used as the substrate and antibodies of IgM, IgG, and IgA isotypes were detected.[8] The researchers compared 57 patients with lupus nephritis, 50 with lupus but no nephritis, 10 controls with nonlupus autoimmune diseases, and 70 healthy controls. They found that the level of AECAs was significantly higher in the lupus nephritis group than in the nonnephritis group and higher in both lupus groups than in controls. Higher levels of AECAs were associated with higher activity scores on renal biopsy in the patients with nephritis, and AECA levels fell after treatment in 16 patients for whom longitudinal data were available.[8] There was no correlation between AECA and anti-dsDNA antibody levels. The researchers therefore proposed that AECAs could be a marker of disease activity separate from anti-dsDNA, although they did not identify the antigen bound by AECAs on the endothelial cells. In fact, AECA measurement has not come into routine use as a measure of disease activity in SLE, perhaps owing to the relative difficulty of carrying out an ELISA on live cultured cells or to the lack of studies comparing disease activity with AECA levels in larger populations of patients with SLE. A later review reiterates that the actual antigens bound by AECAs have not been well characterized.[9]

Because endothelial cells play a crucial role in several organs affected by SLE, it was natural to postulate that AECAs might exert effects on these cells that were relevant to the development of tissue damage in these organs. Tannenbaum, after incubating HUVECs with serum from 16 patients with SLE and 21 healthy controls, found that 14 of the 16 SLE samples stimulated expression of tissue factor (a potent procoagulant).[10] However, it is possible that antiphospholipid (aPL) or anti–beta 2 glycoprotein I antibodies in the samples could have contributed to this effect. In a subsequent experiment, Papa excluded this possibility by studying purified IgG samples from 8 patients with SLE who tested positive for AECAs in the cell-based ELISA but negative for antiphospholipid and anti–beta 2 glycoprotein I antibodies.[11] When HUVECs were cultured with these samples, the response was an increase in expression of adhesion molecules and secretion of interleukin-6. Consistent with the increased adhesion molecule expression, HUVECs cultured with these SLE samples showed increased adhesion of monocytes.[11] Yazici subsequently demonstrated stimulation of the same outcome measures in HUVECs treated with a human monoclonal IgG AECA derived from a B-cell clone from a patient with SLE.[12] Although

Western blot analysis suggested that this monoclonal antibody bound a single 42-kD band in the cell membrane of human microvascular endothelial cells (HMECs), the exact nature of this antigen was not established.

In summary, although there was significant interest in the possible role of AECAs in SLE 10 to 15 years ago, it has not persisted in later work, and exactly which antigen specificities were being detected by the AECA assay is not clear.

References

1. Hahn BH: Should antibodies to high-density lipoprotein cholesterol and its components be measured in all systemic lupus erythematosus patients to predict risk of atherosclerosis? *Arthritis Rheum* 62:639–642, 2010.
2. Delgado Alves J, Ames PR, Donohue S, et al: Antibodies to high-density lipoprotein and beta2-glycoprotein I are inversely correlated with paraoxonase activity in systemic lupus erythematosus and primary antiphospholipid syndrome. *Arthritis Rheum* 46:2686–2694, 2002.
3. Batuca JR, Ames PR, Amaral M, et al: Anti-atherogenic and anti-inflammatory properties of high-density lipoprotein are affected by specific antibodies in systemic lupus erythematosus. *Rheumatology (Oxford, England)* 48:26–31, 2009.
4. O'Neill SG, Giles I, Lambrianides A, et al: Antibodies to apolipoprotein A-I, high-density lipoprotein, and C-reactive protein are associated with disease activity in patients with systemic lupus erythematosus. *Arthritis Rheum* 62:845–854, 2010.
5. Vaarala O, Alfthan G, Jauhiainen M, et al: Crossreaction between antibodies to oxidised low-density lipoprotein and to cardiolipin in systemic lupus erythematosus. *Lancet* 341:923–925, 1993.
6. Gomez-Zumaquero JM, Tinahones FJ, De Ramon E, et al: Association of biological markers of activity of systemic lupus erythematosus with levels of anti-oxidized low-density lipoprotein antibodies. *Rheumatology (Oxford, England)* 43:510–513, 2004.
7. Cines DB, Lyss AP, Reeber M, et al: Presence of complement-fixing anti-endothelial cell antibodies in systemic lupus erythematosus. *J Clin Invest* 73:611–625, 1984.
8. D'Cruz DP, Houssiau FA, Ramirez G, et al: Antibodies to endothelial cells in systemic lupus erythematosus: a potential marker for nephritis and vasculitis. *Clin Exp Immunol* 85:254–261, 1991.
9. Belizna C, Duijvestijn A, Hamidou M, et al: Antiendothelial cell antibodies in vasculitis and connective tissue disease. *Ann Rheum Dis* 65:1545–1550, 2006.
10. Tannenbaum SH, Finko R, Cines DB: Antibody and immune complexes induce tissue factor production by human endothelial cells. *J Immunol* 137:1532–1537, 1986.
11. Papa ND, Raschi E, Moroni G, et al: Anti-endothelial cell IgG fractions from systemic lupus erythematosus patients bind to human endothelial cells and induce a pro-adhesive and a pro-inflammatory phenotype in vitro. *Lupus* 8:423–429, 1999.
12. Yazici ZA, Raschi E, Patel A, et al: Human monoclonal anti-endothelial cell IgG-derived from a systemic lupus erythematosus patient binds and activates human endothelium in vitro. *Int Immunol* 13:349–357, 2001.

PART D Anti-C1q Antibodies
C.G.M. Kallenberg

Antibodies to components of the innate immune system are frequently detected in the sera of patients with SLE. Among these are antibodies against various components of the complement system. Antibodies to C1q have drawn particular attention because they have been suggested to be involved in the pathogenesis of lupus nephritis and to serve as markers of renal disease activity in SLE. This section focuses on the clinical associations and pathogenic potential of anti-C1q autoantibodies (anti-C1q) in SLE.

ANTIGENIC SPECIFICITY AND METHODS OF DETECTION OF ANTI-C1q

C1q is a complex molecule consisting of collagenous portions ending up with globular heads; one molecule is composed of six copies of three different chains each, so giving the impression of a bundle of tulips. Anti-C1q bind to the collagenous portions, which apparently

TABLE 20-2 Autoantibodies to C1q: Clinical Associations

CLINICAL SYNDROME	% OF PATIENTS POSITIVE	NUMBER OF PATIENTS STUDIED
Hypocomplementemic urticarial vasculitis	100%	(n = 174)
Felty syndrome	76%	(n = 21)
SLE	33%	(n = 591)
Lupus nephritis*	63%	(n = 95)
Rheumatoid vasculitis	77%	(n = 31)
Sjögren syndrome	13%	(n = 39)
Membranoproliferative glomerulonephritis	54%	(n = 68)
Immunoglobulin A nephropathy	31%	(n = 36)
Healthy individuals	5%	(n = 140)

*More frequently in proliferative lupus nephritis.

are the main immunogenic region of the molecule. Complexed IgG, as part of an immune complex, binds mainly to the globular portions of C1q, and C1q-binding assays have extensively been used for the detection of circulating immune complexes. In these assays, purified C1q is coated to a solid phase, immune complexes in serum or plasma samples are allowed to bind, and bound complexed IgG is detected with heterologous anti-IgG antibodies. The autoantibodies to C1q bind to neoepitopes only exposed on bound C1q and not present on soluble C1q and, as mentioned, map to different regions of the collagenous portions of C1q.[1,2] Therefore, tests for measuring anti-C1q are, generally, solid-phase ELISAs using whole human C1q as a substrate. In order to inhibit binding of immune complexes, high–ionic strength conditions (0.5-1.0 M NaCl) should be used. The assay allows detection of classes and subclasses of anti-C1q.

CLINICAL ASSOCIATIONS

Anti-C1q antibodies have been described in many conditions (Table 20-2). As such, their specificity for SLE is low. Anti-C1q are invariably present in sera from patients with hypocomplementemic urticarial vasculitis (HUV).[3] This finding suggests that anti-C1q play a pathogenic role in the latter disease, although this possibility has not been proven experimentally. Studies on subclasses and epitopes of anti-C1q in HUV and SLE suggest almost identical anti-C1q in the two diseases despite many differences in clinical presentation.[4]

Anti-C1q have been found to be far more prevalent in patients with who have (proliferative) lupus nephritis than in those without nephritis. Sinico observed that 60% of patients with SLE and nephritis tested positive for anti-C1q, in contrast to only 14% of patients without nephritis; during active nephritis, 89% of patients tested positive, whereas none of the patients with inactive disease tested positive.[5]

Trendelenburg described anti-C1q in 36 of 38 (97.2%) patients with active lupus nephritis; in contrast, only 35% of patients (8 of 26) with inactive lupus nephritis and 25% (9 of 36) with nonrenal lupus tested positive for anti-C1q.[6] Also Meyer found anti-C1q in all (15 of 15) patients in whom lupus nephritis developed, compared with a prevalence of 45% (15 out of 33) in patients without renal disease.[7] However, not all series showed such notable results. Marto found that 75% of their 77 patients with active SLE nephritis tested positive for anti-C1q, compared with 53% of the patients with nonactive nephritis.[8] The autoantibodies were present in 33 of 83 patients (39%) without a history of renal disease, but interestingly, lupus nephritis developed in 9 of these 33 patients after a median interval of 10 months, and one had hypocomplementemic urticarial vasculitis, demonstrating, in accordance with results reported by Meyer,[7] the predictive value of anti-C1q for lupus nephritis in SLE. Comparable prevalences of anti-C1q in lupus nephritis were found by

Grootscholten (65% in 52 patients)[9] and Fang (56% in 150 Chinese patients).[10] In the latter study, higher prevalence (72%) and higher values of anti-C1q were found in patients with class IV lupus nephritis than in those with other classes.

Another study from China described a high prevalence of anti-C1q (58 of 73 patients, or 80%) in lupus nephritis, with the highest levels detected in patients with class IV nephritis.[11] However, a study from Japan did not confirm the association of anti-C1q with active lupus nephritis.[12] The antibodies were detected in 63% (79 of 126) of patients with active SLE and correlated with disease activity, anti-dsDNA antibodies, and complement levels. No significant correlation was found with active lupus nephritis (n = 21), but only 5 patients had active class IV lupus nephritis in this study.

Taken together, anti-C1q are present in various (auto)immune conditions. They are highly sensitive for hypcomplementemic urticarial vasculitis. In SLE, anti-C1q are particularly present in (diffuse) proliferative lupus nephritis in strong association with active disease.

DO LEVELS OF ANTI-C1q FOLLOW DISEASE ACTIVITY IN LUPUS (NEPHRITIS)?

The previously summarized data suggest that levels of anti-C1q follow (renal) disease activity in SLE. A longitudinal study on 43 patients with SLE related levels of anti-C1q to disease activity, in comparison with levels of anti-dsDNA and complement components C3 and C4, by scoring disease activity and sampling plasma every month.[13] No change in autoantibody levels occurred over time in patients with inactive disease. Anti-C1q and anti-dsDNA were both present in 82% of patients with a renal relapse (n = 17) and rose significantly prior to the relapse in 58% and 65% of patients, respectively. During nonrenal relapses (n = 16), anti-C1q was detected in 38% of patients, and levels rose prior to relapse in only 19%. In contrast, nonrenal relapses were accompanied by anti-dsDNA in 94% of patients, and levels rose in 56% of patients prior to relapse. Thus, changes in levels of anti-C1q particularly follow renal disease activity. Also another study by Moroni observed that changes in anti-C1q levels are strongly associated with renal disease activity in SLE, reaching a sensitivity of 87% and a specificity of 92%.[14] Together with other studies showing the predictive value of anti-C1q for renal flares,[7-11,15] the current data suggest that anti-C1q are involved in the pathogenesis of lupus nephritis.

PATHOGENIC ROLE OF ANTI-C1q AUTOANTIBODIES

Mannik extracted antibodies from autopsy kidneys from SLE patients and found anti-C1q activity in extracts from 4 out of 5 kidneys.[16] In addition, anti-C1q were strongly enriched in glomeruli in comparison with serum, as the anti-C1q/IgG ratio in the glomerular extract was more than 50 times higher than the ratio in serum. A strong argument for a pathogenic role of anti-C1q in lupus nephritis comes from the study by Trouw.[17] Injection of a monoclonal antibody to C1q in normal (BALB-c) mice led to depletion of C1q from the circulation and deposition of both C1q and anti-C1q along the glomerular basement membrane (GBM) with, however, only mild granulocyte influx and no proteinuria. Injection with a subnephritogenic dose of complement-fixing rabbit anti–mouse GBM antibody together with the anti-C1q monoclonal antibody led to strong granulocyte influx and massive proteinuria. Apparently, the anti-GBM antibody binds to the GBM, fixes C1q, events that are followed by binding of anti-C1q and inflammation. The investigators concluded that anti-C1q are pathogenic only in the context of immune complex renal disease as occurs in lupus nephritis. This conclusion may also explain why renal lesions do not develop in hypocomplementemic urticarial vasculitis despite the presence of anti-C1q. Otherwise, Bigler,[18] using the MRL/MpJ[+/+] lupus mouse strain, could not demonstrate a correlation between the presence of anti-C1q and overall survival or severity of nephritis in these mice.

Finally, anti-C1q may be involved in an inflammatory clearance of apoptotic cells. Bigler observed that the antibodies particularly target C1q bound on early apoptotic cells.[19] The uptake of anti-C1q by macrophages involves Fc-receptor engagement, resulting in activation of the phagocytic cells.[20]

CONCLUSION

Anti-C1q are most sensitive for hypocomplementemic urticarial vasculitis. They are neither sensitive nor specific for SLE but show an increased prevalence in lupus nephritis, although not in all studies. Rises in levels of anti-C1q may predict ensuing renal relapses. In vivo experimental studies suggest a pathogenic role for anti-C1q in the development of (lupus) glomerulonephritis, although this role could not be substantiated in an animal model of lupus nephritis. Currently, a positive test result for anti-C1q cannot replace a renal biopsy in a patient in whom lupus nephritis is suspected.

References

1. Kallenberg CGM: Anti-C1q autoantibodies. *Autoimmun Rev* 7:612–615, 2008.
2. Schaller M, Bigler C, Danner D, et al: Autoantibodies against C1q in systemic lupus erythematosus are antigen-driven. *J Immunol* 183:8225–8231, 2009.
3. Wisnieski JJ, Naff GB: Serum IgG antibodies to C1q in hypocomplementemic urticarial vasculitis syndrome. *Arthritis Rheum* 32:119–127, 1989.
4. Wisnieski JJ, Jones SM: Comparison of autoantibodies to the collagen-like region of C1q in hypocomplementemic urticarial vasculitis syndrome and systemic lupus erythematosus. *J Immunol* 148:1396–1403, 1992.
5. Sinico RA, Radice A, Ikehata M, et al: Anti-C1q autoantibodies in lupus nephritis: prevalence and clinical significance. *Ann NY Acad Sci* 1050:193–200, 2005.
6. Trendelenburg M, Lopez-Frascasa M, Potlerkova E, et al: High prevalence of anti-C1q antibodies in biopsy-proven active lupus nephritis. *Nephrol Dial Transplant* 21:3115–3121, 2006.
7. Meyer OC, Nicaise-Roland P, Cadoulal N, et al: Anti-C1q antibodies antedate patent active glomerulonephritis in patients with systemic lupus erythematosus. *Arthritis Res Ther* 11:R87, 2009.
8. Marto N, Bertolaccini M, Calabring E, et al: Anti-C1q antibodies in nephritis: correlation between titres and renal disease activity and positive predictive value in systemic lupus erythematosus. *Ann Rheum Dis* 64:444–448, 2005.
9. Grootscholten C, Dieker JW, McGrath FD, et al: A prospective study of anti-chromatin and anti-C1q autoantibodies in patients with proliferative lupus nephritis treated with cyclophosphamide pulses or azathioprine/methylprednisolone. *Ann Rheum Dis* 66:693–696, 2007.
10. Fang QY, Yu F, Tan Y, et al: Anti-C1q antibodies and IgG subclass distribution in sera from Chinese patients with lupus nephritis. *Nephrol Dial Transplant* 24:172–178, 2009.
11. Cai X, Yang X, Lian F, et al: Correlation between serum anti-C1q antibody levels and renal pathological characteristics and prognostic significance of anti-C1q antibody in lupus nephritis. *J Rheumatol* 37:759–765, 2010.
12. Katsumata Y, Miyake K, Kawaguchi Y, et al: Anti-C1q antibodies are associated with systemic lupus erythematosus global activity, but not specifically with nephritis: a controlled study of 126 consecutive patients. *Arthritis Rheum* 63:2436–2444, 2011.
13. Coremans IE, Spronk PE, Bootsma H, et al: Changes in antibodies to C1q predict renal relapses in systemic lupus erythematosus. *Am J Kidney Dis* 26:595–601, 1995.
14. Moroni G, Trendelenburg M, Del Papa N, et al: Anti-C1q antibodies may help in diagnosing a renal flare in lupus nephritis. *Am J Kidney Dis* 37:490–498, 2001.
15. Matrat A, Veysseyre-Balter C, Frolliet P, et al: Simultaneous detection of anti-C1q and anti-double stranded DNA autoantibodies in lupus nephritis: predictive value for renal flares. *Lupus* 20:28–34, 2011.
16. Mannik M, Wener M: Deposition of antibodies to the collagen-like region of C1q in renal glomeruli of patients with proliferative lupus glomerulonephritis. *Arthritis Rheum* 40:1504–1511, 1997.
17. Trouw LA, Groeneveld TW, Seelen MA, et al: Anti-C1q autoantibodies deposit in glomeruli but are only pathogenic in combination with glomerular C1q-containing immune complexes. *J Clin Invest* 114:679–688, 2004.
18. Bigler C, Hopfer H, Danner D, et al: Anti-C1q autoantibodies do not correlate with the occurrence or severity of experimental lupus nephritis. *Nephrol Dial Transplant* 26:1220–1228, 2011.

19. Bigler C, Schaller M, Perahud I, et al: Autoantibodies against complement C1q specifically target C1q bound on early apoptotic cells. *J Immunol* 183:3512–3521, 2009.
20. Reefman E, Limburg PC, Kallenberg CGM, et al: Fcγ receptors in the initiation and progression of systemic lupus erythematosus. *Ann NY Acad Sci* 1051:52–63, 2005.

PART E Antibodies against the Extractable Nuclear Antigens RNP, Sm, Ro/SSA, and La/SSB

Gabriela Riemekasten and Falk Hiepe

Autoantibodies against extractable nuclear antigens (ENAs) describe a subgroup of ANAs that do not react with chromatin. They are directed against nuclear proteins that were isolated by salt extraction. ENAs are mainly recognized by sera from patients with SLE, mixed connective tissue disease (MCTD), and Sjögren syndrome. Classic autoantigens are Sm, ribonucleoprotein (RNP), Sjögren syndrome antigen A (Ro/SSA), and Sjögren syndrome antigen B (La/SSB), which are all detectable in sera from patients with SLE. It is recommended to use the specific antibody designation instead of the global term *anti-ENA*.

STRUCTURE OF THE ANTIGENS
Sm/RNP Complex
Anti-Sm and anti-(RNP antibodies are directed to small nuclear ribonucleoprotein (snRNP) complexes, which are localized in the nucleus and are involved in pre-messenger RNA (pre-mRNA) processing and synthesis of nearly all proteins by conserving coding regions (exons) and removing noncoding regions (introns) within the spliceosome. The five snRNPs each consist of a unique small (less than 190 nucleotides) nuclear RNA molecule, termed U1, U2, U4, U5, or U6, specific associated proteins, and seven common core proteins called Smith (Sm) proteins Sm B, B', D1, D2, D3, Sm-E, Sm-F, and Sm-G, with molecular weights from 9 to 29 kd and named after the patient in whose serum the antibody reactivity was first detected.

Anti-RNP antibodies precipitate only the U1 RNA and the associated proteins called U1 RNP-70, -A, and -C, but not the other unique RNA molecules. Several shared B- and T-cell epitopes exist between U1-RNP-70 and U1-RNP-A proteins, especially in the RNA-binding region (e.g., U1 A epitope 103-108 amino acid [aa] region and U1-RNP-70 epitope 68-72 aa region).[1] The x-ray crystal structure of U1-RNP has now been determined.[2,3]

Anti-Sm antibodies precipitate all snRNP RNA molecules but are predominantly directed against the Sm B/B' and SmD1 proteins.[1] Because SmB/B' and U1-specific RNPs share the cross-reactive epitope motif PPPGMRPP, SmD1 is regarded as the most specific ENA in SLE. The major SmD1 epitope was localized in the C-terminus of SmD1 within the SmD1 83-119 aa region.[4] Minor responses are also directed to SmD2, D3, E, F, and G core proteins as well as to A' or A'' proteins of the U2-snRNP complex.

Ro/SSA and La/SSB RNP Complex
The Ro/SSA and La/SSB RNP complex, located in the nucleus and the cytoplasm, constitutes one of the four small, uridine-rich so-called hY RNAs (human cYtoplasmic RNAs) that are noncovalently associated with at least three proteins, the Ro/SSA52, La/SSB, and Ro/SSA60 autoantigens. Additionally, the proteins calreticulin and nucleolin are also associated. Ro/SSA52 belongs to the tripartite motif (TRIM) or RING-B-box-coiled-coil (RBCC) protein family and shows RING-dependent E3 ligase activity. The major Ro/SSA52 epitope is localized in the middle coiled-coil region, and almost all anti-Ro/SSA52–positive sera have been found to react with the 190-245 aa region independent of the associated disease.

Ro/SSA60 consists of two distinct domains: a von Willebrand factor A domain and a doughnut-shaped domain composed of *Hun*tingtin, elongation factor 3 (*EF*3), protein phosphatase 2A (PP2*A*), and the yeast PI3-kinase *TOR*1 (HEAT) repeats. This domain contains a positively charged central hole, which binds ssRNA. The function of Ro/SSA60 has been related to the quality control or discard pathway for nascent transcripts synthesized by RNA polymerase III. Furthermore, it promotes cell survival after ultraviolet irradiation. The major Ro/SSA60 epitope has been identified within the central part of the molecule. The epitope 169-190 aa region is mainly recognized by anti-Ro/SSA positive sera from patients with SLE, and the epitope 211-232 aa region by sera from patients with Sjögren syndrome.

The La/SSB antigen is a phosphoprotein that binds a variety of small RNAs, including 5S cellular RNA, transfer RNA (tRNA), 7S RNA, and hY RNAs, all of which are transcribed by RNA polymerase III. La/SSB is also involved in the termination of RNA polymerase II transcription. Anti-La/SSB antibodies react with an epitope spanning the sequence 349-364 aa with a sensitivity and specificity of more than 90%.[5]

ASSAYS FOR MEASURING ANTI-ENA ANTIBODIES
Because the anti-ENA antibodies are a subgroup of ANAs, it is recommended that tests for anti-ENA be performed if ANA screening with the indirect IF on human epithelial-2 (HEp2) cells has a positive result. Anti-Ro/SSA and anti-La/SSB show a finely speckled nucleoplasmic fluorescence pattern, whereas anti-Sm and anti-RNP antibodies reveal a granular pattern. As is typically seen in SLE, multiple specificities of ANAs can be present in one patient's serum (e.g., anti-dsDNA, antihistone, antinucleosome plus anti-ENA). Therefore, a specific anti-ENA pattern may be masked. A positive anti-Sm, anti-RNP, or anti-La/SSB test result should be questioned in cases of a negative ANA IF test result. It is most likely a false-positive anti-ENA result, and there are only rare cases of ANA-negativity in which the anti-Ro/SSA test shows a truly positive signal.

Originally, double-radial immunodiffusion (Ouchterlony technique) was employed to detect anti-ENA antibodies using thymic and/or splenic extracts as an antigen source. This method is still considered the gold standard because it is highly specific. However, it is also time and serum consuming, costly, less sensitive, and not automatable. Radioimmunoprecipitation and immunoblotting are suited to identify new antigens and possible subunits. In routine laboratories, these techniques are replaced by ELISA and multiplex assays, including line immunoassays (LIA), addressable laser bead immunoassays (ALBIA), and microarray technology. These sensitive tests allow the simultaneous detection of different autoantibodies in a small sample size and in a large number of patients, making the industrialized detection of antibodies by large laboratories more cost-effective. ELISA and ALBIA yield quantitative results, whereas LIA is a qualitative test, distinguishing only positive and negative results. The test quality may be influenced by the purity and source of the antigen used. In addition to purified native antigens, recombinant proteins and synthesized peptides are employed. The variability of the assay methods and antigen sources prevents a standardization and comparability of the results. Standard and reference sera are available from the U.S. Centers for Disease Control and Prevention (CDC) in Atlanta, Georgia, United States. More information is available on the website of the Autoantibody Standardization Committee in Rheumatic and Related Disorders (www.AutoAb.org), which operates as a subcommittee of the Quality Assessment and Standardization Committee of the International Union of Immunological Societies (IUIS) and reports to parent organizations including the World Health Organization (WHO), the Arthritis Foundation (AF), and the CDC.

TABLE 20-3 Approximate Prevalence and Clinical Associations of Different Anti-ENA Antibodies

ANTIBODIES TO	APPROXIMATE PREVALENCE (RANGE)	REPORTED CLINICAL ASSOCIATIONS
Sm (Smith antibody)	30% (7.5-70%)	Marker antibody of SLE, more common in black patients with SLE,* serositis,* lupus nephritis,* CNS diseases* such as psychoses and schizophrenia, increased mortality, pulmonary fibrosis, leukopenia,* arthritis,* malar or discoid rash,* vasculitis,* elevated systolic pulmonary arterial pressure, antihemoglobin antibodies,* oral ulcers,* chronic active disease in juvenile nonwhite patients with SLE *
U1-RNP	25% (13-47%)	Interstitial lung disease,* rapid progression of pulmonary damage,* pleuritis, CNS involvement,* Raynaud phenomenon,* leukopenia,* meningitis,* higher age at disease onset,* lower prevalence of urinary casts* and reduced risk for nephritis especially in those patients having antibody reactivity towards different U1RNP components,* arthritis,* fever,* myositis,* erosive joint disease
Ro/SSA	25% (25-60%)	Photosensitive skin rash,* subacute cutaneous lupus,* pneumonitis and shrinking lung syndrome,* thrombocytopenia,* lymphopenia,* nephritis, homozygous patients with C2 and C4 complement deficiency,* HLA-DQ1/2, T-cell receptor β gene, vasculitis,* thrombocytopenic purpura,* ocular damage,* secondary Sjögren syndrome,* neonatal lupus syndromes,* lower frequency of pediatric lupus, rheumatoid factor,* CAVB,* especially in the case of high antibody levels and when directed to Ro52/SSA epitope 200-239 aa leucine zipper region, heart rhythm disorders such as prolongation of the QT interval and life-threatening ventricular arrhythmias in adult patients
La/SSB	20% (6-35%)	SCLE,* secondary Sjögren's syndrome,* rheumatoid factor,* pericarditis, lower prevalence of nephritis,* seizures, and anti-dsDNA, rarely found in old male SLE patients and pediatric lupus
Ro/SSA and La/SSB	15% (10-25%)	SCLE,* neonatal lupus erythematosus (NLE),* secondary Sjögren syndrome,* positive rheumatoid factor,* hypergammaglobulinemia*
Ro/SSA, Sm, RNP	15% (10-40%)	Lower percentages in elderly patients, more photosensitivity,* malar and discoid rush,* Raynaud phenomenon,* leukopenia*
No ENAs	26-32%	Lower percentage of adult SLE, absence of alopecia

CAVB, complete atrioventricular block; CNS, central nervous system; ENA, extractable nuclear antigen; La/SSB, Sjögren syndrome antigen B; RNP, ribonucleoprotein; Ro/SSA, Sjögren syndrome antigen A; SCLE, subacute cutaneous lupus erythematosus; SLE, systemic lupus erythematosus,
*Widely agreed-on association.

PREVALENCE AND CLINICAL ASSOCIATIONS IN SLE

With the exception of anti-Sm antibodies, which are constituents of the American College of Rheumatology (ACR) classification criteria for SLE owing to their high disease specificity, anti-ENA antibodies can also be detected in other autoimmune diseases. The prevalence of the different antibodies, their diagnostic and predictive values, as well as their disease associations vary with the assay used. In addition, patient characteristics, such as age at disease onset, ethnic background, hormonal status, and disease activity, are important. Patients 50 years or older at disease onset have a lower frequency of anti-RNP and anti-Sm antibodies. Afro-Caribbean patients show the highest prevalence of anti-Ro/SSA, anti-La/SSB, anti-Sm, and anti–U1-RNP antibodies.[6]

Anti-ENA antibodies are often present in specific clusters reflecting the nature of the antigens. Nearly all patients with anti-Sm antibodies also have anti–U1-RNP antibodies. In contrast, anti–U1-RNP antibodies may occur as the sole specificity. Another cluster of antibodies is formed by Ro/SSA52, Ro/SSA60, and La/SSB. Anti-La/SSB antibodies are usually found in association with anti-Ro/SSA, and serum samples with anti-La/SSB antibodies but without anti-Ro/SSA reactivity are rare. All anti-Ro/SSA–positive sera react with Ro/SSA60, but sera from some anti-Ro/SSA60 antibody–positive patients also bind the Ro/SSA52 autoantigen.

The relationship between disease activity and anti-ENA antibodies still is a matter of debate.[1] Anti-Sm antibodies seem to have the best association between peak SLEDAI score and the levels of antibodies, although this association is weak. There are also divergent results concerning the capacity of anti-ENA antibodies to predict or indicate organ damage. In addition, there still is some discussion about the relationship between anti-ENA and clinical manifestations as well as disease mortality. Anti-ENA antibodies, notably anti-Sm, seem to be a predictor of flare after B-cell depletion therapy with rituximab.[7]

Table 20-3 summarizes the prevalence and the reported clinical associations obtained from different publications.[1,8-13]

Anti-ENA antibodies can also be detected in other compartments, such as in pleural fluid and cerebrospinal fluid (CSF). Presence of anti–U1-RNP antibodies in CSF with an increased anti–U1-RNP CSF/serum index (>2 adjusted for serum dilution) is suggestive of central neuropsychiatric SLE with a sensitivity of 64% and a specificity for 93%.[11]

When anti-ENA reactivity is followed for several years in the same patients, a longitudinal fluctuation of the antibodies can be detected. Anti-Ro/SSA antibodies are the most stable, with 47% of the patients always testing positive for these antibodies. Anti–U1-RNP and anti-La/SSB antibody levels remain stable in 36% and 11% of the patients, respectively. In contrast, only 17% of the sera testing positively for anti-Sm antibodies remain stably positive. Therefore, a periodic reappraisal may be appropriate.[14]

Anti-Ro/SSA60 antibodies appear before or simultaneously with anti-La/SSB and anti-Ro/SSA52 autoantibodies, on average 3.4 years before diagnosis. Anti–U1-RNP antibodies are detected closer to the time of clinical disease onset.[1] In one study, anti–U1-RNP-A antibodies appeared before or simultaneously with anti–U1-RNP-70 antibodies. In another study, the first IgG autoantibodies to appear were directed against U1-RNP-70 and SmB/B′, followed by anti–U1-RNP-A, anti–RNP-C, and anti-SmD1 antibodies.[1] A proline-rich SmD1 cross-reacting octapeptide PPPGMRPP of the carboxyl terminal regions of SmB/B′ was among the first targets of the anti-Sm responses.[15]

VIRUS INFECTIONS AS TRIGGERS FOR AUTOIMMUNITY

Viruses accomplish transcription of their own genes by interaction with the host RNA-processing machinery, and therefore, viral antigens are in close contact with the snRNP complex. Among several viruses, Epstein-Barr virus (EBV) is one of the best investigated candidates for triggering autoimmunity through molecular mimicry of ENA, although this hypothesis has not been proven. Viral antigens present several epitopes cross-reacting to immunodominant epitopes within the Ro/SSA60, SmD1, and U1-RNP autoantigens. Interestingly, the initial autoantigenic epitope for some patients with SLE testing positive for Ro/SSA60 directly cross-reacts with a peptide from Epstein-Barr nuclear antigen 1 (EBNA-1). Rabbits immunized with either the first epitope of Ro/SSA60 or the cross-reactive EBNA-1 epitope progressively develop autoantibodies recognizing multiple Ro/SSA epitopes and Sm antigens. Immunization of mice with EBNA-1 has revealed anti-Sm and anti-DNA antibody production. Immunization with vesicular stomatitis virus nucleocapsid protein induces anti-Ro/SSA60 antibodies in NZW mice. The antibodies bound to five of six shared sequences between Ro/SSA and VSV N-protein (vesicular stomatitis virus nucleocapsid protein). In 10% to 15% of patients with early EBV infection, anti-ENA antibodies are transiently detectable. A higher prevalence of EBV seroconversion has been found in pediatric and adult patients with SLE than in matched controls.[16] Intrinsic defects in the control of EBV infections are also associated with the abnormal immune response in patients with SLE.[17] Studies suggest that the amount of immunizing antigen plays a critical role in triggering autoimmunity, because overstimulation with certain antigens or virus proteins can affect the integrity of the immune system and induce autoimmunity.[18] However, further regulatory mechanisms are necessary to maintain and spread autoimmunity.

SEQUENTIAL PRESENTATION OF ANTI-ENA ANTIBODIES AND RELATIONSHIP OF ANTI-ENA TO OTHER LUPUS-SPECIFIC AUTOANTIBODIES

As shown in animal studies, immunization with a particular ENA can also induce antibodies to other ENAs. Rabbits immunized with the U1-RNP-A epitope spanning aa 44-56 also developed antibodies to U1-RNP-70, U1-RNP-C, SmB/B', SmD1, Ro/SSA, and partially to dsDNA and demonstrated typical clinical lupus symptoms such as renal insufficiency and thrombocytopenia.[19] In line with this finding, spontaneous autoimmunity in patients with SLE starts from single autoantigens and spreads to autoantigens of the same macromolecular complex (intramolecular spreading) or related macromolecular complexes (intermolecular spreading. However, spread of autoimmunity is no random process[1] and seems to be tightly controlled by the antigen or by T-cell reactivity and regulation.[20] Thus, the C-terminus of SmD1 has also been shown to provide T-cell help for the production of anti-dsDNA antibodies in an animal model of lupus.[21]

Antibodies against RNP, Sm, Ro/SSA, and La/SSB are directed against proteins associated with RNA. The often positively charged autoantigens, for example, from the C-terminus of SmD1, may interact with DNA and the anti-dsDNA response.[4] As described in one study, switching from anti-dsDNA to an anti-Sm response was associated with the onset of more severe disease and central nervous system (CNS) involvement.[22]

ROLE OF APOPTOSIS FOR THE GENERATION OF ANTI-ENA ANTIBODIES

Proteins modified during apoptosis could bypass tolerance to self-proteins through different mechanisms, such as cleavage by caspases or granzymes, interferon-inducible expression of untolerized forms of self-antigens, alternative mRNA splicing, and protein modification such as phosphorylation or oxidation. The important role of type I interferon (IFN) is exemplified by the lack of anti-RNP autoantibodies in mice deficient for type I IFN. During ultraviolet (UV) light–induced apoptosis, autoantigens cluster in the surface membrane of distinct apoptotic blebs containing snRNP. Apoptosis-specific modifications have been described for the U1-RNP-70. Sera from patients with Raynaud phenomenon recognize oxidative fragments of the U1-RNP-70, suggesting that reactive oxygen species modify the autoantigen during ischemia-reperfusion.[1] This finding

fits the associations reported between the presence of Raynaud phenomenon and the occurrence of anti-RNP antibodies. No apoptosis-related modifications have been described for other RNP proteins.

TOLL-LIKE RECEPTORS AS KEY MOLECULES FOR THE GENERATION OF ANTI-ENA ANTIBODIES

Toll-like receptors TLR 9 and TLR 7 interact directly with DNA and RNA molecules, respectively, as well as with DNA- and RNA-containing autoantigens. Ligation of these receptors results in the activation of MyD88 and transcription factors of the nuclear factor kappa b (NF-κB) and IFN regulatory factor family members. TLR strongly determine the anti-ENA and anti-dsDNA autoantibody generation and class-switching to the pathogenic IgG2 isotype. The production of anti-Sm/RNP antibodies requires both TLR 7 and engagement of the B-cell receptor (BCR). TLR 7–deficient lupus-prone MRL(lpr/lpr) mice fail to generate anti-Sm/RNP antibodies in vivo but exhibit anti-dsDNA antibodies. These mice have reduced T- and B-cell activation and isotype-switched antibodies, decreased lymphadenopathy, ameliorated immune complex deposition, and renal disease.[23]

TLR 9–deficient MRL(lpr/lpr) mice develop increased hypergammaglobulinemia, lymphocyte activation, and glomerulonephritis despite the absence of anti-dsDNA antibodies, suggesting that anti-dsDNA antibodies are dispensable for the pathology in this model.[23] MyD88-deficient mice as well as TLR 7/9–deficient mice show no ANA reactivity and ameliorated disease. In NZB/W lupus-prone mice, the development of SLE is markedly suppressed by a dual inhibitor of TLR 7 and TLR 9, too, but TLR 9 deficiency alone results in an accelerated development of lupus nephritis and is associated with an increased production of autoantibodies against dsDNA and RNA-related autoantibodies via increased TLR 7 activation.[24]

Other studies suggest that TLR 9 suppresses TLR 7–dependent anti-RNA–associated autoantibodies and is, therefore, an upstream regulator of anti-RNA antibodies. In addition, the paradigm of TLR 7 recognizing exclusively RNA and TLR 9 recognizing exclusively DNA has been questioned.[23]

GENETIC RISKS AND ANTI-ENA ANTIBODIES

The complex genetic inheritance of SLE is also reflected by the presence or absence of different anti-ENA antibodies. HLA class II genes influence the autoantibody repertoire in SLE and its clinical manifestations, whereas the onset of SLE is more likely the consequence of a cooperation of many other non-HLA genes.[25] Reactivity to individual U1-RNP components has been shown to be associated with different HLA class II alleles.[20] HLA-DR3 was found to be associated with the presence of anti-La/SSB antibodies in Jamaican patients.[25] Patients carrying the DRB1*03 and the closely linked DQB1*0201 allele show genetic predisposition to the production of autoantibodies against Ro/SSA and La/SSB and a predisposition for pulmonary involvement, pleuritis, and psychosis. Patients carrying the DQB1*0502 allele are prone to development of anti-Ro/SSA antibodies without anti-La/SSB, renal disease, discoid lupus, and livedo reticularis. T cells recognizing U1-RNP-70 peptides show restriction to HLA-DRB1*0401.[1]

Genome-wide association studies have identified SLE susceptibility variations and single-nucleic polymorphisms associated with the presence of anti-Sm, anti-Ro/SSA, and anti-La/SSB antibodies, such as in the *STAT4* gene mediating the effects of several cytokines, T-helper 1 and T-helper 17 cell differentiation, monocyte activation, or IFN-γ production. Other polymorphisms have been found in the IFN-α pathway genes and for phosphoinositide-3-kinase (PIK 3C3) linked to a simultaneous occurrence of anti-Sm and anti-Ro/SSA antibodies. The latter polymorphism was also found to be associated with a susceptibility to schizophrenia and high IFN-α levels, especially in African American patients.[26]

In addition, a DNase IV polymorphism is reported to be associated with the presence of anti-Sm antibodies, further fostering the hypothesis that impaired RNA degradation combined with decreased clearance of apoptotic cell debris might stimulate the development of autoantibodies against Sm and RNP.[27]

PATHOGENIC IMPORTANCE OF ANTI-RNP AND ANTI-Sm ANTIBODIES

The associations between autoantibody levels and disease activity as well as clinical symptoms suggest a contribution of the antibodies to disease pathogenesis, but such associations were not a consistent finding.[1] In addition, the occurrence of some autoantibodies just before disease onset, such as the anti-SmD1, raises the question of whether some autoantibodies are more pathogenic than others. The important role of autoimmunity to the C-terminal SmD1 peptide 83-119 is suggested by amelioration of murine lupus by tolerance induction to this peptide.[28] In line with this finding, break of autoantigen-specific tolerance by immunizations with the SmD1 83-119 peptide accelerates murine lupus. In addition, immunization with Sm protein induces antibodies to murine hemoglobin in lupus-prone mice.[29]

Convincing data about the pathogenic role of anti-RNP antibodies also come from animal studies. Mice normally resistant to lung damage received anti-RNP–containing serum and were subjected to ischemia/reperfusion-induced lung injury. They exhibited lung damage in a dose-dependent manner, suggesting a contribution of the anti-RNP antibodies to tissue damage.[1,10] Associations between lung injury, high IFN gene signature, and the presence of anti-RNP antibodies in human lupus are in line with this observation.

The pathogenic role of autoimmunity against snRNP is also suggested by tolerance experiments. Muller identified a phosphorylation modification within the U1-RNP-70 131-151aa epitope and used this modified peptide (P140) to induce tolerance in murine and human lupus. In mice, administration of this peptide decreased anti-dsDNA antibody responses as well as proteinuria and increased survival. In a phase 2 clinical trial in human SLE, administration of this peptide improved disease activity and anti-dsDNA autoantibodies in some but not all patients, a finding that needs to be confirmed in a controlled setting.[30]

PATHOGENIC ROLE OF ANTI-Ro/SSA AND ANTI-La/SSB ANTIBODIES

Neonatal lupus erythematosus (NLE) provides the strongest clinical evidence of a pathogenic role for autoantibodies directed to the regularly intracellular located anti-Ro/SSA antigens, because the passive transplacental transfer of maternal autoantibodies induces clinical symptoms in the fetus and neonate, and reversible clinical signs resolve with their clearance from the neonatal circulation. Of note, symptoms similar to those characteristic of neonatal lupus occur in SLE and are found to be associated with anti-Ro/SSA and anti-La/SSB. Examples are photosensitive rash, thrombocytopenia, cerebral white matter lesions, and heart rhythm disorders. The characteristic deposition of immunoglobulins and complement at the epidermal junction in patients with SLE was experimentally reproduced by infusing anti-Ro/SSA antibodies into human skin-grafted mice. For this purpose, the intracellular Ro/SSA antigen must be accessible to autoantibodies in order to be pathogenic. Several studies revealed that Ro/SSA is expressed on the surfaces of keratinocytes after exposure to UV light, estradiol, cytotoxic prostaglandins, viral infections, oxidative stress, heat shock, phorbol 12-myristate 13-acetate, and tumor necrosis factor alpha (TNF-α).[3] Ro/SSA expression on the cell surfaces of blood cells was also described, providing an explanation for how anti-Ro/SSA-associated cytopenia may arise.

Immunization of Balb/c mice with Ro/SSA and La/SSB antigens can induce the corresponding autoantibodies and congenital heart block in pups. In vitro and in vivo data demonstrate that maternal anti-Ro/SSA and/or anti-La/SSB antibodies opsonize fetal apoptotic cardiomyocytes, which in turn induce a proinflammatory and profibrotic response by phagocytosing macrophages, ultimately leading to

tissue injury.[5] Data demonstrate an involvement of TLR 7 by ligation of Ro/SSA60-associated ssRNA that may link inflammation with fetal cardiac fibrosis.[31] Anti-Ro/SSA antibodies may be directly arrhythmogenic. There is evidence that anti-Ro/SSA antibodies block calcium ion channels regulating the bioelectric activity of the atrioventricular (AV) and sinoatrial (SA) node cells.[9]

Anti-Ro/SSA and anti-La/SSB antibodies are also present in lupus models such as the MRL lpr/lpr and the New Zealand Black/White F1 mice, and the levels rise during spontaneous disease development. Mice lacking the Ro/SSA60 protein develop signs of autoimmunity resembling human SLE. They exhibit antiribosome and antichromatin antibodies, photosensitivity, and glomerulonephritis and are susceptible to UV damage.[32] Mice lacking Ro/SSA52 appear phenotypically normal if left unmanipulated. However, they demonstrate severe dermatitis extending from the site of tissue injury induced by ear tags. Furthermore, they show other SLE signs, including hypergammaglobulinemia, anti-dsDNA antibodies, and nephritis. The mice have an enhanced production of proinflammatory cytokines that are regulated by interferon regulatory factor (IRF) transcription factors such as IL-17. Therefore, Ro/SSA52 is an important regulator of proinflammatory cytokine production because it has been identified as E3 ligase, which mediates ubiquitination of several members of the IRF family. This means that a defective Ro/SSA52 function can lead to tissue inflammation and systemic autoimmunity.[33]

Autoantibodies against Sm, RNP, Ro/SSA, and La/SSB, which are often detectable years before the onset of SLE, may contribute in another way to the pathogenesis. They are often resistant to immunosuppression and B-cell depletion therapy, indicating that they are secreted by long-lived plasma cells in the bone marrow. Immune complexes consisting of these autoantibodies and the RNA-containing antigens induce release of type I IFN by plasmacytoid dendritic cells that in turn may activate disease.[34] This process may also explain the observation that anti-ENA antibodies at baseline were identified as the only independent predictor of flares after B-cell depletion therapy with rituximab.[7]

References

1. Kattah NH, Kattah MG, Utz PJ: The U1-snRNP complex: structural properties relating to autoimmune pathogenesis in rheumatic diseases. *Immunol Rev* 233:126–145, 2010.
2. Pomeranz Krummel DA, Oubridge C, Leung AK, et al: Crystal structure of human spliceosomal U1 snRNP at 5.5 A resolution. *Nature* 458:475–480, 2009.
3. Gerl V, Hostmann B, Johnen C, et al: The intracellular 52-kd Ro/SSA autoantigen in keratinocytes is up-regulated by tumor necrosis factor alpha via tumor necrosis factor receptor I. *Arthritis Rheum* 52:531–538, 2005.
4. Riemekasten G, Marell J, Trebeljahr G, et al: A novel epitope on the C-terminus of SmD1 is recognized by the majority of sera from patients with systemic lupus erythematosus. *J Clin Invest* 102:754–763, 1998.
5. Routsias JG, Tzioufas AG: Autoimmune response and target autoantigens in Sjogren's syndrome. *Eur J Clin Invest* 40:1026–1036, 2010.
6. Croca SC, Rodrigues T, Isenberg DA: Assessment of a lupus nephritis cohort over a 30-year period. *Rheumatology (Oxford)* 50:1424–1430, 2011.
7. Ng KP, Cambridge G, Leandro MJ, et al: B cell depletion therapy in systemic lupus erythematosus: long-term follow-up and predictors of response. *Ann Rheum Dis* 66:1259–1262, 2007.
8. Kariuki SN, Franek BS, Mikolaitis RA, et al: Promoter variant of PIK3C3 is associated with autoimmunity against Ro and Sm epitopes in African-American lupus patients. *J Biomed Biotechnol* 2010:826434, 2010.
9. Lazzerini PE, Capecchi PL, Acampa M, et al: Arrhythmogenic effects of anti-Ro/SSA antibodies on the adult heart: more than expected? *Autoimmun Rev* 9:40–44, 2009.
10. Mittoo S, Gelber AC, Hitchon CA, et al: Clinical and serologic factors associated with lupus pleuritis. *J Rheumatol* 37:747–753, 2010.
11. Sato T, Fujii T, Yokoyama T, et al: Anti-U1 RNP antibodies in cerebrospinal fluid are associated with central neuropsychiatric manifestations in systemic lupus erythematosus and mixed connective tissue disease. *Arthritis Rheum* 62:3730–3740, 2010.

12. Tang X, Huang Y, Deng W, et al: Clinical and serologic correlations and autoantibody clusters in systemic lupus erythematosus: a retrospective review of 917 patients in South China. *Medicine (Baltimore)* 89:62–67, 2010.

13. Jaeggi E, Laskin C, Hamilton R, et al: The importance of the level of maternal anti-Ro/SSA antibodies as a prognostic marker of the development of cardiac neonatal lupus erythematosus: a prospective study of 186 antibody-exposed fetuses and infants. *J Am Coll Cardiol* 55:2778–2784, 2010.

14. Faria AC, Barcellos KS, Andrade LE: Longitudinal fluctuation of antibodies to extractable nuclear antigens in systemic lupus erythematosus. *J Rheumatol* 32:1267–1272, 2005.

15. James JA, Gross T, Scofield RH, et al: Immunoglobulin epitope spreading and autoimmune disease after peptide immunization: Sm B/B'-derived PPPGMRPP and PPPGIRGP induce spliceosome autoimmunity. *J Exp Med* 181:453–461, 1995.

16. Poole BD, Templeton AK, Guthridge JM, et al: Aberrant Epstein-Barr viral infection in systemic lupus erythematosus. *Autoimmun Rev* 8:337–342, 2009.

17. Kang I, Quan T, Nolasco H, et al: Defective control of latent Epstein-Barr virus infection in systemic lupus erythematosus. *J Immunol* 172:1287–1294, 2004.

18. Tsumiyama K, Miyazaki Y, Shiozawa S: Self-organized criticality theory of autoimmunity. *PLoS One* 4:e8382, 2009.

19. McClain MT, Lutz CS, Kaufman KM, et al: Structural availability influences the capacity of autoantigenic epitopes to induce a widespread lupus-like autoimmune response. *Proc Natl Acad Sci U S A* 101:3551–3556, 2004.

20. Kaneko Y, Suwa A, Hirakata M, et al: Clinical associations with autoantibody reactivities to individual components of U1 small nuclear ribonucleoprotein. *Lupus* 19:307–312, 2010.

21. Riemekasten G, Langnickel D, Ebling FM, et al: Identification and characterization of SmD183–119-reactive T cells that provide T cell help for pathogenic anti-double-stranded DNA antibodies. *Arthritis Rheum* 48:475–485, 2003.

22. Ishii M, Muramoto Y, Kosaka H, et al: A serological switching from anti-dsDNA to anti-Sm antibodies coincided with severe clinical manifestations of systemic lupus erythematosus (hemophagocytosis, profundus and psychosis). *Lupus* 16:67–69, 2007.

23. Nickerson KM, Christensen SR, Shupe J, et al: TLR9 regulates TLR7- and MyD88-dependent autoantibody production and disease in a murine model of lupus. *J Immunol* 184:1840–1848, 2010.

24. Santiago-Raber ML, Dunand-Sauthier I, Wu T, et al: Critical role of TLR7 in the acceleration of systemic lupus erythematosus in TLR9-deficient mice. *J Autoimmun* 34:339–348, 2010.

25. Sebastiani GD, Galeazzi M: Immunogenetic studies on systemic lupus erythematosus. *Lupus* 18:878–883, 2009.

26. Salloum R, Franek BS, Kariuki SN, et al: Genetic variation at the IRF7/PHRF1 locus is associated with autoantibody profile and serum interferon-alpha activity in lupus patients. *Arthritis Rheum* 62:553–561, 2010.

27. Kim I, Hur NW, Shin HD, et al: Associations of DNase IV polymorphisms with autoantibodies in patients with systemic lupus erythematosus. *Rheumatology (Oxford)* 47:996–999, 2008.

28. Riemekasten G, Langnickel D, Enghard P, et al: Intravenous injection of a D1 protein of the Smith proteins postpones murine lupus and induces type 1 regulatory T cells. *J Immunol* 173:5835–5842, 2004.

29. Bhatnagar H, Kala S, Sharma L, et al: Serum and organ-associated anti-hemoglobin humoral autoreactivity: association with anti-Sm responses and inflammation. *Eur J Immunol* 41:537–548, 2011.

30. Muller S, Monneaux F, Schall N, et al: Spliceosomal peptide P140 for immunotherapy of systemic lupus erythematosus: results of an early phase II clinical trial. *Arthritis Rheum* 58:3873–3883, 2008.

31. Clancy RM, Alvarez D, Komissarova E, et al: Ro60-associated single-stranded RNA links inflammation with fetal cardiac fibrosis via ligation of TLRs: a novel pathway to autoimmune-associated heart block. *J Immunol* 184:2148–2155, 2010.

32. Xue D, Shi H, Smith JD, et al: A lupus-like syndrome develops in mice lacking the Ro 60-kDa protein, a major lupus autoantigen. *Proc Natl Acad Sci U S A* 100:7503–7508, 2003.

33. Espinosa A, Dardalhon V, Brauner S, et al: Loss of the lupus autoantigen Ro52/Trim21 induces tissue inflammation and systemic autoimmunity by disregulating the IL-23-Th17 pathway. *J Exp Med* 206:1661–1671, 2009.

34. Hiepe F, Dörner T, Hauser AE, et al: Long-lived autoreactive plasma cells drive persistent autoimmune inflammation. *Nat Rev Rheumatol* 7:170–178, 2011.

Chapter 21

Autoantigenesis and Antigen-Based Therapy and Vaccination in SLE

Ram Raj Singh, Julia Pinkhasov, Priti Prasad, and Shweta Dubey[1]

The discovery in the early 1990s that self-antigen–reactive T cells can be tolerized to prevent systemic lupus erythematosus (SLE) in animal models[1] eventually led to clinical trials of autoantigenic peptides in patients with SLE.[2-4] In fact, the U.S. Food and Drug Administration (FDA) has granted the "fast track" approval to start a phase 3 trial of Lupuzor, a posttranslationally modified peptide analog derived from U1-70K small nuclear ribonucleoprotein (snRNP).[2] Although this development is encouraging, the identity of true autoantigen-reactive T cells and their exact role in SLE remains to be fully understood. Advances in use of in situ tetramer staining to identify human antigen–specific T cells in the affected organs of patients[5] provide hope for identification of autoantigen-specific T cells that infiltrate the diseased organs in humans. Such T cells and their autoantigens can be true targets for therapy. In the meantime, growing evidence supports a role for apoptosis, posttranslational and other modifications in the antigens themselves, and determinant spreading as possible sources of autoantigens in SLE.[6,7] Antigen mimicry has long been considered a mechanism of autoantigenesis. Molecular mimicry at the T-cell epitope level was detected between lupus-associated autoantigen Sm-D and microbial peptides.[8] Exposure to naturally occurring hydrocarbon oils in otherwise normal mouse strains elicits chronic inflammation, which eventuates in a plethora of autoimmune manifestations, including nephritis, arthritis, pulmonary vasculitis, and lupuslike autoantibodies.[9-12] Development of inflammation long before the onset of autoimmunity in these mice is believed to trigger the autoantigenicity of a variety of nuclear and cytoplasmic antigens.

Major autoantigens in SLE include DNA-associated antigens, namely, nucleosome, which is made up of double-stranded DNA (dsDNA) bound to the five histone molecules, H1, H2A, H2B, H3, and H4, and high-mobility group box 1 (HMGB1) protein, and RNA-associated antigens such as U1 small nuclear ribonucleoprotein (U1 snRNP), Ro/la complex, and ribosome.[7] Studies suggesting a key role for dsDNA in eliciting inflammation in the pathogenesis of SLE have also rekindled interest in manipulating DNA structure using topoisomerase I inhibition, administration of DNase I, or modification of histones using heparin or histone deacetylase inhibitors as possible therapeutic options.[13]

In this chapter, we describe mechanisms of *autoantigenesis*, mechanisms by which autoantigens might contribute to the pathogenesis of SLE, common autoantigens in SLE, and ingenious and arduous approaches to mapping of T-cell epitopes in these autoantigens. Peptides containing these autoantigenic epitopes have been administered in ways that can prevent disease in animal models of lupus via a myriad of proposed mechanisms. Finally, we discuss progress and problems in translating these findings from model systems into human disease to develop antigen-specific therapies.

AUTOANTIGENESIS: MECHANISMS THAT MAKE AN ANTIGEN AN AUTOANTIGEN

That only certain self-proteins frequently elicit an autoimmune response has intrigued many investigators to speculate that autoimmunity might occur as a result of altered self or modified self.[14,15] In

this section, we describe mechanisms—defective apoptosis, impaired removal of apoptotic cells, somatic mutations, genetic polymorphisms, alternative splicing, and posttranslational modifications—that could generate epitopes for which the immune system is not tolerized.[16] See Box 21-1 for a summary of characteristics of autoantigens. The modified antigens can be taken up, processed, and presented by antigen-presenting cells (APCs) and recognized by existing potentially self-reactive B and T cells, resulting in breakage of tolerance and induction of autoimmunity. Defects in this pathway, that is, sensing and uptake and processing of antigens, can also lead to autoantigenesis. Finally, a bystander enrollment as an autoantigen can occur during epitope spreading of immune responses and as a result of mimicry with a foreign antigen.

Defective Apoptosis

Defective apoptosis can result in the generation of neoepitopes.[13] Proteolytic cleavage of lupus-associated autoantigens, like poly (ADP-ribose) polymerase and a catalytic subunit of DNA-dependent protein kinase (DNA-PKCs), has been shown to disturb homeostasis and cause increased apoptosis. As a result of nuclear fragmentation and membrane blebbing in apoptosis, autoantigens that are targeted in SLE are reorganized and transported to cell surfaces.[17] Secondary necrosis can also be an additional source of proteolytically modified forms of specific autoantigens.[18] For example, during the initial apoptotic stages, several autoantigens, including poly ADP-ribose, are cleaved into apoptosis fragments. The apoptotic cells then undergo secondary necrosis in the absence of phagocytosis with additional modifications of autoantigens.[18] A misguided immune response to these modified nuclear and cytoplasmic antigens is believed to be a major mechanism underlying autoantibody production in SLE.

Impaired Removal of Apoptotic Cells

Impaired removal of apoptotic cells could contribute to an overload of autoantigens (particularly nucleosomes) in circulation or in target tissues that could become available to initiate an autoimmune response. Nucleosomes are formed during apoptosis by organized cleavage of chromatin. These nucleosomes together with other autoantigens cluster in apoptotic bodies at the surfaces of apoptotic cells. Systemic release of these autoantigens is normally prevented by swift removal of apoptotic cells. However, if excessive apoptosis exceeds the rate of removal of apoptotic bodies, nucleosomes are released. A number of studies have identified abnormalities that lead to impairment of apoptotic debris removal in patients with SLE and in mouse models. These include deficiencies in complement components, particularly C1q, C2, and C4[19] as well as macrophage proteins that are pertinent to clearance of debris, including scavenger receptor A (SR-A), macrophage receptor and collagenous structure (MARCO),[20] and mer tyrosine kinase.[21]

Mutations

Mutations in self-antigens, which may create a neoepitope, might trigger autoimmunity. For example, in a complementary DNA (cDNA) library made from peripheral blood lymphocytes (PBLs) of

Box 21-1 Some Common Features of Autoantigens Described in Lupus*

1. Ubiquitously present[14,162]
2. Evolutionarily conserved[14,15]
3. Genetically polymorphic[24,162]
4. Expressed in apoptotic blebs[160]
5. Restricted polyclonality, i.e., against autoantigens that are structurally or functionally related[152]
6. Restricted polyclonality through shared T-cell determinants among variable regions of different autoantibodies[76,77]
7. Posttranslationally modified[29,168]
8. Substrates of apoptotic enzymes (caspases)[30,32]
9. Mutated somatically[22,23,157]
10. Charged or coil-coil structure[162]
11. Molecular mimics of infectious agents[33,34]
12. Able to interact with TLR or other receptors[46,47,156]

*Superscript numbers indicate chapter references.

a patient with primary Sjögren syndrome, one study identified a deletion of an (A)-residue in a cDNA encoding for the nuclear autoantigen La (SSB). This leads to a frame shift mutation in one of the major autoepitope regions of the La antigen.[22,23] The modified La peptide shared homology with (1) La protein itself and (2) a series of DNA-binding proteins, including other autoantigens, and viral proteins such as topoisomerase I, RNA-dependent RNA polymerase of influenza virus, and reverse transcriptase. The mutant La peptide represents a putative neoepitope that could be involved in triggering of the autoimmune response.

Genetic Polymorphisms

Genetic polymorphisms may create autoantigens.[24] Analysis of sequence variability has revealed significantly more single-nucleotide polymorphisms (SNPs) within coding regions of known human autoantigens (n = 348) than of other human genes (n = 14,881). Autoantigens had 7.2 SNPs per gene, compared with 3.6 SNPs per control gene. As an example, human Ro52, a major autoantigen in rheumatic diseases, contains two synonymous and three nonsynonymous SNPs, and one of the nonsynonymous SNPs is located in the central immunodominant region of the autoantigen.[25] Further, an intronic SNP that leads to aberrant splicing of Ro52 messenger RNA (mRNA), resulting in the generation of a shortened version of the Ro52 protein, is strongly associated with anti-Ro52 autoantibodies in primary Sjögren syndrome.[26]

Alternative Splicing

Alternative splicing can create autoantigens.[16] A bioinformatics analysis revealed alternative splicing in 100% transcripts of 45 randomly selected autoantigens, which is significantly higher than the approximately 42% rate of alternative splicing observed in 9554 randomly selected human gene transcripts. Within the isoform-specific regions of the autoantigens, 92% and 88% encoded major histocompatibility complex (MHC) class I– and class II–restricted T-cell antigen epitopes, respectively, and 70% encoded antibody-binding domains. Furthermore, 80% of the autoantigen transcripts underwent noncanonical alternative splicing, a rate that is also significantly higher than the less than 1% rate observed in randomly selected gene transcripts.

Posttranslational Modifications

Posttranslational modifications in a protein could also act as a means to promote autoreactivity.[6,7,15] Between 50% and 90% of the proteins in the human body acquire posttranslational modification. Many of these modifications are necessary for the biological functions of proteins. Some posttranslational modifications, however, can create new self-antigens by altering immunologic processing and presentation. Because these modifications occur after the lymphocyte has

undergone negative selection, the existing B and T lymphocytes can recognize the modified antigens, thus causing tolerance breakdown. For example, the spontaneous conversion of asparagine or aspartic acid residues to isoaspartyl residue renders cytochrome *c* and snRNP D peptides immunogenic in murine models of SLE. Mice develop T-cell responses to the isoaspartic acid–containing peptides but not to the native aspartic acid–containing peptides. Autoantibodies in these mice, however, recognize both the isoaspartic peptides and the native aspartic acid peptides. Isoaspartic acid residues have also been detected in histone H2B, a common autoantigen in spontaneous and drug-induced lupus.[27] In other examples of a likely role of posttranslational modification in autoimmunity, patients with SLE have been found to have autoantibodies against the C-terminus of snRNP that contains symmetrical dimethyl arginines,[28] and phosphorylated serine/arginine–rich residues of the SR protein (a family of pre-mRNA splicing factors). Interestingly, some autoantibodies are directed at dephosphorylated SR proteins that normally would exist in a phosphorylated state.[29]

Altered Antigen Processing

Altered antigen processing can lead to generation of new autoantigens for which the immune system is not tolerized. In xenobiotic models of lupuslike autoimmunity, cell death following exposure to autoimmunity-inducing agents leads to generation of novel protein fragments that may activate self-reactive T lymphocytes.[30] During apoptosis, interaction of several autoantigens with granzyme B has been shown to generate unique protein fragments that are not observed during any other form of cell death. Interestingly, nonautoantigens are either not cleaved by granzyme B or are cleaved to generate fragments identical to those formed in other forms of apoptosis. Therefore the ability of granzyme B to generate unique fragments appears to be an exclusive property of autoantigens.[31,32]

Molecular Mimicry

Molecular mimicry has been proposed to explain the role of microbial antigens in inducing and/or exacerbating autoimmune diseases. Association between the development of SLE and viruses such as Epstein-Barr virus (EBV), Coxsackie virus, and retroviruses like human T-lymphocyte virus (HTLV) has been described.[33] For example, analysis of autoantibody responses in patients with SLE prior to the onset of clinical disease led to identification of an initial autoantigenic epitope that appears in some patients who have antibodies to 60-kDa Ro antigen. This initial epitope cross-reacts with a peptide from the latent viral protein Epstein-Barr virus nuclear antigen 1 (EBNA-1). Animals immunized either with the initial epitope of 60-kDa Ro or with the cross-reactive EBNA-1 epitope progressively develop autoantibodies binding to multiple epitopes of Ro and spliceosomal autoantigens. The immunized animals eventually demonstrate clinical symptoms of lupus, thus providing a strong evidence for association of EBV infection and development of SLE.[34] One study has demonstrated molecular mimicry at the T-cell epitope level between lupus-associated autoantigen Sm-D and microbial peptides (Table 21-1). The researchers found that distinct autoreactive T-cell clones were activated by different microbial peptides, suggesting a role for molecular mimicry at the T-cell epitope level for activation of autoantibody augmenting autoreactive T cells.[8]

Defective Sensing and Uptake of Autoantigen

Accumulating evidence suggests that under autoimmune conditions, DNA fragments alone are able to induce signaling cascades that promote inflammation. Pathways through which self-DNA is able to induce proinflammatory reactions are distinct from those activated by microbial nucleic acids.[13] The dsDNA-containing immune complexes undergo endocytosis after engaging the B-cell receptor (BCR) on B cells or Fc receptors (FcRs) on dendritic cells (DCs), macrophages, and glomerular cells. Additionally, dsDNA can be internalized after binding to LL-37 (cathelicidin), or through the HMGB1-RAGE (receptor for advanced glycation end-products)

TABLE 21-1 Potential T-Cell Epitopes That Are Implicated in SLE

REFERENCE	MODEL	METHOD OF IDENTIFICATION	PEPTIDE SOURCE	PEPTIDES	PEPTIDE SEQUENCE/COMMENT
Studies in Mouse Models					
Singh et al., 1995a[1]; Singh et al., 1998b[77]; Singh et al., 1995b[42]	(NZB×NZW)F1	T-cell pepscan using >400 overlapping peptides	V_H regions of 4 anti-dsDNA mAbs	A6 p34 A6 p58 A6 p84 ds3 p33 Others	MNWVKQSHGKSL FYNQKFKGKATL SEDSALYYCARD FITWVKQRTGQGLEW
Kaliyaperumal et al., 1999[121]; Kaliyaperumal et al., 1996[86]	(SWR×NZB)F1	T-cell cloning, and deducing peptides that activate T-cell clones	Core histones of nucleosomes	H2B$_{10-33}$ H4$_{16-39}$ H4$_{71-94}$	PKKGSKKAVTKAQKKDGKKRKRSR KRHRKVLRDNIQGITKPAIRRLAR TYTEHAKRKTVTAMDVVYALKRQG
Brosh et al., 2000b[95]; Waisman et al., 1997[93]	Anti-DNA mAb–induced SLE in mice	Selected CDR-based peptides	Anti-DNA mAb	pCDR1 pCDR3	TGYYMQWVKQSPEKSLEWIG YYCARFLWEPYAMDYWGQGS
Hahn et al., 2001[120]; Singh et al., 1998a[119]	(NZB×NZW)F1	Statistical analysis of 439 peptides from anti-DNA V_H	Artificial	Consensus	FIEWNKLRFRQGLEW
Brosh et al., 2000c[159]	(NZB×NZW)F1	Selected CDR-based peptide	Anti-DNA mAb	pCDR3	YYCARFLWEPYAMDYWGQGS
Freed et al., 2000[163]	MRL-lpr	Eluting MHC class II–bound peptides from lymph nodes	Histones (H2A.2), ribosomal proteins (60S, 40S), RNA splicing factor (Srp 20), 26S proteasome, Ig γ1-chain, Ig γ2b-chain, RNA editase-1, C1r, ferritin, axin, lysozyme c, saposin D, nucleoporin NUP155, 14-3-3 protein (see reference for sequences)		
Monneaux et al., 2000[99]; Monneaux et al., 2001[40]; Monneaux et al., 2004[169]	MRL-lpr, (NZB×NZW) F1		U1-70K snRNP	p131-151 P140	RIHMVYSKRSGKPRGYAFIEY RIHMVYSKRS(P)GKPRGYAFIEY
Fan and Singh, 2002[18]	(NZB×NZW)F1	Bioinformatics and cell-binding assays	Identified multiple epitopes that have high proteolytic cleavage scores, dissociation half-time scores, and MHC class I-binding		
Kaliyaperumal et al., 2002[166]	(SWR×NZB)F1	Eluting MHC class II–bound peptides from an APC line fed with crude chromatin	H1' 22-42 Brain transcription factor BRN-3		
Suen et al., 2004[89]; Suen et al., 2001[88]	(NZB×NZW)F1	Pulsing bone marrow–derived DCs with the protein and detecting T-cell responses to epitopes	T-cell epitope located at the C-terminus of U1A protein Several epitopes in H2A, H2B, H3, and H4		
Fournel et al., 2003[87]	(NZB×NZW)F1	T-cell proliferation and cytokine responses upon ex vivo stimulation	Histone H4	Overlapping—11 peptides	No response
			Histone H3	Peptides 53-70, 64-78, and 68-85	Proliferation, IL-2, IL-10, and IFN-γ
				Peptide 56-73	IFN-γ, but no proliferation
				Peptide 61-78	IL-10, but no proliferation
Rai et al., 2006[171]; Yang et al., 2009[178]	Rabbit	Autoantibody and clinical disease after immunization	"SM" peptide: PPPGMRPP (from nuclear protein Sm B/B'); "GR" peptide: DEWDYGLP (rabbit 2b subunit of neuronal postsynaptic NMDAR)		ANA and anti-dsDNA in >50% rabbits; some with anti-Sm/RNP Two rabbits had seizure-like events and one had nystagmus
Studies in Human SLE					
Williams et al., 1995[106]	In vitro culture with PBMCs	Selected V region peptides	Human anti-DNA mAbs, B3 and 9G4	16-mer peptides	See reference
Linker-Israeli, 1996[107]	PBMCs	Epitope mapping	Human anti-DNA mAb	12-mer overlapping	Sequence not published

TABLE 21-1 Potential T-Cell Epitopes That Are Implicated in SLE—cont'd

REFERENCE	MODEL	METHOD OF IDENTIFICATION	PEPTIDE SOURCE	PEPTIDES	PEPTIDE SEQUENCE/COMMENT
Lu et al., 1999[105]	T-cell clones, lines and fresh PBMCs	Epitope mapping	Histones	$H2B_{10-33}$ $H4_{16-39}$ $H4_{71-94}$ $H2A_{34-48}$ $H3_{91-105}$ $H4_{49-63}$	Same as in mice (see Kaliyaperumal et al., 1996[86]) LRKGNYAERVGAGAP QSSAVMALQEASEAY LIYEETRGVLKVFLE
Talken et al., 1999a[114]	T-cell clones	Epitope mapping	Sm-B	$Sm\text{-}B2_{48-96}$	See reference
Davies et al., 2002[116]	PBMC stimulation	T-cell proliferation by overlapping 15-mer peptides	Human La antigen	La 49-63	Similar T-cell response in HLA-DR3$^+$ patients and controls
Dayan et al., 2000[110]; Shoeger et al., 2003[4]	PBL	T-cell proliferation and/or IL-2 production	Human or murine anti-DNA peptides		Fewer patients than controls show proliferative response Peptides inhibit 16/6 Id–induced proliferation and IL-2 production, increase TGF-β production
Kalsi et al., 2004[108]	PBMC stimulation	Cytokine release in response to 7 peptides	Human anti-DNA mAb	7 V_H region peptides	IFN-γ/IL-10 release frequent in SLE; HLA-DQB1*0201/DRB1*0301 among "responders"
Monneaux et al., 2005[117]	PBMC stimulation	T-cell proliferation and cytokine release	U1-70K snRNP	p131-151 P140	RIHMVYSKRSGKPRGYAFIEY RIHMVYSKRS(P)GKPRGYAFIEY
Kosmopoulou et al., 2006[167]	Homology modeling based on the crystal structure	Common/similar candidate T-cell epitopes identified by 3 approaches: Taylor's sequence pattern, TEPITOPE matrices, MULTIPRED artificial neural network		Six T-cell epitopes were predicted for HLA-DQ7 and nine for HLA-DQ2 in the human La/SSB autoantigen The binding efficiency of predicted epitopes was tested by potential interaction energy, binding affinity, and IC$_{50}$ values
Deshmukh et al., 2011[8]	Immunization of HLA-DR3 Tg mice; stimulation of T-cell clones	Cytokines, proliferation, and autoantibodies	Lupus-associated autoantigen Sm-D protein		Identified Sm-D79-93 as a dominant HLA-DR3 restricted T-cell epitope of Sm-D protein Demonstrated mimicry at T-cell epitope level between Sm-D79-93 and peptides from *Vibrio cholerae*, *Streptococcus agalactiae*, and La protein

ANA, antinuclear antibody; CDR, complementarity-determining region; ds, double-stranded; IC$_{50}$, half maximal inhibitory concentration; IFN, interferon; Ig, immunoglobulin; IL, interleukin; mAb, monoclonal antibody; MHC, major histocompatibility complex; NMDAR, *N*-methyl-D-aspartate receptor; PBL, peripheral blood lymphocyte; PBMCs, peripheral blood mononuclear cells; RNP, ribonucleoprotein; sn, small nuclear; Tg, transgenic; TGF-β, transforming growth factor beta; V_H, variable heavy chain.

pathway. These routes result in localization of DNA to endosomes. The dsDNA-sensing pathways activated differ according to the structure of the DNA. CpG-rich dsDNA activates Toll-like receptor 9 (TLR9), whereas AT-rich dsDNA signals through DAI (DNA-dependent activator of interferons) or RNA polymerase III. These signaling pathways all lead to production of type I interferon (IFN) and inflammation. A fourth dsDNA-sensing pathway involves the AIM2 inflammasome and results in activation of interleukin-1 beta (IL-1β) and induction of pyroptosis. It is logical to hypothesize that defects in these pathways may trigger autoantigenicity of DNA,[13] although little is known about the exact role these pathways play in the pathogenesis of SLE.

Chronic Inflammation as a Trigger of Autoantigenesis

Exposure to naturally occurring hydrocarbon oils, such as the medium-length alkane 2,6,10,14-tetramethyl pentadecane (TMPD, also known as pristane), is associated with the development of chronic inflammation and a variety of pathologic findings in humans and animal models.[9,35] Depending on the genetic background, persistent inflammation in otherwise normal strains of mice eventuates in a cascade of events leading to a plethora of autoimmune manifestations, including glomerulonephritis, arthritis, pulmonary vasculitis, and autoantibodies against a variety of nuclear and cytoplasmic antigens, which mimics human SLE syndrome more closely than the genetically susceptible strains of mice.[9-11]

Data suggest that different autoantibody subsets and organ injury are mediated through different pathways, and both innate and adaptive immune responses participate in the development of full lupuslike syndrome in TMPD-injected mice.[12] The initial response to TMPD is orchestrated by major components of the innate immune system. It starts with the infiltration of neutrophils and Ly6C^{hi} inflammatory monocytes into the peritoneal cavity, which lasts for several months.[35] Type I IFN (IFN-I) production downstream of TLR7 signaling and CCR2 (chemokine [C-C motif] receptor 2) plays a role in the influx of monocytes, whereas IL-1α and CXCL5 (chemokine [C-X-C motif] ligand 5) play a role in neutrophil recruitment to the peritoneal cavity. The adaptor molecules MyD88, IL-1R–associated kinase 4 (IRAK-4), IRAK-1, and IRAK-2 play a role in the recruitment of both monocytes and neutrophils. Deficiency of IL-6, TLR9, and TLR4 attenuate organ injury and production of anti-dsDNA and/or anti-RNP autoantibodies. Although the exact cascade of events that lead to autoantigenicity of lupus autoantigens is not known, studies in this model suggest a role for chronic inflammation in autoantigenesis.

MECHANISMS BY WHICH AUTOANTIGENS MAY CONTRIBUTE TO THE DEVELOPMENT OF DISEASE
Induction of Effector T cells

Autoantigen-specific T cells can contribute to pathogenesis of SLE by helping B cells produce autoantibodies or by directly infiltrating the tissues. Ample evidence also supports the requirement of T-cell help for pathogenic autoantibody production.[36,37] This help is provided by T cells that react with peptides derived from various autoantigens.[37-43] One study has shown that MRL-lpr mice that have no secreted immunoglobulin (Ig) develop spontaneous T-cell activation and some disease,[44] suggesting a direct, antibody-independent role for T cells in the development of SLE-like disease. "Autoantigen-specific" T cells, however, have not yet been demonstrated in the target tissues of humans and mice with lupus. In one study, the use of in situ tetramer staining has allowed identification of human antigen–specific T cells in the affected organs, such as the pancreases of patients with autoimmune diabetes.[5] Both single and multiple T-cell autoreactivities were detected within individual islets in a subset of patients up to 8 years after clinical diagnosis. Use of such technology has potential to identify tissue-infiltrating autoantigen-specific T cells that can be true targets for treatment in patients with SLE.

Reduced Activation of Regulatory, Inhibitory, or Suppressor T Cells

Immunization with self-Ig peptides induces T cells that can suppress anti-DNA antibodies in healthy strains of mice.[45] Induction of such "self-reactive" regulatory T cells is impaired in lupus-prone mice that mount mostly pathogenic T-helper (Th) cell response.

Activation of Toll-Like Receptors

Activation of TLRs by autoantigens can amplify the autoimmune response by activating the innate immune component. Chromatin-containing CpG motif–rich DNA or RNP antigens containing dsRNA can potentially trigger lupuslike autoimmune responses by providing accessory signals through TLR9 on DCs, macrophages, or B cells, or through TLR3 on DCs.[46,47] Further, immune complexes containing IgG bound to chromatin can activate murine DCs through both TLR9-dependent and TLR9-independent pathways,[48] a feature that may affect autoimmune responses. Indeed, TLR9 deficiency specifically reduces the generation of anti-dsDNA and antichromatin autoantibodies in MRL-lpr mice.[49] Viral dsRNA can also activate DCs via TLR3 to induce the production of IFN-I and cytokines associated with disease activity in SLE. Furthermore, TLR3 expression is increased in infiltrating APCs as well as in glomerular mesangial cells in kidney sections of MRL-lpr mice.[50]

HMGB1, a nuclear DNA-binding protein, can trigger a proinflammatory response by interacting with receptors TLR2, TLR4, and RAGE on macrophages and DCs.[51] HMGB1 can also stimulate innate immune responses by acting as a universal sentinel for nucleic acids and facilitating their interaction with a number of receptors, including TLR3, TLR7, and TLR9.[52] Importantly, in patients with SLE, serum HMGB1 and anti-HMGB1 autoantibody concentrations are elevated and correlate with disease activity.[53] A number of reports have linked the activation of TLRs with autoimmune diseases primarily through their ability to drive the induction of autoreactive T and B cells.[54] Furthermore, there is evidence that TLR activation can block T-regulatory (Treg) cell responses, thereby breaking tolerance to self-antigens.

Autoantigens as Chemoattractants

Autoantigens may serve as chemoattractants that recruit innate immune cells to sites of tissue damage.[55] A variety of autoantigens has been shown to induce leukocyte migration by interacting with various chemoattractant Gi protein–coupled receptors (GiPCRs). For instance, myositis autoantigen, histidyl-tRNA synthetase, are chemotactic for the CCR5 and CCR3, thereby recruiting T lymphocytes and immature DCs. Fibrillarin (U3-RNP) and topoisomerase I, which are autoantigens associated with scleroderma, have been shown to serve as chemoattractants for monocytes. In some cases, such as in SLE, a complex of two autoantigens has been found to be chemotactic for immature DCs. Thus, autoantigens not only may attract immune cells to a given tissue but also can activate B cells,[56] DCs,[57,58] and neutrophils[59] via their ability to interact with cell membrane receptors.

Altered Recognition of Autoantigens

Altered recognition of autoantigens in endomembrane traffic might elicit autoimmunity.[60] The RNA transcription termination factor La,

a frequent target of Sjögren autoantibodies, appears in the acinar cell cytoplasm and plasma membranes during viral infection and after in vitro exposure to cytokines. The endomembrane compartments where proteolysis occurs contain La, galactosyltransferase, cathepsin B, and cathepsin D. MHC class II molecules cycle through this compartment. This traffic may permit trilateral interactions in which B cells recognize autoantigens at the surface membranes, CD4+ T cells recognize peptides presented by MHC II, the B cells provide accessory signals to CD4+ T cells, and CD4+ T cells provide cytokines that activate B cells.

Autoantigen Ro52

Autoantigen Ro52 is an E3 ligase that may regulate proliferation and cell death. Increased apoptosis in patients with SLE may result in greater expression of intracellular autoantigen Ro52, which may mediate ubiquitination in survival genes induced during CD40-mediated activation.[61] Ro52 may also enhance functions of genes mediating apoptosis and cell death by relieving them from endogenous repression. Intriguingly, Ro52-deficient mice develop autoimmunity, suggesting that this E3 ligase may also act as a negative regulator.

COMMON AUTOANTIGENS IN LUPUS

Autoimmunity in SLE is directed to some highly conserved intracellular molecules particularly against nuclear and cell membrane phospholipid components.[14] Nuclear antigens include DNA-associated autoantigens such as nucleosome and HMGB1 and RNA-associated autoantigens such as U1 snRNP, Ro/La complex, and ribosomes.[7] Most studies have focused on autoantibody responses to functionally related nucleic acid–containing macromolecules such as chromatin and RNP particles, because autoantibodies to dsDNA and Sm antigens of the U-1 snRNP complex are considered pathognomonic of SLE. These and other autoantibodies are described in detail in other chapters.

In brief, high-affinity antibodies to dsDNA are hallmarks of SLE. Some subsets of these autoantibodies cause renal and vascular injury.[62,63] The common features of such pathogenic autoantibodies, such as class-switched IgGs and somatic mutation, indicate that anti-dsDNA antibodies arise as a result of an antigen-driven process. The antigenic stimuli driving the production of anti-dsDNA autoantibodies remain elusive, but some studies provide possible candidates. Because nucleic acids are poor or not immunogenic, DNA-binding protein in complex with DNA is purported to break tolerance to DNA.[64] One possible explanation is that some peptides can serve as surrogate anti-dsDNA epitopes, thus activating T-cell help for the production of anti-dsDNA antibodies.[65,66] Another possibility supports a hapten carrier–like mechanism, in which T cells specific for peptides derived from the DNA-binding proteins (such as histones) provide help to DNA-specific B cells. For example, immunization of animals with DNA-protein complexes, rather than with protein-free DNA, induces robust anti-dsDNA antibody response.[64] A third possibility is that anti-dsDNA antibody response could occur during the autoantibody response toward the protein constituent of the RNP autoantigens such as nucleosomes or snRNPs.[14]

Autoantibody against the Sm autoantigens of the snRNP complex is also pathognomonic of SLE. The snRNPs are ubiquitous self-antigens that are components of the spliceosome complex that normally functions to excise intervening introns and generate mature mRNA transcripts. In most snRNP particles, seven core proteins—B, D1, D2, D3, E, F, and G—form a heptamer ring, with the snRNA passing through the center. The Sm epitopes are distributed on the outside surface of the ring. A previous study used overlapping octapeptides spanning the full length of the B/B′ protein to identify an epitope, PPPGMRPP, within the C-terminus of SmB′/B, that is recognized very early in animal models and in some patients with SLE.[67] Over time, the immune response spreads beyond this initial epitope to other snRNP autoantigens, including U1-specific RNP epitopes frequently targeted by antibodies present in patients with mixed connective tissue disease.[67] Most Sm-precipitin–positive lupus sera, however, recognize certain Sm-D polypeptides, such as the glycine-arginine (GR)–rich carboxyl region of Sm-D1.[68,69] The levels of the anti–Sm-D83-119 strongly correlate (as does that of antinucleosome) with disease activity. High levels of anti–dsDNA and anti–Sm-D183-119 strongly correlate with lupus nephritis.[70,71]

HMGB1-nucleosome complexes from apoptotic cells activate APCs via TLRs and induce proinflammatory responses. HMGB1 is a ubiquitously expressed, structural chromosomal protein that is highly conserved across species.[72] In the cell nucleus, HMGB1 binds indiscriminately to the minor groove of DNA and induces strong bends. In addition, HMGB1 is able to bind to highly structured noncanonical or damaged DNA and participates in DNA-related processes, including DNA repair, chromatin remodeling, and transcription. HMGB1 facilitates the formation of multiple nucleoprotein complexes by protein-protein interaction. Initial studies demonstrated the prevention of HMGB1 release during early stages of apoptotic cell death. Hypoacetylation of chromosomal proteins and phosphorylation of histone H2B during apoptotic cell death tightens HMGB1 binding to the chromatin and prevents HMGB1 from being released. By contrast, HMGB1 in necrotic cells is loosely bound to chromatin and is allowed to diffuse into the extracellular space of cells, thereby acting as an endogenous alarmin.[73] Evidence now suggests that HMGB1 release also occurs late in the apoptotic cell death process, known as *secondary necrosis*, in which fragmented HMGB1 is released as a complex with chromatin. Additionally, oxidation of HMGB1 during apoptotic and necrotic cell death may lead to immunogenic neoepitopes that may further exacerbate disease progression.[51] HMGB1 itself has been reported to interact with receptors on APCs, including TLR2, TLR4, and RAGE. Interaction with these receptors leads to activation of nuclear factor kappa B (NF-κB), inducing the transcription of proinflammatory genes and the production of inflammatory cytokines. Moreover, HMGB1 induces maturation and migration of DCs. HMGB1 has also been reported to act as a sentinel for virtually all nucleic acids, especially those of viral and microbial origins, thereby aiding in triggering TLR3, TLR7, and TLR9 immune responses by their cognate nucleic acid.[52] HMBG1 in complex with nucleosomes from apoptotic cells can activate APCs via a TLR2-dependent pathway, thereby breaking immunologic tolerance against chromatin. Thus, growing evidence suggests a role for HMGB1 in the pathogenesis of SLE.

Some common features of autoantigens are summarized in Box 21-1. In addition to their being evolutionarily conserved and ubiquitously expressed, lupus autoantigens are highly diverse, yet this diversity is restricted to certain sets of autoantigens, causing a "restricted polyclonality" of autoimmune responses in lupus. Several mechanisms have been proposed to explain this phenomenon; they have been reviewed elsewhere.[74-76] According to a unique mechanism that we have suggested (Singh et al., 1998b),[77] T-cell epitopes (amino acid sequences that can serve as T-cell determinants) are shared among variable regions of different lupus-related autoantibodies but not among other antibodies. Thus, a T-cell epitope present in an anti-DNA Ig may activate T cells that can deliver help to B cells specific for antiphospholipid or anti–red blood cells or other related autoantigens, but not to B cells specific for an unrelated antigen. This is one explanation why lupus autoantibodies are polyclonal yet restricted to a recurring set of autoantigens. The shared T-cell epitopes in autoantibodies may originate as a result of replacement mutations in mutationally "cold" framework regions, which do not affect the binding of antibody to its antigen but create T-cell epitopes.[78,79] In fact, although mutations in normal Ig involve hotspot areas, mutations in lupus Ig occur in non-hotspot areas, which might be responsible for creating T-cell epitopes.[80]

The lupus autoantigens are presumed to initiate and perpetuate the autoimmune response in T and B cells, but exactly how and when this occurs are still not understood. The mechanisms are discussed in other sections of this and other chapters. In brief, autoreactive T cells such as nucleosome-specific T cells have been identified in patients with SLE that drive the formation of anti-dsDNA and anti-histone antibodies.[81,82]

IDENTIFICATION OF AUTOANTIGENIC EPITOPES IN LUPUS
Studies in Animal Models
Work in the late 1980s suggested that autoantibody production in humans and mice with SLE is antigen-driven and depends on Th cells that are mostly CD4+.[36,83-85] To identify the nature and specificity of such autoreactive Th cells, several laboratories have used diverse approaches, including T-cell pepscanning of candidate autoantigens, isolating autoreactive T-cell clones and deducing potential autoantigens, screening phage display libraries, and eluting naturally processed self-peptides from MHC class II molecules. These approaches have led to identification of epitopes that activate autoreactive Th cells in humans and mice with lupus and modulate disease in lupus mice (see Table 21-1).

Nucleosome Core Histone Peptides as Th Autoepitopes
Using lupus-prone SWR/NZB F1 mice, one group cloned Th cells that can initiate and sustain the production of pathogenic autoantibodies and induce lupus nephritis, and recognize nucleosomes.[39] Stimulation of these autoreactive lupus Th cells with 145 overlapping peptides spanning the four core histones H2A, H2B, H3, and H4 led the researchers to localize the critical lupus epitopes in the core histones of nucleosomes at amino acid positions 10 through 33 of H2B and 16 through 39 and 71 through 94 of H4 (see Table 21-1).[86] Autoimmune T cells of SWR/NZB F1 mice are spontaneously primed to these epitopes from early life. Moreover, immunization of preautoimmune SWR/NZB F1 mice with these peptides precipitates lupus nephritis.[86]

In another study, a panel of overlapping peptides spanning the whole sequences of H4 and H3 were cultured with CD4+ T cells from unprimed (NZB/NZW)F1 lupus mice.[87] None of the 11 H4 peptides stimulated CD4+ T cells in these mice, whereas several H3 peptides representing sequences 53 through 70, 64 through 78, and 68 through 85 elicited proliferation and induced secretion of IL-2, IL-10, and IFN-γ. The H3 peptides 56 through 73 and 61 through 78 induced the production of IFN-γ and IL-10, respectively, without detectable proliferation, suggesting that they may act as partial agonists of the TCR. Moreover, the study found that this conserved region of H3, which is accessible at the surfaces of nucleosomes, is targeted by antibodies from (NZB/NZW)F1 mice and patients with lupus, and contains motifs recognized by several distinct HLA-DR molecules. This region might thus be important in the self-tolerance breakdown in lupus.

Pulsing bone marrow–derived DCs with lupus autoantigens U1A protein[88] or nucleosome[89] and then testing in vitro recall T-cell responses to individual epitopes was found to be highly efficient for mapping T-cell epitopes using freshly isolated T cells from unprimed (NZB/NZW)F1 mice. Several potential auto–T-cell epitopes of core histone proteins (H2A, H2B, H3, and H4) were identified with use of this approach.

Self-Ig Peptides as Autoantigenic Epitopes
Early work in the late 1980s and early 1990s suggested that human or murine B cells can process Ig molecules and present Ig-derived peptides in the context of their surface MHC class I and class II molecules. Moreover, Ig-derived peptides are eluted from MHC class II molecules, suggesting that they are naturally processed. T cells from mice expressing a transgene encoding a TCR specific for an Ig-derived peptide provided help for B-cell production of antibodies. Furthermore, Ig peptide–reactive T cells follow rules of conventional T-cell tolerance and activation. It is believed that normal as well as lupus-prone mice generally attain T-cell tolerance to germline-encoded antibody sequences[78,90,91] whereas somatically mutated antibody sequences can activate T-cell help because they arise in rare B cells at a late stage of T and B differentiation, thus creating

neoepitopes.[78] The preceding observations led our group to postulate that SLE B cells process their endogenous or surface Ig into peptides that are presented on MHC class II molecules. These peptide-MHC complexes then activate autoreactive Th cells, which, in turn, stimulate B cells for the increased production of autoantibodies.[1,42,77,92]

Several lines of evidence support the role of these peptides in autoantibody production and lupus. First, many peptides increased anti-dsDNA antibody production in vitro when cultured with syngeneic splenocytes.[77] Second, adoptive transfer of peptide-specific T cell lines or immunizations with peptide/adjuvant emulsions raised serum IgG anti-dsDNA antibody levels, accelerated nephritis, and decreased survival.[42]

SLE-like disease can be induced in normal mice by injecting human or murine anti-DNA monoclonal antibodies that bear a 16/6 idiotype (Id) that is frequently present on Ig of mice and humans with SLE. Using this model, a previous study found that two peptides representing regions of FR1/CDR1/FR2 (termed pCDR1) and FR3/CDR3 (termed pCDR3) of the heavy chain region (V_H) of a monoclonal antibody (mAb), 5G12, stimulated T-cell proliferation in BALB/c and SJL mice and induced proteinuria, leukopenia, and glomerular Ig deposits (see Table 21-1).[93] A T-cell line reactive with pCDR3 also induces experimental lupus in naïve mice.[94,95] These findings indicate an important role for Ig-derived peptides in the development of lupus.

T-Cell Pepscan of U1-70K snRNP Autoantigen
Muller and colleagues tested a series of overlapping peptides recapitulating the sequence of spliceosomal U1-70K snRNP and identified an epitope present in residues 131 through 151 that is recognized very early by IgG antibodies and CD4+ lymph node T cells in lupus-prone MRL-lpr and (NZB/NZW)F1 mice.[96-98] The ability of this peptide to stimulate T cells from mice bearing different MHC haplotypes (H-2^k of MRL-lpr and H-2$^{d/z}$ of [NZB/NZW]F1) correlated with its binding to I-A^k, I-E^k, I-A^d, and I-E^d murine MHC molecules. Interestingly, an analog of peptide 131 through 151 sequence phosphorylated on Ser^{140} (named peptide P140) was more strongly recognized by lymph node and peripheral CD4+ T cells and by IgG antibodies from MRL-lpr mice than the native peptide.[75,99] Subcutaneous administration of P140 in Freund adjuvant accelerated lupus nephritis, demonstrating the pathogenic role of a posttranslationally modified epitope.

Screening Phage Display Library to Identify Peptidomimetics That Bind Anti-DNA Antibody
An entirely different approach was used by Gaynor to identify nephritogenic peptides.[100] The group screened a peptide display phage library with mouse monoclonal antibodies that bind dsDNA and cause nephritis, and identified a decapeptide DWEYSVWLSN that specifically binds an anti-dsDNA monoclonal antibody, R4A. Immunization with this peptide induced IgG antibodies that bind DNA, cardiolipin, and Sm/RNP and caused Ig deposition in glomeruli.[66,101]

Identification of Self-Epitopes in Human SLE
Human T cells reactive with several lupus autoantigens, including DNA-histones, the snRNP antigenic proteins Sm-B, Sm-D, U1-70kD, and U1-A, and heterogeneous RNP (hnRNP) A2, have been isolated from the peripheral blood of patients with SLE.[102] Datta's group first described T-cell lines from patients with SLE, which augmented the production of IgG anti-DNA antibodies ex vivo[103] and antihistone.[104] These autoantibody-promoting T cells are usually CD4+ T cells that use restricted CDR3 characteristic of antigen selection.[104] To identify antigenic epitopes for these T cells, they used 154 peptides spanning the entire length of core histones of nucleosomes to stimulate an anti-DNA antibody–inducing Th clone, CD4+ T cell lines, and freshly isolated T cells in peripheral blood mononuclear cells (PBMCs) from 23 patients with SLE.[105] In contrast to normal T cells, lupus T cells responded vigorously to certain histone peptides, irrespective of the

patient's disease status (see Table 21-1). Interestingly, most of the peptides that activated human T cells from patients with lupus were previously identified as T-cell epitopes in lupus-prone mice (see Table 21-1). Several additional epitopes, including peptides 34 through 48 of H2A, 91 through 105 and 100 through 114 of H3, and 49 through 63 of H4, were also found to activate human T cells from patients with lupus. Most of these sequences are located in the regions of histones that are accessible at the surfaces of nucleosomes and that contain B-cell epitopes targeted by lupus autoantibodies. Importantly, most T-cell epitopes have multiple HLA-DR binding motifs, that is, they are promiscuous with regard to their binding to HLA molecules. Thus, peptides containing these epitopes could potentially be used to treat many patients, obviating the development of individualized therapy.

To determine whether Ig-derived peptides activate T cells from patients with SLE, Williams cultured PBMCs from 28 patients with lupus and 13 healthy individuals with selected 16-mer peptides from two anti-DNA autoantibodies, B3 and 9G4.[106] Three of the 13 healthy individuals (23%) versus 17 of the 28 patients with SLE (61%) had T cells that proliferated in response to at least one V region peptide. In another study, Linker-Israeli cultured 12-mer overlapping peptides from the V_H of two anti-dsDNA antibodies, B3 and F51, with PBMCs from patients with SLE, their first-degree relatives, or unrelated healthy individuals.[107] The expressions of the early T-cell activation markers CD25 and CD69 and of cytokines were determined by flow cytometry. Patients with SLE had significantly increased T-cell activation markers and IL-4–secreting cells than either first-degree relatives or unrelated controls. A subsequent study by these investigators in a larger cohort (31 patients and 20 matched healthy controls) analyzed cytokine release by PBMCs in response to seven peptides from the CDR1/FR2 to CDR2/FR3 V_H regions of human anti-DNA monoclonal antibodies.[108] PBMCs from significantly higher proportions of patients with SLE than controls responded to V_H peptides by generating IFN-γ and IL-10. Three peptides were more stimulatory in patients with SLE than in controls. There was a skewing of the immune response to Th2 bias as the disease progressed from early to later stage. Although none of the peptides was restricted by any particular MHC class II allele, among "responders" there was greater prevalence of HLA-DQB1*0201 and/or DRB1*0301, alleles known to predispose to SLE. Thus, responses to some V_H peptides are more common in SLE and vary with disease duration. Increased peptide presentation by SLE-predisposing HLA molecules might permit brisker increased T-cell responses to autoantibody peptides, thus increasing risk for disease.

Guided by observations in the 16/6 Id murine model described earlier, a previous study examined immune responses of patients with SLE to peptides encompassing complementarity-determining regions (CDRs) of a monoclonal anti-DNA antibody with a 16/6 Id.[109] In contrast to the preceding data showing increased responses to anti-DNA–derived peptides,[106-108] this group found that peripheral blood lymphocytes (PBLs) from significantly fewer patients (37%) than controls (59%) proliferated in response to one of the anti-DNA peptides.[110] A subsequent study by the same group reported in vitro proliferation of PBLs from 24 of the 62 patients with SLE tested after stimulation with the human 16/6 Id.[4] Interestingly, peptides from both the human and murine anti-DNA autoantibodies specifically inhibited the 16/6 Id–induced proliferation and IL-2 production. The latter inhibitions correlated with increased production of TGF-β. Findings of this study suggested that certain anti-DNA peptides may downregulate autoreactive T-cell responses in patients with SLE. Indeed, treatment of severe combined immunodeficient (SCID) mice engrafted with PBLs of patients with SLE by repeated intraperitoneal administration of a human monoclonal anti-DNA autoantibody peptide (hCDR1) suppressed human anti-dsDNA antibodies but not anti–tetanus toxoid antibodies.[111] Such treatment also reduced proteinuria and renal deposits of human IgG and murine complement C3 in the engrafted SCID mice.

Human T cells reactive with various snRNP antigens, including Sm-B, Sm-D, U1-70kD, and U1-A, have been identified and characterized.[102] Subsequent studies on snRNP-reactive human T-cell clones showed that they typically exhibit T-cell receptor alpha/beta–positive ($TCR\alpha\beta^+$) $CD4^+$ $CD45RO^+$ phenotype, recognize antigen in the context of HLA-DR, and produce substantial amounts of IFN-γ, moderate quantities of IL-2, and variable amounts of IL-4 and IL-10.[112] Further, these cells can also provide help for relevant autoantibody production in vitro.[113] Talken established two sets of T-cell clones from patients with connective tissue diseases: one set reacted with Sm-B autoantigen and the others recognized U1-70kD polypeptide.[114,115] Both sets of T-cell clones had a highly restricted TCR CDR3 β- or α-chain gene usage, respectively. Further analysis revealed that the Sm-B–reactive T-cell clones recognized a peptide, Sm-B$_{48-96}$, in the context of HLA-DR. Subsequent T-cell epitope mapping studies of human T-cell clones reactive with the snRNPs U1-70kD, Sm-B, and Sm-D revealed that there are limited T-cell epitopes on these proteins and that almost all reside within functional regions of the protein—either within the Sm motifs for Sm-B and Sm-D or within the RNA binding domain for U1-70kD.

In another study, synthetic 15-mer overlapping peptides spanning the entire La sequence were cultured with PBMCs from patients with SLE and controls with a goal to identify T-cell epitopes in the La antigen. The researchers found a significant, albeit low-level, T-cell proliferative response to a peptide (La 49-63) in HLA-DR3$^+$ patients or healthy controls.[116] This study highlights difficulties in identifying relevant pathogenic T-cell epitopes using PBMC-based T-cell proliferation readout experiments. The findings further suggest that the presence of self peptide–reactive T cells in the peripheral blood of healthy individuals is not uncommon. It is unclear why these Th cells promote autoantibody production only in certain individuals.

As described previously, Muller and colleagues identified a CD4$^+$ T-cell epitope in peptide sequence encompassing residues 131 through 151 of the spliceosomal U1-70K snRNP protein (RIHMVYSKRSGKPRGYAFIEY) and its analog phosphorylated at Ser^{140} (called P140; RIHMVYSKRS(P)GKPRGYAFIEY) in MRL-lpr and (NZB/NZW)F1 mice.[40,117] Importantly, administration of the phosphorylated peptide P140 ameliorates the clinical manifestations of treated MRL-lpr mice.[40,99] Because this peptide sequence, which is completely conserved in the mouse and human U1-70K protein, contains an RNA-binding motif often targeted by antibodies from patients with lupus and mice, the group investigated these peptides as potential candidates for the treatment of patients with lupus.[117] Binding assays with soluble HLA class II molecules and molecular modeling experiments indicate that both peptides behave as promiscuous epitopes and bind to a large panel of human DR molecules. In contrast to normal T cells and T cells from patients with non-SLE autoimmune disease, PBMCs and/or CD4$^+$ T cells from 40% of patients with SLE proliferate in response to peptide 131-151. Interestingly, the phosphorylated analog peptide P140 prevents CD4$^+$ T-cell proliferation but not secretion of regulatory cytokine IL-10. Thus, P140 can serve as a "universal" immunomodulatory T-cell epitope.

In summary, patients with SLE have circulating T cells that recognize diverse sets of autoantigenic peptides, which include core histone peptides, Sm-B, U1-70kD, and peptides derived from the V region of autoantibodies. The significance of these T cells in the pathogenesis of SLE remains to be fully understood.

AUTOANTIGEN-BASED VACCINATION AND PEPTIDE THERAPIES IN LUPUS
Preclinical Animal Studies

A promise to avoid adverse, nonspecific effects of therapies currently used in lupus has led many investigators to test the therapeutic potential of autoantigenic peptides that specifically activate autoreactive T cells and promote pathogenic autoantibody production. Indeed, treatment with many such peptides tolerizes pathogenic Th cells, suppresses autoantibody production, and ameliorates lupus in

murine models.[1,37,118] A summary of these peptide and related therapies is provided in Table 21-2.

Initial studies on T cell–based peptide therapies to induce tolerance in lupus were conducted with the use of self-Ig peptides. Intravenous (IV) treatment with high doses of a combination of three peptides derived from an anti-DNA antibody significantly decreased levels of anti-DNA antibody, serum creatinine, and proteinuria and improved survival in (NZB×NZW)F1 mice.[1] The idea was subsequently confirmed by another study that showed that neonatal administration of peptides derived from the CDR of an anti-DNA antibody that carries a promiscuous idiotype prevented anti-DNA antibody production in an induced model of SLE.[93]

Our initial studies to induce therapeutic tolerance used three major anti-DNA–augmenting peptides.[1] The therapeutic effect was limited, however, and the treatment was ineffective when given to animals with full-blown disease. We soon realized that T-cell responses to peptides in anti-DNA V$_H$ regions spread to multiple epitopes as the disease progresses.[77] Hence, on the basis of our studies of more than 500 peptides, we designed a consensus "superdeterminant"[119] that strongly promoted autoantibody production. This peptide, termed *pConsensus* (pCons), also had a more robust and longer-standing therapeutic effect on disease than peptides given individually or in combination in (NZB×NZW)F1 mice.[120]

The next set of studies on immune tolerance in lupus used histone peptides. A brief therapy with the nucleosomal core histone peptides, administered IV to 3-month-old prenephritic mice already producing pathogenic autoantibodies, markedly delayed the onset of severe lupus nephritis. Long-term therapy with these peptides injected into 18-month-old mice with established glomerulonephritis prolonged survival and halted the progression of renal disease.[121] In another study, intradermal immunization with a histone-derived peptide, H3(111-130), which is preferentially processed by bone marrow–derived DCs, suppressed anti-dsDNA and anti-ssDNA IgG levels and delayed the progression of glomerulonephritis in lupus-prone (NZB/NZW)F1 mice.[89]

As discussed previously, a phosphorylated analog of peptide 131-151 (named peptide P140) derived from spliceosomal U1 snRNP is a strong T-cell epitope in MRL-lpr mice.[75,99] Intravenous treatment of young MRL-lpr mice with P140 peptide in saline reduces proteinuria and dsDNA IgG antibody levels and enhances survival.[122] The therapeutic effect of IV-administered P140 correlates with transient abolition of T-cell intramolecular spreading to other regions of the U1-70K protein,[75] a finding that is important because the conserved T-cell epitope sequence contains an RNA-binding motif called RNP1 that is also present in other sn/hn (heterogeneous nuclear) RNPs and often targeted by antibodies from patients with lupus and mice.[75,97] Thus, modifying responses to this promiscuous and conserved epitope may target a broad autoreactive Th cell repertoire in different models and patients.

Initial studies on antigen-based therapies in murine lupus mostly used parenteral routes of peptide administration. Mucosal delivery of peptides by oral feeding or nasal instillation can also induce strong peptide-specific tolerance in Th cells and suppress autoimmune diseases. The efficacy of mucosal tolerance has also been tested in lupus-prone mice.[123] Nasal instillation of a histone peptide H471 that expresses a dominant T-cell epitope in the histone protein H4 of mononucleosome induces a dose-dependent tolerance to the peptide H471 as well as to the whole mononucleosomes in lupus-prone SNF1 mice. This effect is accompanied by an increase in IL-10 and suppression of IFN-γ production by lymph node cells. Furthermore, long-term nasal instillation of mice with the H471 peptide suppresses the development of autoantibodies and reduces the severity of glomerulonephritis in lupus-prone SNF1 mice. Such nasal tolerance restores the numbers of CD4$^+$CD25$^+$ Treg cells, which the researchers found to be reduced in lupus-prone (NZB/NZW)F1 and SNF1 mice.[124]

In preceding sections, we describe induction of tolerance in Th cells that mostly augment production of autoantibodies against nuclear and nucleoprotein antigens. Humans and mice with lupus

TABLE 21-2 Peptide-Based Vaccination and Therapies for SLE: Studies in Animal Models (Mice, Rabbit, and Pigs)

REFERENCE	MODEL	STAGE OF DISEASE	PEPTIDES	METHOD OF DELIVERY	EFFECT OF TREATMENT
Singh et al., 1995a[1] and 1998	(NZB×NZW)F1	Prenephritic	Cocktail of 3 V_H peptides (A6.1 V_H p34, p58, and p84)	IV, soluble	Decreased anti-DNA and nephritis, and prolonged survival
Singh et al., 1996[134]	(NZB×NZW)F1	Neonatal	A6.1 V_H p58-69	IP, IFA	"Split" T-cell tolerance; increased anti-DNA Abs
Waisman et al., 1997[93]	Induced SLE in normal mice	Neonatal	pCDR1, pCDR3	IP, soluble	Decreased anti-DNA Abs
Gaynor et al., 1997[100]	SCID mice		A decapeptide that bound anti-DNA	IP, soluble	Decreased renal Ig deposition
Kaliyaperumal et al., 1999[121]	(SWR×NZB)F1	Prenephritic Diseased	$H2B_{10-33}$, $H4_{16-39}$, $H4_{71-94}$	IV, soluble	Delayed onset of nephritis Prolonged survival; halted progression of nephritis
Jouanne et al., 1999[165]	(NZB×NZW)F1	Prenephritic	V_H CDR3 of a natural polyreactive autoAb	Soluble	Delayed proteinuria and improved survival
Eilat et al., 2000[161]	(NZB×NZW)F1	Prenephritic	pCDR3 from a mAb anti-DNA	IV, soluble	Decreased disease
Hahn et al., 2001[120]	(NZB×NZW)F1	Prenephritic Diseased	Consensus V_H	IV, soluble	Decreased anti-DNA and nephritis Dramatically prolonged survival
Fan and Singh, 2002[18]	(NZB×NZW)F1	Prenephritic and diseased	MHC class I-binding V_H epitopes	Minigenes	Killed B cells, reduced anti-DNA and nephritis, and prolonged survival
Singh et al., 2002[45]; Hahn et al., 2005[137]; Singh et al., 2007[140]; Singh et al., 2008[139]; Skaggs et al., 2008[176]	(BALB/c×NZW) F1, (NZB×NZW) F1		Ig-derived peptides, Ig peptide–based artificial consensus peptide (pCons)		Induced T cells (CD4+/CD8+) that downregulated anti-DNA Ab production; such regulatory cells express FoxP3
Wu and Staines, 2004[124]; Wu et al., 2002[123]	(SWR×NZB)F1	Prenephritic	Histone peptide H471	Intranasal soluble	Suppressed autoantibody production and reduced the severity of nephritis
Monneaux et al., 2003[122]	MRL-lpr	Predisease	P140, a phosphorylated analog of U1-70K $snRNP_{131-151}$	IV, soluble	Reduced IgG anti-dsDNA Ab and proteinuria and enhanced survival
Shen et al., 2003[125]	NZB	Pre-autoimmune	Anion channel protein band 3 peptide 861-874	Intranasal	Th2 deviation, and reduced severity of autoimmune hemolytic anemia
Suen et al., 2004[89]	(NZB×NZW)F1	Prenephritic	$H3_{111-130}$	ID	Suppressed anti-DNA and delayed nephritis
Riemekasten et al., 2004[143]	(NZB×NZW)F1	Prenephritic	$Sm-D1_{83-119}$	600-1000 µg IV	Delayed autoantibody production and lupus nephritis, and prolonged survival
Fujio et al., 2004[129]	(NZB×NZW)F1	Prenephritic	Engineered nucleosome-specific Treg cells	Multiple gene transfer	Suppressed autoantibody production and nephritis
Amital et al., 2005[127]	MRL-lpr	Prenephritic	Laminin peptide agonists		Prevented renal Ab deposition and reduced renal disease
Sharabi et al., 2006[173]	(NZB×NZW)F1 females	8-mo-old mice with nephritis	Syngeneic spleen cells from hCDR1-treated young mice	Adoptive transfer, IP	Reduced disease manifestations, and IFN-γ and IL-10 levels; increased Treg cells and TGF-β
Voitharou et al., 2008[177]	Rabbit	Complementary peptide epitopes, derived from complementary RNA sequences, Cpep349-364, of the T/B-cell epitope of La/SSB, pep349-364, coupled to sequential oligopeptide carrier			Induced neutralizing anti-cpep349-364 Abs in immunized rabbits
Mozes and Sharabi, 2010[109]	Pig immunized with anti-DNA mAbs	Induced lupus	hCDR1	Wkly treatment × 10 wks	Reduced antinuclear and anti-dsDNA Abs, erythrocyte sedimentation rates, and renal immune complex depositions
Kang et al., 2011[132]	SNF1 females, 12-wk-old	AutoAb+, but prenephritic	$H4_{71-94}$	1 µg SC every 2 wks × 3	Induces "tolerance spreading" and Treg cells that suppress pathogenic autoantibodies and lupus nephritis

TABLE 21-2 Peptide-Based Vaccination and Therapies for SLE: Studies in Animal Models (Mice, Rabbit, and Pigs)—cont'd

REFERENCE	MODEL	STAGE OF DISEASE	PEPTIDES	METHOD OF DELIVERY	EFFECT OF TREATMENT
Skaggs et al., 2011[175]	BWF1 females, 11-wk-old	Prenephritic	pCons; L-MAP or D-MAP forms	Oral 100 µg × 3 in the 1st wk, then wkly × 30	Reduced cumulative proteinuria and serum anti-dsDNA Ab, improved survival, increased serum TGF-β
Shapira et al., 2011[172]	MRL/lpr mice	Early stage of disease (12-wk-old) Advanced disease (24-wk-old)	H2A histone fragment, termed IIIM1	Oral, 10 mg/kg, twice a wk	Reduced proteinuria and serum anti-dsDNA Ab Prolonged survival, decreased lymphadenopathy, and reduced CD4⁻CD8⁻B220⁺ T cells

Ab, antibody; CDR, complementarity-determining region; D-MAP, D form of multiple antigenic peptides; ID, intradermal; IFA, incomplete Freund adjuvant; Ig, immunoglobulin; IV, intravenous(ly); IP, intraperitoneal(ly); L-MAP, L form of multiple antigenic peptides; mAb, monoclonal antibody; MHC, major histocompatibility complex; PBMC, peripheral blood mononuclear cell; TGF-β, transforming growth factor beta; Th, T-helper cell; Treg, T-regulatory cell; V_H, variable heavy chain.

also develop autoantibodies and T cells against cell- or tissue-specific protein antigens. For example, CD4⁺ T cells from NZB mice respond to the anion channel protein band 3, a major target of the pathogenic red blood cell (RBC) autoantibodies in these mice. A band 3 peptide 861-875 is a dominant T-cell epitope recognized by NZB T cells. Injection of NZB mice with the peptide 861-874, which is insoluble, accelerates the development of RBC-bound autoantibodies and auto-immune hemolytic anemia. Inhalation of this peptide also primes T cells for both peptide-specific and whole–band 3 responses. By contrast, inhalation of a soluble analog (Glu861, Lys875) of this peptide deviated the autoimmune response toward a Th2 profile with increased IgG1 RBC–bound IgG, and reduced severity of anemia.[125]

Other groups have tested non–T cell–based peptide therapies for SLE. For example, administration of a DNA surrogate decapeptide, DWEYSVWLSN, in soluble form has been found to protect mice from renal deposition of the anti-DNA antibody in vivo (see Table 21-2).[100] In another study that used anti-dsDNA antibodies to screen a phage peptide display library, purified polyclonal anti-dsDNA antibodies and a monoclonal anti-dsDNA antibody were found to specifically bind a 15-mer peptide, ASPVTARVLWKASHV.[126] This 15-mer peptide can inhibit anti-dsDNA antibodies binding to dsDNA antigen in immunoassays and in the *Crithidia luciliae* assay.

Murine pathogenic lupus autoantibodies also bind to the laminin component of the extracellular matrix. Further analysis revealed reactivity of these autoantibodies with a 21-mer peptide located in the globular part of the α chain of laminin. Immunization of young lupus-prone mice with this peptide accelerated renal disease. Importantly, the binding of lupus autoantibodies to the extracellular matrix could be inhibited in vitro by competitive peptides that cross-react with the antilaminin antibodies. Treatment of MRL-lpr mice with these peptides has been reported to prevent antibody deposition in the kidneys, ameliorate renal disease, and prolong survival of the peptide-treated mice.[127]

Advances in understanding pathways involved in the uptake and sensing of dsDNA by cells have led to increasing evidence that dsDNA constitutes an important pathogenic factor that activates inflammatory responses by itself in autoimmune diseases. Therefore, modifying the structure of DNA to reduce its pathogenicity might be a more targeted approach for the treatment of SLE. Several methods of DNA structure manipulation, including topoisomerase I inhibition, administration of DNase I, and modification of histones using heparin or histone deacetylase inhibitors, are being tested as therapeutic option in mouse models of SLE.[13]

Gene Vaccination for SLE

We have reported that the V_H of anti-DNA antibodies contain epitopes that can be processed efficiently owing to their high cleavage probability score to bind MHC class I molecules.[128] Hence, we hypothesized that CD8⁺ cytotoxic T lymphocytes (CTLs) reactive with such Ig V_H epitopes will recognize and lyse B cells that can process and display the relevant V_H epitope on their surface class I

molecules. We found, however, that it is generally difficult to induce CD8⁺ CTLs in lupus mice. Because antigen delivery via a plasmid DNA or viral vectors generally elicits strong peptide-specific CD8⁺ T-cell response, we surmised that delivery of Ig V_H epitopes via plasmid DNA vectors as minigenes might elicit CTL responses in lupus mice. Indeed, vaccination of (NZB/NZW)F1 mice with plasmid DNA vectors that encode such epitopes activates CTL responses against anti-DNA antibody–producing B cells, inhibits anti-DNA antibody production, retards the development of lupus nephritis, and prolongs survival.[128] Translation of this approach into humans by delivering minigenes to induce anti-V_H CTLs that can ablate autoreactive B cells would represent a novel approach to treat autoantibody-mediated diseases.

One study used autoantigen-specific T cells for the local delivery of therapeutic molecules.[129] The investigators engineered nucleosome-specific regulatory T cells by multiple gene transfer (nucleosome-specific TCR-α, TCR-β, and CTLA4 [cytotoxic T-lymphocyte antigen 4] Ig). Treatment with these engineered cells suppressed pathogenic autoantibody production and nephritis in (NZB/NZW)F1 mice without impairing the T cell–dependent humoral immune responses. Thus, genetically engineered autoantigen-specific Treg cells are a promising strategy to treat autoimmune diseases.

Nanoparticles are being used to deliver peptide vaccines for infectious diseases and cancers. In one study, systemic delivery of nanoparticles coated with type 1 diabetes–relevant peptide MHC complex molecules suppressed the progression of autoimmune disease and restored glucose homeostasis.[130] Such a therapeutic strategy can be used to design antigen-specific nanovaccines for SLE.

Human Studies and Clinical Trials

The encouraging data on the therapeutic potential of antigen-specific T cell tolerance in animal models already discussed are leading to clinical trials of antigen-based therapy in SLE (Table 21-3).[2,3,109,131] Human clinical trials will be further facilitated by findings that the same or similar autoantigenic epitopes that activate T cells in animals with lupus are also recognized by human T cells in most cases.[37,105,117,132] For example, histone peptide H4$_{71-94}$, which effectively suppresses disease in SNF1 mice, is recognized by autoimmune T cells of all patients with lupus tested, irrespective of their HLA type[37,132] and U1-70K peptide P140, which ameliorates lupus in MRL-lpr mice, binds to a large panel of HLA-DR molecules.[117] The three autoantigens discussed in the following paragraphs, two peptides and an autoantigen construct, have been tested in clinical trials.

Excellent results in murine and pig models and in vitro human studies[109] led to a pilot clinical trial of hCDR1 (edratide), a 19-mer synthetic peptide representing the CDR1 of a pathogenic human anti-DNA antibody that bears the 16/6 Id.[131] Nine patients with SLE were treated for 26 weeks with either hCDR1 or placebo. Treatment with hCDR1 significantly downregulated the mRNA expression of the pathogenic cytokines IL-1β, TNF-α, IFN-γ, and IL-10, of BLyS (B-lymphocyte stimulator; also called B cell–activating factor

TABLE 21-3 Modulation of SLE by Peptides: Human Studies

REFERENCE	STUDY DESIGN	STUDY POPULATION	PEPTIDE	OUTCOME	
In Vitro Studies					
Monneaux et al., 2005[117]	In vitro culture using PBMCs or CD4[+] T cells	34 SLE patients, 27 autoimmune controls	P140 (phosphorylated analog of U1-70K snRNP131-151)	Prevents CD4[+] T-cell proliferation, and induces IL-10 production	
Zhang and Reichlin, 2005[126]	In vitro binding by serum	Sera from 22 SLE patient	15-mer peptide DNA surrogate	Inhibited binding of human anti-dsDNA Abs to dsDNA	
Hahn et al., 2008[164]	In vitro culture using PBMCs	36 SLE patients and 32 healthy subjects	Anti-DNA Ig peptides	Increased CD4[+]CD25[high] T cells after culture in patients with SLE, but not in the controls. Expanded cells functioned as Treg cells	
Mozes and Sharabi, 2010[109]	In vitro culture using PBMCs	11 SLE patients and 5 healthy subjects	hCDR1, a complementary-determining region 1 peptide of a human anti-dsDNA Ab	Reduced IL-1β, IFN-γ, and IL-10 gene expression and proapoptotic caspase-3; increased antiapoptotic Bcl-x; increased TGF-β and FoxP3, and CD4[+]CD25[+]FoxP3[+] functional, Treg cells	
Bloom et al., 2011[158]	In vitro/ex vivo binding of human monoclonal anti-dsDNA or lupus sera	Sera or mAb from SLE patients	FISLE-412, a peptidomimetic: molecular scaffolds predicted to have the desired DWEYS mimetic properties	Neutralizes anti-dsDNA/NMDAR lupus autoantibodies and prevents their interaction with tissue antigens; suppresses glomerular deposition and blocks neurotoxicity of SLE autoantibodies	
In Vivo: Humanized Mice					
Mauermann et al., 2004[111]	SCID mice injected IP with PBLs	PBLs from 7 SLE patients	V$_H$ peptide from a human anti-DNA mAb	50 μg once a wk × 8, IP	Suppressed anti-DNA, but not antitetanus, Ab; reduced proteinuria and renal deposition of human IgG
Nikolova et al., 2010[170]	SCID mice reconstituted with PBMCs	PBMCs from SLE patients/healthy donors	DWEYSVWLSN peptide coupled to an anti-CD35 Ab	50 μg IV once a wk × 8	Decreased anti-DNA antibody–secreting B cells from peripheral blood of lupus patients
In Vivo: Clinical Trials					
Sthoeger et al., 2009[131]	Pilot clinical trial	9 SLE patients	Edratide (TV-4710), a human anti-DNA V$_H$ peptide	SC wkly for 26 wks	Reduced inflammatory cytokines, proapoptotic molecules, and disease activity
Muller et al., 2008[3]	Phase 2a clinical trial, dose-ranging, multicenter	20 SLE patients from Europe	P140 (U1-70K 131-151, phosphorylated at Ser140)	200 μg or 1000 μg, SC × 3 doses, every 2 wks	Reduced anti-dsDNA Ab and SLEDAI score at 200-μg dose, and increased IL-10 levels 1 month after treatment
PRELUDE trial Teva[133]	Phase 2 trial in 12 countries	340 SLE patients	Edratide (TV-4710)	0.5 mg, 1.0 mg, 2.5 mg, SC, once a wk for 26 wks	Safe and tolerated, but did not meet its primary end point
Muller, 2011[2]; ImmuPharma PLC	Phase 2b, randomized, placebo-controlled trial	147 patients from Europe and Latin America	P140; Lupuzor	200 μg, SC every 4 wks × 3	Significantly lower SLEDAI score than placebo. Well tolerated, no significant adverse effects. FDA has granted the approval to start a phase 3 trial

Ab, antibody; ds, double-stranded; FDA, U.S. Food and Drug Administration; IFN, interferon; Ig, immunoglobulin; IL, interleukin; IP, intraperitoneal(ly); mAb, monoclonal antibody; NMDAR, N-methyl-D-aspartate receptor; PBL, peripheral blood leukocyte; PBMC, peripheral blood mononuclear cell; PRELUDE, Clinical Trials.gov Identifier:NCT00203151 SC, subcutaneous(ly); SLEDAI, Systemic Lupus Erythematosus Disease Activity Index; snRNP, small nuclear ribonucleoprotein; TGF-β, transforming growth factor beta; Treg, T-regulatory cell; V$_H$, variable heavy chain.

[BAFF]) and of the proapoptotic molecules caspase-3 and caspase-8. In contrast, the treatment upregulated in vivo gene expression of both TGF-β and FoxP3. Furthermore, hCDR1 treatment resulted in a significant decrease in scores on the Systemic Lupus Erythematosus Disease Activity Index 2000 (SLEDAI-2K) (from 8.0 ± 2.45 to 4.4 ± 1.67; $P = 0.02$) and the British Isles Lupus Assessment Group (BILAG) index (from 8.2 ± 2.7 to 3.6 ± 2.9; $P = 0.03$). Although this result was encouraging, edratide did not meet its primary end point, which was lower SLEDAI-2K disease activity score than placebo, in the PRELUDE trial ('A Study to Evaluate the Tolerability, Safety and Effectiveness of Edratide in the Treatment of Lupus'). However, a trend toward a higher number of patients with substantial BILAG index responses in the low-dose (edratide 0.5 mg per week)

treatment arm was observed in the whole group and more so in patients on low dose or no steroid and in those with seropositivity.[133] The peptide was safe and was well tolerated by patients in this randomized, double-blind, placebo-controlled, parallel-assignment, multicenter phase 2 trial that enrolled 340 patients with SLE from 12 countries.

Abetimus sodium (LJP394, Riquent) is a synthetic water-soluble molecule consisting of four double-stranded oligodeoxyribonucleotides each attached to a nonimmunogenic triethylene glycol backbone, a proprietary carrier platform. It was evaluated in a randomized, placebo-controlled, multicenter phase 3 trial by La Jolla Pharmaceuticals (San Diego, California). Abetimus is believed to induce tolerance in B cells directed against dsDNA by cross-linking surface antibodies potentially responsible for lupus nephritis. Although abetimus administered at 100 mg/week for up to 22 months to patients with lupus nephritis significantly reduced anti-dsDNA antibody levels, it did not significantly prolong the time to renal flare in comparison with placebo. Although multiple positive trends in renal end points were observed in the abetimus treatment group, further clinical trials of this drug in lupus have been halted.

Spliceosomal peptide P140 (sequence 131-151 of the U1-70K protein phosphorylated at Ser140) is strongly and reproducibly recognized by lupus CD4+ T cells. An open-label, dose-escalation phase 2 clinical trial of this peptide (Lupuzor) by ImmuPharma (Mulhouse, France) showed that this peptide was safe and well tolerated by patients with SLE. Three subcutaneous (SC) doses of IPP-201101 at 200 μg at 2-week intervals significantly improved the clinical and biologic status of patients with lupus.[2,3] In 2009, ImmuPharma announced the results of a phase 2b trial of P140 peptide (Lupuzor) in patients with active SLE who continued to receive their standard of care during the trial. Lupuzor administered at 200 μg once a month for 3 months achieved a clinically significant improvement in patient response rate in comparison with placebo.[2] As of November 2011, the FDA granted approval to start a phase 3 trial of Lupuzor with a Special Protocol Assessment and Fast Track designation. (Lupuzor has also been called Rigerimod.)

MECHANISMS OF PEPTIDE-BASED THERAPIES IN LUPUS

Neonatal Peptide Tolerance: Can Peptide Vaccines Worsen Lupus?

Our initial attempts to tolerize lupus-prone mice met with difficulty. IP injections of a peptide emulsified in incomplete Freund adjuvant (IFA) were given to newborn mice. Most mice had excellent tolerance of type 1 T-cell responses but had activation of type 2 responses; peptide-specific T cell proliferation, and IL-2 and IFN-γ secretion were suppressed, but peptide-specific IgG antibodies and secretion of IL-4, IL-5, and IL-10 were increased. This type of split T-cell tolerance was associated with increased anti-DNA autoantibody production in (NZB/NZW)F1 mice.[134] Induction of a similar split tolerance in adult mice was also associated with increased peptide-specific antibodies and type 2 cytokine production (RR Singh, unpublished observations, 2000).

Induction of "Direct" Tolerance in Th Cells: Induction of Apoptosis

Subsequently, we found that IV administration of high doses of soluble peptides tolerizes both type 1 and type 2 T-cell responses and strongly suppresses peptide-specific T-cell proliferation and antipeptide antibody responses, presumably through induction of apoptosis (RR Singh, unpublished observations, 2000).[1,135] This strategy successfully suppressed anti-dsDNA antibody production, delayed the onset of nephritis, and prolonged survival in young (NZB/NZW)F1 mice. In contrast to increased apoptosis in effector T cells, treatment with hCDR1 suppressed Fas signaling in CD4+ Tregs via the downregulation of FasL expression, diminished the activity of caspases 3 and 8, and upregulated the survival molecule Bcl-xL.[109] Treatment with hCDR1 also reduced the rate of T-cell apoptosis and modulation of several signaling pathways for apoptosis, including downregulation of the c-Jun NH2-terminal kinase (JNK) that is part of the p21Ras/MAP kinase pathway. Peptide P140, which is in clinical trial in patients with SLE, also increases peripheral blood lymphocyte apoptosis via a mechanism involving γδ T cells.[136]

Modulation of T-Cell Subsets: Increased Regulatory but Decreased Follicular T Helper, Th1, and Th17 Cells

Upon immunogenic challenge, nonautoimmune mice generate self-peptide–reactive CD8+ T cells, termed inhibitory T (Ti) cells, which can inhibit autoantibody production.[45] Further studies have shown that such peptide-induced CD8+ Ti cells are more resistant to

apoptosis than CD8+ T cells from unprimed (NZB/NZW)F1 mice. Ti cells also express regulatory T-cell molecule Foxp3, which mediates the suppression of autoimmune disease,[137-140] whereas peptide-induced CD4+CD25+Foxp3+ Treg cells in this model suppress the production of anti-DNA antibodies in a p38-MAPK (mitogen-activated protein kinase)–dependent fashion.[141] Furthermore, the peptide treatment also facilitates effector T-cell suppression by Treg cells.[142]

Induction of high-dose tolerance to the Sm-D1$_{83-119}$ peptide by IV injections of 600 to 1000 μg per month delays the production of autoantibodies including anti-dsDNA antibodies, postpones the onset of murine lupus nephritis, and prolongs survival.[143] Tolerance to this peptide can be adoptively transferred by CD90+ T cells, which also reduce T-cell help for autoreactive B cells in vitro. The treatment was associated with increased frequencies of IL-10+/IFN-γ+ CD4+ type 1 regulatory T cells, which can also prevent autoantibody generation and anti-CD3–induced proliferation of naïve T cells.

Given possible allergic or anaphylactic reaction to high-zone tolerance, many investigators have attempted low-dose tolerance in lupus mice. For example, treatment with subnanomolar doses of a histone peptide H4$_{71-94}$ effectively delayed nephritis onset and prolonged lifespan in SNF1 mice. This treatment was highly efficient in inducing potent CD8+ Treg cells and stable CD4+CD25+Foxp3+ T cells. The treatment was associated with reduced autoantigen-specific Th1 and Th17 responses, lower frequency of follicular T helper (T$_{FH}$) cells in spleen, and the diminished helper ability of autoimmune T cells to B cells.[132]

Both CD4+ and CD8+ regulatory T cells were also induced in lupus mice treated with hCDR1.[109] Interestingly, although the adoptive transfer of enriched hCDR1-induced CD4+ Tregs into diseased mice resulted in a significant amelioration of disease, adoptive transfer of CD8+ T cells from hCDR1-treated mice into diseased mice had little effect. However, CD8+CD28− Tregs were required for both the optimal expansion and function of CD4+ Tregs induced by hCDR1. Thus, the two subsets of protective T cells might interact with each other to maintain functional tolerance.

Modulation of PD-1

Treatment of (NZB/NZW)F1 mice with the anti-DNA Ig–based peptide pCons is associated with significantly reduced expression of the co-stimulatory molecule PD-1 (programmed death 1) on induced CD8+Foxp3+ Ti cells.[139] In vivo neutralization of PD-1 using an anti–PD-1 antibody in pCons-treated mice prevents the induction of CD8+ Ti cells and abrogates therapeutic tolerance.[144] These data suggest that tightly regulated PD-1 expression is essential for the maintenance of immune tolerance mediated by CD8+ Ti cells that suppress both Th cells and pathogenic B cells.

Role of Dendritic Cells in Facilitating Peptide-Induced Tolerance

Datta and colleagues have shown that SC injections of subnanomolar doses of a nucleosomal histone peptide, H4(71-94), ameliorated disease in SNF1 mice by generating CD4+CD25+ and CD8+ Treg cells. Splenic DCs captured the SC-injected H4(71-94) peptide rapidly and expressed a tolerogenic phenotype. The DCs of the tolerized animal, especially plasmacytoid DCs, produced increased amounts of TGF-β but diminished IL-6 on stimulation via the TLR9 pathway by nucleosome autoantigen; and those plasmacytoid DCs blocked lupus autoimmune disease by simultaneously inducing autoantigen-specific Tregs and suppressing inflammatory Th17 cells that infiltrated the kidneys of untreated lupus mice.[145]

Modulation of Cytokine Production: Reduced Proinflammatory but Increased Regulatory Cytokines

As previously discussed, nonautoimmune mice can curtail pathologic autoimmunity by generation of autoantigenic peptide–reactive CD8+ Ti cells that produce TGF-β.[45] TGF-β produced by these cells appears to be important in their ability to inhibit autoantibody production, because the addition of an anti–TGF-β antibody to cultures abrogates the inhibitory effect. An IFN-inducible gene, *Ifi202b*, also appears to play a role in the suppressive function of CD8+ Treg cells induced anti-DNA Ig peptide based pCons, because the silencing of *Ifi202b* abrogates the suppressive capacity of CD8+ Ti cells.[146] This silencing is associated with decreased expression of Foxp3, TGF-β, and IL-2 but not of IFN-γ, IL-10, or IL-17. TGF-β levels are also increased after treatment of lupus mice with hCDR1 peptide, whereas proinflammatory cytokines IL-1β, TNF-α, IFN-γ, and IL-10 are reduced in hCDR1-treated mice. The hCDR1 treatment also restored the levels of molecules involved in IFN-γ signaling, namely, the suppressor of cytokine signaling-1 (SOCS-1) and pSTAT1 (phosphorylated signal transducer and activator of transcription 1), which are generally impaired in humans and mice with SLE.

Thus, self peptide–mediated suppression in lupus is a complex process that appears to involve interactions among multiple cell types. For example, treatment with histone peptide H4$_{71-94}$ induces stable CD4+CD25+Foxp3+ T cells by decreasing IL-6 and increasing TGF-β production by DCs that induce ALK5 (activin receptor–like kinase 5)–dependent Smad-3 phosphorylation (TGF-β signal) in target autoimmune CD4+ T cells.[132]

Modulation of Molecules Associated with B-Cell Survival and Function

(NZB/NZW)F1 mice treated with hCDR1 peptide had reduced levels of BAFF, along with signaling through both the classical and alternative NF-κB pathways that mediate most of BAFF's functions regulating B-cell maturation and survival.[109] This effect was associated with the reduction in transitional type 1 (T1), transitional type 2 (T2), and marginal zone (MZ) B cells and with a decrease in the expression of integrins lymphocyte function–associated antigen 1 (LFA-1), integrin α4, and integrin β1. Furthermore, the expression of antiapoptotic genes (*Bcl-xL* and *Pim-2*) by B cells was inhibited in hCDR1-treated mice. B lymphocytes from SLE-afflicted mice also express relatively elevated values of CD74 and its ligand macrophage migration inhibitory factor (MIF). Treatment with hCDR1 resulted in the downregulation of MIF and its ligand as well as in reduced B-cell survival.[147] Mechanisms by which self-Ig peptides modulate these molecules in B cells to correct B-cell defects in lupus remain to be determined.

Modulating Determinant Spreading

Kaliyaperumal's group reported that IV administration of histone peptides in 18-month-old (SWR/NZB)F1 mice strongly suppressed autoantibody response to several antigens, a phenomenon they termed "tolerance spreading."[121] The anergy, deletion, suppression, and immune deviation that are classic mechanisms of tolerance induction did not appear to be operative in their system. Instead, they suggested that competition for MHC loading or modulation of some unknown signals involved in T cell–B cell interactions might have been responsible for tolerance induction in their model.[121,132] We have shown that treatment with a consensus anti-DNA variable region–based peptide not only reduced anti-DNA antibody levels but also decreased the production of autoantibodies that bind nucleosome and cardiolipin,[120] a finding suggesting the spreading of tolerance to structurally unrelated lupus autoantigens.

There are also reports in which treatment with autoantigenic peptides accelerated disease spreading of pathogenic T-cell responses to other epitopes or determinants. As a reminder, epitope or determinant spreading has been proposed as an important process, whereby the T-cell responses spontaneously broaden from one part of an autoantigen to other parts of the same autoantigen as well as to other autoantigens during the progression of autoimmune diseases.[76] In the NOD mouse model of autoimmune diabetes, Tian and associates found that treatment of newborn mice with an autoantigenic beta cell peptide (in adjuvant) results in spreading of T-cell response to other beta cell autoantigen determinants, far in advance of when autoimmunity would have naturally arisen to these determinants. Thus,

rather than limiting the loss of self-tolerance, immunotherapy caused the natural spreading hierarchy to be bypassed and autoreactivities to develop precociously.[148] This study further underscores the need for caution in the clinical application of antigen-based immunotherapeutics in autoimmune disorders.

Inhibiting T-Cell Chemotaxis

Lupus mice treated with hCDR1 peptide had reductions in extracellular signal–regulated kinase (ERK) phosphorylation, stromal cell–derived factor-1 alpha (SDF-1α; CXCL12)–induced T-cell adhesion and migration, and expression and function of cell adhesion receptors LFA-1 (αLβ2) and CD44.[149] The peptide-treated mice also had reduced SDF-1α–induced T-cell chemotaxis through fibronectin and collagen type I. SDF-1α is a pleiotropic CXC chemokine that affects the function of various cell types, including T cells, via its interactions with the CXCR4 receptor. SDF-1α also regulates leukocyte proliferation, survival, and entry into sites of inflammation as well as activation of T cells within blood vessels and in extravascular sites. Thus, self-peptides may confer their beneficial effects via modulating chemotaxis and interaction of T cells with extracellular matrix.

Inhibiting Autoantibody Binding to Extracellular Matrix

As described previously, treatment with certain laminin peptide analogs that cross-react with the antilaminin antibodies can suppress lupus in MRL-lpr mice. The investigators of the study suggested that the beneficial effect correlates with the ability of these peptides to directly inhibit the binding of lupus autoantibodies to the extracellular matrix.[127]

Induction of Cytotoxic T Lymphocytes That Ablate Autoreactive B Cells

We identified MHC class I–binding epitopes in the V$_H$ regions of anti-DNA monoclonal antibodies. The CD8+ T cells reactive with these peptides elicit CTL responses against anti-DNA B-cell hybridomas as well as B cells from diseased (NZB/NZW)F1 mice in vitro. This ablation of anti-DNA B cells occurs in a peptide-specific manner, because B cells that do not express Ig containing the relevant V$_H$ epitope are not subjected to killing. Induction of such CTLs in vivo is associated with reduced production of IgG anti-DNA antibody.[128]

Alteration of Autophagic Process and MHC Class II Stability

Peptide P140, the phosphorylated analog of the spliceosomal U1-70K snRNP$_{131-151}$, is protective in MRL-lpr mice and has been deemed successful in a phase 2b clinical trial in patients with SLE. After intravenous administration in MRL-lpr mice, P140 binds both the HSC70/Hsp73 chaperone and MHC class II molecules, which colocalize in splenic MRL/lpr B cells. Expression of HSC70 and MHCII, which is increased in MRL/lpr splenic B cells, is diminished after P140 administration. P140 impairs refolding properties of HSC70 and alters expression of stable MHCII molecules in B lymphocytes. In MRL/lpr B cells, P140 increases the accumulation of the autophagy markers p62/SQSTM1 and LC3-II, consistent with a downregulation of autophagic flux. Thus, P140 peptide may act via this novel mechanism that alters the autophagy pathway, leading to a defect of endogenous (auto)antigen processing in MRL/lpr antigen–presenting B cells and a decrease of T-cell priming and signaling.[136]

WILL PEPTIDE-SPECIFIC TREATMENT EVER BE A REALITY IN PATIENTS WITH SLE?

Ample evidence suggests that autoimmunity is fundamentally a continuously evolving process. The autoimmune responses shift, drift, and diversify with time not only to other epitopes in the original antigen but also to other antigens.[76] Studies in mouse models of autoimmune diabetes indicate that the kinetics and frequency at which beta cell–autoreactive T-cell responses are generated against major beta-cell autoantigens varies greatly in individual diabetic mice.[150] If autoreactive T cells with various specificities also develop in such a stochastic fashion during the course of SLE development in humans, it would be very difficult to determine what antigen-based immunotherapy would be most efficacious for any given individual at a given stage of disease. This possibility suggests that the stochastic development of autoreactive T-cell responses may indeed be a hurdle that must be overcome in the development of autoimmune disease prevention protocols for use in humans.

Unlike humans and mice with many organ-specific autoimmune diseases, those with SLE demonstrate widespread polyclonal T- and B-cell activation.[151] Intriguingly, however, T-cell activation, although polyclonal, is restricted to a set of autoantigens in SLE.[77] Several different mechanisms have been suggested to account for such "restricted polyclonality" in lupus. First, intrastructural organization of the auto-antigenic complex may dictate autoantibody responses to multiple but a restricted set of antigens.[152] Second, a remarkable "promiscuity" in the recognition of lupus autoantigens, such as to histone peptides by T cells, may induce autoantibodies to multiple but a related set of antigens.[153] Third, we reported that Ig-derived T-cell epitope sequences are recurrent among lupus-associated autoantibodies of different specificities but are uncommon in the normal antibody repertoire.[77,154] On the basis of this observation, we hypothesize that such sharing of T-cell epitopes among various autoantibody V region sequences contributes to the restricted polyclonality in lupus. Thus, activation of T cells reactive with one or a few epitopes initially would drive activation of several B cells that display the shared peptide motif.[76]

Degenerate recognition or cross-reactivity based on seemingly different peptides can occur in lupus. Thus, in one study, a single T-cell hybridoma established from an (NZB/NZW)F1 mouse immunized with one self-Ig peptide recognized several Ig-derived determinants, which had little sequence homology with the immunizing peptide.[77] Such T-cell recognition was not completely degenerate, because foreign peptides did not stimulate the self-reactive hybridoma. Such degenerate cross-recognition has also been described in humans with SLE. Therefore, a single TCR on a human snRNP-reactive T-cell clone can recognize two distinct snRNP autoantigenic peptides that have no apparent sequence homology.[155] Similarly, a peptide Sm-D1$_{83-119}$ of Sm-D1 protein (D1 protein of the Smith [Sm] proteins, part of snRNP) activates T-cell help for anti-dsDNA antibody production in (NZB/NZW)F1 mice.[41] The importance of these studies is that tolerogenic treatment with one peptide should lead to tolerance in all cross-reactive T and B cells. For example, we have designed a best-fit "consensus" Ig-based peptide[119] that suppressed reactivity to several different autoantigens.[120]

Further complicating the issue of antigen therapies is the presence of polymorphisms in the HLA regions, thus requiring formulation and testing of expensive individualized therapy. Anticipating this problem, investigators are attempting to develop consensus and/or promiscuous autoantigenic epitopes that can bind many HLA molecules and modulate a broad repertoire of self-reactive T cells. For example, Datta and colleagues have identified a set of highly promiscuous, nucleosomal epitopes that bind many MHC molecules across the species barrier.[121] Similarly, a CD4+ T-cell epitope in the spliceosomal U1-70K snRNP$_{131-151}$ and its phosphorylated analog of this peptide (P140) can bind multiple HLA-DR molecules and can elicit and suppress human T-cell proliferation, respectively.[117] Such "universal" T-cell epitopes could be used to manipulate autoimmune responses in most, if not all, patients. Indeed, treatment with P140 reduced anti-dsDNA antibodies and SLEDAI scores in 147 patients with SLE from several countries on two continents.

It would also be important to rigorously characterize the exquisite T-cell epitopes that activate regulatory and suppressor T cells versus those that stimulate pathogenic Th cells in humans. It is critical to ensure that we do not run into premature disappointment, as seen in some other antigen therapy trials. Complicating the selection of peptides for treatment, our murine studies suggest that suppressor cell and Th-cell epitopes might colocalize or overlap,[154] as if nature has

done a fine balancing act by putting together the "protective" and "pathogenic" epitopes.

Intravenous treatment with the phosphorylated analog P140 peptide, but not with the parent peptide 131-151 derived from autoantigen U1-70K snRNP, ameliorates disease in MRL-lpr mice.[122] This finding highlights the importance of paying attention to posttranslational modifications while screening peptides for clinical studies.[6]

Finally, the route of administration and the dose and form of peptide, including soluble versus with adjuvant, may have enormous consequences for the outcome of tolerance therapy. For example, the same set of peptides can elicit very different immune responses depending on whether the peptide is administered IV, IP, SC, orally, intradermally, and with or without adjuvants (RR Singh, unpublished observations, 2000).[174] Thus, very extensive studies to sort out these issues will be needed before clinical studies in humans can be contemplated.

SYNTHESIS

Immunologists have been fascinated with the idea of using the disease-specific antigen-based therapies and vaccination for autoimmune diseases, infection, and cancers. This task becomes particularly difficult for diseases such as SLE, in which, in contrast to organ-specific autoimmune diseases, there is no organ-specific autoantigen target. Painstaking efforts by several laboratories have led to identification of peptides that activate potentially pathogenic Th cells. A diverse group of self-antigens appears to be the source of these peptides. It is likely that peptides from several different antigens activate autoreactive Th cells that promote autoantibody production and disease in SLE. Probably an interconnected circuitry of reciprocal T cell–B cell recognition drives the spreading of response from one T cell to another until a massive expansion of diverse arrays of T and B cells has occurred. Such T cell–B cell diversification might pose difficulty for the design of antigen-specific therapies. The good news, however, is that tolerogenic treatment with one or just a few peptides appears to quell autoimmune responses against a variety of autoantigens and suppress disease in animal models. Although we have a long way to go to understand these processes in mice and humans with lupus, the initial studies in mice and humans with lupus offer new hope. Remarkably, striking similarities exist between peptides that appear to activate T cells in patients with SLE and peptides that activate Th cells that induce autoantibodies that cause disease in lupus mice. However, experience in other autoimmune diseases, such as type 1 diabetes, has taught us that a rush to clinical trials using autoantigenic peptides must not occur without full realization that the biological basis by which a tolerogenic therapy may suppress disease in an animal model may not be directly translatable to humans. Furthermore, the mechanism of peptide tolerogenic therapy depends on the nature of individual autoantigen or peptide, its form, dose, and route of delivery, and the state of T-cell activation in the host. These variables would have to be individually and carefully worked out for different disease stages and for different autoantigens to avoid unforeseen adverse immune stimulation. Regardless, buoyed by the success of a phase 2b trial, a "fast track" approval has been granted by the FDA to start a phase 3 trial of Lupuzor, a peptide analog derived from U1-70K snRNP autoantigen, in patients with SLE.

References

1. Singh RR, Ebling FM, Sercarz EE, et al: Immune tolerance to autoantibody-derived peptides delays development of autoimmunity in murine lupus. *J Clin Invest* 96:2990–2996, 1995a.
2. Muller S: [Novel strategy in lupus therapy: from the peptide P140 to Lupuzor]. *Ann Pharm Fr* 69:151–154, 2011.
3. Muller S, Monneaux F, Schall N, et al: Spliceosomal peptide P140 for immunotherapy of systemic lupus erythematosus: results of an early phase II clinical trial. *Arthritis Rheum* 58:3873–3883, 2008.
4. Sthoeger ZM, Dayan M, Tcherniack A, et al: Modulation of autoreactive responses of peripheral blood lymphocytes of patients with systemic

lupus erythematosus by peptides based on human and murine anti-DNA autoantibodies. *Clin Exp Immunol* 131:385–392, 2003.

5. Coppieters KT, Dotta F, Amirian N, et al: Demonstration of islet-autoreactive CD8 T cells in insulitic lesions from recent onset and long-term type 1 diabetes patients. *J Exp Med* 209:51–60, 2012.

6. Doyle HA, Mamula MJ: Autoantigenesis: the evolution of protein modifications in autoimmune disease. *Curr Opin Immunol* 24:112–118, 2011.

7. Hoffmann MH, Trembleau S, Muller S, et al: Nucleic acid-associated autoantigens: pathogenic involvement and therapeutic potential. *J Autoimmun* 34:J178–J206, 2010.

8. Deshmukh US, Sim DL, Dai C, et al: HLA-DR3 restricted T cell epitope mimicry in induction of autoimmune response to lupus-associated antigen SmD. *J Autoimmun* 37:254–262, 2011.

9. Reeves WH, Lee PY, Weinstein JS, et al: Induction of autoimmunity by pristane and other naturally occurring hydrocarbons. *Trends Immunol* 30:455–464, 2009.

10. Smith-Bouvier DL, Divekar AA, Sasidhar M, et al: A role for sex chromosome complement in the female bias in autoimmune disease. *J Exp Med* 205:1099–1108, 2008.

11. Smith DL, Dong X, Du S, et al: A female preponderance for chemically induced lupus in SJL/J mice. *Clin Immunol* 122:101–107, 2007.

12. Yang JQ, Singh AK, Wilson MT, et al: Immunoregulatory role of CD1d in the hydrocarbon oil-induced model of lupus nephritis. *J Immunol* 171:2142–2153, 2003.

13. Frese S, Diamond B: Structural modification of DNA-a therapeutic option in SLE? *Nat Rev Rheumatol* 7:733–738, 2011.

14. Riemekasten G, Hahn BH: Key autoantigens in SLE. *Rheumatology (Oxford)* 44:975–982, 2005.

15. Wu CT, Gershwin ME, Davis PA: What makes an autoantigen an autoantigen? *Ann N Y Acad Sci* 1050:134–145, 2005.

16. Ng B, Yang F, Huston DP, et al: Increased noncanonical splicing of autoantigen transcripts provides the structural basis for expression of untolerized epitopes. *J Allergy Clin Immunol* 114:1463–1470, 2004.

17. Casciola-Rosen LA, Anhalt G, Rosen A: Autoantigens targeted in systemic lupus erythematosus are clustered in two populations of surface structures on apoptotic keratinocytes. *J Exp Med* 179:1317–1330, 1994.

18. Wu X, Molinaro C, Johnson N, et al: Secondary necrosis is a source of proteolytically modified forms of specific intracellular autoantigens: implications for systemic autoimmunity. *Arthritis Rheum* 44:2642–2652, 2001.

19. Truedsson L, Bengtsson AA, Sturfelt G: Complement deficiencies and systemic lupus erythematosus. *Autoimmunity* 40:560–566, 2007.

20. Wermeling F, Chen Y, Pikkarainen T, et al: Class A scavenger receptors regulate tolerance against apoptotic cells, and autoantibodies against these receptors are predictive of systemic lupus. *J Exp Med* 204:2259–2265, 2007.

21. Cohen PL, Caricchio R, Abraham V, et al: Delayed apoptotic cell clearance and lupus-like autoimmunity in mice lacking the c-mer membrane tyrosine kinase. *J Exp Med* 196:135–140, 2002.

22. Bachmann M, Hilker M, Grolz D, et al: Different La/SS-B mRNA isoforms are expressed in salivary gland tissue of patients with primary Sjogren's syndrome. *J Autoimmun* 9:757–766, 1996.

23. Grolz D, Bachmann M: The nuclear autoantigen La/SS-associated antigen B: one gene, three functional mRNAs. *Biochem J* 323:151–158, 1997.

24. Stadler MB, Arnold D, Frieden S, et al: Single nucleotide polymorphisms as a prerequisite for autoantigens. *Eur J Immunol* 35:371–378, 2005.

25. Routsias JG, Tzioufas AG, Moutsopoulos HM: The clinical value of intracellular autoantigens B-cell epitopes in systemic rheumatic diseases. *Clin Chim Acta* 340:1–25, 2004.

26. Nakken B, Jonsson R, Bolstad AI: Polymorphisms of the Ro52 gene associated with anti-Ro 52-kd autoantibodies in patients with primary Sjogren's syndrome. *Arthritis Rheum* 44:638–646, 2001.

27. Young AL, Carter WG, Doyle HA, et al: Structural integrity of histone H2B in vivo requires the activity of protein L-isoaspartate O-methyltransferase, a putative protein repair enzyme. *J Biol Chem* 276:37161–37165, 2001.

28. Brahms H, Raymackers J, Union A, et al: The C-terminal RG dipeptide repeats of the spliceosomal Sm proteins D1 and D3 contain symmetrical dimethylarginines, which form a major B-cell epitope for anti-Sm antibodies. *J Biol Chem* 275:17122–17129, 2000.

29. Neugebauer KM, Merrill JT, Wener MH, et al: SR proteins are autoantigens in patients with systemic lupus erythematosus. Importance of phosphoepitopes. *Arthritis Rheum* 43:1768–1778, 2000.

30. Pollard KM, Pearson DL, Bluthner M, et al: Proteolytic cleavage of a self-antigen following xenobiotic-induced cell death produces a fragment with novel immunogenic properties. *J Immunol* 165:2263–2270, 2000.

31. Casciola-Rosen L, Andrade F, Ulanet D, et al: Cleavage by granzyme B is strongly predictive of autoantigen status: implications for initiation of autoimmunity. *J Exp Med* 190:815–826, 1999.

32. Rosen A, Casciola-Rosen L: Autoantigens as substrates for apoptotic proteases: implications for the pathogenesis of systemic autoimmune disease. *Cell Death Differ* 6:6–12, 1999.

33. Stathopoulou EA, Routsias JG, Stea EA, et al: Cross-reaction between antibodies to the major epitope of Ro60 kD autoantigen and a homologous peptide of Coxsackie virus 2B protein. *Clin Exp Immunol* 141:148–154, 2005.

34. McClain MT, Heinlen LD, Dennis GJ, et al: Early events in lupus humoral autoimmunity suggest initiation through molecular mimicry. *Nat Med* 11:85–89, 2005.

35. Lee PY, Kumagai Y, Xu Y, et al: IL-1alpha modulates neutrophil recruitment in chronic inflammation induced by hydrocarbon oil. *J Immunol* 186:1747–1754, 2011.

36. Ando DG, Sercarz EE, Hahn BH: Mechanisms of T and B cell collaboration in the in vitro production of anti-DNA antibodies in the NZB/NZW F1 murine SLE model. *J Immunol* 138:3185–3190, 1987.

37. Datta SK: Major peptide autoepitopes for nucleosome-centered T and B cell interaction in human and murine lupus. *Ann N Y Acad Sci* 987:79–90, 2003.

38. Dumortier H, Monneaux F, Jahn-Schmid B, et al: B and T cell responses to the spliceosomal heterogeneous nuclear ribonucleoproteins A2 and B1 in normal and lupus mice. *J Immunol* 165:2297–2305, 2000.

39. Mohan C, Adams S, Stanik V, et al: Nucleosome: a major immunogen for pathogenic autoantibody-inducing T cells of lupus. *J Exp Med* 177:1367–1381, 1993.

40. Monneaux F, Dumortier H, Steiner G, et al: Murine models of systemic lupus erythematosus: B and T cell responses to spliceosomal ribonucleoproteins in MRL/Fas(lpr) and (NZB x NZW)F(1) lupus mice. *Int Immunol* 13:1155–1163, 2001.

41. Riemekasten G, Langnickel D, Ebling FM, et al: Identification and characterization of SmD183-119-reactive T cells that provide T cell help for pathogenic anti-double-stranded DNA antibodies. *Arthritis Rheum* 48:475–485, 2003.

42. Singh RR, Kumar V, Ebling FM, et al: T cell determinants from autoantibodies to DNA can upregulate autoimmunity in murine systemic lupus erythematosus. *J Exp Med* 181:2017–2027, 1995b.

43. Suh CH, Freed JH, Cohen PL: T cell reactivity to MHC class II-bound self peptides in systemic lupus erythematosus-prone MRL/lpr mice. *J Immunol* 170:2229–2235, 2003.

44. Chan OT, Hannum LG, Haberman AM, et al: A novel mouse with B cells but lacking serum antibody reveals an antibody-independent role for B cells in murine lupus. *J Exp Med* 189:1639–1648, 1999.

45. Singh RR, Ebling FM, Albuquerque DA, et al: Induction of autoantibody production is limited in nonautoimmune mice. *J Immunol* 169:587–594, 2002.

46. Leadbetter EA, Rifkin IR, Hohlbaum AM, et al: Chromatin-IgG complexes activate B cells by dual engagement of IgM and Toll-like receptors. *Nature* 416:603–607, 2002.

47. Viglianti GA, Lau CM, Hanley TM, et al: Activation of autoreactive B cells by CpG dsDNA. *Immunity* 19:837–847, 2003.

48. Boule MW, Broughton C, Mackay F, et al: Toll-like receptor 9-dependent and -independent dendritic cell activation by chromatin-immunoglobulin G complexes. *J Exp Med* 199:1631–1640, 2004.

49. Christensen SR, Kashgarian M, Alexopoulou L, et al: Toll-like receptor 9 controls anti-DNA autoantibody production in murine lupus. *J Exp Med* 202:321–331, 2005.

50. Patole PS, Grone HJ, Segerer S, et al: Viral double-stranded RNA aggravates lupus nephritis through Toll-like receptor 3 on glomerular mesangial cells and antigen-presenting cells. *J Am Soc Nephrol* 16:1326–1338, 2005.

51. Urbonaviciute V, Voll RE: High-mobility group box 1 represents a potential marker of disease activity and novel therapeutic target in systemic lupus erythematosus. *J Intern Med* 270:309–318, 2011.

52. Yanai H, Ban T, Wang Z, et al: HMGB proteins function as universal sentinels for nucleic-acid-mediated innate immune responses. *Nature* 462:99–103, 2009.

53. Abdulahad DA, Westra J, Bijzet J, et al: High mobility group box 1 (HMGB1) and anti-HMGB1 antibodies and their relation to disease

characteristics in systemic lupus erythematosus. *Arthritis Res Ther* 13:R71, 2011.

54. Mills KH: TLR-dependent T cell activation in autoimmunity. *Nat rev Immunol* 11:807–822, 2011.

55. Oppenheim JJ, Dong HF, Plotz P, et al: Autoantigens act as tissue-specific chemoattractants. *Journal of leukocyte biology* 77:854–861, 2005.

56. Lau CM, Broughton C, Tabor AS, et al: RNA-associated autoantigens activate B cells by combined B cell antigen receptor/Toll-like receptor 7 engagement. *J Exp Med* 202:1171–1177, 2005.

57. Decker P, Singh-Jasuja H, Haager S, et al: Nucleosome, the main auto-antigen in systemic lupus erythematosus, induces direct dendritic cell activation via a MyD88-independent pathway: consequences on inflammation. *J Immunol* 174:3326–3334, 2005.

58. Savarese E, Chae OW, Trowitzsch S, et al: U1 small nuclear ribonucleo-protein immune complexes induce type I interferon in plasmacytoid dendritic cells through TLR7. *Blood* 107:3229–3234, 2006.

59. Lindau D, Ronnefarth V, Erbacher A, et al: Nucleosome-induced neu-trophil activation occurs independently of TLR9 and endosomal acidi-fication: implications for systemic lupus erythematosus. *Eur J Immunol* 41:669–681, 2011.

60. Mircheff AK, Gierow JP, Yang T, et al: Sjogren's autoimmunity: how perturbation of recognition in endomembrane traffic may provoke pathological recognition at the cell surface. *J Mol Recognit* 11:40–48, 1998.

61. Espinosa A, Zhou W, Ek M, et al: The Sjogren's syndrome-associated autoantigen Ro52 is an E3 ligase that regulates proliferation and cell death. *J Immunol* 176:6277–6285, 2006.

62. Hahn BH: Antibodies to DNA. *N Engl J Med* 338:1359–1368, 1998.

63. Ohnishi K, Ebling FM, Mitchell B, et al: Comparison of pathogenic and non-pathogenic murine antibodies to DNA: antigen binding and struc-tural characteristics. *Int Immunol* 6:817–830, 1994.

64. Desai DD, Krishnan MR, Swindle JT, et al: Antigen-specific induction of antibodies against native mammalian DNA in nonautoimmune mice. *J Immunol* 151:1614–1626, 1993.

65. Deocharan B, Qing X, Beger E, et al: Antigenic triggers and molecular targets for anti-double-stranded DNA antibodies. *Lupus* 11:865–871, 2002.

66. Putterman C, Diamond B: Immunization with a peptide surrogate for double-stranded DNA (dsDNA) induces autoantibody production and renal immunoglobulin deposition. *J Exp Med* 188:29–38, 1998.

67. James JA, Gross T, Scofield RH, et al: Immunoglobulin epitope spreading and autoimmune disease after peptide immunization: Sm B/B'-derived PPPGMRPP and PPPGIRGP induce spliceosome autoimmunity. *J Exp Med* 181:453–461, 1995.

68. Hoch SO, Eisenberg RA, Sharp GC: Diverse antibody recognition pat-terns of the multiple Sm-D antigen polypeptides. *Clin Immunol* 92:203–208, 1999.

69. James JA, Mamula MJ, Harley JB: Sequential autoantigenic determinants of the small nuclear ribonucleoprotein Sm D shared by human lupus autoantibodies and MRL lpr/lpr antibodies. *Clin Exp Immunol* 98:419–426, 1994.

70. Jaekel HP, Klopsch T, Benkenstein B, et al: Reactivities to the Sm auto-antigenic complex and the synthetic SmD1-aa83-119 peptide in sys-temic lupus erythematosus and other autoimmune diseases. *J Autoimmun* 17:347–354, 2001.

71. Riemekasten G, Marell J, Trebeljahr G, et al: A novel epitope on the C-terminus of SmD1 is recognized by the majority of sera from patients with systemic lupus erythematosus. *J Clin Invest* 102:754–763, 1998.

72. Sessa L, Bianchi ME: The evolution of High Mobility Group Box (HMGB) chromatin proteins in multicellular animals. *Gene* 387:133–140, 2007.

73. Scaffidi P, Misteli T, Bianchi ME: Release of chromatin protein HMGB1 by necrotic cells triggers inflammation. *Nature* 418:191–195, 2002.

74. Deshmukh US, Gaskin F, Lewis JE, et al: Mechanisms of autoantibody diversification to SLE-related autoantigens. *Ann N Y Acad Sci* 987:91–98, 2003.

75. Monneaux F, Muller S: Epitope spreading in systemic lupus erythema-tosus: identification of triggering peptide sequences. *Arthritis Rheum* 46:1430–1438, 2002.

76. Singh RR, Hahn BH: Reciprocal T-B determinant spreading develops spontaneously in murine lupus: implications for pathogenesis. *Immunol Rev* 164:201–208, 1998.

77. Singh RR, Hahn BH, Tsao BP, et al: Evidence for multiple mechanisms of polyclonal T cell activation in murine lupus. *J Clin Invest* 102:1841–1849, 1998b.

78. Wysocki LJ, Zhang X, Smith DS, et al: Somatic origin of T-cell epitopes within antibody variable regions: significance to monoclonal therapy and genesis of systemic autoimmune disease. *Immunol Rev* 162:233–246, 1998.

79. Zhang X, Smith DS, Guth A, et al: A receptor presentation hypothesis for T cell help that recruits autoreactive B cells. *J Immunol* 166:1562–1571, 2001.

80. Manheimer-Lory AJ, Zandman-Goddard G, Davidson A, et al: Lupus-specific antibodies reveal an altered pattern of somatic mutation. *J Clin Invest* 100:2538–2546, 1997.

81. Filaci G, Grasso I, Contini P, et al: dsDNA-, nucleohistone- and DNASE I-reactive T lymphocytes in patients affected by systemic lupus erythe-matosus: correlation with clinical disease activity. *Clin Exp Rheumatol* 14:543–550, 1996.

82. Voll RE, Roth EA, Girkontaite I, et al: Histone-specific Th0 and Th1 clones derived from systemic lupus erythematosus patients induce double-stranded DNA antibody production. *Arthritis Rheum* 40:2162–2171, 1997.

83. Cawley D, Chiang BL, Naiki M, et al: Comparison of the requirements for cognate T cell help for IgG anti-double-stranded DNA antibody production in vitro: T helper-derived lymphokines replace T cell cloned lines for B cells from NZB.H-2bm12 but not B6.H-2bm12 mice. *J Immunol* 150:2467–2477, 1993.

84. Datta SK, Patel H, Berry D: Induction of a cationic shift in IgG anti-DNA autoantibodies. Role of T helper cells with classical and novel pheno-types in three murine models of lupus nephritis. *J Exp Med* 165:1252–1268, 1987.

85. Deusch K, Fernandez-Botran R, Konstadoulakis M, et al: Autoreactive T cells from MRL-lpr/lpr mice secrete multiple lymphokines and induce the production of IgG anti-DNA antibodies. *J Autoimmun* 4:563–576, 1991.

86. Kaliyaperumal A, Mohan C, Wu W, et al: Nucleosomal peptide epitopes for nephritis-inducing T helper cells of murine lupus. *J Exp Med* 183:2459–2469, 1996.

87. Fournel S, Neichel S, Dali H, et al: CD4+ T cells from (New Zealand Black x New Zealand White)F1 lupus mice and normal mice immunized against apoptotic nucleosomes recognize similar Th cell epitopes in the C terminus of histone H3. *J Immunol* 171:636–644, 2003.

88. Suen JL, Wu CH, Chen YY, et al: Characterization of self-T-cell response and antigenic determinants of U1A protein with bone marrow-derived dendritic cells in NZB x NZW F1 mice. *Immunology* 103:301–309, 2001.

89. Suen JL, Chuang YH, Tsai BY, et al: Treatment of murine lupus using nucleosomal T cell epitopes identified by bone marrow-derived den-dritic cells. *Arthritis Rheum* 50:3250–3259, 2004.

90. Guo W, Smith D, Guth A, et al: T cell tolerance to germline-encoded antibody sequences in a lupus-prone mouse. *J Immunol* 175:2184–2190, 2005.

91. Snyder CM, Zhang X, Wysocki LJ: Negligible class II MHC presentation of B cell receptor-derived peptides by high density resting B cells. *J Immunol* 168:3865–3873, 2002.

92. Ebling FM, Tsao BP, Singh RR, et al: A peptide derived from an autoan-tibody can stimulate T cells in the (NZB x NZW)F1 mouse model of systemic lupus erythematosus. *Arthritis Rheum* 36:355–364, 1993.

93. Waisman A, Ruiz PJ, Israeli E, et al: Modulation of murine systemic lupus erythematosus with peptides based on complementarity deter-mining regions of a pathogenic anti-DNA monoclonal antibody. *Proc Natl Acad Sci U S A* 94:4620–4625, 1997.

94. Brosh N, Dayan M, Fridkin M, et al: A peptide based on the CDR3 of an anti-DNA antibody of experimental SLE origin is also a dominant T-cell epitope in (NZBXNZW)F1 lupus-prone mice. *Immunol Lett* 72:61–68, 2000a.

95. Brosh N, Eilat E, Zinger H, et al: Characterization and role in experi-mental systemic lupus erythematosus of T-cell lines specific to peptides based on complementarity-determining region-1 and complementarity-determining region-3 of a pathogenic anti-DNA monoclonal antibody. *Immunology* 99:257–265, 2000b.

96. Monneaux F, Muller S: Laboratory protocols for the identification of Th cell epitopes on self-antigens in mice with systemic autoimmune dis-eases. *J Immunol Methods* 244:195–204, 2000.

97. Monneaux F, Muller S: Key sequences involved in the spreading of the systemic autoimmune response to spliceosomal proteins. *Scand J Immunol* 54:45–54, 2001.

98. Monneaux F, Muller S: Peptide-based immunotherapy of systemic lupus erythematosus. *Autoimmun Rev* 3:16–24, 2004.

99. Monneaux F, Briand JP, Muller S: B and T cell immune response to small nuclear ribonucleoprotein particles in lupus mice: autoreactive CD4(+)

T cells recognize a T cell epitope located within the RNP80 motif of the 70K protein. *Eur J Immunol* 30:2191–2200, 2000.

100. Gaynor B, Putterman C, Valadon P, et al: Peptide inhibition of glomerular deposition of an anti-DNA antibody. *Proc Natl Acad Sci U S A* 94:1955–1960, 1997.

101. Putterman C, Deocharan B, Diamond B: Molecular analysis of the autoantibody response in peptide-induced autoimmunity. *J Immunol* 164:2542–2549, 2000.

102. Hoffman RW: T cells in the pathogenesis of systemic lupus erythematosus. *Clin Immunol* 113:4–13, 2004.

103. Rajagopalan S, Zordan T, Tsokos GC, et al: Pathogenic anti-DNA autoantibody-inducing T helper cell lines from patients with active lupus nephritis: isolation of CD4-8-T helper cell lines that express the gamma delta T-cell antigen receptor. *Proc Natl Acad Sci U S A* 87:7020–7024, 1990.

104. Desai-Mehta A, Mao C, Rajagopalan S, et al: Structure and specificity of T cell receptors expressed by potentially pathogenic anti-DNA autoantibody-inducing T cells in human lupus. *J Clin Invest* 95:531–541, 1995.

105. Lu L, Kaliyaperumal A, Boumpas DT, et al: Major peptide autoepitopes for nucleosome-specific T cells of human lupus. *J Clin Invest* 104:345–355, 1999.

106. Williams WM, Staines NA, Muller S, et al: Human T cell responses to autoantibody variable region peptides. *Lupus* 4:464–471, 1995.

107. Linker-Israeli M, Ebling F, Wallace DJ, et al: T cells of SLE patients recognize VH determinants of anti-dsDNA autoantibodies. *Arthritis Rheum* 39:S267, 1996.

108. Kalsi JK, Grossman J, Kim J, et al: Peptides from antibodies to DNA elicit cytokine release from peripheral blood mononuclear cells of patients with systemic lupus erythematosus: relation of cytokine pattern to disease duration. *Lupus* 13:490–500, 2004.

109. Mozes E, Sharabi A: A novel tolerogenic peptide, hCDR1, for the specific treatment of systemic lupus erythematosus. *Autoimmun Rev* 10:22–26, 2010.

110. Dayan M, Segal R, Sthoeger Z, et al: Immune response of SLE patients to peptides based on the complementarity determining regions of a pathogenic anti-DNA monoclonal antibody. *J Clin Immunol* 20:187–194, 2000.

111. Mauermann N, Sthoeger Z, Zinger H, et al: Amelioration of lupus manifestations by a peptide based on the complementarity determining region 1 of an autoantibody in severe combined immunodeficient (SCID) mice engrafted with peripheral blood lymphocytes of systemic lupus erythematosus (SLE) patients. *Clin Exp Immunol* 137:513–520, 2004.

112. Holyst MM, Hill DL, Hoch SO, et al: Analysis of human T cell and B cell responses against U small nuclear ribonucleoprotein 70-kd, B, and D polypeptides among patients with systemic lupus erythematosus and mixed connective tissue disease. *Arthritis Rheum* 40:1493–1503, 1997.

113. Greidinger EL, Gazitt T, Jaimes KF, et al: Human T cell clones specific for heterogeneous nuclear ribonucleoprotein A2 autoantigen from connective tissue disease patients assist in autoantibody production. *Arthritis Rheum* 50:2216–2222, 2004.

114. Talken BL, Holyst MM, Lee DR, et al: T cell receptor beta-chain third complementarity-determining region gene usage is highly restricted among Sm-B autoantigen-specific human T cell clones derived from patients with connective tissue disease. *Arthritis Rheum* 42:703–709, 1999a.

115. Talken BL, Lee DR, Caldwell CW, et al: Analysis of T cell receptors specific for U1-70kD small nuclear ribonucleoprotein autoantigen: the alpha chain complementarity determining region three is highly conserved among connective tissue disease patients. *Hum Immunol* 60:200–208, 1999b.

116. Davies ML, Taylor EJ, Gordon C, et al: Candidate T cell epitopes of the human La/SSB autoantigen. *Arthritis Rheum* 46:209–214, 2002.

117. Monneaux F, Hoebeke J, Sordet C, et al: Selective modulation of CD4+ T cells from lupus patients by a promiscuous, protective peptide analog. *J Immunol* 175:5839–5847, 2005.

118. Kang HK, Michaels MA, Berner BR, et al: Very low-dose tolerance with nucleosomal peptides controls lupus and induces potent regulatory T cell subsets. *J Immunol* 174:3247–3255, 2005.

119. Singh RR, Ebling F, Hahn BH, et al: Designing consensus "super-determinants" that strongly influence autoantibody production in lupus. *J Invest Med* 46:230A, 1998a.

120. Hahn BH, Singh RR, Wong WK, et al: Treatment with a consensus peptide based on amino acid sequences in autoantibodies prevents T cell activation by autoantigens and delays disease onset in murine lupus. *Arthritis Rheum* 44:432–441, 2001.

121. Kaliyaperumal A, Michaels MA, Datta SK: Antigen-specific therapy of murine lupus nephritis using nucleosomal peptides: tolerance spreading impairs pathogenic function of autoimmune T and B cells. *J Immunol* 162:5775–5783, 1999.

122. Monneaux F, Lozano JM, Patarroyo ME, et al: T cell recognition and therapeutic effect of a phosphorylated synthetic peptide of the 70K snRNP protein administered in MR/lpr mice. *Eur J Immunol* 33:287–296, 2003.

123. Wu HY, Ward FJ, Staines NA: Histone peptide-induced nasal tolerance: suppression of murine lupus. *J Immunol* 169:1126–1134, 2002.

124. Wu HY, Staines NA: A deficiency of CD4+CD25+ T cells permits the development of spontaneous lupus-like disease in mice, and can be reversed by induction of mucosal tolerance to histone peptide autoantigen. *Lupus* 13:192–200, 2004.

125. Shen CR, Youssef AR, Devine A, et al: Peptides containing a dominant T-cell epitope from red cell band 3 have in vivo immunomodulatory properties in NZB mice with autoimmune hemolytic anemia. *Blood* 102:3800–3806, 2003.

126. Zhang W, Reichlin M: A peptide DNA surrogate that binds and inhibits anti-dsDNA antibodies. *Clin Immunol* 117:214–220, 2005.

127. Amital H, Heilweil M, Ulmansky R, et al: Treatment with a laminin-derived peptide suppresses lupus nephritis. *J Immunol* 175:5516–5523, 2005.

128. Fan GC, Singh RR: Vaccination with minigenes encoding V(H)-derived major histocompatibility complex class I-binding epitopes activates cytotoxic T cells that ablate autoantibody-producing B cells and inhibit lupus. *J Exp Med* 196:731–741, 2002.

129. Fujio K, Okamoto A, Tahara H, et al: Nucleosome-specific regulatory T cells engineered by triple gene transfer suppress a systemic autoimmune disease. *J Immunol* 173:2118–2125, 2004.

130. Clemente-Casares X, Tsai S, Yang Y, et al: Peptide-MHC-based nanovaccines for the treatment of autoimmunity: a "one size fits all" approach? *J Mol Med (Berl)* 89:733–742, 2011.

131. Sthoeger ZM, Sharabi A, Molad Y, et al: Treatment of lupus patients with a tolerogenic peptide, hCDR1 (Edratide): immunomodulation of gene expression. *J Autoimmun* 33:77–82, 2009.

132. Kang HK, Chiang MY, Liu M, et al: The histone peptide H4 71-94 alone is more effective than a cocktail of peptide epitopes in controlling lupus: immunoregulatory mechanisms. *J Clin Immunol* 31:379–394, 2011.

133. Urowitz M, Isenberg D, Wallace DJ, et al: PRELUDE—Edratide phase II study outcome—from predefined analyses to more recent assessment approaches. *Ann Rheum Dis* 70 (S3):315, 2011.

134. Singh RR, Hahn BH, Sercarz EE: Neonatal peptide exposure can prime T cells and, upon subsequent immunization, induce their immune deviation: implications for antibody vs. T cell-mediated autoimmunity. *J Exp Med* 183:1613–1621, 1996.

135. Liblau RS, Tisch R, Shokat K, et al: Intravenous injection of soluble antigen induces thymic and peripheral T-cells apoptosis. *Proc Natl Acad Sci U S A* 93:3031–3036, 1996.

136. Page N, Gros F, Schall N, et al: A therapeutic peptide in lupus alters autophagic processes and stability of MHCII molecules in MRL/lpr B cells. *Autophagy* 7:539–540, 2011.

137. Hahn BH, Singh RP, La Cava A, et al: Tolerogenic treatment of lupus mice with consensus peptide induces Foxp3-expressing, apoptosis-resistant, TGFbeta-secreting CD8+ T cell suppressors. *J Immunol* 175:7728–7737, 2005.

138. Singh RP, Dinesh R, Elashoff D, et al: Distinct gene signature revealed in white blood cells, CD4(+) and CD8(+) T cells in (NZB x NZW) F1 lupus mice after tolerization with anti-DNA Ig peptide. *Genes Immun* 11:294–309, 2010.

139. Singh RP, La Cava A, Hahn BH: pConsensus peptide induces tolerogenic CD8+ T cells in lupus-prone (NZB x NZW)F1 mice by differentially regulating Foxp3 and PD1 molecules. *J Immunol* 180:2069–2080, 2008.

140. Singh RP, La Cava A, Wong M, et al: CD8+ T cell-mediated suppression of autoimmunity in a murine lupus model of peptide-induced immune tolerance depends on Foxp3 expression. *J Immunol* 178:7649–7657, 2007.

141. Lourenco EV, Procaccini C, Ferrera F, et al: Modulation of p38 MAPK activity in regulatory T cells after tolerance with anti-DNA Ig peptide in (NZB x NZW)F1 lupus mice. *J Immunol* 182:7415–7421, 2009.

142. Yu Y, Liu Y, Shi FD, et al: Tolerance induced by anti-DNA Ig peptide in (NZB×NZW)F1 lupus mice impinges on the resistance of effector T cells to suppression by regulatory T cells. *Clin Immunol* 142:291–295, 2011.

143. Riemekasten G, Langnickel D, Enghard P, et al: Intravenous injection of a D1 protein of the Smith proteins postpones murine lupus and induces type 1 regulatory T cells. *J Immunol* 173:5835–5842, 2004.

144. Wong M, La Cava A, Singh RP, et al: Blockade of programmed death-1 in young (New Zealand black x New Zealand white)F1 mice promotes the activity of suppressive CD8+ T cells that protect from lupus-like disease. *J Immunol* 185:6563–6571, 2010.

145. Kang HK, Liu M, Datta SK: Low-dose peptide tolerance therapy of lupus generates plasmacytoid dendritic cells that cause expansion of autoantigen-specific regulatory T cells and contraction of inflammatory Th17 cells. *J Immunol* 178:7849–7858, 2007.

146. Dinesh R, Hahn BH, La Cava A, et al: Interferon-inducible gene 202b controls CD8(+) T cell-mediated suppression in anti-DNA Ig peptide-treated (NZB x NZW) F1 lupus mice. *Genes Immun* 12:360–369, 2011.

147. Lapter S, Ben-David H, Sharabi A, et al: A role for the B-cell CD74/macrophage migration inhibitory factor pathway in the immunomodulation of systemic lupus erythematosus by a therapeutic tolerogenic peptide. *Immunology* 132:87–95, 2011.

148. Tian J, Olcott AP, Kaufman DL: Antigen-based immunotherapy drives the precocious development of autoimmunity. *J Immunol* 169:6564–6569, 2002.

149. Sela U, Mauermann N, Hershkoviz R, et al: The inhibition of autoreactive T cell functions by a peptide based on the CDR1 of an anti-DNA autoantibody is via TGF-beta-mediated suppression of LFA-1 and CD44 expression and function. *J Immunol* 175:7255–7263, 2005.

150. Serreze DV, Chen YG: Of mice and men: use of animal models to identify possible interventions for the prevention of autoimmune type 1 diabetes in humans. *Trends Immunol* 26:603–607, 2005.

151. Klinman DM: Polyclonal B cell activation in lupus-prone mice precedes and predicts the development of autoimmune disease. *J Clin Invest* 86:1249–1254,1990.

152. Craft J, Fatenejad S: Self antigens and epitope spreading in systemic autoimmunity. *Arthritis Rheum* 40:1374–1382, 1997.

153. Shi Y, Kaliyaperumal A, Lu L, et al: Promiscuous presentation and recognition of nucleosomal autoepitopes in lupus: role of autoimmune T cell receptor alpha chain. *J Exp Med* 187:367–378, 1998.

154. Singh RR: Prevention and control of reciprocal T-B cell diversification: implications for lupus-like autoimmunity. *Mol Immunol* 40:1137–1145, 2004.

155. De Silva-Udawatta M, Kumar SR, Greidinger EL, et al: Cloned human TCR from patients with autoimmune disease can respond to two structurally distinct autoantigens. *J Immunol* 172:3940–3947, 2004.

156. Anders HJ, Zecher D, Pawar RD, et al: Molecular mechanisms of autoimmunity triggered by microbial infection. *Arthritis Res Ther* 7:215–224, 2005.

157. Bachmann M, Grolz D, Bartsch H, et al: Analysis of expression of an alternative La (SS-B) cDNA and localization of the encoded N- and C-terminal peptides. *Biochim Biophys Acta* 1356:53–63, 1997.

158. Bloom O, Cheng KF, He M, et al: Generation of a unique small molecule peptidomimetic that neutralizes lupus autoantibody activity. *Proc Natl Acad Sci U S A* 108:10255–10259, 2011.

159. Brosh N, Zinger H, Fridkin M, et al: A peptide based on the sequence of the CDR3 of a murine anti-DNA mAb is a better modulator of experimental SLE than its single amino acid-substituted analogs. *Cell Immunol* 205:52–61, 2000c.

160. Cocca BA, Cline AM, Radic MZ: Blebs and apoptotic bodies are B cell autoantigens. *J Immunol* 169:159–166, 2002.

161. Eilat E, Zinger H, Nyska A, et al: Prevention of systemic lupus erythematosus-like disease in (NZBxNZW)F1 mice by treating with CDR1- and CDR3-based peptides of a pathogenic autoantibody. *J Clin Immunol* 20:268–278, 2000.

162. Eisenberg R: Do autoantigens define autoimmunity or vice versa? *Eur J Immunol* 35:367–370, 2005.

163. Freed JH, Marrs A, VanderWall J, et al: MHC class II-bound self peptides from autoimmune MRL/lpr mice reveal potential T cell epitopes for autoantibody production in murine systemic lupus erythematosus. *J Immunol* 164:4697–4705, 2000.

164. Hahn BH, Anderson M, Le E, et al: Anti-DNA Ig peptides promote Treg cell activity in systemic lupus erythematosus patients. *Arthritis Rheum* 58:2488–2497, 2008.

165. Jouanne C, Avrameas S, Payelle-Brogard B: A peptide derived from a polyreactive monoclonal anti-DNA natural antibody can modulate lupus development in (NZBxNZW)F1 mice. *Immunology* 96:333–339, 1999.

166. Kaliyaperumal A, Michaels MA, Datta SK: Naturally processed chromatin peptides reveal a major autoepitope that primes pathogenic T and B cells of lupus. *J Immunol* 168:2530–2537, 2002.

167. Kosmopoulou A, Vlassi M, Stavrakoudis A, et al: T-cell epitopes of the La/SSB autoantigen: prediction based on the homology modeling of HLA-DQ2/DQ7 with the insulin-B peptide/HLA-DQ8 complex. *J Comput Chem* 27:1033–1044, 2006.

168. Mamula MJ, Gee RJ, Elliott JI, et al: Isoaspartyl post-translational modification triggers autoimmune responses to self-proteins. *J Biol Chem* 274:22321–22327, 1999.

169. Monneaux F, Parietti V, Briand JP, et al: Intramolecular T cell spreading in unprimed MRL/lpr mice: importance of the U1-70k protein sequence 131-151. *Arthritis Rheum* 50:3232–3238, 2004.

170. Nikolova K, Mihaylova N, Voynova E, et al: Re-establishing tolerance to DNA in humanized and murine models of SLE. *Autoimmun Rev* 9:499–502, 2010.

171. Rai G, Ray S, Shaw RE, et al: Models of systemic lupus erythematosus: development of autoimmunity following peptide immunizations of non-inbred pedigreed rabbits. *J Immunol* 176:660–667, 2006.

172. Shapira E, Proscura E, Brodsky B, et al: Novel peptides as potential treatment of systemic lupus erythematosus. *Lupus* 20:463–472, 2011.

173. Sharabi A, Zinger H, Zborowsky M, et al: A peptide based on the complementarity-determining region 1 of an autoantibody ameliorates lupus by up-regulating CD4+CD25+ cells and TGF-beta. *Proc Natl Acad Sci U S A* 103:8810–8815, 2006.

174. Singh RR: The potential use of peptides and vaccination to treat systemic lupus erythematosus. *Curr Opin Rheumatol* 12:399–406, 2000.

175. Skaggs BJ, Lourenco EV, Hahn BH: Oral administration of different forms of a tolerogenic peptide to define the preparations and doses that delay anti-DNA antibody production and nephritis and prolong survival in SLE-prone mice. *Lupus* 20:912–920, 2011.

176. Skaggs BJ, Singh RP, Hahn BH: Induction of immune tolerance by activation of CD8+ T suppressor/regulatory cells in lupus-prone mice. *Hum Immunol* 69:790–796, 2008.

177. Voitharou C, Krikorian D, Sakarellos C, et al: A complementary La/SSB epitope anchored to Sequential Oligopeptide Carrier regulates the anti-La/SSB response in immunized animals. *J Pept Sci* 14:1069–1076, 2008.

178. Yang J, Pospisil R, Ray S, et al: Investigations of a rabbit (*Oryctolagus cuniculus*) model of systemic lupus erythematosus (SLE), BAFF and its receptors. *PLoS One* 4:e8494, 2009.

Chapter

22

Overview and Clinical Presentation

Andrea Hinojosa-Azaola and Jorge Sánchez-Guerrero

Systemic lupus erythematosus (SLE) is considered the most clinically and serologically diverse autoimmune disease because it can affect almost any organ and display a broad spectrum of manifestations.[1] It may manifest as a mild disease with skin or joint involvement only or may be severe, affecting vital organs such as the kidney, central nervous system (CNS), and heart. This is why SLE has been addressed as a constellation of different clinical variants, or better, as a *galaxy,*[2] considering that clinical manifestations not only differ from patient to patient but also show considerable geographic and ethnic variation. This diversity is related to the role of genetic and environmental factors as well as abnormalities of the immune system that influence both susceptibility and clinical expression.[3,4]

This chapter presents an overview of the clinical presentation of SLE; the following chapters detail its involvement in specific organs.

HISTORY

Considering the broad spectrum of clinical and immunologic manifestations displayed by patients with SLE, it is important to cover the items presented in Table 22-1, which reviews the cumulative incidence of clinical manifestations in several SLE cohorts.

Regardless of their age and gender, Hispanics, African Americans, and Asians tend to have more hematologic, serosal, neurologic, and renal manifestations and to accrue more damage and at a faster pace than Caucasians.[5] Africans progress more commonly to end-stage renal disease (ESRD), show higher activity at diagnosis and in disease course, and are more commonly affected by discoid rash than Europeans (they present more frequently with malar rash and photosensitivity). Asian and Arab patients show higher frequency of renal disease and damage than Europeans.[6] On the other hand, Hispanics are more heterogeneous in their disease manifestations, with their clinical profile depending on their African, European, or mestizo ethnicity.[7] This heterogeneity reflects genetic, environmental, socioeconomic, and access to medical care differences.[8]

CHIEF COMPLAINT

The presenting complaint varies in patients with SLE. Table 22-2 lists the manifestations noted at the diagnosis of SLE in several studies, and Figure 22-1 shows the preceding factors, onset, and progression of the disease.

In the LUpus in MInorities, NAture vs. Nurture (LUMINA) study's multiethnic cohort, the most common initial manifestation of SLE was arthritis (34.5%), followed by photosensitivity (18.8%) and antinuclear antibody (ANA) positivity (14.2%).[9] In addition, Cervera compared early and late manifestations in a cohort of 1000 patients

and found that the majority of manifestations occurred more frequently during the first 5 years.[10] It is useful to identify the initial SLE manifestations because the long-term prognosis differs with respect to them.[11]

One of the most challenging issues in attributing clinical manifestations to SLE is to define when the disease begins. The lag time between the onset of SLE and its diagnosis reported in major cohorts was almost 50 months before 1980, 28 months in the years 1980 to 1989, 15 months in the years 1990 to 1999, and 9 months after 2000.[12] This difference results from the introduction of ANA testing and advances in the knowledge of autoimmune diseases over time.

Although currently there are no reliable clinical or serologic predictors that allow the identification of SLE at an early stage, there is evidence that at least one autoantibody (more frequently an ANA) is present during a mean time of 3.3 years before the diagnosis of SLE in 88% of patients.[13]

Mariz tested for ANAs in 918 healthy individuals and in 153 patients with autoimmune rheumatic diseases, and found positive results in 118 (13%) of the former group and in 138 (90%) of the latter group, with higher titers and distinctive patterns present in patients with autoimmune rheumatic diseases.[14] When 40 of the ANA-positive healthy individuals were reevaluated after 3.6 to 5 years, all remained healthy and 73% continued testing ANA positive.

VARIATIONS IN CLINICAL PRESENTATION
Incomplete Lupus

It is common for rheumatologists to care for patients who are thought to have SLE but do not meet criteria. These patients are considered by some to have "incomplete," "subclinical," "incipient," "possible," "mild," "latent," or "variant" SLE.[9,15] It is likely, however, that some of these cases are part of the disease spectrum.

The most accepted terms are incomplete lupus and latent lupus, defined as the presence of symptoms related to one organ system plus the presence of ANAs.

In a multicenter European study involving 122 patients with incomplete lupus, SLE developed in 22 patients according to the ACR criteria in the first year, and in 3 additional patients within 3 years. These patients presented with cutaneous and musculoskeletal activity as well as leukopenia.[16]

Ganczarczyk followed 22 patients with latent lupus prospectively for at least 5 years and found that they differed from patients with SLE in the lack of renal and central nervous system involvement as well as the lower frequency of anti-DNA antibody and depressed

TABLE 22-1 Cumulative Incidence of SLE Manifestations

MANIFESTATION	Cumulative Incidence (%)						
	Dubois and Tuffanelli (520 cases; 1964)[31]	Estes and Christian (150 cases; 1971)[46]	Hochberg et al (150 cases; 1985)[47]	Pistiner et al (464 cases; 1991)[27]	Cervera et al (Euro-Lupus; 1000 cases; 1993)[26]	Font et al (600 cases; 2004)[1]	Pons-Estel et al (GLADEL; 1214 cases; 2004)[7]
Systemic:							
Fever	84	77	—	41	52	42	57
Weight loss	51	—	—	—	—	—	27
Musculoskeletal:							
Arthritis and arthralgia	92	95	76	91	84	83	93
Myalgias	48	5	5	79	9	7	18
Aseptic bone necrosis	5	7	24	5	—	—	1
Cardiorespiratory:							
Pericarditis	31	19	23	12	—	—	17
Myocarditis	8	8	—	3	—	2	3
Hypertension	25	46	—	25	—	—	27
Pleural effusion	30	40	57	12	—	28	22
Cutaneous-vascular:							
Skin lesions, all types	72	81	88	55	—	—	90
Butterfly area lesions	57	39	61	34	58	54	61
Alopecia	21	37	45	31	—	18	58
Oral/nasal ulcers	9	7	23	19	24	30	42
Photosensitivity	33	—	45	37	45	41	56
Urticaria	7	13	—	—	—	—	—
Raynaud	18	21	44	24	34	22	28
Discoid lesions	29	14	15	23	10	6	12
Neurologic:							
CNS damage, all types	26	59	39	—	27	18	26
Peripheral neuritis	12	7	21	—	—	—	1
Psychosis	12	37	16	5	—	12	4
Seizures	14	26	13	6	—	12	8
Ocular:							
Cytoid bodies	10	—	—	—	—	—	—
Uveitis	1	—	—	—	—	—	1
Renal:							
Proteinuria /abnormal sediment	46	53	31	31	39	34	46
Nephrotic syndrome	23	26	13	14	—	—	7
Gastrointestinal:							
Diarrhea	6	—	—	—	—	—	—
Ascites	—	—	—	—	—	—	1
Abdominal pain	19	—	—	—	—	—	—
Bowel hemorrhage	6	—	—	—	—	—	—
Hemic-lymphatic:							
Adenopathy	59	36	—	10	12	1	15
Anemia (<11 g hemoglobin per dL)	57	73	57	30	—	20	—
Hemolytic anemia	—	14	27	8	8	8	12
Leukopenia (<4500 leukocytes/mL)	43	66	41	51	—	66	42
Thrombocytopenia (<100,000 platelets/mL)	7	19	30	16	22	31	19

Continued

TABLE 22-1 Cumulative Incidence of SLE Manifestations—cont'd

	Cumulative Incidence (%)						
MANIFESTATION	Dubois and Tuffanelli (520 cases; 1964)[31]	Estes and Christian (150 cases; 1971)[46]	Hochberg et al (150 cases; 1985)[47]	Pistiner et al (464 cases; 1991)[27]	Cervera et al (Euro-Lupus; 1000 cases; 1993)[26]	Font et al (600 cases; 2004)[1]	Pons-Estel et al (GLADEL; 1214 cases; 2004)[7]
Serologic*:							
False-positive VDRL result	—	24	26	30	—	—	—
LE cell preparation	76	78	71	42	—	—	—
ANA	—	87	94	96	96	99	98
Low C3	—	—	59	39	—	31	49
Anti-DNA	—	—	28	40	78	90	71
Anti-Sm	—	—	17	6	10	13	48
Anti-SSa (Ro)	—	—	32	18	25	23	49
Anti-RNP	—	—	34	14	13	14	51
Anticardiolipin IgG/IgM	—	—	—	38 (any)	24/13	15/9	51/41

ANA, antinuclear antibody (test); CNS, central nervous system; GLADEL, Grupo Latino Americano de Estudio de Lupus; Ig, immunoglobulin.
*In this section, the manifestation is a positive result of the test listed unless otherwise specified.

TABLE 22-2 Main Initial Manifestations of SLE

	Incidence (%)			
MANIFESTATION	Dubois and Tuffanelli (520 cases; 1964)[31]	Cervera et al (Euro-Lupus; 1000 cases; 1993)[26]	Font et al (600 cases; 2004)[1]	Pons-Estel et al (GLADEL; 1214 cases) 2004[7]
Arthritis and arthralgia	46	69	64	67
Myositis	2	4	3	8
Any cutaneous involvement	—	—	57	46
Discoid lupus	11	6	—	5
Malar rash	6	40	—	24
Photosensitivity	1	29	—	25
Oral ulcers	—	11	—	11
Raynaud phenomenon	2	18	—	10
Fatigue	4	—	—	—
Fever	4	36	—	29
Lymphadenopathy	1	7	—	5
Serositis	1	17	—	4
Lung involvement		3	1	0.5
Renal involvement	3	16	12	5
Neurologic involvement	1	12	7	4
Thrombocytopenia	—	9	—	5
Hemolytic anemia	2	4	—	2
Thrombosis	—	4	1	1

GLADEL, Grupo Latino Americano de Estudio de Lupus.

complement levels.[17] Seven patients (32%) eventually had SLE, and no predictive factors distinguished them from the 15 who did not.

In a Swedish study of 28 patients with incomplete lupus identified between 1981 and 1992, SLE developed in 16 patients (57%) in a median time of 5.3 years. Malar rash and anticardiolipin antibodies were predictors of SLE, and patients in whom the disease developed were more prone to organ damage.[18]

Late-Onset Lupus

Late-onset SLE, which has been defined as age of onset at or after 50 years, is an uncommon condition that occurs with a frequency of 12% to 18%.[19] The less awareness of its occurrence, insidious onset, and fewer classic manifestations have led to a delay between the onset and diagnosis. Table 22-3 summarizes the main characteristics of patients with late-onset SLE in large studies.

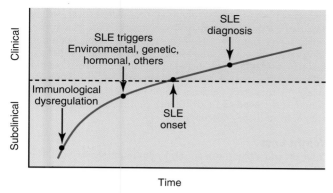

FIGURE 22-1 Preceding factors, onset, and progression of systemic lupus erythematosus (SLE).

Age is known to have an important effect on the clinical expression of the disease.[20] Although it has been recognized that patients with late-onset SLE have lower levels of activity and less major organ involvement, other studies have identified increasing age as an independent factor for poor outcome in terms of damage accrual and mortality.[5,20-23] Factors associated with age (i.e., comorbidities) may explain these findings, rather than true differences in disease phenotype.

Male Lupus

Systemic lupus erythematosus is often considered a "woman's disease" because of the striking differences in prevalence related to sex. Nevertheless, males with SLE have their own distinguishing characteristics in terms of clinical manifestations and outcome.

Data accumulated in the literature account for approximately 4% to 22% of male patients in lupus series, but up to 30% in studies

TABLE 22-3 Frequency of Clinical Features in Patients with Late-Onset SLE*

MANIFESTATION	Frequency (%)		
	Euro-Lupus (93 Cases; 1993)[26]	LUMINA Cohort (73 Cases; 2006)[22]	1000 Faces of Lupus Study (161 Cases; 2010)[19]
Any cutaneous	—	69	—
Malar rash	33	—	51
Photosensitivity	29	—	55
Discoid lesions	7	—	18
Oral/nasal ulcerations	20	—	58
Arthritis	73	—	84
Myositis	10	74	4
Nephropathy	22	29	24
Proteinuria	—	—	38
Neurologic (any)	16	53	4
Seizures	—	—	20
Psychosis	—	—	25
Hematologic	—	—	68
Thrombocytopenia	28	—	34
Hemolytic anemia	9	—	13
Serositis	38	—	32
Pericarditis	—	—	45
Fever	51	—	8
Raynaud phenomenon	22	—	47
Lymphadenopathy	3	—	—
ANAs	97	—	97
Anti–double-stranded DNA	77	—	79
Anti-Sm	—	18	11
Low complement	—	—	25
Anti-Ro (SSa)	16	23	28
Anti-La (SSb)	6	—	11
Anti–U1-RNP	5	—	14
ACL IgG/IgM	13/15	—	55 (any)

ACL, anticardiolipin (antibody); ANA, antinuclear antibody; Ig, immunoglobulin; LUMINA, LUpus in MInorities, NAture versus nurture study;
*Late-onset defined as onset at or after 50 years of age.

considering familial aggregation. Lupus is 8 to 15 times more common in women at childbearing age than in age-matched men; before puberty this ratio is 2:1 to 6:1, and after menopause 3:1 to 8:1.[24]

In a cohort of 107 Latin American male patients with SLE, there was a higher prevalence of renal disease, vascular thrombosis, and anti-dsDNA antibodies, as well as a greater use of moderate to high doses of corticosteroids, in comparison with female patients.[25] Other large studies have confirmed the finding of greater renal involvement in men.[26-28] Furthermore, in the LUMINA study, men accrued damage early, predisposing them to accrue more damage subsequently.[29,30] Additional clinical manifestations found to be more common among males with lupus include serositis, neurologic and cutaneous manifestations, hepatosplenomegaly, cardiovascular manifestations, fever and weight loss at onset, hypertension, and vasculitis.[24]

CONSTITUTIONAL SYMPTOMS

The constitutional symptoms fever, weight loss, malaise, fatigue, and lymphadenopathy are common in patients with SLE and do not fit into any organ-system classification; therefore, they are discussed here.

Fever

Fever is a common manifestation of active SLE and is also a frequent cause of hospital admission. Fever occurred in 84% of patients in a report by Dubois[31] and in 42% in the report by Font[1]; whereas in the Euro-Lupus cohort it was observed in 36% of patients at onset and in 52% during evolution.[26] Fever was present in more patients with early-onset versus late-onset disease in a large Canadian study[19] and was more common in whites than mestizos in a multiethnic cohort.[7] The reported prevalence of fever attributed to SLE has declined progressively, perhaps resulting from a frequent use of nonsteroidal anti-inflammatory drugs.

The attribution of fever to SLE holds only after other causes, such as infections, are excluded. Some definitions for this condition include the one by Rovin, as follows: in the absence of infection despite extensive testing, presence of an illness typical of active SLE accompanying the fever, and no evidence for infection despite the increase in or addition of steroid therapy.[32]

In a retrospective analysis of 160 hospitalized patients with SLE, Stahl identified 83 febrile episodes in 63 patients.[33] Of these, 60% were attributed to active SLE, 23% to infections, and 17% to miscellaneous causes. In the patients with active SLE without infection, the peak temperature range was 38 °C to 40.6 °C, with an intermittent pattern. Other SLE manifestations associated with fever were dermatitis, arthritis, and pleuropericarditis.

In comparison with patients with SLE and fever of infectious etiology, patients with fever due to lupus are more likely to have lower C3 and higher levels of disease activity.[34] A close correlation between serum concentrations of interferon alpha (but not interleukin-1 or tumor necrosis factor alpha) and fever was observed in 25 untreated patients with SLE, suggesting the possible involvement of interferon alpha in its pathogenesis.[35]

Lymphadenopathy

Lymphadenopathy in SLE represents a benign finding, with a mononucleosis-like behavior, and it can be seen in any phase of the disease.[36]

In the study by Dubois generalized adenopathy was observed in 59% of patients, and localized (cervical) adenopathy in 24%.[31] As an initial manifestation, adenopathy was reported in 7% of the patients from the Euro-Lupus cohort[26]; in the multiethnic Grupo Latino Americano de Estudio de Lupus (GLADEL) cohort, it was present in 5% of subjects at disease onset, and in 15% during evolution.[7]

Lupus lymphadenopathy involves mainly the cervical and axillary regions, and the lymph nodes are soft, mobile, painful, and nonadherent to deep planes. Other clinical manifestations, such as malar erythema, photosensitivity, alopecia, oral ulcers, fever, weight loss, nocturnal diaphoresis, and hepatosplenomegaly, are usually present.[36]

In cases of significant lymphadenopathy, lymph node biopsy is indicated to rule out infectious and lymphoproliferative disorders.[37,38] Histopathologic findings include coagulative necrosis with hematoxylin bodies, reactive follicular hyperplasia, and a Castleman's disease–like pattern.[39] Of these, lymph node necrosis with hematoxylin bodies is considered a distinctive finding for SLE, although it is rarely seen in biopsy specimens.[40]

Weight Loss

Anorexia and weight loss are also manifestations of SLE. The incidence of weight loss in large series was found to range from 17% to 51%,[31] showing variations among different ethnic groups.[6,7] The extent of weight loss almost always is less than 10% and precedes the diagnosis of SLE.

Lom-Orta reported five patients with SLE who presented with severe protein-calorie malnutrition.[41] In these patients, malnutrition overshadowed other manifestations of SLE, and in some, it delayed the diagnosis. Corticosteroid treatment and proper food intake resulted in prompt improvement of both SLE and malnutrition. An interesting finding in these patients was that of a significant hypergammaglobulinemia as well as high titers of ANA and rheumatoid factor. Some immunologic alterations are common to patients with primary malnutrition and SLE, such as diminished T lymphocyte levels and a reduction in the capacity to generate spontaneous suppressor T cells.

Malaise and Fatigue

Fatigue is one of the most common symptoms experienced by patients with SLE, affecting up to 80%, and often the most disabling symptom.[42] In the majority of cases several confounding factors, such as disease activity, mood disorders, poor sleeping patterns, low levels of aerobic exercise, medications, and fibromyalgia, concur. Fatigue is a primary contributor to functional disability and visits to health care providers, and its association with disease activity is controversial.[43]

Tench reported fatigue in 81% and poor sleep quality in 60% of 120 patients with SLE.[42] Fatigue correlated negatively with all measures of functioning, was higher in patients with active disease, and was associated with anxiety and depression. On the other hand, Jump found that active disease or therapy did not predict self-reported levels of fatigue in 127 patients with SLE, but pain and depression did.[43] A report by Bruce of 81 patients with SLE supports the finding of no correlation between fatigue and activity or damage of the disease.[44]

In the LUMINA multiethnic cohort, fatigue was reported in 92% of patients. The variables significantly associated with this symptom were Caucasian ethnicity, constitutional symptoms (fever, weight loss), higher levels of pain, abnormal illness-related behaviors, and helplessness.[45]

References

1. Font J, Cervera R, Ramos-Casals M, et al: Clusters of clinical and immunologic features in systemic lupus erythematosus: analysis of 600 patients from a single center. *Semin Arthtitis Rheum* 33:217–230, 2004.
2. Meroni PL, Shoenfeld Y: systemic lupus erythematosus and SLE galaxy. *Autoimmun Rev* 10:1–2, 2010.
3. Gualtierotti R, Biggioggero M, Penatti AE, et al: Updating on the pathogenesis of systemic lupus erythematosus. *Autoimmun Rev* 10:3–7, 2010.
4. Crow MK: Developments in the clinical understanding of lupus. *Arthritis Res Ther* 11:245–255, 2009.
5. Pons-Estel GJ, Alarcón GS, Scofield L, et al: Understanding the epidemiology and progression of systemic lupus erythematosus. *Semin Arthritis Rheum* 39:257–268, 2008.
6. Borchers AT, Naguwa SM, Shoenfeld Y, et al: The geoepidemiology of systemic lupus erythematosus. *Autoimmun Rev* 9:A277–A287, 2010.
7. Pons-Estel BA, Catoggio LJ, Cardiel MH, et al: The GLADEL Multinational Latin American prospective inception cohort of 1,214 patients with systemic lupus erythematosus. Ethnic and disease heterogeneity among "Hispanics." *Medicine* 83:1–17, 2004.

8. Alarcón GS: Of ethnicity, race and lupus. *Lupus* 10:594–596, 2001.
9. Alarcón GS, McGwin G, Jr, Roseman JM, et al: systemic lupus erythematosus in three ethnic groups. XIX. Natural history of the accrual of the American College of Rheumatology criteria prior to the occurrence of criteria diagnosis. *Arthritis Rheum* 51:609–615, 2004.
10. Cervera R, Khamashta MA, Font J, et al: Morbidity and mortality in systemic lupus erythematosus during a 10-year period. A comparison of early and late manifestations in a cohort of 1,000 patients. *Medicine* 82:299–308, 2003.
11. Tokano Y, Morimoto S, Amano H, et al: The relationship between initial clinical manifestations and long-term prognosis of patients with systemic lupus erythematosus. *Mod Rheumatol* 15:275–282, 2005.
12. Doria A, Zen M, Canova M, et al: SLE diagnosis and treatment: when early is early. *Autoimmun Rev* 10:55–60, 2010.
13. Arbuckle MR, McClain MT, Rubertone MV, et al: Development of autoantibodies before the clinical onset of systemic lupus erythematosus. *N Eng J Med* 349:1526–1533, 2003.
14. Mariz HA, Sato EI, Barbosa SH, et al: Pattern of the antinuclear antibody-HEp-2 test is a critical parameter for discriminating antinuclear antibody-positive healthy individuals and patients with autoimmune rheumatic diseases. *Arthritis Rheum* 63:191–200, 2011.
15. Calvo-Alén J, Bastian HM, Straaton KV, et al: Identification of patient subsets among those presumptively diagnosed with, referred, and/or followed up for systemic lupus erythematosus at a large tertiary care center. *Arthritis Rheum* 38:1475–1484, 1995.
16. Swaak AJG, Van de Brink H, Smeenk RJT, et al: Incomplete lupus erythematosus: results of a multicenter study under the supervision of the EULAR Standing Committee on International Clinical Studies Including Therapeutic Trials (ESCISIT). *Rheumatology* 40:89–94, 2001.
17. Ganczarczyk L, Urowitz MB, Gladman DD: "Latent lupus." *J Rheumatol* 16:475–478, 1989.
18. Hallengren CS, Nived O, Sturfelt G: Outcome of incomplete systemic lupus erythematosus after 10 years. *Lupus* 13:85–88, 2004.
19. Lalani S, Pope J, de León F, et al: Clinical features and prognosis of late-onset systemic lupus erythematosus: results from the 1000 Faces of Lupus Study. *J Rheumatol* 37:38–44, 2010.
20. Appenzeller S, Pereira DA, Costallat LTL: Greater accrual damage in late-onset systemic lupus erythematosus: a long-term follow-up study. *Lupus* 17:1023–1028, 2008.
21. Reveille JD, Bartolucci A, Alarcón GS: Prognosis in systemic lupus erythematosus. Negative impact of increasing age at onset, black race, and thrombocytopenia, as well as causes of death. *Arthritis Rheum* 33:37–48, 1990.
22. Bertoli Am, Alarcón GS, Calvo-Alén J, et al: systemic lupus erythematosus in a multiethnic US cohort. Clinical features, course, and outcome in patients with late-onset disease. *Arthritis Rheum* 54:1580–1587, 2006.
23. Studenski S, Allen NB, Caldwell DS, et al: Survival in systemic lupus erythematosus. A multivariate analysis of demographic factors. *Arthritis Rheum* 30:1326–1332, 1987.
24. Lu LJ, Wallace DJ, Ishimori ML, et al: Male systemic lupus erythematosus: a review of sex disparities in this disease. *Lupus* 19:119–129, 2010.
25. Molina JF, Drenkard C, Molina J, et al: systemic lupus erythematosus in Males: a study of 107 Latin American patients. *Medicine* 75:124–130, 1996.
26. Cervera R, Khamashta MA, Font J, et al: systemic lupus erythematosus: clinical and immunologic patterns of disease expression in a cohort of 1,000 patients. *Medicine* 72:113–124, 1993.
27. Pistiner M, Wallace DJ, Nessim S, et al: Lupus Erythematosus in the 1980s: a survey of 570 patients. *Semin Arthritis Rheum* 21:55–64, 1991.
28. Cooper GS, Parks CG, Treadwell EL, et al: Differences by race, sex and age in the clinical and immunologic features of recently diagnosed systemic lupus erythematosus patients in the southeastern United States. *Lupus* 11:161–167, 2002.
29. Andrade RM, Alarcón GS, Fernández M, et al: Accelerated damage accrual among men with systemic lupus erythematosus: XLIV. Results from a multiethnic US cohort. *Arthritis Rheum* 56:622–630, 2007.
30. Alarcón GS, Calvo-Alén J, McGwin G, et al: systemic lupus erythematosus in a multiethnic cohort: LUMINA XXXV. Predictive factors of high disease activity over time. *Ann Rheum Dis* 65:1168–1174, 2006.
31. Dubois EL, Tuffanelly DL: Clinical manifestations of systemic lupus erythematosus. Computer analysis of 520 cases. *JAMA* 190:104–111, 1964.
32. Rovin BH, Tang Y, Sun J, et al: Clinical significance of fever in the systemic lupus erythematosus patient receiving steroid therapy. *Kidney Int* 68:747–759, 2005.
33. Stahl NI, Klippel JH, Decker JL: Fever in systemic lupus erythematosus. *Am J Med* 67:935–940, 1979.
34. Zhou WJ, Yang CD: The causes and clinical significance of fever in systemic lupus erythematosus: a retrospective study of 487 hospitalized patients. *Lupus* 18:807–812, 2009.
35. Kanayama Y, Kim T, Inariba H: Possible involvement of interferon alpha in the pathogenesis of fever in systemic lupus erythematosus. *Ann Rheum Dis* 48:861–863, 1989.
36. Salles N, Rossi K, Manente F, et al: Lymphadenopathy and systemic lupus erythematosus. *Bras J Rheumatol* 50:96–101, 2010.
37. Melikoglu MA, Melikoglu M: The clinical importance of lymphadenopathy in systemic lupus erythematosus. *Acta Reumatol Port* 33:402–406, 2008.
38. Shapira Y, Weinberger A, Wysenbeek AJ: Lymphadenopathy in systemic lupus erythematosus. Prevalence and relation to disease manifestations. *Clin Rheumatol* 5:335–338, 1996.
39. Kojima M, Nakamura S, Morishita Y, et al: Reactive follicular hyperplasia in the lymph node lesions from systemic lupus erythematosus patients: a clinicopathological and immunohistological study of 21 cases. *Pathol Int* 50:304–312, 2000.
40. Kojima M, Motoori T, Asano S, et al: Histological diversity of reactive and atypical proliferative lymph node lesions in systemic lupus erythematosus patients. *Pathol Res Pract* 203:423–431, 2007.
41. Lom-Orta H, Díaz-Jouanen E, Alarcón-Segovia D: Protein-caloric malnutrition and systemic lupus erythematosus. *J Rheumatol* 7:178–182, 1980.
42. Tench CM, McCurdie I, White PD, et al: The prevalence and associations of fatigue in systemic lupus erythematosus. *Rheumatology* 39:1249–1254, 2000.
43. Jump RL, Robinson ME, Armstrong AE et al: Fatigue in systemic lupus erythematosus: contributions of disease activity, pain, depression, and perceived social support. *J Rheumatol* 32:1699–1705, 2005.
44. Bruce IN, Mak VC, Hallett DC, et al: Factors associated with fatigue in patients with systemic lupus erythematosus. *Ann Rheum Dis* 58:379–381, 1999.
45. Burgos PI, Alarcón GS, McGwin G, Jr, et al: Disease activity and damage are not associated with increased levels of fatigue in systemic lupus erythematosus patients from a multiethnic cohort: LXVII. *Arthritis Rheum* 61:1179–1186, 2009.
46. Estes D, Christian CL: The natural history of systemic lupus erythematosus by prospective analysis. *Medicine* 50:85–95, 1971.
47. Hochberg MC, Boyd RE, Ahearn JM, et al: systemic lupus erythematosus: a review of clinic-laboratory features and immunogenetic markers in 150 patients with emphasis on demographic subsets. *Medicine* 64:285–295, 1985.

Chapter 23

Pathomechanisms of Cutaneous Lupus Erythematosus

Jan P. Dutz

Abnormal cutaneous reactivity to sunlight is such a seminal clinical feature of lupus erythematosus (LE) that it is one of the 11 criteria proposed by the American Rheumatism Association in 1982 for a case definition of systemic lupus erythematosus (SLE).[1] Photosensitivity is also a cardinal feature of the cutaneous and neonatal forms of lupus erythematosus. This strong clinical association has led to the postulate that abnormal photoreactivity participates in the pathogenesis of cutaneous lesions in lupus erythematosus. This chapter summarizes the evidence for abnormal photoreactivity in lupus erythematosus and reviews critical and newer data on the cellular, molecular, and genetic factors that may underlie this abnormality. To enable an understanding of the potential mechanisms underlying the development of cutaneous lupus, the chapter discusses the possible interrelated roles of ultraviolet light–mediated induction of apoptosis and inflammation as well as immunomodulation. In addition, the role and importance of humoral and cellular factors in the disease process are considered. Finally, the chapter describes the participation of soluble cytokines and cofactors of inflammation in lesion induction. A model of the pathophysiology of cutaneous lupus is constructed with an incorporation of advances in the fields of photobiology, immunology, cell biology, and genetics.

CLINICAL PHOTOSENSITIVITY IN LUPUS

Skin lesions are common in SLE, being found in up to 90% of patients with the disease.[2] Lupus-specific cutaneous findings such as malar rash (acute cutaneous lupus erythematosus [ACLE]) and discoid lupus (chronic cutaneous lupus erythematosus [CCLE]) were found in 64% and 31% of patients in a large cohort, respectively.[2] Skin disease is the first symptom of disease in 23% to 28% of patients with SLE. There is a clear relationship between sunlight exposure and the manifestations of cutaneous LE, and cutaneous lesions tend to occur in sun-exposed skin. This association was first demonstrated in 1965, when Epstein used a repeated light exposure technique to show that ultraviolet (UV) radiation could induce skin lesions in patients with LE.[3]

Action Spectrum of Cutaneous Lupus Erythematosus

Ultraviolet light is commonly divided into germicidal UV light (UVC), midrange UV light or sunburn UV light (UVB), and longwave UV light (UVA), also termed near-UV or black light (Figure 23-1). This separation is important because the differing wavelengths have varying biologic effects (see later). Although UVC has been used in many in vitro studies of the cellular response to UV irradiation, this spectrum of UV light is completely blocked by the earth's atmosphere and is of dubious pathophysiologic relevance. Early investigators defined an action spectrum in the UVB range (290 to 320 nm) for the cutaneous forms of LE.[4] Subsequent studies demonstrated that UVA (320 to 400 nm) also can contribute to the induction of skin lesions.[5] Multicenter studies have confirmed these results.[6] Although UVA-induced erythema in normal skin requires 1000 times more energy than UVB-induced erythema, daily exposure to UVA is much greater than that to UVB, and at the level of the dermal capillaries,

the effect of UVA effect, as a result of greater penetrance, is much stronger than that of UVB (Figure 23-2). In formal phototesting protocols, lesions occur in a delayed fashion after UV exposure (from days to weeks) and last for weeks to months.[7] In these studies, photoinducible lesions are most common in subacute cutaneous lupus erythematosus (SCLE), followed by lupus tumidus (LT) and discoid lupus erythematosus (DLE) or CCLE.[6]

Role of Ultraviolet Light in the Exacerbation of SLE

It is often stated that sunlight not only aggravates cutaneous LE but induces or worsens systemic features of the disease. Up to 73% of patients with SLE report photosensitivity.[8] However, phototesting with standardized protocols correlates poorly with patient-reported photosensitivity,[9] likely owing to the delayed nature of the lesions induced by phototesting. Repeated single patient observations indicate that sunlight may precipitate disease de novo or may aggravate existing disease. For example, use of tanning beds (a source of predominant UVA) has been reported to exacerbate SLE.[10] Geographic clustering of SLE mortality has been linked to ambient solar radiation levels.[11] Outdoor work, with a strongest effect among people reporting a blistering sunburn following midday sun (odds ratio [OR] = 7.9), was associated with the development of SLE in a large case-control study.[12]

A Selective Sensitivity to Ultraviolet Light in LE?

Clinical observations suggestive of a role for UV light in the pathogenesis of SLE and lupus skin disease have been supported by mechanistic studies. Repeated exposure to UV light can accelerate the spontaneous onset of systemic lupus in murine models. Exposure of BXSB autoimmune lupus mice to UVB has been shown to induce the release of autoantigens, to promote antibody production, and to promote early death.[13] Likewise, repeated UVB exposure can induce antinuclear antibody (ANA) in autoimmune-prone NOD mice.[14] UV-mediated DNA damage induces growth arrest, and DNA damage induces 45α (*gadd45*A) transcript expression in T cells.[15] The molecule *gadd45*A lowers epigenetic silencing of genes by reducing methylation. The resulting hypomethylation of DNA and expression of CD11a and CD70 on T cells promotes T-cell autoreactivity and B-cell stimulation.

RESPONSES TO ULTRAVIOLET LIGHT IN CUTANEOUS LUPUS ERYTHEMATOSUS

Ultraviolet light has multiple effects on living tissue. Potential molecular targets of UV light include not only DNA but RNA, proteins, and lipids. The biologic effects of UV light on the skin are summarized in Table 23-1. In addition to alteration of DNA, cytoskeletal reorganization was noted in keratinocytes (skin cells) after UV irradiation.[16] An early study by LeFeber revealed that UV light induces the binding of antibodies to selected nuclear antigens on cultured human keratinocytes.[17] The specificity of these antibodies was not defined, but it is now known that they are commonly directed against Ro/SSA (anti–Sjögren syndrome antigen A), La/SSB (anti–Sjögren syndrome antigen B), ribonucleoprotein (RNP), and Smith (Sm)

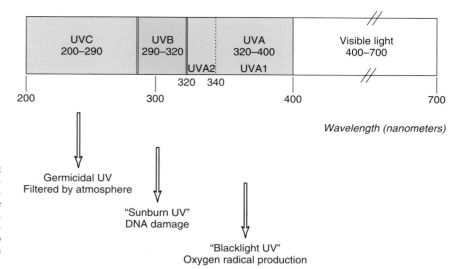

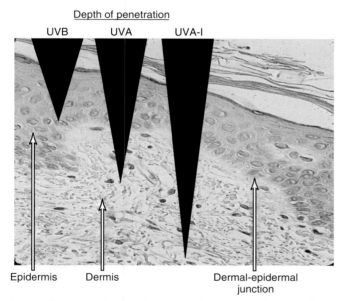

FIGURE 23-1 The spectrum of ultraviolet (UV) light irradiation by wavelength. Ultraviolet light is commonly divided into germicidal UV light (UVC), mid-range UV light or sunburn light (UVB), and long-wave UV light (UVA), also termed near-UV or black light. Both UVB and UVA can induce skin lesions in photosensitive lupus erythematosus. UVA-1 is light limited to the longer wavelength spectrum of UVA and has been used therapeutically in SLE.

FIGURE 23-2 **Photomicrograph of normal skin depicting the depth of penetration of the various forms of ultraviolet radiation (UVR).** The skin is formed by an epidermal compartment that comprises the stratum corneum (horny layer), the epidermis proper, and a basement membrane zone. Keratinocytes (skin cells), melanocytes (pigment cells), and Langerhans cells (dendritic cells) are found in this compartment. The dermal compartment contains the vasculature of the skin and connective tissue. Penetration of UVR is directly proportional to the wavelength of the radiation. UVB is absorbed primarily in the epidermis. UVA penetrates the dermis and can affect the skin vasculature. UVA-1 has the potential to penetrate the skin more deeply than UVA of shorter wavelength.

TABLE 23-1	Biologic Effects of Ultraviolet Radiation	
CHARACTERISTIC	**ULTRAVIOLET B**	**ULTRAVIOLET A**
Absorption by molecules	DNA, amino acids, melanin, urocanic acid	Melanin
Direct DNA damage	Increased	Minimal
Free radical production	Minimal	Increased
Depth of penetration	Epidermal	Dermal
Epidermal effects	Stratum corneum thickening, intermediate and delayed apoptosis, keratinocyte cytokine transcription and release	Immediate apoptosis
Langerhans cell effects	Inactivation, emigration	Minimal

antigens and are the antibodies associated with SLE and photosensitivity. These results could be explained by UV-induced translocation of antigens to the cell surface with or without the death of the cell, or by other alterations in the antigens that allow the binding of autoantibodies taken up by the living cell. In 1995, Casciola-Rosen demonstrated that when keratinocytes grown in cell culture are irradiated with UVB, they actively cleave their DNA and die by a process termed *apoptosis*.[18] During this process, the antigens recognized by autoantibodies, such as Ro/SSA, and calreticulin are concentrated in structures termed *blebs* or apoptotic bodies found at the cell surface. Larger blebs arise from the nucleus and harbor Ro/SSA, La/SSB, and other nuclear material. The bleb-associated antigens are then phagocytosed, packaged, and presented to dendritic cells, thereby stimulating autoimmune responses.

Ultraviolet Light, Cell Death, and the Skin
Apoptosis and necrosis are the two major mechanisms of cell death. Apoptosis is an ordered means of noninflammatory cell removal in which a central biochemical program initiates the dismantling of cells by nuclear fragmentation, formation of an apoptotic envelope, and shrinking of the cell into fragments leading to phagocytosis by parenchymal cells as well as phagocytes. In necrosis, cells are passive targets of extensive membrane damage leading to cell lysis and release of contents. UV light has long been known to induce apoptotic death in suprabasilar keratinocytes; such cells were called "sunburn cells" by morphologists.[19] UV light is now known to induce such apoptosis by multiple mechanisms (for review see reference 20).

Cell Death in Cutaneous Lupus Erythematosus
Using terminal deoxynucleotidyl transferase–mediated deoxyuridine triphosphate nick-end labeling (TUNEL) staining to detect nuclei with DNA damage, Norris demonstrated the presence of an increased number of apoptotic keratinocytes in the basal zones of CCLE lesions and in the suprabasal zones of SCLE lesions.[21] The increased number of apoptotic cells could be a result of a higher rate of apoptosis induction mediated directly by UV light or as a consequence of UV-induced cytokine release. Apoptosis also can be induced by cellular cytotoxic mechanisms. Cytotoxic T lymphocytes (CTLs) and natural killer (NK) cells can induce apoptosis through multiple

mechanisms (reviewed in reference 22), including the release of perforin and granzymes, cytokine release (interferon gamma [IFN-γ], tumor necrosis factor alpha [TNF-α], TNF-β, interleukin-1 [IL-1]); and triggering of Fas by FasL. The presence of leukocytes in proximity to the apoptotic cells and of FasL-positive macrophages in proximity to apoptotic cells in lesional hair follicles suggests a role for such cellular apoptotic mechanisms in established lesions. Although detection of a higher number of apoptotic cells in LE epidermis may underlie an increase in apoptosis, either an increase in the rate of apoptotic death or a decrease in the rate of clearance of apoptotic debris could lead to the observed rise in apoptotic cell number. An accumulation of apoptotic cells in the skin of patients with CLE after UV has been associated with delayed clearance.[23] Apoptotic cells are normally cleared rapidly by macrophages, and the cause of this delayed clearance in patients with CLE is still unclear. A potential role for C1q in the clearance of apoptotic debris and in the genesis of cutaneous LE is suggested by two observations. First, patients with C1q deficiency experience LE-like photosensitive eruptions.[24] Second, mice with C1q deficiency demonstrate an SLE-like disease associated with an accumulation of apoptotic cells in the kidney.[25]

An increased number of apoptotic cells are noted in lesional LE skin. Can this finding have systemic as well as local consequences? There is evidence that the biochemical processes of apoptosis generate novel antigens that are uniquely targeted by autoantibodies. Casciola-Rosen has shown that the caspases activated during apoptosis cleave intracellular proteins into fragments that are bound by autoantibodies from some patients with LE.[26] Patients with LE skin disease have more autoantibodies that preferentially recognize apoptotic-modified U1-70-kd RNP antigen than patients without skin disease.[27] This finding provides further in vivo evidence that immune recognition of modified forms of self-antigen occur in

cutaneous LE and suggests that this immune recognition and the processing of apoptosis-derived antigens may participate in the pathogenesis of the disease. The appearance of autoantibodies to skin-specific antigens such as desmoglein 4 in patients with "pre-SLE" suggests that the skin is an early site in the breakdown of tolerance in SLE.[28]

Necrosis is a cell death process characterized by the rapid depletion of adenosine triphosphate (ATP) stores and subsequent loss of cell membrane integrity that can also result from UV light injury. For example, high doses of UVB preferentially induce keratinocyte necrosis.[29] Necrotic cells release potent proinflammatory mediators such as high mobility group box 1 (HMGB 1) protein[30] and uric acid.[31] Another form of cell death that may release antigenic material is a unique form that occurs principally in neutrophils but also in mast cells and has been termed "NETosis." In this form of cell death, chromatin and cytoplasmic granules are released during the formation of bacteriocidal neutrophil extracellular traps (NETs). The NETs contain not only DNA but also the antimicrobial peptide LL37, which enables self DNA and RNA to engage Toll-like receptors TLR9 and TLR7 to activate plasmacytoid dendritic cells.[32,33] Thus, these substances promote type 1 IFN release and autoimmunity (reviewed in reference 34). NETs are abundant in the dermis of lesional lupus skin.[35] In a mouse model of lupuslike skin inflammation, neutrophil depletion results in a decrease in cytokine release following skin injury.[36] An abundance of apoptotic cells and possibly necrotic cells, either from excessive amount of death induction by UV light or from a defect in clearance, could permit tolerance to self-antigens to be broken. Cells of the early inflammatory response such as neutrophils could then amplify the immune response to self-antigens. The potential role of apoptotic mechanisms in the initiation and perpetuation of photosensitive LE is summarized in Figure 23-3.

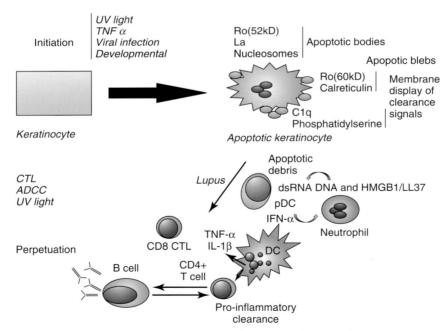

FIGURE 23-3 Potential role of keratinocyte apoptosis in the pathogenesis of photosensitive lupus erythematosus. Apoptosis is an ordered means of cell death. Apoptosis can be initiated in keratinocytes by ultraviolet (UV) radiation (UVB as well as UVA), by viruses, by cytokines (tumor necrosis factor alpha [TNF-α]), by growth factor withdrawal, by differentiation, and by cytotoxic cellular assault. Apoptosis leads to formation of small blebs in which Ro antigen and calreticulin are concentrated. Larger apoptotic bodies contain other potential autoantigens, including Ro antigen (60 kd), La, nucleosomes, and 70-kd ribonucleoprotein (RNP) antigen. Apoptosis leads to the exposure of phosphatidylserine on the cell surface and to the binding of C1q. Apoptosis, delayed apoptosis, and necrosis lead to the release of DNA and double-stranded RNA (dsRNA), which binds to HMGB1 (high-mobility group box-1 protein) or LL37 (cathelicidin) to activate Toll-like receptors (TLRs) within plasmacytoid dendritic cells, initiating the release of interferon alpha (IFN-α). The release of IFN-α activates neutrophils to release neutrophil extracellular traps (NETs), which contain more TLR activators of plasmacytoid dendritic cells, amplifying interferon production. The presence of apoptotic cells in this proinflammatory environment leads to uptake and processing by antigen-presenting cells, resulting in the priming and boosting of T cells and B cells to self-antigen.

Ultraviolet Light as Inflammatory Stimulus

Erythema (redness), a normal response to UV light, is mediated by multiple eicosanoids, vasoactive mediators, neuropeptides, and cytokines released from keratinocytes, mast cells, endothelial cells, and fibroblasts. (The wide range of mediators released by UV light in the skin is listed in Table 23-2.) UV light is not only an executioner, killing keratinocytes by apoptosis/necrosis, but it also is a generator of neoantigens (such as UV-DNA) and inflammation.

UV light can induce cutaneous inflammation by promoting the release of inflammatory mediators and cytokines, by inducing adhesion molecule display, and by releasing chemokines to attract inflammatory cells into the skin (reviewed in reference 37). Both UVB and UVA can participate in lesion induction and act by differing mechanisms. UVB induces the release of the primary cytokines IL-1α and TNF-α from the epidermis, initiating a cascade of inflammatory events. IL-1α and TNF-α are "primary cytokines" that induce the release of a number of other proinflammatory cytokines from the epidermis. For example, IL-1α and TNF-α induce the secondary release of IL-6, prostaglandin E2, IL-8, and granulocyte-monocyte colony-stimulating factor (GM-CSF) by keratinocytes. Chemokines are chemoattractive proteins that are associated with inflammatory cell recruitment. UVB irradiation of primary human keratinocytes in the presence of proinflammatory cytokines such as IL-1 and TNF-α significantly enhances the expression of the inflammatory chemokines CCL5, CCL20, CCL22, CCL27, and CXCL8.[38]

UVA upregulates IL-8 and IL-10 production in keratinocytes and FasL expression in dermal mononuclear cells. The longer wavelength of UVA allows it to penetrate into the dermis and to upregulate vascular endothelial intracellular adhesion molecule 1 (ICAM-1) and E selectin, thereby increasing leukocyte-vascular adhesion. Acute administration of low-dose UVA, but not UVB, results in IL-12 production by keratinocytes in vivo. UVA also results in a rapid increase in IFN-γ levels in the skin, the source of which may be resident epidermal T cells.[39]

HUMORAL FACTORS IN CUTANEOUS LUPUS ERYTHEMATOSUS

Autoantibody production is a sine qua non of SLE, and the autoantibodies can be pathogenic. Autoantibodies can initiate cellular cytotoxicity and activate the complement cascade and also can promote the recognition of epitopes related to the original autoantigens through a process termed *epitope spreading*. Autoantibodies are also detected in CLE.

Immunopathology of Cutaneous Lupus Erythematosus

Immunofluorescence studies of cutaneous LE lesions show lesional deposition of immunoglobulins (Figure 23-4). In 80% to 90% of skin specimens from patients with CCLE or ACLE, and in 50% to 60% of specimens from those with SCLE, a thick band of immunoglobulins and complement components is deposited along the dermoepidermal junction (DEJ). Because these deposits are also found in clinically normal skin of patients with SLE, their role in the local induction of cutaneous tissue injury is still unclear.

Ro/SSA Autoantibodies and LE Photosensitivity

SCLE was recognized as a distinct and uniquely photosensitive subset of cutaneous LE by Sontheimer.[40] Ro/SSA antibodies have been observed in frequencies ranging from 40% to 100% of SCLE patients by immunodiffusion techniques.[41] The deposition pattern is identical to "dustlike particles" of immunoglobulin deposition over the cytoplasm and nuclei of cells in the lower epidermis and upper dermis seen in adults with SCLE and babies with NLE and first described by Nieboer[42] (see also Figure 23-3). Interestingly, the 60-kd Ro and 52-kd Ro antibody responses are among the first to appear in human lupus autoimmunity and may appear many years before disease onset.[43]

The originally described Ro/SSA antigen is a protein of 60 kd that may be bound in vivo to four small RNA molecules called "Y RNA" or "hY RNA." This complex is also associated with the La/SSB antigen, an epitope targeted by sera from patients with Sjögren syndrome or congenital heart block. The function of the 60-kd antigen still is unknown but it has been shown to act as a receptor for beta 2–glycoprotein I on apoptotic cells.[44] Reactivity against a 52-kd polypeptide is another antibody specificity commonly found in anti-Ro/SSA–positive sera, although it is structurally unrelated to the so-called 60-kD Ro/La complex.[45] UV induces upregulation of 52-kd Ro/SSA expression in keratinocytes and in photoprovoked CLE lesions.[46] 52-kd Ro/SSA is an E3 ligase that mediates the ubiquitination of several members of the IFN regulatory factor (IRF) family. Loss of

TABLE 23-2 Mediator Release by Ultraviolet Radiation*

SOURCE OF MEDIATOR	ULTRAVIOLET B	ULTRAVIOLET A
Keratinocyte	IL-1α, tumor necrosis factor alpha (TNF-α) GM-CSF, IL-6, IL-8 IL-10 Transforming growth factor beta PGE₂, PGF₂α	IL-8 IL-10, IL-12 PGE₂, PGF₂α
Mast cell	TNF-α LTC4, LTD4, PGD Histamine	
Endothelial cell	TNF-α, PCI₂	PCI₂
Langerhans cell		IL-12

*Ultraviolet radiation results in the release of interleukins (ILs), prostaglandins (PGs), prostacyclin (PCs), leukotrienes (LTs), and other mediators.

SCLE

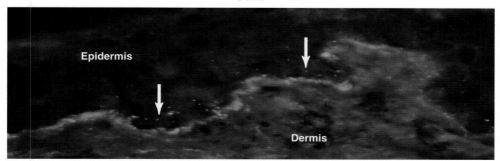

Figure 23-4 Immunopathology of subacute cutaneous lupus. Direct immunofluorescence analysis for the presence of immunoglobulin (Ig) G reveals a "dustlike" distribution of IgG deposits in the suprabasilar keratinocytes (*arrowheads* mark specific IgG "dust" deposits). There is also IgG deposition in the basement membrane zone.

Ro52 (also termed TRIM 21) in mice results in severe skin inflammation at sites of trauma via the IL23/Th17 pathway.[47]

The functions and cellular redistribution of the 52-kd and 60-kd Ro/SSA polypeptides and the La antigen all have been associated with the heat-shock response.[48] Recombinant heat-shock protein 10 (HSP10; chaperonin 10) specifically prevents cutaneous disease in MRL/lpr mice.[49] The pathogenic role of these antibodies is still unclear because not all antibody-positive patients have skin disease. Further, although the anti-Ro/SSA response is clearly associated with SCLE, another clinical type of cutaneous lupus, CCLE, is not exquisitely photosensitive. The majority of patients with CCLE do not have anti-Ro/SSA responses as detected by standard immunodiffusion techniques.

CELLULAR FACTORS
Immunogenetics
Anti-Ro/SSA antibody responses have been linked to susceptibility loci associated with class II major histocompatibility complex (MHC) alleles. There is a strong association between SCLE, anti-Ro/SSA antibodies, and the HLA-A1, HLA-B8, DR-3, DRw52, and C4 null haplotypes.[50] This association would imply the participation of Ro/SSA antigen–specific T cells in the generation of the Ro/SSA antibody response. However, antigen-specific T cells have not yet been identified. SCLE in Caucasians is associated with the DRB1*0301-B*08.6 haplotype that includes a 308A TNFα polymorphism associated with increased TNF-α production by keratinocytes following UV exposure.[51] Genome-wide studies have identified a number of genes associated with a predilection to CLE: Polymorphisms in integrin alpha M (*ITGAM*, also known as CD11b) have been associated with CCLE.[52] Genes of the type 1 IFN and TLR pathways, such as *IRF5* and *TYK2*, are associated with serum IFN-α activity, CCLE, SCLE, and serologic associations, including anti-Ro antibodies.[53,54] Polymorphisms in *FCGR2A* are specifically associated with skin disease (ACLE) in SLE.[55]

Immune Cells and Murine Models of Cutaneous Lupus Erythematosus
Murine models of cutaneous LE include the spontaneously occurring and UV-accelerated forms of disease in MRL/lpr mice, graft-versus-host disease, and NZB/NZW mice (reviewed in reference 56). None of these models accurately recapitulates the cutaneous pathology seen in human disease. They nevertheless have been useful in a dissection of the potential cellular mechanisms of autoimmune inflammation.

MRL/lpr mice demonstrate alopecia and scab formation associated with histopathologic changes similar to cutaneous lupus, including DEJ immunoglobulin deposition. These lesions are characterized by a T-cell inflammatory infiltrate. Both conventional (αβ) and nonclassical (γδ) T cells have been shown to participate in the MRL/lpr disease phenotype, including the skin disease, and autoantigen-specific αβ T cells are absolutely required for full penetrance of disease. The spontaneous activation of T cells in MRL/lpr mice is highly B cell–dependent but is dissociated from antibody production, suggesting that antigen processing and presentation to T cells by B cells are important.

Observations in the MRL/lpr mouse model include correlation of the overexpression of colony-stimulating factor 1 (CSF-1) in the skin with the development of cutaneous lesions. CSF-1 is induced by UV light and promotes macrophage infiltration of the skin.[57] In lupus-prone (NZW/NXB) F1 mice, skin injury by tape-stripping induces skin lesions with the characteristics of CLE.[36] These lesions are characterized by a persistent type 1 IFN signature and depletion of either plasmacytoid dendritic cells (pDCs) or neutrophils or inhibition of TLR7/9 limits disease.

Mutations in RNAse H2 and 3′ repair exonuclease 1 (Trex1) predispose to Aicardi-Goutières syndrome (a disease of unbridled type 1 IFN expression manifesting as chilblains and spastic paraparesis), SLE, and familial chilblain LE.[58] Trex1-deficient mice demonstrate SLE-like systemic autoimmunity. Trex1-deficient mice that lack type 1 IFN receptors are completely protected from disease, demonstrating that IFNs are crucial for disease expression. Trex1 is a negative regulator of the STING (stimulator of interferon genes)–dependent antiviral response to single-stranded DNA.[59] Autoimmune disease begins in nonhematopoietic cells in Trex1-deficient animals, is mediated by T cells, and is aided by B cells. In a study using a reporter gene for IFN release, initiation of inflammation in keratinocytes and other stromal cells was found. Collectively, these observations suggest that tissue-specific deregulation of type 1 IFN expression and the activation of pDCs and neutrophils may underlie a predisposition to cutaneous lupus.

Role of Activated T Cells in Human Cutaneous Lupus Erythematosus
The pathology of cutaneous lupus is one of a lichenoid tissue reaction in which the basal keratinocytes are the primary focus of injury (Figure 23-5). This injury is associated with keratinocyte hyperproliferation, with normal early differentiation and premature terminal differentiation. The inflammatory cell infiltrate is characterized by mononuclear cells at the DEJ as well as around blood vessels and dermal appendages. Inflammatory cells in the infiltrates of established cutaneous LE lesions are predominantly CD3⁺ cells with CD4⁺ cells present in higher numbers than CD8⁺ cells. The study of photo-induced lesions has allowed an analysis of early histologic changes and their evolution. In early lesions, this analysis has demonstrated CD4⁺ T cells predominantly at the DEJ in association with rare HLA class II expression by keratinocytes. Scarring CCLE has now been

SCLE

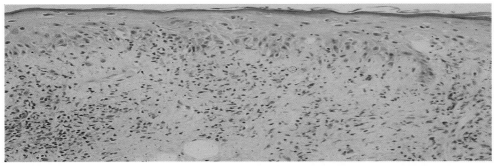

FIGURE 23-5 Photomicrograph of a biopsy of subacute cutaneous lupus. There is disarray in the maturation pattern of the keratinocytes as well as evidence of hyperkeratosis (increased thickness of the horny cell layer). The basement membrane zone is thickened and disorganized with a mononuclear cell infiltrate. There is a dermal mononuclear cell infiltrate that is predominantly perivascular. The mononuclear cells are predominantly CD4 T cells, many showing an activation phenotype, and macrophages.

associated with the presence of lesional and circulating CD8⁺ T cells that express CCR4, the receptor for CCL17, implicating cytotoxic CD8⁺ T cells in the scarring subtype of CCLE.[60] Regulatory T cells, which normally have a homeostatic function, are reduced in cutaneous lupus lesions in comparison with other inflammatory skin diseases.[61]

COFACTORS IN CUTANEOUS LUPUS ERYTHEMATOSUS

Ultraviolet Effects on Cutaneous Vasculature

Dermal blood vessels are involved in all forms of cutaneous lupus as targets for the cytokines and other mediators released from keratinocytes. These vessels also are affected directly by UV light. The potential importance of UV light in contributing to dermal and perivascular inflammation is underscored by the exquisite photosensitivity of lupus tumidus, a dermal variant of cutaneous LE without epidermal or interface changes.[62]

Vascular Activation

Enhanced expression of adhesion molecules on the surfaces of endothelial cells is an essential point of control for leukocyte attachment and migration through the endothelial barrier into cutaneous tissues. The role of molecular interactions in facilitating leukocyte migration into the skin is summarized in Figure 23-6. Chemokines are induced by UV light and are upregulated in lupus skin. The T-helper-1 (Th1) cell–associated CXCR3 ligands CXCL10 and, to a lesser extent, CXCR9 and CXCL11 are expressed at DEJ in CCLE and are the most abundantly expressed chemokine family members in cutaneous LE.[38] A functional role for these ligands is suggested by the expression of CXCR3 by infiltrating dermal T cells. The CXCR3 ligands cooperate with the homeostatic chemokine CXCL12 to recruit cutaneous lymphocyte–associated antigen (CLA)-positive memory T cells into the skin. The functional relevance of lymphocyte CCR4 expression and tissue expression of CCL17 in patients with scarring CCLE has likewise been confirmed by in vitro migration assays.[60]

The clinically normal-appearing skin of patients with active SLE demonstrates elevations of inducible nitric oxide synthase (iNOS) in both the epidermis and adjacent vascular endothelium.[63] Aberrant regulation of iNOS expression also has been noted in photoinduced lesions of cutaneous lupus.[64] Synthesis of iNOS leads to nitric oxide (NO) production, which is known to promote apoptosis and have multiple proinflammatory effects.

Cytokines

An appropriate cytokine *milieu* can facilitate and modulate immune responses. Abnormalities in the production and function of cytokines could underlie the abnormal photoreactivity noted in

cutaneous LE. Analysis of interleukins 2, 4, 5, and 10 and IFN-γ mRNA levels in lesions of cutaneous LE has revealed increased local levels of IL-5 and significant levels of IL-10 and IFN-γ.[65] These results indicate a mixed cytokine pattern favoring cell adhesion and cellular inflammation via IFN-γ–induced intracellular adhesion molecule 1 expression and a T-helper-2 cell response, favoring antibody production, with IL-5 and IL-10.

TNF-α and IL-18

TNF-α is a primary cytokine that can be induced in keratinocytes and in dermal fibroblasts by UVB. A polymorphic variant in the TNF-α promoter in humans (TNF-α 308A) is associated with increased production of TNF-α. The presence of this promoter is associated with an increased risk of SLE in African Americans.[66] The TNF-α 308A promoter polymorphism associated with increased TNF-α production has been shown to be highly associated with photosensitive SCLE.[51] IL-18 is a cytokine in the IL-1 family that is highly expressed in the lesional skin of patients with CLE, promoting TNF-α release from keratinocytes and the apoptotic death of keratinocytes.[67]

IL-17

The IL-17 cytokine family includes IL-17A to IL-17F. Th17 CD4⁺ T cells are the main source of these cytokines. A substantial proportion of T cells in the skin lesions of patients with SLE,[68] SCLE, and DLE express this cytokine.[69]

Type 1 and Type 3 Interferons

Gene array studies have demonstrated that type 1 IFNs (IFN-α and β) play an important role in the pathophysiology of SLE: IFN-inducible protein transcripts have been found to be upregulated in pediatric and adult patients with SLE and the levels of these transcripts correlate with disease activity. Curiously, natural IFN-α–producing cells, also termed pDCs, are found in the skin (but not the peripheral blood) of patients with LE and in the cutaneous lesions of LE and are also found in association with the presence of type 1 IFN–inducible proteins such as Mx.[70] This finding suggests that local IFN-α production by these cells promotes Th1-biased inflammation. In favor of this suggestion, the number of infiltrating CXCR3+ lymphocytes correlates closely with the expression of Mx and the type 1 IFN–inducible chemokine CXCL10, and IFN-α has been shown to potently induce CXCR3 ligand expression by keratinocytes, endothelial cells, and dermal fibroblasts in vitro. IFN-α has also been shown to confer a proinflammatory function to IL-10, resulting in the enhanced production of CXCL10 and CXCL9. The potential central role of pDC-derived IFN-α production in cutaneous LE is underscored by the further observations that immune complexes

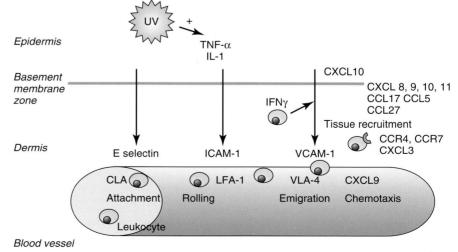

Figure 23-6 Ultraviolet (UV)–induced leukocyte migration into the skin. UV radiation induces cytokine release in cutaneous tissues. These cytokines then induce adhesion molecule expression on endothelial cells and leukocytes, promoting inflammatory cell recruitment to the skin. Likewise, cytokines released by the inflammatory cells can enhance and perpetuate this recruitment. The selectins and adhesion molecules depicted all have been shown to be upregulated in cutaneous lupus erythematosus.

containing nucleic acid released by necrotic or late apoptotic cells and opsonized by lupus immunoglobulin (Ig) G potently induce IFN-α production by pDCs, thereby potentially promoting ongoing disease activity.[71]

The role of pDCs activated by TLR ligands in skin lesions is underlined by the fact that experimental skin lesions in murine models heal more rapidly in the presence of TLR7/9 inhibitors.[36] Although pDCs are the prime source of type 1 IFNs, epithelial cells are the prime source of type 3 IFNs and novel type 1 IFNs. IFN-κ is a type 1 IFN expressed in the skin, and polymorphisms of the IFN κ gene have been correlated with serum type 1 IFN activity as well as the incidence of SLE in males.[72] Both IFN-λ, a type 3 IFN, and its receptor are expressed in CLE skin, and serum levels correlate with skin disease activity.[73] Given the demonstration that tissue expression of IFNs may precipitate autoimmune disease,[59] it is possible that these novel IFNs represent the first step in the pathogenesis of cutaneous lesions.

A MODEL OF PATHOGENESIS OF CUTANEOUS LUPUS ERYTHEMATOSUS

Clinical and experimental data suggest that apoptosis may be an important mechanism leading to autoantigen display in cutaneous LE and that UV light may be an important initiator of apoptosis and possibly necrosis. Abnormalities may exist in either apoptosis

induction or in apoptotic cell clearance that result in a greater load of apoptotic and necrotic cells. Type 1 and type 3 interferons may provide the initial stimulus to initiate inflammation and cell death. In addition to promoting cell death and neoantigen generation (such as UV-DNA), UV light induces and modulates inflammatory mediator release. Genetic abnormalities in TNF-α, IL-1 receptor antagonist, and IL-10 have been linked tentatively to SLE.[74] The dysregulation of such cytokines may allow the upregulation of adhesion molecules, chemokines, and co-stimulatory molecules to allow the recognition of self-antigen and the initiation of an immune response in genetically predisposed individuals. The autoantibodies linked with cutaneous LE are directed at antigens involved in cellular stress responses and in the heat-shock response. These autoantibodies perpetuate type 1 interferon production by plasmacytoid dendritic cells, leading to a positive feedback loop. Autoantibody production and directed T-cell responses may perpetuate and amplify autoantigen recognition as well as keratinocyte toxicity, leading to the clinical hallmarks of cutaneous LE disease. The salient points of a model incorporating observational and mechanistic findings are shown in Figure 23-7.

ACKNOWLEDGMENTS

The author was supported by Senior Scientist Awards from the Michael Smith Foundation and the Child and Family Research Institute.

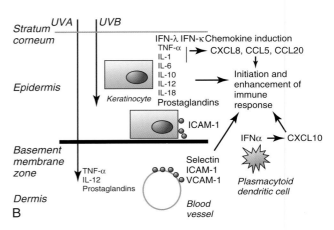

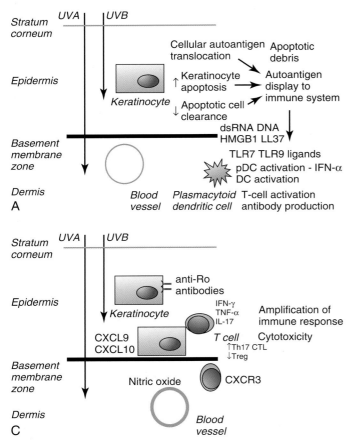

FIGURE 23-7 A model of the pathogenesis of photosensitive cutaneous lupus erythematosus. A, An increased number of apoptotic keratinocytes have been noted in both established lesions and photo-provoked lesions of cutaneous lupus. Either increased apoptosis/necrosis or a delay in the clearance of apoptotic cells could result in an increase in autoantigen packaging and processing in a form accessible to the immune system. **B,** Ultraviolet radiation can induce keratinocyte apoptosis and necrosis and can also stimulate local cytokine release (type 1 and type 3 interferons or other cytokines). This cytokine release can then lead to the observed increase in local mediators of inflammation, including selectins, adhesion molecules, chemokines, and prostanoids. These molecules serve to recruit and activate dendritic cells and T cells. **C,** The end result is a stimulation of the immune system to produce antibodies and to activate dendritic cells to prime T cells directed against stress-induced or stress-altered molecules (Ro antigen, La antigen). These agents of the immune system then act to promote further inflammation and tissue damage by processes such as epitope spreading, mediated by antibodies and B cells, and cellular cytotoxic mechanisms, mediated by T cells, natural-killer cells, and monocyte-macrophages.

References

1. Tan EM, Cohen AS, Fries JF, et al: The 1982 revised criteria for the classification of systemic lupus erythematosus. *Arthritis Rheum* 25:1271–1277, 1982.

2. Petri M: Dermatologic lupus: Hopkins Lupus Cohort. *Semin Cutan Med Surg* 17:219–227, 1998.

3. Epstein JH, Tuffanelli D, Dubois EL: Light sensitivity and lupus erythematosus. *Arch Dermatol* 91:483–485, 1965.

4. Freeman RG, Knox JM, Owens DW: Cutaneous lesions of lupus erythematosus induced by monochromatic light. *Arch Dermatol* 100:677–682, 1969.

5. Lehmann P, Holzle E, Kind P, et al: Experimental reproduction of skin lesions in lupus erythematosus by UVA and UVB radiation. *J Am Acad Dermatol* 22:181–187, 1990.

6. Kuhn A, Wozniacka A, Szepietowski JC, et al: Photoprovocation in cutaneous lupus erythematosus: a multicenter study evaluating a standardized protocol. *J Invest Dermatol* 131:1622–1630, 2011.

7. Kuhn A, Ruland V, Bonsmann G: Photosensitivity, phototesting, and photoprotection in cutaneous lupus erythematosus. *Lupus* 19:1036–1046, 2010.

8. Wysenbeek AJ, Block DA, Fries JF: Prevalence and expression of photosensitivity in systemic lupus erythematosus. *Ann Rheum Dis* 48:461–463, 1989.

9. Walchner M, Messer G, Kind P: Phototesting and photoprotection in LE. *Lupus* 6:167–174, 1997.

10. Geara AS, Torbey E, El-imad B: Lupus cerebritis after visiting a tanning salon. *Bull NYU Hosp Jt Dis* 67:391–393, 2009.

11. Walsh SJ, Gilchrist A: Geographical clustering of mortality from systemic lupus erythematosus in the United States: contributions of poverty, Hispanic ethnicity and solar radiation. *Lupus* 15:662–670, 2006.

12. Cooper GS, Wither J, Bernatsky S, et al: Occupational and environmental exposures and risk of systemic lupus erythematosus: silica, sunlight, solvents. *Rheumatology (Oxford)* 49:2172–2180, 2010.

13. Ansel JC, Mountz J, Steinberg AD, et al: Effects of UV radiation on autoimmune strains of mice: increased mortality and accelerated autoimmunity in BXSB male mice. *J Invest Dermatol* 85:181–186, 1985.

14. O'Brien BA, Geng X, Orteu CH, et al: A deficiency in the in vivo clearance of apoptotic cells is a feature of the NOD mouse. *J Autoimmun* 26:104–115, 2006.

15. Li Y, Zhao M, Yin H, et al: Overexpression of the growth arrest and DNA damage-induced 45alpha gene contributes to autoimmunity by promoting DNA demethylation in lupus T cells. *Arthritis Rheum* 62:1438–1447, 2010.

16. Zamansky GB, Chou IN: Disruption of keratin intermediate filaments by ultraviolet radiation in cultured human keratinocytes. *Photochem Photobiol* 52:903–906, 1990.

17. LeFeber WP, Norris DA, Ryan SR, et al: Ultraviolet light induces binding of antibodies to selected nuclear antigens on cultured human keratinocytes. *J Clin Invest* 74:1545–1551, 1984.

18. Casciola-Rosen LA, Anhalt G, Rosen A: Autoantigens targeted in systemic lupus erythematosus are clustered in two populations of surface structures on apoptotic keratinocytes. *J Exp Med* 179:1317–1330, 1994.

19. Daniels F, Jr, Brophy D, Lobitz WC, Jr: Histochemical responses of human skin following ultraviolet irradiation. *J Invest Dermatol* 37:351–357, 1961.

20. Kulms D, Schwarz T: Molecular mechanisms involved in UV-induced apoptotic cell death. *Skin Pharmacol Appl Skin Physiol* 15:342–347, 2002.

21. Norris DA, Whang K, David-Bajar K, et al: The influence of ultraviolet light on immunological cytotoxicity in the skin. *Photochem Photobiol* 65:636–646, 1997.

22. Henkart PA: Lymphocyte-mediated cytotoxicity: two pathways and multiple effector molecules. *Immunity* 1:343–346, 1994.

23. Kuhn A, Herrmann M, Kleber S, et al: Accumulation of apoptotic cells in the epidermis of patients with cutaneous lupus erythematosus after ultraviolet irradiation. *Arthritis Rheum* 54:939–950, 2006.

24. Bowness P, Davies KA, Norsworthy PJ, et al: Hereditary C1q deficiency and systemic lupus erythematosus. *Qjm* 87:455–464, 1994.

25. Botto M, Dell'Agnola C, Bygrave AE, et al: Homozygous C1q deficiency causes glomerulonephritis associated with multiple apoptotic bodies. *Nat Genet* 19:56–59, 1998.

26. Casciola-Rosen LA, Anhalt GJ, Rosen A: DNA-dependent protein kinase is one of a subset of autoantigens specifically cleaved early during apoptosis. *J Exp Med* 182:1625–1634, 1995.

27. Greidinger EL, Casciola-Rosen L, Morris SM, et al: Autoantibody recognition of distinctly modified forms of the U1-70-kd antigen is associated with different clinical disease manifestations. *Arthritis Rheum* 43:881–888, 2000.

28. Li QZ, Karp DR, Quan J, et al: Risk factors for ANA positivity in healthy persons. *Arthritis Res Ther* 13:R38, 2011.

29. Caricchio R, McPhie L, Cohen PL: Ultraviolet B radiation-induced cell death: critical role of ultraviolet dose in inflammation and lupus autoantigen redistribution. *J Immunol* 171:5778–5786, 2003.

30. Scaffidi P, Misteli T, Bianchi M. E: Release of chromatin protein HMGB1 by necrotic cells triggers inflammation. *Nature* 418:191–195, 2002.

31. Shi Y, Evans JE, Rock KL: Molecular identification of a danger signal that alerts the immune system to dying cells. *Nature* 425:516–521, 2003.

32. Lande R, Ganguly D, Facchinetti V, et al: Neutrophils activate plasmacytoid dendritic cells by releasing self-DNA-peptide complexes in systemic lupus erythematosus. *Sci Transl Med* 3:73ra19, 2011.

33. Garcia-Romo GS, Caielli S, Vega B, et al: Netting neutrophils are major inducers of type I IFN production in pediatric systemic lupus erythematosus. *Sci Transl Med* 3:73ra20, 2011.

34. Bosch X: Systemic lupus erythematosus and the neutrophil. *N Engl J Med* 365:758–760, 2011.

35. Villanueva E, Yalavarthi S, Berthier CC, et al: Netting neutrophils induce endothelial damage, infiltrate tissues, and expose immunostimulatory molecules in systemic lupus erythematosus. *J Immunol* 187:538–552, 2011.

36. Guiducci C, Tripodo C, Gong M, et al: Autoimmune skin inflammation is dependent on plasmacytoid dendritic cell activation by nucleic acids via TLR7 and TLR9. *J Exp Med* 207:2931–2942, 2010.

37. Kuhn A, Beissert S: Photosensitivity in lupus erythematosus. *Autoimmunity* 38:519–529, 2005.

38. Meller S, Winterberg F, Gilliet M, et al: Ultraviolet radiation-induced injury, chemokines, and leukocyte recruitment: an amplification cycle triggering cutaneous lupus erythematosus. *Arthritis Rheum* 52:1504–1516, 2005.

39. Shen J, Bao S, Reeve VE: Modulation of IL-10, IL-12, and IFN-gamma in the epidermis of hairless mice by UVA (320-400 nm) and UVB (280-320 nm) radiation. *J Invest Dermatol* 113:1059–1064, 1999.

40. Sontheimer RD, Thomas JR, Gilliam JN: Subacute cutaneous lupus erythematosus: a cutaneous marker for a distinct lupus erythematosus subset. *Arch Dermatol* 115:1409–1415, 1979.

41. Lee LA, Roberts CM, Frank MB, et al: The autoantibody response to Ro/SSA in cutaneous lupus erythematosus. *Arch Dermatol* 130:1262–1268, 1994.

42. Nieboer C, Tak-Diamand Z, Van Leeuwen-Wallau HE: Dust-like particles: a specific direct immunofluorescence pattern in sub-acute cutaneous lupus erythematosus. *Br J Dermatol* 118:725–729, 1988.

43. Heinlen LD, McClain MT, Ritterhouse LL, et al: 60 kD Ro and nRNP A frequently initiate human lupus autoimmunity. *PLoS One* 5:e9599, 2010.

44. Reed JH, Giannakopoulos B, Jackson MW, et al: Ro 60 functions as a receptor for (beta2glycoprotein) I on apoptotic cells. *Arthritis Rheum* 60:860–869, 2009.

45. Lindop R, Arentz G, Thurgood LA, et al: Pathogenicity and proteomic signatures of autoantibodies to Ro and La. *Immunol Cell Biol* 90:304–309, 2012.

46. Oke V, Vassilaki I, Espinosa A, et al: High Ro52 expression in spontaneous and UV-induced cutaneous inflammation. *J Invest Dermatol* 129:2000–2010, 2009.

47. Espinosa A, Dardalhon V, Brauner S, et al: Loss of the lupus autoantigen Ro52/Trim21 induces tissue inflammation and systemic autoimmunity by disregulating the IL-23-Th17 pathway. *J Exp Med* 206:1661–1671, 2009.

48. Furukawa F, Ikai K, Matsuyoshi N, et al: Relationship between heat shock protein induction and the binding of antibodies to the extractable nuclear antigens on cultured human keratinocytes. *J Invest Dermatol* 101:191–195, 1993.

49. Kulkarni OP, Ryu M, Kantner C, et al: Recombinant chaperonin 10 suppresses cutaneous lupus and lupus nephritis in MRL-(Fas)lpr mice. *Nephrol Dial Transplant* 27:1358–1367, 2011.

50. Millard TP, McGregor JM: Molecular genetics of cutaneous lupus erythematosus. *Clin Exp Dermatol* 26:184–191, 2001.

51. Werth VP, Zhang W, Dortzbach K, et al: Association of a promoter polymorphism of tumor necrosis factor-alpha with subacute cutaneous lupus erythematosus and distinct photoregulation of transcription. *J Invest Dermatol* 115:726–730, 2000.

52. Jarvinen TM, Hellquist A, Koskenmies S, et al: Polymorphisms of the ITGAM gene confer higher risk of discoid cutaneous than of systemic lupus erythematosus. *PLoS One* 5:e14212, 2010.

53. Niewold TB, Kelly JA, Kariuki SN, et al: IRF5 haplotypes demonstrate diverse serological associations which predict serum interferon alpha activity and explain the majority of the genetic association with systemic lupus erythematosus. *Ann Rheum Dis* 71:463–468, 2011.

54. Jarvinen TM, Hellquist A, Koskenmies S, et al: Tyrosine kinase 2 and interferon regulatory factor 5 polymorphisms are associated with discoid and subacute cutaneous lupus erythematosus. *Exp Dermatol* 19:123–131, 2010.

55. Sanchez E, Nadig A, Richardson BC, et al: Phenotypic associations of genetic susceptibility loci in systemic lupus erythematosus. *Ann Rheum Dis* 70:1752–1757, 2011.

56. Ghoreishi M, Dutz JP: Cutaneous lupus erythematosus: recent lessons from animal models. *Lupus* 19:1029–1035, 2010.

57. Menke J, Hsu MY, Byrne KT, et al: Sunlight triggers cutaneous lupus through a CSF-1-dependent mechanism in MRL-Fas(lpr) mice. *J Immunol* 181:7367–7379, 2008.

58. Stetson DB, Ko JS, Heidmann T, et al: Trex1 prevents cell-intrinsic initiation of autoimmunity. *Cell* 134:587–598, 2008.

59. Gall A, Treuting P, Elkon KB, et al: Autoimmunity Initiates in nonhematopoietic cells and progresses via lymphocytes in an interferon-dependent autoimmune disease. *Immunity* 36:120–131, 2012.

60. Wenzel J, Henze S, Worenkamper E, et al: Role of the chemokine receptor CCR4 and its ligand thymus- and activation-regulated chemokine/CCL17 for lymphocyte recruitment in cutaneous lupus erythematosus. *J Invest Dermatol* 124:1241–1248, 2005.

61. Franz B, Fritzsching B, Riehl A, et al: Low number of regulatory T cells in skin lesions of patients with cutaneous lupus erythematosus. *Arthritis Rheum* 56:1910–1920, 2007.

62. Kuhn A, Sonntag M, Richter-Hintz D, et al: Phototesting in lupus erythematosus tumidus—review of 60 patients. *Photochem Photobiol* 73:532–536, 2001.

63. Belmont HM, Levartovsky D, Goel A, et al: Increased nitric oxide production accompanied by the up-regulation of inducible nitric oxide synthase in vascular endothelium from patients with systemic lupus erythematosus. *Arthritis Rheum* 40:1810–1816, 1997.

64. Kuhn A, Fehsel K, Lehmann P, et al: Aberrant timing in epidermal expression of inducible nitric oxide synthase after UV irradiation in cutaneous lupus erythematosus. *J Invest Dermatol* 111:149–153, 1998.

65. Stein LF, Saed GM, Fivenson DP: T-cell cytokine network in cutaneous lupus erythematosus. *J Am Acad Dermatol* 36:191–196, 1997.

66. Sullivan KE, Wooten C, Schmeckpeper BJ, et al: A promoter polymorphism of tumor necrosis factor alpha associated with systemic lupus erythematosus in African-Americans. *Arthritis Rheum* 40:2207–2211, 1997.

67. Wang D, Drenker M, Eiz-Vesper B, et al: Evidence for a pathogenetic role of interleukin-18 in cutaneous lupus erythematosus. *Arthritis Rheum* 58:3205–3215, 2008.

68. Yang J, Chu Y, Yang X, et al: Th17 and natural Treg cell population dynamics in systemic lupus erythematosus. *Arthritis Rheum* 60:1472–1483, 2009.

69. Tanasescu C, Balanescu E, Balanescu P, et al: IL-17 in cutaneous lupus erythematosus. *Eur J Intern Med* 21:202–207, 2010.

70. Wenzel J, Zahn S, Tuting T: Pathogenesis of cutaneous lupus erythematosus: common and different features in distinct subsets. *Lupus* 19:1020–1028, 2010.

71. Obermoser G, Pascual V: The interferon-alpha signature of systemic lupus erythematosus. *Lupus* 19:1012–1019, 2010.

72. Harley IT, Niewold TB, Stormont RM, et al: The role of genetic variation near interferon-kappa in systemic lupus erythematosus. *J Biomed Biotechnol article 706825*, 2010.

73. Zahn S, Rehkamper C, Kummerer BM, et al: Evidence for a pathophysiological role of keratinocyte-derived type III interferon (IFNlambda) in cutaneous lupus erythematosus. *J Invest Dermatol* 131:133–140, 2011.

74. Lopez P, Gutierrez C, Suarez A: IL-10 and TNFalpha genotypes in SLE. *J Biomed Biotechnol* 2010:838–390, 2010.

Chapter 24

Skin Disease in Cutaneous Lupus Erythematosus

Benjamin F. Chong and Victoria P. Werth

Lupus erythematosus (LE) is a multisystem disorder that prominently affects the skin. Cutaneous lesions have a profound effect on quality of life, occur about 50% of the time in the absence of SLE, and can be an indicator of internal disease.[1,2]

HISTORY

The word *lupus* means "wolf" in Latin, signifying that the destructive injuries caused by the disease were similar to wolf bites. Cazenave coined the term "lupus erythematosus" in 1833 and differentiated between lupus erythematosus and lupus vulgaris, a clinical variant of cutaneous tuberculosis. Owing in part to observations of Hutchinson, it was recognized that cutaneous lesions of lupus erythematosus may be associated with significant systemic disease.[3] Starting in 1964, Dubois developed the concept of lupus as a spectrum of disease, ranging from cutaneous disease to life-threatening systemic disease. Gilliam also developed the concept of a spectrum of disease, and, in 1979, described a subset of cutaneous disease, termed "subacute" cutaneous lupus erythematosus (SCLE).[4] The description was virtually identical to that of "ANA-negative" lupus reported by Maddison in 1981.[5]

Hargrave's description of the LE-cell factor in 1948[6] and Friou's subsequent description of the antinuclear antibody assay in 1957[7] ushered in the era of serologic-clinical correlation in LE. The lupus band test by Burnham, Neblett, and Fine in 1963[8] and the association of specific autoantibodies, including associations of anti-Ro (also known as anti-SSA anti–Sjögren syndrome antigen A) autoantibodies with neonatal lupus by Franco in 1981[9] and with subacute cutaneous lupus by Sontheimer in 1982,[10] are noteworthy.

In 1951, the synthetic antimalarial quinacrine[11] and corticosteroids[12] were introduced for the treatment of LE.

EPIDEMIOLOGY

Patients with cutaneous lupus have a lower female-to-male ratio, around 3:1, than that seen in patients with SLE. One study found the incidence of CLE to be 4.3 per 100,000 in a predominantly Caucasian population, with a prevalence of 73.24 per 100,000, close to that found for SLE. Twelve percent of the patients with CLE progressed to having SLE, and the average time to progression was 8.2 years.[2] Of the various forms of chronic cutaneous lupus erythematosus, discoid lupus erythematosus (DLE) is the most common. Several studies have shown an incidence of 0.6 per 100,000 for SCLE, with lupus panniculitis and bullous LE present at much lower rates, 0.03 to 0.06 per 100,000.[2,13] DLE skin lesions are present in 15% to 30% of variously selected study populations with SLE.[14] Approximately 5% to 10% of SLE populations have DLE skin lesions as the presenting disease manifestation.[15] Patients with SCLE are frequently Caucasian and more predominantly female.[13,16]

The most common age at onset of DLE is between 20 and 40 years in both males and females.[17] DLE lesions, however, can appear in infants as well as the elderly. Patients with SCLE tend to be a bit older, with a mean age of around 60 years.

TRIGGERS OF CLE

There are a number of genetic, environmental, and drug-related triggers of cutaneous lupus. Partial C2 and C4 complement deficiencies have been reported in SCLE and chronic cutaneous LE, including DLE and LE panniculitis. Genetic association studies have identified numerous gene polymorphisms that increase the risk for CLE, including genes related to proinflammatory cytokines, tyrosine kinase 2, Fc receptor II (FcRII) and T-cell receptor loci, adhesion molecules, antioxidant enzymes, and apoptosis genes, as well as mutation in *TREX1* in familial chilblain lupus.[18] The genetics of SCLE are distinct, given the strong association with the HLA-DR3 extended haplotype.[19] Ultraviolet (UV) light and visible light can be strong triggers of CLE, and lesions can be induced after natural or experimentally applied light.[20]

The potential role of medication should be considered in all cases of SCLE, but other forms of CLE are much less frequently due to drugs.[21] A number of drugs have been implicated in inducing SCLE (Table 24-1). Ro/SSA autoantibodies have been found in many reported cases of drug-induced SCLE.[21] The skin lesions begin as early as 3 days and as late as 11 years, with a median of 6 weeks, after the medication is started, and the lesions typically improve 6 to 12 weeks after the offending agent is withdrawn.[21] Smoking raises the risk of CLE, especially DLE.[22]

CLINICAL FEATURES
Classification of Cutaneous LE

Gilliam developed a classification for cutaneous lupus based on the clinical characteristics of the skin lesions.[23] This is the most commonly used classification system at the current time. The skin lesions are separated into lupus-specific and lupus-nonspecific cutaneous lesions (see Boxes 24-1 and 24-2). The lupus-specific lesions are pathognomonic of cutaneous LE, whereas lupus-nonspecific lesions are seen with increased frequency in cutaneous LE but are not always associated with lupus. Lupus-specific skin lesions are separated into acute cutaneous, subacute cutaneous, and chronic cutaneous LE (see Box 24-1). Interestingly, lupus-nonspecific skin lesions are more frequently associated with SLE,[24] whereas the presence of lupus-specific skin lesions is relatively protective against severe SLE. Neonatal lupus and bullous lupus are additional cutaneous variants that can be seen in LE.

Lupus-Specific Skin Lesions
Acute Cutaneous LE

The typical lesion of acute cutaneous lupus (ACLE) is the bilateral malar erythema ("butterfly rash"; Figure 24-1). The lesions tend to be transient, to follow sun exposure, and to resolve occasionally with dyspigmentation but without scarring. Patients presenting with this type of eruption must be evaluated carefully for evidence of internal disease.

The morphology of the lesions ranges from mild erythema to intense edema. The presence of telangiectasias, dyspigmentation, and

TABLE 24-1 Drugs That May Precipitate or Exacerbate LE-Specific Skin Disease

SCLE	Acebutolol, angiotensin-converting enzyme inhibitors (captopril, cilazapril), antihistamines (cinnarizine, ranitidine, thiethylperazine), calcium channel blockers* (diltiazem, nifedipine, nitrendipine, verapamil), carbamazepine, griseofulvin, hydrochlorothiazide,* interferon-alpha and -beta, leflunomide, naproxen, oxprenolol, D-penicillamine, phenytoin, piroxicam, procainamide, proton pump inhibitors (lansoprazole, omeprazole), spironolactone, statins (pravastatin, simvastatin), sulfonylureas (glyburide), tamoxifen, Taxotere (docetaxel injection), terbinafine,* tiotropium, tumor necrosis factor blockers
DLE	Etanercept, infliximab, uracil-tegafur, voriconazole
Chilblain LE	Tumor necrosis factor blockers, terbinafine
Lupus tumidus	Angiotensin-converting enzyme inhibitors, bupropion, antiretroviral therapy, hydrochlorothiazide

*Common causes.

Box 24-1 Classification of LE-Specific Skin Disease

I. Chronic cutaneous lupus erythematosus (CCLE)
  A. Classic discoid lupus erythematosus (DLE)
    1. Localized DLE
    2. Generalized DLE
  B. Hypertrophic/verrucous DLE
  C. Lupus panniculitis/lupus profundus
  D. Mucosal DLE
    1. Oral DLE
    2. Conjunctival DLE
    3. Nasal DLE
    4. Genital DLE
  E. LE tumidus/papulomucinous LE
  F. Chilblain LE
  G. Lichenoid DLE (LE-lichen planus overlap)
II. Subacute cutaneous lupus erythematosus (SCLE)
  A. Annular SCLE
  B. Papulosquamous/psoriasiform
  C. Vesiculobullous annular SCLE
  D. Toxic epidermal necrolysis–like SCLE
III. Acute cutaneous lupus erythematosus (ACLE)
  A. Localized ACLE (malar rash)
  B. Generalized ACLE (morbilliform)
  C. Toxic epidermal necrolysis-like ACLE
  D. Bullous LE

Modified from the Gilliam classification scheme.[4]

Box 24-2 Classification of LE-Nonspecific Skin Disease

I. LE-nonspecific cutaneous lesions that serve (or served) as classification criteria for SLE
  A. Photosensitivity
  B. Mucosal ulceration
  C. Alopecia
II. LE-nonspecific cutaneous vascular reactions
  A. Vasculitis
    1. Small vessels
      a. Dependent palpable purpura
      b. Urticarial vasculitis
    2. Medium and large vessels
      a. Purpuric plaques with or without cutaneous necrosis and ulceration
      b. Subcutaneous nodules
  B. Vasculopathies
    1. Ischemic
      a. Raynaud phenomenon
    2. Thromboembolic
      a. Antiphospholipid antibodies
        (1) Livedo reticularis
        (2) Superficial thrombophlebitis
        (3) Cutaneous ulcers
        (4) Purpura/ecchymoses
        (5) Subungual splinter hemorrhages
        (6) Digital gangrene
      b. Cryoglobulins
        (1) Purpura/ecchymoses
        (2) Hemorrhagic skin necrosis
        (3) Cutaneous ulcers
      c. Cholesterol crystals
        (1) Purpuric infarction of toe tips and/or fingertips
      d. Calciphylaxis
        (1) Necrotic plaques
        (2) Cutaneous ulcers
  C. Other cutaneous vascular reactions
    1. Urticaria
    2. Periungual telangiectasia
    3. Erythromelalgia/palmar erythema
III. Other LE-nonspecific cutaneous lesions
  A. Cutaneous mucinosis
  B. Calcinosis cutis
  C. Nail changes
  D. Interstitial granulomatous dermatitis/palisaded neutrophilic granulomatous dermatitis

Modified from the Gilliam classification scheme.[4]

epidermal atrophy (i.e., poikiloderma) may help distinguish the malar erythema of acute cutaneous lupus from that of common facial eruptions such as seborrheic dermatitis and the vascular type of rosacea. Occasionally, there is a papular component, and sometimes lesions develop scale or crust. The duration may range from a few hours to several weeks. The face, particularly the malar area, is most commonly affected, with sparing of the nasolabial fold area. Lesions may be more widespread in distribution, with involvement of widespread morbilliform eruption, often in a photoexposed distribution (Figure 24-2). When lesions occur on the hands, the knuckles are typically spared. It is not unusual for the acute cutaneous eruption to be accompanied by oral ulcerations.

Rarely, patients with lupus experience an acute eruption clinically similar to that of toxic epidermal necrolysis (TEN) or erythema multiforme major (Figure 24-3). A TEN-like presentation can occur in patients with LE from extensive interface dermatitis causing epidermal basal cell layer damage. Widespread sloughing of the skin and mucous membranes and full-thickness epidermal necrosis are visualized in biopsy specimens. The presence in patients with lupus of erythema multiforme–like lesions has been termed Rowell syndrome.[25] These lesions may represent a severe variant of acute cutaneous lupus or, in some cases, subacute cutaneous lupus.

The three major types of cutaneous lupus are not mutually exclusive. In about 10% of patients, more than one type of cutaneous lesion may occur. Localized ACLE facial lesions can be seen in patients with SCLE.

Subacute Cutaneous LE

SCLE, defined by Gilliam in 1977, is a distinct subset of cutaneous LE, having characteristic clinical, serologic, and genetic features.[23] SCLE is typically photosensitive, although the midfacial skin is usually spared while the sides of the face, V of the neck, and extensor

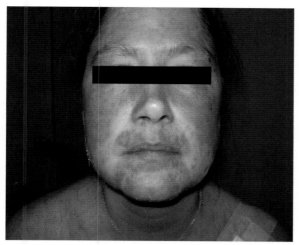

FIGURE 24-1 Butterfly rash with erythema and scale in malar area, sparing nasolabial fold.

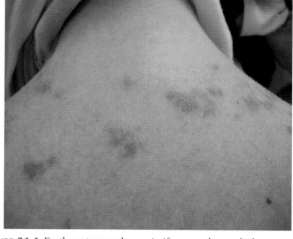

FIGURE 24-4 Erythematous scaly psoriasiform patches and plaques on the upper back of patient with subacute cutaneous lupus erythematosus.

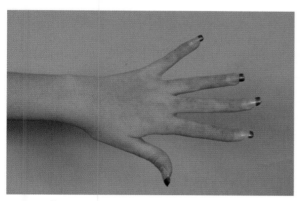

FIGURE 24-2 Photoexposed erythema in patient with acute cutaneous lupus erythematosus. ACLE that manifests both above and below the neck is classified as generalized. Note the macular erythema over the extensor aspect of the wrist that becomes confluent over the dorsal aspect of the hand and interphalangeal areas.

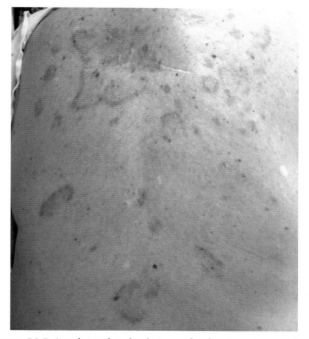

FIGURE 24-5 Annular polycyclic lesions of subacute cutaneous lupus erythematosus.

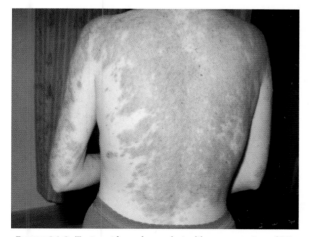

FIGURE 24-3 Toxic epidermal necrolysis–like presentation of LE.

aspects of the upper extremities are commonly involved (Figure 24-4).[26] In some patients, the disease may be mild, with only a few small scaly patches appearing after sun exposure.

Lesions of SCLE may have an annular configuration, with raised red borders and central clearing (Figure 24-5), or a papulosquamous presentation, with an eczematous or psoriasiform appearance. Both types of lesions can be present in the same patient, although papulosquamous lesions are more common overall. SCLE lesions characteristically have a relatively sparse, superficial inflammatory infiltrate, and consequently, there is usually no induration. Lesions often resolve with dyspigmentation but do not scar. Patients can rarely get blisters in association with SCLE.

In some instances, lesions of SCLE are associated with use of certain medications (see Table 24-1). Drug-induced SCLE is clinically indistinguishable from other forms of SCLE. About one third of these patients have associated antihistone antibodies.[21] The lesions normally clear once the medication is discontinued.

Over time, significant internal disease develops in around 10% to 15% of patients with SCLE. Because anti-Ro autoantibodies are associated with Sjögren syndrome as well as about 70% of cases of SCLE, it is not surprising that some patients have features of both conditions and that some may have serious internal manifestations of Sjögren syndrome such as pulmonary or neurologic disease.

Chronic Cutaneous LE

Discoid LE. The most common form of chronic cutaneous LE is classic DLE. Discoid lesions are found most often on the face, scalp, and ears, and lesions above the neck are termed "localized DLE." The scalp is involved in 60% of patients with DLE and is the only area involved in about 10%. Lesions present both above and below the neck are called "generalized DLE" (Figure 24-6). Patients with generalized DLE have a higher likelihood of meeting criteria for SLE. DLE lesions begin as flat or slightly elevated, well-demarcated, red-purple macules or papules with a scaly surface. Early DLE lesions most commonly evolve into larger, coin-shaped (i.e., "discoid") erythematous plaques covered by a prominent, adherent scale that extends into dilated hair follicles (Figure 24-7). Involvement of hair follicles is a prominent clinical feature of DLE lesions. Scales accumulate in dilated follicular openings, which soon become devoid of hair. When the adherent scale is peeled back from more advanced lesions, follicle-sized keratotic spikes similar in appearance to carpet tacks can be seen to project from the undersurface of the scale (i.e., the carpet-tack sign). These discoid plaques can enlarge and merge to form even larger, confluent, disfiguring plaques.

A symmetric, butterfly-shaped DLE plaque occasionally is found over the malar areas and bridge of the nose. Such a DLE lesion is different from the more transient, edematous-erythema reactions that occur over the same distribution in ACLE lesions. As with ACLE, DLE usually spares the nasolabial folds. Discoid lesions can occur on mucosal surfaces, including the lips, other oral mucosal surfaces, nasal mucosa, conjunctivae, and genital mucosa. DLE can masquerade as blepharitis and chronic blepharoconjunctivitis and has manifested as periorbital edema and erythema, madarosis (loss of eyelashes), and cicatrizing conjunctivitis.

Some patients with discoid lesions exhibit a photodistribution, and sun exposure appears to have a role in lesion development. However, many patients have discoid lesions in sun-protected skin, and there is no clear association between sun exposure and their development.

Discoid lesions have the potential for scarring, and with time, a substantial proportion of patients experience disfiguring scarring. Dyspigmentation is to be expected in long-standing lesions, typically with hypopigmentation, with or without central atrophic scarring in the central area and with hyperpigmentation at the periphery. Perioral DLE lesions can occur and often resolve with a striking acneiform pattern of pitted scarring. Rarely, squamous cell carcinoma develops in a long-standing discoid lesion.

Hypertrophic/Verrucous DLE. An unusual variant of DLE is hypertrophic DLE, characterized by thick scaling overlying the discoid lesion or occurring at its periphery. The intensely hyperkeratotic lesions are often prominent on the extensor surfaces of the arms, but the face and upper trunk may also be involved (Figure 24-8). Frequently, typical discoid lesions are also present in other locations. Hypertrophic DLE lesions can easily be mistaken for keratoacanthoma, squamous cell carcinoma, prurigo nodularis, or hypertrophic lichen planus. Thus, a skin biopsy is important to establish the diagnosis.

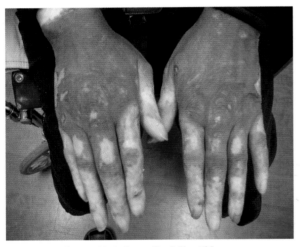

FIGURE 24-6 Generalized discoid lupus.

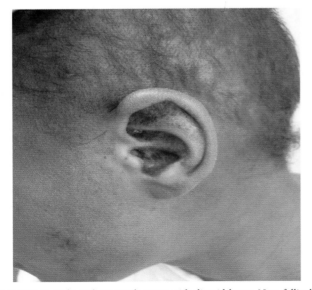

FIGURE 24-7 Scalp and ear involvement with discoid lupus. Note follicular plugging in the ear and scalp.

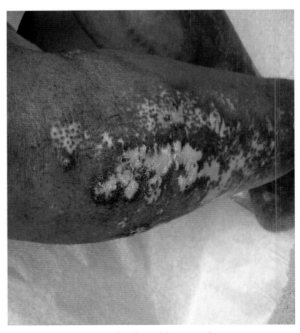

FIGURE 24-8 Hypertrophic discoid lupus erythematosus on arm.

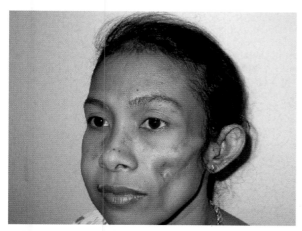

FIGURE 24-9 Lupus panniculitis showing lipoatrophy on cheek, an overlying dyspigmentation from discoid lupus erythematosus.

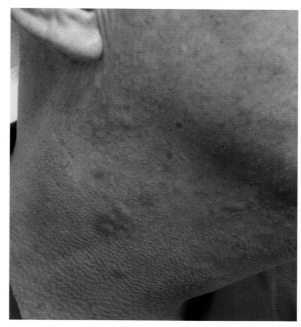

FIGURE 24-10 Tumid lupus erythematosus. Erythematous papules on neck and cheek.

Lupus Panniculitis/Lupus Profundus. Intense inflammation in the fat leads to indurated plaques that can evolve into disfiguring, depressed areas. Lesions of lupus panniculitis have a distinctive distribution, occurring predominantly on the face, upper arms (Figure 24-9), upper trunk, breasts, buttocks, and thighs. Some patients have discoid lesions overlying the panniculitis, and, in those cases, the condition is sometimes referred to as lupus profundus.

The differential diagnosis of patients with lupus panniculitis includes Weber-Christian panniculitis, factitial panniculitis, pentazocine-induced panniculitis, pancreatic panniculitis, traumatic panniculitis, morphea profundus, eosinophilic fascitis, sarcoidosis, subcutaneous granuloma annulare, subcutaneous T-cell lymphoma, and rheumatoid nodules. Deep excisional biopsy often is required to distinguish LE panniculitis from these other disorders, particularly when overlying classic DLE lesions are not present. The most useful histologic criteria for differentiating LE panniculitis from subcutaneous panniculitis–like T-cell lymphoma are the presence of epidermal involvement, lymphoid follicles with reactive germinal centers, clusters of B lymphocytes, mixed cell infiltrate with plasma cells and polyclonal T-cell receptor γ gene rearrangement. It is helpful to have biopsy specimens reviewed by dermatopathologists, because diagnosis can be difficult, and lupus panniculitis can rarely progress to panniculitic T-cell lymphoma.[27]

Mucosal DLE. Mucosal discoid lesions can occur in the mouth most frequently but can also involve the conjunctiva, nose, and genitals. The prevalence of mucous membrane involvement in chronic, cutaneous LE is about 25%. Within the mouth, the buccal mucosa is most commonly involved, and the palate, alveolar processes, and tongue are less frequently involved. The center of an older lesion can become depressed and occasionally undergoes painful ulceration. Well-defined chronic DLE plaques also can appear on the vermilion border of the lips. At times, DLE involvement of the lips can manifest as a diffuse cheilitis, especially on the more sun-exposed lower lip. Although lesions can appear on the tongue, this location is quite uncommon. Chronic oral-mucosal DLE lesions occasionally can degenerate into squamous cell carcinoma, like cutaneous DLE lesions. Any area of asymmetric nodular induration within a mucosal DLE lesion should be carefully evaluated for the possibility of malignant degeneration. Conjunctival DLE lesions begin as small areas of nondescript inflammation most commonly affecting the palpebral conjunctivae or the margin of the eyelid. The lower lid is affected more often than the upper lid. As the early lesions progress, scarring becomes more evident and can produce permanent loss of eyelashes and ectropion. DLE involvement of the eyelid can produce considerable disability. Lid deformities trichiasis, and symblepharon formation can also occur as a result of DLE ocular involvement.[81]

LE Tumidus/Papulomucinous LE. Some patients with cutaneous lupus have lesions characterized by induration and erythema but no scale or follicular plugging. Lesions can be common on the face and trunk and can be edematous (Figure 24-10). Morphologically, the lesions are similar, if not identical, to those of Jessner lymphocytic infiltrate and may have central clearing. The epidermis typically is uninvolved in the disease process, lacks the liquefactive degeneration and basement membrane thickening typically seen in DLE and SCLE, but has an intense dermal inflammatory infiltrate.[28] These lesions are called LE tumidus, or tumid LE.

The very low prevalence of SLE and the relatively low prevalence of immunoglobulin deposition within the cutaneous lesions in patients reported to have tumid lupus have made it difficult to determine whether tumid lupus is actually a variant of lupus erythematosus or an independent entity. The presence of tumid lupus lesions in patients with other specific types of cutaneous lupus is evidence in favor of its being classified as a form of cutaneous lupus. Tumid lupus has been reported to be reproducible by phototesting in the majority of patients.[29] The lesions tend to resolve without scarring or atrophy.

Chilblain LE

Chilblain lupus consists of red or dusky purple papules and plaques on the toes, fingers, and, sometimes, the nose, elbows, knees, and lower legs. The lesions are brought on or exacerbated by cold, particularly moist cold climates. These lesions may represent the concurrence of ordinary chilblains with lupus, and over time the lesions may develop a gross and microscopic appearance consistent with that of a discoid lesion. Chilblain LE must be distinguished from idiopathic chilblains, and the presence of cryoglobulins or cold agglutinins should be ruled out. Patients with chilblain LE frequently have evidence of LE (e.g., autoantibodies, DLE, neutropenia) and Raynaud phenomenon, and their chilblain lesions are more likely than idiopathic chilblains to persist into warmer weather months.

Lichen Planus–Lupus Erythematosus Overlap. Overlap between lupus erythematosus and lichen planus has been observed in a small number of patients. This overlap syndrome is characterized by the presence of clinical, histologic, and/or immunopathologic features of both diseases in the same patient. Such patients have had mainly painful, bluish red plaques with atrophy and scaling as well as hyperkeratotic papules and nodules that favor extremities.[30] Pathologic differences can help differentiate the two entities, with colloid bodies in the dermis and basement membrane clefts seen in lichen planus, and basement zone thickening observed in lupus. Patients with this overlap syndrome may have an autoimmune, viral, and/or genetic predisposition. Successful treatments have included acitretin and cyclosporine.[30]

Additional Variants

Bullous LE. In some patients, vacuolar alteration at the dermal-epidermal junction (DEJ) is so severe that blisters develop in areas of DLE, SCLE, or acute LE. However, there is a separate variant known as bullous LE. Bullous SLE (BSLE) is an autoantibody-mediated subepidermal vesiculobullous skin disease that is LE-nonspecific because the histology is not that of a lichenoid dermatitis at the DEJ. A diagnosis of BSLE requires (1) SLE, (2) vesiculobullous eruption, (3) histologic demonstration of subepidermal blister and neutrophilic upper dermal infiltrate, and (4) immunoglobulin and complement deposition at the basement membrane zone with direct immunofluorescence (immune reactants on or beneath the lamina densa ultrastructurally).[31,32] The clinical, histopathologic, and immunologic patterns seen in BSLE can resemble those of epidermolysis bullosa acquisita (EBA), dermatitis herpetiformis (DH), and bullous pemphigoid (BP), but patients with BSLE have features that are not consistent with any single primary bullous disease. One report argues that BSLE is a vague term that includes a heterogeneous group of vesiculobullous lesions and recommends using immunologic and histologic characteristics to divide BSLE into the following categories: dermatitis herpetiformis–like vesiculobullous LE, epidermolysis bullosa acquisita–like vesiculobullous LE, and bullous pemphigoid–like vesiculobullous LE.[33]

Neonatal LE. A neonatal form of SCLE may occur in infants whose mothers have anti-Ro/SSA autoantibodies. In babies who have neonatal lupus erythematosus (NLE), the SCLE-like lesions are histologically identical to those of SCLE in adults and are associated with anti-Ro/SSA antibodies.[34] NLE lesions frequently occur on the face, especially the periorbital region (Figure 24-11). Photosensitivity is very common in NLE, but sun exposure is not required for lesions to form, because it is possible for them to be present at birth. Neonatal lupus skin lesions typically resolve without scarring, although

dyspigmentation may persist for many months and some children have residual telangiectasias.

Children who have the cutaneous lesions of NLE may also exhibit congenital heart block (with or without cardiomyopathy), hepatobiliary disease, and thrombocytopenia. Cardiac NLE has a mortality rate of approximately 20%, and about two thirds of children with the disease require pacemakers.[35]

Hepatobiliary disease and thrombocytopenia may be present at birth in a child with NLE or may develop within the first few months of life.[34] Hepatobiliary disease has been reported to manifest as liver failure during gestation or in the neonatal period, conjugated hyperbilirubinemia in the first few weeks of life, or mild elevations of aminotransferases occurring at 2 to 3 months of life.

Relationship with Systemic Disease Features

Lupus nonspecific skin lesions are more frequently associated with SLE,[24] whereas the presence of lupus-specific skin lesions is relatively protective against severe SLE. More than 80% of patients with SLE have skin manifestations at some point, and 20% to 25% have cutaneous manifestations as a presenting sign.[36] DLE has been seen in 15% to 25% of patients with SLE. Systemic LE is more frequently diagnosed in those with skin lesions of acute LE (70% or more), followed by SCLE (50%), and DLE. The diagnosis of SLE in patients with DLE is made 20% of the time in those with generalized DLE but just 5% of the time in those with localized DLE. The risk of progression to SLE in patients with CLE is thought to be as high as 20% in 20 years.[2,37] The diagnosis of SLE is frequently made on the basis of whether the patient's findings fulfill four or more criteria for the classification of SLE. Because four of the American College of Rheumatology (ACR) criteria for SLE are dermatologic, patients with CLE frequently meet the criteria for having SLE but without significant systemic disease.[38,39] One study showed that 69% of patients with SLE met the criteria for photosensitivity, 53% had malar rash, 35% had oral ulcers, and 18% had discoid lesions.[36] Thus, clinical judgment is needed to determine whether the designation of SLE based on clinical criteria is meaningful.

PATHOLOGY

Normally, obtaining histologic confirmation of a possible case of cutaneous lupus is important to confirm the diagnosis and guide appropriate therapy. In some cases, transient facial lesions may not be helpful, and the biopsy may not be performed, given the risk of scarring. Histologic findings in cutaneous LE depend on the subtype. In practice, there is overlap of histologic findings among clinical phenotypes of cutaneous lupus, particularly ACLE, SCLE, and DLE lesions. Some of the more distinctive histologic features of cutaneous lupus are basal cell damage, lymphohistiocytic inflammatory infiltrates, and, primarily in discoid lesions, periadnexal inflammation, follicular plugging, and scarring. In lupus panniculitis, in which there is deep inflammation in the fat, a skin biopsy down to fat shows a lobular lymphocytic panniculitis. Interpretation of biopsy specimens can be difficult, and it is recommended that a skilled dermatopathologist read such specimens, particularly because subcutaneous T-cell lymphoma is in the differential diagnosis.

IMMUNOPATHOLOGY

For cases in which routine histology is not diagnostic, further testing by direct immunofluorescence (DIF) to determine the presence or absence of autoantibodies or complement components in the skin can be helpful.[40] In lupus panniculitis, immunoglobulin deposits at the DEJ may or may not be present, depending on the site sampled, the presence or absence of accompanying SLE, and the presence or absence of overlying changes of DLE at the DEJ. Some patients may have false-positive DIF responses, particularly in specimens from the face.

Immunoblotting and indirect immunofluorescence on sodium chloride-split skin show that some patients with BSLE have serum antibodies to type VII collagen.

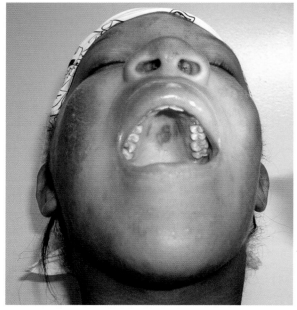

FIGURE 24-11 Ulceration on hard palate in a patient with SLE.

LABORATORY FINDINGS

Patients with cutaneous lupus can lack lupus autoantibodies, including antinuclear antibodies (ANAs), in the blood. Patients with cutaneous lupus should be screened with blood and urine testing for evidence of hematologic or renal disease, ANAs, and SLE-specific autoantibodies. Often the erythrocyte sedimentation rate (ESR) and complement levels are measured. Autoantibodies to double-stranded DNA (dsDNA), Sm, and possibly also ribosomal P are relatively specific for SLE, and are therefore helpful indicators of a high likelihood of systemic disease. Autoantibodies to Ro/SSA, La/SSB (Sjögren syndrome antigen B), U1 ribonucleoprotein (RNP), and histones are common in patients with SLE, but they are not disease-specific. An ANA test is helpful if the result is negative, because it is quite unusual for patients with SLE to have a negative ANA result. A positive ANA result is common in patients with cutaneous lesions, and a positive result does not indicate systemic disease or lupus. Anti-Ro/SSA and anti-La/SSB autoantibodies are frequently seen in high titer in patients with SCLE and those with SCLE/Sjögren overlap.

DIFFERENTIAL DIAGNOSIS

There are mimickers for each subtype of cutaneous lupus. The differential diagnosis for acute cutaneous lupus/malar rash includes rosacea, eczema, acne vulgaris, dermatomyositis, seborrheic dermatitis, sunburn, and photosensitivity due to medications. That for subacute cutaneous lupus consists of eczema, psoriasis, annular erythemas, fungal infection, and granuloma annulare. The differential diagnosis for discoid lupus includes lichen planus or lichen planopilaris, sarcoidosis, polymorphous light eruption, Jessner lymphocytic infiltrate, lymphocytoma cutis, lymphoma cutis, and granuloma faciale. That for tumid lupus lesions consists of polymorphous light eruption, Jessner lymphocytic infiltrate, and reticular erythematous mucinosis; some authorities think of the last two entities as part of the spectrum of tumid LE.

TREATMENT

Because UV light is a common trigger of cutaneous lupus, patients should be counseled on avoidance of sun, use of sunscreens, and use of clothing to protect the skin from the sun. The impact of sun avoidance on quality of life is independent of the severity of cutaneous disease.[41] Patients should be instructed to apply sunscreen 30 minutes before sun exposure in adequate amounts (2 mg/cm²) and to reapply it every 2 to 3 hours. The sunscreen should preferably contain a photostable broad-spectrum protective agent such as Mexoryl SX (ecamsule), titanium dioxide, or zinc oxide in the United States. Outside of the United States, Mexoryl XL, Tinosorb M (bisoctrizole), and Tinosorb S (bemotrizinol) are also suitable and available agents. Patients with CLE and SLE should also be counseled to use sunscreen with the highest sun protection factor (SPF) possible to minimize the effects of application error. In a randomized, blinded, side-to-side comparison study of SPF 85 and SPF 50, SPF 85 statistically outperformed SPF 50 under conditions of normal use.[42] A randomized double-blind controlled study showed that application of broad-spectrum sunscreen effectively prevented CLE lesion formation after UV irradiation of the backs of 25 CLE patients in comparison with vehicle-only application.[43] Photosensitive patients benefit from UV filters for car windows, and fluorescent bulbs should be covered with a cover or shade.[44] Tightly woven clothing can be worn for additional protection, with darker fabrics providing greater UV absorbance. Several apparel companies offer special clothing with high SPF values.

Topical Therapy

Potent topical steroids are helpful in the treatment of cutaneous lupus. Class I steroids may be needed initially, but tapering to topicals with lower strength should be done as soon as possible to minimize side effects, including skin atrophy. There is good evidence supporting the use of potent topical steroids in the treatment of DLE.[45] Another option is calcineurin inhibitors, which have been shown to

help, particularly on thinner skin such as in the face. One study showed that pimecrolimus 0.1% cream is not inferior to betamethasone 17-valerate 0.1% cream.[46] There is evidence that 0.1% tacrolimus ointment is as efficacious as a potent topical steroid in the treatment of DLE with less risk of cutaneous side effects.[47]

Systemic Therapy

There have been few randomized trials to systematically examine the treatment of cutaneous lupus.[48] Case reports and case series generally report subjective improvement by the investigator. The inability to measure outcomes has made multicenter trials and systematic reviews impossible to conduct. In 2005, the Cutaneous Lupus Erythematosus Disease Area and Severity Index (CLASI) was introduced and partially validated as an outcome instrument for CLE.[49] The CLASI reports two separate numerical scores: one for disease activity and one for damage. It is a validated measure for both dermatologists and rheumatologists,[50] and later studies have examined responsiveness, minimal clinically significant response, and correlation with quality of life.[51] The CLASI is being used in a number of international trials and should improve the level of evidence for current and new therapies.

The mainstay of oral therapy is oral hydroxychloroquine, which is normally given at a dose of less than 6.5 mg/kg ideal body weight/day. Randomized controlled trials comparing its antimalarial efficacy with that of acitretin revealed that 50% of patients receiving hydroxychloroquine improved at 8 weeks. Approximately 82% of patients receiving chloroquine improved by 6 months.[47] These percentages are supported by a large case series of patients with CLE treated with antimalarials. Although chloroquine may be more efficacious than hydroxychloroquine, chloroquine is less well tolerated. Addition of quinacrine to either hydroxychloroquine or chloroquine appears to be helpful for refractory cases.[52] Patients receiving hydroxychloroquine or chloroquine should have eye examinations every 6 to 12 months. The American Academy of Ophthalmology recommends that yearly eye screening begins after 5 years, or sooner for patients with risk factors for eye toxicity, while recognizing that rare patients may experience eye toxicity before 5 years. Chloroquine is associated with greater eye toxicity than hydroxychloroquine, but high cumulative doses of either are associated with increased risk.

Patients with significant disease that does respond to or who cannot tolerate antimalarials may need either immunosuppressives or thalidomide. The most frequently used immunosuppressives are mycophenolate mofetil, methotrexate, and azathioprine.[53] Cyclophosphamide can help the skin when required for treatment of other systemic symptoms.

Bullous LE can be treated with dapsone. If disease is severe, then glucocorticoids with or without an immunosuppressive may be required. Rituximab may provide an alternative for resistant cases.

Patients whose disease is refractory to all therapies are more frequently smokers.[16]

LUPUS-NONSPECIFIC SKIN LESIONS

A large number of cutaneous lesions that are found in patients with LE are not exclusive to LE. These lupus-nonspecific lesions do not have the distinctive histologic features seen in LE-specific disease that were described earlier. Nonspecific skin findings in LE include vasculitis, photosensitivity reactions, alopecia, Raynaud phenomenon, livedo reticularis, soft tissue calcification, bullous lesions, urticaria, cutaneous mucinosis, skin necrosis, ulcerations, and nail changes (see Box 24-2).

Several of these findings have been linked with higher activity scores in patients with SLE. Patients with lupus-nonspecific lesions have higher disease activity than both those with only LE-specific lesions and those with both kinds of lesions.[24] In addition, lupus-nonspecific disease may portend the advent of SLE in patients with CLE. Vila discovered that incomplete lupus in patients who had photosensitivity, oral ulcers, and Raynaud phenomenon was more likely to evolve into complete SLE.[54]

The significance of LE-nonspecific lesions is underscored by the fact that two such manifestations, photosensitivity and oral ulcers, are part of the ACR diagnostic criteria for SLE.

PHOTOSENSITIVITY

Photosensitivity is defined clinically as an exaggerated response to UV light, eliciting symptoms such as burning, itching, and redness. Although these responses can include LE-specific skin lesions, they can also manifest as sunburn reactions that are not specific to LE. Photosensitivity can be induced by UVA and/or UVB radiation. For some patients, sun exposure can induce not only cutaneous but also systemic symptoms, including weakness, fatigue, fever, and joint pain. The clinician should rule out other mimics, including medication-induced photosensitivity and rosacea.

Photosensitivity appears to be a relatively sensitive indicator of SLE. Up to 69% of patients with SLE have photosensitivity, which has been noted to be the most common skin-related finding in various studies of patients with SLE.[36,55] In 19 patients with active LE, as defined as having a Systemic Lupus Activity Measure (SLAM) score of 10 or higher, photosensitivity was observed most frequently of all mucocutaneous findings (63%).[56] Photosensitivity could also portend systemic spread of lupus. In a study of 79 patients with incomplete lupus, who have at least one but less than four ACR criteria for SLE diagnosis, the eight patients whose disease evolved to SLE had a higher percentage of photosensitivity at initial presentation than those whose LE remained incomplete (62.5% vs. 25.3%).[54]

Various studies have disagreed over whether photosensitivity in SLE is associated with anti-Ro antibodies. Ioannides found that Ro and La antigen expressions in skin biopsy specimens were four-fold to ten-fold higher in 14 patients with LE and photosensitivity than 12 patients with LE but no photosensitivity.[57] However, a later study of 169 patients with SLE showed no correlation of Ro and La autoantibodies with photosensitivity.[58]

ALOPECIA

Because of its widespread prevalence in patients with SLE, alopecia was an original criterion for the diagnosis of SLE. However, owing to its low sensitivity and specificity, it was not incorporated in the 1982 revised criteria.

Alopecia can either be scarring, which is associated with LE-specific lesions, or nonscarring, which typically falls into the LE-nonspecific category. LE-nonspecific alopecia can have multiple manifestations. "Lupus hair" manifests as coarse, dry hair with increased fragility. It often results in broken hairs and may be more prominent in the periphery of the scalp during a systemic lupus flare 2 to 3 months later (Figure 24-12). Alopecia areata, another cause of nonscarring alopecia, is reported in 10% of patients with LE.[59] Its pathogenesis, histology, and course are distinct from LE-specific alopecia. Last, hair loss due to commonly prescribed medications for LE, including cyclophosphamide and methotrexate, should be considered in the differential diagnosis of LE-nonspecific alopecia. Assessing prevalence of LE-nonspecific alopecia is difficult, because many studies do not clearly delineate between LE-specific and LE-nonspecific alopecia. Of those that have, the percentages of patients with SLE who have LE-nonspecific alopecia have ranged from 9% to 40%.[36,55,60]

LE-nonspecific alopecia is typically self-limited. Because it correlates with disease activity, hair regrowth eventually occurs with disease control using treatments such as antimalarials. There may be accelerated regrowth of hair with use of topical or intralesional corticosteroids.

CUTANEOUS VASCULAR REACTIONS

Reactions that involve the cutaneous vasculature are important to recognize in patients with SLE because they can frequently indicate underlying systemic vascular pathology. Furthermore, it is crucial to differentiate between vasculitis and vasculopathy, because the treatments for the two conditions are distinct (i.e., anticoagulants for vasculopathy and immunosuppressants for vasculitis). *Vasculopathy*

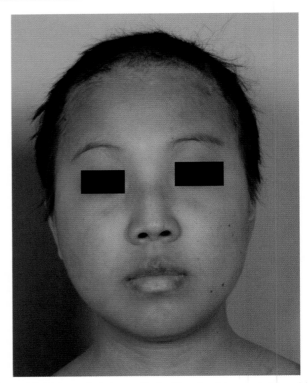

FIGURE 24-12 Lupus hair in a patient with active lupus nephritis and low complement levels.

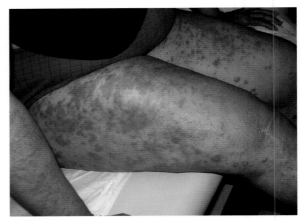

FIGURE 24-13 Palpable purpura on the lower extremities in a patient with leukocytoclastic vasculitis and SLE.

is defined as narrowing of vascular walls resulting in ischemia or noninflammatory vascular lumen occlusion resulting from thromboembolic disease. Vasculitis is caused by primary inflammation (usually immune complex–mediated) of vessel walls with secondary occlusion of lumina by fibrin.

Vasculitis

Seen in 8% to 11% of patients with SLE,[36,55,61] vasculitis most commonly manifests in the skin. Specifically, a study of 670 patients with SLE revealed that of the 76 subjects with vasculitis, 89% had cutaneous involvement, with the remaining 11% having visceral vasculitis.[61] Small vessels, such as the postcapillary venules, are most commonly affected. The most common small vessel vasculitis in patients with SLE, leukocytoclastic vasculitis (LCV), usually manifests as palpable petechiae or purpura in dependent areas (Figure 24-13).[61] Before

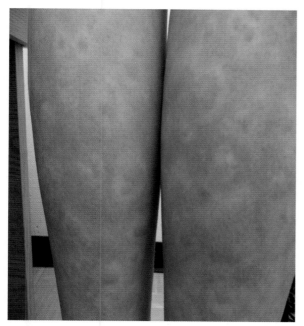

FIGURE 24-14 Urticarial vasculitis in a patient with SLE.

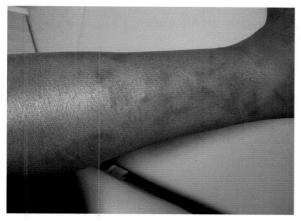

FIGURE 24-15 Medium-sized vessel vasculitis with large retiform purpura and smaller ulcerations in a patient with SLE.

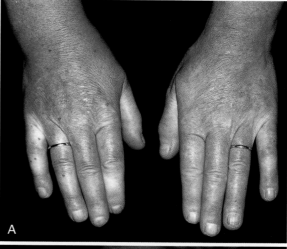

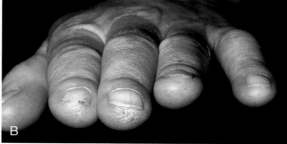

FIGURE 24-16 Patient with Raynaud' phenomenon, tapered fingers, and LE-specific skin lesions on the fingers.

LCV is attributed to SLE, other major causes of LCV, including drugs and infection, need to be ruled out. Urticarial vasculitis, which also involves small vessels, consists of hivelike painful lesions lasting at least 24 hours that leave postinflammatory hyperpigmentation and demonstrate LCV-like pathologic features (Figure 24-14). Low complement levels have been found in patients with SLE who have urticarial vasculitis.[62] Involvement of medium and/or large vessels may manifest as purpuric plaques with stellate or retiform borders with or without cutaneous necrosis and ulceration, or as subcutaneous nodules (Figure 24-15).

Cutaneous vasculitis can often be effectively managed with antiinflammatory medications, including colchicine, dapsone, and antimalarials. Severe or refractory cutaneous vasculitis may require glucocorticoids and/or immunosuppressives. No randomized controlled trials have been conducted to explore the efficacy of specific treatments with vasculitis. Targeted treatments for vasculitis are under investigation and could provide better efficacy.

Vasculopathy

Vasculopathic processes are multifactorial, with some being caused by vascular lumen narrowing (i.e., ischemic) and others being caused by occlusion with bland thrombi in the absence of primary vascular inflammation (i.e., thromboembolic). Box 24-2 lists the several different causes of vasculopathy in patients with SLE.

Ischemic Vasculopathy
Raynaud Phenomenon
Triggered by cold and stress, Raynaud phenomenon has an underlying ischemic process due to the intimal hyperplasia in the vasculature. White discoloration develops, followed by cyanosis and erythema in the digits of the hands and feet (Figure 24-16). The white phase results from vasoconstriction of the digital arteries and arterioles, whose blood flow is already compromised by vessel wall narrowing. Patients may also experience numbness, pain, and paresthesias. The blue phase is a manifestation of decreased blood perfusion in digital capillaries and venules, and the final red phase represents blood reperfusion. Raynaud phenomenon is either a primary (without underlying disease) or secondary (with underlying disease, such as SLE) syndrome. Seen in 25% to 60% of patients with SLE, Raynaud phenomenon has been observed to be the most common LE-nonspecific cutaneous manifestation in different studies of such patients.[36,60] Additionally, the condition may herald a worse prognosis and is associated with higher disease activity scores.[54,56] Chronic severe Raynaud phenomenon can manifest as focal ulcerations on the fingertips and periungual areas that resolve as pitted scarring, prominent nailfold capillary ectasia and drop-out, punctate cuticular hemorrhage due to incompetent nailfold capillaries, fingertip tuft atrophy, digital calcinosis, and pterygium inversum unguium.

Treatment of Raynaud phenomenon is designed to decrease recurrence and prevent complications such as ulcerations. All patients should be instructed to wear gloves with exposure to cold and to avoid other triggers, such as stress and vasoconstrictive medications (i.e., serotonin agonists). Calcium channel blockers are often used in refractory cases because of their vasodilatory properties. Nifedipine

(10-30 mg PO tid) and amlodipine (5-20 mg PO qd) are among the commonly used calcium channel blockers. Calcium channel blockers have been often combined with drugs that inhibit platelet aggregation, such as aspirin. Other vasodilators such as nitrates (e.g., nitroglycerin) and prostaglandins, including iloprost, have been used for severe cases.[63]

Thromboembolic Vasculopathy and Antiphospholipid Antibodies

Antiphospholipid antibodies induce a prothrombotic state through the activation of endothelial cells, monocytes, and platelets and subsequent production of tissue factor and thromboxane A_2.[64] Patients with SLE and antiphospholipid antibodies frequently present with cutaneous symptoms. These include livedo reticularis, superficial thrombophlebitis, retiform purpuric plaques, which may later become necrotic and ulcerate, lower extremity ulcers, purpura, ecchymoses, digital gangrene, and subungual splinter hemorrhages. Lesions are often present in acral locations, because smaller vessels are more likely to become occluded. Other rare skin changes associated with antiphospholipid antibodies are atrophie blanche–like lesions (painful, ivory-colored stellate scars on the lower extremities), Degos-like lesions (small, porcelain-white circular atrophic lesions with peripheral erythema and telangiectasias) and lesions of primary anetoderma (focal loss of dermal elastic tissue, resulting in localized areas of flaccid or herniated saclike skin).[65]

Livedo reticularis manifests as erythematous to violaceous, fishnet-like, mottled, blanchable patches on the extremities and, less commonly, on the trunk and buttocks, resulting from impeded flow of blood through dilated vessels (Figure 24-17). The netlike discoloration is likely due to low flow of hypooxygenated blood in dermal venules. The broken form of livedo reticularis (i.e., livedo racemosa) is thought to be a more severe form of livedo reticularis due to the process of cholesterol and fibrin thrombi and calcification in vessels. The presence of livedo reticularis in a patient with SLE and antiphospholipid syndrome may forecast central nervous system involvement

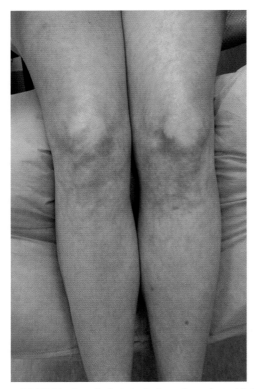

Figure 24-17 Livedo reticularis in the legs of a patient with SLE.

by lupus.[66] Sneddon syndrome, present in 41% of patients with antiphospholipid antibodies, is characterized by widespread livedo reticularis and ischemic cerebrovascular disease, often accompanied by labile hypertension.[67]

Treatment varies by skin manifestation. Cutaneous necrosis and digital gangrene require the anticoagulant heparin, with conversion to warfarin for long-term preventive therapy. Ulcers can be treated with wound care, antimalarials, and low-dose aspirin or dipyridamole, which could be used long term for prevention. There are no specific treatments for livedo reticularis and splinter hemorrhages. Reduction of other exacerbators, including smoking and oral contraceptive use, is also recommended.[67]

Cryoglobulins

Cryoglobulins, which precipitate at lower temperatures in cutaneous vessels, have been observed in 25% of patients with SLE. The vast majority of patients with SLE and cryoglobulinemia have either type II or type III cryoglobulinemia.[68] Mixed cryoglobulins, which are found in type II cryoglobulinemia, produce a small vessel cutaneous vasculitis manifesting as dependent palpable purpura. Severe cases can result in necrosis and ulceration. Cutaneous vasculitis, hepatitis C virus, rheumatoid factor, and low complement were more frequently present in patients with SLE and cryoglobulinemia than those without cryoglobulinemia.[68] Treatment is focused on reducing cold exposure.

Cholesterol Crystals

Cholesterol crystals from spontaneous breakup of atherosclerotic plaques or intravascular procedural manipulation can travel to smaller vessels and impede blood flow. Embolization to the digits can result in purpuric infarction of the tips of toes and/or the fingertips. This condition can be confused with SLE vasculitis or antiphospholipid antibody–associated vasculopathy affecting digital vessels. Supportive treatment is the mainstay, but treatments such as the prostacyclin analog iloprost may have potential in the future for patients with SLE and cholesterol crystals.[69]

Calcium Deposits

Calcium deposits in blood vessels causing calciphylaxis have been observed in patients with SLE and end-stage renal disease.[70] These lesions typically manifest as painful indurated areas of cutaneous hemorrhage that rapidly become necrotic and then ulcerate. Calcium deposits in the walls of blood vessels causes fibrosis and thrombosis, with secondary ischemia and necrosis of tissues. Prognosis is poor, with mortality rates between 60% and 80%. Although the cause is unknown, altered calcium-phosphorous metabolism has been implicated. Treatments include diets with low phosphate intake, phosphate binders, parathyroidectomy, calcimimetics, such as cinacalcet and sodium thiosulfate, and low-calcium dialysis. Wound care involving hydrocolloid dressing is essential for proper healing.

Other Cutaneous Vascular Reactions
Urticaria

Urticaria is sometimes associated with LE and is thought to be a manifestation of the disease process's immune dysregulation. In one study 44% of 73 patients with SLE had been reported to have urticaria, although some of those patients may have had urticarial vasculitis.[55] Urticaria typically manifests as an acute onset of edematous, pruritic, erythematous papules and plaques. It must be differentiated from urticarial vasculitis (see earlier), which tends to be painful and nonblanching, and lasts longer (>24 hours) than urticarial lesions. A skin biopsy can be performed to confirm diagnosis of either condition.

Before urticaria can be attributed to SLE, other causes, such as medications, chronic infections, and malignancies, should be ruled out. Thyroid function tests and thyroid autoantibody tests should be ordered in these patients, because autoimmune thyroid disease is associated with urticaria. First-line treatment of urticaria involves antihistamines and other antipruritics such as doxepin. In addition, antiinflammatory medications commonly used to treat SLE, such as hydroxychloroquine, have demonstrated some efficacy in chronic urticaria.[71]

Periungual Telangiectasias

The most common presentation of periungual telangiectasias in patients with SLE consists of tortuous, meandering, glomerular-like vessels. Dilated capillaries ("megacapillaries") of the nail folds and capillary loop dropout, which are the hallmarks of "scleroderma-pattern" capillaroscopic changes, have also been found in patients with LE but less frequently than in patients with dermatomyositis and systemic sclerosis. In patients with SLE, this pattern of nail fold changes appears to correlate strongly with Raynaud phenomenon and anti–U1-RNP antibodies.[72] Periungual telangiectasias have been proposed to be a risk factor for SLE development in patients with DLE, because 76% of patients who had DLE with SLE (N = 19) versus 0% of those who had DLE without SLE (N = 16) had this finding.[60] No treatment is indicated for these asymptomatic lesions.

Erythromelalgia and Palmar Erythema

Erythromelalgia (i.e., erythermalgia) is characterized by intense burning pain in the feet and hands, accompanied by local macular erythema and warmth. It differs from Raynaud phenomenon, in that it worsens with exposure to heat instead of cold. It can be either primary (without underlying disease) or secondary (with underlying disease such as SLE). Erythromelalgia appears to be caused by microvascular arteriovenous shunting. Gabapentin, tricyclic antidepressants, and selective serotonin reuptake inhibitors have been employed to alleviate pain in patients with erythromelalgia, and calcium channel blockers and pentoxifylline have been prescribed to combat vasculopathy. Aspirin has been also effective for erythromelalgia but particularly only for patients with blood dyscrasias such as polycythemia vera.[73]

Palmar erythema over the hyperthenar and hypothenar eminences in patients with SLE can be differentiated from erythromelalgia by the former's asymptomatic nature (Figure 24-18). One study documented that 4% of a group of 73 patients with SLE had chronic palmar erythema.[55] Reticulated palmar erythema can also be a sign of vasculopathy associated with antiphospholipid antibodies. No treatments are necessary for this condition.

OTHER LE-NONSPECIFIC SKIN LESIONS
Cutaneous Mucinosis

Mucin deposits are frequently found on skin biopsy in LE-specific skin lesions. However, some patients with LE present with asymptomatic skin-colored papules and nodules with abundant amounts of

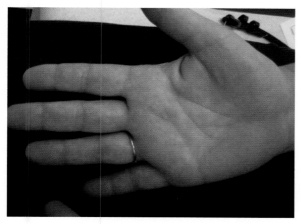

FIGURE 24-18 Palmar erythema in the hands of a patient with SLE.

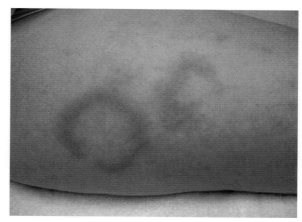

FIGURE 24-19 Papular and nodular dermal mucinosis in a patient with SLE, including pleural effusions and glomerulonephritis.

dermal mucin in the absence of the interface dermatitis or perivascular and perifollicular inflammation seen in LE-specific skin disease (Figure 24-19).[74] Such lesions can be differentiated from those of tumid lupus erythematosus, which appear as indurated erythematous papules, nodules, or plaques, typically on the trunk and/or arms. Histopathologic examination of the lesions of cutaneous mucinosis reveals diffuse dermal mucin deposits.

Treatments include antimalarials, although only 20% of treated cases have been documented to respond well. The addition of oral corticosteroids have been prescribed with some success for refractory cases.[74]

Calcinosis Cutis

The dystrophic form of calcinosis cutis has been observed in patients with SLE, but less so than juvenile dermatomyositis and systemic sclerosis. Calcinosis cutis is commonly found on the extremities and buttocks as asymptomatic subcutaneous nodules and is sometimes found as an incidental radiologic finding. Sometimes the overlying skin can ulcerate and permit the extrusion of a white toothpaste-like or pebble-like material composed of calcium salts. Calcinosis in SLE occurs in the setting of normal calcium metabolism and renal function. The mechanism behind the generation of calcium deposits in SLE is unknown. Several hypotheses have been centered on necrotic and apoptotic cells formed from tissue damage or trauma. Increases in calcium concentration have been noted with the presence of these necrotic and apoptotic cells.[75]

Therapies for calcinosis cutis, including aluminum hydroxide, calcium channel blockers, colchicine, probenecid, low-dose warfarin, bisphosphonates, and surgical excision, have had variable success. Patients with superficial lesions should protect the areas from trauma with padded bandages.[75]

Nail Changes

A wide variety of nail changes have been noted in patients with LE. Nail findings include nail ridging, leukonychia, onycholysis, blue-black bands, nail fold erythema, red lunulae, splinter hemorrhages, and nail fold hyperkeratosis (Figure 24-20). Patients with SLE have altered keratinization of the nail matrix resulting in punctate or striate leukonychia, nail pitting or ridging, and onycholysis or onychomadesis.[76] Blue-back discoloration has been mostly observed in the nails of African-American patients with SLE. One study reported diffuse, dark blue-back nail dyschromia in 52% of 33 African American patients with SLE, which was apparently from increased melanin deposition.[77] These dark bands of nail pigmentation may also be caused by medications such as antimalarials, cyclophosphamide, and methotrexate and can mimic this unique presentation in SLE.[76]

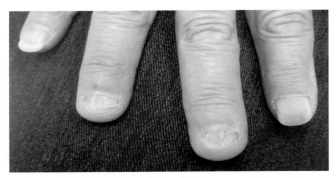

FIGURE 24-20 Nail ridging in the hands of a patient with discoid lupus.

Splinter hemorrhages have been observed in the setting of patients with SLE and antiphospholipid antibodies.[65] No treatments have been specified for these nail changes.

Anetoderma

Anetoderma, which is focal loss of dermal elastic tissue that results in localized areas of flaccid or herniated saclike skin, can also occur in patients with lupus. There has been speculation that loss of elastic fibers may be the result of small thromboses causing ischemia, because patients with lupus and anetoderma frequently have antiphospholipid antibodies, with associated increased hypercoagulable disorders.[78] There is no effective treatment for anetoderma.

Interstitial Granulomatous Dermatitis

Over the past decade, a spectrum of aseptic dermal granulomatous histopathologic changes referred to as *interstitial granulomatous dermatitis* has been increasingly described in the skin of patients with lupus erythematosus. This histopathologic reaction pattern has a number of synonyms: arthritis and interstitial granulomatous dermatitis (Ackerman syndrome), interstitial granulomatous dermatitis with cords, interstitial granulomatous dermatitis with arthritis, interstitial granulomatous dermatitis with plaques and arthritis, rheumatoid papules, Churg-Strauss granuloma, cutaneous extravascular necrotizing granuloma, superficial ulcerating rheumatoid necrobiosis, and palisaded neutrophilic and granulomatous dermatitis of immune complex disease. The pathophysiology of this reaction pattern has been speculated to relate to immune complex deposition.[79]

Interstitial granulomatous dermatitis has a range of cutaneous manifestations, including erythematous papules, plaques, and rope-like cords. Erythematous plaques are often annular, and the rope-like cords are typically unilateral. They have a predilection for the lateral trunk, axillae, thighs, and buttocks. Such lesions can simulate superficial thrombophlebitis but do not affect veins. The interstitial granulomatous dermatitis pathologic pattern is accompanied by fragmented collagen and elastic fibers.[79]

There has been limited success in treating interstitial granulomatous dermatitis lesions with hydroxychloroquine, dapsone, and systemic corticosteroids. Offending medications that could cause this distinct histologic and clinical pattern, such as calcium channel blockers, angiotensin-converting enzyme inhibitors, beta-blockers, lipid-lowering agents, and antihistamines, should be screened for and discontinued before further treatment is initiated.[80]

CONCLUSION

Classification of skin LE lesions depends on the presence or absence of lupus-specific histologic findings of interface dermatitis and perivascular and periappendageal lymphocytic infiltrate. LE-specific lesions are divided into acute, subacute, and chronic cutaneous lupus. LE-nonspecific lesions have a wider range of presentations that affect hair, nails, mucous membranes, and cutaneous vasculature. The ability of the clinician to recognize all potential cutaneous manifestations of lupus facilitates diagnosis and directs appropriate treatment that could potentially limit cutaneous and systemic spread of this troublesome disease.

References

1. Klein R, Moghadam-Kia S, Taylor L, et al: Quality of life in cutaneous lupus erythematosus. *J Am Acad Dermatol* 64:849–858, 2011.
2. Durosaro O, Davis MD, Reed KB, et al: Incidence of cutaneous lupus erythematosus, 1965-2005: a population-based study. *Arch Dermatol* 145:249–253, 2009.
3. Mallavarapu RK, Grimsley EW: The history of lupus erythematosus. *South Med J* 100:896–898, 2007.
4. Sontheimer RD, Thomas JR, Gilliam JN: Subacute cutaneous lupus erythematosus: a cutaneous marker for a distinct lupus erythematosus subset. *Arch Dermatol* 115:1409, 1979.
5. Maddison PJ, Provost TT, Reichlin M: Serological findings in patients with "ANA-negative" systemic lupus erythematosus. *Medicine Baltimore* 60:87–94, 1981.
6. Hargraves M, Richmond H, Morton R: Presentation of two bone marrow elements: the "tart" cell and the "LE" cell. *Mayo Clin Proc* 23:25–28, 1948.
7. Friou GJ: Clinical application of lupus serum: nucleoprotein reaction using fluorescent antibody technique (abstract). *J Clin Invest* 36:890, 1957.
8. Burnham TK, Fine G: The immunofluorescent "band" test for lupus erythematosus. I. Morphologic variations of the band of localized immunoglobulins at the dermal-epidermal junction in lupus erythematosus. *Arch Dermatol* 99:413–420, 1969.
9. Franco HL, Weston WL, Peebles C, et al: Autoantibodies directed against sicca syndrome antigens in the neonatal lupus syndrome. *J Am Acad Dermatol* 4:67–72, 1981.
10. Sontheimer RD, Maddison PJ, Reichlin M, et al: Serologic and HLA associations in subacute cutaneous lupus erythematosus, a clinical subset of lupus erythematosus. *Ann Intern Med* 97:664–671, 1982.
11. Page E: Treatment of lupus erythematosus with mepacrine. *Lancet* ii:755–758, 1951.
12. Hench PS: The reversibility of certain rheumatic and nonrheumatic conditions by the use of cortisone or of the pituitary adrenocorticotrophic hormone. *Ann Intern Med* 36:1–38, 1952.
13. Popovic K, Nyberg F, Wahren-Herlenius M: A serology-based approach combined with clinical examination of 125 Ro/SSA-positive patients to define incidence and prevalence of subacute cutaneous lupus erythematosus. *Arthritis Rheum* 56:255–264, 2007.
14. Vlachoyiannopoulos PG, Karassa FB, Karakostas KX, et al: Systemic lupus erythematosus in Greece. Clinical features, evolution and outcome: a descriptive analysis of 292 patients. *Lupus* 3:303–312, 1993.
15. Dubois EL, Tuffanelli DL: Clinical manifestations of systemic lupus erythematosus. Computer analysis of 520 cases. *JAMA* 190:104–111, 1964.
16. Moghadam-Kia S, Chilek K, Gaines E, et al: Cross-sectional analysis of a collaborative Web-based database for lupus erythematosus-associated skin lesions: prospective enrollment of 114 patients. *Arch Dermatol* 145:255–260, 2009.
17. Shrank AB, Doniach D: Discoid lupus erythematosus. Correlation of clinical features with serum auto-antibody pattern. *Arch Dermatol* 87:677–685, 1963.
18. Rice G, Newman WG, Dean J, et al: Heterozygous mutations in TREX1 cause familial chilblain lupus and dominant Aicardi-Goutieres syndrome. *Am J Hum Genet* 80:811–815, 2007.
19. Provost TT, Talal N, Bias W, et al: Ro(SS-A) positive Sjögren's/lupus erythematosus (SC/LE) overlap patients are associated with the HLA-DR3 and/or DRw6 phenotypes. *J Invest Dermatol* 91:369, 1988.
20. Sanders CJ, van Weelden H, Kazzaz GA, et al: Photosensitivity in patients with lupus erythematosus: a clinical and photobiological study of 100 patients using a prolonged phototest protocol. *Br J Dermatol* 149:131, 2003.
21. Lowe G, Henderson CL, Grau RH, et al: A systematic review of drug-induced subacute cutaneous lupus erythematosus. *Br J Dermatol* 164:465–472, 2011.
22. Koskenmies S, Jarvinen TM, Onkamo P, et al: Clinical and laboratory characteristics of Finnish lupus erythematosus patients with cutaneous manifestations. *Lupus* 17:337–347, 2008.

23. Gilliam JN, Sontheimer RD: Distinctive cutaneous subsets in the spectrum of lupus erythematosus. *J Am Acad Dermatol* 4:471, 1981.
24. Zecevic RD, Vojvodic D, Ristic B, et al: Skin lesions—an indicator of disease activity in systemic lupus erythematosus? *Lupus* 10:364–367, 2001.
25. Rowell NR, Beck JS, Anderson Jr: Lupus erythematosus and erythema multiforme-like lesions. *Arch Dermatol* 88:176–180, 1963.
26. Sontheimer RD: Subacute cutaneous lupus erythematosus. *Clin Dermatol* 3:58–68, 1985.
27. Pincus LB, LeBoit PE, McCalmont TH, et al: Subcutaneous panniculitis-like T-cell lymphoma with overlapping clinicopathologic features of lupus erythematosus: coexistence of 2 entities? *Am J Dermatopathol* 31:520–526, 2009.
28. Weber F, Schmuth M, Fritsch P, et al: Lymphocytic infiltration of the skin is a photosensitive variant of lupus erythematosus: evidence by phototesting. *Br J Dermatol* 144:292, 2001.
29. Kuhn A, Sonntag M, Richter-Hintz D, et al: Phototesting in lupus erythematosus tumidus—review of 60 patients. *Photochem Photobiol* 73:532, 2001.
30. Inaloz HS, Chowdhury MM, Motley RJ: Lupus erythematosus/lichen planus overlap syndrome with scarring alopecia. *J Eur Acad Dermatol Venereol* 15:171–174, 2001.
31. Gammon WR, Briggaman RA: Bullous SLE: a phenotypically distinctive but immunologically heterogeneous bullous disorder. *J Invest Dermatol* 100:28S, 1993.
32. Yell JA, Allen J, Wojnarowska F, et al: Bullous systemic lupus erythematosus: revised criteria for diagnosis. *Br J Dermatol* 132:921, 1995.
33. Ting W, Stone MS, Racila D, et al: Toxic epidermal necrolysis-like acute cutaneous lupus erythematosus and the spectrum of the acute syndrome of apoptotic pan-epidermolysis (ASAP): a case report, concept review and proposal for new classification of lupus erythematosus vesiculobullous skin lesions. *Lupus* 13:941–950, 2004.
34. Lee LA: The clinical spectrum of neonatal lupus. *Arch Dermatol Res* 301:107–110, 2009.
35. Buyon JP, Hiebert R, Copel J, et al: Autoimmune-associated congenital heart block: demographics, mortality, morbidity and recurrence rates obtained from a national neonatal lupus registry. *J Am Coll Cardiol* 31:1658–1666, 1998.
36. Gronhagen CM, Gunnarsson I, Svenungsson E, et al: Cutaneous manifestations and serological findings in 260 patients with systemic lupus erythematosus. *Lupus* 19:1187–1194, 2010.
37. Gronhagen CM, Fored CM, Granath F, et al: Cutaneous lupus erythematosus and the association with systemic lupus erythematosus: a population-based cohort of 1088 patients in Sweden. *Br J Dermatol* 164:1335–1341, 2011.
38. Tan EM, Cohen AS, Fries JF, et al: The 1982 revised criteria for the classification of systemic lupus erythematosus. *Arthritis Rheum* 25:1271, 1982.
39. Albrecht J, Berlin JA, Braverman IM, et al: Dermatology position paper on the revision of the 1982 ACR criteria for systemic lupus erythematosus. *Lupus* 13:839–849, 2004.
40. Reich A, Marcinow K, Bialynicki-Birula R: The lupus band test in systemic lupus erythematosus patients. *Ther Clin Risk Manag* 7:27–32, 2011.
41. Foering K, Okawa J, Rose M, et al: Prevalence of self-report photosensitivity in cutaneous lupus erythematosus. *J Am Acad Dermatol* 66:220–228, 2011.
42. Russak JE, Chen T, Appa Y, et al: A comparison of sunburn protection of high-sun protection factor (SPF) sunscreens: SPF 85 sunscreen is significantly more protective than SPF 50. *J Am Acad Dermatol* 62:348–349, 2010.
43. Kuhn A, Gensch K, Haust M, et al: Photoprotective effects of a broad-spectrum sunscreen in ultraviolet-induced cutaneous lupus erythematosus: a randomized, vehicle-controlled, double-blind study. *J Am Acad Dermatol* 64:37–48, 2011.
44. Klein RS, Werth VP, Dowdy JC, et al: Analysis of compact fluorescent lights for use by patients with photosensitive conditions. *Photochem Photobiol* 85:1004–1010, 2009.
45. Roenigk HH, Jr, Martin JS, Eichorn P, et al: Discoid lupus erythematosus. Diagnostic features and evaluation of topical corticosteroid therapy. *Cutis* 25:281–285, 1980.
46. Barikbin B, Givrad S, Yousefi M, et al: Pimecrolimus 1% cream versus betamethasone 17-valerate 0.1% cream in the treatment of facial discoid lupus erythematosus: a double-blind, randomized pilot study. *Clin Exp Dermatol* 34:776–780, 2009.
47. Kuhn A, Ruland V, Bonsmann G: Cutaneous lupus erythematosus: update of therapeutic options Part I. *J Am Acad Dermatol* 65:e195–e213, 2010.
48. Jessop S, Whitelaw DA, Delamere FM: Drugs for discoid lupus erythematosus. *Cochrane Database Syst Rev* (4):CD002954, 2009.
49. Albrecht J, Taylor L, Berlin JA, et al: The CLASI (Cutaneous Lupus Erythematosus Disease Area and Severity Index): an outcome instrument for cutaneous lupus erythematosus. *J Invest Dermatol* 125:889–894, 2005.
50. Krathen MS, Dunham J, Gaines E, et al: The Cutaneous Lupus Erythematosus Disease Activity and Severity Index: expansion for rheumatology and dermatology. *Arthritis Rheum* 59:338–344, 2008.
51. Klein R, Moghadam-Kia S, LoMonico J, et al: Development of the CLASI as a tool to measure disease severity and responsiveness to therapy in cutaneous lupus erythematosus. *Arch Dermatol* 147:203–208, 2011.
52. Chang AY, Werth VP: Treatment of cutaneous lupus. *Curr Rheumatol Rep* 13:300–307, 2011.
53. Kuhn A, Ruland V, Bonsmann G: Cutaneous lupus erythematosus: update of therapeutic options Part II. *J Am Acad Dermatol* 65:e195–e213, 2011.
54. Vila LM, Mayor AM, Valentin AH, et al: Clinical outcome and predictors of disease evolution in patients with incomplete lupus erythematosus. *Lupus* 9:110–115, 2000.
55. Yell JA, Mbuagbaw J, Burge SM: Cutaneous manifestations of systemic lupus erythematosus. *Br J Dermatol* l 135:355–362, 1996.
56. Parodi A, Massone C, Cacciapuoti M, et al: Measuring the activity of the disease in patients with cutaneous lupus erythematosus. *Br J Dermatol* 142:457–460, 2000.
57. Ioannides D, Golden BD, Buyon JP, et al: Expression of SS-A/Ro and SS-B/La antigens in skin biopsy specimens of patients with photosensitive forms of lupus erythematosus. *Arch Dermatol* 136:340–346, 2000.
58. Paz ML, Gonzalez Maglio DH, Pino M, et al: Anti-ribonucleoproteins autoantibodies in patients with systemic autoimmune diseases. Relation with cutaneous photosensitivity. *Clin Rheumatol* 30:209–216, 2011.
59. Werth VP, White WL, Sanchez MR, et al: Incidence of alopecia areata in lupus erythematosus. *Arch Dermatol* l 128:368–371, 1992.
60. Cardinali C, Caproni M, Bernacchi E, et al: The spectrum of cutaneous manifestations in lupus erythematosus—the Italian experience. *Lupus* 9:417–423, 2000.
61. Ramos-Casals M, Nardi N, Lagrutta M, et al: Vasculitis in systemic lupus erythematosus: prevalence and clinical characteristics in 670 patients. *Medicine (Baltimore)* 85:95–104, 2006.
62. Davis MD, Daoud MS, Kirby B, et al: Clinicopathologic correlation of hypocomplementemic and normocomplementemic urticarial vasculitis. *J Am Acad Dermatol* l 38:899–905, 1998.
63. Garcia-Carrasco M, Jimenez-Hernandez M, Escarcega RO, et al: Treatment of Raynaud's phenomenon. *Autoimmun Rev* 8:62–68, 2008.
64. Ruiz-Irastorza G, Crowther M, Branch W, et al: Antiphospholipid syndrome. *Lancet* 376:1498–1509, 2010.
65. Frances C: Dermatological manifestations of Hughes' antiphospholipid antibody syndrome. *Lupus* 19:1071–1077, 2010.
66. Karassa FB, Ioannidis JP, Touloumi G, et al: Risk factors for central nervous system involvement in systemic lupus erythematosus. *QJM* 93:169–174, 2000.
67. Frances C, Piette JC: The mystery of Sneddon syndrome: relationship with antiphospholipid syndrome and systemic lupus erythematosus. *J Autoimmun* 15:139–143, 2000.
68. Garcia-Carrasco M, Ramos-Casals M, Cervera R, et al: Cryoglobulinemia in systemic lupus erythematosus: prevalence and clinical characteristics in a series of 122 patients. *Semin Arthritis Rheum* 30:366–373, 2001.
69. Elinav E, Chajek-Shaul T, Stern M: Improvement in cholesterol emboli syndrome after iloprost therapy. *BMJ* 324:268–269, 2002.
70. Sakr SH, Russell EB, Jasin HE: Systemic lupus erythematosus and calciphylaxis. *J Rheumatol* 31:1851–1853, 2004.
71. Reeves GE, Boyle MJ, Bonfield J, et al: Impact of hydroxychloroquine therapy on chronic urticaria: chronic autoimmune urticaria study and evaluation. *Intern Med J* 34:182–186, 2004.
72. Cutolo M, Sulli A, Secchi ME, et al: Nailfold capillaroscopy is useful for the diagnosis and follow-up of autoimmune rheumatic diseases. A future tool for the analysis of microvascular heart involvement? *Rheumatology Oxford)* 45 (Suppl 4):iv; 43–46, 2006.
73. Cohen JS: Erythromelalgia: new theories and new therapies. *J Am Acad Dermatol* 43:841–847, 2000.
74. Lowe L, Rapini RP, Golitz LE, et al: Papulonodular dermal mucinosis in lupus erythematosus. *J Am Acad Dermatol* l 27:312–315, 1992.

75. Boulman N, Slobodin G, Rozenbaum M, et al: Calcinosis in rheumatic diseases. *Semin Arthritis Rheum* 34:805–812, 2005.

76. Trueb RM: Involvement of scalp and nails in lupus erythematosus. *Lupus* 19:1078–1086, 2010.

77. Vaughn RY, Bailey JP, Jr., Field RS, et al: Diffuse nail dyschromia in black patients with systemic lupus erythematosus. *J Rheumatol l* 17:640–643, 1990.

78. Sparsa A, Piette JC, Wechsler B, et al: Anetoderma and its prothrombotic abnormalities. *J Am Acad Dermatol* 49:1008–1012, 2003.

79. Verneuil L, Dompmartin A, Comoz F, et al: Interstitial granulomatous dermatitis with cutaneous cords and arthritis: a disorder associated with autoantibodies. *J Am Acad Dermatol* 45:286–291, 2001.

80. Magro CM, Crowson AN, Schapiro BL: The interstitial granulomatous drug reaction: a distinctive clinical and pathological entity. *J Cutan Pathol* 25:72–78, 1998.

81. Gupta T, Beaconsfield M, Rose GE, et al: Discoid lupus erythematosus of the periorbita: clinical dilemmas, diagnostic delays. *Eye* 26:609–12.

Chapter 25

The Musculoskeletal System and Bone Metabolism

Sandra V. Navarra and Tito P. Torralba

Musculoskeletal manifestations involving the joints, muscle, bone, and supporting structures are common among patients with systemic lupus erythematosus (SLE) at diagnosis and throughout the course of illness.[1-3] Although the pathomechanisms are less extensively described than for other lupus organ involvement and diseases like rheumatoid arthritis (RA), pain and fatigue are among the predominant health issues from the patients' perspective.[4]

With long-standing SLE, chronic complications like avascular necrosis and disturbances in bone metabolism, particularly osteoporosis, become increasingly relevant and significantly affect quality of life. In these conditions, medications, notably glucocorticoids, are as contributory as the disease itself, and preventive measures play a vital role in the management approach.

ARTHRITIS

Arthritis is a dominant manifestation of active lupus. The 1971 American Rheumatism Association (ARA) preliminary criteria for the classification of SLE defined it as arthritis without deformity involving one or more peripheral joints characterized by pain on motion, tenderness, effusion, or periarticular soft tissue swelling. The 1982 revised criteria further increased specificity by defining it as nonerosive arthritis. In a subsequent comparison of the relative sensitivities of the 1971 and 1982 criteria in a cohort of patients with SLE, 88% met the preliminary criteria, and 83% met the revised criteria when arthritis was strictly classified as nonerosive arthritis. However, when arthritis was loosely defined as nondeforming arthritis without requiring radiographs, 91% met the revised criteria.[5] These differences were not statistically significant, and variations in the sensitivities of the preliminary and revised definitions of arthritis when tested in various populations illustrate that in clinical practice, arthritis is a major though liberally defined feature of SLE.

Erosions visible on radiographs develop in only a minority of cases, but joint space narrowing, subluxation, malalignment, and instability of joints often ensue even in the setting of relatively indolent arthritis. Studies of hand radiographs of patients with SLE and deforming arthropathy show only mild signs of bony pathology.[6-8] Jaccoud's arthropathy (JA), consisting of progressive rheumatoid-like deformities of the hands and feet, occurs in 3% to 43% of patients with lupus and can be clinically difficult to distinguish from RA, especially in the absence of extraarticular features (Figure 25-1). These joint deformities are usually due to a tenosynovitis rather than synovial hypertrophy. Histopathology reveals synovial membrane hyperplasia, microvascular changes, fibrin deposition, hematoxylin bodies, scant cellular infiltrates, and erosion of cartilage, but without the inflammatory pannus that plays a pivotal role in the cartilage and bone destruction in RA. Magnetic resonance imaging (MRI in a patient with JA demonstrates characteristic signs of soft tissue pathology, such as capsular swelling, edematous and proliferative tenosynovitis, synovial hypertrophy, and occasional bony alterations, for example, erosions, some of which are missed by conventional radiography.[9-11] Rarely, erosive symmetric polyarthritis with deformities similar to those in RA, named *rhupus,* can occur in SLE and may represent a distinct lupus subset.[7,12] In a study that classified patients

with rhupus as fulfilling American College of Rheumatology (ACR) criteria for both SLE and RA, the presence of anti–cyclic citrullinated peptides (anti-CCPs) clearly distinguished patients with rhupus from those with lupus arthropathy whether deforming, nondeforming, or erosive. A strong association has further been observed between the presence of anti-CCP and the presence of erosive arthritis and major histocompatibility complex (MHC) class II alleles among patients with lupus.[13]

The management of arthritis includes background antimalarial drugs and glucocorticoids in appropriate doses for systemic flares. Nonsteroidal anti-inflammatory drugs (NSAIDs) should be used with caution in the presence of renal or cardiovascular involvement. The use of immunosuppressives and disease-modifying antirheumatic drugs like azathioprine, leflunomide, and cyclosporin to treat chronic arthritis is largely based on experience in RA. Methotrexate (MTX) is beneficial for the extrarenal involvement in lupus, having been shown to decrease overall disease activity and steroid requirement.[14,15] The usual precautions apply, particularly the consideration of increased risk for MTX-induced adverse events in patients with renal impairment. Accelerated nodulosis induced by MTX similar to that seen in patients with RA has also been reported in patients with SLE and JA.[16] Mycophenolate mofetil, proven effective for induction and maintenance therapy in lupus nephritis, has shown efficacy in ameliorating nonrenal manifestations of SLE[17] and provides a suitable alternative in the treatment of lupus arthritis.

Despite the established efficacy of biologic agents directed against tumor necrosis factor (TNF) in RA and spondylopathies, their use in lupus arthritis has been restricted by reports of the development of autoantibodies and lupus-like syndromes.[18,19] Nonetheless, an open-label experience with their use[20] suggests that TNF blockade is effective in patients with SLE and arthritis, nephritis, and skin disease, and may be considered in lupus arthritis refractory to other therapies. Precautionary measures and vigilance must be exercised in monitoring for adverse events, including baseline screening and prophylaxis for infections like tuberculosis. Rituximab, a monoclonal antibody targeted against CD20 on B cells, has shown efficacy in RA but did not show any difference from placebo in a large clinical trial for active extrarenal lupus.[21] Belimumab, which neutralizes B-lymphocyte stimulator (BLyS), is a newly approved biologic agent for SLE, having demonstrated benefit across organ systems including the musculoskeletal system.[22,23] Other biologic agents, such as abatacept, which blocks T-lymphocyte co-stimulation, and the interleukin-6 (IL-6) receptor inhibitor tocilizumab have shown benefit in RA trials and are currently under clinical investigation for SLE.

Box 25-1 outlines the key features and general management of joint involvement in SLE.

SOFT TISSUE DISORDERS AND OTHER PAIN SYNDROMES

Patients with lupus may be at increased risk for localized soft tissue disorders owing to weakness, fatigue, and deconditioning, which occur with disease flares and long-term high-dose steroid treatment. There is a general laxity in connective tissue structures in patients

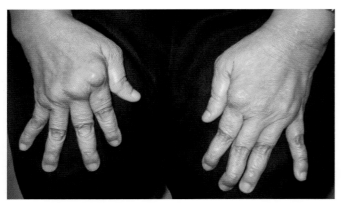

FIGURE 25-1 Jaccoud's arthropathy of the hands in a patient with lupus.

Box 25-1 Joint Involvement in Systemic Lupus Erythematosus

- Arthritis is typically non-deforming and non-erosive in the majority of patients with SLE
- Jaccoud's arthropathy (JA) consists of progressive rheumatoid-like deformities of hands and feet due to tenosynovitis rather than synovial inflammation and pannus formation
- "Rhupus" is characterized by erosive arthritis and a strong association with positive anti–cyclic citrullinated peptides (CCPs)
- Management includes analgesic and antiinflammatory medications. Disease-modifying antirheumatic drugs (DMARDs) and biologic agents may be useful in some cases.

---

with SLE,[24,25] with anecdotal reports of spontaneous tendon ischemia, necrosis, and rupture associated with high-dose systemic corticosteroid therapy.[26-28] Subcutaneous nodules are found in 5% to 12% of patients with SLE, generally in association with active disease. The nodules typically occur along the extensor surfaces of the upper extremities but may occasionally be found overlying the finger joints and along Achilles tendons. Although histologically similar to "rheumatoid" nodules, these nodules have no clear correlation with severe or erosive articular involvement and may be associated with MTX treatment.[16,29]

Generalized pain syndromes typified by fibromyalgia are particularly common in SLE, significantly contributing to poor quality of life. This topic is discussed in more detail in Chapter 52.

MUSCLE INVOLVEMENT

Muscle pain, tenderness, and weakness are common manifestations during SLE disease exacerbations and usually reflect overall disease activity. On the other hand, inflammatory myopathy with muscle enzyme elevation or typical changes on muscle biopsy develops in 5% to 10% of patients and is indistinguishable from idiopathic inflammatory myopathy (IIM).[30,31] In these patients, weakness, or less frequently, tenderness occurs primarily in the proximal limb-girdle muscle groups. Weakness is usually insidious in onset; patients experience easy fatigability manifesting as progressive difficulty in rising from a seated position or combing the hair. Most consistent with an active inflammatory myopathy is the elevation of serum muscle enzymes—creatine kinase (CK), aldolase, aminotransferases, and lactate dehydrogenase (LDH). The pattern of enzyme elevation varies among patients, making it necessary to measure all enzymes at baseline and serially monitor the abnormal levels to determine response to therapy. On the other hand, low creatine kinase levels may signal increased extramuscular active lupus.[32]

There is also a wide variation in electromyography (EMG) and muscle biopsy findings in SLE, depending on the population, selected test site, observer interpretation, and presence or absence of muscle symptoms. In patients with active symptomatic myositis, EMG demonstrates polyphasic motor unit potentials of small amplitude and short duration similar to those of IIM. Muscle biopsy is less sensitive in detecting muscle pathology among patients with SLE and is not routinely performed in clinical practice except in refractory cases or when other causes, such as drugs, need to be excluded. The findings have been described to vary from normal to interstitial inflammation, fibrillar necrosis, and degeneration. Immunopathologic staining studies further show evidence of vascular deposits of immunoglobulin, complement, or immune complexes in about a third of patients. Vacuolization and fibrosis are late occurrences and may signify irreversibility, although vacuolization may occasionally be found in reversible drug-induced myopathy.[33-35] Among the histopathologic findings, lymphocytic vasculitis correlates with high erythrocyte sedimentation rates, arthritis, and Sjögren syndrome.[36] In a study that compared clinical and laboratory features in 10 patients with SLE complicated by biopsy-proven myositis and those in 290 patients with SLE without myositis, those with myositis were more likely to have alopecia, oral ulcers, erosive joint disease, Sjögren syndrome, and presence of anti-ribonucleoprotein (RNP) autoantibodies, but less likely to have renal disease.[37]

The differential diagnoses in a patient with lupus presenting with muscle weakness include drug-induced myopathy (e.g., steroids, anti-malarials, statins[38-40]), concurrent endocrinopathies such as thyroid disease, and neurologic involvement such as chronic inflammatory demyelinating polyneuropathy.[41] A thorough search for relevant clinical clues in combination with muscle enzyme measurements, judicious use of EMG, and muscle biopsy could prove useful in distinguishing inflammatory myopathy from these other conditions. Table 25-1 outlines the clinical features, pathomechanisms, and muscle biopsy findings in some causes of myopathy.

Therapy of muscle involvement in SLE depends on assessment of the overall disease activity and possible contributory factors, such as drugs and infection. As for IIM, high-dose corticosteroids, including pulse therapy, provide dramatic benefit during acute inflammation in lupus myositis but may lead to secondary myopathy with long-term high-dose use. Methotrexate, azathioprine, and other immunosuppressives, and some biologic agents (discussed previously) provide steroid-sparing ability and may be used with similar therapeutic efficacy as in IIM. Drug-induced myopathy due to statins and antimalarials is generally reversible upon discontinuation of the offending drug.

MUSCULOSKELETAL INFECTIONS

The range of musculoskeletal infections in SLE includes cellulitis, septic arthritis, osteomyelitis, pyomyositis, and other deep-seated soft tissue infections. The challenge posed by these infections lies in the difficulty of early recognition because the manifestations tend to be masked by immunosuppressive therapy, with tendency for involvement of multiple sites.[42] Particularly difficult are chronic infections like those caused by mycobacteria that affect tendons, muscle, bone, and joints, sometimes mimicking or triggering active lupus disease.[43] Although the management principles for these conditions are no different from those in the general population, the atypical presentation could cause undue delay in diagnosis and adversely affect outcomes. See Chapter 52 for a more detailed discussion on infections in SLE.

AVASCULAR NECROSIS OF BONE

Avascular necrosis (AVN), also known as osteonecrosis, aseptic necrosis, or ischemic necrosis of bone, is reported in 5% to 30% of patients with SLE.[44-52] It is a major source of morbidity especially among young patients with SLE. The terminology reflects its mainly vascular pathomechanisms, with the initial pathology described as interruption of the blood supply to the epiphysis, followed by reactive hyperemia and bone necrosis leading to subchondral fractures. Healing is characterized by new vessel formation and incongruous bony repair. With repeated microfractures and continued weight-bearing, the original fracture does not heal completely and new

TABLE 25-1 Clinical Features, Pathomechanisms, and Muscle Biopsy Findings of Myopathic Conditions

CONDITION	CLINICAL PRESENTATION	PATHOMECHANISM	MUSCLE BIOPSY
Idiopathic inflammatory myopathy (IIM)	Typically proximal muscle weakness; with distal muscle involvement in inclusion body myositis (IBM). Rarely, problems of swallowing and difficulty breathing due to involvement of throat and thoracodiaphragmatic muscles. Muscle enzymes usually elevated.	Immune (cell-mediated and humoral) and nonimmune (endoplasmic reticulum stress, hypoxia) mechanisms play a role in muscle fiber damage and dysfunction. Proinflammatory nuclear factor kappa B pathway connects the immune and nonimmune components contributing to muscle damage.	Variable degrees of inflammation, necrosis, and atrophic changes. Diffuse, perivascular, and interstitial inflammatory infiltrates with occasional vacuolization and fibrosis. Vascular immunoglobulin and complement deposition. Capillary basement thickening reflects impaired microvascular circulation.
SLE myopathy[30-37]	Muscle pain, tenderness, and weakness common during disease flares. Muscle enzymes normal or elevated. Proximal muscle weakness with muscle enzyme elevation indicates inflammatory myopathy, usually associated with anti-ribonucleoprotein (RNP).	Inflammatory mechanisms in lupus myositis similar to but generally less severe than IIM.	Findings vary from normal to interstitial inflammation, fibrillar necrosis, and degeneration. Vascular deposits of immunoglobulin, complement, or immune complexes.
Steroid-induced myopathy[38]	Proximal muscle weakness especially of lower extremities, occurring weeks to months after start of or after an increase in steroid dosage. Occurs almost exclusively in patients treated with high dosage. Muscle enzymes normal.	Catabolic muscle proteolysis through ubiquitin-proteasome system. Antianabolic action by blunting of muscle protein synthesis resulting from decreased production of insulin growth factor 1 and increased production of myostatin, contributing to muscle atrophy.	Atrophy of type II fibers with absence of inflammation.
Statin-induced myopathy[40]	Myalgia, lassitude and fatigue, occasional frank proximal muscle weakness, occurring weeks to years after start of statin therapy. Muscle enzymes normal or elevated.	Apoptosis likely stimulated by isoprenoid depletion, leading to decreased protein geranyl-geranylation and/or farnesylation, and elevation of cytosolic calcium with activation of mitochondrium-mediated apoptotic signaling.	Vary from mild, discrete, and nonspecific findings to muscle fiber necrosis, mononuclear cell infiltration myophagocytosis, and regeneration.
Antimalarial myopathy[39]	Insidious onset of proximal muscle weakness. Muscle enzymes normal.	Exact mechanism unclear. Antimalarials accumulate in lysosomes and raise intralysosomal pH, causing inhibition of cathepsin B, mucopolysaccharidases, acid phosphodiesterases, and hydrolases—which may lead to amyloid, phospholipid, and glycogen accumulation with curvilinear body formation.	Curvilinear bodies and muscle fiber atrophy with vacuolar changes.

fractures occur, resulting in flattening of the surface and subsequent degenerative changes of the bone and adjacent structures (Figure 25-2).[53,54] The epiphysis of the femoral head is particularly vulnerable to ischemic damage because of the undersupply of functional collateral end-arterial circulation.[55] However, osteonecrosis can develop in other bones, including those at the knees, shoulders, wrists, and ankles, with a tendency to occur at multiple sites among patients with SLE.[56-59] The lesions typically show on radiographs as bone infarcts characterized by serpiginous well-defined densities with sclerotic borders surrounding areas of bone necrosis (Figures 25-3 and 25-4).

Conditions associated with AVN include trauma, drugs, cigarette smoking, alcohol consumption, metabolic disorders, connective tissue disease, and organ transplantation. GC use is the most consistent risk factor for development of AVN in SLE.[51,52,60-65] The pathomechanisms are postulated to be based on lipid-altering effects of GCs due to greater adipogenesis and fatty infiltration of osteocytes with increased apoptosis. The increases in femoral fat content and intracortical pressure compromise interosseous microcirculation, leading to bony necrosis.[66-70] GC-induced AVN is usually dose related, with greater risk of AVN in patients receiving higher steroid doses, especially in the first year of treatment and with longer duration of therapy.[63,64,71] The time interval between steroid use and the development of osteonecrosis varies among individuals, ranging from 1 to 16 months.[71,72] Other contributory factors in the development of AVN in SLE are vasculitis, Raynaud phenomenon, cytotoxic treatment, production of inflammatory mediators, defects in fibrinolysis, gene polymorphisms, antiphospholipid syndrome, and other hypercoagulable states.[64,73-79]

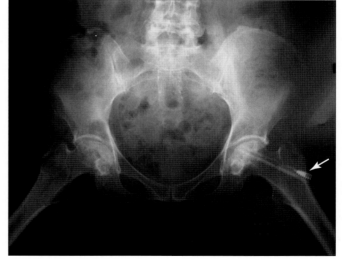

FIGURE 25-2 Bilateral hip osteonecrosis showing flattened femoral heads with preserved joint spaces and no acetabular involvement (Ficat-Arlet stage III). Core decompression with vascularized fibular bone graft (*arrow*) is shown at the left hip.

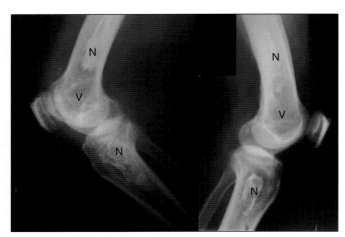

FIGURE 25-3 Osteonecrosis of femur and tibia on both lower extremities showing intramedullary bone infarcts. Dense serpiginous linear margins separate central necrotic zones (N) from adjacent viable bone (V).

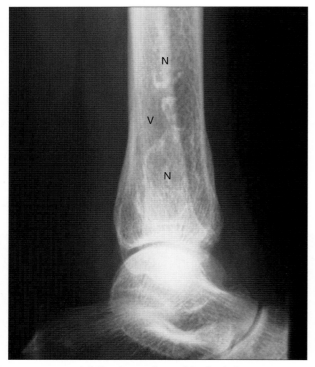

FIGURE 25-4 Intramedullary bone infarcts of the distal tibia in osteonecrosis. Note the central necrotic areas (N) of unaltered density separated from adjacent viable bone marrow (V) by irregular linear margins of increased density.

The diagnosis of AVN should be considered in any patient with SLE who has persistent pain in one or a few joints even without evidence of disease activity in other systems, especially if GCs have been used as treatment. The pain is often insidious in onset and aggravated by weight-bearing and ambulation. In advanced disease, the pain is persistent even at rest. Limitation of range of motion that is not attributable to pain is usually a progressive and late symptom. The risk for development of osteonecrosis in the contralateral hip when one side is affected ranges from 31% to 55%.[53]

In a patient with suspected AVN, the diagnosis is confirmed by imaging studies. Plain radiographs can be completely normal in very early stages of AVN. In stage I of the widely used scale developed by Ficat and Arlet,[80] routine radiographs are normal and the patient is usually asymptomatic or may experience only minimal pain. In stage II, radiographs show cystic or osteosclerotic lesions but no subchondral fracture. Stage III radiographs are characterized by the "crescent sign" resulting from structural collapse of a necrotic segment of subchondral trabecular bone; joint space remains intact. Stage IV represents end-stage disease and osteoarthritic changes are seen on radiographs. These last two stages connote irreversibility, with most patients remaining symptomatic and eventually requiring surgery.

The use of bone scintigraphy or technetium-labeled radionuclide bone scan in the early diagnosis of AVN is based on the increased osteoblastic activity and blood flow in the early stages of AVN. Computed tomography (CT) allows more detailed examination and can demonstrate the characteristic "asterisk sign" of a sclerotic rim surrounding a mottled area of osteolysis and sclerosis. Magnetic resonance imaging (MRI) has the greatest utility in the early diagnosis of AVN in a variety of anatomic locations. It is possible to detect bone marrow edema, an early feature of AVN, on MRI that is not visible on radiography or CT in early stages. Over time, the Ficat classification system has been modified by other groups to include these other imaging modalities and to assist therapeutic decisions. The Steinberg classification includes bone scan and MRI as well as volumetric assessment of the femoral head,[81] and the Association of Research Circulation Osseous (ARCO) modification adds a stage 0 for patients in whom imaging findings are normal but who are at high risk for development of AVN.[82]

Early diagnosis is crucial to the successful treatment of AVN. The critical management decisions are whether to intervene surgically and which procedure to deploy. Conservative medical treatment options are advocated when the involvement is less than 15% of the articular margin and remote from the weight-bearing region.[83] These measures are limited to load reduction on the affected region, such as the use of crutches, and physiotherapy to maintain muscle strength and prevent contractures. Unfortunately, these approaches do not generally prevent disease progression, and most patients eventually require surgical intervention.

Surgical management of femoral head AVN includes core decompression, structural bone grafting, vascularized fibula grafting, osteotomy, resurfacing arthroplasty, hemiarthroplasty, and total hip replacement.[53,83] The timing and type of surgical intervention depends on the involved site and the stage of AVN, with little disagreement about the benefit of joint arthroplasty in stage III and IV AVN. The indications for surgery, including core decompression in the earlier stages, are controversial and based on the limited literature regarding the natural history of the disease. Among the identified risk factors for rapid progression of AVN, age younger than 40 years, abnormal lipid levels, and bilateral femoral head involvement identify patients who may benefit from early aggressive surgical intervention.[84,85]

OSTEOPOROSIS

Osteoporosis with consequent increased fracture risk is an important clinical problem in SLE. A summary of various studies suggests a generalized reduction in bone mineral density (BMD), with the prevalence of osteoporosis ranging from 4.0% to 48.8%, that of osteopenia from 1.4% to 68.7%, and that of fractures from 5.0% to 21.4%,[86] commonly occurring at the leg, foot, arm, vertebrae, and hip.[87] The summary also identified an inverse correlation between BMD and chronic damage measured by the Systemic Lupus International Collaborating Clinics (SLICC) damage index instrument.[88]

Several factors contribute to the development of osteoporosis in SLE. These include chronic inflammation or active disease, GC treatment, renal dysfunction, vitamin D deficiency, ovarian failure, concomitant thyroid disease, and drugs such as anticonvulsants.

Glucocorticoids affect bone metabolism by influencing aspects of the bone remodeling cycle, with disproportionate reduction in bone formation. The decreased bone formation is due both to direct effects on cells of osteoblastic lineage and to indirect effects related to inhibition of the release of gonadotrophins. Enhanced osteocyte apoptosis has also been implicated as an important mechanism of GC-induced

Box 25-2 Mechanisms of Osteoporosis in Systemic Lupus Erythematosus

Chronic Inflammation[86,88]
- Cytokines, e.g., interleukin-1 (IL-1), IL-6, tumor necrosis factor alpha induce osteoclastogenesis
- Decreased osteocalcin, bone-specific alkaline phosphatase, and propeptide of procollagen type 1 with carboxy terminal

Glucocorticoid (GC)–Induced Osteoporosis[89,90,91,93,95,96]
- Decreased insulin growth factor 1 (IGF-1) synthesis in osteoblasts and inhibition of IGF-2 receptor expression
- Decreased messenger RNA levels encoding for osteoblast products such as osteocalcin
- Preferential differentiation of bone marrow stromal cells toward adipocyte instead of osteoblastic cell lineage
- Suppression of osteoblastic function associated with alteration of Wnt signaling pathway
- Enhanced osteocyte apoptosis resulting in failure to direct bone remodeling at trabecular surface with consequent degradation of bone microarchitecture

- Decreased calcium absorption from the gastrointestinal tract and decreased renal tubular reabsorption of calcium leading to secondary hyperparathyroidism
- Inhibition of release of gonadotrophins with resulting hypogonadism
- Altered vitamin D metabolism

Other Factors That Contribute to Bone Loss[86]
- Photosensitivity in SLE with recommendations to avoid sun exposure, thus inducing vitamin D deficiency
- Renal insufficiency with consequent alterations in bone metabolism
- Increase in testosterone oxidation with a decrease in dehydroepiandrosterone
- Chronic pain and fatigue resulting in inactivity
- Concomitant medications, e.g., cyclosporine, methotrexate, heparin, anticonvulsants
- Ovarian dysfunction

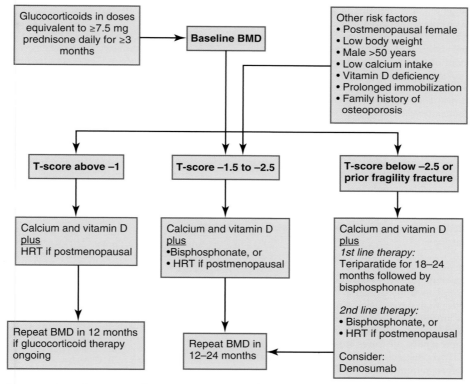

FIGURE 25-5 Algorithm for prevention and treatment of osteoporosis in systemic lupus erythematosus. BMD, bone mineral density testing; HRT, hormone replacement therapy.

osteoporosis.[89,90] These agents also decrease intestinal calcium absorption and renal tubular calcium reabsorption, with consequent secondary hyperparathyroidism. Bone resorption is increased during the first 6 to 12 months of GC therapy as a result of increased osteoclast activity secondary to greater expression of the receptor activator of nuclear factor kappa beta (NF-κB) ligand (RANK-L) and reduced osteoclast apoptosis. With long-term use of these agents, bone turnover is reduced.[91]

A negative association between bone mass and GC use was documented in approximately 60% of patients with SLE. However, vertebral fractures due to GCs occur at higher BMD values than those observed in other types of osteoporosis. This is likely due to the fewer remodeling cycles with less osteoblastic activity and accelerated osteocyte apoptosis, leading to major loss of trabecular connectivity—suggesting that degradation of microarchitecture is just as important as loss of absolute bone mass in determining fracture risk of GC therapy.[92] The fracture threshold is further decreased in postmenopausal women, implying that use of these agents and menopause are independent risk factors for osteoporosis. Most clinical guidelines thus suggest an intervention threshold T-score of −1.5 in GC-induced osteoporosis, compared with to −2.5 in postmenopausal osteoporosis.[93]

Vitamin D levels have been shown to correlate with BMD at the total hip, femoral neck, and spine.[94] There is a high prevalence of vitamin D deficiency among patients with SLE, with significantly lower levels among African Americans than in Caucasians. In addition to decrease in sun exposure, patients with SLE are often taking medicines, such as glucocorticoids, that are known to alter vitamin D metabolism and impair bone health.[95,96] Vitamin D status has also been associated with fall risk owing to its effect on lower extremity muscle function. Thus, vitamin D deficiency may place patients with SLE at a higher fracture risk than that due to low BMD alone. Furthermore, the high prevalence of vitamin D deficiency has been found to correlate with greater SLE disease activity and higher levels of proinflammatory cytokines, consistent with the immunomodulatory effect of vitamin D.[97]

Box 25-2 summarizes some of the mechanisms for osteoporosis in SLE. The management of osteoporosis in SLE entails the identification of all possible risk factors for osteoporosis and fractures in the patient. A baseline BMD measurement, generally by dual-energy x-ray absorptiometry (DXA), is recommended at the start of GC therapy, with repeat scans at 12-month intervals if the patient continually receives high GC doses. Lifestyle risk factors, such as smoking, low dietary calcium, high dietary salt intake, and vitamin D deficiency, must be effectively addressed. Individualizing exercise programs and minimizing physical impediments such as muscle weakness, neurologic involvement, and visual impairment are essential preventive measures against falls and fractures. Calcium, vitamin D, bisphosphonates, and teriparatide have shown demonstrable benefit in the management of GC-induced osteoporosis.[93,98] Denosumab, a human recombinant monoclonal antibody that inhibits bone resorption by binding to RANK-L, has been approved for postmenopausal osteoporosis and is a promising agent for other diseases associated with bone loss, including RA and GC-induced osteoporosis.[99] Hormone replacement therapy (HRT), with estrogen or progesterone either singly or in combination, is more controversial in the setting of SLE. However, there are sufficient data showing potential benefit and safety of these drugs and that of the weak androgen dehydroepiandrosterone (DHEA) in selected patients.[100] Figure 25-5 illustrates an algorithmic approach to osteoporosis in SLE. Regardless of the choice of therapy, utmost consideration must be given to primary prevention and adequate control of the overall SLE disease activity, including the use of antimalarials and steroid-sparing drugs.

SUMMARY

Musculoskeletal involvement in SLE ranges from acute inflammatory conditions like arthritis and myositis of active disease to chronic conditions associated with progressive organ damage like AVN and osteoporosis. The former are generally responsive to antiinflammatory and immunosuppressive therapy with potential benefit from biologic agents, whereas preventive measures are essential to retard the development of the latter. Regardless of the specific musculoskeletal condition, early recognition, timely management, attenuation of risk factors, and adequate control of overall lupus activity are crucial to the prevention of the morbidity, disability, and long-term sequelae of these conditions.

References

1. Hopkinson N, Doherty M, Powell R: Clinical features and race-specific incidence/prevalence rates of systemic lupus erythematosus in a geographically complete cohort of patients. *Ann Rheum Dis* 53:675–680, 1994.
2. Tikly M, Navarra S: Lupus in the developing world—is it any different? *Best Pract Res Clin Rheumatol* 22:643–655, 2008.
3. Navarra S, Ishimori M, Uy E, et al: Studies of Filipino patients with systemic lupus erythematosus: autoantibody profile of first-degree relatives. *Lupus* 20:537–543, 2011.
4. Robinson DJ, Aguilar D, Schoenwetter M, et al: Impact of systemic lupus erythematosus on health, family and work: the patient perspective. *Arthritis Care Res* 62:266–273, 2010.
5. Levin R, Weinstein A, Peterson M, et al: A comparison of the sensitivity of the 1971 and 1982 American Rheumatism Association criteria for the classification of systemic lupus erythematosus. *Arthritis Rheum* 27:530–538, 1984.
6. Alarcon-Segovia D, Abud-Mendoza C, Diaz-Jouanen E, et al: Deforming arthropathy of the hands in systemic lupus erythematosus. *J Rheumatol* 15:65–69, 1988.
7. van Vugt R, Derksen R, Kater L, et al: Deforming arthropathy or lupus and rhupus hands in systemic lupus erythematosus. *Ann Rheum Dis* 57:540–544, 1998.
8. Weissman B, Rappoport A, Sosman J, et al: Radiographic findings in the hands in patients with systemic lupus erythematosus. *Radiology* 126:313–317, 1978.
9. Molina J, Molina J, Gutierrez S, et al: Deforming arthropathy of the hands (Jaccoud's) in systemic lupus erythematosus (SLE): an independent subset of SLE? *Arthritis Rheum* 38:S347, 1995 (abstract).
10. Sierra-Jimenez G, Sanchez-Ortiz A, Aceves-Avila F, et al: Tendinous and ligamentous derangements in systemic lupus erythematosus. *J Rheumatol* 35:2187–2191, 2008.
11. Ostendorf B, Scherer A, Specker C, et al: Jaccoud's arthropathy in systemic lupus erythematosus: differentiation of deforming and erosive patterns by magnetic resonance imaging. *Arthritis & Rheumatism* 48:157–165, 2003.
12. Fernandez A, Quintana G, Matterson E, et al: Lupus arthropathy: historical evolution from deforming arthropathy to rhupus. *Clin Rheumatol* 23:523–526, 2004.
13. Chan M, Owen P, Dunphy J, et al: Associations of erosive arthritis with anti-cyclic citrullinated peptide antibodies and MHC class II alleles in systemic lupus erythematosus. *J Rheumatol* 35:77–83, 2008.
14. Fortin PR, Abrahamowicz M, Ferland D, et al: Steroid-sparing effects of methotrexate in systemic lupus erythematosus: a double-blind, randomized, placebo-controlled trial. *Arthritis Rheum* 59:1796–1804, 2008.
15. Carneiro J, Sato E: Double blind, randomized, placebo controlled clinical trial of methotrexate in systemic lupus erythematosus. *J Rheumatol* 26:1275–1279, 1999.
16. Rivero M, Salvatore A, Gomez-Puerta J, et al: Accelerated nodulosis during methotrexate therapy in a patient with systemic lupus erythematosus and Jaccoud's arthropathy. *Rheumatology* 43:1587–1588, 2004.
17. Ginzler E, Wofsy D, Isenberg DA, et al: Nonrenal disease activity following mycophenolate mofetil or intravenous cyclophosphamide as induction treatment for lupus nephritis: findings in a multicenter, prospective, randomized, open-label, parallel-group clinical trial. *Arthritis Rheum* 62:211–221, 2010.
18. De Rycke L, Baeten D, Kruithof E, et al: Infliximab, but not etanercept, induces IgM anti-double-stranded DNA autoantibodies as main antinuclear reactivity: biologic and clinical implications in autoimmune arthritis. *Arthritis Rheum* 52:2192–2201, 2005.
19. Williams EL, Gadola S, Edwards CJ: Anti-TNF-induced lupus. *Rheumatology* 48:716–720, 2009.
20. Aringer M, Graninger WB, Steiner G, et al: Safety and efficacy of tumor necrosis factor α blockade in systemic lupus erythematosus: an open-label study. *Arthritis Rheum* 50:3161–3169, 2004.
21. Merrill JT, Neuwelt MC, Wallace DJ, et al: Efficacy and safety of rituximab in moderately-to-severely active systemic lupus erythematosus. The randomized, double-blind, phase II/III systemic lupus erythematosus. Evaluation of rituximab trial. *Arthritis Rheum* 62:222–233, 2010.
22. Navarra S, Guzman R, Gallacher A, et al: Efficacy and safety of belimumab in patients with active systemic lupus erythematosus: a randomised, placebo-controlled phase 3 trial. *Lancet* 377:721–731, 2011.
23. Manzi S, Sánchez-Guerrero J, Merrill JT, et al: Effects of belimumab, a B-lymphocyte stimulator-specific inhibitor, on disease activity across multiple organ domains in patients with systemic lupus erythematosus. *Ann Rheum Dis* 2012. doi:10.1136/annrheumdis-2011-200831. in press.
24. Nakamura K, Tajima Y, Takai O. Generalized laxity of connective tissue as a possible syndrome in systemic lupus erythematosus. *Mod Rheumatol* 20:522–527, 2010.
25. Guma M, Olive A, Roca J, et al: Association of systemic lupus erythematosus and hypermobility. *Ann Rheum Dis* 61:1024–1026, 2002.
26. Babini S, Cocco J, Babini J, et al: Atlantoaxial subluxation in systemic lupus erythematosus: further evidence of tendinous alterations. *J Rheumatol* 17:173–177, 1990.
27. Wallace DJ: The musculoskeletal system. In Wallace DJ, Hahn BH, editors: *Dubois' lupus erythematosus*, ed 7, Philadelphia, 2007, Lippincott Williams & Wilkins, pp 647–662.

28. Chiou Y, Lan J, Hsieh T, et al: Spontaneous Achilles tendon rupture in a patient with systemic lupus erythematosus due to ischemic necrosis after methylprednisolone pulse therapy. *Lupus* 14:321–325, 2005.

29. Dubois E, Friou G, Chandor S: Rheumatoid nodules and rheumatoid granulomas in systemic lupus erythematosus. *JAMA* 220:515–518, 1972.

30. Isenberg DA, Snaith M: Muscle disease in systemic lupus erythematosus: a study of its nature, frequency and cause. *J Rheumatol* 8:917–924, 1981.

31. Foote R, Kimbrough S, Stevens J: Lupus myositis. *Muscle Nerve* 5:65–68, 1982.

32. Font J, Ramos-Casals M, Vilas A, et al: Low values of creatine kinase in systemic lupus erythematosus. Clinical significance in 300 patients. *Clin Exp Rheumatol* 20:837–840, 2002.

33. Finol H, Montagnani S, Marquez A, et al: Ultrastructural pathology of skeletal muscle in systemic lupus erythematosus. *J Rheumatol* 17:210–219, 1990.

34. Oxenhandler R, Hart M, Bickel J, et al: Pathologic features of muscle in systemic lupus erythematosus: a biopsy series with comparative clinical and immunopathologic observations. *Hum Pathol* 13:745–757, 1982.

35. Vizjak A, Perkovic T, Rozman B, et al: Skeletal muscle immune deposits in systemic lupus erythematosus. Correlation with histologic changes, autoantibodies, and clinical involvement. *Scan J Rheumatol* 27:207–214, 1998.

36. Lim K, Lowe J, Powell R: Skeletal muscle lymphocytic vasculitis in systemic lupus erythematosus: relation to disease activity. *Lupus* 4:148–151, 1995.

37. Dayal N, Isenberg DA: SLE/myositis overlap: are the manifestations of SLE different in overlap disease? *Lupus* 11:293–298, 2002.

38. Schakman O, Gilson H, Thissen JP: Mechanisms of glucocorticoid-induced myopathy. *J Endocrinol* 197:1–10, 2008.

39. Casado E, Gratacos J, Tolosa C, et al: Antimalarial myopathy: an under-diagnosed complication? Prospective longitudinal study of 119 patients. *Ann Rheum Dis* 65:385–390, 2006.

40. Soininen K, Niemi M, Kilkki E, et al: Muscle symptoms associated with statins: a series of twenty patients. *Basic Clin Pharmacol Toxicol* 98:51–54, 2006.

41. Zoilo M, Eduardo B, Enrique F, et al: Chronic inflammatory demyelinating polyradiculoneuropathy in a boy with systemic lupus erythematosus. *Rheumatol Int* 30:965–968, 2010.

42. Cuchacovich R, Gedalia A: Pathophysiology and clinical spectrum of infections in systemic lupus erythematosus. *Rheum Dis Clin North Am* 35:75–93, 2009.

43. Victorio-Navarra S, Dy E, Arroyo C, et al: Tuberculosis among Filipino patients with systemic lupus erythematosus. *Semin Arthritis Rheum* 26:628–634, 1996.

44. Pistiner M, Wallace DJ, Nessim S, et al: Lupus erythematosus in the 1980s: a survey of 570 patients. *Semin Arthritis Rheum* 21:55–64, 1991.

45. Abeles M, Urman J, Weinstein A, et al: Systemic lupus erythematosus in the younger patient: survival studies. *J Rheumatol* 7:515–522, 1980.

46. Diaz-Jouanen E, Abud-Mendoza C, Inglesias-Gamarra A, et al: Ischemic necrosis of bone in systemic lupus erythematosus. *Orthop Rev* 14:303–309, 1985.

47. Gladman D, Charudhry-Ahluwalia V, Ibanez D, et al: Outcomes of symptomatic osteonecrosis in 95 patients with systemic lupus erythematosus. *J Rheumatol* 28:2226–2229, 2001.

48. Rascu A, Manger K, Kraetsch H, et al: Osteonecrosis in systemic lupus erythematosus, steroid-induced or a lupus-dependent manifestation? *Lupus* 5:323–327, 1996.

49. Tektonidou M, Malagari K, Vlachoyiannopoulos P, et al: Asymptomatic avascular necrosis in patients with primary antiphospholipid syndrome in the absence of corticosteroid use: a prospective study by magnetic resonance imaging. *Arthritis Rheum* 48:732–736, 2003.

50. Zizic T, Marcoux C, Hungerford D, et al: The early diagnosis of ischemic necrosis of bone. *Arthritis Rheum* 29:1177–1186, 1986.

51. Cozen L, Wallace DJ: Avascular necrosis in systemic lupus erythematosus: clinical associations and a 47-year perspective. *Am J Orthop (Belle Mead NJ)* 27:352–354, 1998.

52. Mok C, Lau C, Wong R: Risk factors for avascular bone necrosis in systemic lupus erythematosus. *Br J Rheumatol* 37:895–900, 1998.

53. Chang C, Greenspan A, Gershwin M: Osteonecrosis: current perspectives on pathogenesis and treatment. *Semin Arthritis Rheum* 23:47–69, 1993.

54. Assouline-Dayan Y, Chang C, Greenspan A, et al: Pathogenesis and natural history of osteonecrosis. *Semin Arthritis Rheum* 32:94–124, 2002.

55. Bluemke D, Petri M, Zerhouni E. Femoral head perfusion and composition: MR imaging and spectroscopic evaluation of patients with systemic lupus erythematosus and at risk for avascular necrosis. *Radiology* 197:433–438, 1995.

56. Klippel J, Gerber L, Pollak L, et al: Avascular necrosis in systemic lupus erythematosus: silent symmetric osteonecroses. *Am J Med* 67:83–87, 1979.

57. Klipper A, Stevens M, Zizic T, et al: Ischemic necrosis of bone in systemic lupus erythematosus. *Medicine* 55:251–257, 1976.

58. Fishel B, Caspi D, Eventov I, et al: Multiple osteonecrotic lesions in systemic lupus erythematosus. *J Rheumatol* 14:601–604, 1987.

59. Guillaume M, Brandelet B, Peretz A: Unusual high frequency of multifocal lesions of osteonecrosis in a young patient with systemic lupus erythematosus. *Br J Rheumatol* 37:1248–1249, 1998.

60. Cooper C, Steinbuch M, Stevenson R, et al: The epidemiology of osteonecrosis: findings from the GPRD and THIN databases in the UK. *Osteoporos Int* 21:569–577, 2010.

61. Mont M, Glueck C, Pacheco I, et al: Risk factors for osteonecrosis in systemic lupus erythematosus. *J Rheumatol* 24:654–662, 1997.

62. Zizic T, Marcoux C, Hungerford D, et al: Corticosteroid therapy associated with ischemic necrosis of bone in systemic lupus erythematosus. *Am J Med* 79:596–604, 1985.

63. Weiner E, Abeles M: Aseptic necrosis and glucocorticosteroids in systemic lupus erythematosus: a reevaluation. *J Rheumatol* 16:604–608, 1989.

64. Milgliaresi S, Picillo U, Ambrosone L, et al: Avascular necrosis in patients with SLE: relation to corticosteroid therapy and anticardiolipin antibodies. *Lupus* 3:37–41, 1994.

65. Massardo L, Jacobelli S, Leissner M, et al: High-dose intravenous methylprednisolone therapy associated with osteonecrosis in patients with systemic lupus erythematosus. *Lupus* 1:401–405, 1992.

66. Cui Q, Wang G, Balian G: Steroid-induced adipogenesis in a pluripotential cell line from bone marrow. *J Bone Joint Surg Am* 79:1054–1063, 1997.

67. Wang G, Cui Q, Balian G: The Nicolas Andry award. The pathogenesis and prevention of steroid-induced osteonecrosis. *Clin Orthop Relat Res* 370:295–310, 2000.

68. Yin L, Li Y, Wang Y: Dexamethasone-induced adipogenesis in primary marrow stromal cell cultures: mechanism of steroid-induced osteonecrosis. *Chin Med J (Engl)* 119:581–588, 2006.

69. Weinstein R, Nicholas R, Manolagas S: Apoptosis of osteocytes in glucocorticoid-induced osteonecrosis of the hip. *J Clin Endocrinol Metab* 85:2907–2912, 2000.

70. Kerachian M, Seguin C, Harvey E: Glucocorticoids in osteonecrosis of the femoral head: A new understanding of the mechanism of action. *J Steroid Biochem Mol Biol* 114:121–128, 2009.

71. Oinuma K, Harada Y, Nawata Y, et al: Osteonecrosis in patients with systemic lupus erythematosus develops very early after starting high dose corticosteroid treatment. *Ann Rheum Dis* 60:1145–1148, 2001.

72. Koo K, Kim R, Kim Y, et al: Risk period for developing osteonecrosis of the femoral head in patients on steroid treatment. *Clin Rheumatol* 21:299–303, 2002.

73. Hamijoyo L, Llamado L, Navarra S: Risk factors for avascular necrosis among Filipino patients with systemic lupus erythematosus. *Int J Rheum Dis* 11:141–147, 2008.

74. Sheikh J, Retzinger G, Hess E: Association of osteonecrosis in systemic lupus erythematosus with abnormalities in fibrinolysis. *Lupus* 7:42–48, 1998.

75. Cervera R, Piette JC, Font J, et al: Antiphospholipid syndrome: clinical and immunologic manifestations and patterns of disease expression in a cohort of 1,000 patients. *Arthritis Rheum* 46:1019–1027, 2002.

76. Jones L, Mont M, Le T, et al: Procoagulants and osteonecrosis. *J Rheumatol* 30:783–791, 2003.

77. Calvo-Alen J, McGwin G, Toloza S, et al: Systemic lupus erythematosus in a multiethnic US cohort (LUMINA): XXIV. Cytotoxic treatment is an additional risk factor for the development of symptomatic osteonecrosis in lupus patients: results of a nested matched case-control study. *Ann Rheum Dis* 65:785–790, 2006.

78. Koo K, Lee J, Lee Y, et al: Endothelial nitric oxide synthase gene polymorphisms in patients with nontraumatic femoral head osteonecrosis. *J Orthop Res* 24:1722–1728, 2006.

79. Amin Kerachian M, Cournoyer D, Harvey E, et al: New insights into the pathogenesis of glucocorticoid-induced avascular necrosis: microarray analysis of gene expression in a rat model. *Arthritis Res Ther* 12:R124, 2010.

80. Ficat R, Arlet J: Functional investigation of bone under normal conditions. In Hungerford D, editor: *Ischemia and necrosis of bone*, Baltimore, 1980, Williams & Wilkins, pp 171–182.

81. Steinberg M, Hayken G, Steinberg D: A new method for evaluation and staging of avascular necrosis of the femoral head. In Arlet J, Ficat R, Hungerford D, editors: *Bone circulation*, Baltimore, 1984, Williams & Wilkins, pp 398–403.

82. Gardeniers J: ARCO international classification of osteonecrosis. *ARCO Newsletter* 5:79, 1993.

83. Mont M, Jones L, Seyler T, et al: New treatment approaches for osteonecrosis of the femoral head: an overview. *Instr Course Lect* 56:197–212, 2007.

84. Araon R, Lennox D, Stulberg G. The natural history of osteonecrosis of the femoral head and risk factors for rapid progression. In Urbaniak J, Jones JJ, editors: *Osteonecrosis: etiology, diagnosis and treatment*, 1997, American Academy of Orthopaedic Surgeons, pp 261–265.

85. Lee M, Chang Y, Chao E, et al: Conditions before collapse of the contralateral hip in osteonecrosis of the femoral head. *Chang Gung Med J* 25:228–237, 2002.

86. Garcia-Carrasco M, Mendoza-Pinto C, Escarcega R, et al: Osteoporosis in patients with systemic lupus erythematosus. *Isr Med Assoc J* 11:486–491, 2009.

87. Ramsey-Goldman R, Dunn J, Huang C, et al: Frequency of fractures in women with systemic lupus erythematosus: comparison with United States population data. *Arthritis Rheum* 42:882–890, 1999.

88. Becker A, Fisher R, Scherbaum W, et al: Osteoporosis screening in systemic lupus erythematosus: impact of disease duration and organ damage. *Lupus* 10:809–814, 2001.

89. Canalis E, Mazziotti G, Giustina A, et al: Glucocorticoid-induced osteoporosis: pathophysiology and therapy. *Osteoporos Int* 18:1319–1328, 2007.

90. Lane N, Yao W: New insights into the biology of glucocorticoid-induced osteoporosis. *IBMS BoneKEy* 8:229–236, 2011.

91. Pereira R, Carvalho J, Canalis E: Glucocorticoid-induced osteoporosis in rheumatic diseases. *Clinics (Sao Paulo)* 65:1195–1205, 2010.

92. Chappard D, Legrand E, Basle M, et al: Altered trabecular architecture induced by corticosteroids: a bone histomorphometric study. *J Bone Miner Res* 11:676–685, 1996.

93. Sambrook P: Glucocorticoid-induced osteoporosis. In Hochberg M, Silman A, Smolen JS, et al, editors: *Rheumatology*, ed 5, Philadelphia, 2011, Mosby Elsevier.

94. Bischoff-Ferrari H, Dietrich T, Orav E, et al: Positive association between 25-hydroxy vitamin D levels and bone mineral density: a population-based study of younger and older adults. *Am J Med* 116:634–639, 2004.

95. Kamen D, Aranow C: Vitamin D in systemic lupus erythematosus. *Curr Opin Rheumatol* 20:532–537, 2008.

96. Shoenfeld N, Amital H, Shoenfeld Y: The effect of melanism and vitamin D synthesis on the incidence of autoimmune disease. *Nat Clin Pract Rheumatol* 5:99–105, 2009.

97. Alele J, Kamen D: The importance of inflammation and vitamin D status in systemic lupus erythematosus associated osteoporosis. *Autoimmun Rev* 9:137–139, 2010.

98. Grossman JM, Gordon R, Ranganath VK, et al: American College of Rheumatology 2010 recommendations for the prevention and treatment of glucocorticoid-induced osteoporosis. *Arthritis Care Res* 62:1515–1526, 2010.

99. Dore RK, Cohen SB, Lane NE, et al: Effects of denosumab on bone mineral density and bone turnover in patients with rheumatoid arthritis receiving concurrent glucocorticoids or bisphosphonates. *Ann Rheum Dis* 69:872–875, 2010.

100. Merrill JT, Buyon JP: Hormones and gender related issues. In Wallace DJ, Hahn BH, editors: *Dubois' lupus erythematosus*, Philadelphia, 2007, Lippincott Williams & Wilkins, pp 1249–1261.

Chapter 26

Pathogenesis and Treatment of Atherosclerosis in Lupus

Maureen McMahon, Brian Skaggs, and Jennifer Grossman

INTRODUCTION

Premature atherosclerosis is a major comorbid condition in systemic lupus erythematosus (SLE). Although typical features of SLE, such as nephritis and vasculitis, have been the traditional focus of treatment, the identification of comorbid conditions such as atherosclerosis has become more important as the treatments for SLE improve and patients live longer. In a landmark study, the higher risk of cardiovascular disease in SLE was first recognized in 1976 by Urowitz, who described a bimodal pattern of mortality in a Toronto SLE cohort.[1] Of the 11 deaths in the cohort, 6 deaths occurred within 1 year of diagnosis and were attributed to active SLE disease. Five patients died at a mean of 8.6 years, all of whom had had a recent myocardial infarction (MI), with 4 of the 5 deaths attributed to fatal MI.[1] This bimodal pattern of mortality due to cardiovascular disease has been confirmed in subsequent studies[2] and appears to have remained constant despite improvements in overall lupus mortality. For example, the mortality rate from atherosclerosis in patients with SLE has been between 6% and 16% in various later series.[3] Data from a large international cohort suggests that although standardized all-cause mortality rates for SLE decreased from 4.9 in 1970 through 1979 to 2.0 in 1990 through 2001, the standardized all-cause mortality rates for cardiovascular disease in lupus did not decrease over the same period.[4]

The overall prevalence of clinical coronary heart disease is also elevated in patients with SLE and has ranged from 6% to 10% in various cohorts.[5-7] This risk is higher than that in the general population; for example, in a Swedish lupus population, the risk of coronary artery disease (CAD) in patients with SLE was ninefold higher than in the age-matched general population.[8] The age of onset of cardiovascular disease in SLE also appears to be younger that in the general population; Manzi found that women with SLE in the 35- to 44-year age group were more than 50 times more likely to have an MI than women of similar age in the Framingham Offspring Study.[5] Cardiovascular events may also result in greater morbidity and mortality in patients with SLE; such patients have higher risk of in-hospital mortality and prolonged length of hospitalizations than both diabetic patients and patients without SLE and diabetes.[9]

SUBCLINICAL MEASURES OF ATHEROSCLEROSIS

Our ultimate goal as treating physicians is to detect increased risk of cardiovascular disease in our patients prior to the onset of cardiovascular events, so that treatment strategies can be initiated to prevent morbidity and mortality. The detection of subclinical atherosclerosis using surrogate measurements can predict cardiovascular morbidity and mortality in the general population.[10] Using a variety of surrogate measurements, several groups have also found that the incidence of subclinical atherosclerosis is increased in patients with SLE. In a cross-sectional study using carotid ultrasound as a surrogate measure, Roman found that carotid plaque was present in 37% of patients with SLE, compared with 15% of controls.[11] In a short-term longitudinal follow-up study of the patients with SLE in this cohort, atherosclerosis developed or progressed at an average rate of 10% per year. Further studies using carotid plaque as a surrogate measure have reflected similar prevalences[12-14] and rates of progression[15] of subclinical atherosclerosis in SLE. Electron-beam computed tomography (EBCT) has also been used as a screening instrument; in one study, coronary calcification was present in 31% of patients with SLE but only 9% of controls.[11] In a study using dual-isotope single-photon emission computed tomographic (SPECT) myocardial perfusion imaging, 38% of patients with SLE had perfusion defects indicating subclinical atherosclerosis.[16] When endothelial dysfunction, another marker of subclinical atherosclerosis, was evaluated by ultrasound in another study, 55% of patients with SLE had impaired flow-mediated dilation, compared with 26.3% of control subjects.[17]

Evidence also exists that in addition to abnormalities of the macrovasculature in SLE, there is abnormal coronary microvascular function as well. In one study, abnormal coronary flow reserve (CFR) (measured by means of positron emission tomography [PET]) was seen even in patients with SLE whose coronary arteries were normal.[18] Further, evidence has now revealed a 44% prevalence of abnormal stress myocardial perfusion as shown by adenosine stress cardiac magnetic resonance imaging (MRI) in the absence of obstructive CAD in patients with SLE and angina chest pain; quantitative myocardial perfusion reserve index (MPRI) was observed to be lower in patients with SLE than in controls, and the presence of SLE was a significant predictor of myocardial perfusion reserve index.[19] It should be noted, however, that although these measures of subclinical atherosclerosis are significantly linked to coronary events in the general population,[10] only abnormal myocardial perfusion has been shown to predict future cardiovascular events in SLE.[16]

TRADITIONAL AND SLE-SPECIFIC RISK FACTORS FOR ATHEROSCLEROSIS IN SLE

Traditional Risk Factors

What factors explain the increased risk of cardiovascular disease in SLE? The mechanisms of the increased and accelerated atherosclerotic risk for patients with SLE remain to be determined. It is likely that multiple mechanisms are operative, with the greater risk of atherosclerosis in SLE resulting from a complex interplay between traditional cardiac risk factors and SLE-driven inflammation.

The traditional Framingham cardiac risk factors—hypertension,[3,6,7] hypercholesterolemia,[1,5,7] diabetes mellitus,[1,7] older age,[3,5,7] tobacco use, and postmenopausal status[3,5]—have all been associated with atherosclerotic disease in patients with SLE (Table 26-1). Assessment of cardiovascular risk factors in the Hopkins Lupus Cohort demonstrated that 53% of patients with SLE had at least three traditional risk factors.[7] Although the frequency of some traditional risk factors, like diabetes and hyperlipidemia, may be increased as secondary effects of glucocorticoid therapy,[20] there is also evidence that traditional risk factors may be directly influenced by SLE disease activity. For example, high levels of very-low-density lipoprotein (VLDL) and triglycerides and low levels of high-density lipoprotein (HDL) have been described as the "lupus pattern," and are more strikingly noted in patients with active disease.[21]

Although traditional cardiac risk factors clearly play a role in the pathogenesis of atherosclerosis in SLE, they do not fully explain the increased risk. For example, after data were controlled for gender,

TABLE 26-1 Traditional and Nontraditional Cardiac Risk Factors in Patients with SLE

RISK FACTOR	STUDIES DEMONSTRATING SIGNIFICANT ASSOCIATION WITH OVERT CLINICAL OR SUBCLINICAL ATHEROSCLEROSIS	STUDIES DEMONSTRATING NO ASSOCIATION
Traditional Risk Factors		
Age	5-7,11,12,14,28,37,116,185,186	
Body mass index	37 Association with increased intima-media thickness (IMT) in children: 36	11,14
Diabetes mellitus	6,186	
Dyslipidemia	13 37	11,14
Homocysteine	12 28	
Hypertension	6,7,17,35,37,187,188	
Menopausal status	5	
Tobacco Use	35	11,14
Nontraditional (SLE-Specific) Risk Factors		
Corticosteroid therapy	Inverse association: 11 High and low doses with increased IMT: 36 13,29,34,37,44 Moderate (0.15-0.4 mg/kg/day) doses with decreased IMT in children: 36	
Renal disease	28 27,33,34,36	37
SLE disease activity	Higher disease activity: 11-13,26,28 Lower disease activity: 13	12,16,27
SLE duration	27, 12,13,26	189
SLE damage	12,13,29	189

blood pressure, diabetes, cholesterol, smoking, and left ventricular hypertrophy in a Canadian cohort, Esdaile found the relative risk attributed to SLE for MI was 10.1 and 7.9 for stroke.[22] In a separate cohort, Chung found that 99% of patients with SLE were identified as having low risk using the Framingham risk calculator, with a 10-year risk estimate of less than 1%; however, EBCT demonstrated coronary calcium in 19% of patients with SLE in the cohort.[23] Similarly, in an SLE cohort from Toronto, the mean Framingham 10-year risk of a cardiac event did not differ in 250 patients with SLE and 250 controls.[24] This study did, however, reveal a higher prevalence of nontraditional cardiac risk factors in patients with SLE, including premature menopause, sedentary lifestyle, and increased waist-to-hip ratio.[24] Thus, although patients with SLE are subject to the same traditional risk factors as the general population,[22,25,26] these factors do not adequately account for the significantly higher level of cardiovascular disease.

SLE-Specific Risk Factors
Disease Activity, Duration, and Damage

The association between SLE disease activity and atherosclerosis has been poorly understood to date. Romero-Diaz reported that higher mean disease activity scores were significantly associated with increased coronary calcium scores[27]; however, Manzi found an inverse relationship between SLE activity and carotid plaque,[13] and several other groups found no association between disease activity and progression of atherosclerosis.[12,28] The association between atherosclerosis and disease duration and damage in SLE has been more consistent; several cross-sectional cohort studies have observed significant associations between longer disease duration and either carotid plaque[13] or coronary calcium scores.[27,29] In a UK study, Haque found that subjects with clinical coronary heart disease were more likely to have higher SLICC (Systemic Lupus International Collaborative Clinics) damage index scores than matched patients with SLE without CHD.[30] Similarly, Roman found through multivariate analysis that longer disease duration and higher SLICC damage index scores were independent predictors of carotid plaque in both a cross-sectional study[11] and a longitudinal study.[12]

Renal Disease

Renal disease also appears to be a risk factor for atherosclerosis in patients with SLE; in one large study, both pediatric and adult patients with end-stage renal disease (ESRD) and SLE had significantly higher mortality due to cardiovascular disease than age-matched patients with ESRD but no SLE.[31] In another study of renal transplant recipients with SLE, 82% had evidence of coronary calcium on EBCT.[32] Active renal disease, including proteinuria[33,34] and elevated serum creatinine,[35,36] has been associated with early atherosclerosis in patients with SLE. A history of previous nephritis has also been associated with subclinical atherosclerosis in some[29,35,37] but not all studies.[11,38] Although the exact mechanisms of the greater cardiovascular disease in patients with SLE nephritis has not been indentified, hypertension[39] and dyslipidemia[40] may contribute to the increased risk, because both are frequently seen in patients with proteinuria. Patients with proteinuria also have an increased risk of thrombosis.[41,42]

Glucocorticoid Therapy

Glucocorticoid use may impact traditional cardiac risk factors such as hypertension, obesity, and diabetes.[43] Additionally, prednisone doses higher than10 mg/day have been shown to independently predict hypercholesterolemia in SLE.[7] Conflicting data exist, however, regarding the overall risk of glucocorticoid therapy: Both longer duration of corticosteroid treatment[13,44] and a higher accumulated corticosteroid dose[13,30,35,38,45] have been associated with a higher incidence of atherosclerosis in various cohorts of patients with SLE. In the APPLE (Atherosclerosis Prevention in Pediatric Lupus Erythematosus) study of pediatric lupus patients, however, the highest and lowest cumulative doses of corticosteroids were associated with increased carotid artery intima media thickness (IMT), and moderate doses were associated with decreased carotid artery IMT.[37] Roman also found that former or current use of prednisone and average dose of prednisone were significantly less in patients with carotid plaque,[11] implying that there may be a threshold dose at which the antiinflammatory effects of glucocorticoids may be atheroprotective, whereas higher doses may be atherogenic.

Antiphospholipid Antibodies

Given the strong relationship of antiphospholipid antibodies (aPLs) with arterial and venous clotting complications in patients with SLE, there has been considerable interest in aPLs' possible involvement in accelerated atherosclerosis. However, the role of aPLs in the development of atherosclerosis in patients with lupus remains controversial. Interestingly, there have been numerous reports of aPLs linked with atherosclerosis in non-lupus populations. Antiphospholipid antibodies have been associated with an increased risk of MI in men in several studies[46,47]; however, the presence of anticardiolipin antibodies (aCLs) in the Physician's Health Study was not linked to an increased risk of ischemic stroke.[48] In a population-based, case-control study in a population of Dutch women younger than 50 years, lupus anticoagulant positivity, although seen in only 3% of women with MIs and 17% with ischemic stroke on the basis of a single determination, was associated with an increased risk of (MI (odds ratio [OR] = 5.3) and ischemic stroke (OR = 43.1) In this study, anti–beta 2 glycoprotein I (β_2-GPI) was associated with an increased risk of stroke but not MI, whereas the presence of aCLs did not increase the risk of either stroke or MI.[49]

There has also been variability in the association between aPLs and subclinical atherosclerosis. Two small case-control series using carotid ultrasound in antiphospholipid syndrome (APS) did not find increased plaque prevalence.[50,51] However, four case-control studies have found that IMT is greater in patients with APS than in healthy controls,[52-54] and one case-control study also found impaired flow-mediated dilation in patients with APS.[55]

Likewise, the associations with aPLs in patients with SLE have been variable. Several studies have demonstrated an association between the presence of aPLs and atherosclerosis in SLE. In the LUpus in MInorities, NAture versus nurture (LUMINA) study, aPLs were an independent risk factor for a cardiovascular or cerebrovascular event after a subject's entry into the cohort.[56] In a univariate analysis, the lupus anticoagulant was the only antiphospholipid associated with MI in the Hopkins Lupus Cohort.[57] However, neither lupus anticoagulant (LAC) nor aCL was associated with subclinical atherosclerosis as assessed by carotid ultrasound.[58] In another study, coronary calcification scores were associated with aPL positivity in a univariate analysis; however, the association was no longer significant when data were adjusted for age and sex.[14] Three studies using carotid ultrasound to detect atherosclerosis did not find any association of plaque with aPL.[11,13,59] In a later study of an inception cohort of 1249 patients with SLE who had 22 atherosclerotic events, there was no association of aPLs with the events.[60]

Animal studies evaluating the role of aPLs in atherosclerosis likewise remain contradictory. George and colleagues immunized LDL receptor–deficient mice with β_2-GPI and found that fatty streak formation was accelerated.[61] The group were also able to accelerate atherosclerosis by passively transferring β_2-GPI–reactive lymphocytes. In a follow-up study, the researchers fed β_2-GPI to LDL receptor–deficient mice to induce oral tolerance. They were able to show that the mice that received the β_2-GPI had less atherosclerosis and that the oral tolerance was successful as assessed by a inhibition of lymph node proliferation to β_2-GPI in these mice.[62]

Other investigators, however, have suggested the aPLs may play a protective role in the pathogenesis of atherosclerosis. Immunization of rabbits,[63] LDL receptor–deficient mice,[64] and apolipoprotein E (apo E)–deficient mice[65] with LDL and/or oxidized LDL (ox-LDL) inhibited the progression of atherosclerotic lesions. Furthermore, passive administration of a monoclonal immunoglobulin (Ig) G cardiolipin–reactive antibody to LDL receptor–deficient mice reduced plaque formation.[66] Further studies are needed to explore the contributions of antiphospholipid antibodies to atherosclerosis.

NOVEL BIOMARKERS/"NON-TRADITIONAL" CARDIAC RISK FACTORS

Several novel biomarkers have been implicated in the pathogenesis of atherosclerosis in SLE. Before a discussion of these novel biomarkers, however, it may be helpful to clarify the relationship between inflammation and the development of atherosclerotic plaques in SLE, a description of which follows.

Inflammation and the Pathogenesis of Atherosclerosis

For many years, atherosclerosis was regarded as a passive accumulation of lipids in the vessel wall. It has been realized, however, that inflammation plays a role not only in the development of the atherosclerotic lesion but also in the acute rupture of plaques that occurs during acute myocardial ischemic events.[67] As in the pathogenesis of SLE itself, the interplay of multiple inflammatory mediators, including leukocytes, cytokines, chemokines, adhesion molecules, complement, and antibodies, results in the formation of atherosclerotic plaques.[67]

Monocyte and T-Cell Recruitment to the Arterial Wall

Changes in the vascular endothelium can accelerate the formation of the atherosclerotic plaque. For example, in response to hemodynamic stress, as in cases of hypertension,[68] or when exposed to inflammatory mediators such as ox-LDL or cytokines such as interleukin-1 (IL-1) and tumor necrosis factor (TNF), the vascular endothelium undergoes a series of inflammatory changes, resulting in endothelial cell activation (ECA).[67] When ECA occurs, there is an up-regulation of leukocyte adhesion molecules such as vascular cell adhesion molecule 1 (VCAM-1), intercellular adhesion molecule 1 (ICAM-1), and E-selectin.[68] Chemoattractant cytokines such as monocyte chemoattractant protein 1 (MCP-1), IL-6, and IL-8 are also expressed,[68] thus inducing a cascade of proinflammatory, proatherogenic changes in the endothelium that results in migration of monocytes into the subendothelial space. T cells are also recruited to the subendothelial by similar mechanisms, although at lower numbers. These T cells are generally T-helper 1 (Th1) CD4[+] cells that secrete proinflammatory and proatherogenic interferon gamma (IFN-γ).[67]

Low-Density Lipoproteins and the Development of Foam Cells

Next, LDLs are transported in a concentration-dependent manner into artery walls, where they become trapped and seeded with reactive oxygen species (ROS) produced by nearby artery wall cells.[69] These LDL phospholipids become oxidized (ox-LDL), and in turn stimulate endothelial cells to release cytokines such as MCP-1, macrophage colony-stimulating factor (M-CSF), and GRO, resulting in further monocyte binding, chemotaxis, and differentiation into macrophages.[67] HDL cholesterol is capable of inhibiting the transmigration of leukocytes in response to ox-LDL.[70] The ox-LDLs are phagocytized by infiltrating monocytes/macrophages, which then become the foam cells around which atherosclerotic lesions are built.[69]

Monocytes and T cells infiltrate the margin of the plaque formed by foam cells. Muscle cells from the media of the artery are stimulated to grow.[67] These muscle cells encroach on the lumen of the vessel and ultimately lead to fibrosis, which can render the plaques brittle. The occlusion that results in MI can occur when one of these plaques ruptures or when platelets aggregate in the narrowed area of the artery.[67]

HDL Clears Ox-LDL from the Endothelium

There are many mechanisms designed to clear ox-LDL from the subendothelial space, such as macrophage engulfment using scavenger receptors and enhanced reverse cholesterol transport mediated by HDL.[71] Both HDL and its major apolipoprotein constituent, apo A-I, have also been shown to prevent and reverse LDL oxidation.[71] In addition to apo A-I, HDL contains several enzymes that can prevent or destroy the formation of the oxidized phospholipids in ox-LDL that induce the inflammatory response; these include paraoxonase, platelet-activating factor acetylhydrolase (PAF-AH), and lecithin : cholesterol acyltransferase (LCAT) (Figure 26-1).[71] HDLs

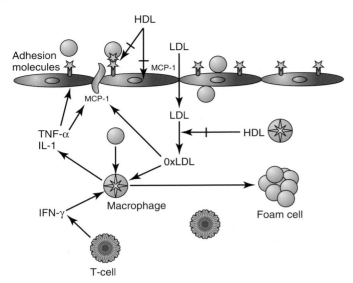

FIGURE 26-1 Atherosclerosis is an inflammatory disorder that is initiated by the interplay of cytokines, lipids, oxidation products, and leukocytes. The process begins when low-density lipoprotein (LDL) enters and is trapped in the arterial intima. LDL is oxidized and transformed into oxidized LDL (OxLDL). OxLDL then activates endothelial cells to express monocyte chemotactic protein 1 (MCP-1), which attracts monocytes from the vessel lumen and into the subendothelial space. OxLDL then promotes the differentiation of monocytes into macrophages. Macrophages in turn release a variety of chemicals, including cytokines. Of these cytokines, tumor necrosis factor alpha (TNF-α) and interleukin-1 (IL-1) activate endothelial cells to express adhesion molecules that bind monocytes, making them available for recruitment into the subendothelial space by MCP-1. Normally functioning high-density lipoprotein (HDL) inhibits the formation of oxidized LDL as well as the expression of endothelial cell adhesion molecules and MCP-1, and promotes the efflux of cholesterol from foam cells. IFN-γ, interferon gamma.

are also capable of inhibiting the expression of cell surface adhesion molecules.[71]

Thus, it is not solely the amount of HDL present that determines atherosclerotic risk, because HDL function is equally significant.[71] However, during the acute-phase response, such as in the postoperative period or during influenza infection, HDLs can be converted from their usual antiinflammatory state to proinflammatory (piHDL). In piHDL, levels of antiinflammatory components of HDL such as apo A-I and HDL-associated paraoxonase activity are reduced.[72] Additionally, acute-phase HDL is greatly enriched in acute-phase reactants such as serum amyloid A.[72] Thus, HDL can be described as a "chameleon-like lipoprotein"—antiinflammatory in the basal state and proinflammatory during the acute-phase response.[71] This acute-phase response, however, can also become chronic and may be a mechanism for HDL dysfunction in SLE.[73]

Innate Immunity in Atherosclerosis
In contrast to adaptive immunity, the components of innate immunity are present at birth and allow for immediate host defenses against pathogens. The receptors of innate immunity are known as pattern recognition receptors (PRRs); these receptors bind to preserved motifs on various pathogens termed pathogen-associated molecular patterns (PAMPs). Toll-like receptors (TLRs) are one type of PRR that respond to various PAMPs by activating their intracellular signaling pathway, leading to the upregulation of immune responsive genes.[74] The ligands for TLRs include microbial ligands, a possibility that may explain some of the connections that have been postulated to exist between infectious organisms such as *Chlamydia pneumoniae* and the development of atherosclerosis. Endogenous ligands can also trigger TLR signaling like microbial ligands do. For

example, minimally oxidized LDL interacts with TLR4 and with the scavenger receptors CD14 and CD36.[75] When ox-LDL binds to the CD14 receptor on macrophages, an inhibition of phagocytosis of apoptotic cells and enhanced expression of the scavenger receptor CD36 occur, leading to increased uptake of ox-LDL. Both of these effects are thought to be proinflammatory and proatherogenic.[69] Activation of TLRr7 and TLR9, resulting in the upregulation of IFN-α, has also been shown to play a major role in lupus disease activity.[76] This pathway may also have implications in atherogenesis, because IFN-α plays a crucial role in premature vascular damage in SLE by altering the balance between endothelial cell apoptosis and vascular repair.[77] High IFN-α levels have been associated with endothelial dysfunction in patients with SLE.[78]

POTENTIAL BIOMARKERS FOR ATHEROSCLEROSIS IN SLE
Many of the inflammatory mediators previously described are also actively involved in the pathogenesis of SLE and are thus likely to play a role in early atherogenesis. Several of these inflammatory factors, as well as traditional risk factors, have been demonstrated in patients with SLE.

Oxidized Low-Density Lipoproteins
As already noted, the oxidation of LDLs is a triggering mechanism in the pathogenesis of atherosclerosis. In fact, high levels of circulating ox-LDL are strongly associated with documented CAD in the general population.[79] There is some speculation that the increased risk of thrombotic and atherosclerotic events associated with ox-LDL may be due in part to a cross-reactivity between aCL and ox-LDL.[80] Cardiolipin is a component of LDL, and anticardiolipin and anti–ox-LDL antibodies have been shown to be cross-reactive.[80] Additionally, β₂-GPI has been shown to bind directly and stably to ox-LDL.[81] Elevations of circulating ox-LDL have been described in patients with SLE and are associated in some reports with a history of cardiovascular disease.[45,82] Levels of the oxidized phospholipid 1-palmitoyl-2-arachidonyl-sn-phosphtidylcholine (ox-PAPC) have also been associated with thickened IMT on carotid ultrasound.[35] ox-LDL–β₂-GPI complexes are also associated with a risk of arterial thrombosis.[83] Interestingly, renal manifestations of SLE have been associated with both higher levels of circulating ox-LDL[82] and circulating ox-LDL/β₂-GPI complexes.[84]

Circulating antibodies to ox-LDL (anti–ox-LDL) have also been described, although their relationship with the development and progression of atherosclerosis is unclear. Antibodies that recognize ox-LDL are generally considered to be protective against atherosclerosis in murine models,[67] but one human study demonstrated a positive association between autoantibodies to ox-LDL and a history of cardiovascular disease in patients with SLE.[45] Conversely, another study demonstrated that antibody titers to one phospholipid component of ox-LDL, phosphorylcholine (anti-PC antibodies), were inversely correlated with the presence of vulnerable carotid plaques in SLE.[85] In two other studies, anti–ox-LDL and arterial disease were not associated.[86,87] Titers of antibodies to ox-LDL have also been associated with disease activity in SLE.[88]

Lipoprotein(a)
In addition to oxidized LDL, lipoprotein(a) (Lp[a]) has also been implicated in the pathogenesis of atherosclerosis in both the general and SLE populations.[79] Lp(a) is structurally related to LDL but also contains apolipoprotein(a), which is covalently linked to apolipoprotein B-100.[89] Lp(a) has been shown to physically associate with both proinflammatory ox-LDL[89] and β₂-GPI.[89] Circulating plasma levels of Lp(a) have been associated with CAD in the general population[90] and in rheumatoid arthritis.[89] Several researchers have also found elevations of Lp(a) in patients with SLE.[91-93] One study reported that serum Lp(a) levels were increased in patients with lupus who also had renal disease and hypoalbuminemia and that treatment with corticosteroids reduced the elevations.[93] Another group reported,

however, that Lp(a) levels are not influenced by corticosteroids or disease activity.[92] Lp(a) can also become oxidized (ox-Lp[a]), and levels of ox-Lp(a) and Lp(a)–β_2-GPI complexes are also higher in subjects with SLE than in controls.[89,94] Higher Lp(a) levels were associated on univariate analysis with increased carotid IMT in a pediatric cohort of subjects with SLE[37] but were not associated with plaque in one adult cohort.[95]

High-Density Lipoproteins: Function and Structure
Proinflammatory HDL
Although quantities of HDL partially determine atherosclerotic risk (low levels are associated with increased risk), HDL function is equally significant.[71] For example, as described, during the acute-phase response, HDLs can be converted from their usual antiinflammatory state to proinflammatory and can actually cause increased oxidation of LDL.[72] This acute-phase response can also become chronic[71] and may be a mechanism for HDL dysfunction in SLE. Indeed, our group has found that HDL function is abnormal in many women with SLE; 45% of women with SLE in our study, compared with 20% of patients with rheumatoid arthritis and 4% of controls, had piHDL that not only was unable to prevent oxidation of LDL but also caused increased levels of oxidation.[73] In this study, four of four patients with SLE with a history of documented atherosclerosis had piHDL, further suggesting that HDL play an important role in the pathogenesis of atherosclerosis. Subsequent studies have indicated that 85% of women SLE with in whom plaque is demonstrated on carotid ultrasound have piHDL, indicating that piHDL may be a biomarker of risk for atherosclerosis in SLE.[38] In addition, HDL appears to be dysfunctional in primary APS, in that HDL isolated from women with APS had blunted beneficial effects on VCAM-1 expression, superoxide production, and monocyte adhesion following activation of human aortic endothelial cells.[55]

In a previous study, our group reported that abnormalities in any one of the measurable components of HDL does not appear to fully explain the piHDL function seen in subjects with SLE.[94] There is evidence, however, that some of the functional components of HDL may also individually contribute to the pathogenesis of atherosclerosis in SLE, as described in detail here.

Apolipoprotein A-I and Antibodies to It
As noted previously, apo A-I, the major apolipoprotein component of HDL, exerts its beneficial effects by enhancing reverse cholesterol transport and preventing the oxidation of LDL and subsequent recruitment of inflammatory mediators.[71] Reduced levels of both HDL and apo A-I have been found in patients with SLE who have IgG anticardiolipin antibodies.[96] Treatment of a murine model of accelerated atherosclerosis and lupus with an apo A-I–mimetic peptide resulted in improvements in proteinuria, glomerulonephritis, osteopenia, and anti–oxidized phospholipid titers.[97] In addition, although overall aortic plaque size was increased in treated animals, a less atherogenic plaque phenotype was seen, with decreases in macrophage infiltration, smooth muscle content, and proatherogenic chemokines.[97]

In the general population, antibodies to apo A-I have been found in up to 21% of patients with acute coronary syndromes who have no other features of autoimmune disease.[98] Antibodies to apo A-I have also been described in SLE; in one study, antibodies to apo A-I were found in 32.5% of patients with SLE and 22.9% of patients with primary APS.[99] It is unclear, however, how the presence of these antibodies affects the function of apo A-I in patients with either SLE or acute coronary syndrome.

Paraoxonase
Serum paraoxonase 1 (PON1) is a serum esterase that is secreted primarily by the liver and is associated with HDL in plasma. PON1 has been identified as one of the important components of HDL that prevents lipid peroxidation and blocks the proinflammatory effects of mildly oxidized LDL.[71] Decreased levels of PON activity have also

been associated with atherosclerosis in the general population.[100] Altered levels of PON activity have also been seen in patients with SLE. In one study, PON activity was lower in patients with SLE and APS than in controls, although there was no reduction in the total antioxidant capacity of the plasma.[101] In that study, antibodies against HDL and β_2-GPI were associated with the reduction in PON1 activity.[101] Similarly, in patients with aCLs, PON1 activity was lower than in healthy controls.[102] Although further investigation is necessary, it is possible that the antibodies against HDL and β_2-GPI contribute to the oxidation of LDL through a cross-reactive, inhibitory effect on PON activity.[101] Decreased PON activity has been associated with increased carotid artery IMT and abnormal flow-mediated dilation in patients with primary APS[55] and also with atherosclerotic events in patients with SLE.[103]

Adipocytokines
White adipose tissue has been recognized as an endocrine organ that secretes adipokines that regulate energy homeostasis and metabolism. The adipokine leptin is an anorectic peptide that acts on the hypothalamus to modulate food intake, body weight, and fat stores.[104] Obese patients have high circulating leptin levels, but they develop resistance to leptin similar to insulin resistance in type 2 diabetes.[104] Hyperleptinemia in the general population is associated with hypertension, metabolic syndrome, and atherosclerosis.[104] In addition, leptin has been linked to increased ox-LDL levels and greater oxidative stress in endothelial cells and cardiomyocytes.[105] Conversely, adiponectin is the most abundant adipocytokine in human plasma, and its levels are inversely correlated with adipose tissue mass.[106] Adiponectin levels are reduced in type 2 diabetes and cardiovascular disease.[106]

Several small cohort studies have shown elevated leptin values in adult[107-109] and pediatric[110] patients with SLE. In our cohort, mean leptin levels were significantly higher in the patients with SLE who had carotid plaque than in those without plaque, and also weakly correlated with carotid IMT.[94] In another cohort, adiponectin levels were significantly and independently associated with carotid plaque in SLE.[111] However, Chung found no significant relationship between leptin or adiponectin levels and coronary calcification.[112]

Markers of Endothelial Dysfunction
A number of abnormalities of the vascular endothelium have been described in association with SLE. Endothelial function can be measured by examining endothelium-dependent dilation, or flow-mediated dilation (FMD), of the brachial artery in response to reactive hyperemia.[68] Endothelial dysfunction has been described as an early abnormality in the development of atherosclerosis and is predictive of subsequent cardiovascular events in the general population.[113] Increased endothelial dysfunction has been described in several adult and pediatric SLE cohorts.[17,114] One pediatric population with SLE, however, demonstrated normal endothelial function.[96] Markers of endothelial cell activation are also associated with atherosclerosis in SLE. In one study, von Willebrand factor, VCAM-1, and fibrinogen were significantly associated with cardiovascular events.[115] In separate cohorts, E-selectin and VCAM-1 were associated with increased coronary calcium[116] and carotid plaque.[111] Antibodies to endothelial cells have also been described in up to 63% of subjects with SLE.[117] Patients with these anti–endothelial cell antibodies were also found to have an increased prevalence of vascular lesions (including arterial and venous thrombosis and vasculitis), lupus nephritis, and anticardiolipin antibodies.[117]

C-Reactive Protein
C-reactive protein (CRP) is an acute-phase reactant that is synthesized in the liver in response to IL-6. It has been well established as a predictor of cardiovascular events in the general population; high levels of both CRP and cholesterol levels are high increase the overall risk for development of a future cardiovascular event up to ninefold.[118] There is evidence that CRP is not solely a marker of systemic

inflammation but, rather, may play a direct role in the pathogenesis of atherosclerosis. For example, CRP has been shown in vitro to activate endothelial cells to express ICAM, VCAM, and E-selectin.[119] CRP has also been shown to activate complement,[120] induce endothelial cells to produce MCP-1,[121] and mediate macrophage uptake of LDL.[122] In subjects with SLE, however, the role of CRP as a predictor of atherosclerosis is less clear. In one cross-sectional study, Manzi found that CRP was significantly associated with focal plaque, although this effect did not persist in the logistic regression models[13]; in a separate cross-sectional study, the same group found that high CRP levels, that is, greater than 4 mg/mL, were independent determinants of IMT.[36] Another group found positive high-sensitivity CRP test results to be associated with longitudinal progression of carotid IMT.[28] Several other studies, however, did not find an association between atherosclerosis and CRP in SLE.[11,38,59]

Homocysteine

Homocysteine is another predictor of atherosclerosis in the general population.[124] A metabolite in methionine production, homocysteine may play a direct role in the pathogenesis of SLE through its toxic effects on the endothelium.[125] Homocysteine is also prothrombotic[126] and decreases the availability of nitric oxide.[127] High levels stimulate monocytes to secrete MCP-1 and IL-8.[128] The thiolactone metabolite of homocysteine combines with LDL to enhance foam cell formation in vessel walls.[129] The molecule releases free oxygen radicals that can damage tissue,[130] and there are several prothrombotic actions on platelets and endothelial cells.[131] Hyperhomocysteinemia can result from increased age, medications such as methotrexate, genetic, and/or dietary factors.[132] Renal insufficiency is also a known cause of homocysteine elevations,[133] but the exact mechanism of hyperhomocysteinemia in SLE has not been fully established and will need to be further elucidated in future studies.

In several studies, elevations of homocysteine in SLE correlated with cross-sectional[24,29,44,45,134] and longitudinal progression[12,135] of subclinical atherosclerosis in SLE. In other studies of SLE, however, homocysteine did not correlate with atherosclerosis.[11,14,34]

STRATEGIES FOR PREVENTION OF CARDIOVASCULAR COMPLICATIONS IN SLE
Minimizing Framingham Risk Factors

In the future, it is likely that novel "SLE-specific" risk prediction panels will be developed and validated for identification of high-risk patients who should be targeted for therapeutic interventions to prevent cardiovascular complications. Currently, expert panels in both the United States and Europe recommend that patients with SLE be annually screened for traditional modifiable risk factors for cardiovascular disease, including smoking status, blood pressure, body mass index (BMI), diabetes, and serum lipids (including total cholesterol, HDL, LDL, and triglycerides)[136,137]; however, once risk factors have been identified, there are no randomized clinical trials for the prevention of atherosclerosis in SLE to guide clinicians, and potential difficulties with recruitment and retention of subjects may act as future significant barriers to performing such trials in patients with SLE.[138] Thus, our current screening and treatment strategies are extrapolated from the best available evidence in the general population. There are some lupus-specific issues to consider in the management of traditional cardiac risk factors and disease activity, as described here.

Hypertension

Because of the high relative risk for cardiovascular morbidity and mortality in SLE, some researchers have advocated that SLE should be considered a cardiac risk equivalent similar to diabetes.[123] Therefore patients with SLE should be treated to the target blood pressure levels of 130 mm Hg systolic/80 mm Hg diastolic, as recommended by the Seventh Report of the Joint National Committee on Prevention, Detection, Evaluation, and Treatment of High Blood Pressure (JNC 7) for those with other high-risk comorbid conditions.[139,140] No

optimum SLE-specific atheroprotective medication regimen has been established[141]; however, angiotensin-converting enzyme (ACE) inhibitors are generally the drug of choice in patients with SLE with renal disease,[142] and the European League Against Rheumatism (EULAR) guidelines also recommend these agents as first-line therapy in patients with inflammatory arthritis because of the potential favorable effects on inflammatory markers and EC function in rheumatoid arthritis.[143] In high-risk patients in the general population, ACE inhibitors do reduce risk of MI, stroke, and death.[144] Angiotensin receptor blockers (ARBs) can also be considered in patients who cannot tolerate ACE inhibitor therapy.[145] Thiazide diuretics are recommended by as first-line therapy for hypertension in the general population by JNC 7 and would generally also be a safe choice in subjects with SLE (although caution should be used, as thiazide diuretics also have dyslipidemic and diabetogenic effects).[140] Beta-blockers have been shown to precipitate Raynaud phenomenon[146] and thus should be used with caution in subjects with SLE.

Dyslipidemia: Statin Use

Statins are competitive inhibitors of hydroxymethylglutaryl–coenzyme A (HMG-CoA) reductase, the rate-limiting step in cholesterol biosynthesis,[147] and are now used widely in the general population to reduce cardiovascular morbidity.[148-150] In addition to their lipid-lowering properties, statins have a variety of direct antiinflammatory and immunomodulatory effects, including diminished secretion of proinflammatory, proatherogenic cytokines and chemokines such as IL-6, IL-8, TNF-α, MCP-1, IFN-γ, IL-2, and IL-12,[151-154] and increased secretion of antiatherogenic cytokines such as IL-4 and IL-10.[155-157] These findings, however, have not been consistently demonstrated in all studies.[152,158] Statins also inhibit adhesion molecules, formation of ROS, activation of T cells, and upregulation of nitric oxide synthesis.[159]

Although there is an abundance of data to support the use of statins in primary and secondary prevention of atherosclerosis in the general population,[148,160,161] the data in lupus have been much less consistent. Several studies have also examined the efficacy of statins in prevention of atherosclerosis in rheumatic diseases. In one study using a rat model of adjuvant-induced arthritis, fluvastatin reversed aortic endothelial dysfunction although it did not affect the severity of arthritis or serum cholesterol concentrations.[162] The statins also decreased ROS production in the aorta.[162] Another study examined the effect of statins in a mouse model of SLE and atherosclerosis, the gld.apoE$^{-/-}$ mouse.[163] Although simvastatin therapy did not alter cholesterol levels, it did decrease atherosclerotic lesion area in both the gld.apoE$^{-/-}$ and apoE$^{-/-}$ mice. In addition, simvastatin reduced lymphadenopathy, renal disease, and proinflammatory cytokine production in the double-knockout mouse.[163] Further studies are necessary, but these findings raise the possibility that statins may be beneficial in reducing not only the increased atherosclerosis of rheumatic disease but also the disease-related inflammation.

There are some data to support the use of statins in patients with SLE as well. In a trial of 64 women with SLE, atorvastatin 20 mg daily for 8 weeks improved endothelium-dependent vasodilation, even after the presence of traditional cardiac risk factors were accounted for.[164] In a 2-year randomized controlled trial of atorvastatin in 200 women with SLE, however, statins did not significantly prevent progression of coronary calcium, IMT, or disease activity.[165] Similarly, in a trial of 33 post–renal transplant patients with lupus, those randomly assigned to fluvastatin therapy had a 73% lower rate of cardiac events, although this difference did not quite reach statistical significance ($P = 0.06$). Many trials that have demonstrated a preventive effect of statins in the general population have larger sample sizes and a longer follow-up duration,[166] so it is possible that larger sample sizes and longer study duration in studies of subjects with SLE might have resulted in positive results. Further investigations are needed to clarify the role that statins could play in the prevention of atherosclerosis in rheumatic disease populations. Until further studies are conducted to determine the safety and efficacy of statin therapy in a broader population of patients with SLE, this therapy should be limited to use according to published guidelines such as the National Cholesterol Education Panel.[167]

MODULATORS OF LUPUS DISEASE ACTIVITY
Antimalarial Therapy

Hydroxychloroquine is thought to be cardioprotective,[168] and in fact, Selzer noted that nonuse of hydroxychloroquine was associated with higher aortic stiffness[169] and plaque on carotid ultrasound in patients with SLE.[11] Additionally, antimalarials have been shown to minimize steroid-induced hypercholesterolemia[170] and to lower fasting blood glucose concentrations.[171] Multiple retrospective cohort studies have shown a reduced incidence of thrombotic events[172-175] and improved overall survival[174,176] in patients with SLE treated with antimalarial agents. The understanding that one mechanism of action of hydroxychloroquine is the antagonism of TLR7 and TLR9 signaling is also intriguing, given the postulated roles of IFN-α in endothelial dysfunction and abnormal vascular repair.[177] Prospective studies demonstrating a cardioprotective effect of hydroxychloroquine in patients with SLE are needed.

Azathioprine

One retrospective case-control study of patients with SLE who had documented CAD found that patients with CAD were more likely to have been treated with azathioprine.[30] Azathioprine use was also associated with cardiac events in the multiethnic LUMINA cohort[178] and with increased carotid IMT in the pediatric SLE APPLE cohort.[37] Further studies will be needed to determine whether these associations are due to a direct effect of azathioprine or to the inability of azathioprine to overcome the inflammation that leads to atherosclerosis.

Glucocorticoids

As discussed previously, glucocorticoid use has been associated with atherosclerosis in patients with SLE,[38] although it is unclear whether steroid use is atheroprotective or contributes to added cardiovascular disease risk in such patients. In a pediatric lupus cohort, moderate doses of prednisone (0.15-0.4 mg/kg/day) were associated with decreased carotid artery IMT, whereas high- and low-dose prednisone regimens were associated with increased IMT,[37] suggesting a narrow "therapeutic window" for the atheroprotective effects of glucocorticoid therapy. Until such a threshold is determined, we recommend following the EULAR recommendations that the lowest possible dose of corticosteroids be used in individual patients.[143]

Mycophenolate Mofetil

Mycophenolate mofetil (MMF) has several potential antiatherogenic effects. In animal models, MMF inhibits nicotinamide adenine dinucleotide phosphate (NADPH) oxidase, thereby inhibiting oxidative stress.[179] In LDLr⁻⁻⁻ mice reconstituted with SLE-prone bone marrow, MMF treatment significantly reduced atherosclerotic burden and recruitment of CD4⁺ T cells to atherosclerotic plaques.[180] In patients with carotid artery stenosis, 2 weeks of MMF therapy resulted in increased numbers of regulatory T cells and decreased plaque expression of inflammatory genes.[181] In addition, a retrospective study found 20% lower cardiovascular mortality among diabetic renal transplant recipients who were treated with MMF than in those who underwent immunosuppressive regimens without MMF.[182] A small prospective observational study from our own group suggests that 12-week treatment with MMF and hydroxychloroquine, but not azathioprine, results in significant improvement of proinflammatory HDL function (2011). In a 2011 longitudinal SLE cohort study, however, exposure of subjects to MMF was not associated with a reduction in IMT or coronary calcium progression.[183] Larger, prospective studies must be undertaken to clarify the potential role of MMF in prevention of progression of atherosclerosis in SLE.

SUMMARY

Atherosclerosis is a complicated inflammatory process characterized by the interactions of numerous different moieties, including lipids, enzymes, endothelial cells, cytokines, and peripheral blood mononuclear cells. The prevalence of atherosclerosis is higher in SLE and occurs at an earlier age. The lupus-related factors that account for this increased risk are likely numerous and related to the factors described in this chapter. Expanding our understanding of the pathogenesis of atherosclerosis in SLE is critical if we are to improve both the quality of care for and the mortality in this vulnerable population.

References

1. Urowitz MB, Bookman AA, Koehler BE, et al: The bimodal mortality pattern of systemic lupus erythematosus. *Am J Med* 60:221–225, 1976.
2. Abu-Shakra M, Urowitz MB, Gladman DD, et al: Mortality studies in systemic lupus erythematosus. Results from a single center. II. Predictor variables for mortality. *J Rheumatol* 22:1265–1270, 1995.
3. Aranow C, Ginzler EM: Epidemiology of cardiovascular disease in systemic lupus erythematosus. *Lupus* 9:166–169, 2000.
4. Bernatsky S, Boivin JF, Joseph L, et al: Mortality in systemic lupus erythematosus. *Arthritis Rheum* 54:2550–2557, 2006.
5. Manzi S, Meilahn EN, Rairie JE, et al: Age-specific incidence rates of myocardial infarction and angina in women with systemic lupus erythematosus: comparison with the Framingham Study. *Am J Epidemiol* 145: 408–415, 1997.
6. Gladman DD, Urowitz MB: Morbidity in systemic lupus erythematosus. *J Rheumatol* 14(Suppl 13):223–226, 1987.
7. Petri M, Perez-Gutthann S, Spence D, et al: Risk factors for coronary artery disease in patients with systemic lupus erythematosus. *Am J Med* 93:513–519, 1992.
8. Jonsson H, Nived O, Sturfelt G: Outcome in systemic lupus erythematosus: a prospective study of patients from a defined population. *Medicine (Baltimore)* 68:141–150, 1989.
9. Shah MA, Shah AM, Krishnan E: Poor outcomes after acute myocardial infarction in systemic lupus erythematosus. *J Rheumatol* 36:570–575, 2009.
10. Folsom AR, Kronmal RA, Detrano RC, et al: Coronary artery calcification compared with carotid intima-media thickness in the prediction of cardiovascular disease incidence: the Multi-Ethnic Study of Atherosclerosis (MESA). *Arch Intern Med* 168:1333–1339, 2008.
11. Roman MJ, Shanker BA, Davis A, et al: Prevalence and correlates of accelerated atherosclerosis in systemic lupus erythematosus. *N Engl J Med* 349:2399–2406, 2003.
12. Roman MJ, Crow MK, Lockshin MD, et al: Rate and determinants of progression of atherosclerosis in systemic lupus erythematosus. *Arthritis Rheum* 56:3412–3419, 2007.
13. Manzi S, Selzer F, Sutton-Tyrrell K, et al: Prevalence and risk factors of carotid plaque in women with systemic lupus erythematosus. *Arthritis Rheum* 42:51–60, 1999.
14. Asanuma Y, Oeser A, Shintani AK, et al: Premature coronary-artery atherosclerosis in systemic lupus erythematosus. *N Engl J Med* 349:2407–2415, 2003.
15. Thompson T, Sutton-Tyrrell K, Wildman RP, et al: Progression of carotid intima-media thickness and plaque in women with systemic lupus erythematosus. *Arthritis Rheum* 58:835–842, 2008.
16. Nikpour M, Gladman DD, Ibanez D, et al: Myocardial perfusion imaging in assessing risk of coronary events in patients with systemic lupus erythematosus. *J Rheumatol* 36:288–294, 2009.
17. El-Magadmi M, Bodill H, Ahmad Y, et al: Systemic lupus erythematosus: an independent risk factor for endothelial dysfunction in women. *Circulation* 110:399–404, 2004.
18. Recio-Mayoral A, Mason JC, Kaski JC, et al: Chronic inflammation and coronary microvascular dysfunction in patients without risk factors for coronary artery disease. *Eur Heart J* 30:1837–1843, 2009.
19. Mariko L, Ishimori RM, Daniel SB, et al: Noel Bairey Merz: Myocardial Ischemia in the Absence of Obstructive Coronary Artery Disease in Systemic Lupus Erythematosus Original Research Article. *JACC: Cardiovascular Imaging* 4:27–33, 2011.
20. Henkin Y, Como JA, Oberman A: Secondary dyslipidemia. Inadvertent effects of drugs in clinical practice. *JAMA* 267:961–968, 1992.
21. Borba EF, Bonfa E: Dyslipoproteinemias in systemic lupus erythematosus: influence of disease, activity, and anticardiolipin antibodies. *Lupus* 6:533–539, 1997.

22. Esdaile JM, Abrahamowicz M, Grodzicky T, et al: Traditional Framingham risk factors fail to fully account for accelerated atherosclerosis in systemic lupus erythematosus. *Arthritis Rheum* 44:2331–2337, 2001.

23. Chung CP, Oeser A, Avalos I, et al: Cardiovascular risk scores and the presence of subclinical coronary artery atherosclerosis in women with systemic lupus erythematosus. *Lupus* 15:562–569, 2006.

24. Bruce IN, Urowitz MB, Gladman DD, et al: Risk factors for coronary heart disease in women with systemic lupus erythematosus: the Toronto Risk Factor Study. *Arthritis Rheum* 48:3159–3167, 2003.

25. Petri M: Hopkins Lupus Cohort. 1999 update. *Rheum Dis Clin North Am* 26:199–213, 2000. v.

26. Cervera R, Khamashta MA, Font J, et al: Morbidity and mortality in systemic lupus erythematosus during a 5-year period. A multicenter prospective study of 1,000 patients. European Working Party on Systemic Lupus Erythematosus. *Medicine (Baltimore)* 78:167–175, 1999.

27. Romero-Diaz J, Vargas-Vorackova F, Kimura-Hayama E, et al: Systemic lupus erythematosus risk factors for coronary artery calcifications. *Rheumatology (Oxford)* 51:110–119, 2012.

28. Kiani AN, Post WS, Magder LS, et al: Predictors of progression in atherosclerosis over 2 years in systemic lupus erythematosus. *Rheumatology (Oxford)* 50:2071–2079, 2011.

29. Von Feldt JM, Scalzi LV, Cucchiara AJ, et al: Homocysteine levels and disease duration independently correlate with coronary artery calcification in patients with systemic lupus erythematosus. *Arthritis Rheum* 54:2220–2227, 2006.

30. Haque S, Gordon C, Isenberg D, et al: Risk factors for clinical coronary heart disease in systemic lupus erythematosus: the lupus and atherosclerosis evaluation of risk (LASER) study. *J Rheumatol* 37:322–329, 2010.

31. Sule S, Fivush B, Neu A, et al: Increased risk of death in pediatric and adult patients with ESRD secondary to lupus. *Pediatr Nephrol* 26:93–98, 2011.

32. Norby GE, Gunther A, Mjoen G, et al: Prevalence and risk factors for coronary artery calcification following kidney transplantation for systemic lupus erythematosus. *Rheumatology (Oxford)* 50:1659–1664, 2011.

33. Theodoridou A, Bento L, D'Cruz DP, et al: Prevalence and associations of an abnormal ankle-brachial index in systemic lupus erythematosus: a pilot study. *Ann Rheum Dis* 62:1199–1203, 2003.

34. Manger K, Kusus M, Forster C, et al: Factors associated with coronary artery calcification in young female patients with SLE. *Ann Rheum Dis* 62:846–850, 2003.

35. Doria A, Shoenfeld Y, Wu R, et al: Risk factors for subclinical atherosclerosis in a prospective cohort of patients with systemic lupus erythematosus. *Ann Rheum Dis* 62:1071–1077, 2003.

36. Selzer F, Sutton-Tyrrell K, Fitzgerald SG, et al: Comparison of risk factors for vascular disease in the carotid artery and aorta in women with systemic lupus erythematosus. *Arthritis Rheum* 50:151–159, 2004.

37. Schanberg LE, Sandborg C, Barnhart HX, et al: Premature atherosclerosis in pediatric systemic lupus erythematosus: risk factors for increased carotid intima-media thickness in the atherosclerosis prevention in pediatric lupus erythematosus cohort. *Arthritis Rheum* 60:1496–1507, 2009.

38. McMahon M, Grossman J, Skaggs B, et al: Dysfunctional proinflammatory high-density lipoproteins confer increased risk of atherosclerosis in women with systemic lupus erythematosus. *Arthritis Rheum* 60:2428–2437, 2009.

39. Mak A, Mok CC, Chu WP, et al: Renal damage in systemic lupus erythematosus: a comparative analysis of different age groups. *Lupus* 16:28–34, 2007.

40. Leong KH, Koh ET, Feng PH, et al: Lipid profiles in patients with systemic lupus erythematosus. *J Rheumatol* 21:1264–1267, 1994.

41. Nickolas TL, Radhakrishnan J, Appel GB: Hyperlipidemia and thrombotic complications in patients with membranous nephropathy. *Semin Nephrol* 23:406–411, 2003.

42. Ordonez JD, Hiatt RA, Killebrew EJ, et al: The increased risk of coronary heart disease associated with nephrotic syndrome. *Kidney Int* 44:638–642, 1993.

43. Liang MH, Mandl LA, Costenbader K, et al: Atherosclerotic vascular disease in systemic lupus erythematosus. *J Natl Med Assoc* 94:813–819, 2002.

44. Petri M: Detection of coronary artery disease and the role of traditional risk factors in the Hopkins Lupus Cohort. *Lupus* 9:170–175, 2000.

45. Svenungsson E, Jensen-Urstad K, Heimburger M, et al: Risk factors for cardiovascular disease in systemic lupus erythematosus. *Circulation* 104:1887–1893, 2001.

46. Wu R, Nityanand S, Berglund L, et al: Antibodies against cardiolipin and oxidatively modified LDL in 50-year-old men predict myocardial infarction. *Arterioscler Thromb Vasc Biol* 17:3159–3163, 1997.

47. Vaarala O, Manttari M, Manninen V, et al: Anti-cardiolipin antibodies and risk of myocardial infarction in a prospective cohort of middle-aged men. *Circulation* 91:232–237, 1995.

48. Ginsburg KS, Liang MH, Newcomer L, et al: Anticardiolipin antibodies and the risk for ischemic stroke and venous thrombosis. *Ann Intern Med* 117:997–1002, 1992.

49. Urbanus RT, Siegerink B, Roest M, et al: Antiphospholipid antibodies and risk of myocardial infarction and ischaemic stroke in young women in the RATIO study: a case-control study. *Lancet Neurol* 8:998–1005, 2009.

50. Bilora F, Boccioletti V, Girolami B, et al: Are antiphospholipid antibodies an independent risk factor for atherosclerosis? *Clin Appl Thromb Hemost* 8:103–113, 2002.

51. Jimenez S, Garcia-Criado MA, Tassies D, et al: Preclinical vascular disease in systemic lupus erythematosus and primary antiphospholipid syndrome. *Rheumatology (Oxford)* 44:756–761, 2005.

52. Medina G, Casaos D, Jara LJ, et al: Increased carotid artery intima-media thickness may be associated with stroke in primary antiphospholipid syndrome. *Ann Rheum Dis* 62:607–610, 2003.

53. Veres K, Papp K, Lakos G, et al: Association of HELLP syndrome with primary antiphospholipid syndrome–a case report. *Clin Rheumatol* 27:111–113, 2008.

54. Margarita A, Batuca J, Scenna G, et al: Subclinical atherosclerosis in primary antiphospholipid syndrome. *Ann N Y Acad Sci* 1108:475–480, 2007.

55. Charakida M, Besler C, Batuca JR, et al: Vascular abnormalities, paraoxonase activity, and dysfunctional HDL in primary antiphospholipid syndrome. *JAMA* 302:1210–1217, 2009.

56. Toloza SM, Roseman JM, Alarcon GS, et al: Systemic lupus erythematosus in a multiethnic US cohort (LUMINA): XXII. Predictors of time to the occurrence of initial damage. *Arthritis Rheum* 50:3177–3186, 2004.

57. Petri M: Update on anti-phospholipid antibodies in SLE: the Hopkins' Lupus Cohort. *Lupus* 19:419–423, 2010.

58. Petri M: The lupus anticoagulant is a risk factor for myocardial infarction (but not atherosclerosis): Hopkins Lupus Cohort. *Thromb Res* 114:593–595, 2004.

59. McMahon M, Grossman J, Skaggs B, et al: Dysfunctional pro-inflammatory high density lipoproteins confer increased risk for atherosclerosis in women with systemic lupus erythematosus. *Arthritis Rheum* 60:2428–2437, 2009.

60. Urowitz MB, Gladman D, Ibanez D, et al: Atherosclerotic vascular events in a multinational inception cohort of systemic lupus erythematosus. *Arthritis Care Res (Hoboken)* 62:881–887, 2010.

61. George J, Harats D, Gilburd B, et al: Adoptive transfer of beta-glycoprotein I-reactive lymphocytes enhances early atherosclerosis in LDL receptor-deficient mice. *Circulation* 102:1822–1827, 2000.

62. George J, Yacov N, Breitbart E, et al: Suppression of early atherosclerosis in LDL-receptor deficient mice by oral tolerance with beta 2-glycoprotein I. *Cardiovasc Res* 62:603–609, 2004.

63. Ameli S, Hultgardh-Nilsson A, Regnstrom J, et al: Effect of immunization with homologous LDL and oxidized LDL on early atherosclerosis in hypercholesterolemic rabbits. *Arterioscler Thromb Vasc Biol* 16:1074–1109, 1996.

64. Freigang S, Horkko S, Miller E, et al: Immunization of LDL receptor-deficient mice with homologous malondialdehyde-modified and native LDL reduces progression of atherosclerosis by mechanisms other than induction of high titers of antibodies to oxidative neoepitopes. *Arterioscler Thromb Vasc Biol* 18:1972–1982, 1998.

65. George J, Afek A, Gilburd B, et al: Hyperimmunization of apo-E-deficient mice with homologous malondialdehyde low-density lipoprotein suppresses early atherogenesis. *Atherosclerosis* 138:147–152, 1998.

66. Nicolo D, Goldman BI, Monestier M: Reduction of atherosclerosis in low-density lipoprotein receptor-deficient mice by passive administration of antiphospholipid antibody. *Arthritis Rheum* 48:2974–2978, 2003.

67. Hansson GK, Hermansson A: The immune system in atherosclerosis. *Nat Immunol* 12:204–212, 2011.

68. Hunt BJ: The endothelium in atherogenesis. *Lupus* 9:189–193, 2000.

69. Moore KJ, Tabas I: Macrophages in the pathogenesis of atherosclerosis. *Cell* 145:341–355, 2011.

70. Navab M, Imes SS, Hama SY, et al: Monocyte transmigration induced by modification of low density lipoprotein in cocultures of human aortic wall cells is due to induction of monocyte chemotactic protein 1

synthesis and is abolished by high density lipoprotein. *J Clin Invest* 88:2039–2046, 1991.

71. Navab M, Reddy ST, Van Lenten BJ, et al: HDL and cardiovascular disease: atherogenic and atheroprotective mechanisms. *Nat Rev Cardiol* 8:222–232, 2011.

72. Van Lenten BJ, Hama SY, de Beer FC, et al: Anti-inflammatory HDL becomes pro-inflammatory during the acute phase response. Loss of protective effect of HDL against LDL oxidation in aortic wall cocultures. *J Clin Invest* 96:2758–2767, 1995.

73. McMahon M, Grossman J, FitzGerald J, et al: Proinflammatory high-density lipoprotein as a biomarker for atherosclerosis in patients with systemic lupus erythematosus and rheumatoid arthritis. *Arthritis Rheum* 54:2541–2549, 2006.

74. Pisetsky DS: The role of innate immunity in the induction of autoimmunity. *Autoimmun Rev* 8:69–72, 2008.

75. Miller YI, Viriyakosol S, Binder CJ, et al: Minimally modified LDL binds to CD14, induces macrophage spreading via TLR4/MD-2, and inhibits phagocytosis of apoptotic cells. *J Biol Chem* 278:1561–1568, 2003.

76. Avalos AM, Busconi L, Marshak-Rothstein A: Regulation of autoreactive B cell responses to endogenous TLR ligands. *Autoimmunity* 43:76–83, 2010.

77. Denny MF, Thacker S, Mehta H, et al: Interferon-alpha promotes abnormal vasculogenesis in lupus: a potential pathway for premature atherosclerosis. *Blood* 110:2907–2915, 2007.

78. Lee PY, Li Y, Richards HB, et al: Type I interferon as a novel risk factor for endothelial progenitor cell depletion and endothelial dysfunction in systemic lupus erythematosus. *Arthritis Rheum* 56:3759–3769, 2007.

79. Tsimikas S, Brilakis ES, Miller ER, et al: Oxidized phospholipids, Lp(a) lipoprotein, and coronary artery disease. *N Engl J Med* 353:46–57, 2005.

80. Vaarala O, Alfthan G, Jauhiainen M, et al: Crossreaction between antibodies to oxidised low-density lipoprotein and to cardiolipin in systemic lupus erythematosus. *Lancet* 341:923–925, 1993.

81. Hasunuma Y, Matsuura E, Makita Z, et al: Involvement of beta 2-glycoprotein I and anticardiolipin antibodies in oxidatively modified low-density lipoprotein uptake by macrophages. *Clin Exp Immunol* 107:569–573, 1997.

82. Frostegard J, Svenungsson E, Wu R, et al: Lipid peroxidation is enhanced in patients with systemic lupus erythematosus and is associated with arterial and renal disease manifestations. *Arthritis Rheum* 52:192–200, 2005.

83. Kobayashi K, Kishi M, Atsumi T, et al: Circulating oxidized LDL forms complexes with beta2-glycoprotein I: implication as an atherogenic autoantigen. *J Lipid Res* 44:716–726, 2003.

84. Bassi N, Zampieri S, Ghirardello A, et al: oxLDL/beta2GPI complex and anti-oxLDL/beta2GPI in SLE: prevalence and correlates. *Autoimmunity* 42:289–291, 2009.

85. Anania C, Gustafsson T, Hua X, et al: Increased prevalence of vulnerable atherosclerotic plaques and low levels of natural IgM antibodies against phosphorylcholine in patients with systemic lupus erythematosus. *Arthritis Res Ther* 12:R214, 2010.

86. Romero FI, Amengual O, Atsumi T, et al: Arterial disease in lupus and secondary antiphospholipid syndrome: association with anti-beta2-glycoprotein I antibodies but not with antibodies against oxidized low-density lipoprotein. *Br J Rheumatol* 37:883–888, 1998.

87. Hayem G, Nicaise-Roland P, Palazzo E, et al: Anti-oxidized low-density-lipoprotein (OxLDL) antibodies in systemic lupus erythematosus with and without antiphospholipid syndrome. *Lupus* 10:346–351, 2001.

88. Gomez-Zumaquero JM, Tinahones FJ, De Ramon E, et al: Association of biological markers of activity of systemic lupus erythematosus with levels of anti-oxidized low-density lipoprotein antibodies. *Rheumatology (Oxford)* 43:510–513, 2004.

89. Zhang C, Li K, Shi B, et al: Detection of serum beta-GPI-Lp(a) complexes in patients with systemic lupus erythematosus. *Clin Chim Acta* 411:395–399, 2010.

90. Virani SS, Brautbar A, Davis BC, et al: Associations between Lipoprotein(a) Levels and Cardiovascular Outcomes in African Americans and Caucasians: The Atherosclerosis Risk in Communities (ARIC) Study. *Circulation* 125:241–249, 2012.

91. Sari RA, Polat MF, Taysi S, et al: Serum lipoprotein(a) level and its clinical significance in patients with systemic lupus erythematosus. *Clin Rheumatol* 21:520–524, 2002.

92. Borba EF, Santos RD, Bonfa E, et al: Lipoprotein(a) levels in systemic lupus erythematosus. *J Rheumatol* 21:220–223, 1994.

93. Okawa-Takatsuji M, Aotsuka S, Sumiya M, et al: Clinical significance of the serum lipoprotein(a) level in patients with systemic lupus

94. McMahon M, Skaggs BJ, Sahakian L, et al: High plasma leptin levels confer increased risk of atherosclerosis in women with systemic lupus erythematosus, and are associated with inflammatory oxidised lipids. *Ann Rheum Dis* 70:1619–1624, 2011.

95. Kiani AN, Vogel-Claussen J, Magder LS, et al: Noncalcified coronary plaque in systemic lupus erythematosus. *J Rheumatol* 37:579–584, 2010.

96. Soep JB, Mietus-Snyder M, Malloy MJ, et al: Assessment of atherosclerotic risk factors and endothelial function in children and young adults with pediatric-onset systemic lupus erythematosus. *Arthritis Rheum* 51:451–457, 2004.

97. Woo JM, Lin Z, Navab M, et al: Treatment with apolipoprotein A-1 mimetic peptide reduces lupus-like manifestations in a murine lupus model of accelerated atherosclerosis. *Arthritis Res Ther* 12:R93, 2010.

98. Vuilleumier N, Reber G, James R, et al: Presence of autoantibodies to apolipoprotein A-1 in patients with acute coronary syndrome further links autoimmunity to cardiovascular disease. *J Autoimmun* 23:353–360, 2004.

99. Dinu AR, Merrill JT, Shen C, et al: Frequency of antibodies to the cholesterol transport protein apolipoprotein A1 in patients with SLE. *Lupus* 7:355–360, 1998.

100. Navab M, Hama SY, Anantharamaiah GM, et al: Normal high density lipoprotein inhibits three steps in the formation of mildly oxidized low density lipoprotein: steps 2 and 3. *J Lipid Res* 41:1495–1508, 2000.

101. Delgado Alves J, Ames PR, Donohue S, et al: Antibodies to high-density lipoprotein and beta2-glycoprotein I are inversely correlated with paraoxonase activity in systemic lupus erythematosus and primary antiphospholipid syndrome. *Arthritis Rheum* 46:2686–2694, 2002.

102. Lambert M, Boullier A, Hachulla E, et al: Paraoxonase activity is dramatically decreased in patients positive for anticardiolipin antibodies. *Lupus* 9:299–300, 2000.

103. Kiss E, Seres I, Tarr T, et al: Reduced paraoxonase1 activity is a risk for atherosclerosis in patients with systemic lupus erythematosus. *Ann N Y Acad Sci* 1108:83–91, 2007.

104. Sweeney G: Cardiovascular effects of leptin. *Nat Rev Cardiol* 7:22–29, 2010.

105. Beltowski J: Leptin and the regulation of endothelial function in physiological and pathological conditions. *Clin Exp Pharmacol Physiol* 39:168–178, 2012.

106. Anderson PD, Mehta NN, Wolfe ML, et al: Innate immunity modulates adipokines in humans. *J Clin Endocrinol Metab* 92:2272–2279, 2007.

107. Garcia-Gonzalez A, Gonzalez-Lopez L, Valera-Gonzalez IC, et al: Serum leptin levels in women with systemic lupus erythematosus. *Rheumatol Int* 22:138–141, 2002.

108. Wislowska M, Rok M, Stepien K, et al: Serum leptin in systemic lupus erythematosus. *Rheumatol Int* 28:467–473, 2008.

109. Sada KE, Yamasaki Y, Maruyama M, et al: Altered levels of adipocytokines in association with insulin resistance in patients with systemic lupus erythematosus. *J Rheumatol* 33:1545–1552, 2006.

110. Al M, Ng L, Tyrrell P, et al: Adipokines as novel biomarkers in paediatric systemic lupus erythematosus. *Rheumatology (Oxford)* 48:497–501, 2009.

111. Reynolds HR, Buyon J, Kim M, et al: Association of plasma soluble E-selectin and adiponectin with carotid plaque in patients with systemic lupus erythematosus. *Atherosclerosis* 210:569–574, 2010.

112. Chung C, Long A, Solus J, et al: Adipocytokines in systemic lupus erythematosus: relationship to inflammation, insulin resistance and coronary atherosclerosis. *Lupus* 18:799–806, 2009.

113. Schachinger V, Britten MB, Zeiher AM: Prognostic impact of coronary vasodilator dysfunction on adverse long-term outcome of coronary heart disease. *Circulation* 101:1899–1906, 2000.

114. Boros CA, Bradley TJ, Cheung MM, et al: Early determinants of atherosclerosis in paediatric systemic lupus erythematosus. *Clin Exp Rheumatol* 29:575–581, 2011.

115. Gustafsson J, Gunnarsson I, Borjesson O, et al: Predictors of the first cardiovascular event in patients with systemic lupus erythematosus - a prospective cohort study. *Arthritis Res Ther* 11:R186, 2009.

116. Rho YH, Chung CP, Oeser A, et al: Novel cardiovascular risk factors in premature coronary atherosclerosis associated with systemic lupus erythematosus. *J Rheumatol* 35:1789–1794, 2008.

117. Navarro M, Cervera R, Font J, et al: Anti-endothelial cell antibodies in systemic autoimmune diseases: prevalence and clinical significance. *Lupus* 6:521–526, 1997.

118. Ridker PM: High-sensitivity C-reactive protein: potential adjunct for global risk assessment in the primary prevention of cardiovascular disease. *Circulation* 103:1813–1818, 2001.

erythematosus: its elevation during disease flare. *Clin Exp Rheumatol* 14:531–536, 1996.

119. Yeh ET: CRP as a mediator of disease. *Circulation* 109(Suppl 1):II11–II14, 2004.

120. Torzewski J, Torzewski M, Bowyer DE, et al: C-reactive protein frequently colocalizes with the terminal complement complex in the intimva of early atherosclerotic lesions of human coronary arteries. *Arterioscler Thromb Vasc Biol* 18:1386–1392, 1998.

121. Pasceri V, Cheng JS, Willerson JT, et al: Modulation of C-reactive protein-mediated monocyte chemoattractant protein-1 induction in human endothelial cells by anti-atherosclerosis drugs. *Circulation* 103:2531–2534, 2001.

122. Zwaka TP, Hombach V, Torzewski J: C-reactive protein-mediated low density lipoprotein uptake by macrophages: implications for atherosclerosis. *Circulation* 103:1194–1197, 2001.

123. Haque S, Bruce IN: Therapy insight: systemic lupus erythematosus as a risk factor for cardiovascular disease. *Nat Clin Pract Cardiovasc Med* 2:423–430, 2005.

124. Malinow MR, Nieto FJ, Szklo M, et al: Carotid artery intimal-medial wall thickening and plasma homocyst(e)ine in asymptomatic adults. The Atherosclerosis Risk in Communities Study. *Circulation* 87:1107–1113, 1993.

125. Wall RT, Harlan JM, Harker LA, et al: Homocysteine-induced endothelial cell injury in vitro: a model for the study of vascular injury. *Thromb Res* 18:113–121, 1980.

126. Hajjar KA: Homocysteine-induced modulation of tissue plasminogen activator binding to its endothelial cell membrane receptor. *J Clin Invest* 91:2873–2879, 1993.

127. Upchurch GR, Jr, Welch GN, Fabian AJ, et al: Homocyst(e)ine decreases bioavailable nitric oxide by a mechanism involving glutathione peroxidase. *J Biol Chem* 272:17012–17017, 1997.

128. Poddar R, Sivasubramanian N, DiBello PM, et al: Homocysteine induces expression and secretion of monocyte chemoattractant protein-1 and interleukin-8 in human aortic endothelial cells: implications for vascular disease. *Circulation* 103:2717–2723, 2001.

129. McCully KS: Homocysteine and vascular disease. *Nat Med* 2:386–389, 1996.

130. Stamler JS, Osborne JA, Jaraki O, et al: Adverse vascular effects of homocysteine are modulated by endothelium-derived relaxing factor and related oxides of nitrogen. *J Clin Invest* 91:308–318, 1993.

131. Woo KS, Chook P, Lolin YI, et al: Hyperhomocyst(e)inemia is a risk factor for arterial endothelial dysfunction in humans. *Circulation* 96:2542–2544, 1997.

132. Gerhard GT, Duell PB: Homocysteine and atherosclerosis. *Curr Opin Lipidol* 10:417–428, 1999.

133. Potter K, Hankey GJ, Green DJ, et al: Homocysteine or renal impairment: which is the real cardiovascular risk factor? *Arterioscler Thromb Vasc Biol* 28:1158–1164, 2008.

134. Refai TM, Al-Salem IH, Nkansa-Dwamena D, et al: Hyperhomocysteinaemia and risk of thrombosis in systemic lupus erythematosus patients. *Clin Rheumatol* 21:457–461, 2002.

135. Rua-Figueroa I, Arencibia-Mireles O, Elvira M, et al: Factors involved in the progress of preclinical atherosclerosis associated with systemic lupus erythematosus: a two year longitudinal study. *Ann Rheum Dis* 69:1136–1139, 2009.

136. Yazdany J, Tonner C, Trupin L, et al: Provision of preventive health care in systemic lupus erythematosus: data from a large observational cohort study. *Arthritis Res Ther* 12:R84, 2010.

137. Mosca M, Tani C, Aringer M, et al: Development of quality indicators to evaluate the monitoring of SLE patients in routine clinical practice. *Autoimmun Rev* 10:383–388, 2011.

138. Costenbader KH, Brome D, Blanch D, et al: Factors determining participation in prevention trials among systemic lupus erythematosus patients: a qualitative study. *Arthritis Rheum* 57:49–55, 2007.

139. Chobanian AV, Bakris GL, Black HR, et al: The Seventh Report of the Joint National Committee on Prevention, Detection, Evaluation, and Treatment of High Blood Pressure: the JNC 7 report. *JAMA* 289:2560–2572, 2003.

140. Graham I, Atar D, Borch-Johnsen K, et al: European guidelines on cardiovascular disease prevention in clinical practice: executive summary. *Atherosclerosis* 194:1–45, 2007.

141. Costenbader KH, Karlson EW, Gall V, et al: Barriers to a trial of atherosclerosis prevention in systemic lupus erythematosus. *Arthritis Rheum* 53:718–723, 2005.

142. Duran-Barragan S, McGwin G, Jr, Vila LM, et al: Angiotensin-converting enzyme inhibitors delay the occurrence of renal involvement and are associated with a decreased risk of disease activity in patients with systemic lupus erythematosus–results from LUMINA (LIX): a multi-ethnic US cohort. *Rheumatology (Oxford)* 47:1093–1096, 2008.

143. Peters MJ, Symmons DP, McCarey D, et al: EULAR evidence-based recommendations for cardiovascular risk management in patients with rheumatoid arthritis and other forms of inflammatory arthritis. *Ann Rheum Dis* 69:325–331, 2010.

144. Sleight P, Yusuf S, Pogue J, et al: Blood-pressure reduction and cardiovascular risk in HOPE study. *Lancet* 358:2130–2131, 2001.

145. Kitamura N, Matsukawa Y, Takei M, et al: Antiproteinuric effect of angiotensin-converting enzyme inhibitors and an angiotensin II receptor blocker in patients with lupus nephritis. *J Int Med Res* 37:892–898, 2009.

146. Coffman JD: Raynaud's phenomenon. An update. *Hypertension* 17:593–602, 1991.

147. Goldstein JL, Brown MS: Regulation of the mevalonate pathway. *Nature* 343:425–430, 1990.

148. Shepherd J, Cobbe SM, Ford I, et al: Prevention of coronary heart disease with pravastatin in men with hypercholesterolemia. West of Scotland Coronary Prevention Study Group. *N Engl J Med* 333:1301–1307, 1995.

149. Shepherd J, Cobbe SM, Ford I, et al: West of Scotland Coronary Prevention Study Group. Prevention of coronary heart disease with pravastatin in men with hypercholesterolemia. 1995. *Atheroscler Suppl* 5:91–97, 2004.

150. Downs JR, Clearfield M, Weis S, et al: Primary prevention of acute coronary events with lovastatin in men and women with average cholesterol levels: results of AFCAPS/TexCAPS. Air Force/Texas Coronary Atherosclerosis Prevention Study. *JAMA* 279:1615–1622, 1998.

151. Chen CH, Jiang W, Via DP, et al: Oxidized low-density lipoproteins inhibit endothelial cell proliferation by suppressing basic fibroblast growth factor expression. *Circulation* 101:171–177, 2000.

152. Leung BP, Sattar N, Crilly A, et al: A novel anti-inflammatory role for simvastatin in inflammatory arthritis. *J Immunol* 170:1524–1530, 2003.

153. Xu ZM, Zhao SP, Li QZ, et al: Atorvastatin reduces plasma MCP-1 in patients with acute coronary syndrome. *Clin Chim Acta* 338:17–24, 2003.

154. Aktas O, Waiczies S, Smorodchenko A, et al: Treatment of relapsing paralysis in experimental encephalomyelitis by targeting Th1 cells through atorvastatin. *J Exp Med* 197:725–733, 2003.

155. Youssef S, Stuve O, Patarroyo JC, et al: The HMG-CoA reductase inhibitor, atorvastatin, promotes a Th2 bias and reverses paralysis in central nervous system autoimmune disease. *Nature* 420:78–84, 2002.

156. Neuhaus O, Strasser-Fuchs S, Fazekas F, et al: Statins as immunomodulators: comparison with interferon-beta 1b in MS. *Neurology* 59:990–997, 2002.

157. Hakamada-Taguchi R, Uehara Y, Kuribayashi K, et al: Inhibition of hydroxymethylglutaryl-coenzyme a reductase reduces Th1 development and promotes Th2 development. *Circ Res* 93:948–956, 2003.

158. Cherfan P, Tompa A, Wikby A, et al: Effects of simvastatin on human T cells in vivo. *Atherosclerosis* 193:186–192, 2007.

159. Forrester JS, Libby P: The inflammation hypothesis and its potential relevance to statin therapy. *Am J Cardiol* 99:732–738, 2007.

160. Salonen R, Nyyssonen K, Porkkala E, et al: Kuopio Atherosclerosis Prevention Study (KAPS). A population-based primary preventive trial of the effect of LDL lowering on atherosclerotic progression in carotid and femoral arteries. *Circulation* 92:1758–1764, 1995.

161. Grundy SM, Cleeman JI, Merz CN, et al: Implications of recent clinical trials for the National Cholesterol Education Program Adult Treatment Panel III guidelines. *Circulation* 110:227–239, 2004.

162. Haruna Y, Morita Y, Yada T, et al: Fluvastatin reverses endothelial dysfunction and increased vascular oxidative stress in rat adjuvant-induced arthritis. *Arthritis Rheum* 56:1827–1835, 2007.

163. Aprahamian T, Bonegio R, Rizzo J, et al: Simvastatin treatment ameliorates autoimmune disease associated with accelerated atherosclerosis in a murine lupus model. *J Immunol* 177:3028–3034, 2006.

164. Ferreira GA, Navarro TP, Telles RW, et al: Atorvastatin therapy improves endothelial-dependent vasodilation in patients with systemic lupus erythematosus: an 8 weeks controlled trial. *Rheumatology (Oxford)* 46:1560–1565, 2007.

165. Petri M, Kiani A, Post W, et al: Lupus atherosclerosis prevention study (LAPS): a randomized double blind placebo controlled trial of atorvastatin versus placebo. *Arthritis Rheum* 54:S520, 2006.

166. Kang S, Wu Y, Li X: Effects of statin therapy on the progression of carotid atherosclerosis: a systematic review and meta-analysis. *Atherosclerosis* 177:433–442, 2004.

167. Stone NJ, Bilek S, Rosenbaum S: Recent National Cholesterol Education Program Adult Treatment Panel III Update: Adjustments and Options. *Am J Cardiol* 96:53–59, 2005.

168. Chen HW, Leonard DA: Chloroquine inhibits cyclization of squalene oxide to lanosterol in mammalian cells. *J Biol Chem* 259:8156–8162, 1984.

169. Selzer F, Sutton-Tyrrell K, Fitzgerald S, et al: Vascular stiffness in women with systemic lupus erythematosus. *Hypertension* 37:1075–1082, 2001.

170. Rahman P, Gladman DD, Urowitz MB, et al: The cholesterol lowering effect of antimalarial drugs is enhanced in patients with lupus taking corticosteroid drugs. *J Rheumatol* 26:325–330, 1999.

171. Petri M: Hydroxychloroquine use in the Baltimore Lupus Cohort: effects on lipids, glucose and thrombosis. *Lupus* 5(Suppl 1):S16–S22, 1996.

172. Wallace DJ: Does hydroxychloroquine sulfate prevent clot formation in systemic lupus erythematosus? *Arthritis Rheum* 30:1435–1436, 1987.

173. Jung H, Bobba R, Su J, et al: The protective effect of antimalarial drugs on thrombovascular events in systemic lupus erythematosus. *Arthritis Rheum* 62:863–868, 2010.

174. Ruiz-Irastorza G, Egurbide MV, Pijoan JI, et al: Effect of antimalarials on thrombosis and survival in patients with systemic lupus erythematosus. *Lupus* 15:577–583, 2006.

175. Kaiser R, Cleveland CM, Criswell LA: Risk and protective factors for thrombosis in systemic lupus erythematosus: results from a large, multiethnic cohort. *Ann Rheum Dis* 68:238–241, 2009.

176. Alarcon GS, McGwin G, Bertoli AM, et al: Effect of hydroxychloroquine on the survival of patients with systemic lupus erythematosus: data from LUMINA, a multiethnic US cohort (LUMINA L). *Ann Rheum Dis* 66:1168–1172, 2007.

177. Sun S, Rao NL, Venable J, et al: TLR7/9 antagonists as therapeutics for immune-mediated inflammatory disorders. *Inflamm Allergy Drug Targets* 6:223–235, 2007.

178. Toloza SM, Uribe AG, McGwin G, Jr, et al: Systemic lupus erythematosus in a multiethnic US cohort (LUMINA). XXIII. Baseline predictors of vascular events. *Arthritis Rheum* 50:3947–3957, 2004.

179. Bravo Y, Quiroz Y, Ferrebuz A, et al: Mycophenolate mofetil administration reduces renal inflammation, oxidative stress, and arterial pressure in rats with lead-induced hypertension. *Am J Physiol Renal Physiol* 293:F616–F523, 2007.

180. van Leuven SI, Mendez-Fernandez YV, Wilhelm AJ, et al: Mycophenolate mofetil but not atorvastatin attenuates atherosclerosis in lupus-prone LDLr-/- mice. *Ann Rheum Dis* 71:408–414, 2011.

181. van Leuven SI, van Wijk DF, Volger OL, et al: Mycophenolate mofetil attenuates plaque inflammation in patients with symptomatic carotid artery stenosis. *Atherosclerosis* 211:231–236, 2010.

182. David KM, Morris JA, Steffen BJ, et al: Mycophenolate mofetil vs. azathioprine is associated with decreased acute rejection, late acute rejection, and risk for cardiovascular death in renal transplant recipients with pre-transplant diabetes. *Clin Transplant* 19:279–285, 2005.

183. Kiani AN, Magder LS, Petri M: Mycophenolate mofetil (MMF) does not slow the progression of subclinical atherosclerosis in SLE over 2 years. *Rheumatol Int* July 27, 2011 (epub ahead of print).

184. Wolak T, Todosoui E, Szendro G, et al: Duplex study of the carotid and femoral arteries of patients with systemic lupus erythematosus: a controlled study. *J Rheumatol* 31:909–914, 2004.

185. Kiani AN, Magder L, Petri M: Coronary calcium in systemic lupus erythematosus is associated with traditional cardiovascular risk factors, but not with disease activity. *J Rheumatol* 35:1300–1306, 2008.

186. Bessant R, Duncan R, Ambler G, et al: Prevalence of conventional and lupus-specific risk factors for cardiovascular disease in patients with systemic lupus erythematosus: A case-control study. *Arthritis Rheum* 55:892–899, 2006.

187. Kiani AN, Petri M: Quality-of-life measurements versus disease activity in systemic lupus erythematosus. *Curr Rheumatol Rep* 12:250–258, 2010.

188. Nikpour M, Urowitz MB, Gladman DD: Epidemiology of atherosclerosis in systemic lupus erythematosus. *Curr Rheumatol Rep* 11:248–254, 2009.

Chapter 27

Cardiopulmonary Disease in SLE

Guillermo Ruiz-Irastorza and Munther Khamashta

CARDIOPULMONARY MANIFESTATIONS

The heart and the lungs can frequently be affected during the course of systemic lupus erythematosus (SLE), because of either the disease itself or the unwanted effects of lupus therapies (Boxes 27-1 and 27-2). The true prevalence of involvement of both systems is unknown, given the protean clinical presentation and the lack of well-designed epidemiologic and/or necropsy studies. In a study of 90 necropsies in Argentina, some degree of pulmonary involvement was found in almost 99% of patients, with pleural disease and infections being the most common.[1] However, clinically apparent disease is much less frequent in large observational cohorts.[2]

Cardiovascular disease is one of the main prognostic predictors in SLE.[2] Patients with lupus are prone to the development of early atherosclerosis, which is specifically covered in another chapter of this book. In addition, the hearts of patients with lupus can be involved in other ways, from the pericardium to the endocardium.[3]

Serositis: Pleurisy and Pericarditis

Pleurisy and pericarditis are the most frequent pulmonary and cardiac manifestations of SLE. The Euro-Lupus (European Working Party on Systemic Lupus Erythematosus) observational cohort found a prevalence of serositis at disease onset of 17% with a cumulative incidence of 36%.[2] Pleuritic chest pain may occur during the course of lupus in up to 60% of patients.[4]

The clinical features of lupus serositis are indistinguishable from those of pleurisy and pericarditis from other causes. Pleuritic chest pain may be unilateral or bilateral and is usually located at the costophrenic margins, either anterior or posterior. Attacks of pleuritic pain often last for several days and may persist for weeks, often accompanied by cough and dyspnea. Pericarditis usually manifests as precordial pain aggravated by deep breathing and decubitus, typically improving with sitting up. Fever and other clinical signs of lupus activity, such as arthralgia/arthritis and rashes, are common. On physical examination, friction rubs may be heard. A decreased intensity of cardiac and respiratory sounds is typical in the presence of large effusions. Respiratory compromise and pericardial tamponade are distinctly unusual in lupus serositis.[3,4]

Pleural and pericardial effusions may or may not occur during the course of serositis, so their presence is not necessary for the diagnosis, which is often based on clinical grounds. They can be apparent in radiographic studies, affecting one or both sides of the pleural cavity with variable intensity (Figure 27-1) and/or showing as an enlarged cardiac silhouette if a significant amount of pericardial fluid is present. Computed tomography (CT) scan and echocardiography have higher sensitivity to detect small effusions (Figure 27-2). Electrocardiographic findings in pericarditis include PR segment depression and widespread ST segment elevation.

The differential diagnoses of pleural and pericardial effusions in SLE include infections—mainly tuberculosis—cardiac failure, nephrotic syndrome, and cancer. Moreover, the differential diagnosis of pleuritic pain in a patient with lupus should always include pulmonary embolism, especially in the presence of antiphospholipid antibodies.

Analysis of the pleural fluid is frequently required to complete the diagnosis. Pericardiocentesis, on the other hand, is a complex invasive procedure, so it is most often not performed. The pleural fluid in SLE is almost always exudative. Both lymphocyte and polymorphonuclear predominance can be seen. In most patients with lupus pleuritis, the pleural fluid glucose concentration is greater than 60 mg/dL. This contrasts with the finding of low glucose levels in the pleural fluid of patients with rheumatoid pleurisy, in whom the glucose concentration is less than 30 mg/dL in 75% of cases.[5] Low pleural fluid glucose concentrations may also occur in malignant effusions, empyema, and tuberculosis.[5]

The presence of antinuclear antibodies (ANAs) in the pleural fluid may be a useful diagnostic test for lupus. Most investigators agree that the negative predictive value of ANAs in pleural fluid is very high for SLE, that is, an ANA-negative pleural effusion is very unlikely to be due to lupus, even in a patient with known SLE, in whom alternative causes should be pursued.[6-8] On the other hand, ANA-positive pleural fluid can be found in patients without lupus. In those cases, malignancy should be put first in the list of possible causes.[7,8] The serum-to–pleural fluid ANA ratio does not seem to improve the performance of ANA testing at titers over 1:160; thus the use of this ratio is not recommended in clinical practice.[7,8] Limited data point to similar performance of ANA testing in pericardial fluid.[7]

Acute Lupus Pneumonitis

Acute lupus pneumonitis is a rare manifestation of lupus, with an incidence ranging between 1% and 12%.[9] Unfortunately, in more than 50% of cases, acute lupus pneumonitis is the presenting manifestation of SLE, making early diagnosis and treatment more difficult.[10]

The histopathology of the lung in acute lupus pneumonitis has been examined in a few patients. Alveolar hyaline membranes and persistent cell infiltrates have been found. Other findings at the autopsy included acute alveolitis, interstitial edema, and arteriolar thrombosis. Granular deposits of immunoglobulin (Ig)G, complement component C3, and DNA have been seen in the alveolar septa of patients with acute lupus pneumonitis.[10]

Patients with acute lupus pneumonitis usually present with fever, dyspnea, cough productive of scanty sputum, tachypnea, and pleuritic chest pain.[9] Physical findings commonly include basal crackles, and, when severe, central cyanosis may be present. Chest radiographs and CT scans show diffuse alveolar infiltrates with a predilection for the bases in all patients (Figure 27-3). Pleural effusion can be present in up to 50% of patients.[10] Respiratory insufficiency is the rule, with many patients having a fulminant course. Adult respiratory distress syndrome may occur with acute lupus pneumonitis, greatly increasing mortality. Anti-DNA antibodies are usually present along with other data revealing lupus activity. Anti-Ro antibodies are also frequently found.[10]

Acute lupus pneumonitis is clinically similar to alveolar hemorrhage (see later). The differential diagnosis should always include pulmonary infections; thus, bronchoalveolar lavage, including specific cultures of the fluid, can be very useful in this setting.[9] Acute

Box 27-1 Respiratory Involvement in Systemic Lupus Erythematosus

Pleural Disease
Pleurisy (with and without effusion)

Parenchymal Lung Disease
Acute lupus pneumonitis
Alveolar hemorrhage
Chronic diffuse interstitial lung disease
Airway obstruction

Vascular Disease
Pulmonary hypertension
Pulmonary thromboembolism
Acute reversible hypoxemia

Diaphragmatic Dysfunction
Shrinking lung syndrome

Secondary
Infection
Drug toxicity

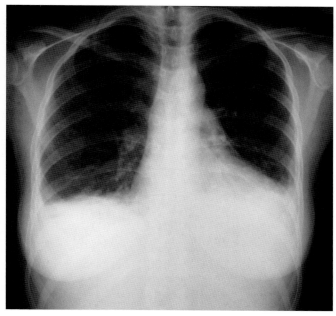

FIGURE 27-1 Bilateral pleural effusion in a woman with SLE.

Box 27-2 Cardiac Involvement in Systemic Lupus Erythematosus

Pericardium
Pericarditis

Myocardium
Myocarditis
Myocardiopathy:
 Ischemic
 Hypertensive
 Toxic (antimalarials, cyclophosphamide)

Endocardium
Valvular disease

Conduction System
Congenital heart block
Conduction abnormalities

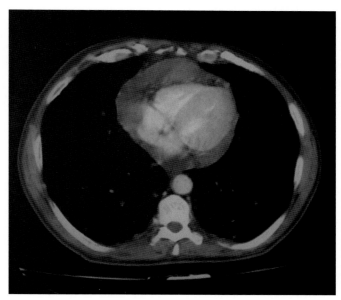

FIGURE 27-2 CT scan showing large pericardial effusion in a patient with SLE.

lupus pneumonitis should be suspected in patients with known SLE and an acute pulmonary picture in the context of high disease activity. Tests for ANAs, anti-DNA antibodies, and complement levels as well as a search for specific clinical manifestations of lupus should be included in the diagnostic routine for young patients presenting with fever and alveolar infiltrates of noninfectious origin.

Owing in part to the frequent delay in the diagnosis, the mortality rate for acute lupus pneumonitis may approach 50%, although prompt and aggressive therapy may substantially improve the prognosis.[9]

Pulmonary Hemorrhage

Pulmonary hemorrhage is a rare, devastating, and frequently fatal manifestation of SLE.[4] The histopathology of the lung is nonspecific, showing diffuse, intraalveolar hemorrhage with intact erythrocytes, and hemosiderin-laden macrophages in the alveoli. Pulmonary capillaritis can be seen in up to 80% of lung tissue specimens, although its presence varies among different series.[11]

The clinical presentation of alveolar hemorrhage closely resembles that of acute lupus pneumonitis. Fever, dyspnea, and cough are

common presenting features. Blood-stained sputum and, eventually, frank hemoptysis can appear in more than 50% of patients, so their absence does not exclude the diagnosis. The clinical course is rapidly progressive over hours or days, with increasing tachypnea, arterial hypoxemia, tachycardia, and acute respiratory distress. The hemoglobin concentration usually drops suddenly, and chest radiographs show bilateral pulmonary infiltrates, with a predominantly alveolar pattern, often extending to the bases but occasionally unilateral in distribution. CT may help confirm radiographic findings and exclude alternative conditions such as infection and cancer. In the absence of hemoptysis, a rapidly falling hemoglobin and diffuse lung infiltrates should alert the clinician to the possibility of lung hemorrhage. Single-breath diffusing capacity for carbon monoxide (CO) is typically raised owing to the presence of blood in the alveolar spaces,

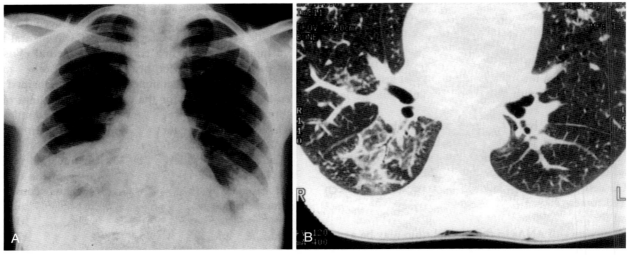

FIGURE 27-3 **A,** Chest CT scan in a patient with acute lupus pneumonitis. **B,** CT scan in this patient shows right-sided interstitial shadowing.

although most patients are too ill to undergo this investigation.[12] Bronchoalveolar lavages are almost universally hemorrhagic, with the presence of hemosiderin-laden macrophages as an indirect sign of alveolar bleeding.[11,12] Open lung biopsy is not generally needed to establish the diagnosis.

Pulmonary hemorrhage is not a common presenting feature of SLE. In a series from Mexico, one third of patients with lupus and alveolar hemorrhage had no previous diagnosis of SLE.[13] Interestingly, most other researchers report that more than 80% of patients with pulmonary hemorrhage have known lupus, usually of recent diagnosis.[11,12] In fact, multisystem disease is almost the rule, with renal and neurologic disease as the most frequent accompanying features.[11,13]

The prognosis of massive pulmonary hemorrhage in patients with SLE is grave, despite aggressive treatment, with mortality rates exceeding 50% in most published series.[11-14] The presence of thrombocytopenia, renal failure, and infection and the need for mechanical ventilation have all been identified as adverse prognostic factors.[11-13]

Chronic Diffuse Interstitial Lung Disease

Diffuse interstitial lung disease (ILD) is a well-recognized pulmonary manifestation of systemic autoimmune diseases, particularly systemic sclerosis and dermatomyositis; however, it is much less common in SLE. The prevalence of symptomatic ILD in SLE has been calculated to be approximately 3% to 8%, being more frequent as disease duration increases.[15]

The classification of idiopathic interstitial pneumonias has been updated.[16] According to this classification, nonspecific interstitial pneumonia (NSIP) is the most common histologic pattern found in patients with SLE.[15] Lung biopsies show interstitial inflammation, fibrosis, or a combination of the two.[16] Usual interstitial pneumonia (UIP) shows a fibrotic pattern, whose more characteristic associated condition is idiopathic pulmonary fibrosis, although UIP can appear in connective tissue diseases, including SLE.[16] Other patterns are lymphocytic interstitial pneumonia (LIP), most common in Sjögren syndrome but also seen in a few patients with SLE, and organizing pneumonia[15] (for the latter, see later discussion of airway obstruction).

The presentation of ILD in SLE resembles that of lung disease in systemic sclerosis and rheumatoid arthritis. ILD can occur at any time during the course of SLE, but in most cases it develops in patients with long-standing disease. The most common clinical manifestations are slowly progressing dyspnea on exertion and

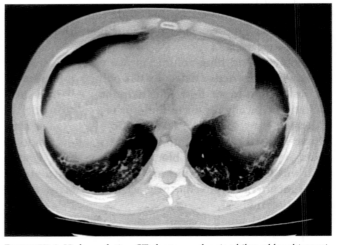

FIGURE 27-4 High-resolution CT chest scan showing bilateral basal interstitial fibrosis with honeycombing.

nonproductive cough. Inspiratory crackles are evident as disease advances. Other lupus features may be present as well in variable combinations. An association of anti-Ro and anti–U1 ribonucleoprotein (anti–U1-RNP) antibodies with ILD has been suggested by some authorities, although this relationship is disputed.[4]

Chest radiographic findings may range from almost normal to severe honeycombing, most frequently showing reticulonodular patterns.[16] Lower lobe disease is the usual finding. The common pattern of nonspecific interstitial pneumonia on CT is a ground-glass appearance, whereas UIP manifests as a reticulonodular infiltrate with variable fibrosis along with parenchymal destruction and volume loss (Figure 27-4).[16] Pulmonary function tests typically show a restrictive pattern with a reduced diffusing capacity for CO.[9] A lung biopsy is not always necessary to establish the diagnosis, but it may be indicated to exclude infection or cancer in selected cases.

The prognosis of ILD in lupus is marked by the histologic type and the degree of lung fibrosis at the time of diagnosis. LIP and organizing pneumonia rarely progress to severe fibrosis. The course of NSIP is usually milder than that of UIP. The chance of reverting established fibrosis is virtually zero, so every effort should be made to detect ILD in earlier stages in order to initiate effective treatment (see later).

Pulmonary Embolism

Pulmonary embolism should always be considered in the setting of chest pain, dyspnea, and respiratory insufficiency, especially if antiphospholipid antibodies are present. Spiral CT scan should be performed in cases of clinical suspicion.[17] The lungs are commonly involved in catastrophic antiphospholipid syndrome, with the usual presentation of acute respiratory distress syndrome. Bucciarelli reported pulmonary involvement in 150 of 220 (68%) patients with catastrophic antiphospholipid syndrome; 47 (21%) patients were diagnosed as having acute respiratory distress syndrome. Prognosis was poor, and 19 (40%) of these patients died. Histologic analysis showed that 7 of 10 patients had a thrombotic microangiopathy (see Chapter 42 for a further discussion of thrombosis and antiphospholipid antibodies).[18]

Reversible Hypoxemia

A relatively rare syndrome of acute reversible hypoxemia in acutely ill patients with SLE without evidence of parenchymal lung involvement may occur.[19] Although some patients have mild pleuropulmonary symptoms, chest radiographic and CT findings are typically normal. Patients present with hypoxemia and hypocapnia with a wide alveolar-arterial gradient. The pathogenesis of the syndrome is unclear. A relationship with disease activity has been noted.[20] Complement activation may lead to diffuse pulmonary injury with leukocyte–endothelial cell adhesion and leukoocclusive vasculopathy within pulmonary capillaries.[17] Indeed, most cases respond to immunosuppression, with rapid improvement of gas exchange within a few days.[17]

Pulmonary Hypertension

Pulmonary hypertension (PH) is characterized by the progressive increase in pulmonary vascular resistance eventually leading to right ventricular failure and premature death. It is defined as a resting mean pulmonary arterial pressure (mPAP) higher than 25 mm Hg measured by right heart catheterization.[21] According to the latest classification of PH—now known as the Dana Point classification, from the location of the 4th World Symposium on Pulmonary Hypertension, at Dana Point, California, in 2008 at which the update was adopted—this condition can be secondary to a number of disorders, including pulmonary diseases and/or hypoxemia, left heart disease, thromboembolic disease of the pulmonary arteries, and a miscellanea of other causes, such as sarcoidosis and lymphangiomyomatosis.[22] For the diagnosis of the subclass known as pulmonary arterial hypertension (PAH), a pulmonary arterial wedge pressure lower than 15 mm Hg is required.[22]

PAH associated with systemic autoimmune diseases is included within group I of the Dana Point classification. PAH is a recognized complication of this group of diseases, particularly systemic sclerosis and, to a much lesser degree, SLE, mixed connective tissue disease, inflammatory myopathies, and Sjögren syndrome.[22] In addition, PH may be secondary to other complications, such as interstitial lung disease, valvular heart disease, and pulmonary thromboembolism, that may occur during the course of lupus.

Plexiform lesions of the pulmonary arteries are the hallmark of PAH, whether or not it is secondary to SLE or other connective tissue disorders.[1] Medial hypertrophy and intimal fibrosis of the branches of the pulmonary artery may be seen. Thrombosis and vasculitis have also been reported in a few patients.[9]

The pathogenesis of PAH in SLE is likely to be multifactorial. Several factors have been implicated, such as recurrent vasospasm, vasculitis, and thrombotic vascular occlusion. In addition, PH can be secondary to pulmonary fibrosis, chronic thromboembolic disease, and left ventricular dysfunction. Increased levels of endothelin-1 have been proposed as a possible mechanism for PAH in patients with lupus.[23] A number of clinical and immunologic variables have been reported as potential markers of an increased risk for PAH: Raynaud phenomenon,[24,25] disease activity,[26,27] and presence of antiphospholipid antibodies[28,29] and anti–U1-RNP antibodies.[27,30]

The actual prevalence of PH in patients with lupus is unknown, ranging from less than 0.5% to 14%,[23] depending on the series. Such discordant results actually reflect the varying definitions of PH. In some series, the diagnosis has been established following a single echocardiographic calculation of systolic pulmonary arterial pressure, with a cutoff point between 30 and 40 mm Hg, depending on the study. This diagnostic strategy, which does not fulfill current recommendations,[21] may well overestimate PH prevalence and also bias the identification of clinical and immunologic predictors. In a necropsy series of 90 patients with SLE, histologic evidence of PAH was found in 4%.[1]

The symptoms of PAH in SLE are nonspecific and similar to those of patients with other forms of this condition. The most common complaints are dyspnea on exertion, chest pain, and chronic nonproductive cough.[9] Weakness, palpitations, edema, and/or ascites may also gradually occur as disease progresses and the right ventricle becomes involved. The physical findings include a loud second pulmonary heart sound, systolic murmurs, and right ventricular lift. Chest radiographic findings include prominent pulmonary arteries and clear lung fields, with cardiomegaly in more advanced cases. Electrocardiography may show changes of right ventricular hypertrophy. Pulmonary function tests in PAH typically show a diminished CO diffusion with normal lung volumes. A restrictive pattern is seen in PH secondary to lung fibrosis. Echocardiogram is considered the best screening test for PH. Calculated PAP values exceeding 40 mm Hg warrant further investigations.[31] Cardiac catheterization is the definitive diagnostic test for PAH, demonstrating the elevation of the mean pulmonary artery pressure to more than 25 mm Hg at rest with a normal wedge pressure, without evidence of intracardiac or extracardiac shunting. For therapeutic purposes, a vasodilator test would be included in the procedure, because a positive response identifies those few cases that can respond to calcium-antagonist drugs (see section on treatment).

PAH has been identified as a predictor of morbidity and mortality in SLE.[2,24] Cardiac failure and sudden death, presumably due to arrhythmias, are the most common causes of death. The survival of patients with lupus and PAH has been considered poor.[9] However, a British national registry of PH starting in 2001 has shown 1- and 3-year survival rates of 78% and 74%, respectively, for PAH secondary to SLE, significantly higher than those of systemic sclerosis–associated PAH.[32] These figures may reflect the availability of new, effective therapies for PAH, but also the differential, specific characteristics of SLE-associated PAH.

Shrinking Lung Syndrome

Shrinking lung syndrome refers to a condition typical of SLE that consists of a purely restrictive respiratory disease with normal lung parenchyma and markedly decreased lung volumes usually evident in radiographic studies, which show elevated hemidiaphragms and basal atelectasis (Figure 27-5).

Diaphragmatic dysfunction has been advocated as the main pathogenetic mechanism of shrinking lung syndrome.[33] However, Laroche found no evidence of isolated weakness of the diaphragm in 12 patients with SLE and this syndrome.[34] Evidence of chronic pleural disease has not been demonstrated either.[33] Anti-Ro antibody positivity has been also linked with the occurrence of shrinking lung syndrome.[35]

Shrinking lung syndrome usually manifests as exertional dyspnea of variable severity, which can progress over a period of weeks or months. Orthopnea may also occur, attributed to diaphragmatic weakness.[33] Pleuritic chest pain is reported frequently, and a previous history of pleurisy and pericarditis is common.[36] Anti-Ro antibodies may be present, although they do not offer an additional diagnostic aid. Physical examination is remarkably normal.

Chest radiography typically shows elevated hemidiaphragms, although this is not a universal finding and its absence does not exclude the diagnosis.[33] Pleural effusions, pleural thickening, and atelectasis may be also evident on plain films or CT scans. Pulmonary

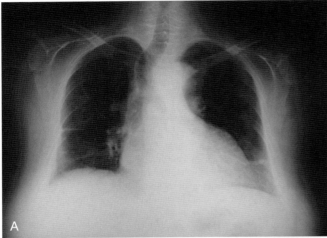

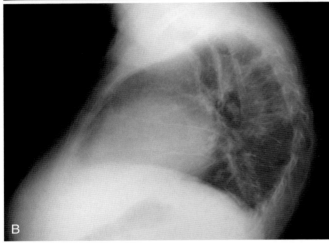

FIGURE 27-5 Shrinking lung in a woman with SLE and associated Jaccoud arthropathy. **A,** Posteroanterior view; **B,** lateral view.

function tests show a marked restrictive pattern, with decreased forced vital capacity (FVC). Carbon monoxide diffusion corrected by lung volumes is typically normal.

The prognosis of this syndrome is usually good, with most patients showing long-term stabilization.[33]

Airway Obstruction

Airway obstruction can be found in a substantial proportion of patients with lupus, up to 20% depending on the series, but severe forms are rare in the absence of other concomitant causes such as smoking.[4] Specific, lupus-related obstructive airway disease is much more uncommon and is caused mainly by bronchiolitis.[33]

Bronchioles are small airways that do not have cartilage in their walls. The term *bronchiolitis* is applied to a variety of inflammatory disorders involving the bronchioles.[37] Two types of primary bronchiolitis can be seen in patients with lupus. The first one is constrictive bronchiolitis, also known as obliterative bronchiolitis or bronchiolitis obliterans.[38] The distinctive pathologic pattern of constrictive bronchiolitis consists of peribronchiolar fibrosis, which surrounds the lumen, resulting in extrinsic compression and obliteration of the airway. Lupus is a rare cause of this type of bronchiolitis, which is most often idiopathic or due to drugs—such as penicillamine—inhalation injury, chronic transplant rejection, or, among autoimmune disorders, rheumatoid arthritis.[38] The clinical picture is that of cough and progressive dyspnea. Physical examination may reveal wheezing and inspiratory crackles. Chest radiographic findings are distinctively normal. On the other hand, CT shows a pattern of mosaic attenuation, with heterogeneous lung density due to decreased perfusion of areas with bronchiolar obstruction and blood flow redistribution to normal areas. Pulmonary function tests typically show a nonreversible obstructive pattern, with predominant involvement of distal airways.[39]

The second type of bronchiolitis that can be seen in patients with lupus is bronchiolitis obliterans organizing pneumonia, also known as cryptogenetic organizing pneumonia.[16] Actually, bronchiolar involvement is not predominant in this entity, which consists of universal polypoid intraluminal plugs of proliferating fibroblasts and myofibroblasts within alveolar ducts and spaces, and occasional signs of organization within the bronchioles.[16] This makes a major difference with obliterative bronchiolitis, in which the fibrosing reaction is peribronchiolar.[38]

Clinical findings include cough and dyspnea of acute/subacute onset, often with prominent systemic symptoms such as fever, myalgia, and weight loss. Occasionally, the clinical presentation may resemble adult respiratory distress syndrome.[38] Chest radiography and CT demonstrate prominent alveolar consolidation with bronchogram. Lung function tests show a restrictive ventilatory pattern with usually moderately reduced CO diffusion. Airflow obstruction is present in a few patients.[16]

The prognosis of these two conditions is also radically different. Although organizing pneumonia usually responds well to immunosuppressive therapy, constrictive bronchiolitis is often a gradually worsening disease with a high mortality rate within a few months.[38]

Infections and the Lung in SLE

Pulmonary infections are common in patients with lupus, especially in those taking corticosteroids and immunosuppressive therapies. Oral prednisone and restrictive lung diseases have been identified as risk factors for serious respiratory infections.[40] Responsible organisms include viruses, bacteria, mycobacteria, parasites, and opportunistic fungal infections, depending on the degree of immunosuppression. For a more thorough review of infectious complications in SLE, see Chapter 42.

Myocardiac Involvement

Myocarditis is a rare manifestation of SLE, occurring in less than 10% of patients, although subtle subclinical disease may be more frequent.[3] This prevalence seems to have decreased since the availability of corticosteroid therapy.[3] Later studies strongly link the occurrence of myocarditis with high disease activity at the time of diagnosis of SLE.[41] Moreover, patients suffering myocarditis in early disease are more likely to accrue organ damage, not only at the cardiac level, during follow-up.[41] This likelihood reflects the frequent occurrence of myocarditis in the context of widespread active lupus, often close to the time of presentation of disease. Up to 85% of patients with lupus myocarditis suffer this complication in early disease.[41] Anti-Ro positivity has been suggested as a risk factor for myocarditis,[42] but this association has not been seen in later cohort studies.[41] African-American ethnicity seems to confer a higher risk of suffering lupus myocarditis.[42]

Lupus myocarditis usually manifests as tachycardia, dyspnea, orthopnea, edema, and other symptoms and signs reflecting heart failure.[43] Chest pain mimicking angina can be the presenting sign. The clinical presentation may vary according to the severity of myocardial dysfunction. Jugular venous distention and gallop rhythm may be found. Myocardial enzymes can be either elevated or normal. Electrocardiographic changes are nonspecific and may include ST-T changes, premature atrial or ventricular complexes, arrhythmias, and conduction abnormalities. In severe cases, the chest radiograph can reveal an enlarged cardiac silhouette and signs of left ventricular failure. Echocardiography can show global hypokinesis, which is strongly suggestive, although not diagnostic, of myocarditis.[3] Pericarditis may accompany myocarditis.

The main differential diagnoses for lupus myocarditis are other causes of myocardial dysfunction, such as hypertensive and ischemic myocardiopathy, as well as idiopathic or other forms of dilated myocardiopathy. All of these conditions manifest in a subacute or chronic rather than acute way. Other clinical features, such as a history of uncontrolled hypertension, angina, and heavy alcohol consumption, may give a clue. Echocardiography may show left ventricular thickening or focal rather than global hypokinesis. Heart failure secondary to severe valvular disease is also easily revealed by echocardiogram.

Myocarditis has been associated to increased mortality, both short and long term.[41,43] Patients surviving the acute onset are more prone to development of damage and to have a statistically decreased survival after 5 years of disease.[41] These features may reflect in part a more severe type of lupus in this subgroup.[41]

Drug-induced myocardial dysfunction should also be taken into account in patients with lupus. Cyclophosphamide can cause myocardial damage, with acute symptoms that may include arrhythmia, conduction disorders, acute fulminant heart failure, and even hemorrhagic myopericarditis with pericardial effusions, cardiac tamponade, and even death. However, this kind of toxicity is seen with the use of high doses of the drug, more than 120 to 200 mg/kg, and usually depending on single rather than cumulative doses.[44]

Antimalarials, particularly hydroxychloroquine, are today considered the cornerstone of SLE therapy.[45] Rather infrequently, antimalarials can also cause myocardiopathy.[46] As with antimalarial-related side effects, chloroquine has been implicated in myocardiopathy more frequently than hydroxychloroquine.[46] Typically, this is an infiltrative form of myocardiopathy, with a restrictive clinical pattern, being characterized by the presence of myocyte vacuolization on optical microscopy and lamellar lysosomal inclusions and curvilinear bodies on electron microscopy.[47] Concomitant similar alterations are common in skeletal muscle biopsy specimens. High cumulative doses of antimalarials are common in affected patients. In cases in which clinical suspicion of antimalarial infiltrative cardiomyopathy exists, generally in patients who have received long-term antimalarial therapy, an endomyocardial biopsy should be performed, unless an affected skeletal muscle exhibits typical histologic changes, in which case the diagnosis can be assumed. Although treatment interruption is mandatory, most cases do not improve, with death being reported in a significant proportion of affected patients.[46] Apart from infiltrative myocardiopathy, other forms of cardiac toxicity have been reported in patients taking antimalarials, largely conduction defects including complete atrioventricular block and, with short-term use of chloroquine, QT prolongation and torsades de pointes.[46,47] Two studies have specifically looked for cardiotoxicity secondary to antimalarials, involving 70 and 28 patients with SLE treated with hydroxychloroquine and chloroquine, respectively.[48,49] No cases of clinically relevant cardiotoxicity, including atrioventricular block, heart conduction disorders, and heart failure, were reported in any patients. Thus, antimalarial-related toxicity should be included in the differential diagnosis of patients with lupus and rhythm abnormalities, with the fact that this is a rather infrequent complication of this group of drugs taken into account.

Indeed, conduction system abnormalities have been described in SLE. The most characteristic clinical picture is congenital heart block secondary to neonatal lupus syndrome (see Chapter 42). Adult patients with SLE can also suffer arrhythmias and conduction disturbances. These are often secondary to myocardial damage due to myocarditis or ischemic heart disease.[50] Sinus tachycardia is closely related with clinical and laboratory features of lupus activity.[51] Thus, persistent sinus tachycardia in the absence of a clear precipitant cause should be considered a warning sign of impending lupus activity. The presence of anti-Ro antibodies has been also related with sinus bradycardia and QT interval prolongation.[52]

Valvular Heart Disease

Valvular heart disease is prevalent in SLE. A classic autopsy series of 36 patients with SLE found heart valve abnormalities in half of them.[53] Later echocardiographic studies have shown variable data, but the prevalence of valve involvement has always been high. Two systematic reviews have analyzed this issue. In the first review, 20 studies published between 1990 and 2007 were selected, involving 1593 patients with lupus.[54] The global prevalence of valvular heart disease was 31%, with individual study prevalence ranging between 7% and 75%. The presence of vegetations, that is, Libman-Sacks endocarditis, was rarer, between 0 and 31%, although the latter prevalence was found in the only study using transesophageal echocardiography.[55] The second systematic review analyzed 23 studies published between 1990 and 2007, with similar results[56]; 508 patients out of a total of 1656 (31%) had some degree of valve involvement. The prevalence of Libman-Sacks endocarditis, specifically shown in a Greek cohort study of 342 patients, was 11%.[57] Thus, it can be said that heart valve abnormalities can be found in one of every three patients with lupus, while valvular vegetations (Libman-Sacks endocarditis) are present in one in every ten patients. However, these figures can be higher if transesophageal echocardiography is used, because this technique has been shown to increase the sensitivity for the detection of valvular vegetations by more than 30% over conventional transthoracic echocardiography.[58]

Several factors may be involved in the development of valve heart disease in lupus, the most consistent predictor being the presence of antiphospholipid antibodies. Both systematic reviews found a clearly higher risk for valvular abnormalities among patients with these antibodies. Fifteen of 20 studies reviewed in the study by Mattos found a significant association between antiphospholipid antibodies and heart valve lesions.[54] Zuily calculated that the odds ratio for heart valve disease was 3.13 for patients with any antiphospholipid antibodies, 5.88 for those with lupus anticoagulant, and 5.63 for those with IgG anticardiolipin antibodies. On the contrary, the presence of IgM anticardiolipin antibodies did not increase the risk for valvular disease.[56] Likewise, the presence antiphospholipid antibodies also conferred a higher risk for Libman-Sacks endocarditis (odds ratio 3.51).[56] Antiphospholipid antibodies seem to be actually involved in the pathogenesis of valvular heart disease in patients with SLE or with primary antiphospholipid syndrome. Deposition of anticardiolipin antibodies has been demonstrated in valve specimens of patients with valvular disease. Binding of antiphospholipid antibodies to valvular endothelium may lead to endocardial damage, superficial thrombosis, subendocardial inflammation, fibrosis, and calcification.[59] Other factors associated with valvular vegetations in lupus include disease duration, a history of pericarditis, and thrombocytopenia.[57] An association of heart valve disease with Jaccoud arthropathy has been suggested in a Brazilian study enrolling 113 patients with lupus.[60] Valvular disease was found in 36% of patients with arthropathy, compared with 9% of those without.

Valvular heart disease is frequently asymptomatic. Mitral involvement is most common, and when valvular dysfunction is seen, insufficiency is more common than stenosis (zuily). Those patients with valvular lesions at the first echocardiography[56] have a less than 10% chance that the lesions will improve over time. On the other hand, a similar proportion of patients with an initially normal echocardiogram eventually experience valve disease.[61] Serious valvular disease requiring surgery is uncommon, occurring in less than 6% of patients.[62] Apart from clinical manifestations derived from valvular dysfunction, mitral valve thickening and regurgitation have shown a strong independent association with cerebrovascular events in patients with SLE.[63]

The diagnosis of heart valve disease should be suspected in patients with significant cardiac murmurs, heart failure, peripheral arterial embolic disease, or cerebrovascular disease. Heart valve lesions should also be actively sought in patients with lupus who have persistently present antiphospholipid antibodies.[56] In cases of high clinical suspicion in which the thoracic echocardiogram is normal, a transesophageal echocardiography should be performed.[58] Differential diagnosis should be made from bacterial endocarditis, especially in the presence of fever. Negative blood culture results in the absence of antibiotic therapy reinforce the nonbacterial origin of vegetations. Despite the clinical association with thromboembolic disease, the prognostic implications of asymptomatic valvular disease in lupus are not yet established.[64]

DIAGNOSTIC CHALLENGES

Achieving the correct and early diagnosis in patients with SLE and cardiorespiratory symptoms is often a difficult task. The presence of dyspnea is always a warning sign. Sudden dyspnea, with or without chest pain, should make the clinician consider the diagnosis of pulmonary embolism. The probability of the clinical diagnosis can be calculated through the use of validated scores such as the Geneva score, which takes into account items such as age, history of venous thromboembolism, and signs of acute venous thrombosis, among others.[65] In the case of patients with lupus, positivity for antiphospholipid antibodies also increases the chance of a pulmonary embolism. For hemodynamically stable patients with a low or intermediate clinical probability, a negative D-dimer test excludes the diagnosis. For the remaining patients, a spiral CT scan is indicated.[66]

Dyspnea can also have a cardiac origin. Signs of heart failure must be sought in patients with lupus who have shortness of breath as well as auscultatory data suggestive of valve disease. In the presence of cardiac signs, an echocardiogram should be performed promptly, especially if the heart shadow is enlarged on chest radiography, to look for pericardial effusion or signs of myocarditis with systolic dysfunction.

Subacute dyspnea is also the usual presenting symptom of PAH. Chest pain and syncope are accompanying symptoms in severe disease. Echocardiogram is also indicated in this setting. The finding of a calculated PAP value equal to or higher than 40 mm Hg is suggestive of PH and warrants further studies to confirm the diagnosis, which is established by right cardiac catheterization.[33] In patients with confirmed PH, it is important to exclude the possibility of chronic thromboembolic disease by means of ventilation/perfusion scanning, especially in patients with antiphospholipid antibodies.[9]

In patients with lung infiltrates, diagnoses other than lupus should be also considered. Infections are first on the list in patients with fever and/or taking immunosuppressive drugs. In seriously ill patients in whom the possibility of infection exists, empirical broad-spectrum antibiotic coverage along with an aggressive search for the causative agent, including bronchoalveolar lavage, should be initiated. Patients with SLE may be at a higher risk for lung cancer.[67] Furthermore, mucosa-associated lymphoid tissue (MALT) lymphomas, albeit more typical of patients with Sjögren syndrome,[68] may appear in patients with lupus as well (Figure 27-6). Thus, histologic confirmation should be sought in patients with atypical lung infiltrates, insufficient response to therapy or other features suggestive of malignancy—weight loss, night sweats, and hemoptysis.

TREATMENT

As in many other aspects of lupus, treatment of pleuropulmonary manifestations is hampered by the lack of good trials. Moreover, most

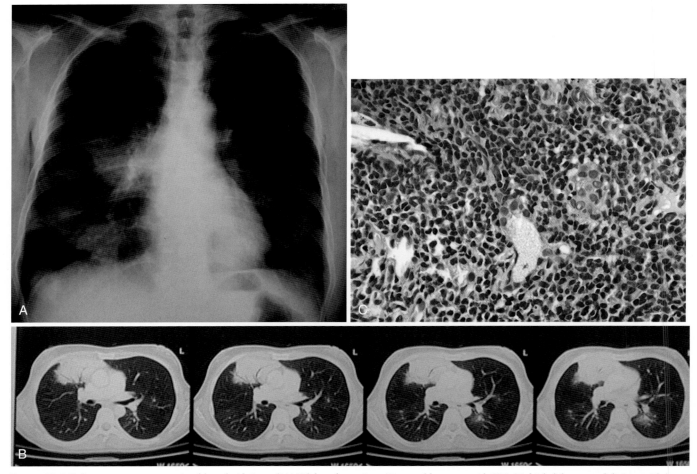

FIGURE 27-6 Pulmonary mucosa-associated lymphoid tissue (MALT) lymphoma in a 40-year-old woman with SLE. Multiple lobar consolidations with bronchogram can be seen in a chest radiograph (**A**) and CT scans (**B**). The patient received antibiotic and immunosuppressive therapy. A CT-guided lung biopsy specimen, which was collected after lack of response to treatment, showed infiltration by B-cell lymphoma (**C**).

TABLE 27-1 Suggested Therapy for Respiratory Manifestations of SLE

MANIFESTATION	THERAPY	COMMENTS
Pleuritis	Hydroxychloroquine Prednisone 5-15 mg/day Pulse methyl-prednisolone 250-500 mg/ day × 3 days in severe cases	Add immunosuppressive drugs (azathioprine, methotrexate, etc.) in cases recurring with maintenance doses of prednisone ≤5 mg/day
Pneumonitis and alveolar hemorrhage	Pulse methylprednisolone 250-500 mg/day × 3 days Prednisone 20-30 mg/day Intravenous cyclophosphamide pulses	Intensive care unit frequently indicated Antibiotic coverage until infection is ruled out Intravenous immunoglobulin indicated if infection is suspected Maintenance therapy with prednisone ≤5 mg/day and oral immunosuppressive drugs (azathioprine)
Interstitial lung disease	Prednisone 20-30 mg/day Intravenous cyclophosphamide pulses	A trial of immunosuppressive therapy is indicated in early stages of the disease Discontinue if no improvement or if established fibrosis
Bronchiolitis obliterans organizing pneumonia	Prednisone 15-30 mg/day Pulse methylprednisolone and intravenous cyclophosphamide pulses in severe cases	Maintenance therapy with prednisone ≤5 mg/day with or without oral immunosuppressive drugs (azathioprine, methotrexate)
Constrictive bronchiolitis		Usually no response to immunosuppressive therapy
Pulmonary thromboembolism	Oral anticoagulation target International Normalized Ratio (INR) 2.0-3.0	Indefinite therapy recommended unless high risk for bleeding
Pulmonary arterial hypertension	Oral anticoagulation target INR 2.0-3.0 Bosentan Ambrisentan Sildenafil Epoprostenol Iloprost	Therapy according to functional class (see text) Calcium antagonists indicated in patients with positive vasodilator test result
Shrinking lung syndrome	Inhaled beta-agonists Theophylline Prednisone 15-20 mg/day	Good prognosis Try to avoid immunosuppressive therapy unless progression is noted

TABLE 27-2 Suggested Therapy for Cardiac Manifestations of SLE

MANIFESTATION	THERAPY	COMMENTS
Pericarditis	Hydroxychloroquine Prednisone 5-15 mg/ day Pulse methylprednisolone 250-500 mg/day × 3 days in severe cases	Add immunosuppressive drugs (azathioprine, methotrexate, etc.) in cases recurring with maintenance doses of prednisone ≤5 mg/ day
Myocarditis	Pulse methyl- prednisolone 250-500 mg/day × 3 days Prednisone 20-30 mg/ day Intravenous cyclophosphamide pulses	Treat heart failure: diuretics, angiotensin- converting enzyme inhibitors
Heart valve disease	Low-dose aspirin Oral anticoagulation if arterial thromboembolism	Efficacy of antiaggregant or anticoagulant therapy not demonstrated

studies focus on lupus nephritis or other common manifestations such as arthritis and rashes. Therefore, most recommendations are based on observational case series and clinical experience (Tables 27-1 and 27-2).

The first important point is to adapt the intensity of treatment to the severity of the clinical manifestations. It should be always kept in mind that immunosuppressive treatment can itself be a source of irreversible damage and serious side effects. In this setting, it is important to avoid doses of prednisone higher than 5 mg/day in the long term.[69] Hydroxychloroquine helps control lupus activity and has other long-term beneficial effects, so it should be used in every patient.[45] The addition of immunosuppressive drugs as steroid-sparing agents is warranted if the combination of an antimalarial and low-dose prednisone is not enough to keep SLE in remission.

Pleuropericarditis

Pleuropericarditis can be treated with low- to medium-dose prednisone.[17] In the rare event of massive pleural effusions or cardiac compromise, pulse methylprednisolone is indicated.[70] Invasive procedures such as chest tube drainage and pericardiocentesis are not needed in the vast majority of patients, given the good response to medical therapy. Long-term therapy with antimalarials is usually effective,[4,71] but immunosuppressive drugs such as azathioprine may be necessary in recurrent cases.[17]

Pneumonitis and Alveolar Hemorrhage

Lupus pneumonitis and alveolar hemorrhage are extremely severe complications with high associated mortality, especially if not treated early. Management is often complicated by the fact that a substantial number of patients do not have a previous diagnosis of lupus and also by the difficulty of ruling out an infectious agent as the cause. Thus, an aggressive approach is warranted, and every effort should be made to confirm or exclude infection (see earlier discussion). Broad-spectrum antibiotic coverage is indicated initially until culture results have proved negative.[17] Admission to an intensive care unit, with or without mechanical ventilation and other supportive measures such as blood transfusions, is frequently needed. Immunosuppressive treatment should be instituted early, with pulse methylprednisolone treatment as the first line of therapy.[14] In the presence of fever or when infection is still a matter of concern, intravenous immunoglobulins should be considered, because they allow bridging to more aggressive immunosuppression without increasing the risk of worsening infection.[72] Intravenous cyclophosphamide and even plasma exchange are indicated in most severe cases once infection is not a concern. The usually recommended associated dose of oral prednisone is 1 mg/kg/day,[14] but it is not supported by any controlled study. The good results seen with lower doses of prednisone in lupus nephritis encourage the use of daily doses not higher than 20 to 30 mg in other patients with acute lupus complications, with rapid tapering to maintenance doses no higher than 5 mg/day.[69] Once remission has been achieved, and with the high frequency of extrapulmonary visceral involvement taken into account, prolonged therapy with oral immunosuppressive drugs such as azathioprine is indicated.

Interstitial Lung Disease

ILD is difficult to treat if the diagnosis is made when irreversible fibrosis is already present. Specific studies in patients with lupus are scarce. The common belief is that immunosuppressive treatment should be commenced in the inflammatory phase of the disease, which is demonstrated by ground-glass infiltrates on high-resolution CT scan. However, only small observational studies suggest that early steroid therapy may halt the progression to lung fibrosis.[73] Analogy with the results obtained in observational studies on scleroderma lung disease has been advocated,[74] although a metaanalysis of clinical trials did not confirm the efficacy of cyclophosphamide in preventing lung function deterioration in patients with systemic sclerosis.[75] However, this negative result may be due to the fact that treatment was started too late, suggesting that this result should be interpreted with caution. Thus, in patients with lupus with early ILD, a trial with intravenous cyclophosphamide pulses is warranted, with close monitoring of toxicity and lung function evolution.[17]

Bronchiolitis

Glucocorticoids are also advocated to treat SLE-related bronchiolitis obliterans organizing pneumonia.[4,39] In general, the response to therapy is good.[38] However, in patients who have severe disease or in whom long-term prednisone therapy is anticipated, an immunosuppressive drug such as cyclophosphamide, azathioprine, or cyclosporine should be considered.[39,76] On the other hand, constrictive bronchiolitis is poorly responsive to steroids and other immunosuppressive drugs.[38]

Pulmonary Thromboembolism

Treatment of pulmonary thromboembolism in patients with SLE follows the recommendations given for the general population.[77] Initial therapy with low-molecular-weight heparin, unfractionated heparin, or fondaparinux is recommended for at least 5 days. In cases with hemodynamic compromise, thrombolytic therapy should be considered. Indefinite therapy with oral anticoagulants to a target International Normalized Ratio (INR) of 2.0-3.0 is recommended in patients with either recurrent disease or first unprovoked venous thromboembolism and a low bleeding risk.[77] The presence of antiphospholipid antibodies does not modify these recommendations, so indefinite therapy with standard-intensity oral anticoagulation is the standard of care in this group. Higher-intensity anticoagulation is recommended for patients with antiphospholipid syndrome and recurrent thromboembolism during anticoagulant therapy.[78]

In the near future, new oral anticoagulant drugs such as rivaroxaban (a factor Xa inhibitor) and dabigatran (a direct thrombin inhibitor) will play a primary role in the management of venous thromboembolism. Clinical trials have now shown that these drugs are at least as effective as, and probably safer and more convenient than, vitamin K inhibitors, without the need for continuous laboratory monitoring.[79,80] The efficacy of these drugs in patients with antiphospholipid syndrome has not been yet studied.[81]

Pulmonary Arterial Hypertension

Recommended therapy for SLE-associated PAH does not differ from those for idiopathic PAH,[82] because no specific clinical trials have been performed in patients with lupus. Oral anticoagulation is recommended irrespective of the presence of antiphospholipid antibodies due to survival benefit in patients with idiopathic PAH, although the indication should be decided on an individual basis.[82,83] For those few patients with a positive vasodilator test result on cardiac catheterization, calcium channel blockers are recommended. However, the response and tolerance to these drugs are decreased in patients with PAH secondary to systemic sclerosis and, perhaps, other connective tissue diseases.[82] In the remaining patients, initial therapy depends on functional status. Those in functional class II should be treated with oral drugs such as bosentan, ambrisentan, and sildenafil. Patients in functional class III can also receive epoprostenol, iloprost, either inhaled or intravenous, or treprostinil. Patients in functional class IV should receive intravenous epoprostenol.[82] Sitaxentan, an endothelin antagonist approved for PAH, was withdrawn in 2010 owing to the occurrence of liver toxicity. Current guidelines also consider combination therapy, recommending its use only in specialized units.[82] For refractory patients, lung transplantation is an option, because the presence of a connective tissue disease is not considered a contraindication per se.

Besides anticoagulant and vasodilator therapy indicated in all forms of PAH, immunosuppressive therapy has been proposed to treat SLE-associated PAH. This recommendation is based on retrospective observational studies,[83,84] so the indication should be individualized according to the clinical profile of the patient.

The largest series included 13 patients with SLE and 10 patients with mixed connective tissue disease and a diagnosis of PAH by cardiac catheterization.[83] Eight of 16 patients showed response to combined therapy with prednisone 0.5 to 1 mg/kg/day with tapering to maintenance doses of 5 to 10 mg/day plus monthly intravenous pulses of cyclophosphamide. Seven additional patients received combined immunosuppressives plus vasodilator therapy, and 4 of them showed response. Global survival was 87.2% at 5 years. A functional class II assignment or a cardiac index higher than 3.1 L/min/m^2 identified cases responding to immunosuppressives. The researchers proposed that patients either in functional class II or in functional class III with a cardiac index higher than 3.1 L/min/m^2 receive initial therapy with prednisone and cyclophosphamide without vasodilators, and that maintenance therapy consist of a regimen containing azathioprine or mycophenolate in responders. Patients showing no response should be started on pulmonary vasodilators. Patients in worse functional classes are candidates for pulmonary vasodilators, with additional immunosuppressive treatment prescribed on an individual basis.

Shrinking Lung Syndrome

Therapy of shrinking lung syndrome includes combinations of prednisone, immunosuppressive drugs, theophylline, and inhaled beta-agonists.[33] Given the good prognosis of this condition, the risk/benefit ratio must be strongly considered, and prolonged regimens with a high potential for toxicity should be avoided.

Myocarditis

Myocarditis is a severe, potentially life-threatening condition that must be diagnosed and treated early. Concomitant severe SLE manifestations are common, which may contribute to long-term irreversible damage. Treatment with different combinations of pulse methylprednisolone, high-dose prednisone, intravenous cyclophosphamide, and immunoglobulins has been proposed.[43] Concomitant therapy to manage heart failure and hypertension, including diuretics and angiotensin-converting enzyme inhibitors, is crucial.[43]

Heart Valve Disease

There are no positive data supporting the efficacy of immunosuppressive therapy in preventing or treating heart valve disease in SLE.[3] Despite the strong relation with antiphospholipid antibodies, there is no evidence that antiaggregant or anticoagulant therapy stops progression of valve lesions.[57] Despite the lack of positive data, aspirin is often given as primary thromboprophylaxis. Should thromboembolic events occur, they would be treated with oral anticoagulation like that given to patients with antiphospholipid syndrome.[81] Severe valve lesions may require surgery, but the frequency of complications, usually thrombotic or hemorrhagic, is high in patients with antiphospholipid antibodies.[85]

References

1. Quadrelli SA, Alvarez C, Arce SC, et al: Pulmonary involvement of systemic lupus erythematosus: analysis of 90 necropsies. *Lupus* 18:1053–1060, 2009.
2. Cervera R, Khamashta MA, Font J, et al; European Working Party on Systemic Lupus Erythematosus: morbidity and mortality in systemic lupus erythematosus during a 10-year period: a comparison of early and late manifestations in a cohort of 1,000 patients. *Medicine* 82:299–308, 2003.
3. Tincani A, Rebaioli CB, Taglietti M, et al: Heart involvement in systemic lupus erythematosus, anti-phospholipid syndrome and neonatal lupus. *Rheumatology (Oxford)* 45(Suppl 4):8–13, 2006.
4. Keane MP, Lynch JP: Pleuropulmonary manifestations of systemic lupus erythematosus. *Thorax* 55:159–166, 2000.
5. Shan SA: The pleura. *Am Rev Respir Dis* 138:184–234, 1988.
6. Porcel JM, Ordi-Ros J, Esquerda A, et al: Antinuclear antibody testing in pleural fluid for the diagnosis of lupus pleuritis. *Lupus* 16:25–27, 2007.
7. Wang DY, Yang PC, Yu WL, et al: Serial antinuclear antibodies titre in pleural and pericardial fluid. *Eur Respir J* 15:1106–1110, 2000.
8. Toworakul C, Kasitanon N, Sukitawut W, et al: Usefulness of pleural effusion antinuclear antibodies in the diagnosis of lupus pleuritis. *Lupus* 20:1042–1046, 2011.
9. Kamen DL, Strange C: Pulmonary manifestations of systemic lupus erythematosus. *Clin Chest Med* 31:479–488, 2010.
10. Cheema GS, Quismorio FP: Interstitial lung disease in systemic lupus erythematosus. *Current Opin Pulmon Med* 6:424–429, 2000.
11. Zamora MR, Warner ML, Tuder R, et al: Diffuse alveolar hemorrhage and systemic lupus erythematosus. Clinical presentation, histology, survival, and outcome. *Medicine (Baltimore)* 76:192–202, 1997.
12. Kwok SK, Moon SJ, Ju JH, et al: Diffuse alveolar hemorrhage in systemic lupus erythematosus: risk factors and clinical outcome: results from affiliated hospitals of Catholic University of Korea. *Lupus* 20:102–107, 2011.
13. Martínez-Martínez MU, Abud-Mendoza C: Predictors of mortality in diffuse alveolar haemorrhage associated with systemic lupus erythematosus. *Lupus* 20:568–574, 2011.
14. Santos-Ocampo AS, Mandell BF, Fessler BJ: Alveolar hemorrhage in systemic lupus erythematosus: presentation and management. *Chest* 118:1083–1090, 2000.
15. Torre O, Harari S: Pleural and pulmonary involvement in systemic lupus erythematosus. *Presse Med* 40:e19–e29, 2011.
16. American Thoracic Society, European Respiratory Society: American Thoracic Society/European Respiratory Society International Multidisciplinary Consensus Classification of the Idiopathic Interstitial Pneumonias. This joint statement of the American Thoracic Society (ATS), and the European Respiratory Society (ERS) was adopted by the ATS board of directors, June 2001, and by the ERS Executive Committee, June 2001. *Am J Respir Crit Care Med* 165:277–304, 2002.
17. Pego-Reigosa JM, Medeiros DA, Isenberg DA: Respiratory manifestations of systemic lupus erythematosus: old and new concepts. *Best Practice & Res Clin Rheumatol* 23:469–480, 2009.
18. Bucciarelli S, Espinosa G, Asherson RA, et al: The acute respiratory distress syndrome in catastrophic antiphospholipid syndrome: analysis of a series of 47 patients. *Ann Rheum Dis* 65:81–86, 2006.
19. Abramson SB, Dobro J, Eberle MA, et al: Acute reversible hypoxemia in systemic lupus erythematosus. *Ann Intern Med* 114:941–947, 1991.
20. Martinez-Taboada VM, Blanco R, Armona J, et al: Acute reversible hypoxemia in systemic lupus erythematosus: a new syndrome or an index of disease activity? *Lupus* 4:259–262, 1995.
21. Badesch DB, Champion HC, Gomez Sanchez MA, et al: Diagnosis and assessment of pulmonary arterial hypertension. *J Am Coll Cardiol* 54:S55–S66, 2009.
22. Simonneau G, Robbins IM, Beghetti M, et al: Updated clinical classification of pulmonary hypertension. *J Am Coll Cardiol* 54:S43–S54, 2009.
23. Pope J: An update in pulmonary hypertension in systemic lupus erythematosus—do we need to know about it? *Lupus* 17:274–277, 2008.
24. Li EK, Tam LS: Pulmonary hypertension in systemic lupus erythematosus: clinical association and survival in 18 patients. *J Rheumatol* 26:1923–1929, 1999.
25. Kasparian A, Floros A, Gialafos E, et al: Raynaud's phenomenon is correlated with elevated systolic pulmonary arterial pressure in patients with systemic lupus erythematosus. *Lupus* 16:505–508, 2007.
26. Shen JY, Chen SL, Wu YX, et al: Pulmonary hypertension in systemic lupus erythematosus. *Rheumatol Int* 18:147–151, 1999.
27. Asherson RA, Higenbottam TW, Dinh Xuan AT, et al: Pulmonary hypertension in a lupus clinic: experience with twenty-four patients. *J Rheumatol* 17:1292–1298, 1990.
28. Asherson RA, Hackett D, Gharavi AE, et al: Pulmonary hypertension in systemic lupus erythematosus: a report of three cases. *J Rheumatol* 13:416–420, 1986.
29. Farzaneh-Far A, Roman MJ, Lockshin MD, et al: Relationship of antiphospholipid antibodies to cardiovascular manifestations of systemic lupus erythematosus. *Arthritis Rheum* 54:3918–3925, 2006.
30. Nishimaki T, Aotsuka S, Kondo H, et al: Immunological analysis of pulmonary hypertension in connective tissue diseases. *J Rheumatol* 26:2357–2362, 1999.
31. McLaughlin VV, Archer SL, Badesch DB, et al; ACCF/AHA: ACCF/AHA 2009 expert consensus document on pulmonary hypertension: a report of the American College of Cardiology Foundation Task Force on Expert Consensus Documents and the American Heart Association: developed in collaboration with the American College of Chest Physicians, American Thoracic Society, Inc., and the Pulmonary Hypertension Association. *Circulation* 119:2250–2294, 2009.
32. Condliffe R, Kiely DG, Peacock AJ, et al: Connective tissue disease-associated pulmonary arterial hypertension in the modern treatment era. *Am J Respir Crit Care Med* 179:151–157, 2009.
33. Karim MY, Miranda LC, Tench CM, et al: Presentation and prognosis of the shrinking lung syndrome in systemic lupus erythematosus. *Semin Arthritis Rheum* 31:289–298, 2002.
34. Laroche CM, Mulvey DA, Hawkins PN, et al: Diaphragm strength in the shrinking lung syndrome of systemic lupus erythematosus. *Q J Med* 265:429–439, 1990.
35. Ishii M, Uda H, Yamagami T, et al: Possible association of shrinking lung and anti-Ro/SSA antibody. *Arthritis Rheum* 43:2612–2613, 2000.
36. Toya SP, Tzelepis GE: Association of the shrinking lung syndrome in systemic lupus erythematosus with pleurisy: a systematic review. *Semin Arthritis Rheum* 39:30–37, 2009.
37. King TE: Overview of bronchiolitis. *Clin Chest Med* 14:607–610, 1993.
38. Ryu JH, Myers JL, Swensen SJ: Bronchiolar disorders. *Am J Respir Crit Care Med* 168:1277–1292, 2003.
39. Wells AU, du Bois RM: Bronchiolitis in association with connective tissue disorders. *Clin Chest Med* 14:655–666, 1993.
40. Ruiz-Irastorza G, Olivares N, Ruiz-Arruza I, et al: Predictors of major infections in systemic lupus erythematosus. *Arthritis Res Ther* 11:R109, 2009.
41. Apte M, Mcgwin G, Vilá LM, et al; LUMINA Study Group: Associated factors and impact of myocarditis in patients with SLE from LUMINA, a multiethnic US cohort (LV). *Rheumatology* 47:362–367, 2008.
42. Logar D, Kveder T, Rozman B, et al: Possible association between anti-Ro antibodies and myocarditis or cardiac conduction defects in with systemic lupus erythematosus. *Ann Rheum Dis* 49:627–629, 1990.
43. Appenzeller S, Pineau C, Clarke A: Acute lupus myocarditis: clinical features and outcome. *Lupus* 20:981–988, 2011.
44. Senkus E, Jassem J: Cardiovascular effects of systemic cancer treatment. *Cancer Treat Rev* 37:300–311, 2011.
45. Ruiz-Irastorza G, Ramos-Casals M, Brito-Zeron P, et al: Clinical efficacy and side effects of antimalarials in systemic lupus erythematosus: a systematic review. *Ann Rheum Dis* 69:20–28, 2010.
46. Nord JE, Shah PK, Rinaldi RZ, et al: Hydroxychloroquine cardiotoxicity in systemic lupus erythematosus: a report of 2 cases and review of the literature. *Semin Arthritis Rheum* 33:336–351, 2004.
47. Newton-Cheh C, Lin AE, Baggish AL, et al: Case records of the Massachusetts General Hospital. Case 11-2011. A 47-year-old man with systemic lupus erythematosus and heart failure. *N Engl J Med* 364:1450–1460, 2011.
48. Costedoat-Chalumeau N, Hulot J, Amoura Z, et al: Heart conduction disorders related to antimalarials toxicity: an analysis of electrocardiograms in 85 patients treated with hydroxychloroquine for connective tissue diseases. *Rheumatology (Oxford)* 46:808–810, 2007.
49. Wozniacka A, Cygankiewicz I, Chudzik M, et al: The cardiac safety of chloroquine phosphate treatment in patients with systemic lupus erythematosus: the influence on arrhythmia, heart rate variability and repolarization parameters. *Lupus* 15:521–525, 2006.

50. Eisen A, Arnson Y, Dovrish Z, et al: Arrhythmias and conduction defects in rheumatological diseases—a comprehensive review. *Semin Arthritis Rheum* 39:145–156, 2009.

51. Guzman J, Cardiel MH, Arce-Salinas A, et al: The contribution of resting heart rate and routine blood tests to the clinical assessment of disease activity in systemic lupus erythematosus. *J Rheumatol* 21:1845–1848, 2004.

52. Lazzerini PE, Acampa M, Guideri F et al: Prolongation of the corrected QT interval in adult patients with anti-Ro/SSA-positive connective tissue diseases. *Arthritis Rheum* 50:1248–1252, 2004.

53. Bulkley BH, Roberts WC: The heart in systemic lupus erythematosus and the changes induced in it by corticosteroid therapy. A study of 36 necropsy patients. *Am J Med* 58:243–264, 1975.

54. Mattos P, Santiago MB: Association of antiphospholipid antibodies with valvulopathy in systemic lupus erythematosus: a systematic review. *Clin Rheumatol* 30:165–171, 2011.

55. Roldan CA, Shively BK, Crawford MH: An echocardiographic study of valvular heart disease associated with systemic lupus erythematosus. *N Engl J Med* 335:1424–1430, 1996.

56. Zuily S, Regnault V, Selton-Suty C, et al: Increased risk for heart valve disease associated with antiphospholipid antibodies in patients with systemic lupus erythematosus: meta-analysis of echocardiographic studies. *Circulation* 124:215–224, 2011.

57. Moyssakis I, Tektonidou MG, Vasilliou VA, et al: Libman-Sacks endocarditis in systemic lupus erythematosus: prevalence, associations, and evolution. *Am J Med* 120:636–642, 2007.

58. Roldan CA, Qualls CR, Sopko KS, et al: Transthoracic versus transesophageal echocardiography for detection of Libman-Sacks endocarditis: a randomized controlled study. *J Rheumatol* 35:224–229, 2008.

59. Soltész P, Szekanecz Z, Kiss E, et al: Cardiac manifestations in antiphospholipid syndrome. *Autoimm Rev* 6:379–386, 2007.

60. Santiago MB, Dourado SMM, Silva NO, et al: Valvular heart disease in systemic lupus erythematosus and Jaccoud's arthropathy. *Rheumatol Int* 31:49–52, 2011.

61. Pardos-Gea J, Ordi-Ros J, Avegliano G, et al: Echocardiography at diagnosis of antiphospholipid syndrome provides prognostic information on valvular disease evolution and identifies two sub- types of patients. *Lupus* 19:575–582, 2010.

62. Nesher G, Ilany J, Rosenmann D, et al: Valvular dysfunction in antiphospholipid syndrome: prevalence, clinical features, and treatment. *Semin Arthritis Rheum* 27:27–35, 1997.

63. Roldan CA, Gelgand EA, Qualls CR, et al: Valvular heart disease as a cause of cerebrovascular disease in patients with systemic lupus erythematosus. *Am J Cardiol* 95:1441–1447, 2005.

64. Cervera R, Tektonidou M, Espinosa G, et al: Task Force on Catastrophic Antiphospholipid Syndrome (APS) and Non-criteria APS Manifestations (I): catastrophic APS, APS nephropathy and heart valve lesions. *Lupus* 20:165–173, 2011.

65. Klok FA, Mos ICM, Nijkeuter M, et al: Simplification of the revised Geneva score for assessing clinical probability of pulmonary embolism. *Arch Intern Med* 168:2131–2136, 2008.

66. Agnelli G, Becattini C: Acute pulmonary embolism. *N Engl J Med* 363:266–274, 2010.

67. Bernatsky S, Boivin JF, Joseph L, et al: An international cohort study of cancer in systemic lupus erythematosus. *Arthritis Rheum* 52:1481–1490, 2005.

68. Papiris SA, Kalomenidis I, Malagari K, et al: Extranodal marginal zone B-cell lymphoma of the lung in Sjögren's syndrome patients: reappraisal of clinical, radiological, and pathology findings. *Resp Med* 101:84–92, 2007.

69. Ruiz-Irastorza G, Danza A, Khamashta M: Glucocorticoid use and abuse in systemic lupus erythematosus. *Rheumatology (Oxford)* 2012 Jan 23 [Epub ahead of print].

70. Badsha H, Edwards CJ: Intravenous pulses of methylprednisolone for systemic lupus erythematosus. *Semin Arthritis Rheum* 32:370–377, 2003.

71. Meinão IM, Sato EI, Andrade LEC, et al: Controlled trial with chloroquine diphosphate in systemic lupus erythematosus. *Lupus* 5:237–241, 1996.

72. Zandman-Goddard G, Blank M, Shoenfeld Y: Intravenous immunoglobulins in systemic lupus erythematosus: from the bench to the bedside. *Lupus* 18:884–888, 2009.

73. Weinrib L, Sharma OP, Quismorio FP: A long-term study of interstitial lung disease in systemic lupus erythematosus. *Semin Arthritis Rheum* 20:48–56, 1990.

74. White B, Moore WC, Wigley FM, et al: Cyclophosphamide is associated with pulmonary function and survival benefit in patients with scleroderma and alveolitis. *Ann Intern Med* 132:947–954, 2000.

75. Nannini C, West CP, Erwin PJ, et al: Effects of cyclophosphamide on pulmonary function in patients with scleroderma and interstitial lung disease: a systematic review and meta-analysis of randomized controlled trials and observational prospective cohort studies. *Arthritis Res Ther* 10:R124, 2008.

76. Schlesinger C, Koss MN: The organizing pneumonias: a critical review of current concepts and treatment. *Treat Respir Med* 5:193–206, 2006.

77. Kearon C, Kahn SR, Agnelli G, et al; American College of Chest Physicians: Antithrombotic therapy for venous thromboembolic disease: American College of Chest Physicians Evidence-Based Clinical Practice Guidelines (8th Edition). *Chest* 133:454S–545S, 2008.

78. Ruiz-Irastorza G, Cuadrado M, Ruiz-Arruza I, et al: Evidence-based recommendations for the prevention and long-term management of thrombosis in antiphospholipid antibody-positive patients: Report of a Task Force at the 13th International Congress on Antiphospholipid Antibodies. *Lupus* 20:206–218, 2011.

79. EINSTEIN Investigators, Bauersachs R, Berkowitz SD, Brenner B, et al: Oral rivaroxaban for symptomatic venous thromboembolism. *N Engl J Med* 363:2499–2510, 2010.

80. Schulman S, Kearon C, Kakkar AK, et al; RE-COVER Study Group: Dabigatran versus warfarin in the treatment of acute venous thromboembolism. *N Engl J Med* 361:2342–2352, 2009.

81. Ruiz-Irastorza G, Crowther MA, Branch W, et al: Antiphospholipid syndrome. *Lancet* 376:1498–1509, 2010.

82. Galiè N, Hoeper MM, Humbert M, et al; ESC Committee for Practice Guidelines (CPG): Guidelines for the diagnosis and treatment of pulmonary hypertension: the Task Force for the Diagnosis and Treatment of Pulmonary Hypertension of the European Society of Cardiology (ESC) and the European Respiratory Society (ERS), endorsed by the International Society of Heart and Lung Transplantation (ISHLT). *Eur Heart J* 30:2493–2537, 2009.

83. Jaïs X, Launay D, Yaici A, et al: Immunosuppressive therapy in lupus- and mixed connective tissue disease-associated pulmonary arterial hypertension: a retrospective analysis of twenty-three cases. *Arthritis Rheum* 58:521–531, 2008.

84. Kato M, Kataoka H, Odani T, et al: The short-term role of corticosteroid therapy for pulmonary arterial hypertension associated with connective tissue diseases: report of five cases and a literature review. *Lupus* 20:1047–1056, 2011.

85. Erdozain J-G, Ruiz-Irastorza G, Segura M-I, et al: Cardiac valve replacement in patients with antiphospholipid syndrome. *Arthritis Care Res (Hoboken)*. 2012 Mar 15 [Epub ahead of print]

Chapter 28

Pathogenesis of the Nervous System

Cynthia Aranow, Betty Diamond, and Meggan Mackay

With greater understanding of the immune abnormalities associated with active lupus, new targets have been identified and new therapies are being developed for the treatment of active disease. However, no new potential agents are on the horizon for the treatment of neuropsychiatric lupus (NPSLE). Understanding the pathophysiologic mechanisms that contribute to NPSLE lupus is critical to the design and evaluation of effective interventions. This chapter discusses what is currently known about the causes of NPSLE and tissue injury.

Lupus affects the nervous system, causing numerous manifestations (see Chapter 29) encompassing both the central nervous system (CNS) and peripheral nervous system (PNS) with symptoms that range from focal thrombotic events to diffuse disorders affecting cognition, mood, and level of consciousness. It is clear that there can be no single pathophysiologic mechanism for all NPSLE, and mechanisms are likely to vary according to the pathoanatomic localization of disease—vascular, CNS, and PNS (Box 28-1). Vascular compromise results in local tissue ischemia and symptoms reflective of the damaged area. CNS symptoms develop from injury to the brain parenchyma, vasculature, and blood-brain barrier (BBB); data now suggest that autoantibodies and cytokines may mediate the insults, causing diffuse or focal effects on the CNS. The PNS is not protected by a BBB and therefore is susceptible to consequences of circulating autoantibodies, immune complexes, and other inflammatory molecules.

Not all neurologic manifestations experienced by patients with lupus arise from lupus, and it is exceedingly important to correctly differentiate lupus from nonlupus causes of neurologic symptoms. CNS lupus can exhibit manifestations similar to those of thrombotic thrombocytopenic purpura, posterior reversible encephalopathy syndrome, and infectious (bacterial, viral, and fungal), metabolic, and hormonal disturbances. Secondary effects of medications, particularly corticosteroids, are an additional possibility that must be considered, especially in the evaluation of emotional and cognitive complaints. Approximately two thirds of neuropsychiatric events occurring in patients with lupus are attributable to other causes.

VASCULAR MECHANISMS

Vascular injury is common in SLE. Postmortem examination of human lupus brain tissue typically shows evidence of microvascular injury with microinfarcts, perivascular lymphocytic infiltrates, and endothelial cell proliferation.[1-3] Microvascular injury leading to ischemia may result in cortical atrophy and ischemic patchy multiple sclerosis–like demyelination observed in lupus brains. Actual vasculitis with an inflammatory infiltrate and fibrinoid necrosis within vessel walls in the brain is rare, although more commonly seen in the PNS.[2,3] Gross infarcts do occur and can stem from the accelerated atherosclerosis associated with lupus or from thrombosis occurring in the context of antiphospholipid antibodies. These autoantibodies—anticardiolipin, anti–beta 2 glycoprotein I (anti–β_2 GPI), and/or the lupus anticoagulant—are associated with a hypercoagulable state that, in combination with a "second hit" such as infection or an inflammatory insult from lupus itself, gives rise to an intravascular clot. Tissue infarction, hemorrhage, or more limited focal neuron

injury results from impaired blood flow, and the actual clinical symptoms that develop from the ischemic insult depend on the location, duration, and degree of vascular compromise. Stroke, transient ischemic attacks, and cognitive decline in association with recurrent microvascular ischemia are manifestations of NPSLE associated with antiphospholipid antibodies. Mechanistically, antiphospholipid antibodies may block β_2 GPI–mediated inhibition of von Willebrand factor–dependent platelet adhesion and aggregation and thus inhibit a physiologic anticoagulant property of β_2 GP1.[4] Antiphospholipid antibodies also contribute to the vascular damage of NPSLE by promoting the development of atherosclerosis independent of the other mechanisms accelerating atherosclerosis in lupus. Antiphospholipid antibodies potentiate the formation of foam cells by facilitating uptake by macrophages of oxidized low-density lipoprotein (LDL).[5] Additionally, they upregulate endothelial cell expression of adhesion molecules, facilitating the egress of circulating monocytes from the blood into the vessel walls, where they subsequently transform into LDL-uptaking macrophages.[6]

CENTRAL NERVOUS SYSTEM MECHANISMS

The brain parenchyma may be the target of autoantibodies, cytokines, and infiltrating cells, resulting in either diffuse or focal injury. Behavioral, cognitive, or mood disorders, psychosis, and an acute confusional state are examples of syndromes attributed to diffuse pathophysiology; focal injury is associated primarily with vascular disease, but focal seizures may also result from parenchymal disease. Brains of young MRL/lpr mice show mononuclear cell infiltrates within the choroid plexus, hippocampus, meninges, and cerebellum.[7,8] As these mice age, CD19+ B cells and CD138+ plasma cells are present, and the brain tissue shows atrophy and decreased branching of neuronal dendritic spines. Cerebrospinal fluid (CSF) from both MRL/lpr mice as well as from patients with SLE may be toxic to neurons.[9,10] However, many of the CNS NPSLE syndromes are not permanent, raising the possibility that neuronal injury may not always be lethal and that neural reparative mechanisms are operative.

Cytokines and Chemokines

Cytokines and chemokines are small molecules which may play a role in the pathophysiology of CNS NPSLE. Elevations of these proteins have been demonstrated within the CSF of patients with CNS NPSLE. They may gain access to the CNS from the peripheral circulation through a permeabilized BBB or be produced within the CNS by astrocytes and microglia. Cytokines have directs effects on endothelial cells and neurons, causing dysfunction and apoptosis. In mice, proinflammatory cytokines are linked to depression, anhedonia, social isolation, and lethargy; in humans, similar associations exist.[11-14]

Examination of CSF of patients with NPSLE has shown the presence of multiple proinflammatory cytokines, including interleukin-6 (IL-6), IL-1, tumor necrosis factor (TNF), interferon alpha (IFN-α), B cell–activating factor (BAFF), and APRIL (a proliferation-inducing ligand) (reviewed in reference 15). Intrathecal elevation of IL-6 is

Box 28-1 Locations of NPSLE Pathophysiology

Vasculature
Brain parenchyma
Peripheral nerve

consistently reported in studies of NPSLE and is present in studies of patients with central NPSLE syndromes. Numerous inflammatory conditions, autoimmune diseases, and neurologic conditions, such as CNS infections, cerebrovascular events, and myelitis, also cause increased levels of intrathecal IL-6 and must be clinically excluded before a CSF IL-6 elevation is attributed to NPSLE. Intrathecal IL-6 in NPSLE is associated with the CSF IgG Index, a measurement of intrathecal immunoglobulin (Ig) G production suggesting that IL-6 in concert with BAFF and APRIL, which are also elevated in CSF from patients with diffuse NPSLE, may increase B-cell activation within the CNS.[16,17] BAFF is a potent B-cell activator that plays a role in the regulation of B-cell proliferation and differentiation.

IFN-α, also demonstrated in the CSF of patients with NPSLE, is of particular interest in the pathophysiology of NPSLE, given its ability to promote an autoimmune response and its recognized role in the etiopathogenesis of SLE.[18,19] Immune complexes created with NPSLE CSF in combination with nucleic acid–containing antigen stimulate release of IFN-α and other proinflammatory molecules (IFN-γ–induced protein 10 [IP-10], IL-8, and monocyte chemoattractant protein-1 [MCP-1]) ex vivo.[19] Indirect support for the role of IFN-α in NPSLE comes from the untoward side effects of this cytokine when used as a therapeutic modality for treatment of hepatitis or malignancy; approximately one third of patients receiving IFN-α exhibit CNS symptoms.[20] The most common feature is depression, but psychosis, confusion, mania, and seizures have also been reported. Of note, IL-6 may potentiate the depressive propensity of IFN-α because high serum levels of IL-6 prior to administration of IFN-α predict the development of depression.[21]

Levels of chemokines such as IL-8, IP-10, fractalkine, RANTES (regulated upon activation, normal T-cell expressed, and secreted), MCP-1, and matrix metalloproteinase 9 (MMP-9) are additionally elevated in NPSLE CSF.[16,22-24] Although these molecules are all capable of triggering inflammatory responses, the pathophysiologic mechanism(s) by which they cause CNS symptoms remains to be elucidated. The intrathecal ratio of IP-10 to MCP-1 is significantly higher in patients with NPSLE than in patients with SLE without CNS symptoms and may be a useful marker of NPSLE.[25] Because multiple cytokines and chemokines are present in the CSF of patients, studying the effects of a single mediator is difficult and may, in fact, not be as informative as the examination of various combinations.

Autoantibodies

Tissue injury in SLE is generally initiated by autoantibodies; thus, the role of autoantibodies in the pathogenesis of CNS NPSLE syndromes continues to be an area of interest. Pathology may potentially result from direct binding of antibodies to cells, from effects of activation of complement and the inflammatory cascade, or from antibody-dependent cellular cytotoxicity. It is likely that numerous antibodies are involved in the pathogenesis of NPSLE.

Antineuronal antibodies were the first autoantibodies identified and studied for a potential pathophysiologic role in NPSLE. However, NPSLE symptoms do not correlate with serum titers of these antibodies, and there are no identified functional effects of antibody binding to neurons in vitro. Immunoproteomic assays that have been used with neuroblastoma lines or brain to probe for specific brain antigens recognized by autoantibodies in lupus sera have identified several neuronal targets.[26,27] Sera from patients with and without NPSLE react with neuronal antigens; however, the specificities of these antineuronal antibodies in the two clinical groups are different.[27] These data suggest that some antineuronal autoantibodies are associated with neuropathology and others are not.

Alpha-tubulin has been recognized as a targeted autoantigen in SLE, particularly in patients with severe CNS manifestations of NPSLE.[28] Longitudinal observational studies of patients with and without these autoantibodies remain to be conducted.

In addition to their prothrombotic properties, earlier studies suggested that antiphospholipid and anti–β$_2$ GPI antibodies have direct effects on brain parenchyma and may influence neuronal function (reviewed in reference 29). In one study, binding of these antibodies to neuronal cell membranes had depolarizing and permeabilizing effects on synaptosomes.[30] However, these reports have not been confirmed or extended, and whether antiphospholipid antibodies are directly neurotoxic remains unclear.

Serum and CSF anti–ribosomal P (anti-P) antibodies occur infrequently in SLE. When first described, they were reported to be associated with lupus psychosis.[31] They are now recognized to occur with multiple features of lupus, including, in some but not all reports, thought and mood disorders.[32,33] Anti-P antibodies have also been shown to disrupt olfaction and cause depression in a mouse model of direct intrathecal injection of the antibodies.[34,35] In these studies, autoantibodies bound to neurons in the hippocampus, cingulate cortex, and olfactory piriform cortex. It is noteworthy that in humans, an impaired sense of smell is associated with lupus disease activity as well as a past history of NPSLE.[36] In vitro, anti-P antibodies are toxic to neurons. They bind a neuronal integral membrane protein, resulting in a rapid and sustained influx in calcium into the neuron with subsequent apoptotic cell death.

Antibodies to the N-methyl-D-aspartate receptor (NMDAR) are likely to play a pathophysiologic role in cognitive and emotional dysfunction in SLE. Anti-NMDAR autoantibodies are a subset of anti–double-stranded DNA (dsDNA) autoantibodies that cross-react with the NR2A and B subunits of the glutamate receptor.[37] Binding of anti-DNA, anti-NMDAR antibodies to neurons can lead to excitatory, apoptotic, and noninflammatory cell death, but the effects of anti-NMDAR antibody binding are concentration dependent. Lower antibody concentration affects synaptic plasticity and results in temporary neuronal dysfunction without death.[38] The NMDAR is found throughout the brain but is most dense in the hippocampus and amygdala, areas associated with learning and affective responses, respectively. Nonautoimmune mice that are immunized to produce anti-DNA, anti-NMDAR antibodies display no behavioral abnormalities and show no neuronal loss despite the presence of circulating anti-NMDAR antibodies.[39] Although seemingly counterintuitive, this observation is consistent with our knowledge of the BBB, which protects the brain parenchyma against potentially toxic substances in the bloodstream (see later). Breach of the BBB in either the hippocampus or the amygdala of these immunized, nonautoimmune mice results in regional loss of neurons in the hippocampus or amygdala, respectively, and leads to associated behavior abnormalities (impaired learning in mice with a breach of the BBB in the hippocampus and attenuated responses to a fear-conditioning paradigm in mice with a breach in the BBB in the amygdala).[39,40] Approximately 25% to 50% of patients with lupus exhibit elevated titers of anti-NMDAR antibody. Although cross-sectional studies have not shown a consistent correlation between serum anti-NMDAR antibodies and cognitive impairment or depression, the antibodies have been detected in CSF of patients with lupus and have been eluted from lupus brain tissue.[37,41-45] Several studies of CSF anti-NMDAR antibody titers show a significant correlation between antibody titers and central, diffuse NPSLE syndromes (seizures, acute confusional state, mood and anxiety disorders, psychosis, severe cognitive dysfunction).[46] Titers subside concomitant with a decrease in symptoms. Furthermore, the presence of CSF anti-NMDAR antibody helps distinguish patients with diffuse NPSLE from patients without NPSLE.

Blood-Brain Barrier

The importance of the BBB in the pathogenesis of central NPSLE symptoms is increasingly recognized.[47,48] The BBB protects the brain parenchyma, and its disruption allows potentially toxic molecules

Accessing the Brain: Two-Step Injury

Circulating autoantibodies or cytokines

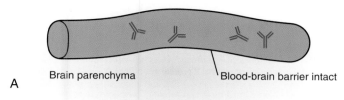

A   Brain parenchyma   Blood-brain barrier intact

Circulating autoantibodies or cytokines and breach in blood-brain barrier

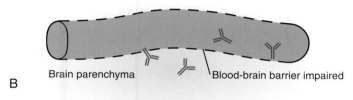

B   Brain parenchyma   Blood-brain barrier impaired

FIGURE 28-1 Circulating autoantibodies or cytokines with neurotoxic potential cannot cause neuronal toxicity unless they have access to the brain parenchyma. **A,** Serum autoantibodies or inflammatory mediators have no pathologic consequences in the brain if the blood-brain barrier (BBB) is intact and unimpaired. An intact BBB sequesters the brain from pathogenic insults. **B,** Circulating autoantibodies or inflammatory mediators may gain access to the brain if there is a breach in the BBB caused by agents such as lipopolysaccharide (LPS; a surrogate for infection), epinephrine, complement activation products, stress, pain, and nicotine. Neuronal damage results when neurotoxic mediators have access to the brain parenchyma because of an impaired BBB.

and cells access to the brain. The BBB additionally serves as a signaling interface between the blood and brain. The components of the BBB are brain endothelial cells, pericytes, astrocytes, and basement membrane. The integrity of the barrier is maintained primarily by tight junctions between brain endothelial cells, so that macromolecules such as antibodies and cells must be transported across the BBB through pinocytosis or active transport.[49] Breach of the BBB allows cells and/or macromolecules direct access to the brain parenchyma (Figure 28-1). Insults such as systemic infection and lipopolysaccharide (LPS) release soluble molecules, including TNF, IL-1, and IL-6, that activate brain endothelial cells, causing upregulation of cell adhesion molecules (intracellular adhesion molecule 1 [ICAM-1], E-selectin, and vascular cell adhesion molecule 1 [VCAM-1]) leading to disruption of the BBB.[50,51] Complement activation is another trigger that alters BBB integrity.[52,53] Exposure of brain endothelial cells to the complement activation product C5a results in increased expression of both inducible nitric oxide synthase (iNOS) and reactive oxygen species (ROS), with cytoskeletal changes and increased BBB permeability.[54] Stress, pain, and nicotine are additional insults that cause BBB dysfunction with alterations in endothelial cell tight junction integrity.[55-58] In lupus, antiphospholipid antibody binding in vitro to brain endothelial cells induces expression of adhesion molecules but has not been shown to alter barrier function.[29]

The response of the BBB to various insults is not uniform, and studies in both mice and humans show regional responses. This might be due to regional microglial activation and an "inside-out" disruption of the BBB, whereby activated microglial cells secrete proinflammatory and immunoregulatory molecules such as TNF-α,

IL-1β, nitric oxide, prostaglandin E_2, transforming growth factor beta (TGF-β), and nerve growth factor, which influence the integrity of the BBB.[48,58] Alternatively, there may be site-specific targets for different agents, owing perhaps to localization of receptors for mediators such as cytokines, C5a, and epinephrine, so that different insults disrupt BBB integrity in characteristic locations. For example, exposure of the brain to LPS causes the BBB of the dorsal hippocampus to become permeable, whereas the amygdala and ventral brain BBBs are susceptible to effects of epinephrine. Therefore, the presence of a pathogenic serum autoantibody is not sufficient to cause brain dysfunction, and serum titers of a neurotoxic autoantibody are not expected to correlate with central NPSLE syndromes. The autoantibody must be able to access brain tissue through a breach in the BBB in order to effect clinical symptoms, and the site of the breach depends on the insulting agent. As predicted by this model, the presence of pathogenic autoantibodies or other toxic substances in the CSF correlates with central NPSLE symptoms.

PERIPHERAL NERVOUS SYSTEM MECHANISMS

Peripheral neuropathies are not uncommon in SLE. Pathogenic mechanisms affecting peripheral nerves differ from those damaging the CNS, because there is no anatomic protective barrier in the periphery, and autoantibodies and other potentially damaging agents such as products of complement activation have direct access to the neural structures. Several autoantibodies have been described in association with peripheral neuropathy in SLE, including lupus-specific antibodies (e.g., anti-Sm) as well as antibodies that are typically associated with other disorders but that have been described in patients with lupus with overlapping neurologic syndromes.[59] These include anti-GM1and anti-GM3 (commonly associated with Guillain-Barré syndrome) and antiacetylcholine receptor (anti-AChR) in patients with overlapping myasthenia gravis.[60,61] The vasculature of the peripheral nerves may also be affected, causing peripheral neurologic symptoms. Nerve biopsy may show vasculitis of the epineural arteries with ischemia and axonal degeneration.[62] The observed response of some cases of peripheral neuropathy to immunosuppressive treatment suggests an inflammation-mediated process.

SUMMARY

Like the pathophysiology of symptoms occurring outside the nervous system, the pathogenesis of many neuropsychiatric syndromes in SLE appears to be mediated by autoantibodies and inflammatory molecules. Several neurotoxic autoantibodies have been clearly associated with CNS manifestations of NPSLE in animal models and human disease, but they do not entirely account for the spectrum of NPSLE symptoms. Our understanding of the processes leading to features of NPSLE affecting the brain is further hindered by our incomplete knowledge of the BBB. Breach of the BBB allows autoantibodies, cells, cytokines, and other potentially neurotoxic substances access to the CNS. The neurologic and behavioral symptoms resulting from neuronal toxicity depend on the anatomic location of the loss of BBB integrity. Additionally, the fact that the BBB generally sequesters the brain from exposure to antibodies or cytokines leads to a relationship between the accumulation of damage and disease activity that is not seen in peripheral organs. Damage in the brain is not directly related to disease activity because systemic disease may often not affect the CNS. Vascular abnormalities resulting from atherosclerotic disease, vasculopathy, and hypercoagulability are other mechanisms contributing to the pathogenesis of NPSLE. Newer imaging modalities may soon permit visualization of neural connectivity and specific patterns of neuronal activation or inhibition, allowing for clearer identification of CNS lupus and better correlations of CSF findings and autoantibodies with symptomatology.

References

1. Johnson RT, Richardson EP: The neurological manifestations of systemic lupus erythematosus. *Medicine (Baltimore)* 47:337–369, 1968.

2. Ellis SG, Verity MA: Central nervous system involvement in systemic lupus erythematosus: a review of neuropathologic findings in 57 cases, 1955-1977. *Semin Arthritis Rheum* 8:212–221, 1979.

3. Hanly JG, Walsh NM, Sangalang V: Brain pathology in systemic lupus erythematosus. *J Rheumatol* 19:732–741, 1992.

4. Hulstein JJ, Lenting PJ, de Laat B, et al: beta2-Glycoprotein I inhibits von Willebrand factor dependent platelet adhesion and aggregation. *Blood* 110:1483–1491, 2007.

5. Kobayashi K, Tada K, Itabe H, et al: Distinguished effects of antiphospholipid antibodies and anti-oxidized LDL antibodies on oxidized LDL uptake by macrophages. *Lupus* 16:929–938, 2007.

6. Simantov R, LaSala JM, Lo SK, et al: Activation of cultured vascular endothelial cells by antiphospholipid antibodies. *J Clin Invest* 96:2211–2219, 1995.

7. Ma X, Foster J, Sakic B: Distribution and prevalence of leukocyte phenotypes in brains of lupus-prone mice. *J Neuroimmunol* 179:26–36, 2006.

8. Sled JG, Spring S, van Eede M, et al: Time course and nature of brain atrophy in the MRL mouse model of central nervous system lupus. *Arthritis Rheum* 60:1764–1774, 2009.

9. Sakic B, Kirkham DL, Ballok DA, et al: Proliferating brain cells are a target of neurotoxic CSF in systemic autoimmune disease. *J Neuroimmunol* 169:68–85, 2005.

10. Maric D, Millward JM, Ballok DA, et al: Neurotoxic properties of cerebrospinal fluid from behaviorally impaired autoimmune mice. *Brain Res* 920:183–193, 2001.

11. Anisman H, Kokkinidis L, Merali Z: Further evidence for the depressive effects of cytokines: anhedonia and neurochemical changes. *Brain Behav Immun* 16:544–556, 2002.

12. Dantzer R: Cytokine, sickness behavior, and depression. *Immunol Allergy Clin North Am* 29:247–264, 2009.

13. Miller DB, O'Callaghan JP: Depression, cytokines, and glial function. *Metabolism* 54:33–38, 2005.

14. Dinan TG: Inflammatory markers in depression. *Curr Opin Psychiatry* 22:32–36, 2009.

15. Okamoto H, Kobayashi A, Yamanaka H: Cytokines and chemokines in neuropsychiatric syndromes of systemic lupus erythematosus. *J Biomed Biotechnol* 268436, 2010.

16. Katsumata Y, Harigai M, Kawaguchi Y, et al: Diagnostic reliability of cerebral spinal fluid tests for acute confusional state (delirium) in patients with systemic lupus erythematosus: interleukin 6 (IL-6), IL-8, interferon-alpha, IgG index, and Q-albumin. *J Rheumatol* 34:2010–2017, 2007.

17. George-Chandy A, Trysberg E, Eriksson K: Raised intrathecal levels of APRIL and BAFF in patients with systemic lupus erythematosus: relationship to neuropsychiatric symptoms. *Arthritis Res Ther* 10:R97, 2008.

18. Winfield JB, Shaw M, Silverman LM, et al: Intrathecal IgG synthesis and blood-brain barrier impairment in patients with systemic lupus erythematosus and central nervous system dysfunction. *Am J Med* 74:837–844, 1983.

19. Santer DM, Yoshio T, Minota S, et al: Potent induction of IFN-alpha and chemokines by autoantibodies in the cerebrospinal fluid of patients with neuropsychiatric lupus. *J Immunol* 182:1192–1201, 2009.

20. Wichers M, Maes M: The psychoneuroimmuno-pathophysiology of cytokine-induced depression in humans. *Int J Neuropsychopharmacol* 5:375–388, 2002.

21. Prather AA, Rabinovitz M, Pollock BG, et al: Cytokine-induced depression during IFN-alpha treatment: the role of IL-6 and sleep quality. *Brain Behav Immun* 23:1109–1116, 2009.

22. Okamoto H, Kobayashi A, Yamanaka H: Cytokines and chemokines in neuropsychiatric syndromes of systemic lupus erythematosus. *J Biomed Biotechnol* 2010:268436, 2010.

23. Trysberg E, Blennow K, Zachrisson O, et al: Intrathecal levels of matrix metalloproteinases in systemic lupus erythematosus with central nervous system engagement. *Arthritis Res Ther* 6:R551–R556, 2004.

24. Fragoso-Loyo H, Richaud-Patin Y, Orozco-Narvaez A, et al: Interleukin-6 and chemokines in the neuropsychiatric manifestations of systemic lupus erythematosus. *Arthritis Rheum* 56:1242–1250, 2007.

25. Okamoto H, Iikuni N, Kamitsuji S, et al: IP-10/MCP-1 ratio in CSF is a useful diagnostic marker of neuropsychiatric lupus patients. *Rheumatology (Oxford)* 45:232–234, 2006.

26. Iizuka N, Okamoto K, Matsushita R, et al: Identification of autoantigens specific for systemic lupus erythematosus with central nervous system involvement. *Lupus* 19:717–726, 2010.

27. Lefranc D, Launay D, Dubucquoi S, et al: Characterization of discriminant human brain antigenic targets in neuropsychiatric systemic lupus erythematosus using an immunoproteomic approach. *Arthritis Rheum* 56:3420–3432, 2007.

28. Ndhlovu M, Preuss BE, Dengjel J, et al: Identification of alpha-tubulin as an autoantigen recognized by sera from patients with neuropsychiatric systemic lupus erythematosus. *Brain Behav Immun* 25:279–285, 2011.

29. Brey RL, Muscal E, Chapman J: Antiphospholipid antibodies and the brain: a consensus report. *Lupus* 20:153–157, 2011.

30. Chapman J, Cohen-Armon M, Shoenfeld Y, et al: Antiphospholipid antibodies permeabilize and depolarize brain synaptoneurosomes. *Lupus* 8:127–133, 1999.

31. Bonfa E, Golombek SJ, Kaufman LD, et al: Association between lupus psychosis and anti-ribosomal P protein antibodies. *N Engl J Med* 317:265–271, 1987.

32. Bonfa E, Elkon KB: Clinical and serologic associations of the antiribosomal P protein antibody. *Arthritis Rheum* 29:981–985, 1986.

33. Karassa FB, Afeltra A, Ambrozic A, et al: Accuracy of anti-ribosomal P protein antibody testing for the diagnosis of neuropsychiatric systemic lupus erythematosus: an international meta-analysis. *Arthritis Rheum* 54:312–324, 2006.

34. Katzav A, Ben-Ziv T, Chapman J, et al: Anti-P ribosomal antibodies induce defect in smell capability in a model of CNS-SLE (depression). *J Autoimmun* 31:393–398, 2008.

35. Katzav A, Solodeev I, Brodsky O, et al: Induction of autoimmune depression in mice by anti-ribosomal P antibodies via the limbic system. *Arthritis Rheum* 56:938–948, 2007.

36. Shoenfeld N, Agmon-Levin N, Flitman-Katzevman I, et al: The sense of smell in systemic lupus erythematosus. *Arthritis Rheum* 60:1484–1487, 2009.

37. DeGiorgio LA, Konstantinov KN, Lee SC, et al: A subset of lupus anti-DNA antibodies cross-reacts with the NR2 glutamate receptor in systemic lupus erythematosus. *Nat Med* 7:1189–1193, 2001.

38. Huerta PT, Volpe BT: Transcranial magnetic stimulation, synaptic plasticity and network oscillations. *J Neuroeng Rehabil* 6:7, 2009.

39. Kowal C, DeGiorgio LA, Nakaoka T, et al: Cognition and immunity; antibody impairs memory. *Immunity* 21:179–188, 2004.

40. Huerta PT, Kowal C, DeGiorgio LA, et al: Immunity and behavior: antibodies alter emotion. *Proc Natl Acad Sci U S A* 103:678–683, 2006.

41. Omdal R, Brokstad K, Waterloo K, et al: Neuropsychiatric disturbances in SLE are associated with antibodies against NMDA receptors. *Eur J Neurol* 12:392–398, 2005.

42. Hanly JG, Robichaud J, Fisk JD: Anti-NR2 glutamate receptor antibodies and cognitive function in systemic lupus erythematosus. *J Rheumatol* 33:1553–1558, 2006.

43. Harrison MJ, Ravdin LD, Lockshin MD: Relationship between serum NR2a antibodies and cognitive dysfunction in systemic lupus erythematosus. *Arthritis Rheum* 54:2515–2522, 2006.

44. Lapteva L, Nowak M, Yarboro CH, et al: Anti-N-methyl-D-aspartate receptor antibodies, cognitive dysfunction, and depression in systemic lupus erythematosus. *Arthritis Rheum* 54:2505–2514, 2006.

45. Kowal C, Degiorgio LA, Lee JY, et al: Human lupus autoantibodies against NMDA receptors mediate cognitive impairment. *Proc Natl Acad Sci U S A* 103:19854–19859, 2006.

46. Fragoso-Loyo H, Cabiedes J, Orozco-Narvaez A, et al: Serum and cerebrospinal fluid autoantibodies in patients with neuropsychiatric lupus erythematosus. Implications for diagnosis and pathogenesis. *PLoS One* 3:e3347, 2008.

47. Abbott NJ, Mendonca LL, Dolman DE: The blood-brain barrier in systemic lupus erythematosus. *Lupus* 12:908–915, 2003.

48. Diamond B, Huerta PT, Mina-Osorio P, et al: Losing your nerves? Maybe it's the antibodies. *Nat Rev Immunol* 9:449–456, 2009.

49. Abbott NJ, Patabendige AA, Dolman DE, et al: Structure and function of the blood-brain barrier. *Neurobiol Dis* 37:13–25, 2010.

50. Banks WA, Erickson MA: The blood-brain barrier and immune function and dysfunction. *Neurobiol Dis* 37:26–32, 2010.

51. Verma S, Nakaoke R, Dohgu S, et al: Release of cytokines by brain endothelial cells: a polarized response to lipopolysaccharide. *Brain Behav Immun* 20:449–455, 2006.

52. Gerard C: Complement C5a in the sepsis syndrome—too much of a good thing? *N Engl J Med* 348:167–169, 2003.

53. Ward PA: The dark side of C5a in sepsis. *Nat Rev Immunol* 4:133–142, 2004.

54. Jacob A, Hack B, Chiang E, et al: C5a alters blood-brain barrier integrity in experimental lupus. *FASEB J* 24:1682–1688, 2010.

55. Hawkins BT, Abbruscato TJ, Egleton RD, et al: Nicotine increases in vivo blood-brain barrier permeability and alters cerebral microvascular tight junction protein distribution. *Brain Res* 1027:48–58, 2004.

56. Hossain M, Sathe T, Fazio V, et al: Tobacco smoke: a critical etiological factor for vascular impairment at the blood-brain barrier. *Brain Res* 1287:192–205, 2009.

57. Brooks TA, Hawkins BT, Huber JD, et al: Chronic inflammatory pain leads to increased blood-brain barrier permeability and tight junction protein alterations. *Am J Physiol Heart Circ Physiol* 289:H738–H743, 2005.

58. Carvey PM, Hendey B, Monahan AJ: The blood-brain barrier in neurodegenerative disease: a rhetorical perspective. *J Neurochem* 111:291–314, 2009.

59. Huynh C, Ho SL, Fong KY, et al: Peripheral neuropathy in systemic lupus erythematosus. *J Clin Neurophysiol* 16:164–168, 1999.

60. Matsuki Y, Hidaka T, Matsumoto M, et al: Systemic lupus erythematosus demonstrating serum anti-GM1 antibody, with sudden onset of drop foot as the initial presentation. *Intern Med* 38:729–732, 1999.

61. Valesini G, Pastore R, de Berardinis PG, et al: Appearance of anti-acetylcholine receptor antibodies coincident with onset of myasthenic weakness in patient with systemic lupus erythematosus. *Lancet* (8328):831, 1983.

62. McCombe PA, McLeod JG, Pollard JD, et al: Peripheral sensorimotor and autonomic neuropathy associated with systemic lupus erythematosus. Clinical, pathological and immunological features. *Brain* 110(Pt 2):533–549, 1987.

Chapter 29

Clinical Aspects of the Nervous System

Sterling G. West

Neuropsychiatric manifestations of systemic lupus erythematosus (NP-SLE) are frequent, vary from mild to severe, and are often difficult to diagnose and distinguish from those of other diseases. Any location in the nervous system may be affected, with symptoms and signs ranging from mild cognitive dysfunction to seizures, strokes, and coma. At the initial development of neurologic manifestations, many patients have other medical conditions or are receiving medications that can affect the central nervous system (CNS) or the peripheral nervous system (PNS). The challenge to the clinician is to determine the exact cause of the nervous system dysfunction to institute the appropriate therapy. This chapter describes the classification, clinical signs and symptoms, laboratory and radiographic findings, differential diagnosis, and treatment of SLE involving the nervous system.

CLASSIFICATION

The prevalence of NP manifestations in adult SLE ranges from 6% to 91%, depending on the ascertainment methodology.[1-5] The lower percentages are from studies that reported only patients with NP-SLE who developed *objective* NP manifestations as a result of lupus, whereas the higher percentages come from studies reporting patients with SLE who have either *subjective* or *objective* complaints of NP dysfunction. However, comparing past studies of NP-SLE is often impossible, because many reports are cross-sectional studies that include patients with varying disease durations and do not use a standardized definition or classification system for NP manifestations. In 1999, an international, multidisciplinary committee developed case definitions, including diagnostic criteria and important exclusions, for 19 NP lupus syndromes[5] (Table 29-1). This American College of Rheumatology (ACR) nomenclature is the current standard used to help clinicians classify NP-SLE, as well as help investigators in future studies. The complete case definitions are available on the ACR web site at http://www.rheumatology.org/publications/ar/1999/aprilappendix.asp?aud=mem.

Since the publication of the ACR nomenclature and case definitions for NP lupus syndromes, several investigators have used these criteria in their surveys. In a cross-sectional, population-based study from Finland, Ainala and others[4] found that 42 of 46 (91%) patients with SLE met criteria for NP-SLE using the ACR nomenclature. Many of these were mild syndromes including cognitive dysfunction, headaches, and mood disorders. When these patients were compared with well-matched control subjects, 56% of the latter fulfilled at least one of the ACR criteria.[6] The criteria therefore had a high sensitivity (91%) but a low specificity (46%). If the ACR criteria were revised to exclude syndromes without objective findings such as anxiety, headaches, mild depression, subjective cognitive complaints, and polyneuropathy symptoms with a negative electromyogram and nerve conduction velocities, then the specificity improved to 93%. Other studies also found a high prevalence of NP manifestations using the ACR nomenclature including investigators from San Antonio (80% of 128 patients with SLE), Italy (72% of 61 patients), London and Cagliari, Italy (57% of 323 patients), Canada (37% of 111 patients), China (19% of 518 patients), and Sweden (38% of 117 patients).[7] In 2002 the Systemic Lupus International Collaborating Clinics (SLICC) research network began enrollment of an inception cohort to study prospectively the frequency and clinical features and outcomes of nervous system disease in patients with SLE over a 10-year period. A recent publication from this important ongoing cohort study reported that NP manifestations are common, the majority of symptoms are mild, and only a minority can be attributed to SLE.[2]

In summary, the ACR nomenclature is useful for major NP-SLE syndromes but problematic when applied to subjective syndromes such as headaches, mild cognitive dysfunction, minor psychiatric symptoms (e.g., anxiety, mild depression), and paresthesias without electrophysiologic abnormalities, which are common in patients without SLE. Using a more restrictive nomenclature that excludes these subjective syndromes, only 12% to 30% of patients with SLE will have a clinically evident NP event that can be directly attributed to lupus (primary NP-SLE) during the course of their disease.

CLINICAL PRESENTATIONS

Frequency of Manifestations

Patients with SLE who develop NP manifestations can present with a myriad of diffuse and/or focal symptoms and signs involving the brain, spinal cord, or PNS. Overall, less than 33% to 50% of these manifestations can be attributed to SLE (primary NP-SLE), whereas the remainder are the result of other causes (e.g., infection, metabolic, medications) (secondary NP events). Approximately 40% to 60% of NP events occur at disease onset or within 1 to 2 years of the diagnosis of SLE.[8] The cumulative frequencies of the various NP presentations are reported in Table 29-1 and can be divided into CNS, psychiatric, and PNS presentations. Notably, an individual patient can have more than one neurologic manifestation.

Etiopathogenesis

Several autopsy series have reported detailed neuropathologic analyses of patients with NP-SLE.[9-11] Many of these studies are hampered by the inclusion of patients with secondary causes of CNS dysfunction, as well as patients with prolonged intervals between NP-SLE manifestations and death. Despite the limitations, these studies provide important insights into the pathogenesis of NP-SLE and agree on several important points. First, there is no distinct typical or pathognomonic lesion exists that NP-SLE causes in the brain that is diagnostically specific, similar to the "wire loop" lesion of the kidney or the "onionskin" lesion of the spleen. Notably, vasculitis is unusual (3% to 5%) at autopsy. The most common finding is a small-vessel, bland, noninflammatory, proliferative vasculopathy characterized by hyalinization. These degenerative and proliferative changes in the small cerebral vessels are similar to the vascular changes observed in hypertensive encephalopathy and thrombotic thrombocytopenia purpura. The neuropathologic lesions of SLE, however, are characterized as more focal or more scattered and by the fact that they vary in age from region to region, rather than appearing to have occurred simultaneously. Finally, clinical manifestations may not be readily explained by pathologic findings. Some patients with NP-SLE, particularly those with diffuse manifestations, may have normal or relatively unremarkable brain pathologic characteristics.[11]

TABLE 29-1 Neuropsychiatric Syndromes of Systemic Lupus Erythematosus (SLE)

MANIFESTATION	FREQUENCY (%)*
Central nervous system	
Acute confusional state	4-7
Cognitive dysfunction	
Mild to moderate	11-54
Severe (dementia)	3-5
Headache (overall)	24-72
Pseudotumor cerebri	<1
Aseptic meningitis	<1
Cerebrovascular disease	5-18
Myelopathy	1
Movement disorders	<1
Demyelinating syndromes	<1
Seizures	7-20
Psychiatric disturbances	
Psychosis	2-11
Mood and anxiety disorders (overall)	24-57
Severe depression	10
Anxiety	4-8
Peripheral nervous system	
Cranial neuropathy	1
Peripheral neuropathy	2-21
Acute inflammatory demyelinating polyradiculopathy (Guillain-Barré syndrome)	<1
Mononeuropathy, single or multiplex	<1
Plexopathy	<1
Autonomic neuropathy	<1
Myasthenia gravis	<1

*Estimated cumulative frequencies are based on published studies and reviews. Adapted from references 5 and 8.

Despite these autopsy findings, the pathogenesis of NP-SLE remains unknown. However, it is unlikely that a single pathogenic mechanism is responsible for the myriad of NP manifestations observed in NP-SLE (see Table 29-1). Diffuse cerebral manifestations (e.g., acute confusional state, psychosis, others) that are often transient, reversible on therapy, and not consistently associated with brain pathologic abnormalities, most likely have a different pathogenesis from the focal symptoms (e.g., strokes, others), which are usually acute in onset, permanent even with therapy, and frequently associated with pathologic lesions at autopsy. Many investigators believe that cerebrovascular endothelial dysfunction plays a pivotal role. Primary NP-SLE events tend to occur during active lupus, supporting complement activation as an important contributor to this endothelial dysfunction.[12,13] Endothelial dysfunction and its associated microvasculopathy can disrupt the blood-brain barrier, allowing an influx of cells, autoantibodies, and cytokines into the CNS, which can cause diffuse NP manifestations. Additionally, procoagulant factors (e.g., antiphospholipid antibodies, others) can contribute to endothelial cell activation, predisposing the patient to thrombosis and emboli leading to strokes and other focal manifestations. In any single patient with NP-SLE, a combination of these mechanisms likely contributes to clinical manifestations[14] (see Chapter 28 for a more complete discussion).

CLINICAL MANIFESTATIONS

NP-SLE can involve the CNS, PNS, autonomic nervous system and/or myoneural junction (see Table 29-1). SLE can exhibit diffuse, focal, or a combination of symptoms. Clinical signs and symptoms range from mild and transient dysfunction to severe presentations, resulting in permanent neurologic sequelae and/or death. This diversity of manifestations and severity are the result of several different immunopathogenic mechanisms, which can affect various areas of an anatomically and physiologically complex nervous system. The clinician must always be aware that neurologic abnormalities in SLE may not

Box 29-1 Secondary (Non-Lupus) Causes of Neuropsychiatric Manifestations in Systemic Lupus Erythematosus

Infection
Medications
Thrombotic thrombocytopenia purpura
Hypertension
Posterior reversible leukoencephalopathy syndrome
Metabolic disturbances
  Hyperglycemia or hypoglycemia
  Electrolyte imbalances (Na^{+2}, Ca^{+2})
  Uremia
Hypoxemia
Fever
Thyroid disease
Vitamin B12 deficiency
Atherosclerotic strokes
Subdural hematoma
Berry aneurysm or cerebral hemorrhage
Cerebral lymphoma
Fibromyalgia
Reactive depression
Sleep apnea
Other primary neurologic or psychiatric diseases

be the result of primary NP-SLE but secondary to infection, electrolyte abnormalities, or numerous other causes (Box 29-1). In the prospective SLICC inception cohort study of 890 patients with lupus, 271 (33%) had 407 NP events of which 93% affected the CNS and only 7% involved the PNS.[2] Of those with NP events, 78% were diffuse and 22% were focal manifestations. Notably, one third or less (16% to 33%) of the events could be attributed to SLE with the majority secondary to a non-lupus cause.

Central Nervous System
Acute Confusional State

Acute confusional state, previously called *acute organic brain syndrome* (OBS) or *encephalopathy*, is defined as a disturbance of consciousness or level of arousal characterized by reduced ability to focus, maintain, or shift attention to external stimuli, and accompanied by disturbances of cognition, mood, affect, and/or behavior.[5] This condition has been termed *delirium* in the *Diagnostic and Statistical Manual of Mental Disorders*, fourth edition (DSM IV) and the *International Classification of Diseases*, ninth revision (ICD-9) diagnostic classifications. Disorganized thinking, loss of orientation, agitation, and delusions can be present. Symptoms may fluctuate or progress. An ominous sign is progression to a reduced level of consciousness, such as stupor or coma. Acute confusional state is one of the most common presentations observed in 4% to 7% of all patients with NP-SLE and up to 30% of patients hospitalized for NP-SLE.[15] Vasculitis, leukothrombosis, and autoantibodies have all been described as causes of acute confusion. Notably, this presentation is also common in patients with SLE who have had NP disturbances caused by cerebral infections, hypertension, medications, thrombotic thrombocytopenia purpura (TTP), and metabolic disturbances, which must always be excluded.

Cognitive Dysfunction

Cognitive dysfunction (previously called *chronic OBS* or *encephalopathy*) can range from mild cognitive impairment to dementia, in which neuropsychological testing reveals abnormalities in multiple domains of attention, reasoning, memory, language, visual-spatial processing, psychomotor speed, and executive function.[5] The recommended 1-hour ACR neuropsychological battery of tests is a standardized, validated instrument (sensitivity 80%, specificity 81%) to document cognitive dysfunction, but it must be administered by a trained neuropsychologist.[16] Other screening tests are also available. Over 80% of patients with lupus have subjective complaints of cognitive difficulties, and multiple secondary causes must be excluded (see Box 28-1). As expected, up to 87% of patients with a history of primary NP-SLE events have objective cognitive deficits on NP testing.[17] However, mild cognitive dysfunction (e.g., *lupus fog*) has also been documented in patients with SLE without a history of NP-SLE. A review of 14 cross-sectional studies of cognitive function in SLE without overt neuropsychological symptoms revealed subclinical cognitive impairment in 11% to 54% of patients.[18] This dysfunction includes various deficits, because no specific SLE pattern of abnormalities is observed. Most studies, however, show deficits in areas of verbal learning or memory, attention and mental flexibility, and visual-spatial skills. In the majority of patients, these abnormalities are subclinical and do not significantly affect the quality of life. In a 5-year prospective study involving 47 patients with SLE, Hanly and colleagues[19] reported that only 21% had cognitive impairment on neuropsychological tests at baseline. On follow-up testing, 19% of patients resolved their cognitive dysfunction without therapy, whereas 17% either maintained their cognitive impairment or developed new cognitive abnormalities. Those few patients who showed cognitive decline on serial testing were those who developed clinically overt NP events during the study period. Other investigators have confirmed that cognitive performance remains stable over time in the majority of patients with mild deficits on testing and does not predict the subsequent development in NP-SLE.[20]

The pathogenesis of cognitive dysfunction in SLE is unknown, but several clinical associations have been reported. Most studies have demonstrated an association between cognitive impairment and active or past NP-SLE events, but they have not shown an association with global SLE disease activity or corticosteroid use.[20] Some studies support but others discount that psychological distress can affect cognitive performance. An association has been reported between cognitive abnormalities and certain autoantibodies in the serum or cerebrospinal fluid (CSF) or both. The strongest agreement is the association between cognitive dysfunction, cognitive decline, and persistently positive antiphospholipid antibodies.[20] Recently, Diamond and colleagues[21] reported that a subset of anti–double-stranded DNA (anti-dsDNA) antibodies that cross react with the anti-*N*-methyl-D-aspartate receptor subunit 2A (NR2A) and anti-*N*-methyl-D-aspartate receptor subunit 2B (NR2B) of the *N*-methyl-D-aspartate receptor (NMDAR) is associated with diffuse CNS manifestations including cognitive dysfunction and emotional distress particularly when present within the CSF. This association is notable as this subset of NMDARs is increased in both the hippocampus (learning and memory) and the amygdala (fear-conditioning response). They are receptors for glutamate, the major excitatory neurotransmitter of the brain. Binding of the anti-NMDAR antibodies to their cognate antigen enhances calcium influx into the neuron, resulting in mitochondrial stress, caspase activation, and apoptosis, which could result in cognitive deficits and other NP manifestations. Finally, no association has been found between mild cognitive impairment and antiribosomal P or antineuronal antibodies.[20]

Many patients with SLE (up to 87%) with a history of NP-SLE have significant cognitive dysfunction on neuropsychological testing.[17] Cerebral atrophy and the number and size of white matter lesions or strokes on magnetic resonance imaging (MRI) correlate with the severity of cognitive dysfunction. Some patients progress to dementia (3% to 5%) with global cognitive dysfunction marked by impairment in short- and long-term memory and disturbances in judgment, abstract thinking, and other high cortical functions. The degree of cognitive impairment may be severe, interfering with the patient's ability to live independently. Dementia can be the result of active NP-SLE, of scarring from previously active NP-SLE, or of multiple infarctions from antiphospholipid antibodies.[22]

Most studies of cognitive impairment have used adult study subjects with SLE but not pediatric patients, because no validated battery of neuropsychological tests for children with SLE has been available.

Recently, a pediatric version of the Automated Neuropsychological Assessment Metrics (P-ANAM) had initial validation in a pediatric lupus population and showed neurocognitive impairment in 16 of 27 (59%) childhood patients with lupus without a history of NP-SLE.[23] The future impact of cognitive dysfunction on a child's academic achievement and activities of daily living is unknown but is likely to be significant as the maturing adolescent brain is more vulnerable to disease-associated injury. An additional concern is the potential effect of maternal antineuronal antibodies such as anti-NMDAR on a fetus whose brain lacks a competent blood-brain barrier for much of gestation.

Headache

Headaches are common in patients with SLE, occurring in 24% to 72% of patients.[2-4,7] Migraine and tension headaches make up the majority. Because of the high prevalence of headache in the general population (40%), the association between headache and SLE is controversial.[24] However, some investigators have described a unique headache as a manifestation of primary NP-SLE. This headache is characterized by an acute presentation during a lupus flare, frequent association with other neurologic complications and abnormal laboratory tests, and resolves with corticosteroid therapy as the lupus disease activity improves. Additionally, previous studies have suggested that migraine headache in patients with SLE is associated with Raynaud phenomenon, antiphospholipid antibodies, and/or thrombotic events. However, controlled studies of over 275 patients have failed to confirm these observations.[25] Despite the lack of confirmation, many clinicians will administer a 2-week trial of low–molecular-weight heparin to determine whether treatment-resistant headaches improve in a patient with antiphospholipid antibodies.

Benign intracranial hypertension (i.e., pseudotumor cerebri) can occasionally occur in patients with NP-SLE.[26] Patients' presenting signs include refractory headaches, papilledema, and no focal neurologic symptoms. Lumbar puncture reveals increased intracranial pressure (greater than 200 mm H_2O), normal protein, and no white blood cells in the CSF. Although pseudotumor cerebri can occur in adults, most patients are young, adolescent women with severe SLE. Several patients had rapid corticosteroid withdrawal and one half had cerebral venous sinus thrombosis as a result of hypercoagulability (e.g., nephrotic syndrome, antiphospholipid antibodies) as a potential cause of pseudotumor cerebri. In addition to pseudotumor cerebri, CNS vasculitis, cerebral vein thrombosis, intracranial hemorrhage, and aseptic meningitis can be the result of lupus and manifest with headache. Non-lupus secondary causes must always be ruled out in all patients before ascribing a severe headache to primary NP-SLE. The most common or important secondary causes include severe hypertension, infection, nonsteroidal antiinflammatory medications (e.g., aseptic meningitis), antimalarial therapy, sleep apnea, cerebral venous sinus thrombosis, and subdural hematoma.

Aseptic Meningitis

Aseptic meningitis in SLE is rare (<1%). Patient symptoms include fever, headache, meningeal signs, and CSF pleocytosis with normal CSF glucose and protein less than 100 mg/dL.[1] The pleocytosis is most commonly less than 200 to 300 cells/mm³ and predominantly lymphocytes. Rarely, significantly higher cell counts with a neutrophil predominance can occur in patients who are severely ill. Infectious meningitis of any cause, subarachnoid hemorrhage, carcinomatous meningitis, sarcoidosis, and medication effects from nonsteroidal antiinflammatory drugs (e.g., ibuprofen, others), as well as from intravenous gamma globulin and azathioprine, must be excluded. The cause of aseptic meningitis in NP-SLE is unclear, but patients usually respond to corticosteroid therapy.

Cerebrovascular Disease

Cerebrovascular disease (CVD) occurs in 5% to 18% of patients with SLE and can affect any area of the brain.[27-29] Ischemic strokes account for 80% of the CVD observed. The age- and sex-adjusted relative risk for stroke is reported to be up to eight times that of the general population. Acute presentations include transient ischemic attacks (TIAs), hemiplegia, aphasia, cortical blindness, or other deficits of cerebral function. Strokes usually occur within the first 5 years of the onset of SLE; and between 13% and 64% of patients who have had a stroke will have a recurrent stroke, resulting in significant morbidity and a 12% to 28% mortality rate.[27,30]

Strokes can be from large- or small-vessel disease. Large-vessel strokes can be the result of vasculitis, thrombosis from a coagulopathy, and cardiogenic emboli.[31] Small-vessel strokes and TIAs can be from vasculitis, noninflammatory vasculopathy, leukothrombosis, emboli, and antiphospholipid antibody–associated thrombosis. Patients with stroke from antiphospholipid antibodies frequently have evidence of livedo reticularis (Sneddon syndrome). Hemorrhagic strokes from intraparenchymal or subarachnoid bleeding also can occur. In any patient with SLE who has had a stroke, both hypertension and accelerated atherosclerosis must also be considered.

Several risk factors for strokes in patients with SLE have been identified including advanced age, previous stroke or TIA, cigarette smoking, hypertension, dyslipidemia, diabetes mellitus, antiphospholipid antibodies, cardiac valvular disease, and a Systemic Lupus Erythematosus Disease Activity Index (SLEDAI) score of >6.[8,29] Clinical experience suggests that the use of the specific cyclooxygenase-2 inhibitors in patients with SLE who have these risk factors may contribute to the risk of subsequent clotting, especially in patients with antiphospholipid antibodies. Control of hypertension, of elevated cholesterol and blood glucose levels, as well as smoking cessation, must be part of the treatment plan to prevent stroke or the recurrence of stroke.

The diagnosis of CVD is made clinically and supported by neuroimaging studies. A computed tomographic (CT) scan of the brain is capable of detecting cerebral hemorrhage and large infarctions, making it a useful study in screening patients with SLE who have acute neurologic deterioration. Cranial MRI with contrast is superior to CT scanning in detecting smaller and frequently transient lesions. An MRI typically shows hyperintense gray and white matter lesions on T2-weighted images, which account for the patient's clinical symptoms. Additional lesions in clinically silent areas are also frequently observed. Magnetic resonance angiography (MRA), carotid Doppler ultrasound, and echocardiogram are noninvasive procedures that can be useful in detecting large-vessel vasculitis, thrombosis, or sources of emboli, leading to vascular occlusion and stroke. Angiograms are more likely to show abnormalities in patients with large infarctions. CSF examination may show pleocytosis and high protein in patients with cerebral vasculitis or blood in patients with subarachnoid hemorrhage. Otherwise, the CSF examination is usually normal or demonstrates nonspecific abnormalities, such as a few cells or high protein or both.

Treatment of strokes in patients with SLE is based on the suspected pathogenesis.[8] Patients with suspected vasculitis are treated with corticosteroids and cytotoxic drugs, whereas those with a coagulopathy or cardiac emboli are treated with anticoagulation therapy. Treatment of patients with strokes as a result of a noninflammatory vasculopathy is difficult since the pathogenesis of these vascular lesions is unclear. Although not proven to reduce stroke in patients with SLE, most clinicians prescribe aspirin or other platelet inhibitors and aggressively treat stroke risk factors. The value of corticosteroids in these patients is uncertain and could potentially contribute to stroke risk by increasing hypertension, cholesterol, and blood glucose. Patients, however, are often given corticosteroids to control other accompanying lupus manifestations.

Myelopathy

Patients with SLE with spinal cord myelopathy present with progressive or sudden weakness or paralysis (e.g., paraplegia, quadriplegia), bilateral sensory deficits, and impaired sphincter control.[32] Myelopathy occurs in approximately 1% of patients and can be the initial presentation of SLE. Most patients (80%) are young women between 20 and 40 years of age, although childhood cases have also been reported. CSF is abnormal in the majority of patients, including elevated protein (greater than 80%), pleocytosis (50% to 70%), and decreased glucose levels less than 30 mg% (50%). An MRI of the spinal cord can help confirm the diagnosis and exclude other causes of spinal cord compression, which may benefit from surgery. An MRI of lupus myelopathy typically shows edema with abnormalities of T2-weighted images (up to 93%), which may be accompanied by spinal cord enlargement in 75% of patients. Any level of the spinal cord can be involved. Notably, some patients (up to 30%) may have a normal MRI, especially if the examination is delayed (longer than 5 days) or if the patient has received treatment. The differential diagnosis includes compressive myelopathy (e.g., tumor, abscess, hematoma), epidural lipomatosis, vertebral compression fracture, anterior spinal artery syndrome, infection (e.g., herpes zoster, tuberculosis, polyoma virus including John Cunningham (JC) virus), sarcoidosis, and Guillain-Barré syndrome.

The cause of lupus myelopathy is multifactorial. Vasculitis during an acute exacerbation of lupus leading to ischemic necrosis of the cord has been pathologically documented in a few cases. Some investigators have reported that patients with SLE with myelopathy frequently have antiphospholipid antibodies and clots, whereas other investigators have not. Recently, anti–neuromyelitis optica (NMO) IgG antibodies have been associated with transverse myelitis.[33] The antigenic target of these antibodies is aquaporin-4, which is the most abundant water channel in the CNS. These patients have several features in common, including the development of longitudinally extensive transverse myelitis involving at least three vertebral segments on MRI. This development is distinct from other causes of myelopathy that typically involve a single segment. Additional features that may be present include optic neuritis, coexistent Sjögren syndrome, and anti–Sjögren syndrome antigen A (anti-SSA/Ro) antibodies.[34] Identification of this subset is important because the presence of anti–neuromyelitis optica IgG (anti-NMO-IgG) antibodies indicates a severe disease course with frequent relapses.

Lupus myelopathy tends to have a poor prognosis. Several reports have emphasized that pulsed methylprednisolone and cyclophosphamide may improve the prognosis of these patients. This therapy must be used early, because 50% of patients will reach their peak severity of myelopathy symptoms within 3 to 5 days of onset. Early use of aggressive therapy has resulted in the reversal of symptoms and stabilization in the majority of patients with 50% having a complete recovery and 29% having a partial recovery.[32] Rituximab has also been successfully used.[34] In patients with significant titers of antiphospholipid antibodies, anticoagulation therapy should probably be used, although studies are limited. Recurrences of myelopathy, particularly in patients with anti-NMO-IgG antibodies, are common (50% to 60%). Rehabilitation measures to prevent pressure sores; preserve range of motion, strength, and mobility; and institute appropriate bladder management should be initiated early.

Movement Disorders

Chorea, hemiballismus, cerebellar ataxia, and parkinsonian-like rigidity or tremors are rare manifestations. Chorea is the most common, occurring in <1% (adults) to 4% (pediatric) of patients with SLE.[35] Chorea is characterized by rapid, brief, involuntary, and irregular movements and may be generalized or limited to the extremities, trunk, or face. Choreoathetosis is diagnosed when chorea is accompanied by slow, writhing movements of the affected extremity. Chorea occurs most commonly in young women, children, and during pregnancy (chorea gravidarum) or the postpartum period. It may be the initial presentation of SLE or precede other manifestations of SLE by years. Chorea usually occurs early in the course of SLE, tends to be unilateral, can be recurrent (35%), and is frequently associated with other NP-SLE symptoms such as strokes. Antiphospholipid antibodies are frequently found and may be responsible for basal ganglia infarction. The CSF examination is usually unremarkable. The symptoms of chorea usually last for several weeks but rarely can last for up to 3 years.

A long differential diagnosis of illnesses is rarely associated with chorea. Sydenham chorea, secondary to rheumatic fever, is the most common and can be ruled out by obtaining antistreptococcal antibodies (anti-DNase B). However, the onset of chorea in a young woman with a positive antinuclear antibody (ANA) test result should strongly suggest SLE. The recommended treatment of chorea has been corticosteroids and dopamine antagonists. Some patients spontaneously recover, whereas others fail to respond to immunosuppressive therapy. Cervera and others[35] have recommended aspirin or anticoagulation therapy in patients with chorea and antiphospholipid antibodies.

Infarction of the subthalamic nucleus can result in hemiballismus.[1] It rarely has been reported in SLE. Ballismus may be steroid responsive or related to antiphospholipid antibodies. Cerebellar ataxia is reported in less than 1% of patients with SLE.[1] Patients have an inability to stop or end purposeful movements. The abnormalities may involve the trunk or extremities. Nystagmus is common. The cause is uncertain, but some cases may be caused by cerebellar or brainstem infarction, antiphospholipid antibodies, or associated with Purkinje cell antibodies. In patients with cerebellar atrophy associated with antibodies against Purkinje cells, a paraneoplastic syndrome must be ruled out before attributing it to NP-SLE.

Tremor of all types has been reported in up to 5% of patients with SLE during the course of their disease.[1] However, parkinsonian-like symptoms caused by alterations of the substantia nigra are an extremely rare manifestation of NP-SLE. Patients present with behavioral alterations (e.g., irritability, apathy), rigidity and progressive bradykinesia, and/or akinetic mutism. Single-photon emission CT (SPECT) cerebral scanning can detect decreased regional cerebral blood flow to the basal ganglia. Treatment with dopamine-agonist drugs can lead to recovery.

Demyelinating Syndrome

Syndromes similar to multiple sclerosis (MS), sometimes called *lupoid sclerosis*, have rarely (<1%) been described in patients with SLE.[36] Interestingly, both MS and NP-SLE share many features including clinical presentation, Lhermitte sign, a positive ANA test result (2% to 27% of patients with MS), abnormal CSF with elevated IgG index and oligoclonal bands, and abnormal brain MRIs. Whether both diseases can coexist in one patient or whether lupoid sclerosis is simply an unusual presentation of NP-SLE is unclear. Notably, antiphospholipid antibodies have been demonstrated in a number of patients with an MS-like illness, suggesting these antibodies may be pathogenic in lupoid sclerosis and transverse myelitis.

Another MS-like presentation is Devic disease (NMO-spectrum disorder).[33,34] These patients present with optic neuritis and longitudinally extensive transverse myelitis either simultaneously or separately. They have anti-NMO-IgG antibodies (75%); however, unlike patients with MS, they frequently have anti-SSA/Ro antibodies (see previous discussion under "Myelopathy"). Patients with SLE with antiphospholipid antibodies can mimic this presentation with optic nerve and spinal cord infarction.

The therapy of patients with lupoid sclerosis differs from MS therapy. Both patient populations may respond to immunosuppressive therapy. However, patients with SLE who have lupoid sclerosis or optic nerve or spinal cord infarction caused by vascular occlusion from antiphospholipid antibodies are best treated with anticoagulation therapy. Patients with SLE with NMO-spectrum disorder should receive aggressive immunosuppressive therapy.

Seizures

Seizures occur in 7% to 20% of patients with SLE. They may occur before the development of other symptoms of SLE or at any time during its course.[37] Generalized major motor (67% to 88%) and partial complex seizures are most common, although any kind of seizure can occur. Seizure episodes are usually self-limited, although status epilepticus can occur and frequently signals a preterminal event. Seizures may occur in isolation or accompany other neurologic symptoms.

The cause of seizures in NP-SLE is multifactorial. Antineuronal antibodies, focal ischemia, and infarctions caused by vascular occlusion from thrombosis and emboli, hemorrhage, and cytokine or neuroendocrine effects on the seizure threshold have all been implicated. Several studies have shown an association between antiphospholipid antibodies and seizures in patients with SLE.[38] An increased risk of seizures, seizures with strokes, and recurrence of seizures exists in patients with higher titers of antiphospholipid antibodies. Some investigators have demonstrated a direct effect of these antibodies on neurons, possibly leading to neuronal dysfunction and seizure by a nonthrombotic mechanism.[39] However, most seizures in patients with antiphospholipid antibodies are probably the result of cerebral ischemia from cerebral microinfarctions. Secondary causes of seizures include infections, medication effects, metabolic disturbances, hypoxemia, and hypertension, which must be ruled out in all patients with SLE who have seizures.

Most patients with a single seizure do not need anticonvulsant medications. Risk factors for recurrent seizures requiring anticonvulsant therapy include focal neurologic signs, abnormal brain MRI, and an epileptiform electroencephalogram (EEG). Although some anticonvulsant medications have been shown to cause a positive ANA test result and rarely clinical SLE, this presentation is no reason to withhold these medications when they are indicated for patients with established lupus. Seizure control is important since recurrent seizures increase the vulnerability of neurons to additional injury. Consequently, corticosteroids and other immunosuppressive medications should be used in patients with status epilepticus, recurrent seizures, or other neurologic manifestations. Patients with SLE with high-titer antiphospholipid antibodies and seizures should also receive anticoagulation therapy, especially if the brain MRI shows areas of microinfarction.

Psychiatric Disorders
Psychosis

Psychosis is defined as a severe disturbance in the perception of reality, characterized by delusions and/or hallucinations (usually auditory in NP-SLE). Psychosis occurs in up to 11% of patients with SLE (2% to 4% in most series) with the initial episode occurring within the first year after the diagnosis of SLE in the majority (60% to 80%).[8,40] Most patients have evidence of globally active lupus. Therefore the sudden onset of psychosis in a patient with clinically and serologically active SLE without a psychiatric history or precipitating cause is usually indicative of NP-SLE. Some investigators have reported an association between anti–ribosomal P antibodies and psychosis.[41] Titers of these antibodies reportedly rise with an exacerbation of psychosis and decrease in response to corticosteroid therapy. Other studies have not found a correlation between these antibodies and psychosis[42] (see Chapter 30).

Mood and Anxiety Disorders

Anxiety and depression are common, occurring in 24% to 57% of patients with lupus.[3,4,7] Most of these psychiatric issues are the result of non-lupus causes such as medications, a reaction to a chronic illness, or other psychosocial factors. However, severe affective disorders such as major depression and anxiety and panic disorders can be the result of primary NP-SLE. Some previous studies have included these manifestations under the category of *lupus psychosis*. Anti–ribosomal P antibodies and anti-NMDAR antibodies have been associated with mood disorders in some but not all studies[43] (see Chapter 30).

Peripheral Nervous System
Cranial Neuropathies

Cranial neuropathy occurs in 1% of patients with SLE during the course of the disease.[1] It usually occurs during active SLE, can be transient, and usually responds to corticosteroid therapy. Ptosis, third and sixth nerve palsies, internuclear ophthalmoplegia, trigeminal neuralgia, and facial nerve palsies are the most common. Optic neuropathy causing blindness, anosmia, tinnitus, vertigo, and sensorineural hearing loss are less common symptoms. The causes of cranial neuropathies include vascular occlusion and focal meningitis. Autopsy studies have demonstrated lesions in the brainstem, as well as the peripheral part of the cranial nerves. Some of these neuropathies have been associated with vasculitis and others with thrombosis associated with antiphospholipid antibodies. All patients with optic neuritis should be tested for anti-NMO-IgG antibodies.[33,34]

Peripheral Polyneuropathies

Peripheral nerve involvement occurs in 2% to 27% of adult and pediatric patients with SLE, depending on diagnostic criteria used,[1,44] and can be the initial presentation of SLE. Symptoms can be severe or subtle and overlooked by the clinician. The most common presentation is a distal sensory or sensorimotor neuropathy (66% of patients). Less commonly, patients can have mononeuritis multiplex, acute or chronic polyradiculopathy, and rarely, a plexopathy.

Patients with distal, symmetric, peripheral polyneuropathy can present with mild to evere sensory or less commonly sensorimotor fiber involvement. Patients usually complain of numbness and dysesthesias. Neurologic testing shows cutaneous hypesthesia to pinprick, light touch, and temperature stimuli. Most of these patients have a length-dependent peripheral neuropathy supported by abnormal neurodiagnostic studies. However, a significant number of patients have symptoms suggestive of a peripheral neuropathy but normal nerve conduction studies. Immunohistologic staining of skin biopsies of these patients has demonstrated an involvement of intradermal, small-diameter, nonmyelinated afferent nerve fibers.[45] Patients with significant paresthesias and abnormal nerve conduction tests are treated with glucocorticoid and neuroleptic agents. Patients with mild symptoms or normal electrodiagnostic studies or both are treated symptomatically with neuroleptic medications because 67% will not deteriorate on follow-up.[44]

Less commonly (<1%), a large, myelinated afferent fiber is involved, which exhibits deficits of vibratory and proprioceptive sense, areflexia, and sensory ataxia with variable motor dysfunction.[1] When motor axons are affected, weakness and muscle atrophy are seen. Electrodiagnostic studies usually show features of a mixed axonal and demyelinating neuropathy. The pathogenesis of the peripheral neuropathy is unclear. Antineuronal antibodies and vasculitis from deposition of immune complexes have both been implicated.

Mononeuritis multiplex is the multifocal and random dysfunction of individual, noncontiguous nerve trunks.[1] Patients frequently develop sensorimotor deficits in the upper or lower extremities (wrist- or foodrop) with an asymmetric distribution. Occasionally, it can be widespread and mimic a distal, symmetric, sensorimotor polyneuropathy. Mononeuritis multiplex typically occurs in the setting of active SLE, often with other neurologic abnormalities. Neurodiagnostic studies usually show an axonal pattern with a reduction in amplitude of evoked compound action potentials with relative preservation of nerve conduction velocities. The cause is believed to be a vasculitis of the vasa nervorum, although this can only be demonstrated on sural nerve biopsy in 50% of cases. Aggressive therapy with corticosteroids and pulse intravenous or daily oral cyclophosphamide with or without plasma exchange is recommended. Rituximab or intravenous gamma globulin therapy has also been effectively used. Recovery of nerve function takes up to 1 year.

Few cases of patients with SLE with an inflammatory polyradiculoneuropathy have been reported.[1] There are two forms: the acute form resembles Guillain-Barré syndrome and the chronic form resembles chronic, inflammatory, demyelinating polyradiculoneuropathy. Patients with acute presentation have an ascending, predominantly areflexic motor paralysis, which peaks in 10 to 14 days. Little or no sensory loss occurs. Little loss of cutaneous sensation develops since small, nonmyelinated fibers are not involved.

Involvement of large myelinated afferent fibers leads to the loss of proprioception and vibratory sensation. An associated autonomic dysfunction can develop in some patients. No sphincter disturbance occurs, which helps separate it from transverse myelitis. CSF examination reveals an elevated total protein level with a white blood cell count less than 50 cells/mm^3. Electrodiagnostic studies reveal a demyelinating pattern with a slowing of nerve conduction velocities, dispersion of evoked compound action potentials, conduction block, and significant prolongation of distal latencies. The pathogenesis is unknown. Unlike in Guillain-Barré syndrome without SLE, patients have been successfully treated with corticosteroid agents. Recovery can occur within weeks if no neuronal damage has occurred. Experience with the use of plasmapheresis or intravenous gamma globulin is limited in patients with SLE who have symptoms similar to those of Guillain-Barré syndrome.

Patients with SLE who exhibit chronic demyelinating polyradiculopathy resembling chronic inflammatory demyelinating polyneuropathy (CIDP) can experience recurrent episodes of acute symptoms similar to those with Guillain-Barré syndrome, a mononeuritis multiplex–like pattern, or a symmetric polyradiculopathy evolving over weeks to months. Electrodiagnostic studies frequently are confusing, showing a mixed axonal-demyelinating pattern. Nerve biopsy is usually not helpful but may show inflammation. Therapy includes corticosteroids, plasmapheresis, cyclophosphamide, and intravenous gamma globulin.

Multiple secondary causes of PNS involvement must be ruled out before attributing peripheral nerve dysfunction to NP-SLE. Uremia, diabetes mellitus, drug toxicities, vitamin deficiencies, heavy metal or solvent exposure, cancers and paraproteinemias, viral and other infections, sarcoidosis, alcohol and other toxins, hereditary neurologic diseases, and other causes must be ruled out.

Autonomic Disorders

Acute severe autonomic neuropathy with profound dysfunction of the parasympathetic or sympathetic nervous system or both have rarely (<1%) been reported. Gastrointestinal (constipation), cardiovascular (orthostatic hypotension), genitourinary (sphincter control, sphincteric action, erectile or ejaculatory dysfunction), sweating (anhidrosis and heat intolerance), and pupillary abnormalities are evident and, when severe, respond to corticosteroids.

Sensitive tests of autonomic function show that mild dysfunction may be present, although clinically unappreciated, in up to 20% of patients with lupus.[46] This dysfunction does not correlate with disease duration, lupus activity, or the presence of peripheral neuropathy. The clinical significance, prognosis, and treatment for these mild abnormalities are unknown.

Myasthenia Gravis and Related Disorders

Myasthenia gravis and SLE may coexist in the same patient.[1] Over 50 cases have been reported. Myasthenia typically precedes the onset of SLE in the majority of these patients. In some cases, SLE develops after thymectomy for the treatment of myasthenia gravis.[47] Patients have typical manifestations of myasthenia with neuromuscular fatigue and a weakness of bulbar or other voluntary muscles with repetitive muscular contractions. No impairment of sensation or loss of reflexes occurs. Antibodies to the acetylcholine receptor can be demonstrated in 85% of patients with myasthenia and are believed to cause neuromuscular symptoms by reducing the number of acetylcholine receptors at the neuromuscular junction. Diagnosis is made clinically and confirmed with electromyography (EMG), and repetitive peripheral nerve stimulation at a rate of 2 per second shows a characteristic decremental response that is reversed by the acetylcholinesterase drugs.

Few patients with SLE with Lambert-Eaton myasthenic syndrome have been reported. Presenting symptoms include weakness and hyporeflexia, which improves with exercise. Neurodiagnostic studies show a myopathic EMG with low-amplitude compound muscle action potential, which increases in amplitude after exercise.

High-frequency, repetitive stimulation demonstrates a 50% or more increment in the amplitude of the compound motor action potential. No improvement of clinical or EMG findings occurs with anticholinesterase drugs. The etiopathogenesis is suspected to be an IgG antibody against the voltage-gated calcium channels in the presynaptic neuromuscular junction. Plasmapheresis and immunosuppressive medications are effective therapy.

Neuropsychiatric Systemic Lupus Erythematosus in Children and Older Adults

As in adults, the prevalence of NP manifestations in pediatric SLE varies from 20% to 95%.[48] A literature review of 11 pediatric studies found a 33% incidence in 353 children.[49] A 6-year prospective study of 75 pediatric patients with SLE found that 95% had evidence of NP-SLE at some time using the ACR NP-SLE nomenclature.[50] If only serious manifestations were considered, then the prevalence of NP-SLE fell to 76%. Not surprisingly, NP-SLE was present in twice as many hospitalized patients, compared with SLE outpatients. In those with NP manifestations, over 70% occur within the first year of diagnosis of SLE. Chorea is a more common manifestation in pediatric NP-SLE than adults and is associated with antiphospholipid antibodies. Additionally, adolescent patients with SLE with antiphospholipid antibodies, particularly the lupus anticoagulant, are most at risk for strokes and need life-long anticoagulation therapy to prevent recurrences.[48] In older age groups (>50 years), CNS involvement is reported to be less frequent (6% to 19%), is milder, and has a better prognosis.[51]

SECONDARY CAUSES OF CENTRAL NERVOUS SYSTEM DYSFUNCTION IN SYSTEMIC LUPUS ERYTHEMATOSUS

Secondary causes of CNS dysfunction in patients with SLE must always be ruled out before attributing symptoms to primary NP-SLE (see Box 29-1). Prospective studies point out that 50% to 67% of neurologic events are caused by secondary factors.[2] The most common secondary causes include infections, medications, metabolic disturbances, TTP, and sleep apnea. Equally as important, the clinician must realize that the presence of an ANA in a patient with neurologic symptoms does not imply that the patient has NP-SLE or, for that matter, SLE at all.

Over the past decade, reversible posterior leukoencephalopathy syndrome (RPLS) has been recognized as an important secondary cause of neurologic dysfunction.[52] At onset, patients with SLE typically have seizures (75% to 100%), accelerated hypertension (90% to 95%), acute renal failure (85% to 90%), headache (70%), blurred vision (45% to 50%), and/or cortical blindness (30%). Notably, over 75% have had augmentation of their immunosuppressants (intravenous methylprednisolone, intravenous cyclophosphamide) within an average of 7 days before the development of RPLS. The majority (61%) have evidence of brain MRI abnormalities involving the posterior circulation caused by vasogenic edema. Therapy includes prompt control of the blood pressure. Further increase in immunosuppressive therapy is contraindicated and potentially detrimental. Long-term anticonvulsant use is rarely needed once neuroimaging abnormalities resolve after an average of 25 days. With early recognition and prompt therapy, full neurologic recovery usually occurs.

CLINICAL AND LABORATORY EVALUATION

No single test can diagnose NP-SLE. After excluding secondary causes, the diagnosis of NP-SLE can only be confirmed if a patient's NP symptoms can be corroborated with objective abnormalities in the neuropsychological examination, CSF analysis, neuroimaging studies, EEG, and/or biopsy. Therefore a methodologic work-up is essential for the patient with SLE who complains of NP symptoms.[8,15] A careful and thorough history and physical examination, including a complete neurologic and mental status evaluation, must be performed on each patient. In addition, a variety of laboratory, CSF, and neurodiagnostic studies must be performed; when appropriate,

---

Box 29-2 Laboratory Evaluation and Diagnostic Imaging of Patients with Systemic Lupus Erythematosus and Neuropsychiatric Manifestations

Complete blood count and peripheral blood smear
Chemistries: electrolytes, creatinine, glucose
Liver-associated enzymes
Urinalysis
C3/C4 and/or CH_{50}
Double-stranded DNA (anti-dsDNA) antibodies
Antiphospholipid antibodies (lupus anticoagulant, anticardiolipin, anti–β_2 glycoprotein I)
Cerebrospinal fluid (CSF): cell count, protein, glucose, Q-albumin, IgG index, oligoclonal bands, Venereal Disease Research Laboratory (VDRL), cultures, India ink, and viral polymerase chain reaction (PCR) when indicated
Brain and/or spinal cord magnetic resonance imaging (MRI) (T1/T2, fluid-attenuated inversion recovery [FLAIR], diffusion-weighted imaging [DWI], gadolinium-enhanced T1)
Electroencephalogram
Other tests when indicated:
  C-reactive protein
  Serum and CSF antineuronal antibodies
  Neuromyelitis optica (anti-NMO-IgG) antibodies
  Anti–ribosomal P antibodies
  Computed tomography (CT) of brain
  Echocardiogram
  CT or magnetic resonance angiogram (MRA)
  Cerebral angiography
  Tests for hypercoagulability: protein C, protein S, serum antithrombin III (SAT III), prothrombin 20210A mutation, factor V Leiden, homocysteine
  Cryoglobulins

Adapted from reference 5.

---

cultures of bodily fluids are tested to assess disease activity and to exclude other diseases that can cause neurologic symptoms. Earlier studies emphasized that certain clinical signs, such as retinal and dermal vasculitis or livedo reticularis, were more common in patients with NP-SLE, particularly those with CVD.[1] Furthermore, although NP-SLE can be the initial or sole active manifestation of SLE, many studies have reported that NP-SLE frequently occurs when SLE is clinically and serologically active.[8] However, in all patients with SLE who have NP dysfunction, additional tests will be necessary to confirm an NP-SLE diagnosis and to exclude other causes (Box 29-2) (Tables 29-2 and 29-3). Recommendations of the basic laboratory evaluation and diagnostic imaging that should be obtained on patients suspected of having NP-SLE have been published[5,8] (see Box 29-2) (Figure 29-1).

Clinical Laboratory Tests

A complete blood count and urinalysis should be obtained for disease activity and to rule out infection. If thrombocytopenia is present, the blood smear should be examined for schistocytes to exclude TTP. Chemistries including electrolytes, creatinine, glucose, and liver-associated enzymes are obtained to exclude metabolic abnormalities that can cause neurologic dysfunction. Complement (C3/C4 or CH_{50}) determinations and anti-dsDNA antibodies should be obtained to assess disease activity. The presence of antiphospholipid antibodies (lupus anticoagulant, anticardiolipin antibodies, anti–β_2 glycoprotein I antibodies) should be determined. Other tests for hypercoagulable states, including factor V Leiden, protein C and S levels, serum antithrombin III levels, and prothrombin 20210A mutation, may be indicated in selected patients. Most patients with SLE will have an elevated erythrocyte sedimentation rate and a normal or mildly elevated C-reactive protein. A significantly elevated C-reactive protein

TABLE 29-2 Frequency of Abnormal Laboratory Tests Commonly Used in the Evaluation of Neuropsychiatric Lupus Erythematosus

TEST	FREQUENCY OF ABNORMAL TEST RESULT RANGE (%)*	COMMENT
Serologic		
Antineuronal antibodies	30-92	Diffuse manifestations
Neuromyelitis optica (anti-NMO-IgG) antibodies	75	Transverse myelitis and/or optic neuritis
Anti–ribosomal P antibodies	24-90	Psychosis/depression
Antiphospholipid antibodies	45-80	Strokes and focal manifestations
Cerebrospinal fluid		
Routine		
Pleocytosis	6-34	Rule out infection and nonsteroidal antiinflammatory drug (NSAID) meningitis
Increased protein	22-50	Nonspecific
Low glucose	3-8	Rule out infection, transverse myelitis
Special		
Antineuronal antibodies (IgG)	30-95	Diffuse manifestations (90%-95%), focal manifestations (25%-30%)
Elevated Q-albumin	8-33	Break in blood-brain barrier
Elevated IgG index	25-66	Diffuse manifestations
Oligoclonal bands (≥2 bands)	20-82	Diffuse manifestations

*Frequencies based on those reported in various studies and reviews.

TABLE 29-3 Frequency of Abnormal Diagnostic Tests Commonly Used in the Evaluation of Neuropsychiatric Lupus Erythematosus

TEST	FREQUENCY OF ABNORMAL TEST RESULTS, RANGE (%)	COMMENT
Electroencephalogram	60-91	No specific abnormality is present; patients with SLE without CNS symptoms can have an abnormal EEG.
Neuroimaging procedures		
CT scan	29-59 (atrophy) 10-25 (infarction or hemorrhage)	Atrophy may be the result of corticosteroids; CT scans miss 20%-25% of definite clinical infarctions.
MRI scan		
All patients with NPLE	30-76	No specific lesion is present; atrophy is common.
Patients with NPLE; diffuse symptoms only	Less than 50	Are more likely abnormal if obtained within 48 hr of treatment.
Patients with NPLE; focal symptoms	Up to 80-100	T2-weighted lesions >10 mm in size are mostly diagnostic.
Patients with SLE; no NP manifestations	18-40	Small (2-5 mm) periventricular and subcortical WMHI are present.
SPECT	44-88	Up to 67% of patients with SLE who have CNS events unrelated to NPLE; 50% of patients with SLE without a history of NP events have abnormal scans.
Angiography	10	Are more likely abnormal in embolic or large strokes.
Echocardiography	40	Definite valvular lesions are more common in patients who have had a stroke; may have an association with antiphospholipid antibodies.

CNS, Central nervous system; CT, computed tomographic; EEG, electroencephalogram; MRI, magnetic resonance imaging; NP, neuropsychiatric; NPLE, neuropsychiatric lupus erythematosus; SLE, systemic lupus erythematosus; SPECT, single-photo emission CT; WMHI, white matter hyperintensities.

(>6 mg/dL) usually indicates systemic vasculitis or infection. A fasting lipid profile and homocysteine levels are obtained to establish vascular risk factors.

Autoantibodies

Over 20 autoantibodies in the serum and CSF have been reported to be associated with NP-SLE.[53-55] They have been detected by a variety of methods using multiple different substrates. Over one half of them are autoantibodies that react to brain antigens, whereas the remaining are systemic autoantibodies. Many of these autoantibodies are not clinically available and remain investigational. However, the four that are clinically available (antiphospholipid, anti–ribosomal P, antineuronal, and anti-NMO-IgG antibodies) and one that is investigational (anti-NMDAR) deserve further discussion.

Antiphospholipid Antibodies

Antiphospholipid antibodies make up a heterogeneous group of autoantibodies associated with thromboembolic events. The lupus anticoagulant, anticardiolipin, and anti–β_2 glycoprotein I (GPI) antibodies are the ones best characterized. In a metaanalysis of 29 retrospective studies made up of more than 1000 patients with SLE, the average prevalences of lupus anticoagulants and anticardiolipin antibodies were 34% and 44%, respectively, with an overall incidence of thrombotic complications of 28%.[56] Many studies combine primary antiphospholipid antibody syndrome patients and SLE patients with antiphospholipid antibodies, making interpretation of these studies difficult to apply to patients with SLE only.

Several neurologic syndromes have been associated with antiphospholipid antibodies in patients with lupus.[8] The most common are stroke (OR [odds ratio] 2-7), cerebral venous sinus thrombosis, dementia (OR 2-5) seizures (OR 3-6), chorea (OR10), transverse myelopathy (OR 10), ocular ischemia, and sensorineural hearing loss. Each one is believed to be caused by a thromboembolic event resulting in vascular occlusion. Patients with SLE with the greatest risk are those who have the lupus anticoagulant and/or high-titer IgG (and possibly IgM and IgA) anticardiolipin-β_2 GPI antibodies. Patients with SLE with multiple antiphospholipid antibodies of different specificities have an increased risk of cerebral infarction compared with patients with only a single antiphospholipid antibody. Clinically, patients with antiphospholipid antibodies who have had a thromboembolic event (stroke, OR 16) livedo reticularis, thrombocytopenia, or active lupus (e.g., vasculitis, hypocomplementemia, elevated anti-dsDNA antibodies) are at increased risk for thrombosis. Furthermore,

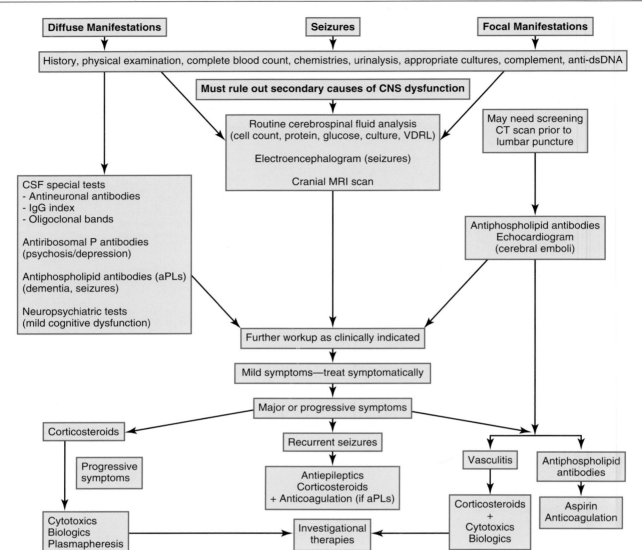

FIGURE 29-1 Algorithm for the evaluation and treatment of patients with systemic lupus erythematosus (SLE) with neuropsychiatric systemic lupus erythematosus (NP-SLE).

approximately one third of patients with antiphospholipid antibodies have abnormal echocardiograms that demonstrate left ventricular valvular lesions, which are a potential source for an embolic stroke. Up to 30% of patients with SLE who develop a thromboembolic event are likely to develop a recurrent episode within 1 year of the initial occurrence.[57] The initial type of thromboembolic event (e.g., arterial versus venous) is the most likely type of event to recur in a given patient, although not usually in the same vascular territory.

The ability of antiphospholipid antibodies to cause thrombosis is the result of a complex interaction among these antibodies, brain endothelial cells, and cerebral hemostasis, which is only partially understood.[12,13,58] Brain endothelial cells display different functional and phenotypic characteristics compared with endothelial cells at other anatomic sites and therefore may be more prone to thromboses. Notably, certain clinical conditions such as surgery and infection can further increase the risk of thrombosis, perhaps through the release of tissue factor. Finally, other cerebrovascular risk factors can be added to the thrombotic risk conferred by antiphospholipid antibodies, including cigarette smoking, hyperlipidemia, hypertension, diabetes mellitus, and hyperhomocysteinemia, which are correctable risk factors that need to be identified and treated.

Anti–Ribosomal P Antibodies

Antibodies to the C-terminal region of cytoplasmic ribosomal P protein are found in 12% to 16% of patients with SLE and their determination is among the most specific tests for SLE.[59] The antibodies may be more prevalent in patients with SLE who are Asian compared with patients with SLE who are Caucasian or African American. Several groups have related anti–ribosomal P antibodies to psychosis and severe depression, whereas others have failed to confirm this association.[41,42] Serum levels of the antibody may correlate with the severity of the psychosis in selected patients, but they also can vary widely over time without any clinical event. Notably, patients with SLE who have mild depression or cognitive dysfunction or both do not have elevated serum anti–ribosomal P antibody levels.[20]

Some investigators have found anti–ribosomal P antibodies associated with NP-SLE in general, as opposed to psychosis in particular.[60] However, an international metaanalysis did not confirm this association, citing limited sensitivity (26%) although good specificity (80%).[42] One explanation for this discrepancy is that the titer of these antibodies can vary over time. Because of this variance, cross-sectional studies may get negative results, whereas all longitudinal and prospective studies have shown a positive association.[60] Because of the high specificity of anti–ribosomal P for SLE, an agreement has been reached that these antibodies are not found in patients with NP conditions who do not have SLE. Some believe that the high specificity of this antibody for SLE makes it particularly useful as a diagnostic test in NP cases without a definite diagnosis of SLE. Furthermore, the titer of antibody may become undetectable with successful therapy in an individual patient who has NP-SLE and anti–ribosomal P antibodies.

Anti–ribosomal P antibodies have been demonstrated in the CSF of patients with NP-SLE. The mechanism explaining how an antibody against a cytoplasmic antigen can cause CNS dysfunction is unclear. Recently, Matus and others[61] demonstrated that anti–ribosomal P antibodies recognize a neuronal surface P antigen (NSPA) that is preferentially distributed in areas of the brain involved in memory, cognition, and emotion. Binding of this antibody to NSPA caused an increase in calcium influx into the neuron, leading to apoptosis and suggesting this as a mechanism.

Antineuronal and Neural Antigen-Specific Antibodies
Serum antineuronal antibodies are more common in patients with NP-SLE (30% to 92%) than in patients with SLE without CNS lupus (4% to 20%).[1,62] They are neither as sensitive nor as specific as CSF antineuronal antibody measurements. Nevertheless, neuroblastoma-binding serum autoantibodies are particularly frequent in patients with NP-SLE with diffuse presentations such as encephalopathy and severe cognitive dysfunction.[15] The antigenic specificity of these serum antineuronal antibodies has not been fully investigated. Recently, two other autoantibodies whose cognate neuronal antigens have been determined were reported. One is the anti-NMO-IgG antibody, which reacts with aquaporin-4 and is associated with manifestations of NMO spectrum disorder (see previous discussion under "Myelopathy"). The other is a subset of anti-dsDNA antibodies that cross-react with the NR2A and NR2B subunits of the NMDA receptor and are associated with psychiatric and cognitive difficulties particularly when present in the CSF (see previous discussion under "Cognitive Dysfunction").

Cerebrospinal Fluid Tests
CSF analysis is useful in all patients with SLE who have had a change in neurologic status, particularly to exclude infection or other secondary causes of CNS dysfunction. In patients with NP-SLE, CSF results may be unremarkable (50%). However, patients with NP-SLE may have abnormalities helpful in confirming the diagnosis and guiding management. Consensus panels recommend that routine CSF tests, IgG index, and oligoclonal bands be determined on all patients suspected of having NP-SLE.[5,8]

Routine Cerebrospinal Fluid Tests
Routine CSF tests include cell count with differential, protein, glucose, Gram stain, other special stains including India ink (*Cryptococcus*), venereal disease research laboratory (VDRL) test, and cultures (including polymerase chain reaction [PCR] for herpes simplex virus [HSV], varicella-zoster virus [VZV], and JC viruses, if indicated). Pleocytosis (<100 cells per high-power field) and elevated protein (70-110 mg/dL) are found in some patients with active NP-SLE. Protein abnormalities are more common (22% to 50%) than pleocytosis (6% to 34%).[1] Neutrophilic pleocytosis with elevated protein suggests cerebral vasculitis with ischemia if infection is ruled out. Patients with antiphospholipid antibodies and neurologic thromboembolic events frequently have elevated protein levels with mild or no pleocytosis.

The CSF glucose level is rarely (3% to 8%) decreased (30 to 40 mg/dL) in NP-SLE. Patients with acute transverse myelopathy have been reported to have hypoglycorrhachia (50%) more than patients with other manifestations of NP-SLE. CSF pleocytosis, elevated protein levels, and low glucose should always raise suspicion of an acute or chronic infection before attributing these abnormalities to NP-SLE.

Cerebrospinal Fluid Immunologic Tests
CSF IgG levels are elevated in 69% to 96% of patients with NP-SLE, and a level greater than 6 mg/dL almost always indicates NP-SLE, although present in only 40% of patients with NP-SLE. An elevated CSF Q-albumin ratio, indicating a break in the blood-brain barrier, has been noted in up to one third of patients, especially those with progressive encephalopathy, transverse myelitis, and strokes.[1,15] Several groups have now confirmed that an elevated IgG index or oligoclonal bands or both are observed in up to 80% of patients, particularly in those with diffuse manifestations, such as encephalopathy and psychosis.[1,15,63] Patients with focal manifestations, such as stroke from antiphospholipid antibodies, typically do not have an elevated IgG index or oligoclonal bands, unless they also have a coexistent encephalopathy (complex presentation).[15] These abnormalities have been shown to normalize in some patients after successful therapy.[15,63]

Cerebrospinal Fluid Antineuronal Antibodies
Using neuroblastoma cells as the antigen source, antineuronal antibodies have been detected in the CSF of 30% to 95% of patients with NP-SLE, compared with only 11% of patients with lupus without CNS disease. Furthermore, 90% of the patients with diffuse manifestations of psychosis, encephalopathy, or generalized seizures had elevated IgG antineuronal antibodies, compared with only 25% of patients with focal manifestations of hemiparesis or chorea. Notably, the antineuronal antibody was concentrated eightfold in the CSF, relative to its concentration in paired serum samples.

Miscellaneous Determinations
Several cytokines (interleukin [IL]-6, IL-8, interferon alpha [IFN-α]), CC chemokine ligands (CCL2, CCL5), CX_3CL chemokines (CXCL1, CXCL8, CXCL10), and matrix metalloproteinase (MMP-9) have been reported to be elevated in the CSF of active patients with NP-SLE and may be important in the pathogenesis.[64] Additionally, levels of glial fibrillary acidic protein and neurofilament-triplet protein are three to seven times higher in the CSF of patients with NP-SLE compared with control subjects. These levels correlated with the degree of abnormalities found on a brain MRI. Measurements of these mediators may be useful in the future for diagnosis and to monitor immunologic activity and neuronal damage.

Summary
When a lumbar puncture is performed in patients with SLE who have CNS dysfunction, the CSF tests that should be ordered are cell count with differential, glucose and protein levels, VDRL, and Gram stain and cultures. In addition, CSF should be sent for antineuronal antibodies and a multiple sclerosis panel, which includes a CSF IgG level, Q-albumin ratio, IgG index, oligoclonal bands, and a calculated IgG synthesis rate. Patients with diffuse manifestations frequently have elevated antineuronal antibodies or an elevated IgG index and oligoclonal bands, suggesting immunologic activity. Patients with only focal manifestations do not usually have antineuronal antibodies, elevated IgG index, or oligoclonal bands, but they may have an elevated Q-albumin ratio caused by a disruption of the blood-brain barrier. Patients with neutrophilic pleocytosis and elevated protein levels with negative cultures frequently have acute inflammation from vasculitis causing their focal symptoms. In contrast, patients with antiphospholipid antibodies, causing thrombosis and focal symptoms, usually have elevated protein levels but mild or no pleocytosis in their CSF. Infection must be ruled out in all patients with CNS dysfunction.

Neuroimaging Studies
Neuroimaging is an important part of the evaluation of patients with SLE who have neurologic dysfunction (see Table 29-3). Currently, conventional MRI (T-1 and T-2 weighted, fluid-attenuated inversion recovery [FLAIR], diffusion-weighted imaging [DWI], and gadolinium-enhanced T1) is the only imaging modality

recommended for the evaluation of NP-SLE.[5,8] A CT scan is useful to rapidly rule out a large infarct or hemorrhage in a patient with SLE and acute neurologic deterioration. MRI is superior to CT scan for detecting edema, infarctions, and hemorrhage. However, no MRI finding is specific for NP-SLE. Furthermore, patients with NP-SLE, particularly those with diffuse manifestations, may have a normal conventional MRI. Conversely, patients with SLE without NP-SLE may have abnormalities on an MRI that may be misinterpreted as NP-SLE. Thus the results of an MRI must be interpreted along with the clinical and other laboratory findings to establish a diagnosis of NP-SLE.[15] Several recent excellent reviews by leaders in the field have summarized the scientific basis for the use of neuroimaging modalities in NP-SLE, have pointed out their limitations, and have made recommendations for their use.[65,66] An in-depth discussion of the various neuroimaging modalities is presented in Chapter 30.

Angiography

Cerebral angiography is frequently normal in patients with NP-SLE, including those with cerebral infarction on MRI. This lack of sensitivity may be explained by the small size of vessels affected by lupus vasculopathy. Occasionally, vasculitis of large-sized arteries or cerebral emboli can be documented. However, angiograms are an invasive procedure with possible morbidity. CT and MRA are noninvasive alternatives that can demonstrate abnormalities in medium to large vessels. In patients with suspected emboli, carotid Doppler and echocardiographic techniques (including transesophageal) should be performed to determine an embolic source.

Electroencephalography

Conventional EEG is abnormal in 60% to 91% of adult and pediatric patients with NP-SLE.[1] The most common finding is diffuse slowing with increased beta and delta background activity. Focal abnormalities and seizure activity can also be seen. Unfortunately, the EEG findings are not specific for NP-SLE, and other disorders, including metabolic encephalopathies and drug effects, can give similar findings. Furthermore, up to 50% of patients with SLE without active NP-SLE can have abnormal EEGs. Consequently, a single abnormal EEG has limited diagnostic value for NP-SLE. On occasion, however, an EEG may be very helpful, revealing unsuspected seizure activity, which was not clinically apparent.

TREATMENT

The therapy of NP-SLE differs, depending on the clinical presentation and suspected pathogenesis.[67] A thorough clinical and diagnostic evaluation of any patient with SLE with new NP symptoms is important to establish the extent of neurologic impairment and brain injury to assess future progression and response to therapy. Secondary causes of CNS dysfunction should be excluded quickly, and all unnecessary medications should be stopped. Therapy should not be delayed pending test results. If it is unclear whether the CNS dysfunction is the result of primary NP-SLE or a secondary cause, then the patient should be treated for both until diagnostic test results return. Recently, recommendations for the treatment of NP-SLE have been published[8] (see Figure 29-1).

Central Nervous System Manifestations

The treatment of NP-SLE is empiric since few controlled clinical trials have been conducted. The therapy should be tailored to the severity of the presentation and suspected etiologic variables. Patients with mild, diffuse manifestations such as headaches, anxiety or dysphoria, paresthesias, or an infrequent seizure may only need analgesics, psychotropic medications and psychological support, neuroleptic agents, or antiseizure medications, respectively, and to be observed closely for any neurologic progression. A particularly difficult clinical situation is the patient with SLE who complains of cognitive dysfunction but has a clinically normal mental status examination. In these

patients, serial psychometric testing may be helpful in establishing the presence, extent, and progression, if any, of impairment. Secondary causes such as medications, thyroid disease, depression, and especially sleep apnea need to be excluded. Treatment should be supportive, including memory aids, and immunosuppressive therapy avoided unless progression can be documented.

Adult and pediatric patients with NP-SLE who have severe or progressive, diffuse or nonthrombotic presentations such as acute confusional state, psychosis, severe depression, aseptic meningitis, and coma may benefit from immunosuppressive medications in addition to their symptomatic therapy (e.g., psychotropic medications). Most clinicians recommend 1 mg/kg/day of prednisone in divided doses. For the most severe cases, pulse intravenous methylprednisolone (pediatric [30 mg/kg]; adults [500 mg to 1 g daily] for 3 days) followed by daily prednisone may be beneficial.[67] Failure to respond within a few days may necessitate doubling the prednisone dose. Switching from prednisone to dexamethasone (12 to 20 mg, once a day) is another alternative, which penetrates the blood-brain barrier more effectively than other corticosteroid preparations. Continued failure to respond is an indication to add cytotoxic medications or a trial of plasmapheresis or both, particularly for a comatose patient. In patients who are corticosteroid-unresponsive, azathioprine and mycophenolate mofetil are less effective than cyclophosphamide. Pulse intravenous cyclophosphamide (0.75 to 1.0 g/m^2) given every 3 to 6 weeks has been reported to be beneficial in both adult and pediatric patients.[67-69] Another successful method of intravenous cyclophosphamide administration, which may have fewer side effects, is the Euro-Lupus regimen of 500 mg every 2 weeks for six doses. Some patients with NP-SLE may not tolerate this regimen or will have contraindications to aggressive immunosuppressive therapy. In these patients, intrathecal methotrexate combined with dexamethasone (10 mg of each, weekly for 3 weeks) has been used successfully in a few patients.[67]

Patients with NP-SLE with focal or thrombotic manifestations demand an immediate and aggressive evaluation. If vasculitis is suspected, then corticosteroids in high doses similar to patients with severe, diffuse, or nonthrombotic manifestations are used. Cytotoxic medications should be administered early to patients with vasculitis. Clinical experience suggests that cyclophosphamide is more effective than other immunosuppressive medications. Plasmapheresis may be beneficial during the first week to allow time for the corticosteroids and cyclophosphamide to take effect. Once the patient's vasculitis is controlled with cyclophosphamide, another cytotoxic medication may be substituted to maintain remission. Whether chronic antiplatelet therapy prevents thrombosis or atheroma formation in the damaged vessel is unknown, but it is often used.

Most strokes caused by NP-SLE are the result of thrombosis associated with antiphospholipid antibodies and not vasculitis. Some are caused by emboli from damaged heart valves. These patients are treated with antiplatelet drugs, hydroxychloroquine for its mild anticoagulant effect, statins, and/or anticoagulation therapy. In patients with large or cardioembolic strokes, excessive heparinization is dangerous and may cause hemorrhage into the infarcted area. Consequently, particularly in patients with an elevated partial thromboplastin time from the lupus anticoagulant agent, heparin levels should be followed, as well as serial brain CT scans ordered to monitor for intracerebral bleeding. The intensity of warfarin therapy is debated. Many experts recommend lifelong warfarin at an international normalized ratio (INR) of 3.0 to 3.5 for cerebral arterial thrombosis.[67] However, two trials comparing different warfarin regimens for secondary prevention of thrombosis did not find a difference between an INR goal of 2.0 to 3.0 and an INR goal of 3.0 to 4.0.[70] Certainly, patients with recurrent stroke, despite warfarin therapy, should have warfarin titrated to maintain the higher INR goal (3.0 to 4.0) and/or be started on combination therapy with an antiplatelet agent. In addition, any patient with recurrent strokes and a lupus anticoagulant should also have periodic factor II and chromogenic factor X levels followed and maintained at 15% to 20% of normal to ensure adequate anticoagulation. Patients who continue to thrombose on appropriate anticoagulation therapy may respond to intravenous immunoglobulin or plasmapheresis with immunosuppressive therapy. The new oral anticoagulants (e.g., thrombin inhibitor, factor Xa inhibitor) have not been adequately studied in this patient population but are an interesting alternative.[71]

Patients with NP-SLE with recurrent seizures should be treated with antiseizure medications. Patients with status epilepticus or frequent seizures should also be treated with high-dose prednisone. Patients with seizures, cerebral infarctions, and moderate to high titers of antiphospholipid antibodies should be started on anticoagulation therapy once seizures are controlled, although they are at increased risk for falls and cerebral trauma. Patients with SLE with seizures should remain on antiseizure medications for at least 1 year. If they have no recurrence of seizures, a normal MRI, and normal EEG, then antiseizure medications can be withdrawn and the patient closely followed. Vehicle driving restrictions should be enforced.

Some patients with NP-SLE will fail to respond or have contraindications to standard immunosuppressive and anticoagulant therapies. In steroid-unresponsive NP-SLE, B-cell depletion therapy with anti-CD20 (rituximab) has been reported to be successful in uncontrolled trials.[72] Belimumab trials excluded patients with severe NP-SLE; consequently, its effectiveness is unknown. Hematopoietic stem cell transplantation or high-dose cyclophosphamide therapy may be considered for patients with severe and resistant NP-SLE.[67]

Difficult Clinical Situations

Several difficult clinical situations warrant further comment. First is the patient who has SLE and is taking corticosteroids who presents with NP symptoms that could be NP-SLE or steroid psychosis.[1] A few caveats concerning steroid psychosis may be clinically helpful: (1) patients are typically not psychotic and usually exhibit a change in mood (mania); (2) most patient are adults, as this condition rarely occurs in children; and (3) steroid psychosis is more likely if the prednisone dose has been increased to more than 30 mg/day in the previous 2 weeks. In the absence of these clinical clues, doubling the dose of corticosteroids for 3 days while awaiting test results is one approach. If the psychotic episode is the result of NP-SLE, then it will respond to this therapy. Failure to improve lessens the likelihood of NP-SLE, and the corticosteroids should be tapered to one half of the original dose. If corticosteroids cannot be tapered, then psychotropic medications such as haloperidol or lithium can be used. Tricyclic antidepressants should be avoided.

A second situation is the young patient (<40 years) with SLE and mild cognitive complaints who is found to have a few (or several) small lesions in the cerebral white matter on T2-weighted brain MRI. Patients in whom cognitive dysfunction is confirmed by formal NP testing should receive antiplatelet therapy (aspirin 75 to 100 mg/day) or hydroxychloroquine or both, especially if antiphospholipid antibodies are present. Patients who fail to respond to this therapy as evidenced by the progression of cognitive dysfunction or the accumulation of brain lesions on an MRI may benefit from oral anticoagulation therapy with warfarin. Another difficult situation is SLE with dementia from prior NP-SLE or from infarctions related to antiphospholipid antibodies. The dementia in these patients will not respond to corticosteroids and, in fact, may worsen. Patients with SLE with stable dementia should not be automatically assumed to have active NP-SLE and therefore should not be treated aggressively with immunosuppressive medications.

Another difficult clinical situation is a patient presenting with acute transverse myelitis. These patients should receive intravenous pulse methylprednisolone, followed by high-dose prednisone. Further treatment is determined by the suspected cause of the myelitis. In patients with probable vasculitis, cyclophosphamide should be instituted and prednisone continued. Patients with myelopathy as a result of thrombosis associated with antiphospholipid antibodies should receive anticoagulation, whereas patients with myelitis as a result of anti-NMO antibodies may benefit from rituximab.

Several other neurologic syndromes, including stroke, transverse myelitis, chorea, seizures, and MS-like syndromes, have been associated with antiphospholipid antibodies and other pathogenic mechanisms. When a patient exhibits one of these manifestations, the antiphospholipid antibody results may take a few days to return. In the interim, these patients can be treated with corticosteroids and antiplatelet drugs until the results of antiphospholipid antibodies return, particularly since vasculitis can coexist with antiphospholipid antibody-associated thrombosis. If the antiphospholipid antibodies are positive, then the next decision is whether to continue with antiplatelet drugs or to treat with anticoagulants. One approach has been to anticoagulate those patients with the lupus anticoagulant or high titer (greater than 40 to 50 IgG phospholipid units) IgG anticardiolipin/anti–β_2 glycoprotein I antibodies, and/or other manifestations of the antiphospholipid antibody syndrome, including livedo reticularis, previous miscarriages, previous thrombotic episodes, and mild thrombocytopenia.

Peripheral Nervous System Manifestations

Patients with SLE and mild, nonprogressive paresthesias require only symptomatic therapy with neuroleptic medications. Patients with cranial or severe peripheral or autonomic neuropathy are initially treated with high-dose corticosteroids. Patients with Guillain-Barré syndrome or CIDP frequently have intravenous immunoglobulin or plasmapheresis as additional therapy. Patients with mononeuritis multiplex as a result of vasculitis should also receive cytotoxic therapy such as cyclophosphamide. When using cyclophosphamide in patients with PNS or autonomic nervous system involvement, determining whether the patient has a neurogenic bladder is important; since failure to eliminate the cyclophosphamide metabolites will lead to hemorrhagic cystitis. Patients with SLE with myasthenia gravis are treated with medications that increase the concentration of acetylcholine at the neuromuscular junction. Other therapy is similar to that for patients without SLE who have myasthenia. The role of thymectomy is controversial since SLE has been reported to flare after the thymus has been removed.

PROGNOSIS

The prognosis for patients with NP-SLE remains guarded. Recent studies have shown that the overall clinical impact of NP-SLE has a negative impact on the quality of life as indicated by lower scores on subscales of the short form (SF)-36, higher damage index scores, and more disability compared with patients with SLE without a history of NP-SLE.[73,74] Although many patients with NP-SLE who have major diffuse symptoms of NP-SLE appear to recover, studies using psychometric testing demonstrate that many patients are left with cognitive dysfunction, suggesting residual CNS damage. Patients with focal manifestations may stabilize but usually do not reverse their deficits during therapy. Notably, individual NP manifestations differ in their prognostic implications.

Few studies have prospectively followed patients with NP-SLE over time. Several studies have shown that mild cognitive deficits detected by formal testing do not appear to progress or adversely affect the quality of life or work capacity over time in the majority of patients.[19,20] However, those patients with the highest number of cognitive domains impaired were more likely to become unemployed. Patients with major NP-SLE manifestations have a less optimistic prognosis. Recurrences of NP-SLE episodes occur in 20% to 40% of pediatric and adult patients with NP-SLE, leading to more residual dysfunction. Residual NP damage was found in 25% of children who had a history of NP-SLE. Patients with seizures, cerebrovascular events, and recurrent episodes of NP-SLE were most at risk for persistent deficits. In a 2-year study of 32 adults with NP-SLE, Karassa and colleagues[75] reported residual deficits in 31%, whereas another prospective study of 44 adult patients with NP-SLE found a higher frequency of work disability compared with patients without a history of NP-SLE.[73] Patients with recurrent episodes of NP-SLE and those with antiphospholipid antibodies generally did worse. Using the

ACR-SLICC damage index, several investigators have reported that NP damage from any cause accumulates over time and develops in 33% to 51% of patients. Notably, the occurrence of NP events, regardless of whether or not they are the result of NP-SLE or a non-lupus cause, is associated with a poorer health-related quality of life.[74]

Some studies have found an increased mortality in adults (7% to 19%) and children (3% to 10%) with NP-SLE, whereas others have not. Status epilepticus, stroke, and coma are poor prognostic signs,[1] demanding aggressive evaluation and treatment to help prevent residual neurologic damage or death. Whether the therapy of NP-SLE improves or contributes to long-term morbidity and mortality from conditions such as atherosclerosis and cancer is unclear. Consequently, the clinician must make every effort to limit the toxicities of therapy by controlling hypertension, treating hyperlipidemia and hyperglycemia, using osteoporosis prophylaxis, administering vaccinations, advising against smoking, treating hyperhomocysteinemia, and using medications for *Pneumocystis jiroveci* prophylaxis.

References

1. West S: The nervous system. In Wallace DJ, Hahn BH, editors: *Dubois' Lupus Erythematosus*, ed 7, Philadelphia, 2007, Lippincott–Williams & Wilkins, pp 707–746.
2. Hanly JG, Urowitz MB, Su L, et al: Short-term outcome of neuropsychiatric events in systemic lupus erythematosus upon enrollment into an international inception cohort study. *Arthritis Rheum* 721–729, 2008.
3. Cervera R, Khamashta MA, Font J, et al: Morbidity and mortality in systemic lupus erythematosus during a 10-year period: a comparison of early and late manifestations in a cohort of 1000 patients 82:299–308, 2003.
4. Ainiala H, Loukkola J, Peltola J, et al: The prevalence of neuropsychiatric syndromes in systemic lupus erythematosus. *Neurology* 57:496–500, 2001.
5. ACR Ad Hoc Committee on Neuropsychiatric Lupus Nomenclature: The American College of Rheumatology Nomenclature and Case Definitions for Neuropsychiatric Lupus Syndromes. *Arthritis Rheum* 42:599–608, 1999.
6. Ainiala H, Hietaharju A, Loukkola J, et al: Validity of the new American College of Rheumatology criteria for neuropsychiatric lupus syndromes: a population-based evaluation. *Arthritis Care & Res* 45:419–423, 2001.
7. Hanly JG: ACR Classification criteria for systemic lupus erythematosus: limitations and revisions to neuropsychiatric variables. *Lupus* 13:861–864, 2004.
8. Bertsias GK, Ioannidis JPA, Aringer M, et al: EULAR recommendations for the management of systemic lupus erythematosus with neuropsychiatric manifestations: report of a task force of the EULAR standing committee for clinical affairs. *Ann Rheum Dis* 69:2074–2082, 2010.
9. Johnson RT, Richardson EP: The neurological manifestations of systemic lupus erythematosus. A clinical-pathological study of 24 cases and review of the literature. *Medicine* 47:337–369, 1968.
10. Ellis SG, Verity MA: Central nervous system involvement in systemic lupus erythematosus: a review of neuropathologic findings in 57 cases, 1955–1977. *Semin Arthritis Rheum* 8:212–221, 1979.
11. Devinsky O, Petito CK, Alonso DR: Clinical and neuropathological findings in systemic lupus erythematosus: the role of vasculitis, heart emboli, and thrombotic thrombocytopenic purpura. *Ann Neurol* 23:380–384, 1988.
12. Belmont HM, Abramson S, Lie JT: Pathology and pathogenesis of vascular injury in systemic lupus erythematosus. Interactions of inflammatory cells and activated endothelium. *Arthritis Rheum* 39:9–22, 1996.
13. Davey R, Bamford J, Emery P: The role of endothelial dysfunction in the pathogenesis of neuropsychiatric systemic lupus erythematosus. *Lupus* 19:797–802, 2010.
14. Abbott NJ, Mendonca LLF, Dolman DEM: The blood-brain barrier in systemic lupus erythematosus. *Lupus* 12:908–915, 2003.
15. West SG, Emlen W, Wener MH, et al: Neuropsychiatric lupus erythematosus: a 10-year prospective study on the value of diagnostic tests. *Am J Med* 99:153–163, 1995.
16. Kozora E, Ellison MC, West S: Reliability and validity of the proposed American College of Rheumatology neuropsychological battery for systemic lupus erythematosus. *Arthritis Rheum* 51:810–818, 2004.
17. Carbotte RM, Denburg SD, Denburg JA: Prevalence of cognitive impairment in systemic lupus erythematosus. *J Nerv Ment Dis* 174:357–364, 1986.
18. Denburg SD, Denburg JA: Cognitive dysfunction and antiphospholipid antibodies in systemic lupus erythematosus. *Lupus* 12:883–890, 2003.
19. Hanly JG, Cassell K, Fisk JD: Cognitive function in systemic lupus erythematosus: results of a 5-year prospective study. *Arthritis Rheum* 40:1542–1543, 1997.
20. Kozora E: Neuropsychological functioning in systemic lupus erythematosus. In Morgan JE, Ricker JH, editors: *Textbook of Clinical Neuropsychology*, New York, 2008, Taylor and Francis, pp 636–649.
21. Faust TW, Chang EH, Kowal C, et al: Neurotoxic lupus autoantibodies alter brain function through two distinct mechanisms. *Proc Natl Acad Sci U S A* 107:18569–18574, 2010.
22. Gómez-Puerta JA, Cervera R, Calvo LM, et al: Dementia associated with the antiphospholipid syndrome: clinical and radiological characteristics of 30 patients. *Rheumatology* 44:95–99, 2005.
23. Brunner HI, Ruth NM, German A, et al: Initial validation of the Pediatric Automated Neuropsychological Assessment Metrics for childhood-onset systemic lupus erythematosus. *Arthritis Rheum* 57:1174–1182, 2007.
24. Mitsikostas DD, Sfikakis PP, Goadsby PJ: A meta-analysis for headache in systemic lupus erythematosus: the evidence and the myth. *Brain* 127:1200–1209, 2004.
25. Fernandez-Nebro A, Palacios-Munoz R, Gordillo J, et al: Chronic or recurrent headache in patients with systemic lupus erythematosus: a case control study. *Lupus* 8:151–156, 1999.
26. Green L, Vinker S, Amital H, et al: Pseudotumor cerebri in systemic lupus erythematosus. *Seminars Arthritis Rheum* 25:103–108, 1995.
27. Futrell N, Millikan C: Frequency, etiology, and prevention of stroke in patients with systemic lupus erythematosus. *Stroke* 20:583–591, 1989.
28. Mok CC, Tang SS, To CH, et al: Incidence and risk factors of thromboembolism in systemic lupus erythematosus: a comparison of three ethnic groups. *Arthritis Rheum* 52:2774–2782, 2005.
29. Mikdashi J, Handwerger B, Langenberg P, et al: Baseline disease activity, hyperlipidemia, and hypertension are predictive factors for ischemic stroke and stroke severity in systemic lupus erythematosus. *Stroke* 38:281–285, 2007.
30. Krishnan E: Stroke subtypes among young patients with systemic lupus erythematosus. *Am J Med* 118:1415.e1–1415.e7, 2005.
31. Roldan CA, Gelgand EA, Qualls CR, et al: Valvular heart disease by transthoracic echocardiography is associated with focal brain injury and central neuropsychiatric systemic lupus erythematosus. *Cardiology* 108:331–337, 2007.
32. Kovacs B, Lafferty TL, Brent LH, et al: Transverse myelopathy in systemic lupus erythematosus: an analysis of 14 cases and review of the literature. *Ann Rheum Dis* 59:120–124, 2000.
33. Pittock SJ, Lennon VA, de Seze J, et al: Neuromyelitis optica and non-organ specific autoimmunity. *Arch Neurol* 65:78–83, 2008.
34. Kolfenbach JR, Horner BJ, Ferucci ED, et al: Neuromyelitis optica spectrum disorder in patients with connective tissue disease and myelitis. *Arthritis Care Res* 63:1203–1208, 2011.
35. Cervera R, Asherson RA, Font J, et al: Chorea in the antiphospholipid syndrome. Clinical, radiologic, and immunologic characteristics of 50 patients from our clinics and the recent literature. *Medicine (Baltimore)* 76:203–212, 1997.
36. Ferreira S, D'Cruz DP, Hughes GR: Multiple sclerosis, neuropsychiatric lupus, and antiphospholipid syndrome: where do we stand? *Rheumatology* 44:434–442, 2005.
37. Appenzeller S, Cendes F, Costallat LTL: Epileptic seizures in systemic lupus erythematosus. *Neurology* 63:1808–1812, 2004.
38. Cimaz R, Meroni PL, Schoenfeld Y: Epilepsy as part of systemic lupus erythematosus and systemic antiphospholipid syndrome (Hughes syndrome). *Lupus* 15:191–197, 2006.
39. Caronti B, Calderaro C, Alessandri C, et al: Serum anti-beta2-glycoprotein I antibodies from patients with antiphospholipid antibody syndrome bind central nervous system cells. *J Autoimmunity* 11:425–429, 1998.
40. Pego-Reigosa JM, Isenberg DA: Psychosis due to systemic lupus erythematosus: characteristics and long-term outcome of this rare manifestation of the disease. *Rheumatology* 47:1498–1502, 2008.
41. Briani C, Lucchetta M, Ghirardello A, et al: Neurolupus is associated with anti-ribosomal P protein antibodies: an inception cohort study. *J Autoimmunity* 32:79–84, 2009.
42. Karassa FB, Afeltra A, Ambrozic A, et al: Accuracy of anti-ribosomal P protein antibody testing for the diagnosis of neuropsychiatric systemic lupus erythematosus. *Arthritis Rheum* 54:312–324, 2006.
43. Stojanovich L, Zandman-Goddard G, Pavlovich S, et al: Psychiatric manifestations in systemic lupus erythematosus. *Autoimmun Rev* 6:421–426, 2007.

44. Omdal R, Loseth S, Torbergsen T, et al: Peripheral neuropathy in systemic lupus erythematosus—a longitudinal study. *Acta Neurol Scand* 103:386–391, 2001.

45. Goransson LG, Tjensvoll AB, Herigstad A, et al: Small-diameter nerve fiber neuropathy in systemic lupus erythematosus. *Arch Neurol* 63:401–404, 2006.

46. Shalimar, Handa R, Deepak KK, et al: Autonomic dysfunction in systemic lupus erythematosus. *Rheumatol Int* 26:837–840, 2006.

47. Omar HA, Alzahrani MA, Al Bshabshe AAA, et al: Systemic lupus erythematosus after thymectomy for myasthenia gravis: a case report and review of the literature. *Clin Exp Nephrol* 14:272–276, 2010.

48. Muscal E, Brey RL: Neurologic manifestations of systemic lupus erythematosus in children and adults. *Neurol Clinics* 28:61–73, 2010.

49. Yancey CL, Doughty RA, Athreya BH: Central nervous system involvement in childhood systemic lupus erythematosus. *Arthritis Rheum* 24:1389–1395, 1981.

50. Sibbitt WL, Jr, Brandt JR, Johnson CR, et al: The incidence and prevalence of neuropsychiatric syndromes in pediatric onset systemic lupus erythematosus. *J Rheumatol* 2002;29:1536–1542.

51. Boddaert J, Huong DLT, Wechsler B, et al: Late-onset systemic lupus erythematosus. *Medicine* 83:348–359, 2004.

52. Mak A, Chan BPL, Yeh IB, et al: Neuropsychiatric lupus and reversible posterior leucoencephalopathy syndrome: a challenging clinical dilemma. *Rheumatology* 47:256–262, 2008.

53. Zandman-Goddard G, Chapman J, Shoenfeld Y: Autoantibodies involved in neuropsychiatric SLE and antiphospholipid syndrome. *Semin Arthritis Rheum* 36:297–315, 2007.

54. Kimura A, Kanoh Y, Sakurai T, et al: Antibodies in patients with neuropsychiatric systemic lupus erythematosus. *Neurology* 74:1372–1379, 2010.

55. Hanley JG, Urowitz MB, Siannis F, et al: Autoantibodies and neuropsychiatric events at the time of systemic lupus erythematosus diagnosis: results from an international inception cohort study. *Arthritis Rheum* 58:843–853, 2008.

56. Love PE, Santora SA: Antiphospholipid antibodies: anticardiolipin and the lupus anticoagulant in systemic lupus erythematosus (SLE) and in non-SLE disorders. Prevalence and clinical significance. *Ann Int Med* 112:682–698, 1990.

57. Levine SR, Brey RL, Joseph CLM, et al: Risk of recurrent thromboembolic events in patients with focal cerebral ischemia and antiphospholipid antibodies. *Stroke* 23(Supp I):I29–I32, 1992.

58. Connor P, Hunt BJ: Cerebral haemostasis and antiphospholipid antibodies. *Lupus* 12:929–934, 2003.

59. Mahler M, Kessenbrock K, Szmyrka M, et al: International multicenter evaluation of autoantibodies to ribosomal P proteins. *Clin Vaccine Immunol* 13:77–83, 2006.

60. Ghirardello A, Briani C, Lucchetta M, et al: Anti-ribosomal P protein antibodies and neuropsychiatric systemic lupus erythematosus: cross-sectional vs. prospective studies. *Lupus* 19:771–773, 2010.

61. Matus S, Burgos PV, Bravo-Zehnder M, et al: Antiribosomal-P autoantibodies from psychiatric lupus target a novel neuronal surface protein causing calcium influx and apoptosis. *J Exp Med* 204:3221–3234, 2007.

62. Kang EH, Shen GQ, Morris R, et al: Flow cytometric assessment of anti-neuronal antibodies in central nervous system involvement of systemic lupus erythematosus and other autoimmune diseases. *Lupus* 17:21–25, 2008.

63. Hirohata S, Taketani T: A serial study of changes in intrathecal immunoglobulin synthesis in a patient with central nervous system systemic lupus erythematosus. *J Rheumatol* 14:1055–1057, 1987.

64. Okamoto H, Kobayashi A, Yamanaka H: Cytokines and chemokines in neuropsychiatric syndromes of systemic lupus erythematosus. *J Biomedicine Biotechnol*; doi: 10.1155/2010/268436.

65. Sibbitt WL, Sibbitt RR, Brooks WM: Neuroimaging in neuropsychiatric systemic lupus erythematosus. *Arthritis Rheum* 42:2026–2038, 1999.

66. Appenzeller S, Pike GB, Clarke AE: Magnetic resonance imaging in the evaluation of central nervous system manifestations in systemic lupus erythematosus. *Clin Rev Allergy Immunol* 34:361–366, 2008.

67. Sanna G, Bertolaccini ML, Khamashta MA: Neuropsychiatric involvement in systemic lupus erythematosus: current therapeutic approach. *Current Pharma Design* 14:1261–1269, 2008.

68. Trevsani VF, Castro AA, Neves Neto JF, et al: Cyclophosphamide versus methylprednisolone for the treatment of neuropsychiatric involvement in systemic lupus erythematosus. *Cochrane Database Syst Rev* CD002265, 2000.

69. Braile-Fabris L, Ariza-Andraca R, Olguin-Ortega L, et al: Controlled clinical trial of IV cyclophosphamide versus IV methylprednisolone in severe neurological manifestations in systemic lupus erythematosus. *Ann Rheum Dis* 64:620–625, 2005.

70. Ruiz-Irastorza G, Hunt BJ, Khamashta MA: A systemic review of secondary thromboprophylaxis in patients with antiphospholipid antibodies. *Arthritis Rheum* 57:1487–1495, 2007.

71. Cohen H, Machin SJ: Antithrombotic treatment failures in antiphospholipid syndrome: the new anticoagulants? *Lupus* 19:486–491, 2010.

72. Ramos-Casals M, Soto MJ, Cuadrado MJ, et al: Rituximab in systemic lupus erythematosus: a systematic review of off-label use in 188 cases. *Lupus* 18:767–776, 2009.

73. Jonsen A, Bengtsson AA, Nived O, et al: Outcome of neuropsychiatric systemic lupus erythematosus within a defined Swedish population: increased morbidity but low mortality. *Rheumatology* 41:1308–1312, 2002.

74. Hanley JG, Su L, Farewell V, et al: Prospective study of neuropsychiatric events in systemic lupus erythematosus. *J Rheumatol* 36:1449–1459, 2009.

75. Karassa FP, Ioannidis JP, Boki JA, et al: Predictors of clinical outcome and radiologic progression in patients with neuropsychiatric manifestations of systemic lupus erythematosus. *Am J Med* 109:628–634, 2000.

Chapter 30

Psychopathology, Neurodiagnostic Testing, and Imaging

John G. Hanly, Antonina Omisade, and John D. Fisk

INTRODUCTION

Involvement of the nervous system by systemic lupus erythematosus (SLE) includes a variety of neurologic and psychiatric manifestations. Neuropsychiatric (NP) events in patients with SLE pose diagnostic and therapeutic challenges because of the lack of specificity of NP events, uncertainty regarding the pathogenic mechanisms, and a paucity of data on therapeutic strategies. This chapter reviews what is currently known about the more common psychiatric syndromes and cognitive impairments in patients with SLE and the role of neurodiagnostic tests, including neuroimaging, in the diagnosis and investigation of NP syndromes.

CLASSIFICATION OF NEUROPSYCHIATRIC SYSTEMIC LUPUS ERYTHEMATOSUS

The central nervous system (CNS) is more commonly involved than either the peripheral or autonomic nervous systems. An NP event may reflect either a diffuse disease process (e.g., psychosis, depression) or focal process (e.g., stroke, transverse myelitis), depending on the anatomic location of the injury. In 1999 the American College of Rheumatology (ACR) research committee produced a standard nomenclature and case definitions for 19 NP syndromes that are known to occur in patients with SLE.[1] For each of the 19 NP syndromes, potential causes other than SLE were identified for either exclusion or recognized as an association, acknowledging that definitive attribution is not possible for some clinical presentations. The identification of other non-lupus causes for NP events is important and has not been adequately addressed in previous classification systems. Specific diagnostic tests were recommended for each syndrome. Although developed primarily to facilitate research studies of neuropsychiatric systemic lupus erythematosus (NP-SLE), the ACR case definitions also provide a practical guide to the assessment of individual patients with SLE who have NP disease.

FREQUENCY AND ATTRIBUTION OF NEUROPSYCHIATRIC SYSTEMIC LUPUS ERYTHEMATOSUS

The overall prevalence of NP disease has varied between 37% and 95% even when using the ACR case definitions.[2-6] The most common are cognitive dysfunction (55% to 80%), headache (24% to 72%), mood disorders (14% to 57%), cerebrovascular disease (5% to 18%), seizures (6% to 51%), polyneuropathy (3% to 28%), anxiety (7% to 24%), and psychosis (0% to 8%). The frequency of other NP syndromes is less than 1% in most studies, emphasizing the rarity of many NP events in patients with SLE.

The attribution of NP events to SLE or non-SLE causes remains a challenge, given the absence of a diagnostic gold standard for most of the syndromes. Thus attribution is determined on a case-by-case basis of exclusion using available clinical, laboratory, and imaging data. For each NP syndrome, the ACR case definitions[1] provide a list of exclusions and associations, the presence of which may indicate a complete or contributing etiologic alternative other than SLE. Using these and other factors,[2] including the temporal relationship between the onset of the NP event and the diagnosis of SLE, recent studies have reported that approximately 66% of all NP events in patients with SLE may be attributed to factors other than lupus.[4,7] Regardless of attribution, the impact of cumulative NP events in patients with SLE is evident from the significant reduction in virtually all domains of the short form (SF)-36, a self-report, health-related, quality-of-life instrument.[4,7]

The substantial variability in the prevalence of NP events may represent inherent differences among study cohorts or a bias in data acquisition. None of the individual NP manifestations is unique to lupus, and some occur with comparable frequency in the general population[2] and in patients with other chronic rheumatic diseases.[8] Thus in research study design, the inclusion of control groups is critical to determine whether the prevalence of NP disease in patients with SLE is in excess of that found in the general population and in other diseases.[9] Because of the rarity of some NP syndromes (<1%), multicenter efforts will be required to study these. Non-SLE factors may likely contribute to a substantial proportion of NP disease in patients with SLE, particularly the softer NP manifestations such as headache, anxiety, and some mood disorders.

PSYCHIATRIC DISORDERS

Prevalence estimates of psychiatric disorders in SLE vary widely.[10] Consistent relations with other SLE manifestations have been lacking, and generalized psychosocial stress is acknowledged as an important factor.[11] Studies of psychiatric disorders in SLE have been hampered by methodologic problems that include selection bias, variations in case ascertainment (e.g., chart reviews, screening instruments, standardized diagnostic interviews), different observation and follow-up periods, failure to account for social and cultural variables, uncertainties regarding psychiatric illness predating SLE, and inadequate comparison groups. Studies including chronic disease control groups, such as rheumatoid arthritis (RA), report comparable prevalence and types of psychiatric disorders,[8] although these comparable factors do not detract from the importance of recognizing and managing psychiatric disorders in SLE. The *Diagnostic and Statistical Manual of Mental Disorders*, fourth edition (DSM-IV), published in 1994 by the American Psychiatric Association, still serves as the basis for the current ACR case definitions[1] describing the psychiatric manifestations of NP-SLE. Importantly, as recognized in DSM-IV, no assumption has been made that states that each category of mental disorder is a completely discrete entity; rather, specific diagnostic criteria included in DSM-IV are meant to serve as guidelines to be informed by clinical judgment. The ACR NP-SLE case definitions[1] include in its taxonomy acute confusional state, anxiety disorder, mood disorders, and psychosis, all of which are consistent with the DSM-IV classifications and are discussed in the text that follows. The concept of cognitive dysfunction, also operationalized in the ACR NP-SLE case definitions, is discussed later in this chapter.

Acute Confusional State (Delirium)

Acute confusional state in the ACR case definitions[1] is synonymous with the term *delirium*, as used in DSM-IV and the *International Classification of Diseases*, ninth revision (ICD-9), and also with the term, *encephalopathy*, which is often preferred by neurologists. It encompasses a state of impaired consciousness or a level of arousal characterized by reduced ability to focus, maintain, and shift attention and is accompanied by disturbances of cognition, behavior, and mood or affect. Other features include disturbed sleep-wake cycles and changes in psychomotor behavior, of which hyperactivity is most easily recognized and lethargy may mask other symptoms.

Incidence and prevalence estimates of delirium in the general population share many of the methodologic problems of NP-SLE previously described. Among older patients, estimates of the incidence of delirium during hospitalization vary from 3% to 42%, whereas estimates of the prevalence of delirium on admission vary from 11% to 33%.[12] Prevalence estimates for delirium among patients with SLE have been lower and in the range of 4% to 7%.[2,4,5] Brey and colleagues[3] found no cases of delirium when they used the ACR case definitions[1] to examine the point prevalence of NP-SLE syndromes in 128 subjects. Distinguishing delirium from persistent cognitive impairment can require an informant's history of acute onset of new symptoms. Because fluctuations in attention and level of arousal are key features of delirium, careful observation over time can be necessary. Mental status screening assessments conducted only once may misdiagnose delirium as dementia. The attribution of delirium to SLE is challenging because doing so requires the exclusion of CNS infection, metabolic disturbances, substance-induced or drug-induced (or withdrawal) delirium, and any mental or neurologic disorder unrelated to SLE.[1] Regardless of its cause or attribution to SLE, delirium is more likely to occur if preexisting cognitive impairment can be associated with an increased risk for dementia. Thus the presentation of delirium in a patient with SLE indicates a need to examine the patient for preexisting cognitive impairment and for careful follow-up of possible residual cognitive or functional impairments.

Anxiety Disorders

Anxiety and depression are common in SLE, occurring in 24% to 57% of patients,[2-6] although uncertainty about their causes and attribution is often present. Anxiety disorders represent prominent generalized anxiety or panic attacks or obsessions or compulsions that result in significant distress or impaired function. However, it is extremely challenging to attribute an anxiety disorder to physiologic changes of the CNS caused by SLE rather than the side effects of a pharmacologic treatment or an adjustment reaction in which anxiety symptoms are the result of the stress of having a medical condition. Although one might presume that clinically significant anxiety symptoms resulting from an adjustment disorder are common in SLE, no studies have directly addressed this presumption.

Variable prevalence estimates of anxiety disorders in SLE have been reported. A retrospective chart review of 518 patients from Hong Kong in which only two cases of anxiety disorders were identified[13] is one extreme. Another study reported 56% lifetime prevalence of phobia and 12% lifetime prevalence of generalized anxiety in patients from Iceland.[14] More typical are prevalence estimates in the range of 7% to 8%,[5] although these estimates may not exceed those of the general population. In more recent studies using the ACR case definitions,[1] Brey and colleagues[3] reported a 24% prevalence of anxiety disorders in 128 patients, and Sibbitt and colleagues[6] reported a 21% lifetime prevalence in 75 patients with symptom onset before age 18 years who were followed for an average of 6 years. Further definitive epidemiologic studies of psychiatric manifestations in SLE using current diagnostic methods are necessary as comparisons among studies remain hampered by case ascertainment differences, possible population base rate differences, and possible cultural and genetic differences in the populations sampled.

As with data derived from self-report instruments for mood and anxiety symptoms, distinguishing between anxiety symptoms and anxiety disorders is important. Based on a prospective study of 23 patients with SLE, Ward and colleagues[15] found that anxiety symptoms varied with global SLE disease activity, whereas Segui and colleagues[16] reported that a decline in anxiety symptoms accompanied the change from active to quiescent disease, suggesting that distress resulting from active lupus may increase anxiety symptoms. Ishikura and colleagues[17] found that anxiety symptoms were associated with the lack of knowledge about SLE and its management at the start of treatment, suggesting that improved knowledge about SLE and its treatment may reduce the likelihood of future emergence of anxiety symptoms.

Mood Disorders

Mood disorders as described in the ACR case definitions for NP-SLE[1] include the equivalent of DSM-IV major depressive disorder (MDD), one or more episodes of 2 or more weeks of depressed mood or loss of interest, plus at least four other symptoms of depression. Mood disorder with depressive features is also included, compatible with the DSM-IV dysthymic disorder (i.e., at least 2 weeks of depressed mood for more days than not, plus additional symptoms of depression not meeting the criteria for MDD). In addition, mood disorders with manic and mixed features are included, compatible with DSM-IV bipolar disorder (i.e., depressive episodes accompanied by manic, mixed, or hypomanic episodes). Such conditions are distinct from substance-induced mood disturbances and from adjustment disorders with depressed mood (i.e., symptoms of depressed mood, tearfulness, and feelings of hopelessness within 3 months of an identifiable precipitating stressor), neither of which has been examined in detail in SLE.

Patten and colleagues noted that "Young people with long-term medical conditions have a particularly high prevalence of mood disorders,"[18] and studies using the ACR case definitions[1] have suggested this to be the case among patients with SLE. Ainiala and colleagues[19] reported a 43% prevalence of mood disorders in their sample of 46 patients. Brey and colleagues[3] reported major depressive-like episodes in 28% and mood disorders with depressive features in 19%, whereas manic (3%) and mixed (1%) features were uncommon. Lower prevalence estimates have been reported by Sanna and colleagues (16.7%),[5] by Hanly and colleagues (14.4%),[4] and by Mok and colleagues (6%).[13]

Despite common acceptance of increased depression among patients with SLE, epidemiologic data remain limited and are complicated by differing case ascertainment methods. Clinical syndromes such as MDD must be distinguished from excessive depressive symptoms alone, although many screening methods do not do so. Commonly used instruments often include symptoms such as fatigue, sleep disturbance, loss of appetite, and worries about health, all of which overlap with autoimmune disorders among other medical conditions. This poor specificity can result in poor positive predictive value when depression-screening instruments are used in patients with SLE. Comparing screening methods can improve the understanding of these instruments, although not necessarily of the prevalence estimates of mood disorders.

A recent study of 111 newly diagnosed patients with SLE illustrates the prevalence of the mood disorders issue. Even when using a screening instrument with fewer somatic items, Petri and colleagues[20] reported an 8.1% prevalence of mood disorder, according to ACR case definition criteria, but a 31% prevalence of depression on the basis of their screen instrument. Using the latter, they found depression to be associated with the presence of fibromyalgia and with poorer cognitive test performance, although not with other demographic or clinical characteristics. Associations between depression and other SLE manifestations have been found by some[21] but not by others.[17] Small samples and differing methodologies make comparisons difficult. Attribution of anxiety and mood disorders to a CNS manifestation of SLE is difficult. For example, in another sample of 111 patients, Hanly and colleagues[4] attributed only three of nine cases of major depression to SLE alone, whereas the remaining cases were attributed either to non-SLE factors or to both. Evidence for a biological basis primarily comes from potential immune system effects on mood states,[22] although complex associations with demographic and social factors, knowledge of disease, social supports, and adjustment to a chronic, unpredictable condition with significant potential morbidity must also be recognized.[17] A disabling autoimmune disease with an unpredictable course is not unique to SLE and is perhaps why patients with RA also frequently experience psychiatric symptoms and respond similarly to screening scales of depression and anxiety symptoms.[8]

Psychosis

Although rare, psychosis (DSM-IV, 293.0) is a dramatic NP-SLE manifestation that must be carefully distinguished from a primary psychiatric illness, delirium, and substance-related disorders. Psychosis in the context of NP-SLE can be associated with predominant symptoms of delusions (DSM-IV, 293.81) or hallucinations (DSM-IV, 293.82) or both, which must be distinguished from delirium. Psychotic features may also be associated with the use of corticosteroids[23] and antimalarial drugs,[24] although substance abuse must also be considered. Prevalence estimates of psychosis vary but have been as high as 8% of patients with SLE.[2-6]

COGNITIVE FUNCTION IN SYSTEMIC LUPUS ERYTHEMATOSUS

Cognition is the sum of mental processes that result in observed behavior. Although conceptually distinct, functional domains of cognition are often used; many, such as attention, memory, or language, are too broad to have simple and well-defined neuroanatomical bases. Cognitive dysfunction may be limited to aspects of particular domains of function or may be more diffuse. Either can result in a relatively global impairment of cognition, although the construct of dementia, a case conceptualization based on Alzheimer disease, has only limited application to SLE. The ACR case definitions[1] acknowledge that even relatively mild cognitive problems still can have significant functional impact for patients with SLE, and recent studies have increasingly emphasized the importance of sensitivity in the detection of cognitive impairments in SLE.

Self-reported cognitive difficulties remain a primary means of identifying patients with possible SLE-associated cognitive dysfunction, but reliance on patients' reports is problematic. Although cognitive complaints are common in SLE, they are also common in many other clinical contexts, and their association with objective cognitive impairment and specific neuropathologies remains unclear. The Cognitive Symptoms Inventory (CSI) questionnaire was designed to assess self-perceived ability to perform everyday activities in patients with rheumatic disease.[25] Higher scores, suggesting greater impairment, have been found for patients with SLE compared with patients with RA,[8] and the CSI may be useful for identifying patients with SLE who are at risk for cognitive impairment.[26] However, validation of subjective complaints with objective measures of cognitive performance is largely lacking. Kozora and colleagues[27] reported increased subjective complaints and objective evidence of impairment among patients with NP-SLE, as well as an association between subjective complaints and impairment among patients with NP-SLE only. However, many of their NP-SLE samples included patients with mood disorders and headache, and strong associations were also found between cognitive impairment and self-reported depression, pain, and fatigue. A large body of literature demonstrates the association of subjective cognitive complaints with stress and disorders of mood and makes distinction among these issues difficult. Indeed, in an 8-week psychoeducational group intervention program for 17 patients with SLE who had subjective cognitive complaints, Harrison and colleagues[28] reported improvements not only in CSI scores and memory test performance but also in self-reported depressive symptoms.

Recognizing and documenting mild yet significant SLE-associated cognitive impairment remains challenging. A review of 14 cross-sectional studies of cognitive function in SLE revealed cognitive impairment that was considered subclinical in 11% to 54% of patients.[29] The ACR case definitions[1] require that cognitive dysfunction be evident on neuropsychological testing with the interpretation

based on normative data appropriate for age, education, sex, and ethnic group, wherever possible. Such neuropsychological assessment typically involves a battery of tests that examine various domains of cognitive functioning—those either identified as problematic by the patient or considered likely to be problematic on the basis of the underlying medical condition, in this case, SLE. The ACR case definitions[1] identify eight domains of cognitive functioning of particular importance: (1) simple attention, (2) complex attention, (3) memory, (4) visual-spatial processing, (5) language, (6) reasoning and problem solving, (7) psychomotor speed, and (8) executive functions. At least one of these domains must be affected, although distinctions among them are blurred as with most such classification systems. For example, psychomotor speed, the speed and efficiency with which mentally demanding tasks can be completed, may well influence a patient's performance on tasks that examine domains such as memory, language, visual-spatial processing, or executive functions. These latter domains, themselves, each have numerous overlapping subcategories of functions. Nonetheless, the ACR case definitions[1] provide a valuable framework that allows operationalization of domains of cognitive functioning and standardization of the content of the neuropsychological assessment.

Standardized neuropsychological test batteries and predetermined thresholds, such as performance as little as one standard deviation below the mean of the general population,[27] allow for an actuarial approach to identifying cognitive impairment. Although this approach has the benefit of standardization for population-based studies, it is not ideal when examining complex multidimensional constructs of cognition, as is required for individual patients in clinical practice. A patient with above-average education and functional level may test at a normal (i.e., average) level, compared with the general population; even for them, the average performance represents a decline in ability; but the opposite may well be true for those with lower premorbid functioning. Although the common practice of combining individual test scores into index variables can serve to mask deficits in specific areas of cognitive functioning, the opposite can occur when multiple tests are simultaneously considered[30] with the result that prevalence estimates of impairment are significantly inflated. Attempts to correct for demographic factors do not fully address issues of sensitivity and specificity of classifications of impairment,[30] and standardization samples differ significantly across various neuropsychological tests. These issues are well illustrated in the study of childhood-onset SLE by Williams and colleagues.[31] For clinical decision making, an individualized approach to patient assessment that accounts for psychosocial, demographic, and clinical characteristics is necessary.

Various neuropsychological testing methods have been used in patients with SLE, and prevalence estimates for cognitive impairment have varied with the threshold for impairment and the clinical and demographic characteristics of the samples. Although many patients are now recognized as having at least mild cognitive impairment even without recent overt signs of CNS disease, prevalence estimates of cognitive impairment determined via neuropsychological assessment have continued to vary from 7% to 80% of patients,[2-6,31] using the ACR case definitions.[1] Clearly, the selection of control groups for comparison and the criteria used for defining impairment remain critical issues,[31] and the need for studies of larger, longitudinal, multicenter efforts remains.

Prospective studies to date have not generally found increasing point prevalence of cognitive impairment,[32,33] although most predate the ACR case definitions.[1] In a 5-year prospective study of 70 patients, Hanly and colleagues[32] found a decline in overall cognitive impairment from 21% to 13% with most either never impaired or with resolution of cognitive impairment and only a minority demonstrating emergent, fluctuating, or persistent impairment (Figure 30-1). Similar relatively benign courses of cognitive impairment have been reported in other prospective studies ranging from 2[33] to 5 years' duration.[34] However, Hanly and colleagues[32] found that patients with clinically overt NP-SLE at any time had a decline in memory test

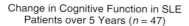

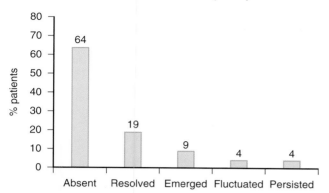

FIGURE 30-1 Change in cognitive impairment in 47 patients with systemic lupus erythematosus (SLE) assessed prospectively on three occasions over 5 years. *(Derived from Hanly JG, Cassell K, Fisk JD: Cognitive function in systemic lupus erythematosus: results of a 5-year prospective study.* Arthritis Rheum *40[8]:1542–1543, 1997.)*

performance over 5 years when compared with patients without such a history. Although the identification of isolated subclinical cognitive impairment may have important current clinical implications, the occurrence of clinically overt NP events may have greater relevance for accumulating cognitive impairment over time. Deterioration may occur in select individuals, but little current evidence suggests that it is inevitable or profound.

The pattern of cognitive impairment typically observed in patients with SLE is neither specific nor unique. Impairments include slowed information-processing speed, reduced working memory, and executive dysfunction (e.g., difficulty with multitasking, organization, and planning), which is a pattern associated with pathologic impairments affecting subcortical brain regions. Impairment is usually observed on tests of immediate memory or recall, verbal fluency, attention, information-processing efficiency, and psychomotor speed. Although Leritz and colleagues[35] reported that 95% of their sample had a subcortical pattern of cognitive dysfunction when screened for cognitive impairment, few actually scored in a range representing impairment on the instrument used. Most problems were on serial sevens tasks that place demands on attention, working memory, and mental tracking. A similar subcortical pattern of cognitive impairments is seen in those with multiple sclerosis (MS), and Shucard and colleagues[36] found that patients with SLE and MS had similar impairments and compensatory strategy use when performing a test requiring information-processing speed and intact working memory.

The common findings of reduced information-processing speed and complex attention deficits in patients with SLE has led to increased interest in and the use of computerized neuropsychological assessment methods as potentially sensitive, reliable, and efficient methods of identifying cognitive impairment among patients with SLE. A study using the recommended ACR neuropsychological test battery in conjunction with a computerized test of cognitive efficiency, the Automated Neuropsychological Assessment Metrics (ANAM),[37] identified cognitive impairment in 78% of patients with SLE, making it one of its most commonly identified NP-SLE syndromes.[3] The identified frequency of cognitive impairment using the ANAM was 69% in these adult patients with SLE[3] and 59% in a study of childhood-onset SLE.[38] In another study of adult patients with SLE studied within 9 months of diagnosis, Petri and colleagues[39] found cognitive impairment in 21% to 61% of cases, depending on the stringency of the definition of impairment. Hanly and colleagues[9] also found a range of cognitive impairment ranging from 11% to 50%, compared with locally recruited healthy control subjects, again

depending on the stringency of the decision rules. However, this frequency was comparable to that observed in patients with RA (9% to 61%) and lower than in patients with MS (20% to 75%) from that same center. Such findings raise some concerns regarding the presumed causes of deficits detected by computerized tests such as ANAM; these measures may not distinguish between nonspecific reduction of sensorimotor efficiency and more specific abnormalities in higher cognitive functions such as working memory and executive abilities. Although computerized tests such as ANAM seem sensitive to reduced cognitive efficiency, this sensitivity may arise from many causes and cannot be used to determine impairment of specific domains of cognitive abilities or be used as a substitute for formal neuropsychological assessment. Future studies are needed to determine the role of computerized testing in screening for cognitive impairment in patients with SLE, as well as its value in the evaluation of changes in cognitive performance over time.

Etiology of Cognitive Impairment in Systemic Lupus Erythematosus

Cognitive Function, Global Systemic Lupus Erythematosus Disease Activity, and Overt Neuropsychiatric Systemic Lupus Erythematosus

Although cognitive impairment may be viewed as a distinct subset of NP-SLE, cognitive functioning may also serve as a surrogate of overall brain health in patients with SLE, one that may be affected by a variety of factors including other NP syndromes. Chronic medical illness provides many potential generic causes of subtle cognitive dysfunction (Box 30-1). Determining whether chronic illness causes or contributes to cognitive dysfunction in patients with SLE requires careful consideration on an individual basis, but the accumulated evidence suggests that such explanations alone are insufficient to account for the entire overall burden of cognitive impairment in SLE. Not surprisingly, the prevalence of cognitive dysfunction in patients with past or current NP-SLE is greater than in those with no such history. However, the relationship between cognitive dysfunction and overall disease activity remains unclear. Some studies[40] have found that patients with active disease had poorer performance on neuropsychological tests than patients with inactive or mildly active disease. Cumulative damage, together with hypertension, antiphospholipid antibodies, and magnetic resonance imaging (MRI) findings (described in further detail in the following text) have also been associated with greater cognitive impairment.[41]

Cognitive Function and Psychiatric Morbidity

Mood and psychological distress can affect cognitive function and performance on neuropsychological tests, although this association is complex. In their sample of 73 patients with SLE, Hay and colleagues[42] found that 21% had a current psychiatric disorder and were more impaired on verbal cognitive tests. Moreover, those whose psychiatric disorders resolved over the intervening year improved their performance, whereas those whose disorders persisted showed no change; those who developed new psychiatric disorders declined.[43] Monastero and colleagues[44] reported an association between the presence and level of depressive symptoms and neuropsychological test performance among patients both with and without NP-SLE. As noted earlier, Kozora and colleagues[27] found associations between cognitive impairment and self-reported depression, fatigue, and pain in one study of patients with NP-SLE. In a subsequent study, they found greater depression and subjective cognitive complaints but no differences in overall cognitive impairment between patients with SLE without NP syndromes and matched control subjects.[45] As previously noted, distinctions between clinical psychiatric syndromes and self-reported psychiatric symptoms are important when considering associations with cognitive functioning; attribution of psychiatric syndromes to SLE remains challenging as well.[4] Although psychiatric morbidity and cognitive dysfunction co-occur in SLE, any clear causal relationship between them should not be expected; both may provide surrogate indicators of overall brain health.

Box 30-1 Nonsystemic Lupus Erythematosus Causes of Cognitive Dysfunction and Examples of Each

Direct Central Nervous System (CNS) Disease or Injury
Ischemia
Traumatic brain injury
Cerebral hemorrhage

Systemic Illness
Hypertension
Hyperthyroidism
Hypothyroidism
Fever

Medication
Beta-blocker medications
Antihistamine agents
Antidepressant medications
Antiepileptic agents
Nonsteroidal antiinflammatory drugs

Psychological or Psychiatric Disturbances
Mania
Depression
Anxiety
Psychosis

Metabolic Disturbances
Hypercalcemia or hypocalcemia
Hypernatremia or hyponatremia
Uremia
Hypoxemia

Pain
Acute or chronic

Fatigue
Acute or chronic

Sleep Disturbances
Fatigue or daytime somnolence
Sleep apnea

(Modified from Hanly JG, Harrison MJ: Management of neuropsychiatric lupus. *Best Pract Res Clin Rheumatol* 19:799–821, 2005.)

Cognitive Function and Medication

Most cross-sectional studies of patients with SLE report no association between cognitive dysfunction and either the use or dose of corticosteroids,[36,46,47] although Denburg and colleagues[48] suggested that brief exposure to low doses has a beneficial effect. Hanly and colleagues[32] compared patients with SLE receiving prednisone at three assessments during a 5-year period with those receiving either no prednisone at any time or intermittent exposure; they found no significant pair-wise differences at any assessment and a group-by-time interaction for only a single neuropsychological test. Medications other than steroids also have the potential to affect cognitive functioning (see Box 30-1), but their potential benefits and risks must be weighed in the clinical context in which each is used.

Cognitive Function and Immunologic Variables

Antineuronal antibodies, determined using human neuroblastoma cell lines as the source of antigen, and brain cross-reactive lymphocytotoxic antibodies have been associated with cognitive impairment in patients with SLE studied at a single tertiary referral center,[49] but these findings have not been confirmed by independent studies.[50]

Furthermore, although the identification of the fine antigenic specificity of antineuronal antibodies has so far not led to more robust clinical-serologic associations, the possibility of specific antibody-induced brain injury in SLE remains an intriguing possibility. In this regard the identification of N-methyl-D-aspartate receptor subunit NR2 antibodies (anti-NR2) and their clear pathogenic potential in animal models for inducing neuronal injury provides a new opportunity to explore this mechanism of brain injury in patients with SLE. However, despite the intriguing results from animal studies, human studies have yielded conflicting evidence in support of the association with NP-SLE and, in particular, with cognitive dysfunction.[51] Measurements of anti-NR2 antibodies in the cerebrospinal fluid (CSF) of patients with SLE may possibly yield a better clinical-serologic association.

Anti–ribosomal P antibodies, which have been associated to a variable extent with psychosis and depression in patients with SLE, have also been examined for their association with cognitive deficits. Although the studies are limited in number,[50] the evidence to date does not support an association.

The strongest association between cognitive impairment and autoantibodies in patients with SLE has been found with antiphospholipid antibodies. For example, in a study of 118 patients with SLE, 33% of whom were positive for the lupus anticoagulant (LA),[52] a significantly greater proportion of individuals with cognitive impairments who were LA positive (50%) were found, compared with patients who were LA negative (25%). The association between cognitive function and anticardiolipin (aCL) antibodies has been examined in a number of cross-sectional and prospective studies. In one study,[53] 51 patients with SLE were divided into those who were persistently aCL antibody–positive or aCL antibody–negative on the basis of up to seven antibody determinations over a 5-year period. The relative change in performance on individual neuropsychological tests was then compared between patients who were antibody positive and negative. Those who were persistently IgG aCL antibody–positive demonstrated a greater reduction in psychomotor speed, compared with those who were aCL antibody–negative. In contrast, patients who were persistently IgA aCL antibody–positive had significantly poorer performance in conceptual reasoning and executive ability. Similar results have been reported by Menon and colleagues[54] in a 2-year prospective study of 45 patients with SLE. These data suggest that IgG and IgA aCL may be responsible for long-term subtle deterioration in cognitive function in patients with SLE.

NEUROIMAGING

Clinical neuroimaging methods, such as computed tomography (CT), MRI, electroencephalogram (EEG), positron emission tomography (PET), and single-photon emission computed tomography (SPECT) have been used to detect structural and functional abnormalities in patients with SLE, particularly those with NP and cognitive manifestations. Other experimental imaging methods have also been used, and each offers unique perspectives on nervous system disease. Current challenges include the need to identify changes that are unique to SLE and to distinguish permanent nervous system damage from disease activity that is potentially reversible with appropriate treatment.

Differences between Brain Structure and Function

Neuroimaging modalities distinguish the observed structure from the function of brain tissue. Structure refers to anatomy that can be observed with the naked eye, microscopically, or on an image that provides a static picture of the brain. Over time, such studies can provide insight into dynamic processes such as the loss in brain volume with age caused by cell loss.

Changes in brain structure, such as tissue loss or atrophy, can be associated with altered cognition and behavior. However, neuroimaging can also reflect brain function through measures of biochemical processes in anatomical regions when patients are either at rest or when they engage in specific cognitive activities or behaviors. These processes are measured as changes in blood flow, brain metabolism, biochemistry, and electrical discharge.

Although brain function is closely tied to structure, no precise mapping of one onto the other exists. For example, although the function of speech production is highly associated with the Broca area (i.e., opercular and triangular sections of the inferior frontal gyrus), expressive language is a complex behavior that involves significantly more than simply the motor act of word production. Numerous other brain regions are implicated in the cognitive processes necessary for the final outcome of speech production.

Clinical Structural Imaging Methods: Computed Tomography and Magnetic Resonance Imaging
Computed Tomography

X-ray CT produces two-dimensional images of the organ of interest. When imaging the brain, contrast between tissues is created by variable x-ray densities produced by different concentrations of electrons in brain tissue. CT is sensitive to cerebral atrophy, which has been detected in 29% to 59% of the patients with NP-SLE.[55] Other pathologic conditions, such as infarction, hemorrhage, and meningeal thickening as a consequence of inflammation, may be detected as well. Although relatively insensitive, CT may detect white matter abnormalities reflecting edema,[55] as well as diffuse neuropathological features associated with NP-SLE, including chronic white matter demyelination and small infarcts.[56] However, CT does not reliably distinguish damage from reversible inflammatory disease in the nervous system.

Magnetic Resonance Imaging

MRI is the preferred method of structural imaging in SLE.[56] It offers a higher spatial resolution than CT and is more sensitive to relatively minor changes in brain tissue.[56] MRI also has the advantage of generating a variety of images, depending on the acquisition sequence used. T1-weighted images are best for differentiating fat from water, with tissue rich in water (e.g., gray matter) appearing darker than tissue rich in fat (e.g., white matter). Abnormalities on MRI scanning have been reported in 19%[57] to 70%[58] of patients with SLE, cortical atrophy on T1-weighted image,[59] being the most commonly reported finding. Correlation between atrophy and cognitive impairment in NP-SLE is well established, highlighting the significance of this finding.

On T2-weighted images, tissues rich in water are brighter than tissues rich in fat, making T2-weighted images particularly sensitive to edema. Applying a fluid-attenuating inversion recovery (FLAIR) pulse to a T2-weighted sequence dampens the CSF signal, thereby further highlighting areas of edema.[60] In subcortical regions, increased signal intensity on T2-weighted imaging is known as white matter hyperintensity (WMHI). WMHIs occur in 20% to 50% of patients with SLE, regardless of clinical NP disease, and in up to 75% of patients with SLE who have antiphospholipid syndrome (APS).[61] In an unselected SLE population, the volume of such T2-weighted image lesions was associated with age, overall disease severity, and disease duration.[62]

Lesion location and appearance can help differentiate NP-SLE from certain other autoimmune disorders, such as MS. Large WMHIs, present in the corpus callosum or periventricular regions and also seen as areas of damage on T1-weighted images, are more characteristic of MS than of SLE.[63] Other abnormalities that may help distinguish damage from active inflammatory disease include acute and reversible lesions that lack clear borders, have a filamentous pattern, and follow the gray-white matter junction along sulci and gyri.[55] Hyperintensities in the gray matter provide further evidence of active inflammatory disease.[55,56] Enhancement of lesions on T1-weighted images after intravenous gadolinium[55] can also be used as an indication of breakdown of the blood-brain barrier and active inflammatory disease.

In SLE, structural changes on MRI may be used as an indication of treatment effects in addition to disease activity. For example, gray matter edema may resolve in 2 to 3 weeks[57] after an acute NP event, especially in patients undergoing corticosteroid therapy.[55] However, the course of clinical symptoms and response to treatment may differ from MRI changes. Kashihara[64] provides an example of a patient with headache, fever, psychosis (e.g., olfactory hallucinations, delusions of persecution, delusions of reference) and psychomotor impairment whose MRI revealed laminar lesions bilaterally in the parietal and temporal cortex. After treatment with corticosteroid therapy, the patient's clinical status resolved over 7 months, whereas the lesions visible on T1- and T2-weighted MRI images resolved in 1 and 5 years, respectively.

Although conventional structural imaging with CT and MRI may identify active nervous system disease in SLE, this is not universally the case. Patients with active NP-SLE often show MRI results similar to those not in the active stage of the disease; and both may have normal MRI images, even when psychiatric symptoms are clearly present.[55,56] NP-SLE syndromes likely to be accompanied by normal structural imaging include delirium, affective disorders, and headaches.[55] Neither CT nor MRI reliably differentiates SLE from non-SLE disorders that have similar behavioral and neurologic presentations, including vascular incidents unrelated to SLE, infectious meningitis, noninflammatory edema, or non–SLE-related infarcts and trauma-related hemorrhage.[62] These limitations are not trivial, because decision making regarding treatment often depends on determining whether the presenting symptoms are caused by active lupus, by preexisting but currently quiescent SLE, or by non-SLE factors.[56]

Clinical Functional Imaging
Electroencephalogram

EEG records spontaneous electrical activity of the brain via electrodes placed along the scalp and is primarily used to diagnose seizure disorders. Seizures[65] occur in approximately 5% of patients with SLE and usually occur early in the disease course, often in the first year after diagnosis. The risk is highest in patients with antiphospholipid antibodies and stroke. Generalized tonic-clonic seizures are the most frequent, followed by complex partial seizures. The most common neuroanatomical site of seizure activity on EEG occurs in the left hemisphere, often affecting the temporal region.[66]

Positron Emission Tomography and Single-Photon Emission Computed Tomography

PET is based on the assumption that blood supply and glucose and oxygen metabolism in a region of the brain vary with changes in neuronal activity in that anatomical region. PET is an effective method of detecting diffuse abnormalities in brain function and for localizing pathologic abnormalities. It uses two technologies that allow for in vivo measurement and the localization of neurologic processes—examination of radiologic tracer kinetics and CT. The former provides information about the compartmental kinetics of glucose metabolism, oxygen metabolism, and blood flow, and can even assist in mapping white matter fibers and axonal projections. The PET scanner is also designed to provide a CT image of the brain, combined with concentration distributions of tracer-labeled products. The disadvantages of PET include exposure of patients to large doses of radiation, the potential limited availability of radiopharmaceutical agents, and its cost.

SPECT operates on similar principles and is a more readily available method to study brain function, but it, too, has drawbacks. As with PET, SPECT requires exposure to radioactive substances via injection or inhalation. Radiotracers used in SPECT often lead to an underestimation of regional cerebral blood flow, and the image resolution is inferior to other tomographic techniques, including CT and PET. As is the case with other functional imaging modalities, SPECT does not provide a direct measure of brain activity; rather, it measures concurrent physiologic changes in brain tissue that are correlated with such activity.

Komatsu and colleagues[67] used PET to compare 12 patients with SLE, with and without psychiatric symptoms. Those with active psychiatric symptoms showed decreased metabolic rates for glucose in prefrontal and inferior parietal lobes and in the anterior cingulate regions bilaterally, whereas those with active SLE but without psychiatric symptoms had normal PET scan results. Similar results have been reported by others using SPECT. Huang and colleagues[68] examined 78 patients with SLE—48 patients with psychiatric symptoms and 30 patients with SLE without NP symptoms. They found that 90% of patients with psychiatric symptoms had regions of hypoperfusion, compared with 20% of patients without such symptoms. These hypoperfused areas were observed mostly in the parietal lobe and, to a lesser extent, in the frontal and temporal lobes and in the regions of distribution of the middle cerebral artery. In general, the literature on SPECT scanning in SLE has found areas of diminished uptake in 86% to 100% of patients with major NP events (e.g., stroke, seizures, psychosis), in 33% to 85% of patients with minor NP events (e.g., headache, subjective memory loss), and in 10% to 50% of patients without apparent NP disease.[62,69]

However, just as with all other imaging techniques, the data obtained using PET and SPECT must be interpreted with caution as abnormalities in glucose absorption, oxygen use, and blood flow may not be indicative of *active* CNS disease. Chronic nervous system damage associated with SLE may cause cell death and consequent decreases in neuronal density that will produce similar results on PET and SPECT to those of active NP-SLE. Furthermore, changes in blood flow and metabolism can also occur in sites distant from those of the pathologic lesion. This phenomenon, known as *diaschisis*, occurs when local neuronal activity is diminished in normal-appearing brain tissue caused by the loss of afferent input from a remote brain region. Thus PET may provide valuable functional information about NP-SLE but has relatively high associated hazards and costs and requires parallel anatomical imaging to be useful on a routine basis.[55] Although SPECT may overcome the issue of cost, abnormalities observed using SPECT have not been found to differentiate patients with major NP-SLE features, such as stroke, seizures, or psychosis, from patients with milder NP-SLE features, such as headaches, dizziness, and mild cognitive impairments.[55] Furthermore, SPECT abnormalities can be seen in patients with SLE without NP disease and may be chronic in some and reversible in others.[55]

Nonconventional Magnetic Resonance Imaging

Although conventional MRI is the most frequently used imaging technique, many other experimental imaging modalities based on the principles of magnetic resonance (MR) are available to provide unique information about brain structure, function, and biochemistry. These include functional magnetic resonance imaging (fMRI), magnetic resonance relaxometry (MRR), magnetization transfer imaging (MTI), diffusion tensor imaging (DTI), and magnetic resonance spectroscopy (MRS).

Functional Magnetic Resonance Imaging

Similar to PET and SPECT, fMRI provides information about brain function by measuring changes in blood flow in brain regions and neural networks either at rest or when performing cognitive tasks. In contrast to PET and SPECT, fMRI does not require the use of radioactive materials. The presence of iron atoms in hemoglobin means that blood has magnetic properties, and that change in blood concentrations in tissues can thereby be detected using MR techniques. As a result, fMRI can be very informative of the functional connectivity of brain regions, and disconnections in such connectivity can be indicative of pathologic abnormalities.

To date, few studies have used fMRI in SLE. Lin and colleagues[70] used resting state fMRI, during which brain function was examined at rest. The study demonstrated attenuation in cerebellar activity in patients with SLE versus control subjects, which was correlated with disease activity. The authors suggest that, since these changes are present even in patients with SLE who have not yet experienced NP changes, screening with fMRI may help determine preclinical NP-SLE.

Studies measuring activation patterns in response to cognitive demands have demonstrated changes in pattern and intensity of activation in SLE. DiFrancesco and colleagues[71] reported expanded and intensified activation in patients with childhood-onset SLE in response to verbal fluency and working memory tasks. During control tasks, patients with SLE demonstrated an undersuppression of brain activity. The authors suggest that these findings demonstrate an imbalance between active and inhibitory responses to cognitive tasks, reflecting deficient connectivity between cortical regions. Intensified and expanded neural activation in SLE have also been reported by Fitzgibbon and colleagues[72] in response to working memory tasks and by Rocca and colleagues[73] in response to completing motor tasks. Such cortical changes may explain the relative preservation of functioning in patients with NP-SLE, despite CNS involvement, and highlight the complex relationship between neural integrity observed on conventional MRI and the performance on standardized assessments of cognition and functioning in those with NP-SLE.

Although fMRI has considerable potential, it also has limitations that must be resolved before its introduction into widespread clinical practice. The signal changes generated by shifts in cognitive states or tasks are relatively small; to detect them, numerous MRI acquisitions and long scanning sessions can be required. Another limitation of fMRI is the absence of clear standards for interpreting hemodynamic responses as indirect measures of neuronal activity. Contributing to this limitation is the lack of knowledge about the exact mechanisms regulating regional blood flow. No clear and consistent relationship exists between excitatory synaptic activity and an increased fMRI signal, perhaps because the contribution of inhibitory synaptic activity to the fMRI signal is variable and still poorly understood. Finally, determining the exact region of neuronal activation is problematic since the increased perfusion of brain tissue that results in the change in fMRI signal occurs on a larger spatial scale than does the electrical activation.

Magnetic Resonance Relaxometry

MRR is a method of quantifying T1- or T2-weighted relaxation times in brain tissue. Relaxation times reflect changes in tissue density or chemical composition; thus relaxometry can add sensitivity to conventional MRI scans and detect abnormalities not observed on conventional images. MRR has been studied in patients with SLE who have active major NP events, such as seizures, psychosis, or coma,[74] with findings of increased T2-weighted relaxation time of otherwise normal-appearing gray matter, suggesting gray matter edema in such patients compared with patients with minor NP-SLE events.

Magnetization Transfer Imaging

MTI is a structural imaging modality that measures the integrity of white matter tracks, which cannot be easily visualized using conventional MRI. The technique is based on quantification of the magnetization exchange between macromolecule-bound protons in myelin and water protons by the generation of a magnetization transfer ratio (MTR), which uses two conventional MRI images—one proton-density or T2-weighted image and another with a saturation pulse. An MTR is directly influenced by the amount of bound protons, which is proportional to the amount of myelin in a specific region of interest (i.e., specific fiber bundle or entire brain). A decrease in the average of an MTR in a region of interest usually signifies demyelination in that region, whereas the distribution of MTR values for individual image pixels can be used as an indicator of tissue integrity. A distribution of MTR values in a region that consists of a single, narrow, high peak indicates homogeneity of the MTR and uniformly healthy tissue. When demyelination is present, the peak on the MTR histogram becomes wider and lower because of increased pixels with lower MTR values.

Studies that have used MTI in patients with SLE[75] have reported global damage in patients with NP-SLE, even in those who are no longer in the active stages of the disease, with normal conventional MRI scans. MTI indices have been found to correlate with indices of neurologic, psychiatric, and cognitive functioning. However, MTI measures continue to demonstrate tissue damage when clinical indicators normalize or improve. Although psychiatric, cognitive, and neurologic symptoms of NP-SLE may resolve, the brain pathologic abnormalities underlying them may not.[76] An MTI may assist in detecting brain abnormalities not seen with conventional MRI and may also be useful in measuring neuropathological functions resulting from NP-SLE even after acute NP symptoms and signs resolve. However, because of a lack of standard interpretation guidelines, MTI is not currently used for clinical purposes.

Diffusion Tensor Imaging

DTI provides an additional method for examining white matter homogeneity and connectivity. DTI is based on the principle of isotropy, *Brownian motion*, which refers to the unrestricted, chaotic movement of proton-containing molecules in free water. In the highly structured tissue of the brain, particularly in white matter fiber tracks, molecules can easily move in the same direction as the myelinated axons, thus creating preferential diffusion or anisotropy. Pathologic conditions that disturb the highly structured integrity of the white matter fibers cause a loss of anisotropy and change the diffusion behavior of the water molecules. The level of fractional anisotropy (FA) can be calculated for individual MRI image pixels in a region of interest or for the whole brain. These results are presented as a histogram with lower FA peaks, indicating more pixels with higher diffusion values that reflect damage or degeneration in white matter tracks.

In studies using DTI, patients with NP-SLE have been found to have more pixels with low FA values than healthy control subjects, particularly in the internal capsule and in the limbic regions.[77] The clinical relevance of these findings is, as yet, unclear.

However, some evidence suggests that mean diffusivity for the whole brain, as well as diffusion parameters in the frontal lobe, corpus callosum, left arm of the forceps major, left anterior corona radiata, and thalamus, can differentiate patients with and without NP-SLE.[78] With further study, DTI changes may conceivably assist in the early diagnosis of NP-SLE and help determine the pathogenesis of NP symptoms.

Magnetic Resonance Spectroscopy

MRS provides a means of evaluating biochemical changes in living brain tissue and is sensitive to the presence of neurochemicals with fairly high concentrations (>1 mm). MRS provides information about the neurochemical composition of tissue in a designated region of interest and displays this information in the form of spectra with peaks that represent concentrations of various brain metabolites. MRS is most often added as a sequence to a conventional MRI scan and can increase the duration of the scan by 7 minutes or longer, depending on the number of regions of interest examined.

Proton magnetic resonance spectroscopy (^{1}H-MRS) is the most commonly used method. As with conventional MRI, ^{1}H-MRS uses the signal provided by hydrogen, which is abundant in human tissue. The metabolites detected using this method typically include *N*-acetylaspartic acid (NAA), choline-containing compounds (Cho), inositol (Ins), lactate, and creatine (Cr). NAA is represented by the highest peak on the spectral profile in healthy adult brains. This metabolite is considered to indicate primarily neuronal integrity, and a reduction in NAA is considered indicative of neuronal loss.

The Cho peak reflects concentrations of phosphocholine and glycerophosphocholine, acetylcholine, and choline. The Cho peak is associated with cell membrane turnover (i.e., loss and replacement of cellular membranes) and with a loss of myelin. The Cho peak is often elevated in patients who have suffered a stroke, brain inflammation, or acute white matter disease, all of which involve membrane metabolism. The Ins peak represents concentrations of myo-inositol and other Ins compounds and reflects membrane stabilization and turnover, especially in glial cells. Concentrations of Ins may permanently

or temporarily increase in conditions where membrane metabolism occurs. Lactate is undetectable in healthy brain tissue, and its presence indicates anaerobic metabolism, usually attributable to ischemia. The Cr peak on the spectral profile reflects concentrations of Cr and phosphocreatine. Cr can either increase or decrease in pathologic conditions such as tumors. All of these metabolites can be observed at the standard clinical MRI field strength of 1.5 T although the Ins peak is only revealed when short (≤35 ms) time-to-echo (TE) is used and is only evident as a single peak.

Biochemical changes that have been noted with ^{1}H-MRS in SLE and linked to neurocognitive dysfunction include reductions of NAA in T2-weighted lesions and in normal-appearing gray and white matter.[56,62] Reduction of NAA has also been associated with psychosis, confusional states, and cognitive dysfunction.[62] Although recovery of NAA levels has been observed,[62,79] the circumstances governing the reversibility of changes in this neurochemical are poorly understood. Clearly, however, reduced NAA is not only observed in active NP-SLE but is also seen in irreversible chronic brain injury.[56]

The Cho peak has also been found to be elevated in NP-SLE in the absence of obvious structural abnormalities on conventional imaging.[80] Elevation in Cho can be a prognostic indicator since it often reflects disease activity or inflammation.[62] Elevation in choline, combined with a reduction in NAA, has been linked to cognitive impairment in patients with NP-SLE.[56,62] Myo-inositol has also been found to be increased in normal-appearing white matter of patients with NP-SLE, particularly in those with major CNS manifestations. Increased myo-inositol is also believed to indicate inflammation. Although ^{1}H-MRS findings cannot be used to diagnose NP-SLE or to reliably differentiate it from disorders with comparable clinical presentations, MRS may be helpful in characterizing brain tissue damage particularly in the presence of otherwise normal imaging results.[55]

Phosphorus-31 magnetic resonance spectroscopy (^{30}P-MRS) is a less commonly used technique that assesses energy metabolism in the tissue and the concentrations of phosphorus-containing compounds involved in membrane synthesis.[62] The principal measures of energy metabolism in tissue include phosphocreatine (PCr) and inorganic phosphate.[62] In a study of NP-SLE, ^{31}P-MRS has been successfully used to demonstrate a reduction of adenosine triphosphate (ATP) and PCr in white matter, which are findings consistent with some of the putative mechanisms underlying NP-SLE, including cerebral ischemia, neuronal death, cell injury, or membrane turnover or degeneration.[55] However, additional research using ^{30}P-MRS is required to determine whether such changes have diagnostic or prognostic utility and whether they are related to specific neuropsychological or psychiatric manifestations.

TREATMENT OF PSYCHIATRIC DISORDERS AND COGNITIVE IMPAIRMENT IN SYSTEMIC LUPUS ERYTHEMATOSUS

Management will need to be tailored according to the individual patient's needs (Box 30-2). A paucity of controlled studies exist to guide treatment decisions. Once a diagnosis of NP-SLE is established, the first step is to identify and treat potential aggravating factors such as hypertension, infection, and metabolic abnormalities. Symptomatic therapy with, for example, antidepressants and antipsychotic medications should be considered if appropriate. Immunosuppressive therapy with high-dose corticosteroids, azathioprine, and cyclophosphamide are used to varying degrees. With one exception,[48] no placebo-controlled studies examining the benefit of either oral or intravenous corticosteroids in NP-SLE have been conducted. Similarly, pulse intravenous cyclophosphamide therapy, which has been used in the treatment of lupus nephritis, has also been reported to be beneficial in NP-SLE, although only one controlled study has been performed. An open-label study of 13 patients with lupus psychosis reported a favorable outcome in all patients treated with oral cyclophosphamide for 6 months, followed by maintenance therapy with azathioprine.[81] Another study by Barile-Fabris and colleagues[82]

Box 30-2 Management of Neuropsychiatric Events in Patients with Systemic Lupus Erythematosus: Treatment Strategies and Examples of Each

Establish Diagnosis of Neuropsychiatric Systemic Lupus Erythematosus (NP-SLE)
Cerebrospinal fluid (CSF) examination primarily to exclude infection
Autoantibody profile (antiphospholipid, anti–ribosomal P)
Neuroimaging to assess brain structure and function
Neuropsychological assessment

Identify Aggravating Factors
Hypertension, infection, metabolic abnormalities

Symptomatic Therapy
Anticonvulsant, psychotropic, anxiolytic agents

Immunosuppression
Corticosteroids, azathioprine, cyclophosphamide, mycophenolate mofetil
B-lymphocyte depletion

Anticoagulation Therapy
Heparin, warfarin

(Modified from Hanly JG: Neuropsychiatric lupus. *Curr Rheumatol Rep* 3:205–212, 2001.)

compared intermittent intravenous cyclophosphamide with intravenous methylprednisolone administered for up to 2 years in patients with SLE who had predominantly neurological disease and reported a significantly better response rate with cyclophosphamide (95%), compared with methylprednisolone (54%) ($P < 0.03$). In virtually all of these studies, immunosuppressive therapy was used in conjunction with corticosteroids in addition to symptomatic therapies, such as antipsychotic medications. More targeted immunosuppressive therapies, such as B-lymphocyte depletion with anti-CD20 (rituximab) used alone or in combination with cyclophosphamide,[83] are promising but require further study. Anticoagulation therapy is strongly indicated for focal disease when antiphospholipid antibodies are implicated, and such therapy will usually be lifelong.[84]

The identification of a potentially reversible cause (see Box 30-1) is the first step in initiating treatment for patients with SLE who have cognitive impairment. Simple causes of new cognitive difficulties are often identified by a review of the patient's history. Recent changes in medication are among the most common. Antidepressants, anticonvulsants, and antihypertensive treatments frequently used in SLE may cause reversible cognitive problems; adjustments in drug selection and dose may result in cognitive improvement. Treatment of even mild anxiety and depression may also improve cognitive symptoms.

At present, any additional attempt to address the issue of treatment of cognitive dysfunction in SLE is at best speculative. Two approaches, pharmacologic treatment and cognitive rehabilitation, can be considered, although neither have yet been systematically attempted in SLE, let alone have established evidence of efficacy. Only one placebo-controlled study of pharmacologic therapy for SLE-associated cognitive dysfunction has been performed.[48] Ten patients with SLE who were not currently using corticosteroids were enrolled in an N of 1 double-blind, controlled trial using 0.5 mg/kg prednisone daily. Except for complaints related to cognition, these patients presumably had inactive SLE at enrollment. The authors reported improvement in cognition in five of the eight participants who completed the trial. The use of antiplatelet or anticoagulant therapy in patients with SLE who have antiphospholipid antibodies for the treatment of cognitive dysfunction without evidence of thromboembolic phenomena has

a theoretical basis but lacks evidence for efficacy and remains controversial. Pharmacologic treatment aimed at cognitive enhancement has not yet been studied in SLE and has only recently been attempted in conditions such as MS. Such treatments may ultimately prove to be efficacious in disorders such as MS and may also have potential applications in SLE. Other pharmacologic agents have been developed for the treatment of cognitive dysfunction associated with conditions such as Alzheimer's disease and attention-deficit disorder. However, both the variability in the presence and persistence of cognitive deficits in patients with SLE, as described earlier in the chapter, and the lack of biological plausibility for efficacy remain major hurdles for the design of clinical trials. Although the actions of such medications are not disease-specific, no data currently support or refute their use in the treatment of SLE-associated cognitive dysfunction.

Cognitive rehabilitation, which typically involves intensive retraining of cognitive skills, suffers from the same problems of variability in the nature, persistence, and biological basis when considering the design and implementation of a trial of program efficacy. Although individualized cognitive rehabilitation programs may indeed prove useful for some patients with SLE, demonstrating the generalized effectiveness of this approach is challenging. Cognitive rehabilitation programs have been used in other conditions (e.g., stroke, dementia, traumatic brain injury, MS) to teach patients with cognitive dysfunction how to adapt functionally to their impairments to maintain, if not regain, some level of independence. Until recently, no cognitive rehabilitation programs specifically intended for patients with SLE have ever been developed. A novel psychoeducational group intervention, which was targeted specifically at patients with SLE who have self-perceived cognitive dysfunction, was designed to improve the performance of common cognitive activities found to be problematic. Results of a pilot study of this program[28] demonstrated that participation may result in improvement in memory self-efficacy, memory function, and ability to perform daily activities that require cognitive function. Although rehabilitation programs similar to this are not generally available, patients with lupus who have verified cognitive dysfunction can be referred for cognitive rehabilitation to a neuropsychologist or occupational therapist with expertise in cognitive retraining.

SUMMARY

NP manifestations of SLE are an important and challenging aspect of the disease because, in part, of the diversity of NP events and their lack of specificity for lupus. Psychiatric disorders and cognitive impairment are among the most frequently reported NP syndromes. The primary pathogenic mechanisms contributing to NP-SLE include microangiopathy, production of autoantibodies, and inflammatory mediators. Neuroimaging is a potentially powerful tool for advancing the understanding of NP-SLE and, in the future, may also facilitate the selection of the most appropriate therapies and objectively document their effectiveness.

ACKNOWLEDGMENTS

Drs. Hanly, Omisade, and Fisk receive grant support from the Canadian Institutes of Health Research.

References

1. The American College of Rheumatology nomenclature and case definitions for neuropsychiatric lupus syndromes. *Arthritis Rheum* 42(4):599–608, 1999.
2. Ainiala H, Hietaharju A, Loukkola J, et al: Validity of the new American College of Rheumatology criteria for neuropsychiatric lupus syndromes: a population-based evaluation. *Arthritis Rheum* 45(5):419–423, 2001.
3. Brey RL, Holliday SL, Saklad AR, et al: Neuropsychiatric syndromes in lupus: prevalence using standardized definitions. *Neurology* 58(8):1214–1220, 2002.
4. Hanly JG, McCurdy G, Fougere L, et al: Neuropsychiatric events in systemic lupus erythematosus: attribution and clinical significance. *J Rheumatol* 31(11):2156–2162, 2004.

5. Sanna G, Bertolaccini ML, Cuadrado MJ, et al: Neuropsychiatric manifestations in systemic lupus erythematosus: prevalence and association with antiphospholipid antibodies. *J Rheumatol* 30(5):985–992, 2003.

6. Sibbitt WL, Jr, Brandt JR, Johnson CR, et al: The incidence and prevalence of neuropsychiatric syndromes in pediatric onset systemic lupus erythematosus. *J Rheumatol* 29(7):1536–1542, 2002.

7. Hanly JG, Urowitz MB, Sanchez-Guerrero J, et al: Neuropsychiatric events at the time of diagnosis of systemic lupus erythematosus: an international inception cohort study. *Arthritis Rheum* 56(1):265–273, 2007.

8. Hanly JG, Fisk JD, McCurdy G, et al: Neuropsychiatric syndromes in systemic lupus erythematosus and rheumatoid arthritis. *J Rheumatol* 32(8):1459–1460, 2005.

9. Hanly JG, Omisade A, Su L, et al: Assessment of cognitive function in systemic lupus erythematosus, rheumatoid arthritis, and multiple sclerosis by computerized neuropsychological tests. *Arthritis Rheum* 62(5):1478–1486, 2010.

10. Wekking EM: Psychiatric symptoms in systemic lupus erythematosus: an update. *Psychosom Med* 55(2):219–228, 1993.

11. Hugo FJ, Halland AM, Spangenberg JJ, et al: DSM-III-R classification of psychiatric symptoms in systemic lupus erythematosus. *Psychosomatics* 37(3):262–269, 1996.

12. Sullivan-Marx EFMD: Delirium. In Maddox GE, editor: *The encyclopedia of aging*, ed 3, New York, 2001, Springer Publishing Company.

13. Mok CC, Lau CS, Wong RW: Neuropsychiatric manifestations and their clinical associations in southern Chinese patients with systemic lupus erythematosus. *J Rheumatol* 28(4):766–771, 2001.

14. Lindal E, Thorlacius S, Steinsson K, et al: Psychiatric disorders among subjects with systemic lupus erythematosus in an unselected population. *Scand J Rheumatol* 24(6):346–351, 1995.

15. Ward MM, Marx AS, Barry NN: Psychological distress and changes in the activity of systemic lupus erythematosus. *Rheumatology (Oxford)* 41(2):184–188, 2002.

16. Segui J, Ramos-Casals M, Garcia-Carrasco M, et al: Psychiatric and psychosocial disorders in patients with systemic lupus erythematosus: a longitudinal study of active and inactive stages of the disease. *Lupus* 9(8):584–588, 2000.

17. Ishikura R, Morimoto N, Tanaka K, et al: Factors associated with anxiety, depression and suicide ideation in female outpatients with SLE in Japan. *Clin Rheumatol* 20(6):394–400, 2001.

18. Patten SB, Beck CA, Kassam A, et al: Long-term medical conditions and major depression: strength of association for specific conditions in the general population. *Can J Psychiatry* 50(4):195–202, 2005.

19. Ainiala H, Loukkola J, Peltola J, et al: The prevalence of neuropsychiatric syndromes in systemic lupus erythematosus. *Neurology* 57(3):496–500, 2001.

20. Petri M, Naqibuddin M, Carson KA, et al: Depression and cognitive impairment in newly diagnosed systemic lupus erythematosus. *J Rheumatol* 37(10):2032–2038, 2010.

21. Omdal R, Husby G, Mellgren SI: Mental health status in systemic lupus erythematosus. *Scand J Rheumatol* 24(3):142–145, 1995.

22. Rogers MP, Fozdar M: Psychoneuroimmunology of autoimmune disorders. *Adv Neuroimmunol* 6(2):169–177, 1996.

23. Chau SY, Mok CC: Factors predictive of corticosteroid psychosis in patients with systemic lupus erythematosus. *Neurology* 61(1):104–107, 2003.

24. Ward WQ, Walter-Ryan WG, Shehi GM: Toxic psychosis: a complication of antimalarial therapy. *J Am Acad Dermatol* 12(5 Pt 1):863–865, 1985.

25. Pincus T SC, Callahan LF: A self-report cognitive symptoms inventory to assess patients with rheumatic diseases: results in eosinophilia-myalgia syndrome (EMS), fibromyalgia, rheumatoid arthritis (RA), and other rheumatic diseases (abstract). *Arthritis Rheum* 39(Suppl 9):S261, 1996.

26. Sanchez M, Alarcón G, Fessler B, et al: Cognitive impairment (CI) in lupus is stable over time and may not be recognized by rheumatologists. Data from a multiethnic cohort. *Arthritis Rheum* 50(9 Suppl):S242, 2004.

27. Kozora E, Ellison MC, West S: Depression, fatigue, and pain in systemic lupus erythematosus (SLE): relationship to the American College of Rheumatology SLE neuropsychological battery. *Arthritis Rheum* 55(4):628–635, 2006.

28. Harrison MJ, Morris KA, Horton R, et al: Results of intervention for lupus patients with self-perceived cognitive difficulties. *Neurology* 65(8):1325–1327, 2005.

29. Denburg SD, Denburg JA: Cognitive dysfunction and antiphospholipid antibodies in systemic lupus erythematosus. *Lupus* 12(12):883–890, 2003.

30. Brooks BL, Iverson GL, Holdnack JA, et al: Potential for misclassification of mild cognitive impairment: a study of memory scores on the Wechsler Memory Scale-III in healthy older adults. *J Int Neuropsychol Soc* 14(3):463–478, 2008.

31. Williams TS, Aranow C, Ross GS, et al: Neurocognitive impairment in childhood-onset systemic lupus erythematosus: measurement issues in diagnosis. *Arthritis Care Res (Hoboken)* 63(8):1178–1187, 2011.

32. Hanly JG, Cassell K, Fisk JD: Cognitive function in systemic lupus erythematosus: results of a 5-year prospective study. *Arthritis Rheum* 40(8):1542–1543, 1997.

33. Hay EM, Huddy A, Black D, et al: A prospective study of psychiatric disorder and cognitive function in systemic lupus erythematosus. *Ann Rheum Dis* 53(5):298–303, 1994.

34. Waterloo K, Omdal R, Husby G, et al: Neuropsychological function in systemic lupus erythematosus: a five-year longitudinal study. *Rheumatology (Oxford)* 41(4):411–415, 2002.

35. Leritz E, Brandt J, Minor M, et al: "Subcortical" cognitive impairment in patients with systemic lupus erythematosus. *J Int Neuropsychol Soc* 6(7):821–825, 2000.

36. Shucard JL, Parrish J, Shucard DW, et al: Working memory and processing speed deficits in systemic lupus erythematosus as measured by the paced auditory serial addition test. *J Int Neuropsychol Soc* 10(1):35–45, 2004.

37. Reeves DL, Kane R, Winter K: *Automated neuropsychological assessment metrics (ANAM V3.11a/96) user's manual: clinical and neurotoxicology subset. (Report No. NCRF-SR-96-01)*, San Diego, Calif. 1996, National Cognitive Foundation.

38. Brunner HI, Ruth NM, German A, et al: Initial validation of the Pediatric Automated Neuropsychological assessment metrics for childhood-onset systemic lupus erythematosus. *Arthritis Rheum* 57(7):1174–1182, 2007.

39. Petri M, Naqibuddin M, Carson KA, et al: Cognitive function in a systemic lupus erythematosus inception cohort. *J Rheumatol* 35(9):1776–1781, 2008.

40. Fisk JD, Eastwood B, Sherwood G, et al: Patterns of cognitive impairment in patients with systemic lupus erythematosus. *Br J Rheumatol* 32(6):458–462, 1993.

41. Tomietto P, Annese V, D'Agostini S, et al: General and specific factors associated with severity of cognitive impairment in systemic lupus erythematosus. *Arthritis Rheum* 57(8):1461–1472, 2007.

42. Hay E, Huddy A, Black D, et al: Psychiatric disorder and cognitive impairment in systemic lupus erythematosus. *Arthritis Rheum* 35(4):411–416, 1992.

43. Hay E, Huddy A, Black D, et al: A prospective study of psychiatric disorder and cognitive function in systemic lupus erythematosus. *Ann Rheum Dis* 53(5):298–303, 1994.

44. Monastero R, Bettini P, Del Zotto E, et al: Prevalence and pattern of cognitive impairment in systemic lupus erythematosus patients with and without overt neuropsychiatric manifestations. *J Neurol Sci* 184(1):33–39, 2001.

45. Kozora E, Arciniegas DB, Filley CM, et al: Cognitive and neurologic status in patients with systemic lupus erythematosus without major neuropsychiatric syndromes. *Arthritis Rheum* 59(11):1639–1646, 2008.

46. Kozora E, Thompson LL, West SG, et al: Analysis of cognitive and psychological deficits in systemic lupus erythematosus patients without overt central nervous system disease. *Arthritis Rheum* 39(12):2035–2045, 1996.

47. Hay EM, Black D, Huddy A, et al: Psychiatric disorder and cognitive impairment in systemic lupus erythematosus. *Arthritis Rheum* 35(4):411–416, 1992.

48. Denburg SD, Carbotte RM, Denburg JA: Corticosteroids and neuropsychological functioning in patients with systemic lupus erythematosus. *Arthritis Rheum* 37(9):1311–1320, 1994.

49. Denburg JA, Carbotte RM, Denburg SD: Neuronal antibodies and cognitive function in systemic lupus erythematosus. *Neurology* 37(3):464–467, 1987.

50. Hanly JG, Walsh NM, Fisk JD, et al: Cognitive impairment and autoantibodies in systemic lupus erythematosus. *Br J Rheumatol* 32(4):291–296, 1993.

51. Hanly JG, Robichaud J, Fisk JD: Anti-NR2 glutamate receptor antibodies and cognitive function in systemic lupus erythematosus. *J Rheumatol* 33(8):1553–1558, 2006.

52. Denburg SD, Carbotte RM, Ginsberg JS, et al: The relationship of antiphospholipid antibodies to cognitive function in patients with systemic lupus erythematosus. *J Int Neuropsychol Soc* 3(4):377–386, 1997.

53. Hanly JG, Hong C, Smith S, et al: A prospective analysis of cognitive function and anticardiolipin antibodies in systemic lupus erythematosus. *Arthritis Rheum* 42(4):728–734, 1999.

54. Menon S, Jameson-Shortall E, Newman SP, et al: A longitudinal study of anticardiolipin antibody levels and cognitive functioning in systemic lupus erythematosus. *Arthritis Rheum* 42(4):735–741, 1999.

55. Sibbitt WL, Jr, Sibbitt RR, Brooks WM: Neuroimaging in neuropsychiatric systemic lupus erythematosus. *Arthritis Rheum* 42(10):2026–2038, 1999.

56. Huizinga TW, Steens SC, van Buchem MA: Imaging modalities in central nervous system systemic lupus erythematosus. *Curr Opin Rheumatol* 13(5):383–388, 2001.

57. McCune WJ, MacGuire A, Aisen A, et al: Identification of brain lesions in neuropsychiatric systemic lupus erythematosus by magnetic resonance scanning. *Arthritis Rheum* 31(2):159–166, 1988.

58. Rovaris M, Viti B, Ciboddo G, et al: Brain involvement in systemic immune mediated diseases: magnetic resonance and magnetisation transfer imaging study. *J Neurol Neurosurg Psychiatry* 68(2):170–177, 2000.

59. Buca A, Perkovic D, Martinovic-Kaliterna D, et al: Neuropsychiatric systemic lupus erythematosus: diagnostic and clinical features according to revised ACR criteria. *Coll Antropol* 33(1):281–288, 2009.

60. Sibbitt WL, Jr, Schmidt PJ, Hart BL, et al: Fluid Attenuated Inversion Recovery (FLAIR) imaging in neuropsychiatric systemic lupus erythematosus. *J Rheumatol* 30(9):1983–1989, 2003.

61. van Swieten JC, van den Hout JH, van Ketel BA, et al: Periventricular lesions in the white matter on magnetic resonance imaging in the elderly. A morphometric correlation with arteriolosclerosis and dilated perivascular spaces. *Brain* 114(Pt 2):761–774, 1991.

62. Sibbitt WL, Jr, Jung RE, Brooks WM: Neuropsychiatric systemic lupus erythematosus. *Compr Ther* 25(4):198–208, 1999.

63. Arnold DL, Matthews PM: MRI in the diagnosis and management of multiple sclerosis. *Neurology* 58(8 Suppl 4):S23–S31, 2002.

64. Kashihara K, Fukase S, Kohira I, et al: Laminar cortical necrosis in central nervous system lupus: sequential changes in MR images. *Clin Neurol Neurosurg* 101(2):145–147, 1999.

65. Bertsias GK, Ioannidis JP, Aringer M, et al: EULAR recommendations for the management of systemic lupus erythematosus with neuropsychiatric manifestations: report of a task force of the EULAR standing committee for clinical affairs. *Ann Rheum Dis* 69(12):2074–2082, 2010.

66. Glanz BI, Laoprasert P, Schur PH, et al: Lateralized EEG findings in patients with neuropsychiatric manifestations of systemic lupus erythematosus. *Clin Electroencephalogr* 32(1):14–19, 2001.

67. Komatsu N, Kodama K, Yamanouchi N, et al: Decreased regional cerebral metabolic rate for glucose in systemic lupus erythematosus patients with psychiatric symptoms. *Eur Neurol* 42(1):41–48, 1999.

68. Huang WS, Chiu PY, Tsai CH, et al: Objective evidence of abnormal regional cerebral blood flow in patients with systemic lupus erythematosus on Tc-99m ECD brain SPECT. *Rheumatol Int* 22(5):178–181, 2002.

69. Govoni M, Castellino G, Padovan M, et al: Recent advances and future perspective in neuroimaging in neuropsychiatric systemic lupus erythematosus. *Lupus* 13(3):149–158, 2004.

70. Lin Y, Zou QH, Wang J, et al: Localization of cerebral functional deficits in patients with non-neuropsychiatric systemic lupus erythematosus. *Hum Brain Mapp* 32(11):1847–1855, 2011.

71. DiFrancesco MW, Holland SK, Ris MD, et al: Functional magnetic resonance imaging assessment of cognitive function in childhood-onset systemic lupus erythematosus: a pilot study. *Arthritis Rheum* 56(12):4151–4163, 2007.

72. Fitzgibbon BM, Fairhall SL, Kirk IJ, et al: Functional MRI in NPSLE patients reveals increased parietal and frontal brain activation during a working memory task compared with controls. *Rheumatology (Oxford)* 47(1):50–53, 2008.

73. Rocca MA, Agosta F, Mezzapesa DM, et al: An fMRI study of the motor system in patients with neuropsychiatric systemic lupus erythematosus. *Neuroimage* 30(2):478–484, 2006.

74. Petropoulos H, Sibbitt WL, Jr, Brooks WM: Automated T2 quantitation in neuropsychiatric lupus erythematosus: a marker of active disease. *J Magn Reson Imaging* 9(1):39–43, 1999.

75. Bosma GP, Middelkoop HA, Rood MJ, et al: Association of global brain damage and clinical functioning in neuropsychiatric systemic lupus erythematosus. *Arthritis Rheum* 46(10):2665–2672, 2002.

76. Bosma GP, Rood MJ, Zwinderman AH, et al: Evidence of central nervous system damage in patients with neuropsychiatric systemic lupus erythematosus, demonstrated by magnetization transfer imaging. *Arthritis Rheum* 2000;43(1):48–54.

77. Emmer BJ, Veer IM, Steup-Beekman GM, et al: Tract-based spatial statistics on diffusion tensor imaging in systemic lupus erythematosus reveals localized involvement of white matter tracts. *Arthritis Rheum* 62(12):3716–3721, 2010.

78. Jung RE, Caprihan A, Chavez RS, et al: Diffusion tensor imaging in neuropsychiatric systemic lupus erythematosus. *BMC Neurol* 10:65, 2010.

79. Steens SC, Bosma GP, ten Cate R, et al: A neuroimaging follow up study of a patient with juvenile central nervous system systemic lupus erythematosus. *Ann Rheum Dis* 62(6):583–586, 2003.

80. Appenzeller S, Li LM, Costallat LT, et al: Neurometabolic changes in normal white matter may predict appearance of hyperintense lesions in systemic lupus erythematosus. *Lupus* 16(12):963–971, 2007.

81. Mok CC, Lau CS, Wong RW: Treatment of lupus psychosis with oral cyclophosphamide followed by azathioprine maintenance: an open-label study. *Am J Med* 115(1):59–62, 2003.

82. Barile-Fabris L, Ariza-Andraca R, Olguin-Ortega L, et al: Controlled clinical trial of IV cyclophosphamide versus IV methylprednisolone in severe neurological manifestations in systemic lupus erythematosus. *Ann Rheum Dis* 64(4):620–625, 2005.

83. Saito K, Nawata M, Nakayamada S, et al: Successful treatment with anti-CD20 monoclonal antibody (rituximab) of life-threatening refractory systemic lupus erythematosus with renal and central nervous system involvement. *Lupus* 12(10):798–800, 2003.

84. Crowther MA, Ginsberg JS, Julian J, et al: A comparison of two intensities of warfarin for the prevention of recurrent thrombosis in patients with the antiphospholipid antibody syndrome. *N Engl J Med* 349(12):1133–1138, 2003.

Chapter 31

Ocular, Aural, and Oral Manifestations

James T. Rosenbaum, Dennis R. Trune, Andre Barkhuizen, and Lyndell Lim

SYSTEMIC LUPUS ERYTHEMATOSUS AND THE EYE

Systemic lupus erythematosus (SLE) may affect any organ or tissue in the body, and the eye is no exception. Although the human eye measures less than 3 cm from cornea to retina, the eye contains a diverse array of structures, almost any of which can be the target of inflammation. The manifestations of SLE in the eye are therefore varied and range from dry eye to infiltrative keratitis, scleritis, episcleritis, retinal vasculitis, optic neuropathy, and orbital inflammation. The eyelid can be involved in cutaneous lupus, and ocular motility can be affected by cranial nerve abnormalities or by orbital myositis.

The most common of the ocular manifestations is dry eye or keratoconjunctivitis sicca (KCS) as a result of secondary Sjögren syndrome (Chapter 32 discusses this topic in detail). Of the other ocular pathologic conditions, retinal vasculopathy in the form of cotton wool spots is the next most common and has ominous systemic implications. Optic neuropathy, although rare, is associated with a poor visual prognosis. Less common manifestations are also briefly discussed in this section. In addition, this chapter discusses the known side effects of antimalarial drugs—a class of common medications used in SLE.

Retinal Vascular Disease

Retinal vascular lesions appearing as localized retinal infarctions at the level of the retinal nerve fiber layer are the most common intraocular manifestations of SLE. These are visible on ophthalmoscopic images as cotton wool spots (Figure 31-1) and are often asymptomatic if located in the periphery of the retina. Occasionally, these cotton wool spots may be associated with intraretinal hemorrhages and may result in a Roth spot (Figure 31-2).

The published prevalence of retinal cotton wool spots in patients with SLE varies from 3% to 29%.[1-3] However, the largest prospective study[4] with more than 15 years of serial observation of 550 patients with SLE found that these lesions were present in 7% of patients with lupus.

Severe, occlusive retinal vasculopathy is far less common but is usually visually devastating, with one series reporting a final acuity of worse than 20/200 (i.e., legal blindness) in 55% of eyes affected by this type of disease.[2] The manifestations seen in this type of vasoocclusive disease include central retinal artery occlusions (Figure 31-3), multifocal retinal arteriolar occlusions (Figure 31-4), capillary bed occlusion resulting in widespread retinal ischemia with secondary retinal and optic disc neovascularization that may lead to vitreal hemorrhage (Figure 31-5) or tractional retinal detachment, and central and branch retinal vein occlusions (Figure 31-6).[2,4-9] Patients with any of these occlusions usually complain of a sudden, painless loss of vision or a loss of visual field or both that classically respects the horizontal meridian. Fortunately, this subtype of retinal vasculopathy is rare with an incidence of less than 1% in the previously mentioned prospective series of 550 patients.[4] Other smaller series have reported an incidence of 2% to 8%.[1,10]

Although retinal vascular involvement is most commonly asymptomatic in patients with SLE, its presence is associated with active SLE in 88% of patients and with lupus cerebritis in 73% of patients.[2,4] A strong correlation between the presence of retinal vascular involvement and lupus anticoagulant or antiphospholipid antibodies has also been found in several studies in addition to a decreased survival time.[2,4,5,10,11] The presence of lupus retinal vascular disease is therefore a marker of poor prognosis for survival.

Choroidal Vascular Disease

Retinal vessels are readily seen with an ophthalmoscope; therefore retinal vascular disease is relatively easy to assess. In contrast, the choroidal vasculature is deep to the retina and usually obscured by the retinal pigment epithelium. Abnormalities of choroidal vessels in SLE are rarely reported but are also significantly more difficult to recognize than retinal vascular disease. A choroidal vasculopathy usually results in multiple foci of serous retinal detachments that eventually resolve with residual scarring of the retinal pigment epithelium and some degree of permanent visual impairment.[5,12]

Optic Neuropathy

Central nervous system (CNS) involvement occurs in up to 39% of patients with SLE.[13,14] Optic nerve involvement is far less common and is estimated to occur in up to 1% of all patients with SLE.[4,15]

The pattern of optic nerve involvement varies in SLE. In some cases, patients present with symptoms and signs consistent with an acute optic neuritis,[15,16] which is characterized by the acute onset of retrobulbar pain aggravated by ocular movement, an afferent pupillary nerve defect, visual field loss or scotomata, and either a normal-appearing or a swollen optic disc (Figure 31-7).

In other patients, the presentation may be more insidious such as a painless loss of vision that may be gradual in its onset[17] with an afferent pupillary defect and an arcuate or altitudinal visual field defect evident on examination.

In both patterns of presentation, the pathogenesis is thought to be the same: microvascular occlusion leading to demyelination of the optic nerve in mild cases and optic nerve infarction in severe cases.[15]

The visual prognosis in individuals with SLE optic neuropathy is poor because it is notoriously difficult to treat. The standard treatment is corticosteroid therapy either orally or pulsed. However, recovery (if any) is slow, with final visual acuities of 20/200 or worse in several series.[18]

More recently, some success has been reported with the use of intravenous cyclophosphamide in addition to steroid treatment. Rosenbaum and colleagues[16] reported a significant improvement in visual acuity and visual function in three patients treated with this regimen; a later series of 10 patients reported similar results with 50% of patients regaining normal visual acuity after treatment.[19]

SLE optic neuropathy is a rare cause of optic nerve disease, in comparison with other causes of optic neuritis, such as multiple sclerosis (MS). Certainly the distinction between SLE optic neuropathy with CNS involvement and MS can be difficult, because both may

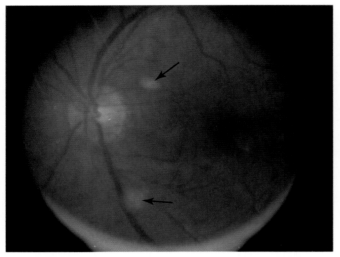

FIGURE 31-1 Color fundus photograph of cotton wool spots *(arrows)*.

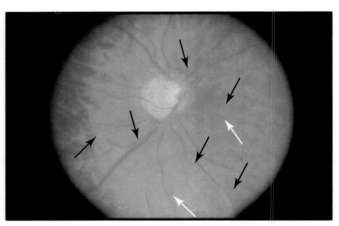

FIGURE 31-4 Multiple arteriolar occlusions *(black arrows)* and intraretinal hemorrhages *(white arrows)* suggest retinal vasculitis in systemic lupus erythematosus (SLE).

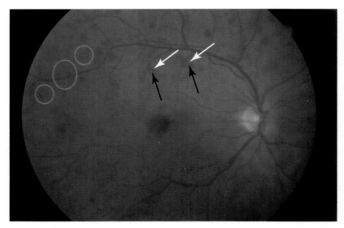

FIGURE 31-2 Roth spot with a central white spot that may represent either fibrin or a retinal infarction *(black arrow)* surrounded by intraretinal hemorrhage *(white arrow)*. Additional Roth spots are shown within the white circles.

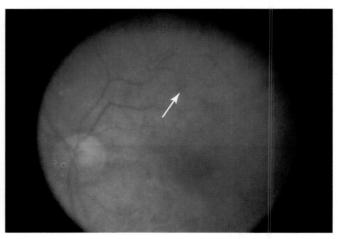

FIGURE 31-5 Neovascularization of the retina *(white arrow)* is depicted.

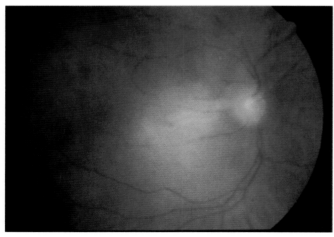

FIGURE 31-3 Central retinal artery occlusion of the right eye. The ischemic, pale, edematous retina is evident.

result in the same signs and symptoms and the two conditions have even been described to coexist.[20] However, the response of SLE optic neuropathy to treatment is slow in comparison with the rapid response of MS-related optic neuritis.[16]

Episcleritis and Scleritis

Both scleritis and episcleritis may occur in patients with SLE[21] and are a result of small vessel vasculitis affecting the tissues of the ocular coat—namely, the sclera and episclera.

Episcleritis is a benign, non–vision-threatening disease that results in ocular injection and mild to moderate periocular discomfort. It usually runs a benign course and often resolves spontaneously after a few weeks. It responds well to topical corticosteroid drops or to oral nonsteroidal antiinflammatory medications. Although it may occur in SLE, the vast majority of patients with episcleritis do not have an underlying systemic inflammatory disease.

Scleritis is a deeper and more severe inflammation than episcleritis and runs a more chronic course. It can result in visually debilitating complications if left untreated. These complications include severe scleral thinning (scleromalacia), resulting in the prolapse of

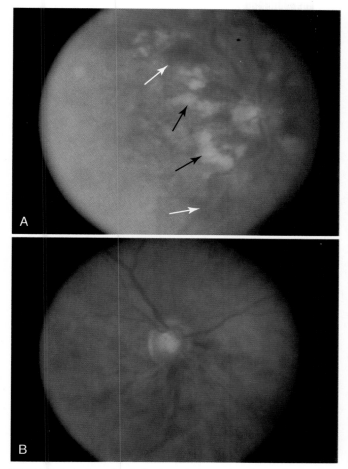

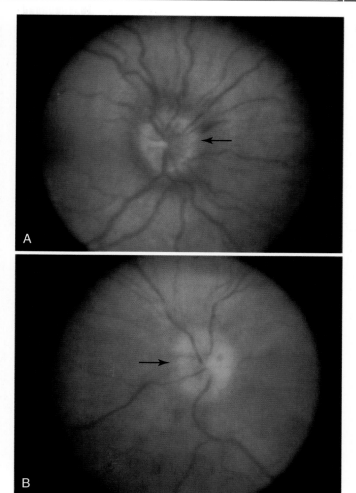

FIGURE 31-6 A, Central retinal vein occlusion with widespread intraretinal hemorrhages *(white arrows)*, dilated tortuous retinal veins, and cotton wool spots *(black arrows)*. Cotton wool spots are not a consistent finding in retinal vein occlusions. **B,** Branch retinal vein occlusion is demonstrated. The sectorial distribution of the hemorrhages distinguishes a branch retinal vein occlusion from a central vein occlusion.

FIGURE 31-7 Swollen optic disc. The blurred margins *(black arrow)* distinguish this abnormality from other causes of a prominent disc such as optic disc drusen.

intraocular structures, corneal scarring, glaucoma, and serous retinal detachments. Clinically, scleritis is often characterized by severe periocular pain, deep ocular injection, and significant tenderness of the affected area to palpation. Less commonly, its presentation may include severe pain and blurred vision without ocular injection if the posterior sclera is involved. More importantly, the development of scleritis is thought to be a serious development in SLE, because it has been described to parallel the degree of disease activity elsewhere.[22-24]

Patients presenting with scleritis are more likely to have an underlying systemic inflammatory disease than those presenting with episcleritis. Rheumatoid arthritis (RA) and granulomatosis with polyangiitis are the two most common systemic inflammations associated with scleritis. SLE is an extremely rare cause of scleritis.

Corneal Disease and Keratitis

As previously mentioned, the most common ocular manifestation in SLE is KCS, which results in a poor tear film and secondary corneal changes such as small dry spots or epithelial erosions (e.g., superficial punctate keratopathy).[1] However, other corneal disease may rarely occur, with a few cases of ulcerative keratitis and deep keratitis or inflammation of the deeper corneal layers (stroma) with secondary impairment of vision being described.[25,26] These presentations are thought to be related to vasculitis affecting the surrounding limbal

vessels. Ulcerative keratitis can also occur in association with scleritis.

Uveitis

Although described, uveitis, or intraocular inflammation, is an extremely rare association with SLE.[22]

Orbital Inflammation

Because SLE may affect any tissue of the body, orbital tissues such as the lacrimal gland (most commonly resulting in sicca), extraocular muscles, and other orbital tissues may also be involved, leading to symptoms of pain, proptosis, lid swelling, and diplopia. Such an orbitopathy from SLE alone is exceedingly rare, with only a handful of case studies being reported.[21]

Chloroquine and Hydroxychloroquine Toxicity

Chloroquine or hydroxychloroquine toxicity is classically characterized by the development of bilateral bull's eye maculopathy that is visible on funduscopy (Figure 31-8). At this stage, observant patients may complain of a paracentral scotoma, whereas others may be asymptomatic. However, should drug exposure continue, further irreversible damage to the retina occurs that is discernible by retinal pigment atrophy, resulting in widespread retinal pigmentary changes

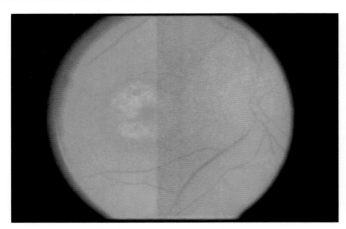

FIGURE 31-8 Bull's eye maculopathy.

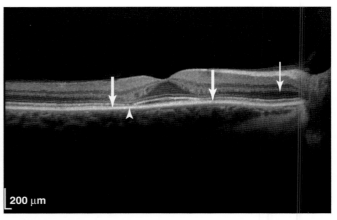

FIGURE 31-9 Ocular coherence tomogram (OCT) of the retina from a patient with hydroxychloroquine-induced retinopathy. Normal thickness of the outer nuclear layer of the retina is shown (thin arrow). This layer locates the nuclei of rods and cones. Areas where this layer is thin (thick arrows) are indicative of the toxicity. The arrowhead points to a focal area of discontinuity in the inner-outer segment junction of photoreceptors in the retina, which is another indication of toxicity.

and retinal vascular attenuation. By this stage, patients have severe visual field loss, decreased visual acuity, and impaired night vision.[27,28]

The first sign of toxicity is thought to be decreased visual function in the paracentral visual field that is detectable before the development of clinically visible bull's eye maculopathy. Cessation of the drug at this early stage is thought to reverse these changes. However, once signs of maculopathy are clinically visible, these changes have been shown to be irreversible.[28] In one recent series,[29] progressive visual field loss or an electroretinographic abnormality was noted even after the medication was stopped.

The risk of retinal toxicity with chloroquine is higher than with hydroxychloroquine and occurs at lower doses (>3 mg/kg/day).[28] A database study included nearly 4000 patients with either RA or SLE who had taken antimalarial medications. The study found that 6.5% of patients discontinued therapy because of ocular complaints. According to this study, weight and daily doses were not important factors in contributing to toxicity, but the duration of use was critical. After taking hydroxychloroquine for 5 years or longer, 1% of users had evidence of retinal toxicity.[30] Several studies have found that ocular toxicity increases with doses greater than 6.5 mg/kg/day.[29]

In addition to dose and duration of therapy, risk factors have also been identified, such as co-existing retinal, renal, and liver disease, obese body habitus, and age older than 60 years.[28] Research has also suggested that carriers of an ABCR-gene polymorphism, which has been linked to Stargardt disease, a form of hereditary maculopathy, may also be prone to developing either chloroquine or hydroxychloroquine toxicity at low doses despite a normal ophthalmic examination before treatment.[31] Therefore the development of hydroxychloroquine (and chloroquine) toxicity may not be purely related to the dose but also to a variety of genetic and environmental factors.

Several recommendations for regular ophthalmic screening of patients treated with chloroquine and hydroxychloroquine have been proposed to detect patients before they develop irreversible, severe vision loss. The American Academy of Ophthalmology currently recommends a baseline ophthalmic examination before commencing treatment. This examination should include a dilated fundal examination and the 10-2 Humphrey visual field test to assess the paracentral visual field.[28] Three relatively recent screening methods have been cited by the American Academy of Ophthalmology for improved sensitivity for screening.[32] These tests are (1) the multifocal electroretinogram, (2) the ocular coherence tomogram (OCT), and (3) autofluorescence imaging. One of these three types of studies should now be included in the assessment. Of the three techniques, OCT is the most standardized and widely available (Figure 31-9).

A repeat examination for individuals at high risk is recommended on a yearly basis. Those not in the high-risk category are screened again at 5 years of hydroxychloroquine use and then annually.

An Amsler grid offers the patient a method to self-assess the visual field. It allows the patient to participate in the screening and has virtually no cost, but it should not be used as a substitute for one of the three studies previously discussed.

Other medications commonly used to treat lupus can also affect the eye. Oral corticosteroids can cause posterior subcapsular cataracts and, occasionally, glaucoma. Immunosuppression, such as cytomegalovirus retinitis, can result in opportunistic infections that affect the eye.

Antiphospholipid Antibody Retinopathy

Retinal vascular disease associated with antiphospholipid antibodies is characterized by diffuse retinal vascular occlusion, often in association with symptoms of a rheumatologic disease.[33] However, the vast majority (>90%) of cases of occlusive retinal vascular diseases (e.g., retinal arterial or venous occlusions) occur in older adults who have other systemic vascular risk factors, such as atherosclerosis or hypertension.[34,35] Therefore primary and secondary antiphospholipid antibody disease accounts for a small proportion of these presentations.

Despite the rarity of this condition, several studies have shown that up to 24% of patients with occlusive retinal vascular disease and no cardiovascular risk factors have high titers of antiphospholipid antibodies. This level is significantly higher than in control populations, in which these antibodies were present in less than 9%.[33,36-38]

Therefore young patients (i.e., younger than 50 years of age) with diffuse occlusive retinal vasculopathy should be investigated for the presence of these antibodies because of the possible ocular and systemic complications that may require prophylactic therapy.

ORAL MANIFESTATIONS

Painless oral ulcers are included in the 1982 classification criteria of SLE and thus were found to be more specific for the recognition of lupus than such common manifestations as alopecia, Raynaud phenomenon, sicca, or fever.[39] Oral ulcers are frequently present during an acute flare of systemic lupus and can occur on any part of the oral mucosa.[40,41] Since lupus-associated oral ulcers usually fluctuate, any persistent ulcer should raise the suspicion for cancer, and, in one case, was found to be caused by squamous cell carcinoma.[42] Lesions on the hard palate may range from patches of erythema to frank ulceration and mucosal hemorrhage. Inclusion of these nonspecific erythematous patches resulted in an estimated frequency as high as 45%, based on a Swedish series of 51 patients with lupus.[43] Additional oral lesions include honeycomb plaques (i.e., silvery white, scarred plaques) and raised keratotic plaques (i.e., verrucous lupus erythematosus). Pathologic features of oral lesions include epithelial acanthosis or hyperplasia, disturbed epithelial maturation, and liquefactive degeneration of basal epithelial cells.[43] Additional features include lichenoid mucositis with vacuolar basal degeneration, basement membrane thickening, and cluster of differentiation 4 (CD4) T lymphocyte predominance with hyperproliferative epithelium on the cytokeratin (CK) profile (i.e., CK5/6 and CK14 on all epithelial layers, CK16 on all suprabasal layers, and CK1 on prickle cell layer only).[44,45] Immunofluorescent testing of the skin and mucosal biopsy tissue frequently shows subepithelial immunoglobulin and complement deposition (i.e., the lupus band). Although its presence is not limited to involved tissue, a lupus band is associated with systemic lupus, as opposed to rarely being associated with chronic cutaneous lupus.[46] Intraoral (sun-protected) and labial (sun-exposed) lupus lesions demonstrated similar cytokine profiles including expression of interferon gamma (IFN-γ), tumor necrosis factor-alpha (TNF-α), and interleukin (IL)-10, indicating that ultraviolet (UV) exposure is not the sole trigger of mucocutaneous lupus lesions.[47] Extensive and diffuse inflammation of the oral cavity, or oral mucositis, is a relatively frequent occurrence in lupus and could be a result of immune-mediated mucosal inflammation. A drug reaction, such as that observed with methotrexate, could have a similar appearance and may require the addition of high doses of folic acid supplementation. A curious syndrome of isolated and extensive oral mucositis exists without any systemic disease; it is antinuclear antibody (ANA) negative using human epithelial-2 (HEp-2) cells but is ANA positive using stratified epithelial cells. The recurrent oral lesions are responsive to hydroxychloroquine and probably share the same pathophysiologic characteristics as the mucositis observed in patients with multisystem disease. Oral candidiasis and herpes simplex viral infection should always be suspected, actively sought, and treated, especially in patients on steroids and other immunosuppressive agents. The only finding of oral candidiasis, especially in patients with xerostomia, may be a burning tongue with a characteristically smooth and red surface. Recurrent aphthous stomatitis and cutaneous lesions with discoid lupus features have been reported in patients with X-linked chronic granulomatous disease. The presence of severe recurrent and chronic infections in childhood is a clue to this rare disorder.[48]

Discoid lesions could occur on mucosal surfaces and are often painful.[43] The lesions frequently involve the labial and buccal mucosa. Lesions have an irregular outline with slightly elevated patches and striated surface, the latter sometimes becoming eroded and transformed into indurated, whitish, raised, scarlike tissue. Biopsy of oral mucosal discoid lesions reveals a similar appearance to that seen in skin. Findings include hyperkeratosis, normal or decreased thickness of the stratum granulosum, irregular acanthosis and atrophic stratum spinosum, focal liquefaction of stratum basale, single-cell keratinization, lymphocytic epithelial inflammation, homogeneous thickening in a bandlike distribution at the basement membrane, and perivascular lymphocytic infiltration with tissue edema.

An association exists between lichen planus of the oral cavity and lupus.[49] Oral lichen planus lesions usually occur on the buccal mucosa, lips, and tongue with lesions rarely found on the palate or gingiva. The lesions may be asymptomatic or may occur with burning or itching. In many cases, oral lichen planus lesions occur without concomitant skin lesions. The lesions may vary from a coalescence of small, pearly gray, hyperkeratotic nodules to a lacelike pattern of hyperkeratotic streaks on an erythematous background with erythema most pronounced at the border. Bullous lichen planus is a rare variant of lichen planus, and ulceration of the tongue and cheeks and less commonly of the gingivae and lips is observed. Bullous lesions are rarely preceded by vesiculation. The ulcers are smooth, and adjacent mucosa is atrophic and erythematous with linear white striae. A biopsy is frequently required to make this diagnosis and needs to be taken from nonulcerated erythematous areas. The histopathologic

examination demonstrates dense subepithelial lymphocytic infiltration with liquefaction of the basal epithelial layers. Bullous SLE is a chronic, widespread, nonscarring, subepidermal, blistering eruption associated with circulating antibodies to type VII collagen. Oral blistering lesions may be found in association with cutaneous disease and can be confused with oral bullous lichen planus. Three cases of Stevens-Johnson syndrome and toxic epidermal necrolysis with mucositis, epidermal detachment, and erosions were reported in lupus without any history of medication or other exposures.

Xerostomia as a result of secondary Sjögren syndrome and is often associated with periodontal disease and poor dentition (see Chapter 32). Therapy of oral mucosal lesions is empiric and includes treatment of the underlying systemic disease with corticosteroids, antimalarial medications, or immunosuppressive agents. Intraoral topical or intralesional steroids may be required for limited oral disease. Oral swish and swallowing antifungal agents for oral candidiasis or tetracycline for aphthous ulceration may be helpful. Avoidance of spicy foods and frequent sips of liquid with meticulous dental hygiene are important ancillary therapies that are often overlooked.

Nasal Septal Disease

The nasal septum is an easily overlooked tissue bed where inflamed blood vessels are easily visualized using an otoscope. Unfortunately, the finding of nasal septal inflammation in lupus is nonspecific and confounded by other causes, such as environmental dryness and airborne irritants, allergic rhinitis, upper respiratory tract infections, excoriations from self-inflicted trauma, and sicca as part of secondary Sjögren syndrome. In association with active lupus, nasal septal inflammation may progress to deep ulceration and rapid destruction of septal cartilage with nasal septal perforation.[50,51] Nasal septal perforation has been reported in 0.8% of patients with the antiphospholipid syndrome. Nasal septal perforation with external nasal swelling and erythema has been reported in a patient with antiphospholipid syndrome and lupus who was successfully treated with intravenous immunoglobulin and anticoagulation therapy.[52] Symptoms of nasal inflammation include stuffiness, hyposmia, epistaxis, or a high-pitched whistling sound, but nasal disease may be totally asymptomatic. The largest study to date is from the University of Toronto Lupus Clinic, in which 40 (4.6%) of 885 patients studied had a nasal septal perforation.[50] This group found an association with involvement of other mucosal beds and with active multisystem disease. Vascular inflammation was a suggested cause.

Overt or occult nasal cocaine use should always be sought in patients with destructive nasal septal disease. A strong association with Raynaud phenomenon was found with nasal septal perforation in a variety of disparate rheumatic diseases including RA, psoriatic arthritis, progressive systemic sclerosis, SLE, and mixed connective tissue disease (MCTD). Other causes of nasal septal perforation include Wegener granulomatosis, sarcoidosis, Behçet disease, lymphoma, tuberculosis, syphilis midline lethal granuloma (probably a form of lymphoma), and cryoglobulinemia.

Nasal biopsies, although frequently obtained, provide limited useful information unless the biopsy specimen includes inflamed blood vessels.[51] Treatment consists of controlling the system disease, active nasal irrigation, and humidification. Closure of the defect, although seemingly an attractive option, may be associated with poor healing of the tissue flap as a result of ongoing vasculitis. A Silastic button may avoid this complication.

Relapsing Polychondritis

Patients with lupus may have a clinical syndrome of inflammation of cartilage including nasal bridge, external ear, and upper airways akin to that observed in relapsing polychondritis. Ultimately, lupus will involve the skin, other organs, and demonstrate characteristic autoantibodies, thus distinguishing it from relapsing polychondritis. In a series of 62 patients with relapsing polychondritis, 22 patients had a total of 27 associated diseases including RA, myeloproliferative syndrome, SLE, or systemic vasculitis (three each), ulcerative colitis, autoimmune thyroiditis, ankylosing spondylitis, or autoimmune hemolytic anemia (two each), Crohn disease, pulmonary fibrosis, or insulin-dependent diabetes mellitus (one each).[53] Catastrophic antiphospholipid syndrome in association with lupus and relapsing polychondritis has been reported.[54] A case report and review of the 16 patients reported in the literature with relapsing polychondritis and SLE provided fairly convincing evidence for a true association rather than two diseases coincidentally occurring together.[55]

Laryngeal Involvement

Hoarseness may occur in patients with lupus and may be caused by laryngeal and pharyngeal edema of obscure origin or inflammatory vocal cord nodules.[56] The incidence of laryngeal involvement in lupus ranges from 0.3% to 30%.[57] The cricoarytenoid joint is a synovial joint and is much less commonly involved in lupus than in RA. Involvement of this joint may lead to vocal cord edema, immobility, and stridor. Several case reports have been published with acute and life-threatening involvement of the cricoarytenoid joint in patients with lupus, requiring treatment with high-dose steroidal medications and a tracheotomy in a particularly severe case.[58,59] Gastroesophageal reflux disease with hoarseness may occur in association with lupus-related motility disorder of the distal esophagus. Oral candidiasis may spread into the larynx and esophagus, resulting in odynophagia and hoarseness.

Temporomandibular Joint

The temporomandibular joint is less frequently involved in lupus than in juvenile idiopathic arthritis, RA, or osteoarthritis, and its presentation may include aural pain, clicking, and difficulty with jaw opening.[60] Panoramic radiographs of the temporomandibular joint followed by multislice computed tomography demonstrated avascular necrosis of the mandibular condyle in 2 out of 26 patients with juvenile lupus and 0 out of 28 healthy control participants.[61] Mild clinical dysfunction and abnormal temporal joint mobility were found in more than one half of the patients with juvenile lupus.[61,62] Because a high rate of fibromyalgia develops in patients with lupus, temporomandibular joint syndrome could be expected in this subset of patients with lupus. The fibromyalgia-associated joint dysfunction may be a result of bruxism or masticatory muscle myofascial pain dysfunction in distinction to structural temporomandibular joint defects observed in temporomandibular degeneration or dysfunction and other inflammatory conditions.

EAR INVOLVEMENT AND LUPUS
Ear Involvement in Lupus

SLE often has a significant effect on the inner ear, causing hearing loss, tinnitus, and vertigo.[63-69] Ear involvement can be unilateral or bilateral; the latter is often asymmetric. Although often reported as predominantly affecting mid to high frequencies, low frequencies are affected as well. Onset of hearing loss can be sudden (hours to days), rapidly progressing (days to weeks), or slowly progressing (weeks to months). Reported prevalence rates of ear manifestations in SLE vary (15% to 67%) and they can be symptomatic or asymptomatic.

Often inner ear dysfunction (e.g., hearing loss, vertigo) is the first manifestation of autoimmune disease before any other systemic symptoms.[63,64,67] Ear problems also commonly occur during a period of lupus remission or inactivity.[65] Thus many patients are initially seen by otolaryngologists and not rheumatologists, which might slow the diagnostic correlation with autoimmune disease. Nevertheless, autoimmune ear problems are generally responsive to glucocorticoid and cytotoxic drug treatment.[63,70] Other common autoimmune diseases have a similar prevalence of hearing loss, vertigo, and tinnitus, including RA, Wegener granulomatosis, Sjögren syndrome, Cogan syndrome, relapsing polychondritis, Behçet disease, and progressive systemic sclerosis.[63,64] Ear manifestations in these other autoimmune diseases imply that a common immune process is responsible for ear pathologic dysfunctions.

Mechanisms of Immune-Mediated Inner Ear Disease

Ear dysfunction, with or without other organ involvement, is often associated with circulating antibodies or immune complexes, but how they impact the inner ear is unknown. Hearing loss in SLE has been inconsistently correlated with circulating autoantibodies to DNA, cardiolipin, phospholipids, endothelial cells, and other serum factors; consequently, no clear cause has been identified.[63-67] In addition, some patients with sudden hearing loss and Ménière disease also have the same elevated autoantibodies but without any other autoimmune disease symptoms.[71,72] These patients may represent those in whom the ear is the first organ affected by disease.

Current theories involve these circulating immune factors compromising cochlear vasculature.[65,67] Endothelial cell tight junctions of the inner ear blood vessels create the blood-labyrinth barrier, which is similar to the blood-brain barrier. The barrier breakdown disrupts critical inner ear ionic transport mechanisms responsible for endolymph production, resulting in hearing loss and vertigo. Further insight into potential mechanisms of immune-mediated inner ear disease has come from studies of mouse models for SLE. All commonly studied autoimmune mice (e.g., MRL/*lpr*, C3H/*lpr*, New Zealand Black, Palmerston North) have inner ear disease and hearing loss.[73] The predominant area affected is the stria vascularis, a vascularized epithelium responsible for ion transport and endolymph homeostasis. Loss of the blood labyrinth barrier that normally protects this region causes a drop in the endocochlear electrical potentials; as a result, hearing declines. As is true in patients, hearing loss in the autoimmune mice can be restored with glucocorticoid treatments. However, mouse hearing loss also responds to mineralocorticoid treatment,[74] providing further evidence for compromised stria vascularis ion transport mechanisms as a result of the disruption of vascular tight junctions. Most clinical glucocorticoids (e.g., prednisone, dexamethasone) also have significant binding affinity for the mineralocorticoid receptor, suggesting that steroid-responsive hearing loss may involve both immunosuppression and restoration of inner ear ion transport.

ACKNOWLEDGMENTS

This work is supported by the National Institutes of Health (NIH): the National Institute on Deafness and Other Communication Disorders (NIDCD) R01 DC 05593, the Stan and Madelle Rosenfeld Family Trust, the William C. Kuzell Foundation, and the William and Mary Bauman Foundation.

References

1. Gold DH, Morris DA, Henkind P: Ocular findings in systemic lupus erythematosus. *Br J Ophthalmol* 56:800–804, 1972.
2. Jabs DA, Fine SL, Hochberg MC, et al: Severe retinal vaso-occlusive disease in systemic lupus erythematosus. *Arch Ophthalmol* 104:558–563, 1986.
3. Lanham JG, Barrie T, Kohner EM, et al: SLE retinopathy: evaluation of fluorescein angiography. *Ann Rheum Dis* 41:473–478, 1982.
4. Stafford-Brady FJ, Urowitz MB, Gladman DD, et al: Lupus retinopathy. Patterns, associations, and prognosis. *Arthritis Rheum* 31:1105–1110, 1988.
5. Snyers B, Lambert M, Hardy JP: Retinal and choroidal vaso-occlusive disease in systemic lupus erythematosus associated with antiphospholipid antibodies. *Retina* 10:255–260, 1990.
6. Silverman M, Lubeck MJ, Briney WG: Central retinal vein occlusion complicating systemic lupus erythematosus. *Arthritis Rheum* 21:839–843, 1978.
7. Graham EM, Spalton DJ, Barnard RO, et al: Cerebral and retinal vascular changes in systemic lupus erythematosus. *Ophthalmology* 92:444–448, 1985.
8. Vine AK, Barr CC: Proliferative lupus retinopathy. *Arch Ophthalmol* 102:852–854, 1984.
9. Read RW, Chong LP, Rao NA: Occlusive retinal vasculitis associated with systemic lupus erythematosus. *Arch Ophthalmol* 118:588–589, 2000.
10. Asherson RA, Merry P, Acheson JF, et al: Antiphospholipid antibodies: a risk factor for occlusive ocular vascular disease in systemic lupus

erythematosus and the "primary" antiphospholipid syndrome. *Ann Rheum Dis* 48:358–361, 1989.

11. Kleiner RC, Najarian LV, Schatten S, et al: Vaso-occlusive retinopathy associated with anti-phospholipid antibodies (lupus anticoagulant retinopathy). *Ophthalmology* 96:896–904, 1989.

12. Jabs DA, Hanneken AM, Schachat AP, et al: Choroidopathy in systemic lupus erythematosus. *Arch Ophthalmol* 106:230–234, 1988.

13. Hochberg MC, Boyd RE, Ahearn JM, et al: Systemic lupus erythematosus: a review of clinico-laboratory features and immunogenetic markers in 150 patients with emphasis on demographic subsets. *Medicine* 64:285–295, 1985.

14. Sheehan KCF, Ruddle NH, Schreiber RD: Generation and characterization of hamster monoclonal antibodies that neutralize murine tumor necrosis factors. *J Immunol* 142:3884–3893, 1989.

15. Jabs DA, Miller NR, Newman SA, et al: Optic neuropathy in systemic lupus erythematosus. *Arch Ophthalmol* 104:564–568, 1986.

16. Rosenbaum JT, Simpson J, Neuwelt EM: Successful treatment of optic neuritis in association with systemic lupus erythematosus using intravenous cyclophosphamide. *Br J Ophthalmol* 81:130–132, 1997.

17. Hayreh SS: Posterior ischemic optic neuropathy. *Ophthalmologica* 82:29–41, 1981.

18. Morrison DC, Jacobs DM: Binding of polymyxin B to the lipid A portion of bacterial lipopolysaccharides. *Immunochemistry* 13:813–818, 1976.

19. Galindo-Rodriguez G, Aviña-Zubieta JA, Pizarro S: Cyclophosphamide pulse therapy in optic neuritis due to systemic lupus erythematosus. *Am J Med* 106:65–69, 1999.

20. Kinnunen E, Müller K, Keto P, et al: Cerebrospinal fluid and MRI findings in three patients with multiple sclerosis and systemic lupus erythematosus. *Acta Neurol Scand* 87:356–360, 1993.

21. Arevalo JF, Lowder CY, Muci-Mendoza R: Ocular manifestations of systemic lupus erythematosus. *Curr Opin Ophthalmol* 13:404–410, 2002.

22. Read RW: Clinical mini-review: systemic lupus erythematosus and the eye. *Ocul Immunol Inflamm* 12:87–99, 2004.

23. Nguyen QD, Foster CS: Systemic lupus erythematosus and the eye. *Int Ophthalmol Clin* 38:33–60, 1998.

24. Hakin KN, Watson P: Systemic associations of scleritis. *Int Ophthalmol Clin* 31:111–129, 1991.

25. Adan CB, Trevisani VF, Vasconcellos M, et al: Bilateral deep keratitis caused by systemic lupus erythematosus. *Cornea* 23:207–209, 2004.

26. Messmer EM, Foster CS: Vasculitic peripheral ulcerative keratitis. *Surv Ophthalmol* 43:379–396, 1999.

27. Hobbs HE, Sorsby A, Freedman A: Retinopathy following chloroquine therapy. *Lancet* 478–480, 1959.

28. Marmor MF, Carr RE, Easterbrook M, et al: Recommendations on screening for chloroquine and hydroxychloroquine retinopathy: a report by the American Academy of Ophthalmology. *Ophthalmology* 109:1377–1382, 2002.

29. Michaelides M, Stover NB, Francis PJ, et al: Retinal toxicity associated with hydroxychloroquine and chloroquine: risk factors, screening, and progression despite cessation of therapy. *Arch Ophthalmol* 129:30–39, 2011.

30. Wolfe F, Marmor MF: Rates and predictors of hydroxychloroquine retinal toxicity in patients with rheumatoid arthritis and systemic lupus erythematosus. *Arthritis Care Res (Hoboken)* 62:775–784, 2010.

31. Shroyer NF, Lewis RA, Lupski JR: Analysis of the ABCR (ABCA4) gene in 4-aminoquinoline retinopathy: is retinal toxicity by chloroquine and hydroxychloroquine related to Stargardt disease? *Am J Ophthalmol* 131:761–766, 2001.

32. Marmor MF, Kellner U, Lai TY, et al: Revised recommendations on screening for chloroquine and hydroxychloroquine retinopathy. *Ophthalmology* 118:415–422, 2011.

33. Dunn JP, Noorily SW, Petri M, et al: Antiphospholipid antibodies and retinal vascular disease. *Lupus* 5:313–322, 1996.

34. Gupta A, Argarwal A, Bansal RK, et al: Ischaemic central retinal vein occlusion in the young. *Eye (Lond)* 7:138–142, 1993.

35. Hayreh SS, Zimmerman MB, Podhajsky P: Incidence of various types of retinal vein occlusion and their recurrence and demographic characteristics. *Am J Ophthalmol* 117:429–441, 1994.

36. Cobo-Soriano R, Sanchez-Ramon S, Aparicio MJ: Antiphospholipid antibodies and retinal thrombosis in patients without risk factors: a prospective case-control study. *Am J Ophthalmol* 128:725–732, 1999.

37. Carbone J, Sánchez-Ramón S, Cobo-Soriano R: Antiphospholipid antibodies: a risk factor for occlusive retinal vascular disorders. Comparison with ocular inflammatory diseases. *J Rheumatol* 28:2437–2441, 2001.

38. Miserocchi E, Baltatzis S, Foster CS: Ocular features associated with anti-cardiolipin antibodies: a descriptive study. *Am J Ophthalmol* 131:451–456, 2001.

39. Tan EM, Cohen AS, Fries JF, et al, The 1982 revised criteria for the classification of systemic lupus erythematosus. *Arth Rheum* 25:1271–1277, 1982.

40. Standefer JA, Mattox DE: Head and neck manifestations of collagen vascular diseases. *Otolaryngol Clin North Am* 19:181–210, 1986.

41. Aliko A, Alushi A, Tafaj A, et al: Oral mucosa involvement in rheumatoid arthritis, systemic lupus erythematosus and systemic sclerosis. *Int Dent J* 60:353–358, 2010.

42. Grimaldo-Carjevschi M, López-Labady J, Villarroel-Dorrego M: Squamous cell carcinoma on the palate in a patient with systemic lupus erythematosus: case report and review of literature. *Lupus* 20:519–522, 2011.

43. Jonsson R, Heyden G, Westberg NG, et al: Oral mucosal lesions in systemic lupus erythematosus. *J Rheumatol* 11:38–42, 1984.

44. López-Labady J, Villarroel-Dorrego M, Gonzalez N, et al: Oral manifestations of systemic and cutaneous lupus erythematosus in a Venezuelan population. *J Oral Pathol Med* 36:524–527, 2007.

45. Lourenço SV, de Carvalho FR, Boggio P, et al: Lupus erythematosus: clinical and histopathological study of oral manifestations and immuno-histochemical profile of the inflammatory infiltrate. *J Cutan Pathol* 34:558–564, 2007.

46. Burge SM, Frith P, Millard PR, et al: The lupus band test in oral mucosa, conjunctiva, and skin. *Br J Dermatol* 121:743–752, 1989.

47. Marques ER, Lourenco SV, Lima DM, et al: Oral lesions in lupus erythematosus-cytokines profiles of inflammatory infiltrate. *J Cutan Pathol* 37:439–445, 2010.

48. Brandrup F, Koch C, Petri M, et al: Discoid lupus erythematosus-like lesions and stomatitis in female carriers of X-linked chronic granulomatous disease. *Br J Dermatol* 104:495–505, 1981.

49. de Jong EM, van der Vleutvan Vlijmen-Willems IM: Differences in extracellular matrix proteins, epidermal growth and differentiation in discoid lupus erythematosus, lichen planus and the overlap syndrome. *Acta Derm Venereol* 77:356–360, 1997.

50. Rahman P, Gladman DD, Urowitz MB: Nasal-septal perforation in systemic lupus erythematosus—time for a closer look. *J Rheumatol* 26:1854–1855, 1999.

51. Lerner DN: Nasal septal perforation and carotid cavernous aneurysm: unusual manifestations of systemic lupus erythematosus. *Otolaryngol Head Neck Surg* 115:163–166, 1996.

52. Kim JE, Amin SH, Fong D, et al: Severe nasal presentation of antiphospholipid syndrome. *Arch Otolaryngol Head Neck Surg* 137:298–301, 2011.

53. Zeuner M, Straub RH, Rauh G, et al: Relapsing polychondritis: clinical and immunogenetic analysis of 62 patients. *J Rheumatol* 24:96–101, 1997.

54. Roux M, Fabre M, Ninet J: Systemic lupus erythematosus and/or relapsing polychondritis with catastrophic antiphospholipid syndrome (article in French). *Rev Med Interne* 25:74–77, 2004.

55. Harisdangkul V, Johnson WW: Association between relapsing polychondritis and systemic lupus erythematosus. *Southern Med J* 87:753–757, 1994.

56. Teitel AD, MacKenzie CR, Stern R, et al: Laryngeal involvement in systemic lupus erythematosus. *Semin Arthritis Rheum* 22:203–214, 1992.

57. Langford CA, Van Waes CV: Upper airway obstruction in the rheumatic diseases: life-threatening complications of autoimmune disease. *Rheum Dis Clin North Am* 23:345–363, 1997.

58. Karim A, Ahmed S, Siddiqui R, et al: Severe upper airway obstruction from cricoarytenoiditis as the sole presenting manifestation of a systemic lupus erythematosus flare. *Chest* 121:990–993, 2002.

59. Nanke Y, Kotake S, Yonemoto K, et al: Cricoarytenoid arthritis with rheumatoid arthritis and systemic lupus erythematosus. *J Rheumatol* 28:624–626, 2001.

60. Jonsson R, Lindvall AM, Nyberg G: Temporomandibular joint involvement in systemic lupus erythematosus. *Arthritis Rheum* 26:1506–1510, 1983.

61. Fernandes EG, Guissa VR, Saviolli C, et al: Osteonecrosis of the jaw on imaging exams of patients with juvenile systemic lupus erythematosus. *Rev Bras Reumatol* 50:3–15, 2010.

62. Fernandes EG, Saviolli C, Siqueira JT, et al: Oral health and the masticatory system in juvenile systemic lupus erythematosus. *Lupus* 16:713–719, 2007.

63. Berrocal JR, Ramirez-Camacho R: Sudden sensorineural hearing loss: supporting the immunologic theory. *Ann Otol Rhinol Laryngol* 111:989–997, 2002.

64. Kastanioudakis I, Ziavra N, Voulgari PV, et al: Ear involvement in systemic lupus erythematosus patients: a comparative study. *J Laryngol Otol* 116:103–107, 2002.

65. Roverano S, Cassano G, Paira S, et al: Asymptomatic sensorineural hearing loss in patients with systemic lupus erythematosus. *J Clin Rheumatol* 12:217–220, 2006.

66. Gomides AP, do Rosário EJ, Borges HM, et al: Sensorineural dysacusis in patients with systemic lupus erythematosus. *Lupus* 16:987–990, 2007.

67. Karatas E, Onat AM, Durucu C, et al: Audiovestibular disturbance in patients with systemic lupus erythematosus. *Otolaryngol Head Neck Surg* 136:82–86, 2007.

68. Agrup C: Immune-mediated audiovestibular disorders in the paediatric population: a review. *Int J Audiol* 47:560–565, 2008.

69. Karabulut H, Dagli M, Ates A, et al: Results for audiology and distortion product and transient evoked otoacoustic emissions in patients with systemic lupus erythematosus. *J Laryngol Otol* 124:137–140, 2010.

70. Rahman MU, Poe DS, Choi HK: Autoimmune vestibulo-cochlear disorders. *Curr Opin Rheumatol* 13:184–189, 2001.

71. Mouadeb DA, Ruckenstein MJ: Antiphospholipid inner ear syndrome. *Laryngoscope* 115:879–883, 2005.

72. Nacci A, Dallan I, Monzani F, et al: Elevated antithyroid peroxidase and antinuclear autoantibody titers in Ménière's disease patients: more than a chance association? *Audiol Neurootol* 15:1–6, 2010.

73. Trune DR: Mouse models for immunologic diseases of the auditory system. In Willott JF, editor: *Handbook of mouse auditory research: from behavior to molecular biology*, Boca Raton, FL, 2001, CRC Press, pp 505–531.

74. Trune DR, Kempton JB, Gross ND: Mineralocorticoid receptor mediates glucocorticoid treatment effects in the autoimmune mouse ear. *Hear Res* 212:22–32, 2006.

Chapter 32

Management of Sjögren Syndrome in Patients with SLE

Hendrika Bootsma, Hjalmar R. Bouma, Frans G.M. Kroese, Arjan Vissink, and Daniel J. Wallace

Sjögren syndrome (SS) is an autoimmune inflammatory disorder of the exocrine glands, which particularly affects the lacrimal and salivary glands. Frequent symptoms are dry mouth and dry eyes, often in conjunction with several nonspecific symptoms, such as malaise and fatigue. In addition, extraglandular manifestations, such as purpura, polyneuropathy, arthritis, and others, can be presenting signs of the disease (Table 32-1). The estimated prevalence of SS in the general population is between 0.5% and 1.0%, which makes SS the most common systemic autoimmune disease after rheumatoid arthritis (RA). SS is more frequent in women than in men, with a female-to-male ratio of 9:1. SS can be a primary idiopathic condition of unknown cause (primary SS [pSS]), but it may also occur in the presence of another autoimmune disorder such as RA, systemic lupus erythematosus (SLE), scleroderma, or mixed connective tissue disease (secondary SS [sSS]). In RA, the prevalence of sSS is approximately 30%; in SLE, approximately 20% of patients fulfill the classification criteria for sSS. Further, SS is associated with organ-specific autoimmune diseases; in particular, autoimmune thyroid disease, primary biliary cirrhosis, and autoimmune gastritis, which underscores the autoimmune nature of the disease.[1,2] Patients with SS may be restricted in their activities and participation in society, resulting in a reduced health-related quality of life and an impaired socioeconomic status.[3]

HISTORY

The first descriptions of SS were reported by European clinicians between 1882 and 1925.[4] In 1892, Mikulicz observed a man with bilateral parotid and lacrimal gland enlargement that was associated with massive round-cell infiltration. In 1925, Gougerot described three patients with salivary and mucous gland atrophy and insufficiency. In 1933, a Swedish ophthalmologist named Henrik Sjögren reported clinical and histologic findings in 19 women with xerostomia and keratoconjunctivitis sicca (KCS), of whom 13 had chronic arthritis. Seminal work by Morgan, Castleman, Bunim, and Talal in New York and at the National Institutes of Health in the 1950s and 1960s established Sjögren syndrome as an autoantibody-associated autoimmune disorder, detailed its clinical features, and recognized its association with lymphoma.[5]

CLINICAL PRESENTATION

Glandular Manifestations

SS affects the exocrine glands, in particular, the lacrimal and salivary glands, resulting in sicca complaints, or dry eyes, and a dryness of the oral cavity. With respect to the eyes, symptoms of burning, sandy sensations with pain, and photophobia and photosensitivity prevail

(Table 32-2). Physical examination reveals chronic irritation and destruction of both corneal and bulbar conjunctival epithelial KCS as a result of disturbed tear production. Accumulation of thick, rope-like secretions along the inner canthus may be the result of decreased tear film and an abnormal mucous component. Progressive keratitis may result in a loss of vision. A common problem in patients with dry eye is blepharitis. Conjunctivitis, as a result of secondary infection with *Staphylococcus aureus*, may also occur.

Reduced saliva production induces the sensation of dry mouth (xerostomia). Typical dryness-related complaints in early SS are predominantly present at rest and during the night. Over time and as SS develops, the dryness is also noted during the day.[6] Physical examination shows a dry mouth and tongue with an adherent, sticky mucus that coats the erythematous mucosa. The tongue may be smooth and reddened with some loss of dorsal papillae, or it may have a fissured appearance (Figure 32-1). The lips often appear cracked, peeling, and atrophic and may even appear furrowed or pebbled. The buccal mucosa may be pale and corrugated in appearance. Dental caries is not uncommon (Figure 32-2), as well as secondary infection of the mucosa with *Candida albicans*. Enlargement of the salivary glands may be present and is, generally, due to the presence of an autoimmune inflammatory process. However, enlargement of the glands might also be the result of lymphoma development or secondary infection caused by stasis of saliva.

Dryness also occurs at the mucosal surfaces in the upper and lower airways where it frequently leads to cough, in the vagina where it is associated with dyspareunia, and at other locations, in particular, the skin (xerosis).

Extraglandular Manifestations

SS is a systemic autoimmune disease in which many different organs may be affected, giving rise to the various extraglandular clinical manifestations[7] (see Table 32-1) (Figures 32-3 and 32-4). The involvement of extraglandular organs can go unrecognized until clinical symptoms become apparent in later stages of the disease. In addition, general systemic symptoms such as fatigue, myalgia, and depression are frequently present.

Lymphoma Development

Lymphomas develop in approximately 7.5% of patients with SS. Moreover, patients with SS have an 18.8 (CI 9.5 to 37.3) times increased risk of developing lymphomas.[8] In most cases these are marginal zone B-cell lymphomas occurring in the salivary glands, in particular the parotid gland, the so-called mucosa-associated lymphoid tissue (MALT) lymphoma. These lymphomas are generally localized and follow an indolent, rather benign, clinical course. In a

TABLE 32-1 Estimated Prevalence of a Particular Extraglandular Manifestation among Patients with Sjögren Syndrome[7,96,97,101]

AFFECTED ORGAN SYSTEM	EXTRAGLANDULAR MANIFESTATIONS	ESTIMATED PREVALENCE (%)*
Joints and muscles	Arthralgia or arthritis	>50
	Myopathy	22
Skin	Xerosis	>50
	Cutaneous vasculitis (purpura)	10
	Other skin lesion (e.g., erythema nodosum, livedo reticularis, lichen planus, vitiligo, cutaneous amyloidosis, and granuloma annulare)	<5
	Raynaud phenomenon vasculitis	13-30
Cardiovascular	Pericarditis	Up to 30
Respiratory tract	Interstitial lung disease (generally mild)	30
	Mucosa-associated lymphoid tissue (MALT) lymphoma	5-9
Gastrointestinal tract	Dysphagia	>50
	Oesophageal involvement	36-90
	Gastritis	20
Nervous system	Peripheral neuropathy	20
	Cranial neuropathy	5
	Central nervous system (CNS) involvement (focal or generalized)	Up to 20
Urogenital tract	Interstitial nephritis with renal tubular acidosis	25
	Glomerulonephritis (associated with cryoglobulinemia)	<10
	Interstitial cystitis	4

*Percentages greatly differ among studies.

TABLE 32-2 Onset and Duration of Symptoms of Eye and Mouth Dryness in Patients with and without Sjögren Syndrome[98]

	pSS (N = 32)	sSS (N = 25)	SS (N = 57)	NON-SS (N = 23)
Onset of first complaints, number (%)				
Eye dryness before mouth dryness	5 (16)	10 (40)	15 (26)	3 (13)
Eye dryness only	1 (3)	2 (8)	3 (5)	2 (9)
Mouth dryness before eye dryness	10 (31)	5 (20)	15 (26)	3 (13)
Mouth dryness only	2 (6)	2 (8)	4 (7)	3 (13)
Simultaneous onset	11 (34)	6 (24)	17 (30)	9 (39)
Neither eye nor mouth dryness	3 (10)	0	3 (5)	3 (13)
Duration at first visit, median, months				
Eye dryness	38	50	43	31
Mouth dryness	44	34	39	31

pSS, Primary Sjögren syndrome; SS, Sjögren syndrome; sSS, secondary Sjögren syndrome.

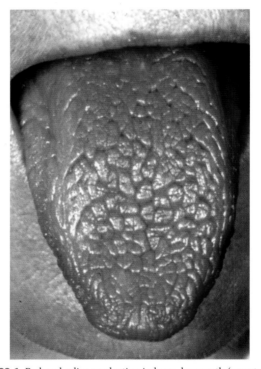

FIGURE 32-1 Reduced saliva production induces dry mouth (xerostomia), which may lead to the development of an arid, furrowed tongue.

minority of patients, aggressive non-Hodgkin lymphoma (NHL) is present and even Hodgkin disease has incidentally been described in SS. Risk factors for the development of lymphoma include the presence of cryoglobulins, low complement C4 levels, and palpable purpura.[9,10] The presence of germinal center–like structures in salivary gland biopsies is highly predictive for the development of lymphoma.[11] Isolated salivary gland enlargement, as well as any persistent lymph node swelling (Figure 32-5), in a patient with SS should raise the suspicion of lymphoma development.

Serologic Findings

The most characteristic autoantibodies in SS are anti–Sjögren syndrome antigen A (anti-SSA/Ro) antibodies, present in 70% of patients, and anti–Sjögren syndrome antigen B (anti-SSB/La) antibodies, present in approximately 50% of patients. High titers of these autoantibodies, in particular anti-SSB/La antibodies, are associated with extraglandular disease. Anti-SSB/La antibodies are considered to be the most specific serologic marker for SS, although they can also be found in 25% to 35% of patients with SLE or other autoimmune connective-tissue disorders and in approximately 5% of healthy individuals. Anti–alph-fodrin autoantibodies occur in approximately 30% of patients with SS and are considered specific for the disease.

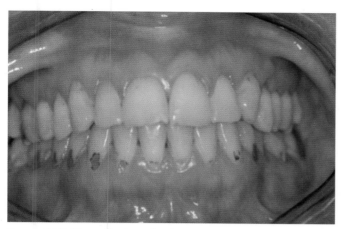

FIGURE 32-2 Hyposalivation-related dental caries. Note the carious destruction of the cervical regions of the teeth, areas that are relatively resistant to caries in patients with normal salivary secretion, because the self-clearance of the oral cavity is reduced.

Autoantibodies to human muscarinic acetylcholine receptor 3 are present in 90% of patients with pSS and 71% of patients with sSS; however, they are not specific for SS, because they are also present in 65% and 68% of patients with RA and SLE, respectively.[12] The rheumatoid factor is present in approximately 50% of patients but has a very low specificity for SS. Between 10% and 20% of patients with SS demonstrate mixed essential cryoglobulins. The presence of cryoglobulins is associated with vasculitic manifestations such as purpura, polyneuropathy/mononeuritis multiplex, and glomerulonephritis, and they constitute a risk factor for the development of lymphoma. Hypergammaglobulinemia, present in 40% of patients, reflects polyclonal B-lymphocyte activation, which is characteristic of SS.[13] In addition, monoclonal gammopathy, reported in 22% of patients, demonstrates excessive clonal B-cell proliferation and is associated with the development of lymphoma.

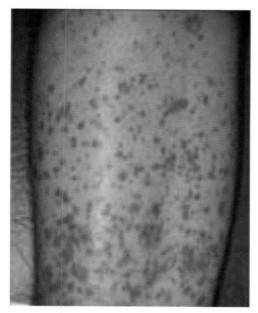

FIGURE 32-3 Purpura as an extraglandular manifestation.

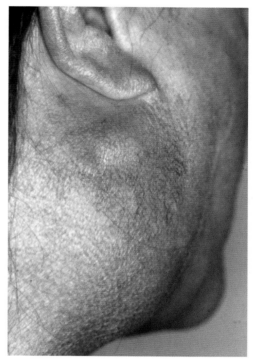

FIGURE 32-5 Swollen parotid gland from the development of mucosa-associated lymphoid tissue (MALT) lymphoma.

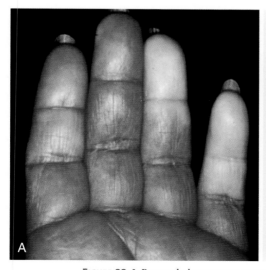
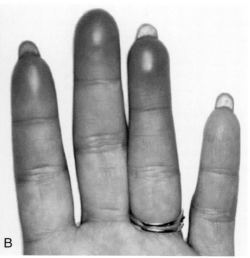

FIGURE 32-4 Raynaud phenomenon occurring in a patient with Sjögren syndrome.

Box 32-1 Revised International Classification Criteria and Revised Rules for Sjögren Syndrome Classification

I. Ocular symptoms—Require a positive response to at least one of the following questions:
　1. Have you had daily, persistent, troublesome dry eyes for more than 3 months?
　2. Do you have a recurrent sensation of sand or gravel in the eyes?
　3. Do you use tear substitutes more than three times a day?
II. Oral symptoms—Require a positive response to at least one of the following questions:
　1. Have you had a daily feeling of dry mouth for more than 3 months?
　2. Have you had recurrently or persistently swollen salivary glands as an adult?
　3. Do you frequently drink liquids to aid in swallowing dry food?
III. Ocular signs (i.e., objective evidence of ocular involvement)—Are defined as a positive result for a least one of the following tests:
　1. Schirmer I test, performed without anesthesia (≤5 mm in 5 minutes)
　2. Rose Bengal score or other ocular dye score (≥4 according to van Bijsterveld scoring system)
IV. Histopathology—In minor salivary glands (obtained through normal-appearing mucosa), focal lymphocytic sialadenitis, evaluated by an expert histopathologist, with a focus score of ≥1, defined as a number of lymphocytic foci (adjacent to normal-appearing mucous acini and contain more than 50 lymphocytes) per 4 mm^2 of glandular tissue
V. Salivary gland involvement—Objective evidence of salivary gland involvement is defined by a positive result to at least one of the following diagnostic tests:
　1. Unstimulated whole salivary flow (≤1.5 mL in 15 minutes)
　2. Parotid sialography showing delayed uptake, reduced concentration, and/or delayed excretion of tracer
　3. Salivary scintigraphy showing delayed uptake, reduced concentration, and/or delayed excretion of tracer

VI. Autoantibodies—Presence in the serum of the following autoantibodies:
　1. Antibodies to Sjögren syndrome antigen A (anti-SSA/Ro) or Sjögren syndrome antigen B (anti-SSB/La) or both

Revised Rules for Classification
For Primary Sjögren Syndrome
Patients without a potentially associated disease, primary Sjögren syndrome (pSS) may be defined as follows:
　a. Presence of any four of the six items is indicative of pSS, as long as either item IV (histopathology) or VI (serology) is positive.
　b. Presence of any three of the four objective criteria items (items III, IV, and VI) is indicative of pSS.
　c. Classification tree procedure represents a valid alternative method for classification, although it should be more properly used in a clinical epidemiologic survey.

Secondary Sjögren Syndrome
Patients with a potentially associated disease (i.e., another well-defined connective tissue disease), the presence of item I or II, and any two among items III, IV, and V may be considered as indicative of secondary SS.

Exclusion Criteria
Previous head and neck radiation treatment
Hepatitis C infection
Acquired immunodeficiency disease (AIDS)
Preexisting lymphoma
Sarcoidosis
Graft-versus-host disease
Anticholinergic drug use (since a time shorter than four-fold the half-life of the drug)

CLASSIFICATION AND DIAGNOSIS OF SJÖGREN SYNDROME

Many classification criteria for SS have been suggested. At present, the revised American-European classification criteria for SS, which were proposed in 2002, are the most widely accepted and validated criteria (Box 32-1). These criteria combine subjective symptoms of dry eyes and dry mouth with the objective signs of KCS and xerostomia.[14]

The subjective ocular and oral symptoms are obtained by history taking. Two tests are used to objectify reduced tear production. In the Schirmer test a piece of filter paper is placed laterally on the lower eyelid, which results in wetting due to tear production. If less than 5 mm of the paper is wetted after 5 minutes, then the test result is considered positive (Figure 32-6). In the rose bengal test, dye stains devitalized areas of the cornea and conjunctiva, which can then be scored using a split lamp. A rose bengal score of ≥4 according to the van Bijsterveld scoring system is considered abnormal. Instead of rose bengal stain, lissamine green can be used, which shows comparable results but is less painful. An additional test, which is not accepted as a diagnostic technique for SS but provides a global assessment of the function of the tear film, is the tear break-up time test. This test is performed by measuring break-up time after the instillation of fluorescein. An interval of less than 10 seconds is considered abnormal.

Currently, the most commonly applied noninvasive objective salivary gland diagnostic test is measuring the flow rate of unstimulated whole saliva. The patient is asked to expectorate once and then collect all saliva into a graduated container during a 15-minute period. Results obtained by sialometry, regardless of the presence of oral

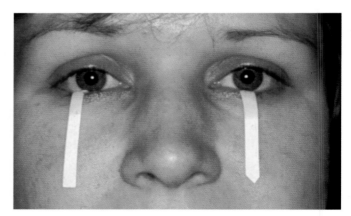

FIGURE 32-6 Schirmer test. A piece of filter paper is placed inside the lower eyelid (conjunctival sac). The eyes are closed for 5 minutes. The paper is then removed, and the amount of moisture is measured. In contrast to what is illustrated in this figure, usually the strips are placed laterally and the patient is asked to look upward so that no corneal abrasion occurs (when the eyes close, the eyeball rotates upward).

complaints, allow monitoring of the disease progression.[6] If more specific functional information is required for a particular gland, for research purposes and for patient-based advice on how best to reduce xerostomia, then individual gland collection techniques can be used (Figures 32-7 and 32-8).

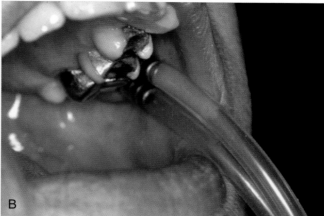

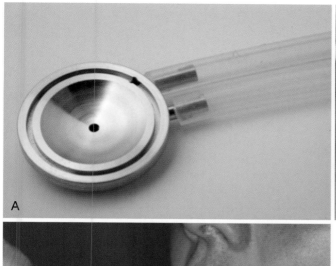

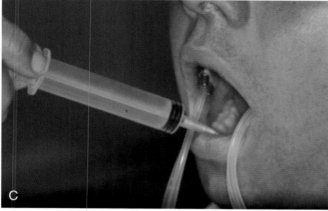

FIGURE 32-7 Collection of glandular saliva. A, A Lashley cup is used to collect parotid saliva. The cup contains a central chamber for collecting the saliva and a peripheral chamber to which a slight underpressure can be applied to keep the cup in place over the orifice of the parotid gland. **B,** The Lashley cup is in place on the orifice of the parotid gland. The secretion of parotid saliva is noted in one of the tubes connected to the cup. The other tube is used for applying slight underpressure. **C,** By blocking both orifices of the parotid gland, saliva collecting on the floor of the mouth can be removed by a syringe to assess submandibular/sublingual flow while collecting parotid saliva.

To confirm the diagnosis of SS histopathologically, usually a biopsy from a labial salivary gland is taken. The diagnosis can be confirmed if this biopsy shows focal lymphocytic sialadenitis with a focus score, defined as an accumulation of 50 or more lymphocytes per 4 mm[2], of ≥1.[15] Recently, it has been shown that parotid biopsies might serve as a proper alternative in the diagnosis of SS. In such biopsies, MALT or NHL pathologic findings are easier to detect because parotid glands are more commonly affected,[16] and the same gland can be biopsied more often.[17] Imaging studies can also be used to evaluate salivary gland involvement. Sialography of the parotid gland has a high diagnostic accuracy. The main characteristic of SS is a diffuse collection of contrast fluid at the terminal acini of the ductal tree, called *sialectasia*.[18,19] With scintigraphy, patients with SS demonstrate decreased uptake and release of technetium (Tc)–99m pertechnetate.[20] Finally, submandibular ultrasound might be a promising, less-invasive alternative to sialography in the classification of SS.[21]

The presence of nonspecific serologic markers of autoimmunity such as antinuclear antibodies, rheumatoid factors, and elevated immunoglobulins (particularly IgG) are important contributors to a definitive diagnosis of SS.[22]

PATHOGENESIS

Most of what is known about the pathogenesis of SS comes from patients with pSS, whereas little specific information is available about the pathogenesis of sSS. Furthermore, much of the work cited in the following text relies on two experimental models of SS: (1) nonobese, diabetic (NOD) mice that are autoimmune prone and diabetic but independent of the usual diabetes and insulinitis in that strain, and (2) B cell–activating factor (BAFF) generated transgenic mice, in which enhanced survival is sufficient to induce disease.

Unfortunately, both of these models lack the autoantibody profile (e.g., anti-SSA/Ro, anti-SSB/La) of the human counterpart.[23]

In the presence of a susceptible genetic background, hormonal and environmental factors are thought to be capable of triggering an autoimmune exocrinopathy. Salivary, lacrimal, and other exocrine glands become infiltrated with cluster of differentiation 4 (CD4+) T cells and large numbers of B cells, and inflamed tissues also contain predominantly IgG (besides IgA) plasma cells. Glandular infiltration can even lead to the formation of germinal center–like structures that contain certain follicular dendritic cells and proliferating B cells. These structures are sites of memory B-cell formation.

Genetic Factors

Human leukocyte antigen (HLA)–DR and HLA-deterodimer (HLA-DQ) class II genes are involved in the pathogenesis of SS but vary with geography and ethnicity.[24] B8, DWw52, DR2, Gla3, and 5 probably each play a role. Anti-SSA/Ro 52 autoantibody production is linked to DRB1*0301, DRB3*0301, DQA1*0501, and DQB1*0201. Genetic-wide association studies have correlated innate immune interferon regulatory factor 5 (IR5) rs2004640 T allele (odds ratio 1.93) polymorphisms, as well as STAT4 (SNP rs7582694), which encodes transcription factors involved with interferon signaling with SS.

Hormonal Factors

SS is far more common among women than men. X-chromosome silencing and sex steroids probably play important roles in the pathogenesis of SS.[25] Many genes on the X chromosome are involved in the immune system, and impaired inactivation of the genes on the X chromosome may contribute to the development of autoimmune

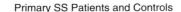

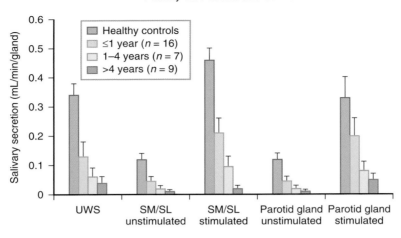

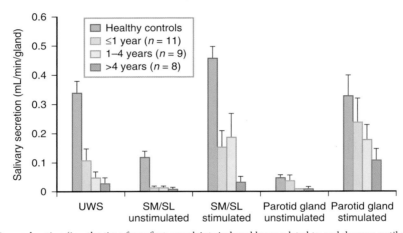

FIGURE 32-8 Relation among disease duration (i.e., the time from first complaints induced by or related to oral dryness until referral), mean salivary flow rates (mean ± SEM), unstimulated whole saliva (UWS), and submandibular/sublingual glands (SM/SL).[16]

disease. Sex hormones have key roles in the function of cells of the immune system. Estrogens appear to have positive effects on the emergence of autoimmune disease, and androgens have a more protective role, although the mechanisms are not well understood. Patients with SS appear to be androgen deficient and have lower serum concentrations of dehydroepiandrosterone (5-DHEA) and its sulfate ester, dehydroepiandrosterone-sulfate (DHEA-S).[26-28] Sex hormones also influence saliva and tear production.

Glandular Infiltration

Epithelial cells in SS glandular tissues are not only targets for the disease, but these cells also exert important immunologic functions. Ductal epithelial cells show enhanced expression of CD40 and adhesion molecules, as well as increased production of lymphoid chemokines, cytokines (including proinflammatory cytokines), and B lymphocyte stimulator (BlyS) or BAFF.[23] Epithelial cells also express Toll-like receptors (TLRs). Glandular viral infections can prompt epithelial cells to activate the innate immune system via TLRs.[29] A high incidence of Epstein-Barr virus reactivation in SS has been reported, and this virus commonly infects salivary epithelial glands and T cells. Binding of viral ligands to TLR3 on ductal cells is believed to be a major source of type I interferons in glandular tissue of patients with SS. One of the important cytokines induced by type I interferons is BAFF. The upregulation of adhesion molecules and

the production of chemokines and cytokines promote the migration of lymphocytes and dendritic cells into epithelial glandular tissues. Epithelial cells derived from patients with SS are probably intrinsically activated. The infiltrating T cells and dendritic cells secreting proinflammatory cytokines, such as interleukin-1 beta (IL-1β), interferon-gamma (IFN-γ), and tumor necrosis factor alpha (TNF-α), promote further activation of the epithelial cells and inflammation of the glands. Through apoptosis and exosomes, epithelial cells present intracellular autoantigens, and anti-SSA/Ro and anti-SSB/La are translocated from apoptotic blebs where they trigger the production of autoantibodies against these antigens by local (infiltrated) B cells. Type I interferon-induced BAFF, produced by the epithelial cells, may well play a role in this B-cell activation. Not only BAFF, but also levels of a proliferation-inducing ligand (APRIL) are increased in patients with pSS. These two cytokines share receptors and play different but essential roles in the regulation of B-cell survival, differentiation, and proliferation. The elevated levels of these cytokines might be, at least partly, responsible for the presence of autoantibodies, hypergammaglobulinemia, oligoclonal B-cell expansion, ectopic germinal center–like structures, and increased risk for developing NHL.

T-helper cell 2 (Th2)-derived cytokines dominate the early phase of SS, whereas Th1-derived cytokines are associated with a later stage of the disease. Mouse studies have consistently supported the role of an activated IL-23–Th17 pathway in the pathogenesis of SS. Finally, CD8+ cytolytic T cells are involved in the pathogenesis by the destruction of glandular tissue. The infiltration of autoreactive B cells and plasma cells, CD4+ T cells, and CD8+ cytolytic T cells all contribute to impaired function and the destruction of the glandular tissue and diminished production of saliva and tears.

SJÖGREN SYNDROME IN PATIENTS WITH LUPUS
The association of SS and SLE was first noted in 1959. Small-scale studies suggested the prevalence of SS in SLE ranging from 7% to 35%. Four recent, large-scale studies have analyzed the influence of SS on SLE. In one study, 9.2% of 283 patients with SLE who were Greek met the American-European classification criteria for SS.[30] Patients with SLE who had SS tended to be older, have a higher prevalence of Raynaud phenomenon, rheumatoid factor, anti-SSA and anti-SSB, and a high frequency for the DRB1*0301 allele. These patients had less renal disease, adenopathy, and thrombocytopenia. Of the patients with SLE who were Norwegian, 81 patients over the age of 70 years were compared with matched individuals with RA and healthy control participants.[31] The SLE group had more fatigue, anti-SSA and anti-SSB antibodies, and a positive Schirmer test. In the Johns Hopkins study, 259 (14%) of the 1531 patients with SLE were found to have SS by clinical evaluation.[32] These patients were generally older, white women with more photosensitivity; oral ulcers; Raynaud phenomenon; less renal disease; and anti-SSA and anti-SSB, anti–double-stranded DNA (anti-dsDNA), and anti-ribonucleoprotein (anti-RNP) antibodies. Approximately 20% of more than 2000 patients with lupus who were of Chinese

descent at Peking Union Medical College also had SS.[33] Significant differences between those with SS/SLE and those with SLE only included older age, female gender, and higher rates of sicca symptoms and signs, renal tubular acidosis, and interstitial lung disease in the former. Patients with SLE only had more rash, nephrosis, central nervous system disease, lower IgG levels, more disease activity, and more immune suppressive and corticosteroid use. Seventy-one percent of the patients with SS/SLE were SSA or SSB positive versus 20% of those with SLE. In summary, patients with SS/SLE who met SS criteria made up approximately 10% of the SLE population, although twice that many have features of SS. These patients tend to be older and, Caucasian, to have a more benign process, and to less frequently require aggressive management.

MANAGEMENT OF GLANDULAR MANIFESTATIONS
Early, accurate diagnosis of SS (Figure 32-9) can help prevent or ensure adequate treatment of many of the complications associated with the disease and may contribute to prompt recognition and treatment of serious systemic complications of SS.[6,7] Management of patients with SS should ideally involve a multidisciplinary team that consists of a specialized rheumatologist, oral and maxillofacial surgeon, and/or dentist, ophthalmologist, pathologist, hematologist, and oral hygienist. (Management strategies are provided in Tables 32-3, 32-4, and 32-5.) Although no curative or causal treatment is available for SS, various symptomatic, supportive, and palliative treatment options are available. Recently, promising results have been reported with some biological agents.

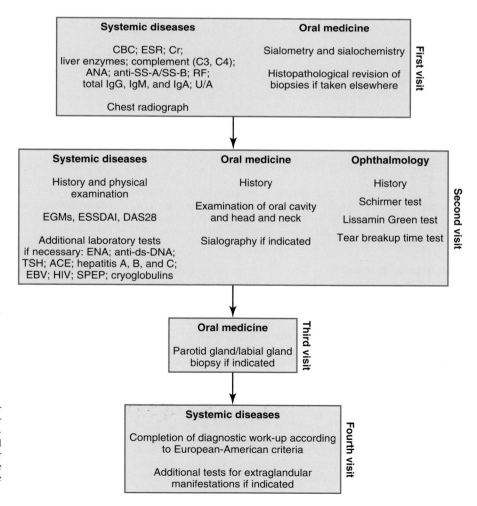

FIGURE 32-9 Diagnostic workup strategy for patients referred to the University Medical Center Groningen, The Netherlands, under clinical suspicion of Sjögren syndrome (SS). The primary referral is done by dentists, general practitioners, or other specialists. Before the first visit, patients receive written information about the diagnostic procedure followed at our institution.

TABLE 32-3 Management Strategies for Ocular Manifestations of Sjögren Syndrome[99,100]

MANAGEMENT STRATEGY	MEASURES
Preventive measures	
Avoid exacerbating factors	Low-humidity atmospheres (e.g., air conditioned stores, centrally heated homes, airplanes, windy locations) Irritants (e.g., dust, cigarette smoke) Activities that provoke tear film instability (e.g., prolonged reading, computer use)
Avoid drugs that may worsen sicca symptoms	Caution when using antidepressants, antihistamines, anticholinergics, antihypertensives (e.g., diuretics, β-blockers), and neuroleptic medications
Treat other medical conditions that result in dry eyes	Eyelid abnormalities (e.g., ectropion), meibomian gland disease, amyloidosis, inflammation (chronic blepharitis or conjunctivitis, pemphigoid, Stevens-Johnson syndrome), neurologic conditions that impair eyelid or lacrimal gland function, sarcoidosis, toxicity (burns or drugs), and a variety of other conditions (corneal anesthesia, blink abnormality, hypovitaminosis A [vitamin A deficiency], trauma)
Symptomatic treatments	
Tear substitution therapy	Low viscous eyedrops (Schirmer test ≤5 mm/5 min) and high mucous secretions in the cul-du-sac High viscous eyedrops (Schirmer test >5 mm/5 min) and low mucous secretions in the cul-du-sac Ophthalmic gels and ointments (at night)
Blepharitis	Daily eyelid rubs with warm water and diluted baby shampoo Topical antibiotics if indicated
Mucous secretions; sticky eyes; mucous filaments	N-acetylcysteine 5% eyedrops (2-3 times/day) as a mucolytic agent
Tear retention measures	Air moisturizers Moisture glasses Lacrimal punctal occlusion (moderately to severely dry eyes)
Topical immunomodulatory agents	Topical nonpreserved corticosteroids (e.g., dexamethasone 0, 1% eyedrops 2 times/day; taper dose or discontinue drops based on clinical findings and eye pressure)
Tear stimulation	
Systemic parasympathomimetic secretagogues	Pilocarpine (5-7.5 mg; 3-4 times/day) Cevimeline (30 mg; 3 times/day)
Treating underlying disorder	
Systemic antiinflammatory or immune modulating therapies to treat the autoimmune exocrinopathy of Sjögren syndrome	Anti-CD20 (rituximab)

Management of Ocular Manifestations
Preventive Measures
Factors that can cause an exacerbation of ocular symptoms should be avoided whenever possible. Several medical conditions that can result in KCS should be ruled out or otherwise promptly treated. In addition, the use of drugs that may worsen sicca symptoms should be avoided (Table 32-3).

Symptomatic Treatment
The most widely used therapy for dry eye disease is tear substitution by topical artificial tears (see Table 32-3).[34] However, natural tears have a complex composition of water, salts, hydrocarbons, proteins, and lipids, which artificial tears cannot completely substitute. In addition, the integrity of the three-layered lipid, aqueous, and mucin structure that is vital to the effective functioning of the tear film cannot be reproduced by these artificial components. Using preservatives may damage the tear film stability and the corneal epithelium; hence, the use of preservative-free, artificial tears is strongly recommended.[35] In addition, if the patient complains of mucous secretions in the eyes or sticky eyes or when mucous filaments are found on an eye examination, a mucolytic agent can be added to the medication (see Table 32-3). When successful, the dose should be tapered; when no effect is seen, application of these drops should be discontinued. Topical preservative-free corticosteroids (e.g., dexamethasone drops) can be used to suppress the associated inflammatory process (see Table 32-3). The use of topical preservative-free corticosteroids should be restricted because of severe side effects, such as glaucoma, cataracts, and increased risk of secondary infections and epithelial defects.

Management of Oral Manifestations
Preventive and General Measures for Oral Complications
Patients with SS require more frequent dental visits and must work closely with their dentist and oral hygienist to maintain optimal dental health[36] (Table 32-4). In dentate patients with SS, frequent radiographs should be taken to follow up carious lesions and to trace new ones. The use of topical fluorides is absolutely critical to control dental caries.[37] The dose chosen and the frequency of application (from daily to once a week) should be based on the severity of the salivary hypofunction and the rate of caries development.[38-40] Patients should be counseled to follow a diet that avoids cariogenic foods, especially fermentable carbohydrates and beverages (see Table 32-4). Polyols such as xylitol are considered to be anticariogenic since they decrease acid fermentation by *Streptococcus mutans*.[41]

Local Salivary Stimulation
Dry mucosal surfaces, difficulty wearing dentures, accumulation of plaque and debris on surfaces normally cleansed by the mechanical washing action of saliva, as well as difficulty speaking, tasting, and swallowing, may all benefit from several techniques available to stimulate salivary secretions (see Table 32-4). Masticatory stimulatory techniques are the easiest to implement and have few side effects. Combined gustatory and masticatory stimulatory techniques, such

TABLE 32-4 Management Strategies for Oral Manifestations of SS[99]

MANAGEMENT STRATEGY	MEASURES
Preventive measures	
Regular dental visits and radiographs	Usually every 3-4 months Intraoral photographs every 6-18 months in dentate patients who frequently develop new and recurrent caries lesions
Optimal oral hygiene	Team of oral health professional guidance (clinical and written instructions)
Topical fluorides and remineralizing solutions	Fluoride mouth rinse (0.1%; weekly) Neutral sodium fluoride gel (depending on the level of oral hygiene and residual level of salivary flow, from once a week to every second day); the gel is preferably applied with a custom-made tray
Diet modifications	Noncariogenic diet Minimize chronic use of alcohol and caffeine Nonfermentable dietary sweeteners (e.g., xylitol, sorbitol, aspartame, saccharine), whenever possible
Avoidance of drugs that may worsen sicca symptoms	Caution when using antidepressants, antihistamines, anticholinergics, antihypertensives, and neuroleptics
Treatment of other medical conditions that result in xerostomia	Endocrine disorders, metabolic diseases, and viral infections
Avoidance of exacerbating factors	Low humidity atmospheres (e.g., air conditioned stores, centrally heated houses, airplanes, windy locations) Irritants such as dust and cigarette smoke (up to date)
Salivary stimulation	
Masticatory stimulatory techniques	Sugar-free gum and mints
Combined gustatory and masticatory stimulatory	Lozenges, mints, and candies Water, with or without a slice of lemon
Parasympathomimetic secretagogues (systemic stimulation)	Pilocarpine (5-7.5 mg; 3-4 times/day) Cevimeline (30 mg; 3 times/day)
Symptomatic treatment	
Relief of oral dryness (nonresponders on systemic salivary stimulation)	Air moisturizers Frequent sips of water Oral rinses, gels, and mouthwashes Saliva substitutes Increased humidification

Oral candidiasis	Topical antifungal drugs:
	  Nystatin oral suspension (100,000 U/mL: 400,000-600,000 units; 4-5 times/day)
	  Clotrimazole cream (1%; 2 times/day)
	  Ketoconazole cream (2%; 1-2 times/day)
	  Amphotericin B lozenge (10 mg; 4 times/day); if not available, an amphotericin B mouth rinse (100 mg/mL) can be used (is less effective than a lozenge because of the reduced contact time in the oral cavity)
	Systemic antifungal drugs:
	  Fluconazole tablets (200 mg on first day, then 100 mg/day for 7-14 days)
	  Itraconazole tablets (200 mg/day for 1-2 weeks)
	  Ketoconazole (200-400 mg/day for 7-14 days)
	  Soak dentures in chlorhexidine solution (2%) at night

Angular cheilitis	Nystatin cream or ointment (100,000 U/g; 4-5 times/day) Clotrimazole cream (1%; 2 times/day) Miconazole cream (2%; 1-2 times/day)
Treating underlying disorder	
Systemic antiinflammatory or immune-modulating therapies to treat the autoimmune exocrinopathy of Sjögren syndrome	Anti-CD20 (rituximab)

as chewing gum, lozenges, mints, and candies, are easy to implement, generally harmless (assuming that they are sugar free), and easy to use by most patients. If an acid is added, malic acid is preferred because it has less harmful effects on tooth substance and oral mucosa.

Systemic Salivary Stimulation

Two secretagogues, pilocarpine[42,43] and cevimeline,[44,45] have been approved by the U.S. Food and Drug Administration (FDA) for the treatment of dry mouth, and these drugs are also found to be effective for dry eye disease (see Table 32-4). Pilocarpine is a nonselective muscarinic agonist, whereas cevimeline is a specific M1/M3-receptor agonist. Therefore fewer cardiac and pulmonary side effects are expected.[46] Unlike in the United States, Canada, and Japan, cevimeline is not yet licensed in Europe.

Symptomatic Treatment

In patients who do not respond to the various stimulation techniques cited in the previous text, several symptomatic treatments are available (see Table 32-4). Water, although less effective than natural

TABLE 32-5 Management Strategies for Extraglandular Manifestations of Sjögren Syndrome[99]

CLINICAL FEATURES	DRUGS
Severe fatigue	NSAIDs Hydroxychloroquine (400 mg/day) Prednisone (7.5-10 mg/day; maximum dose 15 mg)
Anorexia	Hydroxychloroquine (400 mg/day) Prednisone (7.5-10 mg/day; maximum dose 15 mg)
Arthralgia	NSAIDs
Myalgia	NSAIDs
Arthritis	NSAIDs Hydroxychloroquine (400 mg/day) Methotrexate (15 mg/week; maximum dose 25 mg) Prednisone (7.5-10 mg/day; maximum dose 15 mg)
Skin involvement	
Mild vasculitis	Hydroxychloroquine (400 mg/day) and/or Prednisone (7.5-10 mg/day; maximum dose 15 mg)
Polymorphic erythema	Hydroxychloroquine (400/day; maximum dose 800 mg) and/or Prednisone (7.5-10 mg/day; maximum dose 15 mg)
Raynaud phenomenon	Calcium channel blocker
Severe vasculitis	Prednisone (60 mg/day) with or without cyclophosphamide IV (750 mg/m^2; monthly; 6-12 times) Rituximab
Pulmonary involvement	
Pleuritis or serositis	NSAID Prednisone (15-20 mg/day; maximum dose 30 mg)
Interstitial pneumonitis	Prednisone (60 mg/day) with or without cyclophosphamide IV (750 mg/m^2; monthly; 6-12 times)
Esophageal dysfunction	Omeprazole (20-40 mg/day)
Neurologic involvement	
Severe PNS	Prednisone (60 mg/day) with or without cyclophosphamide IV (750 mg/m^2; monthly; 6-12 times) Anti-CD20 (rituximab)
CNS	Prednisone (60 mg/day) with or without cyclophosphamide IV (750 mg/m^2; monthly; 6-12 times) Anti-CD20 (rituximab)
Interstitial cystitis	Pilocarpine (5-7.5 mg, 3 times/day) and/or prednisone (15 mg/day)
Renal involvement	
Interstitial nephritis	Bicarbonate (individual dose) and/or potassium completion (individual dose) Prednisone (15-60 mg/day, depending on severity of proteinuria or renal impairment)
Glomerulonephritis	Prednisone (60 mg/day) with or without cyclophosphamide IV (750 mg/m^2; monthly; 6-12 times) Anti-CD20 (rituximab)
MALT lymphoma With no active SS With symptomatic enlarged parotid gland(s), no active SS With active SS	 Watchful waiting Radiotherapy (2 × 2 Gy) Rituximab IV (375 mg/m^2; weekly; 4 times) Cyclophosphamide IV (750 mg/m^2; 3 weekly; 8 times) Prednisone (100 mg for 5 days after cyclophosphamide infusion (8 times) Rituximab IV (375 mg/m^2; weekly; 4 times) Cyclophosphamide IV (750 mg/m^2; 3 weekly; 8 times) Prednisone (100 mg for 5 days after cyclophosphamide infusion (8 times)

CNS, Central nervous system; IV, intravenous; MALT, mucosa-associated lymphoid tissue; NSAIDs; nonsteroidal antiinflammatory drugs; PNS, peripheral nervous system; SS, Sjögren syndrome.

saliva, is by far the most important fluid supplement for individuals with dry mouth.[47] In addition, numerous oral rinses, mouthwashes, and gels are available for patients with dry mouth.[48-53] Patients should be cautioned to avoid products containing alcohol, sugar, or strong flavorings that may irritate the sensitive, dry oral mucosa. Saliva replacements (i.e., saliva substitutes, artificial salivas) are not well-accepted for long-term use by many patients, particularly when they have not been instructed properly on their uses.

Prevention and Treatment of Oral Candidiasis
Secondary infection of the mucosa with *Candida albicans* is not uncommon in patients with SS. Patients with salivary gland dysfunction may require prolonged treatment to eradicate oral fungal infections. Dentures should be soaked overnight in an aqueous solution of 0.2% chlorhexidine to prevent reinfections of the oral cavity by *Candida* species. Nystatin or clotrimazole cream can be used to treat angular cheilitis (see Table 32-4).

Management of Dry Surfaces Other than the Mouth and Eyes

Sicca symptoms elsewhere are treated symptomatically. Dry lips can be treated with lip salves or petroleum jelly, whereas dryness of the skin may require the use of moisturizing lotions and bath additives. Vaginal dryness can be relieved with lubricant jellies. The use of humidifiers may be helpful for nasal and pharyngeal dryness. Saline nasal sprays are available to resolve blocked nasal passages, which may occur as a result of nasal dryness and can exacerbate oral dryness by stimulating mouth breathing.

OUTCOME MEASURES

After years of inactivity, several clinical trials for SS have been published since 2007 and many more are in development. The best validated methods of ascertainment and outcome measures are the following[54-57]:

1. Salivary gland function (salivary flow rate) and biomarkers (cathepsin D, alpha-enolase, and beta-2 microglobulin)
2. Lacrimal gland function (Schirmer test, lissamine green test, and breakup time)
3. Laboratory assessments (quantitative immunoglobulins and rheumatoid factor)
4. Subjective assessments (fatigue inventories and short form–36 [SF-36])
5. Extraglandular manifestations (scored by organ system)
6. Composite scores (Sjögren Syndrome Disease Activity and Damage Index, the EULAR Sjögren Syndrome Disease Activity Index [ESSDAI], and the EULAR Sjögren Syndrome Patient Reported Index [ESSPRI])

MANAGEMENT OF EXTRAGLANDULAR DISEASE

Most of the traditional antirheumatic drugs used in the treatment of RA and SLE have been tried with pSS with limited results, especially for the glandular manifestations. These drugs, however, may be of benefit in the management of extraglandular manifestations in pSS and sSS. New biological drugs, such as TNF inhibitors and interferon alpha (IFN-α), and B-cell depletion therapy, have been tried in patients with pSS with varying results, and research of their use is ongoing. The current treatment options available for extraglandular manifestations are summarized in Table 32-5.

Antiinflammatory and Disease-Modifying Drugs

Nonsteroidal antiinflammatory drugs (NSAIDs) are the first-line therapy of musculoskeletal and constitutional symptoms in pSS (see Table 32-5). However, tolerance to NSAIDs may be low as a result of dysphagia secondary to decreased salivary flow and esophageal dysmotility.

Corticosteroids are used in the treatment of arthritis, cutaneous symptoms, and severe constitutional manifestations of pSS (see Table 32-5). In a controlled trial, no significant effect on salivary and lacrimal function was found.[58]

Hydroxychloroquine (200 to 400 mg daily) is mostly used for the treatment of cutaneous, musculoskeletal, and constitutional symptoms (see Table 32-5). In some cases it can benefit lupus-like skin manifestations in pSS.[59]

Methotrexate is used for polyarticular inflammatory arthritis in pSS (see Table 32-5), although data on its efficacy regarding arthritis in association with pSS are lacking. Improvement of sicca symptoms was reported in this small study; however, no improvement was recorded on objective parameters without an effect on serologic parameters.

Leflunomide recently showed modest, nonsignificant improvement of salivary and lacrimal gland function in a small open-label study. Although the drug showed an acceptable safety profile in most patients, an exacerbation of leukocytoclastic vasculitis was revealed in some patients.[60]

Azathioprine and *sulfasalazine* failed to show beneficial effects in patients with pSS.

Treatment Strategies in Severe Extraglandular Manifestations

Nephritis

Interstitial nephritis is observed in 30% of patients and leads to clinical symptoms in 5% to 10% of patients. Distal or proximal renal tubular acidosis (RTA) I or II can result in clinical symptoms such as compromised renal function, proteinuria, nephrocalcinosis, renal stones, hypokalemia, hypophosphatemia, polyuria, and nephrogenic diabetes insipidus. An immune complex–mediated mesangial proliferative or membranoproliferative nephritis is seen in 5% to 10% of the patients, leading to clinical findings such as hypertension, proteinuria (mild to nephritic syndrome), and an active urine sediment with erythrocytes and casts. Treatment strategies for SS-associated nephritis are shown in Table 32-5.

Neurologic Manifestations

Central nervous system manifestations associated with SS are treated with high doses of corticosteroids. In patients with diffuse symptoms based on vasculitis, pulse cyclophosphamide is added to high doses of corticosteroids. In an acute setting or when symptoms are worsening, treatment with plasmapheresis or intravenous immunoglobulins (IVIG) or both may be considered. Involvement of the peripheral nervous system affects approximately 10% to 20% of patients with SS, mainly in the form of sensorimotor and sensory polyneuropathies and cranial neuropathies. These manifestations respond poorly to corticosteroids, but stabilization or spontaneous improvements were seen. Axonal neuropathy also responds badly to corticosteroids. Successful treatment with plasmapheresis or IVIG or both was described in anecdotal reports. On the contrary, in multiple mononeuropathies, nerve biopsies revealed vasculitis, and treatment with high doses of corticosteroids and pulse cyclophosphamide was found to be useful.[61]

Vasculitis

Skin lesions based on vasculitis are observed in 10% of patients with pSS. Purpura, polymorphic erythema, urticarial lesions, and ulcers caused by leukocytoclastic vasculitis are seen most often. Systemic vasculitis can lead to neuropathic, renal, pulmonary, and gastrointestinal symptoms. These manifestations are often associated with cryoglobulinemia and low complement levels. Corticosteroids are the first step in treatment, with intravenous cyclophosphamide added in more severe cases. In life-threatening situations, treatment is started with plasmapheresis or IVIG, followed by intravenous corticosteroids and cyclophosphamide. Rituximab, especially in patients with cryoglobulinemia, may be successful, although its efficacy has not yet been proven in controlled trials.[62]

Hematologic Complications

Common hematologic complications are mild autoimmune cytopenias and hyperglobulinemia. No specific therapy is necessary, although these patients require careful follow-up. For more severe cytopenias, aggressive treatment is indicated. Autoimmune hemolytic anemia, thrombocytopenia, and agranulocytosis are treated with corticosteroids. If the response is not sufficient, then cyclophosphamide is added. Treatment with azathioprine is not recommended since it may facilitate the development of lymphoproliferative disorders in patients with pSS, who are already at increased risk for developing B-cell lymphomas. Plasmapheresis, IVIG, and rituximab are second- or third-line options in the treatment of severe hemolytic anemia and thrombocytopenic purpura.

Mucosa-Associated Lymphoid Tissue Lymphoma

Pijpe and others[63,64] showed that rituximab treatment in patients with pSS with MALT lymphoma might result in complete remission of this lymphoma. However, recent studies found that rituximab monotherapy was not sufficient for the treatment of SS-MALT in patients who had an initial high SS disease activity; these patients required retreatment because of a recurrence of MALT lymphoma or the development of SS disease activity or both.[17,65] Pollard and others[17] proposed guidelines for the management and treatment of patients with SS-MALT, based on the treatment experience of 35 patients with pSS and lymphoma (see Table 32-5).

BIOLOGICAL AGENTS IN THE TREATMENT OF SJÖGREN SYNDROME
Interferon-Alpha
IFN-α levels are increased in the plasma of patients with pSS.[66,67] Furthermore, sera from patients with pSS have high type 1 IFN bioactivity.[68] Clinical trials with monoclonal antibodies to IFN-α have not yet been started in pSS. Instead of targeting IFN-α, IFN-α, itself, has been used as a therapeutic agent in pSS. Surprisingly, phase I and II studies showed that IFN-α might increase salivary and lacrimal function in patients with pSS.[69-71] These small studies were followed by a phase III randomized controlled trial showing that IFN-α treatment increased unstimulated whole salivary flow but not stimulated whole salivary flow and oral dryness.[72]

Anti-CD20 Therapy
Rituximab (a monoclonal chimeric humanized CD20 antibody) was shown to be safe and effective in treating RA in controlled studies.[73-77] Relief of ocular and oral symptoms, fatigue, and other extraglandular manifestations was seen after treating SS with rituximab when assessed with both subjective and objective measures.[63,78-82] Although the duration of treatment effect differed among trials, a significant effect occurred between 12 and 24 weeks after treatment in all trials. The effects are transient and treated patients usually experience a relapse of the disease, which parallels the return of B cells in the peripheral blood.[78,81] In contrast to patients with lymphoma or other hematologic malignancies, treating patients with autoimmune disease with rituximab does not appear to be associated with an increased risk for infection.[78,81,83,84] Compared with patients with RA and SLE, patients with pSS develop serum sickness–like disease more frequently (6% to 27%) after treatment with rituximab.[63,78,85] Therefore patients with pSS may need concomitant administration of corticosteroids.[81] To date, the lack of sufficient, long-term data does not allow statements on the efficacy and safety of rituximab monotherapy in pSS to be made definitely.

FUTURE PERSPECTIVES
Novel therapies might consist of a combination of targeting cytokines involved in the regulation of B-cell production by targeting BAFF, which showed significant benefits for patients with SLE,[86] inhibiting the activation of B cells through co-stimulation (i.e., using abatacept, which is currently used as a safe and effective treatment of RA[87]) and/or depleting the circulating B cells by using the anti-CD20 antibody, rituximab. Overexpression of the cytokine BAFF, which is involved in B-cell survival,[88] may result in a less stringent selection of transitional B cells and rescues autoreactive cells from deletion in the periphery.[89,90] Patients with pSS have elevated levels of BAFF in serum, saliva, and salivary glands.[91-94] In addition, salivary gland epithelial cells in pSS express both HLA class II and co-stimulatory molecules and may function as antigen-presenting cells.[95] Abatacept, a fusion molecule of an IgG–fragment specific (IgG-Fc) and a cytotoxic T-lymphocyte antigen 4 (CTLA-4), modulates CD28-mediated T-cell co-stimulation and might be beneficial for patients with SS. A combination therapy that targets CD20 (rituximab) and BAFF may delay B-cell repopulation with autoreactive cells. Targeting co-stimulation with abatacept at some point after rituximab treatment but before the reappearance of B cells in the blood may prevent the activation of autoreactive B cells that either escaped rituximab treatment or were newly generated. To date, data regarding the use of these drugs in the treatment of SS, either alone or combined, are not available yet.

References
1. Fox RI: Sjögren's syndrome. *Lancet* 366(9482):321–331, 2005.
2. Hansen A, Lipsky PE, Dorner T: Immunopathogenesis of primary Sjögren's syndrome: implications for disease management and therapy. *Curr Opin Rheumatol* 17(5):558–565, 2005.
3. Meijer JM, Meiners PM, Huddleston Slater JJ, et al: Health-related quality of life, employment and disability in patients with Sjögren's syndrome. *Rheumatology (Oxford)* 48(9):1077–1082, 2009.
4. Talal N: Sjögren's syndrome: an historical perspective. *Ann Med Interne (Paris)* 149(1):4–6, 1998.
5. Bloch KJ, Buchanan WW, Wohl MJ, et al: Sjoegren's syndrome. A clinical, pathological, and serological study of sixty-two cases. *Medicine (Baltimore)* 44:187–231, 1965.
6. Pijpe J, Kalk WW, Bootsma H, et al: Progression of salivary gland dysfunction in patients with Sjogren's syndrome. *Ann Rheum Dis* 66(1):107–112, 2007.
7. Kassan SS, Moutsopoulos HM: Clinical manifestations and early diagnosis of Sjogren syndrome. *Arch Intern Med* 164(12):1275–1284, 2004.
8. Zintzaras E, Voulgarelis M, Moutsopoulos HM: The risk of lymphoma development in autoimmune diseases: a meta-analysis. *Arch Intern Med* 165(20):2337–2344, 2005.
9. Theander E, Henriksson G, Ljungberg O, et al: Lymphoma and other malignancies in primary Sjögren's syndrome: a cohort study on cancer incidence and lymphoma predictors. *Ann Rheum Dis* 65(6):796–803, 2006.
10. Voulgarelis M, Skopouli FN: Clinical, immunologic, and molecular factors predicting lymphoma development in Sjögren's syndrome patients. *Clin Rev Allergy Immunol* 32(3):265–274, 2007.
11. Theander E, Vasaitis L, Baecklund E, et al: Lymphoid organisation in labial salivary gland biopsies is a possible predictor for the development of malignant lymphoma in primary Sjögren's syndrome. *Ann Rheum Dis* 70(8):1363–1368, 2011.
12. Kovács L, Marczinovits I, György A, et al: Clinical associations of autoantibodies to human muscarinic acetylcholine receptor 3(213–228) in primary Sjögren's syndrome. *Rheumatology (Oxford)* 44(8):1021–1025, 2005.
13. Hansen A, Lipsky PE, Dorner T: B cells in Sjögren's syndrome: indications for disturbed selection and differentiation in ectopic lymphoid tissue. *Arthritis Res Ther* 9(4):218, 2007.
14. Vitali C, Bombardieri S, Jonsson R, et al: Classification criteria for Sjögren's syndrome: a revised version of the European criteria proposed by the American-European Consensus Group. *Ann Rheum Dis* 61(6):554–558, 2002.
15. Daniels TE: Labial salivary gland biopsy in Sjögren's syndrome. Assessment as a diagnostic criterion in 362 suspected cases. *Arthritis Rheum* 27(2):147–156, 1984.
16. Pijpe J, Kalk WW, van der Wal JE, et al: Parotid gland biopsy compared with labial biopsy in the diagnosis of patients with primary Sjögren's syndrome. *Rheumatology (Oxford)* 46(2):335–341, 2007.
17. Pollard RP, Pijpe J, Bootsma H, et al: Treatment of mucosa-associated lymphoid tissue lymphoma in Sjögren's syndrome: a retrospective clinical study. *J Rheumatol* 38(10):2198–2208, 2011.
18. Blatt IM, French AJ, Holt JF, et al: Secretory sialography in diseases of the major salivary glands. *Ann Otol Rhinol Laryngol* 65(2):295–317, 1956.
19. Blatt IM: On sialectasis and benign lymphosialdenopathy. (The pyogenic parotitis, gougerot-Sjoegren's syndrome, Mikulicz's disease complex.) A ten-year study. *Laryngoscope* 74:1684–1746, 1964.
20. Hermann GA, Vivino FB, Goin JE: Scintigraphic features of chronic sialadenitis and Sjögren's syndrome: a comparison. *Nucl Med Commun* 20(12):1123–1132, 1999.
21. Takagi Y, Kimura Y, Nakamura H, et al: Salivary gland ultrasonography: can it be an alternative to sialography as an imaging modality for Sjogren's syndrome? *Ann Rheum Dis* 69(7):1321–1324, 2010.
22. Tzioufas AG, Mitsias DI, Moutsopoulos HM: Sjogren syndrome. In Hochberg MC, Silman AJ, editors: *Rheumatology*, Philadelphia, 2008, Elsevier, pp 1348–1349.
23. Voulgarelis M, Tzioufas AG: Pathogenetic mechanisms in the initiation and perpetuation of Sjogren's syndrome. *Nat Rev Rheumatol* 6(9):529–537, 2010.
24. Cobb BL, Lessard CJ, Harley JB, et al: Genes and Sjögren's syndrome. *Rheum Dis Clin North Am* 34(4):847–868, vii, 2008.
25. Pennell LM, Galligan CL, Fish EN: Sex affects immunity. *J Autoimmun* 2012. (In press.)
26. Valtysdottir ST, Wide L, Hallgren R: Low serum dehydroepiandrosterone sulfate in women with primary Sjögren's syndrome as an isolated sign of impaired HPA axis function. *J Rheumatol* 28(6):1259–1265, 2001.
27. Sullivan DA, Belanger A, Cermak JM, et al: Are women with Sjögren's syndrome androgen-deficient? *J Rheumatol* 30(11):2413–2419, 2003.
28. Hartkamp A, Geenen R, Godaert GL, et al: Effect of dehydroepiandrosterone administration on fatigue, well-being, and functioning in women

with primary Sjögren syndrome: a randomised controlled trial. *Ann Rheum Dis* 67(1):91–97, 2008.

29. Mackay IR: The etiopathogenesis of autoimmunity. *Semin Liver Dis* 25:239–250, 2005.

30. Manoussakis MN, Georgopoulou C, Zintzaras E, et al: Sjögren's syndrome associated with systemic lupus erythematosus: clinical and laboratory profiles and comparison with primary Sjögren's syndrome. *Arthritis Rheum* 50(3):882–891, 2004.

31. Gilboe IM, Kvien TK, Uhlig T, et al: Sicca symptoms and secondary Sjögren's syndrome in systemic lupus erythematosus: comparison with rheumatoid arthritis and correlation with disease variables. *Ann Rheum Dis* 60(12):1103–1109, 2001.

32. Baer AN, Maynard JW, Shaikh F, et al: Secondary Sjögren's syndrome in systemic lupus erythematosus defines a distinct disease subset. *J Rheumatol* 37(6):1143–1149, 2010.

33. Xu D, Tian X, Zhang W, et al: Sjögren's syndrome-onset lupus patients have distinctive clinical manifestations and benign prognosis: a case-control study. *Lupus* 19(2):197–200, 2010.

34. Akpek EK, Lindsley KB, Adyanthaya RS, et al: Treatment of Sjögren's syndrome-associated dry eye: an evidence-based review. *Ophthalmology* 118(7):1242–1252, 2011.

35. Bhojwani R, Cellesi F, Maino A, et al: Treatment of dry eye: an analysis of the British Sjögren's Syndrome Association comparing substitute tear viscosity and subjective efficacy. *Cont Lens Anterior Eye* 34(6):269–273, 2011.

36. Singh M, Palmer C, Papas AS: Sjögren's syndrome: dental considerations. *Dent Today* 29(5):64, 66–64, 67, 2010.

37. Jansma J, Vissink A, Gravenmade EJ, et al: In vivo study on the prevention of postradiation caries. *Caries Res* 23(3):172–178, 1989.

38. Anusavice KJ: Dental caries: risk assessment and treatment solutions for an elderly population. *Compend Contin Educ Dent* 23(10 Suppl):12–20, 2002.

39. Kielbassa AM, Hinkelbein W, Hellwig E, et al: Radiation-related damage to dentition. *Lancet Oncol* 7(4):326–335, 2006.

40. Zero DT: Dentifrices, mouthwashes, and remineralization/caries arrestment strategies. *BMC Oral Health* 15(6 Suppl 1):S9, 2006.

41. Chambers MS, Jones CU, Biel MA, et al: Open-label, long-term safety study of cevimeline in the treatment of postirradiation xerostomia. *Int J Radiat Oncol Biol Phys* 69(5):1369–1376, 2007.

42. Papas AS, Sherrer YS, Charney M, et al: Successful treatment of dry mouth and dry eye symptoms in Sjögren's syndrome patients with oral pilocarpine: a randomized, placebo-controlled, dose-adjustment study. *J Clin Rheumatol* 10(4):169–177, 2004.

43. Petrone D, Condemi JJ, Fife R, et al: A double-blind, randomized, placebo-controlled study of cevimeline in Sjögren's syndrome patients with xerostomia and keratoconjunctivitis sicca. *Arthritis Rheum* 46(3):748–754, 2002.

44. Fife RS, Chase WF, Dore RK, et al: Cevimeline for the treatment of xerostomia in patients with Sjögren syndrome: a randomized trial. *Arch Intern Med* 162(11):1293–1300, 2002.

45. Seror R, Sordet C, Guillevin L, et al: Tolerance and efficacy of rituximab and changes in serum B cell biomarkers in patients with systemic complications of primary Sjögren's syndrome. *Ann Rheum Dis* 66(3):351–357, 2007.

46. Cummins MJ, Papas A, Kammer GM, et al: Treatment of primary Sjögren's syndrome with low-dose human interferon alfa administered by the oromucosal route: combined phase III results. *Arthritis Rheum* 49(4):585–593, 2003.

47. Vissink A, De Jong HP, Busscher HJ, et al: Wetting properties of human saliva and saliva substitutes. *J Dent Res* 65(9):1121–1124, 1986.

48. Regelink G, Vissink A, Reintsema H, et al: Efficacy of a synthetic polymer saliva substitute in reducing oral complaints of patients suffering from irradiation-induced xerostomia. *Quintessence Int* 29(6):383–388, 1998.

49. Epstein JB, Emerton S, Le ND, et al: A double-blind crossover trial of Oral Balance gel and Biotene toothpaste versus placebo in patients with xerostomia following radiation therapy. *Oral Oncol* 35(2):132–137, 1999.

50. Ship JA, McCutcheon JA, Spivakovsky S, et al: Safety and effectiveness of topical dry mouth products containing olive oil, betaine, and xylitol in reducing xerostomia for polypharmacy-induced dry mouth. *J Oral Rehabil* 34(10):724–732, 2007.

51. Fox PC, Brennan M, Pillemer S, et al: Sjögren's syndrome: a model for dental care in the 21st century. *J Am Dent Assoc* 129(6):719–728, 1998.

52. Walsh LJ: Lifestyle impacts on oral health. In Mount G, Hume W, editors: *Preservation and restoration of tooth structure*, Middlesbrough, UK, 2008, Knowledgebooks and Software Ltd., pp 83–110.

53. Turner M, Jahangiri L, Ship JA: Hyposalivation, xerostomia and the complete denture: a systematic review. *J Am Dent Assoc* 139(2):146–150, 2008.

54. Vitali C, Palombi G, Baldini C, et al: Sjögren's Syndrome Disease Damage Index and disease activity index: scoring systems for the assessment of disease damage and disease activity in Sjögren's syndrome, derived from an analysis of a cohort of Italian patients. *Arthritis Rheum* 56(7):2223–2231, 2007.

55. Hu S, Gao K, Pollard R, et al: Preclinical validation of salivary biomarkers for primary Sjögren's syndrome. *Arthritis Care Res (Hoboken)* 62(11):1633–1638, 2010.

56. Seror R, Ravaud P, Bowman SJ, et al: EULAR Sjögren's syndrome disease activity index: development of a consensus systemic disease activity index for primary Sjögren's syndrome. *Ann Rheum Dis* 69(6):1103–1109, 2010.

57. Seror R, Ravaud P, Mariette X, et al: EULAR Sjögren's Syndrome Patient Reported Index (ESSPRI): development of a consensus patient index for primary Sjögren's syndrome. *Ann Rheum Dis* 70(6):968–972, 2011.

58. Dawson LJ, Caulfield VL, Stanbury JB, et al: Hydroxychloroquine therapy in patients with primary Sjögren's syndrome may improve salivary gland hypofunction by inhibition of glandular cholinesterase. *Rheumatology (Oxford)* 44(4):449–455, 2005.

59. Kruize AA, Hene RJ, Kallenberg CG, et al: Hydroxychloroquine treatment for primary Sjögren's syndrome: a two year double blind crossover trial. *Ann Rheum Dis* 52(5):360–364, 1993.

60. van Woerkom JM, Kruize AA, Geenen R, et al: Safety and efficacy of leflunomide in primary Sjögren's syndrome: a phase II pilot study. *Ann Rheum Dis* 66(8):1026–1032, 2007.

61. Gorson KC, Natarajan N, Ropper AH, et al: Rituximab treatment in patients with IVIg-dependent immune polyneuropathy: a prospective pilot trial. *Muscle Nerve* 35(1):66–69, 2007.

62. Ferri C, Mascia MT: Cryoglobulinemic vasculitis. *Curr Opin Rheumatol* 18(1):54–63, 2006.

63. Pijpe J, van Imhoff GW, Spijkervet FK, et al: Rituximab treatment in patients with primary Sjögren's syndrome: an open-label phase II study. *Arthritis Rheum* 52(9):2740–2750, 2005.

64. Pijpe J, van Imhoff GW, Vissink A, et al: Changes in salivary gland immunohistology and function after rituximab monotherapy in a patient with Sjögren's syndrome and associated MALT lymphoma. *Ann Rheum Dis* 64(6):958–960, 2005.

65. Quartuccio L, Fabris M, Salvin S, et al: Controversies on rituximab therapy in Sjögren syndrome-associated lymphoproliferation. *Int J Rheumatol* 2009:424935, 2009.

66. Bave U, Nordmark G, Lovgren T, et al: Activation of the type I interferon system in primary Sjögren's syndrome: a possible etiopathogenic mechanism. *Arthritis Rheum* 52(4):1185–1195, 2005.

67. Zheng L, Zhang Z, Yu C, et al: Association between IFN-alpha and primary Sjögren's syndrome. *Oral Surg Oral Med Oral Pathol Oral Radiol Endod* 107(1):e12–e18, 2009.

68. Wildenberg ME, van Helden-Meeuwsen CG, van de Merwe JP, et al: Systemic increase in type I interferon activity in Sjögren's syndrome: a putative role for plasmacytoid dendritic cells. *Eur J Immunol* 38(7):2024–2033, 2008.

69. Ferraccioli GF, Salaffi F, De VS, et al: Interferon alpha-2 (IFN alpha 2) increases lacrimal and salivary function in Sjögren's syndrome patients. Preliminary results of an open pilot trial versus OH-chloroquine. *Clin Exp Rheumatol* 14(4):367–371, 1996.

70. Shiozawa S, Morimoto I, Tanaka Y, et al: A preliminary study on the interferon-alpha treatment for xerostomia of Sjögren's syndrome. *Br J Rheumatol* 32(1):52–54, 1993.

71. Ship JA, Fox PC, Michalek JE, et al: Treatment of primary Sjögren's syndrome with low-dose natural human interferon-alpha administered by the oral mucosal route: a phase II clinical trial. IFN Protocol Study Group. *J Interferon Cytokine Res* 19(8):943–951, 1999.

72. Smith JK, Siddiqui AA, Modica LA, et al: Interferon-alpha upregulates gene expression of aquaporin-5 in human parotid glands. *J Interferon Cytokine Res* 19(8):929–935, 1999.

73. Tak PP, Kalden JR: Advances in rheumatology: new targeted therapeutics. *Arthritis Res Ther* 13(Suppl 1):S5, 2011.

74. Finckh A, Ciurea A, Brulhart L, et al: B cell depletion may be more effective than switching to an alternative anti-tumor necrosis factor agent in rheumatoid arthritis patients with inadequate response to anti-tumor necrosis factor agents. *Arthritis Rheum* 56(5):1417–1423, 2007.

75. Cohen SB: Updates from B cell trials: efficacy. *J Rheumatol Suppl* 77:12–17, 2006.

76. Emery P, Fleischmann R, Filipowicz-Sosnowska A, et al: The efficacy and safety of rituximab in patients with active rheumatoid arthritis despite methotrexate treatment: results of a phase IIB randomized, double-blind, placebo-controlled, dose-ranging trial. *Arthritis Rheum* 54(5):1390–1400, 2006.

77. Edwards JC, Szczepanski L, Szechinski J, et al: Efficacy of B-cell-targeted therapy with rituximab in patients with rheumatoid arthritis. *N Engl J Med* 350(25):2572–2581, 2004.

78. Dass S, Bowman SJ, Vital EM, et al: Reduction of fatigue in Sjogren syndrome with rituximab: results of a randomised, double-blind, placebo-controlled pilot study. *Ann Rheum Dis* 67(11):1541–1544, 2008.

79. Devauchelle-Pensec V, Pennec Y, Morvan J, et al: Improvement of Sjogren's syndrome after two infusions of rituximab (anti-CD20). *Arthritis Rheum* 57(2):310–317, 2007.

80. Gottenberg JE, Guillevin L, Lambotte O, et al: Tolerance and short term efficacy of rituximab in 43 patients with systemic autoimmune diseases. *Ann Rheum Dis* 64(6):913–920, 2005.

81. Meijer JM, Meiners PM, Vissink A, et al: Effectiveness of rituximab treatment in primary Sjogren's syndrome: a randomized, double-blind, placebo-controlled trial. *Arthritis Rheum* 62(4):960–968, 2010.

82. Chalmers JM: Minimal intervention dentistry: part 1. Strategies for addressing the new caries challenge in older patients. *J Can Dent Assoc* 72(5):427–433, 2006.

83. Kelesidis T, Daikos G, Boumpas D, et al: Does rituximab increase the incidence of infectious complications? A narrative review. *Int J Infect Dis* 15(1):e2–1e6, 2011.

84. US Food and Drug Administration: FDA Public Health Advisory: life-threatening brain infection in patients with systemic lupus erythematosus after Rituxan (rituximab) treatment. 2011. Available at http://www .fda.gov/Drugs/DrugSafety/PostmarketDrugSafetyInformationforPa tientsandProviders/DrugSafetyInformationforHeathcareProfessionals/ PublicHealthAdvisories/ucm124345.htm

85. Meijer JM, Pijpe J, Bootsma H, et al: The future of biologic agents in the treatment of Sjogren's syndrome. *Clin Rev Allergy Immunol* 32(3):292–297, 2007.

86. Wiglesworth AK, Ennis KM, Kockler DR: Belimumab: a BLyS-specific inhibitor for systemic lupus erythematosus. *Ann Pharmacother* 44(12): 1955–1961, 2010.

87. Genovese MC, Schiff M, Luggen M, et al: Efficacy and safety of the selective co-stimulation modulator abatacept following 2 years of treatment in patients with rheumatoid arthritis and an inadequate response to anti-tumour necrosis factor therapy. *Ann Rheum Dis* 67(4):547–554, 2008.

88. Moisini I, Davidson A: BAFF: a local and systemic target in autoimmune diseases. *Clin Exp Immunol* 158(2):155–163, 2009.

89. Thien M, Phan TG, Gardam S, et al: Excess BAFF rescues self-reactive B cells from peripheral deletion and allows them to enter forbidden follicular and marginal zone niches. *Immunity* 20(6):785–798, 2004.

90. Lesley R, Xu Y, Kalled SL, et al: Reduced competitiveness of autoantigen-engaged B cells due to increased dependence on BAFF. *Immunity* 20(4): 441–443, 2004.

91. Groom J, Kalled SL, Cutler AH, et al: Association of BAFF/BLyS over-expression and altered B cell differentiation with Sjogren's syndrome. *J Clin Invest* 109(1):59–68, 2002.

92. Lavie F, Miceli-Richard C, Quillard J, et al: Expression of BAFF (BLyS) in T cells infiltrating labial salivary glands from patients with Sjogren's syndrome. *J Pathol* 202(4):496–502, 2004.

93. Pers JO, d'Arbonneau F, Devauchelle-Pensec V, et al: Is periodontal disease mediated by salivary BAFF in Sjogren's syndrome? *Arthritis Rheum* 52(8):2411–2414, 2005.

94. Pers JO, Daridon C, Devauchelle V, et al: BAFF overexpression is associated with autoantibody production in autoimmune diseases. *Ann N Y Acad Sci* 1050:34–39, 2005.

95. Routsias JG, Tzioufas AG: Autoimmune response and target autoantigens in Sjogren's syndrome. *Eur J Clin Invest* 40(11):1026–1036, 2010.

96. Garcia-Carrasco M, Ramos-Casals M, Rosas J, et al: Primary Sjogren syndrome: clinical and immunologic disease patterns in a cohort of 400 patients. *Medicine (Baltimore)* 81(4):270–280, 2002.

97. Asmussen K, Andersen V, Bendixen G, et al: A new model for classification of disease manifestations in primary Sjogren's syndrome: evaluation in a retrospective long-term study. *J Intern Med* 239(6):475–482, 1996.

98. Vissink A, Kalk WW, Mansour K, et al: Comparison of lacrimal and salivary gland involvement in Sjogren's syndrome. *Arch Otolaryngol Head Neck Surg* 129(9):966–971, 2003.

99. Meiners PM, Meijer JM, Vissink A, et al: Management of Sjögren's syndrome. In Weisman MH, Weinblatt ME, Louie JS, et al, editors: *Targeted treatment of rheumatic diseases*, 2010, Saunders, pp 133–155.

100. Mansour K, Leonhardt CJ, Kalk WW, et al: Lacrimal punctum occlusion in the treatment of severe keratoconjunctivitis sicca caused by Sjogren syndrome: a uniocular evaluation. *Cornea* 26(2):147–150, 2007 Feb.

101. Zufferey P, Meyer OC, Grossin M, et al: Primary Sjögren's syndrome (SS) and malignant lymphoma. A retrospective cohort study of 55 patients with SS. *Scand J Rheumatol* 24(6):342–345, 1995.

Chapter 33

Gastrointestinal and Hepatic Manifestations

David S. Hallegua and Swamy Venuturupalli

GASTROINTESTINAL INVOLVEMENT

Gastrointestinal (GI) manifestations are common in patients with systemic lupus erythematosus (SLE), and the prevalence of their various manifestations is listed in Box 33-1. Abdominal symptoms and signs may be the result of SLE, medications that are used to treat SLE, or intercurrent processes. Historically, William Osler was impressed with the frequency of GI crises in those with lupus and labeled lupus as the new disease that could mimic any other disease.[1]

Prevalence

GI complaints were the initial presentation in 10% of Dubois' patients[2]; 25% to 40% had protracted symptoms. Haserick and colleagues[3] divided the GI symptoms of SLE among 87 patients into three groups: none (63%), minor (29%), and major (8%). Subclinical involvement of the GI tract is also common; chronic mucosal infiltration with inflammatory cells was found in 96% of 26 autopsied children with SLE.[4] Younger patients with lupus are more susceptible. Among 272 patients with SLE, the prevalence of GI manifestations ranged from 10% in children to none in patients over the age of 50 years.[5] A review on GI manifestations in SLE published by Sultan and colleagues[6] found anorexia to be the most common reported manifestation with a prevalence of 36% to 71% in published studies. A recent publication found the cumulative prevalence of GI symptoms in patients with lupus who are of Asian descent to be 3.8% to 18%.[7] In one recent study, patients with lupus who required hospitalization had a higher prevalence of GI symptoms with 39 out of 177 patients being admitted for a GI complaint.[8]

Pharyngitis, Dysphagia, and Esophagitis

Recurrent sore throat is not an infrequent finding, especially in children[9] (see Chapter 23 for discussions on mucous membrane lesions and other features of oral pathologic conditions). Dysphagia and heartburn occur in 1% to 7.3%[2,9,10] and 11% to 50%[9] of patients, respectively. Chong and colleagues[11] found that patients with lupus in comparison with patients with rheumatoid arthritis (RA) had significantly more heartburn. In a literature review, Zizic[12] related that although only 5% of the patients with SLE complained of dysphagia, 25% had impaired esophageal peristalsis, compared with 67% of patients with scleroderma. Several studies using esophageal manometry noted aperistalsis or hypoperistalsis of the esophagus in approximately 10% of patients with SLE.[13-15] Aperistalsis is sometimes correlated with the presence of Raynaud phenomenon. Gutierrez and colleagues[16] compared esophageal motility in 14 patients with SLE and 17 patients with mixed connective-tissue disease (MCTD). A definite correlation was found between Raynaud phenomenon and hypoperistalsis, with the latter being more common in MCTD. The patients in the SLE group had only a slightly decreased lower esophageal sphincter pressure. Esophageal motor dysfunction in SLE can also produce diffuse spasm and result in symptoms of chest pain.

Ramirez-Mata and colleagues[17] performed esophageal manometric studies in a group of unselected patients with SLE and noted abnormalities in 16 patients. An absence of or abnormally low contractions were found at the upper one third in seven patients, at the lower two thirds in three patients, in the entire esophagus in two patients, at the lower esophageal sphincter in two patients, and at the lower two thirds plus the lower sphincter in the remaining two patients. No relationship was found among the presence of esophageal dysfunction and activity, duration, and therapy of SLE. Interestingly, five of the 34 patients who had normal studies complained of dysphagia and heartburn. Esophageal imaging with Gastrografin, computed tomographic (CT) scanning, or endoscopy is required to make the diagnosis of esophageal ulceration or perforation from systemic vasculitis.[10]

The treatment of esophageal symptoms include small and frequent meals, the avoidance of postprandial recumbency, and the administration of antacids, proton-pump inhibitors, histamine-2 (H_2) antagonists, or parasympathomimetic agents. Fungal esophagitis from the use of antibiotics and steroids may need treatment with fluconazole.

Anorexia, Nausea, Vomiting, and Diarrhea

The most common cause of anorexia, nausea, vomiting, and diarrhea in patients with SLE is related to the use of salicylates, nonsteroidal antiinflammatory drugs (NSAIDs), antimalarial drugs, corticosteroids, and cytotoxic agents. Anorexia, nausea, vomiting, and diarrhea symptoms can continue to occur for weeks after therapy is stopped. When caused by the disease, manifestations are persistent and are not explained by other factors.

Anorexia occurs in 49% to 82% of patients,[2,9] especially if untreated. Nausea has been reported in 11% to 38% of patients.[2,9] When medications are excluded as a cause, however, the incidence is approximately 8%.[18] Vomiting and diarrhea can be prominent in patients who are hospitalized with lupus and GI symptoms[2,9,18] and are observed in up to 56.4% and 30.8% of patients, respectively, who are admitted. Children appear to have an increased incidence of all these symptoms.[5]

Motility Disorders

Chronic intestinal pseudoobstruction (CIPO) reflects a dysfunction of the visceral smooth muscle or the enteric nervous system.[19,20] Symptoms and signs of CIPO in patients with SLE include a subacute onset of abdominal pain and distention associated with vomiting and constipation and a distended tender abdomen with hypoactive or absent bowel sounds or a complete lack of bowel sounds. Radiologic examination reveals dilated, fluid-filled bowel loops and occasional bilateral ureteral dilation with a reduced bladder capacity. Antroduodenal manometry demonstrates intestinal and esophageal hypomotility. Nojima and colleagues[20] described two patients with CIPO who had antibodies to proliferating cell nuclear antigen (PCNA) but no other specific antibodies or clinical manifestations of SLE. Treatment of CIPO usually involves high doses of steroids, broad-spectrum antibiotics, and promotility drugs. Perlemuter and colleagues[21] reported the use of octreotide at a dose of 50 µg twice a day subcutaneously in CIPO in SLE and scleroderma. The symptoms of CIPO resolved in the three patients receiving treatment within

Box 33-1 Key Points: Systemic Lupus Erythematosus and the Gastrointestinal Tract

1. Gastrointestinal (GI) symptoms are common in systemic lupus erythematosus (SLE). Secondary causes, such as concurrent disease, stress, and medication, must be ruled out.
2. Sore throat and oral ulcers are common.
3. Dysphagia is present in 1% to 7.3% of patients, especially in association with Raynaud phenomenon.
4. Anorexia, nausea, vomiting, or diarrhea may be prominent in one third of patients when the disease is active. Chronic intestinal pseudoobstruction (CIPO) causes these symptoms and is a disturbance of the enteric nervous system. Inflammatory bowel disease, infection, and concomitant drug administration must be ruled out as other causes.
5. Peptic ulcer disease is found in 6% of patients with acute abdominal pain and is usually caused by antiinflammatory medication.
6. Ascites is found in 8% to 12% of patients. If a result of nephrosis, cirrhosis, or congestive heart failure is present, it is a painless transudate. Exudative causes might be painful and include serosal inflammation. Patients with lupus peritonitis are often responsive to steroids.
7. Pancreatitis is a serious complication of SLE. Pancreatitis is associated with pancreatic vasculitis, activity of SLE in other systems, and, rarely, with subcutaneous fat necrosis. Mild elevation of pancreatic enzyme levels may occur in SLE without pancreatitis; high levels suggest pancreatitis. Steroids are the treatment of choice, but steroids (along with thiazide diuretics, and azathioprine) can induce pancreatitis.
8. Abdominal pain, distention, and tenderness warrant a search for ischemia or bowel ulceration, especially in patients with a SLEDAI score of 4 or higher. In the outpatient setting, abdominal pain, distention, and tenderness may suggest the presence of small intestinal bacterial overgrowth (SIBO).
9. Malabsorption syndromes are rare but do occur.
10. Mesenteric or intestinal vasculitis is a life-threatening complication of SLE, usually associated with multisystem activity. High doses of steroids are required. To reduce mortality, early surgical intervention is indicated if prompt improvement does not occur with steroids. Patients may die from complications of obstruction, perforation, or infarction if surgical exploration is not performed within 48 hours in appropriate patients.

SLEDAI, Systemic Lupus Erythematosus Disease Activity Index.

48 hours. Recurrence of symptoms responded to increasing the dose of octreotide.

Small intestinal bacterial overgrowth (SIBO) may be the result of disordered motility caused by the lack of duration or propagation of migrating motor complex or from the lack of IgG class antibacterial antibodies to indigenous bacteria in the GI tract to neutralize bacteria.[22,23] Albano and colleagues[24] investigated the presence of SIBO in 14 patients with SLE using a lactulose hydrogen breath test. Symptoms of SIBO such as bloating (50%), diarrhea (64%), constipation (42%), and abdominal pain (42%) were present in these patients with SLE without any clear identifiable cause after the history and physical examination were completed. Breath hydrogen above 20 million parts per million (ppm) with two distinct peaks of hydrogen production was diagnostic for SIBO. Twelve patients (86%) were found to have SIBO by predefined criteria.

Abdominal Pain and Acute Abdomen

Abdominal pain is found in 8% to 37% of patients with SLE,[2,7,9,18,25] with the lowest incidence being reported in series that excluded medication-related symptoms. Abdominal pain may be the first symptom of a catastrophic lupus-related complication such as mesenteric vasculitis or may be a non-lupus–related cause such as gluten-sensitive enteropathy or irritable bowel syndrome. A thorough history and physical examination with special attention paid to the activity of lupus in other organs and appropriate imaging can help differentiate between lupus- and non-lupus–related complications. Patients with abdominal pain, even without tenderness, need an aggressive and comprehensive evaluation, including a complete blood count, amylase-level determination, blood-chemistry profiles, and abdominal radiography. If free air, a moderate amount of free fluid, acidosis, and/or hyperamylasemia without pancreatitis are present, then diagnostic laparoscopy should be performed. If pseudoobstruction and/or thumbprinting of the bowel are seen without free peritoneal fluid, then specialized tests, such as an upper GI series, barium enema, CT, magnetic resonance imaging (MRI), gallium and indium white-cell scanning, and visceral angiography, may be necessary.

Intravenous fluids should be administered to patients suspected of having an intraabdominal crisis while undergoing these initial diagnostic evaluations. If peritonitis is suspected, broad-spectrum antibiotics should be administered. Aggressive fluid replacement, antibiotics, and steroid stress dose coverage precede laparoscopic or open surgical exploration. Steroid therapy can mask bowel ischemia and perforation. The best application of diagnostic laparoscopy is in the evaluation of a patient with equivocal findings. In 412 consecutive admissions to Cleveland hospitals for collagen vascular diseases,[25] 63 patients had abdominal complaints; of these, 48 had SLE. Pain was present in 85% of patients, fever was noted on examination in 76% of patients, and peritoneal signs were recorded in 10% of patients. Corticosteroids were administered to 64%. Acute causes, including duodenal or gastric ulcer, gastritis, and pancreatitis, were determined in 33 patients. Mesenteric vasculitis was present in 3 patients, and the pain was of undetermined cause in 16 patients. Surgery was performed on 21 patients; in 11, it was exploratory. Al-Hakeem and colleagues[26] identified 13 patients with a principal diagnosis of abdominal pain out of 88 patients with SLE who were admitted to the hospital during a 15-year period. Diagnoses accounting for abdominal pain included adhesions,[3] diverticulitis,[3] cholecystitis,[2] perforated ulcer and colon, gastroenteritis, duodenitis, and inflammatory bowel disease (1 each). Of the 13 patients in the study, 9 required surgery. In another survey of 63 procedures,[27] 16% morbidity and 6% surgical mortality rates were recorded. Rojas-Serrano[28] evaluated the causes of emergency department consultation for patients with SLE and found that abdominal pain was the third most-frequent reason accounting for 18 out of 180 patients with lupus visiting the emergency department.

Min and colleagues[29] studied the causes of acute abdominal pain in patients visiting the emergency department. Twenty-six patients with SLE and abdominal pain made 44 visits to the emergency department. Twenty-seven (59.1%) of these visits were for ischemic bowel disease. Other diagnoses included pancreatitis, serositis, splenic infarction, angioedema, renal vein thrombosis, pelvic inflammatory disease, upper GI bleeding, and ectopic pregnancy. CT scanning and ultrasound help establish the diagnosis of ischemic bowel disease. Kwok and colleagues[30] studied 706 lupus admissions to the hospital in South Korea from 1990 to 2006; 87 (12.3%) of these patients were admitted for abdominal pain as the main complaint, 41 (47.1%) out of these 87 patients had lupus enteritis as the cause of their abdominal pain. The Systemic Lupus Erythematosus Disease Activity Index (SLEDAI) score and the titers of antiendothelial cell antibodies of patients with enteritis were higher than those admitted for abdominal pain without enteritis.

Peptic Ulcer Disease

The incidence of peptic ulcers in patients with SLE has been reported as being between 4% and 21%,[30,31] but these studies antedate the present era of endoscopy and gastroprotective therapy. In a more recent report, perforated ulcers have been found in 3 (5.8%) out of 55 patients with SLE and acute abdomen.[32] Luo and Chang[33] found that NSAIDs and aspirin were more predictive of developing peptic ulcers compared with *Helicobacter pylori* seropositivity or steroid use in a cohort of 65 patients with lupus who had endoscopies and biopsies performed before and after undergoing pulse steroid therapy.

Helicobacter pylori Infection in Systemic Lupus Erythematosus

Sawalha and colleagues[34] studied the prevalence of seropositivity against *H. pylori* and four other control antigens in 466 patients with SLE and compared them with 466 patients in a control group matched for age (+/− 3 years), sex, and ethnicity. Most of the patients in the control group were from the same pedigree multiplex for SLE. The frequency of seropositivity to *H. pylori* was only lower in the SLE cohort, compared with the control group, and this difference could be explained by the lower prevalence in patients who were African American (38.1 versus 60.2; OR = 0.4, *P* = 0.0009, 95% confidence interval [CI] 0.24-0.69). The mean age of onset of illness in the *H. pylori* group was significantly older (34.4 versus 28, *P* = 0.039), compared with the patients with *H. pylori* seronegative with SLE. Direct biopsies of the gastric antrum were not performed in this study.

Junca and colleagues[35] investigated the prevalence of intrinsic factor and pernicious anemia in 30 patients with SLE and 45 patients in a control group. Pernicious anemia was characterized by the presence of low serum cobalamin concentration and macrocytic anemia; the presence of intrinsic factor antibody was found in only one patient (3.3%), although 23% of patients had low cobalamin levels and 10% patients had intrinsic factor antibody out of the 30 patients with SLE.

Inflammatory Bowel Disease
Ulcerative Colitis

Ulcerative colitis and lupus may occur concurrently in a small number of patients with lupus. Two patients each were found in the large case series of over 400 patients with lupus. Dubois and Wallace[2,10] and Kurlander and Kirsner[36] elegantly documented the clinicopathologic correlations and remarked that lupus colitis and ulcerative colitis can be indistinguishable. In 1965, Alarcón-Segovia and Cardiel[37] reviewed the literature extensively concomitant SLE and ulcerative colitis, adding additional patients in detail from their Mayo Clinic experience. Additionally, 100 patients with ulcerative colitis were evaluated for SLE, which was found in 3 patients. Folwaczny and colleagues[38] found an increased prevalence of positive antinuclear antibody (ANA) in patients with Crohn disease and ulcerative colitis, compared with first-degree relatives and normal control participants. Eighteen percent of patients with Crohn disease and 43% of patients with ulcerative colitis had a positive ANA test, whereas 13% of relatives of patients with Crohn disease and 24% of relatives of patients with ulcerative colitis had a positive test. Of the healthy patients in the control group, 2% had a positive test. Both sulfasalazine and olsalazine have been associated with the development of drug-induced ANA and SLE.

Regional Ileitis

Concurrence of SLE and regional ileitis (i.e., Crohn disease) is surprisingly rare and has been reported in about ten patients.[35,39]

Collagenous Colitis

Collagenous colitis is a distinct disorder that is characterized by colonic lymphocytic infiltration of the surface epithelium. Heckerling and colleagues[40] reported that patients with collagenous colitis have watery diarrhea but a normal endoscopic appearance and radiographic findings. Collagenous colitis rarely overlaps with lupus and may be treated with corticosteroids instead of sulfasalazine when it coexists with lupus.

Celiac Disease in Association with Systemic Lupus Erythematosus

Gluten-sensitive enteropathy is one of the most common autoimmune conditions with a prevalence of 1 in 100 patients. An overlap of this condition with SLE has not been frequently cited. Out of the 246 biopsy-proven patients with celiac disease, 6 fulfilled the American College of Rheumatology (ACR) criteria for lupus. The diagnosis of lupus was made before the diagnosis of the celiac disease in all the patients, and the symptoms of lupus did not improve with the dietary elimination of gluten.[41] Mader and colleagues[42] screened 61 patients fulfilling the ACR criteria for SLE for the presence of antiendomysial antibodies (AEAs) and antigliadin antibodies (AGLAs) and compared the prevalence of seropositivity with 35 healthy controls. None of the patients with lupus or the controls had AEA; however, 27 (44.3%) of the patients with lupus and 6 (17.1%) of the patients in the control group had AGLAs. A positive correlation was found between the presence of AGLAs and arthritis in lupus. The authors concluded that the presence of AGLAs is an epiphenomenon, although small intestinal biopsies were not performed to rule out celiac disease. Mader and colleagues recommend AEA as the preferred screening test for celiac disease in association with SLE.

Protein-Losing Enteropathy and Malabsorption

The presence of severe diarrhea and significant hypoalbuminemia (reported to be as low as 0.8 g/dL) without proteinuria should raise the suspicion of protein-losing enteropathy. A case series of 15 patients with lupus admitted to Peking Union Medical College Hospital from November 2001 to April 2006 showed that the mean age was 40.1 ± 15.4 years (range from 19 to 71 years) with a female-to-male ratio of 4:1.[43] Although all 15 patients had various degrees of peripheral edema, the number of patients with ascites, pleural, and pericardial effusions were 73%, 60%, and 47%, respectively. Fifty-three percent had protein-losing enteropathy as the initial manifestation of lupus and only 40% of the cohort had symptoms of abdominal pain and diarrhea. Patients had significant hypoalbuminemia (100%), hypocomplementemia (80%), hyperlipoproteinemia (67%), and hypocalcemia (40%), but proteinuria and positive double-stranded DNA (dsDNA) antibody status was low. Endoscopy and biopsy showed bowel mucosal edema and chronic inflammation, and technetium-99m (Tc-99) albumin scintigraphy was the diagnostic test used for all the patients. The radiolabeled albumin excretion in the gut resolved in 60% of the patients when they were treated with corticosteroids or immunosuppressive agents. Kim and colleagues[44] showed that hyperlipoproteinemia helps differentiate protein-losing enteropathy in lupus from lupus enteritis and that the level of serum albumin is significantly reduced in lupus-related versus idiopathic protein-losing enteropathy. Hizawa and colleagues[45] described the radiologic findings in protein-losing enteropathy. Lupus enteritis was associated with irregular spiculation and thickening, as well as thumbprinting, which are suggestive of ischemia on double-contrast radiography of the small intestine. Protein-losing enteropathy, by contrast, had thickened folds with nodules that, at biopsy, were shown to be lymphangiectasia. Increased fecal excretion of intravenous radiolabeled albumin is the best quantitative study for following disease activity, although one report[46] has suggested that alpha-1 antitrypsin (α_1-antitrypsin) clearance also can monitor response to therapy.

Response to corticosteroids is nearly universal, but resistant patients may require cyclosporine or intravenous pulse cyclophosphamide. Octreotide, a somatostatin antagonist, is useful in treating protein-losing enteropathy by decreasing intestinal blood flow and by modulating activated inflammatory cells by binding to the surface of the somatostatin receptor. Medium-chain triglycerides are also useful, first because they are carried through the portal system, thereby decreasing lymphatic flow, and second by virtue of being absorbed via the large bowel, thus correcting lipid deficits in this condition. Some patients also may require a gluten-free diet.[47]

Mader and colleagues[48] investigated a cohort of 21 patients with SLE for malabsorption with a screening D-xylose absorption test, examination of the stool for fat droplets, and a histologic examination of a specimen of the duodenum obtained during endoscopy. Two patients (9.5%) had evidence of malabsorption manifested by an abnormal D-xylose absorption and excessive fecal fat excretion. Two other patients showed excessive fecal fat excretion. One of the patients with malabsorption had abnormal small bowel histologic findings of flattened villi and an inflammatory infiltrate. No excessive deposition of immunoglobulins was revealed in the mucosa on immunoperoxidase staining. The cause of the malabsorption remains uncertain.

Ascites and Peritonitis

Ascites can be the initial presentation of SLE. Ascites occurs in 8% to 12% of adult patients with lupus, often as a manifestation of the nephrotic syndrome, and in 36% of children with SLE.[49-51] In an excellent review of ascites in SLE, Schousboe and colleagues[52] classified ascites as either acute or chronic. Acute causes include lupus peritonitis, infarction, perforated viscus, pancreatitis, mesenteric vasculitis, and hemorrhagic and bacterial peritonitis. Chronic causes of ascites include lupus peritonitis, congestive heart failure, pericarditis, nephrotic syndrome, Budd-Chiari syndrome, protein-losing enteropathy, underlying malignancy, cirrhosis, and tuberculosis. Ascitic fluid can be inflammatory or noninflammatory. Jones and colleagues[53] reported that noninflammatory lesions are always painless and associated with transudative fluid, and most patients have nephrotic syndrome. Peritonitis is usually inflammatory, painful, and exudative. Schocket[54] showed that peritoneal tissue can contain immune complex deposits and inflammatory infiltrates. ANA, anti-DNA, and low complement levels can be present in peritoneal fluid. Low and colleagues[55] reported the characteristics of lupus serositis on barium radiographic examination and CT imaging. The small-bowel barium series showed segments of spiculation with tethering, angulation, and obstruction. CT scanning demonstrated ascites and asymmetric thickening of the small bowel wall.

Ascites caused by lupus peritonitis is usually responsive to steroids. Other causes may require additional interventions including azathioprine.[56] Gentle dieresis and paracentesis are important adjunctive measures that often provide symptomatic relief, provided that renal function is not impaired by this approach.

Pancreatitis
Prevalence

Pancreatitis can be the initial manifestation of SLE and may also be caused by non-lupus–related causes. The Johns Hopkins lupus cohort reported that 72 of their 1842 patients with lupus had a diagnosis of acute pancreatitis.[57] Campos and colleagues[58] found acute pancreatitis in 11 out of 263 (4.2%) pediatric patients with lupus seen in their clinic in São Paolo over a period of 26 years.

Clinical Presentation and Etiopathogenesis

Abdominal pain is present in over 80% of patients with pancreatitis associated with SLE and is often accompanied by nausea, vomiting, and fever, although the pain frequently does not radiate to the back.[59] The diagnosis is usually established using amylase and lipase measurements, as well as imaging using ultrasound or CT scanning.[60] The cause was found to be related to lupus in the majority of patients; however, other non-lupus–related causes, such as biliary tract disease, hypertriglyceridemia, alcohol, and drug exposure, each play a role in approximately one half of the patients with lupus-associated pancreatitis.

Corticosteroids are not considered to play a role in causing pancreatitis in patients with SLE. Hernandez-Cruz and colleagues[61] reviewed a database of patients with SLE and found 18 patients with 26 episodes of pancreatitis with an average SLEDAI score of 6.5 at the time of the acute pancreatic episodes. Out of the 26 episodes, 11 were severe and 4 patients died—3 of pulmonary hemorrhage and 1 from septicemia. The most common cause was thought to be medication use (8 episodes), and hypertriglyceridemia, alcohol, and cholelithiasis were thought to be the cause in 4, 2, and 2 patients, respectively. Pascual examined a database of patients with SLE from July 1984 to July 2001 and found 49 separate acute pancreatitis episodes in 35 patients with lupus, giving a prevalence of 3.5%.[62] Of the 49 episodes, 14 (28.5%) patients were considered to have biliary

disease. Alcohol, increased triglycerides, or uremia were considered to be the cause in 10 (20.4%) patients. The remaining 17 (34.7%) patients were considered to be idiopathic or SLE was considered the cause. Steroids and azathioprine did not cause a relapse of the symptoms when patients were challenged with these medications. The Mexican Systemic Lupus Erythematosus Disease Activity Index (Mex-SLEDAI) scores were significantly higher in the idiopathic group (median of 9 [3 to 19] in the idiopathic group versus 5 [0 to 23] in the toxic metabolic group, and 3 [0 to 18] in the biliary group). A case control analysis with a controls-to-cases ratio of 4 : 1 showed an increased prevalence of acute pancreatitis in patients with SLE (46% versus 14%). The odds ratio for the severity of pancreatitis and mortality was significantly higher in pancreatitis associated with SLE than in non-SLE controls (odds ratio [OR] 8.6 versus 7.5). Similar conclusions were drawn by Derk and DeHoratius[63] in their review of all hospital admissions for patients with lupus to Thomas Jefferson University Hospital between 1982 and 2002. Of the 2947 hospitalized patients with SLE, 25 (0.85%) had acute pancreatitis. The majority (76%) of patients had active SLE at the time of admission with an average involvement of 4.4 organs. Of the 25 patients with acute pancreatitis, 18 had an increase in their corticosteroid doses with improvement in their clinical and laboratory parameters. In conclusion, pancreatitis is more often a severe and often fatal manifestation of lupus than an illness from other factors such as biliary disease or from medications including corticosteroids or azathioprine.

Pancreatitis in childhood-onset SLE appeared to coincide with the development of macrophage activation syndrome in 10 out of 11 pediatric patients with lupus.[64] However, the diagnosis was confirmed by bone marrow aspiration in only 3 out of these 10 patients. Yeh and colleagues[65] reported that pancreatitis may occur as a result of thrombi in pancreatic arteries, because of antiphospholipid antibodies.

Mild elevations of serum amylase levels may be noted in patients with SLE in the absence of pancreatitis. Hasselbacher and colleagues[66] studied 25 patients with SLE but without pancreatitis and 15 patients in a non-SLE control group. Amylase levels were elevated in 5 patients, and 6 patients had macroamylasemia, compared with none in the control group. The mean amylase level in the SLE group was 161.7 mg/dL, compared with 116.4 mg/dL in the control group; this difference was statistically significant. Macroamylasemia results from decreased renal clearance of an immunoglobulin-amylase complex. The presence of a pathogenic autoantibody to amylase was proposed. A correlation is present between active SLE and elevated amylase levels without abdominal pain.

Management

Treatment includes immediate discontinuation of nonessential drugs, intravenous hydration, nothing by mouth, antibiotics if needed, and the judicious use of analgesic medications. Mortality is reported to be higher at 61%, compared with 20% when immunosuppressive agents including high-dose steroids are withheld.[60] Careful observation is essential on high-dose steroids in lupus-related pancreatitis for clinical features of increased mortality.

The prognosis of pancreatitis associated with SLE is very poor especially with those patients with active SLE and involvement of multiple systems (40% versus 0%) and hypocalcemia (55% versus 17%), as well as when steroids are withheld.[60] The presence of pancreatitis complications such as infection, renal or respiratory failure, ascites, pseudocyst, or shock also increased the mortality rate (45% versus 3%).

Mesenteric and Intestinal Vasculitis, Melena, and Bowel Hemorrhage
Prevalence

Ju and colleagues[67] reported that the global prevalence of lupus mesenteric vasculitis ranges from 0.2% to 9.7% of all patients with lupus and 29% to 65% of patients with lupus and acute abdominal pain. The prevalence is probably lower in the United States at 0.9%,[68] compared with a 2.2% to 9.7% prevalence in patients with lupus who are Asian.[30] Nadorra and colleagues[4] noted ischemic bowel disease in 60% of 26 necropsies on children.

Clinical Presentation and Etiopathogenesis

The presentation of most patients with mesenteric vasculitis is with cramping or constant abdominal pain, vomiting, and fever.[59] Patients with severe bowel necrosis have critical GI bleeding or an acute surgical abdomen. Other symptoms associated with mesenteric vasculitis include postprandial fullness, hematemesis, diarrhea, and melena. Diffuse direct and rebound tenderness are not always present.

Inflammatory vasculitis or thrombosis triggered by immune complexes deposited in the walls of the mesenteric vessels appears to cause the syndrome.[30] The presence of anticardiolipin antibodies and antiendothelial antibodies is associated with a high risk for mesenteric vasculitis in patients with lupus. Macroscopically, the bowel is swollen and has variable degrees of ulceration, perforation, or gangrene.[59] Fibrinoid necrosis, leukocytoclasis microthrombi, and a diffuse inflammatory infiltrate are found on microscopic examination.

Zizic and colleagues[69] detailed five patients with large bowel perforation. All had active SLE and mesenteric or intestinal vasculitis. The presentation was insidious with lower abdominal pain. Abdominal rigidity was present in only one patient. Most of these patients had nausea, vomiting, diarrhea, and bloody stools. All had tenderness, and most had rebound tenderness and distention. Bowel sounds were diminished or absent. Previous or concurrent steroid administration masked the symptoms in some of the patients and may have promoted thinning of the bowel wall, which led to perforation.

Shapeero and colleagues[70] reviewed the hospital records of 141 patients with SLE who were admitted to the Hospital of the University of Pennsylvania over a 20-year period. Of these patients, 68 had abdominal symptoms and 20 were thought to have ischemic abdominal disease. In nine patients, ischemic abdominal disease was radiographically confirmed by pseudoobstruction of the gastric outlet, duodenal stasis, effacement of mucosal folds, spasticity, and thumbprinting. Of these 20 patients, most had anorexia, nausea, vomiting, postprandial fullness, and abdominal pain. Only 10 patients had melena, 35 had fevers, and 50 had guarding. In addition, 20 patients had leukocytosis and 65 were anemic. All responded to steroidal therapy.

Laboratory, Pathogenetic, and Radiographic Findings

Laboratory evaluations are not particularly helpful. Acute-phase reactants and general indicators of active SLE are usually present. Radiographic changes include pseudoobstruction of the gastric outlet, duodenal stasis, effacement of the mucosal folds, and thumbprinting. Thumbprinting represents bowel submucosal edema or hemorrhage on a barium or Gastrografin enema; this finding is relatively specific for ischemic bowel disease. Similar findings can be found using CT with contrast.[71] CT of the abdomen can identify intraabdominal abscesses, lymphadenopathy, serositis, bowel-wall thickening, edematous and distended loops of bowel, pancreatic pseudocysts, and enlarged liver and spleens in patients with SLE. Ko and colleagues[71] published their findings on radiologic assessment of lupus mesenteric vasculitis. Of the 15 patients with mesenteric vasculitis, CT scans performed within 3 to 4 days of the onset of abdominal pain revealed the characteristic palisade and comblike pattern of mesenteric blood vessels, which were suggestive of vasculitis in 11 out of 15 patients. Peritoneal enhancement of ascitic fluid (11 patients), small-bowel wall thickening (10 patients), and a double halo or target sign (8 patients) were other common signs of mesenteric vasculitis (Figure 33-1). Shiohira showed that abdominal ultrasounds can demonstrate bowel-wall thickening.[72]

Treatment and Outcome

Medina and colleagues[73] studied the relationship between SLEDAI scores and the sources of an acute abdomen in 51 patients with SLE.

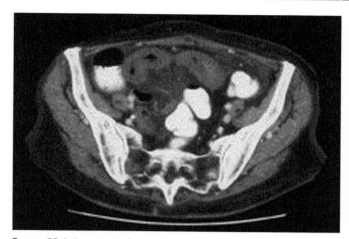

FIGURE 33-1 Lupus vasculitis involving mesenteric arteries causes bowel edema and necrosis of the small and large intestines. Histologic examination shows vasculitis with small-vessel thrombosis. *(Courtesy of Cedars-Sinai Medical Center, Los Angeles.)*

Patients with intraabdominal vasculitis (19 patients) or thrombosis (3 patients) had higher SLEDAI scores than 14 patients with active SLE with non-SLE–related acute abdomens (mean 17.5 [range, 13 to 24] versus 8.2 [range, 5 to 11]). Fifteen patients with inactive SLE (SLEDAI 1.7, range, 0 to 4) had intraabdominal pathologic symptoms that were diverse and not related to lupus. Of the 11 patients with mesenteric vasculitis who were surgically treated after 48 hours, 10 died; whereas none of the 33 patients died who were surgically treated within the first 24 to 48 hours.

Buck and colleagues[68] found that SLEDAI scores greater than 8 appeared to indicate bowel vasculitis in patients with SLE admitted to the hospital for abdominal pain without peritoneal signs. The authors also emphasize imaging and early laparotomy of patients with active SLE and with high SLEDAI scores, whether or not an acute abdomen is present. When all patients with SLE who are hospitalized are evaluated, patients with lupus who have GI vasculitis differed from patients with SLE who were hospitalized for abdominal pain without vasculitis only with regard to having leukopenia at the time of perforation.[74] Lian[75] reported that patients with lupus who had a GI syndrome with abdominal pain, vomiting, and diarrhea as a result of serositis and bowel involvement often resolve with immunosuppressive therapy without surgical intervention. SLEDAI scores in this cohort group requiring hospitalization were lower, at 4 or above.

The treatment of choice for lupus enteritis is 1 to 2 mg/kg/day of parenteral methylprednisolone or its equivalent, in addition to complete bowel rest. If a rapid response is not noted, then surgical intervention is mandatory.[76] Mesenteric vasculitis has a high mortality rate with a reported estimate of up to 50% mortality, depending on the timing and institution of corticosteroid treatment and surgery.[30,73] The surgical experience of 77 patients with lupus and severe abdominal pain after admission to the emergency department in an 11-year period was reported by Vergara-Fernandez and colleagues.[77] The most common cause of abdominal pain was pancreatitis (29%). Intestinal ischemia, gallbladder disease, and appendicitis were each present in approximately 14% to 16% of the patients. Most of the causes of the abdominal pain in patients with SLE were not related to the disease. Acute Physiology and Chronic Health Evaluation (APACHE) II score greater than 12 was statistically associated with the diagnosis of intestinal ischemia, compared with other causes and was predictive of increased mortality. Morbidity and mortality in this series were 57% and 11%, respectively. Box 33-1 presents the key points of SLE and the GI tract.

LIVER MANIFESTATIONS OF SYSTEMIC LUPUS ERYTHEMATOSUS

Liver enzyme abnormalities are frequently seen during the course of lupus. Liver enzyme abnormalities have been reported as frequently as 25% to 50% during the lifetime of a patient with lupus.[78,79] The causes of liver enzyme abnormalities are multifactorial and include drug toxicity and coincident disease activity (Box 33-2).

Enlargement of the liver was present in 10% to 32% of patients with lupus as reported by several studies. However, these studies focused on palpable livers and not measurements of enlargement; consequently, the true incidence of hepatomegaly is not known. Tenderness of the liver is uncommon unless viral hepatitis or peritonitis is present, although it must be noted that hepatomegaly and tenderness may be present with normal liver function tests in SLE. Additionally, an enlarged liver can be histologically normal. Jaundice is observed in 1% to 4% of the patients with lupus, and the most common causes of jaundice in SLE are hemolytic anemia and viral hepatitis; cirrhosis and obstructive jaundice from a biliary or pancreatic mass are rarely seen.

Hepatic arteritis is a rare feature of liver involvement in SLE. Dubois described the first case of hepatic arteritis in 1953. Other case series described this finding as being very rare. However, in a pathologic study of liver specimens from patients with autoimmune diseases that was performed in Japan,[80] the incidence of hepatic arteritis in patients with lupus was reported at 15%. The findings of this study have not been replicated in other more recent studies of liver pathologic complications in lupus, suggesting that hepatic arteritis is indeed a rare complication of SLE and can be associated with ruptured hepatic aneurysms.

Five specific complications are attributable to antiphospholipid antibodies: (1) Budd-Chiari syndrome, (2) hepatic venoocclusive disease, (3) nodular regenerative hyperplasia, (4) liver infarction, and (5) transient elevation of hepatic enzymes resulting from multiple fibrin thrombi. Budd-Chiari syndrome is the occlusion of the hepatic veins with secondary cirrhosis and ascites, which is almost always caused by thromboses in patients with antiphospholipid antibodies.[81] This syndrome usually leads to portal hypertension, which is rarely seen by itself.[4] The diagnosis of nodular regenerative hyperplasia may be missed on clinical grounds, as well as by ultrasound or CT imaging, but will show up as high signal on T1-weighted images and isointense on T2-weighted MRI images.[82]

Liver Function Test Abnormalities: Clinicopathologic Correlates

Liver function tests are usually obtained incidentally as part of a blood chemistry panel. In SLE, nonspecific liver enzyme elevations are seen in a minority of patients and are usually of little significance. The significance of elevated liver enzymes has been a matter of controversy, and several studies have tried to address their importance (Table 33-1). In the authors' experiences, most liver function test abnormalities in SLE are the result of the administration of NSAIDs or methotrexate, or they are elevated because of increased muscle enzyme levels. Pathologic changes are also nonspecific and mild. Table 33-1 summarizes the important studies that reported pathologic findings of liver involvement in SLE.[79,80,83-86]

Based on the studies in Table 33-1, fatty liver is very common in SLE. Additionally, nodular lesions are frequently reported. Fatty livers are usually associated with corticosteroid therapy, and several additional reports in the literature have commented on the presence of nodular regeneration and hyperplasia in SLE. The patients in these reports had normal liver function test results. This underdiagnosed finding could be secondary to steroid or Danazol administration. Concentric membranous bodies in hepatocytes are found in hepatomas but are occasionally seen in lupus, and they reflect increased protein synthesis during regeneration. End-stage liver disease is not common in SLE unless accompanied by other diseases such as nonalcoholic fatty liver disease, autoimmune hepatitis (AIH), or viral hepatitis. Additionally, recent studies seem to suggest that autoimmune liver disease (see the following section for a full discussion) is more prevalent in SLE than previously thought. In summary, pathologic studies of liver specimens in SLE reveal the presence of fatty changes, mild portal fibrosis, nodular changes, and periportal inflammation as a result of autoimmune liver disease.

Another rare finding in lupus is peliosis hepatis. In this condition, blood-filled spaces occur in the liver from diverse causes including injury from drugs and infections on the flow of blood from the sinusoids to the centrilobular veins. Langlet[87] reported on three patients associated with lupus that improved with immunosuppressive treatment.

The association of liver abnormalities in SLE with disease activity remains unclear. Miller and colleagues[78] undertook a prospective study in 260 patients with SLE and 100 control subjects for 12 months. Of the 60 patients with SLE and abnormal liver function testing, 41 were traced to an identifiable cause (e.g., aspirin in 27 patients, alcohol in 6 patients, other causes in 7 patients). Thus they found a high incidence of subclinical liver disease; only 2% of patients had clinical liver disease. Moreover, in 12 of 15 patients with elevated transaminase levels, changes in serum glutamic-pyruvic transaminase (SGPT) corresponded to active lupus. A study by Petri and colleagues[88] aimed to correlate lupus activity with elevations in liver function tests. One third of 216 patients with SLE at Johns Hopkins had abnormal liver function tests over 1717 visits, and their elevated liver enzymes correlated with disease activity. On the other hand, the same authors reported that severe liver disease can be present in patients with SLE with only minimal laboratory abnormalities. In another survey,[89] elevations in liver function tests were associated with disease activity and liver membrane autoantibodies.

Tsuji and colleagues[90] reviewed the records of hospitalized patients with lupus over a decade and found 73 patients with

---

Box 33-2 Key Points: Systemic Lupus Erythematosus and the Liver

1. Hepatomegaly is observed in 10% to 31% of patients with systemic lupus erythematosus (SLE) and in 50% of patients at necropsy. Jaundice is present in 1% to 4% of patients, and is secondary to hemolysis, hepatitis, or pancreatitis.
2. Hepatic vasculitis is uncommon.
3. Budd-Chiari syndrome is associated with the presence of antiphospholipid antibody syndrome.
4. Elevated liver enzymes are observed in 30% to 60% of patients with SLE at some point in the patient's clinical course. Most elevated liver enzymes are caused by infections, salicylates, and nonsteroidal antiinflammatory steroidal drugs (NSAIDs). Enzyme levels >3 times the upper limit of normal are rare.
5. Lupus hepatitis is usually insidious at onset, varying in severity, and frequently associated with ribosomal P antibody. Patients with lupus hepatitis usually fulfill the criteria for SLE and have biopsy findings of periportal infiltration of lymphocytes and isolated degeneration of hepatocytes.
6. Autoimmune hepatitis (lupoid hepatitis) is a form of chronic active hepatitis with malaise, arthralgia, fever, anorexia, jaundice, and negative hepatitis viral studies. Antimitochondrial and anti–smooth muscle antibodies are often present. Abnormalities associated with SLE, such as lupus erythematosus cells and antinuclear antibody, are found. Most of these patients should be classified as being in a subset of chronic active hepatitis. Only 10% fulfill the American College of Rheumatology (ACR) criteria for SLE. Biopsy findings include piecemeal necrosis and are identical to chronic active viral hepatitis B and C.
7. The prevalence of hepatitis B and C infection in patients with SLE is not different from the prevalence in the general population.

TABLE 33-1 Summary of Important Studies of Liver Involvement in Lupus

STUDY	SUBJECTS	LIVER PATHOLOGIC FINDINGS
Ropes M (1976)[83]	Necropsies were identified in 58 patients with lupus.	Enlarged liver: 50% Fatty liver: 44% Portal congestion: 44% Hematoxylin bodies: 3 patients Arteritis: 1 patient Hemosiderosis: 1 patient
Gibson T, Myers AR (1980)[84]	Of the 206 patients with SLE who were tested: Abnormal liver enzyme values were identified in 124 patients. Liver disease was identified in 43 patients. Biopsies were performed on 33 patients.	Steatosis: 12 patients Cirrhosis: 4 patients Chronic active hepatitis: 3 patients Chronic granulomatous hepatitis: 3 patients Centrilobular necrosis: 3 patients Chronic persistent hepatitis: 2 patients Microabscess: 2 patients
Gibson T, Myers AR (1981)[84]	Reviewed liver disease in 81 patients with SLE. Of these patients: 45 (55%) had abnormal liver function tests at some point. 27% had enlarged livers. These abnormalities were accounted for by nonhepatic sources in 9 patients, were drug-induced in 14 patients, and were the result of congestive heart failure in 3 patients.	Nineteen biopsies that were reviewed: Normal: 7 patients Portal-inflammatory infiltrates: 5 patients Fatty liver: 1 patient Chronic active hepatitis: 1 patient Transaminase levels exceeding 100 mg/dL: 3 of the 81 patients
Matsumoto T, Kobayashi S, Shimizu H, and colleagues (2000)[80]	Livers from 160 patients (120 autopsies and 40 liver biopsies) were pathologically examined, 73 with SLE were found.	The following pathologic findings were reported: Arteritis: 11 patients (15.1%) PBC: 2 patients (2.7%) NRH: 5 patients (6.8%) AIH: 2 patients (2.7%) Fatty liver: 53 patients (72.6%) Hepatic congestion: 52 patients (71.2%) NRH: 6 patients (8.2%) Viral chronic hepatitis or cirrhosis: 3 patients (4.1%) Drug-induced hepatitis or cholangitis: 2 patients (2.7%)
Chowdhary VR, Crowson CS, Poterucha JJ, and colleagues (2008)[85]	Retrospective chart review was conducted on a cohort group of patients with SLE who had end-stage liver disease (n = 40).	Major clinical groups studied were: Drug induced: 4 Viral hepatitis: 8 NAFLD: 8 AIH: 6 PBC: 3 Miscellaneous: 8 Infection: 2 Cryptogenic cirrhosis: 2 Lymphoma: 1 Indeterminate: 6
Efe C, Purnak T, Ozaslan E, and colleagues (2011)[86]	Thirty-six patients with lupus had persistent abnormalities of liver function tests.	The following pathologic findings were reported: NAFLD: 12 patients (33.3%) Viral hepatitis: 8 patients (22.2%) HBV: 5 patients (13.8%) HCV: 3 patients (8.4%) AILD: 7 patients (8.4%) AIH: 4 patients (11.1%) PBC: 2 patients (5.5%) Indeterminate causes: 7 patients (19.4%) NRH: 2 patients (5.5%) Viral hepatitis: 8 patients (22.2%)

AIH, Autoimmune hepatitis; AILD, autoimmune liver disease; HBV, hepatitis B virus; HCV, hepatitis C virus; NAFLD, nonalcoholic fatty liver disease; NRH, nodular regenerative hyperplasia; PBC, primary biliary cirrhosis; SLE, systemic lupus erythematosus.

elevated transaminases. Of these patients, 43 (58.9%) did not have an identifiable cause of elevated transaminases and was attributed to active SLE. Of the identifiable cause of elevated liver enzymes, 7 (9.6%) patients were identified to have hemophagocytic syndrome on the basis of a significant elevation of serum ferritin levels (mean, 14,671 mg/dL; range, 370 to 84,651). This group of patients also had the highest elevation in liver enzymes. Viral infections were not ruled out as the cause of hemophagocytic syndrome in this retrospective review.

Van Hoek[91] reviewed the causes of elevated liver enzymes in SLE and found that medications such as NSAIDs, aspirin, and azathioprine were the most common causes. Liver function test abnormalities may result from non–liver-related causes such as unconjugated hyperbilirubinemia, hemolysis, or hepatitis, resulting from immunologic, infectious, or drug-related causes. Hepatitis resulting from SLE was most likely to be lobular and associated with autoantibodies such as anti–double stranded DNA (anti-dsDNA) and anti–ribosomal P antibodies. In contrast, AIH was more likely to be periportal (chronic active hepatitis) with rosetting of liver cells and dense lymphoid infiltrates, and often AIH has specific auto-antibodies to anti–liver-specific protein or have anti–liver-kidney-microsomal antibodies. Both conditions are associated with features of autoimmunity such as polyarthralgia, hypergammaglobulinemia, and a positive ANA.

In summary, most patients with SLE and elevated liver function tests have liver biopsy specimens that reveal nodules, mild fatty changes, or mild fibrosis. Rarely, features of chronic active hepatitis are found.

Autoimmune Liver Disease in Lupus
Lupus Hepatitis—Is there a Distinct Entity of Lupus Hepatitis?
Ohira and colleagues[92] found that 15 (44.1%) of the 34 patients with SLE with liver dysfunction were positive for ribosomal P protein antibody. Of these 34 patients, 16 had SLE-associated hepatitis and 11 out of 16 (68.8%) were positive for ribosomal P protein antibody, whereas a control group of 20 patients with AIH were negative for the antibody. Thus a link seems to exist between anti–ribosomal P antibody and the development of SLE-associated hepatitis. This finding needs to be confirmed through larger studies. No evidence supports the premise that anti–ribosomal P antibody plays a pathogenic role in the development of hepatitis.

The authors of this text found evidence for AIH among 22 of 464 patients with SLE (4.7%) who fulfilled ACR criteria for SLE.[10] Other studies showed that in a cohort of chronic active hepatitis, SLE was rarely seen.

Based on this evidence, a distinct clinical entity of lupus hepatitis appears to exist and it may be defined as an insidious, rarely acute onset of transaminitis in patients who fulfill ACR criteria for SLE and frequently have a positive test for ribosomal P antibody, as well as biopsy findings of lymphocytic infiltration of periportal areas with isolated areas of necrosis[91] (Figure 33-2).

Patients usually have nonspecific symptoms of fatigue, malaise, and anorexia. Jaundice is present in fulminant hepatitis. Mild liver enlargement, jaundice, or ascites in severe cases and other joint- and organ-threatening manifestations of SLE are found on physical examination. Similar to AIH, lupus hepatitis also seems to be responsive to steroid treatment.

Elevations in serum glutamic-oxaloacetic transaminase (SGOT) and SGPT are usually less than twofold to threefold; but in severe cases, significant elevation in transaminases (more than tenfold) with a mild increase in bilirubin and alkaline phosphatase levels may be seen. Antibodies such as a positive ANA, dsDNA, Smith, and hypergammaglobulinemia are seen, and as previously noted, antibody to ribosomal P protein is a strong marker for lupus hepatitis.

Autoimmune Hepatitis and Its Relationship to Lupus
AIH was first described by Waldenström in 1950. Subsequently, because of the recognition of association of this disease with other autoimmune manifestations and the ANA test, the term *lupoid hepatitis* was applied to AIH. Mackay's 1990 review is useful in understanding the historical aspects of this nomenclature and the early studies of this topic.[93]

AIH is characterized by a loss of tolerance to liver tissue. In the 1990s, diagnostic criteria for the classification of AIH were proposed and later revised (Table 33-2). An association with extrahepatic autoimmune diseases, such as RA, autoimmune thyroiditis, ulcerative colitis, and diabetes mellitus, and a family history of autoimmune or allergic disorders are both frequent. Autoantibodies are one of the distinguishing features of AIH; using this approach, AIH type 1 is characterized by the presence of ANA and/or anti–smooth muscle antibodies (anti-SMAs) directed predominantly against smooth muscle actin. AIH type 2 is characterized by anti–liver-kidney-microsomal type 1 autoantibodies (anti-LKM1) directed against cytochrome P450 (CYP) 2D6 and with lower frequency against uridine 5′-diphospho (UDP)–glucuronosyltransferases (UGT). AIH type 3 is characterized by autoantibodies against a soluble liver antigen/liver pancreas (SLA/LP) while identified as UGA suppressor serine tRNA-protein complex.[94]

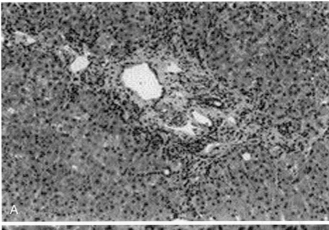

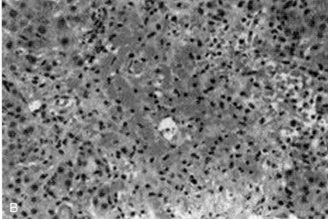

FIGURE 33-2 Biopsy of the liver in a 14-year-old girl of Asian descent with classic systemic lupus erythematosus. Patient had a subacute onset of severe hepatitis (transaminases greater than tenfold) with negative hepatitis virus on serologic studies and other hepatic autoantibodies, as well as strongly positive antiribosomal P antibody. Patient had a complete recovery with high-dose steroids and azathioprine (hematoxylin and eosin [H&E] stain; 1:200). *(Courtesy of Cedars-Sinai Medical Center, Los Angeles.)*

TABLE 33-2 Simplified Diagnostic Criteria for Autoimmune Hepatitis According to Hennes and Colleagues[98]

VARIABLE	CUTOFF	POINTS
ANA or SMA	≥1:40	1
ANA or SMA	≥1:80	2
Anti-LKM1	≥1:40	2
Anti-SLA	Positive	2
IgG	>UNL	1
IgG	>1.1 times the UNL	2
Liver histology	Compatible with AIH	1
Liver histology	Typical of AIH	2
Absence of viral hepatitis	Yes	2

Proceed by adding points achieved for all autoantibodies; the maximum is two points

Interpretation of aggregate points: ≥6 points (probable AIH); ≥7 points (definitive AIH)

AIH, Autoimmune hepatitis; ANA, antinuclear antibody; anti-LKM1, anti–liver-kidney-microsomal antibody; IgG, immunoglobulin G; SMA, smooth muscle antibody; UNL, upper normal limit.

Type I autoimmune (lupoid) hepatitis is defined serologically and histologically and is a subset of chronic active hepatitis. Histologic hepatic changes include periportal piecemeal necrosis, dense lymphoid infiltrates, and prominence of plasma cells. Serologically, patients are positive for ANA and have high levels of gamma (γ) globulins and antibodies to smooth muscle may be found. Chronic active hepatitis is associated with human leukocyte antigen (HLA)-B8, DR3, and DR4, and it has many causes, including viral hepatitis A, B, or C; drug-induced hepatitis; Wilson disease; alcoholism; primary biliary cirrhosis (PBC); and α_1-antitrypsin deficiency, all of which must be ruled out.[94] The incidence of AIH in patients with lupus is somewhat controversial. Some studies suggest that AIH is only rarely seen in patients with lupus.[95] However, more recent studies suggest that AIH is fairly frequent in lupus.[86,87] Because of biochemical similarities between AIH and SLE, AIH could be considered probable by using both the International Autoimmune Hepatitis Group (IAIHG) scoring system and simplified criteria. For definitive diagnosis of AIH, liver biopsy should be performed in all patients with SLE and chronic enzyme abnormalities. The response to therapy is favorable in these patients, and early diagnosis is important for preventing advanced liver disease.[87] The other interesting finding in patients with AIH/PBC overlap syndrome is high anti-dsDNA seropositivity, which is known as a specific marker for SLE. Similar to the study conducted by the authors of this text, Muratori and colleagues[96,97] reported that a prevalence of anti-dsDNA seropositivity of 60% in a patient with AIH/PBC overlap syndrome.

AIH has an insidious onset. Generally found in a young or middle-aged woman with symptoms of fatigue, malaise, anorexia, and low-grade fevers, no physical findings are usually evident at first. Hepatosplenomegaly, jaundice, and signs of cirrhosis or liver failure occur later.

Liver enzymes, γ-globulin, alkaline phosphatase, and bilirubin levels are elevated, the albumin level is decreased, and the prothrombin time may be prolonged. The ANA of AIH has specificities for histones and granulocytes. Lupus erythematosus preparations are usually positive, and some reports suggest they may become negative with clinical improvement. ANAs are positive in approximately 10% to 20% of patients with nonautoimmune, chronic active hepatitis.[93] Anti–single stranded DNA (anti-ssDNA) is found in less than 15% of patients with chronic active hepatitis and other autoantibodies, such as anti-dsDNA, anti-Smith, anti-ribonucleoprotein (anti-RNP), anti–Sjögren syndrome antigen A (anti-SSA/Ro), anti–Sjögren syndrome antigen B (anti-SSB/La), and anticardiolipin antibodies, are found in less than 5% of patients.

Smooth-muscle antibodies and antimitochondrial antibodies are frequently present in AIH. Antimitochondrial antibodies to M5 may cross-react with antibodies to phospholipids and yield false-positive readings in SLE. Hennes and others[98] suggested diagnostic criteria for AIH (see Table 33-2).

Patients with AIH and PBC rarely fulfill the criteria for SLE. Of 89 patients with lupoid hepatitis who were followed at the Mayo Clinic, 43 had arthritis, 10 had thrombocytopenia, 9 had pleurisy, and 8 had leukopenia. Malar rash, pericarditis, neuritis, hemolytic anemia, and proteinuria were observed in two patients or less. Only nine patients fulfilled the ACR criteria for SLE.[99] The overwhelming majority of patients are women, and an increased association with HLA haplotypes B8 and DR3 has been noted. In a comparison of 50 patients with SLE and 50 patients with chronic active hepatitis, 95% of the SLE group and 20% of the chronic active hepatitis group fulfilled ACR criteria for SLE.

AIH responds well to treatment in a majority of patients, irrespective of the histologic type. Steroids remain the mainstay of treatment, prolonging life and making the patient more comfortable. Azathioprine is used as a steroid-sparing agent but is not recommended for the induction of remission. Several small clinical trials support the use of budesonide in the management of AIH, making this drug an attractive alternative to steroid use for AIH treatment.[100] Other alternative agents, which have limited data supporting their use in this disease, include cyclosporine A, mycophenolate, deflazacort, tacrolimus, cyclophosphamide, and ursodeoxycholic acid. Liver transplantation is reserved for refractory cases, although recent studies highlighted the possibility of recurrence of AIH in transplanted livers.

Overlapping Syndromes in Autoimmune Hepatitis

Approximately 20% of patients with AIH have antimitochondrial antibodies; some patients (10%) may have histologic features of mild bile duct injury and a more pronounced biochemical cholestasis; however, they respond to immunosuppressive treatment similarly to those with classical AIH. Any or all of these features suggest an overlap syndrome with PBC. Similarly, 16% of patients with AIH have concurrent inflammatory bowel disease; 10% (adults) to 50% (children) have biliary changes reminiscent of primary sclerosing cholangitis (PSC) by MRI or retrograde endoscopic cholangiography, and approximately 13% of patients fail to respond to corticosteroid treatment. Any or all of these features suggest an overlap syndrome with PSC. The treatment of overlap syndromes is somewhat arbitrary and is based on the predominant clinical feature at presentation.[101]

Other Causes of Hepatitis in Systemic Lupus Erythematosus
Hepatitis B Infection

AIH is rarely observed in patients who are hepatitis B surface–antigen positive. Lu and colleagues[102] investigated the prevalence of hepatitis B viral (HBV) infection in patients with SLE in Taiwan, which is a hyperendemic area for HBV infection. The study also examined the level of interferons (IFNs) in these disorders, which has been found to be low in both. The prevalence of HBV infection was lower than in the general population (3.5% versus 14.7%). The 6 patients out of the 173 patients with SLE who had coexisting HBV infection and SLE had less active SLE with a lesser degree of proteinuria and lower autoantibody levels than patients with SLE but no evidence of HBV infection. These patients and patients with HBV infection had near normal levels of IFN-γ levels when compared with patients with SLE. However, their levels of IFN-α were lower than those in the normal control groups, as well as patients with SLE. This finding suggests that patients with low IFN-α levels are at increased risk for HBV infection and that IFN-γ, which is probably induced by the HBV infection, ameliorates the activity of patients with SLE who have coexistent HBV infection. Abu-Shakra and colleagues[103] found no evidence of HBV infection in 96 patients with SLE in Israel where the prevalence of HBV infection in the general population is 2%.

Hepatitis C

Some AIH may be associated with the hepatitis C virus (HCV) autoantibodies that are specific for AIH, such as anti–SMA, and are seen in up to 66% of patients with HCV infection. Nonspecific antibodies such as low-titer ANA (30%), anticardiolipin antibody (22%), and rheumatoid factor (76%) also are found in chronic HCV infection, prompting the investigation of the prevalence of HCV infection in patients with SLE. Several studies failed to demonstrate an increased incidence of SLE in patients who were afflicted with HBV or HCV, and no available literature supports a distinct or worse phenotype of lupus in patients who are infected with HBV or HCV. In summary, no clear relationship has been found between HBV or HCV infection and systemic lupus. The picture can be confusing (without liver biopsy), especially because patients with lupus can develop viral hepatitis, as can any otherwise healthy person.

Drug-Induced Autoimmune Hepatitis

Drug-induced AIH has been reported after ingestion of the laxative oxyphenisatin or after taking chlorpromazine. Aspirin and NSAIDs are used to treat SLE but are hepatotoxic, and their effects can mimic those of chronic active hepatitis. Perihepatitis has been reported in patients with lupus. Additionally, minocycline use has been reported to be associated with drug-induced lupus and AIH in several patients.[104]

BILIARY ABNORMALITIES: CHOLECYSTITIS, CHOLANGITIS, AND BILIARY CIRRHOSIS

Gallbladder disease is no more common in patients with SLE than it is in the general population. Cholecystitis and serositis can be difficult to distinguish. Cystic duct artery vasculitis is commonly seen in patients with polyarteritis, but only a few reports have noted this in those with SLE. Acalculous cholecystitis can be seen in patients with lupus, and the presence of gallbladder distention should prompt surgical treatment. Rare case reports of sclerosing cholangitis complicating PBC and sclerosing cholangitis are discussed in the section dealing with autoimmune liver disease.

References

1. Osler W: On the visceral complications of erythema exudativum multiforme. *Am J Med Sci* 271(1):106–117, 1976.
2. Dubois EL, Tuffanelli DL: Clinical manifestations of systemic lupus erythematosus. Computer analysis of 520 cases. *JAMA* 190:104–111, 1964.
3. Brown CH, Shirey EK, Haserick JR: Gastrointestinal manifestations of systemic lupus erythematosus. *Gastroenterology* 31:649–666, 1956.
4. Nadorra RL, Nakazato Y, Landing BH: Pathologic features of gastrointestinal tract lesions in childhood-onset systemic lupus erythematosus: study of 26 patients, with review of the literature. *Pediatr Pathol* 7:245–259, 1987.
5. Costallat LTL, Coimbra AMV: Systemic lupus erythematosus: clinical and laboratory aspects related to age at disease onset. *Clin Exp Rheumatol* 12:603–607, 1994.
6. Sultan SM, Ionnou Y, Isenberg DA: A review of gastrointestinal manifestations of systemic lupus erythematosus. *Rheumatol* 38:917–932, 1999.
7. Chng HH, Tan BE, Teh CL, et al: Major gastrointestinal manifestations in lupus patients in Asia: lupus enteritis, intestinal pseudo-obstruction, and protein-losing gastroenteropathy. *Lupus* 19(12):1404–1413, 2010.
8. Xu D, Yang H, Lai CC, et al: Clinical analysis of systemic lupus erythematosus with gastrointestinal manifestations. *Lupus* 19(7):866–869, 2010.
9. King KK, Kornreich HK, Bernstein BH, et al: The clinical spectrum of systemic lupus erythematosus in childhood. Proceedings of the Conference on Rheumatic Diseases of Childhood. *Arthritis Rheum* 20(Suppl):287–294, 1977.
10. Pistiner M, Wallace DJ, Nessim S, et al: Lupus erythematosus in the 1980s: a survey of 570 patients. *Semin Arthritis Rheum* 21:55–64, 1991.
11. Chong VH, Wang CL: Higher prevalence of gastrointestinal symptoms among patients with rheumatic disorders. *Singapore Med J* 49(5):419–424, 2008.
12. Zizic TM: Gastrointestinal manifestations. In Schur P, editor: *The Clinical Management of Systemic Lupus Erythematosus*, New York, 1983, Grune & Stratton, pp 153–166.
13. Fitzgerald RC, Triadafilopoulos G: Esophageal manifestations of rheumatic disorders. *Semin Arthritis Rheum* 26:641–666, 1997.
14. Tatelman M, Keech MK: Esophageal motility in systemic lupus erythematosus, rheumatoid arthritis, and scleroderma. *Radiology* 86:1041–1046, 1966.
15. Turner R, Lipshutz W, Miller W, et al: Esophageal dysfunction in collagen disease. *Am J Med Sci* 265:191–199, 1973.
16. Gutierrez F, Valenzuela JE, Ehresmann GR, et al: Esophageal dysfunction in patients with mixed connective tissue diseases and systemic lupus erythematosus. *Dig Dis Sci* 27:592–597, 1982.
17. Ramirez-Mata M, Reyes PA, Alarcón-Segovia D, et al: Esophageal motility in systemic lupus erythematosus. *Am J Dig Dis* 19:132–136, 1974.
18. Fries J, Holman H: *Systemic Lupus Erythematosus: A Clinical Analysis.* Philadelphia, 1975, WB Saunders.
19. Dwyer KM, Power DA: Chronic intestinal pseudoobstruction in systemic lupus erythematosus due to smooth muscle myopathy. *Lupus* 9:458–463, 2000.
20. Nojima Y, Mimura T, Hamasaki K, et al: Chronic intestinal pseudoobstruction associated with autoantibodies against proliferating cell nuclear antigen. *Arthritis Rheum* 39:877–879, 1996.
21. Perlemuter G, Cacoub P, Chaussade S, et al: Octreotide treatment of chronic intestinal pseudoobstruction secondary to connective tissue diseases. *Arthritis Rheum* 42:1545–1549, 1999.
22. Pimentel M, Soffer EE, Chow EJ, et al: Lower frequency of MMC is found in IBS subjects with abnormal lactulose breath test, suggesting bacterial overgrowth. *Dig Dis Sci* 47(12):2639–2643, 2002.
23. Apperloo-Renkema HZ, Bootsma H, Mulder BI, et al: Host-microflora interaction in systemic lupus erythematosus (SLE): colonization resistance of the indigenous bacteria of the intestinal tract. *Epidemiol Infect* 112(2):367–373, 1994.
24. Albano S, Hallegua DS, Wallace DJ, et al: Small intestinal bacterial overgrowth in systemic lupus erythematosus. *Arthritis Rheum* 42(Suppl):S305, 1999.
25. Flanigan RC, McDougal WS, Griffen WO: Abdominal complications of collagen vascular disease. *Am Surg* 49(5):241–244, 1983.
26. Al-Hakeem MS, McMillen MA: Evaluation of abdominal pain in systemic lupus erythematosus. *Am J Surg* 176(3):291–294, 1998.
27. Takahashi T, De la Garza L, Ponce de Leon S, et al: Risk factors for operative morbidity in patients with systemic lupus erythematosus: an analysis of 63 surgical procedures. *Am Surg* 3:260–264, 1995.
28. Rojas-Serrano J, Cardiel MH: Lupus patients in an emergency unit. Causes of consultation, hospitalization and outcome. A cohort study. *Lupus* 9(8):601–606, 2000.
29. Min J, Park J, Kim S, et al: Acute abdominal pain in patients with systemic lupus erythematosus entered in emergency room. *Arthritis Rheum* 40:S106, 1997.
30. Kwok SK, Seo SH, Ju JH, et al: Lupus enteritis: clinical characteristics, risk factor for relapse and association with anti-endothelial cell antibody. *Lupus* 16(10):803–809, 2007.
31. Dubois EL, Bulgrin JG, Jacobson G: The corticosteroid-induced peptic ulcer: a serial roentgenological survey of patients receiving high dosages. In Mills LC, Moyer JH, editors: *Inflammation and Diseases of Connective Tissue, A Hahnemann Symposium.* Philadelphia, 1961, WB Saunders, pp 648–660.
32. Medina F, Ayala A, Jara LJ, et al: Acute abdomen in systemic lupus erythematosus: the importance of early laparotomy. *Am J Med* 103:100–105, 1987.
33. Luo JC, Chang FY, Chen TS, et al: Gastric mucosal injury in systemic lupus erythematosus patients receiving pulse methylprednisolone therapy. *Br J Clin Pharmacol* 68(2):252–259, 2009.
34. Sawalha AH, Schmid WR, Binder SR, et al: Association between systemic lupus erythematosus and *Helicobacter pylori* seronegativity. *J Rheumatol* 31:8:1546–1550, 2004.
35. Junca J, Cuxart A, Olive A, et al: Anti-intrinsic factor antibodies in lupus erythematosus. *Lupus* 2:111–114, 1993.
36. Kurlander DJ, Kirsner JB: The association of chronic nonspecific inflammatory bowel disease with lupus erythematosus. *Ann Intern Med* 60:799–813, 1964.
37. Alarcón-Segovia D, Cardiel MA: Connective tissue disorders and the bowel. *Baillieres Clin Rheumatol* 3(2):371–392, 1989.
38. Folwaczny C, Noehl N, Endres SP, et al: Antinuclear antibodies in patients with inflammatory bowel disease. High prevalence in first-degree relatives. *Dig Dis Sci* 42:1593–1597, 1997.
39. Sanchez-Burson J, Garcia-Porrua C, Melguizo MI, et al: Systemic lupus erythematosus and Crohn's disease: an uncommon association of two diseases. *Clin Exp Rheumatol* 22(1):133, 2004.
40. Heckerling P, Urtubey A, Te J: Collagenous colitis and systemic lupus erythematosus. *Ann Intern Med* 122:71–72, 1994.
41. Freeman HJ: Adult celiac disease followed by onset of systemic lupus erythematosus. *J Clin Gastroenterol* 42(3):252–255, 2008.
42. Mader R, Adawi M, Mussel Y, et al: Celiac disease antibodies in systemic lupus erythematosus. *Arthritis Rheum* 48:S586, 2003.
43. Zheng WJ, Tian XP, Li L, et al: Protein-losing enteropathy in systemic lupus erythematosus: analysis of the clinical features of fifteen patients. *J Clin Rheumatol* 13(6):313–316, 2007.
44. Kim YG, Lee CK, Byeon JS, et al: Serum cholesterol in idiopathic and lupus-related protein-losing enteropathy. *Lupus* 17(6):575–579, 2008.
45. Hizawa K, Iida M, Aoyagi K, et al: Double-contrast radiographic assessment of lupus-associated enteropathy. *Clin Radiol* 53:925–929, 1998.
46. Benner KG, Montanaro A: Protein-losing enteropathy in systemic lupus erythematosus. Diagnosis and monitoring immunosuppressive therapy by alpha-1-antitrypsin clearance in stool. *Dig Dis Sci* 34:132–135, 1989.
47. Ossandon A, Bombardieri M, Coari G, et al: Protein losing enteropathy in systemic lupus erythematosus: role of diet and octreotide. *Lupus* 11:465–466, 2002.
48. Mader R, Adawi M, Schonfeld S: Malabsorption in systemic lupus erythematosus. *Clin Exp Rheumatol* 15:659–661, 1997.
49. Man BL, Mok CC: Serositis related to systemic lupus erythematosus: prevalence and outcome. *Lupus* 14(10):822–826, 2005.

50. Estes D, Christian CL: The natural history of systemic lupus erythematosus by prospective analysis. *Medicine (Baltimore)* 50(2):85–95, 1971.

51. Richer O, Ulinski T, Lemelle I, et al: Abdominal manifestations in childhood-onset systemic lupus erythematosus. *Ann Rheum Dis* 66(2):174–178, 2007.

52. Schousboe JT, Koch AE, Chang RW: Chronic lupus peritonitis with ascites: review of the literature with a case report. *Semin Arthritis Rheum* 18:121–126, 1988.

53. Jones PE, Rawcliffe P, White N, et al: Painless ascites in systemic lupus erythematosus. *Br Med J* 1:1513, 1977.

54. Schocket AL, Lain D, Kohler PF, et al: Immune complex vasculitis as a cause of ascites and pleural effusions in systemic lupus erythematosus. *J Rheumatol* 5:33–38, 1978.

55. Low VH, Robins PD, Sweeney DJ: Systemic lupus erythematosus serositis. *Australas Radiol* 39(3):300–302, 1995.

56. Kaklaminis P, Vayopoulos G, Stamatelos G, et al: Chronic lupus peritonitis with ascites. *Ann Rheum Dis* 50:176–177, 1991.

57. Makol A, Petri M: Pancreatitis in systemic lupus erythematosus: frequency and associated factors—a review of the Hopkins Lupus Cohort. *J Rheumatol* 37(2):341–345, 2010.

58. Campos LM, Omori CH, Lotito AP, et al: Acute pancreatitis in juvenile systemic lupus erythematosus: a manifestation of macrophage activation syndrome? *Lupus* 19(14):1654–1658, 2010.

59. Tian XP, Zhang X: Gastrointestinal involvement in systemic lupus erythematosus: insight into pathogenesis, diagnosis and treatment. *World J Gastroenterol* 16(24):2971–2977, 2010.

60. Breuer GS, Baer A, Dahan D, et al: Lupus-associated pancreatitis. *Autoimmun Rev* 5(5):314–318, 2006.

61. Hernandez-Cruz B, Pascual V, Villa AR, et al: Twenty six episodes of acute pancreatitis in 18 patients with systemic lupus erythematosus. *Arthritis Rheum* 4:S329, 1998.

62. Pascual-Ramos V, Duarte-Rojo A, Villa AR, et al: Systemic lupus erythematosus as a cause and prognostic factor of acute pancreatitis. *J Rheumatol* 31:707–712, 2004.

63. Derk CT, DeHoratius RJ: Systemic lupus erythematosus and acute pancreatitis: a case series. *Clin Rheumatol* 23(2):147–151, 2004.

64. Campos LM, Omori CH, Lotito AP, et al: Acute pancreatitis in juvenile systemic lupus erythematosus: a manifestation of macrophage activation syndrome? *Lupus* 19(14):1654–1658, 2010.

65. Yeh T-S, Wang C-R, Lee Y-T, et al: Acute pancreatitis related to anticardiolipin antibodies in lupus patients visiting an emergency department. *Am J Emerg Med* 11:230–232, 1993.

66. Hasselbacher P, Myers AR, Passero FC: Serum amylase and macroamylase in patients with systemic lupus erythematosus. *Br J Rheumatol* 27:198–201, 1988.

67. Ju JH, Min JK, Jung CK, et al: Lupus mesenteric vasculitis can cause acute abdominal pain in patients with SLE. *Nat Rev Rheumatol* 5(5):273–281, 2009.

68. Buck AC, Serebro LH, Quinet RJ: Subacute abdominal pain requiring hospitalization in a systemic lupus erythematosus patient: a retrospective analysis and review of the literature. *Lupus* 10:491–495, 2001.

69. Zizic TM, Classen JN, Stevens MB: Acute abdominal complications of systemic lupus erythematosus and polyarteritis nodosa. *Am J Med* 73:525–531, 1982.

70. Shapeero LG, Myers A, Oberkircher PE, et al: Acute reversible lupus vasculitis of the gastrointestinal tract. *Radiology* 112:569–574, 1974.

71. Ko SF, Lee TY, Cheng TT, et al: CT findings at lupus mesenteric vasculitis. *Acta Radiol* 38:115–120, 1997.

72. Shiohira Y, Uehara H, Miyazato F, et al: Vasculitis-related acute abdomen in systemic lupus erythematosus ultrasound appearances in lupus patients with intra-abdominal vasculitis. *Ryumachi* 33(3):235–241, 1993.

73. Medina F, Ayala A, Jara LJ, et al: Acute abdomen in systemic lupus erythematosus: the importance of early laparotomy. *Am J Med* 103(2):100–105, 1997.

74. Lee CK, Ahn EY, Lee EY, et al: Acute abdominal pain in systemic lupus erythematosus: focus on lupus enteritis (gastrointestinal vasculitis). *Ann Rheum Dis* 61:547–550, 2002.

75. Lian TY, Edwards CJ, Chan SP, et al: Reversible acute gastrointestinal syndrome associated with active systemic lupus erythematosus in patients admitted to hospital. *Lupus* 12:612–616, 2003.

76. Einhorn S, Horowitz Y, Einhorn M: Ischemic colitis and disseminated systemic lupus erythematosus. Value of corticosteroid treatment [article in French]. *Rev Rheum Mal Osteoartic* 53:669, 1986.

77. Vergara-Fernandez O, Zeron-Medina J, Mendez-Probst C, et al: Acute abdominal pain in patients with systemic lupus erythematosus. *J Gastrointest Surg* 13(7):1351–1357, 2009.

78. Miller MH, Urowitz MB, Gladman DD, et al: The liver in systemic lupus erythematosus. *Q J Med* 53(211):401–409, 1984.

79. Runyon BA, LaBrecque DR, Anuras S: The spectrum of liver disease in systemic lupus erythematosus: report of 33 histologically-proved cases and review of the literature. *Am J Med* 69:187–194, 1980.

80. Matsumoto T, Kobayashi S, Shimizu H, et al: The liver in collagen diseases: pathologic study of 160 cases with particular reference to hepatic arteritis, primary biliary cirrhosis, autoimmune hepatitis and nodular regenerative hyperplasia of the liver. *Liver* 20(5):366–373, 2000.

81. Sciascia S, Mario F, Bertero, MT: Chronic Budd-Chiari syndrome, abdominal varices, and caput medusae in 2 patients with antiphospholipid syndrome. *J Clin Rheumatol* 16(6):302, 2010.

82. Perez Ruiz F, Orte Martinez FJ, Zea Mendoza AC, et al: Nodular regenerative hyperplasia of the liver in rheumatic diseases: report of seven cases and review of the literature. *Semin Arthritis Rheum* 21(1):47–54, 1991.

83. Ropes M: *Systemic Lupus Erythematosus*, Cambridge, MA, 1976, Harvard University Press.

84. Gibson T, Myers, AR: Subclinical liver disease in systemic lupus erythematosus. *J Rheumatol* 8(5):752–759, 1981.

85. Chowdhary VR, Crowson CS, Poterucha JJ, et al: Liver involvement in systemic lupus erythematosus: case review of 40 patients. *J Rheumatol* 35(11):2159–2164, 2008.

86. Efe C, Purnak T, Ozaslan E, et al: Autoimmune liver disease in patients with systemic lupus erythematosus: a retrospective analysis of 147 cases. *Scand J Gastroenterol* 46(6):732–737, 2011.

87. Langlet P, Karmali R, Deprez C, et al: Severe acute pancreatitis associated with peliosis hepatis in a patient with systemic lupus erythematosus. *Acta Gastroenterol Belg* 64(3):298–300, 2001.

88. Petri M, Baker C, Goldman D: Liver function test (LFT) abnormalities in systemic lupus erythematosus (SLE) (abstract). *Arthritis Rheum* 35:S329, 1992.

89. Kushimoto K, Nagasawa K, Ueda A, et al: Liver abnormalities and liver membrane autoantibodies in systemic lupus erythematosus. *Ann Rheum Dis* 48(11):946–952, 1989.

90. Tsuji T, Ohno S, Ishigatsubo Y: Liver manifestations in systemic lupus erythematosus: high incidence of hemophagocytic syndrome. *J Rheumatol* 29(7):1576–1577, 2002.

91. van Hoek B: The spectrum of liver disease in systemic lupus erythematosus. *Neth J Med* 48(6):244–253, 1996.

92. Ohira H, Takiguchi J, Rai T, et al: High frequency of anti-ribosomal P antibody in patients with systemic lupus erythematosus-associated hepatitis. *Hepatol Res* 28(3):137–139, 2004.

93. Mackay IR: Auto-immune (lupoid) hepatitis: an entity in the spectrum of chronic active liver disease. *J Gastroenterol Hepatol* 5(3):352–359, 1990.

94. Strassburg CP: Autoimmune hepatitis. *Best Pract Res Clin Gastroenterol* 24(5):667–682, 2010.

95. Irving KS, Sen D, Tahir H, et al: A comparison of autoimmune liver disease in juvenile and adult populations with systemic lupus erythematosus—a retrospective review of cases. *Rheumatology (Oxford)* 46(7):1171–1173, 2007.

96. Efe C, Purnak T, Ozaslan E, et al: The serological profile of the autoimmune hepatitis/primary biliary cirrhosis overlap syndrome. *Am J Gastroenterol* 105(1):226; author reply 226–227, 2010.

97. Muratori L, Granito A, Pappas G, et al: The serological profile of the autoimmune hepatitis/primary biliary cirrhosis overlap syndrome. *Am J Gastroenterol* 104(6):1420–1425, 2009.

98. Hennes EM, Zeniya M, Czaja AJ, et al: Simplified criteria for the diagnosis of autoimmune hepatitis. *Hepatology* 48(1):169–176, 2008.

99. Hall S, Czaja AJ, Kaufman DK, et al: How lupoid is lupoid hepatitis? *J Rheumatol* 13(1):95–98, 1986.

100. Manns MP, Woynarowski M, Kreisel W, et al: Budesonide induces remission more effectively than prednisone in a controlled trial of patients with autoimmune hepatitis. *Gastroenterology* 139(4):1198–1206, 2010.

101. Muratori L, Muratori P, Granito A, et al: Current topics in autoimmune hepatitis. *Dig Liver Die* 42(11):757–764, 2010.

102. Lu CL, Tsai ST, Chan CY, et al: Hepatitis B infection and changes in interferon-alpha and -gamma production in patients with systemic lupus erythematosus in Taiwan. *J Gastroenterol Hepatol* 12(4):272–276, 1997.

103. Abu-Shakra M, El-Sana S, Margalith M, et al: Hepatitis B and C viruses serology in patients with SLE. *Lupus* 6(6):543–544, 1997.

104. Angulo JM, Sigal LH, Espinoza LR: Minocycline induced lupus and autoimmune hepatitis. *J Rheumatol* 26(6):1420–1421, 1999.

Chapter 34

Hematologic and Lymphoid Abnormalities in SLE

George A. Karpouzas

Hematologic abnormalities are common in systemic lupus erythematosus (SLE) and are often presenting manifestations of the disease. Sometimes their features may mimic those of primary blood dyscrasias, and the nature of the underlying disorder can be overlooked unless SLE is considered in the differential diagnosis and specific diagnostic studies performed.

ANEMIA

Most patients with SLE will develop anemia at some point throughout the course of the disease (eFig 34-1). The most prevalent type is anemia of chronic disease (ACD); however, iron deficiency anemia (IDA), autoimmune hemolytic anemia (AIHA), drug-induced myelotoxicity, and anemia of chronic renal failure are not uncommon. Box 34-1 illustrates the types of anemias in SLE by decreasing order of frequency.

Anemia of Chronic Disease

A large, single-center prospective study of 132 anemic patients with SLE identified ACD as the most prevalent variant, accounting for 37% of all patients.[1] Although generally mild (mean hemoglobin [Hgb] 9.9 ± 1.3 g/dL), 50% of patients with Hgb less than 8 g/dL from the entire cohort fell in the category of ACD. The same study reported that patients with ACD had higher disease activity as measured by European Consensus Lupus Activity Measurement (ECLAM) scores, compared to those with other types of anemias ($P = 0.01$). This study speculated that higher ECLAM scores might reflect the higher prevalence of lupus nephritis in the ACD group (57%). This type of anemia is likely to persist for prolonged periods in contrast to others; over 50% of patients may still be anemic after 3 years of follow-up.[1]

ACD in SLE represents a hypoproliferative state with several dimensions (Figure 34-1):

(a) Abnormal iron metabolism with sequestration in macrophages, leading to hypoferremia and unavailability to erythropoietic progenitors for Hgb synthesis
(b) Decreased erythropoietin (EPO) supply to red cell progenitors
(c) Increased resistance of responder cells to the proliferative actions of EPO
(d) Potentially reduced erythrocyte survival span

Iron metabolism was investigated in 11 patients with SLE using radioactive iron (^{59}Fe).[2] Iron use was decreased in 7 patients, with increased uptake over the spleen and liver where it was stored, instead of use for Hgb synthesis. Plasma iron turnover, on the other hand, was elevated in most patients. Additionally, the life span of erythrocytes was reduced in the absence of hemolysis. Iron metabolism in ACD at large is currently accepted as mainly altered by an overproduction of the acute phase protein, hepcidin.[3] This cysteine-rich cationic peptide is the main negative regulator of intestinal iron absorption, transport across the placenta, and iron release from macrophages. Its production is mainly driven by interleukin-6 (IL-6).

Although IL-6 levels are reportedly higher in anemic compared to nonanemic SLE subjects, and an inverse correlation between IL-6 and Hgb levels was shown,[4] the contribution of the hepcidin pathway in SLE-associated ACD has not been explored. Prohepcidin levels have been evaluated and shown to have no association with Hgb levels in anemic patients with SLE.[5] However, prohepcidin levels, it is argued, may not associate with serum iron status and may not accurately reflect mature circulating hepcidin.[5]

Insufficient EPO supply to hematopoietic progenitors and enhanced resistance of those cells to the proliferative effects of EPO are the main culprits in SLE-associated ACD (see Figure 34-1). A decreased EPO supply may reflect lower production or enhanced turnover. Impaired production of EPO has been reported in patients with SLE-associated ACD; 42% showed at least 25% lower EPO levels, compared with controls for levels of Hgb, and the slope of EPO response to anemia was significantly blunted ($P = 0.01$).[1] Lower EPO production may be the result of the inhibitory action of cytokines such as interleukin-1 alpha (IL-1α), IL-6, tumor necrosis factor-alpha (TNF-α), interferon alpha (IFN-α), interferon beta (IFN-β), interferon gamma (IFN-γ), and transforming growth factor–beta (TGF-β), all of which are largely implicated in SLE. Specifically, Faquin and colleagues[6] reported that IL-1, TNF-α, and TGF-β inhibited EPO production from the hepatoma line of Hep3B cells at the level of EPO messenger ribonucleic acid (mRNA). Jelkmann and others[7] additionally showed that IL-1β inhibited EPO production in isolated serum-free perfused rat kidneys. In patients with lupus nephritis, effector cluster of differentiation 4 (CD4$^+$) T lymphocytes and macrophages infiltrate the renal interstitium and produce cytokines with inhibitory effects on EPO production.[8] Since such patients frequently display ACD, this mechanism can certainly explain suppressed EPO levels in this subset.

The presence of antibodies against EPO (anti-EPO antibodies) constitutes an alternative explanation for impaired EPO supply; they may bind and neutralize EPO before binding its receptors on target hematopoietic cells. The prevalence of anti-EPO antibodies in unselected patients with SLE is 15%; this is significantly higher in patients with Hgb less than 10 g/dL, compared with nonanemic patients (29% versus 9%; $P < 0.05$), and in those with ACD-related SLE (38%).[1] Additionally, anti-EPO antibody titers are higher in patients with severe anemia, compared with those with moderate anemia, and patients with such antibodies have higher disease activity compared to those without them.[1] The presence of ACD and the severity of ECLAM scores independently predicted the prevalence of anti-EPO antibody (odds ratio [OR] = 3.1, $P = 0.04$ for the presence of ACD, and 1.27 per each ECLAM point, $P = 0.055$).[1] Despite these observations indirectly supporting a neutralizing effect of these antibodies on EPO, it remains unclear whether antibodies to endogenous EPO have a direct pathogenic role in the induction of ACD in SLE. No correlation between anti-EPO antibodies and EPO levels has been demonstrated; however, the possibility of interference of such antibodies in the measurement of EPO cannot be excluded as a major confounder. Anti-EPO antibodies binding to EPO in the form of immunoglobulin G (IgG) complexes may stabilize and prolong EPO half-life, which explains its accumulation, despite the fact that it may not be biologically active.[9] A rare scenario, in which an inverse association between antibodies to endogenous EPO, EPO levels, and Hgb has been reported, is pure red cell aplasia (PRCA) in SLE. In these patients, immunosuppression decreases antibody titers and corrects Hgb levels.[9] Another similar scenario is the induction of secondary PRCA in patients with end-stage renal disease who receive exogenous EPO; temporary withdrawal and immunosuppression successfully decrease antibody levels and treat the anemia.

Box 34-1 Classification of Anemia in Systemic Lupus Erythematosus

Causes of Anemia in Systemic Lupus Erythematosus (SLE)
- Iron deficiency anemia (IDA) (menorrhagia, gastrointestinal loss)
- Nutritional deficiencies (iron, vitamin B12, folate)
- Immune-mediated disorders
  - Autoimmune hemolytic anemia (AIHA)
    - Warm antibody AIHA (IgG)
    - Cold antibody AIHA (IgM)
  - Immune-mediated hematopoietic failure
    - Aplastic anemia
    - Pure red cell aplasia (PRCA)
  - Hemophagocytosis
  - Pernicious anemia
- Anemia of chronic renal insufficiency
- Treatment-induced anemia (cyclophosphamide, azathioprine)
- Microangiopathic hemolytic anemia (MAHA)
  - Disseminated intravascular coagulation (DIC)
  - Thrombotic thrombocytopenia purpura (TTP)
  - Drugs
- Myelofibrosis
- Myelodysplasia
- Hypersplenism
- Infection

Despite the ability of SLE-associated ACD to respond well to EPO, little rationale exists for such use given the reasons previously stated. Additionally, prior in vitro studies on T and B cells in dialysis patients receiving recombinant human erythropoietin (rHuEPO) suggested that it might augment immune responses.[8]

Enhanced resistance of red cell precursors to the proliferative effects of EPO has also been incriminated in the pathogenesis of SLE-associated ACD (see Figure 34-1). Downregulation of surface EPO receptors and the induction of apoptosis in erythroid precursors have been demonstrated by IL-1, TNF-α, and IFN-γ. Proinflammatory cytokines and chemokines exert direct effects on erythropoiesis beyond their involvement in EPO elaboration, amplifying the risk of ACD (see Figure 34-1). TNF-α acts directly on the less mature burst-forming units–erythroid (BFU-E), whereas its effect on colony-forming units–erythroid (CFU-E) is indirect, via the induction of IFN-β release from bone marrow (BM) stromal cells.[10] IL-1 inhibits colony formation of CFU-E indirectly by upregulating the production of IFN-γ by T cells.[10] IFN-α inhibits BFU-E directly and CFU-E indirectly through accessory cells.[10]

ACD is a normochromic, normocytic anemia that is generally mild. Reticulocyte count is low, indicating an underproduction of red cells. A definitive diagnosis may be hampered by coexistent blood loss or medication effects. The evaluation of ACD must include the determination of whole-body iron status to rule out coexistent IDA (usually hypochromic and macrocytic).

Iron Deficiency Anemia

IDA is the second most common type of anemia in SLE; it is usually a result of menorrhagia or gastrointestinal blood loss secondary to the chronic use of NSAIDs and corticosteroids. It can complicate and or coexist with ACD.

Laboratory parameters and an algorithm differentiating ACD, IDA, or a true coexistence of IDA with ACD are provided in eTable 34-1 and eFig 34-2, respectively.

IMMUNE-MEDIATED HEMOLYTIC ANEMIAS
Autoimmune Hemolytic Anemia

Antibody-mediated erythrocyte damage by complement-dependent or complement-independent mechanisms is the third most common cause of anemia in SLE; it is reported in 5% to 14% of patients with this disease.[11] Approximately two thirds of patients with

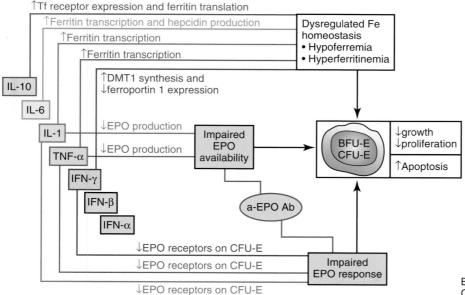

FIGURE 34-1 Pathogenesis of anemia of chronic disease (ACD) in systemic lupus erythematosus.

SLE-associated AIHA exhibit symptoms at the onset of SLE,[12] and 41% to 90% may already be taking immunosuppressive medications at the time of diagnosis. AIHA corresponds with large acute decreases in Hgb levels. The severity of anemia is highest in AIHA, compared with other types in SLE; in a large prospective study, mean Hgb with AIHA was 8.99 ± 1.5 g/dL, compared with 10.9 ± 0.9 for IDA, 9.94 ± 1.3 for ACD, and 9.64 ± 1.8 for the group of other causes ($P <$ 0.001).[1] Interestingly, the severity of anemia correlated with disease activity (ECLAM) only among patients with IDA but not among those with AIHA or ACD in the same report. Median time to remission with therapy is 3 months, and recurrence is unlikely in steroid responders; 85% are recurrence-free after 5 years and 73% remain so after 15 years of follow-up.[1]

Diagnosis

The diagnosis of AIHA is established in a step-wise fashion; a mechanistic algorithm is provided in eFig 34-3 and additional details in Box 34-2.

The first step is to demonstrate that the anemia is, in fact, hemolytic. Generally, hemolytic anemias are normocytic or macrocytic as a result of significant reticulocytosis or concomitant folate deficiency. Anisocytosis and spherocytes may be observed in the blood smear. Low serum haptoglobin and increased reticulocyte count indicate hemolysis. Increased indirect bilirubin, urine urobilinogen, and lactate dehydrogenase (LDH), albeit nonspecific, corroborate hemolytic anemia. LDH reflects the severity of hemolysis and serves as a marker of the therapeutic responses.

The second step is the differentiation between immune and non-immune hemolysis. This is best predicated by the direct antiglobulin test (DAT), Coombs test. A positive test confirms the presence of bound antibodies (particularly IgG, but also immunoglobulin A [IgA] or immunoglobulin M [IgM]) and/or complement (C3d or C3c) on the surface of red cells through red cell precipitation, upon the addition of antihuman IgG antibody. A positive DAT in the context of established hemolytic anemia (step one) generally confirms the diagnosis of AIHA. The prognostic significance of antibody titers remains an unresolved question; patients with weak-positive DAT results may have severe hemolysis, whereas others with a strong-positive DAT result may be without overt anemia. In general, however, a strong-positive DAT result is more likely to be associated with severe AIHA.[13]

The third step is the identification of the type of antibody responsible for hemolysis. AIHA is classified into two major categories based on the optimal temperature of antierythrocyte antibody reactivity with antigens on the red cell surface. The warm antibody type (WA-AIHA) is mediated by antibodies optimally reacting with red blood cell (RBC) antigens at 37° C and causing hemolysis at 37° C. The cold antibody type (CA-AIHA) is mediated by IgM, a complement-fixing antibody that optimally binds RBC antigens at 4° C but mediates hemolysis at 37° C. SLE-associated AIHA is almost

---

Box 34-2 Step-Wise Approach in the Diagnosis of Autoimmune Hemolytic Anemia in Systemic Lupus Erythematosus

Step 1: Is the Anemia Hemolytic?

In certain scenarios, haptoglobin or reticulocyte count may not reflect active hemolysis; haptoglobin is an acute phase reactant and may therefore be normal or even elevated, despite hemolysis in the presence of chronic inflammation or a co-existing tumor. Conversely, haptoglobin may be low in the absence of hemolysis in patients with chronic liver disease or with intramedullary hemolysis. A rare cause of low haptoglobin is congenital ahaptoglobinemia or hypohaptoglobinemia. The Hp0/Hp0 genotype is associated with undetectable serum haptoglobin and is relatively common in those of Korean descent (4%) but rare in Europe and North America (1:4000). Patients with the Hp2/Hp0 or Hp1/Hp0 genotype have low-serum haptoglobin.[1,2] Likewise, reticulocytosis may be absent at diagnosis of hemolytic anemias. In one study, 25% of patients with proven hemolytic anemia had a normal reticulocyte count at presentation.[3] The main reason may be a delayed bone marrow response; in the majority of patients, reticulocytosis can be demonstrated several days later. The absence of reticulocytosis may also be observed with reduced bone marrow function, such as autoimmune hemolytic anemia (AIHA) occurring during or after chemotherapy, and in patients with underlying infiltrating bone marrow disease similar to leukemia, lymphoma, or pure red cell aplasia (PRCA).

Step 2: Is it Autoimmune?

The significance of a positive or negative direct antiglobulin test (DAT) must be evaluated by the clinician. A positive DAT alone without active hemolysis is not sufficient for the diagnosis of AIHA, because 0.007% to 0.1% of the healthy population and 0.3% to 8% of patients who are hospitalized and without hemolytic anemia have a positive DAT result.[5] In systemic lupus erythematosus (SLE), 18% to 65% of patients may have a positive DAT result without evident hemolysis.[4] One reason for a false-positive DAT is hypergammaglobulinemia, for example, after high-dose immunoglobulin therapy. In the case of a negative DAT, the presence of immune hemolysis is unlikely but cannot be excluded. A false-negative DAT may occur in 1% to 10% of all patients with AIHA. A major reason, at least in the past, has been low sensitivity of the laboratory assay,

which is no longer the case.[5] Scenarios with a truly negative DAT include (1) patients with AIHA after treatment with rituximab who become DAT-negative, despite ongoing hemolysis; (2) AIHA in the context of chronic lymphocytic leukemia (CLL) after therapy with fludarabine, cyclophosphamide, or rituximab[5]; and (3) AIHA in the context of solid tumors.[5]

Step 3: What Antibody is Responsible for Aiha?

Cold antibody–AIHA (CA-AIHA) with high cold antibody titer (1:4096) and anti-I specificity has been reported only once in SLE.[6] At large, the antibody is an IgM, measured by the "cold agglutinin assay,"[5] and coated red cells are cleared by the liver. The DAT is positive with complement alone in 74% of patients with IgG and C3 in 22.4%, as well as with IgG alone in 3.4%. Both titer and thermal amplitude of cold agglutinin are clinically relevant. Patients with high titers and narrow amplitude have intermittent attacks of severe hemolysis. Conversely, hemolysis may occur at much lower titers when the thermal amplitude is high. CA-AIHA is generally characterized by extravascular hemolysis and considerably lower response rates to corticosteroids and cytotoxics, compared with IgG warm antibody-AIHA (WA-AIHA).

References

1. Park KU, Song J, Kim JQ: Haptoglobin genotypic distribution (including Hp0 allele) and associated serum haptoglobin concentrations in Koreans. *J Clin Pathol* 57(10):1094–1095, 2004.
2. Delanghe J, Langlois M, De Buyzere M: Congenital anhaptoglobinemia versus acquired hypohaptoglobinemia. *Blood* 91(9):3524, 1998.
3. Liesveld JL, Rowe JM, Lichtman MA: Variability of the erythropoietic response in autoimmune hemolytic anemia: analysis of 109 cases. *Blood* 69(3):820–826, 1987.
4. Voulgarelis M, Kokori SI, Ioannidis JP, et al: Anaemia in systemic lupus erythematosus: aetiological profile and the role of erythropoietin. *Ann Rheum Dis* 59(3):217–222, 2000.
5. Valent P, Lechner K: Diagnosis and treatment of autoimmune haemolytic anaemias in adults: a clinical review. *Wien Klin Wochenschr* 120(5-6):136–151, 2008.
6. Nair K, Pavithran K, Philip J, et al: Cold haemagglutinin disease in systemic lupus erythematosus. *Yonsei Med J* 38(4):233–235, 1997 Aug.

exclusively WA-AIHA.[14] Conversely 6% of patients with WA-AIHA have SLE. RBCs coated by warm IgG undergo membrane alteration in vivo with each pass through the spleen, resulting in the formation of spherocytes; they are ultimately removed from circulation through phagocytosis, predominantly by splenic macrophages and, to a lesser extent, by sinus endothelial cells. The DAT is positive with IgG in 20% to 66% of patients with IgG plus complement (C3d) in 24% to 64% and with complement alone in 7% to 14% of all patients.

Two older studies reported AIHA in the presence of both warm IgG and cold IgM antibodies in the context of SLE. Sokol and colleagues[15] found that 7% of 865 patients with AIHA had warm IgG and cold IgM anti–RBC antibodies, both of which contributed to hemolysis; of those two groups, 20% had SLE. Shulman and others[16] reported that 5 of 12 patients (42%) with combined warm and cold AIHA had SLE. Patients with this type of AIHA have severe hemolysis but good response to corticosteroid therapy, similarly to IgG WA-AIHA.

Antigen Specificity of Antierythrocyte Antibodies

Antierythrocyte antibodies in SLE are mainly warm-type IgG, usually with non-rhesus specificity, otherwise undefined.[1] In primary AIHA, such antibodies react with either Band 3 anion transporter protein on the RBC membrane or an epitope formed by Band 3 protein and glycophorin A. New Zealand black (NZB), lupus-prone mice produce anti-Band 3–specific antibodies.[17] Interestingly, anti-Band 3 IgG antibodies are naturally formed in healthy patients, possibly functioning as eliminators of senescent erythrocytes, which, with aging, express Band 3 protein–derived neoantigens.[18] The relationship between the naturally occurring and pathologic anti-Band 3 autoantibodies, as well as their differences in the context of SLE-associated AIHA, remains unknown.

Several studies in SLE described associations between antiphospholipid antibodies (APLA) and Coombs-positive hemolytic anemia, whereas others suggested that APLA may participate in the pathogenesis of immune hemolysis as antierythrocyte antibodies. Specifically:

(a) Anticardiolipin (aCL) IgG and IgM antibodies were highly prevalent (74%) in patients with SLE-associated AIHA, compared with both unselected patients with SLE[19] and patients with SLE associated with IDA or ACD.[1]

(b) Mean IgG and IgM aCL titers were significantly higher in SLE-associated AIHA, compared with both unselected subjects with SLE and controls.[20]

(c) The presence of both APLA and AIHA in patients with SLE has been correlated with DAT positivity, as well as the reduction of complement receptor 1 (CR1) levels on the RBC surface that regulates C3 fragment deposition; both parallel disease activity.[21]

(d) Certain IgG and IgM APLA antibodies have been shown to bind erythrocytes and fix complement in vivo, accounting for the observed association of these antibodies with positive DAT results.[22] The ability of this binding to decrease erythrocyte survival and cause AIHA was demonstrated in three patients with SLE; the antierythrocyte binding activity of eluted autoantibodies was totally inhibited by absorption with phospholipid micelles.

An interesting, yet unexplained, finding in patients with SLE-associated AIHA is an acquired deficiency in erythrocyte expression of CD55, or decay acceleration factor (DAF), and/or CD59, also known as a membrane inhibitor of reactive lysis (MIRL); compared to SLE subjects without AIHA, who may normally express such molecules. These are glycosylphosphatidylinositol-anchored membrane proteins, serving as complement regulators that protect erythrocyte membranes against complement activation and deposition leading to cell lysis. One study showed that the mean fluorescence intensity (MFI) of both CD55 and CD59 on erythrocytes of patients with SLE-associated AIHA is significantly reduced, compared with those without AIHA and with control patients.[23] Interestingly, the underexpression of CD55 and CD59 has been reported on other formed elements in SLE and is likewise associated with autoimmune thrombocytopenia and lymphopenia.[23] Since all three cytopenias do not always coexist in the same patients, a common mechanism affecting the expression in all three lineages is unsustainable. The fact that the underexpression of CD55 and CD59 may independently exist in different lineages insinuates the presence of lineage-specific pathophysiologic processes; not being an inherited defect, cell-specific antibodies appear as the most plausible alternative.[23] However, the presence of anti-CD55 or anti-CD59 antibodies in SLE and their capacity to induce hemolysis has not yet been reported.

Treatment

General Considerations

In the era of evidence-based medicine, a paucity of succinct guidelines is available for the management of AIHA at large, as well as within the context of SLE:

(a) No established definitions of remission, complete or partial, are available. Certain reports have used benchmarks such as Hgb >12 g/dL and no hemolysis for complete remission; Hgb between 10 and 12 g/dL, or Hgb increase >2 g/dL, or hematocrit (Hct) >30% have been used as descriptors of partial remission. but without universal acceptance. Others have considered the reduction of reticulocyte counts, absence of hemolysis, or decreased need for transfusion as a benchmark for partial remission.

(b) No clinical trials address the efficacy and durability of first-line therapies (e.g., corticosteroids).

(c) No consensus of opinion is offered on when or what decides transition to second-line therapies (e.g., rituximab, splenectomy).

(d) No clinical trials exist that explore the effectiveness and longevity of second-line treatments.

(e) Especially in patients with SLE, AIHA frequently coexists with other manifestations such as nephritis, which may dominate therapeutic decisions. Consequently, most insight on the natural course and treatment of isolated AIHA in SLE is extrapolated from studies in idiopathic AIHA. As such, recommendations stem from retrospective studies, small series of (probably selected) patients or single cases (evidence level V), or a few prospective phase II trials, or are largely based on experience. As a general rule, AIHA occurs at the outset of SLE in two thirds of patients and generally recurs infrequently. The median time to remission with therapy is 3 months, 75% of patients respond to first-line therapy, 85% of responders are recurrence-free after 5 years, and 73% remain so after 15 years of follow-up.[1]

First-Line Therapies

For most cases of idiopathic and secondary AIHA including SLE, prednisone at a dose of 1 mg/kg/day is the first-line treatment of choice.[24] Hgb response usually takes a few days; therefore some patients may require transfusion support. Transfusions should be avoided whenever possible, since patients with SLE develop isoantibodies against RBCs, as well as higher titers of isohemagglutinin antibodies more frequently than control patients. The efficacy of pretransfusion plasma exchange to decrease antierythrocyte antibody mass and to improve transfusion yield has not been validated.[25] Approximately 80% to 90% of patients demonstrate a clear response (Hgb > 10.0 g/dL) within the first 3 weeks of treatment. Nonresponders, at that point, are unlikely to improve on steroids alone and should be considered for second-line therapy.[26] After 3 months, two thirds are in complete remission and approximately 21% to 23% are in partial remission.[27] Approximately 10% of all patients are nonresponders. When a response is achieved, the prednisone dose should be slowly tapered. Although not evidence-based, reducing the dose by 20 mg/day every 2 weeks down to a daily dose of 20 mg/day is generally recommended. In those who maintain response, the dose should be slowly reduced further by 5 mg or 2.5 mg/day every month. Considering the long half-life of erythrocytes, time is required to ascertain that a given dose of prednisone is sufficient to maintain Hgb within an acceptable target range, thus the reason for this strategy. Approximately 20% of adults remain in remission without further therapy, 40% to 50% require low-dose maintenance therapy, and 15% to 20% need a high maintenance dose of prednisone.

Eligibility for second-line therapy is based on the following: (1) Patients refractory to initial steroid treatment after 3 weeks of therapy and those who need more than 15 mg/day prednisone for maintenance are absolute candidates for such treatments; (2) patients in the 15 to 0.1 mg/kg/day prednisone equivalent should be encouraged to proceed to a second-line therapy; (3) patients with the requirement of 0.1 mg/kg/day or less may do well with a long-term, low-dose steroid alone.

Second-Line Therapies

In patients with idiopathic AIHA, anti-CD20 monoclonal antibody (rituximab) and splenectomy are the only second-line therapies with proven short-term efficacy. In eight studies addressing rituximab in patients with AIHA at large, a clinical response was observed in 62 of 76 patients, based on the reduction in reticulocyte count, the absence of hemolysis, the decreased need for transfusion, or a normalization of Hgb.[28] Similarly, in a Belgian retrospective study, 53 patients with primary and secondary AIHA were given rituximab after failing at least one previous therapy—including splenectomy in 19% of patients—and showed an overall response rate of 79% in a median follow-up of 15 months. Progression-free survival at 1 and 2 years were 72% and 56%, respectively.[29] However, the reported experience with rituximab efficacy in adults with SLE-associated AIHA is limited (three case reports). As such, its use in SLE is reserved for severe or recalcitrant disease and perhaps patients with CA-AIHA or mixed WA-AIHA and CA-AIHA. The role of splenectomy is controversial in SLE-associated AIHA. Rivero and others[30] compared the clinical course of 15 patients undergoing splenectomy for SLE-associated AIHA and/or immune thrombocytopenia and 15 SLE patients who were treated medically. Splenectomy produced short-term benefits, but, at follow-up, no difference between the two groups was observed. The splenectomy group had a significantly higher frequency of cutaneous vasculitis and serious infections after surgery. More patients undergoing splenectomy eventually required immunosuppressive therapy, compared with the medically treated group at follow-up.

AIHA represents a *forme fruste* (i.e., incomplete manifestation) of SLE and commonly coexists with other visceral manifestations that may dominate the choice of second-line immunosuppressive agents. These scenarios include the concomitant use of azathioprine (AZA) (2 to 2.5 mg/kg/day), mycophenolate mofetil (MMF), or cyclophosphamide (Cytoxan) in patients with associated renal or central nervous system disease; in such instances recurrence rates of AIHA are rather low (e.g., 3 subjects per 100 patient years, 73% event free at 180 months). However, the utility and steroid-sparing properties of these agents in isolated SLE-associated AIHA have never been interrogated.

Danazol in conjunction with corticosteroids has been reported as useful in WA-AIHA, including that associated with SLE.[31] High-dose intravenous immunoglobulin (IVIG) has been used as a second-line agent after or concurrently with steroids but with low and transient efficacy. It was effective in 40 of 73 patients with WA-AIHA; thus IVIG is not recommended as a standard therapy but may be useful as an adjunct therapy for selected patients, such as those with toxicity to other treatments.[32]

Bone Marrow and Immune-Mediated Hematopoietic Failure in Systemic Lupus Erythematosus

The concept of hematopoietic failure as a result of an immune-mediated BM damage gained momentum in light of BM biopsy studies in patients with SLE-associated cytopenias. The largest study to date reported the histopathologic features in 40 patients with SLE and unexplained cytopenias from a single center[33]; hypocellularity, necrosis, and stromal changes such as edema and fibrosis along with vascular changes were frequently present.

BM was hypocellular in 58% of patients, normocellular in 17%, and hypercellular in 25%. Erythroid lineage was increased, normal, or decreased in 70%, 17%, and 13%, respectively, and myeloid lineage was increased in 13% and decreased in 17% of patients. Megakaryocytes were increased in 65% and decreased in 10% of patients.[33] Dyserythropoiesis was uniformly observed and involved immature erythroid precursors; multinucleation, bizarre nuclear shapes, and budding were common, whereas nuclear karyorrhexis in erythroblasts was less prominent. Erythrophagocytosis was observed in 20% of patients. In addition, disruption of normal BM architecture was a prominent feature, affecting immature cells of all three lineages. In the normal human BM, myeloid precursors reside near the trabecular region, whereas erythroid and megakaryocytic precursors are located in the intertrabecular region. This distribution may be reversed in SLE, with erythroid and megakaryocytic precursors in the trabecular regions designated as abnormal localization of immature precursors (ALIP), which was present in 58% of patients and inversely correlated with Hgb ($P = 0.01$). These observations highlight the BM as a main target organ in SLE.

BM necrosis was present in 90% of patients with SLE and graded as mild in 58%, moderate in 22%, and severe in 10% of patients.[33] Its morphologic features were distinctive—a smooth homogeneous basophilic background protein staining was often present. In addition, an increase in eosinophilic granular stroma was identified, along with the ghosts of many dead hematopoietic cells. The usual mechanism of BM necrosis is vascular obstruction, leading to ischemia. However, microvascular thrombosis or vasculitis was not seen, rendering the pathogenesis of BM necrosis unclear in patients with SLE. However, sinusoidal dilation and destruction of the lining endothelium was present in 20% of patients and was associated with the presence of moderate to severe necrosis ($P = 0.008$).[33]

With regard to the immune system contribution to hematopoietic failure in SLE, evidence points to autoantibodies, immune complexes, and cytotoxic T cells as common effector mechanisms of progenitor growth arrest, inhibition of differentiation, apoptotic death, or BM stromal cell dysfunction (Figure 34-2). Complement-dependent or independent autoantibodies were found to suppress both erythroid- and granulocytic-colony formation by hematopoietic colony-forming units (CFU).[34,35,36] IgG fractions of patients with active SLE cytopenias directly bound CD34+ CFU, causing growth arrest in vitro.[37] However, no correlation was established between the severity of peripheral cytopenias and autoantibody inhibitory capacity, and the nature of respective antigen(s) remains elusive.[37] Such antibodies culminate in syndromes similar to aplastic anemia, PRCA, myeloid hypoplasia, or amegakaryocytic thrombocytopenia and can be suppressed by immunomodulatory therapy.

Homing of autoreactive T cells in the BM has been well-documented in SLE; T- and B-cell aggregates were reported in 58% of patients, mainly in a central perivascular location.[33] Autoreactive T cells were shown to inhibit CFU formation, damage hematopoietic stem cells through direct cytotoxic destruction, or induce apoptosis.[8] In a series of 25 patients with SLE and anemia attributed to T-cell suppressor activity, Yamasaki and colleagues[38] showed that such T cells inhibited autologous or allogeneic BM erythroid colony formation in vitro. T-cell depletion from SLE marrow samples significantly increased the clonogenic potential of progenitor cells.[8] Patients with SLE display low numbers of BM CD34+ cells, compared with controls as a result of the induction of apoptosis by resident autoreactive T cells. Such T cells in the BM are the source of Fas ligand (FasL), IFN-γ, and TNF-α, which result in the upregulation of Fas and apoptosis of CD34+ cells.[39] CD40 ligand (CD40L) upregulation on BM homing T cells facilitates FasL-mediated apoptosis of CD34+ cells; CD40 expression on CD34+ cells shows a significant inverse

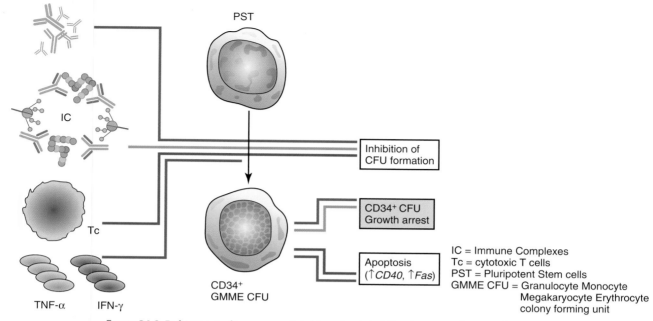

FIGURE 34-2 Pathogenesis of immune-mediated hematopoietic failure in systemic lupus erythematosus.

correlation with Hgb levels, and soluble CD40L inversely correlates with BM CD34$^+$ reserve.[39] A recent study reported allogeneic BM CD34$^+$ cell apoptosis after exposure to serum samples from patients with active SLE, suggesting the possible involvement of humoral factors as well. Interestingly, apoptosis was found to be complement-, Fas-, and IgG-independent; however, the exact mechanisms remain unclear.[40]

Evidence for the culpability of BM stroma in SLE hematopoietic failure is derived from culture experiments in which SLE stromal cells failed to support allogeneic progenitor cell growth.[8] The production of hematopoietic growth factors by BM fibroblasts is insufficient as a result of diminished activity of monocytes, which can further explain hematologic abnormalities in SLE.[41]

Reactive Hemophagocytic Syndrome

Reactive hemophagocytic syndrome (RHPS) is a clinicopathologic entity characterized by increased proliferation and activation of benign macrophages with phagocytosis throughout the reticuloendothelial system. It is classified as primary or familial and secondary or reactive in the context of malignancy, systemic autoimmunity, infection, or drug-hypersensitivity reaction (eBox 34-1). In the framework of systemic autoimmunity, the term *autoimmune-associated hemophagocytic syndrome* (AAHS) has been proposed and accepted. In the largest published series of RHPS, the prevalence of autoimmune disease was 2% to 5%; the reported RHPS incidence in large SLE series is 2.4%.[42] In SLE, RHPS can be observed as two different scenarios: (1) SLE-specific RHPS at the onset of SLE or during a flare without evidence of coexisting infection; and (2) infection-associated RHPS, mostly associated with viral infections. A recent review of 38 patients in the English language literature disclosed that RHPS occurred at onset or during a flare of SLE in 23 patients (61%); onset was related to infection in 8 patients (21%); and RHPS was associated with both infection and SLE onset or flare in 5 patients (13%).[43] By contradistinction, infection constitutes the major trigger of RHPS in other autoimmune syndromes (88%) versus disease onset or during a flare (25%, $P = 0.03$).[42] At the time of RHPS diagnosis, 58% of patients were already on corticosteroids, and 20% received additional immunosuppressive agents.[42]

AAHS carries a mortality rate of 38%[42]; 21% of patients with SLE-associated RHPS died. Factors associated with mortality included the absence of lymphadenopathy (OR = 15, $P = 0.01$), thrombocytopenia $<50 \times 10^9$/L (OR = 28, $P = 0.002$), immunosuppression at the time of diagnosis ($P = 0.009$), or corticosteroids alone (OR = 15, $P = 0.01$).[42]

Proposed mechanisms in SLE-associated RHPS that are not mutually exclusive include the following:

(a) Autoantibody-mediated phagocytosis of hematopoietic cells;
(b) Immune complex deposition on hematopoietic precursors; and
(c) Overproduction of cytokines (IL-1, IL-6, IFN-γ, TNF-α) by primary uncontrolled T-cell activation.

Autoantibodies and immune complexes sensitize BM cells to macrophages that subsequently engage in uncontrolled phagocytosis. T cell–derived cytokines enhance the inappropriate activation of macrophages.

Diagnosis

Prolonged high fever, hepatosplenomegaly, and cytopenias are the cardinal features of RHPS. Lymphadenopathy, icterus, and neurologic symptoms such as cranial nerve palsies or seizures may also be prevalent. Characteristic laboratory findings include high triglycerides, ferritin, LDH, serum soluble IL-2 receptors, transaminases, bilirubin, and low fibrinogen. BM aspiration and biopsy are pivotal; histologic studies typically reveal activated histiocytes or macrophages engulfing leukocytes, erythrocytes, platelets, and their precursors. Similar findings may be present in the lymph nodes, spleen, and liver. A biopsy should be repeated if these findings are absent on the initial specimen. Diagnostic guidelines for RHPS at large are described in eBox 34-2. Given the clinical peculiarities of AAHS, these criteria were subsequently adapted to reflect important points in its diagnosis (eBox 34-3).[44]

Treatment of Autoimmune-Associated Hemophagocytic Syndrome

Given its rare incidence, treatments for AAHS are not well established. The specific clinical setting and the presence of poor prognostic factors should be carefully evaluated when choosing the optimal strategy. In SLE, in which RHPS is primarily driven by disease activity and in the absence of obvious infection, immunosuppressive therapy should be escalated, which includes corticosteroids at high doses, cyclophosphamide (Cytoxan), or cyclosporine.[42] In the context

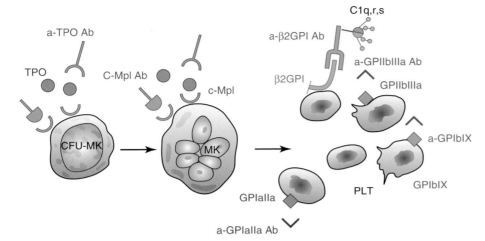

FIGURE 34-3 Pathogenesis of thrombocytopenia in systemic lupus erythematosus.

of contemporaneous infection, IVIG in addition to antiinfectious agents should be considered along with steroids. IVIG improved clinical outcomes in a few pediatric patients with RHPS as early as 24 to 72 hours. It may control both viral replication and lymphohistiocytic dysregulation induced by the infection.[43] In the case of obvious infection triggering AAHS, antibiotics should be promptly instigated and immunosuppressives decreased as much as possible.

THROMBOCYTOPENIA AND QUALITATIVE PLATELET DISORDERS

Thrombocytopenia is defined as platelets fewer than 100,000/µL and is a common clinical manifestation in SLE, ranging from 7% to 30% of patients in large series (eFig 34-4). It is uncommonly severe, and bleeding rates are generally low but can be detrimental. In a large single-center cohort study of 632 patients, 54% of patients with SLE thrombocytopenia had platelet counts of 50,000 to 100,000/µL, 18% had counts between 20,000 and 50,000/µL, and 28% had a platelet count less than 20,000/µL.[45] In 58% of patients, thrombocytopenia was present at the onset of SLE; these patients did not have clinical or serologic differences from those who developed low platelet counts later in their disease. The degree of thrombocytopenia is strongly associated with the severity of hemorrhagic complications ($P < 0.001$).[45] Grade II (gastrointestinal or genitourinary) and grade III (central nervous and pulmonary systems), bleed was observed in 15% of patients with a platelet count of 50,000 to 100,000/µL, 11% in those with a count of 20,000 to 50,000/µL, and 42% of those with a count less than 20,000/µL. The presence of thrombocytopenia in SLE correlates with higher disease activity, morbidity, cumulative organ damage accrual, and mortality; high disease activity (ECLAM score of 4 or higher) correlated with an increased risk of thrombocytopenia (OR = 2.46, $P = 0.03$). End-organ damage accrual, according to measurements of Systemic Lupus International Collaborating Clinics (SLICC), was higher in patients with thrombocytopenia than in those without thrombocytopenia (median of 2 versus 1, respectively, $P < 0.001$). Renal disease and treatment-related complications were higher in thrombocytopenia SLE subjects compared to those without thrombocytopenia (12% versus 0%, $P < 0.001$). Moreover, in two large studies of survivorship, thrombocytopenia was a significant risk factor of mortality.[46] Thrombocytopenia relapse (i.e., platelet count less than 100,000/µL) after successful treatment has been reported in 44% of patients with SLE over the course of their disease.[45]

Pathogenesis of Thrombocytopenia in Systemic Lupus Erythematosus

The unique pathogenesis of thrombocytopenia in SLE has been the subject of a few recently published series.[45,47-49] The most common

mechanism is believed to be peripheral platelet clearance mediated by antiplatelet antibodies, similar to immune thrombocytopenic purpura (ITP) (eBox 34-4). APLAs with or without the full antiphospholipid syndrome (APS), thrombotic thrombocytopenic purpura (TTP), and disseminated intravascular coagulation (DIC) constitute alternative mechanisms of peripheral clearance. Hemophagocytosis largely associates with intramedullary consumption of platelets, whereas amegakaryocytic thrombocytopenia (AMT) or hypomegakaryocytic thrombocytopenia reflects antibody or T cell–mediated suppression of megakaryocyte proliferation and platelet production.[45,48]

Antigen specificity of antiplatelet antibodies in SLE largely segregates on glycoprotein IIb/IIIa (GpIIb/IIIa) membrane glycoprotein ($\alpha_{IIa}\beta_3$ integrin), similar to ITP and secondarily on GpIa/IIa and GPIbIX (Figure 34-3). Megakaryocyte proliferation and differentiation are under the auspices of thrombopoietin (TPO), a protein constitutively synthesized in the liver. TPO binds to its receptor c-Mpl on megakaryocytes and their precursors, signals through Jak-STAT, Ras-Raf-MAPK, PI3K pathways, and induces their proliferation and maturation. In addition, it increases the number, size, and ploidy of megakaryocytes but has no effects on platelet count. Antibodies against c-Mpl have been reported in patients with SLE to antagonize TPO-c-MPL interaction, leading to high TPO levels, compared with control patients. Antibodies to TPO itself also have been reported; however, their relative contribution to the degree and pathophysiology of thrombocytopenia remain unclear.

The prevalence, clinical significance, and associations of antiplatelet and anti–c-Mpl responses in SLE thrombocytopenia have been compared with those in ITP and healthy control groups.[47,49] Anti–GpIIb/IIIa-producing B cells were highly enriched in patients with SLE thrombocytopenia, compared to SLE subjects without it (88% versus 17%, respectively, $P < 0.0001$) and were similar in magnitude to those with ITP (86%).[48] Such responses were absent in healthy controls. In a different study, anti-GpIIb/IIIa antibodies were absent (0%) in patients recovering from thrombocytopenia in response to treatment, compared to actively thrombocytopenic ones (45%, $P = 0.006$), highlighting perhaps their relevance in its pathogenesis.[47] Anti-GpIIb/IIIa antibodies bind circulating platelet and facilitate Fc-γ receptor–mediated clearance of opsonized platelets by reticuloendothelial phagocytes. BM examination in SLE thrombocytopenia discloses increased megakaryocyte levels in 25%, normal levels in 53%, and decreased levels in 22% of patients. This distribution is similar to patients with ITP (20%, 66%, and 14%, respectively). Another report corroborated these findings and disclosed normal or high BM megakaryocytes in 93% of thrombocytopenic

SLE patients, thus highlighting peripheral platelet destruction as the pivotal mechanism in SLE thrombocytopenia.[47]

The prevalence of anti–c-Mpl antibodies in unselected patients with SLE is 12% and similar to that in chronic ITP (8%); no clinical or serologic differences are present in antibody-positive versus antibody-negative SLE, except for a higher prevalence of thrombocytopenia in the former (88% versus 18%, $P = 0.0002$). Such antibody specificity is absent in the healthy control group. The presence of c-Mpl antibodies is enriched in patients with thrombocytopenic versus nonthrombocytopenic SLE (39% versus 2%, $P = 0.0002$)[49]; however, the severity of thrombocytopenia is not different in positive versus negative subjects with low platelet counts. c-Mpl antibody positivity predicts significantly higher frequency of megakaryocyte hypoplasia in the BM (86% versus 4%, $P < 0.0001$).[49] This association appears independent of anti-GpIIb/IIIa antibody status. By contrast, none of the patients who were c-Mpl antibody–negative or anti-GpIIb/IIIa antibody- positive had megakaryocyte hypoplasia. Similarly in ITP, megakaryocyte hypoplasia was more frequent in patients who were c-Mpl antibody–positive versus c-Mpl antibody–negative (79% versus 7%, $P < 0.0001$). These data suggest that c-Mpl antibodies block TPO signaling through c-Mpl, resulting in the inhibition of megakaryogenesis in the BM. In fact, c-Mpl antibodies from patients with SLE were shown to block TPO ligation to c-Mpl on human hematopoietic stem cells in vitro, confirming their pathogenic role in megakaryocyte hypoplasia.[49] Concordantly, patients with c-Mpl antibody–positive thrombocytopenia have higher serum TPO levels, compared with those who were negative ($P = 0.007$). Interestingly, patients with c-Mpl antibody–positive thrombocytopenia demonstrate poor clinical response to corticosteroids and IVIG, compared with those who were negative (86% versus 12%, $P = 0.0006$ for steroids and 100% versus 10% for IVIG, $P = 0.002$, respectively). Since interactions between the Fc portion of the infused immunoglobulins and the Fc receptors on the target cells are thought to be the primary action of IVIG, it is not surprising that IVIG would have little effect on the TPO signal blockade through the variable region of the antibodies.

Anti-TPO antibodies were reported in 39% of unselected patients with SLE.[47] Their prevalence in thrombocytopenic and postthrombocytopenic individuals does not differ from those without thrombocytopenia, which suggests that anti-TPO antibodies may be a feature of SLE that remains stable over time. Remarkably, however, patients who were positive for anti-TPO antibodies exhibited significantly lower circulating TPO levels, compared with patients who were negative.[47] Whether anti-TPO antibodies are truly blocking with physiologic importance or simply an epiphenomenon interfering with the detection of TPO/anti-TPO complex is a matter of debate. Their contribution to thrombocytopenia may occur in a bimodal fashion—first by engendering an immune complex, a nonspecific mechanism that enhances peripheral platelet consumption, and second by decreasing the effective TPO concentration for stimulating megakaryopoiesis.[47]

Thrombocytopenia has been reported in the context of both APS and APLA without symptoms in patients with SLE; 31% of patients (491 of 1588) with associated (or secondary) APS and 25% of patients (360 of 1455) with idiopathic APS have thrombocytopenia (less than 100,000/μL).[50] Cumulative data from four separate studies in ITP have shown that 34% of patients (160 of 474) had positive APLA as described in the laboratory APS criteria,[50a] and 21% of those (33 of 160) developed thrombosis over 3.3 years.[50] APLAs bind directly to platelets via beta 2–glycoprotein I (β_2-GPI) and promote platelet activation. High titers of IgG aCL antibodies had a 77% predictive value for thrombocytopenia.[50] It would then appear that certain patients with APLA-positive ITP make up a subset that eventually develops into full-blown APS; the patients with positive lupus anticoagulant (LA) are more prone to thrombosis. LA-positivity in ITP thrombosis-free patients confers a 4.5% person per year risk of thrombosis.

The measurement of antiplatelet and c-Mpl antibodies in routine clinical practice is controversial, given their limited availability, cost,

and time lapse until a result is obtained. Predicting a response to therapy in different subsets is theoretically useful, particularly in severe thrombocytopenia. By contrast, screening for all subsets and isotypes of APLA is mandatory since they constitute, as a class, one of the diagnostic criteria for SLE, and their presence may be associated with APS.

Acquired Abnormalities of Platelet Function

Activation of normal platelets is induced upon adhesion to collagen and by soluble agonists such as epinephrine and adenosine diphosphate (ADP); it leads to platelet aggregation and granule secretion. In a study by Regan and colleagues,[51] platelets failed to aggregate in response to collagen, ADP, and epinephrine in 57% of patients with SLE; the effects were similar to those induced by aspirin. Additionally, concentration of serotonin and ADP nucleotides in platelet-dense granules was shown to be reduced in patients with acquired-platelet defects, including those with SLE.[52] In fact, a low-platelet serotonin concentration was shown to correlate with disease activity and indicate platelet activation in SLE. However, these functional abnormalities did not translate to specific clinical phenotypes such as bleeding; therefore their clinical relevance and significance remain unknown.

Treatment of Thrombocytopenia in Systemic Lupus Erythematosus

Although the prevalence of thrombocytopenia in SLE is well described, the literature addressing its treatment is based mainly on small case series or extrapolated from that of ITP. In principle, thrombocytopenia with platelets greater than 50×10^9/L does not generally require specific therapy, unless the patients are symptomatic or other organ manifestations coexist that merit therapeutic intervention. Corticosteroids are generally considered first-line therapy. Concrete evidence for their short- and long-term efficacy is largely derived from a single, large, retrospective cohort study of 59 patients with severe thrombocytopenia as the cardinal manifestation of SLE.[53] Mean platelet count at diagnosis was $20 \pm 17 \times 10^9$/L. Platelets greater than 150×10^9/L were considered a complete remission, whereas platelets greater than 50×10^9/L constituted a partial remission. Oral prednisone (1 ± 0.2 mg/kg/day) was used as first-line therapy. The initial response was observed in 40 of 50 evaluable patients (80%) with a complete remission in 28 (56%) and a partial remission in 12 (24%). A sustained response was observed in 11 patients (22%, complete remission $n = 7$; partial remission $n = 4$), over 78 ± 63 months, after a mean treatment of 23 ± 24 months. At the end of the study, 8 of 11 patients were steroid-free, after 13 ± 14 months of therapy and a mean follow-up of 77 ± 61 months after withdrawal. The long-term response was not observed in 39 patients (78%); fifteen (30%) were resistant to the starting dose, and 21 patients (42%) initially responded but relapsed while still receiving a high dose (mean 0.7 ± 0.3 mg/kg/day). Three patients (6%) with a sustained response relapsed 4, 16, and 48 months, respectively, after withdrawal.

High-dose methylprednisolone pulse (HDMP) was administered at a mean dose of 15 mg/kg/day to 10 patients and a transient response was achieved in 6 patients (complete remission in 4 patients [40%]; partial remission in 2 [20%]). Mean time to partial remission after HDPM was 7.2 ± 8.8 days. No sustained response was observed, even in the 2 patients who received monthly HDMP infusions (4 and 5 infusions, respectively).[53]

Danazol was reported as helpful in some patients with thrombocytopenic SLE. In the French study, representing the largest exposure in SLE,[53] 18 patients received danazol; the agent was added to a mean oral prednisone dose of 0.7 mg/kg/day after the steroids failed. Twelve patients had previously received other treatments without a sustained response, including IVIG, immunosuppressants, hydroxychloroquine (HCQ), HDMP, and splenectomy. A sustained long-term response to danazol was observed in 9 patients (50%) (complete remission in 7 [39%] and partial remission in 2 [11%]) with a mean follow-up of 28 ± 30 months. The duration of danazol treatment for the 9 responders was 20 ± 12 months.

In the same study,[53] HCQ proved beneficial in the treatment of thrombocytopenia; HCQ (mean dose 400 mg/day) was combined with oral prednisone at a mean dose of 0.7 mg/kg in 11 patients after prednisone alone failed. Seven patients had previously received other treatments without long-term success, including IVIG, immunosuppressants, HDMP, danazol, or splenectomy. Sustained response was observed in 7 patients (64%) (complete remission in 4 [36%]; partial remission in 3 [27%]) with a follow up of 31 ± 16 months, and prednisone was tapered below 0.2 mg/kg/day. The duration of treatment with HCQ in the responders was 31 ± 17 months, and all remained on the drug by the end of the study.

IVIG has been used in SLE-associated thrombocytopenia with variable and transient successes. In the study by Arnal,[53] the largest experience in SLE, IVIG was administered at 2 g/kg for 2 to 5 days in 31 patients. A transient response was seen in 20 patients (65%) (complete remission in 12 [39%] and partial remission in 8 [26%]). Mean time to partial remission was 4.6 ± 2.8 days. Unfortunately, no sustained response was observed, even in the 4 patients treated with repeated (3 to 12) infusions. A prospective, randomized, clinical trial showed that IVIG offers no advantage over corticosteroids as the primary therapy in untreated patients with ITP, including patients with SLE.[54] Consequently, such therapy may be entertained in cases of life-threatening bleed or patient preparation for surgery.

The experience with immunosuppressive medications targeting specifically SLE thrombocytopenia has been fairly limited. In most cases, such therapy is predicated by coexistent severe visceral manifestations. Nevertheless, pulsed intravenous cyclophosphamide (Cytoxan) was effective in 7 patients refractory to splenectomy, steroids, or requiring excessive doses of steroids.[55,56] Limited success has been reported with AZA, cyclosporine, dapsone, vincristine, and mycophenolate.[57] The French experience, however, was less exciting[53]; 14 patients received one or several immunosuppressants for thrombocytopenia. A total of 22 periods of treatment were observed over 8 ± 11 months. A transient response was seen in 7 of the 22 patients' (32%) treatment periods (complete remission in 3 [14%], partial remission in 4 [18%]). Only 2 patients (14%) who received vinblastine had sustained partial remission in 7 and 25 months after treatment, respectively. Long-term failure was observed in the other 12 patients (86%).

Rituximab has been increasingly evaluated in ITP but only in case reports in SLE-associated thrombocytopenia; complete remission (platelets greater than 100×10^9/L or 150×10^9/L) among 19 case series including 375 treated patients was 44%.[58] Some controlled trials have been performed; one showed 31% success rate.[58] In another study, 63% achieved stable counts greater than 150×10^9/L for 4 to 30 months without additional therapy.[58] In an additional trial, including 60 candidates for splenectomy, 40% patients achieved platelet counts of at least twice their baseline and greater than 50,000/μL.[58] In most studies, relapses after complete response occur in approximately 50% of cases. Future subset analysis of the EXPLORER and LUNAR trials of rituximab in SLE may yield additional information on effectiveness in treatment of thrombocytopenia.

The role of splenectomy in the treatment of SLE thrombocytopenia remains a matter of debate; several authors have reported that it may be less effective in SLE than in ITP and that a significantly higher rate of cutaneous vasculitis and serious infections occur in patients with SLE who undergo splenectomy.[30,59] However, the French experience was quite different: 17 patients with a mean platelet count of $19 \pm 16 \times 10^9$/L underwent splenectomy. A sustained response was observed in 11 patients (65%) (complete remission in 10 [59%]; partial remission in 1 [6%]) with a mean follow-up of 64 ± 108 months. The SLE flare occurred 33 ± 22 months after the splenectomy in 39% of patients. This incidence was no different from those observed who did not undergo a splenectomy (27%, $P = 0.4$) during similar follow-up periods (65 ± 93 months after splenectomy versus 68 ± 57 months without a splenectomy).

Novel approaches have targeted the c-Mpl receptor on megakaryocytes to increase their differentiation and augment platelet counts in ITP. A weekly, subcutaneously administered TPO-receptor agonist named *romiplostim* (AMG 531) is now licensed for the treatment of chronic refractory ITP. It consists of an IgG-1 Fc linked to a peptide domain with four binding sites for Mpl. Romiplostim has no sequence homologic traits with TPO; hence, less risk of developing antibodies against endogenous TPO exists. Response peaks at days 12 through 15.[60] In two phase III placebo-controlled randomized trials, romiplostim was administered to 125 patients with ITP and mean baseline platelet counts of 16×10^9/L for 24 weeks; 63 of the 125 patients underwent splenectomies and 62 of the 125 patients did not. Sustained platelet response was observed in 38% of the splenectomized group receiving romiplostim and none in the placebo arm. Similarly, 56% of those in the nonsplenectomized group who received romiplostim, compared with 5% of patients receiving placebo, experienced sustained platelet responses.[61] This agent has not yet been tested in SLE.

Thrombotic Thrombocytopenic Purpura

Idiopathic TTP is classically characterized by a pentad of microangiopathic hemolytic anemia (MAHA), thrombocytopenic purpura, fever, neurologic abnormalities, and renal disease. The disease is rare, affecting 3.7 cases per million, with significant morbidity, mortality (approximately 10%), and frequent relapses in survivors (30% to 60%).[62] It is currently recognized that the sensitivity of the full pentad is low and anticipation of its full evolution may culminate in detrimental delays. Therefore thrombocytopenia (platelet count less than 100×10^9/L) and MAHA defined by schistocytes in peripheral smears are now accepted as sufficient grounds to diagnose TTP clinically, provided no other causes such as AIHA, DIC, cancer, eclampsia, drug toxicity, stem cell transplantation, or malignant hypertension are present. Patients with SLE are more susceptible to the development of secondary TTP; a single-center study reported that high-disease activity (Systemic Lupus Erythematosus Disease Activity Index [SLEDA] score greater than 10) and coexistent nephritis were independent risk factors for the development of secondary TTP in patients with SLE ($P = 0.006$ and $P = 0.004$, respectively).[63] Incidence of secondary TTP is 1% to 4%, the diagnosis is significantly delayed (19.5 days in secondary TTP versus 7.7 in idiopathic TTP), response to therapy is poorer, and mortality is higher in secondary TTP, averaging 34% to 62%.[64] The presence of infection was the only independent predictor of mortality in secondary TTP (OR = 14.3, $P = 0.035$).[63] Delayed recognition may reflect either a low index of suspicion or delayed symptom evolution as a result of a prior use of steroids and immunosuppressive therapies. Despite more aggressive therapy in secondary TTP with multiorgan involvement from SLE, response to therapy is poor. Time to complete remission was also long in patients with secondary TTP (31.3 ± 26.4 versus 16.8 ± 6.1 days in idiopathic TTP), suggesting a more refractory and severe disease.[64] Acute TTP episodes develop when high shear stress in the microcirculation and von Willebrand factor (vWF) are present.

vWF and platelets are prone to form aggregates. This propensity of vWF and platelets to form microvascular thrombi is mitigated by a disintegrin and metalloprotease with thrombospondin type 1 motif, member 13 (ADAMTS13), which cleaves vWF. Deficiency of ADAMTS13, which is due, in part, to autoimmune inhibitors in patients with acquired TTP and mutations of the ADAMTS13 gene in hereditary cases, leads to ultra-large vWF multimers that aggregate with platelets to cause microvascular thrombi.[62] A study of the specific role of ADAMTS13 in secondary TTP of autoimmune disease suggested that SLE, in particular, is not associated with the trend to low ADAMTS13 activity reported in idiopathic TTP. Furthermore, despite reports of ADAMTS13 antibodies being present in SLE, an overall increase in neutralizing antibodies to ADAMTS13 does not appear to exist. However, when present, the outcomes may be worse. The possibility of neutralizing antibodies being important in the inhibition of ADAMTS13 and the development of a relative deficiency of the protease has been the justification for the use of rituximab in refractory, secondary TTP in lupus. Although rituximab has been used successfully to treat secondary TTP in SLE unresponsive to other interventions, the numbers are small and large series have not been published because of the rarity of the disease. It therefore remains to be seen whether B cell–targeting strategies will be uniformly effective in secondary TTP of SLE.

WHITE BLOOD CELL DISORDERS

Leukopenia is a typical feature of SLE and may encompass lymphopenia, neutropenia, or both. Defined as a white blood cell (WBC) count of less than 4000 cells/mL, it has been reported in roughly 50% of patients with SLE. Generally, counts less than 2000/mL are uncommon; however, a study by Michael and colleagues[65] in 111 hospitalized patients with SLE reported WBC counts of 500/μL in 66 patients (60%) at some time. Leukopenia has been significantly associated with skin rash, lymphopenia, and high anti-DNA titer.

Lymphopenia is one of the most common hematologic findings of SLE. Rivero and colleagues[66] reported a 75% prevalence of absolute lymphopenia at diagnosis in 158 patients with SLE and a cumulative frequency of 93%. Lymphopenia was found to be independent of but contributory to leukopenia. Absolute lymphopenia was correlated with disease activity, and patients with lymphocyte counts less than 1500/μL at diagnosis had a higher frequency of fever, polyarthritis, and central nervous system involvement.[67] Nevertheless, life-table analysis showed no adverse effect of lymphopenia on the survival of patients with lupus. Pathogenic mechanisms contributing to lymphopenia in SLE are synopsized in eBox 34-5.

Granulocytopenia occurs frequently in SLE. A prospective study showed a 62% prevalence at some time during the course of disease, although it was severe (less than 1000/μL) in only 5% of patients studied.[67] Causes may reflect primary disease-associated mechanisms (see eBox 34-5), severe coexisting infection, or treatment-related side effects. A detailed drug history is essential, accounting both for drugs prescribed directly for SLE and for its complications, such as statins, antibiotics, and angiotensin-converting enzyme (ACE) inhibitors. Leukopenia may complicate the use of cyclophosphamide (Cytoxan), azathioprine, methotrexate, and, rarely, cyclosporine A, mycophenolate mofetil, or HCQ. Hemophagocytic syndrome should be considered if cytopenia develops rapidly, especially in juvenile SLE. BM aspiration and biopsy should be considered in severe cases.

Severe neutropenia in SLE is responsive to corticosteroids.[68] In such patients (counts less than $0.1 \times 10^9/L$), treatment with recombinant human granulocyte–colony-stimulating factor (rhG-CSF) should also be contemplated.[69] However, limited literature addresses its use in lupus-associated neutropenia. In one study, rhG-CSF was administered subcutaneously to nine patients with SLE and neutropenia with refractory infections.[61] A rapid increase in neutrophil count was observed, but disease flared in three patients. Others also reported lupus flares with the use of rhG-CSF.[70] Further, the effect on neutrophil counts may be only temporary and, as such, a rationale for concurrent immunosuppression therapy exists.[61]

To understand the importance of granulocyte function as a factor in the susceptibility of patients with SLE to infections, studies explored the phagocytic, opsonizing, chemotactic, and oxidative functions of neutrophils and monocytes. Most concluded that, in general, granulocyte function in SLE is abnormal, but the specific qualitative and quantitative abnormalities reported were either inconsistent or contradictory. The inconsistencies probably reflect differences in methodology and patient selection. Additionally, they emphasize the importance of other factors affecting these tests, such as the use of steroids and other drugs, activity of SLE, and the presence of inhibitory factors in the serum. Although the clinical significance of in vitro functional abnormalities is not entirely clear, in vivo studies using the Rebuck skin window technique have shown abnormalities in granulocyte functions.[71] Whether these abnormalities are primary cellular defects or secondary to the disease is again unclear.

LYMPHADENOPATHY IN SYSTEMIC LUPUS ERYTHEMATOSUS

Lymphadenopathy, a common manifestation of SLE, can be generalized or regional, especially in the cervical and axillary groups. Dubois and Tuffanelli[57] observed adenopathy in 59% of their 520 patients; axillary and cervical adenopathy was present in 42% and 24% of patients, respectively. Similar frequencies were reported in 698 adult patients with SLE collected from six large series in the literature.[57] Generalized adenopathy was the initial manifestation of SLE in 1% of patients. The nodes were usually nontender and discrete, and their size varied from shotty to 3 to 4 cm in diameter. The glandular enlargement was so pronounced in some patients that malignant lymphoma was suspected. Lymphadenopathy is more frequent in children than in adults and most common among African-American patients. The characteristic finding in the lymph nodes in SLE is a diffuse, reactive lymphoid follicular hyperplasia with varying degrees of coagulative necrosis.[72] Hyperplastic germinal centers with plasmacytosis and varying numbers of immunoblasts in the interfollicular areas are found. Three histologic patterns of reactive follicular hyperplasia have been described in SLE[73]: (1) histologic findings of multicentric Castleman disease, (2) T-zone dysplasia with hyperplastic follicles, and (3) nonspecific follicular hyperplasia. In the necrotic areas and within the sinuses are occasional extracellular amorphous bodies, 5 to 12 μm in diameter, that stain intensely with hematoxylin. These "hematoxylin bodies" contain aggregates of DNA, immunoglobulins, and polysaccharides[72] and, when present, are considered characteristic of SLE lymphadenitis.

Kikuchi-Fujimoto disease (KFD), or histiocytic necrotizing lymphadenitis, is a self-limited lupus-like illness of unknown cause in young women that is characterized by cervical adenopathy, fever, weight loss, and a prodrome of an upper respiratory tract infection. Other than a mild leukopenia in 50% of patients, laboratory investigations generally are unremarkable. The disease may be clinically confused with SLE and histologically with malignant lymphoma. The presence of hematoxylin bodies, prominent plasma cells, and the deposition of DNA in the blood vessel wall in lupus lymphadenitis help differentiate it from KFD. Before a diagnosis of nodal KFD is made, serologic tests are necessary to exclude SLE. Coexistent KFD and SLE have been reported in a few patients.[57] Of the 108 patients with KFD who were examined retrospectively, 2 developed SLE. Of the 61 patients from China with KFD, 2 developed SLE 1 month and 5 years later, respectively.

Castleman disease, or angiofollicular lymph node hyperplasia, is a rare lymphoproliferative disorder of unknown cause characterized by lymphadenopathy with or without constitutional symptoms, clinically resembling malignant lymphoma. It should be considered in a patient with a lupus-like presentation with persistent lymphadenopathy despite corticosteroid therapy.

THE SPLEEN IN SYSTEMIC LUPUS ERYTHEMATOSUS

Splenomegaly is common in SLE with a prevalence of 9% to 46% in large series. When present, splenomegaly is often associated with hepatomegaly. Its histopathologic characteristic in SLE is periarterial fibrosis or onionskin lesion, which is defined as the presence of 3 to as many as 20 separated layers of the normally densely packed periarterial collagen of the penicillary or follicular arteries, producing the appearance of concentric rings. Larson[74] found the lesion in 40 of 51 SLE spleens examined at autopsy. Kaiser[75] examined the specificity of the splenic lesion in 18 patients with SLE and 1679 control cases at autopsy; 15 patients with SLE (83%) and 53 of the control subjects (3%) with various diagnoses (especially ITP) were positive.

Functional asplenia is a condition that is characterized by the failure of the splenic uptake of radiolabeled sulfur colloid and the presence of Howell-Jolly bodies, Pappenheimer bodies, spherocytes, and poikilocytes in the peripheral blood smear. Its prevalence in SLE is 4.3%.[57] It does not seem to be related to disease activity in SLE, and it may clinically manifest as an overwhelming infection in a patient who is in disease remission.

References

1. Voulgarelis M, Kokori SI, Ioannidis JP, et al: Autoimmune hemolytic anemia in patients with systemic lupus erythematosus. *Am J Med* 108(3):198–204, 2000.
2. Burger T, Brasch G, Keszthelyi B: Iron metabolism and anaemia in systemic lupus erythematosus and rheumatoid arthritis. *Acta Med Acad Sci Hung* 23(2):96–104, 1967.
3. Ganz T: Molecular pathogenesis of anemia of chronic disease. *Pediatr Blood Cancer* 46(5):554–557, 2006.
4. Ripley BJ, Goncalves B, Isenberg DA, et al: Raised levels of interleukin 6 in systemic lupus erythematosus correlate with anaemia. *Ann Rheum Dis* 64(6):849–853, 2005.
5. Koca SS, Isik A, Ustundag B, et al: Serum pro-hepcidin levels in rheumatoid arthritis and systemic lupus erythematosus. *Inflammation* 31(3):46–153, 2008.
6. Faquin WC, Schneider TJ, Goldberg MA: Effect of inflammatory cytokines on hypoxia-induced erythropoietin production. *Blood* 79(8):1987–1994, 1992.
7. Jelkmann W, Pagel H, Wolff M, et al: Monokines inhibiting erythropoietin production in human hepatoma cultures and in isolated perfused rat kidneys. *Life Sci* 50(4):301–308, 1992.
8. Giannouli S, Voulgarelis M, Ziakas PD, et al: Anaemia in systemic lupus erythematosus: from pathophysiology to clinical assessment. *Ann Rheum Dis* 65(2):144–148, 2006.
9. Tzioufas AG, Kokori SI, Petrovas CI, et al: Autoantibodies to human recombinant erythropoietin in patients with systemic lupus erythematosus: correlation with anemia. *Arthritis Rheum* 40(12):2212–2216, 1997.
10. Means RT Jr, Dessypris EN, Krantz SB: Progress in understanding the pathogenesis of the anemia of chronic disease. *Blood* 80(7):1639–1647, 2006.
11. Giannouli S, Voulgarelis M, Ziakas PD, et al: Anaemia in systemic lupus erythematosus: from pathophysiology to clinical assessment. *Ann Rheum Dis* 65(2):144–148, 2006.
12. Kokori SI, Ioannidis JP, Voulgarelis M, et al: Autoimmune hemolytic anemia in patients with systemic lupus erythematosus. *Am J Med* 108(3):108–204, 2005.
13. Wikman A, Axdorph U, Gryfelt G, et al: Characterization of red cell autoantibodies in consecutive DAT-positive patients with relation to in vivo haemolysis. *Ann Hematol* 84(3):150–158, 2005.
14. Valent P, Lechner K: Diagnosis and treatment of autoimmune haemolytic anaemias in adults: a clinical review. *Wien Klin Wochenschr* 120(5-6):136–151, 2008.
15. Sokol RJ, Hewitt S, Stamps BK: Autoimmune haemolysis: an 18-year study of 865 cases referred to a regional transfusion centre. *Br Med J (Clin Res Ed)* 282(6281):2023–2027, 1981.
16. Shulman IA, Branch DR, Nelson JM, et al: Autoimmune hemolytic anemia with both cold and warm autoantibodies. *JAMA* 253(12):1746–1748, 1985.
17. Barker RN, de Sá Oliveira GG, Elson CJ, et al: Pathogenic autoantibodies in the NZB mouse are specific for erythrocyte band 3 protein. *Eur J Immunol* 23(7):1723–1726, 1993.
18. Kay MM, Marchalonis JJ, Hughes J, et al: Definition of a physiologic aging autoantigen by using synthetic peptides of membrane protein band 3: localization of the active antigenic sites. *Proc Natl Acad Sci U S A* 87(15):5734–5738, 1990.
19. Sturfelt G, Nived O, Norberg R, et al: Anticardiolipin antibodies in patients with systemic lupus erythematosus. *Arthritis Rheum* 30(4):382–388, 1987.
20. Lang B, Straub RH, Weber S, et al: Elevated anticardiolipin antibodies in autoimmune haemolytic anaemia irrespective of underlying systemic lupus erythematosus. *Lupus* 6(8):652–655, 1997.
21. Ross GD, Yount WJ, Walport MJ, et al: Disease-associated loss of erythrocyte complement receptors (CR1, C3b receptors) in patients with systemic lupus erythematosus and other diseases involving autoantibodies and/or complement activation. *J Immunol* 135(3):2005–2014, 1985.
22. Arvieux J, Roussel B, Ponard D, et al: Reactivity patterns of antiphospholipid antibodies in systemic lupus erythematosus sera in relation to erythrocyte binding and complement activation. *Clin Exp Immunol* 84(3):466–471, 1991.
23. Ruiz-Argüelles A, Llorente L: The role of complement regulatory proteins (CD55 and CD59) in the pathogenesis of autoimmune hemocytopenias. *Autoimmun Rev* 6(3):155–161, 2007.
24. Pirofsky B: Clinical aspects of autoimmune hemolytic anemia. *Semin Hematol* 13(4):251–265, 1976.
25. Ruivard M, Tournilhac O, Montel S, et al: Plasma exchanges do not increase red blood cell transfusion efficiency in severe autoimmune hemolytic anemia: a retrospective case-control study. *J Clin Apher* 21(3):202–206, 2006.
26. Murphy S, LoBuglio AF: Drug therapy of autoimmune hemolytic anemia. *Semin Hematol* 13(4):323–334, 1976 Oct.
27. Serrano J: [Autoimmune hemolytic anemia. Review of 200 cases studied in a period of 20 years] (1970–1989). *Article in Spanish Sangre (Barc)* 37(4):265–274, 1992.
28. Gürcan HM, Keskin DB, Stern JN, et al: A review of the current use of rituximab in autoimmune diseases. *Int Immunopharmacol* 9(1):10–25, 2009.
29. Dierickx D, Verhoef G, Van Hoof A, et al: Rituximab in auto-immune haemolytic anaemia and immune thrombocytopenic purpura: a Belgian retrospective multicentric study. *J Intern Med* 266(5):484–491, 2009.
30. Rivero SJ, Alger M, Alarcón-Segovia D: Splenectomy for hemocytopenia in systemic lupus erythematosus. A controlled appraisal. *Arch Intern Med* 139(7):773–776, 1979.
31. Ahn YS, Harrington WJ, Mylvaganam R, et al: Danazol therapy for autoimmune hemolytic anemia. *Ann Intern Med* 102(3):298–301, 1985.
32. Flores G, Cunningham-Rundles C, Newland AC, et al: Efficacy of intravenous immunoglobulin in the treatment of autoimmune hemolytic anemia: results in 73 patients. *Am J Hematol* 44(4):237–242, 1993.
33. Voulgarelis M, Giannouli S, Tasidou A, et al: Bone marrow histological findings in systemic lupus erythematosus with hematologic abnormalities: a clinicopathological study. *Am J Hematol* 81(8):590–597, 2006.
34. Bailey FA, Lilly M, Bertoli LF, et al: An antibody that inhibits in vitro bone marrow proliferation in a patient with systemic lupus erythematosus and aplastic anemia. *Arthritis Rheum* 32(7):901–905, 1989.
35. Fitchen JJ, Cline MJ, Saxon A, et al: Serum inhibitors of hematopoiesis in a patient with aplastic anemia and systemic lupus erythematosus. Recovery after exchange plasmapheresis. *Am J Med* 66(3):537–542, 1979.
36. Brooks BJ Jr, Broxmeyer HE, Bryan CF, et al: Serum inhibitor in systemic lupus erythematosus associated with aplastic anemia. *Arch Intern Med* 144(7):1474–1477, 1984.
37. Liu H, Ozaki K, Matsuzaki Y, et al: Suppression of haematopoiesis by IgG autoantibodies from patients with systemic lupus erythematosus (SLE). *Clin Exp Immunol* 100(3):480–485, 1995.
38. Yamasaki K, Niho Y, Yanase T: Erythroid colony forming cells in systemic lupus erythematosus. *J Rheumatol* 11(2):167–171, 1984.
39. Pyrovolaki K, Mavroudi I, Sidiropoulos P, et al: Increased expression of CD40 on bone marrow CD34+ hematopoietic progenitor cells in patients with systemic lupus erythematosus: contribution to Fas-mediated apoptosis. *Arthritis Rheum* 60(2):543–552, 2009.
40. Tiefenthaler M, Bacher N, Linert H, et al: Apoptosis of CD34+ cells after incubation with sera of leukopenic patients with systemic lupus erythematosus. *Lupus* 12(6):471–478, 2003.
41. Otsuka T, Nagasawa K, Harada M, et al: Bone marrow microenvironment of patients with systemic lupus erythematosus. *J Rheumatol* 20(6):967–971, 1993.
42. Dhote R, Simon J, Papo T, et al: Reactive hemophagocytic syndrome in adult systemic disease: report of twenty-six cases and literature review. *Arthritis Rheum* 49(5):633–669, 2003.
43. Qian J, Yang CD: Hemophagocytic syndrome as one of main manifestations in untreated systemic lupus erythematosus: two case reports and literature review. *Clin Rheumatol* 26(5):807–810, 2007.
44. Kumakura S, Ishikura H, Kondo M, et al: Autoimmune-associated hemophagocytic syndrome. *Mod Rheumatol* 14(3):205–215, 2004.
45. Ziakas PD, Giannouli S, Zintzaras E, et al: Lupus thrombocytopenia: clinical implications and prognostic significance. *Ann Rheum Dis* 64(9):1366–1369, 2005.
46. Pistiner M, Wallace DJ, Nessim S, et al: Lupus erythematosus in the 1980s: a survey of 570 patients. *Semin Arthritis Rheum* 21(1):55–64, 1991.
47. Ziakas PD, Routsias JG, Giannouli S, et al: Suspects in the tale of lupus-associated thrombocytopenia. *Clin Exp Immunol* 145(1):71–80, 2006.
48. Kuwana M, Kaburaki J, Okazaki Y, et al: Two types of autoantibody-mediated thrombocytopenia in patients with systemic lupus erythematosus. *Rheumatology (Oxford)* 45(7):851–854, 2006.
49. Kuwana M, Okazaki Y, Kajihara M, et al: Autoantibody to c-Mpl (thrombopoietin receptor) in systemic lupus erythematosus: relationship to thrombocytopenia with megakaryocytic hypoplasia. *Arthritis Rheum* 46(8):2148–2159, 2002.
50. Cervera R, Tektonidou MG, Espinosa G, et al: Task Force on Catastrophic Antiphospholipid Syndrome (APS) and Non-criteria APS Manifestations

(II): thrombocytopenia and skin manifestations. *Lupus* 20(2):174–181, 2011.

50a. Miyakis S, Lockshin MD, Atsumi T, et al: International consensus statement on an update of the classification criteria for definite antiphospholipid syndrome (APS). *J Thromb Haemost* 4(2):295–306, 2006 Feb.

51. Regan MG, Lackner H, Karpatkin S: Platelet function and coagulation profile in lupus erythematosus. Studies in 50 patients. *Ann Intern Med* 81(4):462–468, 1974.

52. Parbtani A, Frampton G, Yewdall V, et al: Platelet and plasma serotonin in glomerulonephritis. III: The nephritis of systemic lupus erythematosus. *Clin Nephrol* 14(4):164–172, 1980.

53. Arnal C, Piette JC, Léone J, et al: Treatment of severe immune thrombocytopenia associated with systemic lupus erythematosus: 59 cases. *J Rheumatol* 29(1):75–83, 2002.

54. Jacobs P, Wood L, Novitzky N, et al: Intravenous gammaglobulin has no advantages over oral corticosteroids as primary therapy for adults with immune thrombocytopenia: a prospective randomized clinical trial. *Am J Med* 97(1):55–59, 1994.

55. Boumpas DT, Barez S, Klippel JH, et al: Intermittent cyclophosphamide for the treatment of autoimmune thrombocytopenia in systemic lupus erythematosus. *Ann Intern Med* 112(9):674–677, 1990.

56. Roach BA, Hutchinson GJ: Treatment of refractory, systemic lupus erythematosus-associated thrombocytopenia with intermittent low-dose intravenous cyclophosphamide. *Arthritis Rheum* 36(5):682–684, 1993.

57. Quismorio F: Hematologic and lymphoid manifestations of SLE. In Wallace DJ, Hahn BH: *Dubois' lupus erythematosus*, ed 7, Baltimore, 2007, Lippincott Williams & Wilkins.

58. Sailler L: Rituximab off label use for difficult-to-treat auto-immune diseases: reappraisal of benefits and risks. *Clinic Rev Allerg Immunol* 34(1):103–110, 2008.

59. Hall S, McCormick JL, Jr, Greipp PR, et al: Splenectomy does not cure the thrombocytopenia of systemic lupus erythematosus. *Ann Intern Med* 102(3):325–328, 1985.

60. Wang B, Nichol JL, Sullivan JT: Pharmacodynamics and pharmacokinetics of AMG 531, a novel thrombopoietin receptor ligand. *Clin Pharmacol Ther* 76(6):628–638, 2004.

61. Hepburn AL, Narat S, Mason JC: The management of peripheral blood cytopenias in systemic lupus erythematosus. *Rheumatology (Oxford)* 49(12):2243–2254, 2010.

62. Lansigan F, Isufi I, Tagoe CE: Microangiopathic haemolytic anaemia resembling thrombotic thrombocytopenic purpura in SLE: the role of ADAMTS13. *Rheumatology (Oxford)* 50(5):824–829, 2011.

63. Kwok SK, Ju JH, Cho CS, et al: Thrombotic thrombocytopenic purpura in SLE: risk factors and outcome: a single center study. *Lupus* 18(1):16–21, 2009.

64. Letchumanan P, Ng HJ, Lee LH, et al: A comparison of TTP in an inception cohort of patients with and without SLE. *Rheumatology (Oxford)* 48(4):399–403, 2009.

65. Michael SR, Vural IL, Bassen FA, et al: The hematologic aspects of disseminated (systemic) lupus erythematosus. *Blood* 6(11):1059–1072, 1951.

66. Rivero SJ, Díaz-Jouanen E, Alarcón-Segovia D: Lymphopenia in systemic lupus erythematosus. Clinical, diagnostic, and prognostic significance. *Arthritis Rheum* 21(3):295–305, 1978.

67. Katsanis E, Hsu E, Luke KH, et al: Systemic lupus erythematosus and sickle hemoglobinopathies: a report of two cases and review of the literature. *Am J Hematol* 25(2):211–214, 1987.

68. Kondo H, Date Y, Sakai Y, et al: Effective simultaneous rhG-CSF and methylprednisolone "pulse" therapy in agranulocytosis associated with systemic lupus erythematosus. *Am J Hematol* 46(2):157–158, 1994.

69. Capsoni F, Sarzi-Puttini P, Zanella A: Primary and secondary autoimmune neutropenia. *Arthritis Res Ther* 7(5):208–214, 2005.

70. Vasiliu IM, Petri MA, Baer AN: Therapy with granulocyte colony-stimulating factor in systemic lupus erythematosus may be associated with severe flares. *J Rheumatol* 33(9):1878–1880, 2006.

71. Gewurz H, Page AR, Pickering RJ, et al: Complement activity and inflammatory neutrophil exudation in man. Studies in patients with glomerulonephritis, essential hypocomplementemia and agammaglobulinemia. *Int Arch Allergy Appl Immunol* 32(1):64–90, 1967.

72. Case records of the Massachusetts General Hospital: Weekly clinicopathological exercises. Case 42–1979. *N Engl J Med* 301(16):881–887, 1979.

73. Kojima M, Nakamura S, Morishita Y, et al: Reactive follicular hyperplasia in the lymph node lesions from systemic lupus erythematosus patients: a clinicopathological and immunohistological study of 21 cases. *Pathol Int* 50(4):304–312, 2000.

74. Larson DL: *Systemic lupus erythematosus*. Boston, 1961, Little, Brown.

75. Kaiser IH: Specificity of periarterial fibrosis of the spleen in disseminated lupus erythematosus. *Bull Johns Hopkins Hosp* 71:31–42, 1942.

Chapter 35

Clinical and Epidemiologic Features of Lupus Nephritis

Mary Anne Dooley

INTRODUCTION

Renal involvement in systemic lupus erythematosus (SLE) remains the strongest predictor of overall patient morbidity and mortality.[1] Clinical features of lupus glomerulonephritis have been recognized since the 1920s with the first pathologic findings described by 1935. Before the development of corticosteroid therapy and nitrogen mustard in the late 1940s and hemodialysis in the 1960s, the onset of lupus nephritis was associated with a significant risk of death within 2 years.[2]

Survival in lupus has improved with greater than 90% 10-year survival in many cohorts; the survival in patients with lupus nephritis lags behind at 83% over 10 years. Although mortality rates from SLE have been relatively stable among Caucasians, deaths have increased among African-American patients, particularly women ages 45 to 64 years, since the 1970s.[3] Renal involvement remains more frequent and severe among patients with African ancestry, children, and male patients.[4,5] In a London cohort of 156 patients with lupus nephritis followed for 30 years (1975 to 2005), the 5-year mortality rate (60%) significantly decreased among patients identified in the first and second decades, but the rate has not changed in the last 10 years.[6] The 5-year survival rate for end-stage renal disease (ESRD) remained constant through the study. Similarly, a long-term study of 100 patients of Dutch descent diagnosed with lupus nephritis between 1971 and 1995 found no decrease in the risk of ESRD over the study. The authors observed excess mortality with standardized mortality ratios (SMRs) of 9.0, 6.2, and 6.6 among patients diagnosed in the 1970s, 1980s, and 1990s, compared with national age-, sex-, and calendar year–matched death rates.[7] In the United States, the incidence of ESRD from lupus nephritis from 1996 to 2004 did not decline, despite the evolution of treatment and management of important co-morbidities.[8]

This chapter discusses the epidemiologic and clinical features and reviews the general management concepts of renal lupus. Detailed discussions of specific treatment modalities for renal disease are covered separately.

CLINICAL DEFINITION OF LUPUS NEPHRITIS

Active lupus nephritis can be defined clinically and histopathologically. Clinical evaluation for lupus nephritis includes dipstick and microscopic urinalysis, urinary protein and creatinine excretion, serum creatinine determinations, and serologic studies—anti–double stranded DNA (anti-dsDNA) antibody titers and serum complement components C3 and C4. The disease may further be defined as nephrotic by low serum albumin and elevated cholesterol levels. The urinary sediment is useful to characterize disease activity. The presence of glomerular hematuria, leukocyturia, or casts is typical only during periods of disease activity. The most common abnormal sediment findings are leukocyturia, hematuria, and granular casts. Chronic changes observed with nephrotic syndrome include waxy casts, oval fat bodies, and lipid droplets. In one series of 128 patients with SLE nephritis, red cell casts were present in only 39 (7.5%) of the patients.[9] Active lupus nephritis is often preceded by rising anti-DNA antibody titers and hypocomplementemia, especially low complement C3.

CLASSIFICATION CRITERIA

Lupus renal disease may also be defined immunohistopathologically. Tissue obtained by renal biopsy should be evaluated by light microscopy (LM), immunofluorescence (IF), and electron microscopy (EM). A correlation exists between the pathologic class of lupus nephritis and its clinical features.[10,11] Despite this association, patients with so-called silent lupus nephritis have normal urinalyses, an absence of proteinuria, and normal serum creatinine; however, on renal biopsy, they also have anywhere from mesangial to proliferative nephritis.[12] Fortunately, progressive loss of renal function typically does not occur without changes in urinary sediment and protein excretion. Lupus glomerulonephritis is now defined by the International Society of Nephrology (ISN); its classification was developed by nephropathologists in conjunction with rheumatologists and nephrologists.[13] Because prognosis and therapeutic guidelines from many clinical trials have been based on the prior system, the ISN classification (discussed in Chapter 49) must be compared with the preexisting World Health Organization (WHO) classification system and the activity and chronicity indices developed by the National Institutes of Health (NIH). The activity and chronicity indices are no longer scored numerically in the ISN classification, but the features are described. Patients with prior biopsies may have WHO staging to compare with ISN classification on subsequent biopsies. Studies have validated the relationship of the ISN scoring system with clinical outcomes to date and have shown improved inter-rater reliability.[14]

HISTOPATHOLOGIC CLASSIFICATIONS OF LUPUS NEPHRITIS

Lupus nephritis is extremely pleomorphic. All four renal compartments—glomeruli, tubules, interstitium, and blood vessels—may be affected. Adjacent glomeruli from a single biopsy may show variable involvement, as may the biopsies from patients with similar clinical manifestations. Over time, glomerular lesions may transform from one pattern to another. Throughout the years, investigators have sought to define and quantify the many morphologic lesions of lupus nephritis in a comprehensive, systematic fashion. The earliest classifications of renal involvement in patients with SLE divided glomerular changes only into mild forms (lupus glomerulitis), severe proliferative forms (active lupus glomerulonephritis), and membranous glomerulopathy.[15,16]

Three major classification systems have been proposed over the last three decades. The original WHO classification was formulated in 1974 and recognized five major classes of lupus nephritis.[17,18] In 1982, a modified WHO classification was promulgated by the International Study of Kidney Disease in Children (ISKDC) with further revisions in 1995.[19,20] It defines six major classes of lupus nephritis and a large number of subclasses with an emphasis on distribution, activity, and chronicity of the lesions. Although significantly more detailed and precise than the original classification, the modified WHO classification has not been as widely accepted because of its greater complexity with excessive reliance on subclasses. Moreover, its treatment of mixed or overlapping classes of lupus nephritis has been controversial. A third classification, proposed in 2004 by a consensus conference organized jointly by the ISN and the Renal Pathology Society (RPS), retains the simplicity of the original WHO classification but incorporates some of the refinements introduced by the modified WHO classification.[13,21] The ISN/RPS classification has the advantage of standardizing pathologic criteria and defining the distinctions among the classes more precisely.

PATHOLOGIC FEATURES OF LUPUS NEPHRITIS ACCORDING TO THE INTERNATIONAL SOCIETY OF NEPHROLOGY/RENAL PATHOLOGY SOCIETY CLASSIFICATION

Class I: Minimal Mesangial Lupus Nephritis

Class I denotes normal glomeruli by LM with mesangial immune deposits detected by IF or EM or both. The original WHO class I, defined as an entirely normal renal biopsy, was rarely if ever encountered because such patients typically have no clinical renal abnormalities and are not subjected to renal biopsy. Therefore the "normal" category was eliminated from the ISN/RPS classification. By LM the glomeruli are normocellular (Figure 35-1). By IF, immune deposits are limited to the mesangium. The mesangial deposits tend to be small and vary from segmental to global in distribution. By EM, corresponding electron-dense deposits are present in the mesangium but without involvement of the peripheral glomerular capillary walls.

Class II: Mesangial Proliferative Lupus Nephritis

Class II is defined as pure mesangial hypercellularity of any degree and/or mesangial matrix expansion by LM with mesangial immune deposits. Mesangial hypercellularity is defined as three or more mesangial cells in mesangial areas away from the vascular pole, assessed in 3-micron-thick histologic sections. The mesangial proliferation is usually mild to moderate and does not compromise the glomerular capillary lumina (Figure 35-2). By IF, granular mesangial immune deposits are visualized. The pattern by IF outlines the axial framework of the glomerulus, corresponding to the mesangial stalk.

By EM, electron-dense deposits are revealed within the mesangial matrix. Strictly speaking, pure class II lupus nephritis should have no detectable subendothelial or subepithelial deposits. However, in practice, some cases of purely mesangial proliferative lupus nephritis will manifest rare, small subendothelial electron-dense deposits, particularly extending out from the adjacent mesangium. Lupus nephritis with severe but purely mesangial hypercellularity and without obliteration of the capillary lumina may pose difficulties in classification. If EM and IF confirm that the immune deposits are limited to the mesangium, then even cases of severe diffuse mesangial proliferation should be classified as class II. If significant subendothelial deposits are observed by IF or EM or if they are visible by LM, then the case should be classified as focal proliferative (class III) or diffuse proliferative (class IV), depending on their distribution.

Class III: Focal Lupus Nephritis and Class IV: Diffuse Lupus Nephritis

Most investigators consider class III and class IV lupus nephritis to be qualitatively similar glomerular lesions that differ only in severity and distribution. Therefore these two related classes are described together. Class III lupus nephritis is defined as focal segmental and/or global endocapillary and/or extracapillary glomerulonephritis affecting less that 50% of the total glomeruli sampled (Figure 35-3). Class IV is defined as diffuse segmental and/or global endocapillary and/or extracapillary glomerulonephritis affecting 50% or more of the total glomeruli (Figure 35-4). Both class III and class IV manifest subendothelial immune deposits (relatively focal in class III and diffuse in class IV), with or without mesangial alterations. The ISN/RPS classification subdivides lupus nephritis class IV into those cases with diffuse segmental and those with diffuse global proliferation (Table 35-1). The designation IV-S is used if more than 50% of the affected glomeruli have segmental lesions (Figure 35-5); the designation IV-G is used if more than 50% of the affected glomeruli have global lesions (see Figure 35-4). This subdivision was proposed to facilitate future

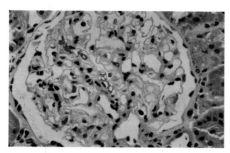

FIGURE 35-1 Lupus nephritis class I. Glomerular tuft is normocellular with patent capillaries and glomerular basement membranes of normal thickness (hematoxylin and eosin, ×400).

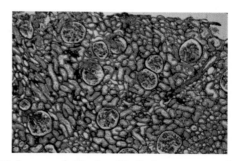

FIGURE 35-3 Lupus nephritis class III. On low-power examination, focal and segmental proliferation of the glomeruli is demonstrated. Overall, endocapillary or extracapillary proliferation affected less than 50% of the total glomeruli in this biopsy, qualifying this case as class III (Jones methenamine silver stain, ×4).

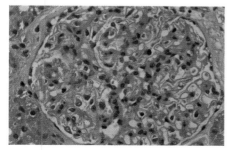

FIGURE 35-2 Lupus nephritis class II. Mild global mesangial hypercellularity is present (hematoxylin and eosin, ×400).

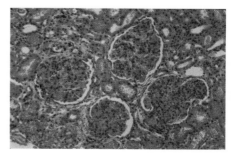

FIGURE 35-4 Lupus nephritis class IV-G. Pattern of diffuse and global endocapillary proliferation is demonstrated. All four glomeruli illustrate a similar degree of glomerular involvement (hematoxylin and eosin, ×80).

TABLE 35-1 International Society of Nephrology and Renal Pathology Society Classification of Lupus Nephritis (2004)

Class I	Minimal mesangial LN Normal glomeruli by LM, but mesangial immune deposits by LF
Class II	Mesangial proliferative LN Purely mesangial hypercellularity of any degree of mesangial matrix expansion by LM with mesangial immune deposits Possibly a few isolated subepithelial or subendothelial deposits visible by IF or EM but not by LM
Class III	Focal LN* Active or inactive focal, segmental and/or global endocapillary and/or extracapillary GN involving <50% of all glomeruli, typically with focal subendothelial immune deposits, with or without mesangial alterations
Class III (A)	Purely active lesions: focal proliferative LN
Class III (A/C)	Active and chronic lesions: focal proliferative and sclerosing LN
Class III (C)	Chronic inactive with glomerular scars: focal sclerosing LN
Class IV	Diffuse LN* Active and inactive diffuse, segmental and/or global endocapillary and/or extracapillary GN involving ≥50% of all glomeruli, typically with diffuse subendothelial immune deposits, with or without mesangial alterations Divided into diffuse segmental proliferative (IV-S), in which >50% of the involved glomeruli have segmental lesions, and diffuse global proliferative (IV-G), in which >50% of the involved glomeruli have global lesions Segmental is defined as a glomerular lesion that involves less than one half of the glomerular tuft
Class IV-S (A) or IV-G (A)	Purely active lesions; diffuse segmental or global proliferative LN
Class IV-S (A/C) or IV-G (A/C)	Active and chronic lesions; diffuse segmental or global proliferative and sclerosing LN
Class IV-S (C) or IV-G (C)	Inactive with glomerular scars: diffuse segmental or global sclerosing LN
Class V	Membranous LN† Global or segmental subepithelial immune deposits or their morphologic sequelae by LM and by IF or EM, with or without mesangial alterations
Class VI	Advanced sclerosing LN ≥90% of glomeruli globally sclerosed without residual activity

Definitions of pathologic terms: *Diffuse*, lesion involving most (≥50%) glomeruli; *endocapillary proliferation*, endocapillary hypercellularity as a result of an increased number of mesangial cells, endothelial cells, and infiltrating monocytes, causing a narrowing of the glomerular capillary lumina; *extracapillary proliferation or cellular crescent*, extracapillary cell proliferation of more than two cell layers occupying one fourth or more of the glomerular capsular circumference; *focal*, lesion involving <50% of glomeruli; *global*, lesion involving more than one half of the glomerular tuft; *hyaline thrombi*, intracapillary eosinophilic material of a homogeneous consistency that, by IF, has been shown to consist of immune deposits; *karyorrhexis*, presence of apoptotic, pyknotic, and fragmented nuclei; *mesangial hypercellularity*, ≥3 mesangial cells per mesangial region in a 3 μg-thick section; *necrosis*, lesion characterized by fragmentation of nuclei or disruption of the basement membrane and often associated with the presence of fibrin-rich material; *segmental*, lesion involving less than one half of the glomerular tuft.
Proportion of involved glomeruli indicates the percentage of total glomeruli affected by lupus nephritis, excluding ischemic glomeruli with inadequate perfusion as a result of vascular pathologic features separate from LGN.
Combination of class III and class V requires membranous involvement of at least 50% of the glomerular capillary surface area of at least 50% of glomeruli by LM or IF.
Combination of class IV and class V requires membranous involvement of at least 50% of the glomerular capillary surface area of at least 50% of glomeruli by LM or IF.
In the report, active lesions have to be specified; the percentage of glomeruli with capillary wall disruption (necrosis) and crescents should be included in the diagnostic line.
*Indicates the proportion of glomeruli with active and sclerotic lesions.
Indicates the proportion of glomeruli with fibrinoid necrosis and with cellular crescents.
Indicates the grade (e.g., mild, moderate, severe) tubular atrophy, interstitial inflammation and fibrosis, severity of arteriosclerosis, or other vascular lesions.
†May occur in combination with class III or IV, in which case both will be diagnosed; may show advanced sclerosis.
EM, Electron microscopy; GN, glomerulonephritis; IF, immunofluorescence; LGN, lupus glomerulonephritis; LM, light microscopy; LN, lupus nephritis.

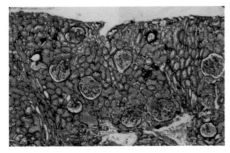

FIGURE 35-5 Lupus nephritis class IV-S. Low-power examination of the biopsy shows a pattern of diffuse glomerular proliferation involving more than 50% of the glomeruli with a predominantly segmental distribution and involving a portion of each glomerular tuft (Jones methenamine silver stain, ×4).

studies addressing possible differences in outcome and pathogenesis among these subgroups.

Both class III and class IV may have active (proliferative) or inactive (sclerosing) lesions or both. In determining the percentage of total glomeruli affected by glomerulonephritis, both the proliferative

and sclerosing lesions must be taken into account. Although most active glomerular lesions are endocapillary proliferative in nature, both class III and class IV factor in glomerular lesions that are membranoproliferative or extracapillary proliferative, or consist of wire-loop deposits without associated proliferation. For these reasons, the ISN classification prefers the broader terms *focal lupus nephritis* and *diffuse lupus nephritis* over the more restrictive terms *focal proliferative lupus nephritis* and *diffuse proliferative lupus nephritis*, which are used in the original WHO classification.

The endocapillary proliferative lesions in class III tend to be relatively segmental (involving only a portion of the glomerular tuft), although some glomeruli may be affected globally. In class IV, the endocapillary proliferation is typically more diffuse and global. However, some examples of class IV have a diffuse and segmental distribution (designated IV-S in the ISN/RPS classification). The glomerular lesions in class III and class IV are qualitatively similar. Common light microscopic features include wire-loop deposits, hyaline thrombi, leukocyte infiltration, necrosis, hematoxylin bodies, cellular crescents, and glomerular scarring, each of which is described in the following text.

In class III and class IV lupus nephritis, subendothelial immune deposits may be large enough to detect with LM, forming wire-loop thickenings of the glomerular capillary walls. Special stains reveal the deposits to be entirely or largely subendothelial, with preservation of an outer peripheral layer of glomerular basement membrane. In some cases, the subendothelial deposits are incorporated into the glomerular capillary wall by a subendothelial layer of neomembrane, producing a double contour. This may be accompanied by mesangial interposition, giving a membranoproliferative appearance. Some cases of class II or class IV exhibit large intracapillary deposits forming *hyaline thrombi*. This term is actually a misnomer; these represent not true fibrin thrombi but massive intracapillary immune deposits with the same composition by IF as the neighboring subendothelial immune deposits.

In most cases of class III and class IV lupus nephritis, the endocapillary hypercellularity results from the proliferation of glomerular endothelial and mesangial cells, as well as by leukocyte infiltration, including neutrophils, monocytes, and lymphocytes. However, several morphologic variants of class IV lack the typical picture of florid endocapillary proliferation with leukocyte infiltration. The first is the membranoproliferative variant. In this form, the endocapillary proliferation has a distinctly membranoproliferative aspect, with extensive mesangial interposition and duplication of glomerular basement membranes resembling membranoproliferative glomerulonephritis type 1. Other histologic variations include diffuse wire-loop deposits without glomerular hypercellularity or diffuse wire-loop deposits accompanied by mesangial proliferation. In each of these histologic variants, the *sine qua non* of active class IV is the presence of diffuse subendothelial deposits, albeit with variable patterns of glomerular proliferation.

Glomerular necrosis is a feature of active class III and class IV lupus nephritis and consists of foci of smudgy fibrinoid degeneration of the glomerular tuft. Necrosis may be accompanied by the deposition of intracapillary fibrin, glomerular basement membrane (GBM) rupture, and apoptosis of infiltrating neutrophils, producing pyknotic or karyorrhectic nuclear debris, referred to as *nuclear dust*. Necrotizing lesions are typically segmental in distribution, but more than one glomerular lobule may be affected, particularly in diffuse proliferative lupus nephritis.

Hematoxylin bodies are the only truly pathognomonic lesion of lupus nephritis. However, they are extremely uncommon, affecting less than 2% of biopsy specimens of lupus nephritis.[22] They consist of smudgy lilac-staining structures that may be smaller or larger than normal nuclei. They may be isolated or clustered and usually occur in glomeruli with very active proliferative and necrotizing lesions. Hematoxylin bodies are the tissue equivalent of the lupus erythematosus body and consist of naked nuclei whose chromatin has been altered after cell death with the extrusion of the nucleus and binding to ambient circulating antinuclear antibodies (ANAs).

Cellular crescents are a feature of active lupus nephritis that may be frequently encountered in both class III and class IV lupus nephritis. They are common overlying necrotizing lesions. Glomerular scarring is a feature of chronic glomerular injury in class III and class IV lupus nephritis. In class III, the glomerular scarring is often initially focal and segmental. Associated fibrous crescents may form synechiae to the sclerotic segments. In chronic class IV lupus nephritis, the glomerular scarring is typically more global and diffuse.

By IF, in class III and IV lupus nephritis, subendothelial immune deposits generally follow the distribution of the endocapillary proliferation. Thus subendothelial deposits tend to be relatively focal and segmental in class III and more diffuse and global in class IV lupus nephritis. These subendothelial deposits are typically superimposed on generalized mesangial immune deposits. Hyaline thrombi form occlusive intracapillary globular deposits. Scattered subepithelial deposits are not uncommon in class III or class IV and usually have a more finely granular quality. However, according to the ISN/RPS classification, the presence of regular subepithelial deposits involving over 50% of the glomerular capillary surface area of at least 50% of glomeruli exceeds what is acceptable in class III or class IV alone and would warrant an additional diagnosis of membranous lupus

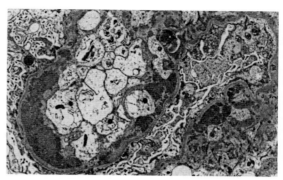

FIGURE 35-6 Lupus nephritis class IV. Electron microscopy (EM) shows a representative glomerular capillary with a large subendothelial electron-dense deposit located between the endothelium and the overlying glomerular basement membrane. Smaller electron-dense deposits are present in the adjacent mesangium at the bottom (×3000).

nephritis class V. By EM, class III and class IV lupus nephritis typically display subendothelial electron-dense deposits that tend to be focal and segmental in class III and more diffuse and global in class IV, superimposed on a substratum of mesangial deposits (Figure 35-6). The extent and distribution of deposits observed by EM usually parallels that visualized with IF. Rare cases of class III or class IV lupus nephritis have relatively sparse subendothelial deposits, relative to the extent and severity of the active necrotizing lesions. Such cases resemble examples of pauci-immune focal segmental necrotizing glomerulonephritis, and some may be associated with antineutrophil cytoplasmic antibodies (ANCAs).

Class V: Membranous Lupus Nephritis

Class V designates membranous lupus nephritis, as defined by subepithelial immune deposits or their morphologic sequelae. The membranous alterations may be present alone or on a background of mesangial hypercellularity and mesangial immune deposits. IF or EM or both, but not LM, may identify a few small subendothelial immune deposits.

In the modified WHO classification, membranous lupus nephritis was subdivided into four subclasses, designated Va through Vd. Being familiar with these categories is important, because older outcome studies frequently used these designations. Class Va denotes pure membranous lupus nephritis without associated mesangial deposits or mesangial proliferation. Class Vb includes the typical peripheral capillary wall features of membranous glomerulopathy, together with mesangial alterations, either mesangial deposits alone or with mesangial hypercellularity. The modified WHO classification also recognizes class Vc (combined class Va and class III), in which the typical features of focal and segmental endocapillary proliferative glomerulonephritis are superimposed on the membranous pattern, and class Vd (combined class Va and class IV), in which superimposed diffuse endocapillary proliferative and membranous lupus nephritis is evident. A major disadvantage of this system is that it places undue emphasis on the membranous component rather than on the more serious proliferative component. According to the ISN classification, the designation mixed class III and class V replaces the Vc lesion, and the designation mixed class IV and class V replaces the Vd lesion. In this schema, the additional designation of class V in the setting of class III or class IV requires membranous involvement of at least 50% of glomerular capillary surface area of at least 50% of glomeruli visualized by LM or IF or both. This approach is amply supported by clinical pathologic studies that demonstrate that class Vd has an extremely poor prognosis, even worse than that of pure diffuse proliferative class IV.[23]

By LM, the peripheral glomerular capillary wall alterations display a spectrum and evolution similar to those of idiopathic membranous glomerulopathy. In the early stages, the glomerular capillary walls may appear normal in thickness and texture by LM, but subepithelial deposits are detected by IF and EM. At this stage, the glomerular capillaries often have a rigid, ecstatic appearance with visceral epithelial cell swelling. Well-established membranous lesions are typically characterized by uniform and diffuse thickening of glomerular capillary walls (Figure 35-7) with well-developed spikes of the GBM that are best demonstrated with the silver stain. As the lesions evolve, the deposits may become largely resorbed and overlaid by neomembrane formation, producing a vacuolated GBM profile.

Patients with lupus nephritis class V are at risk for developing renal vein thrombosis. Examination of the renal biopsy may provide clues to the occurrence of superimposed renal vein thrombosis. Suspicious findings include erythrocyte congestion and focal fibrin thrombosis of the glomerular capillaries, as well as diffuse interstitial edema. In chronic renal vein thrombosis, there may be diffuse tubular atrophy and interstitial fibrosis out of proportion to the degree of glomerular sclerosis.

A diagnosis of class V is based on the presence of global or segmental continuous granular subepithelial immune deposits by IF. A background of mesangial immune deposits is commonly observed. By EM, electron-dense subepithelial deposits range from small to large but involve the majority of capillaries. As the disease progresses, the same ultrastructural stages observed in idiopathic membranous glomerulopathy may evolve. GBM spikes often separate the subepithelial deposits. In more chronic cases, the deposits become overlaid by neomembrane and later become resorbed and relatively electron lucent. Extensive foot process effacement is exhibited in the distribution of the subepithelial deposits. Mesangial electron-dense deposits are commonly observed. Sparse, small subendothelial electron-dense deposits also may be found but are not accompanied by endocapillary proliferation.

Class VI: Advanced Sclerosing Lupus Nephritis

Class VI is defined by global glomerular sclerosis affecting more than 90% of glomeruli without residual activity. Most such cases likely represent advanced class IV disease. However, patients with class V or repeated flares of class III also may progress to end-stage and manifest this pattern late in their course. By LM, extensive global glomerular sclerosis involves over 90% of glomeruli without significant ongoing activity. Some glomeruli may be segmentally sclerotic. Glomeruli with less advanced sclerosis may display residual hypercellularity or thickenings of the GBMs. Vestiges of old crescents may be discernible with the periodic acid–Schiff (PAS) stain as subcapsular fibrous proliferations with disruptions of the Bowman capsule. Severe tubular atrophy, interstitial fibrosis inflammation, and arteriosclerosis usually accompany the glomerular sclerosis. In some cases, the process is so end-stage that a diagnosis of chronic lupus nephritis is difficult on morphologic grounds. By IF, some residual immune deposits are usually discovered in the few nonsclerotic glomeruli, as well as in the obsolescent glomeruli. Granular deposits may also be detected in the tubulointerstitial compartment or vessel walls.

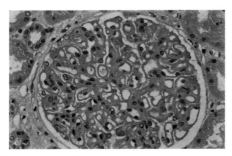

FIGURE 35-7 Lupus nephritis class V. Membranous lupus nephritis displays a global thickening of the glomerular capillary walls, which have a rigid aspect. Several mesangial areas also appear mildly hypercellular (hematoxylin and eosin, ×500).

EPIDEMIOLOGIC FEATURES

The renal criteria for the American College of Rheumatology (ACR) are defined as persistent proteinuria (>0.5 g/day or ≤3+), or cellular casts of any kind[24] (see Chapter 1). By these criteria, the prevalence of renal disease in eight large cohort studies consisting of 2649 patients with SLE varied from 31% to 65%.[2] Tertiary referral centers tended to have higher percentages of patients with renal disease, as did studies that were published before 1965 (when ANAs became widely available and identified more mild cases of patients with SLE). The mean age at disease onset in patients with nephritis is younger than in those patients with SLE but without nephritis (Wallace and colleagues[9] reported disease onset at 4 years younger [27 versus 31 years of age] and 230 versus 379 patients, respectively). Nossent and associates[7] also observed a similar difference in 110 patients of Dutch descent. Most patients develop nephritis early in their disease course; the onset of renal disease can occur at any point in the patient's disease course. Nephritis is present in most children. Although it was once thought rare in older adults, subsequent studies have shown that race confounded the relationship of lupus nephritis with age of onset of disease.[25] When race is controlled, patients with older-onset lupus do not have *milder* features, and the outcome of lupus is worse as a result of the increased prevalence of co-morbidities.[26]

The incidence and prevalence of SLE nephritis differ among patients of different racial and ethnic backgrounds. Despite much investigative attention, these differences in lupus expression remain poorly understood. African Americans have a threefold increased incidence of SLE, develop the disorder at younger ages, more frequently develop nephritis, and more frequently express anti-Smith (anti-Sm) and ribonucleoprotein (RNP) autoantibodies.[2] African-American patients develop nephritis earlier in the course of their SLE. In an inception cohort of 265 lupus patients in the southeastern United States, 31% of African-American patients versus 13% of Caucasian patients met ACR renal criteria within 18 months of diagnosis[27] (Table 35-2). Patients of Hispanic ethnicity develop nephritis more frequently than Caucasians.[28] Once they have nephritis, African Americans and Hispanics are more likely to progress to ESRD than Caucasians.[27,28] These findings have also been reported in cohorts based in London and Toronto with National Health Care systems.[29,30] Patients of Asian descent also have greater frequency and severity of nephritis compared with Caucasians. However, Asians generally have good outcomes of cytotoxic therapy.[31] Patients with lupus and nephritis are more likely than patients without renal involvement to have a family history of diabetes, hypertension, and renal disease (Table 35-3). The annual incidence of nephritis in 384 patients with

TABLE 35-2 Findings in Patients with Systemic Lupus Erythematosus and Nephritis (*n* = 128) Compared with Those without Nephritis (*n* = 336)*

MORE FREQUENT	LESS FREQUENT
Family history of SLE	Other CNS symptoms
Anemia	Seizures
High sedimentation rate	Thrombocytopenia
High serum cholesterol	Fibromyalgia
High serum triglycerides	
Positive ANAs	
High anti-dsDNA	
Low C3 complement	
Low C4 complement	

*$p < 0.01$
ANAs, Antinuclear antibodies; anti-dsDNA, anti–double stranded DNA; CNS, central nervous system; SLE, systemic lupus erythematosus.

TABLE 35-3 History of Kidney Disease, Hypertension, and Diabetes in First-Degree Relatives (Parents or Siblings)*

	NEW RECRUITED PATIENTS WITH LUPUS NEPHRITIS (N = 93)	PATIENTS WITH LUPUS BUT WITHOUT NEPHRITIS (N = 147)	ODDS RATIO (95% CI)†		ALL PATIENTS WITH LUPUS NEPHRITIS (N = 140)	COMPARISON OF PATIENTS WITH LUPUS BUT WITHOUT NEPHRITIS OR (95% CI)†
Kidney Disease						
No	68 (73)	129 (90)	1.0 (referent)	1	109 (78)	1.0 (referent)
Yes	25 (27)	15 (10)	4.7 (2.1, 10.8)		31 (22)	3.6 (1.7, 7.9)
	(0 missing)	(3 missing)			(0 missing)	
Dialysis						
No	86 (93)	140 (97)	1.0 (referent)		129 (93)	1.0 (referent)
yes	6 (7)	4 (3)	3.3 (0.71, 15.2)		10 (7)	3.7 (0.94, 14.7)
	(1 missing)	(3 missing)			(1 missing)	
Hypertension						
No	27 (29)	64 (44)	1.0 (referent)		50 (36)	1.0 (referent)
yes	65 (71)	80 (56)	2.2 (1.2, 4.2)		89 (64)	1.7 (1.0, 3.0)
	(1 missing)	(3 missing)			(1 missing)	
Diabetes						
No	56 (61)	93 (65)	1.0 (referent)		91 (65)	1.0 (referent)
yes	36 (39)	51 (35)	1.3 (0.71, 2.5)		48 (35)	0.98 (0.56, 1.7)
	(1 missing)	(3 missing)			(1 missing)	

*Southeastern United States inception cohort[27] with an additional 93 patients with biopsy-defined lupus nephritis with onset during the study period.
†Patients with CLU (follow-up): Did any of these relatives ever have…? If yes, specific questions are asked of specific relatives.
†Patients with lupus nephritis: Specific questions are asked of the mother, father, and each sibling.
CI, Confidence interval; CLU, Carolina Lupus Study; OR, odds ratio.

established lupus followed at the Johns Hopkins Medical Center between 1992 and 1994 was 10%.[32]

Important co-morbidities such as diabetes, hypertension, patient compliance with medical regimens, and socioeconomic and psychosocial variables may also influence renal outcomes. In several studies, however, the worse outcome for African-American patients with lupus nephritis was independent of health care access, compliance with medications, and socioeconomic status. Others have shown a strong impact of poverty on renal outcomes. Although African-American patients had more frequent or uncontrolled hypertension, hypocomplementemia, and higher chronicity indices including interstitial fibrosis in some patient series, other series report poorer response to intravenous cyclophosphamide (IVC), independent of these factors. In a series of 86 patients with class IV nephritis, renal survival after NIH protocol intermittent IVC was 95% at 5 years in Caucasians but 79% at 1 year and 58% at 5 years in African-American patients.[33] Similarly, the Lupus Nephritis Collaborative Study Group reported that African-American race significantly affected renal and patient survival in the Lewis plasmapheresis trial. In black patients, renal survival was 38% at 10 years compared with 68% in whites; overall patient survival was 38% in black compared to 68% in white patients.[34] A retrospective study of a cohort of 213 patients with lupus nephritis noted that black patients and Hispanic patients had significantly greater frequency of ESRD or doubling of serum creatinine than the non-Hispanic whites from the cohort (31% black, 18% Hispanic patients compared with 10% white patients).[35] The influence of race and ethnicity on response to therapy with IVC and mycophenolate mofetil (MMF) was striking in the global Aspreva Lupus Management Study (ALMS) induction trial[36] (Figure 35-8).

Lupus nephritis is only one of many kidney diseases in which African-American patients suffer more frequent adverse consequences. African ancestry may also be associated with a non–lupus-related predisposition to kidney failure after renal injury. African-American patients with hypertension, diabetes mellitus, focal segmental sclerosis, or human immunodeficiency viral (HIV)

nephropathy develop renal failure significantly more often than Caucasian patients. Although variants of myosin heavy chain 9 (MYH9) have been associated with focal segmental glomerulosclerosis (FSGS) in African Americans, its frequency is not increased in patients with lupus nephritis.[37]

Inheritance of the DR2 and B8 genes is associated with an increased risk of developing nephritis in some populations, and this risk is amplified if certain DQ-beta genes also are present (see Chapter 4, Genetics of Human Systemic Lupus Erythematosus). Inheritance of the DR4 gene reduces the risk for lupus nephritis.[2] Several studies have shown that allelic variants of the immunoglobulin G (IgG) fragmented, crystallizable gamma receptors (FcγR) RIIA and RIIIA, associated with poor binding and phagocytosis of IgG1 and IgG2, increase the risk for lupus nephritis in several populations. However, the association has not been found in all populations. In recent metaanalyses including data on over 3000 patients with lupus, the population-attributable fractions of SLE cases from the FcγRIIA-R131 allele were 13%, 40%, and 24% in patients of European, African, and Asian descents, respectively. These findings were not a risk for lupus nephritis. Other researchers have noted an angiotensin-converting enzyme gene that may be associated with lupus. An interferon alpha (IFN-α) signature has been reported in patients with SLE, although not uniformly associated with disease activity or manifestations.[2]

CLINICAL AND LABORATORY PRESENTATIONS

Klippel[38] described five clinical types of lupus nephritis: occult, chronic active nephritis, rapidly progressive nephritis, nephrotic syndrome, and progressive renal insufficiency in patients with repeatedly normal urinalyses. Glomerulosclerosis, hypertension, diabetes, and, occasionally, medications—especially nonsteroidal antiinflammatory drugs (NSAIDs)—are likely the cause of renal insufficiency in the last group. Patients in this group, along with those with occult disease and chronic active nephritis, are often asymptomatic. These five clinical subtypes reflect the extraordinary range of expression of

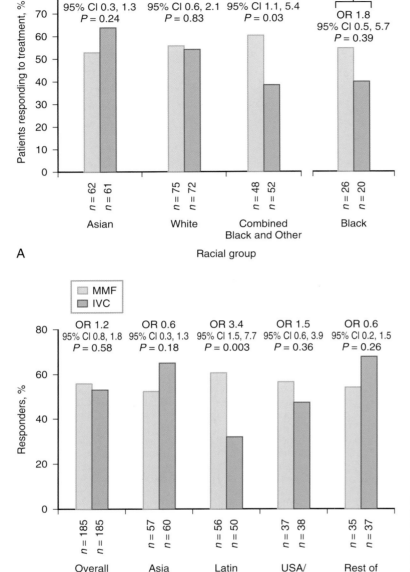

FIGURE 35-8 A, Percentage of patients in the induction study of the Aspreva Lupus Management Study (ALMS) responding to therapy by race and treatment group; African American is a subset of the "other" racial group. **B,** Percentage of patients responding to therapy by region and treatment group (intent-to-treat populations). *(From Isenberg D, Appel GB, Contreras G, et al: Influence of race/ethnicity on response to lupus nephritis treatment: the ALMS study. Rheumatology 49:128–140, 2010.)*

lupus nephritis. Mesangial lupus nephritis is often accompanied by normal diagnostic findings or a mild degree of proteinuria but not typically by hypertension or abnormal urinary sediment. Focal and diffuse proliferative lupus glomerulonephritis are often associated with the worst prognosis for renal survival. Both can be accompanied by nephrotic syndrome, significant hypertension, and abnormal urine sediment. Presentation with acute renal failure was observed in 36 of 196 (18.4%) patients with SLE who were admitted to the hospital in the group monitored by Yeung and others.[39] Infection and lupus activity, including central nervous system disease, were frequently associated. Recovery of renal function with aggressive management was reported in 76% of patients. Others have confirmed these findings, even in patients requiring dialysis at presentation.[33]

Membranous lupus nephritis often exhibits moderate-to-severe proteinuria without hematuria or casts and often in the absence of hypertension. The majority of these patients have a good prognosis and relative preservation of renal function. However, in up to one third of patients with membranous lupus nephritis, decreased renal function and ESRD may occur.[40]

Nephrotic syndrome (defined as a serum albumin less than 2.8 g/dl with greater than 3.5 g/24 hr of urine protein) was observed in 13% to 26% of patients in eight well-detailed series.[2] Patients who were mildly proteinuric may only have ankle edema on examination; frankly nephrotic states are associated with ascites and presacral edema, as well as pleural and pericardial effusions. Serositis as a result of lupus may be distinguished from uremia because inflammatory effusions will have exudative rather than transudative features. Physical examinations are often deceptively normal except for blood pressure measurements in patients with isolated lupus nephritis. Indeed, as these patients are often young, blood pressure measurements may well be lower than 140/90 mm Hg but are hypertensive for the age of the patient. Patients with SLE have an increased incidence of renal tubular dysfunction, characterized by a proximal or distal renal tubular acidosis. This dysfunction is particularly evident in patients with Sjögren syndrome.

Serologic Indicators Associated with Lupus Nephritis

Usually, no one test result allows the practitioner to take any particular course of action unless it is consistently abnormal or supported by the clinical picture and other confirmatory laboratory tests.

Antinuclear Antibodies

ANA tests are a sensitive screening tool; more than 95% of patients with lupus will be positive when the test is performed using a substrate containing human nuclei such as human epithelial-2 (HEp-2) cells. Increasingly, large commercial laboratories are abandoning tissue-based IF assays for the enzyme-linked immunosorbent assay (ELISA) or bead assays. Although these tests are less expensive and less subjective, concern has been raised that some positive ANA results may be missed. In a patient with a strong clinical picture for lupus and a negative ANA result, the test should be repeated in a reliable laboratory using a human cell line. A positive test for ANA is not specific for those with SLE; positive ANA results may also occur in other rheumatic diseases, with treatment using certain biologic agents, in infections, or in malignancies—especially lymphoreticular malignancies. Approximately 15% of normal aging individuals above age 65 years will have positive ANA tests. The majority of these individuals are women, and the antibody levels are low titer. Many healthy family members of patients with lupus have detectable serum antinuclear and other autoantibodies. Increased incidence of positive ANA tests in spouses of patients with lupus and in laboratory workers handling lupus sera have been observed.[2]

Complement

Various tests of complement available in the clinical laboratory are relevant to lupus nephritis: C3, C4, total hemolytic complement, antibodies to complement 1q (C1q), and C3d:C4d ratios. (See Chapters 14, Complement and Systemic Lupus Erythematosus, and 43, Clinical Application of Serologic Tests, Serum Protein Abnormalities, and Other Clinical Laboratory Tests in Systemic Lupus Erythematosus, for a review of the biologic and clinical importance of complement). A low C3 level correlates with activity indices on biopsy, and the long-term normalization of complement is associated with a better prognosis. Conversely, low complement levels also may denote congenital or acquired deficiencies of various components, and some patients have persistently low complement levels with no clinical evidence of disease activity. Recently, long-term follow-up has confirmed continued serologic activity but clinical quiescence for 15 years in patients taking no medications.[41]

Anti–Double Stranded DNA

Anti-dsDNA antibody levels are elevated in most patients with active nephritis. Test methods include the *Crithidia luciliae* test, the ELISA, bead assays, or the Farr assay to quantitate its presence. Anti-DNA is found in 50% to 75% of patients with active nephritis but may be absent in patients with pure membranous disease. Anti-dsDNA antibodies, once thought to be highly specific for diagnosing SLE, may occur in patients receiving a number of biologic therapies including anti–necrosis factor alpha (anti–TNF-α) inhibitors and INF-α. Typically, these drug-induced dsDNA antibody titers are low, and renal involvement is rare. The presence of anti-Smith (anti-Sm) antibodies is highly specific for those with SLE. However, it is detected in only 15% to 30% of patients, more frequently in African-American patients than in Caucasians.

Other Tests

Other clinical correlates useful in reflecting renal disease activity have been sought. These include cryoglobulins, autoantibodies to poly(adenosine diphosphate [ADP]-ribose) polymerase inhibition, circulating immune complexes, interleukin (IL) 2 receptor levels, ANA patterns, antiendothelial-cell antibody levels, plasma thrombomodulin, and measurement of the activation and degradation components of complement (see Chapter 14, Complement and Systemic Lupus Erythematosus). These tests are not universally available or are less reliable than those discussed earlier in this chapter.

Measurements of Renal Function

The principal tests to evaluate renal function are blood urea nitrogen (BUN), serum creatinine, and creatinine clearance. The utility of the BUN is limited by its alteration with hydration status, bleeding, and hepatic and dietary conditions. In clinical practice, the most convenient serial measurement of renal function is the serum creatinine. Serum creatinine levels can vary with body weight, muscle mass, and state of hydration. Measurements of serum creatinine tend to overestimate renal function by as much as 20% because they do not account for proximal tubular creatinine secretion. Creatinine is hypersecreted by injured tubules in patients with glomerulopathy. Administering cimetidine (400 mg) tablets four times a day for 2 days blocks tubular secretion of creatinine and provides a more reliable measure of the glomerular filtration rate (GFR). Because creatinine is calculated on a logarithmic scale, a rise from 1 to 2 mg/dL represents a 50% change, whereas a rise from 6 to 7 mg/dL reflects only a 3% change. Often, clinical investigators must use the ratio 1:creatinine value for statistical analysis.

Because determining accurate renal function is vital in SLE clinical research, GFR measurements have become the gold standard. GFRs may be calculated using standard formulas including the Modification of Diet in Renal Disease (MDRD) or the Cockcroft-Gault formula in adults or the Schwartz formula in children. GFRs that are derived by insulin clearance, iothalamate clearance, chromium 51(^{51}Cr)–labeled ethylenediaminetetraacetic acid (EDTA)–GFR, and technetium 99m with diethyleneaminopentaacetic acid (Tc99-DTPA) clearance have proved to be reliable but expensive and inconvenient. The MDRD-calculated GFR predicted long-term renal outcome more accurately than serum creatinine in a re-examination of data from the Lewis plasmapheresis trial.[42]

Twenty-Four Hour Urine Proteins

Twenty-four hour urine proteins are valuable to follow only when they are elevated. Levels below 250 mg per 24 hours are normal; values up to 1000 mg may not require significant interventions and can be observed in healthy patients after vigorous exercise. Nephrotic syndromes include urine protein values higher than 3500 mg per 24 hours and are observed when proteinuria, edema, hypertension, and hyperlipidemia are present. Anasarca can be observed in patients who have urine protein values in excess of 7000 mg per 24 hours. Patients with membranous disease may have continuous nephrotic-range proteinuria for longer than 20 years and still have normal serum creatinine levels. However, nephrosis is associated with greater risks of thrombosis and cardiovascular mortality.[43] Rapid decrease in proteinuria is associated with better renal response to therapy in the Euro-Lupus and Plasmapheresis trials.[44] Many patients and settings have difficulty acquiring a valid 24-hour urine collection; reports have suggested that a random spot urine collection for urine protein:creatinine ratio (UPC) (corrected for a body surface area [BSA] of 1.75 m^2) correlates with and may be more reliable than a 24-hour urine collection.[45] Others have reported greater reliability with a spot UPC taken from a 24-hour collection.[46] Decreases in 24-hour urine protein values usually correlate with clinical improvement unless associated with declining glomerular filtration. In this latter circumstance, dropping levels are a sign of renal failure.

Urinary Proteins and Sediment

Although the urinalysis may be normal despite abnormal findings on a renal biopsy, nearly all patients with clinically important renal disease have abnormal microscopic urine findings. Reports in patients with nephritis have found microscopic hematuria in 33% to 78%, fat bodies in 33% to 48%, cellular casts in 34% to 40%, and greater than 1 g/24 hr of urinary protein in 26% to 87%. The appearance of five or more leukocytes or red cells in a clean midstream urine specimen without infection, renal stones, or other causes, especially with at least a trace of albumin, suggests active nephritis. As the process progresses, the amount of albumin generally increases, as do the numbers of leukocytes and erythrocytes. Confusing the picture, young female patients with lupus who are menstruating may be erroneously considered to have urinary infections or hematuria. Many have been given multiple courses of antibiotics before the diagnosis of lupus nephritis. As lupus damage advances, fine granular casts may appear. Later in the disease process, coarse granular casts, red-cell casts, and white-cell casts are found. If a nephrotic syndrome is present, urinary protein may be as high as 30 g/24 hr with good renal function. The other classic findings of nephrosis, such as oval fat bodies in the urine, hypoalbuminemia, hyperlipidemia, and anasarca, may also be present. With further progression of renal disease, the numbers of all types of casts increase; waxy casts, broad renal failure casts, and telescoped sediment become evident. Herbert and associates[47] found that a relapse of lupus nephritis can be best predicted by cellular casts, followed by hematuria and white cells in the urine; these were more reliable than a drop in C3 complement.

Analysis of Urine Protein Components

Urine protein can be separated into albumin and gamma globulin fractions. Measurements of urinary albumin excretion by radioimmunoassay can pick up larger amounts than normally would be detected. These are not generally clinically helpful, although diminution in albumin excretion correlates with clinical response to treatment. Microalbuminuria is associated with mesangial disease and does not predict the development of nephritis, whereas polymeric albumin is associated with more serious disease. Urinary protein electrophoresis demonstrates increased gamma globulin levels during active disease; levels decrease with therapeutic response. No specific patterns are observed in patients with SLE.[2]

Other Urinary Findings

Bacterial cystitis or pyelonephritis is common in patient cohorts; Dubois[9] observed this in 22.5% of his 520 patients. Autoantibodies may also be detected. Positive urinary ANAs in have been found in 32% of patients with HEp-2 cells. Anti-Sm, antiribonucleoprotein (anti-RNP), anti–Sjögren syndrome antigen A (anti-SSA/Ro), and anti-dsDNA also were detected. The presence of anti-dsDNA and ANAs correlated with increased clinical severity. ANAs might appear in the urine as a result of decreased tubular reabsorption, antigen deposition, or genitourinary tract inflammation, but they probably represent glomerular leakage. Numerous reports have suggested that numerous urinary substances are increased with active lupus nephritis and are good markers of clinical activity. These include ferritin, anti–RNA polymerase I antibodies, neopterin, acid mucopolysaccharides, histuria, fibrin-degradation products, several gastrointestinal enzymes, IL-6, anti-DNA soluble IL-2 receptors, urinary C4, monocyte chemotactic and activating factor, retinal-binding protein, tumor necrosis factor-alpha (TNF-α) and adhesion molecules, low–molecular-weight C3 fragments, monocyte chemoattractant protein 1 (MCP-1), and complement receptor 1 (CR1).[2]

Urinary prostaglandins, renal-tubular acidosis, aldosterone, the syndrome of inappropriate antidiuretic hormone, and renin activity measurements are discussed in Chapter 38.

Renal Vein Thrombosis

Thrombosis of the renal veins complicating lupus nephritis was first reported in 1968 and has been described in numerous cases since. It should be strongly considered in patients with nephrotic syndrome and/or antiphospholipid antibodies (APLAs) with flank pain and fever, thrombophlebitis, or pulmonary emboli.[2] Renal vein thrombosis should be differentiated from renal arteriolar thrombi observed on biopsy not associated with APLAs but with a thrombotic microangiopathic picture. The clinical scenarios of accelerated or malignant hypertension or superimposed thrombotic thrombocytopenic purpura (TTP) may produce these findings.

Although the APLAs predispose one to renal vein thrombosis, their presence is not mandatory. Renal vein thrombosis has also been reported in patients with SLE who have received renal allografts.[48] Renal vein thrombosis must be promptly treated with anticoagulants. Renal failure and pulmonary emboli are its most serious complications. Thrombolytic therapies should also be considered in the appropriate clinical setting.

Clinicopathologic Laboratory Correlates

The six major parameters used to assess lupus nephritis disease activity are: (1) serum creatinine, (2) assessment of daily protein excretion, (3) creatinine clearance, (4) C3 complement, (5) urine sediment, and (6) anti-dsDNA.[49] Because each of these tests reveals different aspects of the disease, therapeutic decisions are based on the combined results. Clinical trials also use other outcome criteria, criteria that may be less important in a community practice. These include rigorous definitions for remissions, flares, relapses, exacerbations, and lupus activity scores. Serum creatinine is an insensitive measure of the level of renal function. Because the proximal tubule actively reabsorbs creatinine until the mechanism is saturated, a patient may lose 50% of creatinine clearance with an increase in serum creatinine that remains within the normal range. Normalization of the creatinine level is associated with a favorable prognosis. A creatinine clearance of less than 10 mL/hr, or a serum creatinine of over 7 mg/dL, with uremic symptoms is usually an indication for dialysis. As mentioned earlier, hydration status, obstruction, severe infection, acute tubular necrosis, contrast-induced nephropathy, and certain medications (especially NSAIDs) can temporarily raise serum creatinine levels.

When Should a Renal Biopsy Be Performed?

An important issue in the evaluation and treatment of lupus renal disease is the necessity and timing of a renal biopsy. The strongest argument for a renal biopsy is the likelihood that the histopathologic findings will influence initiation, selection, or discontinuation of therapeutic agents. Many patients may have renal disease from other causes than lupus (e.g., drug-induced interstitial nephritis, hypertensive nephrosclerosis, diabetes, acute tubular necrosis [ATN]). A repeat renal biopsy may be required in patients with a changing clinical course in whom additional, more aggressive therapy is being considered. Dubois[2] noted two primary reasons to obtain a renal biopsy: (1) confirmation of the diagnosis in equivocal cases and (2) determination, in advanced cases, whether further treatment is indicated. Diffuse scarring with little or no inflammation would prompt conservative management alone.

Several advances have increased the frequency and safety of renal biopsies. The availability of an improved renal biopsy needle and real-time ultrasound guidance decreases the risk of significant bleeding. Recent recommendations from a committee tasked with providing the ACR with guidelines advise that all patients who fulfill the definition of lupus nephritis undergo an initial biopsy.

Histologic evidence of substantial interstitial fibrosis, glomerulosclerosis, and tubular atrophy are predictors of subsequent progression to ESRD. The patterns of injury previously described correlate, to some degree, with a spectrum of clinical presentations of lupus nephritis. The mesangial pattern is typically associated with subnephrotic proteinuria, microscopic hematuria, and the preservation of GFR. As in idiopathic membranous nephropathy, a predominantly subepithelial accumulation of immune complexes is associated with nephrotic proteinuria and the preservation or gradual reduction in GFR. In contrast, the endothelial pattern of injury is frequently associated with dysmorphic erythrocyturia, red-cell casts, sterile pyuria, various degrees of proteinuria, and an acute loss of GFR. Despite these general correlations, substantial overlap exists in the clinical presentation of patients with the various histopathologic findings, and ascertaining the type or severity of renal disease based on clinical grounds alone is very difficult. Renal disease may constitute the initial presentation of SLE in 3% to 6% of patients. For this reason, a renal biopsy is useful, if not essential, in the management of patients with suspected lupus nephritis. It provides an invaluable guide to therapy by clarifying the clinicopathologic syndrome and assessing the relative degrees of active inflammation and chronic scarring. It may also identify unsuspected causes for an acute worsening in renal function, such as the development of a thrombotic microangiopathy or drug-induced tubulointerstitial nephritis.

Thrombotic microangiopathy has increased frequency in SLE and is sometimes associated with APLAs or with an overlap syndrome such as systemic sclerosis. TTP is also increased in frequency in SLE. This complication is characterized by subendothelial expansion in glomerular capillaries, fibrinoid necrosis of arterioles, and edematous intimal expansion in arteries. The resultant narrowing of lumina, as well as superimposed thrombosis, may cause severe and rapid renal failure and a microangiopathic hemolytic anemia. Another difficulty in managing patients with lupus nephritis lies in the fact that the pathologic lesions may change from one form of glomerular injury to another. The progression of a class III lesion to class IV lupus nephritis is common. Both class III and class IV lesions can transform into membranous (class V) lupus nephritis, either spontaneously or with immunosuppressive therapy. It is less common but possible, however, for membranous lesions to transform into more proliferative lesions. Even repetitive clinical evaluations may not be sufficiently insightful in detecting these changes, and repeated renal biopsies are sometimes necessary. Follow-up biopsies are indicated if therapy would be significantly altered as a result of the findings.

MANAGEMENT OF LUPUS NEPHRITIS

Therapeutic decisions for individual patients with lupus nephritis should be based on a consideration of the patient's demographic background, clinical presentation, laboratory features, and histologic findings on biopsy. The principal goal of therapy is to improve or prevent the progressive loss of renal function. Prevention of ESRD is important because of the morbidity and mortality associated with its treatment. Mortality rates among patients on dialysis with lupus do not differ from the overall dialysis population (10% per year in the United States), but the patients with lupus are younger, are more frequently women, and have fewer co-morbidities such as diabetes. ESRD can be managed by dialysis or transplantation; therefore the treatment of lupus nephritis should aim for improved overall survival, not simply renal preservation. Box 35-1 lists the toxicities of various therapies.

Renal Transplantation in Patients with Systemic Lupus Erythematosus

Recent studies addressing the outcome of renal transplantation in patients with SLE, compared with those without the disease, have reported improved graft survival in patients with lupus. Data from the United States Renal Data System compared the outcomes of 772

Box 35-1 Toxicities of Aggressive Regimens Used to Treat Proliferative Nephritis*

I. Prolonged high-dose oral prednisone therapy (1 mg/kg/day equivalent for >6 weeks)
   Accelerated development of cataracts, glaucoma, hypertension, osteoporosis
   Diabetes mellitus
   Avascular necrosis of bone
   Diffuse ecchymoses
   Weight gain and significant cushingoid facies
   Diplopia
   Emotional lability, mood changes
   Dyspepsia, ulcer risk
   Increased infection risk
   Menstrual irregularities
II. Cyclophosphamide (more common in oral doses)
   Alopecia
   Amenorrhea, infertility
   Hemorrhagic cystitis
   Risk of malignancy
   Severe nausea and vomiting
   Increased risk of infection
   Teratogenicity
   Anemia, leukopenia, thrombocytopenia
III. Azathioprine
   Nausea and vomiting
   Abnormal liver function tests
   Increased risk of infection
   Anemia, leukopenia, thrombocytopenia

*These toxicities may occur at least 5% of the time.

adults with ESRD from lupus nephritis and 32,644 adults with ESRD as a result of other causes who received a transplant between 1987 and 1994.[50] After adjustment for potential confounding factors, the risk of graft failure or patient mortality was not increased in patients with SLE after first cadaveric or first living-related renal transplant. The reported rates of recurrent SLE disease after transplantation have also improved; recurrent lupus nephritis accounts for graft loss in less than 10 % of cases.[2]

The general concepts and specific therapies outlined in this text have evolved over a nearly 40-year period with increasing rapidity as new data become available. The evolution of current therapeutic approaches is best understood by reviewing the important clinical trials summarized in Table 35-4. The initial NIH randomized, controlled trial for lupus nephritis included 106 predominately Caucasian patients with all classes of lupus nephritis. Patients had nephritis for a mean of 11 months before entry, renal insufficiency was an exclusion criteria (serum creatinine [sCr] concentration of higher than 2 g/24 hr), and IVC dosing was given quarterly alone.[51] These factors favored less aggressive disease and a longer time to achieve end points. The trial included five arms with IVC, oral CyX, combined oral CyX and azathioprine (AZA), and AZA alone versus prednisone alone. At 15 years, the trial showed improved renal but not overall patient survival. Considering the lack of improvement in patient survival, concern for the toxicities versus the benefits of immunosuppressive therapy led to the design of two additional clinical trials. Boumpas and associates[52] compared the use of intermittent pulse methylprednisolone (MP) versus two courses of IVC-short (6 monthly doses) versus IVC-long (6 monthly doses, followed by quarterly doses to complete 24 months). The majority of patients had class IV disease and more severe nephritis. The trial also included African-American patients (28 of the 65 patients). The IVC-containing arms were superior to MP alone. Within 5 years, 48% of the patients treated with MP had a doubling of serum creatinine

TABLE | 35-4 Important Clinical Trials Informing the Treatment of Lupus Nephritis

NIH trials			
Austin HA	$n = 106$	6 monthly doses IVC	3-year results doubling sCr in IVC arms 25%
Boumpas D	$n = 65$ (28 AA)	*versus*	vs 48% in MP alone
Gourley MF	sCr 1.6-2.0 mg/dL	6 monthly doses IVC every 3 mo for	Renal relapse higher in short course than
	$n = 82$	24 mo	long course IVC arms
		Monthly doses of MP 1 g/m² IV for 1 yr	11-year follow-up
		versus	Doubling of sCr
		6 monthly doses IVC, then every 3 mo for	15/24 MP arm, 13/21 IVC arm, 1/20 in
		24 mo	combination arm
		versus	*but*
		6 monthly doses of combination IVC and	Mortality rate in the IVC arms was 18% vs
		pulse MP, then every 3 mo for 24 mo	4% in MP arm
Contreras G	$n = 59$		6-year results
			Doubling of sCr
			24-mo NIH regimen 15%
			6-7 mo IVC, then MMF 5%
			6-7 mo IVC, then AZA 5%
Euro-Lupus Nephritis trial	$n = 90$	All received pulse MP 750 mg/day IV for 3 days, then prednisone tapered, all	No differences in treatment failure (16% vs 20% in high dose arm)
	Predominately Caucasian Europeans	received AZA 2 mg/kg/day after IVC	Renal remission (71% vs 54%)
	60% class IV on biopsy	IVC 500 mg for 6 doses every 2 wk	Renal flares (27% vs 29%)
	Mean baseline sCr 1.15 mg/dL	*versus*	
		IVC 0.5 g/m² every month for 6 mo and 2 quarterly doses	
Dutch Working Party[57]	$n = 87$	IVC 6 monthly doses and 7 quarterly doses	
	Predominately Caucasian	*versus*	
	Predominately class IV on biopsy	AZA 2 mg/kg/day	
	Mean baseline sCr 1.2 mg/dL		
ALMS induction trial[60]	$n = 350$		
	One third Asian		
	Class III, IV, V		
ALMS maintenance trial[61]	$n = 227$	AZA 2 mg/kg/day vs MMF 1 g/day	3-year results treatment failure (renal relapse, doubling of sCr, death, or increased TX)
	Responded to induction		MMF more effective than AZA 16% vs 32% $P = 0.003$
Maintain[62]	$n = 105$	All received pulse MP 750 mg/day IV for 3 days, then prednisone tapered	3-year results showed no difference in renal relapse (nephrotic proteinuria, increased
	83 Caucasians	IVC 500 mg every 2 wk	sCr by 33%, or 3 times increased
	Class III 33	AZA 2 mg/kg/day vs MMF 2 g/day	proteinuria and hematuria)
	Class IV 61		MMF 19% vs 25% AZA
	Class V 11		

AA, African American; ALMS, the Aspreva Lupus Management Study; AZA, azathioprine; IV, intravenous; IVC, intravenous cyclophosphamide; MMF, mycophenolate mofetil; MP, methylprednisolone; NIH, National Institutes of Health; sCr, serum creatinine; TX, Transplantation.

versus 25% of the patients in the IVC arms. Renal relapse was more frequent in the IVC-short course, compared with the IVC-long course. African-American patients did worse, with 80% of those in the MP arm doubling serum creatinine within 5 years. Gourley and colleagues[53] reported a third trial comparing 12 months of MP versus the combination of MP and IVC monthly for 6 months and then quarterly to complete 2 years versus IVC alone as 6 monthly doses followed by quarterly doses to complete 2 years. Some patients cycled through more than 1 course of monthly IVC, depending on response to therapy. The IVC-containing arms were superior, with 11-year follow-up showing 15 of 24 patients in the MP arm versus 13 of 21 in the IVC arm versus 1 of 20 patients in the combined arm experiencing a renal relapse. However, the mortality in the IVC arms was 18% versus 4% in the MP arm.

This study sparked interest in alternatives to IVC therapy. In 2005, Contreras and others[54] published a pivotal trial comparing induction with six or seven doses of IVC, followed by a three-arm maintenance trial using the completion of IVC for 2 years (NIH protocol) versus AZA or MMF mofetil over 5 years. A clear superiority of maintenance with AZA or MMF was observed in this largely African-American and Hispanic population, leading many clinicians to

shorten their use of IVC to 6 months and following it AZA or MMF as a maintenance therapy.

In Europe, two groups addressed the use of IVC for lupus nephritis in different ways. Houssiau and associates[55] compared the 2-year NIH regimen of IVC to a shortened course consisting of 500 mg IVC every 2 weeks for 6 months. Both arms received pulse MP followed by a prednisone taper, and both arms transitioned to AZA as a maintenance regimen. Patients were predominately Caucasian Europeans, 60% had class IV nephritis confirmed by biopsy, and few had abnormal serum creatinine levels. No difference was observed in treatment failure in the low-dose IVC compared with high-dose IVC (16% versus 20%). Although renal remission was more frequent in the high-dose arm (71% versus 54%), renal flares were similar (27% versus 29%). Long-term follow-up of this cohort to 15 years continues to show comparability in outcomes.[56] The Dutch Working Party[57] compared the NIH regimen with AZA at 2 mg/kg alone in 87 predominately Caucasian patients. The mean serum creatinine was 1.2 mg/dL and proteinuria 4 g/24 hr. Again, no clinical differences between the arms were reported, although renal biopsies at 2 years in a subset of patients showed greater chronicity in patients receiving AZA alone.

The ALMS trial included 350 patients with proliferative or membranous nephritis. Although the trial was a global study, one third of the patients were of Asian descent. The trial included an induction arm comparing IVC versus MMF over 24 weeks. MMF was not superior to IVC.[58] Patients were required to meet response criteria to enter the 3-year maintenance arm. Few African-ancestry patients were included (10%), because few met these criteria. Patients were rerandomized to MMF at 2 g/day versus AZA at 2 mg/kg adjusted for white cell count. MMF was significantly more effective than AZA in preventing treatment failure (i.e., doubling of serum creatinine, renal relapse death, or need for increased immunosuppressive medication). Only 16% of patients in the MMF arm versus 32% in the AZA arm had treatment failure.[58] This result was independent of induction therapy received, race, or ethnicity. An open-label study comparing MMF with AZA in 105 patients after Euro-lupus IVC induction did not record a difference in the rate of renal relapse, with 19% in the MMF versus 25% in the AZA arm.[59] Finally, the importance of achieving a remission with therapy for lupus nephritis was highlighted by a recent re-examination of the Lupus Nephritis Collaborative Network Plasmapheresis study.[34] The risk of ESRD in this cohort with over 10 years of follow-up was 8% in complete responders versus 57% in partial responders and 87% in nonresponders. In the ALMS induction trial, only 8.6% of patients receiving MMF versus 8.1% receiving IVC attained a complete remission; just over 50% of patients in both arms reached either a complete or a partial response. In the maintenance trial, 62% of patients in the MMF arm versus 59% in the AZA arm reached remission. Thus new or additional therapies are certainly needed to improve the response to the treatment of lupus nephritis.

General Information on the Therapeutic Agents Used to Treat Lupus Nephritis

Pulse Methylprednisolone
Typically, treatment for severe class III or class IV lupus nephritis is initiated with pulse MP (7 mg/kg/day for 3 days at the author's institution), followed by oral prednisone. Oral prednisone may be started at a dose of 1 mg/kg/day for the first month (not to exceed 60 mg per day), followed by a gradual taper over the following 3 to 4 months. The goal is to minimize exposure to prednisone, decreasing to 15 mg or less per day as needed for the treatment of extrarenal disease.

Intravenous Cyclophosphamide
IVC is administered once a month for 6 consecutive months, starting at a dose of 0.5 to 0.75 g/m^2 and increasing by 0.25 g/m^2 BSA on successive treatments (not to exceed 1 g/m^2 BSA), provided that the 2-week leukocyte count remains above 3000 cells/mm^3. Patients with significant renal impairment need a reduction in the dose of parenteral CyX to avoid increased risk of bone marrow toxicity. In the NIH protocol after the first 6 months, pulse IVC was administered every 3 months for a total of 24 months.

Azathioprine
The role of AZA in the treatment of proliferative lupus nephritis is less well established than that of IVC. Early studies have suggested improved outcomes with the use of AZA in combination with corticosteroids over corticosteroids alone. However, AZA has less gonadal toxicity than CyX and may be considered for patients with focal proliferative nephritis (ISN class III) without markers associated with a greater risk of ESRD, such as histologic findings of necrosis or cellular crescents. In recent years, AZA has also been proposed as an effective maintenance regimen for patients with lupus nephritis after 6 months of therapy with IVC (see Table 35-4). Recently, measurement of AZA metabolites has become clinically available, allowing titration of the dose for individual patients to maximize therapeutic response and minimize the risk of toxicity. Dosing in excess of 2 mg/kg may be considered for greater efficacy, if metabolite levels are monitored for the risk of toxicity. In addition, patients lacking gene *MtPT6* can be spared exposure to the drug.

Mycophenolate Mofetil
Because of its favorable safety profile when compared with CyX, the use of MMF has gained great interest for the treatment of lupus nephritis. Results of the ALMS trial, the largest trial reported to date with 350 patients with lupus nephritis, did not show superiority of CyX over MMF. However, response to MMF was significantly increased in patients of African ancestry and in patients with Hispanic ethnicity.[36] Sufficient data support the use of MMF as a first-line drug in the treatment of lupus nephritis. The recently published ALMS maintenance trial demonstrated the superiority of MMF to AZA over a 3-year follow-up. Further research is needed to determine the optimum duration of MMF therapy required and because long-term outcomes beyond 3 years are lacking.

Calcineurin Inhibitors
Cyclosporin A has been shown to be effective in reducing clinical and histologic activity in proliferative lupus nephritis. Autoantibody formation and hypocomplementemia do not uniformly improve, and the frequent occurrence of hypertension and nephrotoxicity limit the utility of this therapy. Concern for progression of renal activity on repeat biopsy, despite apparent clinical response, has also been raised. Recently, trials evaluating tacrolimus therapy for lupus nephritis have been reported (see Chapter 51). Adverse effects similar to those observed with cyclosporin A exist, as well as an increased risk of diabetes and neuropathy.

Intravenous Gamma Globulin
Case reports of efficacy in refractory features of severe lupus, including pulmonary hemorrhage, leukocytoclastic vasculitis, and polyradiculopathy, have been noted.[2] Unfortunately, the outcome of this therapy has not always been beneficial. Severe exacerbation of lupus and the development of vasculitis have been described as toxicities after intravenous immunoglobulin (IVIG). Nephrotoxicity can be a serious rare complication of IVIG therapy because of osmotic nephrosis when sucrose is used in the preparation. Preexisting renal disease, volume depletion, and older age are risk factors for such toxicity. In addition, hyperviscosity complicated by neurologic events may occur. Previous variable results of IVIG treatment in patients with SLE could be related to variable enrichment of different lots of IVIG in suppressive anti–pathogenic idiotype antibodies.

Plasmapheresis
Plasmapheresis has been used in the treatment of lupus nephritis to eliminate pathogenic antibodies and circulating immune complexes. However, a large-scale, prospective controlled clinical trial showed no additional benefit of plasmapheresis, compared with corticosteroids and short-course oral CyX therapy alone.[11] Plasmapheresis may, however, have a role in the treatment of patients with overwhelming disease in whom standard therapy is failing. The incidence of TTP is increased in those with SLE. In the Glomerular Disease Collaborative Network (GDCN) nephropathologic database, TTP occurs in 10% of patients with severe class IV lupus nephritis. In this disorder, plasmapheresis is lifesaving.

Biologic Agents
The last few years have witnessed the advent of a number of biologic agents targeting specific inflammatory pathways. Several are currently under investigation for the treatment of SLE or lupus nephritis or both. These include monoclonal antibodies directed against co-stimulatory molecules including B-lymphocyte stimulator (BLyS), B cell–activating factor (BAFF), and cytotoxic T-lymphocyte antigen 4–immunoglobulin (CTLA4-Ig). Rituximab (Rituxan) targeting B lymphocyte–expressed CD-20 has been used in refractory lupus. Two randomized trials, one in lupus and one in lupus nephritis, failed to show a significant response. Nonetheless, some clinicians have criticized the design of the trials, and numerous anecdotal series have reported significant response to Rituxan. Epratuzumab, an anti-CD 22, is also under study with initial phase

studies showing positive results. Monoclonal antibodies targeting complement components are also of interest. So far, none has been sufficiently evaluated to warrant their use outside of controlled clinical trials. The use of available biologic agents to improve the response to therapy for lupus nephritis is also an area of active interest. CTLA4-Ig is under study in a trial using the Euro-lupus regimen in patients with lupus nephritis in the United States. A previous trial using this agent with MMF is under evaluation to inform future trials.

Clinical Guidelines for the Evaluation and Treatment of Lupus Nephritis

1. All patients with lupus who develop glomerulonephritis should have a renal biopsy, providing no contraindications exist (e.g., severe thrombocytopenia, refusal of blood products, coagulopathy) and a physician who is an expert in biopsy is available. Because therapy often differs greatly for different histopathologic classes, tissue evaluation is essential. In addition to classifying the lesion activity and chronicity, indices should be described with attention to high-risk features such as crescent formation, karyorrhexis, or necrosis.

2. Evaluating renal activity should include the following: urine sediment appearance, serum creatinine, blood pressure, serum albumin, C3-complement determination, anti-dsDNA antibody level, proteinuria (often estimated by protein-to-creatinine ratio), and creatinine clearance. These values may be monitored as the clinical situation dictates. Daily measurement of the serum creatinine level may be useful in rapidly progressive disease; other parameters require 1 to 2 weeks to change.

3. Patients with APLAs and lupus nephritis have a poorer renal outcome, more histologic thrombotic microangiopathy, and increased complications with dialysis and transplantation. At a minimum, low-dose aspirin should be administered; individuals with a history of a thrombotic event should be on a life-long warfarin regimen or an equivalent thromboprophylactic agent. This therapy may complicate renal biopsy because an anticoagulation regimen is typically suspended for up to 2 weeks after biopsy to decrease the risk of bleeding at the biopsy site.

4. Hypertension must be aggressively treated. With lupus nephritis, the goal should be age-appropriate blood pressure (especially important in young patients). The target blood pressure for patients with a history of glomerulonephritis should be 120/80 mm Hg or lower.

5. The following parameters are essential to monitor toxicity associated with corticosteroids, diuretics, and cytotoxic agents: blood pressure, complete blood count, platelet count, potassium, glucose, cholesterol, liver function tests, weight, muscle strength, gonadal function, and bone density. These parameters are closely monitored as the clinical situation requires.

6. Patients are instructed to avoid therapeutic doses of salicylates and NSAIDs because they may impair renal function, exacerbate edema and hypertension, and increase the risk of gastrointestinal toxicity, particularly in combination with corticosteroids and immunosuppressive agents. Topical NSAID formulations are available as patches, gels, or liquids with low systemic absorption. If absolutely necessary during the course of treatment for nephritis, oral NSAIDs should be administered for short periods at low doses with careful supervision. The cardiovascular risks with NSAIDs are currently unknown.

7. Pregnancy should be discouraged in patients with active nephritis; the risks for maternal and fetal morbidity and mortality, including renal failure, are increased. Pregnancy in a patient requiring dialysis is high risk to both the mother and the fetus with a low rate of success, despite daily dialysis treatments.

8. Antimalarial medications may be given or continued for active skin disease or to reduce risks of APLA syndrome. Reports of improved response to immunosuppressive therapy for nephritis continue to remain an area of active investigation.

Treatment of lupus nephritis requires an understanding of the immunopathogenesis, the risk stratification by ISN classification on renal biopsy, and a familiarity with the specific therapeutic modalities. Discussing the various therapeutic agents in the context of the specific ISN class of lupus renal disease is useful. The following therapies are advised for specific biopsy patterns (Figure 35-9): For issues in the treatment of lupus nephritis in children, see Chapter 40.

1. ISN class I or class II (WHO class I and class II): Many mesangial lesions do not need specific therapy. In patients with ISN class I or class II, hydroxychloroquine and prednisone are usually administered in accordance with the degree of extrarenal clinical activity.

2. ISN class III or class IV (WHO class III and class IV): These classifications are treated similarly because they have similar prognoses. Because the risk of ESRD in 10 years may exceed 50%, unless a complete remission is attained, aggressive management is advised. The following recommendations are offered:

   A. One mg/kg/day of prednisone equivalent is administered for at least 4 weeks, depending on clinical response. The age of the patient will affect steroidal therapy; children and young adults into their early 20s may require higher doses of prednisone than older patients. Pediatric rheumatologists commonly prescribe high-dose prednisone (2 mg/kg/day). Cytotoxic drugs often take months to become effective, and glucocorticoidal medications stabilize the patient in the interim. Prednisone is tapered over 3 to 4 months. Doses are then decreased or tapered to a maintenance level of 15 mg/day or less of prednisone equivalent for extrarenal activity. Individual patient circumstances, such as uncontrollable diabetes or hypertension, multiple sites of painful avascular necrosis, severe osteoporosis, or steroid psychosis, may accelerate this taper.

   B. Unless contraindicated by infection or other compelling clinical circumstances, cytotoxic drugs should be added at the onset of therapy. The results of the ALMS trial have supported the use of either MMF or IVC therapy for 6 months as an induction therapy. IVC is administered monthly for 6 months, per the NIH regimen beginning with 0.5 to 0.75 gr/m^2 up to 1 g/m^2 while maintaining the patient's white blood cell count above 3000/mm^3 for 7 to 10 days; therapy is not currently administered consecutively for more than 6 months. Sodium 2–mercaptoethane sulfonate (MESNA) can be administered with each infusion to minimize bladder toxicity, and ondansetron or granisetron can be given to minimize nausea. Patient circumstances, such as refractory hemorrhagic cystitis despite MESNA therapy, severe nausea and/or vomiting, refusal to accept the possibility of infertility, prior radiation therapy, history of malignancy, and cytopenia as a result of marrow suppression (cytopenias as a result of peripheral destruction are not contraindications), may preclude IVC.

   C. The dosing of MMF may be started at 250 to 500 mg twice daily, advancing by 500 mg every few days to 1 week (between 2 and 3 g/day). Because MMF is tightly protein bound, patients with severe nephrosis will have a higher free drug fraction and more gastrointestinal side effects unless started at lower doses. Based on the Contreras study, which demonstrated improved 5-year outcomes with 6 months of IVC therapy, followed by one of two agents for up to 5 years—MMF (2 g/day) or AZA (2 mg/kg/day), we follow induction with one of these agents. The ALMS maintenance trial demonstrated the superiority of MMF to AZA in this global trial. The length of maintenance is not clear, but at least 2 to 5 years is supported by the NIH and ALMS trials. The risk of relapse with discontinuing immunosuppression should encourage a slow taper.

3. Acute flares with renal deterioration can be managed with pulse MP and consideration of a new immunosuppressive regimen. Apheresis may be useful only if the patient has cryoglobulinemia, hyperviscosity, catastrophic APLA syndrome, or TTP.

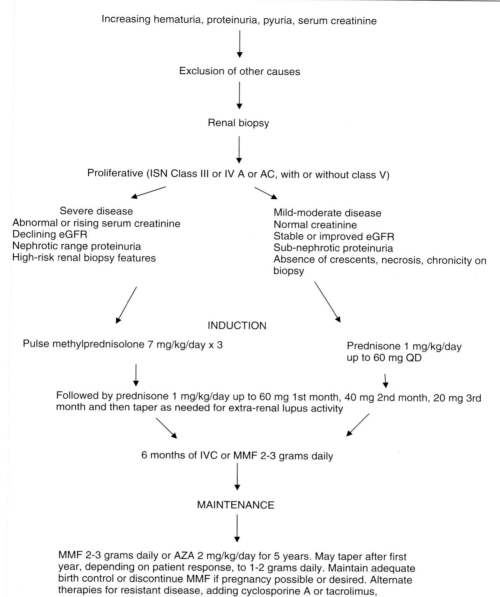

Increasing hematuria, proteinuria, pyuria, serum creatinine

↓

Exclusion of other causes

↓

Renal biopsy

↓

Proliferative (ISN Class III or IV A or AC, with or without class V)

Severe disease
Abnormal or rising serum creatinine
Declining eGFR
Nephrotic range proteinuria
High-risk renal biopsy features

Mild-moderate disease
Normal creatinine
Stable or improved eGFR
Sub-nephrotic proteinuria
Absence of crescents, necrosis, chronicity on biopsy

INDUCTION

Pulse methylprednisolone 7 mg/kg/day x 3

Prednisone 1 mg/kg/day up to 60 mg QD

Followed by prednisone 1 mg/kg/day up to 60 mg 1st month, 40 mg 2nd month, 20 mg 3rd month and then taper as needed for extra-renal lupus activity

6 months of IVC or MMF 2-3 grams daily

↓

MAINTENANCE

↓

MMF 2-3 grams daily or AZA 2 mg/kg/day for 5 years. May taper after first year, depending on patient response, to 1-2 grams daily. Maintain adequate birth control or discontinue MMF if pregnancy possible or desired. Alternate therapies for resistant disease, adding cyclosporine A or tacrolimus, rituximab

FIGURE 35-9 Algorithm for the treatment of proliferative (the International Society of Nephrology [ISN] class III or class IV) lupus nephritis.

4. Somewhere between 20% and 40% of cases especially in patients of minority descent (e.g., African American, Hispanic) and those with nephritic urinary sediment, will be refractory to prednisone plus IVC or MMF. Among this subset, the following options are available:
   A. Switch the patient to the alternative induction agent (IVC or MMF). Although African-American and Hispanic patients responded better to MMF in the ALMS trial, the response of the individual patient may differ. Monthly pulse doses of MP may be added but should not be substituted for immunosuppressive therapy.
   B. Change to oral immunosuppressive with MMF, cyclosporine A, or tacrolimus, or to a combination of these drugs. Recently, the combination of tacrolimus and MMF has been reported efficacious in treating lupus nephritis.
   C. Consideration of experimental therapies including B-cell depletion with rituximab (anti-CD20), intravenous gamma globulin, addition of CTLA4-Ig to CyX therapy, or bone marrow transplantation.

5. Class V: Patients may be treated with 1 mg/kg/day of prednisone equivalent for 6 to 12 weeks, followed by its discontinuation if no response occurs or tapering to a maintenance level of 10 mg/day prednisone equivalent for 1 to 2 years if a response occurs. Others may use the Ponticelli protocol of alternate day prednisone. Cytotoxic drugs are not generally used unless patients have severe nephrosis (more than 10 g proteinuria daily) or developing renal insufficiency is present. Pure membranous lesions are approximately 15% to 20% of all lupus biopsies. Reports of MMF, cyclosporin A, and tacrolimus efficacy in managing membranous nephritis remain controversial.
   A. Aggressive immunosuppressant management is usually not advised unless a high activity index is also present or extra-renal disease is evident, which would warrant cytotoxic therapy.

B. Patients may be maintained on 5 to 10 mg/day of prednisone equivalent if needed to control extrarenal lupus, bearing in mind the increased risk of infection if the patient requires a peritoneal or hemodialysis catheter rather than a shunt or graft for dialysis access.

6. Patients who should not be treated include those with significant renal scarring or other evidence of irreversible disease. Little benefit is realized in aggressively managing patients with a stable creatinine level above 5 mg/dL; it frequently produces more harm than good. Planning for dialysis or transplantation or both is preferable. Chronic renal insufficiency evaluation should include measurements of erythropoietin, vitamins D1 and D25, calcium, parathyroid hormone (PTH), and phosphorus levels.

The reader is referred to Chapter 5, Nonpharmacologic Therapeutic Methods, for a discussion of the management of patients with lupus and ESRD (i.e., dialysis and transplantation).

Adjunctive and Supportive Care

Active supportive care is crucial in maintaining the benefits of aggressive immunosuppression in preserving renal function and in minimizing short- and long-term side effects of therapy. Compulsive attention must be paid to the early detection and aggressive treatment of infections, because they account for approximately 20% of deaths among patients with SLE. Whenever corticosteroids are used, measures must be taken to minimize the development of osteoporosis (following ACR guidelines to prevent steroid-induced osteoporosis). These measures include calcium and vitamin D supplementation, weight-bearing exercise as tolerated, and potential therapy with pharmacologic agents including calcitonin in a renally impaired patient, bisphosphonates (unless contraindicated by azotemia or gastrointestinal toxicity), or recombinant PTH. (See Chapter 52, Adjunctive Measures and Issues: Allergies, Antibiotics, Vaccines, Osteoporosis, and Disability.) The entire spectrum of antihypertensive agents has been used in patients with lupus, but interest is ongoing in the benefits of angiotensin-converting enzyme (ACE) inhibitors, especially in patients with persistent proteinuria. ACE inhibitors may have renal protective properties. The use of an angiotensin-receptor blocker (ARB) alone or in combination with ACE inhibitors is also commonly used. With appropriate electrolyte monitoring, loop diuretics are administered to diminish edema and control hypertension when necessary. With nephrosis and hypoalbuminemia, torsemide may be more effective than furosemide. However, whenever possible, thiazide diuretics should be used because they avoid the increased calciuria produced by loop diuretics, which helps prevent osteoporosis.

Hypercholesterolemia may accompany the nephrotic syndrome and may also be a complication of long-term steroid therapy. Although no prospective controlled studies have, as yet, been published that demonstrate improved outcomes in patients with lupus, such studies are underway. The American Heart Association's new guidelines of serum cholesterol below 180 mg/dL, rather than 200 mg/dL, should be the target for therapy, considering the increase in cardiovascular disease associated with SLE. Clinically, it is recommended that patients follow a low-cholesterol, low-fat diet, and receive lipid-lowering agents such as the hydroxymethylglutaryl–coenzyme A (HMG-CoA) reductase inhibitors when hyperlipidemia is persistent. Many clinicians, recognizing the increased risk of atherosclerosis in patients with lupus, will advise patients to take an aspirin daily and folic supplementation of 1 to 5 mg/day. Plaquenil has also been associated with fewer cardiovascular events, particularly in patients who have APLA syndrome.

Contraception, fertility, and pregnancy are important issues in this predominately female patient population. Advice on the choice of contraceptive method should be given, keeping in mind the additive thrombotic risk factors including the presence of APLAs, hypertension, and nephrotic syndrome. Clinical trials of estrogen-containing oral contraceptives in APLA-negative premenopausal women with SLE have recently been published, showing no increase in lupus flares. In postmenopausal women, an increase risk of 10% for mild-to-moderate, but not severe, flares was noted with hormone replacement therapy. In small pilot studies of women with SLE, the use of the gonadotropin-releasing hormone (GnRH) agonist leuprolide acetate appeared to prevent CyX-induced ovarian failure. However, because this agent is an agonist, levels of estrogen may be increased in the first few days, raising the risks of ovarian hyperstimulation syndrome, multiple birth if pregnancy occurs, and possible blood clots. These risks must be carefully reviewed with the patient and referring physicians. In young women with multiple risks or with a history of clotting, subcutaneous heparin should be considered until the estrogen production is suppressed. Of course, bone density must also be assessed and maintained.

RECENT AND CUMULATIVE INSIGHTS

Therapeutic advances in the management of lupus nephritis have focused on defining prognostic subsets of patients who respond differently to various treatment modalities. Nephrotic syndrome, biopsy-defined class IV lesions, high chronicity indices, thrombocytopenia, African-American race, Hispanic ethnicity, and childhood onset of nephritis are associated with poorer outcome. Despite all these advances, however, certain subsets of patients with focal or diffuse proliferative lesions and scarring of glomerular and tubulointerstitial regions still have a 50% chance of having ESRD within 5 years, and aggressive management appears to be warranted.

SUMMARY AND FUTURE DIRECTIONS

Lupus nephritis has evolved from a frequently terminal process to one in which a fairly normal quality of life and good outcome are possible. First, the treating physician must accurately stage the disease with laboratory and tissue evaluations. Next, therapy is fashioned for the specific disease subsets that are involved. Third, both side effects and the complications of treatment must be managed, along with frequent assessments and modifications of therapy, depending on the patient's response. At present, many centers are reassessing the traditional 2-year NIH regimen of IVC for severe lupus nephritis, reducing exposure to this toxic therapy and using long-term maintenance with AZA or MMF. Currently, more than eight clinical trials of agents for the treatment of lupus, including biologic therapies, have been conducted. These include monoclonal antibodies directed against anti-CD40 ligand, BLyS, BAFF, complement component C5, B-cell depletion with anti-CD20 chimeric antibody, and T-cell tolerogen CTLA4-Ig and anti-DNase (see Chapter 56, Experimental Therapies in Systemic Lupus Erythematosus). It is critical for expert clinicians to interpret this rapidly changing field to best advise individual physicians and their patients on the optimal therapeutic course.

References

1. Danila MI, Pons-Estel GJ, Zhang J, et al: Renal damage is the most important predictor of mortality within the damage index: data from LUMINA LXIV, a multiethnic US cohort. *Rheumatology (Oxford)* 48(5):542–545, 2009.
2. Dooley MA: Clinical and epidemiologic features of lupus nephritis. In Wallace DJ, Hahn B, Dubois EL, editors: *Dubois' lupus erythematosus*, ed 7, Philadelphia, 2007, Lippincott Williams & Wilkins, pp 1112–1130.
3. Walsh SJ, Algert C, Gregorio DI, et al: Divergent racial trends in mortality from systemic lupus erythematosus. *J Rheumatol* 22:1663–1668, 1995.
4. Pistiner M, Wallace DJ, Nessim S, et al: Lupus erythematosus in the 1980s: a survey of 570 patients. *Semin Arthritis Rheum* 21:55–64, 1991.
5. Contreras G, Lenz O, Pardo V, et al: Outcomes in African Americans and Hispanics with lupus nephritis. *Kidney Int* 69:1846–1851, 2006.
6. Croca SC, Rodrigues T, Isenberg DA: Assessment of a lupus nephritis cohort over a 30-year period. *Rheumatology (Oxford)* 50(8):1424–1430, 2011.
7. Nossent JC, Bronsveld W, Swaak AJ: Systemic lupus erythematosus. III. Observations on clinical renal involvement and follow up of renal function: Dutch experience with 110 patients studied prospectively. *Ann Rheum Dis* 48:810–816, 1989.

8. Ward MM: Changes in the incidence of endstage renal disease due to lupus nephritis in the United States, 1996-2004. *J Rheumatol* 36:63–67, 2009.

9. Wallace DJ, Podell T, Weiner J, et al: Systemic lupus erythematosus—survival patterns. Experience with 609 patients. *JAMA* 245:934–938, 1981.

10. Appel GB, Cohen DJ, Pirani CL, et al: Long-term follow up of patients with lupus nephritis. A study based on the classification of the world health organization. *Am J Med* 83:877–885, 1987.

11. Moroni G, Pasquali S, Quaglini S, et al: Clinical and prognostic variables of serial renal biopsies in lupus nephritis. *Am J Kidney Dis* 34:530–539, 1999.

12. Eiser AR, Katz SM, Swartz C: Clinically occult diffuse proliferative lupus nephritis: an age related phenomenon. *Arch Intern Med* 139:1022–1025, 1979.

13. Weening JJ, D'Agati VD, Schwartz MM, et al: The classification of glomerulonephritis in systemic lupus erythematosus revisited. *J Am Soc Nephrol* 15:241–250, 2004.

14. Hwang J, Kim HJ, Oh JM, et al: Outcome of reclassification of World Health Organization (WHO) class III under International Society of Nephrology-Renal Pathology Society (ISN-RPS) classification: retrospective observational study. *Rheumatol Int* 2011. [Epub ahead of print]

15. Baldwin DS, Lowenstein J, Rothfield NF, et al: The clinical course of the proliferative and membranous forms of lupus nephritis. *Ann Intern Med* 73:929–942, 1970.

16. Pollak VE, Pirani CL, Schwartz FD: The natural history of the renal manifestations of systemic lupus erythematosus. *J Lab Clin Med* 63:537–550, 1964.

17. Appel GB, Silva FG, Pirani CL, et al: Renal involvement in systemic lupus erythematosus (SLE): a study of 56 patients emphasizing histologic classification. *Medicine (Baltimore)* 57:371–410, 1978.

18. McCluskey R: *Lupus nephritis.* East Norwalk, Conn, 1975, Appleton-Century Crofts.

19. Churg J, Sobin L: *Renal Disease: classification and atlas of glomerular diseases,* New York, 1982, Igaku-Shoin.

20. Churg J, Bernstein J, Glassock R: *Renal disease: classification and atlas of glomerular diseases,* New York, 1995, Igaku-Shoin.

21. Weening JJ, D'Agati VD, Schwartz MM, et al: The classification of glomerulonephritis in systemic lupus erythematosus revisited. *Kidney Int* 65:521–530, 2004.

22. Silva F: *The nephropathies of systemic lupus erythematosus,* New York, 1983, Churchill Livingstone.

23. Schwartz MM, Lan SP, Bonsib SM, et al: Clinical outcome of three discrete histologic patterns of injury in severe lupus glomerulonephritis. *Am J Kidney Dis* 13:273–283, 1989.

24. Tan EM, Cohen AS, Fries JF, et al: The 1982 revised criteria for the classification of systemic lupus erythematosus. *Arthritis Rheum* 25:1271–1277, 1982.

25. Ward MM, Studenski S: Age associated clinical manifestations of systemic lupus erythematosus: a multivariate regression analysis. *J Rheumatol* 17:476–481, 1990.

26. Maddison P, Farewell V, Isenberg D, et al: The rate and pattern of organ damage in late onset systemic lupus erythematosus. *J Rheumatol* 29:913–917, 2002.

27. Cooper GS, Parks CG, Treadwell EL, et al: Differences by race, sex and age in the clinical and immunologic features of recently diagnosed systemic lupus erythematosus patients in the southeastern United States. *Lupus* 11:161–167, 2002.

28. Bastian HM, Roseman JM, McGwin G Jr, et al: Systemic lupus erythematosus in three ethnic groups. XII. Risk factors for lupus nephritis after diagnosis. *Lupus* 11:152–160, 2002.

29. Adler M, Chambers S, Edwards C, et al: An assessment of renal failure in an SLE cohort with special reference to ethnicity, over a 25-year period. *Rheumatology (Oxford)* 45:1144–1147, 2006.

30. Johnson SR, Urowitz MB, Ibañez D, et al: Ethnic variation in disease patterns and health outcomes in systemic lupus erythematosus. *J Rheumatol.* 33:1990–1995, 2006.

31. Chan TM, Li FK, Tang CS, et al: Efficacy of mycophenolate mofetil in patients with diffuse proliferative lupus nephritis. Hong Kong-Guangzhou Nephrology Study Group. *N Engl J Med* 343:1156–1162, 2000.

32 Petri M: Lupus in Baltimore: evidence-based 'clinical pearls' from the Hopkins Lupus Cohort. *Lupus* 14:970–973, 2005.

33. Dooley MA, Hogan S, Jennette C, et al: Cyclophosphamide therapy for lupus nephritis: poor renal survival in black Americans. Glomerular Disease Collaborative Network. *Kidney Int* 51:1188–1195, 1997.

34. Chen YE, Korbet SM, Katz RS, et al; Collaborative Study Group: Value of a complete or partial remission in severe lupus nephritis. *Clin J Am Soc Nephrol* 3:46–53, 2008.

35. Contreras G, Pardo V, Cely C, et al: Factors associated with poor outcomes in patients with lupus nephritis. *Lupus* 14:890–895, 2005.

36. Isenberg D, Appel GB, Contreras G, et al: Influence of race/ethnicity on response to lupus nephritis treatment: the ALMS study. *Rheumatology (Oxford)* 49:128–140, 2010.

37. Lin CP, Adrianto I, Lessard CJ, et al: Role of MYH9 and APOL1 in African and non-African populations with lupus nephritis. *Genes Immun* 13:232–238, 2012.

38. Klippel JH: Predicting who will get lupus nephritis. *J Clin Rheumatol* 1:257–259, 1995.

39. Yeung CK, Ng WL, Wong WS, et al: Acute deterioration in renal function in systemic lupus erythematosus. *Q J Med* 56:393–402, 1985.

40. Balow JE, Austin HA 3rd: Therapy of membranous nephropathy in systemic lupus erythematosus. *Semin Nephrol* 23:386–391, 2003.

41. Steiman AJ, Gladman DD, Ibañez D, et al: Prolonged serologically active clinically quiescent systemic lupus erythematosus: frequency and outcome. *J Rheumatol* 37:1822–1827, 2010.

42. Patel SB, Korbet SM, Lewis EJ: The prognosis of severe lupus nephritis based on the Modification of Diet in Renal Disease (MDRD) study estimated glomerular filtration rate. *Lupus* 20:256–264, 2011.

43. Zhang W, Aghdassi E, Reich HN, et al: Glomerular filtration rate predicts arterial events in women with systemic lupus erythematosus. *Rheumatology (Oxford)* 50:799–805, 2011.

44. Houssiau FA, Vasconcelos C, D'Cruz D, et al: Early response to immunosuppressive therapy predicts good renal outcome in lupus nephritis: lessons from long-term followup of patients in the Euro-Lupus Nephritis Trial. *Arthritis Rheum* 50:3934–3940, 2004.

45. Sessions S, Mehta K, Kovarsky J: Quantitation of proteinuria in systemic lupus erythematosus by random, spot urine collection. *Arthritis Rheum* 26:918–920, 1983.

46. Ardoin S, Birmingham DJ, Hebert PL, et al: An approach to validating criteria for proteinuric flare in systemic lupus erythematosus glomerulonephritis. *Arthritis Rheum* 63:2031–2037, 2011.

47. Herbert LA, Dillon JJ, Middendorf DF, et al: Relationship between appearance of urinary red cell/white blood cell casts and the onset of renal relapse in systemic lupus erythematosus. *Am J Kidney Dis* 26:432–438, 1995.

48. Liaño F, Mampaso F, Garcia Martin F, et al: Allograft membranous glomerulonephritis and renal vein thrombosis in a patients with a lupus anticoagulant factor. *Nephrol Dial Transplant* 3:684–689, 1988.

49. Dubois EL: *Lupus erythematosus: a review of the current status of discoid and systemic lupus erythematosus and their variants,* ed 2, Los Angeles, 1976, USC Press.

50. Ward MM: Outcomes of renal transplantation among patients with endstage renal disease caused by lupus nephritis. *Kidney Int* 57:2136–2143, 2000.

51. Austin HA 3rd, Klippel JH, Balow JE, et al: Therapy of lupus nephritis. Controlled trial of prednisone and cytotoxic drugs. *N Engl J Med* 314:614–619, 1986.

52. Boumpas DT, Austin HA 3rd, Vaughn EM, et al: Controlled trial of pulse methylprednisolone versus two regimens of pulse cyclophosphamide in severe lupus nephritis. *Lancet* 340:741–745, 1992 Sep 26.

53. Gourley MF, Austin HA 3rd, Scott D, et al: Methylprednisolone and cyclophosphamide, alone or in combination, in patients with lupus nephritis. A randomized, controlled trial. *Ann Intern Med* 125:549–557, 1996.

54. Contreras G, Pardo V, Leclercq B, et al: Sequential therapies for proliferative lupus nephritis. *N Engl J Med* 350:971–980, 2004.

55. Houssiau FA, Vasconcelos C, D'Cruz D, et al: Immunosuppressive therapy in lupus nephritis: the Euro-Lupus Nephritis Trial, a randomized trial of low-dose versus high-dose intravenous cyclophosphamide. *Arthritis Rheum* 46:2121, 2002.

56. Houssiau FA, Vasconcelos C, D'Cruz D, et al: The 10-year follow-up data of the Euro-Lupus Nephritis Trial comparing low-dose and high-dose intravenous cyclophosphamide. *Ann Rheum Dis* 69:61–64, 2010.

57. Grootscholten C, Ligtenberg G, Hagen EC, et al; Dutch Working Party on Systemic Lupus Erythematosus: Azathioprine/methylprednisolone versus cyclophosphamide in proliferative lupus nephritis. A randomized controlled trial. *Kidney Int* 70:732–742, 2006.

58. Grootscholten C, Bajema IM, Florquin S, et al; Dutch Working Party on Systemic Lupus Erythematosus: Treatment with cyclophosphamide delays the progression of chronic lesions more effectively than does

treatment with azathioprine plus methylprednisolone in patients with proliferative lupus nephritis. *Arthritis Rheum* 56:924–937, 2007.

59. Arends S, Grootscholten C, Derksen RH, et al; on behalf of the Dutch Working Party on Systemic Lupus Erythematosus: Long-term follow-up of a randomised controlled trial of azathioprine/methylprednisolone versus cyclophosphamide in patients with proliferative lupus nephritis. *Ann Rheum Dis* 2011 Nov 29. [Epub ahead of print]

60. Appel GB, Contreras G, Dooley MA, et al: Mycophenolate mofetil versus cyclophosphamide for induction treatment of lupus nephritis. *J Am Soc Nephrol* 20:1103–1112, 2009.

61. Dooley MA, Jayne D, Ginzler EM, et al: Mycophenolate versus azathioprine as maintenance therapy for lupus nephritis. *N Engl J Med* 365:1886–1895, 2011.

62. Houssiau FA, D'Cruz D, Saugle S, et al: Azathioprine versus mycophenolate mofetil for long-term immunosuppression in lupus nephritis: results from the maintain nephritis trial. *Ann Rheum Dis* 69:2083–2089, 2010.

Chapter

36

Pregnancy in Women with SLE

Megan E. B. Clowse

Systemic lupus erythematosus (SLE) primarily affects women of childbearing age; pregnancy is therefore a dilemma frequently encountered in this patient population that requires prudent clinical guidance. In the past, because of concerns related to high maternal and fetal mortality rates, medical professionals generally recommended that women with SLE avoid pregnancy. Over the last few decades, however, advances in managing SLE in the context of pregnancy have improved the landscape of risk, and the majority of SLE pregnancies result in a healthy infant and mother.[1]

Barring previous exposure to cyclophosphamide, women with SLE experience normal fertility rates, and many will become pregnant easily (and sometimes unexpectedly).[2] For these reasons, to avoid unwanted or ill-timed pregnancies, addressing contraception with young women with SLE is essential. A small group of women are best advised to avoid pregnancy altogether—those with severe pulmonary hypertension or interstitial lung disease and those with a history of myocardial infarction or arterial thrombosis.

Approximately 4500 pregnancies occur annually in this patient population in the United States.[3,4] In some of these patients, pregnancy will lead to a dramatic intensification of symptoms that can be life threatening, but most will experience only a modest increase in symptoms, which may exacerbate the discomforts of pregnancy but will not affect long-term survival.[5] For a significant minority, pregnancy is complicated by SLE activity, preterm delivery, preeclampsia, and/or pregnancy loss. With current methods of managing SLE, however, mitigating these risks is possible. Indeed, with careful management and timing of pregnancy, most women with SLE can expect to deliver a child in good health.

IMMUNOBIOLOGIC IMPLICATIONS OF PREGNANCY

Physiologic Alterations of Pregnancy

Pregnancy is heralded by significant physiologic alterations in the mother's cardiovascular, renal, and immune systems that can have particular bearing on women with SLE. Maternal blood volume increases by 50%, elevating the heart rate, cardiac output, and renal and pulmonary blood flow. Women whose previous disease activity resulted in a damaged cardiopulmonary system may not be able to manage this increased blood volume in pregnancy and may also have particular difficulty with the rapid postpartum loss of volume. Vascular resistance decreases in pregnancy, leading to a mild decrease in blood pressure that may precipitate presyncopal episodes in some women.[6]

In women who have suffered renal damage, which is not uncommon among women with SLE, escalations in renal blood flow may lead to increased proteinuria. Although a 24-hour urine protein level of 300 mg is considered normal in any pregnancy and less than a two-fold increase in proteinuria is not unexpected, more dramatic levels require immediate attention, because they may signal the onset of either lupus nephritis or preeclampsia.[6] In the latter half of pregnancy, alterations in salt concentrations mediated by the kidneys may promote lower extremity edema. For the majority of women, this edema is uncomfortable but not a cause for concern; it can be managed by decreasing salt intake, elevating the legs, and wearing support hose. For some women, however, lower extremity edema may be a symptom of preeclampsia. If it is unilateral, a deep vein thrombosis must be considered.

Even among healthy women, thrombotic risk increases two- to three-fold during pregnancy, which is, in itself, a hypercoagulable condition.[7] Women with SLE are at high risk for thrombosis during pregnancy with 1% experiencing deep vein thrombosis, 0.4% experiencing pulmonary embolism, and 0.32% experiencing stroke.[4] Moreover, the risk for thrombosis continues for 6 weeks after delivery.

Immunologic Mechanisms of Pregnancy

A significant, yet poorly understood immunologic shift is required to maintain a pregnancy. Because the fetus is an allograft, the maternal immune system must have mechanisms that suppress its typical response to new antigens. The available data suggest that this happens along several routes, including the presentation of unique human leukocyte antigen G (HLA-G) proteins on fetal cells, the production of modified antibodies that selectively bind paternal antigens without stimulating a maternal immune reaction, and increases in the number and activity of regulatory T cells.[8,9] How these shifts interact with SLE is unclear. The possibilities vary widely in their implications. The mechanisms that improve maternal-fetal tolerance may also decrease rheumatologic disease; the new antigens might, on the other hand, intensify the production of maternal autoantibodies, or the SLE immune system may be more likely to result in fetal rejection due to impaired tolerance mechanisms. An understanding of these processes is currently too limited to apply them to the management of SLE in pregnancy.

SYSTEMIC LUPUS ERYTHEMATOSUS ACTIVITY IN PREGNANCY

Types of Systemic Lupus Erythematosus Activity and Their Impact on Pregnancy Outcomes

An estimated 50% of women with SLE will experience a flare during pregnancy.[10-17] In most, the flare will be mild, involve the skin or joints, and will not have a major impact on the pregnancy outcome or fetus. Up to 20% of women with SLE will have a more severe flare, involving the kidneys, hematologic disease, serositis, and/or severe arthritis, which can increase the risks for pregnancy loss, preterm birth, and preeclampsia.[11,12,15]

If SLE is active or platelet counts are low in the first trimester, then the risk for pregnancy loss is increased three- to five-fold (with a 44% rate of pregnancy loss among women with active SLE).[18] Women with active SLE are twice as likely to deliver prematurely as a result of medical intervention to protect the health of the mother, preeclampsia, and spontaneous preterm labor.[12]

Predictors of Systemic Lupus Erythematosus Activity

The three best predictors of SLE activity in pregnancy are the following:

1. Increased SLE activity in the 3 to 6 months before conception
2. Discontinuation of needed immunosuppressive agents during pregnancy
3. History of frequent and significant flares

Having minimal lupus activity in the 6 months before becoming pregnant lowers the chances of a significant SLE flare during pregnancy. Women with mild SLE in the 6 months before conception had an 8% risk of increased SLE activity in pregnancy, compared with a 56% risk among women with active SLE in this same period—a more than seven-fold increase.[12] Among women with active SLE at the time of conception, a two-fold increase in the risk for a lupus flare exists during pregnancy.[11,17] Because SLE activity is a primary cause of preterm birth and pregnancy loss in this population, preventing pregnancy in the months after a significant SLE flare through patient education and a prescription of contraception is important to avoid adverse maternal and fetal outcomes. Women with a history of multiple severe flares are at increased risk for flares in pregnancy. In addition, discontinuation of hydroxychloroquine (HCQ) before or during pregnancy increases the risk for SLE flares.[13,19]

To decrease the risk of SLE activity in pregnancy requires not only careful planning but also a willingness to modify, yet continue, immunosuppressive therapy. For women with a history of a significant flare, particularly lupus nephritis or significant cytopenias, the discontinuation of immunosuppression for pregnancy may be counterproductive. Although cyclophosphamide and mycophenolate mofetil (MMF)—and probably mycophenolic acid, although no published data is available—pose significant risks for pregnancy loss and for teratogenic effects on the fetus, other immunosuppressants are much safer. Azathioprine has been well documented in large studies of women with solid organ transplants and inflammatory bowel disease and has been determined to be safe and to have limited, if any, teratogenic risk.[20]

Considering the 40% risk of pregnancy loss, the 66% risk of preterm birth, and the increased maternal morbidity associated with significant SLE activity in pregnancy, it is difficult to overlook the advantages of continuing immunosuppressive therapy with azathioprine, HCQ, or cyclosporin, all of which are associated with no or minimal increase in pregnancy loss, preterm birth, and teratogenicity. If possible, MMF or cyclophosphamide should be switched to azathioprine or cyclosporin at least 3 to 6 months before conception to determine whether SLE will flare on the revised regimen.

PREGNANCY OUTCOMES IN SYSTEMIC LUPUS ERYTHEMATOSUS WITH MEDIATORS OF COMPLICATIONS

Whether or not SLE is active, women with SLE often have complicated pregnancies: One third will result in a cesarean section, another one third will result in preterm birth, and up to 20% will be affected by preeclampsia.[21-23] Offspring outcomes are generally positive, although low birth weight and small-for-gestational-age (SGA) status are not uncommon. Rates of maternal mortality do not appear to exceed those of women with SLE who are not pregnant. Although an SLE pregnancy can present a range of challenges requiring careful medical management, overall outcomes are good even when complications arise.

Pregnancy Loss

Approximately 20% of SLE pregnancies result in miscarriage or stillbirth.[1] Although the risk of miscarriage, which, by definition, occurs before 20 weeks' gestation, is not significantly elevated in patients with SLE relative to that of the general population, the risk of stillbirth, which occurs after 20 weeks' gestation, is elevated by approximately eight-fold to 5% to 10% of pregnancies, according to several studies[12,23] (Table 36-1).

Increased lupus activity and antiphospholipid syndrome (APS) appear to be the two most important predictors of pregnancy loss. Among a Greek cohort, fetal loss occurred in 75% of pregnancies of women with highly active SLE, compared with 14% of pregnancies in those without active lupus and 5% of non-SLE pregnancies.[24] Although lupus activity did not affect rates of miscarriage, it resulted in a three-fold increase in the stillbirth rate in the Hopkins lupus pregnancy cohort study.[12] Careful consideration must also be given to the timing of SLE activity; it directly correlates with the rates of pregnancy loss, with early pregnancy activity presenting the greatest cause for concern. When lupus activity is present at the time of conception and in the first trimester, the risk of pregnancy loss, particularly stillbirth, increases by up to three-fold.[5] Moreover, first-trimester proteinuria, thrombocytopenia, and hypertension each represent an independent risk factor for pregnancy loss, introducing a 30% to 40% chance of pregnancy loss.[18] Managing disease activity is therefore

TABLE 36-1 Pregnancy Outcomes in Prospective Cohorts of Pregnancies in Women with Systemic Lupus Erythematosus

	NUMBER OF PREGNANCIES	PREGNANCY LOSS	PRETERM BIRTH[1]	LOW BIRTH WEIGHT[1]	PREECLAMPSIA
Cortés-Hernández and colleagues, 2002[13]	103	34.0%	27.9%	35.3%	1.9%
Clowse and colleagues, 2005[12]	267	14.2%	46.3%	22.7%	Not reported
Cavallasca and colleagues, 2008[25]	72	15.3%	45.9%	39.3%	11.1%
Kwok and colleagues, 2011[26]	55	10.9%	49.0%	38.8%	20.0%
Smyth and colleagues, 2010[2,23]	1847	22.1%	39.4%	12.7%	7.6%

[1]Percentage of live births with complications.
[2]Metaanalysis included 12 prospective studies, including the first 3 cohorts in this table, and 25 retrospective studies of pregnancies in women with systemic lupus erythematosus (SLE).

essential to achieve clinical remission and thus reduce the risk of fetal loss.

Preterm Birth

Women with lupus are more likely to deliver prematurely, before 37 weeks' gestation. In one population-based study,[27] preterm deliveries occurred at a rate of 21% for women with SLE, almost six-fold higher than in healthy women. Cohorts at tertiary referral centers, however, suggest a more dramatic risk, with rates ranging from 20% to 54%.[10-17,21,28] Again, active SLE during pregnancy is the primary risk factor.[12] Although the rate of preterm birth is estimated to be 33% in women with quiescent SLE, it dramatically increases to 66% in pregnant women with an SLE flare.[21] Other risk factors for preterm birth include lupus activity in the months before pregnancy, higher prednisone doses, and hypertension.

Although a substantial proportion of early deliveries are medically induced to preserve maternal and fetal health (e.g., as in the context of preeclampsia), the majority of early deliveries result from spontaneous processes.[14,21] A prominent immediate cause of preterm birth among patients with lupus is the premature rupture of membranes (PROM).[14,29] In pregnant women without SLE, approximately one third of spontaneous preterm births are associated with chorioamnionitis, an infection in the uterus. The inflammation associated with chorioamnionitis leads to the dissolution of the fetal membranes, a ripening of the cervix, and uterine contractions, all of which induce premature delivery. At this time, no data have been published concerning the rate of chorioamnionitis in SLE pregnancies, but placenta studies have not demonstrated increased rates of infection or pathologic abnormalities.[30] Although the inflammation typical of active lupus may affect the uteroplacental unit in ways similar to chorioamnionitis, research has yet to clarify the role of inflammation in preterm birth.

Preeclampsia

Preeclampsia is defined as a combination of hypertension (blood pressure [BP] higher than 140/90 mm Hg) and proteinuria (more than 300 mg serum protein in the urine in 24 hours) that occurs in the third trimester and resolves postpartum. A dangerous pregnancy complication, preeclampsia places a woman and her fetus at considerable risk for stroke, preterm birth, and even death. Severe preeclampsia can be accompanied by a range of symptoms, including extreme hypertension (BP of 160/110 mm Hg); microangiopathic hemolytic anemia with thrombocytopenia, anemia, and an elevated lactate dehydrogenase level; liver damage with elevated liver enzymes and epigastric pain; ischemia of the central nervous system, leading to headaches, visual changes, and stroke; and renal pathologic disorders with nephritic-range proteinuria and an increasing serum creatinine level. In the most dramatic episodes, preeclampsia may evolve into eclampsia, which is characterized by the addition of maternal grand mal seizures. When preeclampsia occurs, the definitive treatment is delivery; hypertension, proteinuria, and the associated risks subside once the fetus and the placenta have been removed.

Women with SLE are at particularly high risk for developing preeclampsia in pregnancy. Although preeclampsia affects 5% to 8% of all pregnancies in the United States, it is far more common in SLE pregnancies with an estimated 7% to 35% rate of occurrence.[3,11,23,31,32] According to research, not only will an average of one in four women with SLE develop preeclampsia, but the risks are even greater for women with preexisting hypertension or a history of lupus nephritis.[3,4,33] Other risks include first pregnancy, a history of preeclampsia, active SLE at conception, positive anti–double stranded DNA (anti-dsDNA) or antiribonucleoprotein antibodies, low complement levels, and obesity.[11,14,31,32]

The cause of preeclampsia remains under investigation. Preeclampsia is generally thought to arise from vascular dysfunction in the placenta, possibly the result of poor implantation and diminished trophoblast invasion of the uterine spiral arteries.[34] Several experimental markers for preeclampsia, including soluble Fms-like tyrosine kinase 1 (sFlt-1) and placental growth factor (PGF), have been found to correspond to preeclampsia in patients with lupus, as they do in women without SLE.[35]

Daily low-dose aspirin may decrease the risk for preeclampsia, premature delivery, and fetal loss, especially among those already at high risk for such complications. Aspirin minimizes two factors that contribute to preeclampsia: (1) the vasoconstrictor thromboxane and (2) platelet activation. In a Cochrane Review[36] of aspirin in pregnancy, which included 57 trials, none of which specifically enrolled patients with autoimmune disease, and over 37,000 women, low-dose aspirin was found to be safe and even potentially beneficial for both mother and baby. For women at high risk for preeclampsia, daily low-dose aspirin can decrease the risk for preeclampsia by 25% and the risk for pregnancy loss by 31%.[36] Considering the particularly high risk for preeclampsia in SLE pregnancies, 81 mg of aspirin per day should be considered for all pregnant women with lupus.

Offspring Outcomes

Preterm birth is perhaps the greatest risk faced by offspring of mothers with SLE, because infants born before 28 weeks' gestation are more likely to endure long-term medical complications or die soon after birth. SLE activity during pregnancy greatly increases the probability of a dangerously early delivery. In the Hopkins lupus pregnancy cohort,[12] delivery between 24 and 28 weeks' gestation occurred in 17% of all pregnancies with active SLE, whereas delivery during this high-risk period occurred in only 6% of those pregnancies in which SLE was quiescent.

Whether low birth weight is a higher risk for offspring of women with SLE than it is in women without SLE is still a matter of debate. Because high rates of preterm birth complicate any study of birth weight, especially among lupus pregnancies, weight is generally corrected according to gestational age. Infants who weigh less than the tenth percentile based on national norms are considered SGA. On average, of all SLE pregnancy cohort births, 9.4% were SGA, which is comparable to expectations in the general population.[21] However, certain cohorts had SGA rates as high as 35%.[12,14]

Because the risk for SGA is relatively low, clear risk factors have not been identified. Placental insufficiency could lead to slow fetal growth and inadequate weight gain. Accordingly, with placental studies reporting a higher incidence of thrombosis among SLE pregnancies, some of these pregnancies can be expected to produce growth-restricted infants.[30]

Maternal Mortality Rate

The maternal mortality rate for women with SLE—325 per 100,000 pregnancies—is estimated to be twenty-fold higher than it is for average women.[4] However, when the annual death rate for all women with SLE is taken into consideration—approximately 1000 per 100,000 patient years—it appears that pregnancy probably does not increase the risk of death for women with SLE.[37] However, women with SLE who have had previous arterial thrombosis, a weakened heart from myocarditis, previous myocardial infarction or valve disease, uncontrolled hypertension, pulmonary hypertension, or a previous severe SLE flare during pregnancy may be placed at a higher risk for death by becoming pregnant.

TYPES OF DISEASE ACTIVITY

Fortunately, most pregnant women with SLE experience only mild disease activity. The most common presenting symptoms include skin, joint, and constitutional disorders. Depending on the severity measured, the risk for skin disorders ranges from 25% to 90%.[10,24,38] Similarly disparate rates have been reported for arthritis symptoms during SLE pregnancy, again based on the degree of severity assessed. Although a 20% risk of significant arthritis exists, according to two large cohort studies, many more women will experience an increase in joint pain that is less severe.[10] The risk of developing hematologic disease during pregnancy, in particular, thrombocytopenia, ranges from 10% to 40%.[10,24]

TABLE 36-2 Factors That Distinguish Systemic Lupus Erythematosus Activity, Pregnancy Symptoms, and Preeclampsia

	SLE ACTIVITY	PREGNANCY SYMPTOMS	PREECLAMPSIA
Timing in pregnancy	Any time during or after pregnancy	Any time during pregnancy, varies with each trimester	Second half of pregnancy, after 20 weeks More typically after 30 weeks Resolution within weeks of delivery
Extremities	Pain localized over joints	Mild-to-moderate pitting edema in the lower extremities, particularly in the second half of pregnancy	Rapid onset of lower extremity edema
Hands	Pain localized over joints Possible improvement in Raynaud phenomenon	Diffuse swelling Carpal tunnel syndrome	
Pulmonary system	Increased pulmonary embolism risk Pleurisy	Tachypnea in first trimester as a result of progesterone Dyspnea in third trimester as a result of increasing uterine size	
Cardiovascular system	Pericarditis	Tachycardia Orthostatic hypotension	Hypertension with blood pressure >140/90 mm Hg Chest pain
Gastrointestinal system		Nausea and vomiting in the first half of pregnancy	
Renal system	Proteinuria; can double if baseline is not normal Active urinary sediment Rising creatinine	Fall in creatinine levels Mild proteinuria <300 mg/24 hr	Proteinuria >300 mg/24 hr Bland urinary sediment Rising creatinine
Hematologic considerations	Thrombocytopenia Rare hemolytic anemia Lymphopenia	Thrombocytopenia to 100 k/mm² can be normal Mild anemia from hemodilution Elevated WBC count	Significant thrombocytopenia, hemolytic anemia
Lupus-associated laboratory tests	Complement low Positive dsDNA in activity	Possible increase in complement	No dramatic changes in complement and dsDNA
Other laboratory tests			Increasing uric acid Decreased urine calcium

dsDNA, double-stranded DNA; HELLP, hemolysis, elevated liver enzymes, low platelet count; SLE, systemic lupus erythematosus; WBC, white blood cell.

Lupus Nephritis
Frequency in Pregnancy
Depending on the characteristics of a given cohort and how lupus nephritis is defined in a given study, the overall risk for developing lupus nephritis ranges from 4% to 30%.[13,16,28,38] A history of lupus nephritis increases the risk of relapse during pregnancy to 20% to 30% among women with SLE.[13,16] For women whose renal function has been impaired by SLE nephritis during the course of pregnancy, an estimated 25% will endure ongoing postpartum renal damage, even when an aggressive course of therapy is prescribed.[13-15] Very few patients, however, will require life-long dialysis.

Impact on Pregnancy Outcomes
Although a history of lupus nephritis does not preclude pregnancy, the risks for reactivation of lupus activity, preeclampsia, and pregnancy loss are increased. Research suggests that among patients with a history of lupus nephritis before becoming pregnant, overall rates of nonelective pregnancy loss range from 8% to 36%.[31,39,40] However, if creatinine levels remain stable and proteinuria is minimal, only 11% to 13% of pregnancies among patients with previous lupus nephritis result in fetal loss.[31,41] Fetal loss occurs in 36% to 52% of pregnancies complicated by active lupus nephritis.[31,39] Prematurity rates of 35% to 40% are reported in most studies of women with lupus nephritis in pregnancy.[31,39,40]

Differentiating Lupus Nephritis from Preeclampsia
Distinguishing preeclampsia from a lupus nephritis flare is one of the greatest challenges faced by medical professionals caring for patients with SLE during pregnancy; at times, it is impossible. Previous lupus nephritis increases the risk for both a renal flare during pregnancy and for preeclampsia, further complicating efforts to discriminate between the two conditions. Although the presentations for both conditions include proteinuria, hypertension, and lower extremity edema, treatment is different for each of these conditions. For preeclampsia, immediate delivery is indicated and results in complete remission; lupus nephritis requires immunosuppressive therapy.

The breadth of symptoms associated with severe preeclampsia makes it necessary to assess specific risk factors, as well as laboratory and physical findings that may clarify the diagnosis (Table 36-2). Although preeclampsia is often accompanied by an increase in serum uric acid or a decline in urine calcium, lupus nephritis may be accompanied by falling complement, rising anti-dsDNA titers, and other signs or symptoms of active lupus, such as arthritis, elevated body temperatures, and rash. Thrombocytopenia, hemolysis, and elevated liver tests occur in both severe preeclampsia and in lupus nephritis, which precludes these tests from serving as reliable factors for distinguishing the two conditions.

When the pregnancy is near full term and the cause for illness remains indeterminate, delivery may be the best option. If symptoms continue for longer than 48 hours after delivery, then aggressive treatment for SLE should be started immediately. If the condition occurs in earlier stages of pregnancy, however, a better approach may be to administer high-dose steroids, which could improve the medical situation and thus prolong the opportunity for in utero fetal development.[5]

Antiphospholipid Syndrome
Etiologic and Pathophysiologic Characteristics
APS is characterized by the presence of antiphospholipid antibodies (APLAs) in the setting of either vascular thrombosis or pregnancy

TABLE 36-3 Pregnancy Outcomes in Randomized Controlled Trials of Treatments for Antiphospholipid Syndrome

STUDY	Heparin Plus Aspirin			Aspirin Alone			
	NUMBER OF PREGNANCIES	NUMBER OF PREGNANCY LOSSES	PREGNANCY LOSS RATE	NUMBER OF PREGNANCIES	NUMBER OF PREGNANCY LOSSES	PREGNANCY LOSS RATE	P-VALUE
Kutteh, 1996[47]	25	5	20%	25	14	56%	<0.05
Farquharson and colleagues, 2002[48]	51	11	22%	47	13	28%	0.29
Rai and colleagues, 1997[49]	45	13	29%	45	26	58%	<0.05

complications.[42] Among the proposed mechanisms for APS-induced pregnancy loss is APLA interaction with platelet membrane phospholipids; inhibition of annexin-V, a cell-surface protein that inhibits tissue factor; direct inhibition of protein S; and an altered regulation of the complement cascade.[43,44] Recent insights into the pathophysiologic characteristics of APS suggest that poor pregnancy outcomes may be related not only to thrombosis but also to inflammation via the complement cascade.

Pregnancy Outcomes
Pregnancy complications associated with APS include recurrent first trimester loss, second and third trimester fetal loss, or early development of severe preeclampsia. If APS remains untreated, then fetal loss will occur in 45% to 90% of pregnancies.[45] The chance of pregnancy loss decreases to less than 30% when treatment is administered[46] (Table 36-3).

Maternal Outcomes
The maternal risks associated with pregnancy for women with APS are often overlooked. Preeclampsia and the more severe HELLP (**H**emolysis, **E**levated **L**iver enzymes, **L**ow **P**latelet count) syndrome are both increased in women with APS. The risk for these complications does not appear to be significantly decreased with anticoagulation therapy.[50] Both arterial thrombosis (including myocardial infarction and stroke) and venous thrombosis are also risks that are not completely eliminated by anticoagulation therapy. The risk for thrombosis is particularly elevated in the days after delivery; consequently, resuming anticoagulation therapy as soon as possible after delivery is important. This risk persists for 6 weeks postpartum, and anticoagulation therapy should not be discontinued until this period has passed.[51]

Impact of Medications
Several studies have assessed a range of potential therapeutic regimens for women with obstetric APS, defined as the presence of APLAs and recurrent miscarriage or at least one fetal loss, in the absence of SLE or previous thrombosis. The following current treatment guidelines are based on expert opinion and the best available data.
1. For patients with APLAs but with no history of thrombosis or pregnancy complications, either no treatment or treatment with low-dose aspirin is recommended.
2. For women with APLAs and a history of pregnancy complication, treatment with a prophylactic dose of low-molecular-weight heparin (LMWH) in combination with low-dose aspirin is recommended.
3. In women with APLAs and history of vascular thrombosis, treatment with a full dose of LMWH and low-dose aspirin is recommended.[52]

Although unfractionated heparin is less expensive than LMWH and has been used to prevent coagulation in patients with APS, LMWH is the preferred treatment because it introduces less risk for osteoporosis, heparin-induced thrombocytopenia, and bruising.[53] At this time, no studies support long-term anticoagulation therapy with

warfarin after pregnancy in patients with APS with only obstetric complications.

MEDICATIONS IN SYSTEMIC LUPUS ERYTHEMATOSUS PREGNANCY
Considering the risks of active SLE to both mother and fetus outlined earlier in this chapter, the prevention of SLE activity during pregnancy is of primary importance. The risks of some medications are minimal and should not dissuade a patient from taking immunosuppressant medications when warranted (Table 36-4).

In the absence of signs or symptoms of active SLE, women with lupus require no specific treatment during pregnancy. Although the prophylactic use of corticosteroids was formerly considered good practice, that recommendation has been rescinded because of increased rates of hypertension, preterm birth, and low birth weight associated with the excessive use of this medication.

Nonsteroidal Antiinflammatory Drugs and Acetaminophen
Women should avoid taking nonsteroidal antiinflammatory drugs (NSAIDs) around the time of implantation; women who take NSAIDs may be more likely to suffer an early miscarriage.[54] Preliminary evidence suggests that cyclooxygenase (COX) enzymes, which NSAIDs inhibit, are necessary for embryo implantation.[20,54,55] During the latter part of the first trimester and during the second trimester, occasional use of NSAIDs is considered fairly safe, although they may decrease fetal renal excretion and therefore lead to a deficiency in the levels of amniotic fluid.[56] In the third trimester, however, women should avoid taking NSAIDs; they can prolong labor and promote premature closure of the ductus arteriosus.[20] Low-dose aspirin (less than 100 mg per day) does not increase the risk of closure of the ductus arteriosus and is considered safe through to delivery.

Corticosteroids
Corticosteroid use is relatively safe in pregnancy and is a cornerstone of treatment for rheumatic disease during this time. For most pregnant women with SLE, inflammation related to accelerated autoimmune activity places the pregnancy at higher risk than steroids, even at higher doses. When treating the mother with a corticosteroid is necessary, prednisone and prednisolone are recommended; less than 10% of the dose will cross the maternal-fetal membranes.[20] Mild SLE activity is easily treated with prednisone in low doses (less than 20 mg per day). Although limiting daily prednisone to less than 20 mg is optimal, the mother can be treated with higher doses of corticosteroids, including pulse-dose steroids, in the presence of more severe lupus activity.

As in women who are not pregnant, the side effects associated with corticosteroids include increased maternal risk for hypertension and diabetes. Systemic corticosteroid use carries a two- to three-fold increase in the risk for cleft lip or palate, although the absolute risk remains low (approximately 3 per 1000 infants exposed to corticosteroids).[57] Fluorinated glucocorticoids, such as dexamethasone and betamethasone, easily cross the placenta and can be helpful in treating the fetus, in particular to address congenital heart blocks or to

TABLE 36-4 Medications for Women with Systemic Lupus Erythematosus in Pregnancy and Lactation

	FDA PREGNANCY CLASSIFICATION[1]	PREGNANCY	LACTATION
acetaminophen	C	Minimal risk at therapeutic doses	AAP approved
NSAIDs	C (first and second trimester) D (third trimester)	Occasional use in first and second trimesters; avoided in third trimester because of the closure of the ductus arteriosus	AAP approved; ibuprofen preferred
prednisone	C	Best medication to control SLE in pregnancy; may increase risk of cleft lip or palate (first trimester), preeclampsia, and preterm birth	AAP approved; acceptable if dose is less than 20 mg/day
hydroxychloroquine	C	Well tolerated; low teratogenic risk; discontinuation increases risk of SLE flare	AAP approved
methotrexate	X	Avoid; teratogenic risk (10%)	Contraindicated
azathioprine	D	Well tolerated; low teratogenic risk	Generally avoided
cyclosporin	C	Low teratogenic risk	Generally avoided
mycophenolate mofetil	D	Avoid; high risk of pregnancy loss; teratogenic risk (25%)	Avoided
cyclophosphamide	D	Avoid; teratogenic in first trimester (>20%)	Avoided
belimumab	C	Unknown	Unknown
rituximab	C	Unknown	Unknown
abatacept	C	Unknown	Unknown

AAP, American Academy of Pediatrics; NSAIDs, nonsteroidal antiinflammatory drugs; SLE, systemic lupus erythematosus.

[1]U.S. Food and Drug Administration (FDA) pregnancy classification: A: Human studies show no risk to the fetus in any trimester. B: Animal reproductive studies show no risk to the fetus; no adequate or well-controlled human studies have been conducted; OR animal studies show an adverse effect, but human studies show no risk to the fetus in any trimester. C: An adverse effect is shown in animal studies, but no adequate or well-controlled human studies have been conducted; drugs should only be given if potential benefits outweigh the risks. D: Adverse effects in human studies show positive evidence of risk to the fetus, but potential benefits may warrant use in pregnancy to treat serious disease, despite the risks. X: Animal and human studies demonstrate adverse effects, and the risks clearly outweigh the potential benefits; use is contraindicated in pregnancy.

promote fetal lung maturity before a preterm delivery. However, they have also been associated with lasting adverse effects on the offspring, including increased blood pressure and possibly cognitive deficits.[58] In addition, fetal exposure to ongoing dexamethasone or high-dose prednisone treatments may result in newborn adrenal insufficiency.[20] Dexamethasone and betamethasone therefore should not be administered to manage SLE flares during pregnancy.

Hydroxychloroquine

HCQ, a well-tolerated medication, is often prescribed to patients with SLE who are not pregnant to decrease the risk of an SLE flare, improve the prognosis of SLE nephritis, and prevent death.[59] A panel of international leaders[20] in the research and care of women with SLE recently recommended that patients with SLE continue to take HCQ during pregnancy.

HCQ has perhaps the best side-effect profile of all available SLE medications. In studies of more than 300 offspring with in utero exposure to HCQ, no overall elevation of fetal anomalies was identified, nor did a specific pattern of anomalies emerge.[19,60] Although chloroquine may result in ocular or auditory damage when taken in supratherapeutic doses, no instances of such damage were reported among 133 infants with fetal exposure to HCQ.[60] Indeed, infants exposed to HCQ in utero have normal electrocardiographic results at delivery, as well as normal results for ophthalmic and auditory examinations after birth.[60-62] In addition, HCQ has been shown to decrease the need for high-dose corticosteroids.[19]

When patients with SLE who are not pregnant discontinue treatment with HCQ, their risk for elevated SLE activity increases twofold for the 6 months that follow.[59] Likewise, pregnant patients with SLE who stop taking HCQ increase their risk for flares. In the Hopkins lupus pregnancy cohort,[19] 56 patients with lupus maintained their HCQ regimen throughout pregnancy, whereas 38 patients ceased taking HCQ just before pregnancy or early in pregnancy because of concerns about fetal exposure. Among those 38 women, the risk for lupus flare—whether measured by the physician's estimate

of activity, by changes in this scale, or by the Systemic Lupus Erythematosus Disease Activity Index (SLEDAI)—increased substantially, and more of these women required corticosteroids at higher doses than did women who maintained treatment. As in other studies, the Hopkins lupus pregnancy cohort reported no increase in fetal abnormalities after HCQ exposure. Pregnancy outcomes were similar among all women in the study, which may reflect that the type of SLE activity suffered by women who discontinued treatment largely involved fatigue and joint symptoms, rather than more serious complications such as lupus nephritis, anemia, or thrombocytopenia. Although the symptoms these women experienced were not life threatening and did not require cytotoxic therapy, they did at times necessitate the commencement or increase of corticosteroid use during pregnancy.

Azathioprine

Despite being listed in the U.S. Food and Drug Administration (FDA) pregnancy category D, azathioprine may in fact be the safest immunosuppressant medication for use during pregnancy. Initial reports noted immunosuppressive activity in offspring, but more recent studies have provided evidence of its relative safety. Not only has it been shown that azathioprine crosses the maternal-fetal membranes largely in the form of thiouric acid, an inactive metabolite, but no significant increase in congenital anomalies were documented in case-control studies that compared pregnancies with and without azathioprine exposure.[63] The enzyme required to metabolize azathioprine into its active form cannot be produced by the fetal liver.[20]

Among pregnant women who were treated with azathioprine for inflammatory bowel disease or after renal transplant, no significant increase in fetal abnormalities was detected.[20] However, up to 40% of the offspring of patients who had a renal transplant were SGA; whether SGA status was the result of underlying illness, corticosteroids, or azathioprine is unclear.[20,64]

Few data are available concerning the use of azathioprine in women with SLE during pregnancy. In one cohort study,[65] 31 pregnancies were exposed to azathioprine. Of the 13 women who continuously took azathioprine, from before conception and for the duration of pregnancy, 2 women had pregnancy loss, both of whom had experienced SLE flares. All 10 women whose lupus activity remained low and who were treated with azathioprine throughout pregnancy had successful, near-term deliveries. Continuation of azathioprine treatment through all three trimesters is therefore recommended for women who require it to manage lupus symptoms before pregnancy. Switching from MMF to azathioprine therapy before conception is also advisable to avoid the teratogenic repercussions of the former.

Mycophenolate Mofetil

MMF, marketed as CellCept and Myfortic, is an immunosuppressant medication often used to treat lupus nephritis, but it should be strictly avoided during pregnancy. The data on MMF in pregnancy are limited but worrisome, suggesting an elevated risk for both fetal anomalies and pregnancy losses.[20] A report of 21 pregnancies in women with renal transplants who took MMF during pregnancy found a high rate of pregnancy loss (42%) and, of fetuses born alive, a high rate of fetal anomalies (26%). Three of the four abnormal infants had ear anomalies and one died as a result of severe malformations.[66] For this reason, the FDA pregnancy warning was increased from C to D, and it is recommended that the drug be discontinued before pregnancy. Women taking MMF before pregnancy may benefit from switching to azathioprine before conception to prevent an SLE flare during pregnancy.

Cyclosporin

Many pregnancies in women with solid organ transplants have been successful after treatment with cyclosporin.[66] Although the rates of premature delivery and SGA infants are increased in these patients, it is unclear whether these increases are the result of the medications or the underlying disease. A few case reports support the safe use of cyclosporin to treat SLE during pregnancy.[67,68]

Cyclophosphamide

Although cyclophosphamide (Cytoxan) is a known teratogen, particularly when exposure occurs during the first trimester, no significant pregnancy loss or congenital anomalies have been documented among women treated for breast cancer in the latter half of pregnancy.[69] In SLE pregnancy, however, cyclophosphamide use has been less successful, with only three reported cases resulting in a live birth; in utero fetal death occurred soon after the administration of the drug in the other two patients.[70-71] It remains unclear whether these pregnancy losses were the result of the use of cyclophosphamide or the severity of the lupus activity that prompted such treatment. Nevertheless, avoiding conception during cyclophosphamide therapy is advisable; consequently, contraception should be prescribed and pregnancy tests administered for the duration of treatment. Cyclophosphamide should be considered a treatment of last resort and should not be pursued until the medical caregiver has had a candid discussion with the mother about the risk for pregnancy loss.

Intravenous Immunoglobulin

Intravenous immunoglobulin (IVIG) is considered relatively safe for the management of moderate to severe SLE activity during pregnancy, since the fetus is already exposed to maternal immunoglobulin during the latter half of pregnancy. IVIG can be particularly helpful in the context of hematologic and renal diseases.[72]

Although further validation is needed, a preliminary study of 12 patients with SLE indicated that IVIG diminishes SLE activity and promotes a successful pregnancy.[73] The literature on the offspring effects of IVIG is limited, but cell count levels appear to remain stable and no congenital anomalies have been reported in infants with in utero exposure to the drug. Sucrose-containing IVIG can lead to maternal renal insufficiency, but sucrose-containing IVIG has not materially affected the treatment of lupus nephritis in women who

are not pregnant.[72] Severe side effects are rare with IVIG therapy, but some women will experience minor effects such as headaches, rigors, or elevated body temperatures.

Rituximab

Although the randomized pharmaceutical-sponsored trials of rituximab did not show efficacy in the treatment of SLE, rituximab is still used by some clinicians. Data supporting the use of rituximab in pregnancy are limited but reassuring. It is classified by the FDA as class C for pregnancy because studies in monkeys during organogenesis were associated with dose-dependent decreases in fetal B cells that persisted for up to 6 months after birth. No teratogenic effects were noted, however.[74]

Over 150 pregnancies with known exposure to rituximab either during or before pregnancy have been reported. In data accumulated by the drug maker, 60% of 153 pregnancies resulted in a live birth with almost one half of the losses the result of elective termination.[74] Of the live births, 24% resulted in a preterm birth, all delivered between 30 and 37 weeks' gestation, and two births had congenital anomalies (1 clubfoot, 1 cardiac defect). A subset of 20 pregnancies with the administration of rituximab during pregnancy for maternal disease demonstrated improved outcomes: no pregnancy losses, no maternal deaths, and no congenital anomalies; 55% delivered at term. However, significant neonatal lymphopenia was reported in 7 of the 11 infants in which it was measured.[74]

Belimumab

Belimumab is classified by the FDA as class C, likely as a result of decreases in B cell and immunoglobulin levels in infant monkeys exposed to the drug in utero. No congenital anomalies or increase in pregnancy loss was noted in these studies.[75] In data released to the FDA, eight reported pregnancies occurred during randomized trials of belimumab for SLE: one in the placebo group that ended in a spontaneous abortion and seven in the belimumab group, five of which ended in a spontaneous abortion. Based on the available data, establishing the safety of belimumab in pregnancy is not possible; however, the drug maker is collecting a registry of exposed pregnancies.

DISCUSSION

Lupus activity can be instigated by the hormonal and physiologic changes associated with pregnancy. In turn, significant pregnancy complications can be precipitated by the elevated inflammatory responses of a lupus flare. Because discriminating between SLE symptoms and the signs of pregnancy can be difficult, whether healthy or with pathologic abnormalities, pregnant women with SLE are best served by including a rheumatologist and a high-risk obstetrician on their medical teams. Although they may require skilled guidance and care, most women with lupus can remain healthy during pregnancy and successfully deliver babies.

References

1. Clark CA, Spitzer KA, Laskin CA: Decrease in pregnancy loss rates in patients with systemic lupus erythematosus over a 40-year period. *J Rheumatol* 32(9):1709–1712, 2005.
2. Mitchell K, Kaul M, Clowse ME: The management of rheumatic diseases in pregnancy. *Scand J Rheumatol* 39(2):99–108, 2010.
3. Chakravarty EF, Nelson L, Krishnan E: Obstetric hospitalizations in the United States for women with systemic lupus erythematosus and rheumatoid arthritis. *Arthritis Rheum* 54(3):899–907, 2006.
4. Clowse ME, Jamison M, Myers E, et al: A national study of the complications of lupus in pregnancy. *Am J Obstet Gynecol* 199(2):127, e1–e6, 2008.
5. Clowse ME: Lupus activity in pregnancy. *Rheum Dis Clin North Am* 33(2):237–252, v, 2007.
6. Maynard SE, Karumanchi SA, Thadhani RI: Hypertension and kidney disease in pregnancy. In Brenner B, editor: *Brenner and Rector's the kidney*, ed 8, Philadelphia, 2007, Saunders Elsevier.
7. James AH, Brancazio LR, Ortel TL: Thrombosis, thrombophilia, and thromboprophylaxis in pregnancy. *Clin Adv Hematol Oncol* 3(3):187–197, 2005.

8. Hunt JS, Langat DL: HLA-G: a human pregnancy-related immunomodulator. *Curr Opin Pharmacol* 9(4):462–469, 2009.

9. Munoz-Suano A, Hamilton AB, Betz AG: Gimme shelter: the immune system during pregnancy. *Immunol Rev* 241(1):20–38, 2011.

10. Carmona F, Font J, Cervera R, et al: Obstetrical outcome of pregnancy in patients with systemic lupus erythematosus. A study of 60 cases. *Eur J Obstet Gynecol Reprod Biol* 83(2):37–142, 1999.

11. Chakravarty EF, Colón I, Langen ES, et al: Factors that predict prematurity and preeclampsia in pregnancies that are complicated by systemic lupus erythematosus. *Am J Obstet Gynecol* 192(6):1897–1904, 2005.

12. Clowse ME, Magder LS, Witter F, et al: The impact of increased lupus activity on obstetric outcomes. *Arthritis Rheum* 52(2):514–521, 2005.

13. Cortés-Hernández J, Ordi-Ros J, Paredes F, et al: Clinical predictors of fetal and maternal outcome in systemic lupus erythematosus: a prospective study of 103 pregnancies. *Rheumatology (Oxford)* 41(6):643–560, 2002.

14. Lima F, Buchanan NM, Khamashta MA, et al: Obstetric outcome in systemic lupus erythematosus. *Semin Arthritis Rheum* 25(3):184–192, 1995.

15. Rubbert A, Pimer K, Wildt L, et al: Pregnancy course and complications in patients with systemic lupus erythematosus. *Am J Reprod Immunol*, 28(3-4):205–207, 1992.

16. Tincani A, Faden D, Tarantini M, et al: Systemic lupus erythematosus and pregnancy: a prospective study. *Clin Exp Rheumatol* 10(5):439–446, 1992.

17. Urowitz MB, Gladman DD, Farewell VT, et al: Lupus and pregnancy studies. *Arthritis Rheum* 36(10):1392–1397, 1993.

18. Clowse ME, Madger LS, Witter F, et al: Early risk factors for pregnancy loss in lupus. *Obstet Gynecol* 107(2 Pt 1):293–299, 2006.

19. Clowse ME, Madger LS, Witter F, et al: Hydroxychloroquine in lupus pregnancy. *Arthritis Rheum* 54(11):3640–3647, 2006.

20. Østensen M, Khamashta M, Lockshin M, et al: Anti-inflammatory and immunosuppressive drugs and reproduction. *Arthritis Res Ther* 8(3):209, 2006.

21. Clark CA, Spitzer KA, Nadler JN, et al: Preterm deliveries in women with systemic lupus erythematosus. *J Rheumatol* 30(10):2127–2132, 2003.

22. Clowse ME, Jamison M, Myers E, et al: A national study of the complications of lupus in pregnancy. *Am J Obstet Gynecol* 199(2):127, e1–e6, 2008.

23. Smyth A, Oliveira GH, Lahr BD, et al: A systematic review and meta-analysis of pregnancy outcomes in patients with systemic lupus erythematosus and lupus nephritis. *Clin J Am Soc Nephrol* 5(11):2060–2068, 2010.

24. Georgiou PE, Politi EN, Katsimbri P, et al: Outcome of lupus pregnancy: a controlled study. *Rheumatology (Oxford)* 39(9):1014–1019, 2000.

25. Cavallasca JA, Laborde HA, Ruda-Vega H, et al: Maternal and fetal outcomes of 72 pregnancies in Argentine patients with systemic lupus erythematosus (SLE). *Clin Rheumatol* 27(1):41–46, 2008.

26. Kwok LW, Tam LS, Zhu T, et al: Predictors of maternal and fetal outcomes in pregnancies of patients with systemic lupus erythematosus. *Lupus* 20(8):829–836, 2011.

27. Yasmeen S, Wilkins EE, Field NT, et al: Pregnancy outcomes in women with systemic lupus erythematosus. *J Matern Fetal Med* 10(2):91–96, 2001.

28. Wong KL, Chan FY, Lee CP: Outcome of pregnancy in patients with systemic lupus erythematosus. A prospective study. *Arch Intern Med* 151(2):269–273, 1991.

29. Johnson MJ, Petri M, Witter FR, et al: Evaluation of preterm delivery in a systemic lupus erythematosus pregnancy clinic. *Obstet Gynecol* 86(3):396–399, 1995.

30. Magid MS, Kaplan C, Sammaritano LR, et al: Placental pathology in systemic lupus erythematosus: a prospective study. *Am J Obstet Gynecol* 179(1):226–234, 1998.

31. Moroni G, Ponticelli C: The risk of pregnancy in patients with lupus nephritis. *J Nephrol* 16(2):161–167, 2003.

32. Qazi UM, Petri M: Autoantibodies, low complement, and obesity predict preeclampsia in SLE: a case-control study. *Arthritis Rheum* 54(9 Suppl): S264, 2006.

33. Carmona F, Font J, Moga I, et al: Class III-IV proliferative lupus nephritis and pregnancy: a study of 42 cases. *Am J Reprod Immunol* 53(4):182–188, 2005.

34. Lamarca B: The role of immune activation in contributing to vascular dysfunction and the pathophysiology of hypertension during preeclampsia. *Minerva Ginecol* 62(2):105–120, 2010.

35. Qazi U, Lam C, Karumanchi SA, et al: Soluble Fms-like tyrosine kinase associated with preeclampsia in pregnancy in systemic lupus erythematosus. *J Rheumatol* 35(4):631–634, 2008.

36. Duley L, Henderson-Smart DJ, Meher S, et al: Antiplatelet agents for preventing pre-eclampsia and its complications. *Cochrane Database Syst Rev* (2):CD004659, 2007.

37. Cervera R, Khamashta MA: Epidemiology of systemic lupus erythematosus at the change of the millennium: lessons from the Euro-Lupus and the LUMINA projects. *Lupus* 15(1):1–2, 2006.

38. Petri M, Howard D, Repke J, et al: The Hopkins Lupus Pregnancy Center: 1987–1991 update. *Am J Reprod Immunol* 28(3-4):188–191, 1992.

39. Rahman FZ, Rahman J, Al-Suleiman SA, et al: Pregnancy outcome in lupus nephropathy. *Arch Gynecol Obstet* 271(3):222–226, 2005.

40. Wagner SJ, Craici I, Reed D, et al: Maternal and foetal outcomes in pregnant patients with active lupus nephritis. *Lupus* 18(4):342–347, 2009.

41. Jungers P, Dougados M, Pélissier C, et al: Lupus nephropathy and pregnancy. Report of 104 cases in 36 patients. *Arch Intern Med* 142(4):771–776, 1982.

42. Miyakis S, Lockshin MD, Atsumi T, et al: International consensus statement on an update of the classification criteria for definite antiphospholipid syndrome (APS). *J Thromb Haemost* 4(2):295–306, 2006.

43. Bick RL: Antiphospholipid syndrome in pregnancy. *Hematol Oncol Clin North Am* 22(1):107–120, vii, 2008.

44. Salmon JE, Girardi G: Antiphospholipid antibodies and pregnancy loss: a disorder of inflammation. *J Reprod Immunol* 77(1):51–56, 2008.

45. Rai RS, Clifford K, Cohen H, et al: High prospective fetal loss rate in untreated pregnancies of women with recurrent miscarriage and antiphospholipid antibodies. *Hum Reprod* 10(12):3301–3304, 1995.

46. Empson M, Lassere M, Craig JC, et al: Recurrent pregnancy loss with antiphospholipid antibody: a systematic review of therapeutic trials. *Obstet Gynecol* 99(1):135–144, 2002.

47. Kutteh WH: Antiphospholipid antibody-associated recurrent pregnancy loss: treatment with heparin and low-dose aspirin is superior to low-dose aspirin alone. *Am J Obstet Gynecol* 174(5):1584–1589, 1996.

48. Farquharson RG, Quenby S, Greaves M: Antiphospholipid syndrome in pregnancy: a randomized, controlled trial of treatment. *Obstet Gynecol* 100(3):408–413, 2002.

49. Rai R, Cohen H, Dave M, et al: Randomised controlled trial of aspirin and aspirin plus heparin in pregnant women with recurrent miscarriage associated with phospholipid antibodies (or antiphospholipid antibodies). *BMJ* 314(7076):253–257, 1997.

50. Clark EA, Silver RM, Branch DW: Do antiphospholipid antibodies cause preeclampsia and HELLP syndrome? *Curr Rheumatol Rep* 9(3):219–225, 2007.

51. Branch DW, Silver RM, Porter TF: Obstetric antiphospholipid syndrome: current uncertainties should guide our way. *Lupus* 19(4):446–452, 2010.

52. Derksen RH, Khamashta MA, Branch DW: Management of the obstetric antiphospholipid syndrome. *Arthritis Rheum* 50(4):1028–1039, 2004.

53. Bates SM, Greer IA, Hirsh J, et al: Use of antithrombotic agents during pregnancy: the Seventh ACCP Conference on Antithrombotic and Thrombolytic Therapy. *Chest* 126(3 Suppl):627S–644S, 2004.

54. Li DK, Liu L, Odouli R: Exposure to non-steroidal anti-inflammatory drugs during pregnancy and risk of miscarriage: population based cohort study. *BMJ* 327(7411):368, 2003.

55. Scherle PA, Ma W, Lim H, et al: Regulation of cyclooxygenase-2 induction in the mouse uterus during decidualization. An event of early pregnancy. *J Biol Chem* 275(47):37086–37092, 2000.

56. Topuz S, Has R, Ermiş H, et al: Acute severe reversible oligohydramnios induced by indomethacin in a patient with rheumatoid arthritis: a case report and review of the literature. *Clin Exp Obstet Gynecol* 31(1):70–72, 2004.

57. Park-Wyllie L, Mazzotta P, Pastuszak A, et al: Birth defects after maternal exposure to corticosteroids: prospective cohort study and meta-analysis of epidemiological studies. *Teratology* 62(6):385–392, 2000.

58. Costedoat-Chalumeau N, Amoura Z, Le Thi Hong D, et al: Questions about dexamethasone use for the prevention of anti-SSA related congenital heart block. *Ann Rheum Dis* 62(10):1010–1012, 2003.

59. No author. A randomized study of the effect of withdrawing hydroxychloroquine sulfate in systemic lupus erythematosus. The Canadian Hydroxychloroquine Study Group. *N Engl J Med* 324(3):150–154, 1991.

60. Costedoat-Chalumeau N, Amoura Z, Duhaut P, et al: Safety of hydroxychloroquine in pregnant patients with connective tissue diseases: a study of one hundred thirty-three cases compared with a control group. *Arthritis Rheum* 48(11):3207–3211, 2003.

61. Klinger G, Morad Y, Westall CA, et al: Ocular toxicity and antenatal exposure to chloroquine or hydroxychloroquine for rheumatic diseases. *Lancet* 358(9284):813–814, 2001.

62. Motta M, Tincani A, Faden, D, et al: Follow-up of infants exposed to hydroxychloroquine given to mothers during pregnancy and lactation. *J Perinatol* 25(2):86–89, 2005.

63. Polifka JE, Friedman JM: Teratogen update: azathioprine and 6-mercaptopurine. *Teratology* 65(5):240–261, 2002.

64. Miniero R, Tardivo I, Curtoni ES, et al: Pregnancy after renal transplantation in Italian patients: focus on fetal outcome. *J Nephrol* 15(6):626–632, 2002.

65. Clowse MEB, Magder LS, Witter F, et al: Azathioprine use in lupus pregnancy. *Arthritis Rheum* 52(9 Suppl):S386–S387, 2005.

66. Armenti VT, Daller JA, Constantiescu S, et al: Report from the National Transplantation Pregnancy Registry: outcomes of pregnancy after transplantation. *Clin Transpl* 57–70, 2006.

67. Hussein MM, Mooij JM, Roujouleh H: Cyclosporine in the treatment of lupus nephritis including two patients treated during pregnancy. *Clin Nephrol* 40(3):160–163, 1993.

68. Doria A, Di Lenardo L, Vario S, et al: Cyclosporin A in a pregnant patient affected with systemic lupus erythematosus. *Rheumatol Int* 12(2):77–78, 1992.

69. Gwyn KM, Theriault RL: Breast cancer during pregnancy. *Curr Treat Options Oncol* 1(3):239–243, 2000.

70. Clowse ME, Magder L, Petri M: Cyclophosphamide for lupus during pregnancy. *Lupus* 14(8):593–597, 2005.

71. Kart Köseoglu H, Yücel AE, Künefeci G, et al: Cyclophosphamide therapy in a serious case of lupus nephritis during pregnancy. *Lupus* 10(11):818–820, 2001.

72. Rauova L, Lukac J, Levy Y, et al: High-dose intravenous immunoglobulins for lupus nephritis—a salvage immunomodulation. *Lupus* 10(3):209–213, 2001.

73. Perricone R, De Carolis C, Kröegler B, et al: Intravenous immunoglobulin therapy in pregnant patients affected with systemic lupus erythematosus and recurrent spontaneous abortion. *Rheumatology (Oxford)* 47(5):646–651, 2008.

74. Chakravarty EF, Murray ER, Kelman A, et al: Pregnancy outcomes after maternal exposure to rituximab. *Blood* 117(5):1499–1506, 2011.

75. Auyeung-Kim DJ, Devalaraja MN, Migone TS, et al: Developmental and peri-postnatal study in cynomolgus monkeys with belimumab, a monoclonal antibody directed against B-lymphocyte stimulator. *Reprod Toxicol* 28(4):443–455, 2009.

Chapter 37

Neonatal Lupus Erythematosus

Marie Wahren-Herlenius, Sven-Erik Sonesson, and Megan E. G. Clowse

The association of neonatal cardiac and skin disease with maternal systemic lupus erythematosus (SLE) was first identified through case reports in the 1950s and 1960s.[1,2] Since then, several clinical manifestations, most importantly congenital heart block (CHB), but also neonatal skin lesions, transient hematologic and a liver abnormalities, central nervous system (CNS) involvement, and rare bone disease, have all been linked to in utero exposure to maternal anti–Sjögren syndrome antigen A (anti-SSA/Ro) or anti–Sjögren syndrome antigen B (anti-SSB/La) antibodies[3] (Table 37-1).

Maternal IgG antibodies of all subclasses are transported across the placenta, starting at approximately 16 weeks' gestation. Although the complete spectrum of maternal IgG specificities, including autoantibodies, cross the placenta, the vast majority of cases of neonatal lupus erythematosus (NLE) are associated with anti-SSA/Ro and anti-SSB/La antibodies, with a few cases associated with antiribonucleoprotein (anti-RNP) or antihistone antibodies.[4-6] Infants born to women with these antibodies are expected to have circulating maternal autoantibodies at decreasing levels for the first 3 to 6 months of life.[7,8]

The majority of infants born to women with anti-SSA/Ro antibodies are born without obvious abnormalities or illnesses. Cutaneous disease occurs in up to 25% of infants exposed to anti-SSA/Ro antibodies, but it is mild and resolves without diagnosis or significant acknowledgment in many patients.[9] Complete CHB occurs in up to 2% of infants exposed to SSA/Ro antibodies, with a recurrence rate between 12% and 20%.[10-13] The occurrence of CHB in infants born to women with a prior infant with NLE involving the skin has been reported as 13%.[14] Hematologic manifestations often go unnoticed in an otherwise healthy infant but can be found in up to 50% of tested infants.[15] Mild elevations of transaminase enzymes typically remain asymptomatic but can be identified in 25% of tested infants.[15,16] Neurologic abnormalities, including hydrocephalus and nonspecific white matter changes, which are visualized with brain computed tomography (CT), have been reported in fewer than 10% of exposed infants, often without symptoms.[17,18] A rare skeletal disorder, chondrodysplasia punctata, may also be associated with in utero exposure to maternal autoantibodies.[3,19]

Maternal disease manifestations before and during pregnancy do not appear to have a significant impact on neonatal outcomes. The mothers may be diagnosed with Sjögren syndrome (SS) or SLE; however, fewer than 20% of the women fulfill the criteria for a rheumatic disease at the time that CHB is detected in the fetus, although many mothers display symptoms of an undifferentiated connective tissue disease and have complaints such as dry eyes, dry mouth, fatigue, or photosensitivity.[20,21] Approximately one half of the women without a diagnosis will progress to rheumatologic disease over the subsequent 3 to 6 years, most commonly SS or SLE.[21,22]

ETIOLOGIC FACTORS AND PATHOGENESIS

The close association of NLE with maternal SSA/Ro and SSB/La antibodies rather than manifest clinical rheumatic disease led to the hypothesis that the antibodies have a direct role in disease pathogenesis. The histopathologic examination of the hearts of fetuses who died of CHB support antibody involvement and an inflammatory reaction as part of the process leading to conduction failure, with the presence of Ro-specific immunoglobulin and complement deposits, inflammatory cells dominated by macrophages, and cytokine expression, including tumor necrosis factor–alpha (TNF-α) and transforming growth factor–beta (TGF-β).[23-25] Calcification and fibrosis denote end-stage destruction of the atrioventricular (AV) node and will clinically correspond to complete, third-degree AV block (AVB) (Figure 37-1). Of note, antibodies, complement deposits, and signs of fibrosis and calcification can be observed not only at the AV node but also in the entire myocardium, suggesting a potential involvement of maternal autoantibodies in other cardiac manifestations of CHB, such as sinus bradycardia and cardiomyopathy.

Maternal Autoantibodies in Congenital Heart Block

The association between maternal SSA/Ro and SSB/La autoantibodies and CHB was described in the early 1980s.[26,27] The observation that the SSA/Ro autoantigen consists of two unrelated proteins, Ro52 and Ro60,[28,29] and subsequent studies of the CHB association with maternal antibodies have led to efforts determine the serum profile of mothers of affected children regarding the three components, Ro52, Ro60, and La. Although the data vary among the different studies, depending on the methods used for antibody detection, as well as the definition of CHB, the enrollment criteria for pregnancies, most of the attempts demonstrate that anti-Ro and especially anti-Ro52 antibodies are present in a high proportion of mothers of children with CHB.[4-6,30-32] The close correlation between maternal anti-Ro52 antibodies and CHB in combination with the fact that only 1% to 2% of children born to women who are anti-Ro positive develop heart block, has prompted a search for a specific profile within the pool of maternal anti-Ro52 antibodies. Dominant epitopes within the central part of the Ro52 protein have been described in the context of SLE and SS,[33,34] and epitope mapping using overlapping peptides covering this region revealed a significant association between maternal antibodies to amino acids 200-239 of Ro52 (denoted p200) and the risk for CHB.[6,30,35] In a prospective study of women who were anti-Ro52 positive during weeks 18 through 24 of pregnancy, maternal antibodies to Ro52/p200 were shown to correlate to longer AV time intervals in the fetuses.[36]

As anti-Ro60 and anti-La antibodies are most often found with anti-Ro52 antibodies, assessing their individual contribution to the development of CHB is difficult. In addition, most studies still rely on clinical assays that do not distinguish between Ro52 and Ro60 to investigate the presence of anti-Ro antibodies in maternal sera. In two studies, the levels of anti-La antibodies were found to be higher in mothers of children with cutaneous NLE than in women giving birth to a child with CHB.[37,38] However, another study suggested that the risk for CHB was increased in the presence of anti-La antibodies.[39] The current consensus is that antibodies to Ro60 and La may contribute to the inflammatory reaction that leads to AV block but CHB may develop in their absence.

Considering the low risk for fetal heart block in an anti-Ro–positive pregnancy (2%), a search for other antibodies associated with heart block has been undertaken by different research groups and has yielded some candidates. However, this small number of studies has often involved too few infants to demonstrate a reliable association between the presence of antibodies and pregnancy outcomes. Thus antibodies to calreticulin, a protein involved in calcium storage, have been found more frequently in sera from mothers of children with CHB than in sera from mothers of healthy children.[40] Antibodies recognizing the muscarinic acetylcholine receptor M_1 have also been associated with the development of CHB, and in vitro studies suggest a functional role for these antibodies through binding to and interfering with the function of their target in the neonatal myocardium.[41,42] In addition, antibodies recognizing a cleavage product of α-fodrin have been proposed as an additional serologic marker for heart block.[43] Similarly, reactivity to the α_{1D} calcium channel subunit was recently found in sera from mothers of children with CHB; however, such reactivity was limited to approximately 14% of all mothers of infants with CHB who were tested.[44]

To date, anti-Ro52 antibodies seem to remain the maternal autoantibodies that correlate to the development of CHB to the greatest extent, despite the low penetrance of the condition in anti-Ro–positive pregnancies. It is possible that not only the presence but also the levels of maternal anti-Ro52 antibodies are of importance in predicting fetal outcome, as is suggested in a recent study in which cardiac conduction disturbances were associated with moderate to high levels of anti-Ro antibodies but not with low levels.[38]

Clues to Pathogenic Mechanisms in Congenital Heart Block from Experimental Models

Direct evidence of a pathogenic role of maternal anti-Ro and anti-La antibodies in CHB come from experimental in vitro and in vivo studies of heart block. In vitro studies on rat or human hearts perfused with the Langendorff technique have demonstrated a direct pathogenic role of antibodies from mothers of children with CHB, because maternal IgG containing anti-Ro or anti-La antibodies induced bradycardia and complete AV block within 15 minutes.[45,46] Affinity-purified anti-Ro52 antibodies had the same effects, showing the individual pathogenic potential of anti-Ro52 antibodies. Similar results were obtained in Langendorff-perfused rabbit hearts exposed to anti-Ro or anti-La antibodies purified from mothers of children with CHB.[47,48]

Evidence for the pathogenicity of anti-Ro or anti-La antibodies in vivo has been gathered from animal models based on the passive transfer of antibodies or active immunization of women before gestation. Transfer of affinity-purified anti-Ro or anti-La antibodies from mothers of children with CHB into pregnant female BALB/c mice induced first-degree AV block and sinus bradycardia in the offspring.[49] Immunization models of CHB, in which female rats, mice, or rabbits were injected with a particular antigen before gestation, made it possible to investigate separately the pathogenic potential of antibodies toward Ro52, Ro60, or La. Immunization of BALB/c mice with Ro60 or La led to the development of first-degree AV block in 19% or 7% of the offspring, respectively,[50] and similar results were observed in C3H/HEJ mice.[51] Immunization of mice, rats, or rabbits with the human or mouse Ro52 protein induced first-degree AV block in 9% to 45% of the offspring[45,50,52,53] but also higher degrees of AV block and rates of neonatal deaths.[45,50,52] The AV block–inducing capacity of Ro52 antibodies and the fine specificity of the Ro52 antibodies inducing block have been further confirmed by both immunization with the Ro52-p200 peptide[36] and the passive transfer of monoclonal antibodies targeting different epitopes in different domains of the Ro52 protein.[54] In the transfer of Ro52 monoclonal antibodies to pregnant rats, only antibodies targeting amino acids

TABLE 37-1 Frequency of Different Organ Manifestations in Children Born to Mothers Who Are Positive for Anti–Sjögren Syndrome Antigen A

ORGAN AND TYPE OF MANIFESTATION	REPORTED FREQUENCY	REFERENCE
Heart		
First-degree atrioventricular block[1]	10%-14%	70, 100
Third-degree atrioventricular block	2%	10
Skin	25%	
Liver	9%-26%	15, 16
Elevated transaminase enzymes	25%	15
Hematologic manifestations	27%-50%	15
Neutropenia	23%	15
Anemia	5%	15
Thrombocytopenia	4%	15
Nervous system		
Hydrocephalus (transient)	10%	17
Nonspecific white matter changes	8%	
Bone		
Chondrodysplasia punctata	Rare	91, 92

[1]Observed by postnatal electrocardiographic examination.

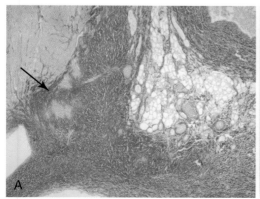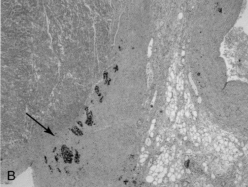

FIGURE 37-1 Histopathologic examination of a fetal heart affected by congenital heart block (CHB). Formalin-fixed, paraffin-embedded cardiac tissue, including the atrioventricular (AV) nodal area *(arrows)* from a fetus that died from CHB during gestational week 36 was sectioned and stained with Sirius red stain (A) and hematoxylin stain (B) to visualize fibrosis and calcification, respectively.

200-239 of Ro52 induced AV block, which was observed in 100% of exposed pups.[54]

Targets for Maternal Antibodies in the Fetal Heart

The intracellular localization of the Ro52, Ro60, and La proteins has proven a major stumbling block in the elucidation of the molecular mechanisms leading to CHB. How can the antibodies exert a pathogenic effect if their target antigens are not within their reach? Two schools of thought, not mutually exclusive and each supported by experimental data, have emerged: the *apoptosis hypothesis* and the *cross-reactivity hypothesis*.

The apoptosis hypothesis postulates that maternal antibodies gain access to their target antigen when it is exposed on the surface of apoptotic cells. The presence of Ro60 or La has indeed been reported on apoptotic cardiac myocytes.[50] Ro52 has also been detected on the surface of apoptotic but not live cardiac cells in one study, although only one out of the five anti-Ro52 monoclonal antibodies tested bound apoptotic cells and did so to a lesser extent than did anti-Ro60 or anti-La antibodies.[55]

The apoptosis hypothesis fails, however, to explain the rapid electrophysiologic effects of maternal anti-Ro or anti-La antibodies on Langendorff-perfused hearts and the specificity of the reaction in targeting the AV node. The cross-reactivity hypothesis therefore suggests that maternal anti-Ro and anti-La antibodies, or at least a subset of these, bind to cardiac membrane proteins involved in the control of electric signal generation or conduction or both, interfering with their function. The involvement of maternal anti-Ro52 antibodies cross-reacting with the serotoninergic 5-hydroxytryptamine (5-HT_4) receptor was suggested after Eftekhari and colleagues[56] found that antibodies to the Ro52 peptide 365-382 recognized residues 165-185 of the cardiac 5-HT_4 receptor and that affinity-purified 5-HT_4 antibodies could antagonize the serotonin-induced calcium channel activation in atrial cells.[57] However, only 16% of the sera from mothers of children with CHB were shown to be positive for anti–5-HT_4 antibodies, indicating that cross-reactivity to the serotoninergic 5-HT_4 receptor, if indeed involved in the development of CHB, may only represent a small subset of cases.[58]

Calcium channels constitute another group of molecules investigated for an involvement in CHB. IgG purified from mothers of children with CHB inhibits L-type and T-type calcium currents in ventricular myocytes, as well as in sinoatrial node cells and exogenous expression systems.[46,52,59-61] Experimental data supporting a possible cross-reactivity of maternal anti-Ro or anti-La antibodies with the α_{1C} and α_{1D} calcium channel subunits have also been provided.[60,61] Further, mouse pups transgenic for the L-type calcium channel, voltage-dependent, α_{1C} subunit (Ca_v 1.2) were found to develop AV block and sinus bradycardia at a lower frequency than nontransgenic littermates after in utero exposure to anti-Ro or anti-La antibodies in an immunization model.[44] In addition, mouse pups in which the Ca_v1.3 subunit of the L-type calcium channel has been genetically knocked out exhibit first-degree AV block, and the occurrence of AV block is increased after immunization of the female mice with the Ro and La protein before gestation.[62] A specific effect of Ro52 antibodies targeting the p200 epitope was demonstrated as p200-specific monoclonal antibodies that induced AV block in vivo also dysregulated calcium oscillations of spontaneously beating primary neonatal cardiomyocytes in culture.[54] Although these studies do not prove that maternal anti-Ro and anti-La antibodies directly cross-react with subunits of the L-type calcium channel, they support the hypothesis that maternal autoantibodies exert their pathogenic effects at least in part by affecting calcium homeostasis in the heart and disrupting the cardiac electric and contractile functions. Prolonged disruption of cardiac calcium homeostasis may possibly lead to increased apoptosis in the fetal heart,[36] which would then be accompanied by exposure of the intracellular Ro and La proteins and allow for the establishment and amplification of an inflammatory reaction as described in the apoptosis hypothesis, leading to irreversible damage and complete CHB (Figure 37-2).

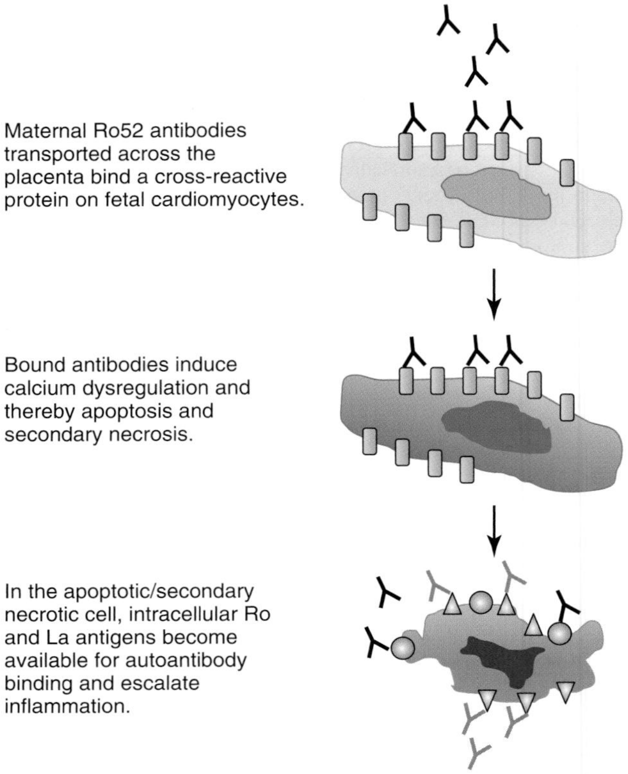

Maternal Ro52 antibodies transported across the placenta bind a cross-reactive protein on fetal cardiomyocytes.

Bound antibodies induce calcium dysregulation and thereby apoptosis and secondary necrosis.

In the apoptotic/secondary necrotic cell, intracellular Ro and La antigens become available for autoantibody binding and escalate inflammation.

FIGURE 37-2 How Ro52 autoantibodies may induce congenital heart block (CHB). Schematic illustrations visualize the binding of maternal Ro52 antibodies to a cross-reactive fetal cardiac cell surface antigen, inducing calcium regulation (Karnabi, Salomonsson), followed by apoptosis and secondary necrosis, thereby exposing intracellular antigens and making them accessible for direct binding Ro and La antibodies (Clancy) and escalating cardiac inflammation.

Additional Risk Factors in Congenital Heart Block Development

A risk of 2% for CHB in an anti-Ro–positive pregnancy and a reported recurrence rate of only 12% to 20%,[10-13] despite persisting maternal antibodies, indicate that additional factors are critical for the establishment of heart block. Epidemiologic, environmental, and genetic factors have been investigated in this respect (Table 37-2).

Although neither fetal gender nor maternal disease severity has been associated with CHB,[13,32,63] it has been proposed that maternal age or parity or both may have an influence on the outcome of anti-Ro52–positive pregnancies.[8] An analysis of risk factors for the development of heart block in a population-based Swedish cohort demonstrated that the risk for CHB increased with maternal age but was not influenced by parity.[13] In addition, the seasonal timing of the pregnancy influenced the outcome, with an increased proportion of affected pregnancies when the susceptibility weeks (18 to 24 weeks' gestation) fell in the late winter season. An association of the winter season with decreased sun exposure and vitamin D levels readily comes to mind; in addition, however, other events linked to the winter season such as viral infections may provide the mechanistic explanation for the seasonal influence on the development of heart block.

Genetic polymorphisms influencing fetal susceptibility to CHB in anti-Ro– and anti-La–positive pregnancies were first investigated in a group of 40 children with CHB using a candidate-gene approach and focusing on two known polymorphisms of the genes encoding the proinflammatory and profibrotic cytokines TNF-α and TGF-β. The TGF-β polymorphism assessed was found significantly more

TABLE 37-2 Factors Examined and Influencing or Not Influencing the Risk for Congenital Heart Block

PARAMETER	INFLUENCES	REFERENCE
Maternal Ro/La antibodies	Yes	5, 6, 26, 27, 112
Maternal age[1]	Yes	8, 13
Previous congenital heart block (CHB) pregnancy[2]	Yes	11-13
Increasing parity	No	13
Maternal disease activity	No	32, 63
Fetal gender	No	13
Season of birth[3]	Yes	13
Maternal histocompatibility complex (MHC)[4]	Yes	53, 113
Fetal MHC[5]	Yes	53, 65, 114

[1]The odds ratio for CHB increases by four in women 35 years of age and older, compared with women 24 years of age or younger.
[2]The risk for CHB increases six- to ten-fold in pregnancies after a CHB pregnancy in mothers who are positive for Ro/La antibodies.
[3]The risk for CHB increases in gestational weeks 18 to 24.
[4]Maternal human leukocyte antigen (HLA)–DRB1*03 is more frequently observed in mothers of children with CHB than in the general population.
[5]Fetal MHC genes influence the risk for the development of CHB, with the tumor necrosis factor–alpha (TNF-α) polymorphism and HLA-Cw3 identified as genetic factors.

frequently in children with CHB, whereas the TNF-α polymorphism studied was found at an increased frequency in both children with CHB or rash, compared with those in the healthy control group.[64] These findings have, however, not yet been replicated in a large group of infants with CHB. More recently, a genome-wide association study of infants with CHB born to anti-Ro– and anti-La–positive mothers was performed and a significant association with polymorphisms in the HLA region and at the location 21q22 reported, compared with those in the healthy control group.[65] Although the association with the major histocompatibility complex (MHC) locus is supported by experimental studies in an animal model,[53] one should be careful in the interpretation of the genetic associations because the studies presented so far were performed by comparing infants with CHB with healthy control infants from the general population. The associations may therefore reflect the genetic bias present in the mothers who may have SLE or SS or, even if asymptomatic, have autoantibodies to the Ro/La autoantigens.

CARDIAC MANIFESTATIONS

An isolated AVB without any associated cardiac malformation is most frequently detected at 18 to 24 weeks' gestation[66,67] when the block is already complete and results in sustained fetal bradycardia with a regular ventricular rate between 35 and 80 beats per minute (bpm). Recent fetal magnetocardiographic observations do not only provide support that the onset of complete AVB appears to be an early and rapid progress, but they also confirm a more complex disease process, including more diverse rhythm and conduction abnormalities such as junctional ectopic tachycardia or ventricular tachycardia, than previously appreciated.[68]

The authors of this text and other investigators have reported a 10% to 14% prevalence of first-degree AVB at birth, remaining stable or normalizing before 1 year of age.[69,70] In addition to AVB, both transient sinus bradycardia and QT prolongation, resolving without complications, have been observed after birth in small cohort groups of fetal antibody–exposed infants,[10,71] but these have not been consistently demonstrated by other studies.[72]

The postnatal progression from normal sinus rhythm and first- and second-degree AVB (with or without a history of successful fetal steroid treatment of second-degree AVB) to a higher degree of block has been described in infants exposed to maternal anti-Ro and anti-La antibodies.[73,74] The progression of incomplete AVB has also been observed in fetuses initially diagnosed with second-degree AVB progressing to a complete AVB.[75,76]

Maternal anti-Ro and anti-La antibodies have not only been demonstrated to affect the tissue of the cardiac conduction system, but they have also induced a more diffuse reaction within the endo-myocardium, with an echocardiographic presentation of ventricular dilation and systolic dysfunction, myocardial hypertrophy, and, in addition, a frequent increased echogenicity of the endocardium—endocardial fibroelastosis (EFE).[77,78] Fetal EFE is observed in close to 15% of fetuses with AVB,[67] usually when detecting the block, and frequently progresses to end-stage heart failure and death.[67,78] Fatal cases of fetal EFE have also been observed in the absence of AVB,[77] but most reported cases of isolated EFE seem to have a better prognosis. EFE located to papillary muscles has also been associated with the rupture of the valve tensor apparatus of the AV valves, resulting in severe regurgitation.[79]

Complete AVB has a significant risk of perineonatal demise, ranging from 10% to 30%, particularly in association with heart rates below 50 to 55 bpm, fetal hydrops, EFE, and poor ventricular function.[66,67,75,80] In addition, approximately 5% to 10% of neonatal survivors with normal cardiac function at birth develop a life-threatening dilated cardiomyopathy during the childhood years.[81-83] The wide spectrum of neonatal outcomes in CHB is illustrated in three different fetuses in Figure 37-3.

CUTANEOUS MANIFESTATIONS

The cutaneous manifestations of NLE are common and frequently benign. Up to 25% of infants exposed to SSA/Ro antibodies in utero will develop neonatal lupus skin lesions, which are histopathologically similar to subacute cutaneous lupus erythematosus (SCLE).[3] Similar to SCLE lesions, they are typically erythematous, slightly scaly, and usually annular with the middle of each lesion somewhat faded. They have a predilection for the face, although not particularly in a malar distribution, and can also occur on the trunk, diaper area, or extremities. Confluence of the lesions in the periorbital area gives the appearance of a "raccoon mask" or "owl eye."[84,85] In addition, similar to SCLE, the lesions are photosensitive but can also occur in areas without sun exposure.[9] On rare occasions, the rash can have a bullous appearance, particularly on the soles of the feet.

The lesions are most frequently noticed within the first 2 months of life and can be present at birth. They resolve within 6 months after birth as the maternal autoantibodies dissipate. When present, they typically last for 4 to 5 months.[8] The majority of lesions (80% to 90%) resolve without scarring, but they may leave hyperpigmentation or telangiectasias that can be long lasting.[8]

Skin abnormalities are common in infants, the majority of which resolve without specific intervention. Other diagnoses to consider in an infant with an erythematous rash include psoriasis, atopic dermatitis, neonatal acne, tinea corporis, urticaria, erythema multiforme, seborrheic dermatitis, granuloma annulare, annular erythema of infancy, and congenital infections. Antibody testing in the mother can help clarify the diagnosis. A skin biopsy is not typically required for diagnosis,[85] but, if performed, the findings may include damaged keratinocytes with vacuolar changes; a superficial mononuclear cell infiltrate may be present, and IgG deposition in a particulate pattern may be found in the epidermis on immunofluorescence.[9]

Most infants with cutaneous NLE respond to low-potency topical steroids, resolving within 2 weeks after treatment is initiated. Breast-feeding, which prolongs the exposure of the infant to maternal autoantibodies, does not appear to influence the development of NLE skin lesions.[86,87] Avoiding sun exposure may be helpful. Oral medications are not indicated; systemic corticosteroids are not required and antimalarial medications are too slow to be effective for this transient condition.[9] Laser therapy may resolve residual telangiectasias once the primary skin lesion is gone.[85]

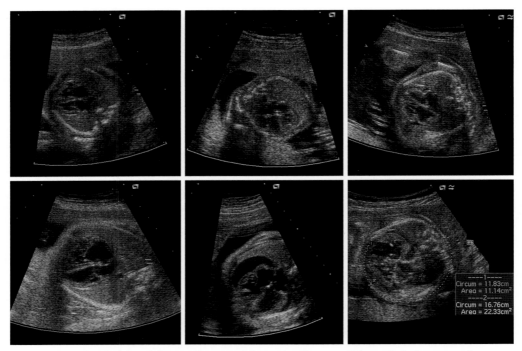

FIGURE 37-3 **Complete atrioventricular block (AVB) diagnosed at 20 weeks' gestation illustrates different clinical courses and outcomes.** Echocardiographic recordings were obtained in a transverse projection of the thorax, showing the ventricles and atrias of the hearts in three fetuses. Examinations performed at the time of diagnosis *(top row)* show a more or less normal-sized heart with normal thickness and echogenicity of the ventricular walls and septum in all three fetuses. At follow-up, the first fetus *(bottom, left)* still appeared normal. The second fetus *(bottom, middle)* had a severely dilated, hypertrophic heart with pericardial effusion that did not respond to treatment and resulted in fetal demise at 32 weeks' gestation. The third fetus *(bottom, right)* had junctional tachycardia at 21 weeks and thereafter developed a dilated cardiomyopathy with poor ventricular function and patchy echogenic changes, typical for endocardial fibroelastosis. In addition, these abnormalities were resistant to transplacental treatment and resulted in an intrauterine death.

OTHER MANIFESTATIONS
Hematologic Abnormalities

Most hematologic abnormalities caused by NLE go unnoticed, are asymptomatic, and resolve within several weeks after birth. Of 124 infants with in utero exposure to anti-SSA/Ro antibodies, 27% developed a hematologic anomaly.[15] The most common finding was neutropenia (23%), followed by anemia (5%) and thrombocytopenia (4%). Among the infants with blood levels monitored periodically through the first year of life, hematologic abnormalities were most commonly found between 1 and 2 months of life (50%) and least commonly at birth (13%). Despite low neutrophil levels, sepsis was not reported.

Liver Abnormalities

NLE involvement in the liver is a generally unappreciated consequence of in utero antibody exposure. In a prospective study in which liver function tests were routinely assessed in 120 infants with in utero exposure to anti-SSA/Ro antibodies, 26% had at least one liver test abnormality.[15] In a subset of these infants with serial laboratory testing (e.g., alanine aminotransferase [ALT], aspartate aminotransferase [AST], gamma-glutamyl transferase [GGT] from birth through the first year of life), 16 of 19 infants (84%) had abnormal results at birth, compared with 11 of 17 infants (65%) between 3 and 5 months of age. The most common finding was an elevated GGT, signifying cholestasis, which was found in 11% of infants. All of the abnormalities revealed in this study were described as mild, and no infants displayed any clinical symptoms, even though five infants continued to have abnormal levels at 1 year of age.

In contrast, more serious liver disease was observed in a retrospective review of the Research Registry for Neonatal Lupus. The authors found liver abnormalities attributed to NLE in 19 of 219 infants,[16] most likely an underestimate of the actual incidence because the majority of the 180 infants without reported liver disease did not undergo liver testing or evaluation. Of the 19 children, 6 died from fulminant liver failure, 4 of whom were found to have dramatically increased iron storage in the liver (i.e., neonatal hemochromatosis). Of the infants who died, 4 also had CHB and the other 2 were siblings without other manifestations of NLE. Of the remaining infants, one half had cholestasis with increased conjugated bilirubin levels but normal transaminases, and the other one half had elevated transaminase levels but normal bilirubin. Based on this study, three patterns of hepatic involvement with NLE have been described: (1) fulminant liver failure with iron storage, (2) transient mild cholestasis, and (3) transient transaminitis.

Neurologic Abnormalities

The blood-brain barrier is not completely formed in utero, leading to potential exposure of maternal SSA/Ro antibodies to the fetal central nervous system, which may lead to pathologic manifestations. Neuroimaging in the first 5 weeks of life may uncover abnormalities, including echogenic lenticulostriate vessels, which are a nonspecific indicator of prenatal brain injury. In a series of 10 infants with cutaneous NLE with or without hematologic and hepatic disease, 3 infants had these changes and an additional 6 infants had cerebral white matter changes. Despite these findings, the infants appeared to be neurologically intact. Transient hydrocephalus has been reported in 7 of 87 infants (8%) born to women with anti-SSA/Ro antibodies. Of these, only 1 had clinical consequences and required neurosurgical intervention.[17]

Parent-reported neuropsychiatric diagnoses were not significantly higher in children with NLE when compared with unaffected siblings and friends.[88] However, an increased frequency of attention-deficit disorder in boys with CHB was suggested. Studies have uncovered a higher prevalence of learning disabilities and attention-deficit disorder in boys born to mothers with SLE.[89] A study of children exposed to both SSA/Ro antibodies and high doses of dexamethasone, however, did not reveal an increased rate of neuropsychiatric difficulties.[90]

Chondrodysplasia Punctata

Chondrodysplasia punctata (CDP) is a rare congenital anomaly that exhibits bone and cartilage anomalies. Punctate calcifications are found with x-ray examination in the epiphyses of the long bones, nasal bone, trachea, larynx, and vertebrae, leading to malformation of the face and limbs. It has been linked to a variety of genetic abnormalities including peroxisomal disorders, disorders of cholesterol biogenesis, teratogen exposures, and congenital infections.[91] CDP also appears to be associated with maternal SLE, mixed connective tissue disease, and scleroderma with more than a dozen cases reported in the literature. Although a specific autoantibody has not been consistently reported in these patients, suspected pathophysiologic characteristics include the maternal autoantibody targeting a protein in the fetal cartilage, leading to inflammation and damage.[92]

FETAL SCREENING AND SURVEILLANCE
Cardiac Involvement

Fetal monitoring during pregnancy may identify CHB early (Table 37-3). Fetal echocardiography with m-mode and Doppler techniques remains the dominating modality for prenatal diagnosis of fetal cardiac rhythm, conduction, and function.

Recent advances in signal processing have improved the acquisition of transabdominal fetal electrocardiography (ECG), but atrial depolarizations (p waves) are still difficult to detect.[93] Magnetocardiography, which provides significantly better signal quality than fetal ECG, is probably the most accurate technique for the evaluation of fetal AVB, but it is expensive, requires a magnetically shielded room, and is available in few centers.

Assuming that AVB is a gradually progressing and preventable disease, starting during a critical period in midgestation with a less abnormal AV conduction before progressing to a complete AVB, ultrasound Doppler methods have been developed and reference values established to detect first-degree AVB.[93-97] Using standard ultrasound equipment, atrial and ventricular depolarizations are identified indirectly by their mechanical or hemodynamic consequences.[98,99] A specific schedule has not yet been tested or established, but most experts recommend repeated fetal ECG examinations between weeks 16 and 18, between weeks 24 and 26, and even into the third trimester.

The authors' experience of using these techniques for the surveillance of SSA/Ro52 antibody–exposed fetuses is that almost 30% display abnormal AV conduction, the majority normalizing before or shortly after birth; however, less than 5% develop second- or third-degree AVB.[69] Interestingly, a mechanical component of the time interval contributes to the transient prolongation of AV time intervals, suggesting that the fetal hearts not only have a disturbed electrical conduction but also a decrease in systolic cardiac performance.[100] This observation can explain, at least in part, why midtrimester Doppler has the potential to identify almost all fetuses with first-degree AVB with an ECG examination at birth but with a low positive-predictive value of approximately 45%, as well as to exclude conduction disturbances in the newborn period with a negative predictive value close to 100%.[69]

From a basic science perspective, the observation of a transient, spontaneously reversible prolongation of AV conduction, also observed by other investigators,[101] is interesting because it may serve as a marker of subclinical disease giving insight into the pathophysiologic implications of congenital AVB. However, from a clinical perspective, identifying an early marker of irreversible cardiac damage and progression to AVB is a more urgent need; however, to date, no prospective controlled studies have been performed to address this issue. In the multicenter PR Interval and Dexamethasone Evaluation (PRIDE) prospective study,[101] made up of 98 SSA/Ro antibody–positive pregnancies, 2 fetuses developed AV time prolongation exceeding 150 ms (i.e., three z-scores above normal mean), reverting to normal conduction during transplacental dexamethasone treatment. In the authors' single-center study of 95 fetuses, 3 with mitral A-wave/aortic outflow time intervals exceeding 150 ms spontaneously normalized their AV conduction, 1 before birth and 2 after birth and in another 2 infants, second-degree AVB reverted to first-degree AVB during transplacental betamethasone treatment.[69] Combining data from these two studies, an abnormal AV time interval was documented in only 1 of 7 infants before progressing to second- or third-degree AVB. Two infants had normal AV time intervals 1 week before the block was diagnosed; and in 4 more infants, some time had elapsed from a previous normal examination, suggesting that weekly examinations might be insufficient to identify an early marker of irreversible progression to complete AVB. In another prospective multicenter study using a somewhat different technique, estimating AV time intervals from tissue instead of blood flow velocity recording, 6 of 70 infants had an AV time interval exceeding two z-scores above the normal mean.[97] All 6 infants were transplacentally treated with dexamethasone and had normalized AV conduction within 3 to 14 days.

Screening for Other Features of Neonatal Lupus Erythematosus

The majority of infants with noncutaneous, noncardiac manifestations of NLE remains asymptomatic and has a resolution of findings without specific intervention. For this reason, screening for hematologic, hepatic, or neurologic changes is not recommended. When an infant of a mother with anti-SSA/Ro antibodies becomes ill, however, consideration of NLE may guide the diagnosis and treatment.

PREVENTION AND THERAPY

Several intrauterine regimens for the prevention and treatment of CHB have been tried, most with the rationale to diminish the inflammatory insult or to eliminate the maternal autoantibodies or both.

Steroids

Notably, prednisone is metabolized by the placenta, whereas fluorinated steroids are only partially so and may reach the fetus in active form. Early transplacental treatment with fluorinated steroidal agents has been observed to inhibit progression or even reverse first- and second-degree AVB.[69,76,97,101,102] A complete AVB is, however, commonly considered irreversible, a concept challenged by one recent study demonstrating improved conduction in two infants with third-degree AVB with an unusually good escape rhythm of 97 bpm.[103] Transplacental steroid treatment may also resolve cavity effusions and diminish endomyocardial echogenic changes.[76,102] A standardized treatment protocol including dexamethasone plus sympathomimetic drugs for fetuses with heart rates lower than 55 bpm has been demonstrated to increase 1-year survival from

TABLE 37-3 Fetal Surveillance and Evaluation Methods for Identifying Congenital Heart Block

METHOD	ADVANTAGES	DISADVANTAGES
Echocardiography: Doppler flow velocity Doppler tissue velocity	Uses standard equipment Is available at most clinics	Requires high experience with fetal echocardiographic techniques Uses indirect hemodynamic or mechanical markers of electrical events
Electrocardiography	Records electrical signals	Has a poor signal-to-noise ratio
Magnetocardiography	Records electromagnetic signals Has a high signal-to-noise ratio	Is expensive Requires a magnetically shielded room Is available at only a few centers

46% to 90% and significantly decrease the number of infants with postnatal cardiomyopathy.[104] Other investigators have, however, not been able to confirm these observations.[76,105]

Maternal risks related to treatment with fluorinated steroids include infection, hypertension, glucose intolerance, preeclampsia, insomnia, and osteoporosis, whereas the major concerns for the fetus are neurologic development, growth retardation, and oligohydramnios, discussed in a recent review.[106] Some reports of repeated high-dose dexamethasone treatment to promote fetal lung development suggest lasting neurocognitive effects on children. These concerns were not confirmed in a study of 14 children exposed to high-dose dexamethasone for CHB; none of these children had a low intelligence quotient (IQ) or learning disability.[90] Regardless, the infant must be monitored for adrenal insufficiency at birth and may require a slow prednisone taper during the first months of life to allow for adrenal recovery.

Intravenous Immunoglobulin

Transplacental and postnatal treatment with intravenous immunoglobulin (IVIG) might hold some promise for the treatment of EFE and dilated cardiomyopathy, but further studies are needed to answer this question.[103] Several trials of IVIG during pregnancy failed to prevent the development of congenital heart block in fetuses exposed to antibodies in utero in mothers with a prior infant with NLE.[107,108]

Hydroxychloroquine

A case-control study of infants with NLE has demonstrated a potential protective effect of hydroxychloroquine (HCQ) for CHB. Of 50 children with CHB, only 7 (14%) were exposed to HCQ during pregnancy, compared with 56 of the 151 children (37%) with non-cardiac NLE ($P < 0.05$).[14]

Sympathomimetic Medications

Treatment with sympathomimetic agents can be expected to increase ventricular rate by 5 to 10 bpm,[102,106] but it has not been documented to improve survival.

LONG-TERM OUTCOMES

Few long-term follow-up studies of patients with CHB beyond childhood have been published, but the high mortality and cardiac morbidity rates reported by Michaelsson and colleagues[109] led to their recommendation of pacemaker treatment for all adolescent patients with third-degree CHB. Even if the mortality rate is by far the highest before birth and during the first month of life, approximately 5% to 10% of neonatal survivors with CHB develop a life-threatening dilated cardiomyopathy during childhood years.[81-83] In a study by Villan and colleagues,[81] close to 30% of 56 infants with CHB and antibody-positive mothers developed dilated cardiomyopathy, and 10% died at 4 to 12 years of age, despite pacemaker treatment. In another group of 55 infants with CHB and anti-Ro– or anti-La–negative mothers, in which 53 were treated with a pacemaker, no child developed cardiomyopathy or died. Still, long-term studies assessing the potentially different effect of the increase in pacemaker implants in children with CHB of Ro/La antibody–positive and of Ro/La antibody–negative mothers, respectively, are lacking.

A future risk of autoimmune disease in infants with NLE has been suggested, but conclusive evidence is lacking. Case reports of SLE developing at an early age in infants born with CHB have been presented,[110] but studies, to date, and follow-up with a larger set of individuals with NLE point in different directions. In a study of children over the age of 8 years with NLE, a sibling with NLE, or a friend with NLE, the incidence of maternally reported arthritis was similar in each group. However, 6 of the 49 children (12%) with prior NLE developed a rheumatologic disease, compared with none of the 45 siblings or 53 friends.[111] A subsequent similar study did not demonstrate an increased risk for rheumatologic disease. In this study, 5 of 33 children with CHB (15%), 2 of 20 with neonatal rash (10%), 5 of 51 unaffected siblings (10%), and 1 of 22 friends (4.5%) developed

a rheumatologic disease by an average age of 14 years.[88] The autoimmune diseases reported in this study were wide and varied and included hypothyroidism, inflammatory bowel disease, juvenile inflammatory arthritis, Hashimoto thyroiditis, minimal change in kidney disease, psoriasis, and type I diabetes but not SLE or SS.

References

1. McCuiston CH, Schoch EP, Jr: Possible discoid lupus erythematosus in newborn infant; report of a case with subsequent development of acute systemic lupus in mother. *AMA Arch Derm Syphilol* 70:782–785, 1954.
2. Hull D, Binns BA, Joyce D: Congenital heart block and widespread fibrosis due to maternal lupus erythematosus. *Arch Dis Child* 41:688–690, 1966.
3. Silverman E, Jaeggi E: Non-cardiac manifestations of neonatal lupus erythematosus. *Scand J Immunol* 72(3):223–225, 2010.
4. Buyon JP, Winchester RJ, Slade SG, et al: Identification of mothers at risk for congenital heart block and other neonatal lupus syndromes in their children. Comparison of enzyme-linked immunosorbent assay and immunoblot for measurement of anti-SS-A/Ro and anti-SS-B/La antibodies. *Arthritis Rheum* 36(9):1263–1273, 1993.
5. Julkunen H, Miettinen A, Walle TK, et al: Autoimmune response in mothers of children with congenital and postnatally diagnosed isolated heart block: a population based study. *J Rheumatol* 31(1):183–189, 2004.
6. Salomonsson S, Dzikaite V, Zeffer E, et al: A population-based investigation of the autoantibody profile in mothers of children with atrioventricular block. *Scand J Immunol* 74(5):511–517, 2011.
7. Cimaz R, Meroni PL, Brucato A, et al: Concomitant disappearance of electrocardiographic abnormalities and of acquired maternal autoantibodies during the first year of life in infants who had QT interval prolongation and anti-SSA/Ro positivity without congenital heart block at birth. *Arthritis Rheum* 48:266–268, 2003.
8. Skog A, Wahren-Herlenius M, Sundstrom B, et al: Outcome and growth of infants fetally exposed to heart block-associated maternal anti-Ro52/SSA autoantibodies. *Pediatrics* 121(4):e803–e809, 2008.
9. Lee LA: Cutaneous lupus in infancy and childhood. *Lupus* 19(9):1112–1117, 2010.
10. Brucato A, Frassi M, Franceschini F, et al: Risk of congenital complete heart block in newborns of mothers with anti-Ro/SSA antibodies detected by counterimmunoelectrophoresis: a prospective study of 100 women. *Arthritis Rheum* 44(8):1832–1835, 2001.
11. Julkunen H, Eronen M: The rate of recurrence of isolated congenital heart block: a population-based study. *Arthritis Rheum* 44(2):487–488, 2001.
12. Solomon DG, Rupel A, Buyon JP: Birth order, gender and recurrence rate in autoantibody-associated congenital heart block: implications for pathogenesis and family counseling. *Lupus* 12(8):646–647, 2003.
13. Ambrosi A, Salomonsson S, Eliasson H, et al: Development of heart block in children of SSA/SSB-autoantibody-positive women is associated with maternal age and displays a season-of-birth pattern. *Ann Rheum Dis* 71(3):334–340, 2011.
14. Izmirly PM, Kim MY, Llanos C, et al: Evaluation of the risk of anti-SSA/Ro-SSB/La antibody-associated cardiac manifestations of neonatal lupus in fetuses of mothers with systemic lupus erythematosus exposed to hydroxychloroquine. *Ann Rheum Dis* 69(10):1827–1830, 2010.
15. Cimaz R, Spence DL, Hornberger L, et al: Incidence and spectrum of neonatal lupus erythematosus: a prospective study of infants born to mothers with anti-Ro autoantibodies. *J Pediatr* 142(6):678–683, 2003.
16. Lee LA, Sokol RJ, Buyon JP: Hepatobiliary disease in neonatal lupus: prevalence and clinical characteristics in cases enrolled in a national registry. *Pediatrics* 109(1):e11, 2002.
17. Boros CA, Spence D, Blaser S, et al: Hydrocephalus and macrocephaly: new manifestations of neonatal lupus erythematosus. *Arthritis Rheum* 57(2):261–266, 2007.
18. Cabañas F, Pellicer A, Valverde E, et al: Central nervous system vasculopathy in neonatal lupus erythematosus. *Pediatr Neurol* 15(2):124–126, 1996.
19. Shanske AL, Bernstein L, Herzog R: Chondrodysplasia punctata and maternal autoimmune disease: a new case and review of the literature. *Pediatrics* 120(2):e436–e441, 2007.
20. Press J, Uziel Y, Laxer RM, et al: Long-term outcome of mothers of children with complete congenital heart block. *Am J Med* 100(3):328–332, 1996.
21. Julkunen H, Eronen M: Long-term outcome of mothers of children with isolated heart block in Finland. *Arthritis Rheum* 44(3):647–652, 2001.

22. Rivera TL, Izmirly PM, Birnbaum BK, et al: Disease progression in mothers of children enrolled in the Research Registry for Neonatal Lupus. *Ann Rheum Dis* 68:828–835, 2009.

23. Litsey SE, Noonan JA, O'Connor WN, et al: Maternal connective tissue disease and congenital heart block. Demonstration of immunoglobulin in cardiac tissue. *N Engl J Med* 312(2):98–100, 1985.

24. Lee LA, Coulter S, Erner S, et al: Cardiac immunoglobulin deposition in congenital heart block associated with maternal anti-Ro autoantibodies. *Am J Med* 83(4):793–796, 1987.

25. Clancy RM, Kapur RP, Molad Y, et al: Immunohistologic evidence supports apoptosis, IgG deposition, and novel macrophage/fibroblast crosstalk in the pathologic cascade leading to congenital heart block. *Arthritis Rheum* 50(1):173–182, 2004.

26. Scott JS, Maddison PJ, Taylor PV, et al: Connective-tissue disease, antibodies to ribonucleoprotein, and congenital heart block. *N Engl J Med* 309(4):209–212, 1983.

27. Taylor PV, Taylor KF, Norman A, et al: Prevalence of maternal Ro (SS-A) and La (SS-B) autoantibodies in relation to congenital heart block. *Br J Rheumatol* 27(2):128–312, 1988.

28. Wolin SL, Steitz JA: The Ro small cytoplasmic ribonucleoproteins: identification of the antigenic protein and its binding site on the Ro RNAs. *Proc Natl Acad Sci U S A* 81(7):1996–2000, 1984.

29. Ben-Chetrit E, Chan EK, Sullivan KF, et al: A 52-kD protein is a novel component of the SS-A/Ro antigenic particle. *J Exp Med* 167(5):1560–1571, 1988.

30. Salomonsson S, Dörner T, Theander E, et al: A serologic marker for fetal risk of congenital heart block. *Arthritis Rheum* 46(5):1233–1241, 2002.

31. Fritsch C, Hoebeke J, Dali H, et al: 52-kDa Ro/SSA epitopes preferentially recognized by antibodies from mothers of children with neonatal lupus and congenital heart block. *Arthritis Res Ther* 8(1):R4, 2006.

32. Eronen M, Miettinen A, Walle TK, et al: Relationship of maternal autoimmune response to clinical manifestations in children with congenital complete heart block. *Acta Paediatr* 93(6):803–809, 2004.

33. Blange I, Ringertz NR, Pettersson I: Identification of antigenic regions of the human 52kD Ro/SS-A protein recognized by patient sera. *J Autoimmun* 7(2):263–274, 1994.

34. Kato T, Sasakawa H, Suzuki S, et al: Autoepitopes of the 52-kd SS-A/Ro molecule. *Arthritis Rheum* 38(7):990–998, 1995.

35. Strandberg L, Winqvist O, Sonesson SE, et al: Antibodies to amino acid 200–239 (p200) of Ro52 as serological markers for the risk of developing congenital heart block. *Clin Exp Immunol* 154(1):30–37, 2008.

36. Salomonsson S, Sonesson SE, Ottosson L, et al: Ro/SSA autoantibodies directly bind cardiomyocytes, disturb calcium homeostasis, and mediate congenital heart block. *J Exp Med* 201(1):11–17, 2005.

37. Silverman ED, Buyon J, Laxer RM, et al: Autoantibody response to the Ro/La particle may predict outcome in neonatal lupus erythematosus. *Clin Exp Immunol* 100(3):499–505, 1995.

38. Jaeggi E, Laskin C, Hamilton R, et al: The importance of the level of maternal anti-Ro/SSA antibodies as a prognostic marker of the development of cardiac neonatal lupus erythematosus: a prospective study of 186 antibody-exposed fetuses and infants. *J Am Coll Cardiol* 55(24):2778–2784, 2010.

39. Gordon P, Khamashta MA, Rosenthal E, et al: Anti-52 kDa Ro, anti-60 kDa Ro, and anti-La antibody profiles in neonatal lupus. *J Rheumatol* 31(12):2480–2487, 2004.

40. Orth T, Dörner T, Meyer Zum Buschenfelde KH, et al: Complete congenital heart block is associated with increased autoantibody titers against calreticulin. *Eur J Clin Invest* 26(3):205–215, 1996.

41. Borda E, Sterin-Borda L: Autoantibodies against neonatal heart M1 muscarinic acetylcholine receptor in children with congenital heart block. *J Autoimmun* 16(2):143–150, 2001.

42. Bacman S, Sterin-Borda L, Camusso JJ, et al: Circulating antibodies against neurotransmitter receptor activities in children with congenital heart block and their mothers. *FASEB J* 8(14):1170–1176, 1994.

43. Miyagawa S, Yanagi K, Yoshioka A, et al: Neonatal lupus erythematosus: maternal IgG antibodies bind to a recombinant NH2-terminal fusion protein encoded by human alpha-fodrin cDNA. *J Invest Dermatol* 111(6):1189–1192, 1998.

44. Karnabi E, Qu Y, Wadgaonkar R, Mancarella S, et al: Congenital heart block: identification of autoantibody binding site on the extracellular loop (domain I, S5-S6) of alpha(1D) L-type Ca channel. *J Autoimmun* 34(2):80–86, 2010.

45. Boutjdir M, Chen L, Zhang ZH, et al: Arrhythmogenicity of IgG and anti-52-kD SSA/Ro affinity-purified antibodies from mothers of children with congenital heart block. *Circ Res* 80(3):354–362, 1997.

46. Boutjdir M, Chen L, Zhang ZH, et al: Serum and immunoglobulin G from the mother of a child with congenital heart block induce

47. Garcia S, Nascimento JH, Bonfa E, et al: Cellular mechanism of the conduction abnormalities induced by serum from anti-Ro/SSA-positive patients in rabbit hearts. *J Clin Invest* 93(2):718–724, 1994.

conduction abnormalities and inhibit L-type calcium channels in a rat heart model. *Pediatr Res* 44(1):11–19, 1998.

48. Hamilton RM, Lee-Poy M, Kruger K, et al: Investigative methods of congenital complete heart block. *J Electrocardiol* 30(Suppl):69–74, 1998.

49. Mazel JA, El-Sherif N, Buyon J, et al: Electrocardiographic abnormalities in a murine model injected with IgG from mothers of children with congenital heart block. *Circulation* 99(14):1914–1918, 1999.

50. Miranda-Carus ME, Boutjdir M, Tseng CE, et al: Induction of antibodies reactive with SSA/Ro-SSB/La and development of congenital heart block in a murine model. *J Immunol* 161(11):5886–5892, 1998.

51. Suzuki H, Silverman ED, Wu X, et al: Effect of maternal autoantibodies on fetal cardiac conduction: an experimental murine model. *Pediatr Res* 57(4):557–562, 2005.

52. Xiao GQ, Qu Y, Hu K, et al: Down-regulation of L-type calcium channel in pups born to 52 kDa SSA/Ro immunized rabbits. *FASEB J* 15(9):1539–1545, 2001.

53. Strandberg LS, Ambrosi A, Jagodic M, et al: Maternal MHC regulates generation of pathogenic antibodies and fetal MHC-encoded genes determine susceptibility in congenital heart block. *J Immunol* 185(6):3574–3582, 2010.

54. Ambrosi A, Dzikaite V, Park J, et al: Anti-Ro52 monoclonal antibodies specific for amino acid 200–239, but not other Ro52 epitopes, induce congenital heart block in a rat model. *Ann Rheum Dis* 71(3):448–454, 2012.

55. Clancy RM, Neufing PJ, Zheng P, et al: Impaired clearance of apoptotic cardiocytes is linked to anti-SSA/Ro and -SSB/La antibodies in the pathogenesis of congenital heart block. *J Clin Invest* 116(9):2413–2422, 2006.

56. Eftekhari P, Salle L, Lezoualc'h F, et al: Anti-SSA/Ro52 autoantibodies blocking the cardiac 5-HT4 serotoninergic receptor could explain neonatal lupus congenital heart block. *Eur J Immunol* 30(10):2782–2790, 2000.

57. Eftekhari P, Roegel JC, Lezoualc'h F, et al: Induction of neonatal lupus in pups of mice immunized with synthetic peptides derived from amino acid sequences of the serotoninergic 5-HT4 receptor. *Eur J Immunol* 31(2):573–579, 2001.

58. Kamel R, Eftekhari P, Clancy R, et al: Autoantibodies against the serotoninergic 5-HT4 receptor and congenital heart block: a reassessment. *J Autoimmun* 25(1):72–76, 2005.

59. Xiao GQ, Hu K, Boutjdir M: Direct inhibition of expressed cardiac l- and t-type calcium channels by igg from mothers whose children have congenital heart block. *Circulation* 103(11):1599–1604, 2001.

60. Qu Y, Xiao GQ, Chen L, et al: Autoantibodies from mothers of children with congenital heart block downregulate cardiac L-type Ca channels. *J Mol Cell Cardiol* 33(6):1153–1163, 2001.

61. Qu Y, Baroudi G, Yue Y, et al: Novel molecular mechanism involving alpha1D (Cav1.3) L-type calcium channel in autoimmune-associated sinus bradycardia. *Circulation* 111(23):3034–3041, 2005.

62. Karnabi E, Qu Y, Mancarella S, et al: Rescue and worsening of congenital heart block-associated electrocardiographic abnormalities in two transgenic mice. *Journal of Cardiovascular Electrophysiology* 22(8):922–930, 2011.

63. Llanos C, Izmirly PM, Katholi M, et al: Recurrence rates of cardiac manifestations associated with neonatal lupus and maternal/fetal risk factors. *Arthritis Rheum* 60(10):3091–3097, 2009.

64. Clancy RM, Backer CB, Yin X, et al: Cytokine polymorphisms and histologic expression in autopsy studies: contribution of TNF-alpha and TGF-beta 1 to the pathogenesis of autoimmune-associated congenital heart block. *J Immunol* 171(6):3253–3261, 2003.

65. Clancy RM, Marion MC, Kaufman KM, et al: Identification of candidate loci at 6p21 and 21q22 in a genome-wide association study of cardiac manifestations of neonatal lupus. *Arthritis Rheum* 62(11):3415–3424, 2010.

66. Buyon JP, Hiebert R, Copel J, et al: Autoimmune-associated congenital heart block: demographics, mortality, morbidity and recurrence rates obtained from a national neonatal lupus registry. *J Am Coll Cardiol* 31(7):1658–1666, 1998.

67. Jaeggi ET, Hamilton RM, Silverman ED, et al: Outcome of children with fetal, neonatal or childhood diagnosis of isolated congenital atrioventricular block. A single institution's experience of 30 years. *J Am Coll Cardiol* 39(1):130–137, 2002.

68. Zhao H, Cuneo BF, Strasburger JF, et al: Electrophysiological characteristics of fetal atrioventricular block. *J Am Coll Cardiol* 51(1):77–84, 2008.

69. Bergman G, Wahren-Herlenius M, Sonesson SE. Diagnostic precision of Doppler flow echocardiography in fetuses at risk for atrioventricular block. *Ultrasound Obstet Gynecol* 36(5):561–566, 2010.

70. Motta M, Rodriguez-Perez C, Tincani A, et al: Outcome of infants from mothers with anti-SSA/Ro antibodies. *J Perinatol* 27:278–283, 2007.

71. Cimaz R, Stramba-Badiale M, Brucato A, et al: QT interval prolongation in asymptomatic anti-SSA/Ro-positive infants without congenital heart block. *Arthritis Rheum* 43(5):1049–1053, 2000.

72. Costedoat-Chalumeau N, Amoura Z, Lupoglazoff JM, et al: Outcome of pregnancies in patients with anti-SSA/Ro antibodies: a study of 165 pregnancies, with special focus on electrocardiographic variations in the children and comparison with a control group. *Arthritis Rheum* 50(10): 3187–3194, 2004.

73. Askanase AD, Friedman DM, Copel J, et al: Spectrum and progression of conduction abnormalities in infants born to mothers with anti-SSA/Ro-SSB/La antibodies. *Lupus* 11(3):145–151, 2002.

74. Gordon PA, Khamashta MA, Hughes GR, et al: A normal ECG at birth does not exclude significant congenital cardiac conduction disease associated with maternal anti-Ro antibodies. *Rheumatology (Oxford)* 40(8):939–940, 2001.

75. Breur JM, Kapusta L, Stoutenbeek P, et al: Isolated congenital atrioventricular block diagnosed in utero: natural history and outcome. *J Matern Fetal Neonatal Med* 21(7):469–476, 2008.

76. Saleeb S, Copel J, Friedman D, et al: Comparison of treatment with fluorinated glucocorticoids to the natural history of autoantibody-associated congenital heart block: retrospective review of the research registry for neonatal lupus. *Arthritis Rheum* 42(11):2335–2345, 1999.

77. Nield LE, Silverman ED, Smallhorn JF, et al: Endocardial fibroelastosis associated with maternal anti-Ro and anti-La antibodies in the absence of atrioventricular block. *J Am Coll Cardiol* 40(4):796–802, 2002.

78. Nield LE, Silverman ED, Taylor GP, et al: Maternal anti-Ro and anti-La antibody-associated endocardial fibroelastosis. *Circulation* 105(7):843–848, 2002.

79. Cuneo BF, Fruitman D, Benson DW, et al: Spontaneous rupture of atrioventricular valve tensor apparatus as late manifestation of anti-Ro/SSA antibody-mediated cardiac disease. *Am J Cardiol* 107(5):761–766, 2011.

80. Groves AM, Allan LD, Rosenthal E: Outcome of isolated congenital complete heart block diagnosed in utero. *Heart* 75(2):190–194, 1996.

81. Villain E, Coastedoat-Chalumeau N, Marijon E, et al: Presentation and prognosis of complete atrioventricular block in childhood, according to maternal antibody status. *J Am Coll Cardiol* 48(8):1682–1687, 2006.

82. Moak JP, Barron KS, Hougen TJ, et al: Congenital heart block: development of late-onset cardiomyopathy, a previously underappreciated sequela. *J Am Coll Cardiol* 37(1):238–242, 2001.

83. Udink ten Cate FE, Breur JM, Cohen MI, et al: Dilated cardiomyopathy in isolated congenital complete atrioventricular block: early and long-term risk in children. *J Am Coll Cardiol* 37(4):1129–1134, 2001.

84. Weston WL, Morelli JG, Lee LA: The clinical spectrum of anti-Ro-positive cutaneous neonatal lupus erythematosus. *J Am Acad Dermatol* 40(5 Pt 1):675–681, 1999.

85. Perez MF, Torres MEd, Buján MM, et al: Lupus eritematoso neonatal: reporte de cuatro casos. *An Bras Dermatol* 86(2):347–351, 2011.

86. Askanase AD, Miranda-Carus ME, Tang X, et al: The presence of IgG antibodies reactive with components of the SSA/Ro-SSB/La complex in human breast milk: implications in neonatal lupus. *Arthritis Rheum* 46(1):269–271, 2002.

87. Klauninger R, Skog A, Horvath L, et al: Serologic follow-up of children born to mothers with Ro/SSA autoantibodies. *Lupus* 18(9):792–798, 2009.

88. Askanase AD, Izmirly PM, Katholi M, et al: Frequency of neuropsychiatric dysfunction in anti-SSA/SSB exposed children with and without neonatal lupus. *Lupus* 19(3):300–306, 2010.

89. Ross G, Sammaritano L, Nass R, et al: Effects of mothers' autoimmune disease during pregnancy on learning disabilities and hand preference in their children. *Arch Pediatr Adolesc Med* 157(4):397–402, 2003.

90. Brucato A, Astori MG, Cimaz R, et al: Normal neuropsychological development in children with congenital complete heart block who may or may not be exposed to high-dose dexamethasone in utero. *Ann Reum Dis* 65:1422–1426, 2006.

91. Tim-aroon T, Jaovisidha S, Wattanasirichaigoon D: A new case of maternal lupus-associated chondrodysplasia punctata with extensive spinal anomalies. *Am J Med Genet A* 155A(6):1487–1491, 2011.

92. Chitayat D, Keating S, Zand DJ, et al: Chondrodysplasia punctata associated with maternal autoimmune diseases: expanding the spectrum from systemic lupus erythematosus (SLE) to mixed connective tissue disease

(MCTD) and scleroderma report of eight cases. *Am J Med Genet A* 146A(23):3038–3053, 2008.

93. Nii M, Hamilton RM, Fenwick L, et al: Assessment of fetal atrioventricular time intervals by tissue Doppler and pulse Doppler echocardiography: normal values and correlation with fetal electrocardiography. *Heart* 92(12):1831–1837, 2006.

94. Glickstein JS, Buyon J, Friedman D: Pulsed Doppler echocardiographic assessment of the fetal PR interval. *Am J Cardiol* 86(2):236–239, 2000.

95. Andelfinger G, Fouron JC, Sonesson SE, et al: Reference values for time intervals between atrial and ventricular contractions of the fetal heart measured by two Doppler techniques. *Am J Cardiol* 88(12):1433–1436, A8, 2001.

96. Van Bergen AH, Cuneo BF, Davis N: Prospective echocardiographic evaluation of atrioventricular conduction in fetuses with maternal Sjogren's antibodies. *Am J Obstet Gynecol* 191(3):1014–1018, 2004.

97. Rein AJJT, Mevorach D, Perles Z, et al: Early diagnosis and treatment of atrioventricular block in the fetus exposed to maternal anti-SSA/Ro-SSB/La antibodies. *Circulation* 119(14):1867–1872, 2009.

98. Sonesson SE: Diagnosing foetal atrioventricular heart blocks. *Scand J Immunol* 72(3):205–212, 2010.

99. Eliasson H, Wahren-Herlenius M, Sonesson SE: Mechanisms in fetal bradyarrhythmia: 65 cases in a single center analyzed by Doppler flow echocardiographic techniques. *Ultrasound Obstet Gynecol* 37(2):172–178, 2011.

100. Bergman G, Eliasson H, Bremme K, et al: Anti-Ro52/SSA antibody-exposed fetuses with prolonged atrioventricular time intervals show signs of decreased cardiac performance. *Ultrasound Obstet Gynecol* 34(5):543–549, 2009.

101. Friedman DM, Kim MY, Copel JA, et al: Utility of cardiac monitoring in fetuses at risk for congenital heart block: the PR Interval and Dexamethasone Evaluation (PRIDE) prospective study. *Circulation* 117(4): 485–493, 2008.

102. Cuneo BF, Lee M, Roberson D, et al: A management strategy for fetal immune-mediated atrioventricular block. *J Matern Fetal Neonatal Med* 23(12):1400–1405, 2010.

103. Trucco SM, Jaeggi E, Cuneo B, et al: Use of intravenous gamma globulin and corticosteroids in the treatment of maternal autoantibody-mediated cardiomyopathy. *J Am Coll Cardiol* 57(6):715–723, 2011.

104. Jaeggi ET, Fouron JC, Silverman ED, et al: Transplacental fetal treatment improves the outcome of prenatally diagnosed complete atrioventricular block without structural heart disease. *Circulation* 110(12):1542–1548, 2004.

105. Rosenthal E, Gordon PA, Simpson JM, et al: Letter regarding article by Jaeggi et al, "Transplacental fetal treatment improves the outcome of prenatally diagnosed complete atrioventricular block without structural heart disease." *Circulation* 111(18):e287–e288, 2005.

106. Hutter D, Silverman ED, Jaeggi ET: The benefits of transplacental treatment of isolated congenital complete heart block associated with maternal anti-Ro/SSA antibodies: a review. *Scand J Immunol* 72(3):235–241, 2010.

107. Friedman DM, Llanos C, Izmirly PM, et al: Evaluation of fetuses in a study of intravenous immunoglobulin as preventive therapy for congenital heart block: results of a multicenter, prospective, open-label clinical trial. *Arthritis Rheum* 62(4):1138–1146, 2010.

108. Pisoni CN, Brucato A, Ruffatti A, et al: Failure of intravenous immunoglobulin to prevent congenital heart block: findings of a multicenter, prospective, observational study. *Arthritis Rheumat* 62(4):1147–1152, 2010.

109. Michaelsson M, Jonzon A, Riesenfeld T: Isolated congenital complete atrioventricular block in adult life. A prospective study. *Circulation* 92(3):442–449, 1995.

110. Feist E, Keitzer R, Gerhold K, et al: Development of systemic lupus erythematosus in a patient with congenital heart block. *Arthritis Rheumat* 48(9):2697–2698, 2003.

111. Martin V, Lee LA, Askanase AD, et al: Long-term followup of children with neonatal lupus and their unaffected siblings. *Arthritis Rheumat* 46(9):2377–2383, 2002.

112. Buyon JP, Ben-Chetrit E, Karp S, et al: Acquired congenital heart block. Pattern of maternal antibody response to biochemically defined antigens of the SSA/Ro-SSB/La system in neonatal lupus. *J Clin Invest* 84(2):627–634, 1989.

113. Siren MK, Julkunen H, Kaaja R, et al: Role of HLA in congenital heart block: susceptibility alleles in mothers. *Lupus* 8(1):52–59, 1999.

114. Siren MK, Julkunen H, Kaaja R, et al: Role of HLA in congenital heart block: susceptibility alleles in children. *Lupus* 8(1):60–67, 1999.

Chapter 38

Reproductive and Hormonal Issues in Women with Autoimmune Diseases

Eliza F. Chakravarty

INTRODUCTION

Because systemic lupus erythematosus (SLE) commonly affects women during the childbearing years, reproductive issues are of utmost importance to patients and their families. Furthermore, the delicate interplay between female sex steroids and SLE can make caring for women throughout their lifespan a challenging task for the clinician.

The underlying causes of SLE are, without a doubt, multifactorial, evolving from several alternative triggering events that impair the orderly balance of immune responses in susceptible hosts. The strong female predominance of SLE, changes in disease activity observed with changes in the levels of endogenous female sex steroids, and known immunologic effects of sex hormones strongly suggest a role for estrogens in the initiation and possible maintenance of disease. Because of concerns surrounding the use of exogenous estrogen-based therapies in women with SLE, their use has been avoided in the past. However, hormonal imbalance need not dictate that all exogenous hormone combinations are necessarily toxic. The perceived advantages of hormonal use in select clinical situations (e.g., effective contraception, osteoporosis prevention, ovulation induction, preservation of fertility in patients receiving cyclophosphamide) suggest a need to determine whether such therapies can be used safely or at least within a rational therapeutic window. Aside from cyclophosphamide-induced ovarian failure, fertility is not reduced in women with SLE, and conception during periods of active underlying disease or while taking potentially teratogenic medications underscores the necessity for effective contraception in this population. Additionally, osteoporosis remains a significant problem for patients with SLE, and exogenous estrogens may prove beneficial in the prevention of glucocorticoid-induced bone mineral density (BMD) loss, particularly in premenopausal women who may not be optimal candidates for bisphosphonate therapy.

HORMONES AND REPRODUCTIVE IMMUNOLOGY
Gonadal Hormones and the Immune System

Gonadal hormones clearly play a role in immune homeostasis. Specific hormones, including estrogen, progesterone, and prolactin, exhibit direct effects on numerous immune cells, cytokines, and apoptosis; and clinical experience suggests that changes in gonadal hormones may modulate disease activity.[1] During young adulthood (i.e., childbearing years) the female-to-male ratio for lupus is 9:1; however, this female preponderance is not so striking in children and in older adults.[2] Furthermore, men with Klinefelter syndrome (47,XXY) appear to have an increased prevalence of SLE, suggesting a role of the X chromosome in the pathogenesis of SLE.[3] Different studies have suggested that increased levels of female sex hormones—use of exogenous estrogens as oral contraceptives or postmenopausal

hormone therapy and pregnancy—in women with SLE may exacerbate disease.

Female Hormones and Inflammatory Mediators

The regulation of the menstrual cycle or invasion and implantation of the uterine wall by an embryo requires an ebb and flow of inflammatory mediators that are unique to the adult female environment. The need to protect the semiallograft fetus from immune attack without initiating rejection or graft-versus-host disease, while still maintaining an effective immune surveillance and response to infection, indeed sets a high bar for carefully regulated immune response throughout implantation, pregnancy, and parturition. Thus it makes sense that many systemic inflammatory and immunologic responses are mediated, at least in part by female sex steroids—predominantly estrogen, progesterone, and prolactin. For example, progesterone is important in suppressing the inflammatory reaction that would be expected in response to the presence of a foreign body, in this case an embryo. Sex hormones play an influential role on systemic cytokine production and release, largely mediated through the nuclear factor–kappa B (NF-κB). In general, estrogens stimulate a T-helper (Th) cell 2 response and activate antibody production. The production of interleukin (IL)-1, IL-4, IL-6, and IL-10 in macrophages is stimulated by estrogen, as is the production of IL-4, IL-5, IL-6, and IL-10 by Th 2 cells. In contrast, androgens stimulate a Th cell 1 response with the production of IL-1 and IL-12 and activate cluster of differentiation 8 (CD8$^+$) T cells.[1] Progesterone may also suppress IL-8 and cyclooxygenase-2 expression, suggesting that progesterone withdrawal at the time of menstruation might promote these inflammatory mediators in preparation for the increased tissue inflammation that accompanies the extrusion process.[4]

Complex Effects of Sex Hormones on Inflammation

Estrogen replacement in postmenopausal women may increase C-reactive protein[5,6] while decreasing a number of other inflammatory mediators.[6,7] In the context of the rapidly evolving literature, hormones produced during the ovulatory cycle may normally regulate the complex network of endometrial cytokines.[8] However, signal cascades may have counterregulatory effects such that inflammatory mediators that will impact the levels of circulating hormones. For example, lipopolysaccharide, a potent stimulator of monocytes, induces a lengthening of the follicular phase and is associated with decreased estradiol concentrations and increased pituitary release of the luteinizing hormone (LH) and the follicle-stimulating hormone (FSH).[9] Complex relationships among female sex hormones, inflammatory mediators, and systemic vasculature are intrinsic to the development of sexual maturity, to the maintenance of the ovulatory cycle in preparation for implantation of the conceptus, and to the maintenance of a healthy pregnancy leading to successful reproduction. However, it is precisely this complicated interplay of female sex hormones and the immune system that sets the stage for the female preponderance of autoimmune diseases including SLE.

Sex Hormones and the Immune and Vascular Systems

Estrogen receptors are found on human monocytes, B cells, and T cells, indicating a direct role for estrogens in the regulation of immune cell activation.[10] Overall, estrogen appears to enhance B-cell activation while, at the same time, suppressing T-cell reactivity. Importantly, different circulating levels of estradiol may have differing effects on the immune system; for example, low doses of 17β-estradiol have been found to inhibit IL-6 secretion by human endothelial cells.[11] Progesterone is also known as the *hormone of pregnancy*, because of its profound influence on the cellular, immunologic, and tissue-remodeling changes that are necessary during pregnancy.[12] Progesterone induces and hones uterine natural killer (uNK) cells, a variant of NK cells with low spontaneous cytotoxic activity that function locally to induce tolerance to self or fetal antigens. Additionally, progesterone acts to differentiate T-cells into Th2-dominanat cells and the production of IL-3, IL-4, and IL-10. Many of these actions are mediated by a progesterone-induced blocking factor (PIBF).

Inflammation and inflammation-induced coagulation mechanisms are sometimes predictors of future cardiovascular events.[13] Because of this, sex steroids may have indirect effects on the risk of vascular thrombosis through immune-modulating effects. For example, estrogen can improve markers of fibrinolysis and vascular inflammation in the arteries of postmenopausal women,[7] as well as having other antiinflammatory properties that may have beneficial effects on cardiovascular risk.[14] At the same time, estrogen has been shown to increase C-reactive protein,[7] a marker of subclinical inflammation independently associated with the increased risk of cardiovascular disease. Many inflammatory cytokines induce adhesion molecules in blood vessel walls, augmenting inflammatory cell adhesion, which may lead to the development of atherosclerosis. One study observed a statistically significant increase in several such adhesion molecules; men and untreated postmenopausal women with coronary artery disease were compared with postmenopausal women with coronary artery disease who were receiving estrogen therapy.[15] Clearly, the role of estrogen is multifactorial, with some effects promoting or inhibiting systemic inflammation, as well as the expression of endothelial adhesion molecules of vessel walls. Reasons for this discrepancy may include dose-dependent effects, multiple signaling pathways, and local hormonal and cytokine milieux.

Increased knowledge of the roles of sex steroids in the immune system raises concerns and questions regarding the safety of surges of exogenous or endogenous (during pregnancy) female sex hormones in terms of the diseases of the immune system including SLE. Past observational studies have suggested increased rates of SLE flares with the use of estrogen-containing oral contraceptives or postmenopausal hormone therapy, as well as the use of sex steroids during pregnancy or ovulation induction.[16] However, pregnancy and child-rearing are an important part of a full and complete life for many women with SLE, and effective contraception is essential for women with SLE to be able to plan pregnancies during times of relative disease quiescence and to avoid fetal exposure to potentially teratogenic medications. Improved understanding concerning how underlying autoimmune disease may affect a women's reproductive health and how changes in female sex hormones over the reproductive life affects underlying SLE are critical to caring for and counseling women with chronic autoimmune disorders.

Maternal-Fetal Immunology

The normal relationship between mother and fetus promotes growth and maturation in contrast to an allogeneic model of destruction of foreign antigens.[17] To enable the fetal semiallograft to survive and grow during 40 weeks of exposure to the maternal immune system, that system must undergo a complex modulation of its innate and humoral components, much of which is not well understood. Pregnancy has long been understood as a Th2-predominant condition, during which a shift of Th cells toward a Th2-dominant state, possibly induced by increasing levels of progesterone, is necessary to establish and maintain a normal pregnancy. This theory is consistent with earlier observations that SLE (a Th2-predominant disease) may be exacerbated by pregnancy, whereas Th1-mediated autoimmune diseases (e.g., rheumatoid arthritis, multiple sclerosis, psoriasis) appear to be characterized by clinical improvement during pregnancy.[17] More recently, however, it is becoming increasingly clear that many more components of both the innate and adaptive immune systems are involved in normal pregnancy.[18] Furthermore, many of the immunologic changes during pregnancy may be preferentially located at the maternal-fetal interface and may not be accurately sampled using peripheral blood. Before conception, endometrial stromal cells transform into decidual cells that contain T-cell subtypes with immunosuppressive activity. One Th cell subset secretes cytokines that are beneficial or neutral to the fetus, whereas another is thought to prevent colonization with microbial pathogens.[18] uNK cells (also known as decidual NK cells) reside in the endometrium in the nonpregnant state but grow in numbers during the late secretory phase of the menstrual cycle and early pregnancy and make up the most abundant proportion of decidual leukocytes.[19] These cells appear to lack the level of cytotoxicity toward trophoblasts that is seen in peripheral NK cells toward infected or malignant cells and serve as a source of local inflammatory and regulatory cytokines and angiogenic growth factors that regulate trophoblast invasion.[19]

The trophoblast and placenta, once considered passive mediators of maternal-fetal immune trafficking, have been increasingly recognized as playing active roles in mediating inflammation while simultaneously maintaining effective host defense.[20,21] Villous cytotrophoblasts and syncytiotrophoblasts escape immune-mediated destruction because both express nonclassical major histocompatibility complex (MHC) antigens that prevent trophoblast destruction through the inhibition of lysis by activated NK cells, as well as limit leukocyte cytotoxic activity, suppress proinflammatory cytokine production, and induce T-cell death. Nonclassical MHC antigens also promote trophoblast proliferation and invasion. Altered expression of nonclassical MHC antigens has been linked to recurrent pregnancy loss (RPL) and preeclampsia. Placental expression of Fas ligand (FasL) may also play a role in pregnancy success through the selective deletion of antifetal T-cell clones. In animal studies, binding to the FasL causes death and removal of autoreactive T cells.

Taken together, a complete understanding of the immune regulation of a healthy pregnancy remains elusive, and an understanding of how pregnancy-related immunologic changes interplay with an abnormal immune system stemming from preexisting autoimmunity is even less evident. Many disorders of pregnancy, including RPL, preeclampsia, intrauterine growth restriction, and prematurity, have been attributed, at least in part, to defects in the tightly regulated systemic and local immunologic changes necessary to support a healthy pregnancy.

Embryologic Development of the Immune System

The development of the immune system begins at conception and continues throughout the pregnancy and into the newborn period. During weeks 2 and 3 of gestation, pluripotent yolk sac stem cells are the precursors for all blood cell components. The thymus develops in the human embryo at 6 weeks' gestation, and lymphocyte differentiation proceeds in the absence of foreign antigens. Small lymphocytes appear in the peripheral blood at 7 weeks' gestation and lymphocyte plexuses by week 8. As early as 13 weeks' gestation, the human fetus has the ability to respond to congenital infections by producing plasma cells and antibodies (although in low numbers).

Although not a completely protected barrier, the presence of an intact trophoblastic cellular barrier prevents the movement of large numbers of immunocompetent cells into or out of the fetus during pregnancy. In contrast, maternal immunoglobulin G (IgG), by virtue of fragment-specific (Fc) receptors in the placenta, is specifically selected for transplacental transfer. Fetal concentrations of IgG subclass 1 exceed those of other IgG subclasses at all time points. Very little IgG is seen in fetal circulation during the first trimester of pregnancy. Levels slowly rise during the second trimester and reach maternal serum concentrations by approximately 26 weeks' gestation. Maximum IgG transfer across the maternal-fetal interface occurs during the last 4 weeks of gestation, and fetal concentration often exceeds maternal concentration at term delivery.[22] Adequate humoral immunity in the neonatal period depends on the circulating immunoglobulins that have crossed the placenta, and fetal blood levels of IgG reflect maternal levels and specificities. Of course, the placenta is unable to differentiate between helpful and pathologic IgG antibodies; consequently, potentially harmful maternal autoantibodies (including anti–Sjögren syndrome antigen A [anti-SSA/Ro], anti–Sjögren syndrome antigen B [anti-SSB/La], and anticardiolipin antibodies [aCL] will pass into fetal circulation and have the potential to exert pathologic effects on the fetus. Additionally, maternal exposure to IgG-based pharmaceutical agents will lead to passage to fetal circulation.

REPRODUCTIVE ISSUES IN WOMEN WITH SYSTEMIC LUPUS ERYTHEMATOSUS AND RELATED AUTOIMMUNE DISORDERS
Contraception

Effective and safe contraception is important for women of childbearing age to be able to avoid unplanned pregnancies; this control is even more critical for women with underlying SLE because of the additional need to plan pregnancies around periods of relative disease quiescence and to avoid antenatal exposure to potentially teratogenic medications commonly used for the treatment of disease, including mycophenolate mofetil, warfarin, methotrexate, and angiotensin-converting enzyme (ACE) inhibitors. In the absence of cyclophosphamide-induced premature ovarian failure (POF), women with lupus have normal fertility and are at risk for unintended pregnancy without the use of effective contraception. Because of concerns about exacerbating the disease with the use of exogenous estrogens, estrogen-containing contraceptives have been considered relatively contraindicated in women with lupus

until fairly recently.[16] Two large multicenter trials have recently demonstrated that estrogen-containing oral contraceptives may be used with low risk of disease flares in women with quiescent to -mild disease activity and without antiphospholipid antibodies (APLAs).[23,24]

Irrespective of the decision to use or to avoid using estrogen-containing contraceptives, many other safe and effective options are available for women with SLE; however, patients continue to be at increased risk for unintended pregnancy because of the inconsistent use of contraceptive methods or the use of contraceptive methods that are unreliable. Even in the general population, approximately 50% of pregnancies are unintended,[25] and women taking potentially teratogenic medications do not necessarily use effective contraception more consistently than women without medication exposure. A study of nearly 500,000 reproductive-aged women in northern California found that 77,378 were prescribed a potentially teratogenic medication (U.S. Food and Drug Administration [FDA] pregnancy category D or X) over a single year. Of these women, approximately 50% had no contraceptive method dispensed (e.g., prescription of hormonal contraception, insertion of intrauterine device [IUD], surgical sterilization), and fewer than 50% had any documentation of contraceptive counseling.[26] Fortunately, women prescribed category D or X medications were less likely to become pregnant than women prescribed category A or B medications (1.0% versus 1.4% prescriptions). Among a cohort of 222 women with SLE of reproductive age, 42% were at potential risk for becoming pregnant (they were sexually active, premenopausal, and not surgically sterile).[27] Of these, 59% reported no contraceptive counseling in the past year. The majority of women in this study reported consistent use of contraception; however, most relied on barrier methods rather than the more effective hormonal contraceptives or IUDs. These results were not changed when the cohort was limited to women taking potentially teratogenic medications.[27] Another questionnaire-based study of women with SLE found that 46% of women attending a lupus clinic in the United States were at risk of becoming pregnant; of these, 23% reported routine unprotected sex, and 55% reported at least one occasion of unprotected sex.[28] The minority of women (35%) were using hormonal contraceptives or an IUD. Taken together, it is clear that women with SLE require contraceptive counseling concerning the risks of unintended pregnancy, as well as the risks and benefits of different contraceptive options. A summary of contraceptive options is presented in Table 38-1.

TABLE 38-1 Contraceptive Options for Women with Systemic Lupus Erythematosus

	BENEFITS	RISK	BOTTOM LINE
Contraceptive counseling	Decreases the risk of unintended pregnancies. Corrects misinformation. Improves compliance.	Has no risks.	Should be offered to all patients during childbearing years.
Estrogen-containing contraception	Is highly effective when used correctly. Has additional benefits for bone. Reduces excessive menstrual blood loss. Protects against medication-induced ovarian failure.	Exacerbates SLE (is widely believed but not proven). Increases the risk for thrombosis.	May be considered in patients with mild (or no) disease activity and no APLAs. Risk of flare is very small.[23,24]
Progestin-only contraception	Is highly effective if used regularly. May reduce the risk for iron deficiency.	Increases irregular menstrual bleeding. Increases BMD loss (is not seen with implantable progestins).	Is a very good choice for many patients with SLE.
Intrauterine device	Is highly effective. Bypasses issues of compliance.	Requires contact with health care provider. (Numerous studies have failed to find evidence for the increased risk for infection.)	Is a very good choice for many patients with SLE.
Barrier method	Protects against infection. Has no hormonal risks or side effects. Is inexpensive. Does not require health care contact. Is available any time of the day.	Is not very reliable. Has no benefit for menstrual bleeding.	Is reasonable for women with infrequent sexual encounters and/or those who do not accept risks with other contraceptives.

APLAs, Antiphospholipid antibodies; BMD, bone marrow density; SLE, systemic lupus erythematosus.

Estrogen-Containing Contraception

The use of estrogen-containing contraceptive methods has, in the past, been very controversial. Benefits of these methods include positive effects on bone density, contraceptive efficacy, reduction of excessive menstrual blood loss, and protection against cyclophosphamide-induced ovarian failure; however, these benefits need to be considered in the context of possible risks of increased thrombotic potential and the theoretical risks of exacerbating disease activity.[16] Two recent randomized clinical trials have been published to help define the safety and efficacy of estrogen-containing combined oral contraceptives. The Safety of Estrogens in Lupus Erythematosus–National Assessment (SELENA) trial, conducted in the United States, randomized 183 women with SLE of childbearing potential to oral combined contraceptives or placebo for 12 months. To be eligible, women needed to have clinically quiescent or mild, stable disease (i.e., Systemic Lupus Erythematosus Disease Activity Index [SLEDAI] < 4) and agree to use barrier methods of contraception throughout the study.[23] Important exclusion criteria included moderate to high titer anticardiolipin (aCL) antibodies, lupus anticoagulant (LA), or any history of thromboses. In this noninferiority study, the primary endpoint of the study was severe SLE flares. Results showed that in this group of women with mild disease, the rates of severe flares over 12 months were not different among those on estrogen-containing contraception and placebo (7.7% versus 7.6%); in addition, the rates of mild to moderate flares were no different between the two groups (1.40 versus 1.44 flares per person per year). One case of deep-venous thrombosis occurred in each group, as did low numbers of pregnancies.[23] Similarly, a single-center randomized study of three contraceptive methods was performed in Mexico. In this study, 162 women with SLE were randomized to either estrogen-containing combined contraceptives, progestin-only pill, or a copper IUD for 12 months.[24] This study was also designed to compare disease activity among the three groups; exclusion criteria included active disease (SLEDAI score higher than 30) and any history of thrombosis. Rates of SLE flares were similar among the three groups (incidence density rates of 0.86, 1.14, and 0.91 for combined oral contraceptives, progestin-only pill, and IUD, respectively). The incidence of severe flares was similar among groups—two, four, and two flares in estrogen, progestin, and IUD groups, respectively). Two deep-venous thromboses occurred in each of the hormone-containing arms (all of whom had low positive APLAs), and one to two pregnancies occurred in each group.[24] These data provide convincing evidence that overall and severe flare rates do not appear to be significantly increased in women using estrogen-containing oral contraceptives. Guidelines for the use of oral contraceptives in women with SLE, based on these studies, are listed in Box 38-1. The important caveat is that women with active disease, renal disease, and antiphospholipid antibody syndrome (APS) were excluded from the study—arguably the very patients who are in the greatest need of pregnancy prevention.

Box 38-1 Guidelines for the Use of Oral Contraceptives in Women with Systemic Lupus Erythematosus

1. Inactive or stable or moderate disease activity
2. No history of venous or arterial thrombosis
3. IgG APLAs < 40; IgM APLAs < 40; IgA APLAs < 50; no circulating lupus anticoagulant (unknown if presence of low to moderate titer of APLAs in the absence of a previous thrombosis is contraindicated)
4. Nonsmoker
5. Normotensive
6. Lowest dose of ethinylestradiol (30-35 μg) for combined pill
7. Patient without migraine headaches
8. Addition of low-dose aspirin therapy to hormone regimen if risk factors are a concern

APLAs, Antiphospholipid antibodies.

Progestin-Only Hormonal Contraception

In women who may not be considered safe for the use of estrogen-containing contraceptives, hormonal contraception using progestin-only compounds remains another option for effective pregnancy prevention.[29] Progestin-only contraceptives come in a variety of delivery methods including oral, every-3-month intramuscular injections, a 3-year subcutaneous implantable device, and a levoprogesterone-containing IUD. No data are available that suggest an increase in disease activity with the use of any progestin-only hormonal contraceptive device, including in the Sanchez-Guerrero[24] randomized trial of hormonal or implantable contraceptives. Additionally, progestin-only contraceptives do not confer an increased risk for thromboses; therefore they may be safer alternatives than estrogen-containing compounds among women with APS or women with a history of cardiovascular disease. All forms of progestin-only contraceptives are considered highly effective if used regularly. Implantable progestin contraceptives have the additional benefit of 3 years of efficacy that avoids problems of compliance with pills or with quarterly injections performed in office settings. Because progestins work by thickening cervical mucus and thinning the endometrial lining, continued use may lead to reduced menstrual bleeding or amenorrhea in some patients,[30] thus potentially reducing iron deficiency anemia in susceptible women.

Potential adverse effects of progestin-only contraceptives include irregular menstrual bleeding that lasts beyond the initial few months of use. Additionally, some women experience weight gain that may lead to the discontinuation of use; large-scale studies have been inconsistent as to whether there is, indeed, a causal relationship.[30] An additional potential concern of relative importance in the SLE population is the risk of BMD loss during the use of progestin-only pills or injections as a result of reduced levels of serum estradiol. Fortunately, BMD loss appears to be reversible on the discontinuation of use in the general population, although it has not been studied in patients with SLE. Implantable progestins do not carry the risk of BMD loss because endogenous estrogen levels return to baseline after initial decrease.[30]

Intrauterine Devices

IUDs are inserted into the uterus, generally by a gynecologist, with contraceptive effects lasting 5 to 10 years. Worldwide, IUDs are the most widely used reversible method of contraception.[28] Two types of IUDs are currently available in the United States: copper-containing devices and a hormone-containing device that releases progesterone. Copper IUDs (ParaGuard) remain effective for up to 10 years; because these devices do not contain hormones, they do not cause changes in menstrual bleeding or other symptoms of premenstrual syndrome. Perhaps the more commonly used type is the progesterone-releasing IUD (Merena). This device is effective for up to 5 years.[29] In response to the local release of progesterone, the endometrial lining thins dramatically, leading to a reduction or a loss of menstrual bleeding, which again may provide additional benefits to the patient with SLE by preventing menses-related blood loss. Currently available IUDs are excellent options for women with SLE who need effective, long-term contraception but may be reluctant to add another pill to an already complicated medical regimen. IUDs offer the benefit of completely bypassing issues of compliance and require an active process (i.e., scheduled visit to gynecologist) to remove the device and to restore fertility. As with hormone-releasing contraception, fertility is restored shortly after discontinuation, and devices can be used in both nulliparous and parous women.[28] These devices do not carry potential risks of BMD loss or thromboses as observed in other hormone-containing contraceptives.

Because of concerns of increased risk of infections and pelvic inflammatory disease with the use of IUDs in decades past, misperceptions persist of the safety of IUDs in immunosuppressed women.[28] Numerous studies have since been performed in several populations at high risk for sexually transmitted diseases without evidence of increased infections, compared with women not using IUDs. These studies include women with human immunodeficiency virus,[31] women with a history of sexually transmitted diseases, and women with multiple sexual partners.[28]

Barrier Methods

Barrier methods of contraception, including condoms and diaphragms with or without spermicide, are among the least effective forms of contraception. They rely on consistent and proper use at every occurrence of sexual intercourse and are fraught with problems of compliance. Additionally, they do not offer any benefits regarding the reduction in menstrual bleeding but avoid all risks associated with the administration of exogenous hormones or device failure. However, barrier methods offer a few distinct advantages. They are among the only contraceptive methods that provide protection against infection with sexually transmitted diseases, a particular concern in women who are likely to be taking long-term immunosuppressive therapies and therefore may be at increased risk of contracting infectious diseases. Additionally, condoms and spermicide are inexpensive, do not require a physician office visit or prescription, and are widely available at any time of day. Thus they may be reasonable options for women with infrequent sexual encounters who do not wish to accept the risks associated with hormonal or implantable contraception. Regular use of spermicide with barrier methods will increase the efficacy of barrier forms of contraception.[29]

Infertility and Protection against Premature Ovarian Failure

Fertility in women with SLE is thought to be equivalent to that of the general population. Likewise, disease activity does not appear to affect fertility.[32] Perhaps the greatest risk to fertility among women with SLE is the potential for POF caused by cyclophosphamide, which is one of several medications commonly used to treat lupus nephritis and other severe manifestations of the disease.[33] Cyclophosphamide appears to be the only commonly used immunosuppressive therapy for SLE that carries a risk of POF. The majority of data on sustained amenorrhea or POF comes from retrospective studies of cohorts of women exposed to oral or intravenous cyclophosphamide. Although no absolute threshold levels have been established, the risk of POF increases with cyclophosphamide exposure at an older age and with a larger cumulative dose of cyclophosphamide.[33]

The possibility of POF is a significant concern for young patients with SLE who have not completed their families, and women may decline or delay cyclophosphamide therapy because of these concerns, even in the setting of worse disease-related outcomes. Because estrogen-containing oral contraceptives that prevent ovulation have not been studied in women with severe SLE (the very patients who may require cyclophosphamide therapy), their use cannot be advocated without adequate safety data. However, an increasing body of literature has grown to support the use of gonadotropin-releasing hormone (GnRH) agonists to protect against POF in women undergoing cyclophosphamide-based therapy for malignant disease or SLE. To maintain normal menstrual cycles, the endogenous GnRH is secreted by the hypothalamus in a pulsatile fashion. Continuous exposure, via exogenous GnRH agonist therapy, suppresses ovulation and reduces the levels of estrogen and progesterone. GnRH agonists are often used for the treatment of endometriosis. Although much data are derived from observational studies, an analysis of 40 women treated with a standard regimen of cyclophosphamide for severe SLE found 1 woman among 20 women (5%) developed amenorrhea who also underwent therapy with GnRH agonists, compared with 6 of 20 women (30%) who did not receive GnRH agonist therapy.[34] A meta-analysis of nine studies comparing POF and subsequent pregnancy rates after GnRH agonist therapy for women undergoing chemotherapy for SLE or malignant disease found a 68% overall increased rate of preserved ovarian function among GnRH users, compared with unexposed women.[35] Additionally, 22% of women receiving GnRH agonist therapy later achieved pregnancy, compared with 14% of women who did not receive GnRH agonist therapy.[35]

The benefit of preservation of ovarian function with the use of GnRH agonists must be balanced against the potential risks of therapy. Initiation of GnRH agonist therapy may lead to an initial surge of estrogen levels for a few days, which raises the theoretical possibility of increasing the risk of estrogen-related flares of underlying disease, worsening hypertension, and increasing thrombotic risk.[33] Additionally, extended use of GnRH agonists is associated with BMD loss; however, this loss may be offset by the protection against decreases in BMD associated with POF.

Newer regimens for the treatment of lupus nephritis and other severe organ-threatening manifestations are increasingly minimizing the cumulative dose of cyclophosphamide with the increased use of maintenance therapies that are less toxic (e.g., the Euro-Lupus regimen with 500 mg every other week for 3 months for lupus nephritis), which will additionally help reduce the risk of POF. A retrospective analysis found that women who received five to seven monthly intravenous treatments of cyclophosphamide, followed by maintenance with mycophenolate mofetil, had significantly lower rates of sustained amenorrhea than women receiving prolonged cyclophosphamide therapy (4% versus 51%, $P = 0.05$).[36]

Assisted Reproductive Technologies

Even in the absence of cyclophosphamide-induced POF, many women with SLE may experience subfertility and may require assisted reproductive technologies (ARTs) to achieve desired pregnancies. This situation may be largely the result of the fact that many women with SLE delay pregnancy for reasons of controlling active disease or the inability to replace potentially teratogenic medications with drugs that may be safer during pregnancy. Even in the general population, ARTs are being increasingly used for infertile or subfertile couples. ARTs are made up of a series of surgical, hormonal, or gamete manipulations that increase the chance of conception and implantation of an embryo. Many of these technologies involve ovarian stimulation and ovulation induction through the manipulation of female sex hormones including GnRH agonists, human chorionic gonadotropin, and progesterone.

Just as increased risks may exist with an initial surge of estrogen after the initiation of GnRH therapy, many ARTs involve hormonal manipulation that carries a risk of disease flare or thromboses.[37] Indeed, many case reports have been published that describe serious adverse effects in women with SLE undergoing ovulation induction therapy; however, these reports must be balanced by the many case reports describing successful and uneventful ovarian stimulation and pregnancy in patients with SLE.[37] Women at highest risk for ART-associated complications mirror those for use of exogenous estrogens and pregnancy itself—active disease, uncontrolled hypertension, smoking, and APS.[38] Ovarian-stimulation regimens should be tailored to avoid the induction of high estradiol levels wherever possible. Patients with APLAs without prior thrombotic or obstetric events do not appear to be at an increased risk for infertility or ART-associated thromboses than the general population, although controlled studies have not been performed.[38] Infertile women who are at high risk for ART- or pregnancy-related morbidity may decide on a healthy egg donor to undergo ovarian stimulation and egg retrieval or a female surrogate to carry the pregnancy to term or both.

Recurrent Pregnancy Loss

Most pregnancy losses are sporadic, nonconsecutive spontaneous abortions that occur as an isolated event in the reproductive career of women with other successful pregnancies. Approximately 10% to 20% of pregnant women experience sporadic loss of a clinically recognized pregnancy.[39] The diagnosis of recurrent pregnancy loss (RPL) is three or more consecutive miscarriages, affecting less than 3% of women. Patients with primary RPL who have had successive pregnancy losses without a prior healthy pregnancy have a poorer prognosis regarding future pregnancies than women with secondary RPL, that is, women who have had recurrent losses after at least one live birth. In the majority of patients, pregnancies are lost during the preembryonic or embryonic period (10 weeks' gestation).[40] An etiologic factor of RPL is identified in fewer than 50% of pregnancies, and known causes include uterine structural anomalies, genetic disorders, endocrine dysfunction, environmental factors, and thrombophilia.[41] Other risk factors may include smoking, moderate alcohol use, and advanced maternal age. Immunologic mechanisms of RPL have generated considerable interest, and both antibody-mediated and cellular-mediated mechanisms have been proposed. Thus far, human studies of such mechanisms have yielded inconsistent results, as have the uses of immune-based therapies for treating women with RPL.

Antiphospholipid Antibody–Mediated Recurrent Pregnancy Loss

To date, the only scientifically validated humoral cause for RPL remains APS, mediated by APLAs including LA and aCL antibodies. APS may occur secondary to autoimmune diseases including SLE, but it may also occur in women without other immunologic diseases and is referred to as *primary APS*. The revised 2006 criteria for APS include the following: (1) laboratory criteria: LA and aCL antibodies or anti–beta 2 glycoprotein I (anti–β_2 GPI) positive on two or more occasions at least 12 weeks apart; (2) vascular thromboses: at least one unequivocal episode of arterial, venous, or small-vessel thrombosis; and (3) obstetric criteria: one or more unexplained deaths of a morphologically healthy fetus after 10 weeks' gestation; one or more births before 34 weeks' gestation as a result of preeclampsia or placental insufficiency; or three or more consecutive spontaneous abortions before 10 weeks' gestation without chromosomal, anatomical, hormonal, or other causes to explain the RPL.[42] Women with *obstetric APS* without a history of vascular thromboses in the nonpregnant state are not uncommon.

APLAs are not frequently associated with sporadic pregnancy loss; these losses are more commonly the result of chromosomal and other causes. The original description of APS included only women with fetal death rather than earlier pregnancy loss. Subsequent series reported that positive tests for LA or IgG or IgM aCL antibodies are found in up to 20% of women with RPL.[43] It should be noted that some investigators believe that women with APS identified in the setting of recurrent preembryonic or embryonic loss, without a history of other clinical manifestations of APS, represent a different population from those identified because of thromboembolic disease, SLE, or adverse second- or third-trimester obstetric outcomes. Women with LA or medium-to-high positive IgG aCL antibodies have been shown to have losses more specific to the fetal period.[44] In one study of 366 women with two or more consecutive pregnancy losses, investigators found that women with moderate to high levels of APLAs had significantly different histories of pregnancy losses, compared with women with low levels or absence of APLAs.[44] Although the overall rates of prior losses were similar in the two groups (84%), 50% of the prior losses in women with moderate-to-high APLA levels were fetal deaths, compared with less than 15% in women without APLAs. In another prospective, large case series that included women with SLE, prior thromboses, and other medical conditions, women with APS experienced high rates of preterm birth secondary to gestational hypertension–preeclampsia and uteroplacental insufficiency as manifested by fetal growth restriction, oligohydramnios, and nonreassuring fetal surveillance findings.[45]

The causes of APLA-related adverse preembryonic and embryonic outcomes (e.g., RPL) and later APLA-related fetal complications are thought to be the same by some experts.[46] The implication is that APLA-mediated inflammation operates along the continuum of gestation to cause either preembryonic and embryonic or fetal damage. Other investigators question this theory, suggesting that women with recurrent preembryonic and embryonic losses and APLAs represent a largely different patient population than those who experience fetal death and other late pregnancy complications.[47] The International Congress on Antiphospholipid

Antibodies included both preembryonic and embryonic losses and the fetal-neonatal complications in their 1999 criteria, dividing them into three categories:

1. One or more unexplained deaths of a morphologically normal fetus at or beyond 10 weeks' gestation
2. One or more premature births of a morphologically normal neonate at or before 34 weeks' gestation
3. Three or more unexplained consecutive spontaneous abortions before 10 weeks' gestation

A recent observational study evaluated late pregnancy outcomes in 83 pregnancies among 67 women with APS into three clinical categories: (1) recurrent early embryonic loss, (2) late fetal loss or premature delivery, and (3) thrombotic complications.[48] All women with thrombotic APS underwent anticoagulation with low–molecular-weight heparin (LMWH) throughout pregnancy. Results showed that women with thrombotic APS had higher rates of most adverse pregnancy outcomes. Early embryonic losses were not captured in this dataset.

Treatment of Antiphospholipid Antibody–Mediated Recurrent Pregnancy Loss

Treatment strategies for women with obstetric APS have been designed to suppress the immune system (with corticosteroids and intravenous immunoglobulin [IVIG]), to prevent thromboses (with heparin and aspirin), and to improve placental blood flow by decreasing the thromboxane-to-prostacyclin ratio (with aspirin). Over time, it has become clear that heparin or low-dose aspirin or both are the treatments of choice for preventing or reducing pregnancy loss in women with APLA-mediated RPL. Several metaanalyses compared heparin with aspirin to aspirin alone among women with RPL and APS or patients with RPL and positive for APLAs.[49,50] They evaluated studies of RPL only and did not include obstetric patients with APS with only fetal or neonatal complications. Both metaanalyses concluded that combination therapy with unfractionated heparin or LMWH, in addition to aspirin, was superior to aspirin alone for the prevention of first-trimester pregnancy losses and to increase live birth rates. However, one metaanalysis separately evaluated late-pregnancy losses and found no significant differences between combination therapies with heparin or aspirin alone.[49] The use of prophylactic versus treatment doses of heparins may depend on individual patient history, including the history of thromboses. Experts generally agree that low-dose aspirin should be instituted during the preconception period, with the addition of once daily subcutaneous LMWH or unfractionated heparin on confirmation of pregnancy.[48,51]

Pregnancy losses continue to occur in up to 30% of patients even when heparin prophylaxis is administered.[52,53] Several alternative therapies have been tried in such patients who are refractory to treatment. Glucocorticoid agents, often in high doses, have sometimes been added to regimens of heparin and low-dose aspirin. Although anecdotal successes have been reported, this practice has never been studied in appropriately designed trials, and the combination of glucocorticoids and heparin may increase the risk for preeclampsia and osteoporotic fracture.[53] IVIG has also been tried during pregnancy in women with APS who have continued to have poor obstetric outcomes despite heparin therapy. However, two randomized, controlled trials found no benefit of this expensive therapy, compared with heparin and low-dose aspirin.[54] Newer experimental evidence strongly suggests a critical role of tissue factor and activated complement in APS-mediated pregnancy loss.[55] Inhibitors of these factors have yet to be studied in the clinical setting (see Table 36-3, "Pregnancy Outcomes in Randomized Controlled Trials of Treatments for Antiphospholipid Syndrome" in Chapter 36.)

Menopause and Disease Activity

The corollary to concerns about increased disease activity related to increases in female sex steroids (e.g., menarche, pregnancy, estrogen-containing contraceptives) is the possibility that disease activity may abate after menopause when the level of endogenous female sex hormones drops. This abatement is supported by studies of animal data in which ovariectomy ameliorates disease activity in lupus-prone mice.[56] Indeed, Mok and colleagues[57] demonstrated that women with cyclophosphamide-induced POF had fewer flares and a reduced number of severe flares than women with preserved ovarian function. A study of 30 women of Mexican descent with SLE followed before and after natural menopause found a slight, but statistically significant, reduction in maximum disease activity after menopause, compared with the years preceding menopause; most women in the cohort study had relatively low disease activity throughout the period of observation.[58] A more recent study evaluated the role of menopause in disease activity in three ways.[59] In part one, women diagnosed with SLE while premenopausal had less active disease than women initially diagnosed in the postmenopausal period. The second phase of the study compared disease activity of women for 3 years before and 3 years after menopause (mean age of menopause was 45.5 years). Results were consistent in this phase, with the adjusted mean disease activity being lower after menopause in these women. This level of disease activity was found to be unrelated to disease duration at enrollment into the study (Systemic Lupus Erythematosus Disease Activity Index–2K [SLEDAI-2K]). However, in the third phase of the study, 193 women with SLE with 6 years of observation before menopause were compared with 76 patients who were followed for 6 years during the postmenopausal period. Results concluded that the postmenopausal decrease in disease activity may be more of a factor of disease duration than a change in hormonal status per se. From this three-part study, the authors concluded that disease activity appears to be greater in premenopausal women; however, the decrease in disease activity after menopause may be more attributable to changes in disease over time.[59]

Postmenopausal Hormone Replacement

Once women become postmenopausal, from cyclophosphamide-induced POF, surgical oophorectomy, or natural menopause, the issue of hormone therapy naturally arises as the loss of estrogen through the cessation of ovarian function leads to uncomfortable vasomotor symptoms, accelerated loss of BMD, and increases in risks for atherosclerotic vascular disease. In the era after the publication of the *Women's Health Initiative* (WHI), which found that the use of postmenopausal hormone therapy was associated with increased risks of breast cancers and cardiovascular disease, the appropriate use of hormone therapy has been difficult to determine, even among women without underlying SLE.[60] Currently, the use of postmenopausal hormone therapy should be restricted to the lowest dose and shortest duration of therapy to achieve control of vasomotor symptoms. Its use for the prevention of chronic diseases cannot be advocated at this time[60] (Box 38-2).

Box 38-2 Management of Menopause in Women with Systemic Lupus Erythematosus

Hormonal treatment
Benefits
- Effectively controls vasomotor symptoms
- Prevents the loss of bone mineral density

Risks
- Increases the risk for thromboembolic disease
- Increases the risk for breast cancer
- Increases the risk for cardiovascular disease

Bottom line
Should be restricted to the lowest dose and shortest duration to control vasomotor symptoms.

Hormone Therapy and Cardiovascular Disease and Thromboses

The decision to use postmenopausal hormone therapy, even for the treatment of vasomotor symptoms, is even more complicated in women with SLE who may have increased risks of both osteoporosis and cardiovascular disease at baseline. Although the initial results of the WHI did not find hormone therapy to be protective against cardiovascular disease, many women entered the trial longer than 10 years after menopause. Subsequent analyses have suggested a slight protective effect of estrogen-containing hormone therapy in women who begin its use shortly after the onset of menopause. Prospective, randomized controlled trials are currently under way to directly test this hypothesis,[60] which may be of particular relevance to patients with SLE and with premature menopause. However, to better understand the complicated relationship between hormone therapy and cardiovascular disease, other analyses of the WHI results found that women with increased baseline risks for cardiovascular disease (including elevated low-density lipoprotein/high-density lipoprotein [LDL/HDL] ratio) may be a subset of women at higher risk for cardiovascular events after the initiation of menopausal hormone therapy.[61] These considerations are of considerable importance to patients with SLE, given the mounting evidence that accelerated development of atherosclerosis is a significant risk for morbidity and mortality in these patients.[62] One recent observational study[63] sought to understand the effects of menopausal hormone therapy on the development of incident cardiovascular disease in postmenopausal patients with lupus. This study compared 114 postmenopausal women who had taken hormone therapy with 227 who had not. All patients had no history of cardiovascular disease and were similar with respect to APLA status, traditional cardiovascular risk factors, and prednisone use. The proportion of patients who developed incident cardiovascular disease was similar among those who used hormone therapy (11.4%) and those who did not (13.7%), and the time to develop cardiovascular disease was not different between the two groups.[63,64] However, this study was much smaller than studies of hormone therapy in the general population, and it cannot be concluded that hormonal therapy in patients with SLE is safe.

The subset of patients with the APS with a history of thromboses may be a group for whom hormone therapy is contraindicated. Its use in women with positive APLAs without a history of arterial or venous events should proceed with caution. Several biologic properties of estrogens and APLAs may contribute to similar pathways leading to thrombogenetic potential. Synthetic estrogens are more *procoagulant* than natural preparations, and oral estrogen formulations influence coagulation to a greater degree than transdermal preparations, since the latter avoids the first-passage effect of oral estrogens. The use of oral estrogen therapy is associated with an increased risk of 2.5 (95% confidence interval [CI] 1.9 to 3.4) of first-time deep venous thrombosis; the increased risk did not meet statistical significance among users of transdermal preparations (relative risk 1.2, 95% CI 0.9 to 1.7).[65]

Effect of Menopausal Hormone Replacement on Disease Activity

Like the use of estrogen-containing contraceptives, with concerns about their leading to flares of underlying SLE, the use of estrogen for menopausal hormone replacement had been relatively contraindicated in lupus populations until formal studies had been undertaken.[66,67] It must be kept in mind that the doses of estrogen are substantially lower in postmenopausal hormone therapy, compared with oral contraceptives. The SELENA group published results of a randomized, placebo-controlled study of the effects of hormone therapy on the rates of disease flares in a U.S. population.[66] Investigators randomized 351 postmenopausal patients with SLE to receive either 0.625 mg conjugated estrogen daily with discontinuous progesterone or matched placebo for 12 months. Participants were at an average age of 50 years at enrollment, had a range of disease activity, and were excluded for a history of thrombosis, uncontrolled hypertension, and high-titer aCL antibodies or LA. Severe flares were infrequent in both groups and were not significantly increased in the women who were taking hormone therapy. They had more mild to moderate flares than those taking the placebo (1.14 versus 0.86 flares per person per year), although the clinical significance of this finding was not considered to be a concern. Four women taking hormones and one woman in the placebo group suffered thromboembolic events, although the difference was not statistically significant. Shortly after publication of the hormone therapy trial in the United States, a group from Mexico published the results of a randomized, placebo-controlled trial of the effects of hormone therapy or placebo on disease activity in postmenopausal women with SLE.[67] This study randomized 106 postmenopausal women with SLE to either placebo or 0.625 mg conjugated equine estrogen plus discontinuous progesterone for 24 months. Relevant exclusions included age older than 65 years, the use of estrogens within 3 months, severe lupus activity (SLEDAI score higher than 30), and a history of thrombosis within 6 months. Participants had a mean age of 48.8 years, with a mean age at menopause of 41.5 years. SLEDAI scores at study entry were lower than 15. Only one severe flare occurred during the 24-month study, in a participant receiving the placebo. Otherwise, the overall flare rates were not statistically distinguishable between the two groups, with a median time to first flare of 3 months in both groups. One thrombosis occurred in the placebo group in contrast to three in the hormone therapy group. On the basis of these data, it was concluded that adding a short course of hormone therapy might be associated with a small risk for increasing the flare rate of lupus, but most of the flares recorded were mild to moderate, and in many or even most patients, the contained risks observed in the studies might be favorably weighed against the potential amelioration of perimenopausal symptoms. However, rates of thromboses were numerically larger in women taking hormone therapy than placebo in both studies and may limit the enthusiasm for use in high-risk populations.

Bone Health and Osteoporosis

Estrogen elicits both direct and indirect effects on bone metabolism. Positive changes in calcium homeostasis are achieved by enhancing synthesis of 1,25(OH)2D and absorption of calcium in the intestines.[68] Additionally, the bone-resorbing cytokines IL-1 and IL-6 are inhibited by estrogens.[69,70] The net effect is not only to prevent bone loss but also to increase bone mass in individuals with osteopenia.[71] Most of the increase in bone mass occurs during the first 12 months of therapy,[72] which is consistent with the model that the primary mechanism is inhibition of bone resorption, allowing the ongoing complementary process of bone formation to reinstitute the bone mass over a prolonged period.

Many endogenous and exogenous factors contribute to the development of osteoporosis, including genetics, caffeine, alcohol, smoking, body stature, physical activity, renal disorders, thyroid disease, chronic inflammation, sun avoidance, and treatment with glucocorticoids.[73] Glucocorticoid use contributes significantly to the risk of osteoporosis in women with SLE. Ramsey-Goldman and colleagues[74] surveyed the frequency of fractures and associated risk factors in 702 women with SLE who had been followed for 5951 person-years and found that fractures occurred in 12.3% of the patients, an almost five-fold increase compared with a background population. Older age at diagnosis and longer duration of steroidal use were important variables. Two recent studies have addressed BMD loss in premenopausal women with SLE. Sinigaglia and others[75] reported osteoporosis in 22.6% of 84 premenopausal patients, with both disease duration and glucocorticoid use being associated risks. Gilboe and colleagues[76] observed similar results in a study of 75 patients with SLE (combined premenopausal and postmenopausal) and concluded that premenopausal patients taking glucocorticoids were at particularly high risk. Other variables that have been found to be associated with osteoporosis and fractures among women with SLE include older age at SLE diagnosis and SLE severity.[73] Because of the high rates of osteoporosis and fractures among patients with SLE and the clear association with glucocorticoids, it is imperative that preventative measures including behavior modifications or pharmaceutical interventions be instituted as early as possible.[77] Additionally, one small study has been published that evaluates the effect of transdermal estrogen therapy in postmenopausal osteopenic women with SLE.[78] This study randomized 43 women to therapy with transdermal estrogen therapy (50 mg transdermal 17β-estradiol) or placebo for 1 year. Results showed an increase in BMD loss and markers of bone turnover in the hormone therapy group, compared with the placebo group without significant changes in disease activity; however, more than one half of the women in the active group terminated therapy before 1 year, raising concerns about the viability of this therapy for long-term use (Table 38-2).

Prevention of Osteoporosis

Because of the myriad of risks of cardiovascular disease and malignancy associated with long-term use of oral postmenopausal hormone therapy, it should no longer be prescribed for the prevention or treatment of chronic diseases, including osteoporosis. Indeed, any reduction in hip or vertebral fractures with the use of hormonal therapy does not last far beyond the cessation of therapy.[60] Therefore alternative strategies need to be used in postmenopausal women with SLE. Many strategies have been studied in women with SLE. A great deal of evidence supports adequate calcium and vitamin D

TABLE 38-2 Recommendations for Women with Systemic Lupus Erythematosus

	BENEFITS	RISKS	BOTTOM LINE
Behavior modification (e.g., smoking cessation, weight-bearing activity)	Offers clear benefits.	Has no risks.	Is recommended for all patients.
Estrogen-replacement therapy	Improves bone-mineral density while under treatment (see Box 38-2).	Increases cardiovascular and malignancy risks (see Box 38-2).	Is no longer recommended.
Bisphosphonates	Are effective in many randomized trials for both postmenopausal and corticosteroid-induced osteoporosis.	Have teratogenic potential.	Are appropriate for most postmenopausal patients at risk for osteoporosis.
Raloxifene (selective estrogen-receptor modulator)	Is effective in randomized trials for both postmenopausal and corticosteroid-induced osteoporosis.	Has no major risks. Has no increased risk for SLE flares.	Is appropriate for many postmenopausal patients at risk for osteoporosis.
5-DHEA	Is supported by theory and animal data. Has mixed results in trials. Has no proven benefits for SLE itself or other health aspects.	Lowers HDL cholesterol levels.	Is not recommended.

5-DHEA, dehydroepiandrosterone; HDL, high-density lipoproteins; SLE, systemic lupus erythematosus.

supplementation in all women, irrespective of bone density or menopausal status. Other options that have been studied in women with SLE include bisphosphonates, selective estrogen-receptor modulators (raloxifene), and adrenal androgen therapy with dehydroepiandrosterone (5-DHEA).

Bisphosphonates, analogs of pyrophosphate, are deposited under osteoclasts and increase bone mass by reducing bone turnover.[79] They have been shown to reduce the rate of vertebral and nonvertebral fractures in large studies of postmenopausal women. Few studies have specifically addressed the use of bisphosphonates in women with SLE. One placebo-controlled study[80] evaluated the use of oral pamidronate disodium for the prevention of glucocorticoid-induced bone loss in 30 premenopausal patients with active connective tissue diseases (70% with SLE) on background calcium and vitamin D supplementation. After 1 year of therapy, this study found that both groups sustained loss in BMD at the hip, but that BMD loss in the lumbar spine observed in the placebo group was averted in the pamidronate group.[80] A second study evaluated the effects of alendronate and calcitriol combination treatment and placebo on background calcium supplementation on the loss of BMD in premenopausal women with SLE on long-term glucocorticoids.[81] Ninety-eight patients were randomized to one of the three treatment arms for 2 years. Participants receiving alendronate plus calcium had a mean increase in BMD in both the lumbar spine and hip; those receiving calcitriol plus calcium did not show significant change in BMD; and those receiving calcium alone had a small decrease in BMD at the hip only. A more recent study evaluated ibandronate in both premenopausal and postmenopausal women with SLE on corticosteroids.[82] Forty patients were randomized to receive either monthly oral ibandronate or placebo on background calcium supplementation for 12 months. Although no significant changes were seen in BMD in either group at 12 months, improvements in bone microarchitecture assessed by quantitative computed tomography were seen only in the ibandronate group. Thus bisphosphonates may be very reasonable options to prevent corticosteroid-induced bone loss among women with SLE. It must be remembered, however, that bisphosphonates have teratogenic potential and should not be used in women who are or may become pregnant.

Although straightforward hormone therapy cannot be advocated for the prevention or treatment of osteoporosis, other hormone-based options may be available for the patient with SLE at risk for or diagnosed with osteoporosis. However, as with all steroid-based therapies, concerns may arise regarding possible effects on disease activity. Raloxifene is one of the selective estrogen-receptor modulators, a class of agents that bind to estrogen receptors with different specificities in different tissues. A large trial in postmenopausal osteoporotic women found a significant reduction in vertebral fractures when compared with placebo.[83] A small placebo-controlled trial of raloxifene was performed with 33 postmenopausal patients with SLE and osteopenia taking low-dose prednisone[84] and addressed its effects on BMD and disease activity. As in other studies of hormone-based therapies, women with active SLE, a history of thromboses, or APLAs were excluded. Thirty-three women were randomized to raloxifene or placebo for 12 months. Significant decreases in BMD observed in the placebo group were not seen in the raloxifene group, and overall disease activity was similar in the two groups. Four flares were observed in raloxifene-treated participants, compared to six in the placebo arm.[84]

Androgen Therapy with Dehydroepiandrosterone

Deficiencies in 5-DHEA and its primary metabolite, 5-DHEA sulfate, have been reported in SLE,[85] and 5-DHEA may have an impact on a number of immunologic functions relevant to SLE. Endogenous-circulating 5-DHEA levels vary widely by gender, age, and ethnicity and can be affected by changes in corticosteroid levels, alcohol intake, smoking, body mass index, medications, and thyroid function. With this level of complexity in 5-DHEA metabolism, it is not surprising that clinical confirmation of efficacy in SLE activity has been inconsistent and controversial, hampering drug development for this theoretically promising treatment.

It remains unclear whether low 5-DHEA levels in patients with SLE are truly pathogenic or simply reflective of chronic disease, considering the many disorders, including normal aging, in which 5-DHEA levels drop. In the past, there was considerable enthusiasm for the use of 5-DHEA for the treatment of active SLE, and several randomized controlled trials were performed. Unfortunately, most studies did not meet primary outcomes, although reduced corticosteroid requirements were suggested in several studies.[85]

Despite disappointing results in clinical trials for the treatment of SLE itself, 5-DHEA has been studied for potentially beneficial effects of improved bone health and cardiovascular disease. Following data in a randomized control trial for disease activity that found significant differences in BMD loss in 5-DHEA-treated versus placebo groups, several trials were designed and performed to address the effects of 5-DHEA specifically on BMD in women receiving chronic glucocorticoids with mixed results.[86,87] Furthermore, 5-DHEA was found to reduce HDL levels without beneficial effects of vascular function or markers of bone turnovers in a study of 13 premenopausal women with SLE.[88] Thus although murine models and epidemiologic data suggested a role for 5-DHEA in ameliorating the deleterious effects of SLE, randomized clinical trials do not show a convincing positive effect on disease or on bone or cardiovascular health and show possible evidence of harm. Therefore the use of 5-DHEA for the treatment or prevention of disease in the SLE population cannot be advocated at this time.

REPRODUCTIVE HEALTH CARE AND SCREENING

Since treatment and management of acute disease has improved dramatically over the past few years with increasing survival rates of patients, treatment and prevention of chronic co-morbid conditions become increasingly important in the care of patients with SLE. Women with SLE require health care screening and maintenance arguably more frequently than in the general population since they may be at increased risk for osteoporosis and certain reproductive malignancies as a result of chronic active inflammatory disease, as well as long-term steroid and immunosuppressive therapy. Unfortunately, the focus of most health care for the patient with SLE is on the acute management of disease flares, and preventative measures are often relegated to the prevention of specific therapy-induced toxicity. Two groups have recently published guidelines for the care of patients with SLE.[89,90] In addition to guidelines for monitoring disease activity and damage accrual, both reports outline the importance of contraceptive counseling and routine screening for malignancies including breast, cervical, and colon cancers. Epidemiologic studies of preventative health care screening in the lupus population have shown mixed results. One study of a community-based population of 685 patients with SLE found that cervical cancer screening (70%) and mammography (70%) rates were no different from those seen in the general population.[91] Older age, higher socioeconomic status, and involvement of a generalist in health care were predictive of receiving appropriate screening. In another study from Canada, mammography and cervical cancer screening rates were substantially lower than in the general Canadian population.[92] Again, lower educational attainment was associated with suboptimal cancer screening, as were nonwhite race and higher damage scores.

Similar to reproductive health care screening, screening for and the prevention of osteoporosis remain suboptimal, despite known increased risks in the SLE population and its importance highlighted in recent quality of care guidelines.[89,90] A study of bone health care in a U.S. community-based population of patients with SLE found low rates of BMD testing, calcium and vitamin D supplementation, or the use of antiresorptive therapy among all patients with SLE and those receiving chronic glucocorticoid therapy.[93] Similar results were reported in a sample of patients with SLE in an academic rheumatology practice: 59% of patients had received appropriate BMD screening, 62% received calcium and vitamin D supplementation, and 86% with documented osteoporosis received antiresorptive or anabolic therapy.[94]

Clearly, much work needs to be done to prevent or reduce the risk of co-morbid conditions including osteoporosis and reproductive malignancies. Increasing awareness on the part of patients, primary care physicians, and rheumatologists will serve to enhance adherence to screening guidelines.

References

1. González DA, Díaz BB, Rodríguez Pérez Mdel C, et al: Sex hormones and autoimmunity. *Immunol Lett* 133:6–13, 2010.
2. Rahman P, Gladman DD, Urowitz MB, et al: Early damage as measured by the SLICC/ACR damage index is a predictor of mortality in systemic lupus erythematosus. *Lupus* 10:93–96, 2001.
3. Scofeld RH, Bruner GR, Namjou B, et al: Klinefelter's syndrome (47,XXY) in male systemic lupus erythematosus patients. *Arthritis Rheum* 58:2511–2517, 2008.
4. Critchley HO, Kelly RW, Brenner RM, et al: The endocrinology of menstruation—a role for the immune system. *Clin Endocrinol* 55:701–710, 2001.
5. Cushman M, Meilahn EN, Psaty BM, et al: Hormone replacement therapy, inflammation, and hemostasis in elderly women. *Arterioscler Thromb Vasc Biol* 19:893–899, 1999.
6. Langer RD, Pradhan AD, Lewis CE, et al: Baseline associations between postmenopausal hormone therapy and inflammatory, haemostatic, and lipid biomarkers of coronary heart disease. The Women's Health Initiative Observational Study. *Thromb Haemost* 93:1108–1116, 2005.
7. Koh KK, Cardillo C, Bui MN, et al: Vascular effects of estrogen and cholesterol-lowering therapies in hypercholesterolemic postmenopausal women. *Circulation* 99:354–360, 1999.
8. Taylor RN, Ryan IP, Moore ES, et al: Angiogenesis and macrophage activation in endometriosis. *Ann NY Acad Sci* 828:194–207, 1997.
9. Xiao E, Xia-Zhang L, Barth A, et al: Stress and the menstrual cycle: relevance of cycle quality in the short- and long-term response to a 5-day endotoxin challenge during the follicular phase in the rhesus monkey. *J Clin Endocrinol Metab* 25:1305–1312, 1998.
10. Suenaga R, Evans MJ, Mtiamura K, et al: Peripheral blood T cells and monocytes and B cell lines derived from patients with lupus express estrogen receptor transcripts similar to those of normal cells. *J Rheumatol* 12:1305–1312, 1998.
11. Keck C, Herchenbach D, Pfisterer J, et al: Effects of 17beta-estradiol and progesterone on interleukin-6 production and proliferation of human umbilical vein endothelial cells. *Exp Clin Endocrinol Diabetes* 106:334–339, 1998.
12. Szekeres-Bartho J, Halasz M, Palkovics T: Progesterone and pregnancy; receptor-ligand interaction and signaling pathways. *J Repro Endocrin* 83:60–64, 2009.
13. Kullo IJ, Gau GT, Tajik AJ: Novel risk factors for atherosclerosis. *Mayo Clin Proc* 75:369–380, 2000.
14. Suzuki A, Mizuno K, Asada Y, et al: Effects of 17beta-estradiol and progesterone on the adhesion of human monocytic THP-1 cells to human female endothelial cells exposed to minimally oxidized LDL. *Gynecol Obstet Invest* 44:47–52, 1997.
15. Caulin-Glaser T, Farrell WJ, Pfau SE, et al: Modulation of circulating cellular adhesion molecules in postmenopausal women with coronary heart disease. *J Am Coll Cardiol* 31:1555–1560, 1998.
16. Petri M, Robinson C: Oral contraceptives and systemic lupus erythematosus. *Arthritis Rheum* 40:797–803, 1997.
17. Silver RM, Branch DW: The immunology of pregnancy. In: Creasy R, Resnik R, editors: *Maternal fetal medicine*, ed 4, Philadelphia, 2004, WB Saunders.
18. Bansal AS: Joining the immunological dots in recurrent miscarriage. *Am J Reprod Immunol* 64:307–315, 2010.
19. Lash GE, Robson SC, Bulmer JN: Review: functional role of uterine natural killer (uNK) cells in human early pregnancy decidua. *Placenta* 31(Suppl):S87–S92, 2010.
20. Chanute G, Ledée-Bataille N, Dubanchet S: Immune cells in uteroplacental tissues throughout pregnancy: a brief review. *Reprod Biomed Online* 14:256–266, 2007.
21. Manaster I, Mandelboim O: The unique properties of uterine NK cells. *Am J Reprod Immunol* 63:434–444, 2010.
22. Saji F, Samejima Y, Kamiura S, et al: Dynamics of immunoglobulins at the feto-maternal interface. *Rev Reproduct* 4:81–89, 1999.
23. Petri M, Kim MY, Kalunian KC, et al: Combined oral contraceptives in women with systemic lupus erythematosus. *New Eng J Med* 353:2550–2558, 2005.
24. Sanchez-Guerrero J, Uribe AG, Jimenez-Santana L, et al: A trial of contraceptive methods in women with systemic lupus erythematosus. *New Eng J Med* 353:2539–2549, 2005.
25. Finer LB, Henshaw SK: Abortion incidence and services in the United States in 2000. *Perspect Sex Reprod Health* 35:6–15, 2003.
26. Schwartz EB, Postlethwaite DA, Hung YY, et al: Documentation of contraception and pregnancy when prescribing potentially teratogenic medications for reproductive-age women. *Ann Int Med* 147:370–376, 2007.
27. Yazdany J, Trupuin L, Kaiser R, et al: Contraceptive counseling and use among women with systemic lupus erythematosus: a gap in health care quality. *Arthritis Care Res* 63:358–365, 2011.
28. Schwartz EB, Manzi S: Risk of unintended pregnancy among women with systemic lupus erythematosus. *Arthritis Rheum* 59:863–866, 2009.
29. Clowse MEB: Managing contraception and pregnancy in the rheumatologic diseases. *Best Pract Res Clin Rheumatol* 24:373–385, 2010.
30. Spencer AL, Bonnema R, McNamara MC: Helping women choose appropriate hormonal contraception: update on risks, benefits, and indications. *Am J Med* 122:497–506, 2009.
31. Sivin I, Batar I: State-of-the-art of non-hormonal methods of contraception: III. Intrauterine devices. *Eur J Contracept Reprod Health Care* 15:96–112, 2010.
32. Kaufman RL, Kitrodou RC: Pregnancy in mixed connective tissue disease: comparison with systemic lupus erythematosus. *J Rheumatol* 549–555, 1982.
33. Mersereau J, Dooley MA: Gonadal failure with cyclophosphamide therapy for lupus nephritis: advances in fertility preservation. *Rheum Dis Clin North Am* 36:99–108, 2010.
34. Somers EC, Marder W, Cristman GM, et al: Use of a gonadotropin-releasing hormone analog for protection against premature ovarian failure during cyclophosphamide therapy in women with severe lupus. *Arthritis Rheum* 52:2761–2767, 2005.
35. Clowse ME, Behera MA, Anders CK, et al: Ovarian preservation by GnRH agonists during chemotherapy: a meta-analysis. *J Womens Health (Larchmt)* 18:311–319, 2009.
36. Laskari K, Zintzaras E, Tzioufas AG: Ovarian function is preserved in women with severe systemic lupus erythematosus after a 6-month course of cyclophosphamide followed by mycophenolate mofetil. *Clin Exp Rheumatol* 28:83–86, 2010.
37. Costa M, Colia D: Treating infertility in autoimmune patients. *Rheumatology* 47:iii38–iii41, 2008.
38. Bellver J, Pellicer A: Ovarian stimulation for ovulation induction and in vitro fertilization in patients with systemic lupus erythematosus and antiphospholipid antibody syndrome. *Fertil Steril* 92:1803–1810, 2009.
39. Salat-Baroux J: Recurrent spontaneous abortions. *Reprod Nutr Dev* 28:1555, 1988.
40. Goldstein SR: Embryonic death in early pregnancy: a new look at the first trimester. *Obstet Gynecol* 84:294–297, 1994.
41. Toth B, Jeschke U, Rogenhofer N, et al: Recurrent miscarriage: current concepts in diagnosis and treatment. *J Reprod Immunol* 85:25–32, 2010.
42. Miyakis S, Lockshin MD, Atsumi T, et al: International consensus statement on an update of the classification criteria for definite antiphospholipid antibody syndrome (APS). *Thromb Haemost* 4:295–306, 2006.
43. Rai RS, Regan L, Clifford K, et al: Antiphospholipid antibodies and beta 2-glycoprotein-I in 500 women with recurrent miscarriage: results of a comprehensive screening approach. *Human Reprod* 10:2001–2005, 1995.
44. Oshiro BT, Silver RM, Scott JR, et al: Antiphospholipid antibodies and fetal death. *Obstet Gynecol* 87:489–493, 1996.
45. Lockshin MD, Druzin ML, Goei S, et al: Antibody to cardiolipin as a predictor of fetal distress or death in pregnant patients with systemic lupus erythematosus. *N Engl J Med* 313:152–156, 1985.
46. Clark CA, Spitzer KA, Laskin CA: The spectrum of the antiphospholipid syndrome: a matter of perspective. *J Rheumatol* 28:1939–1941, 2001.
47. Branch DE: Antiphospholipid antibodies and fetal compromise. *Thromb Res* 114:415–418, 2004.
48. Bramham K, Hunt BJ, Germain S, et al: Pregnancy outcome in different clinical phenotypes of antiphospholipid antibody syndrome. *Lupus* 19:58–64, 2010.
49. Ziakas PD, Pavlou M, Voulgarelis M: Heparin treatment in antiphospholipid syndrome with recurrent pregnancy loss: a systematic review and meta-analysis. *Obstet Gynecol* 115:1256–1262, 2010.
50. Mak A, Cheung MW, Cheak AA, et al: Combination of heparin and aspirin is superior to aspirin alone in enhancing live births in patients with recurrent pregnancy loss and positive anti-phospholipid antibodies:

a meta-analysis of randomized controlled trials and meta-regression. *Rheumatology* 49:281–288, 2010.

51. Ruiz-Irastorza G, Growther M, Branch W, et al: Antiphospholipid syndrome. *Lancet* 376:1498–1509, 2010.

52. Erkan D, Merrill JT, Yazici Y, et al: High thrombosis rate after fetal loss in antiphospholipid syndrome: effective prophylaxis with aspirin. *Arthritis Rheum* 44:1466–1467, 2001.

53. Cowchock FS, Reece EA, Balaban D, et al: Repeated fetal losses associated with antiphospholipid antibodies; a collaborative randomized trial comparing prednisone with low-dose heparin treatment. *Am J Obstet Gynecol* 166:1318–1323, 1992.

54. Practice Committee of the American Society for Reproductive Medicine. Intravenous immunoglobulin (IVIG) and recurrent spontaneous pregnancy loss. *Fertil Steril* 82(Suppl 1):S199–S200, 2004.

55. Pierangeli SS, Erkan D: Antiphospholipid syndrome treatment beyond anticoagulation: are we there yet? *Lupus* 19:475–485, 2010.

56. Roubinian JR, Talal N, Greenspan JS, et al: Effect of castration and sex-hormone treatment on survival, anti-nucleic acid antibodies, and glomerulonephritis in NZB/NZW F1 mice. *J Exp Med* 147:1568–1583, 1978.

57. Mok CC, Wong RWS, Lau CS: Ovarian failure and flares of systemic lupus erythematosus. *Arthritis Rheum* 42:1274–1280, 1999.

58. Sanchez-Guerrero J, Villegas A, Mendoza-Fuentes A, et al: Disease activity during the premenopausal and postmenopausal periods in women with systemic lupus erythematosus. *Am J Med* 111:464–468, 2001.

59. Urowitz MB, Ibanez D, Jerome D, et al: The effect of menopause on disease activity in systemic lupus erythematosus. *J Rheumatol* 33:2192–2198, 2006.

60. Taylor HS, Manson JE: Update in hormone therapy use in menopause. *J Clin Endocrinol Metab* 96:255–264, 2011.

61. Bray PF, Larson JC, Lacroix AZ, et al: Usefulness of baseline lipids and C-reactive protein in women receiving menopausal hormone therapy as predictors of treatment-related coronary events. *Am J Cardiol* 101:1599–1605, 2008.

62. Sherer Y, Zinger H, Shoenfeld Y: Atherosclerosis in systemic lupus erythematosus. *Autoimmunity* 43:98–102, 2010.

63. Hochman J, Urowitz MB, Ibañez D, et al: Hormone replacement therapy in women with systemic lupus erythematosus and risk of cardiovascular disease. *Lupus* 18:313–317, 2009.

64. Schwartz J, Freeman R, Frishman W: Clinical pharmacology of estrogens: cardiovascular actions and cardioprotective benefits of replacement therapy in postmenopausal women. *J Clin Pharmacol* 35:314–329, 1995.

65. Canonico M, Plu-Bureau G, Lowe GD, et al: Hormone replacement therapy and risk of venous thromboembolism in post-menopausal women: systematic review and meta-analysis. *BMJ* 336:1227–1231, 2008.

66. Buyon JP, Petri MA, Kim MY, et al: The effect of combined estrogen and progesterone hormone replacement therapy on disease activity in systemic lupus erythematosus: a randomized trial. *Ann Intern Med* 142:953–962, 2005.

67. Sánchez-Guerrero J, González-Pérez M, Durand-Carbajal M, et al: Menopause hormonal therapy in women with systemic lupus erythematosus. *Arthritis Rheum* 56:3070–3079, 2007.

68. Gallagher JC, Riggs BL, Deluca HF: Effect of estrogen on calcium absorption and serum vitamin D metabolites in postmenopausal osteoporosis. *J Clin Endocrin Metab* 51:1359–1364, 1980.

69. Pacifici R, Rifas L, McCracken R, et al: Ovarian steroid treatment blocks a postmenopausal increase in blood monocyte interleukin-1 release. *Proc Natl Acad Sci USA* 86:2398–2402, 1989.

70. Jilda RL, Hangoc G, Girasole F, et al: Increased osteoclast development after estrogen loss-mediation by interleukin-6. *Science* 257:88–91, 1992.

71. Ettinger B, Genant HK, Conn CE: Long-term estrogen replacement therapy prevents bone loss and fractures. *Ann Intern Med* 102:319–324, 1985.

72. The Writing Group for the PEPI Trial. Effects of hormone therapy on bone mineral density: results from the postmenopausal estrogen/progestin interventions (PEPI) trial. *JAMA* 276:1389–1396, 1996.

73. Sinigaglia L, Varenna M, Girasole G, et al: Epidemiology of osteoporosis in rheumatic diseases. *Rheum Dis Clin North Am* 32:631–658, 2006.

74. Ramsey-Goldman R, Dunn JE, Huang CF, et al: Frequency of fractures in women with systemic lupus erythematosus: comparison with United States population data. *Arthritis Rheum* 42:882–890, 1999.

75. Sinigaglia L, Varenna M, Binelli L, et al: Determinants of bone mass in systemic lupus erythematosus: a cross sectional study on premenopausal women. *J Rheumatol* 26:1280–1284, 1999.

76. Gilboe IM, Kvien TK, Haugeberg G, et al: Bone mineral density in systemic lupus erythematosus: comparison with rheumatoid arthritis and healthy controls. *Ann Rheum Dis* 59:110–115, 2000.

77. Compston JE: Emerging consensus on prevention and treatment of glucocorticoid-induced osteoporosis. *Curr Rheum Reports* 9:78–84, 2007.

78. Bhattoa HP, Bettembuk P, Balogh A, et al: The effect of 1-year transdermal estrogen replacement therapy on bone mineral density and biochemical markers of bone turnover in osteopenic postmenopausal systemic lupus erythematosus patients: a randomized, double-blind, placebo-controlled trial. *Osteoporosis Int* 15:396–404, 2004.

79. Reszka AA, Rodan GA: Bisphosphonate mechanism of action. *Curr Rheum Rep* 5:65–74, 2003.

80. Nzeussu Toukap AN, Depresseux G, Devogelaer JP, et al: Oral pamidronate prevents high-dose glucocorticoid-induced lumbar spine bone loss in premenopausal connective tissue disease (mainly lupus) patients. *Lupus* 14:517–520, 2005.

81. Yeap SS, Fauzi AR, Kong NCT, et al: A comparison of calcium, calcitriol, and alendronate in corticosteroid-treated premenopausal patients with systemic lupus erythematosus. *J Rheumatol* 35:2344–2347, 2008.

82. Li EK, Zhu TY, Hung VY, et al: Ibandronate increases cortical bone density in patients with systemic lupus erythematosus on long-term glucocorticoid. *Arthritis Res Ther* 12:R198, 2010.

83. Ettinger B, Black DM, Mitlak BH, et al: Reduction of vertebral fracture risk in postmenopausal women with osteoporosis treated with raloxifene: results from a 3-year randomized clinical trial. *JAMA* 282:637–645, 1999.

84. Mok CC, To CH, Mak A, et al: Raloxifene for postmenopausal women with systemic lupus erythematosus. *Arthritis Rheum* 52:3997–4002, 2005.

85. Sawalha AH, Kovats S: Dehydroepiandrosterone in systemic lupus erythematosus. *Curr Rheum Reports* 10:286–291, 2008.

86. Mease PJ, Ginzler EM, Gluck OS, et al: Effects of prasterone on bone mineral density in women with systemic lupus erythematosus receiving chronic glucocorticoid therapy. *J Rheumatol* 32:616–621, 2005.

87. Sanchez-Guerrero J, Fragoso-Loyo HE, Neuwelt CM, et al: Effects of prasterone on bone mineral density in women with active systemic lupus erythematosus receiving chronic glucocorticoid therapy. *J Rheumatol* 35:1567–1575, 2008.

88. Marder W, Somers EC, Kaplan MJ, et al: Effects of prasterone (dehydroepiandrosterone) on markers of cardiovascular risk and bone turnover in premenopausal women with systemic lupus erythematosus: a pilot study *Lupus* 19:1229–1236, 2010.

89. Yazdany J, Panopalis P, Gillis JZ, et al: A quality indicator set for systemic lupus erythematosus. *Arthritis Rheum* 61:370–377, 2009.

90. Mosca M, Tani C, Aringer M, et al: European League Against Rheumatism recommendations for monitoring patients with systemic lupus erythematosus in clinical practice and in observational studies. *Ann Rheum Dis* 69:1269–1274, 2010.

91. Yazdany J, Tonner C, Trupin L, et al: Provision of preventive health care in systemic lupus erythematosus: data from a large observational cohort study. *Arthritis Res Ther* 12:R84, 2010.

92. Bernatsky SR, Cooper GS, Mill C, et al: Cancer screening in patients with systemic lupus erythematosus. *J Rheumatol* 33:45–49, 2006.

93. Schmajuk G, Yelin E, Chakravarty E, et al: Osteoporosis screening, prevention, and treatment in systemic lupus erythematosus: application of the systemic lupus erythematosus quality indicators. *Arthritis Care Res* 62:993–1001, 2010.

94. Demas KL, Keenan BT, Solomon DH, et al: Osteoporosis and cardiovascular disease care in systemic lupus erythematosus according to new quality indicators. *Semin Arthritis Rheum* 40:193–200, 2010.

SECTION

VI

SPECIAL
CONSIDERATIONS,
SUBSETS OF SLE
AND LUPUS-RELATED
SYNDROMES

Chapter

39

Drug-Induced Lupus: Etiology, Pathogenesis, and Clinical Aspects

Dipak Patel and Bruce Richardson

Lupus flares when genetically predisposed people encounter drugs or environmental agents that trigger the disease. Although the agents triggering idiopathic lupus remain incompletely defined and the mechanisms involved are unclear, drug-induced lupus erythematosus (DIL) provides an opportunity to study defined agents and analyze the pathways involved. This chapter compares the initiating agents and pathogenic mechanisms implicated in causing DIL and idiopathic lupus, reviews how studies of DIL have provided insights into the mechanisms contributing to idiopathic lupus, and compares the clinical presentations of idiopathic lupus and DIL. Areas of uncertainty are also highlighted with the hope that future studies may provide new and therapeutically important insights into the pathogenesis and treatment of idiopathic human lupus.

ETIOLOGY
Drugs Implicated

More than 80 drugs and recombinant therapeutic agents have been associated with lupus-like autoimmunity.[1-3] For many, the evidence is based on case reports of lupus developing in patients receiving a drug and improving after its discontinuation. However, lupus is a chronic relapsing disease; therefore the relationship of drug ingestion to disease onset, flare, or remission may be coincidental, and some of the drugs reported to cause DIL may represent chance associations. Causality can be supported by documenting disease remission after the discontinuation of a drug and recurrence with repeat administration, which has been done for hydralazine,[4] procainamide,[5] isoniazid,[6] chlorpromazine,[7] quinidine,[8] and minocycline.[9] Prospective and case-control studies have provided additional confirmatory evidence for some of these and other drugs. Prospective studies support roles for procainamide,[10] hydralazine,[11] isoniazid,[12] methyldopa,[13] and levodopa[14] as well as estrogen and progesterone,[15] in initiating lupus flares. Similarly, a matched case-control study of 875 participants with incident lupus in the United

Kingdom General Practice Research Database reveals a significantly increased risk of lupus for patients receiving hydralazine, minocycline, and carbamazepine.[16] Another case-control study confirms a significant lupus risk for estrogen/progesterone contraceptives[17]; this may be considered a form of DIL. These agents are listed in Table 39-1 together with their lupus risk or odds ratio, and the structures of the nonhormonal drugs are shown in Figure 39-1. Although methyldopa and levodopa have similar chemical structures and hydralazine and isoniazid share a hydrazine side chain, the other molecules have little in common, suggesting that no single chemical structure is responsible for inducing autoimmunity and that these drugs may induce autoimmunity by multiple mechanisms.

Nearly all of these drugs cause a positive antinuclear antibody (ANA) test more frequently than clinically overt DIL, and the duration of drug exposure required to develop DIL typically ranges from 1 to 3 years.[10,11] Of these drugs, procainamide and hydralazine induce DIL most frequently with a 20% incidence after an average of 10 months of treatment with procainamide[18] and 7% after 3 years with hydralazine.[19] Oral contraceptives containing high doses of estrogens were also implicated in causing autoantibodies as well as clinical lupus in early reports. However, the more recent use of lower estrogen doses in combination pills may have decreased the incidence of DIL somewhat.[20] Postmenopausal estrogen replacement has also been reported to cause lupus flares, but the flares are of mild to moderate severity.[21] How estrogen influences autoimmunity is discussed in other sections of this textbook.

Finally, some recombinant biological agents, such as the tumor necrosis factor (TNF) antagonists and interferon-alpha (IFN-α), have been shown to cause lupus-like autoimmunity in prospective studies. These agents are also listed in Table 39-1. Like the lupus-inducing drugs, the TNF antagonists and IFN-α also cause ANAs more frequently than clinical lupus.[2,22]

TABLE 39-1 Confirmed Lupus-Inducing Drugs

DRUG	ANA PREVALENCE (%)	DIL PREVALENCE (%)	DIL ODDS RATIO	REFERENCES
Procainamide	75	15-20		5,10
Hydralazine	15-45	5-10	6.62	16
Isoniazid	22	<1		12
Chlorpromazine	20-50	<1		7
Minocycline			4.23	16
Carbamazepine			1.88	16
Methyldopa	19	<2		13
Levodopa	11	<2		14
Estrogens/progesterones	<2	<2		17
TNF antagonists	11-53	<1		81,114
IFN-α	18-72	0.1-2.1		81

ANA, Antinuclear antibody; DIL, drug-induced lupus erythematosus; IFN-α, interferon-alpha; TNF, tumor necrosis factor.

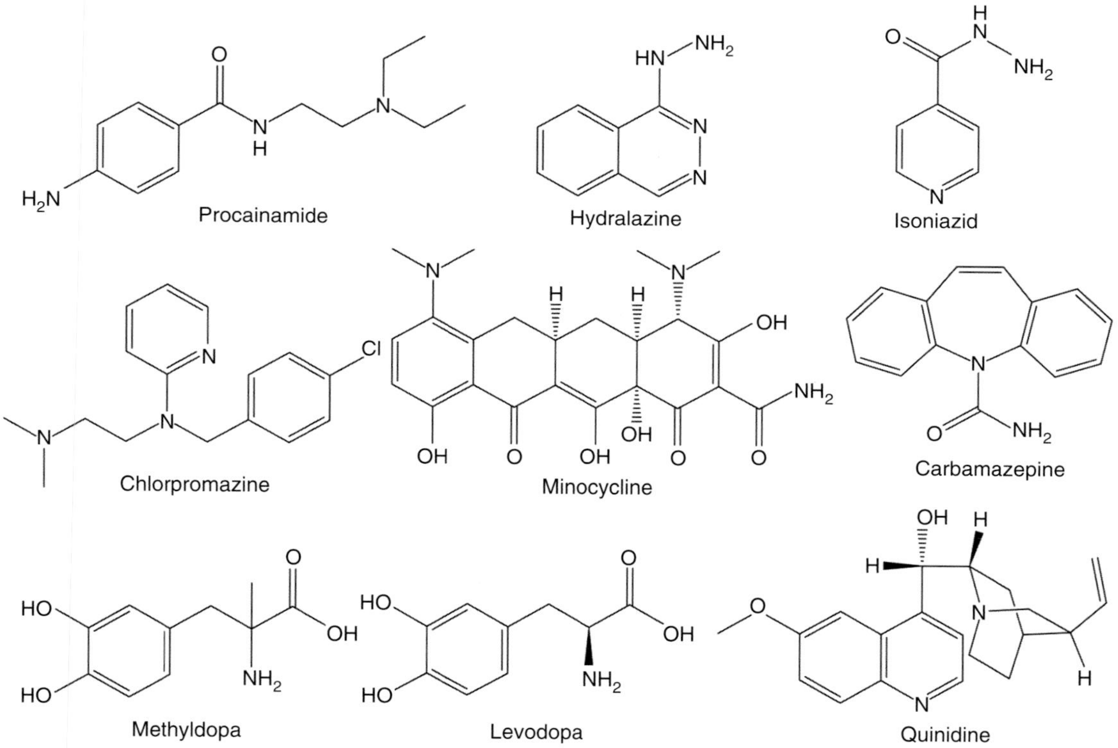

FIGURE 39-1 Structures of confirmed lupus-inducing drugs.

Genetic Contributions to Drug-Induced and Idiopathic Lupus

DIL and idiopathic lupus both require a genetic predisposition for disease to develop in response to the triggering agents. Genome-wide association studies (GWASs) have identified multiple genetic loci predisposing an individual to idiopathic lupus, whereas the genes contributing to DIL are only minimally defined. Conversely, although the nature and identity of the environmental agents triggering idiopathic lupus remain incompletely understood, DIL provides an excellent example of defined exogenous agents causing lupus-like autoimmunity in genetically predisposed people.

Current evidence indicates that multiple genes are required for idiopathic lupus to develop. Those with a higher total genetic risk tend to develop lupus at an earlier age than those with a lower genetic risk, and those with a higher total genetic risk also develop anti–double stranded DNA (anti-dsDNA) antibodies and hematologic disorders (e.g., hemolytic anemia, lymphopenia, leukopenia, thrombocytopenia), as well as immunologic disorders (e.g., anti-Smith antibodies, antiphospholipid antibodies) more often than those with lower total genetic risk.[23,24] This evidence suggests that people with even a lower total genetic risk are either unaffected or may develop ANAs only in response to environmental agents. Proposed environmental agents include infections, smoking, insecticides, silica, and ultraviolet (UV) light, among others.[25-28]

As with idiopathic lupus, drugs also activate lupus in genetically predisposed people, although the genetic associations with DIL are less well studied. Certain class II major histocompatibility complex (MHC) alleles predispose a person to idiopathic lupus,[29] and a susceptibility to hydralazine-induced lupus has been associated with the human leukocyte antigen (HLA)–DR4 allele,[30] although this observation was not confirmed by a second group.[31] Unfortunately, the other genetic loci confirmed in idiopathic lupus are largely unstudied in DIL, and future studies could prove informative. Importantly, though, at least one genetic difference distinguishes DIL and idiopathic lupus. People who metabolize drugs slowly because of genetically determined slow acetylator status, perhaps as a result of N-acetyltransferases 1 (NAT1) or 2 (NAT2) polymorphisms,[32] are more likely to develop DIL in response to drugs including hydralazine and procainamide than those who rapidly metabolize these drugs. In contrast, slow acetylator status does not predispose a person to idiopathic lupus.[32]

Age and Gender Contributions to Drug-Induced and Idiopathic Lupus

Age and gender also influence the susceptibility to DIL and idiopathic lupus. Although idiopathic lupus is usually considered a disease of young women, a recent study of more than 1600 patients with lupus in the British health care system demonstrates that the incidence of idiopathic lupus increases steadily up to approximately 75 years of age in men. In contrast, the incidence of lupus increases to approximately the age of menopause (50 to 54 years of age) in women but then declines, perhaps reflecting the decrease in estrogen after menopause, although some women still develop lupus well into their 80s.[33]

The age dependency in both men and women raises the possibility that environmental exposures have a cumulative effect in people genetically predisposed to lupus. As previously noted, those with a greater number of lupus genes develop lupus at an earlier age than those with fewer predisposing genes and have a more severe phenotype,[23,24] supporting a gene-environment interaction in which a greater genetic predisposition permits lupus development with a lesser total cumulative environmental contribution; those with a lesser genetic predisposition require a more prolonged exposure. Interestingly, ANAs develop with age[34] and often precede the development of clinical lupus by several years,[35] also suggesting that cumulative effects of environmental exposures occurring over time in people with a lower genetic predisposition contribute to the development of ANAs and sometimes lupus later in life. The roles of age and the environment are discussed further in "Pathogenesis."

In contrast to idiopathic lupus, drug exposure is required for DIL; consequently, the demographics of DIL differ from those of idiopathic lupus in part by reflecting the age of people receiving the drugs. With the exceptions of antiseizure medications more commonly used in younger people[36] and minocycline used to treat acne in young women,[37] older individuals tend to receive most of the drugs listed in Table 39-1. Perhaps, then, it is not surprising that DIL usually affects older adults more often than younger individuals.[38] A case-control study reveals that patients developing minocycline-induced lupus were an average of 8.5 years younger than control participants developing idiopathic lupus.[16] In contrast, the same study also found that people with hydralazine-induced lupus were approximately 25 years older at the time of disease diagnosis than patients with idiopathic lupus.[16] Another factor potentially contributing to the increased incidence of DIL in older people is that drug metabolism slows with age,[39] prolonging drug exposure in older adults, possibly analogous to slow acetylator status in procainamide- and hydralazine-induced lupus.[40]

Gender is also genetically determined, and women are affected by idiopathic lupus approximately nine times more often than men. Estrogen likely contributes to this female predisposition,[20,21] as does having two X chromosomes.[41] In contrast to idiopathic lupus, though, some forms of DIL occur only modestly more frequently in women.[30,42] However, people receiving many of these drugs also tend to be older, and the decreased female-to-male ratio could also reflect declining estrogen levels in postmenopausal women.

Summary

The etiologic variables of both idiopathic lupus and DIL involve genetic and exogenous factors. Aging contributes another variable that impacts the metabolism of exogenous agents and drugs as well as exposure to lupus-inducing drugs; these exposures may have cumulative effects as well. The gender distribution of DIL includes a somewhat higher percentage of men than is commonly seen in idiopathic lupus. This fact may reflect the effect of age, as the incidence of idiopathic lupus becomes somewhat closer in older men and women, as well as gender-specific differences in the use of certain drugs and declining estrogen levels in women. Finally, a dose-dependent genetic contribution to lupus exists, with some suggestion of commonality in the MHC for idiopathic lupus and DIL, but detailed genetic analyses have not been performed in DIL, and acetylator status is clearly different between idiopathic lupus and DIL. Thus etiologic variables contributing to DIL include exposure, age, gender, rates of drug metabolism, and genetic predisposition, and some of these variables could contribute to idiopathic lupus as well.

PATHOGENESIS

The mechanisms by which most of the drugs listed in Table 39-1 cause autoimmunity are poorly understood. A number of possibilities have been considered, including drug metabolites acting as haptens to modify self-antigens and induce autoantibodies through epitope spreading; drug-induced cytotoxicity, releasing self-macromolecules; nonspecific lymphocyte activation; and a disruption of central tolerance in the thymus by the drugs themselves or by their reactive metabolites generated during inflammatory responses.[1,43] However, although in vitro and in vivo models have been devised to support the feasibility for some of the mechanisms proposed, evidence that these mechanisms actually contribute to human DIL has been difficult to obtain for most of these drugs, and how the mechanisms might be relevant to idiopathic lupus remains unclear. Studies of procainamide and hydralazine, though, have provided important insights into epigenetic mechanisms contributing to both DIL and idiopathic lupus, whereas IFN-α and the TNF antagonists highlight important roles for these cytokines in the pathogenesis of idiopathic lupus. These mechanisms are discussed in the text that follows.

Epigenetics and Gene Expression

Epigenetics is defined as heritable changes in gene expression that do not involve a change in the DNA sequence. Epigenetic mechanisms include DNA methylation, a variety of covalent histone modifications that include acetylation, methylation, and phosphorylation, and microRNAs (miRNAs). DNA methylation and histone modifications regulate gene expression by altering chromatin structure to promote or suppress gene transcription, whereas miRNAs modify gene expression through effects on messenger RNA stability. Of these mechanisms, DNA methylation is the most strongly implicated in the pathogenesis of DIL and idiopathic lupus, and DNA methylation, together with histone acetylation, plays an essential role in regulating gene expression through effects on chromatin structure. Since epigenetic mechanisms are reviewed in detail elsewhere in this textbook, the relationships among DNA methylation, histone acetylation, chromatin structure, and gene expression are briefly reviewed here.

Epigenetics, Chromatin Structure, and Gene Expression

DNA is packaged into the nucleus as chromatin, the basic subunit of which is the nucleosome. Each nucleosome consists of two turns of DNA wrapped around a protein core containing two molecules each of histones H2a, H2b, H3, and H4. The nucleosomes are then arranged into higher order structures to form chromatin fibers. Histone tails protrude from the nucleosome, and positively charged lysines in the histone tails bind negatively charged phosphates in the DNA, stabilizing chromatin in a tightly compressed configuration (Figure 39-2). Chromatin in this configuration is inaccessible to transcription-factor binding and the messenger RNA (mRNA)

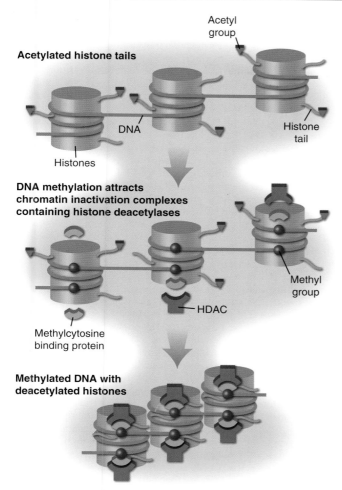

Acetylated histone tails

Acetyl group

Histones

DNA

Histone tail

DNA methylation attracts chromatin inactivation complexes containing histone deacetylases

Methyl group

HDAC

Methylcytosine binding protein

Methylated DNA with deacetylated histones

FIGURE 39-2 DNA methylation, histone acetylation, and chromatin structure. DNA is packaged as chromatin, a polymer of nucleosomes, each consisting of two turns of DNA wrapped around a core of histone proteins, the tails of which protrude. Transcriptionally active chromatin is characterized by unmethylated DNA and acetylated *(green triangles)* histone tails. The DNA is exposed and accessible to transcription-factor binding *(top panel)*. Methylation of cytosine bases in the DNA *(red dots)* attracts methylcytosine-binding proteins, which in turn attract and tether chromatin inactivation complexes containing histone deacetylases and other proteins *(middle panel)*. These complexes deacetylate the histones and promote condensation of the chromatin into a compressed structure inaccessible to the transcription-initiation complexes *(bottom panel)*.

transcription complexes responsible for gene expression. Gene expression thus first requires localized remodeling of the chromatin to make the DNA accessible, and these changes are replicated during cell division, making them *heritable*. The mechanisms regulating these changes in chromatin structure, which cause a heritable change in gene expression without a change in the DNA sequence, are referred to as *epigenetic*.[44]

Histone Modifications

One important epigenetic mechanism in chromatin remodeling is acetylation of lysines in the histone tails, referred to as *histone acetylation*. Acetylation of these lysines neutralizes their positive charge, releasing the histone tails from the negatively charged DNA and permitting localized remodeling of the chromatin into a transcription-permissive configuration open to transcription-factor binding (see Figure 39-2). Histone acetylation regulates gene expression in most

if not all eukaryotic cells. Methylation, phosphorylation, ubiquitination, and other moieties also covalently modify the histone tail lysines to form a *histone code* that regulates other chromatin functions.[45]

Different cell lineages can express overlapping sets of transcription factors, potentially causing an expression of genes inappropriate for the function of different cell types. Histone modifications such as acetylation and deacetylation serve, in part, to facilitate appropriate gene responses and suppress inappropriate gene expression by permitting or preventing transcription-factor binding. However, this system is sensitive to the environment. Maintaining chromatin structure involves a dynamic balance in the activities of histone acetyltransferases (HATs), which add acetyls to histones, and histone deacetylases (HDACs), which remove them (see Figure 39-2), as well as the availability of acetyl groups, provided by acetyl-coenzyme A (acetyl-CoA). This process is potentially unstable because acetylation reactions are susceptible to environmental agents that affect the levels and activity of the HATs and HDACs, as well as intracellular acetyl-CoA levels, affecting gene expression. In higher eukaryotes and in particular vertebrates, chromatin is further stabilized in a condensed, transcriptionally silent configuration by DNA methylation.

DNA Methylation

DNA methylation refers to methylation of carbon 5 in cytosines to form deoxymethylcytosine (d^mC). Methylated cytosines are found in mammals almost exclusively in cytosine-guanine (CpG) pairs. Methylcytosine-binding proteins such as MeCP2, MBD1, MBD2, and MBD3 bind d^mC and tether HDAC-containing chromatin inactivation complexes to the methylated sequences, stabilizing the adjacent chromatin in a transcriptionally silent structure.[46] The carbon-carbon bond between the methyl group and the deoxycytosine (dC) base is strong and resistant to enzymatic cleavage, providing a stable repressive mark on the DNA. The role of DNA methylation in silencing gene expression is also shown in Figure 39-2.

DNA methylation patterns are established during development by the *de novo* DNA methyltransferase 3a (Dnmt3a) and DNA methyltransferase 3b (Dnmt3b) and then replicated each time a cell divides by DNA methyltransferase 1 (Dnmt1), the *maintenance* methyltransferase. As cells enter mitosis, signals transmitted through the extracellular-regulated protein kinase (ERK) and jun-N-terminal kinase (JNK) pathways upregulate Dnmt1, which binds the replication fork in the dividing cells and reads CpG pairs. If a dC in the parent DNA strand is methylated, then Dnmt1 catalyzes transfer of the methyl group from *S*-adenosylmethionine (SAM) to the corresponding dC in the daughter strand, replicating the methylation pattern and producing SAM[47] (Figure 39-3). This step is crucial, because if DNA methylation is inhibited, either by preventing Dnmt1 upregulation or by interfering with the transmethylation reaction, then the methylation patterns will not be replicated in the daughter cell. Consequently, genes that are normally silent can become demethylated and expressed. Further, since the changes are heritable, the errors will be replicated during subsequent cell divisions and will accumulate over time and, hence, with aging. Thus DNA methylation and, consequently, gene expression become sensitive to the environment at this point. *Therefore drugs or chemicals that interfere with Dnmt1 levels or enzymatic activity and dietary or metabolic abnormalities that decrease SAM or increase S-adenosylhomocysteine (SAH) levels can inhibit DNA methylation, activating gene expression in a stable, heritable fashion; these errors will accumulate with age.*[48]

Table 39-2 lists some of the recognized DNA demethylating agents and their mechanisms of action. These agents may affect gene expression in a wide variety of cells. However, T cells are particularly dependent on DNA methylation to regulate gene expression, and T cell DNA demethylation can contribute to lupus-like autoimmunity.

T Cells, DNA Methylation, and Drug-Induced Lupus

DNA methylation plays a critical role in regulating T lymphocyte effector and other functions. CD4+ T cells differentiate throughout

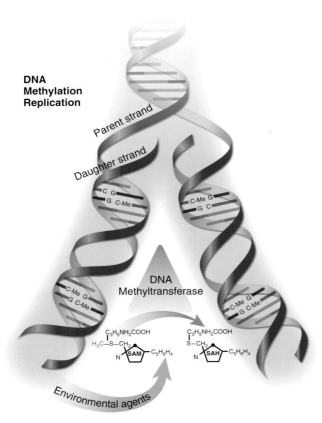

DNA
Methylation
Replication

Parent strand

Daughter strand

DNA
Methyltransferase

Environmental agents

FIGURE 39-3 Replication of DNA-methylation patterns. DNA-methylation patterns are replicated during mitosis by Dnmt1, which binds the replication fork and *reads* CpG pairs. If a deoxycytosine (dC) base in the parent strand is methylated (C-Me), then Dnmt1 catalyzes transfer of the methyl group from *S*-adenosylmethionine (SAM) to the corresponding dC in the daughter strand, replicating the methylation pattern and producing *S*-adenosylhomocysteine (SAH).[47] This chemical reaction is susceptible to environmental agents such as procainamide, hydralazine, dietary abnormalities that affect SAM and SAH levels, and others.

TABLE 39-2 Exogenous Agents and Proposed Mechanisms

DRUG	MECHANISM	REFERENCES
Hydralazine	ERK pathway inhibitor	67
Procainamide	Dnmt1 inhibitor	115
Ultraviolet light	ERK pathway inhibitor	72,116
Aging	ERK/JNK pathway inhibitor	116
Diet	Modifies transmethylation reactions	117

Dnmt1, DNA methyltransferase 1; ERK, extracellular-regulated protein kinase; JNK, jun-N-terminal kinase.

life into multiple subsets, such as naive to memory, and T-helper 0 (Th0) to Th1, Th2, Th17, and T-regulator (Treg) cells. Although differentiation into these subsets is regulated by key transcription factors such as GATA-3 for Th2, T-bet for Th1, and FoxP3 for Treg, expression of many of the effector molecules, and therefore effector functions specific to these subsets, is regulated by a set of transcription factors that are expressed in more than one subset, potentially leading to inappropriate gene expression and cellular functions. Effector and other genes inappropriate for each subset are silenced by a repressive chromatin structure, stabilized by methylation of CpGs in their regulatory elements. Since DNA methylation patterns must be replicated

each time T cells divide, interfering with DNA methylation during mitosis will induce expression of those genes normally suppressed by DNA methylation but for which the transcription factors are present. For example, treating dividing T cells with the irreversible Dnmt1 inhibitor 5-azacytidine (5-azaC) induces interferon-gamma (IFN-γ) in Th2 cells, interleukin 4 (IL-4) in Th1 cells, perforin in CD4+ T cells, FoxP3 in CD4+CD25− T cells, and killer-cell immunoglobulin-like receptors in CD4+ and CD8+ T cells.[49,50]

Inhibiting DNA methylation in CD4+ T cells also makes them autoreactive. CD4+ T cells normally recognize antigenic foreign peptides presented by self-class II MHC molecules on antigen-presenting cells (APC). Early studies demonstrate that DNA methylation inhibitors convert normal, antigen-specific CD4+ T cells into autoreactive cells that respond specifically to self class II MHC molecules on APC without the appropriate peptide in the antigen-binding cleft.[51] The autoreactivity is caused by an overexpression of the adhesion molecule lymphocyte-function–associated antigen 1 (LFA-1) (CD11a/CD18). LFA-1 normally binds intercellular adhesion molecule 1 (ICAM-1) on APC and surrounds the T-cell receptor–MHC complex, forming the *immunologic synapse*. This binding stabilizes the T cell receptor–MHC interaction and provides additional co-stimulatory signals that result in T-cell activation when the T-cell receptor recognizes both the antigenic peptide and the MHC determinants. Treating CD4+ T cells with DNA methylation inhibitors, such as 5-azaC, increases LFA-1 expression. This allows the T cells to respond to the lower affinity interaction between the T-cell receptor and self-class II MHC molecules without the appropriate antigen, making the T cells autoreactive. Identical autoreactivity develops when T cells are transfected with LFA-1.[52] Thus causing LFA-1 overexpression by treating with DNA methylation inhibitors or transfection is sufficient to break tolerance and cause MHC-specific T-cell autoreactivity.

Functionally, the autoreactive T cells recognize and respond to the self-class II MHC molecules on B cells, overstimulating antibody production through effects on both cell surface co-stimulatory molecules, as well as by secreting stimulatory cytokines similar to IFN-γ.[53,54] The autoreactive T cells also respond to the self-class II MHC molecules on macrophages, but they kill them by inducing apoptosis, causing the release of apoptotic chromatin from the dying macrophages.[55] Importantly, apoptotic chromatin is antigenic. Genetic deletion of any of the molecules involved in clearing apoptotic material causes lupus-like autoantibodies to nuclear antigens, including chromatin and DNA, as does overwhelming the clearance mechanisms by injecting apoptotic cells.[56,57] Further, since macrophages are responsible for removing and degrading apoptotic chromatin, macrophage apoptosis will prevent clearance of the apoptotic debris left behind, augmenting autoantibody responses. The importance of macrophage apoptosis in autoimmunity was confirmed by experiments demonstrating that clodronate liposomes, which selectively deplete macrophages by apoptosis in vivo, cause lupus-like autoantibodies when injected into normal mice and accelerate nephritis in lupus-prone mice.[58] Thus T cells made autoreactive by DNA methylation inhibition can generate both a source of antigenic chromatin by stimulating macrophage apoptosis, as well as overstimulating B cell responses to the nuclear antigens, contributing to the development of lupus-like autoimmunity.

The pathologic relevance of demethylated, autoreactive CD4+ T cells was first demonstrated in experiments during which murine CD4+ T cells were made autoreactive by treatment with the DNA methylation inhibitor 5-azaC and then injected into genetically identical mice. The modified cells caused anti-DNA antibodies and an immune complex glomerulonephritis.[59] More recent studies used a transgenic mouse model to confirm that inducing T cell DNA demethylation in vivo causes lupus-like autoimmunity.[60]

The observation that CD4+ T cells treated with a DNA methylation inhibitor cause lupus-like autoimmunity prompted studies testing whether drugs that cause lupus-like autoimmunity are DNA-methylation inhibitors. Procainamide and hydralazine, the two drugs causing DIL most often (see Table 39-1), were found to be

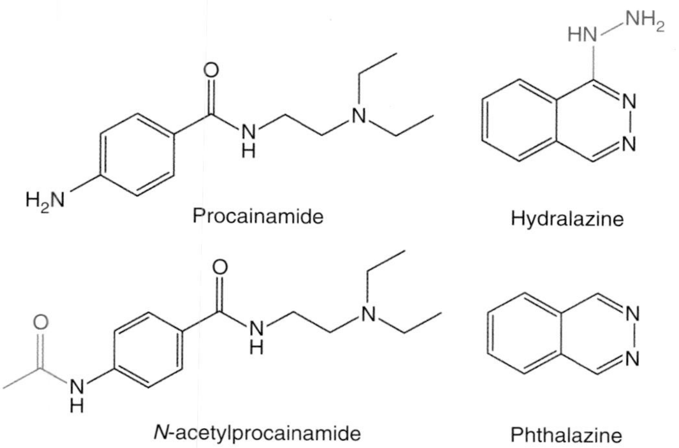

FIGURE 39-4 **Structures of lupus-inducing DNA methylation inhibitors and inactive derivatives.** Procainamide is a competitive Dnmt1 inhibitor and causes DIL. In contrast, N-acetylprocainamide is a poor inhibitor of Dnmt1 and does not induce DIL. Hydralazine also inhibits DNA methylation, whereas phthalazine does not. Structural differences are shown in *red*.

DNA-methylation inhibitors, and treating CD4+ T cells with procainamide or hydralazine caused an LFA-1 overexpression and made CD4+ T cells autoreactive like 5-azaC. Procainamide was found to inhibit Dnmt1 enzymatic activity,[61] whereas hydralazine was found to prevent Dnmt1 upregulation during mitosis by inhibiting ERK pathway signaling.[62] Interestingly, N-acetylprocainamide, the acetylated metabolite of procainamide (Figure 39-4), does not cause DIL flares in patients with previous procainamide-induced lupus,[63] is less potent in causing T-cell LFA-1 overexpression and autoreactivity in vitro, and has a reduced ability to cause autoimmunity in animal models.[64] Other structure-function studies have compared hydralazine with phthalazine. Hydralazine is a phthalazine derivative with a hydrazine side chain (see Figure 39-4), and phthalazine is less potent than hydralazine in causing T-cell LFA-1 overexpression and autoreactivity and has reduced the ability to cause autoimmunity in animal models, suggesting that the hydrazine side chain may play a role.[64]

Whether the other drugs listed in Table 39-1 also affect DNA methylation is unknown, although isoniazid also has a hydrazine side chain (see Figure 39-1). It is unclear whether the effects of DNA methylation inhibitors on cells other than T lymphocytes also contribute to DIL. Nonetheless, the adoptive transfer and transgenic mouse models demonstrate that T-cell DNA demethylation alone, caused by procainamide, hydralazine, or in a transgenic model, is sufficient to cause lupus-like autoimmunity.

T Cells, DNA Methylation, and Idiopathic Lupus

The relationship between T-cell DNA demethylation and DIL suggests that T-cell DNA demethylation might also contribute to idiopathic lupus in humans. The first report examining DNA methylation in autoimmunity used high-pressure liquid chromatography (HPLC) to compare methylcytosine content in T-cell DNA from patients with lupus and rheumatoid arthritis with control participants. This study demonstrated lower DNA methylation levels in lupus and rheumatoid arthritis T cells, relative to T cells from healthy age-matched control participants; it also demonstrated that patients with active lupus had lower DNA methylation levels than patients with inactive lupus.[65] The DNA demethylation was traced to low Dnmt1 levels in patients with lupus, caused by decreased ERK pathway signaling.[66] Subsequent studies traced the ERK pathway signaling defect to protein kinase C delta (PKCδ), which is also inhibited by hydralazine, suggesting a common mechanism between idiopathic and hydralazine-induced lupus.[67] Interestingly, PKCδ-deficient mice developed lupus.[68] The significance of T-cell DNA demethylation in

rheumatoid arthritis is unclear, but it may reflect different sequences affected or a lack of lupus-predisposing genes or both.

Other studies demonstrated that CD4+ T cells from patients with active lupus also overexpress LFA-1, similar to experimentally demethylated T cells; that the LFA-1–overexpressing T cells from patients with lupus kill autologous macrophages by apoptosis, similar to experimentally demethylated T cells[55]; and that patients with active but not inactive lupus have circulating apoptotic monocytes,[69] suggesting similar autoreactive monocyte or macrophage killing in vivo. Overexpression of other genes normally suppressed by DNA methylation in CD4+ T cells, including perforin, CD40L on the inactive X in women, and the killer cell immunoglobulin-like receptor (KIR) gene family were also found to be overexpressed on experimentally demethylated CD4+ T cells and CD4+ T cells from patients with active lupus, all the result of demethylation of the same DNA regulatory sequences in lupus as in the in vitro models.[49,70,71] Similarly, procainamide, hydralazine, and 5-azacytidine caused overexpression of the B-cell co-stimulatory molecule CD70 on CD4+ T cells by demethylating a region just upstream of the transcription start site, and CD4+ T cells from patients with lupus have identical DNA demethylation and overexpression of CD70.[72] Recent high-throughput sequencing studies demonstrate demethylation of other sequences as well.[73] Together, these studies strongly suggest that demethylation of critical regulatory elements in CD4+ T cells contribute to the development of lupus in animal models and people and that drugs that inhibit DNA methylation, such as procainamide and hydralazine, can induce autoimmunity by the same mechanism.

T Cells, DNA Methylation, and the Environment

The procainamide and hydralazine studies prompted experiments investigating mechanisms that cause T-cell DNA demethylation in idiopathic lupus. Sun exposure triggers lupus flares, and UV light was found to inhibit the T-cell ERK signaling pathway such as hydralazine to cause similar T-cell DNA demethylation, LFA-1 overexpression, and autoreactivity.[74] Since UV light causes oxidative stress,[75] this report suggests a mechanism by which UV light and perhaps other agents that trigger oxidative stress, such as infections, silica, and smoking, may activate systemic lupus erythematosus (SLE) in genetically predisposed people.[25-28]

T-cell DNA also demethylates with age[76] as a result, in part, of decreased ERK pathway signaling causing lower Dnmt1 levels,[77] as well as the accumulation of DNA methylation errors caused by environmental or drug exposures that are then replicated during subsequent mitoses. As previously noted, the incidence of lupus increases in men up to 75 years of age and in women up to menopause, suggesting an aging component.[33] Aging, therefore, possibly contributes to the development of idiopathic lupus through cumulative effects on DNA methylation. Further, replication of DNA methylation patterns during mitosis depends not only on Dnmt1 levels, but also on intracellular pools of the methyl donor SAM and is inhibited by SAH.[77] A recent study demonstrates that age-dependent decreases in Dnmt1 sensitize the replication of T-cell DNA methylation patterns to low SAM or increased SAH levels, causing aberrant expression of genes such as perforin and the KIR gene family on CD4+ T cells from older but not younger people.[77] This conclusion suggests that diet and environmental exposure to some lupus-inducing drugs, UV light, and agents causing oxidative stress such as silica, infections, smoking, and others may combine to demethylate DNA and trigger lupus flares in genetically predisposed people and that these methylation defects can accumulate with age.

Finally, studies performed in identical twins also support a role for age, DNA methylation, and the environment in lupus. The first study compared T-cell DNA methylation in identical twins at ages 3 and 50 years and found highly similar DNA methylation patterns at 3 years of age but a significant disparity in patterns at age 50 years. Interestingly, the methylation patterns differed more if the twins spent less of their lifetime together or had a more different natural health–medical history, or both.[78] The second study compared DNA methylation in identical twins discordant for lupus. This study found that the twin with more demethylated leukocyte DNA had lupus.[79] Since these studies were performed in genetically identical people, they strongly support an environmental component to the DNA demethylation, as well as the importance of DNA demethylation in the development of lupus.

Recombinant Biologic Agents
Interferon-Alpha
IFN-α is an important cytokine in immune responses and is used in the treatment of diseases including viral hepatitis, malignancies such as chronic myelogenous leukemia, non-Hodgkin lymphoma, Kaposi sarcoma, and even some autoimmune diseases.[2] However, as previously noted and in Table 39-1, IFN-α stimulates ANAs in 18% to 72% of people receiving this drug, and DIL develops in 0.1% to 2.1% of these individuals, again suggesting a genetic requirement for full disease development. The ability of this cytokine to cause DIL is interesting and relevant because IFN-α participates in the pathogenesis of idiopathic lupus and may contribute to the development of autoimmunity through similar mechanisms when used to treat other diseases. Evidence supporting a role for IFN-α in idiopathic lupus comes from array studies demonstrating an "interferon signature" in the peripheral blood leukocytes of patients with lupus, as well as studies demonstrating the stimulatory effects of IFN-α on dendritic cell maturation, Treg suppression, and B cell stimulation.[80] IFN-α also stimulates IFN-γ production, and IFN-γ can act as an adjuvant.[25] Interestingly, some lupus-associated genetic variations, such as interferon-regulatory factors 5 (IRF5) and 7 (IRF7), may increase IFN-α levels,[80] suggesting a mechanism by which these alleles may contribute to lupus pathogenesis.

Tumor Necrosis Factor Inhibitors
TNF is a cytokine that induces inflammation and apoptotic cell death, and TNF inhibitors are currently used in the treatment of inflammatory diseases including rheumatoid arthritis, ankylosing spondylitis, psoriatic arthritis, psoriasis, and inflammatory bowel disease. However, the TNF inhibitors frequently cause ANAs in patients receiving them but rarely autoimmune diseases. Infliximab causes a positive ANA in 23% to 53% of patients, but DIL in 0.19%; adalimumab causes a positive ANA in 12.5% to 41.4%, but DIL in 0.41%; and etanercept causes a positive ANA in 11% to 48.8%, but DIL in 0.18%.[81] Interestingly, autoimmune thyroid disease develops more frequently (1.8% to 13.1%) than DIL.[2]

The mechanisms by which TNF inhibitors initiate autoimmunity are unclear. TNF antagonists may induce autoantibodies in part by suppressing C-reactive protein (CRP), which participates in the clearance of apoptotic debris,[82] and, as previously discussed, apoptotic debris can simulate antichromatin and anti-DNA antibodies. These agents can also induce monocyte or macrophage apoptosis, potentially leading to antichromatin antibodies by mechanisms similar to those caused by autoreactive T cells in idiopathic SLE.[58]

Finally, TNF can suppress IFN-α production; consequently, TNF inhibitors may increase IFN-α levels,[83] which can also induce lupus-like autoimmunity as previously discussed.

Summary
Multiple factors likely influence the development of DIL and include the sex, age, and genetic predisposition of people receiving the drugs, as well as the structure of the inciting drug and the rate of metabolism as determined by acetylator status. The two drugs most commonly causing DIL, procainamide and hydralazine, appear to trigger lupus in genetically predisposed people at least in part by inhibiting CD4+ T-cell DNA methylation, causing aberrant expression of genes that convert normal helper T cells into autoreactive, cytotoxic proinflammatory T cells, and a similar mechanism contributes to the development of idiopathic lupus. How the other drugs listed in Table 39-1 induce lupus, though, is unclear. Hormonal supplementation can also contribute to the development of lupus, likely through the same mechanisms by which endogenous estrogens contribute to autoimmunity in women. The TNF antagonists and IFN-α also likely induce autoimmunity through immunologic pathways, although the precise mechanisms are incompletely understood.

CLINICAL ASPECTS
DIL and idiopathic lupus have differences and similarities in patient characteristics, symptoms, and autoantibody patterns. Moreover, these features also differ in idiopathic lupus depending on the age of onset. Since older people receive drugs causing DIL more often than younger individuals, age needs to be considered when comparing the clinical manifestations between idiopathic lupus and DIL. Clinical manifestations of idiopathic lupus in younger individuals, older individuals, and DIL are compared in the following text and in Table 39-3.

Idiopathic Lupus in Younger versus Older Adults
Patient Characteristics
Late-onset lupus has been defined as lupus with age of onset after 50 years and accounts for approximately 12% to 18% of all individuals with lupus.[84-86] Similar to early-onset lupus, late-onset lupus also appears to predominantly affect women. However, the female predominance in older individuals is not as strong as the 9:1 ratio observed in early-onset lupus.[87] In the 13 series reviewed by Lazaro,[88] the female-to-male ratio varied between 18:1 and 2.6:1, and one report found a male predominance with a 4:1 male-to-female ratio.[89] However, the most commonly reported ratio was 5:1 female-to-male.

Clinical and Serologic Features
In contrast to early-onset lupus, patients with late-onset lupus tend to develop arthritis, fevers, serositis, photosensitivity, sicca symptoms, Raynaud phenomenon, lung disease, and neuropsychiatric symptoms more often, whereas malar rash, oral ulcers, discoid

---

TABLE 39-3 Most Common Features of Lupus in Younger and Older Adults, and of Drug-Induced Lupus

GROUP	YOUNGER ONSET (≤50)	OLDER ONSET (>50)	DRUG INDUCED
Gender	Predominantly female (9:1)	Predominantly female but less biased than early onset	Reflects population taking the medication
Symptoms	Malar rash, discoid lesions, oral ulcers, nephritis, CNS involvement	Arthritis, fevers, serositis, photosensitivity, sicca symptoms, Raynaud phenomenon, neuropsychiatric	Arthralgias, myalgias, fevers, serositis, rashes
Laboratory abnormalities	Proteinuria, cytopenias, low complement levels	Normal complement	Normal complement
Autoantibodies	ANA, anti-dsDNA, antihistones, anti-Smith anti-RNP	ANA, variable anti-dsDNA,* anti-SSA/Ro, anti-SSB/La, rheumatoid factor	ANA, antihistone

ANA, antinuclear antibodies; CNS, central nervous system; dsDNA, double-stranded DNA; RNP, ribonucleoprotein.
*Variable anti-dsDNA reflects the fact that different studies show anti-dsDNA antibodies are observed with higher, the same, or lower frequencies than lupus with an onset before age 50 years.

lesions, cytopenias, proteinuria, and nephritis occur less often.[24,84,90] As previously discussed, the differences between early- and late-onset lupus may reflect a lower total genetic risk in the older patients, as well as differences in exposure history and the effects of age.

Like early-onset lupus, late-onset lupus is characterized by a positive ANA. However, it must be kept in mind that ANA titers increase with age; as a result, a positive ANA alone is not specific for lupus.[34] In general, patients with late-onset lupus are also less likely to have anti-ribonucleoprotein (anti-RNP) antibodies, anti-Smith antibodies, or low complement levels.[24,84,90]

Whether anti-dsDNA antibodies are more or less prevalent in late-onset lupus is unclear; multiple small series show that anti-dsDNA antibodies can be found at higher, lower, or the same frequencies as in younger patients.[24,84,87,90] Similar to ANAs, anti-dsDNA antibodies also increase with age. Interestingly, the anti-dsDNA antibodies found in healthy older patients are generally of the IgA subclass and do not fix complement.[91] In general, antibodies to Sjögren syndrome antigen A (SSA/Ro) and Sjögren syndrome antigen B (SSB/La) are more common in late-onset lupus, as is the rheumatoid factor. In contrast, anti-Smith and anti-RNP antibodies are more commonly seen in early-onset lupus.[24,84,90]

Overall, late-onset lupus is considered to have a more benign course than lupus in younger patients.[92] Formiga compared Systemic Lupus Erythematosus Disease Activity Index (SLEDAI) scores during the first year of disease in older and younger patients, and a benign disease course was seen in 75% of late-onset cases but only 27% of the younger patients,[93] possibly reflecting fewer lupus genes in the older cohort.[23,24] Boddaert similarly found less severe disease in a cohort of 150 French patients, as well as in a metaanalysis involving 5400 patients.[87] In contrast, Lalani found increased disease activity in late-onset lupus, but moderate to severe renal disease was significantly greater in the early-onset group, whereas congestive heart failure and peptic ulcer disease were more common in the older group.[90]

Despite having a generally more benign course, late-onset lupus has a higher mortality than early-onset lupus. In one study, 10-year survival was 95% in young patients and 71% in patients with late-onset disease.[87] However, infection, malignancy, and cardiovascular disease are the most common causes of death in late-onset lupus, whereas flares of the disease more commonly cause death in younger patients.[87,90,94,95] Increased time to diagnosis in older patients could also contribute to the increased mortality. Font found that 3 years elapsed before lupus was diagnosed in patients under age 50 years, compared with 5 years in patients over age 50 years.[89] Mak also found that late-onset lupus was diagnosed more slowly than early-onset disease.[96]

Drug-Induced Lupus versus Idiopathic Lupus
Patient Characteristics

DIL has more characteristics in common with late-onset lupus than early-onset lupus, perhaps consistent with DNA demethylation in older people. Up to 10% of cases of SLE are drug induced, and an estimated 15,000 to 30,000 cases of DIL occur in the United States every year.[97,98] No standard criteria exist for DIL. The standard 4 out of 11 diagnostic criteria for idiopathic lupus are not always met in patients with DIL. Some consider one symptom and one lupus-associated autoantibody sufficient. The diagnosis of DIL is usually based on a clinical picture consistent with lupus and the history of the disease demonstrating a causal relationship with the suspect drug.[99]

There are three forms of DIL. The systemic form of DIL, affecting multiple organs, is extensively discussed in the following text. The subacute cutaneous form of DIL is more common in women, and its presentation is generally with an ANA and antibodies to histones, SSA/Ro, and SSB/La. Considerable debate has been waged regarding whether drug-induced subacute cutaneous lupus differs from the idiopathic form.[100,101]

As previously noted, DIL has a male-to-female ratio that mirrors that of the population receiving the drug in question, and more men

than women take drugs such as procainamide; consequently, lupus secondary to procainamide occurs more frequently in men compared with women. DIL also occurs more frequently in older patients. Again, this reality can be attributed at least in part to the fact that older patients take more of the drugs that can cause lupus, compared with younger patients.

Clinical Features

The clinical features of DIL are similar to those of late-onset lupus. In general, arthralgias, myalgias, fevers, and serositis are more common in DIL. In contrast, renal involvement, central nervous system disease, malar rash, discoid rash, photosensitivity, and oral ulcers occur less frequently in DIL.[1,102]

In the specific case of hydralazine-induced lupus, leukopenia, neuropsychiatric symptoms, pericarditis, skin vasculitis, and renal involvement are also less likely to occur than in idiopathic lupus. Patients with hydralazine DIL are also more likely to be older and male, compared with patients with idiopathic lupus.[1,103] In procainamide-induced lupus, arthralgias, myalgias, constitutional symptoms, and serositis are the most common symptoms,[104] also as in late-onset disease.

Lupus induced by TNF inhibitors is most commonly characterized by a rash. Williams recently reported lupus secondary to etanercept in a 62-year-old woman with rheumatoid arthritis. It resolved with the discontinuation of the medication and did not recur after golimumab was started for the 6-month period reported.[105] In contrast, Subramanian reported 13 patients with inflammatory bowel disease who developed lupus induced by infliximab. Eight patients were switched to either certolizumab or adalimumab. Six patients remained asymptomatic, but one patient each with certolizumab or adalimumab developed DIL again.[106]

Speculating that the different manifestations of lupus induced by specific drugs could be explained by drug-specific genetic polymorphisms or other drug-specific abnormalities is tempting. Unfortunately, as previously noted, no reports attempt to link clinical manifestations unique to a specific drug with genetic or epigenetic abnormalities.

Autoantibodies

DIL is characterized by a positive ANA, similar to idiopathic lupus and aging. The ANA in DIL tends to have a homogeneous pattern, although a speckled pattern may also be seen.[107] Antihistone antibodies are found in 75% of patients with DIL. However, antihistone antibodies are also found in 75% of patients with idiopathic lupus; therefore it is not a specific test.[108] Notably, antihistone antibodies may persist even after the offending drug has been stopped and the symptoms have resolved. The antihistone antibodies in idiopathic lupus are primarily detected against the H1 and H2B subunits. In contrast, the antihistone antibodies found in most patients with DIL are directed against the H2A and H2B subunits. In the case of hydralazine, the antihistone antibodies are directed against H1 and H3-H4 complex.[109-112]

Antibodies to single-stranded DNA (ssDNA) are similarly not specific for DIL. In contrast, antibodies to double-stranded DNA (dsDNA) are found in approximately one half of patients with idiopathic lupus but in less than 5% of patients with DIL.[1,113] Finally, DIL also tends to be characterized by normal complement levels. However, a recent review reported a more frequent occurrence of elevated anti-dsDNA titers and low complement levels in anti-TNFα–related DIL as compared with non-TNF–related DIL.[114]

SUMMARY

Current evidence indicates that some drugs and certain environmental agents such as UV light, silica, and others can inhibit T-cell DNA methylation, thereby altering gene expression. These epigenetic alterations are heritable and can accumulate over time, resulting in modifications of T-cell function that cause changes varying from a positive ANA test in asymptomatic individuals to formally diagnosable lupus with a wide range of severity. Which situation develops depends at least in part on the number and relative risk of lupus genes in any given individual. Although great strides have been recently made in identifying lupus susceptibility genes and quantifying their relative risk associations, much work still needs to be done to identify completely the genetic and epigenetic changes that increase susceptibility to lupus development. Ultimately, identifying environmental causes of DNA demethylation and measuring the total lupus genetic risk for any given individual may suggest ways to delay onset or even prevent lupus.

References

1. Yung RL, Richardson BC: Drug-induced lupus. *Rheum Dis Clin North Am* 20:61–86, 1994.
2. Gota C, Calabrese L: Induction of clinical autoimmune disease by therapeutic interferon-alpha. *Autoimmunity* 36:511–518, 2003.
3. Niewold TB, Clark DN, Salloum R, et al: Interferon alpha in systemic lupus erythematosus. *J Biomed Biotechnol* ePub 2010:948364, 2010.
4. Reinhardt DJ, Waldron JM: Lupus erythematosus-like syndrome complicating hydralazine (apresoline) therapy. *J Am Med Assoc* 155:1491–1492, 1954.
5. Prockop LD: Myotonia, procaine amide, and lupus-like syndrome. *Arch Neurol* 14:326–330, 1966.
6. Zingale SB, Minzer L, Rosenberg B, et al: Drug induced lupus-like syndrome. Clinical and laboratory syndrome similar to systemic lupus erythematosus following antituberculous therapy: report of a case. *Arch Intern Med* 112:63–66, 1963.
7. Dubois EL, Tallman E, Wonka RA: Chlorpromazine-induced systemic lupus erythematosus: case report and review of the literature. *JAMA* 221:595–596, 1972.
8. Cohen MG, Kevat S, Prowse MV, et al: Two distinct quinidine-induced rheumatic syndromes. *Ann Intern Med* 108:369–371, 1988.
9. Gordon MM, Porter D: Minocycline induced lupus: case series in the West of Scotland. *J Rheumatol* 28:1004–1006, 2001.
10. Blomgren SE, Condemi JJ, Bignall MC, et al: Antinuclear antibody induced by procainamide. A prospective study. *N Engl J Med* 281:64–66, 1969.
11. Condemi JJ, Moore-Jones D, Vaughan JH, et al: Antinuclear antibodies following hydralazine toxicity. *N Engl J Med* 276:486–491, 1967.
12. Rothfield NF, Bierer WF, Garfield JW: Isoniazid induction of antinuclear antibodies. A prospective study. *Ann Intern Med* 88:650–652, 1978.
13. Mackay IR, Cowling DC, Hurley TH: Drug-induced autoimmune disease: haemolytic aneamia and lupus cells after treatment with methyldopa. *Med J Aust* 2:1047–1050, 1968.
14. Cotzias GC, Papavasiliou PS: Autoimmunity in Patients Treated With Levodopa. *JAMA* 207:1353–1354, 1969.
15. Tarzy BJ, Garcia CR, Wallach EE, et al: Rheumatic disease, abnormal serology, and oral contraceptives. *Lancet* 2:501–503, 1972.
16. Schoonen WM, Thomas SL, Somers EC, et al: Do selected drugs increase the risk of lupus? A matched case-control study. *Br J Clin Pharmacol* 70:588–596, 2010.
17. Bernier MO, Mikaeloff Y, Hudson M, et al: Combined oral contraceptive use and the risk of systemic lupus erythematosus. *Arthritis Rheum* 61:476–481, 2009.
18. Rubin RL, Nusinow SR, Johnson AD, et al: Serologic changes during induction of lupus-like disease by procainamide. *Am J Med* 80:999–1002, 1986.
19. Cameron HA, Ramsay LE: The lupus syndrome induced by hydralazine: a common complication with low dose treatment. *Br Med J (Clin Res Ed)* 289:410–412, 1984.
20. Walker S: The importance of sex hormones in systemic lupus erythematosus. In: Wallace DaHB, editor: *Dubois' lupus erythematosus*. Philadelphia, 2007, Lippincott Williams & Wilkins, p 278.
21. Buyon JP, Petri MA, Kim MY, et al: The effect of combined estrogen and progesterone hormone replacement therapy on disease activity in systemic lupus erythematosus: a randomized trial. *Ann Intern Med* 142:953–962, 2005.
22. Haraoui B, Keystone E: Musculoskeletal manifestations and autoimmune diseases related to new biologic agents. *Curr Opin Rheumatol* 18:96–100, 2006.
23. Taylor KE, Chung SA, Graham RR, et al: Risk alleles for systemic lupus erythematosus in a large case-control collection and associations with clinical subphenotypes. *PLoS Genet* 7:e1001311, 2011.
24. Webb R, Kelly JA, Somers EC, et al: Early disease onset is predicted by a higher genetic risk for lupus and is associated with a more severe phenotype in lupus patients. *Ann Rheum Dis* 70:151–156, 2011.
25. Cooper GS, Gilbert KM, Greidinger EL, et al: Recent advances and opportunities in research on lupus: environmental influences and mechanisms of disease. *Environ Health Perspect* 116:695–702, 2008.
26. Parks CG, Walitt BT, Pettinger M, et al: Insecticide use and risk of rheumatoid arthritis and systemic lupus erythematosus in the Women's Health Initiative Observational Study. *Arthritis Care Res (Hoboken)* 63:184–194, 2011.
27. Parks CG, Cooper GS, Nylander-French LA, et al: Occupational exposure to crystalline silica and risk of systemic lupus erythematosus: a population-based, case-control study in the southeastern United States. *Arthritis Rheum* 46:1840–1850, 2002.
28. Harel-Meir M, Sherer Y, Shoenfeld Y: Tobacco smoking and autoimmune rheumatic diseases. *Nat Clin Pract Rheumatol* 3:707–715, 2007.
29. Flesher DL, Sun X, Behrens TW, et al: Recent advances in the genetics of systemic lupus erythematosus. *Expert Rev Clin Immunol* 6:461–479, 2010.
30. Batchelor JR, Welsh KI, Tinoco RM, et al: Hydralazine-induced systemic lupus erythematosus: influence of HLA-DR and sex on susceptibility. *Lancet* 1:1107–1109, 1980.
31. Brand C, Davidson A, Littlejohn G, et al: Hydralazine-induced lupus: no association with HLA-DR4. *Lancet* 1:462, 1984.
32. Cooper GS, Treadwell EL, Dooley MA, et al: *N*-acetyl transferase genotypes in relation to risk of developing systemic lupus erythematosus. *J Rheumatol* 31:76–80, 2004.
33. Somers EC, Thomas SL, Smeeth L, et al: Incidence of systemic lupus erythematosus in the United Kingdom, 1990–1999. *Arthritis Rheum* 57:612–618, 2007.
34. Nilsson BO, Skogh T, Ernerudh J, et al: Antinuclear antibodies in the oldest-old women and men. *J Autoimmun* 27:281–288, 2006.
35. Arbuckle MR, McClain MT, Rubertone MV, et al: Development of autoantibodies before the clinical onset of systemic lupus erythematosus. *N Engl J Med* 349:1526–1533, 2003.
36. Singsen BH, Fishman L, Hanson V: Antinuclear antibodies and lupus-like syndromes in children receiving anticonvulsants. *Pediatrics* 57:529–534, 1976.
37. Schlienger RG, Bircher AJ, Meier CR: Minocycline-induced lupus. A systematic review. *Dermatology* 200:223–231, 2000.
38. Yokoyama T, Usui T, Kiyama K, et al: Two cases of late-onset drug-induced lupus erythematosus caused by ticlopidine in elderly men. *Mod Rheumatol* 20:405–409, 2010.
39. McLean AJ, Le Couteur DG: Aging biology and geriatric clinical pharmacology. *Pharmacol Rev* 56:163–184, 2004.
40. Uetrecht JP, Woosley RL: Acetylator phenotype and lupus erythematosus. *Clin Pharmacokinet* 6:118–134, 1981.
41. Scofield RH, Bruner GR, Namjou B, et al: Klinefelter's syndrome (47,XXY) in male systemic lupus erythematosus patients: support for the notion of a gene-dose effect from the X chromosome. *Arthritis Rheum* 58:2511–2517, 2008.
42. Beernink DH, Miller JJ, 3rd: Anticonvulsant-induced antinuclear antibodies and lupus-like disease in children. *J Pediatr* 82:113–117, 1973.
43. Rao T, Richardson B: Environmentally induced autoimmune diseases: potential mechanisms. *Environ Health Perspect* 107(Suppl 5):737–742, 1999.
44. Bonasio R, Tu S, Reinberg D: Molecular signals of epigenetic states. *Science* 330:612–616, 2010.
45. Berger SL: The complex language of chromatin regulation during transcription. *Nature* 447:407–412, 2007.
46. Bird AP, Wolffe AP: Methylation-induced repression—belts, braces, and chromatin. *Cell* 99:451–454, 1999.
47. Tung JW, Heydari K, Tirouvanziam R, et al: Modern flow cytometry: a practical approach. *Clin Lab Med* 27:453–468, v, 2007.
48. Richardson BC: Role of DNA methylation in the regulation of cell function: autoimmunity, aging and cancer. *J Nutr* 132:2401S–2405S, 2002.
49. Basu D, Liu Y, Wu A, et al: Stimulatory and inhibitory killer Ig-like receptor molecules are expressed and functional on lupus T cells. *J Immunol* 183:3481–3487, 2009.
50. Sawalha AH: Epigenetics and T-cell immunity. *Autoimmunity* 41:245–252, 2008.
51. Richardson B: Effect of an inhibitor of DNA methylation on T cells. II. 5-Azacytidine induces self-reactivity in antigen-specific T4+ cells. *Hum Immunol* 17:456–470, 1986.
52. Yung R, Powers D, Johnson K, et al: Mechanisms of drug-induced lupus. II. T cells overexpressing lymphocyte function-associated antigen 1 become autoreactive and cause a lupuslike disease in syngeneic mice. *J Clin Invest* 97:2866–2871, 1996.

53. Richardson BC, Liebling MR, Hudson JL: CD4+ cells treated with DNA methylation inhibitors induce autologous B cell differentiation. *Clin Immunol Immunopathol* 55:368–381, 1990.

54. Oelke K, Lu Q, Richardson D, et al: Overexpression of CD70 and overstimulation of IgG synthesis by lupus T cells and T cells treated with DNA methylation inhibitors. *Arthritis Rheum* 50:1850–1860, 2004.

55. Richardson BC, Strahler JR, Pivirotto TS, et al: Phenotypic and functional similarities between 5-azacytidine-treated T cells and a T cell subset in patients with active systemic lupus erythematosus. *Arthritis Rheum* 35:647–662, 1992.

56. Mevorach D, Zhou JL, Song X, et al: Systemic exposure to irradiated apoptotic cells induces autoantibody production. *J Exp Med* 188:387–392, 1998.

57. Walport MJ: Lupus, DNase and defective disposal of cellular debris. *Nat Genet* 25:135–136, 2000.

58. Denny MF, Chandaroy P, Killen PD, et al: Accelerated macrophage apoptosis induces autoantibody formation and organ damage in systemic lupus erythematosus. *J Immunol* 176:2095–2104, 2006.

59. Quddus J, Johnson KJ, Gavalchin J, et al: Treating activated CD4+ T cells with either of two distinct DNA methyltransferase inhibitors, 5-azacytidine or procainamide, is sufficient to cause a lupus-like disease in syngeneic mice. *J Clin Invest* 92:38–53, 1993.

60. Sawalha AH, Jeffries M, Webb R, et al: Defective T-cell ERK signaling induces interferon-regulated gene expression and overexpression of methylation-sensitive genes similar to lupus patients. *Genes Immun* 9:368–378, 2008.

61. Scheinbart LS, Johnson MA, Gross LA, et al: Procainamide inhibits DNA methyltransferase in a human T cell line. *J Rheumatol* 18:530–534, 1991.

62. Deng C, Lu Q, Zhang Z, et al: Hydralazine may induce autoimmunity by inhibiting extracellular signal-regulated kinase pathway signaling. *Arthritis Rheum* 48:746–756, 2003.

63. Kluger J, Drayer DE, Reidenberg MM, et al: Acetylprocainamide therapy in patients with previous procainamide-induced lupus syndrome. *Ann Intern Med* 95:18–23, 1981.

64. Yung R, Chang S, Hemati N, et al: Mechanisms of drug-induced lupus. IV. Comparison of procainamide and hydralazine with analogs in vitro and in vivo. *Arthritis Rheum* 40:1436–1443, 1997.

65. Richardson B, Scheinbart L, Strahler J, et al: Evidence for impaired T cell DNA methylation in systemic lupus erythematosus and rheumatoid arthritis. *Arthritis Rheum* 33:1665–1673, 1990.

66. Deng C, Kaplan MJ, Yang J, et al: Decreased Ras-mitogen-activated protein kinase signaling may cause DNA hypomethylation in T lymphocytes from lupus patients. *Arthritis Rheum* 44:397–407, 2001.

67. Gorelik G, Fang JY, Wu A, et al: Impaired T cell protein kinase C delta activation decreases ERK pathway signaling in idiopathic and hydralazine-induced lupus. *J Immunol* 179:5553–5563, 2007.

68. Miyamoto A, Nakayama K, Imaki H, et al: Increased proliferation of B cells and auto-immunity in mice lacking protein kinase Cdelta. *Nature* 416:865–869, 2002.

69. Richardson BC, Yung RL, Johnson KJ, et al: Monocyte apoptosis in patients with active lupus. *Arthritis Rheum* 39:1432–1434, 1996.

70. Kaplan MJ, Lu Q, Wu A, et al: Demethylation of promoter regulatory elements contributes to perforin overexpression in CD4+ lupus T cells. *J Immunol* 172:3652–3661, 2004.

71. Lu Q, Wu A, Tesmer L, et al: Demethylation of CD40LG on the inactive X in T cells from women with lupus. *J Immunol* 179:6352–6358, 2007.

72. Richardson B: Primer: epigenetics of autoimmunity. *Nat Clin Pract Rheumatol* 3:521–527, 2007.

73. Jeffries M, Dozmorov M, Tang Y, et al: Genome-wide DNA methylation patterns in CD4+ T cells from patients with systemic lupus erythematosus. *Epigenetics* 6:593–601, 2011.

74. Richardson B, Powers D, Hooper F, et al: Lymphocyte function-associated antigen 1 overexpression and T cell autoreactivity. *Arthritis Rheum* 37:1363–1372, 1994.

75. Bergamini CM, Gambetti S, Dondi A, et al: Oxygen, reactive oxygen species and tissue damage. *Curr Pharm Des* 10:1611–1626, 2004.

76. Golbus J, Palella TD, Richardson BC: Quantitative changes in T cell DNA methylation occur during differentiation and ageing. *Eur J Immunol* 20:1869–1872, 1990.

77. Gonzalez AV, Li G, Suissa S, et al: Risk of glaucoma in elderly patients treated with inhaled corticosteroids for chronic airflow obstruction. *Pulm Pharmacol Ther* 23:65–70, 2010.

78. Fraga MF, Ballestar E, Paz MF, et al: Epigenetic differences arise during the lifetime of monozygotic twins. *Proc Natl Acad Sci U S A* 102:10604–10609, 2005.

79. Javierre BM, Fernandez AF, Richter J, et al: Changes in the pattern of DNA methylation associate with twin discordance in systemic lupus erythematosus. *Genome Res* 20:170–179, 2010.

80. Salloum R, Niewold TB: Interferon regulatory factors in human lupus pathogenesis. *Transl Res* 157:326–331, 2011.

81. Katz U, Zandman-Goddard G: Drug-induced lupus: an update. *Autoimmun Rev* 10:46–50, 2010.

82. Burlingame RW, Volzer MA, Harris J, et al: The effect of acute phase proteins on clearance of chromatin from the circulation of normal mice. *J Immunol* 156:4783–4788, 1996.

83. Palucka AK, Blanck JP, Bennett L, et al: Cross-regulation of TNF and IFN-alpha in autoimmune diseases. *Proc Natl Acad Sci U S A* 102:3372–3377, 2005.

84. Rovensky J, Tuchynova A: Systemic lupus erythematosus in the elderly. *Autoimmun Rev* 7:235–239, 2008.

85. Maddison PJ: Systemic lupus erythematosus in the elderly. *J Rheumatol Suppl* 14(Suppl 13):182–187, 1987.

86. Baker SB, Rovira JR, Campion EW, et al: Late onset systemic lupus erythematosus. *Am J Med* 66:727–732, 1979.

87. Boddaert J, Huong DL, Amoura Z, et al: Late-onset systemic lupus erythematosus: a personal series of 47 patients and pooled analysis of 714 cases in the literature. *Medicine (Baltimore)* 83:348–359, 2004.

88. Lazaro D: Elderly-onset systemic lupus erythematosus: prevalence, clinical course and treatment. *Drugs Aging* 24:701–715, 2007.

89. Font J, Pallares L, Cervera R, et al: Systemic lupus erythematosus in the elderly: clinical and immunological characteristics. *Ann Rheum Dis* 50:702–705, 1991.

90. Lalani S, Pope J, de Leon F, et al: Clinical features and prognosis of late-onset systemic lupus erythematosus: results from the 1000 faces of lupus study. *J Rheumatol* 37:38–44, 2010.

91. Ruffatti A, Calligaro A, Del Ross T, et al: Anti-double-stranded DNA antibodies in the healthy elderly: prevalence and characteristics. *J Clin Immunol* 10:300–303, 1990.

92. Padovan M, Govoni M, Castellino G, et al: Late onset systemic lupus erythematosus: no substantial differences using different cut-off ages. *Rheumatol Int* 27:735–741, 2007.

93. Formiga F, Moga I, Pac M, et al: Mild presentation of systemic lupus erythematosus in elderly patients assessed by SLEDAI. SLE Disease Activity Index. *Lupus* 8:462–465, 1999.

94. Bertoli AM, Alarcon GS, Calvo-Alén J, et al: Systemic lupus erythematosus in a multiethnic US cohort. XXXIII. Clinical [corrected] features, course, and outcome in patients with late-onset disease. *Arthritis Rheum* 54:1580–1587, 2006.

95. Mok CC, Mak A, Chu WP, et al: Long-term survival of southern Chinese patients with systemic lupus erythematosus: a prospective study of all age-groups. *Medicine (Baltimore)* 84:218–224, 2005.

96. Mak SK, Lam EK, Wong AK: Clinical profile of patients with late-onset SLE: not a benign subgroup. *Lupus* 7:23–28, 1998.

97. Borchers AT, Keen CL, Gershwin ME: Drug-induced lupus. *Ann N Y Acad Sci* 1108:166–182, 2007.

98. Vasoo S: Drug-induced lupus: an update. *Lupus* 15:757–761, 2006.

99. Antonov D, Kazandjieva J, Etugov D, et al: Drug-induced lupus erythematosus. *Clin Dermatol* 22:157–166, 2004.

100. Lowe G, Henderson CL, Grau RH, et al: A systematic review of drug-induced subacute cutaneous lupus erythematosus. *Br J Dermatol* 164:465–472, 2011.

101. Marzano AV, Lazzari R, Polloni I, et al: Drug-induced subacute cutaneous lupus erythematosus: evidence for differences from its idiopathic counterpart. *Br J Dermatol* 165:335–341, 2011.

102. Callen JP: Drug-induced cutaneous lupus erythematosus, a distinct syndrome that is frequently unrecognized. *J Am Acad Dermatol* 45:315–316, 2001.

103. Yokogawa N, Vivino FB: Hydralazine-induced autoimmune disease: comparison to idiopathic lupus and ANCA-positive vasculitis. *Mod Rheumatol* 19:338–347, 2009.

104. Chang C, Gershwin ME: Drug-induced lupus erythematosus: incidence, management and prevention. *Drug Saf* 34:357–374, 2011.

105. Williams VL, Cohen PR: TNF alpha antagonist-induced lupus-like syndrome: report and review of the literature with implications for treatment with alternative TNF alpha antagonists. *Int J Dermatol* 50:619–625, 2011.

106. Subramanian S, Yajnik V, Sands BE, et al: Characterization of patients with infliximab-induced lupus erythematosus and outcomes after retreatment with a second anti-TNF agent. *Inflamm Bowel Dis* 17:99–104, 2011.

107. Chang C, Gershwin ME: Drugs and autoimmunity—a contemporary review and mechanistic approach. *J Autoimmun* 34:J266–J275, 2010.

108. Gomez-Puerta JA, Burlingame RW, Cervera R: Anti-chromatin (anti-nucleosome) antibodies: diagnostic and clinical value. *Autoimmun Rev* 7:606–611, 2008.

109. Rubin RL, Bell SA, Burlingame RW: Autoantibodies associated with lupus induced by diverse drugs target a similar epitope in the (H2A-H2B)-DNA complex. *J Clin Invest* 90:165–173, 1992.

110. Burlingame RW, Rubin RL: Drug-induced anti-histone autoantibodies display two patterns of reactivity with substructures of chromatin. *J Clin Invest* 88:680–690, 1991.

111. Totoritis MC, Tan EM, McNally EM, et al: Association of antibody to histone complex H2A-H2B with symptomatic procainamide-induced lupus. *N Engl J Med* 318:1431–1436, 1988.

112. Yung RL, Johnson KJ, Richardson BC: New concepts in the pathogenesis of drug-induced lupus. *Lab Invest* 73:746–759, 1995.

113. Hang LM, Nakamura RM: Current concepts and advances in clinical laboratory testing for autoimmune diseases. *Crit Rev Clin Lab Sci* 34:275–311, 1997.

114. Costa MF, Said NR, Zimmermann B: Drug-induced lupus due to anti-tumor necrosis factor alpha agents. *Semin Arthritis Rheum* 37:381–387, 2008.

115. Lee BH, Yegnasubramanian S, Lin X, et al: Procainamide is a specific inhibitor of DNA methyltransferase 1. *J Biol Chem* 280:40749–40756, 2005.

116. Chen Y, Gorelik GJ, Strickland FM, et al: Decreased ERK and JNK signaling contribute to gene overexpression in "senescent" CD4+CD28−T cells through epigenetic mechanisms. *J Leukoc Biol* 87:137–145, 2010.

117. Li Y, Liu Y, Strickland FM, et al: Age-dependent decreases in DNA methyltransferase levels and low transmethylation micronutrient levels synergize to promote overexpression of genes implicated in autoimmunity and acute coronary syndromes. *Exp Gerontol* 45:312–322, 2010.

Chapter 40

SLE in Childhood and Adolescence

Thomas J.A. Lehman

Children and adolescents with systemic lupus erythematosus (SLE) represent both a special challenge and a special opportunity. Early onset allows us to observe the natural history of SLE and to investigate potential causes, free from the confounding factors that may be present in older patients.[1] Recognition of the special considerations that relate to ongoing physical and emotional growth directly influences the choice of medications and the likelihood of success. A satisfactory outcome for the child with SLE is not simply a 5- or 10-year survival period but a 50- or 60-year survival period.

Compliance is one of the most profound determinants of outcome for SLE. It cannot be assumed that the child and family will comply. Children and adolescents are extremely vulnerable to the psychological impact of both the chronic illness and the medications that dramatically alter their appearance (Figure 40-1). To offset peer group pressures on both the child and the family, which may be overwhelming, excellent medical care must be coupled with multidisciplinary family education and support. Without compliance, even the best therapeutic regimen is ineffective.

Although childhood-onset SLE often is described as more severe and a large proportion of children and adolescents have significant renal or central nervous system (CNS) involvement at the time of diagnosis,[2,3] the perception of increased severity may arise from delayed diagnosis and poor compliance.

English-language reports of children with SLE appeared as early as 1892. Sequeira and Balean,[4] writing from the London Hospital in 1902, noted that the disease commences early in life in a much larger proportion of patients than was commonly believed. Series of children with SLE began to be published in the 1950s and 1960s. In the era before steroids were available, childhood-onset SLE was a rapidly evolving and usually fatal multisystem disease. SLE is now a common diagnosis in every large pediatric rheumatology program. With proper care, most children and adolescents with SLE now have an excellent prognosis.

EPIDEMIOLOGY

The incidence and prevalence of SLE in childhood have been estimated at 0.5 to 1 in 100,000 and 1 in 10,000, respectively. The influences of sex and racial origin on the occurrence and manifestations of SLE are widely recognized.[5] In childhood, the influence of race is striking. The age- and sex-adjusted prevalences of SLE in African American, Asian, and Hispanic children were more than threefold those of Caucasian children at one large center. Although based on a limited sample, these data suggest a significant variation in the influence of sex hormones and puberty on the predisposition to SLE among different races.

DIAGNOSIS

Although physicians often rely on antinuclear antibody (ANA) testing, which is useful for prompting the consideration of SLE, a positive test is not sufficient for the diagnosis. Conversely, ANA-positive children who fulfill at least one other criterion should be periodically reevaluated. Definite SLE may manifest decades after the initial presentation.[6]

In most ways, diagnosing SLE in childhood is the same as diagnosing SLE in an adult. Confirming the diagnosis of SLE in children and adolescents is based on criteria developed by the American Rheumatism Association (ARA) for use in adults.[7] Classification as definite SLE is based on the fulfillment of four criteria, but the diagnosis should not be automatically discarded in children who meet only three. Although the ARA criteria are useful guidelines, the fulfillment of four criteria does not exclude other diagnoses; similarly, the failure to fulfill four criteria does not exclude SLE. It is not unusual for children to be told that they do not have SLE because they fulfill only two or three of the criteria developed by the American College of Rheumatology (ACR) only to be recognized as having definite SLE within an additional 1 to 2 years. In many patients the initial dismissal of the diagnosis results in a delay in further evaluation or the return to medical care despite progressive symptoms. Physicians evaluating children who do not fulfill all the necessary criteria at the time of the initial evaluation must remain aware that additional findings may evolve and counsel families accordingly.

CLINICAL MANIFESTATIONS

Unexplained elevated body temperature, malaise, and weight loss are the most common manifestations of SLE in children and adolescents. Because these nonspecific symptoms may be associated with many chronic illnesses, the physician should actively seek evidence of arthritis or a photosensitive rash, hematuria or proteinuria, hypergammaglobulinemia, and hypocomplementemia. Any of these findings should prompt consideration of SLE, but one cannot rely on their presence. On the initial evaluation, the patient and family often do not describe findings such as arthritis of the small joints of the hands, alopecia, or photosensitivity unless they are specifically questioned. The reported frequency of many complaints varies widely among series of children with SLE, reflecting selection and referral criteria and the care with which the complaint was sought (Table 40-1).[8]

Some children and adolescents with SLE are acutely ill at presentation. These children may have seizures, psychosis, uremia, profound anemia, pulmonary hemorrhage, or sepsis. Often, the diagnosis of SLE is not considered until the clinician notes that the child is not recovering as expected, despite adequate therapy for the presenting manifestation.

Renal Disease

Renal disease is evident in nearly two thirds of children and adolescents with SLE.[2,3,8] Renal manifestations range from mild glomerulitis to sudden renal failure. Hematuria, proteinuria, and hypertension may be present in any combination. In the absence of nephrotic syndrome, renal involvement may be silent in childhood.

Renal biopsy without regard to clinical manifestations demonstrates varying renal involvement in most children.[9] Children with a normal urine sediment level typically have only mild glomerulitis. Although occasional biopsies demonstrate silent diffuse proliferative glomerulonephritis (DPGN), the significance of silent DPGN is uncertain. Series reporting follow-up of silent nephritis in SLE describe a benign prognosis.[9] Thus the importance of detecting silent DPGN is uncertain. Renal biopsy should be performed if necessary to confirm the diagnosis, to investigate unexplained changes in renal

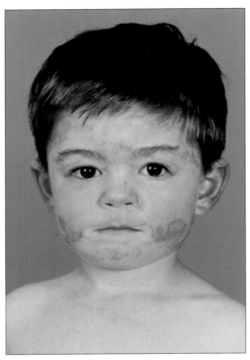

FIGURE 40-1 Altered facial appearance in a young man with systemic lupus erythematosus. *(From Hochberg MC, Silman AJ, Smolen JS, et al. [editors]: Rheumatology, ed 5, Philadelphia, 2010, Mosby.)*

TABLE 40-1 Clinical Manifestations of Systemic Lupus Erythematosus in Children and Adults[a]

	Number of Patients		
PARAMETER	**CASSIDY**[60]	**KING**[3]	**PISTINER**[b]
Renal involvement	86	61	28
Hypertension	28	—	25
Musculoskeletal findings	76	79	91
Cutaneous involvement	76	70	55
Photosensitivity	16	—	37
Hair loss	20	—	31
Oral, nasal ulceration	16	—	19
Cardiac involvement	47	17	12
Pulmonary involvement	36	19	12
Central nervous system involvement	31	13	11
Anemia	47	—	30
Leukopenia	71	—	51
Thrombocytopenia	24	—	16

[a]The findings from Cassidy and others and from King and others represent two large pediatric series; those from Pistiner and colleagues represent a large adult series.
[b]Pistiner M, Wallace DJ, Nessim S, et al: Lupus erythematosus in the 1980s: a survey of 570 patients. *Semin Arthritis Rheum* 21:55-64, 1991.

function, and when the clinician is considering or monitoring the effects of aggressive therapy.

Renal involvement is categorized according to criteria developed by the World Health Organization (WHO). Mild glomerulitis is the most benign form, followed by focal segmental glomerulonephritis and membranous glomerulonephritis.[10] DPGN carries the greatest risk of chronic renal failure and is the most frequent abnormality in children who undergo biopsy because of abnormal urine sediment. However, in a series in which all children with SLE underwent biopsy, only 20% had DPGN.[10] Combined data from several large series showed that 42% of children (108 of 256) had DPGN at the time of initial biopsy, 26% had either mild glomerulitis or no abnormality, 25% had focal glomerulitis, and 6% had membranous glomerulonephritis.

Focal glomerulonephritis and membranous glomerulonephritis are generally benign, but either may progress to DPGN with ultimate renal failure.[10] Repeat renal biopsy should be performed in affected patients if renal function continues to deteriorate or if they develop persistent hypocomplementemia. Long-term studies indicate that renal scarring (i.e., chronicity index) is a better predictor of the ultimate outcome than the WHO classification.[10] In the absence of scarring, active disease (including glomerular crescents) is not automatically associated with a poor prognosis; however, good outcomes for these children are contingent on aggressive management of their renal disease to prevent the development of scarring (see the section on pharmaceutical therapies in this chapter). Most children with SLE do not develop renal disease beyond the first 2 years after diagnosis,[2] but one third of those with significant renal disease lack evidence of renal involvement at presentation.

The sudden onset of renal failure in a child with SLE may result from active nephritis, but alternative explanations must be excluded. Renal vein thrombosis and renal artery thrombosis occur in children with SLE and are more frequent in association with anticardiolipin (aCL) antibodies.[11] Drugs and health food supplements that interfere with glomerular filtration or are directly nephrotoxic must also be considered. A mild rise in the blood urea nitrogen (BUN) level usually follows the initiation of acetylsalicylic acid or other nonsteroidal antiinflammatory drugs (NSAIDs) in patients with renal involvement, but some children with SLE are unusually sensitive to their effects. An unexpectedly sharp rise in the BUN level after the initiation of NSAIDs should prompt further investigation for renal involvement.

Mild clinical manifestations of renal involvement are usually well controlled with corticosteroid and diuretic agents. Persistent renal disease typically requires immunosuppressive therapy. Chronic glomerular scarring is prevented by cyclophosphamide over the intermediate term.[12] The major concern of the physician caring for a child with lupus nephritis is preserving sufficient renal function to support normal growth and development. For female adolescents, this includes the preservation of adequate renal function to support pregnancy. These concerns dictate intervention before significant renal compromise has occurred. Physicians who normally care for adults must be reminded that the normal serum creatinine level of children is much lower. Levels of serum creatinine elevation that might represent minimal impairment in an adult may indicate severe renal compromise in a child.

Current treatment regimens for children and adolescents with lupus nephritis have led to a steady improvement in the survival of 5- and 10-year renal function. However, whether these improvements will result in significantly enhanced survival 20 and 30 years after diagnosis is not yet clear. Maintaining adequate renal function is important for children and adolescents with SLE. In contrast to adults, they progress poorly on long-term dialysis. Children with SLE coming to dialysis with active disease often die of sepsis or other complications within the first year. However, those who have gradually developed global glomerular sclerosis often progress well with dialysis and subsequent renal transplantation.[61]

Children whose proteinuria and hematuria improve with corticosteroid therapy but whose creatinine clearance slowly deteriorates are of particular concern. Often, these children do well over a 5-year period but progress to renal failure between 5 and 10 years after diagnosis. Routine monitoring of creatinine clearance and, if deterioration is evident, early intervention are important. In the event of chronic deterioration, the clinician should aggressively intervene while adequate function can still be preserved. Adult series suggest that maintaining a creatinine clearance of 70 mL/min per 1.75 m² is adequate, but intervention at this point may not preserve sufficient renal function for the satisfactory growth and development of children and adolescents.

Optimal therapy for children and adolescents with lupus nephritis remains uncertain. In large part, this uncertainty is the result of the failure of many investigators to stratify the patients properly in their studies. The systematic use of intermittent intravenous cyclophosphamide has been successful in children with DPGN and useful for children with membranous glomerulonephritis.[12,13] More recently, mycophenolate mofetil has shown early promise, but its efficacy in routine use is limited by poor compliance. When the 10-year renal survival is considered, the systematic use of intravenous cyclophosphamide appears to offer the best outcome.[13] Newer regimens, which intend to minimize the amount of cyclophosphamide by combining it with rituximab, have shown excellent promise in the short term but have not yet completed long-term follow-up study.[14-16]

Some centers restrict the use of cyclophosphamide to children with well-established severe renal disease and elevated serum creatinine levels. Once significant renal scarring has occurred and the creatinine level has become elevated, a poor outcome is typical, despite therapy. The consistent failure of reporting centers to stratify patients according to age, race, sex, and severity of disease, despite the fact that these factors are all recognized to affect survival, and the varied populations served by various centers make comparative analysis of varied treatment regimens difficult.

At present, a large-scale study of criteria for evaluating the response to therapy of children with SLE is under way.[17] The use of these criteria should improve the ability to assess the various therapeutic regimens that have been advocated for children with lupus nephritis. Routine use of intravenous cyclophosphamide has many advantages, including accurate assessment of patient compliance and clinical status at each dosage interval. Poor compliance is a major determinant of poor outcome. In addition, periodic inpatient cyclophosphamide therapy allows the physician to monitor renal function status and clinical status before each immunosuppressive drug dose, thus minimizing complications. New regimens in which the frequency and total dose of cyclophosphamide are substantially reduced are under investigation. Although consistent use of high-dose mycophenolate mofetil has been recommended for the control of lupus nephritis in adults,[18] its sustained benefit is unproven in children and adolescents. Rituximab is a new biologic agent directed against activated B cells bearing the lymphocyte marker CD20. Several case reports regarding its use in SLE and several small series have been published.[16,19,20] Additional agents that block or eliminate activated B cells (such as BLyS antagonists) are under evaluation. Regimens using a combination of conventional agents and the newer biologic agents may hold the greatest promise.

Autologous stem-cell transplantation has been proposed and used for a variety of autoimmune diseases including SLE in some children.[21] Although this technique may hold great promise, it is associated with a significant mortality and the majority of the reported responses have not persisted over time. Whether the beneficial effect is the result of the stem cell transplantation or of the immunosuppressive chemotherapy given at the time of stem cell transplant is under active investigation.

Central Nervous System Manifestations

Psychosis, sudden personality change, seizures, chorea, transverse myelitis, peripheral neuropathy, and pseudotumor cerebri all may be presenting manifestations of SLE in childhood.[3, 22-24] Most series have reported CNS involvement in 20% to 30% of children. If carefully sought, mild evidence of CNS involvement is present in up to 45% of children and adolescents. In every instance, appropriate investigation should be undertaken to exclude stroke as the cause of sudden CNS changes, even in the patient who is not known to be aCL antibody–positive.

Subtle CNS changes, including impaired judgment and poor short-term memory, are the most common CNS manifestations of SLE. These alterations are often ascribed to steroid therapy or situational stress, but they occur with greater frequency in SLE than in other chronic childhood rheumatic diseases that require similar corticosteroid therapy. Adolescents with SLE often have difficulty complying with their medications or appointments, and they often alienate friends and family in ways that are inconsistent with their prior behavior. Physicians must be acutely aware of these changes, because they may have disastrous consequences. A trial of increased corticosteroids may be beneficial in children with SLE whose behavior has become erratic or uncharacteristic, even in the absence of objective findings. Others have argued for reducing the corticosteroids in such circumstances, but this reduction is rarely effective.

Delirium, hallucinations, seizures, and coma are the most common objective neurologic signs in childhood. Psychosis that is unrelated to corticosteroid therapy typically occurs in 4% to 10% of children. The reported frequency of neuropsychiatric manifestations in children and adolescents with SLE is lower than that in adults.[25] This finding may be true, but it more likely represents a decreased appreciation of the neuropsychiatric involvement in childhood.

Chorea is more frequent in children than it is in adults with SLE.[25] Although infrequent, chorea has been documented as being the initial manifestation of childhood SLE in multiple reports, perhaps because it is such a striking finding. Of children with SLE, 4% to 10% are affected by chorea at some point.[22-26] This increased incidence may reflect an increased sensitivity of the basal ganglia to damage by autoreactive antibodies or vascular events accompanying SLE in childhood.

Most often, acute CNS involvement occurs early in the natural history of childhood SLE.[25] Frequently, it first becomes evident during or worsens immediately after the initiation of corticosteroid therapy. The explanation for this is uncertain, but these symptoms frequently resolve with pulse methylprednisolone therapy. Late-onset CNS involvement more often is the result of stroke, uremia, or an infectious process.

Both sudden onset of optic neuritis and acute sensorineural hearing loss may occur in children with SLE.[27,28] However, the most striking CNS damage in children and adolescents with SLE is typically the result of seizures or strokes, including cerebral vein thrombosis. These complications may occur in the presence or absence of aCL antibodies.[22-26]

Cognitive defects and aberrant behavior present a more difficult management problem. Aberrant behavior may have dramatic effects on social acceptance, grades, and compliance, thereby directly affecting both self-image and long-term prognosis. Efforts to ascribe behavioral change to a single cause are rarely successful.[22-25] Unfortunately, this often results in a failure to aggressively treat these problems with resultant progression.

Nonspecific problems in children with diffuse CNS involvement most likely represent the combined effects of SLE, situational factors, and corticosteroid therapy. When such symptoms are present, increasing the corticosteroid dose is more often successful than a dramatic reduction.

No single objective test for the presence of CNS involvement in SLE is accurate in childhood. Computed tomography (CT) of children and adolescents with SLE who have received long-term corticosteroid therapy commonly demonstrates diffuse cortical atrophy. Alterations in cerebrospinal fluid protein or sugar levels or cell count are not reliable, but these studies are often necessary to exclude infection and other explanations for altered CNS function.[25] Single-photon emission CT may be a more sensitive test for cerebral perfusion abnormalities in these children, but other studies suggest that MRI is more sensitive.[23] Antibodies to ribosomal P have been found to correlate with CNS manifestations of SLE in adults, but their presence correlates less reliably with CNS disease in children and adolescents.[25]

Treatment of CNS manifestations in children and adolescents with SLE is a challenge. Because the manifestations may result from corticosteroid therapy, physicians frequently hesitate to increase the dose; nonetheless, this is often the most effective therapy. For severe CNS manifestations, pulse methylprednisolone therapy is often effective. When other measures fail, intravenous cyclophosphamide is frequently beneficial. Children with short-term psychosis or coma often respond to therapy, but when significant impairment has been present for long periods, the prognosis is guarded. Responding aggressively to continuing evidence of CNS deterioration is important. Chronic, mild problems for which intervention is not believed to be warranted may, nonetheless, progress to dementia over time. In children with active CNS manifestations but relatively normal serum complement levels and only minimal evidence of active SLE in other organ systems, consideration may be given to a trial of anticoagulation instead of increased immunosuppressive agents.[29,30]

Psychosocial Concerns

Psychological reactions that relate to the many issues affecting children and adolescents with SLE are often confusing. Children with SLE commonly demonstrate an impaired quality of life that is affected by the activity of their disease.[31,32] Adolescents who are afflicted with chronic disease are caught between their need to establish an independent personality and the dependency of the sick role. Just as they are struggling to assert their independence, they must be taken for doctor's visits, are forced to undergo examinations and blood tests, and are required to take unpleasant medications. This situation is intensified by the almost universal need for doses of corticosteroids that increase acne and produce obvious cushingoid facies. The adolescent who does not rebel under these circumstances is unusual. This rebellion may take the form of noncompliance with scheduled physician visits, overt or covert medication noncompliance, or familial disruption. The physician who expects the adolescent with SLE to act like an adult should expect an unsatisfactory patient-physician relationship, which often results in a poor outcome.

Anger is frequently the adolescent's predominant response to his or her situation. Remembering that no well-defined target exists for this anger is important. The adolescent is obviously angry about having SLE, but the disease has no direct embodiment. The physician, the medications, and the required examinations, however, all are direct manifestations of the disease and thus are easy targets for the adolescent's rage, which may be overtly expressed by refusal to cooperate, but may also be covert and initially go unrecognized.

No single successful method for dealing with adolescent rebellion in the setting of chronic illness is available. Because adolescents frequently believe that important information is being kept from them, emphasizing honesty, trust, and integrity is important. The physician cannot demand these without providing them in return. Many issues that the adolescent is afraid to voice in front of parents or siblings may exist. Directly asking the patient what the physician or family has done to provoke the behavior is often useful. Frequently, it takes only a few minutes of conversation to elicit the recognition that the anger is primarily over being ill. Honestly and directly dealing with this is a key step in developing a healthy patient-physician-family relationship.

For some children, no amount of discussion and reassurance is sufficient. Often, this scenario is a response to unspoken fears or needs in the family of which the physician may not be aware. In these circumstances, family counseling is the best recommendation. Individual counseling of the adolescent without the involvement of other family members furthers the adolescent's feeling of having been singled out and is often counterproductive. Situations in which both honest discussion and family counseling fail are unusual. When they do occur, however, determining whether the adolescent behavior may be a manifestation of unrecognized cerebritis is important.

If a satisfactory patient-family-physician relationship cannot be established despite every possible effort, then referral to another physician or center may be indicated. Because a referral to another health care professional forces the adolescent and family to reevaluate their conduct and initiate new relationships, it may be beneficial even when no additional steps are taken.

Pulmonary Manifestations

Pleurisy and pleural effusions are the most common pulmonary manifestations.[33-35] Severe manifestations, including pneumothorax, pneumonia, chronic restrictive lung disease, pulmonary hypertension, and acute pulmonary hemorrhage, may occur.[35] Pleuritic chest pain, pleural effusions, and chronic interstitial infiltrates affect 10% to 30% of children with SLE. When a series of Canadian children with SLE were reviewed for manifestations of respiratory involvement, 77% of the patients (17 of 24) had evidence of pulmonary involvement.[33]

Chronic pulmonary involvement may result in progressive diaphragmatic dysfunction and restrictive lung disease, which result in progressive malaise with dyspnea on exertion and leads to an increased frequency of infection.[33,34] Noting both pulse and respiration rates as part of the routine examination is useful. Gradual increases in either or both parameters may be a clue to developing cardiac or pulmonary dysfunction.

A study of 15 children with SLE by Trapani and colleagues[36] found pulmonary involvement in 6 patients who were without pulmonary symptoms. Children with dyspnea or tachypnea at rest should be monitored with periodic pulmonary function testing.

The most common fatal complication of pulmonary is pneumonia. At autopsy, pneumonia was the primary cause of death for 9 of the 26 children with SLE in one reported series; pulmonary hemorrhage contributed to the death of 5 others. In contrast, renal failure and CNS involvement were the primary causes of death in only 4 and 3 children, respectively.

Pulmonary hypertension is an ominous finding in children and adolescents with SLE. Once established, it progresses steadily to right ventricular heart failure and death.[34] Pulmonary hemorrhage may occur in the setting of preexisting pulmonary hypertension or in isolation.[32-36] Sudden unexplained pallor and tachypnea may be the first symptoms of pulmonary hemorrhage,[36] which, if left untreated, is rapidly fatal. Children with pulmonary hypertension may benefit symptomatically from the addition of calcium channel–blocking agents or endothelin-1 receptor antagonists to reduce pulmonary vascular resistance. No therapy is known to reverse the course of this complication. Cytotoxic drugs have been ineffective, except in rare anecdotal reports. Pneumonia is a frequent complication in children with established pulmonary hypertension and may progress rapidly to sepsis. Massive pulmonary hemorrhage may respond to large doses of corticosteroids with ventilator support and, perhaps, plasmapheresis or extracorporeal membrane oxygenation.

Minor manifestations of pulmonary involvement normally respond to corticosteroids. Deaths from pneumonia, in which *Escherichia coli*, the genus *Klebsiella*, or *Staphylococcus aureus* were the predominant organisms, illustrate the need for broad-spectrum antibiotic coverage.[35] *Pneumocystis carinii* and other nonbacterial organisms may be present.[35] When pneumonia is superimposed on active pulmonary SLE, the contributions of infection and active SLE cannot be differentiated with certainty. Both antibiotics and increased doses of corticosteroids may be appropriate.

Musculoskeletal Manifestations

Significant arthritis at presentation is found in 40% to 60% of children and adolescents with SLE, and it occurs in over 80% of children with SLE at some point.[3] Usually, the arthritis affects the small joints of the hands and feet, with swelling and pain on motion. Asymptomatic knee effusions are frequently present in children with active disease who may not have arthritis elsewhere.

The arthritis of SLE is generally nondeforming and responds well to antiinflammatory medications. Rarely, children with well-documented juvenile rheumatoid arthritis (JRA) and erosive changes develop definite SLE.[37]

Avascular necrosis is the most significant musculoskeletal complication of SLE in children and adolescents, and it may result from SLE alone, corticosteroid therapy, or their interaction. A cross-sectional radiographic study of 35 children with SLE treated with high-dose corticosteroids found evidence of avascular necrosis in 40%.[38]

Avascular necrosis usually affects the hips and knees of children with SLE. Children report gradual onset of progressive discomfort in the affected joints, and the initial evaluation may prove negative. Magnetic resonance imaging (MRI) and, later, routine radiography ultimately reveal the evidence of osteonecrosis. Although no clear association of avascular necrosis with the total dose of corticosteroids or their mode of administration has been found, the incidence of avascular necrosis is far higher in children who have received corticosteroid therapy for prolonged periods.[38]

Meaningful muscle involvement is rare in children with SLE. Diffuse weakness may be the result of steroid myopathy. Mild elevations of serum creatinine phosphokinase levels are rarely associated with clinical weakness. Antibodies to the acetylcholinesterase receptor may produce a picture similar to myasthenia gravis, and transplacental passage of antibodies to this receptor is reported to have caused weakness in the child of a mother with SLE.[39]

Dermatologic Manifestations

Rashes occur frequently in children with SLE,[3] but only 30% to 50% ever manifest the typical butterfly rash (Figure 40-2). Cutaneous lesions may take the form of recurrent urticaria, bullae, vasculitic nodules, or chronic ulceration. Vasculitic involvement of the hard palate frequently accompanies the facial rash of SLE, and vasculitic lesions are often a manifestation of active disease. Other dermatologic manifestations may wax and wane independently of systemic disease.

Bullous lesions resembling bullous pemphigoid are the predominant manifestations of SLE in some children. Boys with this manifestation predominate and often have mild systemic disease; renal involvement is rare. Dapsone is often helpful for these children.

Most dermatologic manifestations respond to treatment without significant scarring. All the dermatologic lesions of SLE may be aggravated by sun exposure, and children with SLE should be counseled to use sun-blocking agents and to avoid unnecessary sun exposure, which may provoke increased systemic disease activity.

Adolescents often resent being told they cannot go to the beach or other all-day outdoor activities (e.g., theme parks) with their friends. Every effort must be made to accentuate the positive. For example, patients should be encouraged to participate in these activities in the evening when the risk of significant ultraviolet exposure is less. However, long sleeves, hats, and sun block are recommended at all times. Finally, the health care professional also must emphasize the exact nature of the risk. A recent patient of the author of this chapter suffered severe skin irritation after going to a tanning salon. The patient professed not to understand that this, too, was ultraviolet exposure and included in the photosensitivity precautions previously explained.

Discoid lupus erythematosus (DLE) is unusual in childhood. Most children referred for DLE are found to have systemic manifestations when carefully questioned and examined. Although rare, some children with DLE progress to SLE. Isolated DLE is of concern because of associated disfigurement and psychological effects. In the past, dermatologic lesions of SLE in childhood have been treated primarily with topical corticosteroids. However, these agents have adverse effects on the skin with sustained use. More recently, topical ointments containing tacrolimus or related compounds have been found to be effective. However, the risk of skin cancer increases if their use is sustained.[40]

Cardiac Manifestations

Cardiac manifestations are rarely prominent in children and adolescents with SLE.[3] Pericarditis, myocarditis, and mild valvular involvement are common but may be asymptomatic.[41] Clinically evident pericarditis or myocarditis occurs in 10% of children. Clinically evident cardiac tamponade is uncommon. However, severe and recurrent pericarditis may warrant surgical intervention.

Many children with SLE develop flow murmurs secondary to anemia. Libman-Sacks endocarditis may occur, however, which predisposes the patient to bacterial endocarditis. In large series, bacterial endocarditis occurred with a greater-than-expected frequency.[42] All children with significant valvular lesions must receive antibiotic coverage for dentistry and other invasive procedures. Some authorities recommend routine bacterial endocarditis prophylaxis for all patients with SLE.

Circulating lipid abnormalities occur in adolescents and young adults with SLE and may contribute to premature myocardial infarctions and coronary arteritis. These lipid abnormalities are, in part, related to prolonged corticosteroid therapy. Preliminary studies to determine whether statins are safe and effective for children with SLE are under way.[43] The association of prolonged corticosteroid therapy with premature myocardial infarction is well documented.[44]

Gastrointestinal Manifestations

Mild gastrointestinal involvement is common in children and adolescents with SLE; 30% to 40% demonstrate hepatomegaly or splenomegaly at diagnosis.[3] Chronic abdominal pain, anorexia, weight loss, and malaise are also frequent presenting complaints.[3,45] The onset of the abdominal pain may be acute. Abdominal pain that is unresponsive to corticosteroids may be the result of small-vessel vasculitis.[45] These children may respond to a further increase in their

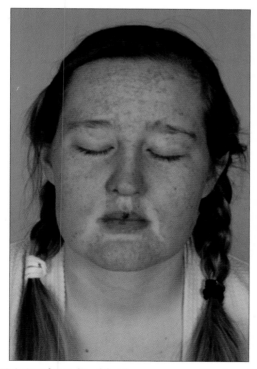

FIGURE 40-2 Significant altered facial appearance resulting from skin manifestations is exhibited in a female teenager with systemic lupus erythematosus. *(From Hochberg MC, Silman AJ, Smolen JS, et al. [editors]: Rheumatology, ed 5, Philadelphia, 2010, Mosby.)*

corticosteroid dose. Retroperitoneal fibrosis is a rare cause of abdominal pain in children with SLE. More often, abdominal pain is the result of pancreatitis that is induced by SLE, corticosteroids, or both.[45] Fulminant pancreatitis resulting in death has also occurred.

Pneumatosis cystoides intestinalis may be the result of chronic ischemia.[46] Clinically evident bowel ischemia is often found at autopsy.[46] Although severe ischemia is probably a terminal event, its frequency suggests that the bowel is often compromised by vascular insufficiency in children with severe SLE. For some children, these conditions may be the reasons for unexplained chronic abdominal pain.

Less frequent gastrointestinal manifestations of SLE include hepatitis and ileitis.[3,45,46] Protein-losing enteropathy and significant hyperlipoproteinemia also occur. Their relationship to SLE is uncertain. Gastrointestinal irritation, secondary to drugs used in treating SLE, is frequent. Severe gastritis and ulcers may occur as well. The simultaneous occurrence of gastrointestinal inflammation and cystitis is reported.

Although infarction of the spleen may produce acute abdominal pain, splenic involvement in SLE usually is asymptomatic. Functional asplenia is associated with increased susceptibility to infection.[47] The presence of Howell-Jolly bodies on the peripheral blood smear should alert the clinician to the possibility of functional asplenia and prompt hospitalization if the child is febrile without adequate explanation.

Infection

Infection is a major cause of both morbidity and mortality for children and adolescents with SLE.[2,3] Platt and colleagues[48] documented 55 separate infections occurring in 70 patients over a mean follow-up of 9 years. Sepsis was a contributing cause in 25% to 85% of deaths in various series, and it was a cited factor in 42% of the deaths (35 of 83) occurring in 374 children collected from six large studies.

The increased frequency of sepsis is most likely the result of the combined effects of SLE and its therapy. The frequency of infection increases with increasing steroid dose.[49] Both bacterial infections and opportunistic infections, as well as infections caused by viruses, fungi, and related organisms, are more common in children with SLE.[31,35] The indiscriminate use of immunosuppressive drugs may also contribute to infections; however, careful use of periodic intravenous cyclophosphamide accompanied by a reduction in the need for corticosteroid therapy often leads to a reduced frequency of infections. In contrast to children taking daily azathioprine or other immunosuppressive agents, children receiving periodic intravenous cyclophosphamide therapy can be intensively screened before receiving each dose. Potentially fatal infections, including both bacterial endocarditis and meningitis, occur with a greater-than-expected frequency in children with SLE.[35] Functional asplenia, decreased phagocytosis, poor complement metabolism, and corticosteroid effects may all contribute to this problem.

Hematologic Manifestations

The most common hematologic manifestation of SLE in children and adolescents is anemia. Usually, this condition is not a Coombs-positive hemolytic anemia with a reticulocytosis; rather, it is a microcytic anemia of chronic disease. Leukopenia and thrombocytopenia are common but not invariably present. Sickle cell anemia is not directly associated with SLE, but it is common in African Americans, who have an increased incidence of SLE. When SLE and sickle cell disease occur together, the similarity of symptoms between the two illnesses may produce confusion. If the physician cannot distinguish the etiology of problems with certainty, he or she may have to treat both conditions as appropriate.

Children who have ANAs and thrombocytopenia are often labeled as having immune thrombocytopenic purpura (ITP). A false-positive biologic test result for syphilis or prolonged partial thromboplastin time (PTT) in this setting may suggest SLE. Children with ITP

TABLE 40-2 Incidence of Serologic Antibodies in 92 Children with Systemic Lupus Erythematosus[a]

ANTIBODY	Incidence (%)	
	OUCHTERLONY METHOD	ELISA
SSA/Ro	16	46
SSB/La	11	17
Sm (RNP)	27	58

[a]The presence of these antibodies did not correlate with disease activity, except that SSA/Ro antibodies in the study by Ouchterlony were significantly more common in children younger than 10 years of age (11 of 28 versus 4 of 64, $P < .001$).[62] Children younger than 10 years of age also had a significantly higher mean ELISA titer of SSA/Ro antibodies. ELISA, Enzyme-linked immunosorbent assay; RNP, ribonucleoprotein; Sm, Smith; SSA/Ro, Sjögren syndrome antigen A; SSB/La, Sjögren syndrome antigen B.

may have antibodies to Smith (Sm), Sjögren syndrome antigen A (SSA/Ro), Sjögren syndrome antigen B (SSB/La), or ribonucleoprotein (RNP). However, all children with any of these serologic markers should be carefully followed and reevaluated for evidence of systemic disease including periodic testing for hypocomplementemia, renal impairment, and proteinuria or hematuria. Some of these patients will ultimately develop SLE (Table 40-2). In the absence of other manifestations of SLE, therapy is similar to that for ITP alone.

Menorrhagia may be the presenting feature of SLE in female teenagers. Prolonged bleeding or a prolonged PTT resulting from the lupus anticoagulant may be the initial manifestation of SLE in a child who is being screened for other reasons. However, these findings alone do not establish the diagnosis of SLE. Management of these complications is the same for children and adolescents as it is for adults.

aCL antibodies occur in children with SLE with a similar frequency to that of adults.[50] They are associated with an increased risk of thrombosis and CNS disease. Children with high-titer aCL, lupus anticoagulant, and thrombocytopenia may be at highest risk of thrombosis. The risk for children with low-titer aCL in the absence of lupus anticoagulant appears to be low. Low-dose aspirin therapy remains controversial. Children who present with aCL antibodies but who initially lack the criteria for a diagnosis of SLE may later develop definite SLE.

LABORATORY EVALUATION

No laboratory feature of SLE is unique to the pediatric age group. For clinicians, the diagnosis of SLE is strongly suggested by the constellation of hypergammaglobulinemia, leukopenia, anemia, and thrombocytopenia. A positive ANA test is confirmatory, but none of these findings is essential.

ANAs are present in over 90% of children and adolescents with SLE.[51] Antibodies to various other nuclear and cytoplasmic antigens also are found.[52] One study that compared the incidence of antibodies to DNA, Smith (Sm), and RNP found a lower frequency in children with SLE than in a simultaneously studied population of adult patients with SLE.[52] Antibodies to SSA/Ro and SSB/La were found in similar numbers of patients of adult and childhood onset. These antibodies are also found with increased frequency in the relatives of children with SLE.[52] Their presence in asymptomatic relatives has been variously interpreted as being evidence of environmental exposure or genetic predisposition.

Antibodies against double-stranded DNA (dsDNA) are both sensitive and specific for active SLE in childhood but may occur in other conditions.[52] Decreased serum levels of the third component of complement correlate well with active SLE in childhood, but neither decreased complement 3 (C3) levels nor antibodies to dsDNA are reliable as specific indicators of active renal disease.

TABLE 40-3 Immunosuppressive Treatment of Childhood Systemic Lupus Erythematosus

DRUG(S)[a]	SUGGESTED DOSAGE	USEFUL FOR	REMARKS
NSAIDs	—	Mild disease	Monitor for idiosyncratic effects of NSAIDs on renal and CNS functions.
Prednisone	1-2 mg/kg/day	More severe or unresponsive disease	Rarely exceeds 80 mg/day; dose may be divided into four daily doses, if necessary.
Methylprednisolone	30 mg/kg/day, IV	Acute manifestations of CNS or renal diseases	Maximum: 1000 mg for 3 days.
Cyclophosphamide	500-1000 mg/m²/mo for 7 mo, then every 3 mo for 30 additional mo	DPGN	May be helpful for some children with severe nephrotic syndrome or CNS disease.

[a]Other agents have been used, with differing reports of efficacy.
CNS, Central nervous system; DPGN, diffuse proliferative glomerulonephritis; IV, intravenous; NSAIDs, nonsteroidal antiinflammatory drugs;

Decreased complement 4 (C4) levels often are correlated with decreases in C3, but they may occur in isolation. Hypergammaglobulinemia is frequently present in children with SLE but also may be found in various chronic inflammatory states.[2,3] Immunoglobulin A (IgA) deficiency is occasionally seen, as is panhypogammaglobulinemia.[3] Panhypogammaglobulinemia is a common complication of cyclophosphamide therapy, but it also occurs in patients with SLE who have not received immunosuppressive agents.[53]

False-positive test results for syphilis were formerly found in many children with SLE,[3] but more recent studies report fewer occurrences. In the United States, the family must be warned that positive results may need to be reported to the public health department. Unwarranted investigation can be halted if questions are referred to the physician. The diagnosis of SLE, however, does not exclude the possibility of treponemal disease. False-positive fluorescent treponemal antibody (FTA) test results may occur because of nonspecific agglutination resulting from hypergammaglobulinemia,[54] but FTA-positive individuals in whom the possibility of treponemal disease cannot be reliably excluded should receive appropriate therapy.

PHARMACEUTICAL THERAPIES

NSAIDs provide useful control of the arthritis and musculoskeletal manifestations of SLE in children and adolescents (Table 40-3). Renal function and blood pressure must be monitored because of NSAIDs' known effects on glomerular filtration, but significant undesired effects are infrequent. Antiinflammatory doses of aspirin (80 mg/kg/day) have been advocated, but children with SLE are very susceptible to salicylate-induced hepatotoxicity. Alternate NSAIDs are preferable.

Hydroxychloroquine (Plaquenil) and chloroquine are routinely used in children and adolescents with SLE.[2,3] They are believed to have a useful steroid-sparing effect at a maximum dose of 7 mg/kg/day (for hydroxychloroquine). Although rare ocular toxicity is a concern, it was not reported in children or adolescents in any of these series (Box 40-1).

Intravenous pulse methylprednisolone (30 mg/kg daily, up to 1 g) given as an intravenous infusion has been used to control flares of nephritis[55] or CNS disease. Therapy was associated with dramatic short-term improvement in renal disease, but it was not superior to daily prednisone over the longer term. Long-term benefit from pulse methylprednisolone is more likely in children with acute CNS involvement and other manifestations of SLE that appear to be the result of an acute event. Although rare, side effects may occur with pulse methylprednisolone, including significant hypotension, hypertension, and pancreatitis. Deaths have occurred.

In the 1970s, most children were treated with high-dose corticosteroids (2 mg/kg/day), followed by gradual tapering once the disease came under control.[2] Children with continuing active disease and evidence of renal involvement received immunosuppressive agents.[6]

Box 40-1 Dosages of Medications Commonly Used for Children with Systemic Lupus Erythematosus and Active Central Nervous System Disease

NSAIDs
Naproxen: 10-15 mg/kg divided into two doses per day (usual maximum dose, 500 mg twice daily)
Diclofenac: 1-3 mg/kg divided into two doses per day (usual maximum dose, 75 mg twice daily)
Ibuprofen: 20-40 mg/kg divided into three or four doses per day (usual maximum dose, 800 mg three times daily); may be associated with idiosyncratic reactions in SLE

Other Drugs
Hydroxychloroquine: 7 mg/kg up to 200 mg/day (maximum dose for some centers, 400 mg/day)
Dapsone: 1 mg/kg up to 100 mg/day

Immunosuppressive Agents
Azathioprine: 1-3 mg/kg/day (usual maximum dose, 100 mg/day)
Cyclophosphamide: See text for intravenous administration under "Therapy"; not recommended orally because of the risk for hemorrhagic cystitis
Methotrexate: 10 mg/m²/wk; safety and efficacy in SLE not yet established

These doses for typical uses only. Full prescribing information provided by the manufacturer should be consulted for possible side effects, interactions, and other consequences of the use of these medications.

Cushingoid facies, cataracts, avascular necrosis, and other complications were common.[6]

In the late 1980s, the systematic use of intravenous cyclophosphamide became common. It has been argued that corticosteroids are preferable to cytotoxic agents, because corticosteroids do not have life-threatening side effects. However, overt suicide resulting from the psychosocial stresses of cushingoid facies and chronic disease has occurred, and covert suicide in the form of noncompliance (e.g., stopped corticosteroids against medical advice) is not uncommon.[48]

Although the therapeutic role of cytotoxic drugs remains controversial, data supporting their safety and efficacy are convincing.[56] Concerns regarding sterility, risk of infections, and risk of neoplasia limit their use to children with significant disease activity that is unresponsive to acceptable doses of corticosteroids. New studies in which lesser doses of cyclophosphamide or other immunosuppressive drugs are combined with agents such as rituximab show great promise for increased efficacy and reduced toxicity.[16,56]

Immunosuppressives have been used in those with CNS disease with varying results.[6] Although a few centers report good results using high-dose prednisone and azathioprine over both 5- and 10-year periods, others have had less success with this regimen. Controlled trials in adult patients with SLE have found cyclophosphamide to be as effective as, and less toxic than, the combination of cyclophosphamide and azathioprine.[57] Proper stratification of patients at study entry may be the key to resolving these issues. Excluding the patients whose CNS symptoms are the result of aCL-associated thrombosis is also important.

The systematic use of cyclophosphamide is associated with a far greater and faster improvement in clinical parameters and sense of well-being, while allowing a more rapid reduction in corticosteroid doses. A large number of children initially treated with systematic intravenous cyclophosphamide for a period of 3 years are now off all immunosuppressive agents and disease free.[12] As noted in the section on nephritis, newer agents such as mycophenolate mofetil and biologic agents are promising. Their ultimate safety and utility in childhood remain uncertain. It is hoped that the combined use of a variety of agents, such as those used in the treatment of childhood neoplasms, will ultimately lead to the development of a regimen with maximum efficacy and minimum toxicity.

For children and adolescents with SLE, the desire to avoid iatrogenic injury must be balanced against the goal of sustained survival. Cyclophosphamides administered with vigorous intravenous hydration and careful inpatient monitoring have proved to be both safe and effective.[12] Although sterility and late-onset neoplasia are theoretical risks, avascular necrosis, cataracts, and cushingoid facies are commonly experienced by children receiving high doses of corticosteroids over a prolonged period.

At the Hospital for Special Surgery in New York City, children who fail to respond adequately to corticosteroid therapy receive a combination of intravenous cyclophosphamide and rituximab according to a well-defined protocol. Children initially receive 750 mg/m² of rituximab (maximum 1 g), followed by 750 mg/m² of cyclophosphamide in 24 hours. Both drugs are repeated 14 days later. If the child does not have significant renal disease, then this regimen is repeated at 24, 26, 76, and 78 weeks. The corticosteroids are rapidly tapered (as tolerated), and hydroxychloroquine is maintained. For children with significant renal disease, additional doses of cyclophosphamide (750 mg/m²) are administered at weeks 6, 12, and 18.

Some of these children initially treated with systematic cyclophosphamide are now well and have their own children more than 20 years later, and are off all medications despite having biopsy-proven DPGN when therapy was initiated. Children with DPGN who received the new combination of cyclophosphamide and rituximab remain well on minimal doses of prednisone 5 years after their last treatment with either medication.

For those with only moderate disease activity but persistent hypocomplementemia, therapy with mycophenolate mofetil (up to 1 g twice daily) may be beneficial. The major risks associated with the aggressive use of cytotoxic agents are bone-marrow suppression (often complicated by infection), hemorrhagic cystitis, infertility, and the induction of neoplastic disease (early or late). Infectious complications can be minimized by careful evaluation before administration of each dose of cyclophosphamide and by a high index of suspicion for infection if the patient experiences difficulty during the period of maximal marrow suppression after each dose. Cystitis, infertility, and the induction of neoplastic disease are the remaining concerns that are substantially reduced by the new regimen, which reduces the total exposure to cyclophosphamide by almost two thirds (6 g/m² total cyclophosphamide dose instead of 17 g/m²).

Studies of older patients with SLE indicate that the risk of sterility after cytotoxic drug therapy increases with age. Premenarchal children may have some protection. In children with amenorrhea that is secondary to active SLE, menses often return during cyclophosphamide therapy. Many successful pregnancies have been reported after cyclophosphamide therapy in adolescents, and one pregnancy that originated during cyclophosphamide therapy (despite counseling) was successfully carried to term without difficulty. (No further

cytotoxic agents were administered after the pregnancy was discovered.) However, no definitive data concerning the risks of infertility or neoplasia are available for children with SLE. Both conditions have occurred in children who received cyclophosphamide as part of multidrug regimens for neoplastic disease. Families should be warned about these concerns before therapy is begun, and patients should be selected accordingly. With corticosteroid therapy alone, many children progress inexorably to renal failure.

Methotrexate, cyclosporine, and intravenous gamma globulin all have been used in small numbers of children with SLE. Sufficient data have not been obtained to judge their efficacy. Methotrexate must be used with great caution in the presence of renal compromise.

Recently, autologous stem cell transplantation has received extensive attention for the treatment of rheumatic diseases including SLE, and some teenagers are included in the reported series.[21] Whether the benefits of autologous stem cell transplantation will endure remains unclear. The early European Bone Marrow Transplant (BMT) consortium results already describe patients after autologous stem cell transplantation. Recognizing that SLE is a chronic, recurrent disease that may require prolonged therapy is increasing, even in the absence of active disease. However, for the patient with continued active disease in spite of intensive chemotherapy, these regimens may be warranted. Significant improvements in the therapy of children with SLE will require careful collaborative studies.

PROGNOSIS

The prognosis for children and adolescents with SLE has dramatically improved over the past 20 years. With improved antiinflammatory therapy and pediatric care, the 10-year survival rates are now approaching 90%.[48] Nonetheless, significant numbers of children continue to progress to chronic renal failure and/or death (Table 40-4 and Box 40-2).

Often, children and adolescents with SLE progress poorly because of the inability of the child and family to cope with the chronic, relapsing nature of the disease. Success requires a sustained relationship between the child and family and the treating facility. Institutions serving stable populations with good socioeconomic status and easy access to care consistently report superior survival rates to those serving disadvantaged populations.[58] Poor understanding of the importance of medications for silent manifestations of SLE,

TABLE 40-4 Incidence of Adverse Outcomes in 72 Children with Systemic Lupus Erythematosus

OUTCOME	INCIDENCE (%)
Renal failure	15
Severe central nervous system disease	11
Stroke	1
Chronic thrombocytopenia	7
Chronic active disease	56
Death	18

Box 40-2 Predictors of Poor Prognosis in Childhood Systemic Lupus Erythematosus

1. Persistent anemia: hemoglobin <10 g/dL for longer than 6 months
2. Persistent hypertension: diastolic blood pressure >90 mm Hg for longer than 6 months
3. Persistent hematuria: >20 red blood cells (RBCs) per high-power field (HPF) for longer than 6 months
4. Pulmonary hypertension
5. Recurrent emergency admissions

such as hypertension, remains a familiar cause of morbidity. These preventable deaths have become increasingly frustrating, since the ability to control the manifestations of SLE has improved.

The quality of survival must be addressed in efforts to improve the outcomes for children and adolescents with SLE. Long-term survival of a cushingoid adolescent with aseptic necrosis who requires dialysis may not be satisfactory to the patient. Platt and colleagues[48] described three young adults who died more than 10 years after diagnosis; two of the three died after they had discontinued their medications against medical advice.

Although end-stage renal failure and dialysis have been associated with decreased SLE activity in some reports, both children and adolescents requiring long-term dialysis often fare poorly. In one series, 9 of 16 children with SLE succumbed within 5 years of beginning dialysis.[59]

For children and adolescents with SLE, a satisfactory outcome is measured in decades. The goal of health care professionals should be to report a 90% 50-year survival. Children without renal disease who have survived 5 years are at low risk. Children with renal disease of any type, however, remain at risk. Gradual progression to renal failure over 5 to 10 years or longer, despite clinically inactive disease, has been reported in both children and adults with SLE.[59] Health care professionals dealing with children and adolescents who have SLE must strive to aid patients and their families through a normally difficult period under even more difficult circumstances. Every effort must be made to guarantee the availability of appropriate services. Not only must medical therapy be aggressive; so should patient and family education to ensure compliance. With the increasing presence of specialized pediatric centers for children with rheumatic diseases and growing numbers of collaborative studies to determine optimal therapy, survival measured in decades should now become the norm.

SUMMARY

The information in this chapter can be summarized as follows:

1. Children and adolescents represent both a special challenge and opportunity. Success in caring for this group requires an awareness of the complex interactions among the children's illness, the needs of their family, and their own needs as developing individuals.

2. Childhood-onset SLE has been recognized since the early 1900s. Although it is frequently described as a more severe disease than adult SLE, this description may be the result of the failure to properly diagnose many mild cases.

3. No thorough epidemiologic studies of SLE in childhood have been completed. It is estimated that the annual incidence is approximately 0.6 per 100,000, and that between 5000 and 10,000 children in the United States currently have SLE. The incidence of SLE is much higher in female children than in male children and in non-Caucasians than in Caucasians.

4. The cause of SLE remains unknown, but the high frequency of immunologic abnormalities among family members of children with SLE suggests that a combination of genetic and environmental factors plays an important role. The presence of SSA/Ro in a large proportion of the mothers of young children with SLE may indicate predisposing genetic factors in the family. SLE is also more frequent in children who have defects of the immune system, suggesting that defective antigen processing may predispose a child to the development of SLE.

5. The most common clinical manifestations of SLE are fever, malaise, and weight loss, but these are nonspecific manifestations of many chronic ailments. The typical butterfly rash is present only in approximately one third of children with SLE.

6. Renal disease occurs in two thirds of children with SLE in most reported series. Although the renal disease may be mild, severe DPGN remains a leading cause of morbidity in childhood SLE. Mild renal disease can often be controlled with corticosteroid therapy, but active renal disease that does not fully respond to corticosteroids and DPGN with a falling creatinine clearance require therapy with cytotoxic agents. Children with active SLE progress poorly on dialysis.

7. All of the CNS manifestations described in adults with SLE also occur in children. Behavioral disturbances, which may be ascribed to acting out by an adolescent with SLE, often represent CNS disease that may respond to increased therapy. Chorea is also seen more commonly among children with SLE.

8. Pulmonary involvement in childhood SLE takes many forms, including pleurisy, pleural effusions, pulmonary fibrosis, and pulmonary hemorrhage. Diaphragmatic dysfunction is common and may be the underlying factor predisposing a child to recurrent episodes of pneumonia. Pulmonary hypertension is often a life-threatening complication. Abnormal pulmonary function may be present despite a normal chest radiograph.

9. Musculoskeletal manifestations of SLE include arthritis and mild inflammatory myopathy, and they are often predominant at presentation. Both are responsive to corticosteroid therapy, however, and rarely contribute to long-term morbidity. Avascular necrosis is the exception, which may occur as a complication of SLE with or without corticosteroid therapy, and ultimately requires joint replacement.

10. Dermatologic involvement is common in childhood SLE but is rarely a significant problem except when the face is prominently disfigured, causing psychological problems (see Figure 40-1). DLE is unusual in childhood.

11. Cardiac manifestations of SLE include pericarditis and myocarditis, sometimes with recurrent effusions, and can usually be controlled with NSAIDs or low-dose corticosteroids. Valvular involvement is common and may predispose the child to bacterial endocarditis. Careful consideration should be given to antibiotic prophylaxis whenever bacteremia is expected. Premature myocardial infarctions have occurred in young adults, with significant atherosclerosis after prolonged corticosteroid therapy.

12. Gastrointestinal manifestations of childhood SLE are varied. Nonspecific findings such as chronic abdominal pain and anorexia are frequent, and significant bowel infarction may occur. Pneumatosis intestinalis may result from recurrent microvascular insults.

13. Infection is a major cause of morbidity and mortality in children and adolescents with SLE. Active SLE predisposes children to infection. Whether a child's rapid deterioration is the result of infection or active SLE is often unclear. In this setting, increased doses of both corticosteroids and antibiotics may be necessary. Reticuloendothelial system overload and functional asplenia may predispose children with active SLE to a rapid progression of sepsis.

14. Hematologic manifestations are common in children and adolescents with SLE; most are nonspecific. Thrombocytopenia is a frequent presenting complaint, particularly in young boys, and menorrhagia may also be a significant problem in adolescent girls. As in adults, the presence of aCL antibodies predisposes children to clotting dysfunction and stroke.

15. Laboratory manifestations of childhood SLE are identical to those of adult SLE. One unique concern is the awareness that a positive serologic result for syphilis in a child or adolescent is reported to the school district and warrants prompt investigation by public welfare authorities. Families should be warned about this possibility, and inquiries should be promptly diverted to the physician.

16. Therapy for childhood-onset SLE is similar to that for adult-onset disease. Because of the increased burdens of growth and development on renal function, however, instituting aggressive intervention earlier in children with DPGN may be important. Developing therapies that provide acceptable 50-year survival, not 5- or 10-year survival, for children and adolescents with SLE must be the goal. The systematic administration of cytotoxic drugs may provide superior quality of life and long-term survival.

References

1. James JA, Kaufman KM, Farris AD, et al: An increased prevalence of Epstein–Barr virus infection in young patients suggests a possible etiology for systemic lupus erythematosus. *J Clin Invest* 100:3019–3026, 1997.
2. Meislin AG, Rothfield N: Systemic lupus erythematosus in childhood. Analysis of 42 cases, with comparative data on 200 adult cases followed concurrently. *Pediatrics* 42:37–49, 1968.
3. King KK, Kornreich HK, Bernstein BH, et al: The clinical spectrum of systemic lupus erythematosus in childhood. Proceedings of the conference on rheumatic diseases of childhood. *Arthritis Rheum* 20(2 Suppl):287–294, 1977.
4. Sequeira JH, Balean H: Lupus erythematosus: a clinical study of seventy-one cases. *Br J Dermatol* 14:367–379, 1902.
5. Singsen BH: Rheumatic diseases of childhood. *Rheum Dis Clin North Am* 16:581–599, 1990.
6. Arbuckle MR, McClain MT, Rubertone MV, et al: Development of autoantibodies before the clinical onset of systemic lupus erythematosus. *N Engl J Med* 349(16):1526–1533, 2003.
7. Tan EM, Cohen AS, Fries JF, et al: Special article: the 1982 revised criteria for the classification of systemic lupus erythematosus. *Arthritis Rheum* 25:1271–1277, 1982.
8. Iqbal S, Sher MR, Good RA, et al: Diversity in presenting manifestations of systemic lupus erythematosus in children. *J Pediatr* 135:500–505, 1999.
9. Stamenkovic I, Favre H, Donath A, et al: Renal biopsy in SLE irrespective of clinical findings: long-term follow-up. *Clin Nephrol* 26:109–115, 1986.
10. Lehman TJA, Mouradian JA: Systemic lupus erythematosus. In Holliday MA, Barrat TM, Avner ED, editors: *Pediatric nephrology*, ed 3, Baltimore, 1994, Williams & Wilkins, pp 849–870.
11. Ostuni PA, Lazzarin P, Pengo V, et al: Renal artery thrombosis and hypertension in a 13 year old girl with antiphospholipid syndrome. *Ann Rheum Dis* 49:184–187, 1990.
12. Lehman TJA, Onel KB: Intermittent intravenous cyclophosphamide arrests progression of the renal chronicity index in childhood systemic lupus erythematosus. *J Pediatrics* 136:243–247, 2000.
13. Wang LC, Yang YH, Lu MY, et al: Retrospective analysis of the renal outcome of pediatric lupus nephritis. *Clin Rheumatol* 23(4):318–323, 2004.
14. Macdermott EJ, Adams A, Lehman TJ: Systemic lupus erythematosus in children: current and emerging therapies. *Lupus* 16:677–683, 2007.
15. Marks SD, Patey S, Brogan PA, et al: B lymphocyte depletion therapy in children with refractory systemic lupus erythematosus. *Arthritis Rheum* 52(10):3168–3174, 2005.
16. Podolskaya A, Stadermann M, Pilkington C, et al: B cell depletion therapy for 19 patients with refractory systemic lupus erythematosus. *Arch Dis Child* 93(5):401–406, 2008.
17. Brunner HI, Higgins GC, Wiers K, et al: Prospective validation of the provisional criteria for the evaluation of response to therapy in childhood-onset systemic lupus erythematosus. *Arthritis Care Res* 62:335–344, 2010.
18. Sinclair A, Appel G, Dooley MA, et al: Mycophenolate mofetil as induction and maintenance therapy for lupus nephritis: rationale and protocol for the randomized, controlled Aspreva Lupus Management Study (ALMS). *Lupus* 16:972–980, 2007.
19. Edelbauer M, Jungraithmayr T, Zimmerhackl LB: Rituximab in childhood systemic lupus erythematosus refractory to conventional immunosuppression. Case report. *Pediatr Nephrol* 20(6):811–813, 2005.
20. van Vollenhoven RF, Gunnarsson I, Welin-Henriksson E, et al: Biopsy-verified response of severe lupus nephritis to treatment with rituximab (anti-CD20 monoclonal antibody) plus cyclophosphamide after biopsy-documented failure to respond to cyclophosphamide alone. *Scand J Rheumatol* 33(6):423–427, 2004.
21. Burt RK: BMT for severe autoimmune diseases: an idea whose time has come. *Oncology (Williston Park)* 11(7):1001–1014, 1997.
22. Muscal E, Brey RL: Neurologic manifestations of systemic lupus erythematosus in children and adults. *Neurol Clin* 28:61–73, 2010.
23. Klein-Gitelman M, Brunner HI: The impact and implications of neuropsychiatric systemic lupus erythematosus in adolescents. *Curr Rheumatol Rep* 11:212–217, 2009.
24. Levy DM, Ardoin SP, Schanberg LE: Neurocognitive impairment in children and adolescents with systemic lupus erythematosus. *Nat Clin Pract Rheumatol* 5:106–114, 2009.
25. Benseler SM, Silverman ED: Neuropsychiatric involvement in pediatric systemic lupus erythematosus. *Lupus* 16(8):564–571, 2007.
26. Olfat MO, Al-Mayouf SM, Muzaffer MA: Pattern of neuropsychiatric manifestations and outcome in juvenile systemic lupus erythematosus. *Clin Rheumatol* 23(5):395–399, 2004.
27. Ahmadieh H, Roodpeyma S, Azarmina M, et al: Bilateral simultaneous optic neuritis in childhood systemic lupus erythematosus. *J Neuroophthalmol* 14:84–86, 1994.
28. Hisashi K, Komune S, Taira T, et al: Anticardiolipin antibody-induced sudden profound sensorineural hearing loss. *Am J Otolaryngol* 14:275–277, 1993.
29. Avcin T, Benseler SM, Tyrrell PN, et al: A followup study of antiphospholipid antibodies and associated neuropsychiatric manifestations in 137 children with systemic lupus erythematosus. *Arthritis Rheum* 59:206–213, 2008.
30. Bertsias GK, Ioannidis JP, Aringer M, et al: EULAR recommendations for the management of systemic lupus erythematosus with neuropsychiatric manifestations: report of a task force of the EULAR standing committee for clinical affairs. *Ann Rheum Dis* 69:2074–2082, 2010.
31. Moorthy LN, Peterson MG, Hassett A, et al: Impact of lupus on school attendance and performance. *Lupus* 19:620–627, 2010.
32. Moorthy LN, Peterson MG, Hassett AL, et al: Relationship between health-related quality of life and SLE activity and damage in children over time. *Lupus* 18:622–629, 2009.
33. Delgado EA, Malleson PN, Pirie GE, et al: Pulmonary manifestations of childhood onset systemic lupus erythematosus. *Semin Arthritis Rheum* 29:285–293, 1990.
34. de Jongste JC, Neijens HJ, Duiverman EJ, et al: Respiratory tract disease in systemic lupus erythematosus. *Arch Dis Child* 61:478–483, 1986.
35. Nadorra RL, Landing BH: Pulmonary lesions in childhood onset systemic lupus erythematosus: analysis of 26 cases, and summary of literature. *Pediatr Pathol* 7(1):1–18, 1987.
36. Trapani S, Camiciottoli G, Ermini M, et al: Pulmonary involvement in juvenile systemic lupus erythematosus: a study on long function in patients asymptomatic for respiratory disease. *Lupus* 7:545–550, 1998.
37. Ragsdale CG, Petty RE, Cassidy JT, et al: The clinical progression of apparent juvenile rheumatoid arthritis to systemic lupus erythematosus. *J Rheumatol* 7:50–55, 1980.
38. Bergstein J, Wiens C, Fish AJ, et al: Avascular necrosis of bone in systemic lupus erythematosus. *J Pediatr* 85:31–35, 1974.
39. Rider LG, Sherry DD, Glass ST: Neonatal lupus erythematosus simulating transient myasthenia gravis at presentation. *J Pediatr* 118:417–419, 1991.
40. Kreuter A, Gambichler T, Breuckmann F, et al: Pimecrolimus 1% cream for cutaneous lupus erythematosus. *J Am Acad Dermatol* 51(3):407–410, 2004.
41. Guevara JP, Clark BJ, Athreya BH: Point prevalence of cardiac abnormalities in children with systemic lupus erythematosus. *J Rheumatol* 28(4):854–938, 2001.
42. Lehman TJ, Palmeri ST, Hastings C, et al: Bacterial endocarditis complicating systemic lupus erythematosus. *J Rheumatol* 10:655–658, 1983.
43. Schanberg LE, Sandborg C: Dyslipoproteinemia and premature atherosclerosis in pediatric systemic lupus erythematosus. *Curr Rheumatol Rep* 6(6):425–433, 2004.
44. Schanberg LE, Sandborg C, Barnhart HX, et al: Atherosclerosis Prevention in Pediatric Lupus Erythematosus Investigators. Premature atherosclerosis in pediatric systemic lupus erythematosus: risk factors for increased carotid intima-media thickness in the atherosclerosis prevention in pediatric lupus erythematosus cohort. *Arthritis Rheum* 60:1496–1507, 2009.
45. Richer O, Ulinski T, Lemelle I, et al: Abdominal manifestations in childhood-onset systemic lupus erythematosus. *Ann Rheum Dis* 66:174–178, 2007.
46. Nadorra RL, Nakazato Y, Landing BH: Pathologic features of gastrointestinal tract lesions in childhood-onset systemic lupus erythematosus: study of 26 patients, with review of the literature. *Pediatr Pathol* 7:245–259, 1987.
47. Malleson P, Petty RE, Nadel H, et al: Functional asplenia in childhood onset systemic lupus erythematosus. *J Rheumatol* 15:1648–1652, 1988.
48. Platt JL, Burke BA, Fish AJ, et al: Systemic lupus erythematosus in the first two decades of life. *Am J Kidney Dis* 2(Suppl 1):212–222, 1982.
49. Ginzler E, Diamond H, Kaplan D, et al: Computer analysis of factors influencing frequency of infection in systemic lupus erythematosus. *Arthritis Rheum* 21:37–44, 1978.
50. Campos LM, Kiss MH, D'Amico EA, et al: Antiphospholipid antibodies and antiphospholipid syndrome in 57 children and adolescents with systemic lupus erythematosus. *Lupus* 12(11):820–826, 2003.
51. Gillespie JP, Lindsley CB, Linshaw MA, et al: Childhood systemic lupus erythematosus with negative antinuclear antibody test. *J Pediatr* 98:578–581, 1981.

52. Lehman TJA, Hanson V, Singsen BH, et al: The role of antibodies directed against double-stranded DNA in the manifestations of systemic lupus erythematosus in childhood. *J Pediatr* 96:657–661, 1980.

53. Cronin ME, Balow JE, Tsokos GC: Immunoglobulin deficiency in patients with systemic lupus erythematosus. *Clin Exp Rheumatol* 7:359–364, 1989.

54. McKenna CH, Schroeter AL, Kierland RR, et al: The fluorescent treponemal antibody absorbed (FTA-ABS) test beading phenomenon in connective tissue diseases. *Mayo Clin Proc* 48:545–548, 1973.

55. Brunner HI, Klein-Gitelman MS, Ying J, et al: Corticosteroid use in childhood-onset systemic lupus erythematosus—practice patterns at four pediatric rheumatology centers. *Clin Exp Rheumatol* 27:155–162, 2009.

56. Marks SD, Tullus K: Modern therapeutic strategies for paediatric systemic lupus erythematosus and lupus nephritis. *Acta Paediatr* 99:967–974, 2010.

57. Balow JE, Austin HA, 3rd, Muenz LR, et al: Effect of treatment on the evolution of renal abnormalities in lupus nephritis. *N Engl J Med* 311:491–495, 1984.

58. Kamphuis S, Silverman ED: Prevalence and burden of pediatric-onset systemic lupus erythematosus. *Nat Rev Rheumatol* 6:538–546, 2010.

59. McCurdy DK, Lehman TJA, Bernstein B, et al: Lupus nephritis: prognostic factors in children. *Pediatrics* 89:240–246, 1992.

60. Cassidy JT, Sullivan DB, Petty RE, et al. Lupus nephritis and encephalopathy. Proceedings of the conference of rheumatic diseases in childhood. *Arthritis Rheum.* 20(2 Suppl):315–322, 1977.

61. Kimberly AA, Lockshin MD, Sherman RL, Beary JF, Mouradian J, Cheigh JS. Medicine (Baltimore). Jul;60(4):277–87, 1981.

62. Kostiala RP, Kostiala I. Enzyme-linked immunosorbent assay (ELISA) for IgM, IgG and IgA class antibodies against Candida albicans antigens: development and comparison with other methods. Sabouraudia. Jul;19(2):123–34, 1981.

Chapter

41

Mixed Connective Tissue Disease and Undifferentiated Connective Tissue Disease

Robert W. Hoffman and Eric L. Greidinger

MIXED CONNECTIVE TISSUE DISEASE

Historical Perspective

The first full-length publication describing what the authors called *mixed connective tissue disease* (MCTD) was reported from Stanford by Sharp and colleagues in 1972.[1] The patients described in this publication were proposed to be distinct, based on the presence of high levels of antibodies against an extractable nuclear antigen (ENA) that was ribonuclease (RNase)- and trypsin-sensitive. Subsequently, it was shown that ENA contained both the RNase- and trypsin-sensitive ribonucleoprotein (RNP) antigen, and the RNase- and trypsin-resistant Smith (Sm) antigens. Current knowledge recognizes that the RNP antigen consists of a complex containing a series of small nuclear RNPs (snRNP) including three polypeptides (70kD, 70kA, and 70kC) that associate noncovalently with U1-RNA as part of the spliceosome complex.[2,3] The spliceosome is found in the nucleus of eukaryotic cells and has the physiologic function of assisting in the excision of introns and the processing of premessenger RNA to mature messenger RNA (mRNA). The RNP antigen is also known by a variety of other names including nuclear RNP (nRNP), U1-snRNP, and U1-RNP.[3]

Clinically, the patients initially reported by Sharp and colleagues[1] were described as having overlapping features of systemic lupus erythematosus (SLE), scleroderma, and polymyositis. The patients were believed to be distinctive, based on the absence of serious renal or central nervous system involvement and their favorable clinical response to treatment with corticosteroids.[1] The initial studies on MCTD that were begun at Stanford continued at the University of Missouri–Columbia by Sharp and colleagues, beginning in 1969. Sharp's collaborative studies with five other academic medical centers, including the University of Missouri–Columbia, Stanford University, the Mayo Clinic, the University of Cincinnati, and Northwestern University, resulted in a seminal paper in 1976 describing patients with MCTD.[4] Numerous studies on MCTD by Sharp and colleagues followed in the ensuing decades from the University of Missouri–Columbia, including prospective longitudinal studies on a large cohort of patients, some of whom had been followed for as long as 30 years.[5-9] Dr. Sharp has published a historical review describing the collective body of this work.[10] The work of a large number of additional individuals has substantially advanced the understanding of the clinical, immunologic, and genetic features of MCTD since its original description, now over 3 decades ago.

Definition

Four widely recognized criteria for the classification of patients with MCTD have been published.[11-13] Some authors currently favor the criteria proposed by Alarcon-Segovia and Villarreal, and later validated by Alarcon-Segovia and Cardiel, because of its simplicity and perceived general applicability.[11,12] This proposed classification algorithm is shown in Box 41-1. The other published classification criteria are substantially more cumbersome to apply outside of a clinical research setting. Unfortunately, no international consensus conference has addressed the topic of disease classification criteria in MCTD since the international conference on MCTD held in Japan in 1986.[11] Recently, however, new research on the classification of MCTD has been published using Rasch analysis, which is an alternative statistical approach applied to the complex issue of disease classification.[14] This and other new approaches to the challenges of disease classification may help inform the selection of patients for future clinical trials.

Acknowledging that the controversy exists in the literature over the nomenclature of MCTD is important. Although most critics accept that a recognizable group of patients have *MCTD* a dispute continues over the nomenclature and whether MCTD should be considered a distinct disease rather than a syndrome on the continuum of another rheumatic disease, such as SLE or scleroderma. Some have used the eponym *Sharp's syndrome* for MCTD, in part to avoid confusion between the general concept of rheumatic overlap syndromes and the more specific diagnosis of MCTD, in which autoimmunity to RNP determinants is required.

Since the initial description of MCTD by Sharp and others,[1] the concept of MCTD has evolved.[1,5-10] In the last 2 decades, considerable advances have been made in areas that assist in the classification of rheumatic diseases; these notably include the identification of genetic markers of rheumatic diseases and more extensive characterization of the immunologic profiles associated with particular conditions.[15] Studies using these advances have been of significant importance in clarifying the classification of systemic rheumatic diseases, including MCTD. For example, an increased frequency of human leukocyte antigen (HLA)–DR4 has been shown in patients with MCTD, compared with healthy control subjects in population-based studies performed on several continents, including North America, South America, and Europe,[15-19] a pattern distinct from that observed in SLE or scleroderma. Genome-wide association studies (GWASs) have also suggested that genes outside of the major histocompatibility complex (MHC) on chromosome 6, which encodes a number of key immunologic molecules including those for HLA-DR, may also contribute to a susceptibility to MCTD.[20]

MCTD has likewise been observed to be distinct from SLE regarding the pattern of reactivity to epitopes of the heterogeneous nuclear RNP (hnRNP)-A2/B1 antigen recognized by B and T cells.[21-23] Thus

Box 41-1 Diagnostic Criteria for Mixed Connective Tissue Disease*

Serologic Criterion
Antiribonucleoprotein (anti-RNP) antibody must be present at a moderately high level in serum.
  AND

Clinical Criteria
At least three out of the following five clinical findings must be present:
  1. Edema of the hand
  2. Synovitis
  3. Myositis
  4. Raynaud phenomenon
  5. Acrosclerosis
  This must include either synovitis or myositis

*Anti-RNP was defined in the Alarcon-Segovia and Villarreal[11,12] study using hemagglutination. A titer ≥1:1600 was required in this study to be considered moderate or high. The range and cut-off value for a positive or for a high-positive value depend on the specific assay used.

TABLE 41-1 Clinical Features of Mixed Connective Tissue Disease*

CLINICAL FEATURE	AT DIAGNOSIS (%)	CUMULATIVE FINDINGS (%)
Raynaud phenomenon	89	96
Arthralgia or arthritis	85	96
Swollen hands	60	66
Esophageal dysmotility	47	66
Pulmonary disease	43	66
Sclerodactyly	34	49
Pleuritis or pericarditis	34	43
Rash	30	53
Myositis	28	51
Renal disease	2	11
Neurologic disease	0	17

*From Burdt MA, Hoffman RW, Deutscher SL, et al: Long-term outcome in mixed connective tissue disease: longitudinal clinical and serologic findings. *Arthritis Rheum* 42(5):899–909, 1999.

as newer classification criteria of MCTD are developed, they should take full advantage of the advances in methodologic approaches to disease classification, immunologic markers, and genetic markers that might be particularly useful in defining the relationships between MCTD and other rheumatic conditions.[14,15,20]

Finally, studies on disease pathogenesis serve to refine and more clearly delineate the fundamental understanding of MCTD.[22-27] Studies of autoantibodies and T cells in disease pathogenesis have advanced the understanding of the contributions of both B cells and T cells in MCTD, whereas recent studies in an animal model support a direct role for T- and B-cell immunity against the U1-70kD polypeptide of the RNP antigen in disease pathogenesis. Studies in murine models have revealed the importance that the U1-70kD self-antigen may have in driving the disease—in that a single immunization with autologous U1-70kD polypeptide of the RNP antigen plus U1-RNA can induce anti-RNP immunity and autoimmune lung disease characteristic of MCTD.[27] Disease pathogenesis and animal models are discussed in greater detail later in this chapter (see Pathogenesis).

Clinical Features
General Features
In the absence of a universally accepted classification criteria and with the current understanding of MCTD having evolved over the past 3 decades, a review of the literature on MCTD poses some challenges. This is particularly true for rare complications of the disease described as case reports or small series of patients in the literature. Despite these challenges, numerous well-characterized clinical series are now reporting on substantial numbers of patients from across the world that define the clinical features of MCTD.[1,3-9,28-34] A summary of the most common clinical features of MCTD is shown in Table 41-1.[3-9]

The primary clinical features of MCTD are Raynaud phenomenon, swollen fingers or hands, arthralgia with or without associated arthritis, esophageal reflux or dysmotility, acrosclerosis (also known as *sclerodactyly*), mild myositis, and pulmonary involvement of a variety of forms (see Table 41-1). Additional clinical features that have been commonly reported include malar rash, alopecia, anemia, leukopenia, lymphadenopathy, and trigeminal neuralgia. The characteristic serologic findings are a high-titer fluorescent antinuclear antibody (FANA) test result with a speckled pattern and the presence of antibodies to RNP at moderate to high levels in the serum; some authors require the absence of antibodies to Sm to classify patients as having MCTD.[7] In patients with major end-organ

manifestations of SLE that are uncommon in historical MCTD cohorts, such as diffuse proliferative nephritis, MCTD may also frequently be excluded from the diagnosis.

Epidemiologic Characteristics
Currently, a paucity of epidemiologic data exist on MCTD. A nationwide multicenter collaborative survey on MCTD from Japan reported a prevalence of 2.7%.[33] MCTD prevalence has been reported to be appreciably lower elsewhere in the world. Sharp and colleagues[7] have reported that at a tertiary referral center known for its expertise in MCTD observed the disease less frequently than SLE or rheumatoid arthritis (RA) but more commonly than polymyositis, dermatomyositis, or scleroderma. Although ethnic differences have been identified in the rates of development of anti-RNP antibodies and ethnic differences appear to exist in the prevalence of MCTD, the rate at which specific clinical manifestations appear among patients with MCTD from different ethnic groups has been quite consistent.[34]

Sex Distribution
MCTD is more common in women than it is in men. It appears to have a sex distribution similar to that observed in SLE.[7] In a Japanese nationwide survey, MCTD was found to have a female-to-male ratio of 16:1,[33] whereas the longitudinal prospective clinical series of Burdt and others[8] reported an 11:1 ratio of women to men among patients from a tertiary referral center in the midwestern United States. Lundberg and Hedfors[32] reported a 4:1 ratio among patients selected for presence of anti-RNP antibodies rather than MCTD, per se, who were studied at Huddinge University Hospital in Stockholm, Sweden.

Skin
Raynaud phenomenon is one of the most common manifestations of MTCD in all clinical series.[1,3-9,28-34] It has been reported to be present at diagnosis in 90% to 95% of patients.[3-9] It may diminish in severity or resolve over time in some patients. A small number of patients will have associated digital infarcts. Pathologic and radiographic studies have reported the presence of an obliterative vasculopathy in these patients. Digital infarcts appear to correlate with the presence of severe obliterative vasculopathy. As in other organs, the vascular endothelium appears to be a major target of the pathologic process in MCTD.

Swollen fingers or swelling of the hand is very common in patients with MCTD, particularly at the onset of disease.[1,3-9,28-34] Total hand edema can occur but is less common. Acrosclerosis (also known as *sclerodactyly*) occurs with or without proximal scleroderma and is typically a later manifestation of the disease. Nail-fold vascular changes identified by unaided direct visual inspection or by one of several methods of capillary microscopy occur in those with MCTD. These changes are characterized by vascular dilation and vessel loss or *dropout*.

Rashes are present in 50% to 60% of patients.[1,3-9,28-34] Photosensitive and malar rashes similar to those typical of SLE have been reported to be common. Discoid lesions are also occasionally present. The scleroderma-like features of squared telangiectasia over the hands and face or periungual telangiectasia and sclerodactyly with or without calcinosis cutis also occur in some patients with MCTD. In contrast, truncal scleroderma is rare or absent in most series.[1,3-9,28-34]

Gottron papules or a heliotrope rash, typical of dermatomyositis, is also seen in MCTD. Erythema nodosum, hyperpigmentation, or hypopigmentation of the skin is uncommon but has been reported. Nodules appear to be uncommon, despite the fact that arthritis and rheumatoid factor are common features of the disease.

The sicca complex has been found to be present in approximately one fourth to as high as one half of all patients with MCTD.[9] Although many patients with MCTD have anti–**S**jögren syndrome antigen A (anti-SSA/Ro) and anti–Sjögren syndrome antigen B (anti-SSB/La) antibodies, a poor correlation exists between the presence of these antibodies and clinical sicca.[9]

Oral and genital ulcers have been reported to occur in patients with MCTD.[1,3-9,28-34] More severe lesions resulting in nasal septal perforation have also been described.

Joints

Arthralgia, like Raynaud phenomenon, is reported by almost all patients with MCTD.[1,3-9,28-35] Inflammatory arthritis is also very common in MCTD. Arthritis ultimately develops in 50% to 60% of patients. Rheumatoid factor is also common in MCTD, occurring in 50% to 75% of patients. In fact, despite the fact that MCTD was initially observed among patients with overlapping features of SLE (e.g., scleroderma, polymyositis), patients with MCTD are now recognized as also having many features in common with RA. This includes an increased frequency of the HLA-DR4 susceptibility gene and immune responses against serum immune globulin (i.e., rheumatoid factor), as well as immunity against hnRNP in the form of antibodies and T cells.[16-19] Some patients with MCTD may fulfill the classification criteria for RA. In contrast to patients with RA, however, most patients with MCTD have no bony erosions or only small marginal erosions with well-demarcated edges. Occasionally, patients will develop RA-like deformities, including boutonnière and swan neck deformities. More severe erosive arthropathy has been reported to be associated with HLA-DR4. A severe destructive arthritis including arthritis mutilans has been reported in MCTD. A Jaccoud-like arthropathy, similar to that observed in patients with SLE with or without erosions has also been reported.

Muscles

Myalgias are common in MCTD and are reported in 25% to 50% of patients. Myositis has been reported in 20% to 70% of patients.[1,3-9,28-34,36,37] The majority of patients with MCTD, however, do not develop clinical weakness.[3-9] Mild myositis with normal or modest elevation of muscle enzymes and normal electromyographic findings are most common in patients with MCTD; however, patients may be completely asymptomatic.[3-9] In contrast, however, myositis can be severe in some patients and can be indistinguishable from classic dermatomyositis. Patients such as these may meet the criteria for the classification of myositis. Lundberg and others[37] have published findings of a longitudinal study comparing patients with myositis with or without RNP antibodies. They found that patients with anti-RNP antibodies and myositis appeared to respond quickly to treatment with corticosteroids and that their myositis rarely relapsed

after the initial treatment. The pathologic muscle findings reported in MCTD include lymphocytic infiltrates that may be either perivascular (i.e., within the endomysium vessel wall) or perimysial focal fiber necrosis and occasionally perifascicular atrophy.

As in other chronic diseases, patients with MCTD may develop fibromyalgia; in some patients, this condition can be a clinically dominant aspect of the course and management.[38]

Pulmonary System

Pulmonary involvement can be a serious complication of MCTD and is the most common disease-related cause of death in those with MCTD.[1,3-9,28-34,39] Symptoms can include cough, dyspnea on exertion or at rest, and pleuritic chest pain. The physical examination may reveal basilar rales or a cardiac finding compatible with pulmonary hypertension. Often, however, the physical examination of the lungs is normal. More sensitive testing may be required to detect early pulmonary disease, such as pulmonary function testing with measurement of carbon monoxide diffusing capacity (DLCO).[7,8]

Decreased DLCO has been shown to be a helpful measurement for detecting pulmonary involvement in MCTD and appears to be effective when used for periodic screening of patients as an approach to identify those with early pulmonary disease.[7,8] Some patients may have an abnormal chest x-ray result. The most common radiographic findings are small, irregular opacities of the basilar or, less commonly, the middle lung fields, although changes can include interstitial abnormalities, pleural effusions, infiltrative lesions, or pleural thickening.

High-resolution computed tomography of the chest may reveal findings of fibrosis or alveolitis that are not detectable using plain-film radiography of the chest. Pathologic changes that may be found on biopsy or at autopsy include interstitial pneumonitis with or without fibrosis, obliterative vasculopathy of pulmonary vessels with intimal proliferation and medial hypertrophy of the pulmonary arteries and arterioles along with plexiform lesions, and either frank vasculitis or inflammatory perivascular cuffing. Although a diversity of patterns has been reported, clinical patterns of interstitial lung disease have most frequently been characterized as nonspecific interstitial pneumonitis or usual interstitial pneumonitis. Significant fibrosis is observed in only approximately one half of the patients with MCTD lung disease.

Pulmonary hypertension is the most common disease-related cause of death in those with MCTD.[8] In the longitudinal study of Burdt and others,[8] 13% (6 out of 47) of the patients died of pulmonary hypertension. In addition, evidence suggested that treatment of pulmonary hypertension in MCTD can result in prolonged survival in some patients; therefore early identification and proper treatment of pulmonary hypertension are very important (see "Treatment" section later in this chapter).[39] In the REVEAL (**R**andomized **EV**aluation of the **E**ffects of **A**nacetrapib through **L**ipid-modification) trial, pulmonary hypertension in patients with MCTD was found to have features distinct from those of pulmonary hypertension in scleroderma but a mortality rate similar to that of scleroderma-associated pulmonary hypertension.[40] In other studies, however, a subset of patients has been reported that responds to immunosuppressive therapy.[7,8,39,40] Rare pulmonary manifestations that have been reported in MCTD include pulmonary hemorrhage and diaphragm dysfunction.

Gastrointestinal System

Esophageal motility disorders with symptomatic esophageal reflux, including heartburn or regurgitation of food, are very common in patients with MCTD.[1,3-9,28-34,41] Less commonly, patients may experience pain or difficulty swallowing. Uncommon features of gastrointestinal involvement in MCTD that have been reported include pseudodiverticula along the antimesenteric border (similar to that described in scleroderma), mesenteric vasculitis, pancreatitis, bacterial overgrowth syndrome, malabsorption, protein-losing enteropathy, pseudoobstruction, serositis, colonic perforation, and gastrointestinal bleeding. In addition, reports in the literature describe chronic active hepatitis, biliary cirrhosis, and Budd-Chiari syndrome in patients with MCTD.

Cardiac System

Evidence of cardiac abnormalities is not uncommon in those with MCTD and is confirmed with methods such as electrocardiography or echocardiography.[1,3-9,28-34,42] Approximately 20% of patients will have abnormalities when examined with either electrocardiography or echocardiography. As previously discussed, pulmonary involvement is common in MCTD and may result in cardiopulmonary disease, such as pulmonary hypertension. Pulmonary hypertension can result in associated cardiac changes, such as right ventricular hypertrophy, right atrial enlargement, and intraventricular or atrioventricular electrical conduction abnormalities. Pericarditis has been reported to occur in 10% to 30% of patients with MCTD. Myocardial involvement may be found with severe myopathy or when pulmonary hypertension is present. Additional cardiac abnormalities that have been described include septal hypertrophy, various left ventricular abnormalities, mitral valve prolapse, intimal hyperplasia of the coronary arteries, and endocardial abnormalities. Although atherosclerotic heart disease has now been recognized as a significant complication of other rheumatic diseases, including SLE and RA, similar findings have not yet been reported in longitudinal studies on MCTD.

Nervous System

Although MCTD was initially described to be notable for the absence of serious neurologic involvement, practitioners now recognize that neurologic disease can occur in some patients with MCTD.[1,3-9,28-34,43-45] The presence of neuropsychiatric manifestations of MCTD was first emphasized by Bennett and colleagues. They reported that over one half of the 20 patients whom they studied with MCTD had findings including aseptic meningitis, psychosis, seizures, peripheral neuropathy, trigeminal neuropathy, or cerebella ataxia.[43] The prevalence of neuropsychiatric manifestations in MCTD has been reported to be lower in other subsequently reported cohorts.[3-9]

Vascular headaches have been frequently described in MCTD.[44] Aseptic meningitis has been reported to be associated with the use of nonsteroidal antiinflammatory agents, particularly ibuprofen, in patients with MCTD. A peripheral, predominantly sensory polyneuropathy can occur in MCTD.

Rarely, trigeminal neuralgia can be the presenting feature of MCTD.[45] Trigeminal neuralgia can manifest as neuralgic pain or as partial or complete anesthesia over the distribution of one or more branches of the trigeminal nerve. Cerebellar dysfunction, psychosis, and seizure have been infrequently reported in patients with MCTD. Other neurologic problems that have been rarely reported (most often in the form of case reports) in MCTD include cauda equina syndrome, transverse myelitis, stroke, and cerebral hemorrhage. The relationship of these entities with MCTD has not been clearly established.

Renal Disease

Subtle renal involvement can be detected in approximately 25% of patients with MCTD[46] but infrequently leads to significant clinical sequelae. In patients with MCTD who undergo renal biopsy, focal proliferative glomerulonephritis may be observed.[1,3-9,28-34,46,47] Diffuse proliferative glomerulonephritis is uncommon in MCTD. Patients with diffuse renal involvement often initially have or subsequently develop anti-Sm or anti–double stranded DNA (anti-dsDNA) antibodies or both.[3,8] The development of anti-Sm antibodies (particularly against the Sm-D peptide) appears to occur when ongoing immune spreading and more severe disease are observed.

In MCTD, membranous glomerulonephritis (with or without nephrotic syndrome) may rarely occur. Intimal proliferation in arteries and ischemic changes have been observed in MCTD. Scleroderma-like renal crisis has also been infrequently reported to occur in MCTD. Patients with MCTD and concomitant Sjögren syndrome may develop interstitial nephritis and have associated findings such as renal tubular acidosis.

Hematologic Disorders

Hematologic abnormalities are common in MCTD.[1,3-9,28-34] Mild lymphadenopathy occurs in approximately 25% to 50% of patients. Lymphadenopathy is often an initial feature of the disease and tends to decrease over time, although it may re-appear with a flare of disease. The development of massive lymphadenopathy and pseudolymphoma has been observed.

Anemia, lymphopenia, and leukopenia are all common in MCTD, occurring in 50% to 75% of patients. Antilymphocyte antibodies have been found to be common and have been reported to correlate with disease activity. Anemia of chronic disease is one of the most common findings in several series of MCTD. Coombs-positive immune-mediated hemolytic anemia has been reported to be a rare feature of MCTD.

Thrombocytopenia occurs in MCTD but appears less commonly than leukopenia or anemia.[1,3-9,28-34] Finally, case reports describe idiopathic thrombocytopenic purpura, red-cell aplasia, and thrombotic thrombocytopenic purpura in MCTD. Coagulation abnormalities appear to be rare but have been described.

Miscellaneous Systemic Features

Malaise and low-grade fever may occur in MCTD. The disease has been reported to develop an elevated body temperature of unknown origin.[1,3-9,28-34] Rarely, patients may have high-grade fever without an identifiable infection agent as the cause of the elevated temperature. In these patients, the inference is that MCTD is the cause of the fever, recognizing that a careful search for infection should always be completed before an elevated body temperature is attributed to the underlying disease.

Sicca symptoms are common in MCTD, occurring in 25% to 50% of patients.[9] Those with MCTD frequently have antibodies to SSA/Ro, and these may develop after the onset of MCTD. Anti-SSB/La is found in a small number of patients with MCTD, occurring in less than 5%.[1,3-9] However, the presence of SSA/Ro and/or SSB/La antibodies does not correlate with clinical manifestations of sicca in MCTD. Photosensitivity and malar rash appear to be increased among patients with MCTD who are positive for SSA/Ro antibodies.[9] Orofacial and ocular vascular involvement has been described in MCTD,[48] as well as autoimmune thyroiditis and persistent hoarseness.

Children

MCTD in a child was described within 1 year after the initial report of MCTD in adults.[49] Early studies in children helped establish that the disease could occur in any age group, and the examination of pathologic material from children who had died as a result of the disease provided some of the earliest insights into the vascular proliferative lesions that are fundamental to the immunopathologic process underlying MCTD.[30] A more complete understanding of MCTD in children has been gained over the past 3 decades, as clinical series containing larger numbers of children with increasing lengths of follow-up have been published.[5,7,9,30,49,50] Taken together, these studies demonstrate that MCTD can occur at any age and that MCTD in children appears to have clinical manifestations of disease and disease outcomes similar to those observed in adults.[1,3-9,28-34,49,50]

The initial report of MCTD in a child was published in 1973 by Sanders, Huntley, and Sharp.[49] Subsequently, Singsen and others[30] comprehensively described patients with MCTD who were clinically characterized as having arthritis, Raynaud phenomenon, sclerodermatous skin findings, fever, abnormal esophageal motility, and evidence of myositis. Serologically, these children had high levels of antinuclear antibodies (ANAs) exhibiting a speckled pattern and high levels of antibodies against ENA and RNP, as measured by hemagglutination with their specificity against RNP confirmed using immunodiffusion.[30]

Early clinical and serologic studies established that MCTD occurred in children. In contrast to most of the outcome studies recently reported, initial studies from Singsen and colleagues[30] at the Los Angeles Children's Hospital found that renal involvement and thrombocytopenia appeared to be common and that the prognosis was unfavorable in a significant number of the small group of children they studied. More recent studies have challenged these initial observations that MCTD is different in children, although some studies from Japan have also reported that MCTD in that country may have a worse prognosis when the disease has its onset in childhood. Subsequent longitudinal studies from Europe and the United States, however, have found childhood MCTD to have the same core clinical manifestations as observed in adults, including Raynaud phenomenon, swollen hands, arthralgia, arthritis, mild myositis, telangiectasias, and sclerodactyly. These studies have also reported that MCTD in children has a relatively favorable outcome in approximately 70% of patients, with 5% to 20% having complete remission of their disease after treatment.[5,7,9,30,49,50]

As in adults, pulmonary involvement appears to be an important feature of the disease in children and the development of pulmonary hypertension has been reported from the United States and Japan. Thrombocytopenia, as initially reported by Singsen and colleagues, has not been found to be clinically significant in other series.[5,7,9,30,49,50] Infection complicating the disease has been reported as a major cause of death in children with MTCD. Coexisting sicca syndrome has been reported by some to be common in children with MCTD, and neurologic involvement in children with MCTD, which can be severe, is rarely reported.

Pregnancy

A small number of published studies has examined the effects of MCTD on pregnancy.[51,52] Lundberg and Hedfors from Stockholm, Sweden,[51] have retrospectively examined pregnancy outcome in 40 pregnancies among 20 patients with high-titer RNP antibodies. They found fetal and maternal outcomes were excellent with no evidence of flares of disease during pregnancy or the postpartum period. These findings were in contrast to a somewhat less favorable outcome for pregnancy in patients with MCTD reported by Kaufman and Kitridou from Los Angeles[52]; they found parity was decreased and fetal wastage was increased similarly among patients with either MCTD or SLE. Overall, the outcome of pregnancy in MCTD with careful clinical monitoring at medical centers with experience in managing MCTD appears highly favorable.[51]

Patients should be counseled regarding contraception to prevent unplanned pregnancies, especially when taking medications that could be harmful to the fetus. Studies have not examined the potential risk of estrogens in MCTD, but considering that the female predominance in MCTD resembles that of SLE, the concerns raised on the subject of higher doses of estrogen in the context of SLE are viewed as being applicable to MCTD as well.[53]

In the absence of formal studies of cohorts of pregnant patients with MCTD, approaches to the management of pregnancy in MCTD have been adapted from the SLE literature. High-risk obstetric evaluation and care should be provided to the mother before and during a planned pregnancy. Attention should be given to the identification of any additional risk factors that often occur in such patients, such as the presence of anti-SSA/Ro antibodies, which have been associated with congenital cardiac disease including heart block, and antiphospholipid antibodies (APLAs), which have been associated with increased risk for fetal loss. Many drugs used to treat MCTD are not approved for use during pregnancy.

Serologic and Immunologic Studies

Patients with MCTD have ANAs against a series of nuclear antigens.[1,3-9,28-34,54-56] The presence of antibodies against U1-RNP is required for the diagnosis by its original definition and subsequently proposed classification criteria.[11-13] The typical patient with MCTD will have high titers of FANA, exhibiting a speckled pattern of immunofluorescence with the commonly used HEp-2 cell line, as well as with other human or mouse tissue substrates. Patients will have antibodies against ENA and RNP, which typically will be present at high levels in untreated patients at the onset of disease. The development of anti-RNP antibodies occurs in close temporal relationship to the onset of clinical disease, with symptoms developing within 1 year after the appearance of this antibody in most patients. Although in active disease, no close correlation exists between the level of anti-RNP and disease activity or severity, the level of anti-RNP antibodies may diminish or even disappear with treatment over time in some patients, particularly in those treated with cytotoxic drugs such as cyclophosphamide.[8]

To fully understand the typical autoantibodies found in MCTD, reviewing the structure of the spliceosome and its major components is helpful. The spliceosome contains a series of snRNP associated with a series of uridylic acid-rich RNAs. In the normal cell these are involved in the complex process of excising introns during the processing of pre-mRNA to the final mature mRNA molecules.[2]

The primary antigenic components of the spliceosome include uridylic acid-rich RNAs (U1, U2, U4/6, and U5), which are associated with snRNP peptides. The snRNP complex contains both the Sm and RNP antigens.[2,3] The RNP antigen consists of three polypeptides, 70kD, A, and C, noncovalently associated with U1 RNA (Figure 41-1). The Sm antigen consists of eight polypeptides (Sm-D1 to 3, B1 and 2, E, F, and G), which are noncovalently associated with U1, U2, U4/U6, and U5 RNA. The primary reactivity found in MCTD is with the U1-70kD polypeptide (previously called the 68kD polypeptide),[2,3,9] although patient sera may react with the U1-A or less commonly with the U1-C polypeptide of RNP.[8] An individual patient's serum may react with some or all of the U1-associated polypeptides. At the onset of disease, the most common reactivity is with the 70kD polypeptide or with the A polypeptide; over time, immune spreading will occur to other components of the complex.[55-57] In long-standing disease, especially in patients who have received cytotoxic drug

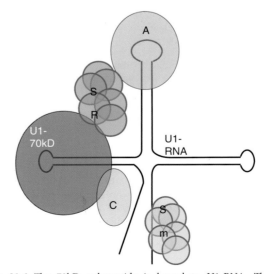

FIGURE 41-1 The 70kD polypeptide is bound to U1-RNA. The other U1-associated polypeptides, A and C, form the complex. The Sm polypeptides B, D, E, F, and G, which bind to U1, U2, U3, and U4/6 RNA, are also illustrated. (*Modified from Greidinger and Hoffman.*[55])

therapies such as cyclophosphamide, so-called epitope contraction may occur, during which antibody reactivity with one or more of these snRNP polypeptides decreases or disappears.[8] A number of studies have found that serologic reactivity with the U1-70kD polypeptide is closely associated with clinical findings of MCTD and is superior to measuring antibodies to RNP alone.[3,5,6-8]

In contrast to the reactivity with RNP typically found in MCTD, the snRNP antibody reactivity characteristically observed in patients with SLE is directed against the Sm antigen and its associated polypeptides. Approximately one third of patients diagnosed with SLE will develop anti-Sm antibodies. The most prevalent antibodies found in sera that are reactive with the Sm antigen are directed against the Sm-B and Sm-D polypeptides, although reactivity with the other Sm polypeptides (e.g., Sm-E, Sm-F, Sm-G) has been described.[3] It appears that immune spreading to develop reactivity with the Sm-D polypeptides occurs later in the anti-snRNP immune response. The presence of anti-Sm-D antibodies is associated with the presence of renal disease and a worse clinical outcome.[8,46]

Reactivity to the U1-specific polypeptides (including 70kD) and to the U1-U6-associated Sm-B and Sm-D polypeptides is observed at the time of initial presentation in a subset of patients. In addition, some patients who initially have reactivity with the U1-specific polypeptides may have immune spreading and develop antibodies against the Sm-B or Sm-D polypeptides or both while under observation. As previously discussed, such patients may develop more typical SLE-like clinical manifestations, have significant renal involvement, and receive a worse prognosis.[3,7,8]

A small group of patients exhibit reactivity with both Sm and RNP at the time of diagnosis. According to some classification criteria, the presence of antibodies against Sm disqualifies these patients from being classified as having MCTD.[7,11] One set of classification criteria proposed by Sharp and colleagues would eliminate any patient with significant levels of antibodies against Sm or double-stranded DNA from being classified as having MCTD.[7,11] Patients with anti-Sm antibodies appear at increased risk for the development of renal involvement and may have a different MHC genotype (HLA-DR2) from patients with isolated reactivity to RNP (HLA-DR4).[7,46]

Thus both genetic and clinical differences appear to exist between patients who have immune reactivity limited to U1-RNP (particularly U1-70kD) and those who exhibit immune spreading and develop immune reactivity against both U1-RNP and Sm polypeptides.

Immune reactivity with U1-RNA, U1-70kD, rheumatoid factor, phospholipids, beta-2-glycoprotein, SSA/Ro, viruses, U1-A, and hnRNP can occur.

Antibodies against U1-RNA are common in MCTD.[6] Antibody levels against U1-RNA have been described as correlating with disease activity in at least one study, although other studies have not been able to confirm a strong correlation between antibody levels and disease activity.[6,8,58] Interestingly, the RNA-binding domain on the 70kD polypeptide has been identified as the dominant T-cell epitope recognized by patients with MCTD, suggesting a link between B- and T-cell responses against U1-RNA.[59] Antibodies against the complex of U-70k and U1-RNA have also been identified in patients with MCTD. Recently, U1-RNA was shown to activate murine and human cells through triggering innate immune receptors, including Toll-like receptors (TLRs) 3 and 7.[56,59-60] These emerging studies support the broader concept that autoimmune diseases may have defects in both the acquired and innate arms of the immune system and that adaptive and innate immunity are potentially important in triggering or sustaining systemic autoimmune disease or both.[59]

Rheumatoid factor is common in MCTD, occurring in 50% to 75% of patients.[1,3-9,28-34] Antibodies to SSA/Ro are also common, occurring in one third of the 55 patients with MCTD followed in a recent longitudinal study. In this study, anti-SSA/Ro and anti-SSB/La were found in 33% and 4% of patients, respectively.[9] Antibodies against phospholipids have been detected in MCTD, occurring in 15% of patients in one study.[61] Unlike in SLE, however, APLAs were not found to be associated with an increased risk of clotting in MCTD.[61]

Many of these ALPAs in MCTD may be directed against beta 2-glycoprotein I (β_2-GPI).[62] Although not associated with clotting, their presence has been reported by some to be associated with an increased risk for the development of pulmonary hypertension.[8]

Antibodies against viruses or their products have been examined in MCTD. A cross-reactive epitope on 70kD and certain retroviral antigens have been reported, although no definitive evidence exists for retroviral triggering of MCTD.[59] An association between past infection or immunization against cytomegalovirus and the development of anti-RNP antibodies has also been found in some but not all studies where this association has been examined.

In addition to antibodies, T cells reactive with U1-70kD, U1-A snRNP, and hnRNP A2 polypeptides have been identified from the peripheral blood of patients with MCTD, as well as in murine models of MCTD.[22,24,25,27,63-66] T-cell clones reactive with U1-70kD and hnRNP from the peripheral blood of patients with MCTD have been extensively characterized. Studies have shown that such T cells can provide help ex vivo to autoantibody-producing B cells. Several features of the autoantibodies identified in MCTD are characteristic of a T cell-dependent B-cell response, suggesting a central role for T cells in the disease.[59] This discussion is expanded in the following text (see Pathogenesis).

Immunopathologic Considerations

Early studies that included autopsy analyses on children reported by Singsen and colleagues[30] provided some of the earliest information on the histopathology of MCTD and supported the concept that MCTD is a distinct entity. They found widespread proliferative vascular lesions, involving small, medium, and large vessels. They reported involvement of the coronary, renal, and pulmonary arteries, as well as the aorta with endothelial proliferation and an obliterative vasculopathy. They found that plasmacyte-containing inflammatory infiltration of tissue was common and that vasculitis was also present. Subsequent studies have confirmed and extended these early findings.[7]

Pathogenesis

An overarching model of disease pathogenesis in MCTD requires the incorporation of a large amount of information on genetics, environmental influences, self-antigen modification, immune-effector cells, immunoregulation, and local tissue injury.[59] A proposed model of disease pathogenesis in MCTD is shown in Figure 41-2. Substantial knowledge gained from clinical observational studies and animal models has helped shape the current understanding of the pathogenesis of MCTD. Genetic and environmental factors both contribute to a susceptibility to MCTD. Immune-effector mechanisms and abnormal immune regulation appear to be important features of the disease. Adaptive and innate immunity may both contribute to MCTD. Immune cells (e.g., T cells, B cells, antigen-presenting cells [APCs]) and their products (e.g., cytokines, chemokines, antibodies) may all be important in the pathogenetic process. Finally, local tissue injury may affect the distinctive clinical manifestations of MCTD.

Genetic Factors

As previously discussed, MHC and non-MHC genes have been identified as having associations with disease susceptibility in MCTD. Within the MHC, the HLA-DR4 has been shown to be associated with anti-RNP antibody responses and with MCTD, per se, in a number of studies among several different populations, including patients from the United States, Mexico, and Europe.[7,16-19] In contrast, the HLA class II phenotype/genotype most closely associated with scleroderma, HLA-DR5, and its subtypes has been shown to have a negative association with MCTD.[7,16-19] Outside the MHC, select immunoglobulin allotypes have been found to be associated with anti-RNP responses and MCTD in some but not all studies.[7,15] Genome-wide association studies have suggested that additional genetic regions associated with anti-RNP antibody production are yet to be fully characterized.[20]

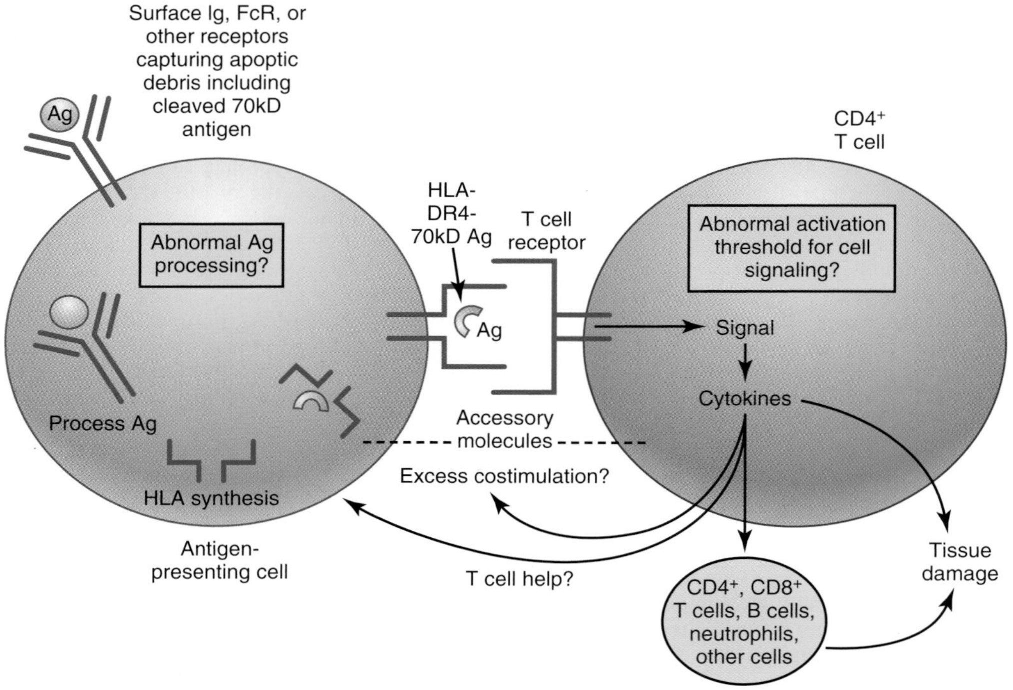

FIGURE 41-2 Hypothetical model of the pathogenesis of mixed connective tissue disease (MCTD). In this model, apoptotic material, including the 70kD polypeptide, is taken up by antigen-presenting cells (APC) and is processed and presented to autoreactive T cells in the context of the major histocompatibility complex (MHC) antigen human leukocyte antigen (HLA)–DR4. Cluster of differentiation 4 (CD4)–positive T cells respond to antigens by producing cytokines that assist in the expansion of themselves in an autocrine fashion, as well as in the differentiation and proliferation of autoantibody-producing cells. Tissue injury may be mediated directly by these cells or by soluble factors released from them. The autoreactive T cells may have an abnormal threshold for T cell–receptor triggering that renders them prone to autoimmunity. *(Modified from Hoffman RW: T cells in the pathogenesis of systemic lupus erythematosus. Clin Immunol 113[1]:4–13, 2004.)*

As for other multigenetic human diseases, the genetic contributions to the development of MCTD appear complex. Although the data are limited, reports of familial MCTD are rare. In longitudinal studies of families of affected individuals, the presence of anti-RNP antibodies was virtually never found among unaffected family members.[7] These findings are also consistent with studies among military personnel in which the development of anti-RNP antibodies was closely associated temporally with the development of clinical disease.[57] These results suggest that the development of anti-RNP autoimmunity is a robust marker for the development of MCTD and that their development is genetically regulated but may be triggered by noninherited environmental factors.

Environmental Factors

Several environmental factors that modify disease susceptibility or trigger disease have been proposed; most convincing among these is the influence of female sex hormones as suggested by the significant female-to-male ratio of the disease and other findings.[59] In addition, studies suggest that Epstein-Barr virus, retroviruses, or other viruses may play a role in triggering disease in some patients. Cytomegalovirus has also been suggested as being able to elicit anti-RNP antibody responses in the absence of disease. Environmental exposure to vinyl chloride has been associated with the development of an MCTD-like syndrome.

B Cells in Pathogenesis

The presence of antibodies against RNP is required for the diagnosis of MCTD, based on the initial description by Sharp and colleagues and as defined by the currently proposed classification criteria (see Box 41-1).[1] The facts that anti-RNP antibodies are present in high levels in patient sera have often undergone isotype switch to the IgG

class and that anti-RNP–producing B cells exhibit nucleotide substitutions that are typical of an antigen-driven immune response have been presented as evidence that anti-RNP immunity in MCTD is an antigen-driven immune process.[55,56,59] Anti-RNP antibodies may be reactive with the U1-70kD, A, or C polypeptides of the U1-snRNP complex.[3,8] Patients may also have antibodies against the Sm-B peptide, which can be complexed to U1 or to another member of the Sm-associated U1-6 RNPs. IgG antibodies directed against U1-70kD appear to be those most closely linked to disease pathogenesis.[55] The presence of antibodies against multiple individual components of the U1-RNA/RNP-snRNP macromolecular complex and the fact that immune spreading to different components of the complex occurs both support the hypothesis that MCTD is an antigen-driven immune process.[59]

Although anti-RNP antibodies are required for the diagnosis of MCTD, their development in serum is closely linked chronologically to the onset of clinical symptoms.[59] Furthermore, the development of anti-RNP antibodies appearing in cerebrospinal fluid has been associated with the development of neuropsychiatric manifestations in MCTD. Anti-RNP antibodies with antiendothelial activity have been reported in MCTD, although they have not been proven to mediate tissue injury directly. Studies in the recently developed animal model of MCTD may allow the potential pathogenic roles of antibodies in MCTD to be examined definitively (see the following text).

T Cells in Pathogenesis

T cells are also believed to play a central role in the pathogenesis of MCTD.[59] As discussed in the previous text, autoantibody-producing B cells produce high levels of IgG antibodies and exhibit features of T cell–derived, cytokine-driven affinity maturation. Epitope mapping of anti-RNP antibodies reveals that epitope spreading, typical of T cell–dependent B-cell responses, is identifiable.[59] T cells may also serve as APCs and produce cytokines or other soluble factors that recruit other cells to sites of inflammation or directly mediate tissue injury.

Antigen-specific T cells may drive both T- and B-cell responses as illustrated in the model shown in Figure 41-2. Autoantigen-reactive human T cells have been identified and characterized from the peripheral blood of patients with MCTD, including T cells reactive with U1-70kD, U1-A, and hnRNP A2.[21,22,63-65] These T cells have been linked to the presence of autoantibody production ex vivo and have been shown to provide help for autoantibody production in vitro.[22]

Substantial evidence suggests that in autoimmunity, T-cell hyperactivity and the presentation of apoptotically modified self-antigen may be important in the pathogenesis of MCTD (see Figure 41-2). Structural modifications of the antigens, such as could occur during apoptosis, may render them more immunogenic and be important in breaking immune tolerance.[59]

Innate Immunity in Pathogenesis

The potential importance of innate immune signaling through a TLR has been recognized in autoimmunity.[59,60] The finding that the dominant T-cell epitope on U1-70kD resides entirely within the RNA-binding domain of the RNP molecule, the fact that U1-RNA antibodies are tightly linked to MCTD, and, finally, the fact that U1-RNA can activate human and murine cells through TLR3 and TLR7 all suggest that innate immune signaling is of substantial potential importance in the pathogenesis of MCTD.[59,60] The schema shown in Figure 41-2 illustrates how this information may be unified in a single model of disease.

As has been described in SLE, levels of interferon-inducible genes are elevated in peripheral blood mononuclear cells of some patients with MCTD. In lupus, this elevation has been interpreted as the result of increased type I interferon secretion by plasmacytoid dendritic cells (pDCs) in response to TLR7 activation. In a murine model of anti-RNP autoimmunity, the induction of MCTD-like lung disease was found to be dependent on dendritic cells that were not pDCs and on TLR3 rather than TLR7, suggesting that pDC pathogenesis via TLR7 and another subset of dendritic cells via TLR3 may potentially contribute to MCTD.[60]

Tissue Injury in Pathogenesis

A central feature of immunopathogenesis in MCTD may be local factors influencing tissue injury. Based on pathologic studies, one of the primary targets of tissue injury is the vascular endothelium. Clinically, this is demonstrated by the almost uniform presence of Raynaud phenomenon in MCTD and the potentially lethal development of pulmonary hypertension that remains the primary disease-related cause of death.[8] Although antiendothelial antibodies have been described, very little information is available on how tissue-specific local responses may participate in the development of pathologic lesions. This important area awaits further investigation.

There is also evidence for differential fragmentation and differential recognition of self-antigen in MCTD, which may also play a role in tissue injury. Differences in the antibody recognition of fragments of the U1-70kD protein have been reported to distinguish patients with anti-RNP with photosensitive skin disease (in whom increased recognition of fragments anticipated to be produced by ultraviolet light–induced keratinocyte apoptosis was noted) from those with Raynaud phenomenon (in whom increased recognition of fragments anticipated to be produced by local ischemia-reperfusion injury were produced).[59]

Course and Prognosis

MCTD can evolve from mild to a more severe disease over time.[8] Patients typically exhibit Raynaud phenomenon, arthralgia, and swollen hands with or without polyarthritis at the outset of their disease. These symptoms often lead to the diagnosis of RA, another connective tissue disease, or undifferentiated connective tissue disease (UCTD) at initial presentation. (See "Undifferentiated Connective Tissue Disease and Overlap Syndromes" later in this chapter.) Prospective studies have shown that pulmonary or esophageal dysfunction may be detectable before the onset of clinical symptoms when sensitive diagnostics, such as pulmonary DLCO and esophageal manometry, are used.[7,8]

Long-term outcome studies by Burdt and colleagues[8] found that with standard immunomodulatory treatments, certain features of the disease, including arthritis, swollen hands, serositis, myositis, erythematosus rash, Raynaud phenomenon, and esophageal hypomotility, are diminished. In contrast, sclerodactyly, diffuse sclerosis, pulmonary dysfunction, nervous system involvement, and pulmonary hypertension were less responsive to treatment and became the dominant residual features of the disease over time.[8] In those unusual patients who develop serious renal involvement, prognosis was less favorable.[8] The patients who develop pulmonary hypertension, occurring in 23% of the 47 patients followed for up to 30 years, had the worst prognosis.[8] Some patients treated with corticosteroids or corticosteroids plus cyclophosphamide had prolonged remission of their disease, and some were able to discontinue all medications. Despite prolonged remission, some patients had a recurrence of their disease, including some who developed membranoproliferative glomerulonephritis.[8] Overall, however, the majority of patients were able to lead functionally normal lives.

Subsequent reports of the treatment of pulmonary hypertension in MCTD have also shown that approximately 50% of patients respond to aggressive immunosuppressive or cytotoxic therapies, which is clearly distinct from scleroderma, in which the likelihood and magnitude of benefit from cytotoxic therapy for pulmonary hypertension has been found to be negligible.[39,40] Patients with MCTD and pulmonary hypertension who have perivascular and interstitial infiltrates as their primary lesion appear to be those likely to respond to immunosuppressive therapy, whereas the remainder develop scleroderma-like fibrotic lesions with endothelial hyperproliferation and are less likely to respond. An ongoing challenge in MCTD is to develop a clinically useful diagnostic test that can predict those who will benefit from aggressive immunosuppressive therapy (Figure 41-3).

Treatment

No large controlled clinical trials in MTCD have been conducted; therefore management must be designed using data from controlled trials of other diseases and observational studies that typically include small numbers of patients.[53] No drugs have been specifically developed for the treatment of MCTD and approved in the United States by the U.S. Food and Drug Administration (FDA).

Arthralgia and mild synovitis can be treated with nonsteroidal antiinflammatory agents and hydroxychloroquine.[53] For patients in whom these measures are ineffective, disease-modifying antirheumatic medications can be used, similar to the approach used in the treatment of RA. However, some specific issues should be considered. Inasmuch as MCTD can have associated lung disease, drugs that also have the potential to induce lung injury such as methotrexate must be monitored closely. As in SLE, antitumor necrosis therapy can potentially exacerbate disease or affect the development of anti-dsDNA antibodies and induce renal disease or central nervous system disease in those with MCTD.

Raynaud phenomenon is treated with protective measures that maintain total body warmth and prevent peripheral cooling. The use of gloves should be encouraged and may assist patients.[53] Calcium-channel blockers are effective at reducing the severity and frequency of episodes of Raynaud phenomenon. More recent measures adopted for the management of scleroderma-associated Raynaud phenomenon, such as the use of angiotensin-receptor blockers or phosphodiesterase 5 inhibitors, may also be useful in patients with MCTD and bothersome Raynaud phenomenon.[53] In patients with severe Raynaud phenomenon and complications such as digital infarctions, other more aggressive measures used in scleroderma, such as prostaglandin

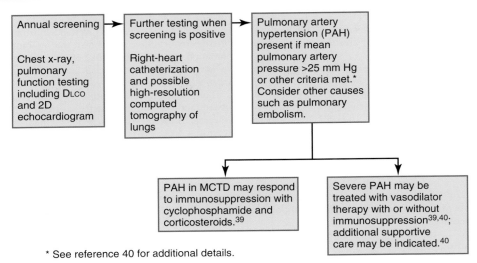

* See reference 40 for additional details.

FIGURE 41-3 Monitoring, diagnosis, and treatment of pulmonary artery hypertension in MCTD.

therapy, may be considered. Other approaches have been tried, such as regional sympathectomy, but it remains unclear how effective these may be. Physical and occupational therapy may be helpful to maintain mobility and facilitate function.

Esophageal reflux symptoms can be effectively controlled in most patients with proton-pump inhibitors. Many patients require long-term therapy to control symptoms and may, like patients with scleroderma, require higher than usual drug doses. Evaluation for Barrett esophagus should be made, although the timing of such an evaluation has not been clearly defined. Dilation of the esophagus may be beneficial for patients with strictures. Case reports of severe, refractory esophageal involvement that responds to aggressive immunotherapy with corticosteroids and with cyclophosphamide are available.[53] Diarrhea in those with MCTD may be related to bacterial overgrowth syndrome and can result in malabsorption.

Clinically significant myopathy in MCTD can be treated in most patients with corticosteroids. The addition of methotrexate should be considered in more severe or refractory cases.[32,37,53] In individuals with the elevation of serum creatine kinase (CK) but without clinical weakness, low-dose corticosteroids or no treatment may be adequate with continued monitoring. Complete normalization of serum CK may not be readily achievable in the patient with myositis or required in patients without symptoms. Finally, fibromyalgia may be the cause of muscle pain in patients with MCTD. As in other rheumatic diseases, fibromyalgia may develop later during the course of the disease.[38]

Pulmonary function should be monitored in MCTD because pulmonary disease is common and the most frequent disease-associated cause of death. Annual pulmonary function testing measuring the DLCO, plain-film radiographic studies of the chest, and two-dimensional echocardiographic images have been empirically recommended. Recent studies have reinforced that these screening measures are still not sufficiently sensitive to detect all cases of pulmonary hypertension. Right-heart catheterization may be required to evaluate pulmonary hypertension when significant abnormalities are detected by echocardiography or by pulmonary imaging studies, or when the clinical picture is suggestive of this diagnosis. High-resolution computed tomography of the chest may be indicated to assess for interstitial lung disease when abnormalities are found on the plain-film radiographs or pulmonary function testing. Intensive immunosuppressive therapy, including high-dose corticosteroids and intravenous cyclophosphamide, may benefit interstitial lung disease and pulmonary hypertension in those with MCTD.[39,40,53] Controlled clinical trial data are lacking, but in addition to intensive

immunosuppression or as an alternative therapy, approaches similar to those used to treat primary pulmonary hypertension may be attempted.[40] Although the presence of APLAs appears to be less clearly linked to clotting in patients with MCTD than it is in those with SLE, their presence has been associated with the development of pulmonary hypertension.[7,8]

Thrombocytopenia may respond to corticosteroids; however, in patients who fail to respond, treatments used in immune thrombocytopenic purpura (ITP) including intravenous immunoglobulin, rituximab, and splenectomy may be beneficial. Patients may also respond to cytotoxic therapy with cyclophosphamide or other agents.[53] Specific treatment is typically not required for mild anemia or leukopenia.

Sicca symptoms are common and can be treated with supportive measures including ocular lubrication, preventative dental care, lubrication for dry skin, and vaginal lubrication for dyspareunia.[53] A trial of antimuscarinic therapy may be indicated in patients with more severe oral symptoms and those who cannot obtain adequate relief with supportive measures alone. Topical tacrolimus may be considered for patients with more severe ocular dryness.

Erectile dysfunction and altered sexual response are now recognized to be common problems, particularly in chronically ill populations. The use of phosphodiesterase 5 inhibitors may benefit such patients after they have had careful evaluation.[53]

UNDIFFERENTIATED CONNECTIVE TISSUE DISEASE AND OVERLAP SYNDROMES

UCTD is said to be present when a patient lacks adequate clinical or diagnostic features to fit a recognizable clinical syndrome. Conceivably, this may range from the presence of a single clinical or laboratory finding, such as a positive ANA antibody test or the presence of arthralgia, to a more complete syndrome with the presence of a number of clinical and serologic features. The term *undifferentiated connective tissue disease* was first used by LeRoy and colleagues[67] in 1980 to describe the early phase of connective tissue diseases when the findings were nonspecific and often indistinct. Subsequent authors have similarly used the acronym *UCTD*, although the criteria for inclusion in later studies have not been uniform.[68-70] In addition, studies that have been reported have not always included laboratory testing for complete serologic characterization of ANAs present in the patients' sera. It should be emphasized that the term UCTD as applied by LeRoy and colleagues was not intended to describe an *overlap syndrome*, which is a condition in patients who have two or more distinctly recognizable rheumatic diseases.[67]

Box 41-2 Autoantibody Specificities and Their Clinical Features

tRNA synthetase	Myositis with arthritis and pulmonary involvement
PM/Scl	Overlapping features of polymyositis and limited scleroderma
Ku antigen	Polymyositis and systemic sclerosis
RNA polymerase II	Systemic lupus erythematosus (SLE) overlap

PM/Scl, Polymyositis and limited scleroderma.

Another approach to classification of rheumatic disease is the use of autoantibodies as disease markers. It has been proposed that manifestations of disease in a single patient reflect the constellation of autoantibodies specifically present and that these may evolve over time.[8,15] If, in fact, the presence of specific autoantibodies is linked to select aspects of disease, then the classification of disease may be useful if primarily based on the autoantibodies present. Studies on immune spreading of autoantibodies and on epitope contraction potentially provide one explanation of how evolving and even fluctuating clinical manifestations may be linked to autoantibody production.[7,15] Box 41-2 summarizes a number of uncommon antibodies that have been associated with systemic rheumatic diseases with protean and often overlapping clinical manifestations. To date, however, efforts to define rheumatic diseases strictly by autoantibody reactivities have failed to be as widely accepted as traditional clinical criteria.

Undifferentiated Connective Tissue Disease

Disease in the patient initially classified as having UCTD may evolve into a recognizable rheumatic disease over time, or the patient may remain without adequate features for classification as a well-recognized rheumatic disease. Alarcon and colleagues have published a series of studies examining the evolution of UCTD and the classification of the rheumatic diseases.[68,69] Their work indicates that over 90% of patients who initially have a well-recognized diagnosis will retain that diagnosis over time and that a moderate percentage of patients with UCTD will evolve into having a recognizable disease, although many will still have UCTD. Mosca and colleagues[70] reported that the cases of UCTD that they studied did not progress into distinctly recognizable rheumatic diseases but remained classified as UCTD when observed over time. Thus UCTD may remain stable over time and appears to have a favorable outcome.[68-70]

In cohorts of patients with UCTD, patients are frequently observed to have manifestations of disease that fall primarily within the constellation of a single well-defined rheumatic syndrome. This has led some commentators to regard these cases as "incomplete" forms of the diseases that they resemble rather than fully undifferentiated disease. Patients with apparently "incomplete" forms of disease share the overall favorable prognosis observed for UCTD. Approximately one third of cases of UCTD will ultimately evolve into a defined rheumatic syndrome. Although clinical and serologic factors of "incomplete" diseases have been reported to be associated with the diseases that emerge in the cases that do differentiate further, instances of differentiation into a rheumatic diagnosis other than the one for which the initial manifestations might have been most evocative have been described. The presence of more clinical and serologic manifestations at baseline appears to increase the risk for differentiation into a defined rheumatic syndrome overall, but protean UCTD and apparently "incomplete" syndromes have yet to be distinguished in terms of their risk of progressing. Until a more complete understanding of the pathogenesis of the rheumatic diseases is obtained and markers more accurately predict organ damage and disease outcomes, controversy in the area of disease classification will continue.[15]

As in most specific rheumatic syndromes, female predominance has been reported in UCTD. Among the most frequent rheumatic manifestations observed in clinical UCTD cohorts are arthralgia, arthritis, ANA positivity, Raynaud phenomenon, sicca manifestations, and photosensitivity. A diagnosis of UCTD has been associated with increased complications of pregnancy and increased risk of flares, suggesting that patients with UCTD should receive close rheumatologic follow-up and high-risk obstetric evaluation like patients with defined rheumatic syndromes.[53]

In some studies, patients with interstitial lung disease have been found to have an increased prevalence of UCTD, occurring in approximately 10% of patients.[71] Those with UCTD-associated interstitial lung disease have been reported to have a more favorable prognosis than those with idiopathic pulmonary fibrosis.

Overlap Syndromes

A number of so-called overlap syndromes have been described.[72-75] Many of these are identifiable by the presence of a specific antibody. Some examples of these syndromes and their associated antibodies are shown in Box 41-2.

Synthetase Syndromes

Synthetase syndromes are immunologically characterized by the presence of antibodies reactive with aminoacyl-transfer RNA (tRNA) synthetases.[72] The first to be reported were characterized by the presence of antibodies against the Jo-1 antigen; these autoantibodies are now known to be directed against histidyl-tRNA synthetase.[72] Clinically, patients possessing anti–Jo-1 antibodies have inflammatory muscle disease plus the presence of additional signs and symptoms of widespread connective tissue disease. Patients may have Raynaud phenomenon, arthralgia, arthritis, sicca symptoms, telangiectasias, dermatomyositis-like rashes, dysphagia, and pulmonary fibrosis.[72]

Polymyositis and Limited Scleroderma

Patients with polymyositis and limited scleroderma (PM/Scl) antibodies are characterized by having features of both polymyositis and scleroderma.[73] The illness may include Raynaud phenomenon, tendon inflammation, and concomitant pulmonary involvement. Although sclerodactyly or mild proximal scleroderma may be present, widespread sclerodermatous skin involvement is seldom present. However, severe renal involvement with scleroderma-like kidney disease has been described to occur in these patients.

Ku Antigen

Patients first described as having antibodies against the Ku antigen were found to have overlapping features of polymyositis and systemic sclerosis.[74] Patients with antibodies against the Ku antigen may also have a wide range of clinical manifestations including features of SLE, MCTD, and Sjögren syndrome.[74]

RNA Polymerase II

Patients with a number of clinical syndromes can have antibodies against one or more of the nuclear enzymes RNA polymerase I, II, and III.[75] A moderate number of patients with diffuse scleroderma or, less commonly, patients with limited scleroderma may have antibodies against RNA polymerase I and RNA polymerase III.[75] Patients classified as having SLE-overlap syndrome have been reported to have antibodies against RNA polymerase II in the absence of antibodies against RNA polymerase I and III. Frequently, these patients also have antibodies reactive with other specificities including Ku, RNP, and topoisomerase I.

Co-Existing Rheumatic Diseases

No evidence supports the theory that having one rheumatic disease protects an individual against having a second independent disease. Indeed, patients with a single autoimmune disease are at increased risk of getting a second independent autoimmune disease. In part, this is likely to be explained by the fact that genetic polymorphisms related to immune regulation are risk factors for autoimmunity that are often shared by multiple autoimmune syndromes. Even if no shared predisposing factors are considered, a patient may spontaneously develop two co-existing rheumatic diseases; their co-existence is not causally related but rather is based on a chance association. This co-existence is statistically more likely for diseases that are relatively common, such as RA and Sjögren syndrome. Such an explanation for co-existing rheumatic diseases is an important alternative consideration when potential overlap syndromes are reported in case reports and small clinical series. Patients who have experienced two or more independent failures of immune regulation leading to co-existing autoimmune syndromes might be anticipated to have more profound defects in immune regulation than patients who develop a single autoimmune disease. However, no systematic analyses have suggested that the prognosis of patients with multiple autoimmune syndromes is worse than would otherwise be expected from each individual diagnosis.

References

1. Sharp GC, Irvin WS, Tan EM, et al: Mixed connective tissue disease—an apparently distinct rheumatic disease syndrome associated with a specific antibody to an extractable nuclear antigen (ENA). *Am J Med* 52(2):148–159, 1972.
2. Pettersson I, Hinterberger M, Mimori T, et al: The structure of mammalian small nuclear ribonucleoproteins. Identification of multiple protein components reactive with anti-(U1)ribonucleoprotein and anti-Sm autoantibodies. *J Biol Chem* 259(9):5907–5914, 1984.
3. Holyst M-M, Hoffman RWU: Small nuclear ribonucleoprotein (RNP)-reactive autoantibodies: diagnostic testing and clinical interpretation. *Clin Immunol Newsletter* 18:53–57, 1998.
4. Sharp GC, Irvin WS, May CM, et al: Association of antibodies to ribonucleoprotein and Sm antigens with mixed connective-tissue disease, systematic lupus erythematosus and other rheumatic diseases. *N Engl J Med* 295(21):1149–1154, 1976.
5. Hoffman RW, Cassidy JT, Takeda Y, et al: U1-70-kd autoantibody-positive mixed connective tissue disease in children. A longitudinal clinical and serologic analysis. *Arthritis Rheum* 36(11):1599–1602, 1993.
6. Hoffman RW, Sharp GC, Deutscher SL: Analysis of anti-U1 RNA antibodies in patients with connective tissue disease. Association with HLA and clinical manifestations of disease. *Arthritis Rheum* 38(12):1837–1844, 1995.
7. Sharp GC, Hoffman RW: Mixed connective tissue disease. In Belch J, Zurier R, editors: *Connective tissue diseases*, London, 1995, Chapman and Hall.
8. Burdt MA, Hoffman RW, Deutscher SL, et al: Long-term outcome in mixed connective tissue disease: longitudinal clinical and serologic findings. *Arthritis Rheum* 42(5):899–909, 1999.
9. Setty YN, Pittman CB, Mahale AS, et al: Sicca symptoms and anti-SSA/Ro antibodies are common in mixed connective tissue disease. *J Rheumatol* 29(3):487–489, 2002.
10. Sharp GC: MCTD: a concept which stood the test of time. *Lupus* 11(6):333–339, 2002.
11. Kasukawa R, Sharp GC, editors: *Mixed connective tissue disease and antinuclear antibodies. Proceedings of the International Symposium on Mixed Connective Tissue Disease and Anti-nuclear Antibodies*, New York, 1987, Excerpta Medica.
12. Alarcon-Segovia D, Cardiel MH: Comparison between 3 diagnostic criteria for mixed connective tissue disease. Study of 593 patients. *J Rheumatol* 16(3):328–334, 1989.
13. Amigues JM, Cantagrel A, Abbal M, et al: Comparative study of 4 diagnosis criteria sets for mixed connective tissue disease in patients with anti-RNP antibodies. Autoimmunity Group of the Hospitals of Toulouse. *J Rheumatol* 23(12):2055–2062, 1996.
14. Perkins K, Hoffman RW, Bezruczko N: A Rasch analysis for classification of systemic lupus erythematosus and mixed connective tissue disease. *J Appl Meas* 9(2):136–150, 2008.
15. Hoffman RW, Sharp GC: Is anti-U1-RNP autoantibody positive connective tissue disease genetically distinct? *J Rheumatol* 22(4):586–589, 1995.
16. Hoffman RW, Rettenmaier LJ, Takeda Y, et al: Human autoantibodies against the 70-kd polypeptide of U1 small nuclear RNP are associated with HLA-DR4 among connective tissue disease patients. *Arthritis Rheum* 33(5):666–673, 1990.
17. Kaneoka H, Hsu KC, Takeda Y, et al: Molecular genetic analysis of HLA-DR and HLA-DQ genes among anti-U1-70-kd autoantibody

18. Gendi NS, Welsh KI, Van Venrooij WJ, et al: HLA type as a predictor of mixed connective tissue disease differentiation. Ten-year clinical and immunogenetic followup of 46 patients. *Arthritis Rheum* 38(2):259–266, 1995.
19. Genth E, Zarnowski H, Mierau R, et al: HLA-DR4 and Gm (1, 3; 5, 21) are associated with U1-nRNP antibody positive connective tissue disease. *Ann Rheum Dis* 46(3):189–196, 1987.
20. Cervino AC, Tsinoremas NF, Hoffman RW: A genome-wide study of lupus: preliminary analysis and data release. *Ann N Y Acad Sci* 1110:131–139, 2007.
21. Skriner K, Sommergruber WH, Tremmel V, et al: Anti-A2/RA33 autoantibodies are directed to the RNA binding region of the A2 protein of the heterogeneous nuclear ribonucleoprotein complex. Differential epitope recognition in rheumatoid arthritis, systemic lupus erythematosus, and mixed connective tissue disease. *J Clin Invest* 100(1):127–135, 1997.
22. Greidinger EL, Gazitt T, Jaimes KF, et al: Human T cell clones specific for heterogeneous nuclear ribonucleoprotein A2 autoantigen from connective tissue disease patients assist in autoantibody production. *Arthritis Rheum* 50(7):2216–2222, 2004.
23. Fritsch-Stork R, Müllegger D, Skriner K, et al: The spliceosomal autoantigen heterogeneous nuclear ribonucleoprotein A2 (hnRNP-A2) is a major T cell autoantigen in patients with systemic lupus erythematosus. *Arthritis Res Ther* 8(4):R118, 2006.
24. Holyst MM, Hill DL, Hoch SO, et al: Analysis of human T cell and B cell responses against U small nuclear ribonucleoprotein 70-kd, B, and D polypeptides among patients with systemic lupus erythematosus and mixed connective tissue disease. *Arthritis Rheum* 40(8):1493–1503, 1997.
25. Greidinger EL, Foecking MF, Schäfermeyer KR, et al: T cell immunity in connective tissue disease patients targets the RNA binding domain of the U1-70kDa small nuclear ribonucleoprotein. *J Immunol* 15:169(6):3429–3437, 2002.
26. Greidinger EL, Foecking MF, Magee J, et al: A major B cell epitope present on the apoptotic but not the intact form of the U1-70-kDa ribonucleoprotein autoantigen. *J Immunol* 172(1):709–716, 2004.
27. Greidinger EL, Zang Y, Jaimes K, et al: A murine model of mixed connective tissue disease induced with U1 small nuclear RNP autoantigen. *Arthritis Rheum* 54(2):661–669, 2006.
28. Reichlin M, Mattioli M: Correlation of a precipitin reaction to an RNA protein antigen and a low prevalence of nephritis in patients with systemic lupus erythematosus. *N Engl J Med* 286(17):908–911, 1972.
29. Homma M: Concepts and clinical pictures of mixed connective tissue disease [article in Japanese]. *Nihon Rinsho* 34(6):1113–1118, 1976.
30. Singsen BH, Bernstein BH, Kornreich HK, et al: Mixed connective tissue disease in childhood. A clinical and serologic survey. *J Pediatr* 90(6):893–900, 1977.
31. Ginsberg WW, Conn DL, Bunch TW, et al: Comparison of clinical and serological markers in systemic lupus erythematosus and overlap syndrome: a review of 247 patients. *J Rheumatol* 10(2):235–241, 1983.
32. Lundberg I, Hedfors E: Clinical course of patients with anti-RNP antibodies. A prospective study of 32 patients. *J Rheumatol* 18(10):1511–1519, 1991.
33. Kotajima L, Aotsuka S, Sumiya M, et al: Clinical features of patients with juvenile onset mixed connective tissue disease: analysis of data collected in a nationwide collaborative study in Japan. *J Rheumatol* 23(6):1088–1094, 1996.
34. Maldonado ME, Perez M, Pignac-Kobinger J, et al: Clinical and immunologic manifestations of mixed connective tissue disease in a Miami population compared to a Midwestern US Caucasian population. *J Rheumatol* 35(3):429–437, 2008.
35. Bennett RM, O'Connell DJ: The arthritis of mixed connective tissue disease. *Ann Rheum Dis* 37(5):397–403, 1978.
36. Oxenhandler R, Hart M, Corman L, et al: Pathology of skeletal muscle in mixed connective tissue disease. *Arthritis Rheum* 20(4):985–988, 1977.
37. Lundberg I, Nennesmo I, Hedfors E: A clinical, serological, and histopathological study of myositis patients with and without anti-RNP antibodies. *Semin Arthritis Rheum* 22(2):127–138, 1992.
38. Bennett RM: The concurrence of lupus and fibromyalgia: implications for diagnosis and management. *Lupus* 6(6):494–499, 1997.
39. Jais X, Launay D, Yaici A, et al: Immunosuppressive therapy in lupus- and mixed connective tissue disease-associated pulmonary arterial hypertension: a retrospective analysis of twenty-three cases. *Arthritis Rheum* 58(2):521–531, 2008.

40. McLaughlin VV, Archer SL, Badesch DB, et al: ACCF/AHA. ACCF/AHA 2009 expert consensus document on pulmonary hypertension: a report of the American College of Cardiology Foundation Task Force on Expert Consensus Documents and the American Heart Association: developed in collaboration with the American College of Chest Physicians, American Thoracic Society, Inc., and the Pulmonary Hypertension Association. *Circulation* 28;119(16):2250–2294, 2009.

41. Marshall JB, Kretschmar JM, Gerhardt DC, et al: Gastrointestinal manifestations of mixed connective tissue disease. *Gastroenterology* 98(5 Pt 1):1232–1238, 1990.

42. Alpert MA, Goldberg SH, Singsen BH, et al: Cardiovascular manifestations of mixed connective tissue disease in adults. *Circulation* 68(6):1182–1193, 1983.

43. Bennett RM, O'Connell DJ: Mixed connective tissue disease: a clinicopathologic study of 20 cases. *Semin Arthritis Rheum* 10(1):25–51, 1980.

44. Bronshvag MM, Prystowsky SD, Traviesa DC: Vascular headaches in mixed connective tissue disease. *Headache* 18(3):154–160, 1978.

45. Searles RP, Mladinich EK, Messner RP: Isolated trigeminal sensory neuropathy: early manifestation of mixed connective tissue disease. *Neurology* 28(12):1286–1289, 1978.

46. Hoffman RW: Mixed connective tissue disease. In Massry SG, Glassock RJ, editors: *Textbook of nephrology*, ed 4, Philadelphia, PA, 2001, Lippincott, Williams & Wilkins.

47. Kitridou RC, Akmal M, Turkel SB, et al: Renal involvement in mixed connective tissue disease: a longitudinal clinicopathologic study. *Semin Arthritis Rheum* 16(2):135–145, 1986.

48. Varga E, Field EA, Tyldesley WR: Orofacial manifestations of mixed connective tissue disease. *Br Dent J* 168(8):330–331, 1990.

49. Sanders DY, Huntley CC, Sharp GC: Mixed connective tissue disease in a child. *J Pediatr* 83(4):642–645, 1973.

50. Michels H: Course of mixed connective tissue disease in children. *Ann Med* 29(5):359–364, 1997.

51. Lundberg I, Hedfors E: Pregnancy outcome in patients with high titer anti-RNP antibodies. A retrospective study of 40 pregnancies. *J Rheumatol* 18(3):359–362, 1991.

52. Kaufman RL, Kitridou RC: Pregnancy in mixed connective tissue disease: comparison with systemic lupus erythematosus. *J Rheumatol* 9(4):549–555, 1982.

53. Hoffman RW, Greidinger EL: Mixed connective tissue disease. In Tsokos GC, Moreland LW, Kamen GM, et al, editors: *Modern therapeutics in rheumatic diseases*, Totowa, NJ, 2001, Humana Press.

54. Greidinger EL, Casciola-Rosen L, Morris SM, et al: Autoantibody recognition of distinctly modified forms of the U1-70-kd antigens is associated with different clinical disease manifestations. *Arthritis Rheum* 43(4):881–888, 2000.

55. Greidinger EL, Hoffman RW: The appearance of U1 RNP antibody specificities in sequential autoimmune human antisera follows a characteristic order that implicates the U1-70 kd and B'/B proteins as predominant U1 RNP immunogens. *Arthritis Rheum* 44(2):368–375, 2001.

56. Greidinger EL, Hoffman RW: Autoantibodies in the pathogenesis of mixed connective tissue disease. *Rheum Dis Clin North Am* 31:437–440, 2005.

57. Arbuckle MR, McClain MT, Rubertone MV, et al: Development of autoantibodies before the clinical onset of systemic lupus erythematosus. *N Engl J Med* 349(16):1526–1533, 2003.

58. Hoet RM, Koornneef I, de Rooij DJ, et al: Changes in anti-U1 RNA antibody levels correlate with disease activity in patients with systemic lupus erythematosus overlap syndrome. *Arthritis Rheum* 35(10):1202–1210, 1992.

59. Hoffman RW, Maldonado ME: Immune pathogenesis of mixed connective tissue disease: a short analytical review. *Clin Immunol* 128(1):8–17, 2008.

60. Hoffman RW, Gazitt T, Foecking MF, et al: U1 RNA induces innate immunity signaling. *Arthritis Rheum* 50(9):2891–2896, 2004.

61. Komatireddy GR, Wang GS, Sharp GC, et al: Antiphospholipid antibodies among anti-U1-70kDa autoantibody positive patients with mixed connective tissue disease. *J Rheumatol* 24(2):319–322, 1997.

62. Mendonca LL, Amengual O, Atsumi T, et al: Most anticardiolipin antibodies in mixed connective tissue disease are beta2-glycoprotein independent. *J Rheumatol* 25(1):189–190, 1998.

63. Hoffman RW, Takeda Y, Sharp GC, et al: Human T cell clones reactive against U-small nuclear ribonucleoprotein autoantigens from connective tissue disease patients and healthy individuals. *J Immunol* 151(11):6460–6469, 1993.

64. De Silva-Udawatta M, Kumar SR, Greidinger EL, et al: Cloned human TCR from patients with autoimmune disease can respond to two structurally distinct autoantigens. *J Immunol* 172(6):3940–3947, 2004.

65. Greidinger EL, Zang YJ, Jaimes K, et al: CD4+ T cells target epitopes residing within the RNA-binding domain of the U1-70-kDa small nuclear ribonucleoprotein autoantigen and have restricted TCR diversity in an HLA-DR4-transgenic murine model of mixed connective tissue disease. *J Immunol* 180(12):8444–8454, 2008.

66. Trivedi S, Zang Y, Culpepper S, et al: T cell vaccination therapy in an induced model of anti-RNP autoimmune glomerulonephritis. *Clin Immunol* 137(2):281–287, 2010.

67. LeRoy EC, Maricq HR, Kahaleh MB: Undifferentiated connective tissue syndromes. *Arthritis Rheum* 23(3):341–343, 1980.

68. Williams HJ, Alarcon GS, Joks R, et al: Early undifferentiated connective tissue disease (CTD). VI. An inception cohort after 10 years: disease remissions and changes in diagnoses in well established and undifferentiated CTD. *J Rheumatol* 26(4):816–825, 1999.

69. Calvo-Alen J, Bastian HM, Straaton KV, et al: Identification of patient subsets among those presumptively diagnosed with, referred, and/or followed up for systemic lupus erythematosus at a large tertiary care center. *Arthritis Rheum* 38(10):1475–1484, 1995.

70. Mosca M, Neri R, Bombardieri S: Undifferentiated connective tissue diseases (UCTD): a review of the literature and a proposal for preliminary classification criteria. *Clin Exp Rheumatol* 17(5):615–620, 1999.

71. Kinder BW, Shariat C, Collard HR, et al: Undifferentiated connective tissue disease-associated interstitial lung disease: changes in lung function. *Lung* 188(2):143–149, 2010.

72. Marguerie C, Bunn CC, Beyon HL, et al: Polymyositis, pulmonary fibrosis and autoantibodies to aminoacyl-tRNA synthetase enzymes. *Q J Med* 77(282):1019–1038, 1990.

73. Treadwell EL, Alspaugh MA, Wolfe JF, et al: Clinical relevance of PM-1 antibody and physiochemical characterization of PM-1 antigen. *J Rheumatol* 11(5):658–662, 1984.

74. Yaneva M, Arnett FC: Antibodies against Ku protein in sera from patients with autoimmune disease. *Clin Exp Immunol* 76(2):366–372, 1989.

75. Chang M, Wang RJ, Yangco DT, et al: Analysis of autoantibodies against RNA polymerases using immunoaffinity-purified RNA polymerase I, II, and III antigen in an enzyme-linked immunosorbent assay. *Clin Immunol Immunopathol* 89(1):71–78, 1998.

Chapter 42

Clinical Aspects of the Antiphospholipid Syndrome

Aisha Lateef and Michelle Petri

INTRODUCTION

The antiphospholipid syndrome (APS), an acquired thrombophilia, is characterized by vascular thrombosis and/or fetal loss in the presence of antiphospholipid antibodies (APLAs). APLAs are mainly directed against plasma proteins with an affinity for anionic phospholipids. Functional assays that measure the prolongation of phospholipid-dependent coagulation assays are used to detect the lupus anticoagulant (LA).[1] Solid-phase assays, such as enzyme-linked immunosorbent assays (ELISAs), detect anticardiolipin (aCL) and anti–beta 2 glycoprotein I (anti–β_2 GPI) antibodies.[1] This chapter focuses on current knowledge of the epidemiology, classification, pathogenesis, clinical features, diagnosis, and management of APS.

EPIDEMIOLOGY

APS is the most common form of acquired thrombophilia. In younger patients with stroke (under 50 years of age), APLAs are frequently present (one out of five patients), compared with older patients in whom other vascular risk factors may play more important roles.[2] APS accounts for 15% to 20% of all episodes of deep-vein thrombosis (DVT), with or without pulmonary embolism. The estimated prevalence of DVT in the general population is approximately 2% to 5%; consequently, APS may be responsible for DVT in 0.3% to 1% of the general population.[3] ALPAs are present in 30% to 40% of patients with systemic lupus erythematosus (SLE), but only one third of them develop clinical manifestations of APS, highlighting the importance of non-APLA contributory factors.[4] Recurrent pregnancy loss occurs in approximately 1% of women, and 10% to 15% of these women are diagnosed with APS.[5,6] In addition, APS is recognized to increase the risk of pregnancy complications such as preeclampsia, placental insufficiency, intrauterine growth restriction, and fetal loss.[7]

CLASSIFICATION CRITERIA

In 1999, an international consensus meeting formulated the first classification criteria—the "Sapporo criteria"—for patients with APS.[8] These criteria were updated during the 11th International Congress on Antiphospholipid Antibodies in November 2004 in Sydney, Australia.[1] According to the original 1999 criteria, a definite classification of APS requires the presence of one of the two major clinical manifestations of APS (pregnancy morbidity or thrombosis) with either aCL or LA on at least two occasions, 6 weeks apart. The revised Sydney criteria (Box 42-1) included anti–β_2 GPI and increased the period for persistence to 12 weeks.

Other noncriteria manifestations, such as thrombocytopenia, cardiac valvular disease, livedo reticularis, neurologic manifestations, and other APLAs, were also discussed during this meeting. It was concluded that although associated with APS, these features were not specific enough for inclusion in the classification criteria.[1]

PATHOGENESIS

Despite the strong association between APLAs and the risk of thrombosis and fetal loss, the pathogenic processes have not been fully elucidated. Multiple mechanisms have been proposed, including interference with hemostatic reactions, cellular activation, and the activation of the complement system. These different pathways are likely contributory rather than mutually exclusive.

The binding of APLAs to negatively charged phospholipids can interfere with multiple hemostatic mechanisms. Reported effects include increased thrombin formation, an inhibition of protein C and S activity, interference with the annexin A5 anticoagulant shield, production of microparticles, and impaired fibrinolysis. The net effect shifts the equilibrium in favor of a prothrombotic state.[7,9-12]

The anti–β_2 GPI complex can also bind to and activate many cell types, including monocytes, endothelial cells, and platelets. Monocytes express increased numbers of adhesion molecules; both monocytes and endothelial cells upregulate the production of tissue factor. Platelets that are activated by the anti–β_2 GPI complex increase the synthesis of thromboxane and the expression of platelet-membrane glycoproteins (GPs), particularly GPIIb/IIIa and GPIIIa, contributing to the heightened thrombotic risk.[7,9,10]

Recently, complement activation has been found to play a significant role in an animal APLA model of thrombosis and pregnancy morbidity. In vitro studies have shown that APLAs induce complement activation, which generates split products that then attract inflammatory cells and initiate thrombosis and tissue injury.[13,14] Lower complement levels have been noted in patients with primary APS, compared with other systemic autoimmune diseases (excluding SLE) or healthy volunteers.[15] The anti–β_2 GPI complexes preferentially target the placenta, activating complement via the classical pathway. The proinflammatory environment can result in trophoblast injury and pregnancy loss.[16-18] In addition, direct cytotoxic effects of APLAs on trophoblast cells may contribute to pregnancy morbidity.[19]

Contributory non-APLA factors serve as the "second hit" leading to thrombosis. Estrogen therapy, smoking, and certain genetic variants of clotting factors have been shown to increase the risk of myocardial infarction and stroke in women with positive APLAs.[7,20]

CLINICAL FEATURES

The majority of clinical manifestations of APS are related to thrombosis, whereas immune mechanisms may contribute to some nonthrombotic manifestations.

Thrombotic Manifestations

In the Euro-Phospholipid project, 37% of the cohort participants had only venous thrombosis, 27% had arterial thrombosis, whereas 15% had both arterial and venous thrombosis.[21] DVT is the most common type of venous thrombosis (~40%), followed by superficial leg vein thrombosis (~12%).[21] Other reported organs include the kidneys (renal vein thrombosis), liver (Budd-Chiari syndrome), brain (cerebral venous thrombosis), and eye (retinal vein thrombosis).[21,22] Arterial thrombosis includes strokes, transient ischemic attacks (TIAs), and myocardial infarction. Digital and limb ischemia, as well as other organ infarctions, have been described.[21,22] Thrombotic events usually occur at single sites, except in catastrophic APS (CAPS), in which multiple sites can be involved simultaneously or in quick succession.[23]

Box 42-1 Revised Classification Criteria for the Antiphospholipid Syndrome

Antiphospholipid antibody syndrome (APS) is defined as the presence of at least one of the following clinical criteria and one of the following laboratory criteria:

Clinical Criteria

1. Vascular thrombosis
   - One or more clinical episodes of arterial, venous, or small-vessel thrombosis are present in any tissue or organ. Thrombosis must be confirmed by objective validated criteria (i.e., unequivocal findings of appropriate imaging studies or histopathologic examination). For histopathologic confirmation, thrombosis should be present without significant evidence of inflammation in the vessel wall.
2. Pregnancy morbidity
   - One or more unexplained deaths of a morphologically normal fetus occurs at or beyond 10 weeks' gestation with normal fetal morphologic features documented by ultrasound or by the direct examination of the fetus.

   or

   - One or more premature births of a morphologically normal neonate occurs before 34 weeks' gestation because of either:
     a. Eclampsia or severe preeclampsia, as defined according to standard definitions; or
     b. Recognized features of placental insufficiency

   or

   - Three or more unexplained consecutive spontaneous abortions that occur before 10 weeks' gestation with maternal anatomic or hormonal abnormalities and paternal and maternal chromosomal causes excluded.

In studies of populations of patients who have had more than one type of pregnancy morbidity, investigators are strongly encouraged to stratify the groups of patients according to one of the above criteria.

Laboratory Criteria

1. Lupus anticoagulant (LA)
   - Is present in plasma on two or more occasions, at least 12 weeks apart, and detected according to the guidelines of the International Society on Thrombosis and Hemostasis (Scientific Subcommittee on LAs/phospholipid-dependent antibodies).
2. Anticardiolipin (aCL) antibodies
   - IgG or IgM isotype or both are present in the serum or plasma in medium or high titer (i.e., >40 GPL or MPL, or greater than the 99th percentile), on two or more occasions, at least 12 weeks apart, and as measured by a standardized ELISA.
3. Anti–beta 2 glycoprotein I antibody
   - IgG or IgM isotype in serum or plasma (in titer greater than the 99th percentile) or both are present on two or more occasions, at least 12 weeks apart, measured by a standardized ELISA, according to recommended procedures.

ELISA, Enzyme-linked immunosorbent assay; GPL, IgG antiphospholipid units; MPL, IgM antiphospholipid units.

Reproduced with permission from Miyakis S, Lockshin MD, Atsumi T, et al: International consensus statement on an update of the classification criteria for definite antiphospholipid syndrome (APS). *J Thromb Haemost* 4(2):295-306, 2006.

Neurologic Manifestations

Although most neurologic manifestations of APS are related to thromboembolism, local inflammation and neurotoxic effects of APLAs may contribute to some manifestations, including seizures, chorea, and myelitis.[24-28]

Cerebrovascular events, strokes, and TIAs are the most frequent neurologic manifestation and are reported to be the initial presenting feature in 18% to 30% of patients with APS.[21,29] Strokes may be recurrent and lead to multi-infarct dementia.[30] Multiple studies have found a strong association of APLAs (especially LA) with cerebrovascular events.[20,24,25,31] The risk of cerebrovascular events was higher in the presence of other concomitant vascular risk factors, such as smoking and the use of oral contraceptives.[20,32] Cardiac valvular lesions may be associated with cerebrovascular events in patients with APS.[33,34] Although valvular thickening is the most common presentation, noninfective vegetations (e.g., Libman-Sack endocarditis) are also well reported. Cardiac echocardiography is recommended in APS patients with cerebrovascular events.[35]

Although cerebrovascular disease is the only neurologic manifestation listed in the APS classification criteria, the linkage between epilepsy and APLAs has been documented by experimental and clinical studies.[26,28,36,37] The prevalence of epilepsy in APS is reported to be approximately 8.6%, which is 20 times higher than in the general population.[21,24,38] Direct neurotoxicity of APLAs may play a significant role, in addition to ischemic insult from cerebral thrombosis.[24,39]

Headaches, including migraine, are a common complaint in APS, but any causative association with APLAs remains unproven. Most prospective studies have not found any association between APLAs and headache.[24,39] An exception would be headache secondary to cerebral vein thrombosis. Movement disorders (e.g., chorea) have been associated with APLAs.[27] The prevalence has been reported to be 1.3% in the Euro-Phospholipid project and 1% to 4% in patients with SLE and APLAs.[21,40] Demyelinating disorders, including myelitis and neuromyelitis optica (e.g., Devic disease), have been associated with APLAs.[41-43]

Ocular Manifestations

Occlusion of the central and branch retinal arteries and veins may lead to visual disturbances. Ischemic optic neuropathy, retinal vessel abnormalities, cilioretinal artery occlusion, and choroidal infarctions have been described.[44]

Cardiovascular Manifestations

Ischemic heart disease is more common in patients with APS than the general population. In the Euro-Phospholipid project, myocardial infarction was noted in 5.5% of the cohort participants.[21] The prevalence of myocardial ischemia was seven times higher in patients with APS.[45] Cardiac valvular lesions are more frequently reported in those with APS. Transthoracic and transesophageal echocardiographic studies reported prevalence rates of 35% to 82% in patients with APS.[35,46,47] The most common lesion is valvular thickening, although vegetations, stenosis, and regurgitation may also be present. The mitral valve is most commonly involved, followed by the aortic valve.[35,47] The majority of the lesions are mild. Symptomatic valvular disease occurs in only 5% of the patients.[35,46,47] An association between cardiac valvular lesions and arterial thrombosis, including cerebrovascular events, has been described in APS and is likely linked by the higher embolic risk in patients with valvular lesions.[33-35]

Dermatologic Manifestations

Livedo reticularis, a purplish discoloration of the skin with a netlike pattern, is the most common abnormality, noted in 16% to 25% of patients with APS.[48,49] Livedo reticularis is reportedly more common in secondary APS and in women. It has been associated with positive immunoglobulin G (IgG) aCL, arterial thrombotic events, and cardiac valvular disease.[35,49,50] It may also occur in a variety of other disorders such as other autoimmune diseases, vasculitis, severe sepsis, cholesterol embolism, and even normal individuals (e.g., livedo rosacea). Livedo racemosa, an irregular branching pattern of finer and more widespread purplish discoloration and often with broken circles, has been associated with APLA-positive Sneddon syndrome.[51]

Cutaneous ulcerations are reported in 4% to 8% of patients with APS and range from ischemic to postphlebitic ulcers.[50] Ischemic ulcers are usually observed on the legs around the pretibial area and feet and are small and painful with central necrotic areas and sharp margins. They are often preceded by recurrent necrotizing purpura and leave whitish atrophic scars on healing. Occasionally, large solitary pyoderma gangrenosum–like ulcers, but without the undermined edges, have been reported in patients with APS.[50] Postphlebitic ulcers can occur in patients with long-standing venous thrombosis of the leg, leading to chronic edema, characteristic skin changes, and ulcerations.[50]

Superficial thrombophlebitis, mainly on the limbs, is noted in a small percentage of patients. Thrombocytopenic purpura is uncommon but may occur when the platelet counts are below 20×10^9/L. Digital gangrene and cutaneous gangrene are rare manifestations, usually preceded by digital cyanosis and extensive painful purpura, respectively.[50]

Pulmonary Manifestations

The predominant pulmonary manifestation is pulmonary embolism in 14% to 40% of patients, with a majority of them having concomitant DVT.[21,52] A small percentage progress to chronic thromboembolic pulmonary hypertension.[52]

Other Manifestations

Thrombocytopenia is a well-recognized feature of APS and is noted in up to 30% of patients in a large European study.[21] It is generally mild, although moderate to severe cases have been described. Thrombocytopenia is more common in secondary APS associated with SLE than with primary APS.[21] The pathogenesis is multifactorial but can include peripheral destruction of platelets, mediated by APLA binding and removal by the reticuloendothelial system. Antibodies directed against platelet GPs may also contribute to thrombocytopenia.[1] Occasionally, ethylenediaminetetraacetic acid (EDTA)–dependent APLAs and antiplatelet antibodies cause platelet clumping, leading to pseudothrombocytopenia.[53] Approximately 10% of patients with APS develop a Coombs-positive hemolytic anemia.[21]

Renal involvement usually takes the form of APS nephropathy with microvessel and glomerular thrombosis, although all levels of vasculature may be involved. Clinical manifestations include hypertension, proteinuria, and renal failure.[54] Rare intraabdominal manifestations include mesenteric ischemia and pancreatic and splenic infarctions.[21,54] An association of APLAs with avascular necrosis of bone has been suggested but remains unproven.[48,55]

PREGNANCY COMPLICATIONS

Pregnancy morbidity is one of the defining characteristics of APS. Both early and late losses occur with increased frequency—35% and 15%, respectively, in the European cohort. Increased rates of intrauterine growth restriction, preeclampsia, placental insufficiency, and preterm delivery have been reported.[21,56] The pregnancy outcomes in patients with APS have significantly improved; successful pregnancy rates of 70% or more can be achieved with appropriate treatment.[57] Multiple pathogenic mechanisms likely contribute to pregnancy loss in APS. In the murine model of APLA-induced pregnancy loss, it has been shown that complement activation plays a causative role and complement inhibition can rescue the pregnancies.[16] It has also been demonstrated that heparin inhibits activation of complement and, as a result, low prophylactic doses can prevent pregnancy loss.[16] Other proposed mechanisms of APLA-induced pregnancy loss include inhibition of trophoblast function, interference with the prostaglandin balance at the endothelial cell level, and placental thrombosis.[19]

CATASTROPHIC ANTIPHOSPHOLIPID SYNDROME

CAPS is a rare (less than 1%) but severe form of APS, associated with the acute onset of accelerated thrombosis in multiple organs. Classification criteria have been developed and validated.[58,59] In addition to the clinical picture of thrombosis in three or more organs in

Box 42-2 Classification Criteria for Catastrophic Antiphospholipid Syndrome

1. Involvement of three or more organs, systems, and/or tissues.[a]
2. Development of manifestations simultaneously or in less than 1 week.
3. Histopathologic confirmation of small-vessel occlusion in at least one organ or tissue.[b]
4. Laboratory confirmation of the presence of APLAs (LA and/or aCL).[c]

Definite CAPS
- All four criteria

Probable CAPS
- Any of the following:
  (a) All four criteria, except for only two organs, systems, and/or tissues involved
  (b) All four criteria, except for the absence of laboratory confirmation (within at least 6 weeks) owing to the early death of a patient never tested for APLA before the CAPS
  (c) Criteria 1, 2, and 4
  (d) Criteria 1, 3, and 4 and the development of a third event between 1 week and 1 month after presentation, despite anticoagulation

[a]Usually, clinical evidence of vessel occlusions, confirmed by imaging techniques when appropriate. Renal involvement is defined by a 50% rise in serum creatinine, severe systemic hypertension (>180/100 mm Hg), and/or proteinuria (>500 mg/24 hr).

[b]For histopathologic confirmation, significant evidence of thrombosis must be present, although vasculitis may coexist occasionally.

[c]If the patient had not been previously diagnosed as having APS, the laboratory confirmation requires that the presence of APLAs must be detected on two or more occasions at least 6 weeks apart (not necessarily at the time of the event), according to the proposed preliminary criteria for the classification of definite APS.

aCL, Anticardiolipin antibodies; ALPAs, antiphospholipid antibodies; CAPS, catastrophic antiphospholipid syndrome; LA, lupus anticoagulant.

Reproduced with permission from Asherson RA, Cervera R, de Groot PG, et al: Catastrophic antiphospholipid syndrome: international consensus statement on classification criteria and treatment guidelines. *Lupus* 12(7):530-534, 2003.

less than a week, these require the demonstration of multiple small-vessel occlusions and laboratory confirmation of the presence of APLAs, usually in high titer[58] (Box 42-2).

CAPS is a distinct subset of APS; small-vessel thrombosis predominate the clinical picture, in contrast to classic APS. The thrombosis is accompanied by a systemic inflammatory response syndrome (SIRS), contributing to the unique clinical presentations of this syndrome.[60]

A large international registry of patients with CAPS was created in 2000. The majority of the CAPS episodes (60%) were preceded by a precipitating event, most commonly infection.[60] The mortality rate remains high (30%), although significant improvement has been reported over the years.[23] The clinical manifestations depend on the location and extent of thrombosis, as well as the severity of SIRS. Kidneys, lungs, bowel, heart, and brain are the most commonly affected organs, but adrenal, testicular, splenic, pancreatic, and skin involvements have also been described. Depending on the organs involved, patients may have hypertension and renal impairment, acute respiratory distress syndrome, alveolar hemorrhage and capillaritis, confusion, and disorientation, or abdominal pain and distention secondary to bowel infarction.[60] Up to 50% of patients with CAPS have thrombocytopenia, one third develop hemolysis, and some may have features of disseminated intravascular coagulation (DIC).[60]

It has recently been suggested that a continuum of conditions may exist in which the presence of APLAs is associated with microangiopathy. The features include small-vessel thrombosis, microangiopathic hemolytic anemia with the presence of schistocytes, and thrombocytopenia. It includes some patients with thrombotic thrombocytopenic purpura (TTP); hemolysis, elevated liver enzymes, low platelet count (HELLP) syndrome; and CAPS. A new term, *microangiopathic APS* (MAPS), has been proposed to describe the disease in this group of patients.[61]

LABORATORY DIAGNOSIS

The laboratory tests used for the detection of APLAs can be divided into two categories: (1) LA assays and (2) solid-phase assays.

Lupus Anticoagulant Test

The LA test measures the ability of the APLAs to prolong phospholipid-dependent clotting reactions. LA detection is based on the following criteria: (1) prolongation of at least one phospholipid-dependent coagulation test, (2) lack of the correction of the prolonged test upon mixing with normal plasma, and (3) correction upon the addition of extra phospholipids. Multiple factors can affect the assays used for detecting LA including the types and titers of APLAs (e.g., presence or absence of anti–β_2 GPI), test methods, phospholipid content of the reagents, and the cut-off values used. The Subcommittee on Lupus Anticoagulant/Antiphospholipid Antibody of the Scientific and Standardization Committee (SSC) of the International Society on Thrombosis and Hemostasis (ISTH) has issued detailed guidelines for the detection of LA.[62] In summary, the recommendations are to perform two different phospholipid-dependent tests—diluted Russell vapor venom test and sensitive partial thromboplastin time—followed by mixing and confirmatory studies. LA has been shown to be more specific than other APLAs in predicting the risk of thrombotic and pregnancy complications of APS.[63-66]

Solid-Phase Assays

Pathogenic aCL are dependent on the phospholipid-binding protein β_2-GPI.[67] A specific ELISA to detect anti–β_2 GPI is also available. Other less commonly described APLAs are directed against prothrombin, annexin A5, phosphatidylserine, thromboplastin, protein S, and protein C.

Low titers of transient APLAs can be detected in other conditions, including infections (e.g., syphilis, Lyme disease, Q fever, hepatitis C, tuberculosis, leprosy, human immunodeficiency virus) and other connective tissue diseases, as well as secondary to drugs. On the other hand, detection of high titers of persistent APLAs confers the greatest risk of APS. International efforts have been taken to improve APLA detection, leading to development of guidelines for APLA testing. Recent revised classification criteria for APS requires the presence of aCL and/or anti–β_2 GPI of IgG and/or IgM isotypes in medium or high titer (i.e., >40 IgG antiphospholipid unit [GPL] or IgM antiphospholipid unit [MPL] or greater than the 99th percentile), on two or more occasions, at least 12 weeks apart, measured by a standardized ELISA.[1]

MANAGEMENT

The main goal of therapy in APS is to prevent thrombosis. After a thrombotic event, long-term anticoagulation therapy remains the therapeutic approach. The role of corticosteroid or immunosuppressive therapies is limited to special situations such as CAPS or severe thrombocytopenia. The management strategies may vary, depending on the clinical situation:

1. Treatment of patients who are APLA positive with prior thrombosis
2. Primary thromboprophylaxis in patients who are APLA positive without prior thrombosis
3. Obstetric APS
4. CAPS

Treatment of Patients with Prior Thrombosis

The risk of recurrent thrombosis in a patient with positive APLAs and a prior thrombosis is between 22% and 69%.[68-70] The risk is highest in the first year after the discontinuation of anticoagulation

therapy.[71,72] Experts recommend life-long anticoagulation for APS patients after a thrombotic event. These recommendations apply to patients with persistently positive APLAs in moderate to high titers or the LA and a definite diagnosis of APS. Patients with prior thrombosis and APLA positivity who do not fulfill the APS criteria (e.g., low titer, transient) should be managed as the general population.[73]

Initial retrospective studies suggested that high-intensity anticoagulation with warfarin with a target international normalized ratio (INR) of 3.0 or higher was more effective than moderate-intensity anticoagulation (target INR of 2.0 to 3.0).[72,74] In contrast, two randomized controlled trials found that high-intensity warfarin was not better than moderate-intensity warfarin (INR of 2.0 to 3.0) in preventing recurrent thrombosis.[75,76] However, patients with arterial thrombosis were not well represented in these studies.

Limited data are available for recommendations in patients who develop recurrences on oral anticoagulation. Special emphasis should be placed on monitoring and achieving the target INR, as the majority of recurrences occur during periods of subtherapeutic INR.[77] If the recurrent event occurred on the target INR, then increasing the target INR to higher than 3.0, adding aspirin, or switching to low–molecular-weight heparin (LMWH) can be considered. These decisions have to be individualized, with the knowledge that supporting evidence is very limited.[72,77,78]

Recently, direct anticoagulants have been developed that target a single step in the coagulation mechanism. Dabigatran etexilate directly binds to both free and clot-associated thrombin. It has been shown to have similar efficacy to warfarin with a reduced need for monitoring and fewer bleeding episodes in patients with venous thromboembolism and atrial fibrillation.[79,80] Currently, however, the U.S. Food and Drug Administration (FDA) has not approved the use of direct anticoagulants in the treatment of APS. More efficacy and safety data are required before any recommendations can be made for the use of these drugs in patients with APS.

Primary Thromboprophylaxis

The risk of thrombosis in asymptomatic carriers of APLAs depends not only on the types and titers of the antibody but also on associated risk factors. Studies suggest that patients with SLE and APLA have a high risk of thrombosis. A large cohort study from Hopkins reported increased risks for arterial and venous thrombosis in patients with SLE and the presence of any APLA (odds ratio, 1.84), but the risk was highest with LA (odds ratio, 4.16).[64] Women with purely obstetric APS are also noted to have a risk of future thrombosis.[81,82] In contrast, the risk in healthy asymptomatic carriers of APLAs is low.[83]

Studies evaluating the benefit of aspirin in asymptomatic carriers of APLAs have reported conflicting results. Earlier retrospective studies have shown a beneficial effect of aspirin in asymptomatic APLA carriers with SLE and in women with obstetric APS.[81,84,85] In contrast, a later randomized trial, Antiphospholipid Antibody Acetylsalicylic Acid (APLASA) study, found no difference in treating asymptomatic APLA carriers with low-dose aspirin versus placebo.[86] However, this study has been criticized for excluding high-risk groups and being underpowered to detect a beneficial effect of aspirin. Low-dose aspirin can be considered as a primary thromboprophylaxis in patients with SLE and persistently positive APLA. Women with obstetric APS and no prior thrombosis can also be considered for long-term aspirin therapy.[81]

Hydroxychloroquine has been shown to reduce the risk of thrombosis in SLE, in addition to its beneficial effects on disease activity.[87] It should be considered in patients with SLE who are APLA positive, in addition to aspirin.

Additional risk factors such as smoking, hypertension, and estrogen therapy further increase the risk of thrombosis. In the APLASA study, the majority of thrombotic events occurred in patients with additional thrombotic risk factors or autoimmune diseases in addition to the presence of APLAs.[86]

Obstetric Antiphospholipid Syndrome

The pharmacologic treatment of obstetric APS depends on the presence or absence of concomitant risk factors and can generally be divided into the following groups:

- **Low-risk patients**: This group includes women with positive APLAs but no prior thrombotic event or prior pregnancy loss. Studies have shown lower live-birth rates in APLA-positive women (range of 62% to 84%) than in APLA-negative women (range of 90% to 98%).[88] Although data are limited, low-dose aspirin is recommended throughout the pregnancy.[88,89]
- **Medium-risk patients**: This group includes women with recurrent early losses or one or more late fetal loss in the presence of APLAs. Studies have evaluated different therapies including aspirin, heparin, corticosteroids, and intravenous immunoglobulin (IVIG). A Cochrane analysis and a recent metaanalysis have summarized the extensive literature in this field.[57,90] Current consensus is that prophylactic doses of heparin, in combination with aspirin, significantly reduce the risk of pregnancy loss.[57,89,90] LMWH has similar efficacy to unfractionated heparin, with fewer adverse effects and ease of monitoring. Some pharmacokinetic studies have suggested that LMWH may require more frequent dosing during pregnancy.[91] Although practices differ, twice daily dosing of LMWH during pregnancy, even for prophylactic doses, are suggested. LMWH may have a prolonged duration of action at the time of delivery, when it may be necessary to reverse anticoagulation rapidly. Therefore before delivery, LMWH must be switched to unfractionated heparin. Heparin should be continued for 6 weeks after delivery.[92] Corticosteroids, in combination with aspirin, have similar efficacy but higher maternal morbidity.[89,93]
- **High-risk patients**: This group can include two types of patients:
  1. Women with recurrent losses despite treatment with heparin and aspirin—no set regimen exists for this clinical scenario. The addition of IVIG to heparin and aspirin did not have any added benefits in two underpowered trials.[94,95]
  2. Patients with previous thrombosis should be given therapeutic doses of heparin throughout pregnancy. Warfarin is contraindicated in pregnancy because of its teratogenic potential.[96] The switch to heparin should be made before conception because the risk of warfarin embryopathy is high, even with a short exposure before a pregnancy is clinically recognized.

Catastrophic Antiphospholipid Syndrome

CAPS is an uncommon but severe form of APS with a very high mortality. The current treatment guidelines include heparin, intravenous methylprednisolone, and plasmapheresis or IVIG.[60] Heparin is preferred because it likely inhibits complement activation (antiinflammatory effect) in addition to anticoagulation. Heparin can be followed by oral anticoagulation. IVIG, instead of plasmapheresis, can be particularly useful in patients with severe thrombocytopenia. Caution should be exercised in the use of IVIG; the risk of increased thromboembolism and renal failure has been described.[60] Rituximab has been suggested for refractory cases.[97,98]

Other Therapies
Statins

Statins inhibit the enzyme hydroxymethylglutaryl–coenzyme A (HMG-CoA) reductase and are involved in the mevalonate pathway of cholesterol synthesis. In addition to their known cholesterol-lowering effects, statins have pleiotropic effects on endothelial function, inflammatory responses, plaque stability, and thrombus formation.[99] This dual ability of statins to lower cholesterol and inhibit inflammation may provide additional benefit in APS. In vitro and animal studies have shown that statins inhibit APLA-induced tissue-factor production, endothelial cell adhesiveness, and thrombus formation.[100,101] In a pilot study of nine patients with APS, fluvastatin at 40 mg per day decreased the concentrations of inflammatory and thrombogenic mediators after 30 days of treatment.[102] In another study of 42 patients with APS and 35 controls, fluvastatin at a dose of 20 mg per day for a month led to alterations in monocyte activity with reduced prothrombotic tendency.[103] Statins reduced miscarriages in an APS pregnancy mouse model, but the clinical use of statins in human pregnancy must be avoided in view of teratogenicity.[104-106] Data from a recent large randomized controlled trial, Justification for the Use of Statin in Prevention: An Intervention Trial Evaluating Rosuvastatin (JUPITER), showed a decreased risk of venous thromboembolism in healthy people with normal cholesterol concentrations given rosuvastatin.[107] Although evidence for the benefit of statins in APS is currently limited to animal models and mechanistic studies in humans, statins are likely to be prescribed to a large number of patients with APS for other clinical indications. Whether statins will provide additional antithrombotic benefits needs to be evaluated further in large-scale clinical studies.

Rituximab

Rituximab is a chimeric anti–cluster of differentiation 20 (CD20) monoclonal antibody that depletes CD20-positive B cells. It has been used in the treatment of B-cell malignancies and in certain autoimmune diseases, including rheumatoid arthritis and immune-mediated thrombocytopenia. Rituximab had shown a high response rate in refractory APS in multiple case reports and series.[108,109] The clinical resolution of symptoms, including thrombosis and hematologic and other noncriteria manifestations, was reported in the majority of these patients. APLA levels became negative or were significantly reduced. In addition, significant reductions in APLAs were also reported in a cohort of 32 patients with SLE who received B-cell depletion therapy.[110]

Future Targets

Current treatment of APS remains ineffective in some patients. Agents with potential benefit in APS include direct anticoagulants, tissue-factor inhibitors, complement-based therapies, and signaling pathway inhibitors. They remain in development phases, and their role in APS management remains to be defined.[109,111]

CONCLUSION

In summary, APS is an acquired thrombophilic state, in which autoantibodies against phospholipid-binding proteins generate a prothrombotic state. Additional second hits are likely necessary to lead to clinical episodes of thrombosis. These antibodies also mediate the pregnancy morbidity associated with the syndrome, as well as other nonthrombotic manifestations. After a thrombotic event, long-term anticoagulation is recommended.

References

1. Miyakis S, Lockshin MD, Atsumi T, et al: International consensus statement on an update of the classification criteria for definite antiphospholipid syndrome (APS). *J Thromb Haemost* 4(2):295–306, 2006.
2. Bushnell CD, Goldstein LB: Diagnostic testing for coagulopathies in patients with ischemic stroke. *Stroke* 31(12):3067–3078, 2000.
3. Ginsburg KS, Liang MH, Newcomer L, et al: Anticardiolipin antibodies and the risk for ischemic stroke and venous thrombosis. *Ann Intern Med* 117(12):997–1002, 1992.
4. Tektonidou MG, Laskari K, Panagiotakos DB, et al: Risk factors for thrombosis and primary thrombosis prevention in patients with systemic lupus erythematosus with or without antiphospholipid antibodies. *Arthritis Rheum* 61(1):29–36, 2009.
5. Rai RS, Regan L, Clifford K, et al: Antiphospholipid antibodies and beta 2-glycoprotein-I in 500 women with recurrent miscarriage: results of a comprehensive screening approach. *Hum Reprod* 10(8):2001–2005, 1995.
6. Yetman DL, Kutteh WH: Antiphospholipid antibody panels and recurrent pregnancy loss: prevalence of anticardiolipin antibodies compared with other antiphospholipid antibodies. *Fertil Steril* 66(4):540–546, 1996.
7. Ruiz-Irastorza G, Crowther M, Branch W, et al: Antiphospholipid syndrome. *Lancet* 376(9751):1498–1509, 2010.

8. Wilson WA, Gharavi AE, Koike T, et al: International consensus statement on preliminary classification criteria for definite antiphospholipid syndrome: report of an international workshop. *Arthritis Rheum* 42(7): 1309–1311, 1999.

9. Arnout J, Vermylen J: Current status and implications of autoimmune antiphospholipid antibodies in relation to thrombotic disease. *J Thromb Haemost* 1(5):931–942, 2003.

10. de Groot PG, Derksen RH: Pathophysiology of the antiphospholipid syndrome. *J Thromb Haemost* 3(8):1854–1860, 2005.

11. Rand JH, Wu XX, Quinn AS, et al: The annexin A5-mediated pathogenic mechanism in the antiphospholipid syndrome: role in pregnancy losses and thrombosis. *Lupus* 19(4):460–469, 2010.

12. Frank M, Sodin-Semrl S, Rozman B, et al: Effects of low-molecular-weight heparin on adhesion and vesiculation of phospholipid membranes: a possible mechanism for the treatment of hypercoagulability in antiphospholipid syndrome. *Ann N Y Acad Sci* 1173:874–886, 2009.

13. Salmon JE, de Groot PG: Pathogenic role of antiphospholipid antibodies. *Lupus* 17(5):405–411, 2008.

14. Pierangeli SS, Girardi G, Vega-Ostertag M, et al: Requirement of activation of complement C3 and C5 for antiphospholipid antibody-mediated thrombophilia. *Arthritis Rheum* 52(7):2120–2124, 2005.

15. Oku K, Atsumi T, Bohgaki M, et al: Complement activation in patients with primary antiphospholipid syndrome. *Ann Rheum Dis* 68(6):1030–1035, 2009.

16. Girardi G, Redecha P, Salmon JE: Heparin prevents antiphospholipid antibody-induced fetal loss by inhibiting complement activation. *Nat Med* 10(11):1222–1226, 2004.

17. Salmon JE, Girardi G: Antiphospholipid antibodies and pregnancy loss: a disorder of inflammation. *J Reprod Immunol* 77(1):51–56, 2008.

18. Salmon JE, Girardi G, Lockshin MD: The antiphospholipid syndrome as a disorder initiated by inflammation: implications for the therapy of pregnant patients. *Nat Clin Pract Rheumatol* 3(3):140–147; quiz 1 p following 187, 2007 Mar.

19. Di Simone N, Meroni PL, D'Asta M, et al: Pathogenic role of anti-beta2-glycoprotein I antibodies on human placenta: functional effects related to implantation and roles of heparin. *Hum Reprod Update* 13(2):189–196, 2007.

20. Urbanus RT, Siegerink B, Roest M, et al: Antiphospholipid antibodies and risk of myocardial infarction and ischaemic stroke in young women in the RATIO study: a case-control study. *Lancet Neurol* 8(11):998–1005, 2009.

21. Cervera R, Boffa MC, Khamashta MA, et al: The Euro-Phospholipid project: epidemiology of the antiphospholipid syndrome in Europe. *Lupus* 18(10):889–893, 2009.

22. Hughes GR: Hughes syndrome (the antiphospholipid syndrome): a disease of our time. *Inflammopharmacology* 19(2):69–73, 2011.

23. Bucciarelli S, Espinosa G, Cervera R: The CAPS Registry: morbidity and mortality of the catastrophic antiphospholipid syndrome. *Lupus* 18(10): 905–912, 2009.

24. Arnson Y, Shoenfeld Y, Alon E, et al: The antiphospholipid syndrome as a neurological disease. *Semin Arthritis Rheum* 40(2):97–108, 2010.

25. Muscal E, Brey RL. Antiphospholipid syndrome and the brain in pediatric and adult patients. *Lupus* 2010;19(4):406–411.

26. Chapman J, Soloveichick L, Shavit S, et al: Antiphospholipid antibodies bind ATP: a putative mechanism for the pathogenesis of neuronal dysfunction. *Clin Dev Immunol* 12(3):175–180, 2005.

27. Cervera R, Asherson RA, Font J, et al: Chorea in the antiphospholipid syndrome. Clinical, radiologic, and immunologic characteristics of 50 patients from our clinics and the recent literature. *Medicine (Baltimore)* 76(3):203–212, 1997.

28. Espinosa G, Cervera R, Font J, et al: Antiphospholipid syndrome: pathogenic mechanisms. *Autoimmun Rev* 2(2):86–93, 2003.

29. Mejia-Romero R, Garcia-Carrasco M, Galarza-Maldonado C, et al: Primary antiphospholipid syndrome in Latin American mestizo patients: clinical and immunologic characteristics and comparison with European patients. *Clin Rheumatol* 27(7):891–897, 2008.

30. Asherson RA, Mercey D, Phillips G, et al: Recurrent stroke and multi-infarct dementia in systemic lupus erythematosus: association with antiphospholipid antibodies. *Ann Rheum Dis* 46(8):605–611, 1987.

31. Janardhan V, Wolf PA, Kase CS, et al: Anticardiolipin antibodies and risk of ischemic stroke and transient ischemic attack: the Framingham cohort and offspring study. *Stroke* 35(3):736–741, 2004.

32. Toloza SM, Uribe AG, McGwin G, Jr, et al: Systemic lupus erythematosus in a multiethnic US cohort (LUMINA). XXIII. Baseline predictors of vascular events. *Arthritis Rheum* 50(12):3947–3957, 2004.

33. Krause I, Lev S, Fraser A, et al: Close association between valvar heart disease and central nervous system manifestations in the antiphospholipid syndrome. *Ann Rheum Dis* 64(10):1490–1493, 2005.

34. Roldan CA, Gelgand EA, Qualls CR, et al: Valvular heart disease as a cause of cerebrovascular disease in patients with systemic lupus erythematosus. *Am J Cardiol* 15;95(12):1441–1447, 2005.

35. Pardos-Gea J, Ordi-Ros J, Avegliano G, et al: Echocardiography at diagnosis of antiphospholipid syndrome provides prognostic information on valvular disease evolution and identifies two subtypes of patients. *Lupus* 19(5):575–582, 2010.

36. Eriksson K, Peltola J, Keranen T, et al: High prevalence of antiphospholipid antibodies in children with epilepsy: a controlled study of 50 cases. *Epilepsy Res* 46(2):129–137, 2001.

37. Tanne D, Hassin-Baer S: Neurologic manifestations of the antiphospholipid syndrome. *Curr Rheumatol Rep* 3(4):286–292, 2001.

38. Cimaz R, Meroni PL, Shoenfeld Y: Epilepsy as part of systemic lupus erythematosus and systemic antiphospholipid syndrome (Hughes syndrome). *Lupus* 15(4):191–197, 2006.

39. Sanna G, Bertolaccini ML, Cuadrado MJ, et al: Central nervous system involvement in the antiphospholipid (Hughes) syndrome. *Rheumatology (Oxford)* 42(2):200–213, 2003.

40. Avcin T, Cimaz R, Silverman ED, et al: Pediatric antiphospholipid syndrome: clinical and immunologic features of 121 patients in an international registry. *Pediatrics* 122(5):e1100–e1107, 2008.

41. Rodrigues CE, de Carvalho JF: Clinical, radiologic, and therapeutic analysis of 14 patients with transverse myelitis associated with antiphospholipid syndrome: report of 4 cases and review of the literature. *Semin Arthritis Rheum* 40(4):349–357, 2011.

42. Birnbaum J, Petri M, Thompson R, et al: Distinct subtypes of myelitis in systemic lupus erythematosus. *Arthritis Rheum* 60(11):3378–3387, 2009.

43. Squatrito D, Colagrande S, Emmi L: Devic's syndrome and primary APS: a new immunological overlap. *Lupus* 19(11):1337–1339, 2010.

44. Utz VM, Tang J: Ocular manifestations of the antiphospholipid syndrome. *Br J Ophthalmol* 95(4):454–459, 2011.

45. Sacre K, Brihaye B, Hyafil F, et al: Asymptomatic myocardial ischemic disease in antiphospholipid syndrome: a controlled cardiac magnetic resonance imaging study. *Arthritis Rheum* 62(7):2093–2100, 2010.

46. Nesher G, Ilany J, Rosenmann D, et al: Valvular dysfunction in antiphospholipid syndrome: prevalence, clinical features, and treatment. *Semin Arthritis Rheum* 27(1):27–35, 1997.

47. Turiel M, Muzzupappa S, Gottardi B, et al: Evaluation of cardiac abnormalities and embolic sources in primary antiphospholipid syndrome by transesophageal echocardiography. *Lupus* 9(6):406–412, 2000.

48. Cervera R, Piette JC, Font J, et al: Antiphospholipid syndrome: clinical and immunologic manifestations and patterns of disease expression in a cohort of 1,000 patients. *Arthritis Rheum* 46(4):1019–1027, 2002.

49. Frances C, Niang S, Laffitte E, et al: Dermatologic manifestations of the antiphospholipid syndrome: two hundred consecutive cases. *Arthritis Rheum* 52(6):1785–1793, 2005.

50. Frances C: Dermatological manifestations of Hughes' antiphospholipid antibody syndrome. *Lupus* 19(9):1071–1077, 2010.

51. Frances C, Papo T, Wechsler B, et al: Sneddon syndrome with or without antiphospholipid antibodies. A comparative study in 46 patients. *Medicine (Baltimore)* 78(4):209–219, 1999.

52. Ford HJ, Roubey RA: Pulmonary manifestations of the antiphospholipid antibody syndrome. *Clin Chest Med* 31(3):537–545, 2010.

53. Bizzaro N, Brandalise M: EDTA-dependent pseudothrombocytopenia. Association with antiplatelet and antiphospholipid antibodies. *Am J Clin Pathol* 103(1):103–107, 1995.

54. Gigante A, Gasperini ML, Cianci R, et al: Antiphospholipid antibodies and renal involvement. *Am J Nephrol* 30(5):405–412, 2009.

55. Jones LC, Mont MA, Le TB, et al: Procoagulants and osteonecrosis. *J Rheumatol* 30(4):783–791, 2003.

56. Tincani A, Bompane D, Danieli E, et al: Pregnancy, lupus and antiphospholipid syndrome (Hughes syndrome). *Lupus* 15(3):156–160, 2006.

57. Mak A, Cheung MW, Cheak AA, et al: Combination of heparin and aspirin is superior to aspirin alone in enhancing live births in patients with recurrent pregnancy loss and positive anti-phospholipid antibodies: a meta-analysis of randomized controlled trials and meta-regression. *Rheumatology (Oxford)* 49(2):281–288, 2010.

58. Asherson RA, Cervera R, de Groot PG, et al: Catastrophic antiphospholipid syndrome: international consensus statement on classification criteria and treatment guidelines. *Lupus* 12(7):530–534, 2003.

59. Cervera R, Font J, Gómez-Puerta JA, et al: Validation of the preliminary criteria for the classification of catastrophic antiphospholipid syndrome. *Ann Rheum Dis* 64(8):1205–1209, 2005.

60. Cervera R: Update on the diagnosis, treatment, and prognosis of the catastrophic antiphospholipid syndrome. *Curr Rheumatol Rep* 12(1): 70–76, 2010.

61. Asherson RA, Cervera R: Microvascular and microangiopathic antiphospholipid-associated syndromes ("MAPS"): semantic or antisemantic? *Autoimmun Rev* 7(3):164–167, 2008.

62. Pengo V, Tripodi A, Reber G, et al: Update of the guidelines for lupus anticoagulant detection. Subcommittee on Lupus Anticoagulant/Antiphospholipid Antibody of the Scientific and Standardisation Committee of the International Society on Thrombosis and Haemostasis. *J Thromb Haemost* 7(10):1737–1740, 2009.

63. Galli M, Luciani D, Bertolini G, et al: Lupus anticoagulants are stronger risk factors for thrombosis than anticardiolipin antibodies in the antiphospholipid syndrome: a systematic review of the literature. *Blood* 101(5):1827–1832, 2003.

64. Petri M: Update on anti-phospholipid antibodies in SLE: the Hopkins' Lupus Cohort. *Lupus* 19(4):419–423, 2010.

65. Roubey RA: Risky business: the interpretation, use, and abuse of antiphospholipid antibody tests in clinical practice. *Lupus* 19(4):440–445, 2010.

66. Ruiz-Irastorza G, Khamashta MA: Antiphospholipid syndrome in pregnancy. *Rheum Dis Clin North Am* 33(2):287–297, vi, 2007.

67. Galli M, Comfurius P, Maassen C, et al: Anticardiolipin antibodies (ACA) directed not to cardiolipin but to a plasma protein cofactor. *Lancet* 335(8705):1544–1547, 1990.

68. Finazzi G, Brancaccio V, Moia M, et al: Natural history and risk factors for thrombosis in 360 patients with antiphospholipid antibodies: a four-year prospective study from the Italian Registry. *Am J Med* 100(5):530–536, 1996.

69. Krnic-Barrie S, O'Connor CR, Looney SW, et al: A retrospective review of 61 patients with antiphospholipid syndrome. Analysis of factors influencing recurrent thrombosis. *Arch Intern Med* 157(18):2101–2108, 1997.

70. Rosove MH, Brewer PM: Antiphospholipid thrombosis: clinical course after the first thrombotic event in 70 patients. *Ann Intern Med* 117(4): 303–308, 1992.

71. Lim W, Crowther MA, Eikelboom JW: Management of antiphospholipid antibody syndrome: a systematic review. *JAMA* 295(9):1050–1057, 2006.

72. Khamashta MA, Cuadrado MJ, Mujic F, et al: The management of thrombosis in the antiphospholipid-antibody syndrome. *N Engl J Med* 332(15):993–997, 1995.

73. Kearon C, Kahn SR, Agnelli G, et al: Antithrombotic therapy for venous thromboembolic disease: American College of Chest Physicians Evidence-Based Clinical Practice Guidelines (8th Edition). *Chest* 133(6 Suppl):454S–545S, 2008.

74. Ruiz-Irastorza G, Khamashta MA, Hunt BJ, et al: Bleeding and recurrent thrombosis in definite antiphospholipid syndrome: analysis of a series of 66 patients treated with oral anticoagulation to a target international normalized ratio of 3.5. *Arch Intern Med* 162(10):1164–1169, 2002.

75. Crowther MA, Ginsberg JS, Julian J, et al: A comparison of two intensities of warfarin for the prevention of recurrent thrombosis in patients with the antiphospholipid antibody syndrome. *N Engl J Med* 349(12): 1133–1138, 2003.

76. Finazzi G, Marchioli R, Brancaccio V, et al: A randomized clinical trial of high-intensity warfarin vs. conventional antithrombotic therapy for the prevention of recurrent thrombosis in patients with the antiphospholipid syndrome (WAPS). *J Thromb Haemost* 3(5):848–853, 2005.

77. Crowther M, Crowther MA: Intensity of warfarin coagulation in the antiphospholipid syndrome. *Curr Rheumatol Rep* 12(1):64–69, 2010.

78. Dentali F, Manfredi E, Crowther M, et al: Long-duration therapy with low molecular weight heparin in patients with antiphospholipid antibody syndrome resistant to warfarin therapy. *J Thromb Haemost* 3(9): 2121–2123, 2005.

79. Giorgi MA, Cohen Arazi H, Gonzalez CD, et al: Changing anticoagulant paradigms for atrial fibrillation: dabigatran, apixaban and rivaroxaban. *Expert Opin Pharmacother* 12(4):567–577, 2011.

80. Schulman S, Kearon C, Kakkar AK, et al: Dabigatran versus warfarin in the treatment of acute venous thromboembolism. *N Engl J Med* 361(24): 2342–2352, 2009.

81. Erkan D, Merrill JT, Yazici Y, et al: High thrombosis rate after fetal loss in antiphospholipid syndrome: effective prophylaxis with aspirin. *Arthritis Rheum* 44(6):1466–1467, 2001.

82. Quenby S, Farquharson RG, Dawood F, et al: Recurrent miscarriage and long-term thrombosis risk: a case-control study. *Hum Reprod* 20(6): 1729–1732, 2005.

83. Vila P, Hernández MC, López-Fernández MF, et al: Prevalence, follow-up and clinical significance of the anticardiolipin antibodies in normal subjects. *Thromb Haemost* 72(2):209–213, 1994.

84. Erkan D, Yazici Y, Peterson MG, et al: A cross-sectional study of clinical thrombotic risk factors and preventive treatments in antiphospholipid syndrome. *Rheumatology (Oxford)* 41(8):924–929, 2002.

85. Hereng T, Lambert M, Hachulla E, et al: Influence of aspirin on the clinical outcomes of 103 anti-phospholipid antibodies-positive patients. *Lupus* 17(1):11–15, 2008.

86. Erkan D, Harrison MJ, Levy R, et al: Aspirin for primary thrombosis prevention in the antiphospholipid syndrome: a randomized, double-blind, placebo-controlled trial in asymptomatic antiphospholipid antibody-positive individuals. *Arthritis Rheum* 56(7):2382–2391, 2007.

87. Jung H, Bobba R, Su J, et al: The protective effect of antimalarial drugs on thrombovascular events in systemic lupus erythematosus. *Arthritis Rheum* 62(3):863–868, 2010.

88. Derksen RH, Khamashta MA, Branch DW: Management of the obstetric antiphospholipid syndrome. *Arthritis Rheum* 50(4):1028–1039, 2004.

89. Petri M, Qazi U: Management of antiphospholipid syndrome in pregnancy. *Rheum Dis Clin North Am* 32(3):591–607, 2006.

90. Empson M, Lassere M, Craig J, et al: Prevention of recurrent miscarriage for women with antiphospholipid antibody or lupus anticoagulant. *Cochrane Database Syst Rev* (2):CD002859, 2005.

91. Sephton V, Farquharson RG, Topping J, et al: A longitudinal study of maternal dose response to low molecular weight heparin in pregnancy. *Obstet Gynecol* 101(6):1307–1311, 2003.

92. Bates SM, Greer IA, Pabinger I, et al: Venous thromboembolism, thrombophilia, antithrombotic therapy, and pregnancy: American College of Chest Physicians Evidence-Based Clinical Practice Guidelines (8th Edition). *Chest* 133(6 Suppl):844S–886S, 2008.

93. Cowchock FS, Reece EA, Balaban D, et al: Repeated fetal losses associated with antiphospholipid antibodies: a collaborative randomized trial comparing prednisone with low-dose heparin treatment. *Am J Obstet Gynecol* 166(5):1318–1323, 1992.

94. Dendrinos S, Sakkas E, Makrakis E: Low-molecular-weight heparin versus intravenous immunoglobulin for recurrent abortion associated with antiphospholipid antibody syndrome. *Int J Gynaecol Obstet* 104(3): 223–225, 2009.

95. Triolo G, Ferrante A, Ciccia F, et al: Randomized study of subcutaneous low molecular weight heparin plus aspirin versus intravenous immunoglobulin in the treatment of recurrent fetal loss associated with antiphospholipid antibodies. *Arthritis Rheum* 48(3):728–731, 2003.

96. Abadi S, Einarson A, Koren G: Use of warfarin during pregnancy. *Can Fam Physician* 48:695–697, 2002.

97. Asherson RA, Espinosa G, Menahem S, et al: Relapsing catastrophic antiphospholipid syndrome: report of three cases. *Semin Arthritis Rheum* 37(6):366–372, 2008.

98. Erre GL: Effect of rituximab on clinical and laboratory features of antiphospholipid syndrome: a case report and a review of literature. *Lupus* 17:50–55, 2008.

99. Abeles AM, Pillinger MH: Statins as antiinflammatory and immunomodulatory agents: a future in rheumatologic therapy? *Arthritis Rheum* 54(2):393–407, 2006.

100. Meroni PL, Raschi E, Testoni C, et al: Statins prevent endothelial cell activation induced by antiphospholipid (anti-beta2-glycoprotein I) antibodies: effect on the proadhesive and proinflammatory phenotype. *Arthritis Rheum* 44(12):2870–2878, 2001.

101. Ferrara DE, Liu X, Espinola RG, et al: Inhibition of the thrombogenic and inflammatory properties of antiphospholipid antibodies by fluvastatin in an in vivo animal model. *Arthritis Rheum* 48(11):3272–3279, 2003.

102. Jajoria P, Murthy V, Papalardo E, et al: Statins for the treatment of antiphospholipid syndrome? *Ann N Y Acad Sci* 1173:736–745, 2009.

103. López-Pedrera C, Ruiz-Limón P, Aguirre MÁ, et al: Global effects of fluvastatin on the prothrombotic status of patients with antiphospholipid syndrome. *Ann Rheum Dis* 70(4):675–682, 2011.

104. Redecha P, van Rooijen N, Torry D, et al: Pravastatin prevents miscarriages in mice: role of tissue factor in placental and fetal injury. *Blood* 113(17):4101–4109, 2009.

105. Girardi G: Pravastatin prevents miscarriages in antiphospholipid antibody-treated mice. *J Reprod Immunol* 82(2):126–131, 2009.

106. Lockshin MD, Pierangeli SS: Statins for the treatment of obstetric complications in antiphospholipid syndrome? *J Reprod Immunol* 84(2):206; author reply 206–207, 2010.

107. Glynn RJ, Danielson E, Fonseca FA, et al: A randomized trial of rosuvastatin in the prevention of venous thromboembolism. *N Engl J Med* 360(18):1851–1861, 2009.

108. Kumar D, Roubey RA: Use of rituximab in the antiphospholipid syndrome. *Curr Rheumatol Rep* 12(1):40–44, 2010.

109. Pierangeli SS, Erkan D: Antiphospholipid syndrome treatment beyond anticoagulation: are we there yet? *Lupus* 19(4):475–485, 2010.

110. Melander C, Sallee M, Trolliet P, et al: Rituximab in severe lupus nephritis: early B-cell depletion affects long-term renal outcome. *Clin J Am Soc Nephrol* 4(3):579–587, 2009.

111. Pericleous C, Ioannou Y: New therapeutic targets for the antiphospholipid syndrome. *Expert Opin Ther Targets* 14(12):1291–1299, 2010.

Chapter

43

Clinical Application of Serologic Tests, Serum Protein Abnormalities, and Other Clinical Laboratory Tests in SLE

Francisco P. Quismorio, Jr., and Karina D. Torralba

One hallmark of systemic lupus erythematosus (SLE) is the wide array of serologic abnormalities, including a polyclonal hypergammaglobulinemia, the presence of antinuclear antibodies (ANAs) and various organ-specific and non–organ-specific autoantibodies, circulating immune complexes, and serum complement changes. The presence of some of these serologic abnormalities is important in corroborating the diagnosis of SLE, whereas others are useful in monitoring disease activity.

This chapter focuses on the clinical application of selected serologic abnormalities in establishing the diagnosis, in assessing disease activity, and in predicting specific organ-system involvement and overall prognosis. Immunoglobulins and other serum protein changes in SLE are also discussed. Serologic and other important laboratory tests that are available in most clinical laboratories and other promising tests are reviewed.

DIAGNOSIS OF SYSTEMIC LUPUS ERYTHEMATOSUS

When the diagnosis of SLE is suspected or made on the basis of clinical data, the following serologic tests are considered to be helpful in corroborating the diagnosis: immunofluorescent ANA test, ANA panel, serum complement level, and antiphospholipid antibodies (APLAs) that include lupus anticoagulant, anticardiolipin antibodies, and Venereal Disease Research Laboratory (VDRL) or other comparable serologic tests for syphilis. In certain situations, other serologic tests are applicable, such as the Coombs test in a patient with hemolytic anemia, or lupus anticoagulant and anticardiolipin antibodies in a patient with thrombosis or pregnancy-related abnormalities.

Virtually all patients with active and untreated SLE test positive for ANAs. Nevertheless, ANAs are prevalent in other rheumatic and nonrheumatic disorders including conditions that mimic the clinical features of SLE. ANAs are also found in healthy children and adults.

Thus, by itself, a positive ANA test result has a low diagnostic specificity for SLE, but its value increases when the patient meets the clinical criteria for SLE.

The indirect immunofluorescent antibody (IFA) test is the most commonly used method for detecting ANAs, and the choice of substrate in this test is important. Most clinical laboratories use human epithelial-2 (HEp-2), a tissue culture cell line, as the substrate and a positive serum titered to give a semiquantitative value to the antibody level. Each clinical laboratory should have normal reference values, although most consider an IFA titer of less than 1:40 as negative.

The indirect IFA test for ANA is useful for screening when the index of suspicion for SLE or other systemic rheumatic diseases such as systemic sclerosis is high. A study in a large teaching hospital revealed a high sensitivity of a positive ANA test for SLE; however, the positive predictive value was low for SLE because many patients with other diagnoses also tested positive for ANAs.[1] The clinician should recognize the limitation of a positive ANA test when the patient in question does not have clinical features consistent with SLE or other connective tissue diseases.

Automated screening methods using bead-based multiplex platforms, enzyme-linked immunosorbent assays (ELISA), and other solid-phase immunoassays for ANAs have been developed and are now used by many hospital and commercial clinical laboratories. Automated tests are less time consuming and less labor intensive; however, only a limited number of purified nuclear antigens are included in these tests. More importantly, no comprehensive or organized study has been conducted that compares these various methods with the immunofluorescent ANA test with regard to sensitivity, specificity, and predictive values. The American College of Rheumatology Antinuclear Antibody Task Force recommends that the immunofluorescent test remain the "gold standard" for ANA testing

Adapted from Solomon DH, Kavanaugh AJ, Schur PH, American College of Rheumatology Ad Hoc Committee on Immunologic Testing Guidelines: Evidence-based guidelines for the use of immunologic tests: antinuclear antibody testing. *Arthritis Rheum* 47(4):434–444, 2002.

> **Box 43-1** Evidence-Based Guidelines for Immunofluorescent Antinuclear Antibody Testing
>
> 1. Immunofluorescent antinuclear antibody (ANA) test results should include the highest titer for which immunofluorescence is detected. The laboratory report should include the percentage of control patients without those ANA-associated diseases who have similar titers.
> 2. Immunofluorescent ANA testing should preferably use human epithelial-2 (HEp-2) cell line or rodent tissue as substrate.
> 3. Immunofluorescent ANA is the best diagnostic test when a strong clinical suspicion exists that a patient has SLE.
> 4. Immunofluorescent ANA tests should be conducted when the diagnosis of systemic sclerosis is suspected. A negative test result should prompt consideration of other fibrosing conditions including eosinophilic fasciitis or linear scleroderma.
> 5. Immunofluorescent ANA testing is useful when the diagnosis of mixed connective tissue disease (MCTD) or drug-induced lupus erythematosus is suspected.
> 6. All patients with known juvenile chronic arthritis should be tested for immunofluorescent ANA to stratify the risk of uveitis.
> 7. ANAs should be tested in patients with Raynaud phenomenon only when signs and symptoms of an underlying connective tissue disease are present.
> 8. Immunofluorescent ANA testing is not useful in establishing the diagnosis of rheumatoid arthritis (RA), polymyositis, dermatomyositis, or fibromyalgia.
> 9. Serial immunofluorescent ANA testing in patients with known positive ANAs, including those with SLE, systemic sclerosis, MCTD, and RA, is not clinically useful in monitoring disease activity.

at this time. Standardization of the ANA test and other autoantibody tests is being undertaken by international ad hoc committees. While waiting for their recommendations, a clinical laboratory using a solid-phase immunoassay should provide data on request by the clinician that the sensitivity and specificity of the test system used are the same as or better than the immunofluorescent ANA test.[2,3] Box 43-1 shows evidence-based guidelines for immunofluorescent ANA testing.[3]

The ANA panel that is available in most clinical laboratories includes ANAs of defined specificity: anti–double stranded DNA (anti-dsDNA), anti-Smith (anti-Sm), anti–U1 ribonucleoprotein (anti–U1-RNP), anti–Sjögren syndrome antigen A (anti-SSA/Ro), anti–Sjögren syndrome antigen B (anti-SSB/La), anticentromere, antiscleroderma 70 kD (anti-Scl-70) (also known as antitopoisomerase I), and anti–tRNA synthetase (anti–Jo-1). Other laboratories offer tests for antinucleosome, antihistone, anti–ribosomal P, and anti–single stranded DNA (anti-ssDNA) antibodies.

When the immunofluorescent ANA test is positive in a patient suspected of having SLE, an ANA panel should be obtained. Anti-dsDNA and anti-Sm antibodies are considered highly diagnostic, and the presence of either or both antibodies confirms the clinical diagnosis of SLE. However, a negative test for either or both does not exclude the diagnosis because anti-dsDNA antibodies are seen in up to 60% of patients, whereas anti-Sm antibodies are present in approximately 30% of the patients with SLE. The other specific types of ANAs in the panel have a lesser value as a diagnostic marker for SLE except in special situations such as positive anti-SSA/Ro antibodies in a patient with subacute cutaneous lupus or neonatal lupus syndrome.

A positive test for APLAs measured as anticardiolipin antibodies, lupus anticoagulant, or a biologic false-positive VDRL is included in the American College of Rheumatology (ACR) criteria for the classification of SLE. These are helpful in delineating a subset of patients with SLE and secondary antiphospholipid syndrome. Moderate to high titers of immunoglobulin G (IgG) and/or immunoglobulin M (IgM) anticardiolipin antibodies on two separate occasions, 12 weeks apart, are the criteria for antiphospholipid syndrome. The clinical significance of low-titered anticardiolipin antibodies is not known.

Serum complement levels are measured as concentration of C3 and/or C4 or as CH50 hemolytic units. Although most commonly used clinically to monitor disease activity, the presence of both hypocomplementemia and elevated titers of anti-dsDNA is highly associated with the diagnosis of SLE. Additionally, genetic deficiencies of early components of classical complement (C1) pathway are associated with increased risk for SLE or lupus-like syndrome. Genetic deficiencies of C1q and C1r/C1s have the highest risk, whereas deficiencies of C4 and C2 have a lower risk. A combination of normal serum C3 and low CH50 should raise the possibility of genetic complement deficiency. In patients with fewer than four of the ACR criteria, the presence of low C4 levels was predictive of subsequent evolution into SLE.[4]

MONITORING DISEASE ACTIVITY IN SYSTEMIC LUPUS ERYTHEMATOSUS

Serologic tests are widely used for assessing disease activity and predicting exacerbations. Determinations of the serum titer of anti-dsDNA and of serum complement are the most common and probably the most useful serologic tests that are readily available to the clinician.

Although applicable to most patients, both tests have important clinical limitations. Elevated titers of anti-dsDNA and hypocomplementemia do not occur in every patient with active SLE, and their correlation with the disease activity is not absolute. A subset of these patients test positive for anti-dsDNA antibodies (i.e., "serologically active") but without evidence of clinical disease activity, even when followed for several months.[5,6] Box 43-2 provides recommendations by the European League Against Rheumatism (EULAR) on laboratory assessment for monitoring SLE in clinical practice.[6]

> **Box 43-2** EULAR Recommendations on Laboratory Assessment for Monitoring Systemic Lupus Erythematosus in Clinical Practice
>
> 1. Changes in anti–double stranded DNA (anti-dsDNA) antibody titers sometimes correlate with disease activity and active renal disease and may be useful in monitoring disease activity.
> 2. Treating patients with anti-dsDNA antibodies in the absence of clinical activity is not recommended.
> 3. Anti–Sjögren syndrome antigen A (anti-SSA/Ro), anti–Sjögren syndrome antigen B (anti-SSB/La), and antiribonucleoprotein (anti-RNP) may have prognostic value in systemic lupus erythematosus (SLE).
> 4. Complement levels are sometimes associated with active disease, although no predictive value for the development of disease flares is available.
> 5. Antiphospholipid antibodies are associated with general disease activity, thrombotic manifestations, damage development, and pregnancy complications.

EULAR, European League Against Rheumatism.
Adapted from Mosca M, Tani C, Aringer M, et al: European League Against Rheumatism recommendations for monitoring patients with systemic lupus erythematosus in clinical practice and in observational studies. *Ann Rheum* 69:1269–1274, 2010.

CLINICAL SIGNIFICANCE OF ANTI–DOUBLE STRANDED DNA ANTIBODIES

Diagnostic Value

Anti-dsDNA should be tested if the screening test for ANAs is positive in a patient suspected of having SLE.[7] The presence of anti-dsDNA is highly characteristic of SLE and is rarely seen in other rheumatic conditions except for drug-induced lupus secondary to anti–tumor necrosis factor agents used for rheumatoid arthritis (RA) and seronegative spondyloarthropathies.[8]

Anti-dsDNA antibodies are listed as an immunologic criterion for the classification of SLE by the ACR. In a large prospective study, the combination of an elevated titer of anti-dsDNA and low serum C3 has a high positive predictive value for the diagnosis of SLE.[9]

Clinical Tests for Anti–Double Stranded DNA

The most commonly available tests for anti-dsDNA in clinical practice are the radioimmunoassays using the Farr or Millipore filter binding technique, *Crithidia luciliae* immunofluorescent test, and ELISA. The Farr technique is a sensitive, highly reproducible method; it provides greater sensitivity for diagnosis and is helpful in monitoring disease activity but may miss low-avidity anti-dsDNA antibodies. Approximately 60% to 70% of patients with SLE will test positive by this method some time along the course of their illness. The immunofluorescent test uses fixed smears of *C. luciliae*, a non-pathogenic hemoflagellate containing a cytoplasmic organelle—called *kinetoplast*—that consists of pure circular dsDNA. The test is simple, has relatively good sensitivity and specificity, and measures both high- and intermediate-avidity anti-dsDNA antibodies. However, a precise serum titer cannot be easily determined. The ELISA test for anti-dsDNA is technically easier to perform, can be automated, and is thus less labor intensive and rapid, as well as avoids the use of radioactive reagents. The serum titer can be readily quantified, and both low- and high-avidity anti-dsDNA antibodies can be detected. False-positive test results can be observed when impure DNA is used as a substrate.

The qualitative properties of anti-dsDNA, including avidity, complement-fixing property, and immunoglobulin class, may affect their pathogenicity. The various clinical tests for anti-dsDNA preferentially measure antibodies of different properties and thus do not necessarily provide identical information on an individual patient.

In general, the highly specific Farr technique or the *C. luciliae* immunofluorescent test is best used for the diagnosis of SLE. The ELISA test can also be used, but using it later to confirm a positive result from either the Farr technique or the *C. luciliae* immunofluorescent test may be preferable. Box 43-3 shows guidelines for anti-dsDNA testing in the rheumatic diseases.[7]

For monitoring the disease course, especially lupus nephritis, quantitative measurement by ELISA or the Farr technique and expressing the results in international units per milliliter (IU/mL) are recommended.[10]

Preemptive Treatment of Serologically Active Systemic Lupus Erythematosus

Prospective controlled studies have examined whether increasing the daily dose of corticosteroids soon after a rise in serum titer of anti-dsDNA antibodies and/or the elevation in serum C3a can prevent clinical relapse. Bootsma and associates[11] reported that early treatment with prednisone as soon as a 25% rise in anti-dsDNA was measured by the Farr technique prevented a clinical relapse in most but not all patients. Tseng and colleagues[12] used a more stringent criterion for a serologic relapse—an elevation in anti-dsDNA level by 25% and an elevated level of serum C3a—and reported that a short-term, moderate dose of prednisone in clinically stable patients with SLE may have averted a severe disease flare. The results of this preliminary study, however, cannot be generalized and recommended to all patients with SLE. Certain limitations in the study design and an estimated positive-predictive value of 40% for the serologic change to predict flares indicated that these were not strong biomarkers for

Box 43-3 Guidelines for Anti–Double Stranded DNA Testing in the Rheumatic Diseases

1. Anti–double stranded DNA (anti-dsDNA) antibodies provide strong support for the diagnosis of systemic lupus erythematosus (SLE) in the correct clinical setting. Patients who are positive for antinuclear antibodies (ANAs) should be tested.
2. A positive anti-dsDNA test result does not necessarily make a diagnosis of SLE because anti-dsDNA antibodies may be found in a small number of patients with other conditions.
3. A negative test result for anti-dsDNA antibodies does not exclude the diagnosis of SLE.
4. Testing for anti-dsDNA antibodies is not useful in establishing the diagnosis of systemic sclerosis, rheumatoid arthritis, and other rheumatic diseases.
5. Anti-dsDNA antibodies correlate with overall disease activity, but the results must be interpreted in the overall clinical context.
6. Anti-dsDNA antibodies correlate with disease activity of lupus nephritis but only to a limited extent.
7. Increasing titers of anti-dsDNA antibodies may antedate or be associated with lupus disease flares.

Adapted from Kavanaugh AF, Solomon DH, American College of Rheumatology Ad Hoc Committee on Immunologic Testing Guidelines: Guidelines for immunologic laboratory testing in the rheumatic diseases: anti-DNA antibody tests. *Arthritis Rheum* 47(5):546–555, 2002.

disease flares.[13] Moreover, disease flares can occur in patients without a rise in anti-dsDNA and/or a lowering of serum C3 or C4 levels. The use of medications other than systemic corticosteroids as preemptive treatments has not been investigated.

Summary

The quantitative determination of anti-dsDNA antibodies does not adequately predict disease flares in every patient, which is not unexpected considering the heterogeneity of the clinical disease and the anti-dsDNA antibodies. The qualitative properties of the anti-dsDNA antibodies, such as the complement-fixing property, avidity, dissociation constant, and immunoglobulin class, as well as the total antibody content are important determinants in the pathogenicity and correlation with disease activity. Most of these measurements, however, are not readily available to the practicing clinician. Meanwhile, the anti-dsDNA antibody titer continues to be widely used as a serologic parameter for assessing disease activity. Combined with serum complement and other renal laboratory parameters, anti-dsDNA antibody titer is a valuable parameter in patients with lupus nephritis. It is especially useful if the patient in question has had a high anti-dsDNA and a low serum complement in past exacerbations of the disease. Anti-dsDNA should be measured at frequent intervals when following the clinical course of the patient.

ANTI-SMITH ANTIBODIES

Anti-Sm antibodies react to multiple antigens in small ribonucleoprotein particles that function in the splicing of precursor messenger RNA. Different methods and antigen preparations are used in the clinical laboratories for measuring anti-Sm antibodies, including immunodiffusion, ELISA, counterimmunoelectrophoresis (CIE), multiplex bead assays, and hemagglutination. The ELISA test, using purified antigens, is more sensitive than immunodiffusion or CIE but less specific; however, it is superior in quantifying the serum antibody titer.

Anti-Sm antibodies are present in only 30% of patients with SLE, but these autoantibodies have considerable diagnostic value because they are rarely found in other rheumatic diseases, such as mixed connective tissue disease (MCTD), systemic sclerosis, and RA. Anti-Sm is included in the ACR criteria for the classification of SLE, and, as an immunologic parameter, it carries the same weight as anti-dsDNA antibodies and APLAs.

As a diagnostic test, anti-Sm has a relatively low sensitivity but a high specificity; thus a positive test result is useful in confirming a diagnosis. However, a negative test result does not exclude the diagnosis of SLE. When patients with SLE were compared with healthy control patients, anti-Sm had a weighted mean sensitivity of 24% and a specificity of 98%. On the other hand, when SLE was compared with other rheumatic conditions, anti-Sm had a mean sensitivity of 30% and a specificity of 96%.[14]

Prevalence

The prevalence of anti-Sm antibodies in SLE varies among the racially different population groups in the world, ranging from 10% to 44%. Both anti-Sm and anti–U1-RNP antibodies are more prevalent in African Americans and Afro-Caribbeans when compared with Caucasians.[14] The test system, antigen used, and selection of patients and controls are different in these studies, which may suggest that the results may not be comparable. In the United States, Arnett and colleagues[15] found anti-Sm and anti–U1-RNP antibodies to be more common in African Americans (25% and 40%, respectively) than in Caucasians (10% and 24%, respectively). Antibodies to SSA/Ro and SSB/La, however, occurred with equal frequencies in the two racial groups.

Anti-Smith Antibody Association with Organ Involvement

Whether the presence of anti-Sm antibodies defines a clinical subset of patients with SLE or carries a prognostic value in SLE remains uncertain. Cross-sectional studies have reported an association with nephritis, neuropsychiatric lupus, serositis, pulmonary fibrosis, and peripheral neuropathy. These associations have not been consistently confirmed by other investigators, and often the purported association has been based on a single serum specimen rather than on a sequential determination in a prospective study.

Anti-Smith Antibodies and Disease Activity

Few longitudinal studies have been performed on the usefulness of anti-Sm antibody titers in monitoring disease activity in patients with SLE. A recent analysis of published investigations concluded that an anti-Sm–positive result is not useful in the diagnosis of nephritis or in predicting renal flares in patients with SLE. Although the analysis found no strong evidence for its utility in predicting neuropsychiatric lupus or other organ system involvement, very few superior evidenced-based medicine articles have been published on the topic.

A prospective quantitative study, conducted over a period of 2 years, of anti–extractable nuclear antigen (anti-ENA) antibodies that included anti–Sm antibodies provided no useful additional information in assessing overall lupus disease activity.[16]

ANTI-U1 RIBONUCLEOPROTEIN

Anti–U1-RNP antibodies react to antigens in small nuclear ribonucleoprotein particles distinct from anti-Sm specificities. Both autoantibodies are measured together using the same test system. Different laboratory methods are available; however, the ELISA is probably most commonly used by clinical laboratories.

Arnett and colleagues[15] found that the prevalence of anti–U1-RNP antibodies measured by the immunodiffusion and CIE tests is higher in African-American patients (40%) than it is in Caucasian patients with SLE (23%). The ELISA test for anti–U1-RNP has a higher sensitivity for SLE and MCTD.[14]

Unlike anti-Sm antibodies, anti–U1-RNP antibodies are not considered specific for SLE. Anti–U1-RNP antibodies can be found in MCTD, RA, Sjögren syndrome, systemic sclerosis, and inflammatory myositis.

Clinical Association of Anti–U1 Ribonucleoprotein Antibodies

The presence of high titers of anti–U1-RNP antibodies is associated with MCTD, a clinical entity that is characterized by overlapping clinical features of SLE, scleroderma, and polymyositis. The diagnosis of MCTD requires the presence of anti–U1-RNP antibodies and the absence of anti-Sm and anti-dsDNA antibodies. Multiple types of ANAs in an individual patient suggest an alternative diagnosis such as SLE instead of MCTD. The issue of whether MCTD is a distinct rheumatic disease or a clinical syndrome that may occur during the course of SLE, systemic sclerosis, or another systemic rheumatic disease remains controversial.

In analyzing published data, Benito-Garcia and associates[14] concluded that a positive anti–U1-RNP test result supports a diagnosis of MCTD in the appropriate clinical setting. On the other hand, a negative anti–U1-RNP result will exclude MCTD, and an alternative diagnosis should be considered.

As a diagnostic test for SLE, anti–U1-RNP has a low sensitivity and moderate specificity. Unlike the anti-Sm test, the anti–U1-RNP test is not useful in supporting a diagnosis of SLE in the appropriate clinical setting. Among patients with SLE, the presence of anti–U1-RNP antibodies does not predict the occurrence of neuropsychiatric manifestations or lupus nephritis.

Serum Antibody Titer

Published data on the utility of serial quantitative testing of anti–U1-RNP antibodies as a measure of SLE disease activity have yielded inconclusive results. The serum titer of anti–U1-RNP antibodies fluctuated with disease activity in some but not all patients, whereas other investigators have reported no correlation either with specific organ involvement or with disease activity. In current clinical practice, a rising serum titer of anti–U1-RNP and/or anti-Sm is not used independently of clinical assessment and other laboratory parameters to predict disease exacerbation or to make changes in drug therapy.

The presence of anti–U1-RNP and/or anti-Sm antibodies does not appear to affect survival in SLE. Patients with undifferentiated connective tissue disease (UCTD) have signs and symptoms suggestive of a systemic autoimmune disease but do not fulfill the classification criteria for SLE, RA, systemic sclerosis, and other disorders. A large proportion of patients with UCTD, who tested positive for anti–U1-RNP antibodies, subsequently developed MCTD.[17] Box 43-4 lists guidelines for anti-Sm and anti–U1-RNP testing in the rheumatic diseases.

ANTI–SJÖGREN SYNDROME ANTIGEN A

Anti-SSA/Ro antibodies are the most common specific ANA type encountered in the clinical laboratory. Anti-SSA/Ro antibodies are

---

Box 43-4 Guidelines for Anti-Smith and Antiribonucleoprotein Testing in Rheumatic Diseases

1. Anti-Smith (anti-Sm) antibodies are very useful for confirming the diagnosis of systemic lupus erythematosus (SLE). A positive test result strongly supports the diagnosis; however, a negative test result cannot exclude the diagnosis.
2. Antiribonucleoprotein (anti-RNP) antibodies are useful in the diagnosis of mixed connective tissue disease but not in the diagnosis of SLE.
3. Neither anti-Sm nor anti-RNP antibodies are useful in establishing the diagnosis of dermatomyositis or polymyositis, rheumatoid arthritis, systemic sclerosis, drug-induced lupus erythematosus, or Sjögren syndrome.
4. Anti-Sm and anti-RNP antibodies are not useful in predicting lupus nephritis or in diagnosing neuropsychiatric lupus or other systemic manifestations of SLE.

Adapted from Benito-Garcia E, Schur PH, Lahita R, American College of Rheumatology Ad Hoc committee on Immunologic Testing Guidelines: Guidelines for immunologic laboratory testing in the rheumatic diseases: anti-Sm and anti-RNP antibody tests. *Arthritis Rheum* 51:1030–1044, 2004.

generally associated with Sjögren syndrome and SLE; however, these autoantibodies may also be seen in RA, polymyositis, systemic sclerosis, and other conditions.

Anti-SSA/Ro antibodies are detected by different methods including ELISA and bead immunoassays, which are the tests most commonly used by clinical laboratories. Different preparations of purified antigen are used by manufacturers. An indirect IFA test using transfected HEp-2 cells that overexpress the human necrosis factor receptor 1 (60-kDa) SSA/Ro antigen is highly sensitive, screening a ring-shaped RNA-binding protein test.

Anti-SSA/Ro antibodies are of two distinct types reacting with different antigens from the ribonucleoprotein complex: 60-kDa and 52-kDa. The 52-kDa autoantigen is a ubiquitin ligase involved in the proteasomal degradation of a variety of proteins, whereas the 60-kDa autoantigen may function in noncoding RNA quality control. Although most patients have both types of autoantibodies, some patients may have a single type of anti-SSA/Ro antibody. In most clinical laboratories, anti-SSA/Ro60 and anti-SSA/Ro52 are not tested separately on a routine basis.

Diagnostic Specificity and Associations

Anti-SSA/Ro antibodies are present in 30% to 40% of patients with SLE and in 60% to 90% of patients with primary Sjögren syndrome, depending on the test method. Anti-SSA/Ro antibodies do not carry a high diagnostic specificity for SLE; however, their presence is associated with photosensitivity and certain clinical subsets including subacute cutaneous lupus, neonatal lupus syndrome, secondary Sjögren syndrome in patients with SLE, homozygous C2 and C4 deficiency with lupus-like disease, and interstitial pneumonitis.

Anti-SSA/Ro antibodies are found in 60% to 90% of patients with subacute cutaneous lupus erythematosus (SCLE), depending on the assay system, and are primarily directed to the 60-kDa Ro antigen, although anti-SSA/Ro 50-kDa antibodies may be concomitantly present. SCLE is a distinct clinical subtype of SLE characterized by recurrent, erythematous, photosensitive, widespread, and non-scarring skin lesions in a typical distribution involving the face, trunk, and arms and by mild systemic disease.[18]

Neonatal lupus syndrome is a rare condition in infants born of mothers with SLE. It is characterized by photosensitive, annular, discoid, or erythematous skin lesions of the face and trunk, which appear at or before 2 months of age and disappear by 6 to 12 months of age. Congenital heart block with or without structural cardiac defects is observed in 50% of patients. Almost all afflicted infants and their mothers have anti-SSA/Ro and/or anti-SSB/La antibodies. Buyon and colleagues[19] found that women with both antibodies, especially if the anti-SSA/Ro antibodies identify the 52-kDA component, have an increased risk of giving birth to an infant with neonatal lupus syndrome. Most of the commercially available tests for anti-SSA/Ro antibodies do not distinguish between antibodies to the 52-kDA and the 60-kDA components.

Genetic deficiencies of the early components of classical pathway C1q, C2, and C4 can clinically exhibit a lupus-like illness. Anti-dsDNA antibodies are absent in affected patients, but a high frequency of anti-SSA/Ro and other anti-ENA antibodies are present. The patients exhibit symptoms of fever, rash, arthritis, and sometimes glomerulonephritis.[20]

ANA-negative SLE refers to the rare patient with clinical features of SLE or SCLE with a negative ANA result by the immunofluorescent test using rodent kidney or liver as substrate. With a sensitive ELISA, these patients uniformly have anti-SSA/Ro and, in addition, some have anti-SSB/La and/or anti–U1-RNP antibodies.[21]

Among Caucasian patients with SLE, photosensitivity is associated with anti-SSA/Ro antibodies. In contrast, the presence of anti-SSA/Ro antibodies in South African black patients has been reported to be negatively correlated with photosensitivity.[22]

Both anti-SSA/Ro and anti-SSB/La are strongly associated with sicca symptoms in patients with SLE. Other features of SLE reported to have a probable association with anti-SSA/Ro antibodies include interstitial pneumonitis, shrinking lung syndrome, and a deforming arthropathy.

Cavazzana and associates[23] reported that 24% of patients with UCTD who test positive for anti-SSA/Ro antibodies progressed within a short period to either SLE or primary Sjögren syndrome.

Serial Measurement of Anti–Sjögren Syndrome Antigen A Titer

Studies on the utility of anti-SSA/Ro and anti-SSB/La antibodies in monitoring disease activity in SLE have yielded discrepant results. A recent 2-year prospective study found a positive correlation between anti-SSA/Ro and anti-Sm antibody titers with disease activity in a minority of patients; however, in the majority of these patients, no such correlation was observed.[15]

In current clinical practice, serial quantitative measurements of anti-SSA/Ro and anti-SSB/La antibodies are not used as biomarkers for overall disease activity or for specific organ involvement such as nephritis.

Summary

Anti-SSA/Ro antibodies are strongly associated with the clinical subsets of SCLE, ANA-negative SLE, and lupus-like syndrome associated with a genetic deficiency of complement. Infants of mothers with SLE with anti-SSA/Ro or anti-SSB/La antibodies have an increased risk of neonatal lupus syndrome. Therefore pregnant patients with SLE should be tested for these antibodies as part of their prenatal assessment. A sensitive ELISA test for anti-SSA/Ro antibodies is useful in the diagnosis of ANA-negative SLE. Well-designed prospective studies are needed to further evaluate the value of anti-SSA/Ro and anti-SSB/La antibodies in monitoring disease activity.

ANTI-SSB/LA ANTIBODIES

Anti-SSA/Ro antibodies react with an intracellular 47-kD phosphoprotein that associates with small RNAs transcribed by RNA polymerase III, protecting them from digestion and regulating their downstream processing. Anti-SSA/Ro antibodies are usually found together with anti-SSB/La antibodies. Whereas anti-SSA/Ro antibodies can be seen alone, it is rare to find anti-SSB/La antibodies alone in the serum of a patient.

Anti-SSA/Ro antibodies are found in 10% to 15% of patients with SLE and 30% to 60% of patients with primary Sjögren syndrome. Anti-SSB/La antibodies are more prevalent (38%) in the patients with SLE who also had secondary Sjögren syndrome than in those without Sjögren syndrome (7%).[24]

Both anti-SSA/Ro and anti-SSB/La should be tested in a female patient with SLE, MCTD, Sjögren syndrome, or other systemic rheumatic conditions who is planning a pregnancy, as well as in a patient with photosensitive cutaneous lesions suggestive of SCLE. Box 43-5

Box 43-5 Clinical Significance of Anti-SSA/Ro and Anti-SSB/La in Systemic Lupus Erythematosus

1. Anti-SSA/Ro antibodies are strongly associated with the clinical subsets of subacute cutaneous lupus erythematosus (SCLE), antinuclear antibody (ANA)–negative systemic lupus erythematosus (SLE), and lupus-like syndrome in genetic deficiency of C1q, C2, or C4.
2. Infants of SLE mothers with anti-SSA/Ro and anti-SSB/La antibodies have an increased risk of neonatal lupus syndrome. Patients with SLE, mixed connective tissue disease (MCTD), Sjögren syndrome, or other systemic rheumatic diseases who are planning a pregnancy should be tested for these autoantibodies during prenatal assessment.
3. Both anti-SSA/Ro and anti-SSB/La antibodies are associated with secondary Sjögren syndrome among patients with SLE.

Anti-SSA/Ro, Anti–Sjögren syndrome antigen A; anti-SSB/La, anti–Sjögren syndrome antigen B.

explains the clinical significance of anti-SSA/Ro and anti-SSB/La in SLE.

ANTIHISTONE ANTIBODIES

Antihistone antibodies make up a heterogeneous group of antibodies that are reactive with a single histone, a histone-DNA complex, or complexes of histones. Although they are primarily found in patients with SLE, drug-induced lupus erythematosus, or RA, these autoantibodies have been reported in patients with other rheumatic diseases, malignancy, and liver disease. In SLE, these antibodies are directed against H1, H2B, H3, and H2A-H2B complex, although other specificities can occur. Histone H1 is the major autoantigen in SLE at the B- and T-cell levels.[25] All isotypes of antihistone antibodies are common in SLE.

Several test systems have been developed for antihistone antibodies, including ELISA, immunoblotting, complement fixation, and immunofluorescence. Antihistone antibodies are found in 21% to 90% of patients with SLE, depending on the method and substrate used and the patient selection.

Antihistone antibodies are of limited diagnostic specificity for idiopathic SLE. The presence of these antibodies does not appear to be any more significant than that of anti-dsDNA or anti-Sm antibodies in corroborating the clinical diagnosis of the disease. Wallace and associates[26] found that antibodies to histone (H2A-H2B) DNA complex in the absence of anti-dsDNA antibodies are found more commonly in MCTD and scleroderma-related conditions than in SLE.

Clinical Association

Several published studies on antihistone antibodies and the clinical features of SLE have reported inconsistent and often discrepant results. Similarly, available data on the association between antihistone antibodies and disease activity are inconclusive. Schett and colleagues[27] have identified antibodies to histone H1, a component of the nucleosome, as the major ANAs responsible for the lupus erythematosus cell phenomenon in SLE.

Summary

Antihistone antibodies are of limited value in corroborating the clinical diagnosis of SLE. Serial determinations of these antibodies do not significantly add to the measurement of anti-dsDNA and other serologic parameters for assessing disease activity in patients with SLE. Further studies on the binding of histone with SLE IgG in circulating immune complexes are needed to fully understand the significance of antihistone antibodies, including pathogenicity and assessment of disease activity.

ANTINUCLEOSOME ANTIBODIES IN SYSTEMIC LUPUS ERYTHEMATOSUS

Nucleosome, the fundamental unit of chromatin, consists of DNA wrapped around a histone octamer with histone H1 bound on the outside. Antinucleosome antibodies are the first specific type of ANAs described and are responsible for the lupus erythematosus cell phenomenon. Antinucleosome antibodies are most commonly measured by an ELISA or a bead-based immunoassay using either H1-stripped chromatic or nucleosome core particle as antigens.

A recent analysis of several published studies on antinucleosome antibodies reported high sensitivity and specificity for SLE and drug-induced lupus erythematosus.[28] The sensitivity for SLE ranged from 48% to 100% and the specificity from 90% to 99%. Antinucleosome antibodies are also found in 40% to 50% of patients with autoimmune hepatitis but only in a small number of patients with MCTD, systemic sclerosis, and Sjögren syndrome. IgG antinucleosome antibodies are most helpful in the diagnosis of SLE in those patients who test negative for anti-dsDNA and anti-Sm antibodies.

Antinucleosome antibodies appear to be associated with lupus disease activity, especially nephritis, in several cross-sectional studies of different ethnicities. However, other investigators have failed to observe a significant correlation. A well-designed prospective longitudinal study on new-onset, biopsy-proven lupus nephritis concluded that antinucleosome antibodies are not better predictors of renal outcome than anti-dsDNA antibodies measured by ELISA.[29]

To summarize, antinucleosome antibodies are prevalent in SLE, and high-serum antibody titers maybe a useful aid in the diagnosis of SLE, especially in patients who test negative for anti-dsDNA and anti-Sm antibodies. Antinucleosome antibodies may be observed in drug-induced lupus erythematosus, MCTD, and systemic sclerosis. Well-designed prospective studies are needed to investigate the utility of antinucleosome antibodies in individual patients with SLE for assessing disease activity and following the response to therapy.

ANTICOMPLEMENT 1Q ANTIBODIES

Anticomplement 1q (anti-C1q) antibodies react with determinants on the collagen-like region of C1q and are measured by ELISA using purified C1q as antigen. The assay is performed under high salt (1 mol/L NaCl) that prevents an interaction among immune complexes that may be present in the patient's serum with the immobilized C1q but will allow high-avidity anti-C1q antibodies to bind.

Anti-C1q antibodies are not specific for SLE. They are found in practically all patients with hypocomplementemic urticarial vasculitis, in 33% of the general SLE population, and in 63% of patients with lupus nephritis. Anti-C1q antibodies are also prevalent in those with Felty syndrome, rheumatoid vasculitis, membranoproliferative glomerulonephritis, and other conditions.[30]

Although not specific, anti-C1q antibodies are associated with disease activity in SLE, and several investigators have shown a positive correlation with active lupus nephritis.[30] Simultaneous detection of anti-dsDNA and anti-C1q provides a 67% predictive value for active lupus nephritis. On the other hand, the absence of both autoantibodies has a very high negative predictive value of 74% for active nephritis,[31] suggesting that anti-C1q antibodies are a promising biomarker for disease activity. Cross-sectional studies on anti-C1q and a combination of autoantibodies need to be validated in large-scale prospective longitudinal studies before these are adopted for routine clinical use.

ANTI–RIBOSOMAL P ANTIBODIES

Anti–ribosomal P antibodies are heterogeneous antibodies that react with three phosphoproteins located within the 60S-ribosomal subunit in the cell cytoplasm. These autoantibodies give rise to cytoplasmic staining in the indirect IFA test using HEp-2 cells.

In the clinical laboratory, ELISA and line or bead immunoassays are commonly used for detecting these antibodies. To date, no standardized assay system, native antigen, synthetic peptide, or recombinant polypeptides are used by manufacturers of test systems.

Anti–ribosomal P antibodies are present in 10% of consecutive patients with SLE and up to 40% in those with active disease. Despite the relatively low prevalence, these autoantibodies are highly specific for SLE (>90% specificity) and can be present even in those who are negative for anti-dsDNA or anti-Sm antibodies.[32,33]

The presence of anti–ribosomal P antibodies has been reported to be associated with neuropsychiatric lupus and especially with psychosis, active lupus nephritis, and SLE-associated hepatitis. Serial determination of anti–ribosomal P antibodies showed a correlation with lupus disease activity. These reported clinical associations have not been uniformly observed, and the discrepant results are, in part, a result of the differences in the test assays, antigens used, and patient selection.

Currently, anti–ribosomal P antibodies are not widely used in clinical practice. Although they are highly specific for SLE, their sensitivity is relatively low when compared with anti-Sm and anti-dsDNA antibodies. Further investigation is required to determine whether anti–ribosomal P antibodies can be used to confirm the diagnosis of SLE in patients who test negative for anti-dsDNA and anti-Sm antibodies. Box 43-6 explains the clinical significance of antihistone, antinucleosome, anti-C1q, and anti–ribosomal P antibodies in SLE.

Box 43-6 Clinical Significance of Antihistone, Antinucleosomes, Anticomplement 1q, and Anti–Ribosomal P

1. Antihistone antibodies are associated with drug-induced lupus erythematosus and are of limited value in establishing the diagnosis of idiopathic SLE. Serial determinations of antihistone antibodies do not significantly add to anti-dsDNA and other serologic parameters for the assessment of lupus disease activity.
2. Antinucleosome antibodies are prevalent in SLE and are responsible for the lupus erythematosus cell phenomenon. High serum antibody titers may be a useful aid in the diagnosis of SLE, especially in patients who test negative for anti-dsDNA and anti-Sm antibodies.
3. Anti-C1q antibodies are not specific for SLE but are associated with disease activity, especially lupus nephritis.
4. Anti–ribosomal P antibodies are found in 10% of patients but are considered highly specific for SLE and appear to be associated with neuropsychiatric lupus, active nephritis, and SLE-associated hepatitis.

ANTICENTROMERE AND ANTISCLEROMA 70-KD ANTIBODIES

Anti–Scl-70 antibodies are considered a specific marker for the diffuse type of systemic sclerosis. However, these autoantibodies can be seen in SLE, ranging from 0% to 25% of patients with a mean of 4.1%.[34] The serum antibody titers in patients with SLE are significantly lower than those observed in patients with systemic sclerosis. Moreover, anti–Scl-70 antibodies in SLE react to antigenic epitopes different from those bound by systemic sclerosis sera. Pulmonary hypertension and renal disease have been observed to be more common among patients with SLE and anti–Scl-70 than those without the autoantibody.[35]

Anticentromere antibodies react with three major proteins, centromere protein (CENP) A (CENP-A), CENP-B, and CENP-C, and are considered a marker for the limited form of systemic sclerosis, although patients with other diagnoses, including SLE, RA, and Sjögren syndrome, may test positive for these autoantibodies.

Anticentromere antibodies are measured by immunofluorescence, immunoblotting, and ELISA using purified CENP-B as the antigen. Approximately 1% to 2% of patients with SLE have anticentromere antibodies; however, these patients do not have concurrent scleroderma features and do not constitute a distinct clinical subset.[36]

To summarize, the presence of anti–Scl-70 (also known as topoisomerase I) and/or anticentromere antibodies does not exclude the diagnosis of SLE.

ERYTHROCYTE SEDIMENTATION RATE

Erythrocyte sedimentation rate (ESR) is a simple and inexpensive laboratory test that is often used to monitor disease activity in SLE. The Westergren method is the recommended test; however, many clinical laboratories now use automated closed systems. These alternative ESR tests should be carefully evaluated and standardized against the Westergren method to establish their own normal reference ranges, sensitivity, and levels of clinical significance.

An elevation in the ESR has been noted in more than 90% of patients with SLE and is associated with fever, fatigue, myalgias, and greater disease activity in general. Mildly, moderately, and significantly elevated ESRs are associated with disease activity and damage accrual. The association with disease activity is particularly strong in the presence of anti-dsDNA antibodies.[37,38]

ESR is helpful when taken in the context of those patients for whom its levels reflect other clinical and laboratory features because ESR can be elevated even in patients with inactive disease, and vice versa. Co-morbid conditions such as infections and malignancy are associated with high ESR. Among hospitalized patients with SLE, the level of the ESR was not different in patients with active lupus flares than in those with infection.[39] ESR can also be influenced by anemia, low serum albumin, macrocytosis, age, and ethnicity of the patient.

C-REACTIVE PROTEIN AND THE IMMUNE SYSTEM

C-reactive protein (CRP), a pentraxin, is an acute-phase protein that is clinically used as a biomarker for inflammation. Its production by hepatocytes is regulated by interleukin (IL)-6, IL-1β, and tumor necrosis factor–alpha (TNF-α). CRP participates in host defense while limiting potentially damaging inflammatory effects of complement activation via an interaction with the classical complement pathway through its interactions with C1q. CRP also inhibits the activation of the C5b-9 complex and the deposition of C3b and mannan-binding lectin–initiated complement cytolysis by this lectin pathway. CRP also functions in the clearance of apoptotic and damaged cells.[40]

Clinical Significance of C-Reactive Protein in Systemic Lupus Erythematosus

Serum CRP levels in patients with active SLE can be elevated but are generally low or modest in amounts when compared with those levels observed in active RA. This is a consequence of modest CRP production rather than a consequence of enhanced clearance or cytokine deficiency. The cause of the lower production rate is not well understood.[41]

CRP levels have been reported to correlate with disease activity, especially with serositis, as well as with musculoskeletal and pulmonary involvement in SLE; however, this correlation remains controversial because other studies have failed to confirm such an association.[39,40,42-44]

CRP can also be elevated in the presence of infection, and several investigators have suggested that a certain level of serum CRP may differentiate the infected from the noninfected patient with SLE. Using a high-sensitivity CRP (hsCRP), Firooz and colleagues[39] confirmed that the hsCRP was significantly lower in hospitalized patients with SLE during a disease flare than in those with active infection. A cutoff level of 5 mg/dL correlated with active infection with a specificity of 80%.

In clinical practice, setting up an arbitrary CRP level to differentiate a flare from infection in an individual patient is not recommended at this time. Significantly elevated CRP levels can be observed during disease flares; however, the absence of an identifiable flare such as serositis should raise the suspicion of an infection in a febrile patient.[45] Infection may also precipitate a lupus flare. Prospective longitudinal studies are needed to determine further the clinical use of CRP in monitoring disease activity. Table 43-1 lists the association between CRP levels and various clinical settings in SLE.[40,45]

C-Reactive Protein and Cardiovascular Risk in Systemic Lupus Erythematosus

Coronary artery disease is the leading cause of mortality among patients with SLE of more than 5-years' duration. The recognized biomarker for the inflammatory component of atherosclerosis is hsCRP, and it is predictive of coronary and cerebrovascular events and peripheral artery disease. Assessing hsCRP levels may be useful in predicting cardiovascular risk in patients with SLE.[42] Attempts to correlate cardiovascular risk factors such as hsCRP and endothelial dysfunction have shown increased hsCRP levels and decreased flow-mediated dilation among patients with SLE, compared with normal subjects.[46]

Studies that examined the predictors of high hsCRP levels among patients with SLE have noted that high hsCRP levels are associated with high body mass index, low socioeconomic and educational status, African-American ethnicity, current or past smoking, diabetes, cumulative prednisone use, high disease activity, increased age, postmenopausal status, and infection; whereas low hsCRP levels are associated with the use of statins and immunosuppressants.[47,48] The

TABLE 43-1 Associations between C-Reactive Protein and Clinical Situations in Systemic Lupus Erythematosus

CLINICAL SETTING	C-REACTIVE PROTEIN (RANGE) *(Note differences in units depending on reference source)*
Infection and severity of inflammation	≥60 mg/L (1-400)*
Mild inflammation and viral infections	10-50 mg/dL[†]
Active inflammation and bacterial infection	50-200 mg/dL[†]
Severe infection and trauma	>200 mg/dL[†]
Disease exacerbation with or without serositis	16.5 mg/L (1-375)
With serositis	76 mg/L (2-375)
Without serositis	16 mg/L (1-53)

*ter Borg EJ, Horst G, Limburg PC, van Rijswijk MH, Kallenberg CG: C-reactive protein levels during disease exacerbations and infections in systemic lupus erythematosus: a prospective longitudinal study. *J Rheumatol* 17(12):1642–1648, 1990.
[†]de Carvalho JF, Hanaoka B, Szyper-Kravitz, Shoenfeld Y: C-reactive protein and its implications in systemic lupus erythematosus. *Acta Reumatol Port* 32(4):317–322, 2007.

variability of hsCRP levels and the effect of different factors pose questions concerning the value of this marker in predicting cardiovascular risk in SLE. Therefore further longitudinal studies are needed to determine its clinical usefulness.

Anti–C-Reactive Protein and Antipentraxin Antibodies

Antibodies to CRP are found in 10% to 40% of patients with SLE.[49,50] They have been proposed to increase cardiovascular risk through their interaction with the monomeric or degraded form of CRP.[49] Antibodies to CRP contribute to an impairment of clearance of damaged and apoptotic cells and have been found to be related to disease activity and renal disease. Anti-CRP antibodies have been found in 51% of patients with SLE and 54% of patients with APLAs, and to be associated with lupus nephritis and clinical features of antiphospholipid antibody syndrome.[51] Pentraxin has been found to play a role in the clearance of apoptotic neutrophils by phagocytes, acting as a neutrophil membrane surface signal, thus assisting in innate resistance against pathogens and regulating inflammation. Antibodies to pentraxin-3 have been found to be increased among patients with SLE when compared with control subjects, and their levels are found to correlate with APLA positivity and the presence of renal disease.[52] The role of pentraxin and its autoantibodies in the pathogenesis and potential treatment of SLE warrants further investigation. (See Box 43-1 for a list of the association between CRP levels and various clinical settings in patients with SLE.[40,45])

SERUM COMPLEMENT

The in vivo activation of the complement system by immune complexes of anti-DNA and other autoantibodies is central to the pathogenesis of the glomerular injury and, possibly, to other tissue damage in patients with SLE.

Acute exacerbations of the disease can often be associated with low serum complement levels. Serial measurements of C3 and C4 levels are routinely ordered in clinical practice, whereas testing for total hemolytic activity (i.e., CH50) is sometimes used to assess lupus disease activity. Box 43-7 lists guidelines on the use of complement levels in SLE.

A prospective study of patients with SLE studied monthly noted that a decrease in the serum levels of C3 and C4 was not consistently associated with global measures of disease activity.[53] Other

Box 43-7 Serum Complement Levels in Systemic Lupus Erythematosus

1. Despite some limitations, serial measurements of serum C3 and C4 remain practical and useful laboratory parameters to assess disease activity in systemic lupus erythematosus (SLE).
2. The plasma concentration of activation products of complement, including C3d, C4d, and C3a, is superior to native C3 and C4 in assessing disease activity.
3. Measurement of activation products is currently not used in standard clinical practice because of certain drawbacks that include short half-life, a need for special and careful handling of specimens, and interference with results by co-morbidities, especially infections.

investigators have also reported that measurements of C3 and C4 levels are not always reliable markers or predictors of lupus disease activity or to separate patients with mild disease from those with severe disease. In a comparison of baseline, preflare, and at-flare values in lupus nephritis, the serum levels of neither C3 nor C4 decreased during preflare, but both decreased significantly at flare when compared with baseline values. The sensitivity of C3 was 75%, but C4 had a sensitivity of only 41%. Both had a specificity of only 71%. Combining C3 and C4 with other parameters including ESR and CRP did not generate a better clinical tool to assess renal flare.[54]

Serum C3 and C4 levels are useful in determining pregnancy risks. During pregnancy, patients with SLE and high clinical activity, as well as hypocomplementemia or positive anti-dsDNA, have the highest risk for pregnancy loss and preterm birth.[55]

Several reasons are cited that explain why serum complement levels are imperfectly associated with lupus disease activity. A wide variation of normal complement protein concentrations is present among individuals partly because of genetic factors. The serum-protein concentrations are controlled by the rate of protein synthesis and catabolism that vary among individual patients. Complement components including C3 and C4 are acute-phase reactants, and synthesis may increase in response to inflammation. Serum levels of complement proteins do not reflect what is occurring at the tissue level.

In vivo activation of complement can be shown by measuring for split products and/or complexes of complement in the plasma. Several studies have shown that the plasma concentration of activation products including C3a, C4a, C3d, C4d, the terminal complex, C5b-9, and serum Ba and Bb, as well as C3d in the urine, can be useful in assessing disease activity and predicting lupus exacerbations. Most of these studies conclude that measurements of the activation products are superior to the determination of serum C3 or C4 values. A drawback of these assays is the need for special and careful handling of the plasma specimen to prevent spurious activation of complement in vitro. In addition, the half-life of these peptides in the serum is short, and co-morbid conditions, especially infections, can activate the complement and release of split products. Cell-bound complement products such as C3d and C4d on erythrocytes appear to be promising biomarkers for diagnosis and disease activity.[56]

Despite its limitations, measurement of native C3 and C4 levels has not been replaced by that of cell-bound or split products of complement in current clinical practice.[57]

PLASMA PROTEINS
Serum Protein Electrophoresis

Serum protein electrophoresis (SPEP) is a widely available and inexpensive laboratory test that examines specific serum proteins based on their physical properties. Albumin and five major globulin fractions are identified. In clinical practice, SPEP is indicated when multiple myeloma, macroglobulinemia, amyloidosis, or other protein disorders are suspected. SPEP does not help in establishing a diagnosis of SLE, but it may be useful in screening for monoclonal protein or hypogammaglobulinemia, which may occasionally be revealed in this disease. An early study of SPEP in SLE showed low albumin in 47% of patients and increased gamma globulin in 58% of patients. The alpha-2 globulin fraction, which includes ceruloplasmin, alpha macroglobulin, and haptoglobin, was increased in 33% of patients. The beta fraction that includes transferrin, C3, and beta-lipoprotein was increased in 11% of patients.[58] Tables 43-2 and 43-3

TABLE 43-2 Alpha Globulins and Their Associations with Systemic Lupus Erythematosus

ALPHA GLOBULINS	ASSOCIATIONS WITH SYSTEMIC LUPUS ERYTHEMATOSUS
α_1-Acid glycoprotein (orosomucoid)	Increased levels in most patients at some time during the course of disease
α_1-Fetoprotein	Increased levels in most pregnant patients without association with neural tube defects
α_1-Antitrypsin	Normal or slightly increased levels Not associated with any phenotype Dominant protease inhibitor in plasma
α_1-Antichymotrypsin	Increased levels in one study
α_2-Macroglobulin	Increased levels in patients
Hemagglutinin (HA) glycoprotein	Protease inhibitor
Lactoferrin and neutrophil elastase	Increased levels in one study
Ceruloplasmin	Increased by 20%-40% in patients in one study
Haptoglobin	Decreased levels in patients with hemolysis

Adapted from Wallace DJ: Serum and plasma protein abnormalities and other clinical laboratory determinations in systemic lupus erythematosus. In Wallace DJ, Hahn BH, editors: *Dubois' lupus erythematosus*, ed 7, Philadelphia, 2007, Lippincott Williams and Wilkins, pp 911–919.

TABLE 43-3 Beta Globulins and Their Associations with Systemic Lupus Erythematosus

BETA GLOBULINS	ASSOCIATIONS WITH SYSTEMIC LUPUS ERYTHEMATOSUS
Transferrin	Increased or normal levels in patients β-globulin carrier molecule
β_2-Macroglycoprotein	Increased levels in patients, higher in active disease Possible presence of autoantibody to thermal β_2-macroglycoprotein in active disease
β_2-Microglobulin	Increased levels with active disease, nephropathy, low-level C3, high-level ESR, anti-dsDNA Increased levels with age 64% sensitivity and 87% specificity for assessing disease activity when compared with healthy patients

Other β-globulins:
- Complement components: Refer to section on "Serum Complement" within this chapter.
- Prothrombin, fibrinogen, plasminogen, and other clotting factors: Refer to Chapter 34, "Hematologic and Lymphoid Abnormalities in Systemic Lupus Erythematosus."

anti-dsDNA, Anti–single stranded DNA; ESR, erythrocyte sedimentation rate.
Yoshizawa S, Nagasawa K, Yoshiaki Y, et al: A thermolabile beta 2-macroglycoprotein (TMG) and the antibody against TMG in patients with systemic lupus erythematosus. *Clin Chim Acta* 264(2):219–225, 1997.
Wallace DJ: Serum and plasma protein abnormalities and other clinical laboratory determinations in systemic lupus erythematosus. In Wallace DJ, Hahn BH, editors: *Dubois' lupus erythematosus*, ed 7, Philadelphia, PA, 2007, Lippincott Williams and Wilkins, pp 911–919.

list selected alpha and beta globulins and their associations with SLE.[59,60]

Albumin

Hypoalbuminemia is common among patients with SLE, occurring in 30% to 50% of patients, and is usually caused by chronic disease with an increased fractional catabolism of albumin in patients with active disease. Hypoalbuminemia is a feature of a variety of clinical manifestations of SLE including nephrotic syndrome, protein-losing enteropathy, and chronic lupus peritonitis with ascites.

Gamma Globulins

Polyclonal gammopathy is observed in the majority of patients with SLE and is a hallmark of an autoimmune reaction. Significant hypogammaglobulinemia is rarely noted and is associated with recurrent infections.

Monoclonal gammopathy is observed in up to 5.4% of patients with SLE. In contrast, the prevalence in the general population is 1% in individuals older than 25 years of age and increases to 3% by 70 years of age. Monoclonal gammopathy of undetermined significance (MGUS) is usually noted as an incidental finding when serum electrophoresis is performed and defined by the presence of a serum monoclonal protein (M-protein) at <3 g/dL, <10% monoclonal plasma cells in bone marrow, and the absence of lytic bone lesions, anemia, renal insufficiency, hypercalcemia, and hyperviscosity related to a lymphoplasmacytic proliferative process. MGUS among patients with SLE appears to be a benign course with no increase toward the development of cancer, mortality rates, disease activity, disease damage, and steroid use.[61]

Serum Immunoglobulins

Measurement of baseline serum immunoglobulin levels is useful to diagnose primary immunodeficiencies associated with SLE, including combined variable immunodeficiency and selective immunoglobulin A (IgA) deficiency, and to identify hypogammaglobulinemia that can occur as a result of treatment or as part of the disease. Hypogammaglobulinemia may be asymptomatic but should be suspected in patients with recurrent, unusual, or opportunistic infections, vaccine-related illnesses, and a family history of immunodeficiency.[62]

Immunodeficiency can occur among patients with SLE as either a primary entity such as rare genetic complement deficiencies that can predispose a patient to SLE or as a secondary deficiency as a result of medications.[63]

Immunoglobulin G

Polyclonal IgG is increased in approximated 91% of patients with SLE, tends to be elevated at diagnosis, but normalizes with treatment. The survival half-life of IgG in these patients is decreased at an average of 8.2 days, compared with 18 days in normal patients with an average of 10.1% of total body IgG catabolized daily compared with a mean of 3.9% in normal patients.[64]

IgG deficiency has been noted to occur in patients with SLE and may be associated with infections. It is theorized that excessive T-cell suppressor and decreased B-cell activity characterized this subset. Total serum IgG levels have no correlation with age, sex, race, or duration of disease.

The serum concentration of IgG subclasses in SLE varies with the elevation of IgG1, IgG2 and IgG3, and normal IgG4. In patients with active disease, the serum concentration of IgG3 is decreased, whereas the other subclasses remain normal. The differential changes of the IgG subclasses during the course of the disease are unclear.[65]

The IgG subclass distribution of pathogenic autoantibodies may be important because of differences in their ability to activate complement. IgG1 and IgG2 subclasses activate complement more efficiently than IgG3, and, in contrast, IgG4 is not complement fixing. The serum titers of IgG1 anti-dsDNA and IgG2 anti-nucleohistone have been noted to rise before a renal relapse and were the predominant subclasses in the serum in patients with active nephritis. In contrast, however, all four IgG subclasses were detected in the renal glomerular deposits.[66]

Immunoglobulin M

Ten percent of serum immunoglobulin is IgM, which has a half-life of 5 to 10 days. Unlike other immunoglobulin isotypes, IgM concentration peaks at 20 to 40 years of life and reaches a plateau at 50 years. The turnover of serum IgM in SLE is normal. Serum IgM levels in SLE have been reported to be increased during the early stages of the disease and during periods of disease activity. The serum IgM concentration can also be decreased especially in patients with SLE of longer duration.[67,68]

Selective IgM deficiency is a rare immunodeficiency that is characterized by an isolated low serum level of IgM (<2 standard deviations below the age-adjusted means). The most common clinical feature is recurrent infections, especially rhinosinusitis and other respiratory infections. Approximately 14% of reported patients with selective IgM deficiency have autoimmune conditions including a few patients with SLE.[69]

Immunoglobulin A

IgA, the second most abundant immunoglobulin, exists in two isotypes—IgA1 and IgA2—with the former as the predominant isotype in the serum. IgA found in secretions consists of polymers of monomeric IgA2 and is vital to mucos defense systems, especially in preventing the binding of viruses to epithelial cells of the respiratory, gastrointestinal, and urogenital tracts. Monomeric IgA1 has anti-inflammatory functions theorized to work via FcαRI-inhibitory signaling.[70]

Selective IgA deficiency is the most common of the primary immunodeficiencies with a frequency ranging from 0.03% to 0.25% in patients who are hospitalized or in clinics and 0.1% in the general community. The frequency varies in different populations. In the majority of patients, IgA deficiency does not cause clinically relevant disease; however, in some patients it can be associated with recurrent bacterial infections, atopic disorders, transfusion reactions, and/or autoimmune diseases including RA and SLE.

Selective IgA deficiency is seen in up to 6.17% of adult patients with SLE and 5.2% of pediatric patients with SLE. However, its significance remains unclear, because the clinical features, laboratory findings, disease activity, and course of patients with SLE and IgA deficiency are not different from those with normal IgA levels.[71,72]

Individuals with selective IgA deficiency frequently have circulating IgG antibodies to IgA. These autoantibodies have been noted in 58% to 100% of patients with SLE and selective IgA deficiency. The presence of these antibodies can cause a severe anaphylactic transfusion reaction.[72,73]

Immunoglobulin E

Elevated serum immunoglobulin E (IgE) levels may correlate with disease activity including nephritis in patients with SLE but without known allergies. High serum IgE concentration is also associated with IgE ANAs but not with the presence of IgE antibodies to allergens. IgE ANA observed in 32% of patients with SLE are heterogeneous with multiple specificities including dsDNA, Sm, SSA/Ro, and SSB/La antigens.[74]

Hyper-IgE syndrome is a heterogeneous group of primary immunodeficiency diseases characterized by significantly elevated serum IgE, eczematous skin rashes, and recurrent infections. Rare cases of SLE developing in this syndrome have been reported.[75]

Common Variable Immunodeficiency

Common variable immunodeficiency (CVID) is a heterogeneous syndrome of primary immunodeficiency marked by the failure of antibody production. Recurrent respiratory and sinus infections are notable among patients with CVID, but they can also develop features of immune dysregulation including lymphadenopathy, inflammatory bowel disease, sarcoidlike disease, thrombocytopenia, autoimmune hemolytic anemia, and thyroid disease.

CVID has been rarely described in patients with SLE after treatment has been initiated, rendering the diagnosis of CVID difficult because other causes of hypogammaglobulinemia need to be excluded. SLE itself is typified by high levels of serum immunoglobulins and circulating autoantibodies. CVID should be suspected in patients with SLE with quiescent disease activity and not on immunosuppressive treatment but with recurrent sinopulmonary infections.[62,73,76] Table 43-4 lists immunoglobulin abnormalities and their association with SLE.

Drug-Related Hypogammaglobulinemia

Box 43-8 lists drugs for the treatment of SLE that have been associated with the development of hypogammaglobulinemia.[62] Drug rash

TABLE 43-4 Immunoglobulin Abnormalities

CONDITION	ASSOCIATION WITH SYSTEMIC LUPUS ERYTHEMATOSUS (PREVALENCE, IF KNOWN)	MOLECULAR DEFECTS	MANIFESTATIONS AND ASSOCIATIONS
Selective IgA deficiency	Strong 6.17% of adult SLE 5.2% of pediatric SLE	Antibodies to IgA or IgA deficiency leads to decreased FcαRI-inhibitory signaling	Majority–asymptomatic Autoimmunity Viral infections
Selective IgM deficiency	18.5%-22% of adult SLE	Unknown mechanism	Majority–asymptomatic Recurrent sinopulmonary infections
Common variable immunodeficiency	Weak	Failure of antibody production; lack of immunoglobulins, variable T-cell dysfunction	Recurrent sinopulmonary infections; cytopenias, lymphadenopathy, inflammatory bowel disease, sarcoidlike disease, autoimmune hemolytic anemia, and thyroid disease
X-linked agammaglobulinemia	Weak	BTK mutation	Chronic arthritis, dermatomyositis, scleroderma
Hyper-IgM syndrome	Weak	Immunoglobulin defects in class-switch recombination; gene mutations that may include CD40/CD40 ligand pathway; decreased IgG and IgA levels; increased IgM levels	Recurrent bacterial infections

BTK, Bruton tyrosine kinase; SLE, systemic lupus erythematosus.

Box 43-8 Systemic Lupus Erythematosus–Related Treatments Associated with Hypogammaglobulinemia

Cyclophosphamide
Mycophenolate mofetil
Azathioprine
Rituximab
Sulfasalazine
Corticosteroid

TABLE 43-5 Significance of Other Clinical Laboratory Tests in Systemic Lupus Erythematosus

	FREQUENCY	CLINICAL SIGNIFICANCE
Rheumatoid factor	33%	Is associated with secondary Sjögren syndrome, erosive inflammatory arthritis ("rhupus"), and late-onset SLE.
Anti-CCP	1%-5%	Is associated with "rhupus." Positive anti-CCP does not exclude the diagnosis of SLE.
ANCA	15%-20%	Has multiple specificities. Correlation with disease activity is modest and not clinically useful. Is used as a monitoring test.
Antiendothelial antibodies	39%-93%	Are not specific for SLE and are seen in other conditions. Are associated with disease activity but are not used in clinical practice. No standardized assay is available.
Cryoglobulins	Variable	Mixed type and presence are associated with disease activity. Are seen in hepatitis C infections. No standardized test assay.

ANCA, Antineutrophil cytoplasmic antibodies; CCP, cyclic citrullinated peptide; SLE, systemic lupus erythematosus

with eosinophilia and systemic symptoms (DRESS) can be associated with transient hypogammaglobulinemia. Other than anticonvulsants, DRESS has been reported with the use of antibiotics, allopurinol, and nonsteroidal antiinflammatory drugs.[77]

Circulating Plasma Cells in Systemic Lupus Erythematosus

The number and frequency of plasma cells in the peripheral blood of patients with SLE are increased and significantly correlated with disease activity and serum titer of anti-dsDNA. These immunoglobulin-secreting plasmablasts expressing CD19 and high levels of CD27 but not CD20 are detected by flow cytometry and may be clinically useful in assessing disease activity. The expansion of these cells implies defective immune regulation, and their capacity to produce anti-dsDNA suggests an important pathogenic role; they may be considered as a target for drug therapy.[78]

Type 1 interferon alpha (IFN-α) has a central role in the pathogenesis of human and murine SLE. Several mechanisms have been proposed by which IFN-α contributes to autoimmunity including its effect on B cells. IFN-α has been shown to induce large numbers of short-lived plasma cells accompanied by high titers of anti-dsDNA and accelerate the onset of the disease in a mouse model of SLE. Whether this mechanism is relevant to human SLE remains to be established.[79]

OTHER SEROLOGIC ABNORMALITIES IN SYSTEMIC LUPUS ERYTHEMATOSUS

Table 43-5 summarizes the significance of other clinical laboratory tests in SLE.

Rheumatoid Factor

Rheumatoid factors (RFs) make up a heterogeneous group of antibodies that are reactive with specific antigenic determinants on the Fc portion of human or animal IgG. Although RFs belonging to the IgM class are the commonly measured isotype in the clinical laboratory, RFs belonging to the IgA, IgG, IgD, and IgE classes have been identified. In the clinical laboratory, IgM RFs are tested most commonly by latex agglutination test, ELISA, and nephelometry. The values are expressed as serum titer or in international units per milliliter (IU/mL). IgG and IgA RFs are not routinely tested in clinical practice.

The prevalence of IgM RFs in large series of patients with SLE measured by latex fixation test ranges from 20% to 60% (mean, 33%). The serum titer is generally lower, compared with those observed in patients with RA. RFs belonging to isotypes other than IgM are not prevalent in SLE, compared with RA.

Several investigators have reported that nephritis is less frequent and with milder morphologic lesions in patients with SLE who test positive for RF, compared with those who are seronegative, suggesting that RFs may have a protective role in vivo. RFs can compete with complement for binding to immune complexes. RFs binding to antigen-antibody complexes may result in a more efficient removal from the circulation by the reticuloendothelial system. However, other investigators have failed to confirm the negative association of RFs and lupus nephritis and have found that the frequency of renal disease and survival rate of patients who are positive for RFs are not different from the general SLE population.[80,81]

Patients with coexistent RA and SLE ("rhupus") test positive for RF and anti–cyclic citrullinated peptide (anti-CCP) antibodies.[82] RFs have been reported to be more prevalent in patients with late-onset SLE than in younger patients, those patients with SLE and sicca syndrome, those with pulmonary hypertension, and those with abdominal vasculitis and/or serositis.[83] The clinical significance of these clinical associations is not clear. The varying results of several studies on the relationship of RFs and lupus nephritis or SLE in general are due to several factors including the differences in measurement of RF, patient population studied, fluctuation of serum titer, and heterogeneity of RF with regard to avidity, complement fixation, and other properties.

Anti–Cyclic Citrullinated Peptide Antibodies

Anti-CCP antibodies are found in RA and considered a diagnostic marker for the disease with high sensitivity and specificity. Commonly measured by an ELISA using synthetic citrullinated peptides as the antigen, anti-CCP antibodies are now widely accepted as superior to RF for diagnosing and is a predictive marker for the severity and prognosis of RA. However, a few patients with other diagnoses, including SLE, Sjögren syndrome, chronic hepatitis, and psoriatic arthritis, test positive for anti-CCP antibodies.

Anti-CCP antibodies in an unselected SLE population are uncommon (1% to 5%) and, in general, the serum titers are lower than those observed in RA. Clinical subsets of patients with SLE based on the clinical characteristics of joint involvement have different prevalence, titer, and citrulline-dependence of anti-CCP antibodies. Anti-CCP antibodies are most prevalent in patients with SLE and erosive and deforming arthritis (38%), and the serum titers can be comparable to those seen in RA. These patients with Jaccoud arthropathy exhibit ulnar deviation, and swan-neck, boutonnière, and Z-deformities. Anti-CCP antibodies also appear to be more prevalent in patients with SLE and severe erosive arthritis indistinguishable from RA ("rhupus"), although this has not been consistently observed in various studies. In contrast, anti-CCP in patients with SLE with nonerosive inflammatory arthritis, including those who fulfill the ACR criteria for RA but without radiographic evidence of erosions, tend to be less prevalent with low serum titers.[84,85]

Anti-CCP tests available in clinical laboratories measure reactivity to the citrullinated peptide and cannot differentiate antibody reactivity to the unmodified peptide containing arginine. Anti-CCP antibodies found in patients with tuberculosis and chronic active hepatitis are citrulline-independent and thus different from the citrulline-dependent anti-CCP antibodies seen in RA. Patients with SLE and erosive-deforming arthropathy have citrulline-dependent anti-CCP antibodies. In contrast, patients with inflammatory nonerosive arthritis have citrulline-independent anti-CCP antibodies.[84]

The presence of anti-CCP antibodies in a patient with inflammatory arthritis may not exclude a diagnosis of SLE. Whether high-titer anti-CCP antibodies can identify a subset of patients with SLE who will develop Jaccoud arthropathy early in the disease course remains to be established.

Cryoglobulins

Cryoglobulins are serum immunoglobulins that precipitate at temperatures below 37° C and redissolve on warming. Cryoglobulins are detected by incubating serums at 4° C usually for 7 days for the presence of cold insoluble precipitate. Immunochemical analysis of the cryoprecipitate identifies three major types of cryoglobulins. Type I consists of a single monoclonal immunoglobulin IgG, IgM, or IgA. Type II consists of mixed cryoglobulins with one of the components a monoclonal immunoglobulin. Monoclonal IgM with RF activity and a polyclonal IgG is the most common combination. Type III cryoglobulins are mixed cryoglobulins with polyclonal components. Type II and III cryoglobulins often contain RF, other autoantibodies, complement components, especially C1q, and fibronectin. Type III is generally associated with infections and autoimmune disorders including SLE, RA, and systemic sclerosis.

Mixed cryoglobulins are considered to represent circulating antigen-antibody complexes and are pathogenic in certain conditions. In hepatitis C infections, mixed cryoglobulins, consisting of viral antigens, polyclonal IgG, and monoclonal IgM RF deposits as immune complexes in small blood vessels, activate the complement system, resulting in inflammation and tissue injury in target organs including leukocytoclastic vasculitis, peripheral neuropathy, and/or glomerulonephritis.[86]

In SLE, mixed cryoglobulins have been found to contain RFs, antinuclear, antilymphocyte, DNA, and other autoantigens. Cryoglobulinemia in SLE is associated with disease activity including nephritis and hypocomplementemia. These observations suggest that cryoglobulins in SLE represent a subset of circulating immune complexes with potential pathogenicity. Glomerular subendothelial deposits of cryoglobulins identified by electron microscopy in a patient with lupus nephritis supports a pathogenic role of cryoglobulins.[87]

The high frequency of cryoglobulinemia in patients with SLE and concomitant hepatitis C infection has been noted.[88] All patients with a diagnosis of SLE should be routinely screened for hepatitis C and B infections.

Despite their association with disease activity in SLE, serum cryoglobulins are not routinely measured in clinical practice. The lack of a standardized test procedure, the lengthy duration to obtain the test results, and the need for careful handling of specimens are some of its disadvantages as a monitoring test.

Antiendothelial Cell Antibodies

Antiendothelial cell antibodies (AECAs) are a heterogeneous group of antibodies that bind to vascular endothelium cell antigens and are found in primary vasculitides, SLE, systemic sclerosis, other connective tissue diseases, as well as several other inflammatory conditions. The target antigens recognized by AECA may differ in these diseases; although some antigens are specific for endothelial cells, many antigens can be found in other cell types. Specific antigens that have been reported include Hsp60, DNA, proteinase 3, adhesion molecules, and many other novel candidate autoantigens identified by molecular cloning.

AECAs are commonly detected by ELISA using cultured human umbilical vein endothelial cells as a substrate. Other laboratory techniques and substrates are also available; however, no standardized assay is available to date.

AECAs are prevalent in SLE, ranging from 39% to 93% of patients.[89] The wide range of prevalence is in part due to differences in the test systems used. The presence of AECAs is associated with lupus nephritis, and the highest titers are seen in those with both nephritis and vasculitis. AECAs are also reported to be associated with lupus psychosis, pulmonary hypertension, and digital vasculitis. An elevated serum level of AECAs during disease activity declines with clinical improvement.

Despite their heterogeneity and presence in many medical conditions, AECAs have biologic properties that suggest a pathogenic role. The clinical association with overall disease activity and specific organ involvement, including vasculitis, nephritis, and neuropsychiatric manifestations, supports a putative pathogenic role in SLE. AECAs from patients with SLE activate endothelial cells followed by the upregulation of adhesion molecules and the production of proinflammatory cytokines and tissue factor in the coagulation cascade. AECAs can induce apoptosis of endothelial cells. This sequence of events leads to a proinflammatory and procoagulant phenotype of endothelial cells that may be important in the pathogenesis of vascular injury.[89,90]

Clinical application of AECAs in monitoring disease activity in individual patients with SLE is not currently recommended. No standardized test is available, and, moreover, it is not known whether measuring AECAs provides additional information to the commonly used laboratory tests in clinical practice.

Antineutrophil Cytoplasmic Antibodies

Antineutrophil cytoplasmic antibodies (ANCAs) are a heterogeneous group of autoantibodies directed against cytoplasmic antigens in neutrophils and monocytes. Several antigens have been identified, and autoantibodies to proteinase 3 and myeloperoxidase are clinically relevant. The indirect immunofluorescent test with ethanol-fixed normal human neutrophils as a substrate is used to screen for ANCAs. Four fluorescent patterns are seen: (1) classic ANCA (c-ANCA), (2) atypical c-ANCA, (3) perinuclear ANCA with or without nuclear extension (p-ANCA), and (4) atypical ANCA. ANAs may interfere with the interpretation of a p-ANCA fluorescent pattern, and performing specific ELISA tests is necessary for antimyeloperoxidase and antiproteinase 3 antibodies in all ANCA-positive sera by the immunofluorescent test.

ANCAs are associated with the primary vasculitides, and c-ANCAs are seen in Wegener granulomatosis and react with proteinase 3, although other antigenic specificities may also be seen. p-ANCAs are generally seen in microscopic polyangiitis, Churg-Strauss granuloma, and idiopathic crescentic glomerulonephritis and react with myeloperoxidase. ANCAs with other specificities include autoantibodies to elastase, cathepsin G, lactoferrin, and azuridin.[91]

A recent analysis of 13 published studies on ANCAs in SLE concluded that 15% to 20% of patients with SLE test positive, predominantly with a p-ANCA pattern and not with a c-ANCA pattern.[92] The antigenic specificities of ANCAs in SLE are primarily directed against lactoferrin, myeloperoxidase, elastase, and cathepsin G.

Various studies on the clinical correlation have yielded inconsistent results. In general, higher disease activity in patients with SLE who are ANCA positive appears to be a trend; however, the correlation is, at best, modest and not clinically important in the management of an individual patient.[92] Patients with active lupus nephritis have higher serum ANCA titers than those with renal disease. Elevated ANCA titers have been described in patients with lupus nephritis showing crescents in the renal biopsy and, in rare cases, co-existent lupus nephritis; ANCA-associated focal, segmental necrotizing, and crescentic glomerulonephritid have also been reported.[93]

Minocycline, which is widely used for the treatment of acne and RA, can occasionally cause a drug-induced lupus characterized serologically by positive ANAs, a high frequency of positive p-ANCAs (67%), and negative antihistone antibodies.[94]

The clinical application of ANCAs in SLE as a marker of disease activity and prognosis needs to be better defined. Routine testing of ANCAs in patients with SLE is not indicated at this time.

CLUSTERING OF AUTOANTIBODIES

By cluster analysis, groups of patients with SLE and a similar autoantibody profile can be identified. The number of clusters in various reports ranges from three to five, and the number partly depends on the ethnicity of the patients, the number of autoantibodies tested, and possibly other influences including genetic and environmental factors.

The cluster—not a single autoantibody—appears to be associated either positively or negatively with certain clinical features, disease severity, and prognosis. An autoantibody cluster characterized by the presence of anti-dsDNA, anti-SSA/Ro, and anti SSB/La was associated with a higher frequency of lupus nephritis.[95] A cluster of anti-SSA/Ro, anti-SSB/La, anti-Sm, and anti-RNP was associated with the absence or a milder form of nephritis in another SLE population studied.[96]

The development and availability of multiplex-antigen arrays and bead-based immunoassays, which can rapidly detect multiple autoantibodies using small volumes of serum, can facilitate studies on clustering in different ethnic populations of patients with SLE. The positivity of ANA, as well as anti-dsDNA, anti-Sm, anti-RNP, anti-SSA/Ro, and anti-SSB/La, remains stable with time.[97]

Longitudinal prospective studies can be instituted to determine whether autoantibody clustering is of value in deciding therapeutic management of patients with lupus.

References

1. Slater CA, Davis RB, Shmerling RH: Antinuclear antibody testing. A study of clinical utility. *Arch Intern Med* 156(13):1421–1425, 1996.
2. Meroni PL, Schur PH: ANA screening: an old test with new recommendations. *Ann Rheum Dis* 69(8):1420–1422, 2010.
3. Solomon DH, Kavanaugh AJ, Schur PH, and American College of Rheumatology Ad Hoc Committee on Immunologic Testing Guidelines: Evidence-based guidelines for the use of immunologic tests: Antinuclear antibody testing. *Arthritis Rheum* 47:434–444, 2002.
4. Vila LM, Mayor AM, Valentin AH, et al: Clinical outcome and predictors of disease evolution in patients with incomplete lupus erythematosus. *Lupus* 9:110–115, 2000.
5. Steiman AJ, Gladman DD, Ibanez D, et al: Prolonged serologically active clinically quiescent systemic lupus erythematosus. Frequency and outcome. *J Rheumatol* 37:1822–1827, 2010.
6. Mosca M, Tani C, Aringer M, et al: European League Against Rheumatism recommendations for monitoring patients with systemic lupus erythematosus in clinical practice and in observational studies. *Ann Rheum* 69:1269–1274, 2010.
7. Kavanaugh AF, Solomon DH, and the American College of Rheumatology Ad Hoc Committee on Immunologic Testing Guidelines: Guidelines for immunologic laboratory testing in the rheumatic diseases: Anti-DNA antibody tests. *Arthritis Rheum* 17(5):546–555, 2002.
8. Costa MF, Said NR, Zimmermann B: Drug-induced lupus due to anti-tumor necrosis factor alpha agents. *Semin Arthritis Rheum* 37(6):381–387, 2008.
9. Weinstein A, Bordwell B, Stone B, et al: Antibodies to native DNA and serum complement (C3) levels. Application to diagnosis and classification of systemic lupus erythematosus. *Am J Med* 74:206–216, 1983.
10. Tozzoli R, Bizzaro N, Tonutti E, et al; Italian Society of Laboratory Medicine Study Group on the Diagnosis of Autoimmune Diseases: Guidelines for the laboratory use of autoantibody tests in the diagnosis and monitoring of autoimmune rheumatic diseases. *Am J Clin Pathol* 117(2):316–324, 2002.
11. Bootsma H, Spronk P, Derksen R, et al: Prevention of relapses in systemic lupus erythematosus. *Lancet* 345(8965):1595–1599, 1995.
12. Tseng CE, Buyon JP, Kim M, et al: The effect of moderate-dose corticosteroids in preventing severe flares in patients with serologically active, but clinically stable, systemic lupus erythematosus: findings of a prospective, randomized, double-blind, placebo-controlled trial. *Arthritis Rheum* 54(11):3623–3632, 2006.
13. Liang MH, Simard JF: The large print giveth and the small print taketh away: preemptive treatment of serologically active, clinically quiet systemic lupus erythematosus. *Arthritis Rheum* 54(11):3378–3380, 2006.
14. Benito-Garcia E, Schur PH, Lahita R: American College of Rheumatology Ad Hoc Committee on Immunologic Testing Guidelines for immunologic laboratory testing in the rheumatic diseases: anti-Sm and anti-RNP antibody tests. *Arthritis Rheum* 51(6):1030–1044, 2004.
15. Arnett FC, Hamilton RG, Roebber MG, et al: Increased frequencies of Sm and nRNP autoantibodies in American blacks compared to whites with systemic lupus erythematosus. *J Rheumatol* 15(12):1773–1776, 1988.
16. Agarwal S, Harper J, Kiely PD: Concentration of antibodies to extractable nuclear antigens and disease activity in systemic lupus erythematosus. *Lupus* 18(5):407–412, 2009.
17. Frandsen PB, Kriegbaum NJ, Ullman S, et al: Follow-up of 151 patients with high-titer U1RNP antibodies. *Clin Rheumatol* 15(3):254–260, 1996.
18. Sontheimer RD: Subacute cutaneous lupus erythematosus: 25-year evolution of a prototypic subset (subphenotype) of lupus erythematosus defined by characteristic cutaneous, pathological, immunological, and genetic findings. *Autoimmunity Rev* 4:253–263, 2005.
19. Buyon JP, Winchester RJ, Slade SS: Identification of mothers at risk for congenital heart block and other neonatal lupus syndromes in their children. *Arthritis Rheum* 36:1263–1273, 1993.
20. Pettigrew HD, Teuber SS, Gershwin ME: Clinical significance of complement deficiencies. *Ann NY Acad Sci* 1173:108–123, 2009.
21. Reichlin M: ANA negative systemic lupus erythematosus sera revisited serologically. *Lupus* 9(2):116–119, 2000.
22. Sutej PG, Gear AJ, Morrison RC, et al: Photosensitivity and anti-Ro(SSA) antibodies in black patients with systemic lupus erythematosus. *Br J Rheumatol* 28(4):321–324, 1989.
23. Cavazzana I, Franceschini F, Belfiore N, et al: Undifferentiated connective tissue disease with antibodies to Ro/SSa: clinical features and follow-up of 148 patients. *Clin Exp Rheumatol* 19(4):403–409, 2001.
24. Manoussakis MN, Georgopoulou C, Zintzaras E, et al: Sjögren's syndrome associated with systemic lupus erythematosus: clinical and laboratory profiles and comparison with primary Sjögren's syndrome. *Arthritis Rheum* 50(3):882–891, 2004.
25. Stumvoll GH, Fritsch RD, Meyer B, et al: Characterization of cellular and humoral autoimmune responses to histone H1 and core histones in human systemic lupus erythematosus. *Ann Rheum Dis* 68:110–116, 2009.
26. Wallace DJ, Lin HC, Shen GQ, et al: Antibodies to histone (H2AH2B)-DNA complexes in the absence of antibodies to double stranded DNA or to (H2A-H2B) complexes are more sensitive and specific for scleroderma-related disorders than for lupus. *Arthritis Rheum* 37:1795–1797, 1994.
27. Schett G, Steiner G, Smolen JS: Nuclear antigen histone H1 is primarily involved in lupus erythematosus cell formation. *Arthritis Rheum* 41:1446–1455, 1988.
28. Gómez-Puerta JA, Burlingame RW, Cervera R: Anti-chromatin (anti-nucleosome) antibodies: diagnostic and clinical value. *Autoimmunity Rev* 7:606–611, 2008.
29. Manson JJ, Ma A, Rogers P, et al: Relationship between anti-ds DNA, anti-nucleosome and anti-alpha-actinin antibodies and markers of renal disease in patients with lupus nephritis. A prospective longitudinal study. *Arthritis Res Ther* 11(5):R154, 2009.
30. Kallenberg CGM: Anti-C1q autoantibodies. *Autoimmunity Rev* 7:612–615, 2008.
31. Matrat A, Veyssetre-Balter C, Trolliet P, et al: Simultaneous detection of anti-C1q and anti-ds DNA autoantibodies in lupus nephritis: predictive value for renal flares. *Lupus* 20:28–34, 2011.
32. Toubi E, Shoenfeld Y: Clinical and biological aspects of anti-P-ribosomal protein autoantibodies. *Autoimmunity Rev* 6:119–125, 2007.
33. Barkhudarova F, Dahnrich C, Rosemann A, et al: Diagnostic value and clinical laboratory associations of antibodies against recombinant ribosomal P0, P1 and P2 proteins and their native heterocomplex in a Caucasian cohort with systemic lupus erythematosus. *Arthritis Res Therapy* 13:R20–R30, 2011.
34. Mahler M, Silverman ED, Schulte-Pelkum J, et al: Anti-Scl-70 (topo-1) antibodies in SLE. Myth or reality. *Autoimmunity Rev* 9:756–760, 2010.
35. Gussin HAE, Ignat GP, Varga J, et al: Anti-topoisomerase I (anti-Scl-70) antibodies in patients with systemic lupus erythematosus. *Arthritis Rheum* 44(2):376–383, 2001.
36. Respaldiza N, Wichmann I, Ocaña CG, et al: Anti-centromere antibodies in patients with systemic lupus erythematosus. *Scand J Rheumatol* 35:290–294, 2006.
37. Vila LM, Alarcon GS, McGwin G, Jr, et al: Systemic lupus erythematosus in a multiethnic cohort (LUMINA): XXIX. Elevation of erythrocyte sedimentation rate is associated with disease activity and damage accrual. *J Rheumatol* 32(11):2150–2155, 2005.

38. Nasiri S, Karimifar M, Bonakdar ZS, et al: Correlation of ESR, C3, C4, anti-DNA and lupus activity based on British Isles Lupus Assessment Group Index in patients of rheumatology clinic. *Rheumatol Int* 30(12): 1605–1609, 2010.

39. Firooz N, Albert DA, Wallace DJ, et al: High sensitivity C-reactive protein and erythrocyte sedimentation rate in systemic lupus erythematosus. *Lupus* 20:588–597, 2011.

40. De Carvalho JF, Hanaoka B, Szyper-Kravitz M, et al: C-reactive protein and its implications in systemic lupus erythematosus. *Acta Reumatol Port* 32(4):317–322, 2007.

41. Gaitonde S, Samols D, Kushner I: C-reactive protein and systemic lupus erythematosus. *Arthritis Rheum* 59(12):1814–1820, 2008.

42. Barnes EV, Narain S, Naranjo A, et al: High sensitivity C-reactive protein in systemic lupus erythematosus: relation to disease activity, clinical presentation and implications for cardiovascular risk. *Lupus* 14(8):576–582, 2005.

43. Bertoli AM, Vila LM, Reveille JD, et al; LUMINA Study Group: Systemic lupus erythematosus in a multiethnic US cohort (LUMINA):LXI. Value of C-reactive protein as a marker of disease activity and damage. *J Rheumatol* 35(12):2355–2358, 2008.

44. Lee SS, Singh S, Link K, et al: High-sensitivity c-reactive protein as an associate of clinical subsets and organ damage in systemic lupus erythematosus. *Semin Arthritis Rheum* 38(1):41–54, 2008.

45. ter Borg EJ, Horst G, Limburg PC, et al: C-reactive protein levels during disease exacerbations and infections in systemic lupus erythematosus: a prospective longitudinal study. *J Rheumatol* 17(12):1642–1648, 1990.

46. Karadag O, Calguneri M, Atalar E, et al: Novel cardiovascular risk factors and cardiac event predictors in female inactive systemic lupus erythematosus patients. *Clin Rheumatol* 26:695–699, 2007.

47. Lee SS, Singh S, Magder LS, et al: Predictors of high sensitivity C-reactive protein levels in patients with systemic lupus erythematosus. *Lupus* 17:114–123, 2008.

48. Nikpour M, Gladman DD, Ibañez D, et al: Variability and correlates of high sensitivity C-reactive protein in systemic lupus erythematosus. *Lupus* 18:966–973, 2009.

49. Meyer O: Anti-CRP antibodies in systemic lupus erythematosus. *Joint Bone Spine* 77(5):384–389, 2010.

50. Shoenfeld Y, Szyper-Kravitz M, Witte T, et al: Autoantibodies against protective molecules—C1q, C-reactive protein, serum amyloid P, mannose-binding lectin, and apolipoprotein A1: prevalence in systemic lupus erythematosus. *Ann N Y Acad Sci* 1108:227–239, 2007.

51. Figueredo MA, Rodriguez A, Ruiz-Yagüe M, et al: Autoantibodies against C-reactive protein: clinical associations in systemic lupus erythematosus and primary antiphospholipid antibody syndrome. *J Rheumatol* 33(10): 1980–1986, 2006.

52. Bassi N, Ghirardello A, Blank M, et al: IgG anti-pentraxin 3 antibodies in systemic lupus erythematosus. *Ann Rheum Dis* 69:1704–1710, 2010.

53. Ho A, Barr SG, Magder LS, et al: A decrease in complement is associated with increased renal and hematologic activity in patients with systemic lupus erythematosus. *Arthritis Rheum* 44:2350–2357, 2001.

54. Birmingham DJ, Irshaid F, Nagaraja HN, et al: The complex nature of serum C3 and C4 as biomarkers of lupus renal flare. *Lupus* 19:1272–1280, 2010.

55. Clowse MEB, Magder LS, Petri M: The clinical utility of measuring complement and anti-ds DNA antibodies during pregnancy in patients with systemic lupus erythematosus. *J Rheumatol* 38:1012–1016, 2011.

56. Liu CC, Manzi S, Kao AH, et al: Cell-bound complement biomarkers for SLE: from benchtop to bedside. *Rheum Dis Clin North Am* 36(1):161–172, 2010.

57. Sturfelt G, Truedsson: Complement and its breakdown products in SLE. *Rheumatol* 44:1227–1232, 2005.

58. Ogryzlo MA, Maclachlan M, Dauphinee JA, et al: The serum proteins in health and disease; filter paper electrophoresis. *Am J Med* 27:596–616, 1959.

59. Wallace DJ: Serum and plasma protein abnormalities and other clinical laboratory determinations in systemic lupus erythematosus. In Wallace DJ, Hahn BH, editors: *Dubois' lupus erythematosus*, ed 7, Philadelphia, PA, 2007, Lippincott Williams and Wilkins, pp 911–919.

60. Yoshizawa S, Nagasawa K, Yoshiaki Y, et al: A thermolabile β2-macroglycoprotein (TMG) and the antibody against TMG in patients with systemic lupus erythematosus. *Clin Chim Acta* 264(2):219–225, 1997.

61. Ali YM, Urowitz MB, Ibanez D, et al: Monoclonal gammopathy in systemic lupus erythematosus. *Lupus* 16:426–429, 2007.

62. Yong PFK, Aslam L, Karim MY, et al: Minocycline-induced lupus: clinical features and response to rechallenge. *Rheumatology (Oxford)* 47:1400–1405, 2008.

63. Karim MY: Immunodeficiency in the lupus clinic. *Lupus* 15:127–131, 2006.

64. Levy J, Barnett EV, MacDonald NS, et al: Altered immunoglobulin metabolism in systemic lupus erythematosus and rheumatoid arthritis. *J Clin Invest* 49(4):708–715, 1970.

65. Lin GG, Li JM: IgG subclass serum levels in systemic lupus erythematosus patients. *Clin Rheumatol* 28(11):1315–1318, 2009.

66. Bijl M, Dijstelbloem HM, Oost WW, et al: IgG subclass distribution of autoantibodies differs between renal and extra-renal relapses in patients with systemic lupus erythematosus. *Rheumatology (Oxford)* 41(1):62–67, 2002.

67. Saiki O, Saweki Y, Tanaka T, et al: Development of selective IgM deficiency in systemic lupus erythematosus patients with disease of long duration. *Arthritis Rheum* 30:1289–1292, 1987.

68. Sivri A, Hasçelik Z: IgM deficiency in systemic lupus erythematosus patients. *Arthritis Rheum* 38(11):1713, 1995.

69. Goldstein MF, Goldstein AL, Dunsky EH, et al: Selective IgM immunodeficiency: retrospective analysis of 36 adult patients with review of the literature. *Ann Allergy Asthma Immunol* 97(6):717–730, 2006.

70. Monteiro RC: The role of IgA and IgA Fc receptors as anti-inflammatory agents. *J Clin Immunol* 30(Suppl 1):S61–S64, 2010.

71. Mantovani APF, Monclaro MP, Skare TL: Prevalence of IgA deficiency in adult systemic lupus erythematosus and the study of the association with its clinical and autoantibody profiles. *Bras J Rheumatol* 50(3):273–282, 2010.

72. Cassidy JT, Kitson RK, Selby CL: Selective IgA deficiency in children and adults with systemic lupus erythematosus. *Lupus* 16:647–650, 2007.

73. Carneiro-Sampaio M, Liphaus BL, Jesus AA, et al: Understanding systemic lupus erythematosus physiopathology in the light of primary immunodeficiencies. *J Clin Immunol* 28(Suppl 1):S34–S41, 2008.

74. Atta AM, Santiago MB, Guerra FG, et al: Autoimmune response of IgE antibodies to cellular self-antigens in systemic lupus erythematosus. *Int Arch Allergy Immunol* 152(4):401–406, 2010.

75. North I, Kotecha S, Houtman P, et al: Systemic lupus erythematosus complicating hyper IgE syndrome. *Br J Rheumatol* 36(2):297–298, 1997.

76. Fernández-Castro M, Mellor-Pita S, Citores MJ, et al: Common variable immunodeficiency in systemic lupus erythematosus. *Semin Arthritis Rheum* 36:238–245, 2007.

77. Boccara O, Valeyrie-Allanore L, Crickx B, et al: Association of hypogammaglobulinemia with DRESS (Drug Rash with Eosinophilia and Systemic Symptoms). *Eur J Dermatol* 16(6):666–668, 2006.

78. Dörner T, Lipsky PE: Correlation of circulating CD27 high plasma cells and disease activity in systemic lupus erythematosus. *Lupus* 13(5):283–289, 2004.

79. Mathian A, Gallegos M, Pascual V, et al: Interferon-α induces unabated production of short-lived plasma cells in pre-autoimmune lupus-prone (NZB×NZW)F1 mice but not in BALB/c mice. *Eur J Immunol* 41(3):863–872, 2011.

80. Estes D, Christian CL: The natural history of systemic lupus erythematosus by prospective analysis. *Medicine* 50:85–96, 1971.

81. Shoenfeld Y, Toubi E: Protective autoantibodies. Role in homeostasis, clinical importance and therapeutic potentials. *Arthritis Rheum* 52:2599–2606, 2005.

82. Amezcua-Guerra LM, Springall R, Marquez-Velasco R, et al: Presence of antibodies against cyclic citrullinated peptides in patients with "rhupus": a cross-sectional study. *Arthritis Res Ther* 8(5):R144, 2006.

83. Quismorio FP, Jr, Sharma O, Koss M, et al: Immunopathologic and clinical studies in pulmonary hypertension associated with systemic lupus erythematosus. *Semin Arthritis Rheum* 13(4):349–359, 1984.

84. Kakumanu P, Sobel ES, Narain S, et al: Citrulline dependence of anti-cyclic citrullinated peptide antibodies in systemic lupus erythematosus as a marker of deforming/erosive arthritis. *J Rheumatol* 36(12):2682–2690, 2009.

85. Qing YF, Zhang QB, Zhou JG, et al: The detecting and clinical value of anti-cyclic citrullinated peptide antibodies in patients with systemic lupus erythematosus. *Lupus* 18:713–717, 2009.

86. Ferri C: Mixed cryoglobulinemia. *Orphanet J Rare Dis* 3:25, 2008.

87. Cohen RA, Bayliss G, Crispin JC, et al: T cells and in situ cryoglobulin deposition in the pathogenesis of lupus nephritis. *Clin Immunol* 128(1):1–7, 2008.

88. García-Carrasco M, Ramos-Casals M, Cervera R, et al: Cryoglobulinemia in systemic lupus erythematosus: prevalence and clinical characteristics in a series of 122 patients. *Semin Arthritis Rheum* 30(5):366–373, 2001.

89. Belizna C, Duijvestijn A, Hamidou M, et al: Antiendothelial cell antibodies in vasculitis and connective tissue disease. *Ann Rheum Dis* 65:1545–1550, 2006.

90. Domiciano DS, Carvalho JF, Shoenfeld Y: Pathogenic role of anti-endothelial cell antibodies in autoimmune rheumatic diseases. *Lupus* 18:1233–1238, 2009.

91. Bosch X, Guilabert A, Font J: Antineutrophil cytoplasmic antibodies. *Lancet* 368:404–417, 2006.

92. Sen D, Isenberg DA: Antineutrophil cytoplasmic autoantibodies in systemic lupus erythematosus. *Lupus* 12:651–658, 2009.

93. Nasr SH, D'Agati VD, Park H-R, et al: Necrotizing and crescentic lupus nephritis with antineutrophil cytoplasmic antibody seropositivity. *Clin Am Soc Nephrol* 3:682–690, 2008.

94. Lawson TM, Amos N, Bulgen D, et al: Minocycline-induced lupus: clinical features and response to rechallenge. *Rheumatology (Oxford)* 40:329–335, 2001.

95. To CH, Petri M: Is antibody clustering predictive of clinical subsets and damage in systemic lupus erythematosus. *Arthritis Rheum* 52(12):4003–4010, 2005.

96. Tápanes FJ, Vásquez M, Ramirez R, et al: Cluster analysis of antinuclear autoantibodies in the prognosis of SLE nephropathy: are anti-extractable nuclear antibodies protective? *Lupus* 9:437–444, 2000.

97. Ippolito A, Wallace DJ, Gladman D, et al: Autoantibodies in systemic lupus erythematosus: comparison of historical and current assessment of seropositivity. *Lupus* 20:250–255, 2011.

Differential Diagnosis and Disease Associations

Meenakshi Jolly, Serene Francis, and Winston Sequeira

Systemic lupus erythematosus (SLE) exhibits a variety of signs and symptoms among patients, which frequently poses diagnostic dilemmas. SLE is frequently referred to as the "great mimicker," and the process of reaching the correct diagnosis is marked by several physician visits, wrongful diagnoses, and a considerable time lag of up to 5 years after the onset of symptoms in its establishment and management. In 1906, Osler and Jadassohn described the systemic features of SLE. Nearly a century later, despite the many innovations in medical science and the easy availability of various investigative modalities available to the modern physician, the diagnosis of SLE remains mainly a clinical one.

The need to come to an accurate diagnosis of SLE is crucial for two main reasons: (1) to allow for timely and appropriate therapeutic interventions (e.g., immunosuppressive therapy) if the patient's condition (e.g., SLE) mandates to control inflammation, limit irreversible organ damage, and optimize health outcomes; and (2) if the patient's diagnosis (e.g., non-SLE) does not warrant immunosuppressive medicines, avoiding unnecessary risks and harm from their use. This chapter puts together a list of differential diagnoses and features of SLE to help the reader differentiate these diseases from SLE, as well as some of its disease associations.

IS IT REALLY SYSTEMIC LUPUS ERYTHEMATOSUS?

Diagnosing SLE involves taking a detailed history, conducting a thorough physical examination, and reviewing pertinent current and past laboratory or imaging evaluations to exclude more common diseases that may explain the current symptoms and to evaluate for evidence of involvement of other organ systems as may occur in SLE. Based on these assessments, if the pretest possibility for SLE is high, then antinuclear antibody (ANA) testing is ordered to support the diagnosis. Guidelines for the clinical use of the ANA test and the algorithm for screening positive ANAs have been formulated and are available.[1,2] With a thorough clinical evaluation, a diagnosis can be made 90% of the time.

The differential diagnosis of SLE is broad and includes but is not restricted to rheumatoid arthritis (RA), mixed connective tissue disorder (MCTD), undifferentiated connective tissue disorder (UCTD), Kikuchi disease, acute viral and reactive syndromes, Behçet disease (BD), familial Mediterranean fever, amyopathic dermatomyositis, drug-induced lupus erythematosus (DIL) (including anti-tumor necrosis factor therapy induced), serum sickness, juvenile idiopathic arthritis (JIA), and fibromyalgia, among others (Box 44-1). For example, the differential diagnosis in a young woman with myalgias, arthralgias, and skin rash and a positive ANA titer is quite vast. Most of the time, the difficulties in diagnosing SLE come from having to make the distinction between SLE and other autoimmune disorders such as MCTD or UCTD. The diagnosis of SLE is complicated by the presence of co-existing autoimmune and nonautoimmune conditions. Co-existent autoimmune diseases with SLE include antiphospholipid syndrome, RA, scleroderma, Sjögren syndrome, myositis, MCTD, relapsing polychondritis, autoimmune hepatitis, vasculitis, psoriasis, primary biliary cirrhosis, autoimmune thrombocytopenia,

thyroid disorders, and diabetes. Thirty percent of patients with SLE have at least one other autoimmune disease,[3] and, in 23% of these patients, the secondary autoimmune disease preceded the diagnosis of SLE.[3] Some of the nonrheumatologic diseases known to occur with SLE are infections (e.g., tuberculosis, leishmania, treponema, hepatitis, human immunodeficiency virus [HIV]), fibromyalgia, depression, myasthenia gravis, ichthyosis, psoriasis, lichen planus, gout, and hematologic abnormalities (e.g., sickle cell disease, anemia). Some of these infections may exhibit symptoms similar to SLE and thus pose diagnostic and treatment dilemmas. The ease with which a physician can make the diagnosis of SLE at first presentation greatly depends on the initial manifestation of the disease. For example, in a patient with renal failure, thrombocytopenia, elevated body temperatures, and a positive ANA test, the diagnosis of SLE may be made more confidently, as opposed to someone who might have fevers, oral ulcers, arthralgias, and a positive ANA test.

Recognizing that SLE symptoms may begin years earlier but may not be as evolved to be clearly ascribable to SLE complicates these diagnostic issues; thus the condition may be categorized under the diagnosis of UCTD. Terms such as *latent lupus* and *incomplete lupus* have been used in the past for UCTD. SLE was diagnosed in 24% of patients with UCTD who were followed longitudinally after a mean period of 54 months.[4]

Why is it necessary to differentiate these conditions? Arriving at a specific diagnosis is necessary to not only understand the course and prognosis of the illness and treat it effectively, but also to avoid unnecessary laboratory and other evaluations, to prevent harm to the patient from immunosuppressive medications, and to optimize health care resource utilization and outcomes. For example, if methotrexate was initiated for a presumed SLE diagnosis in a patient with arthralgias as a result of fibromyalgia, the treatment would not be beneficial and would adversely tip the risk-benefit ratio. However, if this patient truly had SLE (with or without fibromyalgia), then the use of methotrexate for inflammatory arthritis would be considered judicious and beneficial.

Similarly, if the therapy to treat anti-tumor necrosis factor had been instituted in a patient who was thought to have RA, and fatigue, fever, rash, arthralgias, or thrombocytopenia developed, it would be assumed that these changes were reactions to the treatment or to DIL. If ANAs had been initially sought and found, however, antitumor necrosis factor therapy might not have been used, and the changes noted would have been recognized as being evidence for the progression of the underlying SLE.

Misdiagnosis of Lupus

Many people who are told they have or might have SLE actually do not have the disorder. Hochberg and associates[5] noted that only one third of patients who were told they had lupus by a physician actually fulfilled the American College of Rheumatology (ACR) classification criteria for SLE. Of the 149 patients referred to the University of Alabama for the management of and/or consultation for suspected SLE, 60% (90 patients) met the 1982 revised ACR classification criteria, whereas 15% had a diagnosis of clinical SLE but did not meet

Box 44-1 Differential Diagnoses of Systemic Lupus Erythematosus Disease

Connective Tissue Disorders
Rheumatoid arthritis and "rhupus"
Undifferentiated connective tissue disease
Inflammatory myopathy
Scleroderma
Vasculitides
Sjögren syndrome
Juvenile inflammatory arthritis

Infections
Viral
–Parvovirus
–Epstein-Barr virus and infectious mononucleosis
–Human immunodeficiency viral and human T-lymphotropic viral infections

Other Disorders
Bacterial infections
–Salmonella
–Tuberculosis
–Leprosy

Parasitic Disorders

Granulomatous Disorders
Sarcoidosis
Kikuchi disease

Carcinomas

Dermatologic Disorders
Porphyrias
Dermatitis herpetiformis
Psoriasis

Miscellaneous Disorders
Fibromyalgia
Serum sickness
Amyloidosis
Angioimmunoblastic lymphadenopathy with dysproteinemia
Immunoglobulin G4 (IgG4)–related autoimmune fibrosis[285]
Familial Mediterranean fever
Chronic granulomatous disease
Thallium poisoning

the ACR criteria.[6] Another 25% of patients had fibromyalgia-like manifestations, tested positive for ANAs, and very likely did not belong to the SLE spectrum.[6] Of the 263 patients referred to the University of Florida Autoimmune Disease Clinic between 2001 and 2002 with a working diagnosis of SLE, a 49% agreement rate with the referring physicians' working diagnosis of SLE was observed.[7] Of all the referring physicians, rheumatologists were four times more likely to make the correct diagnosis of SLE than non-rheumatologists.[7] Treatment with steroids was administered to 15% of the patients (as high as 60 mg/day) without any autoimmune disease but with positive ANA testing.[7] Misdiagnosing lupus leads to unnecessary, toxic, and expensive treatments, the stigmatization of patients, and pointless lifestyle and dietary restrictions, and affects family relationships and reproductive planning.

Positive Antinuclear Antibody Testing: How Often Is it Systemic Lupus Erythematosus?

To rule out SLE, rheumatologists all too often are referred patients who feel good or have vague symptoms but have a positive ANA test.

The ANA test is sensitive for the diagnosis of SLE (95% to 100% patients with SLE have ANAs), but this test should be ordered only if the pretest possibility of this diagnosis is high. A positive ANA test is often found in patients with other disorders and in seemingly healthy patients. The prevalence of positive ANAs depends on the patient's sex and age; older persons, particularly women older than 65 years of age, more commonly have ANAs. With the use of the HEp-2 substrate, approximately 20% of healthy individuals have an ANA titer of 1:40 or higher and 5% have an ANA titer of 1:160 or higher.[8] Relatives of 25% to 30% of patients with connective tissue disease have titers equal to or higher than 1:40.[2] A positive ANA test has an 11% positive predictive value for SLE.[2] Of note, solid-phase methods, which are being increasingly used for assessing ANAs, have increased false-negative results for SLE; the ACR task force for ANA supports immunofluorescence testing as the "gold standard" method.[9] Of the 471 patients with SLE, ANA levels were the first ACR criterion accrued among 20% of patients.[10] In a study using donated sera from 130 soldiers who were being inducted into the armed forces and who ultimately developed SLE,[11] 115 had at least one SLE autoantibody (78% had ANAs) a mean 3.3 years before diagnosis.

Antinuclear Antibody–Negative Lupus

A positive ANA test is only 1 of 11 criteria that are used to define SLE according to the ACR classification. Of the 11 criteria, 4 must be present to make a diagnosis, but ANA positivity is so central to the current concepts of SLE that many rheumatologists find it inconceivable for SLE to be present without it. Several reports have documented the delayed appearance of ANAs in patients suspected of having SLE. In the view of the authors of this text,[12,13] documenting a mean of 3 to 4 years between onset of symptoms and time of diagnosis is not surprising. Case series of patients with lupus nephritis in whom negative ANAs persisted for years before becoming positive are known.[14,15] Persillin and Takeuchi[16] found ANAs in the urine and pleural fluid of a patient with diffuse proliferative nephritis and nephrotic syndrome for some time before serum ANAs were present. Low antibody concentrations in the serum secondary to a loss in body fluids can be present as noted by Ferreiro and associates.[17]

The concept of ANA-negative SLE was introduced in 1976[18] and has been said to be typical of patients with photosensitivity and antibodies to Sjögren syndrome antigen A (anti-SSA/Ro).[19] With the use of modern microscopes and HEp-2 cells as a source of nuclear antigens, the existence of ANA-negative SLE has been questioned.[20] Reichlin[21] has stated that with a Ketjen Black (KB) or Hep-2 substrate, 98% of all patients with SLE are ANA positive, because non–DNA-containing antigens such as SSA/Ro are better represented when these cell lines are studied. Unfortunately, human cell lines are less specific, although they are more sensitive.

Technical inaccuracy, specimen collection and storage issues, variations in microscope quality, ANAs hidden within circulating immune complexes (CICs), in vivo binding of ANAs by tissues, types of fixation on substrate slides, antiimmunoglobulin-conjugate characteristics (e.g., isotype specificity, fluorescein isothiocyanate–to–protein ratio, antibody-to-protein ratio, specific antibody content and working dilution), and problems with reference sera are causes of negative ANAs in patients with SLE.[8] Wide variations in the reproducibility of ANA tests and difficulties in standardization are also problems that remain unresolved.[8] It needs to be stressed, however, in view of increasing use of quantitative, automated high-volume solid-phase assays, that if the clinician strongly suspects SLE and ANAs are negative, then checking with the laboratory concerning the assay used to assess ANAs is important. The use of an enzyme-linked immunosorbent assay (ELISA) or coated beads increases false-negative rates as do solid-phase substrates that use a limited number of autoantigens.[9] In a study comparing the frequency of ANAs using immunofluorescence and ELISA (BioPlex) among 192 patients with SLE, the latter fared worse than immunofluorescence (75.5% versus 81.3%).[22] BioPlex sensitivity and specificity for SLE were 78.9% and 38.9%, respectively.[22] Therefore confirming with the laboratory which assay was used to measure the ANAs is important; if the ELISA was used and the physician's suspicion for SLE is strong, then a repeat of the ANA test with immunofluorescence assay is recommended.

Undifferentiated Connective-Tissue Disease

The term was first coined by LeRoy in 1980 and is used to refer to a group of systemic autoimmune diseases with signs and symptoms that are not sufficiently evolved to fulfill the accepted classification criteria for the defined connective tissue diseases.[4] In a series of papers written by Williams and colleagues,[23] 213 patients with early UCTD were followed for over 10 years. At 10 years they reported that the presence of malar rash, serositis, or discoid lupus in patients with UCTD suggested an eventual diagnosis of SLE. In another follow-up study of 83 patients with UCTD, 18 patients (22%) developed SLE at a mean period of 54 months,[4] and the presence of anticardiolipin (aCL) antibody was associated with the development of SLE. The authors concluded that the rate of evolution to a connective tissue disease is greatest in the first years of follow-up and then decreases over time. Bodolay and others[24] followed 746 patients with early UCTD and noted the development of SLE in 4.2% and a resolution of symptoms among 12% of the patients. The highest probability of development of a defined connective tissue disease was noted in the first 2 years; 12% of the patients underwent remission and 64.5% remained in the UCTD category. Most of the UCTD studies note that the disease is mild, and most patients remain in the UCTD category; those cases that evolve further into a defined connective tissue disease category do so early on.[4,24,25]

Incomplete Lupus

Incomplete lupus is a misleading term that has appeared in the literature to denote patients who are thought to have SLE but do not fulfill four ACR criteria. Hence, this term could be inappropriately applied to UCTD or to patients with clinical SLE. These individuals range from having biopsy-documented nephritis to idiopathic thrombocytopenic purpura with positive ANAs to fibromyalgia. In a study of 28 Swedish patients with incomplete SLE, 57% developed complete SLE after a median period of 5.3 years.[26] As in the patients with UCTD, the presence of aCL antibodies was found to be a predictor for SLE. Swaak and colleagues[27] noted skin, musculoskeletal, and leukopenia-related disease activity in 122 patients of European descent with incomplete lupus; 27 patients met the full criteria shortly after study entry, and 3 patients met the criteria over the following 3 years. Patients with incomplete SLE have been found to have less frequent disease flares[28] and a good prognosis.[27] Too many patients who carry this label undergo unnecessary treatments and become stigmatized and medicated; hence, this term should not be used in patients meeting the criteria for a UCTD diagnosis.

Rheumatoid Arthritis

Clinical Differentiation

RA is usually easily diagnosed, especially when it occurs in its characteristic form with symmetric, bilateral inflammatory small-joint arthritis, along with a positive rheumatoid factor (RF), positive anticyclic citrullinated peptide (anti-CCP), and, in a majority of cases, ANA negativity. With advances in awareness, early diagnosis, and aggressive treatment for RA, nonerosive disease (rather than advanced erosive disease) is usually encountered today. Therefore the presence of erosions may not be helpful to distinguish early and well-treated RA from usually nonerosive SLE. Furthermore, when RA displays extraarticular involvement or is ANA positive, differentiating RA from SLE is occasionally difficult. When a patient exhibits a new inflammatory arthritis that has overlapping features of both diseases, it may take 6 to 12 months of clinical observation before a definitive diagnosis can be made.

Extraarticular Differentiation

Extraarticular RA may include serositis, Sjögren syndrome, subcutaneous nodules, cutaneous vasculitis, anemia, fatigue, poor sleep,

depression, and other features that are observed in SLE. Turesson and associates[29] in a retrospective study of 609 patients with RA found a 41% occurrence of extraarticular features; a 30-year cumulative incidence of serositis and the Felty syndrome were observed in 2.5% and 1.6% of patients, respectively. Felty syndrome consists of positive ANAs, splenomegaly, arthritis, leukopenia, and an increased incidence of cutaneous vasculitis. Felty syndrome is also characterized by anti-granulocyte (as opposed to anti-lymphocyte) antibodies and elevated complement levels.[30] Close examination, however, reveals that the overwhelming majority of those with Felty syndrome are middle-aged men, in whom anti-DNA is never present and who have circulating cryoglobulins.[31-33] Central nervous system involvement and renal disease are absent. Ropes[34] compared 142 patients with SLE to a cohort of patients with RA. The latter had 1% incidence of sun sensitivity (versus 34% in those with SLE) and a 4% incidence of alopecia (versus 46% in patients with SLE). The incidence of thyroid antibodies is increased in both disorders. Another differentiating feature between RA and SLE is the lack of kidney involvement in those with RA. Davis and colleagues[35] reviewed the records of 5232 patients with RA; only 0.1% had glomerulonephritis. Davis and colleagues' literature review of glomerulonephritis in RA demonstrated that most of the cases could be accounted for by medications (gold or penicillamine in the past), as well as interstitial nephritis, amyloid, or diabetes.

Laboratory and Serologic Differentiation

RF was present in 9% of 166 patients with SLE, with titers of at least 1:40, and was associated with milder disease.[36] Among 302 patients with SLE, RF was present in 20%.[37] The availability of anti-CCP further helped differentiate SLE from RA. However, 14% of 138 patients of Chinese descent with SLE[38] and 8% of the 104 patients from the United Kingdom with SLE[39] tested positive for anti-CCP. In another study of 231 patients with SLE tested for anti-CCP, only 3 patients (less than 1%) were positive.[40] The Euro-Lupus project prospectively studied 1000 patients with SLE from seven European countries for 10 years and reported 18% positivity for RF in their cohort.[41] These patients tended to have sicca syndrome and lesser incidence of nephropathy.

Numerous investigators have looked for ANAs in RA. Icen and colleagues,[42] who followed 603 patients with incident RA, found four or more SLE features in 15.5% of patients within 25 years after the original RA incidence. ANA positivity was reported in 32.3% of patients and anti-dsDNA in 2.3%, whereas anti-Smith (Sm) antibodies were reported in 0.4% patients with RA.[42]

Rhupus

Among the many controversies that exist in rheumatology, the co-existence of SLE and RA is one. When a patient exhibits a new inflammatory arthritis that has overlapping features of both diseases, it may take 6 to 12 months of clinical observation before a definitive diagnosis can be made. The clinical co-existence of RA and SLE was first described in 1969 by Kantor and was termed *rhupus syndrome* by Schur.[43] Cohen and Webb[44] reported the development of SLE in 11 Australian patients with typical RA who were observed over a 17-year period, but the total number of patients with RA followed was not stated. Brand and colleagues[45] presented 11 co-existing cases; most had class II genetic determinations of both disorders. Among 22 patients with rhupus in Mexico City, an increased prevalence of human leukocyte antigen (HLA)–DR1 and DR2 alleles were found.[46]

In an epidemiologic study including approximately 7000 new patients, the prevalence of RA and SLE was 15% and 8.9%, respectively. The expected coincidence of RA and SLE by chance would therefore be 1.2%. However, the observed prevalence of rhupus was 0.09%, less than one tenth of that expected.[47] A Mexican case series[43] studied seven patients with rhupus who fulfilled the ACR criteria for both RA and SLE and compared them with seven patients each with RA and SLE. They concluded that rhupus is an overlap of RA and SLE. Another study[48] examined 34 patients with SLE (14 with and 20 without deforming arthropathy), using 34 patients with RA and 9 patients with rhupus as control subjects. They found patients with SLE (with or without deforming arthropathy) to have normal serum anti-CCP concentrations. In contrast, 97% of the patients with RA were positive for anti-CCP and had 30-fold higher than normal amounts of anti-CCP; the patients with rhupus (100% were positive for anti-CCP) had 23-fold higher than normal amounts of anti-CCP. Patients with SLE and deforming arthropathy were more frequently positive for RF (65%) than patients with nondeforming arthritis (15%).

Juvenile Idiopathic Arthritis

Like healthy adults, healthy children may have ANA positivity. A 2004 study on ANA prevalence among 214 healthy children from Brazil between the ages of 6 months and 20 years (mean age 8.7 years) demonstrated that ANA was observed in 13% of children using the immunofluorescence technique. Although no differences in ANAs were noted by gender, an association of higher frequency of ANA titers ($\geq$1:80) was observed among children between 5 and 10 years of age. Of the 27 healthy children with positive ANAs, 8 were reevaluated 36 months later, and none of them developed any rheumatic diseases, although the sera remained positive in 2 of them. ANAs were present in 42 of 116 patients (36.2%), and the authors concluded that ANA determination should be required only in individuals with clinical signs and symptoms suggestive of autoimmune disease.[49]

Children with JIA also have positive ANAs. Several large-scale studies have observed ANAs in approximately 60% of patients with JIA, particularly oligoarticular disease in young girls with uveitis.[50,51] The following rates of ANA positivity and titers were noted among 153 children of Korean descent with JIA[52]: 1:40 dilution in 33% of patients, >1:40 in 70%, >1:80 in 2%, >1:160 in 16%, >1:320 in 2%, and >1:640 in 10%. ANA seropositivity was associated with female sex, negative HLA-B27, and a persistently elevated erythrocyte sedimentation rate (ESR) at follow-up.[52] Recently, Ravelli and colleagues[53] proposed that ANA-positive patients with JIA by current International League of Associations for Rheumatology (ILAR) criteria constituted a distinct yet homogeneous subgroup of patients characterized by younger age at disease onset, female preponderance, asymmetric arthritis, iridocyclitis, relatively fewer joints affected over time, and a lack of hip involvement, as compared with patients who were ANA-negative with JIA.[53] Another study that sought to describe the patterns and time course of arthritis in patients with ANA-positive JIA in 195 patients found that 72% (including most of those who later developed polyarthritis) had monoarthritis at disease onset.[54] Similar results were noted by Guillaume and associates in 2000.[55] Among patients with oligoarticular onset, polyarticular extension occurred in approximately 50% of patients within the first 3 to 4 years after disease onset and tended to be less likely thereafter.[54]

Vasculitis

Although polyarteritis nodosa (PAN) is relatively rare, it can be mistaken for SLE. In contrast to patients with SLE, those with PAN are usually men and include all age groups equally. A patient with SLE may develop PAN-like vasculitis of renal arteries.[56,57] Cutaneous vasculitis may be more prominent, as may eosinophilia, wheezing, and nerve and bowel symptoms. The ANAs are often negative. Hypersensitivity angiitis may mimic SLE at first but, ultimately, can be distinguished by a self-limited course, an absence of ANAs, and rarity of severe visceral involvement. Ordering antineutrophilic cytoplasmic antibody testing can often differentiate lupus from microscopic polyangiitis and Wegener granulomatosis.[58] One case of SLE in a child with Kawasaki disease has been reported.[59]

Behçet disease (BD) is a condition complicated by recurrent painful oral and genital ulcers, eye manifestations of uveitis, and complications and skin manifestations ranging from a positive pathergy test (rarer in the Western world and more common in Japan and around the Mediterranean) and erythema nodosum to other papulopustular lesions.[60] Some cases also are complicated by the occurrence of vasculitis of small and medium vessels, and venous thrombosis occasionally occurs, more often in men than in women. Arthropathy (seen in 16% to 84% of patients with SLE) is generally mild, mostly with arthralgias; when arthritis (often nonerosive and monoarticular) are the most frequent clinical features of the disease.[61] ANAs are frequently negative. Considering that SLE is a female-predominant disease with painless oral ulcers and positive ANAs in almost 99% of patients, the distinction is relatively easy to make; however, in the rare event that a confusion exists, HLA-B51 testing might help.[62] Among 4800 patients with BD and 16,289 controls from 78 independent studies,[62] the pooled odds ratio (OR) of HLA–B51/B5 allele carriers to develop BD compared with noncarriers was 5.78 (95% confidence interval [CI] of 5.00 to 6.67). The lack of any diagnostic test for BD further complicates the picture, and one case of co-existent disease has been reported.[63]

SLE is a disease of the small arteries and medium-sized arterioles, but it can rarely affect larger-caliber vessels. Large-vessel vasculitis is not associated with autoantibody formation. Older people more commonly develop polymyalgia rheumatica and giant-cell arteritis, however, and SLE is occasionally included in the differential diagnosis because musculoskeletal symptoms are present and age-related positive ANAs may be found.[64] A true concurrence of giant-cell arteritis and SLE has been reported twice.[65,66] Takayasu pulseless arteritis is found in young women who are mostly Japanese but also in other Asian and Hispanic women. Several people have reported case reports and case series of patients with either SLE or Takayasu arteritis that later developed the other disease[67-73]; however, co-existent SLE and Takayasu arteritis is rare.

Polymyositis and Dermatomyositis

In contrast to SLE, patients with polymyositis and dermatomyositis are less often women[74] and rarely have an autoimmune family history. In addition, dermatomyositis and polymyositis are easier to distinguish because they usually exhibit overt muscle weakness, mostly in middle-aged women, and evident elevations of muscle enzymes, with or without skin changes such as Gottron papules, heliotrope lid, shawl sign, periungual erythema, and cuticular thickening. Different co-existing malignancies may also occur; serositis is rare, and nephritis, liver inflammation, and hematologic abnormalities are absent. ANAs overall are observed in approximately 30% of patients with inflammatory myopathies.

A low-grade myositis with muscle enzyme levels two to three times normal may be seen in SLE that responds to low doses of corticosteroids; however, it may be as severe as inflammatory myositis.[74] Amyopathic dermatomyositis may be present with symptoms that closely resemble those of SLE, especially if the classical dermatomyositis rash is not present. Consider a female patient with fever, alopecia, oral ulcers, myalgias, arthritis, and a few macular erythematous plaques on her leg, and laboratory testing has confirmed lymphopenia and anemia but without overt muscle weakness. She would fulfill the ACR criteria for SLE; however, if an ANA test is negative, then diagnostic considerations would point toward another connective tissue disorder. In a review article by Gerami and associates[75] of 291 patients with adult-onset clinically amyopathic dermatomyositis, 63% of the patients had positive ANAs.

Scleroderma and Other Fibrosing Syndromes

Although ANAs are present in most patients with scleroderma, other serologies associated with SLE are observed in a small minority of those with scleroderma. These include antiphospholipid antibodies[76,77] and other nuclear antigens.[78] Anti-topoisomerase antibodies are usually associated with scleroderma but can be found in up to 7.7% of patients with SLE; however, the titers are higher in scleroderma.[79] Scleroderma and SLE fit within the same spectrum of interferon-mediated disease, and a subset of patients with scleroderma, as well as anti-topoisomerase and anti–U1 ribonucleoprotein (anti–U1-RNP) antibodies, show a lupus-like high interferon-inducible–gene expression pattern.[80]

In contrast to SLE, familial occurrence of scleroderma is rare. Clinically, sclerodactyly, telangiectasias, calcinosis, and malignant hypertension with acute renal failure are almost unheard of in patients with SLE. Differentiating SLE, MCTD, and scleroderma is important, because the last rarely is responsive to steroids or cytotoxic agents.

Case reports have appeared of autoimmune hemolytic anemia,[81,82] high levels of anti–native DNA (anti-nDNA), lupus nephritis,[83] and discoid lupus[84-86] occurring in patients with scleroderma. Patients with anti-scleroderma (anti-Scl) antibodies probably have lupus rather than scleroderma if anti–double stranded DNA (anti-dsDNA) is present.[87] Scleroderma may evolve into SLE and vice versa[88]; morphea[89] and linear scleroderma can be seen with SLE.[90] Neonatal SLE with morphea[91] and eosinophilic fasciitis with SLE have also been reported. Although digital ulcers are rarely seen in SLE, they may be the initial manifestation.[92] Similarly, patients with SLE may also develop calcinosis cutis,[93] although this condition is usually seen in scleroderma and myositis.

Retroperitoneal fibrosis in SLE has been noted,[94,95] although rarely. Nephrogenic fibrosing dermopathy is usually seen in patients with impaired renal function, and its occurrence has been reported in SLE.[96]

Serum Sickness

Serum sickness was initially described as a clinical syndrome characterized by fever, lymphadenopathy, cutaneous eruptions, and arthralgias often in association with proteinuria, but without other evidence of glomerulonephritis. Hence, one can see how the features of serum sickness can mimic SLE. Serum sickness has a self-limiting course unlike SLE, and the skin findings are most commonly described as a morbilliform eruption that tends to begin on the trunk as a patchy erythema before spreading to involve the extremities. ANAs are usually negative, as evidenced by the paper by Lawley and colleagues,[97] who studied the immunologic features of serum sickness in 12 patients and found none of the 9 patients who were tested for ANAs to be positive. C3 and C4 levels were both low in all patients, with C4 being significantly reduced, compared with C3.[97] Furthermore, glomerulonephritis is less likely, although patients with severe glomerular and tubular damage as a result of serum sickness have been reported.[98]

Kikuchi Disease

Kikuchi-Fujimoto disease (KFD) is a benign and usually self-limited form of histiocytic-necrotizing lymphadenitis first described by Kikuchi and others and usually affecting young adult women. Clinical features at presentation can include lymphadenopathy involving one or more predominantly posterior cervical lymph nodes and may be associated with fever, myalgias, arthralgias, weight loss, diarrhea, chills, sweating, and/or, less commonly, hepatosplenomegaly.[99,100] Associations with SLE have been reported,[100] and common features are fever, myalgias, and leukopenias. Reports of KFD evolving into SLE have also been reported.[101,102] The diagnosis of KFD is usually based on lymph node histologic findings; therefore obtaining a lymph node biopsy when lymphadenopathy is the dominant feature in a young woman is important. The clinical course of this disease is usually favorable, with spontaneous remission in less than 4 months in almost all patients.

Fibromyalgia

Patients with SLE not in frequently experience chronic fatigue,[103,104] and many symptoms are indistinguishable from fibromyalgia. The prevalence of secondary fibromyalgia in SLE is common and observed in approximately 22% of patients with SLE.[105-107] A study on the prevalence of fibromyalgia in three SLE groups—African Americans, Caucasians, and Hispanics—found a negative correlation with African American ethnicity.[108] Tender points, altered sleep patterns,

and a lack of restorative sleep with the absence of objective parameters of active disease—normal C3, C4, anti-dsDNA, and ESR—makes it difficult to differentiate secondary from primary fibromyalgia. Some of these symptoms may be a result of rapid tapering of steroids or emotional and/or physical stress.

Patients with primary fibromyalgia are commonly referred to the rheumatologist because of weakly positive ANAs. Patients may research these finding over the Internet and convince themselves that they have early SLE. Frequently when ANAs are positive, primary care physicians may also find making the correct diagnosis a challenge. ANAs can be seen in fibromyalgia in low titers; however, their presence is not a predictor of future development of connective tissue disease.[109]

Wolfe and colleagues[110] compared the various co-morbid conditions in RA, SLE, fibromyalgia, and noninflammatory rheumatic diseases (NIRDs) and found depression in 34% of patients with fibromyalgia and SLE. Self-reported diagnosis was a limitation to this study. The LUMINA study group[111] studied the effect of body mass index (BMI) on fibromyalgia in patients with SLE. Obesity and SLE have a component of inflammation with increased levels of tumor necrosis factor–alpha (TNF-α), interleukin (IL)-1 and C-reactive protein (CRP) in both conditions.[112,113] The association of increased BMI and fibromyalgia has been described[114] and was confirmed in this study, but obesity and fibromyalgia had no effect on organ damage accrual in SLE.[111] The association with fibromyalgia, however, results in increased symptoms with poor response to treatment.[111] Factors associated with the quality of life and fibromyalgia seem to have a greater influence on the severity of reported fatigue than the level of SLE disease activity.[115] Increased number of fibromyalgia tender points is also likely to correlate with poor health status.[116] These complaints may be erroneously interpreted as active SLE and treated inappropriately with increased steroids and immunosuppressive agents.

Sleep studies,[117] performed on patients with SLE who had fatigue and daytime sleepiness showed a pattern similar to that observed in fibromyalgia. Patients with disabling tiredness were found to have a poor quality of sleep. Some of these patients were depressed, but daytime sleepiness in SLE was not necessarily associated with depression. Patients with SLE with the worst depressive symptoms complained of tiredness but were not objectively sleepy.

Fatigue in SLE is multidimensional, and a depressed mood contributes to physical and mental tiredness. Physical fatigue has also been associated with poor aerobic capacity in SLE.[118] The treatment needs to be individualized in these patients. Optimizing pain control and managing SLE flares may take care of the physical fatigue, but the mental fatigue may require focusing on alleviating the depressed mood.[118]

Crystal-Induced Arthropathies

Although 29% of patients with SLE are hyperuricemic (usually secondary to nephritis, diuretics, or chemotherapy), clinical gout is rare, which could be the result of a predominance of menstruating women among those with active SLE.

Until 2000, fewer than 20 cases had been described in the literature[119-121]; most were men taking diuretic medications. Recently, however, two groups examined the clinical features of 15 and 10 patients with gout and SLE, respectively. Over 90% had nephritis, many had received transplants, some were taking diuretics and cyclosporine, and the lupus was almost always inactive.[122,123] Wallace and colleagues[124] reviewed the negative association between gout and RA. Only 3 of the 464 patients with idiopathic SLE had clinical gout, including a 25-year-old woman with nephritis who had tophaceous deposits. One report reviewed three young women with SLE and tophaceous deposits; all were underexcretors of uric acid.[120] It has been proposed that patients with SLE (who often have decreased synovial fluid complement levels) have a natural barrier to gout, because urates require the presence of near-normal synovial fluid complement levels to induce inflammation.[125] The rarity of pseudogout in patients with SLE has been reviewed by Rodriquez and colleagues.[126]

Dermatitis Herpetiformis

The association of dermatitis herpetiformis (DH) and SLE is rare but reported.[127] Thomas and Su[128] found nine patients with concomitant DH and SLE who were followed at the Mayo Clinic from 1950 to 1981 and reviewed the literature. Penneys and Wiley[129] reported four patients with SLE with lesions histologically resembling DH, but immunofluorescence testing, was typical of SLE in three of the four patients. Five other reports have appeared, the most important of which are those of Aronson and associates[130] and Davies and colleagues.[131]

Sarcoidosis

SLE and sarcoidosis share many immunologic features. Both manifest hyperglobulinemia, decreased skin test and lymphocyte responsiveness, lymphopenia, impaired antibody-dependent cellular cytotoxicity, and increased levels of CICs. Cryoglobulins and anti-lymphocyte antibodies may be present in both disorders, and up to 29% of patients with sarcoidosis may have positive ANAs.[132] In a retrospective study of 34 patients with sarcoidosis, 10 were ANA positive, and of these, two had dsDNA in addition.[132] SLE did not develop in these patients in the 10- to 15-year follow-up period. Differential diagnosis can be a problem,[133] but despite these similarities, co-existence is infrequent.[134-137]

Amyloid

Patients with SLE would be expected to have an increased incidence of amyloid, as do those with RA or ankylosing spondylitis. Cathcart and Scheinberg[138] enumerated many reasons why SLE and amyloid should co-exist. For example, the two have a common pathogenetic pathway, and polyclonal B-cell proliferation is observed in both. Benson and Cohen[139] found serum levels of amyloid protein A to be elevated in 25 patients of active SLE, although these were one half the levels observed in an RA group. This alpha-globulin is a precursor of the major protein constituent of secondary amyloid fibrils. The serum amyloid P component can also be deposited in lupus tissues without evidence of clinical amyloid[140] and may be protective against lupus.[141] Despite this, fewer than 20 patients with co-existing SLE and amyloidosis have been reported.[142-144] Primary cutaneous nodular amyloidosis has been reported to occur in a patient with SLE.[145]

Seronegative Spondyloarthropathies and Psoriasis

Nashel and associates[146] estimated that 500 concurrent cases of ankylosing spondylitis (AS) and SLE should be present in the United States, but this figure does not take into account the differences in catchment groups (AS—male Caucasians; SLE—women, especially non-Caucasians). They presented the first true case of co-existence and reviewed three cases reported earlier. None of these met both AS and SLE criteria, but few have appeared since.[147,148] Difficulty in determining a differential diagnosis may arise because patients with SLE may exhibit sacroiliitis[149] by bone scan and be HLA-B27 positive. DIL-like illness from the use of anti-TNF treatment in AS has been noted.[150] Only one case of SLE and reactive arthritis and one case of discoid lupus in AS have been reported.[151,152]

Several reviews have drawn attention to the co-existence of psoriasis and SLE.[153-157] A 1980 report presented 23 cases of co-existence at the Mayo Clinic (10 met the ACR criteria for SLE, and 13 were DLE) between 1950 and 1975 and reviewed 15 reports of 33 patients (11 of whom antedated 1960).[155] Of these, 63% were women, SLE and psoriasis each appeared first one half of the time, and 80% had discoid lesions that were usually distinct from psoriatic patches (appearing and disappearing independently), but 7 of 27 biopsied lesions had pathologic features of both disorders. Discoid lupus erythematosus (DLE) can be misdiagnosed as psoriasis,[158] may flare with ultraviolet B or psoralen and ultraviolet A (PUVA) therapy,[153,154] and subacute cutaneous lupus erythematosus (SCLE) can be induced

Box 44-2 Disease Associations

Raynaud phenomenon
HELLP syndrome (hemolysis, elevated liver enzymes, low platelet count)
Primary biliary cirrhosis
Multiple sclerosis
Myasthenia gravis
Thyroiditis
Inflammatory bowel disease
Syphilis
Down syndrome
Klinefelter syndrome
Sickle cell anemia
Autoimmune hemolytic anemia
Thrombocytopenic purpura
Sjögren syndrome
Pemphigus
Chronic active hepatitis
Lysinuric protein intolerance
Moyamoya disease
Hunter syndrome
Osler-Weber-Rendu disease
Amyotrophic lateral sclerosis
Fabry disease
Werner syndrome
Noonan syndrome
Wilson disease
Hermansky-Pudlak syndrome
Osteopoikilosis
Stiff person syndrome
Hemophilia A
Rosai-Dorfman disease
Autoimmune neuromyotonia
Multicentric reticulohistiocytosis

during PUVA treatments in patients who are positive for Sjögren syndrome antigen A (SSA/Ro).[156,157] Despite the not uncommon concurrence of DLE and psoriasis, only one case of psoriatic arthritis and SLE has been reported, and no HLA studies were cited in any of these reports.[158]

ASSOCIATION OF SYSTEMIC LUPUS ERYTHEMATOSUS WITH OTHER DISORDERS

Several disorders have increased or decreased associations with SLE, and others can mimic its presentation and must be considered in the differential diagnosis (Box 44-2). The relationship among Raynaud phenomenon, HELLP (hemolysis, elevated liver enzymes, low-platelet count) syndrome, biliary cirrhosis, multiple sclerosis, myasthenia gravis, thyroiditis, inflammatory bowel disease, syphilis, Klinefelter syndrome, sickle cell anemia, autoimmune hemolytic anemia, Sjögren syndrome, thrombocytopenic purpura, pemphigus, chronic active hepatitis, and SLE are discussed in other chapters. Additional associations and differential diagnostic considerations are reviewed here. The reader is referred to an excellent discussion by Lorber and associates[159] regarding the rationale for such associations.

Porphyria

Both porphyria and SLE are characterized by fever, rash, sun sensitivity, leukopenia, anemia, arthralgias, and central nervous system abnormalities. Two comprehensive evaluations of 55 and 158 patients with porphyria cutanea tarda[160,161] found that none met the ACR criteria for SLE, although 12 were ANA positive. In one review of 38 patients with porphyria,[162] 8 of 15 patients with acute intermittent porphyria were ANA positive and 1 patient had SLE. Filotou and colleagues[163] reviewed 9 patients with acute intermittent porphyria in the literature, of whom 8 had preexisting SLE. In the study by Gibson and McEvoy,[164] 15 of 676 patients with porphyria had concurrent lupus; 9 had DLE, 5 had SLE, and 1 had SCLE. Porphyria was precipitated by hydroxychloroquine therapy in 2 patients. The ability of chloroquine to induce cutaneous porphyria further complicates the differential diagnosis.

Angioimmunoblastic Lymphadenopathy with Dysproteinemia and Autoimmune Lymphoproliferative Syndrome

Angioimmunoblastic lymphadenopathy with dysproteinemia (AILD) is a hyperimmune state that exhibits a rash, polyclonal gammopathy, Coombs-positive hemolytic anemia, hepatosplenomegaly, anergy, and decreased T-cell suppressor levels. It is fatal within months without treatment. AILD can resemble SLE[165-169] in that sicca syndrome, symmetric peripheral polyarthritis, and positive serologies can be observed.[170,171] In their literature review, Rosenstein and associates[169] discussed several patients who followed the pattern of having an established autoimmune disease terminate with AILD, and they speculated that it represents a malignant transformation of immune-mediated disorders. Patients with autoimmune lymphoproliferative syndrome (ALS), characterized by a defect of the Fas-mediated apoptosis pathway, are usually children. Most have antinuclear and antiphospholipid antibodies.[172,173]

Carcinoma

The occurrence of malignancies in those with SLE is discussed in Chapter 57. The initial presentation of a patient with elevated body temperatures, weight loss, adenopathy, and joint pains requires consideration of autoimmune and malignant disorders. Renal cell carcinomas can exhibit necrotizing vasculitis, Raynaud phenomenon, cryoglobulinemia, positive ANAs, false-positive syphilis serologies, and elevated levels of CICs.[174-176] Resection of the tumor usually reverses these findings. Mycosis fungoides can mimic chronic cutaneous lupus.[177] A case of a woman with breast carcinoma and post-radiation pneumonitis and serositis with a positive ANA test and SLE-cell preparation that disappeared after corticosteroid therapy has also been reported. Other malignancies are associated with ANAs.[178] ANAs were detected in 27.7% of 274 Spanish patients with malignancies but in only 6.4% of healthy subjects.[179] Paraneoplastic rheumatic symptoms were observed more often in those who were ANA positive. For example, 31% of 204 patients with hepatocellular carcinoma had a positive ANA test.[176] Patients with immunoblastic sarcoma,[178] lymphoma,[180-183] Burkitt lymphoma,[184] hairy cell leukemia,[185] ovarian carcinoma,[186] adrenal adenoma,[187] myelodysplastic syndromes,[188,189] and Meigs syndrome[190] were thought to have SLE on initial presentation.

Tumor-associated antigen cold antibody (CA) 19-9, which is a fairly specific marker for gastrointestinal adenocarcinomas, was positive in 6 of 19 patients with SLE in one report,[191] and tumor-associated antigen CA 125 was present in active SLE in another study.[192]

Infectious Diseases

The association of SLE and infections is well known. Infections may trigger the development of SLE or SLE flares; however, it is interesting to note that SLE may reduce the susceptibility to malaria.[193] The propensity of patients with SLE to develop infections and specific infectious associations with the disease are discussed in detail in Chapter 45. Problems relating to the differential diagnoses are presented here.

Viral Infections

Viral infections may display overlapping features with those of SLE on the initial presentation; these features include fever, arthralgias, rashes, and intense fatigue. Molecular mimicry, especially between Sm or SSA/Ro autoantigens and Epstein-Barr virus (EBV) nuclear antigen 1 response, as well as the over-expression of type 1 interferon

genes, is among the major contributors to SLE development.[194] In a study of 88 patients with SLE and acute viral infections, 25 of 88 patients were diagnosed with new-onset SLE associated with parvovirus B19 (n = 15), cytomegalovirus (n = 6), EBV (n = 3), and hepatitis A (n = 1).[195] Viral infections in the remaining 63 patients occurred in those with well-established SLE, 18 of whom exhibited symptoms similar to SLE. Park and associates[196] studied 230 recently diagnosed patients with SLE and 276 control subjects for antibodies to EBV capsid antigen and cytotoxic T-lymphocyte antigen 4 (CTLA-4) genotypes. They found EBV immunoglobulin A (IgA) seroprevalence among African Americans to be strongly associated with SLE (OR 5.6), and higher EBV IgG absorbance ratios were observed in patients with SLE with a significant dose response across the units of the international standardized ratio in African Americans. Allelic variations in the CTLA-4 gene promoter significantly modified the association between SLE and EBV.

The chronicity of certain viral infections, such as EBV, herpes virus cytomegalovirus, and viral hepatitis in young women, as well as the tendency of patients with SLE to develop infections, makes differentiation between the two scenarios complex.[197,198] Infections with these viruses can induce a low-titer ANA, aCL antibody, RF, anti-DNA antibodies, and cryoglobulin, among others.[199,200] Similarly, SLE may be associated with immunoglobulin M (IgM) antiviral antibodies.[201-203] Increased antibody titers to EBV capsid antigen, early antigen, and nuclear antigen, as well as polymerase chain reaction (PCR) compared with those of the controls, have been noted in patients with SLE,[204-207] and false-positive Monospot test results have been reported.[208] It has been suggested that EBV can induce SLE[209] and that nearly all patients with SLE had seroconverted. Nearly all adults with SLE (195 of 196 patients) in one study had been exposed to EBV.[210] CD8+ T cells may defectively regulate viral loads in SLE.[211] Fevers, fatigue, adenopathy, and leukopenia can represent EBV or SLE or both, especially in adolescents.[212] Surveys have shown that 5% to 69% of patients with SLE are reactive to cytomegalovirus antibodies representing viral induction or activation of SLE, simultaneous disease, or an immunosuppressive-mediated viral illness.[209,213-215] The high prevalence of varicella zoster in SLE is probably associated with reduced CD4 T-cell responses to the virus.[216] A study of 44 patients with parvovirus B19 infection demonstrated an association with a transient, subclinical autoimmune state, complete with the expression of anti-nDNA and antilymphocyte antibodies in most patients.[217] This association can be confused with SLE or may co-exist with or flare it.[218-221] The measles virus genome, along with elevated antibody titers, has been found in patients with lupus nephritis.[222]

The presentation of human immunodeficiency viral (HIV) infection can mimic that of autoimmune phenomena.[223,224] Fevers, lymphadenopathy, rash, renal dysfunction, neurologic and hematologic disorders, sicca syndrome, and arthralgias can be observed in both and delay appropriate treatment.[225] HIV positivity is associated with the presence of the lupus-circulating anticoagulant (although thrombosis does not occur), hemolytic anemia, ANAs, RF, CICs, immune thrombocytopenia, polyclonal hyperglobulinemia, and leukopenia. Anti–Sjögren syndrome antigen A (anti-SSA/Ro) and anti–Sjögren syndrome antigen B (anti-SSB/La) are not seen.[226-230]

Barthels and Wallace[231] discussed two cases, reviewed the literature, and presented an algorithm for following patients with SLE and false-positive results of acquired immunodeficiency syndrome (AIDS) testing. Approximately 40 cases of concurrent AIDS and SLE have been presented.[224,232-236] Before 2002, 30 cases were reported and reviewed by Palacios and colleagues[237] and Daikh and colleagues;[238] only 18 fulfilled the ACR criteria for SLE. Interestingly, approximately one-half were African American male children with nephritis (especially with congenital AIDS). Aggressive antiretroviral therapy can re-activate lupus,[239,240] whereas cyclophosphamide can reactivate HIV.[241] Kaye[242] hypothesized that SLE may somehow be protective of AIDS. In a retrospective study of 888 inpatients with HIV, SLE was reported in only 3.[243] Assuming that 500,000 Americans have SLE and that 150,000 have AIDS, at least 400 concurrent cases would be expected. This negative correlation becomes more impressive when one considers that if 10% of patients with SLE had autoimmune hemolytic anemia or other complications that required transfusions (e.g., uremia, surgery) between 1978 and 1983 when the U.S. blood supply was unsafe, then up to 50,000 individuals should have been at risk of becoming infected with HIV[242]; however, not a single report has stated that any person converted to HIV seropositivity.[244] Work by Scherl and associates[245] using sera from 88 patients who were HIV negative but had SLE and other autoimmune disorders reported that HIV-1 was directly recognized by 60% of sera from patients with autoimmune disorders. Reduction in viral loads by patient sera correlated with their reactivity in Western blot analysis, suggesting a possible protective role of autoantibodies against HIV infection in patients with SLE. Interestingly, many patients with HIV infections have antibodies to ribonucleoprotein (RNP). It has been suggested that immunization with anti-U1–small nuclear RNP (snRNP) can potentially block HIV infectivity.[246,247] High interleukin (IL)–16 levels associated with SLE also might be protective.[248]

Approximately 10% to 20% of patients with SLE will have indeterminate reactivity patterns against various glycoproteins that are associated with HIV-1, human T-cell lymphotropic virus (HTLV)-1, and HTLV-2.[249-256] Occasional reports of concurrent disease have appeared;[257-261] and in such cases lupus activity may be suppressed in the HIV patient.[262]

Bacterial Infections

Tuberculosis and SLE have overlapping chest and central nervous system features, as well as symptoms of fever, malaise, and weight loss.[263] Feng and Tan[264] found concurrent tuberculosis in 16 of 311 patients with SLE (5%) who were seen in Singapore between 1963 and 1979. Tam and others[265] reported 11% of 526 patients had tuberculosis in a Hong Kong study, and 3.6% of 556 patients of Turkish descent were reported to have co-existent tuberculosis.[266] Previous pleural injury (pleuritis) (not immunosuppressives or steroids) was found to be a risk factor for developing pulmonary tuberculosis ($n = 20$) in 1283 patients with SLE.[267] In another study, co-existence of tuberculosis correlated with steroid dosing and renal involvement and was frequently extrapulmonary.[268] Isoniazid prophylaxis is safe and effective.[268,269]

Salmonella infection can occur in patients with SLE.[270] Four patients with SLE with active disease were diagnosed with salmonellosis, but the diagnosis was delayed as a result of the similarity in symptoms with active SLE. In three of the four patients, salmonella infection localized to a site of clinical SLE involvement.[270]

Leprosy rarely occurs in association with SLE,[271-273] but the presence of deforming arthritis, alopecia, rash, and neuropathy in both conditions can make the differential diagnosis challenging. A positive ANA test or RF is found in 3% to 36% of leprosy cohorts, but other antibody systems are absent.[274-277] Mackworth-Young and colleagues[278] have found a common idiotypic determinant that is shared by patients with SLE and lepromatous leprosy.

Parasites

Additionally, a variety of infections (e.g., toxoplasmosis, schistosomiasis, leishmaniasis) can exhibit symptoms of SLE with autoantibodies.[279-282] *Strongyloides* infection may mimic abdominal vasculitis and diffuse alveolar hemorrhage, which are presentations usually associated with SLE activity.[283]

Miscellaneous Disorders

Glomerulonephritis, hypocomplementemia, and circulating immune complexes, such as those observed in SLE, may be also seen in a recently recognized condition—IgG4-related disease. However, SLE-specific autologous antibodies are not seen in IgG4-related diseases.[284] Kobayashi and colleagues[285] reported the first case of SLE with IgG4-related autoimmune pancreatitis. Familial Mediterranean fever and SLE have similar manifestations with fever and serositis

and may pose a diagnostic dilemma. The co-existence of familial Mediterranean fever and SLE has also been reported in two cases.[286] Skin lesions of chronic granulomatous disease can mimic those of DLE[287-292] and co-exist with SLE.[293,294] Thallium poisoning can result in ANA formation and mimic SLE.[295,296] Down syndrome is associated with an inflammatory arthropathy that sometimes resembles SLE[297-300] and can co-exist with it. Two cases of lysinuric protein intolerance,[301,302] moyamoya disease,[303,304] and prolidase deficiency[305] with SLE have been reported. Concurrent cystinosis and SLE have been reported; however, it is not clear whether the disease was DIL from cysteamine[306] treatment. Patients with Hunter syndrome,[307] Osler-Weber-Rendu disease,[308] amyotrophic lateral sclerosis,[309] Fabry disease,[310] Werner syndrome,[311] Noonan syndrome, Wilson disease, Hermansky-Pudlak syndrome, osteopoikilosis, stiff person syndrome, hemophilia A, Rosai-Dorfman disease, autoimmune neuromyotonia, multicentric reticulohistiocytosis,[312-322] and sickle cell disease[323] with SLE have been described.

KEY POINTS

- Diagnosis of SLE is mainly clinical.
- ANA test is 95% to 100% sensitive but should be ordered only if the pretest probability of SLE is high.
- If SLE is strongly suspected, but the ANA test is negative, then the laboratory should be contacted to determine which assay method was used; immunofluorescence assays are more specific than ELISA.
- ACR classification is useful, but 4 of the 11 criteria need not always be present.
- Appropriate differential diagnoses should be considered before the SLE diagnosis is made.

References

1. Kavanaugh A, Tomar R, Reveille J, et al: Guidelines for clinical use of the antinuclear antibody test and tests for specific autoantibodies to nuclear antigens. *Arch Pathol Lab Med* 124(1):71–81, 2000.
2. Solomon DH, Kavanaugh AJ, Schur PH, American College of Rheumatology Ad Hoc Committee on Immunologic Testing Guidelines: Evidence-based guidelines for the use of immunologic tests: antinuclear antibody testing. *Arthritis Rheum* 47(4):434–444, 2002.
3. McDonagh JE, Isenberg DA: Development of additional autoimmune diseases in a population of patients with systemic lupus erythematosus. *Ann Rheum Dis* 59(3):230–232, 2000.
4. Mosca M, Neri R, Bencivelli W, et al: Undifferentiated connective tissue disease: analysis of 83 patients with a minimum followup of 5 years. *J Rheumatol* 29(11):2345–2349, 2002.
5. Hochberg MC, Perlmutter DL, Medsger TA, et al: Prevalence of self-reported physician-diagnosed systemic lupus erythematosus in the USA. *Lupus* 4(6):454–456, 1995.
6. Calvo-Alén J, Bastian HM, Straaton KV, et al: Identification of patient subsets among those presumptively diagnosed with, referred, and/or followed up for systemic lupus erythematosus at a large tertiary care center. *Arthritis Rheum* 38(10):1475–1484, 1995.
7. Narain S, Richards HB, Satoh M, et al: Diagnostic accuracy for lupus and other systemic autoimmune diseases in the community setting. *Arch Intern Med* 164(22):2435–2441, 2004.
8. Kavanaugh AF, Solomon DH, American College of Rheumatology Ad Hoc Committee on Immunologic Testing Guidelines: Guidelines for immunologic laboratory testing in the rheumatic diseases: anti-DNA antibody tests. *Arthritis Rheum* 47(5):546–555, 2002.
9. Meroni PL, Schur PH: ANA screening: an old test with new recommendations. *Ann Rheum Dis* 69(8):1420–1422, 2010.
10. Alarcón GS, McGwin G, Jr, Roseman JM, et al: Systemic lupus erythematosus in three ethnic groups. XIX. Natural history of the accrual of the American College of Rheumatology criteria prior to the occurrence of criteria diagnosis. *Arthritis Rheum* 51(4):609–615, 2004.
11. Heinlen LD, McClain MT, Merrill J, et al: Clinical criteria for systemic lupus erythematosus precede diagnosis, and associated autoantibodies are present before clinical symptoms. *Arthritis Rheum* 56(7):2344–2351, 2007.
12. Wallace DJ, Podell T, Weiner J, et al: Systemic lupus erythematosus—survival patterns. Experience with 609 patients. *JAMA* 245:934–938, 1981.

13. Wallace DJ, Podell TE, Weiner JM, et al: Lupus nephritis. Experience with 230 patients in a private practice from 1950 to 1980. *Am J Med* 72:209–220, 1982.

14. Gianviti A, Barsotti P, Barbera V, et al: Delayed onset of systemic lupus erythematosus in patients with "full-house" nephropathy. *Pediatr Nephrol* 13(8):683–687, 1999.

15. Cairns SA, Acheson EJ, Corbett CL, et al: The delayed appearance of an antinuclear factor and the diagnosis of systemic lupus erythematosus in glomerulonephritis. *Postgrad Med J* 55(648):723–727, 1979.

16. Persellin RH, Takeuchi A: Antinuclear antibody-negative systemic lupus erythematosus: loss in body fluids. *J Rheumatol* 7:547–550, 1980.

17. Ferreiro JE, Reiter WM, Saldana MJ: Systemic lupus erythematosus presenting as chronic serositis with no demonstrable antinuclear antibodies. *Am J Med* 76(6):1100–1105, 1984.

18. Koller SR, Johnston, CL, Jr, Moncure CW: Lupus erythematosus cell preparation-antinuclear factor incongruity. A review of diagnostic tests for systemic lupus erythematosus. *Am J Clin Pathol* 66(3):495–505, 1976.

19. Maddison PJ, Provost TT, Reichlin M: Serological findings in patients with "ANA-negative" systemic lupus erythematosus. *Medicine (Baltimore)* 60(2):87–94, 1981.

20. Cross LS, Aslam A, Misbah SA: Antinuclear antibody-negative lupus as a distinct diagnostic entity—does it no longer exist? *QJM* 97(5):303–308, 2004.

21. Reichlin M: Diagnostic criteria and serology. In Schur PH, editor: *Clinical management of systemic lupus erythematosus*, New York, 1983, Grune & Stratton.

22. Hanly JG, Thompson K, McCurdy G, et al: Measurement of autoantibodies using multiplex methodology in patients with systemic lupus erythematosus. *J Immunol Methods* 352(1-2):147–152, 2010.

23. Williams HJ, Alarcon GS, Joks R, et al: Early undifferentiated connective tissue disease (CTD). VI. An inception cohort after 10 years: disease remissions and changes in diagnoses in well established and undifferentiated CTD. *J Rheumatol* 26(4):816–825, 1999.

24. Bodolay E, Csiki Z, Szekanecz Z, et al: Five-year follow-up of 665 Hungarian patients with undifferentiated connective tissue disease (UCTD). *Clin Exp Rheumatol* 21(3):313–320, 2003.

25. Vaz CC, Couto M, Medeiros D, et al: Undifferentiated connective tissue disease: a seven-center cross-sectional study of 184 patients. *Clin Rheumatol* 28(8):915–921, 2009.

26. Ståhl HC, Nived O, Sturfelt G: Outcome of incomplete systemic lupus erythematosus after 10 years. *Lupus* 13(2):85–88, 2004.

27. Swaak AJG, van de Brink H, Smeenk RJT, et al: Incomplete lupus erythematosus: results of a multicentre study under the supervision of the EULAR Standing Committee on International Clinical Studies Including Therapeutic Trials (ESCISIT). *Rheumatology (Oxford)* 40(1):89–94, 2001.

28. Laustrup H, Voss A, Green A, et al: SLE disease patterns in a Danish population-based lupus cohort: an 8-year prospective study. *Lupus* 19(3):239–246, 2010.

29. Turesson C, O'Fallon WM, Crowson CS, et al: Extra-articular disease manifestations in rheumatoid arthritis: incidence trends and risk factors over 46 years. *Ann Rheum Dis* 62(8):722–727, 2003.

30. Denko CW, Zumpft CW: Chronic arthritis with splenomegaly and leukopenia. *Arthritis Rheum* 5:478–491, 1962.

31. Goldberg J, Pinals RS: Felty syndrome. *Semin Arthritis Rheum* 10(1):52–65, 1980.

32. Ruderman M, Miller LM, Pinals RS: Clinical and serologic observations on 27 patients with Felty's syndrome. *Arthritis Rheum* 11(3):377–384, 1968.

33. Weisman M, Zvaifler NJ: Cryoimmunoglobulinemia in Felty's syndrome. *Arthritis Rheum* 19(1):103–110, 1976.

34. Ropes MW: *Systemic lupus erythematosus*, Cambridge, MA, 1976, Harvard University Press.

35. Davis JA, Cohen AH, Weisbart R, et al: Glomerulonephritis in rheumatoid arthritis. *Arthritis Rheum* 22(9):1018–1023, 1979.

36. Feldman D, Feldman D, Ginzler E, et al: Rheumatoid factor in patients with systemic lupus erythematosus. *J Rheumatol* 16(5):618–622, 1989.

37. Ippolito A, Wallace DJ, Gladman D, et al: Autoantibodies in systemic lupus erythematosus: comparison of historical and current assessment of seropositivity. *Lupus* 20(3):250–255, 2011.

38. Zhao Y, Li J, Li XX, et al: What can we learn from the presence of anti-cyclic citrullinated peptide antibodies in systemic lupus erythematosus? *Joint Bone Spine* 76(5):501–507, 2009.

39. Chan MT, Owen P, Dunphy J, et al: Associations of erosive arthritis with anti-cyclic citrullinated peptide antibodies and MHC Class II alleles in systemic lupus erythematosus. *J Rheumatol* 35(1):77–83, 2008.

40. Mediwake R, Isenberg DA, Schellekens GA, et al: Use of anti-citrullinated peptide and anti-RA33 antibodies in distinguishing erosive arthritis in patients with systemic lupus erythematosus and rheumatoid arthritis. *Ann Rheum Dis* 60(1):67–68, 2001.

41. Cervera R, Khamashta MA, Hughes GR: The Euro-lupus project: epidemiology of systemic lupus erythematosus in Europe. *Lupus* 18(10):869–874, 2009.

42. Icen M, Nicola PJ, Maradit-Kremers H, et al: Systemic lupus erythematosus features in rheumatoid arthritis and their effect on overall mortality. *J Rheumatol* 36(1):50–57, 2009.

43. Amezcua-Guerra LM, Springall R, Marquez-Velasco R, et al: Presence of antibodies against cyclic citrullinated peptides in patients with "rhupus": a cross-sectional study. *Arthritis Res Ther* 8(5):R144, 2006.

44. Cohen MG, Webb J: Concurrence of rheumatoid arthritis and systemic lupus erythematosus: report of 11 cases. *Ann Rheum Dis* 46(11):853–858, 1987.

45. Brand CA, Rowley MJ, Tait BD, et al: Coexistent rheumatoid arthritis and systemic lupus erythematosus: clinical, serological, and phenotypic features. *Ann Rheum Dis* 51(2):173–176, 1992.

46. Simón JA, Granados J, Cabíedes J, et al: Clinical and immunogenetic characterization of Mexican patients with "rhupus." *Lupus* 11(5):287–292, 2002.

47. Panush RS, Edwards NL, Longley S, et al: "Rhupus" syndrome. *Arch Intern Med* 148(7):1633–1636, 1988.

48. Damián-Abrego GN, Cabiedes J, Cabral AR: Anti-citrullinated peptide antibodies in lupus patients with or without deforming arthropathy. *Lupus* 17(4):300–304, 2008.

49. Hilário MO, Len CA, Roja SC, et al: Frequency of antinuclear antibodies in healthy children and adolescents. *Clin Pediatr* 43(7):637–642, 2004.

50. Cassidy JT, Levinson JE, Bass JC, et al: A study of classification criteria for a diagnosis of juvenile rheumatoid arthritis. *Arthritis Rheum* 29(2):274–281, 1986.

51. Chudwin DS, Ammann AJ, Cowan MJ, et al: Significance of a positive antinuclear antibody test in a pediatric population. *Am J Dis Child* 137(11):1103–1106, 1983.

52. Shin JI, Kim KH, Chun JK, et al: Prevalence and patterns of anti-nuclear antibodies in Korean children with juvenile idiopathic arthritis according to ILAR criteria. *Scand J Rheumatol* 37(5):348–351, 2008.

53. Ravelli A, Varnier GC, Oliveira S, et al: Antinuclear antibody-positive patients should be grouped as a separate category in the classification of juvenile idiopathic arthritis. *Arthritis Rheum* 63(1):267–275, 2011.

54. Felici E, Novarini C, Magni-Manzoni S, et al: Course of joint disease in patients with antinuclear antibody-positive juvenile idiopathic arthritis. *J Rheumatol* 32(9):1805–1810, 2005.

55. Guillaume S, Prieur AM, Coste J, et al: Long-term outcome and prognosis in oligoarticular-onset juvenile idiopathic arthritis. *Arthritis Rheum* 43(8):1858–1865, 2000.

56. Melamed N, Molad Y: Spontaneous retroperitoneal bleeding from renal microaneurysms and pancreatic pseudocyst in a patient with systemic lupus erythematosus. *Scand J Rheumatol* 35(6):481–484, 2006.

57. Vivancos J, Soler-Carrillo J, Ara-del Rey J, et al: Development of polyarteritis nodosa in the course of inactive systemic lupus erythematosus. *Lupus* 4(6):494–495, 1995.

58. Ben Chetrit E, Rahav G: Saved by a test result. *N Engl J Med* 330(5):343–346, 1994.

59. Lawson JP: The joint manifestations of the connective tissue diseases. *Semin Roentgenol* 17(1):25–38, 1982.

60. Alpsoy E, Zouboulis CC, Ehrlich GE: Mucocutaneous lesions of Behçet disease. *Yonsei Med J* 48(4):573–585, 2007.

61. Davatchi F, Shahram F, Chams-Davatchi C, et al: Behçet disease in Iran: analysis of 6500 cases. *Int J Rheum Dis* 13(4):367–373, 2010.

62. de Menthon M, Lavalley MP, Maldini C, et al: HLA-B51/B5 and the risk of Behçet's disease: a systematic review and meta-analysis of case-control genetic association studies. *Arthritis Rheum* 61(10):1287–1296, 2009.

63. Lee WS, Kim SJ, Ahn SK: Behçet's disease as a part of the symptom complex of SLE? *J Dermatol* 23(3):196–199, 1996.

64. Maragou M, Siotsiou F, Sfondouris H, et al: Late-onset systemic lupus erythematosus presenting as polymyalgia rheumatica. *Clin Rheumatol* 8(1):91–97, 1989.

65. Bunker CB, Dowd PM: Giant cell arteritis and systemic lupus erythematosus. *Br J Dermatol* 119(1):115–120, 1988.

66. Scharre D, Petri M, Engman E, et al: Large intracranial arteritis with giant cells in systemic lupus erythematosus. *Ann Intern Med* 104(5):661–662, 1986.

67. Sachetto Z, Fernandes SR, Del Rio AP, et al: Systemic lupus erythematosus associated with vasculitic syndrome (Takayasu's arteritis). *Rheumatol Int* 30(12):1669–1672, 2010.

68. Kitazawa K, Joh K, Akizawa T: A case of lupus nephritis coexisting with podocytic infolding associated with Takayasu's arteritis. *Clin Exp Nephrol* 12(6):462–466, 2008.

69. Sano N, Kitazawa K, Totsuka D, et al: A case of lupus nephritis with alteration of the glomerular basement membrane associated with Takayasu's arteritis. *Clin Nephrol* 58(2):161–165, 2002.

70. Kameyama K, Kuramochi S, Ueda T, et al: Takayasu's aortitis with dissection in systemic lupus erythematosus. *Scand J Rheumatol* 28(3):187–188, 1999.

71. Saxe PA, Altman RD: Takayasu's arteritis syndrome associated with systemic lupus erythematosus. *Semin Arthritis Rheum* 21(5):295–305, 1992.

72. Saxe PA, Altman RD: Aortitis syndrome (Takayasu's arteritis) associated with SLE. *J Rheumatol* 17(9):1251–1252, 1990.

73. Igarashi T, Nagaoka S, Matsunaga K, et al: Aortitis syndrome (Takayasu's arteritis) associated with systemic lupus erythematosus. *J Rheumatol* 16(12):1579–1583, 1989.

74. Garton MJ, Isenberg DA: Clinical features of lupus myositis versus idiopathic myositis: a review of 30 cases. *Br J Rheumatol* 36(10):1067–1074, 1997.

75. Gerami P, Schope JM, McDonald L, et al: A systematic review of adult-onset clinically amyopathic dermatomyositis (dermatomyositis siné myositis): a missing link within the spectrum of the idiopathic inflammatory myopathies. *J Am Acad Dermatol* 54(4):597–613, 2006.

76. Seibold JR, Buckingham RB, Medsger TA, Jr, et al: Cerebrospinal fluid immune complexes in systemic lupus involving the central nervous system. *Semin Arthritis Rheum* 12:68–76, 1982.

77. Rowell NR, Tate GM: The lupus anticoagulant in systemic lupus erythematosus and systemic sclerosis. *Br J Dermatol* 117(32 S):13–14, 1987.

78. Bennett RM: Scleroderma overlap syndromes. *Rheum Dis Clin North Am* 16(1):185–198, 1990.

79. Mahler M, Silverman ED, Schulte-Pelkum J, et al: Anti-Scl-70 (topo-I) antibodies in SLE: myth or reality? *Autoimmun Rev* 9(11):756–760, 2010.

80. Assassi S, Mayes MD, Arnett FC, et al: Systemic sclerosis and lupus: points in an interferon-mediated continuum. *Arthritis Rheum* 62(2):589–598, 2010.

81. Ivey KJ, Hwang YF, Sheets RF: Scleroderma associated with thrombocytopenia and Coombs-positive hemolytic anemia. *Am J Med* 51(6):815–817, 1971.

82. Rosenthal DS, Sack B: Autoimmune hemolytic anemia in scleroderma. *JAMA* 216(12):2011–2012, 1971.

83. Kondo S, Tone M, Teramoto N, et al: [Clinical studies of 15 cases of progressive systemic sclerosis (PSS) associated with positive proteinuria and membranous glomerulonephritis]. [Japanese]. *Nihon Hifuka Gakkai Zasshi* 99(10):1105–1110, 1989.

84. Foster CS: Systemic lupus erythematosus, discoid lupus erythematosus, and progressive systemic sclerosis. *Int Ophthalmol Clin* 37(2):93–110, 1997.

85. Sasaki T, Nakajima H: Systemic sclerosis (scleroderma) associated with discoid lupus erythematosus. *Dermatology* 187(3):178–181, 1993.

86. Hayakawa K, Nagashima M: Systemic sclerosis associated with disseminated discoid lupus erythematosus. *Int J Dermatol* 32(6):440–441, 1993.

87. Warner NZ, Greidinger EL: Patients with antibodies to both PmScl and dsDNA. *J Rheumatol* 31(11):2169–2174, 2004.

88. Roddi R, Riggio E, Gilbert PM, et al: Progressive hemifacial atrophy in a patient with lupus erythematosus. *Plast Reconstr Surg* 93(5):1067–1072, 1994.

89. Ko JY, Kim YS, Lee CW: Multifocal lesions of morphoea in a patient with systemic lupus erythematosus. *Clin Exp Dermatol* 34(8):e676–e679, 2009.

90. Mackel SE, Kozin F, Ryan LM, et al: Concurrent linear scleroderma and systemic lupus erythematosus: a report of two cases. *J Invest Dermatol* 73(5):368–372, 1979.

91. Ohtaki N, Miyamoto C, Orita M, et al: Concurrent multiple morphea and neonatal lupus erythematosus in an infant boy born to a mother with SLE. *Br J Dermatol* 115(1):85–90, 1986.

92. Rosato E, Molinaro I, Pisarri S, et al: Digital ulcers as an initial manifestation of systemic lupus erythematosus. *Intern Med* 50(7):767–769, 2011.

93. Kim MS, Choi KC, Kim HS, et al: Calcinosis cutis in systemic lupus erythematosus: a case report and review of the published work. *J Dermatol* 37(9):815–818, 2010.

94. Granata A, Stella M, Santoro D, et al: [Acute renal failure secondary to retroperitoneal fibrosis as first manifestation of lupus nephritis]. [Italian]. *G Ital Nefrol* 23(1):86–89, 2006.

95. Lichon FS, Sequeira W, Pilloff A, et al: Retroperitoneal fibrosis associated with systemic lupus erythematosus: a case report and brief review. *J Rheumatol* 11(3):373–374, 1984.

96. Obermoser G, Emberger M, Wieser M, et al: Nephrogenic fibrosing dermopathy in two patients with systemic lupus erythematosus. *Lupus* 13(8):609–612, 2004.

97. Lawley TJ, Bielory L, Gascon P, et al: A prospective clinical and immunologic analysis of patients with serum sickness. *N Engl J Med* 311(22):1407–1413, 1984.

98. Cuzić S, Śćukanec-Spoljar M, Bosnić D, et al: Immunohistochemical analysis of human serum sickness glomerulonephritis. *Croat Med J* 42(6):618–623, 2001.

99. Kuo TT: Cutaneous manifestation of Kikuchi's histiocytic necrotizing lymphadenitis. *Am J Surg Pathol* 14(9):872–876, 1990.

100. el Ramahi KM, Karrar A, Muhammad AA: Kikuchi disease and its association with systemic lupus erythematosus. *Lupus* 3(5):409–411, 1994.

101. Alijotas-Reig J, Casellas-Caro M, Ferrer-Oliveras R, et al: Recurrent Kikuchi-Fujimoto disease during pregnancy: report of case evolving into systemic lupus erythematosus and review of published work. *J Obstet Gynaecol Res* 34(4 Pt 2):595–598, 2008.

102. Santana A, Lessa B, Galrao L, et al: Kikuchi-Fujimoto's disease associated with systemic lupus erythematosus: case report and review of the literature. *Clin Rheumatol* 24(1):60–63, 2005.

103. Bruce IN, Mak VC, Hallett DC, et al: Factors associated with fatigue in patients with systemic lupus erythematosus. *Ann Rheum Dis* 58(6):379–381, 1999.

104. Krupp LB, LaRocca NG, Muir J, et al: A study of fatigue in systemic lupus erythematosus. *J Rheumatol* 17(11):1450–1452, 1990.

105. Weir PT, Harlan GA, Nkoy FL, et al: The incidence of fibromyalgia and its associated comorbidities: a population-based retrospective cohort study based on *International Classification of Diseases,* 9th Revision codes. *J Clin Rheumatol* 12(3):124–128, 2006.

106. Morand EF, Miller MH, Whittingham S, et al: Fibromyalgia syndrome and disease activity in systemic lupus erythematosus. *Lupus* 3(3):187–191, 1994.

107. Middleton GD, McFarlin JE, Lipsky PE: The prevalence and clinical impact of fibromyalgia in systemic lupus erythematosus. *Arthritis Rheum* 37(8):1181–1188, 1994.

108. Friedman AW, Tewi MB, Ahn C, et al: Systemic lupus erythematosus in three ethnic groups: XV. Prevalence and correlates of fibromyalgia. *Lupus* 12(4):274–279, 2003.

109. Al-Allaf AW, Ottewell L, Pullar T: The prevalence and significance of positive antinuclear antibodies in patients with fibromyalgia syndrome: 2–4 years' follow-up. *Clin Rheumatol* 21(6):472–477, 2002.

110. Wolfe F, Michaud K, Li T, et al: Chronic conditions and health problems in rheumatic diseases: comparisons with rheumatoid arthritis, noninflammatory rheumatic disorders, systemic lupus erythematosus, and fibromyalgia. *J Rheumatol* 37(2):305–315, 2010.

111. Chaiamnuay S, Bertoli AM, Fernández M, et al: The impact of increased body mass index on systemic lupus erythematosus: data from LUMINA, a multiethnic cohort (LUMINA XLVI). *J Clin Rheumatol* 13(3):128–133, 2007.

112. Ghanim H, Aljada A, Hofmeyer D, et al: Circulating mononuclear cells in the obese are in a proinflammatory state. *Circulation* 110(12):1564–1571, 2004.

113. Grondal G, Gunnarsson I, Ronnelid J, et al: Cytokine production, serum levels and disease activity in systemic lupus erythematosus. *Clin Exp Rheumatol* 18(5):565–570, 2000.

114. McKendall MJ, Haier RJ: Pain sensitivity and obesity. *Psychiatry Res* 8(2):119–125, 1983.

115. Bruce IN, Mak VC, Hallett DC, et al: Factors associated with fatigue in patients with systemic lupus erythematosus. *Ann Rheum Dis* 58(6):379–381, 1999.

116. Akkasilpa S, Goldman D, Magder LS, et al: Number of fibromyalgia tender points is associated with health status in patients with systemic lupus erythematosus. *J Rheumatol* 32(1):48–50, 2005.

117. Iaboni A, Ibanez D, Gladman DD, et al: Fatigue in systemic lupus erythematosus: contributions of disordered sleep, sleepiness, and depression. *J Rheumatol* 33(12):2453–2457, 2006.

118. Da Costa D, Dritsa M, Bernatsky S, et al: Dimensions of fatigue in systemic lupus erythematosus: relationship to disease status and behavioral and psychosocial factors. *J Rheumatol* 33(7):1282–1288, 2006.

119. Lally EV, Parker VS, Kaplan SR: Acute gouty arthritis and systemic lupus erythematosus. *J Rheumatol* 9(2):308–310, 1982.

120. Veerapen K, Schumacher HR, Jr, van Linthoudt D, et al: Tophaceous gout in young patients with systemic lupus erythematosus. *J Rheumatol* (4):721–724, 1993.

121. Frocht A, Leek JC, Robbins DL: Gout and hyperuricaemia in systemic lupus erythematosus. *Br J Rheumatol* 26(4):303–306, 1987.

122. Ho HH, Lin JL, Wu YJ, et al: Gout in systemic lupus erythematosus and overlap syndrome—a hospital-based study. *Clin Rheumatol* 22(4-5):295–298, 2003.

123. Bajaj S, Fessler BJ, Alarcón GS: Systemic lupus erythematosus and gouty arthritis: an uncommon association. *Rheumatology (Oxford)* 43(3):349–352, 2004.

124. Wallace DJ, Klinenberg JR, Morham D, et al: Coexistent gout and rheumatoid arthritis. Case report and literature review. *Arthritis Rheum* 22(1):81–86, 1979.

125. Greenfield DI, Fong JS, Barth WF: Systemic lupus erythematosus and gout. *Semin Arthritis Rheum* 14(3):176–179, 1985.

126. Rodriguez MA, Paul H, Abadi I, et al: Multiple microcrystal deposition disease in a patient with systemic lupus erythematosus. *Ann Rheum Dis* 43(3):498–502, 1984.

127. Kurano TL, Lum CA, Izumi AK: The association of dermatitis herpetiformis and systemic lupus erythematosus. *J Am Acad Dermatol* 63(5):892–895, 2010.

128. Thomas JR, III, Su WP: Concurrence of lupus erythematosus and dermatitis herpetiformis. A report of nine cases. *Arch Dermatol* 119(9):740–745, 1983.

129. Penneys NS, Wiley HE, III: Herpetiform blisters in systemic lupus erythematosus. *Arch Dermatol* 115(12):1427–1428, 1979.

130. Aronson AJ, Soltani K, Aronson IK, et al: Systemic lupus erythematosus and dermatitis herpetiformis: concurrence with Marfan's syndrome. *Arch Dermatol* 115(1):68–70, 1979.

131. Davies MG, Marks R, Waddington E: Simultaneous systemic lupus erythematosus and dermatitis herpetiformis. *Arch Dermatol* 112(9):1292–1294, 1976.

132. Weinberg I, Vasiliev L, Gotsman I: Anti-dsDNA antibodies in sarcoidosis. *Semin Arthritis Rheum* 29(5):328–331, 2000.

133. Soto-Aguilar MC, Boulware DW: Sarcoidosis presenting as antinuclear antibody positive glomerulonephritis. *Ann Rheum Dis* 47(4):337–339, 1988.

134. Wesemann DR, Costenbader KH, Coblyn JS: Co-existing sarcoidosis, systemic lupus erythematosus and the antiphospholipid antibody syndrome: case reports and discussion from the Brigham and Women's Hospital Lupus Center. *Lupus* 18(3):202–205, 2009.

135. Begum S, Li C, Wedderburn LR, et al: Concurrence of sarcoidosis and systemic lupus erythematosus in three patients. *Clin Exp Rheumatol* 20(4):549–552, 2002.

136. Schnabel A, Barth J, Schubert F, et al: Pulmonary sarcoidosis coexisting with systemic lupus erythematosus. *Scand J Rheumat* 25(2):109–111, 1996.

137. Askari A, Thompson P, Barnes C: Sarcoidosis: atypical presentation associated with features of systemic lupus erythematosus. *J Rheumatol* 15(10):1578–1579, 1988.

138. Cathcart ES, Scheinberg MA: Systemic lupus erythematosus in a patient with amyloidosis. Discussion. *Arthritis Rheum* 19:254–255, 1976.

139. Benson MD, Cohen AS: Serum amyloid A protein in amyloidosis, rheumatic, and enoplastic diseases. *Arthritis Rheum* 22(1):36–42, 1979.

140. Breathnach SM, Kofler H, Sepp N, et al: Serum amyloid P component binds to cell nuclei in vitro and to in vivo deposits of extracellular chromatin in systemic lupus erythematosus. *J Exp Med* 170(4):1433–1438, 1989.

141. Queffeulou G, Berentbaum F, Michel C, et al: AA amyoidosis in systemic lupus erythematosus: an unusual complication. *Nephrol Dial Transplant* 13:1840–1848, 1998.

142. Gomez-Puerta JA, Cervera R, Moll C, et al: Proliferative lupus nephritis in a patient with systemic lupus erythematosus and longstanding secondary amyloid nephropathy. *Clin Rheumatol* 28(1):95–97, 2009.

143. Aktas YB, Duzgun N, Mete T, et al: AA amyloidosis associated with systemic lupus erythematosus: impact on clinical course and outcome. *Rheumatol Int* 28(4):367–370, 2008.

144. Huston DP, McAdam KP, Balow JE, et al: Amyloidosis in systemic lupus erythematosus. *Am J Med* 70(2):320–323, 1981.

145. Schwendiman MN, Beachkofsky TM, Wisco OJ, et al: Primary cutaneous nodular amyloidosis: case report and review of the literature. *Cutis* 84(2):87–92, 2009.

146. Nashel DJ, Leonard A, Mann DL, et al: Ankylosing spondylitis and systemic lupus erythematosus: a rare HLA combination. *Arch Intern Med* 142(6):1227–1228, 1982.

147. Jiang L, Dai X, Liu J, et al: Hypoparathyroidism in a patient with systemic lupus erythematosus coexisted with ankylosing spondylitis: a case report and review of literature. *Joint Bone Spine* 77(6):608–610, 2010.

148. Olivieri I, Gemignani G, Balagi M, et al: Concomitant systemic lupus erythematosus and ankylosing spondylitis. *Ann Rheum Dis* 49(5):323–324, 1990.

149. Kohli M, Bennett RM: Sacroiliitis in systemic lupus erythematosus. *J Rheumatol* 21(1):170–171, 1994.

150. Mounach A, Ghazi M, Nouijai A, et al: Drug-induced lupus-like syndrome in ankylosing spondylitis treated with infliximab. *Clin Exp Rheumatol* 26(6):1116–1118, 2008.

151. Aisen PS, Cronstein BN, Kramer SB: Systemic lupus erythematosus in a patient with Reiter's syndrome. *Arthritis Rheum* 26(11):1405–1408, 1983.

152. Singh S, Sonkar GK, Singh U: Coexistence of ankylosing spondylitis and systemic lupus erythematosus. *J Chin Med Assoc* 73(5):260–261, 2010.

153. Eyanson S, Greist MC, Brandt KD, et al: Systemic lupus erythematosus: association with psoralen-ultraviolet-a treatment of psoriasis. *Arch Dermatol* 115(1):54–56, 1979.

154. Kulick KB, Mogavero H, Provost TT, et al: Serologic studies in patients with lupus erythematosus and psoriasis. *J Am Acad Dermatol* 8(5):631–634, 1983.

155. Millns JL, Muller SA: The coexistence of psoriasis and lupus erythematosus: an analysis of 27 cases. *Arch Dermatol* 116(6):658–663, 1980.

156. Dowdy MJ, Nigra TP, Barth WF: Subacute cutaneous lupus erythematosus during PUVA therapy for psoriasis: case report and review of the literature. *Arthritis Rheum* 32(3):343–346, 1989.

157. Mcgrath H, Scopelitis E, Nesbitt LT: Subacute cutaneous lupus erythematosus during psoralen ultraviolet A therapy. *Arthritis Rheum* 33(2):302–303, 1990.

158. Wohl Y, Brenner S: Cutaneous LE or psoriasis: a tricky differential diagnosis. Letter to the Editor. *Lupus* 13(1):72–74, 2004.

159. Lorber M, Gershwin ME, Shoenfeld Y: The coexistence of systemic lupus erythematosus with other autoimmune diseases: the kaleidoscope of autoimmunity. *Semin Arthritis Rheum* 24(2):105–113, 1994.

160. Clemmensen O, Thomsen K: Porphyria cutanea tarda and systemic lupus erythematosus. *Arch Dermatol* 118(3):160–162, 1982.

161. Griso D, Macri A, Biolcati G, et al: Does an association exist between PCT and SLE? Results of a study on autoantibodies in 158 patients affected with PCT. *Arch Dermatol Res* 281(4):291–292, 1989.

162. Allard SA, Charles PJ, Herrick AL, et al: Antinuclear antibodies and the diagnosis of systemic lupus erythematosus in patients with acute intermittent porphyria. *Ann Rheum Dis* 49(4):246–248, 1990.

163. Filiotou A, Vaiopoulos G, Capsimali V, et al: Acute intermittent porphyria and systemic lupus erythematosus: report of a case and review of the literature. *Lupus* 11(3):190–192, 2002.

164. Gibson GE, McEvoy MT: Coexistence of lupus erythematosus and porphyria cutanea tarda in fifteen patients. *J Am Acad Dermatol* 38(4):569–573, 1998.

165. Becker NJ, Borek D, Abdou NI: Angioimmunoblastic lymphadenopathy presenting as SLE with GI protein loss. *J Rheumatol* 15:1452–1454, 1988.

166. Gleichmann E, Van Elven F, Gleichman H: Immunoblastic, lymphadenopathy, systemic lupus erythematosus, and related disorders. *Am J Clin Pathol* 72(Suppl 4):708–723, 1979.

167. Gusterson BA, Fizharris BM: Angio-immunoblastic lymphadenopathy with lupus erythematosus cells. *Br J Haematol* 43:149–150, 1979.

168. Pierce DA, Stern R, Jaffe R, et al: Immunoblastic sarcoma with features of Sjögren's syndrome and systemic lupus erythematosus in a patient with immunoblastic lymphadenopathy. *Arthritis Rheum* 22(8):911–916, 1979.

169. Rosenstein ED, Wieczorek R, Raphael BG, et al: Systemic lupus erythematosus and angioimmunoblastic lymphadenopathy: case report and review of the literature. *Semin Arthritis Rheum* 16(2):146–151, 1986.

170. McHugh NJ, Campbell GJ, Landreth JJ, et al: Polyarthritis and angioimmunoblastic lymphadenopathy. *Ann Rheum Dis* 46:555–558, 1987.

171. Bignon YJ, Janin-Mercier A, Dubos Ult JJ, et al: Angioimmunoblastic lymphadenopathy with dysproteinemia (AILD) and sicca syndrome. *Ann Rheum Dis* 45:519–522, 1986.

172. Pittoni V, Sorice M, Circella A, et al: Specificity of antinuclear and antiphospholipid antibodies in sera of patients with autoimmune lymphoproliferative disease. *Clin Exp Rheumatol* 21(3):377–385, 2003.

173. Sneller MC, Dale JK, Straus SE: Autoimmune lymphoproliferative syndrome. *Curr Opin Rheumatol* 15(4):417–421, 2003.

174. Harisdangkul V, Benson CH, Myers A: Renal cell carcinoma presenting as necrotizing vasculitis with digital gangrene. *Intern Med* 5:108–117, 1984.

175. Marcus RM, Grayzel AI: A lupus antibody syndrome associated with hypernephroma. *Arthritis Rheum* 22(12):1396–1398, 1979.

176. Imai H, Nakano Y, Kiyosawa K, et al: Increasing titers and changing specificities of antinuclear antibodies in patients with chronic liver disease who develop hepatocellular carcinoma. *Cancer* 71(1):26–35, 1993.

177. Friss AB, Cohen PR, Bruce S, et al: Chronic cutaneous lupus erythematosus mimicking mycosis fungoides. *J Am Acad Dermatol* 33(5):891–895, 1995.

178. Stevanovic G, Cramer AD, Taylor CR, et al: Immunoblastic sarcoma in patients with systemic lupus erythematosus. *Arch Pathol Lab Med* 107:589–592, 1983.

179. Solans-Laqué R, Pérez-Bocanegra C, Salud-Salvia A, et al: Clinical significance of antinuclear antibodies in malignant diseases: association with rheumatic and connective tissue paraneoplastic syndromes. *Lupus* 13(3):159–164, 2004.

180. Kitagawa Y, Hanada T, Matsuoka Y, et al: Primary malignant lymphoma of the brain: clinical and pathological investigations. *Jpn J Med* 28(1):2–7, 1989.

181. Asherson RA, Block S, Houssiau FA, et al: Systemic lupus erythematosus and lymphoma: association with an antiphospholipid syndrome. *J Rheumatol* 18:277–279, 1991.

182. Legerton CW, Sergent JS: Intravascular malignant lymphoma mimicking central nervous system lupus. *Arthritis Rheum* 36(1):135, 1993.

183. Zuber M: Positive antinuclear antibodies in malignancies. *Ann Rheum Dis* 51(4):573–574, 1992.

184. Posner MA, Gloster ES, Bonagura VR, et al: Burkitt's lymphoma in a patient with systemic lupus erythematosus. *J Rheumatol* 17(3):380–382, 1990.

185. Strickland RW, Limmani A, Wall JG, et al: Hairy cell leukemia presenting as a lupus-like illness. *Arthritis Rheum* 31(4):566–568, 1988.

186. Freundlich B, Makover D, Maul GG: A novel antinuclear antibody associated with a lupus-like paraneoplastic syndrome. *Ann Intern Med* 109(4):295–297, 1988.

187. Zuber M, Meisel R, Brandl B: A patient with a high titer of antinuclear antibody and a functioning adrenal tumor. *Clin Rheumatol* 14:100–103, 1995.

188. Kuzmich PV, Ecker GA, Karsh J: Rheumatic manifestations in patients with myelodysplastic and myeloproliferative diseases. *J Rheumatol* 21(9):1649–1654, 1994.

189. Kohli M, Bennett RM: An association of polymyalgia rheumatica with myelodysplastic syndromes. *J Rheumatol* 21(7):1357–1359, 1994.

190. Aoshima M, Tanaka H, Takahashi M, et al: Meigs' syndrome due to Brenner tumor mimicking lupus peritonitis in a patient with systemic lupus erythematosus. *Am J Gastroenterol* 90(4):657–658, 1995.

191. Shimomura C, Eguchi K, Kawakami A, et al: Elevation of a tumor associated antigen CA 199 levels in patients with rheumatic diseases. *J Rheumatol* 16:1410–1415, 1989.

192. Moncayo R, Moncayo H: Serum levels of CA 125 are elevated in patients with active systemic lupus erythematosus. *Obstet Gynecol* 77:932–934, 1991.

193. Singh S, Chatterjee S, Sohoni R, et al: Sera from lupus patients inhibit growth of *P. falciparum* in culture. *Autoimmunity* 33(4):253–263, 2001.

194. Doria A, Canova M, Tonon M, et al: Infections as triggers and complications of systemic lupus erythematosus. *Autoimmun Rev* 8(1):24–28, 2008.

195. Ramos-Casals M, Cuadrado MJ, Alba P, et al: Acute viral infections in patients with systemic lupus erythematosus: description of 23 cases and review of the literature. *Medicine* 87(6):311–318, 2008.

196. Parks CG, Cooper GS, Hudson LL, et al: Association of Epstein-Barr virus with systemic lupus erythematosus: effect modification by race, age, and cytotoxic T lymphocyte-associated antigen 4 genotype. *Arthritis Rheum* 52(4):1148–1159, 2005.

197. Bulpitt KJ, Brahn E: Systemic lupus erythematosus and concurrent cytomegalovirus vasculitis: diagnosis by antemortem skin biopsy. *J Rheumatol* 16(5):677–680, 1989.

198. Jones JF, Ray CG, Minnich LL, et al: Evidence for active Epstein-Barr virus infection in patients with persistent, unexplained illnesses: elevated anti-early antigen antibodies. *Ann Intern Med* 102(1):1–7, 1985.

199. Hansen KE, Arnason J, Bridges AJ: Autoantibodies and common viral illnesses. *Semin Arthritis Rheum* 27(5):263–271, 1998.

200. Cainelli F, Betterle C, Vento S: Antinuclear antibodies are common in an infectious environment but do not predict systemic lupus erythematosus. *Ann Rheum Dis* 63(12):1707–1708, 2004.

201. Cannavan FP, Costallat LT, Bertolo MB, et al: False positive IgM antibody tests for human cytomegalovirus (HCMV) in patients with SLE. *Lupus* 7(1):61–62, 1998.

202. Stratta P, Canavese C, Ciccone G, et al: Correlation between cytomegalovirus infection and Raynaud's phenomenon in lupus nephritis. *Nephron* 82(2):145–154, 1999.

203. Bendiksen S, Van Ghelue M, Rekvig OP, et al: A longitudinal study of human cytomegalovirus serology and viruria fails to detect active viral infection in 20 systemic lupus erythematosus patients. *Lupus* 9(2):120–126, 2000.

204. Kitagawa H, Iho S, Yokochi T, et al: Detection of antibodies to the Epstein-Barr virus nuclear antigens in the sera from patients with systemic lupus erythematosus. *Immunol Lett* 17(3):249–252, 1988.

205. Sculley DG, Sculley TB, Pope JH: Reactions of sera from patients with rheumatoid arthritis, systemic lupus erythematosus and infectious mononucleosis to Epstein-Barr virus-induced polypeptides. *J Gen Virol* 67 (Pt 10):2253–2258, 1986.

206. Incaprera M, Rindi L, Bazzichi A, et al: Potential role of the Epstein-Barr virus in systemic lupus erythematosus autoimmunity. *Clin Exp Rheumatol* 16(3):289–294, 1998.

207. Dror Y, Blachar Y, Cohen P, et al: Systemic lupus erythematosus associated with acute Epstein-Barr virus infection. *Am J Kidney Dis* 32(5):825–828, 1998.

208. Al Jitawi SA, Hakooz BA, Kazimi SM: False positive Monospot test in systemic lupus erythematosus. *Br J Rheumatol* 26(1):71, 1987.

209. James JA, Kaufman KM, Farris AD, et al: An increased prevalence of Epstein-Barr virus infection in young patients suggests a possible etiology for systemic lupus erythematosus. *J Clin Invest* 100(12):3019–3026, 1997.

210. James JA, Neas BR, Moser KL, et al: Systemic lupus erythematosus in adults is associated with previous Epstein-Barr virus exposure. *Arthritis Rheum* 44(5):1122–1126, 2001.

211. Kang I, Quan T, Nolasco H, et al: Defective control of latent Epstein-Barr virus infection in systemic lupus erythematosus. *J Immunol* 172(2):1287–1294, 2004.

212. Katz BZ, Salimi B, Kim S, et al: Epstein-Barr virus burden in adolescents with systemic lupus erythematosus. *Pediatr Infect Dis J* (2):148–153, 1920.

213. Sekigawa I, Nawata M, Seta N, et al: Cytomegalovirus infection in patients with systemic lupus erythematosus. *Clin Exp Rheumatol* (4):559–564, 1920.

214. Zhang C, Shen K, Jiang Z, et al: Early diagnosis and monitoring of active HCMV infection in children with systemic lupus erythematosus. *Chin Med J* 114(12):1309–1312, 2001.

215. Stratta P, Colla L, Santi S, et al: IgM antibodies against cytomegalovirus in SLE nephritis: viral infection or aspecific autoantibody? *J Nephrol* 15(1):88–92, 2002.

216. Park HB, Kim KC, Park JH, et al: Association of reduced CD4 T cell responses specific to varicella zoster virus with high incidence of herpes zoster in patients with systemic lupus erythematosus. *J Rheumatol* 31(11):2151–2155, 2004.

217. Soloninka CA, Anderson MJ, Laskin CA: Anti-DNA and antilymphocyte antibodies during acute infection with human parvovirus B19. *J Rheumatol* 16(6):777–781, 1989.

218. Bengtsson A, Widell A, Elmstahl S, et al: No serological indications that systemic lupus erythematosus is linked with exposure to human parvovirus B19. *Ann Rheum Dis* 59(1):64–66, 2000.

219. Tovari E, Mezey I, Hedman K, et al: Self limiting lupus-like symptoms in patients with parvovirus B19 infection. *Ann Rheum Dis* 61(7):662–663, 2002.

220. Hsu TC, Tsay GJ: Human parvovirus B19 infection in patients with systemic lupus erythematosus. *Rheumatology* 40(2):152–157, 2001.

221. Seve P, Ferry T, Koenig M, et al: Lupus-like presentation of parvovirus B19 infection. *Semin Arthritis Rheum* 34(4):642–648, 2005.

222. Filimonova RG, Bogomolova NN, Nevraeva EG, et al: Measles virus genome in patients with lupus nephritis and glomerulonephritis. *Nephron* 67(4):488–489, 1994.

223. de Clerck LS, Couttenye MM, de Broe ME, et al: Acquired immunodeficiency mimicking Sjögren's syndrome and systemic lupus erythematosus. *Arthritis Rheum* 31:272–275, 1988.

224. Kopelman RG, Zolla-Pazner S: Association of human immunodeficiency virus infection and autoimmune phenomena. *Am J Med* 84(1): 82–88, 1988.

225. Chowdhry IA, Tan IJ, Mian N, et al: Systemic lupus erythematosus presenting with features suggestive of human immunodeficiency virus infection. *J Rheumatol* 32(7):1365–1368, 2005.

226. Calabrese LH: The rheumatic manifestations of infection with the human immunodeficiency virus. *Semin Arthritis Rheum* 18(4):225–239, 1989.

227. Cohen AJ, Philips TM, Kessler CM: Circulating coagulation inhibitors in the acquired immunodeficiency syndrome. *Ann Intern Med* 104(2): 175–180, 1986.

228. Stimmler MM, Quismorio FP, Jr, McGehee WG, et al: Anticardiolipin antibodies in acquired immunodeficiency syndrome. *Arch Intern Med* 149(8):1833–1835, 1989.

229. Montero A, Prato R, Jorfen M: [Systemic lupus erythematosus and AIDS. Difficulties in the differential diagnosis]. [Spanish]. *Medicina* 51(4):303–306, 1991.

230. Esteva MH, Blasini AM, Ogly D, et al: False positive results for antibody to HIV in two men with systemic lupus erythematosus. *Ann Rheum Dis* 51(9):1071–1073, 1992.

231. Barthels HR, Wallace DJ: False-positive human immunodeficiency virus testing in patients with systemic lupus erythematosus. *Semin Arthritis Rheum* 23:1–7, 1993.

232. D'Agati V, Seigle R: Coexistence of AIDS and lupus nephritis: a case report. *Am J Nephrol* 10(3):243–247, 1990.

233. Strauss J, Abitbol C, Zilleruelo G, et al: Renal disease in children with the acquired immunodeficiency syndrome. *N Engl J Med* 321(10):625–630, 1989.

234. Lu I, Cohen PR, Grossman ME: Multiple dermatofibromas in a woman with HIV infection and systemic lupus erythematosus. *J Am Acad Dermatol* 32(5 Pt 2):901–903, 1995.

235. Werninghaus K: Lupus-like eruption and human immunodeficiency virus infection. *Cutis* 55(3):153–154, 1995.

236. Bambery P, Deodhar SD, Malhotra HS, et al: Blood transfusion related HBV and HIV infection in a patient with SLE. *Lupus* 2(3):203–205, 1993.

237. Palacios R, Santos J, Valdivielso P, et al: Human immunodeficiency virus infection and systemic lupus erythematosus. An unusual case and a review of the literature. *Lupus* 11(1):60–63, 2002.

238. Daikh BE, Holyst MM: Lupus-specific autoantibodies in concomitant human immunodeficiency virus and systemic lupus erythematosus: case report and literature review. *Semin Arthritis Rheum* 30(6):418–425, 2001.

239. Diri E, Lipsky PE, Berggren RE: Emergence of systemic lupus erythematosus after initiation of highly active antiretroviral therapy for human immunodeficiency virus infection. *J Rheumatol* 27(11):2711–2714, 2000.

240. Drake WP, Byrd VM, Olsen NJ: Reactivation of systemic lupus erythematosus after initiation of highly active antiretroviral therapy for acquired immunodeficiency syndrome. *J Clin Rheumatol* 9:176–180, 2003.

241. Alonso CM, Lozada CJ: Effects of IV cyclophosphamide on HIV viral replication in a patient with systemic lupus erythematosus. *Clin Exp Rheumatol* 18(4):510–512, 2000.

242. Kaye BR: Rheumatologic manifestations of infection with human immunodeficiency virus (HIV). *Ann Intern Med* 111(2):158–167, 1989.

243. Yao Q, Frank M, Glynn M, et al: Rheumatic manifestations in HIV-1 infected in-patients and literature review. *Clin Exp Rheumatol* 26(5):799–806, 2008.

244. Wallace DJ: Lupus, acquired immunodeficiency syndrome, and antimalarial agents. *Arthritis Rheum* 34(3):372–373, 1991.

245. Scherl M, Posch U, Obermoser G, et al: Targeting human immunodeficiency virus type 1 with antibodies derived from patients with connective tissue disease. *Lupus* 15(12):865–872, 2006.

246. Douvas A, Takehana Y, Ehresmann G, et al: Neutralization of HIV type 1 infectivity by serum antibodies from a subset of autoimmune patients with mixed connective tissue disease. *AIDS Res Hum Retroviruses* 12(16):1509–1517, 1996.

247. Gonzalez CM, Lopez-Longo FJ, Samson J, et al: Antiribonucleoprotein antibodies in children with HIV infection: a comparative study with childhood-onset systemic lupus erythematosus. *AIDS Patient Care STDS* 12(1):21–28, 1998.

248. Sekigawa I, Lee S, Kaneko H, et al: The possible role of interleukin-16 in the low incidence of HIV infection in patients with systemic lupus erythematosus. *Lupus* 9(2):155–156, 2000.

249. Soriano V, Ordi J, Grau J: Tests for HIV in lupus. *N Engl J Med* 331(13): 881, 1994.

250. Font J, Vidal J, Cervera R, et al: Lack of relationship between human immunodeficiency virus infection and systemic lupus erythematosus. *Lupus* 4(1):47–49, 1995.

251. Higashi J, Kumagai S, Hatanaka M, et al: The presence of antibodies to p24gag protein of JRA-I in sera of patients with systemic lupus erythematosus. *Virus Genes* 6:357–364, 1992.

252. Herrmann M, Baur A, Nebel-Schickel H, et al: Antibodies against p24 of HIV-1 in patients with systemic lupus erythematosus? *Viral Immunol* 5(3):229–231, 1992.

253. Bermas BL, Petri M, Berzofsky JA, et al: Binding of glycoprotein 120 and peptides from the HIV-1 envelope by autoantibodies in mice with experimentally induced systemic lupus erythematosus and in patients with the disease. *AIDS Res Human Retroviruses* 10(9):1071–1077, 1994.

254. Pinto LA, Dalgleish AG, Sumar N, et al: Panel anti-GP 120 monoclonal antibodies reacts with same nuclear proteins in uninfected cells as those recognized by autoantibodies from patients with systemic lupus erythematosus. *AIDS Res Human Retroviruses* 10:823–838, 1994.

255. Scott TF, Goust JM, Strange CB, et al: SLE, thrombocytopenia, and JRA-1. *J Rheumatol* 17:1565–1566, 1990.

256. Gul A, Inanc M, Yilmaz G, et al: Antibodies reactive with HIV-1 antigens in systemic lupus erythematosus. *Lupus* 5(2):120–122, 1996.

257. Marlton P, Taylor K, Elliott S, et al: Monoclonal large granular lymphocyte proliferation in SLE with JRA-I seroreactivity. *Aust N Z J Med* 22:54–55, 1992.

258. Montero A, Jorfen M, Arpini R: HIV infection in a patient with chronic cutaneous lupus erythematosus. *Medicine* 51:545–547, 1991.

259. Kondo T, Matsui M: Migrating radiculopathy—an unusual complication of systemic lupus erythematosus in a JRA-1 carrier. *Rinsho Shinkeigaku* 34:466–469, 1994.

260. De Maria A, Cimmino MA: Diagnostic approach to possible HIV-1 infection in patients with systemic lupus erythematosus. *J Rheumatol* 24(4):807–808, 1997.

261. Takayanagui OM, Moura LS, Petean FC, et al: Human T-lymphotropic virus type I-associated myelopathy/tropical spastic paraparesis and systemic lupus erythematosus. *Neurology* 48(5):1469–1470, 1997.

262. Byrd VM, Sergent JS: Suppression of systemic lupus erythematosus by the human immunodeficiency virus. *J Rheumatol* 23(7):1295–1296, 1996.

263. Prabu V, Agrawal S: Systemic lupus erythematosus and tuberculosis: a review of complex interactions of complicated diseases. *J Postgrad Med* 56(3):244–250, 2010.

264. Feng PH, Tan TH: Tuberculosis in patients with systemic lupus erythematosus. *Ann Rheum Dis* 41(1):11–14, 1982.

265. Tam LS, Li EK, Wong SM, et al: Risk factors and clinical features for tuberculosis among patients with systemic lupus erythematosus in Hong Kong. *Scandinavian J Rheumatol* 31(5):296–300, 2002.

266. Sayarlioglu M, Inanc M, Kamali S, et al: Tuberculosis in Turkish patients with systemic lupus erythematosus: increased frequency of extrapulmonary localization. *Lupus* 13(4):274–278, 2004.

267. Yun JE, Lee SW, Kim TH, et al: The incidence and clinical characteristics of *Mycobacterium tuberculosis* infection among systemic lupus erythematosus and rheumatoid arthritis patients in Korea. *Clin Exp Rheumatol* 20(2):127–132, 2002.

268. Gaitonde S, Pathan E, Sule A, et al: Efficacy of isoniazid prophylaxis in patients with systemic lupus erythematosus receiving long term steroid treatment. *Ann Rheum Dis* 61(3):251–253, 2002.

269. Mok MY, Lo Y, Chan TM, et al: Tuberculosis in systemic lupus erythematosus in an endemic area and the role of isoniazid prophylaxis during corticosteroid therapy. *J Rheumatol* 32(4):609–615, 2005.

270. Lovy MR, Ryan PF, Hughes GR: Concurrent systemic lupus erythematosus and salmonellosis. *J Rheumatol* 8(4):605–612, 1981.

271. Ohkawa S, Ozaki M, Izumi S: Lepromatous leprosy complicated with systemic lupus erythematosus. *Dermatologica* 170(2):80–83, 1985.

272. Posner DI, Guill MA, III: Coexistent leprosy and lupus erythematosus. *Cutis* 39(2):136–138, 1987.

273. Zorbas P, Kontochristopoulos G, Detsi I, et al: Borderline tuberculoid leprosy coexisting with systemic lupus erythematosus. *J Eur Acad Dermatol Venereol* 12(3):274–275, 1999.

274. Bonfa E, Llovet R, Scheinberg M, et al: Comparison between autoantibodies in malaria and leprosy with lupus. *Clin Exp Immunol* 70(3):529–537, 1987.

275. Chavez-Legaspi M, Gomez-Vazquez A, Garcia-De La Torre I: Study of rheumatic manifestations and serologic abnormalities in patients with lepromatous leprosy. *J Rheumatol* 12(4):738–741, 1985.

276. Lamarre D, Talbot B, de Murcia G, et al: Structural and functional analysis of poly(ADP ribose) polymerase: an immunological study. *Biochim Biophys Acta* 950(2):147–160, 1988.

277. Miller RA, Wener MH, Harnisch JP, et al: The limited spectrum of antinuclear antibodies in leprosy. *J Rheumatol* 14(1):108–110, 1987.

278. Mackworth-Young C, Sabbaga J, Schwartz RS: Idiotypic markers of polyclonal B cell activation. Public idiotypes shared by monoclonal antibodies derived from patients with systemic lupus erythematosus or leprosy. *J Clin Invest* 79(2):572–581, 1987.

279. Rahima D, Tarrab-Hazdai R, Blank M, et al: Anti-nuclear antibodies associated with schistosomiasis and anti-schistosomal antibodies associated with SLE. *Autoimmunity* 17(2):127–141, 1994.

280. Li EK, Cohen MG, Ho AK, et al: *Salmonella* bacteraemia occurring concurrently with the first presentation of systemic lupus erythematosus. *Br J Rheumatol* 32(1):66–67, 1993.

281. Braun J, Sieper J, Schulte KL, et al: Visceral leishmaniasis mimicking a flare of systemic lupus erythematosus. *Clin Rheumatol* 10(4):445–448, 1991.

282. Lyngberg KK, Vennervald BJ, Bygbjerg IC, et al: Toxoplasma pericarditis mimicking systemic lupus erythematosus. *Ann Med* 24:337–340, 1992.

283. Mora CS, Segami MI, Hidalgo JA: *Strongyloides stercoralis* hyperinfection in systemic lupus erythematosus and the antiphospholipid syndrome. *Semin Arthritis Rheum* 36(3):135–143, 2006.

284. Katano K, Hayatsu Y, Matsuda T, et al: Endocapillary proliferative glomerulonephritis with crescent formation and concurrent tubulointerstitial nephritis complicating retroperitoneal fibrosis with a high serum level of IgG4. *Clin Nephrol* 68(5):308–314, 2007.

285. Kobayashi S, Yoshida M, Kitahara T, et al: Autoimmune pancreatitis as the initial presentation of systemic lupus erythematosus. *Lupus* 16(2):133–136, 2007.

286. Yildiz G, Kayatas M, Uygun Y, et al: Coexistence of systemic lupus erythematosus and familial Mediterranean fever. *Intern Med* 49(8):767–769, 2010.

287. Brunsting R, Sillevis Smitt JH, van der Meer JW, et al: Discoid lupus erythematosus and other clinical manifestation in female carriers of chronic granulomatous disease. *Ned Tijdschr Geneeskd* 132:18–21, 1988.

288. Strate M, Brandrup F, Wang P: Discoid lupus erythematosus-like skin lesions in a patient with autosomal recessive chronic granulomatous disease. *Clin Genetics* 30(3):184–190, 1986.

289. Hafner J, Enderlin A, Seger RA, et al: Discoid lupus erythematosus-like lesions in carriers of X-linked chronic granulomatous disease. *Br J Dermatol* 127:446–447, 1992.

290. Stalder JF, Dreno B, Bureau B, et al: Discoid lupus erythematosus-like lesions in an autosomal form of chronic granulomatous disease. *Br J Dermatol* 114(2):251–254, 1986.

291. Sillevis Smitt JH, Weening RS, Krieg SR, et al: Discoid lupus erythematosus-like lesions in carriers of X-linked chronic granulomatous disease. *Br J Dermatol* 122(5):643–650, 1990.

292. Lovas JGL, Issekutz A, Walsh N, et al: Lupus erythematosus-like oral mucosal and skin lesions in a carrier of chronic granulomatous disease. *Radiol Endod* 80:78–82, 1995.

293. Manzi S, Urbach AH, McCune AB, et al: Systemic lupus erythematosus in a boy with chronic granulomatous disease: case report and review of the literature. *Arthritis Rheum* 34(1):101–105, 1991.

294. Cobeta-Garcia JC, Domingo-Morera JA, Monteagudo-Saez I, et al: Autosomal chronic granulomatous disease and systemic lupus erythematosus with fatal outcome. *Br J Rheumatol* 37(1):109–111, 1998.

295. Alarcón-Segovia D, Amigo MC, Reyes PA: Connective tissue disease features after thallium poisoning. *J Rheumatol* 16(2):171–174, 1989.

296. Montoya-Cabrera MA, Sauceda-Garcia JM, Escalante-Galindo P, et al: [Thallium poisoning which stimulated systemic lupus erythematosus in a child]. [Spanish]. *Gac Med Mex* 127(4):333–336, 1991.

297. Franklin CM, Torretti D: Systemic lupus erythematosus and Down's syndrome. *Arthritis Rheum* 28(5):598–599, 1985.

298. Yancey CL, Zmijewski C, Athreya BH, et al: Arthropathy of Down's syndrome. *Arthritis Rheum* 27(8):929–934, 1984.

299. Bakkaloglu A, Ozen S, Besbas N, et al: Down syndrome associated with systemic lupus erythematosus: a mere coincidence or a significant association? *Clinical Genetics* 46(4):322–323, 1994.

300. Dubois EL, Tuffanelli DL: Clinical manifestations of systemic lupus erythematosus. Computer analysis of 520 cases. *JAMA* 190:104–111, 1964.

301. Parsons H, Snyder F, Bowen T, et al: Immune complex disease consistent with systemic lupus erythematosus in a patient with lysinuric protein intolerance. *J Inherited Metab Dis* (5):627–634, 2010.

302. Kamoda T, Nagai Y, Shigeta M, et al: Lysinuric protein intolerance and systemic lupus erythematosus. *European J Pediatr* 157(2):130–131, 1998.

303. Prelipcean V, Koch AE: Systemic lupus erythematosus associated with moyamoya disease. Case report and review of the literature. *J Clin Rheumatol* 4:328–332, 1998.

304. El Ramahi KM, Al Rayes HM: Systemic lupus erythematosus associated with moyamoya syndrome. *Lupus* 9(8):632–636, 2000.

305. Shrinath M, Walter JH, Haeney M, et al: Prolidase deficiency and systemic lupus erythematosus. *Arch Dis Child* 76(5):441–444, 1997.

306. Ahmad ZP, Johnstone LM, Walker AM: Cystinosis and lupus erythematosus: coincidence or causation. *Pediatr Nephrol* 25(8):1543–1546, 2010.

307. Zimmermann B, III, Lally EV, Sharma SC, et al: Severe aortic stenosis in systemic lupus erythematosus and mucopolysaccharidosis type II (Hunter's syndrome). *Clin Cardiol* 11(10):723–725, 1988.

308. Genereau T, Pasquier E, Cabane J, et al: [Disseminated lupus erythematosus associated with Rendu-Osler disease. Antiphospholipid antibodies don't protect from hemorrhage]. [French]. *Presse Med* 21(3):129, 1992.

309. Forns X, Bosch X, Graus F, et al: Amyotrophic lateral sclerosis in a patient with systemic lupus erythematosus. *Lupus* 2(2):133–134, 1993.

310. Rahman P, Gladman DD, Wither J, et al: Coexistence of Fabry's disease and systemic lupus erythematosus. *Clin Exp Rheumatol* 16(4):475–478, 1998.

311. Kogure A, Ohshima Y, Watanabe N, et al: A case of Werner's syndrome associated with systemic lupus erythematosus. *Clin Rheumatol* 14(2):199–203, 1995.

312. Alanay Y, Balci S, Ozen S: Noonan syndrome and systemic lupus erythematosus: presentation in childhood. *Clin Dysmorphol* 13(3):161–163, 2004.

313. Mitsui H, Komine M, Watanabe T, et al: Does Hermansky-Pudlak syndrome predispose to systemic lupus erythematosus? *Br J Dermatol* 146(5):908–911, 2002.

314. Tolusa-Hunt syndrome in a patient with systemic lupus erythematosus. *Eur Radiol* 12:341–344, 2002.

315. Bicer A, Tursen U, Ozer C, et al: Coexistence of osteopoikilosis and discoid lupus erythematosus: a case report. *Clin Rheumatol* 21(5):405–407, 2002.

316. Goeb V, Dubreuil F, Cabre P, et al: Lupus revealing itself after a stiff-person syndrome. *Lupus* 13(3):215, 2004.

317. Saito K: A case of systemic lupus erythematosus complicated with multicentric reticulohistiocytosis (MRH): successful treatment of MRH and lupus nephritis with cyclosporin A. *Lupus* 10(2):129–132, 2001.

318. Kim TY, Lee SH, Kim TJ, et al: [A case of fulminant hepatic failure in Wilson's disease combined with systemic lupus erythematosus]. [Korean]. *Taehan Kan Hakhoe Chi* 8(1):100–104, 2002.

319. Kornfeld S, Beyssier-Berlot C, Vinceneux A, et al: Acquired hemophilia A in a patient with systemic lupus erythematosus. *Ann Dermatol Venereol* 129:316–319, 2002.

320. Ishikawa T, Tsukamoto N, Suto M, et al: Acquired hemophilia A in a patient with systemic lupus erythematosus. *Intern Med* 40(6):541–543, 2001.

321. Taylor PW: Isaacs' syndrome (autoimmune neuromyotonia) in a patient with systemic lupus erythematosus. *J Rheumatol* 32(4):757–758, 2005.

322. Kaur PP, Birbe RC, DeHoratius RJ: Rosai-Dorfman disease in a patient with systemic lupus erythematosus. *J Rheumatol* 32(5):951–953, 2005.

323. Cherner M, Isenberg D: The overlap of systemic lupus erythematosus and sickle cell disease: report of two cases and a review of the literature. *Lupus* 19(7):875–883, 2010.

Chapter 45

SLE and Infections

Judith A. James, Andrea L. Sestak, and Evan S. Vista

Infections in systemic lupus erythematosus (SLE) remain a significant source of morbidity and mortality. Both the disease process itself and the accompanying immunosuppression can lead to infections with a wide variety of pathogens, both typical and exotic, as well as influence the way in which such infections develop. This fact, combined with the varied array of baseline symptoms in patients with SLE, makes distinguishing an acute infection from a lupus flare a common clinical challenge. The balancing act of suppressing the immune system enough to prevent autoimmune complications without making patients overly vulnerable to infection remains a challenge to the practicing rheumatologist. Research into biomarkers distinguishing these two states shows promise but they are not yet available at the bedside. This chapter reviews infections in SLE, emphasizing the effect of infections on lupus morbidity and mortality, potential pathogenic mechanisms, susceptibility factors for infection, the clinical spectrum of infection, and biomarkers or other clinical factors that may assist the clinician when differentiating active infection from a SLE disease flare.

MORTALITY AND INFECTIONS IN SYSTEMIC LUPUS ERYTHEMATOSUS

Infection contributes to excess mortality both early and late in the course of SLE and is responsible for approximately 20% to 55% of all deaths in patients with SLE (Table 45-1). A high standardized mortality ratio of 5 for patients with SLE and infection, influenced by gender, age, and disease duration, was reported by Bernatsky and colleagues.[1] In a 10-year prospective multinational cohort study of patients with SLE, infections and cardiovascular events were the most frequent cause of death.[2] The most frequent infectious complications were pneumonia and sepsis of unknown origin. Pulmonary, abdominal, and genitourinary infections during the first 5 years of follow-up were the leading causes of death in a study by Cervera and associates.[2] Parallel studies among patients of Mexican and South African descent also denote infection as the leading cause of mortality.[3,4]

Multiple factors influence mortality from infection in patients with SLE. African-American, Hispanic-American, North American Indian, Eastern Indian, and black Caribbean patients have increased mortality, compared with Caucasian patients.[5-8] Long-term survival of patients of Chinese descent with SLE is comparable to that reported for Caucasians, but it is influenced by the age of onset. In a long-term survival study of an inception cohort of Chinese patients with SLE, survival was significantly worse in patients with late-onset disease (i.e., patients diagnosed after 50 years of age). Survival rates in 5-, 10-, and 15-year studies were 66%, 44%, and 44%, respectively, compared with 92%, 83%, and 80% in the group overall ($P < 0.0001$).[9] Among juvenile patients with SLE, the mortality rate of those hospitalized was associated with sepsis, and infection was an important cause of admission to intensive care units.[10] A low serum albumin was a predictor of mortality and was also associated with increased infections.[11]

PREVALENCE OF INFECTIONS IN SYSTEMIC LUPUS ERYTHEMATOSUS

The rate of infection in patients with SLE determines a major disease burden and accounts for a significant portion of total morbidity. In a multicenter population study documenting 16,751 hospitalizations of 8670 patients with SLE over a 3-year period, 2123 were considered potentially avoidable. Pneumonia was the major cause of avoidable hospitalization (40.1%), along with cellulitis (19.3%) and pyelonephritis (5.3%).[12] A second large study in Mexico estimates the prevalence of infection at 65% in a series of 473 hospitalized patients with SLE.[13] In the intensive care setting, the cause of admission among 104 patients with SLE was infection (61.5%, $n = 64$), most commonly with pneumonia (67.2%), followed by peritonitis (23.4%), urinary tract infection (17.2%), and central nervous system (CNS) infection (4.7%). Most of these patients (96.9%, $n = 62$) also had signs of lupus activity.[13] Long-term prospective data on 66 patients with SLE, a majority of whom were Caucasian, were collected from a Danish population-based study and recorded 26 patients with infection.[14] From these 26 individuals, 20 patients (77%) developed infections before an SLE disease flare, with 1 patient (4%) developing an infection during an SLE flare, and 5 (19%) developing infections after a disease flare, suggesting that infections may trigger increased SLE disease activity in susceptible patients.

A study by Jeong and associates[15] in 2009 cites the incidence of infectious disease as 4.4 in 100 patient-years, with a total follow-up duration of 954 years in a case control study of 110 patients. This incidence rate is significantly reduced from the overall infection rate of 59 in 100 and 142 in 100 patient-years cited from other studies during the past decade. Forty-two patients (38%) had at least one episode of an infectious disease, with the type of infection similar to that in the other studies presented in this text but with 32 community-acquired infections versus 10 nosocomial infections. Pathogens were identified in 24 patients, of whom 5 were identified with *Streptococcus pneumoniae*.[15]

IDENTIFYING INDEPENDENT RISK FACTORS FOR INFECTION IN SYSTEMIC LUPUS ERYTHEMATOSUS

At this time, no definitive test is available to distinguish SLE disease activity from infection, but several risk factors for infection have been identified (Table 45-2). Yuhara and colleagues[16] noted that a model incorporating a decreased serum albumin level increased serum creatinine, and a prednisolone dose equal to or greater than 60 mg per day predicted infection in hospitalized patients with SLE with a sensitivity and specificity of 65% and 91%, respectively. Usually, fever is also a sign of infection and is otherwise rare in patients with SLE receiving prednisone at maintenance doses or greater. Additional risk factors include hypocomplementemia, active nephritis,[17] neutropenia[18] (although not leukopenia),[19] and lymphopenia.[20] Other independent predictors of infection at the time of SLE diagnosis are an Systemic Lupus Erythematosus Disease Activity Index (SLEDAI) greater than 12 ($p = 0.01$), C3 levels less than 90 mg/dL ($P = 0.01$), and positive anti–double stranded DNA (anti-dsDNA) antibodies ($P < 0.01$).[15] Frequent disease flares ($p = 0.04$) and follow-up disease duration of 8 years or longer ($p = 0.023$) were also significant risk factors for increased infections in patients with SLE.[15] (See Table 45-2 for additional information regarding a

TABLE 45-1 Infection as a Cause of Death in Patients with Systemic Lupus Erythematosus

COUNTRY	NUMBER OF PATIENTS	NUMBER OF DEATHS	DEATHS CAUSED BY INFECTION (%)	YEARS INCLUDED	REFERENCE
United States	138	38	39	1949-1954	S1
United States	223	55	36	1966-1976	S2
United States	609	128	21	1950-1980	S3
United States	1103	222	33	1965-1978	S4
Canada	417	51	28	1970-1983	29
United States	464	26	19	1980-1989	S5
Thailand	537	77	30	1980-1989	S6
Chile	218	48	12	1970-1991	S7
Mexico	65	14	29	1970-1993	S8
Korea	544	43	33	1993-1997	S9
Denmark	513	122	21	1975-1995	S10
China	186	9	67	1975-1999	S11
Puerto Rico	662	161	27	1960-1994	S12
France	87	10	20	1960-1997	26
Korea	110	7	71	1991-2000	15
Brazil*	71	18	52	1994-2003	S13
Europe†	1000	68	25	1990-2000	2
SLICC, CaNIOS‡	9547	1255	3.6	1958-2001	1
China	442	30	60	2000-2006	S14
Britain	470	67	25	1978-2007	28
Spain	705	195	38.6	1980-2008	S15
Philippines*	78	9	77	2004-2008	S16

CaNIOS = Canadian Network for Imporved Oucomes in Systemic Lupus Erythematosus. SLICC = Systemic Lupus International Collaborating Clinics.
*Pediatric SLE study.
†Includes the United Kingdom, Poland, Spain, Turkey, Norway, Italy, and Belgium.
‡Includes North America, the United Kingdom, Iceland, Sweden, and South Korea.
References labeled S are supplementary references that can be found in the online supplementary material for this chapter.

summary of risk factors for infection from a variety of published clinical studies.)[15-18,20-32]

FACTORS THAT INFLUENCE INFECTION SUSCEPTIBILITY IN SYSTEMIC LUPUS ERYTHEMATOSUS

A number of different intrinsic and extrinsic factors are thought to increase patient susceptibility to infection in those with SLE. Patients with SLE have dysregulated immune systems that are often focused on targeting self, rather than protecting against invading pathogens. Defects in macrophages, neutrophils, T cells, natural killer (NK) cells, and B cells may all be critical in the increased risk of infection in SLE patients (Figure 45-1). In addition, select patients with SLE may have defects in immunoglobulin production, complement, and reticuloendothelial pathways that increase the risks for infection. Immunosuppressive actions of a number of standard lupus therapeutic agents also increase the risks for infection. Finally, evolving data suggest that select defects in mannose-binding pathways and fragmented, crystallizable gamma receptor (FcγR) systems may also play roles in the risk for infection in patients with SLE. These issues are briefly discussed in the following text and are reviewed in greater detail in Section two and in the literature.[33,34]

Systemic Lupus Erythematosus Intrinsic Immune Dysfunction

Macrophages

The monocytes of SLE patients have decreased phagocytic activity and impaired ability to engulf apoptotic cells.[35] Superoxide generation is also diminished in these patients after FcγR phagocytosis. Patients with SLE can also have autoantibodies against the FcγRs, as well as genetic polymorphisms within this receptor family, which may decrease the effectiveness of phagocytosis.[35] Any or all of these intrinsic immune defects may decrease pathogen clearance and increase the risk of, as well as the ability to respond to, select infections in patients with SLE.

Neutrophils

Neutropenia is a common finding in patients with SLE. Neutrophils in these patients have been shown to have impaired phagocytosis, and this impairment is more pronounced in patients with active disease.[36] The neutrophils of these patients also have impaired chemotaxis[37] and reduced opsonization.[38] These factors combine to decrease effective immune responses against invading pathogens.

T Cells and Natural Killer Cells

Patients with SLE are known to have a variety of T-cell defects. Significant lymphopenia is commonly observed in untreated patients, which can often correlate with increased disease activity. Lymphopenia has also been correlated with increased infectious risk. T cells in these patients have impaired production of a number of cytokines, such as interferon gamma (IFN-γ), interleukin (IL)-1, IL-2, and tumor necrosis factor–alpha (TNF-α), all of which may increase the risk of infection. Extensive discussion of SLE–T cell abnormalities are presented in Chapter 9. Patients with SLE have also been shown to have decreased numbers of NK cells,[39] and circulating autoantibodies to NK-cell surface antigens may also contribute to decreased

TABLE 45-2 Identified Risk Factors for Infection in Systemic Lupus Erythematosus Patients

TYPE OF INFECTION	RISK FACTORS	REFERENCE
All infections	Active lupus nephritis, disease activity, disease flares, prednisone dose, leukopenia, intravenous steroids and/or immunosuppressive drugs, neutropenia, lymphopenia, complement levels	Ginzler and colleagues, 1978[24] Nived, Sturfelt, Wollheim, 1985[25] Cervera and colleagues, 1999[23] Noel and colleagues, 2001[26] Kang, Park, 2003[51] Bosch and colleagues, 2006[22] Ng and colleagues, 2006[20] Dias and colleagues, 2009[18] Goldblatt and colleagues, 2009[28] Jeong and colleagues, 2009[15] Vargas, King, Navarra, 2009[21] Sayeeda and colleagues, 2010[27]
Major, at time of death	Prednisone dose, cytotoxic drugs, disease activity, disease duration	Rubin, Urowitz, Gladman, 1985[29] Ruiz-Irastorza and colleagues, 2009[17]
Fatal opportunistic	Prednisone dose, cytotoxic drugs, complement levels Disease activity	Hellmann, Petri, Whiting-O'Keefe, 1987[30]
During hospitalization	Disease activity, prednisone dose	Duffy, Duffy, Gladman, 1991[31]
Hospitalization for infection	Disease activity, prednisone or prednisolone dose, cytotoxic drugs	Petri, Genovese, 1992[32] Yuhara and colleagues, 1996[16]

NK-cell activity.[40] Impaired T-cell responses in patients with SLE may diminish the ability to respond to viruses and other intracellular pathogens.

B Cells and Immunoglobulin
Autoantibody production, B-cell hyperactivity, and polyclonal B-cell activation are nearly universal in SLE. B-cell abnormalities are described in greater detail in Chapter 8 and Section 3. Some patients with SLE suffer from hypogammaglobulinemia, immunoglobulin (Ig) G subclass deficiencies, IgA deficiencies, or various combinations that could all lead to increased susceptibility to infections.

Reticuloendothelial System Defects
The spleen is the major component of the reticuloendothelial system (RES), and dysfunction of this organ has been described, leading to severe cases of bacterial sepsis.[41] Disease activity has also been correlated with defective clearance of IgG-sensitized erythrocytes by the RES.[42]

Therapeutic Toxicities
Aggressive immunomodulation with glucocorticoids and cytotoxic drugs has dramatically improved the survival rates of patients with SLE. As a consequence, however, severe infections as a result of the chronic immunodeficient state created by these drugs have become major secondary causes of morbidity and mortality. Additionally, patients with SLE are more susceptible to infections than patients with other systemic rheumatic diseases treated with comparable agents. Immunosuppressive drugs used in the treatment of SLE, such as high-dose cyclophosphamide, azathioprine, mycophenolate mofetil, and repeated rituximab,[43-45] have been implicated in causing

hypogammaglobulinemia, which predisposes patients to a range of infections typically observed in inherited immunodeficiencies.

Glucocorticoids
After 50 years of effective use, glucocorticoids remain a mainstay of lupus therapy. Although their role as powerful immunosuppressants is central to their success as therapeutic agents, the resulting dysregulation of immunity may enhance the susceptibility to the development of infectious disease.[46] Glucocorticoids affect cellular function primarily by altering gene regulation via the direct transmission of signals to the nucleus.[47] Although the resulting decrease of inflammation is, in fact, the desired therapeutic outcome, both autoinflammatory and pathogen specific immune responses are inhibited by steroid treatment. Glucocorticoids decrease the number of circulating dendritic cells,[47] possibly impairing antigen presentation to naive T cells and, subsequently, the responses to new infectious agents. They also inhibit the recruitment of neutrophils and monocyte/macrophages to the inflammatory site and depress monocyte and neutrophil bactericidal activity.

Several studies evaluated the infections in patients with SLE who are receiving glucocorticoid therapy; however, patients with the most active disease usually receive the highest doses of steroids. Prednisolone is a risk factor for the development of CNS infection in patients with SLE if administered at high doses at the onset of infection and high mean doses within the previous year.[48] Tam and colleagues[49] reported that the cumulative dose, maximum oral dose, and administration by pulse therapy were all independent risk factors for tuberculosis (TB) in patients with SLE who are undergoing steroid therapy. Badsha and colleagues[11] showed a high infection rate in the group of patients taking at least 20 mg/day of prednisone for at least 1 month with a history of administration of cyclophosphamide. Low-dose pulse methylprednisolone (1 to 1.5 g over 3 days) was effective in controlling SLE flares and was associated with fewer serious infections than the more traditional high-dose treatment (1 g per day for 3 days). The incidence of infectious complications rises with increased daily doses given for longer than 4 weeks. In one series, a 10 mg per day increase of prednisone increased the risk of serious infection eleven-fold.[17] The relative risk ratio for infection was reported to be 1 to 6 in all patients receiving corticosteroid therapy, compared with those not receiving corticosteroids; in addition, alternate-day steroid use considerably reduces the risk of infection.[17,50]

Other Immunosuppressive Systemic Lupus Erythematosus Therapies
Cyclophosphamide causes neutropenia through both decreased production and increased destruction of neutrophils. Cyclophosphamide use was associated with an increased incidence of herpes zoster infection, and the infection rates in patients receiving the oral and intravenous forms of the drug were found to be comparable.[51,52] The rate of infections in patients with SLE and nephritis who were treated with cyclophosphamide plus low-dose steroids is the same as that observed in patients treated with high-dose steroids alone. Pulse cyclophosphamide therapy for lupus nephritis is associated with rates of infections similar to those of daily oral cytotoxic treatment.[19]

Azathioprine and its metabolite inhibit protein synthesis. Treatment results in lymphopenia and suppressed immunoglobulin synthesis.[53] Neutrophil function seems to remain intact with azathioprine therapy; however, neutropenia may result from bone marrow suppression, thus predisposing the patient to infection. This type of neutropenia seems to be dose dependent. Infections complicating cyclosporine therapy are similar to those associated with defective cell-mediated immunity and are thought to arise from impaired transmission of activation signals from the T-cell receptor by calcineurin. Cyclosporine binds to cyclophilin, an endogenous intracellular protein, resulting in a complex that inhibits the activity of calcineurin.[54] The incidence of infectious complications appears less frequent with mycophenolate mofetil, an inhibitor of inosine-5′-monophosphate that preferentially inhibits B-cell and T-cell

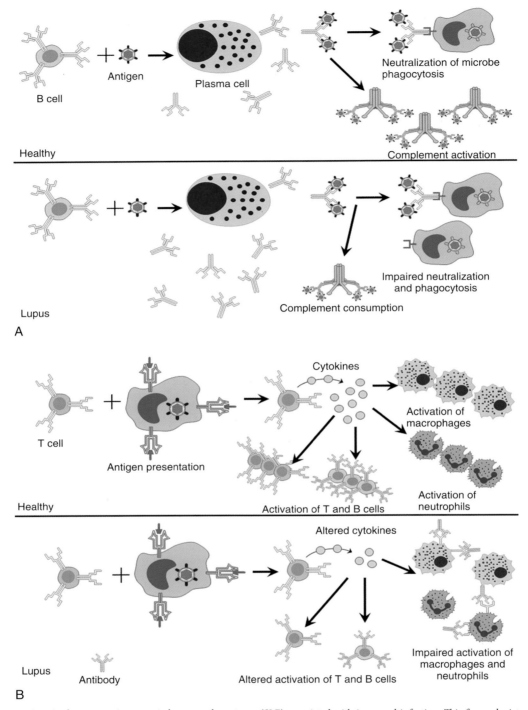

FIGURE 45-1 Common impaired processes in systemic lupus erythematosus (SLE) associated with increased infection. This figure depicts common impaired humoral processes (**A**) and cell-mediated processes (**B**) in SLE that are associated with increased infection risk.

functions, as compared with cyclophosphamide.[51] Herpes zoster is still the most common viral infection in patients with SLE who are treated with cyclophosphamides or mycophenolate mofetil.[51]

Biologic therapies are, by and large, still in the clinical trial phases, and therefore the data on infectious complications from such therapies are limited. A metaanalysis performed by Salliot and associates[55] investigated the risk of serious infections of several biologic treatments in SLE. This study did not reveal a significant increase in the risk of serious infection during treatment with rituximab, a peripheral B cell–depleting anti-CD20 monoclonal antibody. Among

those patients receiving rituximab who experienced serious infections, bacterial respiratory tract infections were the most common.[55] Newer reviews, however, highlight the potential concern for more serious infections with rituximab, including, for example, reactivation of hepatitis B, *Pneumocystis* infection, or rarely progressive multifocal leukoencephalopathy.[56]

Belimumab, an anti–B lymphocyte stimulator (anti-BLyS) and B cell–activating factor (BAFF)–directed therapeutic, is the first drug approved by the U.S. Food and Drug Administration (FDA) for SLE in over 50 years. Because belimumab is a new therapeutic drug, few data exist regarding the infection risks in these patients. In a large phase III study of the drug ($n = 867$), serious infection was reported in 22 patients (8%) receiving 1 mg/kg belimumab, 13 patients (4%) receiving 10 mg/kg belimumab, and 17 patients (6%) receiving a placebo.[57] However, real-world use of the medication is needed to determine the clinical rates of infection in anti-BLyS–treated individuals.

The combined use of steroids and cyclophosphamide presents the strongest risk factor for infectious complications. The magnitude of effect of these agents is dose dependent. Careful monitoring and prompt and appropriate treatment of infections in these individuals are therefore imperative. Although these drugs are valuable tools for the treatment of active disease, the choice of dose, route, and timing should be thoroughly balanced with the risk of infection and other side effects.

Hydroxychloroquine Use and Protection from Infection

Among the therapeutic modalities currently being used for SLE, only hydroxychloroquine is usually considered immunomodulatory without being immunosuppressive. Hydroxychloroquine downregulates the processing of low-affinity antigens, such as self peptides, while preserving the processing of high-affinity antigens, such as foreign peptides derived from infectious agents.[58] In fact, patients taking antimalarial medications are 16 times less likely to suffer a major infection.[17] An antimalarial drug also blocks activation of Toll-like receptors (TLRs) on plasmacytoid dendritic cells and shows a strong inverse association with major infections. In vitro activity of hydroxychloroquine has also been reported against numerous bacteria (e.g., *Tropheryma whipplei*, *Staphylococcus aureus*, *Legionella pneumophila*, *Francisella tularensis*, *Mycobacterium* spp., *Salmonella typhi*, *Escherichia coli*, *Borrelia burgdorferi*), fungi (*Histoplasma capsulatum*, *Cryptococcus neoformans*, *Aspergillus fumigatus*), and viruses, including human immunodeficiency virus (HIV).[59]

Select Genetic Defects and Risk of Infection

Mannose-Binding Lectin

Patients with SLE and homozygous variant alleles for mannose-binding lectin (MBL) have been shown to have significantly increased risk of infection (odds ratio [OR] = 8.6).[60] MBL is structurally similar to complement 1q (C1q), which binds to antibodies and protein structures on bacteria and viruses. Homozygosity for MBL-variant alleles was demonstrated in 7.7% of patients with SLE, compared with 2.8% of patients in a control group. Among homozygotes, the time between SLE diagnosis and first infection was significantly shorter, and the annual number of infections was four times higher than in patients who were heterozygous or homozygous for the normal allele.[60] Patients with SLE and homozygous risk MBL alleles has also been shown to have increased infection risk in general and of respiratory infections in particular.[61] Patients of Chinese descent with MBL-risk haplotypes are also at increased risk of infection.[62]

Fc-Gamma Receptors

Polymorphisms in the inhibitory FcγR RIIB have been associated with SLE and have recently also been shown to protect against malaria.[63] Saturation of Fc receptors on spleen and liver cells by immune complexes or dysfunctional Fc receptors on monocyte cell surfaces may prevent the clearance of opsonized bacteria and increase the susceptibility to overwhelming pneumococcal bacteremia and *Salmonella* carrier state observed in some patients with SLE.

Complement Components

SLE is common in individuals with genetic defects in early aspects of the early complement system (C1q, C1r, C1s, C4, and, to a lesser degree, C2), which increases the risk of infection. Although the majority of patients with SLE do not have congenital defects of complement components, inactive disease consumption of complement, as well as decreased expression of complement receptors on erythrocytes, may also increase the risk of infection.

PROTEAN SPECTRUM OF INFECTION IN SYSTEMIC LUPUS ERYTHEMATOSUS

A broad spectrum of infections has been reported in SLE. In addition to unusual opportunistic fungal and protozoan infections, common pathogens may behave more aggressively and cause more severe infections in patients with SLE. A major obstacle to recognizing infection in these patients stems from the similarities in clinical features of disease flare and infection, as well as atypical presentations of infections.

Bacteria

Bacteria are the most frequent causes of infection, and the urinary tract is the most frequent site in patients with SLE. *E. coli* has been reported as the most frequent uropathogen (23 out of 30 cultures; 76.6%).[64] Some studies suggest that susceptibility to acute pyelonephritis by select *E. coli* strains may have a genetic basis; for example, individuals positive for the P blood group who have low expression of neutrophil-activating chemokine ligand 1 (CXCR1) and TLR 4 were observed to have a higher incidence of *E. coli* pyelonephritis.[64]

S. pneumoniae infections are also common and often severe in patients with SLE. The preponderance of this infection in lupus is attributed to impaired clearance of the encapsulated bacteria.[65] *S. aureus* infections are also common, affecting the lung, sinuses, skin, and bone. *Salmonella* bacteremia is found more frequently in hospitalized patients with SLE than in other patients with chronic disease.[66] *Salmonella enteritidis B* is a common pathogen of SLE septic arthritis.[67] Septic arthritis is a medical emergency, and thus a high index of suspicion is warranted when patients have acute monoarticular pain and swelling. The most common articular predisposing factor for septic arthritis in patients with SLE is avascular necrosis of the hip.[66]

Among patients with SLE, an episode of bacteremia was associated with an unfavorable long-term outcome. The bacterial species significantly influenced short-term survival.[68] Thus initiating empiric antibiotic treatment covering the pathogens suspected at the first sign of infection is recommended.

Mycobacterium

Aside from factors inherent to the disease, endemicity plays an important role in the increased frequency of *Mycobacterium tuberculosis* infections in developing countries. In a summary of published studies on TB in SLE,[69] the incidence of TB among patients with SLE was seven-fold higher than expected in the general population in certain areas. Extrapulmonary involvement was present in 22% to 66% of patients, and mortality was 5% to 31% among Asians with SLE and TB. Deaths were primarily due to disseminated disease, especially among those with concomitant active lupus. Although routine prophylaxis with isoniazid has been proposed in patients with SLE, the efficacy of this practice is not well established. The increased incidence of extrapulmonary TB (in the absence of pulmonary symptoms) may predispose patients to drug resistance when receiving isoniazid prophylaxis rather than the combination treatment for active TB. Cutaneous granulomatous lesions, with ulcerations in particular, appear in patients with established SLE, especially when further enhanced immunosuppressive interventions fail.[70] In a cohort study by Mok and colleagues,[71] soft tissue and skin were the predominant sites of involvement by nontuberculous mycobacterium and clinically manifested as local or disseminated skin nodules or abscesses. Chronic skin ulcers and cellulitis were also occasionally seen and may mimic lupus-related cutaneous vasculitis. One postulate is that the cytokine milieu found in active SLE at disease onset could lead to a functionally immunodeficient state that renders the patient more susceptible to TB infection. Alternatively, the immune factors involved in controlling TB infection, such as IFN-γ, could precipitate the first manifestation of SLE in a susceptible person.

Although CNS infections are not common in patients with SLE, they do account for a significant amount of mortality.[72] Furthermore, the presenting symptoms can resemble those of a lupus flare or neuropsychiatric lupus, making accurate diagnosis and the institution of appropriate therapy difficult. The pathogenic agents responsible for CNS infections in a Chinese cohort of patients with SLE showed that *Mycobacterium tuberculosis* (50%) was the most common cause of CNS infections in that demographic, followed in frequency by *C. neoformans* (31.6%), *Listeria monocytogenes* (7.9%), *Klebsiella pneumoniae* (2.6%), *S. aureus* (2.6%), gram-positive bacteria (2.6%), and *Aspergillus fumigatus* (2.6%).[18] The presentation of tuberculous meningitis in patients with SLE is commonly associated with extrapulmonary or multiorgan involvement and lower levels of serum albumin.[48]

Viruses

Empiric antibiotic therapy is often initiated in a febrile patient with SLE and no clear source of infection while awaiting culture results. This practice can contribute to a higher rate of opportunistic infections, which are a common cause of death in patients with SLE. With the exception of herpes zoster, which is oftentimes somewhat easily diagnosed, the majority of reported opportunistic infections cannot be identified antemortem.[5,15,68,73]

Among viral infections, those caused by herpes zoster are the most common in SLE. Decreased delayed-type skin hypersensitivity against the varicella antigens in patients with SLE suggests impaired herpes zoster cellular immunity.[74] Differentiating SLE from HIV infection can be challenging in HIV-endemic regions because of overlapping clinical features and the prevalence of a positive antinuclear antibody (ANA) test among patients with HIV.

Fungal

Active lupus is also a risk factor for fungal infection in patients with SLE. The most common fungal infection is *Candida*, affecting the pharynx, esophagus, urinary tract, and soft tissues. In a study by Chen and colleagues,[75] patients with SLE and fungal infections had a poorer prognosis than the general SLE population. Disseminated candidiasis and *Nocardia* infections are common fungal infections in steroid-treated patients with SLE, particularly in the lung.[75] Severe lymphopenia, associated either with increased disease activity or with aggressive immunosuppression, is associated with *Pneumocystis jirovecii* pneumonia, leading some experts to support prophylaxis in patients with very low lymphocyte counts.[76]

A few cases of SLE and mucormycosis have been documented, and the combination is associated with higher mortality (61% to 80%).[77] The patient's clinical features typically include sinus disease with concomitant neurologic or pulmonary symptoms or both. Hypocomplementemia, lupus nephritis, and uremia were identified as predisposing factors. *Blastomyces dermatitidis,* an infection usually seen among domesticated animals, should be suspected when acid-fast positive material with no bacilliform organisms is seen on Ziehl-Neelsen skin biopsy preparations for patients with SLE and cutaneous lesions.[78]

Parasitic and Protozoan

Immunocompromised patients also need an early diagnosis and specific treatment, because they are at increased risk of acquiring parasitic diseases and their associated complications.[59] Hyperinfection with *Strongyloides stercoralis* may occur in patients with SLE and is characterized by profound malabsorption, diarrhea, electrolyte abnormalities, and, at times, even superinfection, coma, and death. Visceral leishmaniasis and paragonimiasis have also been reported. Eosinophilia is not a good marker for parasitic infection in patients with SLE; it may not be observed as a result of corticosteroid use.

Toxoplasmosis has also been described in patients with SLE and active disease or aggressive immunosuppression.[79] The CNS symptoms of this infection can mimic lupus cerebritis, and false-positive antibody tests are also found in SLE. In addition, toxoplasma infection may increase autoantibody production, which may interfere with standard immunologic testing for infection.[79]

USING SYSTEMIC LUPUS ERYTHEMATOSUS BIOMARKERS TO DIFFERENTIATE BETWEEN INFECTION AND DISEASE FLARE

Deciding on a course of therapy in a febrile patient with SLE is often difficult, because no definite point of contact laboratory parameters are sufficiently reliable to distinguish a lupus flare from an acute infection. Moreover, these disease processes are not mutually exclusive and commonly occur together. Among the readily available tests, published data suggest that C-reactive protein (CRP) may help differentiate an infectious entity from an SLE exacerbation.[80] With use of a cut-off of high-sensitivity CRP (hsCRP) above 6 mg/dL, hsCRP correlates with infection with a specificity of 84%. In particular, CRP levels greater than 6 mg/dL in a patient without pleuritis strongly suggests the presence of an infection.[81]

Active investigation is ongoing to identify potential biomarkers that can distinguish infection from a lupus flare. Procalcitonin, induced by bacterial endotoxin and a TNF-α pathway mediator, has been investigated as one such potential biomarker for bacterial infection, although it is not useful for TB or viral infection.[82] Another study found that soluble levels of triggering receptor expressed in myeloid cells 1 (sTREM-1) were significantly increased in infection compared with the flare at the onset of fever and days 1 and 2 of a febrile episode.[83] 2′5′-oligoadenylate synthetase (OAS) isoforms have also been reported as potential biomarkers of infection in some microarray gene expression studies.[84] The expression of three isoforms of OAS (OAS1, OAS2, and OASL) was upregulated in a cohort study of newly diagnosed patients with active SLE, and was lower in SLE complicated with infections. These findings offer a new perspective for the application of blood leukocyte expression signatures for the diagnosis and differentiation of SLE disease activity and infectious diseases.[85]

CLINICAL APPROACH TO PATIENTS WITH SYSTEMIC LUPUS ERYTHEMATOSUS AND A SUSPECTED INFECTION

The clinical signs and symptoms of infection may present a mixed picture with the manifestations of SLE, thus making it more difficult to attain effective therapeutic management. Clinical presentations are variable, from fatal sepsis to simple skin or soft-tissue infections. Fever in a patient with SLE requires prompt evaluation. Although fever can be an indicator of autoimmune disease activity, it is rare in those patients of SLE receiving immunosuppressive medications. Therefore a febrile patient with SLE will often have a clinical infection requiring immediate evaluation and prompt therapy. Patients with SLE and clinical infections can also suffer from concurrent disease flares, resulting in the judicious use of concurrent antimicrobial treatment in combination with corticosteroids or other immunomodulatory medications when clinically warranted. Consideration of infections is mandatory to care adequately for patients with SLE who present with fever or other infectious manifestations. Prospective and controlled studies in this group are difficult, and therefore the literature on infectious complications among patients with SLE is full of widely varied reports. These studies demonstrate the global aspect of infection. It transcends individual factors such as socioeconomic background, access to health care, and genetics in becoming a significant predictor of SLE mortality. The need to develop effective disease markers in distinguishing infection from disease flare is therefore preeminent. At present, clinicians must rely on constant vigilance, knowledge of identified risk factors, and optimal judicious use of cytotoxic medications. A full awareness of the wide array of disease pathogens and their diverse clinical presentations will assist with the diagnosis and management of patients with SLE and infectious complications.

SUMMARY

Key points summarized in this chapter include the following:
- Infections remain an important cause of morbidity and mortality in patients with SLE of all races and socioeconomic backgrounds.

- Susceptibility to infection may be increased by at least two major factors: (1) the immune dysregulation that is the hallmark of SLE, and (2) the influence of immunosuppressive therapies in impairing response to infection.
- The long-term use of corticosteroids in increased doses and their combined use with cyclophosphamide present the highest risk for infection, whereas the use of hydroxychloroquine among patients with SLE may decrease the risk of infection.
- Select genetic defects in MBL and complement components promote the risk of infection in SLE.
- The broad spectrum of organisms isolated from infected patients with SLE includes common organisms, as well as exotic pathogens causing opportunistic infections, especially in patients with active SLE and ongoing immunosuppression.
- Bacteria are the most common infectious organisms, mainly infecting the urinary tract for ambulatory patients and causing pneumonia among hospitalized patients.
- Timely differentiation between the presence of active infection and a SLE disease flare, or the concomitant presentation of both, has been a long-standing challenge compromising therapeutic outcomes for patients with SLE. Several independent risk factors have been identified, and potential biomarkers differentiating infection from flare are being developed.

ACKNOWLEDGMENTS

We are grateful to Julie Robertson, PhD, for scientific editing. This work was supported in part by the National Institutes of Health (AI47575, AR45451, AR48045, RR031152, AR48940, RR020143, AR49084, AR053483, and AI082714) and from the Oklahoma Medical Research Foundation (OMRF), Lou C. Kerr, Chair in Biomedical Research and Kirkland Scholar Award Program. The contents of this work in are the sole responsibility of the authors and do not necessarily represent the official views of the NIH or its relevant institutes.

References

1. Bernatsky S, Boivin JF, Joseph L, et al: Mortality in systemic lupus erythematosus. *Arthritis Rheum* 54:2550–2557, 2006.
2. Cervera R, Khamashta MA, Font J, et al: Morbidity and mortality in systemic lupus erythematosus during a 10-year period: a comparison of early and late manifestations in a cohort of 1,000 patients. *Medicine* 82:299–308, 2003.
3. Zonana-Nacach A, Yañez P, Jiménez-Balderas FJ, et al: Disease activity, damage and survival in Mexican patients with acute severe systemic lupus erythematosus. *Lupus* 16:997–1000, 2007.
4. Wadee S, Tikly M, Hopley M: Causes and predictors of death in South Africans with systemic lupus erythematosus. *Rheumatology (Oxford)* 46:1487–1491, 2007.
5. Ippolito A, Petri M: An update on mortality in systemic lupus erythematosus. *Clin Exp Rheumatol* 26:S72–S79, 2008.
6. Fernández M, Alarcón GS, Calvo-Alén J, et al: A multiethnic, multicenter cohort of patients with systemic lupus erythematosus (SLE) as a model for the study of ethnic disparities in SLE. *Arthritis Rheum* 57:576–584, 2007.
7. Trager J, Ward MM: Mortality and causes of death in systemic lupus erythematosus. *Curr Opin Rheumatol* 13:345–351, 2001.
8. Tikly M, Navarra SV: Lupus in the developing world—is it any different? *Best Pract Res Clin Rheumatol* 22:643–655, 2008.
9. Mok CC, Mak A, Chu WP, et al: Long-term survival of southern Chinese patients with systemic lupus erythematosus: a prospective study of all age-groups. *Medicine* 84:218–224, 2005.
10. Chen YS, Yang YH, Lin YT, et al: Risk of infection in hospitalised children with systemic lupus erythematosus: a 10-year follow-up. *Clin Rheumatol* 23:235–238, 2004.
11. Badsha H, Kong KO, Lian TY, et al: Low-dose pulse methylprednisolone for systemic lupus erythematosus flares is efficacious and has a decreased risk of infectious complications. *Lupus* 11:508–513, 2002.
12. Ward MM: Avoidable hospitalizations in patients with systemic lupus erythematosus. *Arthritis Rheum* 59:162–168, 2008.
13. Namendys-Silva SA, Baltazar-Torres JA, Rivero-Sigarroa E, et al: Prognostic factors in patients with systemic lupus erythematosus admitted to the intensive care unit. *Lupus* 18:1252–1258, 2009.
14. Laustrup H, Voss A, Green A, et al: SLE disease patterns in a Danish population-based lupus cohort: an 8-year prospective study. *Lupus* 19:239–246, 2010.
15. Jeong SJ, Choi H, Lee HS, et al: Incidence and risk factors of infection in a single cohort of 110 adults with systemic lupus erythematosus. *Scand J Infect Dis* 41:268–274, 2009.
16. Yuhara T, Takemura H, Akama T, et al: Predicting infection in hospitalized patients with systemic lupus erythematosus. *Intern Med* 35:629–636, 1996.
17. Ruiz-Irastorza G, Olivares N, Ruiz-Arruza I, et al: Predictors of major infections in systemic lupus erythematosus. *Arthritis Res Ther* 11:R109, 2009.
18. Dias AM, do Couto MC, Duarte CC, et al: White blood cell count abnormalities and infections in one-year follow-up of 124 patients with SLE. *Ann N Y Acad Sci* 1173:103–107, 2009.
19. Opastirakul S, Chartapisak W: Infection in children with lupus nephritis receiving pulse and oral cyclophosphamide therapy. *Pediatr Nephrol* 20:1750–1755, 2005.
20. Ng WL, Chu CM, Wu AK, et al: Lymphopenia at presentation is associated with increased risk of infections in patients with systemic lupus erythematosus. *QJM* 99:37–47, 2006.
21. Vargas PJ, King G, Navarra SV: Central nervous system infections in Filipino patients with systemic lupus erythematosus. *Int J Rheum Dis* 12:234–238, 2009.
22. Bosch X, Guilabert A, Pallarés L, et al: Infections in systemic lupus erythematosus: a prospective and controlled study of 110 patients. *Lupus* 15:584–589, 2006.
23. Cervera R, Khamashta MA, Font J, et al: Morbidity and mortality in systemic lupus erythematosus during a 5-year period. A multicenter prospective study of 1,000 patients. European Working Party on Systemic Lupus Erythematosus. *Medicine* 78:167–175, 1999.
24. Ginzler E, Diamond H, Kaplan D, et al: Computer analysis of factors influencing frequency of infection in systemic lupus erythematosus. *Arthritis Rheum* 21:37–44, 1978.
25. Nived O, Sturfelt G, Wollheim F: Systemic lupus erythematosus and infection: a controlled and prospective study including an epidemiological group. *Q J Med* 55:271–287, 1985.
26. Noël V, Lortholary O, Casassus P, et al: Risk factors and prognostic influence of infection in a single cohort of 87 adults with systemic lupus erythematosus. *Ann Rheum Dis* 60:1141–1144, 2001.
27. Sayeeda A, Al Arfaj H, Khalil N, et al: Herpes zoster infections in SLE in a university hospital in Saudi Arabia: risk factors and outcomes. *Autoimmune Dis* 2011:174891, 2010.
28. Goldblatt F, Chambers S, Rahman A, et al: Serious infections in British patients with systemic lupus erythematosus: hospitalizations and mortality. *Lupus* 18:682–689, 2009.
29. Rubin LA, Urowitz MB, Gladman DD: Mortality in systemic lupus erythematosus: the bimodal pattern revisited. *Q J Med* 55:87–98, 1985.
30. Hellmann DB, Petri M, Whiting-O'Keefe Q: Fatal infections in systemic lupus erythematosus: the role of opportunistic organisms. *Medicine (Baltimore)* 66:341–348, 1987.
31. Duffy KN, Duffy CM, Gladman DD: Infection and disease activity in systemic lupus erythematosus: a review of hospitalized patients. *J Rheumatol* 18:1180–1184, 1991.
32. Petri M, Genovese M: Incidence of and risk factors for hospitalizations in systemic lupus erythematosus: a prospective study of the Hopkins Lupus Cohort. *J Rheumatol* 19:1559–1565, 1992.
33. Sjöholm AG, Jönsson G, Braconier JH, et al: Complement deficiency and disease: an update. *Mol Immunol* 43:78–85, 2006.
34. Smith KG, Clatworthy MR: FcgammaRIIB in autoimmunity and infection: evolutionary and therapeutic implications. *Nat Rev Immunol* 10:328–343, 2010.
35. Li Y, Lee P, Reeves W: Monocyte and macrophage abnormalities in systemic lupus erythematosus. *Arch Immunol Ther Exp* 58:355–364, 2010.
36. Yu CL, Chang KL, Chiu CC, et al: Defective phagocytosis, decreased tumour necrosis factor-alpha production, and lymphocyte hyporesponsiveness predispose patients with systemic lupus erythematosus to infections. *Scand J Rheumatol* 18:97–105, 1989.
37. Goetzl EJ: Defective responsiveness to ascorbic acid of neutrophil random and chemotactic migration in Felty's syndrome and systemic lupus erythematosus. *Ann Rheum Dis* 35:510–515, 1976.
38. Nived O, Linder C, Odeberg H, et al: Reduced opsonisation of protein A containing *Staphylococcus aureus* in sera with cryoglobulins from patients with active systemic lupus erythematosus. *Ann Rheum Dis* 44:252–259, 1985.

39. Erkeller-Yüsel F, Hulstaart F, Hannet I, et al: Lymphocyte subsets in a large cohort of patients with systemic lupus erythematosus. *Lupus* 2:227–231, 1993.

40. Nived O, Johanson I, Sturfelt G: Effects of ultraviolet irradiation on natural killer cell function in systemic lupus erythematosus. *Ann Rheum Dis* 51:726–730, 1992.

41. Piliero P, Furie F: Functional asplenia in systemic lupus erythematosus. *Semin Arthritis Rheum* 20:185–189, 1990.

42. Frank MM, Hamburger MI, Lawley TJ, et al: Defective reticuloendothelial system Fc-receptor function in systemic lupus erythematosus. *N Engl J Med* 300:518–523, 1979.

43. Fedor ME, Rubinstein A: Effects of long-term low-dose corticosteroid therapy on humoral immunity. *Ann Allergy Asthma Immunol* 97:113–116, 2006.

44. Edwards JC, Cambridge G, Leandro MJ: B cell depletion therapy in rheumatic disease. *Best Pract Res Clin Rheumatol* 20:915–928, 2006.

45. Bresnihan B, Cunnane G: Infection complications associated with the use of biologic agents. *Rheum Dis Clin North Am* 29:185–202, 2003.

46. Tait AS, Butts CL, Sternberg EM: The role of glucocorticoids and progestins in inflammatory, autoimmune, and infectious disease. *J Leukoc Biol* 84:924–931, 2008.

47. Rozkova D, Horvath R, Bartunkova J, et al: Glucocorticoids severely impair differentiation and antigen presenting function of dendritic cells despite upregulation of Toll-like receptors. *Clin Immunol* 120:260–271, 2006.

48. Yang CD, Wang XD, Ye S, et al: Clinical features, prognostic and risk factors of central nervous system infections in patients with systemic lupus erythematosus. *Clin Rheumatol* 26:895–901, 2007.

49. Tam LS, Li EK, Wong SM, et al: Risk factors and clinical features for tuberculosis among patients with systemic lupus erythematosus in Hong Kong. *Scand J Rheumatol* 31:296–300, 2002.

50. Toussirot E, Streit G, Wendling D: Infectious complications with anti-TNFalpha therapy in rheumatic diseases: a review. *Recent Pat Inflamm Allergy Drug Discov* 1:39–47, 2007.

51. Kang I, Park SH: Infectious complications in SLE after immunosuppressive therapies. *Curr Opin Rheumatol* 15:528–534, 2003.

52. Ramos-Casals M, Cuadrado MJ, Alba P, et al: Acute viral infections in patients with systemic lupus erythematosus: description of 23 cases and review of the literature. *Medicine* 87:311–318, 2008.

53. Segal BH, Sneller MC: Infectious complications of immunosuppressive therapy in patients with rheumatic diseases. *Rheum Dis Clin North Am* 23:219–237, 1997.

54. Schreiber SL, Crabtree GR: The mechanism of action of cyclosporin A and FK506. *Immunol Today* 13:136–142, 1992.

55. Salliot C, Dougados M, Gossec L: Risk of serious infections during rituximab, abatacept and anakinra treatments for rheumatoid arthritis: meta-analyses of randomised placebo-controlled trials. *Ann Rheum Dis* 68:25–32, 2009.

56. Gea-Banacloche JC: Rituximab-associated infections. *Semin Hematol* 47:187–198, 2010.

57. Navarra SV, Guzmán RM, Gallacher AE, et al: Efficacy and safety of belimumab in patients with active systemic lupus erythematosus: a randomised, placebo-controlled, phase 3 trial. *Lancet* 377:721–731, 2011.

58. Ruiz-Irastorza G, Ramos-Casals M, Brito-Zeron P, et al: Clinical efficacy and side effects of antimalarials in systemic lupus erythematosus: a systematic review. *Ann Rheum Dis* 69:20–28, 2010.

59. Mora CS, Segami MI, Hidalgo JA: *Strongyloides stercoralis* hyperinfection in systemic lupus erythematosus and the antiphospholipid syndrome. *Semin Arthritis Rheum* 36:135–143, 2006.

60. Garred P, Madsen HO, Halberg P, et al: Mannose-binding lectin polymorphisms and susceptibility to infection in systemic lupus erythematosus. *Arthritis Rheum* 42:2145–2152, 1999.

61. Garred P, Voss A, Madsen HO, et al: Association of mannose-binding lectin gene variation with disease severity and infections in a population-based cohort of systemic lupus erythematosus patients. *Genes Immun* 2:442–450, 2001.

62. Mok MY, Ip WK, Lau CS, et al: Mannose-binding lectin and susceptibility to infection in Chinese patients with systemic lupus erythematosus. *J Rheumatol* 34:1270–1276, 2007.

63. Willcocks LC, Carr EJ, Niederer HA, et al: A defunctioning polymorphism in FCGR2B is associated with protection against malaria but susceptibility to systemic lupus erythematosus. *Proc Natl Acad Sci USA* 107: 7881–7885, 2010.

64. Wullt B, Bergsten G, Fischer H, et al: The host response to urinary tract infection. *Infect Dis Clin N Am* 17:279–301, 2003.

65. Naveau C, Houssiau FA: Pneumococcal sepsis in patients with systemic lupus erythematosus. *Lupus* 14:903–906, 2005.

66. Huang JL, Huang JJ, Wu KC, et al: Septic arthritis in patients with systemic lupus erythematosus: Salmonella and Nonsalmonella infections compared. *Semin Arthritis Rheum* 36:61–67, 2006.

67. Wu KC, Yao TC, Yeh KW, et al: Osteomyelitis in patients with systemic lupus erythematosus. *J Rheumatol* 31:1340–1343, 2004.

68. Chen MJ, Tseng HM, Huang YL, et al: Long-term outcome and short-term survival of patients with systemic lupus erythematosus after bacteraemia episodes: 6-yr follow-up. *Rheumatology (Oxford)* 47:1352–1357, 2008.

69. Hou CL, Tsai YC, Chen LC, et al: Tuberculosis infection in patients with systemic lupus erythematosus: pulmonary and extra-pulmonary infection compared. *Clin Rheumatol* 27:557–563, 2008.

70. Ye S, Yang CD: Lupus erythematosus and lupus vulgaris: a case report and historical remarks. *Clin Rheumatol* 26:120–121, 2007.

71. Mok MY, Wong SS, Chan TM, et al: Non-tuberculous mycobacterial infection in patients with systemic lupus erythematosus. *Rheumatology (Oxford)* 46:280–284, 2007.

72. Zandman-Goddard G, Berkun Y, Barzilai O, et al: Neuropsychiatric lupus and infectious triggers. *Lupus* 17:380–384, 2008.

73. Cuchacovich R, Gedalia A: Pathophysiology and clinical spectrum of infections in systemic lupus erythematosus. *Rheum Dis Clin North Am* 35:75–93, 2009.

74. Nagasawa K, Yamauchi Y, Tada Y, et al: High incidence of herpes zoster in patients with systemic lupus erythematosus: an immunological analysis. *Ann Rheum Dis* 49:630–633, 1990.

75. Chen HS, Tsai WP, Leu HS, et al: Invasive fungal infection in systemic lupus erythematosus: an analysis of 15 cases and a literature review. *Rheumatology (Oxford)* 46:539–544, 2007.

76. Liam CK, Wang F: *Pneumocystis carinii* pneumonia in patients with systemic lupus erythematosus. *Lupus* 1:379–385, 1992.

77. Mok CC, Que TL, Tsui EYK, et al: Mucormycosis in systemic lupus erythematosus. *Semin Arthritis Rheum* 33:115–124, 2003.

78. Hidron A, Franco-Paredes C, Drenkard C: A rare opportunistic infection in a woman with systemic lupus erythematosus and multiple skin lesions. *Lupus* 18:1100–1103, 2009.

79. Wilcox MH, Powell RJ, Pugh SF, et al: Toxoplasmosis and systemic lupus erythematosus. *Ann Rheum Dis* 49:254–257, 1990.

80. Suh CH, Jeong YS, Park HC, et al: Risk factors for infection and role of C-reactive protein in Korean patients with systemic lupus erythematosus. *Clin Exp Rheumatol* 19:191–194, 2001.

81. Firooz N, Albert D, Wallace D, et al: High-sensitivity C-reactive protein and erythrocyte sedimentation rate in systemic lupus erythematosus. *Lupus* 20:588–597, 2011.

82. Quintana G, Medina YF, Rojas C, et al: The use of procalcitonin determinations in evaluation of systemic lupus erythematosus. *J Clin Rheumatol* 14:138–142, 2008.

83. Kim J, Koh JK, Lee EY, et al: Serum levels of soluble triggering receptor expressed on myeloid cells-1 (sTREM-1) and pentraxin 3 (PTX3) as markers of infection in febrile patients with systemic lupus erythematosus. *Clin Exp Rheumatol* 27:773–778, 2009.

84. Ye S, Guo Q, Tang JP, et al: Could 2'5'-oligoadenylate synthetase isoforms be biomarkers to differentiate between disease flare and infection in lupus patients? A pilot study. *Clin Rheumatol* 26:186–190, 2007.

85. Chaussabel D, Quinn C, Shen J, et al: A modular analysis framework for blood genomics studies: application to systemic lupus erythematosus. *Immunity* 29:150–164, 2008.

Chapter 46

Clinical Measures, Metrics, and Indices

Zahi Touma, Dafna D. Gladman, and Murray B. Urowitz

Systemic lupus erythematosus (SLE) is a protean, multisystem complex disease characterized by remissions and exacerbations. The SLE disease course varies from flares to persistently active disease (PAD), from disease improvements to remissions.[1,2] Patients with SLE may experience events that are related to lupus disease activity, chronic irreversible damage, and adverse events from the medications, all of which impact their quality of life. Monitoring each of these aspects is challenging but essential for the successful management of patients. The use of validated and reliable tools is therefore fundamental for the management of patients with lupus and to allow for comparisons among patients from different centers.

PRINCIPLES FOR ASSESSING PATIENTS WITH LUPUS

The assessment of patients with lupus includes the determination of five domains: (1) disease activity, (2) chronic damage resulting from lupus activity or its treatment, (3) adverse events of drugs, (4) health-related quality of life (HRQoL), and (5) economic impact (Table 46-1).[3] To date, no universal agreement regarding the optimal tools to be used is available to assess each of the five domains in SLE. Whether in research or in clinical care settings, investigators and rheumatologists must identify the appropriate tools suited to the particular research or clinical needs. This chapter focuses on describing the available measures to assess all domains in patients with lupus.

APPROACHES TO CLINICAL MEASUREMENT IN LUPUS

A number of measures have been developed to assess disease activity, damage, and HRQoL in patients with lupus. In some instances, instruments have been specifically developed for lupus, whereas in other scenarios, generic instruments are used that have been developed for other chronic diseases. The following sections describe the development and use of the instruments in SLE.

DISEASE ACTIVITY INDICES

Disease activity can be defined as a reversible clinical or laboratory manifestation, reflecting the immunologic and inflammatory manifestation of organ involvement from lupus at a specific point in time.[4] The ability to quantify and grade disease activity, whether in a clinical practice or in research settings, is important. For this purpose, several measures have been developed and adopted to assess disease activity. Appropriate measures must be shown to be reliable and valid, as well as sensitive to change. In addition, the practical applicability of the measure includes the ease of administration, the low costs of data collection and method of scoring, and the ease of score interpretation.[5] Two types of disease activity measures have been developed. Global indices describe the overall burden of inflammatory disease, whereas organ-specific indices relate to disease activity within each organ system, either individually or incorporated into one summary score.

Global Indices
Systemic Lupus Erythematosus Disease Activity Index and Its Versions

The Systemic Lupus Erythematosus Disease Activity Index (SLEDAI) is a global disease activity index that was initially developed and introduced in 1985. This index was modeled on clinicians' global judgment. A group of experienced rheumatologists with expertise in lupus participated in the development of this index. The use of the nominal group process ensured that the resulting index, SLEDAI, represented the consensus of the developers. From the initial list of 37 descriptors derived from the literature that have been used to describe disease activity in lupus, 24 of the *most important* descriptors were retained for the development of SLEDAI. The elimination of the 13 descriptors occurred in the first phase of development (preconference ratings) and was accomplished by 15 clinicians. SLEDAI is thus based on the presence of 24 descriptors in 9 organ systems. Based on the experts' evaluation of 1400 case scenarios, multiple regression models were used to derive the weighted scores for each descriptor. Most of the definitions of the descriptors were based on the American College of Rheumatology (ACR) glossary of rheumatic disease terms, and they were further refined throughout the development process of SLEDAI.[6,7] The scores of the descriptors were derived from the values obtained through the regression models and ranged from 1 to 8 with a total possible score of 105. The initial validation of SLEDAI was conducted throughout the primary development phase, and descriptors were used to evaluate disease activity on a cohort database from the University of Toronto Lupus Clinic. The descriptors in SLEDAI were precisely defined in the 10-day period before the assessment and within which the manifestation must be recorded.[4] The intrarater and interrater reliability of SLEDAI was shown during the phase of development on a set of case scenarios of patients with lupus across the investigators.[4] Rheumatologists from four countries have successfully used SLEDAI in a multicenter study, confirming its reliability in real patients.[8] Furthermore, SLEDAI reproducibility has been demonstrated when used in routine clinical visits and among less experienced observers (e.g., rheumatologist trainees) in the assessment of disease activity in patients with lupus.[9,10] SLEDAI has been shown to correlate with other validated measures of disease activity.[8,10,11] Moreover, SLEDAI has been used in both research and clinical settings and as a predictive variable and outcome measure in prognostic studies of lupus.[10,12,13] It has also shown sensitivity to change over time and validity in the assessment of childhood lupus.[14-16] Lupus disease activity, as determined by SLEDAI, has been associated with mortality and survival in studies of patients with lupus and has been the major determinant of damage accrual.[17,18] SLEDAI is highly prognostic for mortality in the next 6 months, with increasing relative risks of 1.28 for SLEDAI 1 through 5, 2.34 for SLEDAI 6 through 10, 4.74 for SLEDAI 11 through 19, and 14.11 for SLEDAI higher than 20 (Figure 46-1).[19]

TABLE 46-1 Assessment of Lupus by Five Domains

DOMAINS	TOOLS	WHERE DEVELOPED	SCORE RANGE	TIME FRAME	REFERENCES
Disease Activity					
SLEDAI, and its versions and modifications	SLEDAI	Toronto	0-105	Last 10 days	4
	SLEDAI-2K	Toronto	0-105	Last 10 days	23
	SLEDAI-2K 30 days	Toronto	0-105	Last 30 days	27, 28
	Mex-SLEDAI	Mexico	0-32	Last 10 days	20, 21
	SELENA-SLEDAI*	North America*	0-105	Last 10 days	22
SRI-50	SRI-50	Toronto	0-105	Last 30 days	65, 67, 68
BILAG and its version	BILAG	United Kingdom	Categories A-E	Previous month	24, 37
	BILAG 2004	United Kingdom	Categories A-E	Previous month	43
SLAM and its versions	SLAM	Boston	0-86	Previous month	11
	SLAM-R	Boston	0-81	Previous month	26, 29
	SLAQ		0-44	Previous month	106
ECLAM	ECLAM	Europe	0-17.5	Previous month	25, 32, 33
LAI	LAI	UCSF, Hopkins	0-3	Last 2 weeks	10
SIS	SIS	NIH	0-52	Last week	107
RIFLE	RIFLE				61
Damage					
Physician completed	SDI	SLICC/ACR	0-49	Present for 6 months	75
Patients completed	LDIQ–English Spanish, Portuguese, French			Present for 6 months	84, 85
Health-Related Quality-of-Life Questionnaires					
Generic	SF-36	Boston	0-100	Previous month	92
Specific	LupusQoL	Blackburn, United Kingdom	0-100	Previous month	91, 99, 100
	LupusQoL–United States	Chicago	0-100	Previous month	
	LupusQoL–Spanish, Dutch, French, Greek, Italian, Hyperion, Portuguese, Chinese	Spain	0-100	Previous month	
	SSC–Dutch, English	The Netherlands		Previous month	93
	SLEQoL–English, Portuguese, Chinese	Singapore	0-240	Previous month	94
	L-QoL English, Hungarian, Turkish	United Kingdom		Previous month	95
Adverse Events					
	As reported by patients or determined by physicians (or both)				
Economic Costs and Impact					
	Direct and indirect costs; work productivity				

*The SELENA-SLEDAI, developed by the study investigators in the Safety of Estrogens in Lupus Erythematosus–National Assessment Trial, uses a modified version of SLEDAI and includes flare assessment and physician's global assessment.

ACR, the American College of Rheumatology; BILAG, the British Isles Lupus Assessment Group; ECLAM, the European Consensus Lupus Activity Measurement; HRQoL, health-related quality of life; LAI, lupus activity index; LDIQ, the Lupus Damage Index Questionnaire; LupusQoL, lupus quality of life; Mex-SLEDAI, Mexican version of SLEDAI; NIH, the National Institutes of Health; PGA, physician's global assessment; RIFLE, the Responder Index for Lupus Erythematosus; SDI, the SLICC/ACR Damage Index; SELENA, the Safety of Estrogens in Lupus Erythematosus–National Assessment; SF-36, Short Form 36; SIS, SLE activity index score; SLAM, Systemic Lupus Activity Measure; SLAQ, the Systemic Lupus Activity Questionnaire; SLE, systemic lupus erythematosus; SLEDAI, the Systemic Lupus Erythematosus Disease Activity Index; SLEDAI-2K, SLEDAI 2000; SLEQoL, SLE-specific quality of life; SLICC, the Systemic Lupus International Collaborating Clinics; SRI-50, the SLEDAI-2K Responder Index 50; SSC, SLE system checklist; UCSF, the University of California, San Francisco.

Mexican Version of SLEDAI

In 1992 a modification of SLEDAI was developed in Mexico in an attempt to reduce the cost inherent in a SLEDAI calculation by eliminating the laboratory tests included in SLEDAI.[20] The Mexican version of SLEDAI (Mex-SLEDAI) excludes immunologic descriptors. Moreover, some clinical and laboratory manifestations were added (fatigue, mononeuritis, and myelitis clustered in the descriptor neurologic disorder; peritonitis grouped with serositis; creatinine increase grouped with renal disorders; and hemolysis and lymphopenia grouped with leukopenia) and others were excluded (lupus headache, visual disturbance, and pyuria). The total number of variables in the Mex-SLEDAI was reduced to 10. In addition, investigators modified the definitions for a few descriptors. Different weighted scores were assigned to Mex-SLEDAI, as compared with SLEDAI, with a maximum score of 32.[20] The Mex-SLEDAI was originally validated in Spanish-speaking countries.[20] In 2004, the modifications of SLEDAI 2000 (SLEDAI-2K) were incorporated for the first time into the Mex-SLEDAI version and applied to patients of non-Hispanic descent (Mex-SLEDAI-2K).[21] Mex-SLEDAI-2K was shown to have convergent validity with SLEDAI-2K and the revised systemic lupus activity measure (SLAM-R), as well as moderate correlation (r = 0.54) with physician's global assessment (PGA).[21] Nevertheless, the sensitivity to change of the Mex-SLEDAI needs to be studied further.[20,21] Mex-SLEDAI has not been used extensively in clinical trials and is limited to a few centers in Latin America.

SELENA-SLEDAI

The Safety of Estrogens in Lupus Erythematosus–National Assessment Trial (SELENA) proposed a new modification of SLEDAI to

SLEDAI-2K (30 DAYS)
DATA COLLECTION SHEET

Study No.: _____ Patient Name: _____ Visit Date: _____ _____ _____
d   m   yr

(Enter weight in SLEDAI-2K Score column if descriptor is present at the time of the visit or in the preceding 30 days)

Weight	SCORE	Descriptor	Definition
8	☐	Seizure	Recent onset, exclude metabolic, infections, or drug causes.
8	☐	Psychosis	Altered ability to function in normal activity due to severe disturbance in the perception of reality. Include hallucinations, incoherence, marked loose associations, impoverished thought content, marked illogical thinking, bizarre, disorganized, or catatonic behavior. Exclude uremia and drug causes.
8	☐	Organic brain syndrome	Altered mental function with impaired orientation, memory, or other intellectual function, with rapid onset and fluctuating clinical features, inability to sustain attention to environment, plus at least 2 of the following: perceptual disturbance, incoherent speech, insomnia or daytime drowsiness, or increased or decreased psychomotor activity. Exclude metabolic, infectious, or drug causes.
8	☐	Visual disturbance	Retinal changes of SLE. Include cytoid bodies, retinal hemorrhages, serous exudate or hemorrhages in the choroid, or optic neuritis. Exclude hypertension, infection, or drug causes.
8	☐	Cranial nerve disorder	New onset of sensory or motor neuropathy involving cranial nerves.
8	☐	Lupus headache	Severe, persistent headache; may be migrainous, but must be nonresponsive to narcotic analgesia.
8	☐	CVA	New onset of cerebrovascular accident(s). Exlcude arteriosclerosis.
8	☐	Vasculitis	Ulceration, gangrene, tender finger nodules, periungual infarction, splinter hemorrhages, or biopsy or angiogram proof of vasculitis.
4	☐	Arthritis	≥2 joints with pain and signs of inflammation (i.e., tenderness, swelling, or effusion).
4	☐	Myositis	Proximal muscle aching/weakness, associated with elevated creatine phosphokinase/aldolase or electromyogram changes or a biopsy showing myositis.
4	☐	Urinary casts	Heme-granular or red blood cell casts.
4	☐	Hematuria	>5 red blood cells/high power field. Exclude stone, infection, or other cause.
4	☐	Proteinuria	>0.5 gram/24 hours.
4	☐	Pyuria	>5 white blood cells/high power field. Exclude infection.
2	☐	Rash	Inflammatory type rash.
2	☐	Alopecia	Abnormal, patchy or diffuse loss of hair.
2	☐	Mucosal ulcers	Oral or nasal ulcerations.
2	☐	Pleurisy	Pleuritic chest pain with pleural rub or effusion or pleural thickening.
2	☐	Pericarditis	Pericardial pain with at least 1 of the following: rub, effusion, or electrocardiogram or echocardiogram confirmation.
2	☐	Low complement	Decrease in CH50, C3, or C4 below the lower limit of normal for testing laboratory.
2	☐	Increased DNA binding	Increased DNA binding by Farr assay above normal range for testing laboratory.
1	☐	Fever	>38° C. Exclude infectious cause.
1	☐	Thrombocytopenia	<100,000 platelets/× 10^9/L, exclude drug causes.
1	☐	Leukopenia	<3000 white blood cells/× 10^9/L, exclude drug causes.

FIGURE 46-1 The Systemic Lupus Erythematosus Disease Activity Index 2000 (SLEDAI-2K). *(From Gladman DD, Ibañez D, Urowitz MB: Systemic lupus erythematosus disease activity index 2000. J Rheumatol 29(2):288–291, 2002.)*

which a composite flare outcome—the SELENA-SLEDAI Flare Index (SFI)—was added.[22] In this version of SLEDAI, several descriptors were modified. The definition of the descriptor *seizure* was modified in SELENA-SLEDAI to exclude seizures that were due to past irreversible central nervous system damage, and the descriptor *cerebrovascular accident* was modified to exclude hypertensive causes. However, these modifications were unnecessary; in the original SLEDAI, these two descriptors are scored as present only if the features are attributed to lupus disease activity.[4] The descriptor *visual disturbance* was modified to include scleritis and episcleritis. This modification has not been validated because these features do not reflect the same changes included under "visual" in the original SLEDAI and may not deserve a score of 8. In the descriptor *cranial nerve disorder*, "include vertigo due to lupus" was added to the definition. Nevertheless, vertigo is one of the manifestations of vestibulocochlear cranial nerve involvement and was intended to be reflected in the original SLEDAI, because it is one of the manifestations of the cranial nerve disturbance. The definitions of *pleurisy* and *pericarditis* were modified by adding the phrase "classic and severe" to ensure the attribution of the descriptors to lupus disease activity. More importantly, SLEDAI and SLEDAI-2K mandate the presence of subjective (e.g., pleuritic or pericardial pain) and objective (e.g., rub, effusion, electrocardiographic or echocardiographic confirmation, or pleural thickening) findings for pleurisy and pericarditis to be scored as present.[4,23] In the SELENA-SLEDAI, researchers accepted the presence of either the objective or subjective findings to score the descriptor as present.[22] In the SELENA-SLEDAI, arthritis is scored if more than two joints are active, whereas SLEDAI-2K defined arthritis as two or more actively inflamed joints as in the definition of lupus arthritis in the ACR glossary of terms. The SELENA-SLEDAI defines proteinuria as new onset or recent increase of more than 0.5 gm/24 h as in the original SLEDAI. However, SLEDAI-2K modified the descriptor proteinuria to be >0.5 gm/24 hours.[23] As in the original SLEDAI, the score ranges from 0 to 105 (eFigure 46-2).[22,23] Despite the modifications in some of the descriptors, SELENA-SLEDAI appears similar to SLEDAI-2K. Importantly, no validation of all of the modifications introduced in SELENA-SLEDAI has been made. Thus the SELENA-SLEDAI version lacks the stringent validation steps that are essential before a measure can be used in clinical trials or research settings. The authors of this text believe that the SLEDAI-2K could serve well as the SLEDAI component of the SELENA instrument, which also includes a flare measure.

SLEDAI-2000

SLEDAI-2K was introduced in 2002 and validated.[23] In the glossary of the original SLEDAI, certain descriptors were scored as active only if they were new; thus PADs were not scored. This would lead to an apparent improvement that, in fact, did not occur. Among SLEDAI descriptors, rash, alopecia, and mucosal ulcers had been scored only if they were new or recurrent and, in the case of proteinuria, if new onset or a recent increase of more than 0.5 grams in 24 hours is present. SLEDAI-2K was modified to allow the documentation of ongoing disease activity in the descriptors: rash, alopecia, mucosal ulcers, and proteinuria.[4] Thus SLEDAI-2K includes the presence of any inflammatory rash, alopecia, or mucosal ulcers, and new, recurrent, or persistent proteinuria greater than 0.5 grams in 24 hours. As in the original SLEDAI, all the descriptors in SLEDAI-2K must be attributed to lupus activity.[23] In the validation phase of SLEDAI-2K against SLEDAI, the entire cohort of the University of Toronto Lupus Clinic was used. Of 18,636 visits, 78% of the scores were concordant in SLEDAI-2K and SLEDAI. In the remaining 22% of the visits, the differences were the result of proteinuria, rash, alopecia, and mucosal ulcers. SLEDAI-2K at presentation was equivalent to SLEDAI at presentation as a predictor of mortality. Moreover, SLEDAI-2K described disease activity at different activity levels in a comparable manner with the original SLEDAI. SLEDAI-2K was equivalent to SLEDAI in describing changes in disease activity from one visit to the next (see Figure 46-1).[23]

SLEDAI-2K: 30-Day Version

In the original SLEDAI and its 2000 modification, the time frame for the individual components was a 10-day period before the assessment.[4,23] Other major disease activity indices for SLE measure disease activity in the preceding 30 days.[24-26] Moreover, the usual time frame of observations within a clinical trial is 30 days; thus validating SLEDAI-2K 30 days against SLEDAI-2K 10 days was relevant. The first validation study was conducted on 149 patients who were seen over 9 weeks at the University of Toronto Lupus Clinic. The results showed that SLEDAI-2K 30 days is similar to SLEDAI-2K 10 days in both patients who were in remission and patients with a spectrum of disease activity levels.[27] The second study validated SLEDAI-2K 30 days against SLEDAI-2K 10 days in a group of 41 patients who were followed at monthly intervals for 12 months. These studies confirmed that having a manifestation of active lupus present at 11 to 30 days before a visit and a complete resolution in the 10 days before the visit is unusual. Therefore the 30-day time frame for SLEDAI-2K should now be used in clinical studies and clinical trials to describe disease activity in patients with SLE.[27,28]

One of the drawbacks of SLEDAI-2K is that it can detect only 100% improvement of the active descriptors and thus cannot reflect a partial improvement in disease manifestation. A second drawback is that SLEDAI-2K does not detect a worsening of an already active descriptor; nevertheless, this particular descriptor will continue to be scored as active and thus scored as present. Despite the fact that SLEDAI-2K is a global index and generates a total score reflecting overall disease activity, disease activity in each of the nine organ systems of SLEDAI-2K can be derived if required in clinical trials. The practical applicability of SLEDAI-2K in clinical settings, its ease of administration, and its simplicity in scoring are fundamental properties. These benefits have enabled SLEDAI-2K to be one of the most commonly used global disease activity measures in longitudinal observational studies and clinical trials.

Systemic Lupus Activity Measure

The Systemic Lupus Activity Measure (SLAM) index was introduced in Boston and first published in 1989 to measure global disease activity. The SLAM index uses disease manifestations derived from the American Rheumatology Association Council on SLE and includes 31 items—23 clinical and 7 laboratory—in 11 systems with a total possible score of 86. The SLAM index assesses global disease severity in the previous month.[6,11,26] Most clinical and laboratory items are categorized as present or absent and are then scored from 0 to 3, based on the severity without considering the significance of the organ involved.[11,29] For instance, mild fatigue or oral ulcers are scored similar to lupus headache or seizure. A few items can score only 1 or 2, in particular, fatigue, oral ulcers, headache, alopecia, Raynaud phenomenon, lymphadenopathy, and hepatomegaly or splenomegaly (eFigure 46-3). The revision, SLAM-R index, includes 23 clinical manifestations and the same 7 laboratory parameters and has a possible range of 0 to 81 with a score of 7 being considered clinically significant.[29] The definitions of several items were modified in the SLAM-R index; in particular, pleurisy, pericarditis, and pneumonitis were dropped because of the difficulty in scoring. The definitions and weighting of fatigue, stroke syndrome, seizure, and headache were modified.[29] The SLAM-R index does not include immunologic tests as in SLEDAI-2K. The SLAM index and its updated version, SLAM-R, are reliable and valid in measuring disease activity across cultures and when compared with other disease activity measures.[8,11] Moreover, the SLAM and SLAM-R indices have been shown to capture patients' assessments better than the other indices, and this could be explained by the presence of subjective items in these indices that reflect patients' perceptions of the disease.[30,31] The SLAM-R index is valid for assessing disease activity of childhood lupus.[15,16] A potential drawback in the SLAM-R index is that it includes subjective items, such as fatigue, shortness of breath, chest pain, abdominal pain, myalgia, and arthralgia, which are then scored by their severity. Although these items reflect the patients' perceptions of the disease, as in other indices, these items should only be scored if the assessor believes they are attributed to lupus disease activity. Nevertheless, the assessment of these items has been associated with ambiguity in research settings and clinical trials, and a score of 7 on the SLAM-R index is not unusual for subjective complaints that can be misinterpreted as lupus activity. Although the SLAM and SLAM-R indices have been used in clinical trials and research settings in the assessment of adult and childhood lupus and are sensitive to change, the previously listed drawbacks should be considered.[8,15,16,30]

European Consensus Lupus Activity Measurement

The European Consensus Lupus Activity Measurement (ECLAM) index was first published in 1992 by the Consensus Study Group of the European Workshop for Rheumatology Research. The ECLAM index was developed on the basis of the analysis of 704 patients with lupus from 29 centers in 14 countries.[25,32,33] The 15 items of the ECLAM index were derived through univariate analysis to reflect the best clinical and laboratory features of SLE and weighted according to their respective coefficient as determined using multivariate regression analyses. In the initial development and validation steps of the ECLAM index, the PGA was considered the criterion construct "gold standard" for lupus disease activity. The ECLAM index evaluates disease activity over the previous month, and the maximum possible score is 10 (eFigure 46-4). The ECLAM index has been shown to be reliable, valid, and sensitive to change, when compared against other indices including the SLEDAI and the British Isles Lupus Assessment Group (BILAG) index.[30] The ECLAM index can be used to evaluate disease activity retrospectively in patients from the data provided in clinical charts as shown in a study conducted on 64 patients.[34] The ECLAM index has been validated for the assessment of disease activity in childhood-onset lupus.[15] More important, the ECLAM index has not been extensively used in clinical trials.

Lupus Activity Index

The lupus activity index (LAI) was proposed in 1989 to assess the global disease activity over the previous 2 weeks.[10] The LAI includes five sections, eight organ systems, and three laboratory measures. The PGA, as well as the score for treatment with corticosteroids and immunosuppressive drugs, is part of this index. The severity of the disease is based on the physician's judgment. The overall score reflects the mean of the PGA, physician's judgment of the severity of clinical manifestations, degree of laboratory abnormalities, and treatment. The score of the LAI ranges from 0 to 3.[10] The LAI validity was demonstrated in a study on 150 patients in which the correlation of the LAI was modified (M-LAI) so as not to contain the PGA and was scored at 0.64. The interrater and intrarater reliability of the LAI was shown in a study conducted on six patients in routine practice.[10] The LAI has performed well in assessing disease activity when compared with other disease activity measures and has been sensitive to change; nonetheless its use has been limited as compared with other disease activity measures.[30]

SLE Activity Index Score

The SLE activity index score (SIS) is a global index developed by clinicians at the National Institutes of Health (NIH). The SIS includes 17 clinical items and is based on clinical manifestations and subjective features reflecting the perception of the patients on the disease, in particular, fatigue, arthralgia, and myalgia, as well as laboratory items (eFigure 46-5). The SIS is a weighted index, and the scores range from 0 to 52. The SIS assesses disease activity over the previous week and categorizes disease activity into inactive, mildly active, moderately active, active, and very active. The SIS is a valid index that has been adopted in some clinical trials and research settings.[33,35] The validity of the SIS index has been demonstrated against other disease activity indices, in particular, the SLEDAI, SLAM, and BILAG

indices. In this study, all four indices were closely correlated with each other (r = 0.86 between SIS and SLAM); nevertheless, the SIS has not been used as extensively as the SLEDAI or the BILAG index.[33,36]

Organ-Specific Indices
British Isles Lupus Assessment Group

The BILAG index was proposed by a group of investigators from different centers in the United Kingdom, and its first version was published in 1988.[37] This index was developed using a nominal consensus approach and is based on the principle of the physician's intention to treat. BILAG includes 86 items including clinical signs, symptoms, and laboratory variables in 8 systems. The items recorded must have been attributed to active lupus and present during the 4 weeks before the assessment.[37] Based on the presence of certain features in each system, a system is categorized into one of four levels: A for action; B for beware; C for content; and D for discount (eFigure 46-6).[24] The BILAG index was shown to have good between-rater reliability and to be valid when compared with the "gold standard" criterion (i.e., starting or increasing disease-modifying therapy).[24] Further validation of the BILAG index showed that disease activity in different systems in SLE does not follow a common pattern. This study recommended the use of the individual BILAG components rather than the total BILAG score as a primary endpoint in clinical and epidemiologic studies.[38] The BILAG index sensitivity to change over time was shown in a study on 23 patients who were prospectively followed every 2 weeks for up to 40 weeks, with a standardized response means of 0.57.[30] The BILAG index was adapted and validated in the assessment of SLE in children.[15] The BILAG index has been found to be reliable and valid in several studies conducted by the BILAG group and other investigators and has correlated with other disease activity measures, in particular, the SLEDAI and the SLAM index.[11,14,15,24,30,38,39] The BILAG index has been successfully used in clinical trials and research settings and has been particularly effective for demonstrating new organ flares.[8,15,39-43]

The classic BILAG index has undergone a series of revisions to the current BILAG-2004.[11,24,37] The members of the BILAG proposed the BILAG-2004 index, which included further changes in some divisions of organs and systems; refinements in the definitions of some items, in particular, the neurologic system; the removal of items attributed to damage rather than reflecting lupus disease activity, in particular, avascular necrosis and tendon contracture; and modifications in the glossary and scoring.[43] As in the classic BILAG index, the BILAG-2004 index is based on the physician's intention to treat.[43] The BILAG-2004 index contains 97 items, whereas the classic BILAG index has only 86. The system vasculitis was removed and its items were included in other systems, and the gastrointestinal and ophthalmic systems were added.[43] In the classic BILAG index, all items that are improving can only contribute to a C score, which does not reflect the appropriate level of disease activity for more severe manifestations.[43] In the BILAG-2004 index, features that contribute to an A score when recorded as being the same, worse, or new will contribute to a B score when improving (Figure 46-7).[43]

A complete history and physical examination is required to determine disease activity by the BILAG-2004. The BILAG-2004 index generates a score for each of the nine systems assessed. The scoring of lupus disease activity in each system is graded A through E, based on the assessment of the clinical features and/or the laboratory findings for the appropriate system and representing disease activity. Like the classic BILAG index, the BILAG-2004 is a transitional index that is able to capture changing severity of clinical manifestations. The items in each system are rated using a scale from 0 through 4 (0 = not present, 1 = improving, 2 = same, 3 = worse, and 4 = new), and some items are scored as present or absent, reflecting disease activity over the last 4 weeks, as compared with the previous 4 weeks. The classic BILAG index and its versions, including the BILAG-2004 index, are ordinal scale indices, and an additive numerical scoring

BILAG-2004 INDEX

- Only record manifestations/items <u>due to SLE disease activity</u>
- Assessment refers to <u>manifestations occurring in the last 4 weeks</u> (compared with the previous 4 weeks)
- TO BE USED WITH THE GLOSSARY

Record: NA Not Available
     0 Not present
     1 Improving
     2 Same
     3 Worse
     4 New
     Yes/No OR Value (where indicated)
     *Y/N Confirm this is <u>due to SLE activity</u> (Yes/No)

CONSTITUTIONAL
1. Pyrexia - documented >37.5°C   ( )
2. Weight loss - unintentional >5%   ( )
3. Lymphadenopathy/splenomegaly   ( )
4. Anorexia   ( )

MUCOCUTANEOUS
5. Skin eruption - severe   ( )
6. Skin eruption - mild   ( )
7. Angio-oedema - severe   ( )
8. Angio-oedema - mild   ( )
9. Mucosal ulceration - severe   ( )
10. Mucosal ulceration - mild   ( )
11. Panniculitis/Bullous lupus - severe   ( )
12. Panniculitis/Bullous lupus - mild   ( )
13. Major cutaneous vasculitis/thrombosis   ( )
14. Digital infarcts or nodular vasculitis   ( )
15. Alopecia - severe   ( )
16. Alopecia - mild   ( )
17. Periungual erythema/chilblains   ( )
18. Splinter haemorrhages   ( )

NEUROPSYCHIATRIC
19. Aseptic meningitis   ( )
20. Cerebral vasculitis   ( )
21. Demyelinating syndrome   ( )
22. Myelopathy   ( )
23. Acute confusional state   ( )
24. Psychosis   ( )
25. Acute inflammatory demyelinating polyradiculoneuropathy   ( )
26. Mononeuropathy (single/multiplex)   ( )
27. Cranial neuropathy   ( )
28. Plexopathy   ( )
29. Polyneuropathy   ( )
30. Seizure disorder   ( )
31. Status epilepticus   ( )
32. Cerebrovascular disease (not due to vasculitis)   ( )
33. Cognitive dysfunction   ( )
34. Movement disorder   ( )
35. Autonomic disorder   ( )
36. Cerebellar ataxia (isolated)   ( )
37. Lupus headache - severe unremitting   ( )
38. Headache from IC hypertension   ( )

MUSCULOSKELETAL
39. Myositis - severe   ( )
40. Myositis - mild   ( )
41. Arthritis (severe)   ( )
42. Arthritis (moderate)/tendonitis/tenosynovitis   ( )
43. Arthritis (mild)/Arthralgia/Myalgia   ( )
44. Myocarditis - mild   ( )
45. Myocarditis/endocarditis + cardiac failure   ( )
46. Arrhythmia   ( )
47. New valvular dysfunction   ( )

48. Pleurisy/pericarditis   ( )
49. Cardiac tamponade   ( )
50. Pleural effusion with dyspnoea   ( )
51. Pulmonary haemorrhage/vasculitis   ( )
52. Interstitial alveolitis/pneumonitis   ( )
53. Shrinking lung syndrome   ( )
54. Aortitis   ( )
55. Coronary vasculitis   ( )

GASTROINTESTINAL
56. Lupus peritonitis   ( )
57. Abdominal serositis or ascites   ( )
58. Lupus enteritis/colitis   ( )
59. Malabsorption   ( )
60. Protein-losing enteropathy   ( )
61. Intestinal pseudo-obstruction   ( )
62. Lupus hepatitis   ( )
63. Acute lupus cholecystitis   ( )
64. Acute lupus pancreatitis   ( )

OPHTHALMIC
65. Orbital inflammation/myositis/proptosis   ( )
66. Keratitis - severe   ( )
67. Keratitis - mild   ( )
68. Anterior uveitis   ( )
69. Posterior uveitis/retinal vasculitis - severe   ( )
70. Posterior uveitis/retinal vasculitis - mild   ( )
71. Episcleritis   ( )
72. Scleritis - severe   ( )
73. Scleritis - mild   ( )
74. Retinal/choroidal vaso-occlusive disease   ( )
75. Isolated cotton-wool spots (cytoid bodies)   ( )
76. Optic neuritis   ( )
77. Anterior ischaemic optic neuropathy   ( )

RENAL
78. Systolic blood pressure (mm Hg) value ( ) Y/N*
79. Diastolic blood pressure (mm Hg) value ( ) Y/N*
80. Accelerated hypertension Yes/No ( )
81. Urine dipstick protein (+=1, ++=2, +++=3) ( ) Y/N*
82. Urine albumin-creatinine ratio mg/mg ( ) Y/N*
83. Urine protein-creatinine ratio mg/mg ( ) Y/N*
84. 24-hour urine protein (g) value ( ) Y/N*
85. Nephrotic syndrome Yes/No ( )
86. Creatinine (plasma/serum) μmol/L ( ) Y/N*
87. GFR (calculated) mL/min/1.73 m^2 ( ) Y/N*
88. Active urinary sediment Yes/No ( )
89. Active nephritis Yes/No ( )

HAEMATOLOGICAL
90. Haemoglobin (g/dL) value ( ) Y/N*
91. Total white cell count (x 10^9/L) value ( ) Y/N*
92. Neutrophils (x 10^9/L) value ( ) Y/N*
93. Lymphocytes (x 10^9/L) value ( ) Y/N*
94. Platelets (x 10^9/L) value ( ) Y/N*
95. TTP ( )
96. Evidence of active haemolysis Yes/No ( )
97. Coomb's test positvie (isolated) Yes/No ( )

FIGURE 46-7 The British Isles Lupus Assessment Group (BILAG) 2004 index. *(From Isenberg DA, Rahman A, Allen E, et al: BILAG 2004. Development and initial validation of an updated version of the British Isles Lupus Assessment Group's disease activity index for patients with systemic lupus erythematosus. Rheumatology (Oxford) 44(7):902–906, 2005.)*

scheme for the BILAG-2004 index is available (A grade = 12 points, B = 8, C = 1, D = 0, and E = 0).[44] This scoring system is mainly adopted in studies in which the BILAG-2004 index needs to be compared with other numerical indices or to facilitate the statistical analysis, if required; however, the BILAG-2004 index was not designed to be used in this way.[43,44] The British Lupus Integrated Prospective System (BLIPS) is a computerized program that calculates the BILAG scores with the option to derive the SLEDAI, the SLAM-R index, the Systemic Lupus International Collaborating Clinics (SLICC)/ACR Damage Index, and the Medical Outcomes Study (MOS) Short Form 36 (SF-36).[45] BLIPS has also undergone further refinement to reflect the BILAG-2004 index, and several amendments have been made to the other activity indices.[43,45]

The BILAG-2004 index has been able to discriminate among patients and has shown a good reliability and high levels of physician agreement in almost all systems.[43] The reliability of the BILAG-2004 index was evaluated in a larger study involving 11 centers across the United Kingdom with the participation of 14 raters and 97 patients. This study showed that the BILAG-2004 is a reliable index to assess SLE activity and recommended the training of raters to ensure its optimal performance.[46] More recently, the construct validity of the BILAG-2004 index was confirmed by its association with the erythrocyte sedimentation rate (ESR), C3 level, C4 level, anti–double stranded DNA (anti-dsDNA), and, more importantly, the SLEDAI-2K index.[47] The criterion validity of BILAG-2004, defined as change in therapy, was confirmed by the association between the BILAG-2004 index and the increase in therapy.[47] In this study, higher SLEDAI-2K scores were significantly associated with overall BILAG-2004 scores reflecting higher disease activity. Although the BILAG index has been extensively used in clinical trials, its routine use in long-term studies has some drawbacks, in particular, the practical applicability and the complicated glossary of the clinical features, and the scoring analysis, which requires a specialized computer program.

Renal Outcome Measures

Several renal composite outcome measures have been proposed and adopted in the assessment of lupus nephritis clinical trials and research studies. These measures include the quantitative change in urinary sediments (e.g., hematuria, pyuria, cellular casts), proteinuria (e.g., 24-hour urine protein level, 24-hour urine protein/creatinine ratio, spot urine protein/creatinine ratio), and renal function (e.g., 24-hour creatinine clearance, estimated creatinine clearance, estimated Cockcroft-Gault formula, estimated glomerular filtration rate). The patients' responses, with use of the composite outcomes, can be defined as either improvement (complete, partial response, or no response), reduction in renal flares, or increase time to flare.[48,49] Renal histologic factors can be considered to assess renal response in lupus nephritis trials whenever feasible.[49]

Organ-specific measures concentrate on the findings in one system, and this priority might be critical in a multisystem disease such as lupus, particularly when efficacy for a treatment is sought for a particular system such as renal or skin. If such agents are to be tested in clinical trials, using the organ-specific measures in association with a global disease activity measure is advisable to evaluate lupus activity in all systems. In an effort to standardize the assessment of lupus nephritis and to achieve optimal detection of the response to treatment in clinical trials, the members of the SLICC group in collaboration with nephrologists developed a measure of renal activity in SLE.[50] The measure was then used to develop an SLE renal response index.[50] The renal activity score was computed as follows: proteinuria 0.5 to 1 g/day (3 points), proteinuria >1 to 3 g/day (5 points), proteinuria >3 g/day (11 points), urine red blood cell count >10/high-power field (HPF) (3 points), and urine white blood cell count >10/HPF (1 point). A reasonable agreement was reached among physician ratings in a pilot study. Nevertheless, the developers of the index suggested further refinement, testing, and validation.[50]

Cutaneous Lupus Erythematosus Disease Area and Severity Index

The Cutaneous Lupus Erythematosus Disease Area and Severity Index (CLASI) was developed to facilitate the quantification of disease activity and damage of cutaneous lupus erythematosus and was first published in 2005.[51] The index has separate scores for damage and activity of skin manifestations.[51] Activity is scored as a summary score of erythema, scale, and hypertrophy of the skin, mucous membrane lesions, and nonscarring recent alopecia. Damage is scored in terms of dyspigmentation or scarring that also includes scarring alopecia. Patients' subjective symptoms, in particular, pruritus, pain, or fatigue, are recorded separately on visual 0 to 10 analog scales. The total possible scores for activity and damage are 70 and 56, respectively.[51] The CLASI has good content validity and interrater and intrarater reliability when used by dermatologists. A recent study conducted on 14 patients with cutaneous lupus assessed by academic rheumatologists and dermatologists showed superior results with dermatologists in the use of the CLASI. Moreover, this study recommended that rheumatologists may benefit from incorporating input from dermatologists for the use of the CLASI.[52] The revised CLASI (RCLASI) was proposed to describe accurately all types of cutaneous lupus.[53] The RCLASI is an expanded version of the CLASI, in which the accuracy of the existing parameters was increased—in particular, scaling or hypertrophy and dyspigmentation—and new parameters, such as edema and infiltration and subcutaneous nodules and plaque, were added.[53] The RCLASI validity and reliability were proven among dermatologists only.[53] Notwithstanding, the reliability and validity of CLASI and its versions require further validation and assessment among rheumatologists before it can be adopted in lupus clinical trials.

Measures of Disease Activity over Time
Adjusted Mean SLEDAI-2K

SLEDAI-2K assesses disease activity at a single point in time.[23] To summarize disease activity over time, the Adjusted Mean SLEDAI-2K (AMS) was developed. The AMS calculates the area under the curve of SLEDAI-2K divided by the length of the time interval.[54] The AMS has been used as a predictor of major outcomes in lupus, including mortality, damage, and coronary artery disease (CAD).[54-56] In longitudinal studies, an increase of 1 AMS unit increased the risk for mortality by 16%, for damage by 6%, and for CAD by 12%.[56] A recent study evaluated whether the frequency of visits would affect the accuracy of estimating the AMS. This study showed that when groups of patients are analyzed, the frequency of visits within 1 year (quarterly, semi-annually, or annually) does not have a significant effect on the AMS. However, in individual patients, only visits up to 3 months apart provided an accurate estimation of disease activity over time, and visits beyond 3 months compromised this measure.[57] AMS plays an important role in measuring disease activity over time in addition to its prognostic value, especially in patients with prolonged follow-up in longitudinal studies.

Responder Measures

Improvement and flare are considered clinically meaningful changes in disease activity, as compared with baseline, which can be determined with the use of appropriate tools. Of the validated tools, SLEDAI-2K and its versions and the BILAG index along with other measures have been most adopted in clinical trials to define these concepts.[22-24] Time to flare, the numbers of flares, and the severity of flares—in particular, mild, moderate, and severe flares—have been used as outcome measures in clinical trials.

Flares

The SELENA-SLEDAI Flare Index (SFI) was proposed by the SELENA trials investigators to define SLE flares, which are an important outcome measure in clinical trials.[58] The original SFI proposed mild/moderate and severe flares, and this separation was applied in a number of randomized controlled trials (RCTs).[1,22] SFI is a composite outcome of SELENA-SLEDAI; mild, moderate, and severe flares; and the PGA (0 = none, 1 = mild, 2 = moderate, 3 = severe) of disease activity.[22] In a study conducted on patient scenarios, the reliability of the SFI was substantial (k = 0.65) for severe flares and fair (k = 0.16) for mild/moderate flares.[58] The developers of SFI showed that the training of the examiners on SFI improves its performance, in particular for mild/moderate flares (k = 0.54).[58] Furthermore, a different group evaluated the reliability and validity of the SELENA-SLEDAI, PGA, and SFI retrospectively on patients' charts. This group found that the PGA and SELENA-SLEDAI components of the SFI are more reliable and valid than the SFI. Both intrarater and interrater reliability of PGA and the SELENA-SLEDAI performed better than the SFI.[59] Moreover, PGA and the SELENA-SLEDAI demonstrated adequate agreement with each other; however, the SFI demonstrated poor agreement with PGA-defined and SELENA-SLEDAI–defined flares (see eFigure 46-2). PGA-defined and SELENA-SLEDAI–defined flares also demonstrated poor agreement. This study raises a question regarding the validity of the SFI; nevertheless, the authors explained that the inadequate performance of the SFI could have been related to the method of retrospective chart abstraction and study design.[59] With the advances in treatment in lupus, the SELENA researchers realized that distinguishing between mild and moderate disease activity in clinical trials is important and proposed the revised version of the SFI.[60] The revised SFI suggests specific clinical manifestations for each organ system and categorizes flares (mild, moderate, and severe), based on the treatment decision. In this new version of the SFI, two of the major components of the original SFI—PGA and SELENA-SLEDAI—have been excluded.[60]

Improvement

Responder Index for Lupus Erythematosus. The Responder Index for Lupus Erythematosus (RIFLE) was developed to measure partial and complete responses to therapy, particularly in clinical trials, and has been published only in an abstract in the peer review literature.[61] The RIFLE is able to detect considerable variation in disease activity and is sensitive to change in important disease activity over time.[61] The RIFLE characterized patients on the basis of their SLE manifestations into worsening, present or no change, partial response, resolution, and not present.[61] The RIFLE has been used in a limited number of clinical trials and research studies and needs further validation.[50,62] A recent study evaluated the minimal clinically important differences of validated measures of lupus disease activity in childhood-onset SLE. This study showed that the RIFLE appears to be less useful for the assessment of childhood-onset SLE than it is for adult-onset SLE, as compared with SLEDAI-2K, SLAM-R, ECLAM, and BILAG indices.[63]

SLE Responder Index. Evidence-based exploratory analysis of the B lymphocyte–stimulating factor antagonist belimumab in a phase II SLE trial led to the development of a novel responder index, the SLE Responder Index (SRI), to define a clinically meaningful change in disease activity.[41] The SRI is a composite outcome that incorporates the modification of the SLEDAI, SELENA-SLEDAI, BILAG, and PGA.[4,22,24,38] As proposed by the authors of the SRI, the SELENA-SLEDAI score was used to determine global improvement. The BILAG domain scores were used to ensure that no significant worsening in heretofore unaffected organ systems had occurred. The PGA ensured that improvement in disease activity was not achieved at the expense of the patient's overall condition.[41] The SRI was initially assessed in a subset of 321 patients with serologically active lupus in a phase II placebo-controlled clinical trial evaluating belimumab. In patients with serologically active disease, the addition of belimumab to concomitant standard of care therapy resulted in a statistically significant response in 46% of patients at week 52, compared with 29% of the patients receiving the placebo.[41] More recently, a randomised, placebo-controlled, phase 3 trial used this novel 3 part outcome response measure and demonstrated a statistically significant difference in responders in patients on belimumab as compared

to placebo.[42] In the epratuzumab trial, researchers proposed a modification of the SRI, in which the BILAG index is to be used to define primary improvement, whereas the SLEDAI and PGA are used to indicate that no deterioration in disease activity has occurred.[64]

SLEDAI-2K Responder Index 50. The SLEDAI and its versions record descriptors of disease activity as present or absent.[4,20,22,23,27,28] To demonstrate improvement, a manifestation has to resolve completely. Thus the SLEDAI-2K utility in observational studies and, more importantly, in clinical trials is limited; it does not allow one to discern a signal toward improvement but still incomplete. The recognition of this limitation of the SLEDAI-2K led the SLEDAI developers to consider modifications to capture partial improvement in disease activity. A minimum of 50% improvement was believed by clinicians to reflect a clinically important improvement and gave rise to the concept of the SLEDAI-2K Responder Index 50 (SRI-50).[65] In 2009 the SLEDAI-2K 30 days was used to build the SRI-50.[66] The SRI-50 is made up of the same 24 descriptors as the SLEDAI-2K and covers 9 organ systems. After a review of the literature, the new definitions of the SRI-50 were generated to identify a 50% improvement in each of the 24 descriptors of the SLEDAI-2K. Content and face validity of the SRI-50 definitions were confirmed according to the methodology adopted in the development of the SRI-50. The SRI-50 definitions were developed as a two-page document (Figure 46-8). As in the SLEDAI-2K 30 days, each descriptor in the SRI-50 refers to the preceding 30 days.[27,28] The assigned scores for the descriptors of the SRI-50 were derived by dividing the score of the corresponding SLEDAI-2K by 2. As in the SLEDAI-2K, the score of the SRI-50 can range from 0 to 105.[67] The method of scoring the SRI-50 is simple, cumulative, and intuitive as in the original SLEDAI-2K.[23,67] To familiarize physicians with both the definitions of the SRI-50 and the SRI-50 data retrieval form, a dedicated web site (www.sri-50.com) was developed that offered training and examination modules.

The SRI-50 data retrieval form was developed to standardize the recording of the descriptors in an efficient way to allow the calculation of the SRI-50 scores (Figure 46-9).[67] In the initial validation of the SRI-50, the concurrent construct validity of the SRI-50 and the physician-response assessment were evaluated in 141 patients. The SRI-50 scores decreased more than the SLEDAI-2K scores in patients who improved. A moderate correlation was found between the SRI-50 and the physician-response assessment. More importantly, the decrease in the SRI-50 scores was clinically more important than the decrease in the SLEDAI-2K scores in patients who improved and met the definition of improvement by decreasing by 4 or higher.[2,67] In a multicenter study, the SRI-50 was evaluated on patient profiles and demonstrated both intrarater and interrater reliability with average intraclass correlation coefficients of 0.99 and 1.00, respectively.[68] More recently, the SRI-50 has shown that it enhances the ability of the composite outcome SRI to identify patients with clinically important improvement in disease activity.[40]

Disease Activity in Childhood

The Pediatric Rheumatology International Trial Organization (PRINTO) and the ACR Provisional Criteria for the Evaluation of Response to Therapy for children with childhood SLE attempted to prospectively validate the provisional criteria for the evaluation of response in children with SLE. The PRINTO could not firmly choose the specific disease activity tool for the assessment of global disease activity in lupus. The differences in sensitivity and specificity among the evaluated indices, in particular, the SLEDAI-2K and the ECLAM, SLAM-R, and BILAG indices, were small; all performed equally in evaluating disease activity. Although the BILAG index may have had a slightly higher sensitivity than the other indices, the PRINTO emphasized the complexity of the BILAG scoring system, which could result in considerable measure error when less experienced and trained raters, in particular, did the scoring.[16]

Text continued on p. 575.

SLEDAI-2K Responder Index 50 (SRI-50)© – Definitions

Descriptors are present at the time of the visit or in the preceding 30 days and must be attributable to lupus.

DESCRIPTOR	SLEDAI-2K DEFINITION	DEFINITION OF SRI-50 IMPROVEMENT
Seizure	Recent onset. Exclude metabolic, infectious or drug causes.	≥50% reduction in frequency of baseline seizure days/month.
Psychosis*	Altered ability to function in normal activity due to severe disturbance in the perception of reality. Include hallucinations, incoherence, marked loose associations, impoverished thought content, marked illogical thinking, bizarre, disorganized, or catatonic behavior. Exclude uremia and drug causes.	≥50% improvement of the psychotic manifestations judged by physician.
Organic brain syndrome*	Altered mental function with impaired orientation, memory, or other intellectual function, with rapid onset and fluctuating clinical features. Include clouding of consciousness with reduced capacity to focus, and inability to sustain attention to environment, plus at least 2 of the following: perceptual disturbance, incoherent speech, insomnia or daytime drowsiness, or increased or decreased psychomotor activity. Exclude metabolic, infectious or drug causes.	≥50% improvement of the organic brain manifestations judged by physician.
Visual disturbance	Retinal changes of SLE. Include cytoid bodies, retinal hemorrhages, serous exudate or hemorrhages in the choroid, or optic neuritis. Exclude hypertension, infection, or drug causes.	≥50% improvement of the retinal exam assessed by physician.
Cranial nerve disorder§	New onset of sensory or motor neuropathy involving cranial nerves.	≥50% recovery of motor or sensory function in affected nerve within 1 month from the event on the basis of decrease in lupus disease activity or ≥50% decrease of the severity of pain within 1 month from the event on the basis of decrease in lupus disease activity as determined by patient on numerical scale of 1–10 if applicable with no worsening in either.
Lupus headache#	Severe, persistent headache; may be migrainous, but must be nonresponsive to narcotic analgesia.	≥50% decrease of the severity of pain as determined by patient on numerical scale of 1–10.
CVA§	New onset of cerebrovascular accident(s). Exclude arteriosclerosis.	≥50% recovery of motor or sensory function related to CVA within 1 month from the event on the basis of decrease in lupus disease activity as determined by physician without worsening in either.
Vasculitis†	Ulceration, gangrene, tender finger nodules, periungual infarction, splinter hemorrhages, or biopsy or angiogram proof of vasculitis.	≥50% improvement of the vasculitis lesions present with no new lesion or worsening in either. A ≥50% improvement for ulceration or gangrene is defined as ≥50% decrease in the body surface area; for periungual infarction, splinter hemorrhages or tender finger nodules a ≥50% improvement is defined as ≥50% decrease in the total number of involved digits with periungual infarction, splinter hemorrhages and tender finger nodules. Multiple lesions in a single digit, count only one.

Numerical scale: 1 is mild and 10 is most severe.

To determine body surface area use Rule of Nines for skin scoring: Head 9%, chest 9%, abdomen 9%, back 18%, legs 36%, arms/hands 18% and mucous membrane 1%; physician's palm for 1%.

* Overlap of symptoms will count for only one descriptor: either Psychosis or Organic Brain Syndrome.

Lupus headache improvement will count regardless of whether patient is using narcotic analgesia or not though it has to be part of the baseline lupus headache.

§ CVA and Cranial Nerve improvement will count if it occurs within 1 month from the event on the basis of decrease in lupus disease activity as this is more likely on the basis of decreased disease activity.

† Vasculitis, Rash and Alopecia; if the total BSA ≤1%, a ≥50% improvement is defined by ≥50% decrease in the activity of the most active lesion by decreasing by 2 grades or ≥50% decrease in the number of lesions or decrease in the size of the biggest lesion with no worsening in either.

© University Health Network

FIGURE 46-8 The SLEDAI-2K Responder Index 50 (SRI-50) definitions. *(From Touma Z, Gladman DD, Ibañez D, et al: Development and initial validation of the Systemic Lupus Erythematosus Disease Activity Index 2000 Responder Index 50. J Rheumatol 38(2):275–284, 2011.)*

Continued

SLEDAI-2K Responder Index 50 (SRI-50)© – Definitions

DESCRIPTOR	SLEDAI-2K DEFINITION	DEFINITION OF SRI-50 IMPROVEMENT
Arthritis	≥2 joints with pain and signs of inflammatory (i.e., tenderness, swelling or effusion).	≥50% reduction in the number of joints with pain and signs of inflammation (i.e., tenderness, swelling or effusion).
Myositis	Proximal muscle aching/weakness, associated with elevated creatinine phosphokinase/aldolase or electromyogram changes or a biopsy showing myositis.	≥50% increase in muscles power judged by physician or increase of 1 grade upon a scale of zero to five or ≥50% decrease in the level of creatinine phosphokinase/ aldolase level comparing to previous visit with no worsening in either.
Urinary casts	Hemegranular or red blood cell casts.	Decrease by ≥50% in the total number of casts (hemegranular and red blood cell casts).
Hematuria	>5 red blood cells/high power field. Exclude stone, infection, or other cause.	Decrease by ≥50% in the number of red blood cell/high power field at this visit.
Proteinuria	New onset, recurrent, or persistent proteinuria of >0.5 gram/24 hours.	Decrease by ≥50% in the range of proteinuria.
Pyuria	>5 white blood cells/high power field. Exclude infection.	Decrease by ≥50% in the number of white blood cells/high power field.
Rash†	New onset, recurrent or persistent inflammatory lupus rash. *Activity of skin lesions should be based on the evaluation of the most active lesion.*	Decrease by ≥50% of involved body surface area and/or activity of most active lesion with no worsening in either. Activity of the lesion should be determined by the color of the lesions: 0 – absent 1 – pink, faint erythema 2 – red 3 – dark red/purple/violaceous/crusted/hemorrhagic A ≥50% decrease in the activity of the lesion is defined by decreasing by 2 grades. Dyspigmentation, scarring and atrophy are not active lesions.
Alopecia†	New onset, recurrent, or persistent abnormal, patchy or diffuse loss of hair. *Size of patchy alopecic lesion should be determined based on involved total scalp surface. Total scalp surface is 4.5%.* *Diffuse alopecia is determined by patient on numerical scale of 1–10.* *Activity of alopecia should be based on the evaluation of the most active lesion.*	Decrease by ≥50% of total scalp involved area for patchy alopecic lesion or ≥50% reduction in the diffuse alopecia as determined by patient on numerical scale of 1–10, and/ or activity of the most active alopecic lesions with no worsening in either. Activity of the alopecic lesion should be determined by the color of the most active lesion: 0 – absent 1 – pink, faint erythema 2 – red 3 – dark red/purple/violaceous/crusted/hemorrhagic A ≥50% decrease in the activity of the lesion is defined by decreasing by 2 grades.
Mucosal ulcers	New onset, recurrent, or persistent oral or nasal ulcerations.	Decrease by ≥50% in the number of ulcers at this visit.
Pleurisy	Pleuritic chest pain with pleural rub or effusion, or pleural thickening.	≥50% reduction in the pain severity as determined by patient on numerical scale of 1–10 and or ≥50% reduction in the amount of fluid (on imaging) with no worsening in either.
Pericarditis	Pericardial pain with at least one of the following: Rub, effusion, electrocardiogram or echocardiogram confirmation.	≥50% reduction in the pain severity as determined by patient on numerical scale of 1–10 and/or ≥50% reduction in the amount of fluid (on imaging) with no worsening in either.
Low complement	Decrease in CH50, C3, or C4 below the lower limit of normal for testing laboratory.	≥50% increase in the level of any complement or normalization of one of them without a drop in either.
Increased anti-DNA antibodies levels	Increase in the level of anti-DNA antibodies above normal range for testing laboratory.	≥50% reduction in the level of anti-DNA antibodies.
Fever	>38°C. Exclude infectious causes.	≥50% reduction in the degree of fever above normal.
Thrombocytopenia	<100,000 platelets/x 10⁹/L. Exclude drug causes.	≥50% increase in the level of platelets but <100,000 platelets/mm³.
Leukopenia	<3,000 white blood cells/x 10⁹/L. Exclude drug causes.	≥50% increase in the level of white blood cells but <3,000/mm³.

©The SLEDAI-2K-50 Responder Index (SRI-50) is a licensed work of the University Health Network.

FIGURE 46-8, cont'd

Patient ID: _____

Descriptors are present at the time of the visit or in the preceding 30 days and must be attributable to lupus.

BASELINE VISIT	Score (Circle)	FOLLOW-UP VISIT	Score (Circle) Improvement		
			<50%	≥50%	100%
Visit Date: _____ / _____ / _____		Visit Date: _____ / _____ / _____			
Seizure ☐ Partial (focal, local) seizures 　☐ simple partial seizures (consciousness not impaired) 　☐ complex partial (with impairment of consciousness) 　☐ partial seizures (simple or complex) evolving to secondarily generalized seizures ☐ Generalized seizures 　☐ nonconvulsive (absence) 　☐ convulsive **Days per month** _____	8	**Seizure** ☐ Partial (focal, local) seizures 　☐ simple partial seizures (consciousness not impaired) 　☐ complex partial (with impairment of consciousness) 　☐ partial seizures (simple or complex) evolving to secondarily generalized seizures ☐ Generalized seizures 　☐ nonconvulsive (absence) 　☐ convulsive **Days per month** _____	8	4	0
Psychosis ☐ Altered ability to function in normal activity due to: 　☐ hallucinations ☐ incoherence 　☐ marked loose associations 　☐ impoverished thought content 　☐ marked illogical thinking 　☐ bizarre, disorganized or catatonic behavior	8	**Psychosis** ☐ Altered ability to function in normal activity due to: 　☐ hallucinations ☐ incoherence 　☐ marked loose associations 　☐ impoverished thought content 　☐ marked illogical thinking 　☐ bizarre, disorganized or catatonic behavior **Percentage of improvement of the acute event** _____ %	8	4	0
Organic brain syndrome ☐ Altered mental function (with rapid onset and fluctuating clinical features) with impaired: 　☐ orientation 　☐ memory 　☐ other intellectual function 　☐ clouding of consciousness with reduced capacity to focus and inability to sustain attention to environment 　　☐ perceptual disturbance 　　☐ incoherent speech 　　☐ insomnia or daytime drowsiness 　　☐ increased or decreased psychomotor activity	8	**Organic brain syndrome** ☐ Altered mental function (with rapid onset and fluctuating clinical features) with impaired: 　☐ orientation 　☐ memory 　☐ other intellectual function clinical features 　☐ clouding of consciousness with reduced capacity to focus and inability to sustain attention to environment 　　☐ perceptual disturbance 　　☐ incoherent speech 　　☐ insomnia or daytime drowsiness 　　☐ increased or decreased psychomotor activity **Percentage of improvement of the acute event** _____ %	8	4	0
Visual disturbance ☐ cytoid bodies ☐ retinal hemorrhage ☐ serous exudates in the choroid ☐ hemorrhage in the choroid ☐ optic neuritis	8	**Visual disturbance** ☐ cytoid bodies ☐ retinal hemorrhage ☐ serous exudates in the choroid ☐ hemorrhage in the choroid ☐ optic neuritis **Percentage of improvement of the retinal exam** _____ %	8	4	0
Cranial nerve disorder Nerves involved _____ ☐ motor power _____ ☐ sensory deficit _____ ☐ pain as determined by patient on numerical scale of 1-10 _____	8	**Cranial nerve disorder** Nerves involved _____ ☐ motor power _____ **Percentage of improvement of the acute event** _____ % ☐ sensory deficit _____ **Percentage of improvement of the acute event** _____ % ☐ **pain as determined by patient on numerical scale of 1-10** _____	8	4	0
Lupus headache ☐ pain as determined by patient on numerical scale of 1-10 _____	8	**Lupus headache** ☐ **pain as determined by patient on numerical scale of 1-10** _____	8	4	0
CVA Clinical diagnosis _____ Date of CVA (yyyy/mm/dd) _____ ☐ face ☐ upper extremities ☐ lower extremities ☐ motor power _____ ☐ sensory deficit location _____	8	**CVA** Clinical diagnosis: _____ Date of CVA (yyyy/mm/dd) _____ ☐ face ☐ upper extremities ☐ lower extremities ☐ motor power _____ ☐ sensory deficit location _____ **Percentage of improvement of the acute event** _____ %	8	4	0
Vasculitis ☐ ulceration of _____ ☐ gangrene of _____ Body surface area _____ % Number of lesions: _____ Size of biggest lesion: _____ ☐ periungual infarction # of involved digits _____ ☐ splinter hemorrhages # of involved digits _____ ☐ tender finger nodules # of involved digits _____	8	**Vasculitis** ☐ ulceration of _____ ☐ gangrene of _____ **Body surface area** _____ % **Number of lesions:** _____ **Size of biggest lesion:** _____ ☐ periungual infarction # **of involved digits** _____ ☐ splinter hemorrhages # **of involved digits** _____ ☐ tender finger nodules # **of involved digits** _____	8	4	0

FIGURE 46-9 The SLEDAI-2K Responder Index 50 (SRI-50) data retrieval form. *(From Touma Z, Gladman DD, Ibañez D, et al: Development and initial validation of the Systemic Lupus Erythematosus Disease Activity Index 2000 Responder Index 50. J Rheumatol 38(2):275–284, 2011.)* *Continued*

Data retrieval form of SLEDAI-2K Responder Index-50 (SRI-50)©

BASELINE VISIT	Score (Circle)	FOLLOW-UP VISIT	Score (Circle) Improvement		
			<50%	≥50%	100%
Arthritis Number of joints with pain and signs of inflammation (i.e., tenderness, swelling or effusion) # _____	4	**Arthritis** Number of joints with pain and signs of inflammation (i.e., tenderness, swelling or effusion) # _____	4	2	0
Myositis Motor power _____ creatinine phosphokinase level _____ or aldolase _____	4	**Myositis** Motor power _____ creatinine phosphokinase level _____ or aldolase _____ Percentage of improvement in muscles power___%	4	2	0
Urinary casts Number of hemegranular casts _____ or red blood cells casts _____	4	**Urinary casts** Number of hemegranular casts _____ or red blood cells casts _____	4	2	0
Hematuria: Number of red blood cells/high power field _____	4	**Hematuria:** Number of red blood cells/high power field _____	4	2	0
Proteinuria: Level of proteinuria_____	4	**Proteinuria:** Level of proteinuria_____	4	2	0
Pyuria: Number of white blood cells/high power field_____	4	**Pyuria:** Number of white blood cells/high power field_____	4	2	0
Rash ☐ Head ☐ Chest ☐ Abdomen ☐ Back ☐ Legs ☐ Arms/hands ☐ Mucous membrane Body surface area: _____% Number of lesions: _____ Size of biggest lesion: _____ Activity of most active skin lesion by color: ☐ Absent ☐ Pink, faint erythema ☐ Red ☐ Dark/purple/violaceous/crusted/hemorrhagic Dyspigmentation, scarring and atrophy are not active lesions	2	**Rash** ☐ Head ☐ Chest ☐ Abdomen ☐ Back ☐ Legs ☐ Arms/hands ☐ Mucous membrane Body surface area: _____% Number of lesions: _____ Size of biggest lesion: _____ Activity of most active skin lesion by color: ☐ Absent ☐ Pink, faint erythema ☐ Red ☐ Dark/purple/violaceous/crusted/hemorrhagic Dyspigmentation, scarring and atrophy are not active lesions	2	1	0
Alopecia ☐ Patchy Total scalp area involved: _____% Number of lesions: _____ Size of biggest lesion: _____ ☐ Diffuse alopecia as determined by patient on numerical scale of 1–10: _____ Activity of alopecia by color based on most active lesion: ☐ Absent ☐ Pink, faint erythema ☐ Red ☐ Dark/purple/violaceous/crusted/hemorrhagic	2	**Alopecia** ☐ Patchy Total scalp area involved: _____% Number of lesions: _____ Size of biggest lesion: _____ ☐ Diffuse alopecia as determined by patient on numerical scale of 1–10: _____ Activity of alopecia by color based on most active lesion: ☐ Absent ☐ Pink, faint erythema ☐ Red ☐ Dark/purple/violaceous/crusted/hemorrhagic	2	1	0
Mucosal ulcers: Number of ulcers per month: _____	2	**Mucosal ulcers:** Number of ulcers per month: _____	2	1	0
Pleurisy: ☐ Pain as determined by patient on numerical scale of 1–10: _____ Amount of effusion if determined radiologically: _____	2	**Pleurisy:** ☐ Pain as determined by patient on numerical scale of 1–10: _____ Amount of effusion if determined radiologically: _____	2	1	0
Pericarditis: ☐ Pain as determined by patient on numerical scale of 1–10: _____ Amount of effusion if determined radiologically: _____	2	**Pericarditis:** ☐ Pain as determined by patient on numerical scale of 1–10: _____ Amount of effusion if determined radiologically: _____	2	1	0
Low complement: C3 _____ C4 _____	2	**Low complement:** C3 _____ C4 _____	2	1	0
Anti-DNA antibodies level: _____	2	**Anti-DNA antibodies level:** _____	2	1	0
Fever: T°C (mean) _____	1	**Fever:** T°C (mean) _____	1	0.5	0
Thrombocytopenia: Platelet count _____	1	**Thrombocytopenia:** Platelet count _____	1	0.5	0
Leucopenia: WBC count _____	1	**Leucopenia:** WBC count _____	1	0.5	0
TOTAL SCORE		**TOTAL SCORE**			

FIGURE 46-9, cont'd

Disease Activity in Pregnancy

The assessment of lupus during pregnancy is affected by the physiologic changes that influence the clinical manifestation and laboratory tests of lupus. Since 1999, several lupus activity scales have been adapted for use during pregnancy, in particular, the Systemic Lupus Erythematosus Pregnancy Disease Activity Index (SLEPDAI), the modified SLAM (m-SLAM) index, and the lupus activity index in pregnancy (LAI-P).[69] Nevertheless, demonstrating reliability and validity of these modifications is fundamental before they are used in clinical trials and research studies.[69]

Clinically Meaningful Change in Disease Activity Measures

Improvement

Improvement has been accepted as an important and relevant outcome measure in clinical trials. At present, improvement is defined on the basis of disease activity measures, in particular, the SLEDAI-2K and BILAG index, as follows: improvement is a reduction in SLEDAI-2K of 4 or higher or a reduction in the BILAG scores. A major clinical response by the BILAG index is a BILAG C score or better at 6 months with no new BILAG A or B scores and the maintenance of response with no new BILAG A or B scores between 6 and 12 months.[49] Although the BILAG-2004 index was significantly associated with a decrease in therapy with a major improvement from Grade A or B to C or D, it was not definitively responsive to the improvement in disease activity from very active to moderately active (Grade A to B). In fact, a reduction from Grade A to B is not always reflected by a reduction in therapy. This issue led the authors to recommend that clinical trials using the BILAG-2004 index should use the efficacy criterion of improvement to low-level activity (Grade C or D) as the main outcome, instead of improvement from Grade A to B.[70]

Until recent years, few responder indices have been developed that measure response to treatment in multiple systems. Of the available responder indices, the BILAG index has been the most used in clinical trials, whereas the RIFLE has been the least used. In June 2010, the U.S. Food and Drug Administration (FDA) publication, "Guidance for Industry: Systemic Lupus Erythematosus—Developing Medical Products for Treatment," referred to the BILAG index as being the best available to study the reduction in disease activity in clinical trials.[71] Nevertheless, the ACR expressed the need for the development and validation of new reliable indices that can measure improvement in disease activity in response to new drugs in the treatment of lupus.

Although the SLEDAI-2K has been used to define improvement in disease activity, it is important to highlight that the SLEDAI-2K captures improvement in the descriptors that resolve completely. This led to the development of the SRI-50, a novel index based on the SLEDAI-2K but that measures the clinically important improvement of 50% or greater in disease activity.[66,67,72] The performance of the SRI-50 was evaluated prospectively and retrospectively in longitudinal studies and proved to be superior to the SLEDAI-2K in identifying patients with 50% or greater improvement.[66,67,72] More importantly, the SRI-50 enhances the ability of the composite outcome SRI to identify patients with clinically important improvement in disease activity.[40] Currently, the SRI-50 is being used as the primary and secondary outcomes measure in several therapeutic trials in lupus.

Flare

Flare is considered one of the most commonly used outcome measures of disease activity. Flare is defined as an increase in the SLEDAI-2K of 4 points or more, an increase in the SELENA-SLEDAI score of 3 points or more, or one new category A or two new category B grades on the BILAG index.[13,22,39] In terms of specific flare indices, the SELENA researchers initially proposed the SFI and, more recently, the revised SFI version in an effort to differentiate mild and moderate flares.[58,60] The revised SFI suggested specific clinical manifestations for each organ system and categorized flares (mild, moderate, and severe) on the basis of the treatment decision.[60] A recent study

individually evaluated mild, moderate, and severe flares and showed that the intraclass correlation coefficients are 0.54, 0.21, and 0.18 for a BILAG-2004 flare, SELENA flare, and PGA flare, respectively. The results of this study highlight the difficulty in the distinction between mild and moderate flares, and the results among the examiners were much less consistent, despite use of the new SFI version.[60] Similarly, the separation between mild and moderate flares remains problematic even with the use of the BILAG-2004 index.[70] More importantly, the BILAG-2004 index appears to perform better at detecting increases in disease activity, as compared with improvement in disease activity, leading to the recommendation that the BILAG-2004 index be used in longitudinal studies that aim to determine, in particular, worsening in disease activity. Moreover, the renal scoring in the BILAG-2004 index is powered to detect new-onset lupus nephritis or significant improvement (Grade C or D), and using more specific criteria is advisable to define response in longitudinal studies on lupus nephritis and, ultimately, in clinical trials.[70]

Besides flare, SLEDAI-2K scores are used to define PAD with a SLEDAI-2K score change of 4 or less between visits and a remission as a SLEDAI score of 0. A recent study from the Lupus Clinic in Toronto showed that among 417 patients, one third of the patients had 1 or more flares, whereas nearly one half experienced PAD in a given year. Nearly 60% of the patients had episodes of flare or PAD per year. At least 25% of patients had PAD without achieving the definition of flare, whereas SLEDAI-2K scores at the start of the outcome interval and prior cutaneous or musculoskeletal disease activity predicted PAD.[2] Although flare has been considered the most commonly used outcome measure to describe worsening disease activity, PAD also is a common disease state in patients with active disease and should be used in clinical and research settings.

DAMAGE

The survival of patients has significantly improved, and death is often attributed to accrued damage from lupus, its treatment, and other co-morbidities in those who die late in the course of their disease.[73] The concept of damage was recognized in the initial meeting of the Conference on Prognosis Studies in SLE in 1985, and the initial validation and development of the index were confirmed at a subsequent workshop of the SLICC in 1992.[74] In 1996 the SLICC group, in collaboration with the ACR, developed the SLICC/ACR Damage Index (SDI).[75] The SDI describes the accumulation of damage that has occurred since the onset of lupus in 12 different systems (Figure 46-10). In addition, the SDI includes 41 items that may have resulted from the previous disease activity leading to organ failure (e.g., renal failure), disease therapy (e.g., steroid-induced diabetes), or intercurrent illness (e.g., cancer, surgery) without being attributed to lupus.[75] Items must be present for at least 6 months to be included in the SDI and based on clinical judgment rather than on specialized techniques to allow ease of use.[75] Some items can score between 2 and 3 for recurrent events (e.g., avascular necrosis) or serious damage (e.g., end-stage renal disease), and the total score ranges from 0 to 49, although patients rarely score above 10. The SDI scored at 2.38 ± 2.22, in a group of 146 patients from the University of Toronto Lupus Clinic with a mean disease duration of 21.2 ± 8.4 years.[76] Patients continue to accrue damage over time. In a study on 235 patients, the SDI was 0.47 ± 0.96, at year 1; 0.74 ± 1.19, at year 3; and 0.95 ± 1.27, at year 5.[77] The SDI has been shown to be valid and reliable in several studies[78] and accepted as an independent outcome measure in clinical trials and mainly in longitudinal studies.[79] The SDI has also predicted mortality in patients with lupus and was valid in the assessment of the long-term effect of treatment.[79] Disease activity at presentation and over time predicted the SDI, as well as ethnicities and socioeconomic status and late-onset as compared with early-onset lupus.[55,80-82] In childhood-onset SLE, it was shown that prolonged use of high-dose corticosteroids may further increase the SDI, but the use of immunosuppressive agents may protect against disease damage.[83] In observational longitudinal studies, the presence of damage was not associated with the

Visit Date: _____

SLICC/ACR DAMAGE INDEX and GLOSSARY OF TERMS

Damage occurring since <u>diagnosis</u> of lupus, ascertained by clinical assessment and present for at least <u>6 months</u> unless otherwise stated. Repeat episodes mean at least 6 months apart to score 2. The same lesion cannot be scored twice.

ITEM	SCORE (circle)
OCULAR (Either eye, by clinical assessment)	
Any cataract ever	1
Retinal change OR optic atrophy	1
NEUROPSYCHIATRIC	
Cognitive impairment (e.g., memory deficit, difficulty with calculation, poor concentration, difficulty in spoken or written language, impaired performance level) OR major psychosis	1
Seizures requiring therapy for 6 months	1
Cerebral vascular accident ever (Score 2 if >1) OR resection not for malignancy	1 2
Cranial or peripheral neuropathy (excluding optic)	1
Transverse myelitis	1
RENAL	
Estimated or measured GFR <50%	1
Proteinuria 24 h, ≥3.5 g OR	1
End-stage renal disease (regardless of dialysis or transplantation)	3
PULMONARY	
Pulmonary hypertension (right ventricular prominence, or loud P2)	1
Pulmonary fibrosis (physical and X-ray)	1
Shrinking lung (X-ray)	1
Pleural fibrosis (X-ray)	1
Pulmonary infarction (X-ray) OR resection not for malignancy	1
CARDIOVASCULAR	
Angina OR coronary artery bypass	1
Myocardial infarction ever (Score 2 if >1)	1 2
Cardiomyopathy (ventricular dysfunction)	1
Valvular disease (diastolic murmur, or a systolic murmur >3/6)	1
Pericarditis x 6 months or pericardiectomy	1

Visit Date: _____

SLICC/ACR DAMAGE INDEX - Page 2

ITEM	SCORE
PERIPHERAL VASCULAR	
Claudication x 6 months	1
Minor tissue loss (pulp space)	1
Significant tissue loss ever (e.g., loss of digit or limb, resection) (Score 2 if >1)	1 2
Venous thrombosis with swelling, ulceration, OR venous stasis	1
GASTROINTESTINAL	
Infarction or resection of bowel (below duodenum), spleen, liver or gallbladder ever (Score 2 if >1)	1 2
Mesenteric insufficiency	1
Chronic peritonitis	1
Stricture OR upper gastrointestinal tract surgery ever	1
Pancreatic insufficiency requiring enzyme replacement or with pseudocyst	1
MUSCULOSKELETAL	
Atrophy or weakness	1
Deforming or erosive arthritis (including reducible deformities, excluding avascular necrosis)	1
Osteoporosis with fracture or vertebral collapse (excluding avascular necrosis)	1
Avascular necrosis (Score 2 if >1)	1 2
Osteomyelitis	1
Ruptured tendons	1
SKIN	
Alopecia	1
Extensive scarring or panniculum other than scalp and pulp space	1
Skin ulceration (excluding thrombosis) for more than 6 months	1
PREMATURE GONADAL FAILURE	1
DIABETES (regardless of treatment)	1
MALIGNANCY (Exclude dysplasia)	1 2
TOTAL SCORE	

FIGURE 46-10 The Systemic Lupus International Collaborating Clinics/American College of Rheumatology (SLICC/ACR) Damage Index (SDI). (From Gladman DD, Urowitz MB, Goldsmith CH, et al; The reliability of the Systemic Lupus International Collaborating Clinics/American College of Rheumatology Damage Index in patients with systemic lupus erythematosus. Arthritis Rheum 40(5):809–813, 1997.)

Visit Date: _____

SLICC/ACR DAMAGE INDEX
GLOSSARY OF TERMS

Damage: Non-reversible change, not related to active inflammation, occurring since <u>diagnosis</u> of lupus, ascertained by clinical assessment and present for at least <u>6 months</u> unless otherwise stated. Repeat episodes mean at least 6 months apart to score 2. The same lesion cannot be scored twice.

Cataract: A lens opacity (cataract) in either eye, ever, whether primary or secondary to steroid therapy, documented by ophthalmoscopy.

Retinal change: Documented by ophthalmoscopic examination, may result in field defect, legal blindness.

Optic atrophy: Documented by ophthalmoscopic examination.

Cognitive impairment: Memory deficit, difficulty with calculation, poor concentration, difficulty in spoken or written language, impaired performed level, documented on clinical examination, or by formal neurocognitive testing.

Major psychosis: Altered ability to function in normal activity due to psychiatric reasons. Severe disturbance in the perception of reality characterized by the following features: delusions, hallucinations (auditory, visual), incoherence, marked loose associations, impoverished thought content, marked illogical thinking, bizarre, disorganized or catatonic behavior.

Seizures: Paroxysmal electrical discharge occurring in the brain and producing characteristic physical changes including tonic and clonic movements and certain behavioral disorders. Only seizures requiring therapy for 6 months are counted as damage.

CVA: Cerebral vascular accident resulting in focal findings such as paresis, weakness, etc, OR surgical resection for causes other than malignancy.

Neuropathy: Damage to either a cranial or peripheral nerve, excluding optic nerve, resulting in either motor or sensory dysfunction.

Transverse myelitis: Lower extremity weakness or sensory loss with loss of rectal and urinary bladder sphincter control.

Renal: Estimated or measured GFR <50%, proteinuria ≥3.5 g in 24 hours, or end-stage renal disease (regardless of dialysis or transplantation).

Pulmonary: Pulmonary hypertension (right ventricular prominence, or loud P2), pulmonary fibrosis (physical and X-ray), shrinking lung (X-ray), pleural fibrosis (X-ray), pulmonary infarction (X-ray), a resection for cause other than malignancy.

Cardiovascular: Angina or coronary artery bypass, myocardial infarction (documented by EKG and enzymes) ever, cardiomyopathy (ventricular dysfunction documented clinically), valvular disease (diastolic murmur, or a systolic murmur >3/6), pericarditis x 6 months pericardiectomy.

Peripheral vascular: Claudication, persistent for 6 months, by history.
Minor tissue loss, such as pulp space, ever.
Significant tissue loss, such as loss of digit or limb, or resection, ever.
Venous thrombosis with swelling, ulceration, or clinical evidence of venous stasis.

Gastrointestinal: Infarction or resection of bowel below duodenum, by history.
Resection of spleen, liver or gallbladder ever, for whatever cause.
Mesenteric insufficiency, with diffuse abdominal pain on clinical examination.
Chronic peritonitis, with persistent abdominal pain and peritoneal irritations, on clinical examination.
Oesophageal stricture, shown on endoscopy.
Upper gastrointestinal tract surgery, such as correction of stricture, ulcer surgery, etc., ever, by history.
Pancreatic insufficiency requiring enzyme replacement or with a pseudocyst.

Musculoskeletal: Muscle atrophy or weakness, demonstrated on clinical examination.
Deforming or erosive arthritis, including reducible deformities (excluding avascular necrosis), on clinical examination.
Osteoporosis with fracture or vertebral collapse (excluding avascular necrosis) demonstrated on X-ray.
Avascular necrosis, demonstrated on any imaging technique.
Osteomyelitis, documented clinically, and supported by culture evidence.
Tendon ruptures.

Skin: Scarring, chronic alopecia, documented clinically.
Extensive scarring or panniculum other than scalp and pulp space, documented clinically.
Skin ulceration (excluding thrombosis) for more than 6 months.

Premature gonadal failure: Secondary amenorrhea, prior to age 40.

Diabetes: Diabetes requiring therapy, but regardless of treatment.

Malignancy: Documented by pathology, excluding dysplasias.

FIGURE 46-10, cont'd

patient's sex, the SLEDAI, or an antimalarial agent but was significantly associated with the AMS, age, disease duration, and use of steroids or immunosuppressive medications.[55] In clinical trials, the SDI is used in the stratification of patients and as an independent outcome measure, because an effective drug would be expected to prevent the progression of damage. More recently, a patient self-administered version of the SDI, the Lupus Damage Index Questionnaire (LDIQ), was developed and validated.[84] The developers of this index suggested its use whenever a direct assessment by physicians is not practical. The agreement between the SDI and LDIQ by Spearman's correlation ranged from 0.24 to 0.66 (overall, r = 0.50) and was not distributed equally among all 12 systems, in particular, 0.24 for integument system, 0.25 for gastrointestinal system, and 0.42 for each of the following systems: gonadal, neuropsychiatric, and peripheral vascular.[84] The LDIQ was translated into several languages, and its correlation with the SDI ranged from 0.68 for the Spanish version, to 0.43 for the French version, and 0.37 for the Portuguese version.[85] The LDIQ has not yet been validated for use in longitudinal studies, and its reliability among patients needs to be evaluated. More importantly, the time needed to complete the SDI form for a complex case that is unknown to a physician may take up to 10 to 15 minutes, or less on a follow-up visit. The SDI was accepted among rheumatologists in determining damage; however, what the LDIQ offers over the SDI remains questionable. Caution is advised with the use of the LDIQ to determine damage especially when the damage is used to stratify patients in research and clinical studies, considering its prognostic properties. In summary, the SDI should be the "gold standard" in determining the damage in research and clinical settings. Damage is an independent outcome measure that needs to be determined by experienced and trained physicians on the use of the SDI.

HEALTH-RELATED QUALITY OF LIFE

Survival of patients with SLE has improved significantly over a 36-year period, and new morbidities have emerged, leading to altered patterns of outcome in this disease.[73] HRQoL refers to the impact that a disease and its treatment have on an individual's ability to function and his or her perceived well-being in physical, mental, and social domains of life, in particular, fatigue, functioning, sleep, general appearance, and the inability to plan ahead.[86] HRQoL of patients with SLE seems to be significantly worse and affects all health domains at an earlier age, in comparison with patients with other common chronic diseases.[87,88] HRQoL is an independent outcome measure and is not usually associated with either lupus disease activity or damage.[89] HRQoL is an important outcome measure in the assessment of patients with SLE and can readily be assessed by disease-generic and disease-specific questionnaires.[76,90] Because the SF-36 is a generic questionnaire, it has been suggested that this tool may not be sufficient to characterize the numerous dimensions in which SLE may affect a patient (e.g., infertility, physical appearance) and that it lacks one or more domains pertinent to patients with SLE (e.g., sleep, body image, sexual health).[91] It has therefore been advocated that disease-specific questionnaires be included in the assessment of HRQoL, because they might be more sensitive to change than generic instruments and more appropriate to evaluate specific therapeutic interventions in clinical trials. Both disease-generic and, to a lesser extent, disease-specific questionnaires have been adopted in the assessment of HRQoL in those with lupus.[91,92] Several SLE-specific questionnaires have been published in the literature—the lupus quality-of-life (LupusQoL) instrument and its versions, the SLE symptom checklist (SSC) and the SLE-specific quality-of-life (SLEQoL) instrument.[91,93-95]

Generic Questionnaires

Although several measures of HRQoL have been studied in SLE, the most commonly used and accepted measure is the MOS SF-36, which is a generic measure that is applicable in a variety of conditions and chronic diseases including SLE.[76,86,88,92] The SLICC group has recommended the SF-36 as the measure of HRQoL in SLE.[90] This self-administered SF-36 measures the quality of life in 8 areas of perceived health that are reflected in 36 items. Domain scores are on a scale from 0 to 100. The SF-36 subscales can be further summarized into two component scores: (1) the physical component summary (PCS) and (2) the mental component summary (MCS). Nevertheless, evaluating all domains along the summary scales is advisable to capture change in all of the aspects. Both of these subscales are standardized; therefore they can be easily compared with each population. For SF-36, 0 reflects the worst quality of life and 100 the best quality of life. The SF-36 is a valid and reliable tool that captures the physical, psychological, and social effects of the disease on patients with lupus.[88,89] Studies of HRQoL have shown that the SF-36 is not sensitive to change in SLE in longitudinal studies when administered biannually or annually.[76,96]

The SF-36 in patients with established SLE changes little over an 8-year period, and changes are not affected by disease activity, steroids, or damage accumulation during the interval, but changes are affected by the presence of fibromyalgia.[76] In this study the only domain that showed a decline over time was physical functioning, and changes in this domain were different among ethnicities and were associated with fibromyalgia.[76] The SF-36 assesses the preceding 1-month period; when administered monthly and over 6 to 12 months, the SF-36 scores change with clinically meaningful change in the disease activity.[31,97] Some studies, however, have shown that annual changes in SF-36 scores, in particular those related to mental health, are strongly associated with the clinical outcome of neuropsychiatric events in patients with SLE.[98] Discrepancies between the HRQoL assessment and the physician's judgment on disease activity are not unusual. HRQoL incorporates the patient's perception of the disease, whereas the physician's judgment is based on and driven by clinical and objective findings.

Disease-Specific Questionnaires

Although the SF-36 is the most commonly used HRQoL questionnaire, several new lupus-specific tools have been developed. The Dutch SSC was developed in the Netherlands and translated into English.[93] The SSC has satisfactory psychometric properties, including reliability and responsiveness.[93] The SLEQoL instrument is a 40-item questionnaire in English developed initially in Singapore and then translated into Portuguese and Chinese. The L-QoL instrument was developed in the United Kingdom in English and then translated into Hungarian and Turkish.[95] The LupusQoL was developed and validated in the United Kingdom, underwent cultural adaptation for use in the United States (LupusQoL-US), and then translated into different languages.[99,100] The LupusQoL has 34 items across 8 domains.[91] The potential advantage of the LupusQoL and other disease-specific questionnaires is that they contain items and domains related more specifically to patients with lupus. Published studies have focused on evaluating the validity of LupusQoL and its correlation with disease activity.[91,100] In a cross-sectional analysis, HRQoL was found to be impaired in patients with lupus, and, more importantly, no association could be found among the eight domains of the LupusQoL and clinical or demographic variables.[101] A 2011 study in which 40 patients were followed monthly for 1 year showed that LupusQoL and the SF-36 were equivalent in assessing the quality of life of patients with lupus over time. Moreover, both the SF-36 and LupusQoL showed a small to moderate effect of responsiveness when a clinically significant change in disease activity occurred. Although previous studies demonstrate that HRQoL measures do not change with disease activity, these either were cross-sectional or measured HRQoL at yearly intervals.[76,86,89] The 2011 study confirms that the assessment of HRQoL in patients with lupus should be determined monthly in clinical trials and research studies, in particular, if the objective is to evaluate responsiveness.[97]

Further studies are needed to determine whether the LupusQoL instrument and other disease-specific questionnaires contribute additional information not obtained using the SF-36. However, because the SF-36 is generic, comparisons can be made with other patient groups or, through the standardized PCS and MCS, with the population at large. Therefore the SF-36 might be a better instrument to use.

COSTS AND ECONOMIC IMPACT EVENTS

The economic effect of SLE is substantial. Studies have shown that the economic cost is higher in patients with SLE, compared with the general population, for both hospitalizations and physician visits.[102,103] A recent study showed that health care costs and the loss of productivity are similar among patients with lupus nephritis and those without; the loss of productivity for caregivers is higher for patients with lupus nephritis; and the health care costs are greater in active lupus nephritis than in inactive lupus nephritis.[104] The Economics Working Group of Outcome Measures in Rheumatology (OMERACT) recommended determining the economic impact of the disease in trials and general health care and developed a standardized framework for the conduct of economic evaluation.[103] Several types of economic evaluations have been proposed: cost of illness, cost minimization, cost effectiveness, cost utility, and cost benefit. The economic evaluation estimates the direct and indirect costs of lupus. Direct costs include resources used in providing care to a patient, in particular the cost of therapy and adverse events, and the overall cost of resources used as a result of the disease, therapy, and adverse events. The indirect costs highlight the types of productivity impairments due to lupus, in particular, the time lost from work, an inability to work in the home, childcare costs, travel expenses, and loss in productivity.[102] Several indirect measures, such as the EuroQoL's EQ-5D instrument and the Health Utilities Index Mark III (HUI), are useful in the assessment of quality-adjusted life-years and for policy makers.[105] With the recent advances and emergence of biological treatments for lupus, which greatly impact the cost of treatment, an evaluation is needed to determine whether the benefits of these drugs for patients outweigh their economic burden. Nevertheless, with the presumed effectiveness of new drugs and their positive impact on disease activity, damage, and HRQoL, one would expect that these drugs will diminish the economic impact from the disease itself and allow patients to be more productive, positively affecting their social life.

ADVERSE EVENTS

The FDA and OMERACT recommend assessing the adverse events and the safety profile of new medications, in particular, in the clinical trials of new drugs.[49,103] In these drug trials, participants are monitored for toxicity through the clinical assessment and laboratory evaluation at each study visit and when required. The assessment of adverse events should be reported by the patient or determined by the physician and should include all types of adverse events: unexpected, serious, related to the use of the study drug, possibly related, and unrelated. An adverse event reported by physicians is defined as any clinical or laboratory abnormality that the investigator deems clinically important. In clinical trials the identification of adverse events is subject to the follow-up time, which may be too short to identify all possible events. Thus conducting the assessment of any new drug in marketing and postmarketing phases to gather additional safety information is not unusual, especially for rare and serious adverse events. In addition, the decision regarding the safety profile for any new drug might require the use of available data from registries and longitudinal studies, especially with a chronic disease such as lupus.[49] Participants who discontinue study medication early are still being followed for the duration of the study and evaluated in the same manner as those continuing the study regimen. In addition, the sample size of the patients who are studied is important to ensure that the detection of all types of adverse events is feasible.

References

1. Petri M, Buyon J, Kim M: Classification and definition of major flares in SLE clinical trials. *Lupus* 8(8):685–691, 1999.
2. Nikpour M, Urowitz MB, Ibañez D, et al: Frequency and determinants of flare and persistently active disease in systemic lupus erythematosus. *Arthritis Rheum* 61(9):1152–1158, 2009.
3. Smolen JS, Strand V, Cardiel M, et al: Randomized clinical trials and longitudinal observational studies in systemic lupus erythematosus: consensus on a preliminary core set of outcome domains. *J Rheumatol* 26(2):504–507, 1999.
4. Bombardier C, Gladman DD, Urowitz MB, et al: Derivation of the SLEDAI. A disease activity index for lupus patients. The Committee on Prognosis Studies in SLE. *Arthritis Rheum* 35(6):630–640, 1992.
5. Boers M, Brooks P, Strand CV, et al: The OMERACT filter for outcome measures in rheumatology. *J Rheumatol* 25(2):198–199, 1998.
6. American Rheumatism Association Glossary Committee: Dictionnary of the Rheumatic Diseases. Vol. I: Signs and Symptoms, New York, 1982, Contact Associates International.
7. American Rheumatism Association Glossary Committee: Dictionnary of the Rheumatic Diseases. Vol. II: Diagnostic Testing. New York, 1985, Contact Associates International.
8. Gladman DD, Goldsmith CH, Urowitz MB, et al: Crosscultural validation and reliability of 3 disease activity indices in systemic lupus erythematosus. *J Rheumatol* 19(4):608–611, 1992.
9. Hawker G, Gabriel S, Bombardier C, et al: A reliability study of SLEDAI: a disease activity index for systemic lupus erythematosus. *J Rheumatol* 20(4):657–660, 1993.
10. Petri M, Hellmann D, Hochberg M: Validity and reliability of lupus activity measures in the routine clinic setting. *J Rheumatol* 19(1):53–59, 1992.
11. Liang MH, Socher SA, Larson MG, et al: Reliability and validity of six systems for the clinical assessment of disease activity in systemic lupus erythematosus. *Arthritis Rheum* 32(9):1107–1118, 1989.
12. McLaughlin JR, Bombardier C, Farewell VT, et al: Kidney biopsy in systemic lupus erythematosus. III. Survival analysis controlling for clinical and laboratory variables. *Arthritis Rheum* 37(4):559–567, 1994.
13. Gladman DD, Urowitz MB, Kagal A, et al: Accurately describing changes in disease activity in systemic lupus erythematosus. *J Rheumatol* 27(2):377–379, 2000.
14. Gladman DD, Goldsmith CH, Urowitz MB, et al: Sensitivity to change of 3 systemic lupus erythematosus disease activity indices: international validation. *J Rheumatol* 21(8):1468–1471, 1994.
15. Brunner HI, Feldman BM, Bombardier C, et al: Sensitivity of the Systemic Lupus Erythematosus Disease Activity Index, British Isles Lupus Assessment Group Index, and Systemic Lupus Activity Measure in the evaluation of clinical change in childhood-onset systemic lupus erythematosus. *Arthritis Rheum* 42(7):1354–1360, 1999.
16. Brunner HI, Higgins GC, Wiers K, et al: Prospective validation of the provisional criteria for the evaluation of response to therapy in childhood-onset systemic lupus erythematosus. *Arthritis Care Res (Hoboken)* 62(3):335–344, 2010.
17. Zonana-Nacach A, Yañez P, Jimènez-Balderas FJ, et al: Disease activity, damage and survival in Mexican patients with acute severe systemic lupus erythematosus. *Lupus* 16(12):997–1000, 2007.
18. Becker-Merok A, Nossent HC: Damage accumulation in systemic lupus erythematosus and its relation to disease activity and mortality. *J Rheumatol* 33(8):1570–1577, 2006.
19. Cook RJ, Gladman DD, Pericak D, et al: Prediction of short term mortality in systemic lupus erythematosus with time dependent measures of disease activity. *J Rheumatol* 27(8):1892–1895, 2000.
20. Guzman J, Cardiel MH, Arce-Salinas A, et al: Measurement of disease activity in systemic lupus erythematosus. Prospective validation of 3 clinical indices. *J Rheumatol* 19(10):1551–1558, 1992.
21. Uribe AG, Vila LM, McGwin G, Jr, et al: The Systemic Lupus Activity Measure–revised, the Mexican Systemic Lupus Erythematosus Disease Activity Index (SLEDAI), and a modified SLEDAI-2K are adequate instruments to measure disease activity in systemic lupus erythematosus. *J Rheumatol* 31(10):1934–1940, 2004.
22. Petri M, Kim MY, Kalunian KC, et al: Combined oral contraceptives in women with systemic lupus erythematosus. *N Engl J Med* 353(24):2550–2558, 2005.
23. Gladman DD, Ibañez D, Urowitz MB: Systemic lupus erythematosus disease activity index 2000. *J Rheumatol* 29(2):288–291, 2002.
24. Hay EM, Bacon PA, Gordon C, et al: The BILAG index: a reliable and valid instrument for measuring clinical disease activity in systemic lupus erythematosus. *Q J Med* 86(7):447–458, 1993.
25. Vitali C, Bencivelli W, Isenberg DA, et al: Disease activity in systemic lupus erythematosus: report of the Consensus Study Group of the European Workshop for Rheumatology Research. II. Identification of

the variables indicative of disease activity and their use in the development of an activity score. The European Consensus Study Group for Disease Activity in SLE. *Clin Exp Rheumatol* 10(5):541–547, 1992.

26. Fellows of Harvard College: SLE Activity Measure-Revised (SLAM-R). Revised 1998.

27. Touma Z, Urowitz MB, Gladman DD: SLEDAI-2K for a 30-day window. *Lupus* 19(1):49–51, 2010.

28. Touma Z, Urowitz MB, Ibañez D, et al: SLEDAI-2K 10 days versus SLEDAI-2K 30 days in a longitudinal evaluation. *Lupus* 20(1):67–70, 2011.

29. Bae SC, Koh HK, Chang DK, et al: Reliability and validity of systemic lupus activity measure-revised (SLAM-R) for measuring clinical disease activity in systemic lupus erythematosus. *Lupus* 10(6):405–409, 2001.

30. Ward MM, Marx AS, Barry NN: Comparison of the validity and sensitivity to change of 5 activity indices in systemic lupus erythematosus. *J Rheumatol* 27(3):664–670, 2000.

31. Fortin PR, Abrahamowicz M, Neville C, et al: Impact of disease activity and cumulative damage on the health of lupus patients. *Lupus* 7(2):101–107, 1998.

32. Vitali C, Bencivelli W, Isenberg DA, et al: Disease activity in systemic lupus erythematosus: report of the Consensus Study Group of the European Workshop for Rheumatology Research. I. A descriptive analysis of 704 European lupus patients. European Consensus Study Group for Disease Activity in SLE. *Clin Exp Rheumatol* 10(5):527–539, 1992.

33. Bencivelli W, Vitali C, Isenberg DA, et al: Disease activity in systemic lupus erythematosus: report of the Consensus Study Group of the European Workshop for Rheumatology Research. III. Development of a computerised clinical chart and its application to the comparison of different indices of disease activity. The European Consensus Study Group for Disease Activity in SLE. *Clin Exp Rheumatol* 10(5):549–554, 1992.

34. Mosca M, Bencivelli W, Vitali C, et al: The validity of the ECLAM index for the retrospective evaluation of disease activity in systemic lupus erythematosus. *Lupus* 9(6):445–450, 2000.

35. Aringer M, Graninger WB, Steiner G, et al: Safety and efficacy of tumor necrosis factor alpha blockade in systemic lupus erythematosus: an open-label study. *Arthritis Rheum* 50(10):3161–3169, 2004.

36. Vitali C, Bencivelli W, Mosca M, et al: Development of a clinical chart to compute different disease activity indices for systemic lupus erythematosus. *J Rheumatol* 26(2):498–501, 1999.

37. Symmons DP, Coppock JS, Bacon PA, et al: Development and assessment of a computerized index of clinical disease activity in systemic lupus erythematosus. Members of the British Isles Lupus Assessment Group (BILAG). *Q J Med* 69(259):927–937, 1988.

38. Stoll T, Stucki G, Malik J, et al: Further validation of the BILAG disease activity index in patients with systemic lupus erythematosus. *Ann Rheum Dis* 55(10):756–760, 1996.

39. Gordon C, Sutcliffe N, Skan J, et al: Definition and treatment of lupus flares measured by the BILAG index. *Rheumatology (Oxford)* 42(11):1372–1379, 2003.

40. Touma Z, Gladman DD, Ibañez D, et al: SLEDAI-2K Responder Index (SRI-50) enhances the ability to identify responders in clinical trials. *J Rheumatol* 38(11):2395–2399, 2011.

41. Furie RA, Petri MA, Wallace DJ, et al: Novel evidence-based systemic lupus erythematosus responder index. *Arthritis Rheum* 61(9):1143–1151, 2009.

42. Navarra SV, Guzmán RM, Gallacher AE, et al: Efficacy and safety of belimumab in patients with active systemic lupus erythematosus: a randomised, placebo-controlled, phase 3 trial. *Lancet* 377(9767):721–731, 2011.

43. Isenberg DA, Rahman A, Allen E, et al: BILAG 2004. Development and initial validation of an updated version of the British Isles Lupus Assessment Group's disease activity index for patients with systemic lupus erythematosus. *Rheumatology (Oxford)* 44(7):902–906, 2005.

44. Yee CS, Cresswell L, Farewell V, et al: Numerical scoring for the BILAG-2004 index. *Rheumatology (Oxford)* 49(9):1665–1669, 2010.

45. Isenberg DA, Gordon C: From BILAG to BLIPS—disease activity assessment in lupus past, present and future. *Lupus* 9(9):651–654, 2000.

46. Yee CS, Farewell V, Isenberg DA, et al: Revised British Isles Lupus Assessment Group 2004 index: a reliable tool for assessment of systemic lupus erythematosus activity. *Arthritis Rheum* 54(10):3300–3305, 2006.

47. Yee CS, Farewell V, Isenberg DA, et al: British Isles Lupus Assessment Group 2004 index is valid for assessment of disease activity in systemic lupus erythematosus. *Arthritis Rheum* 56(12):4113–4119, 2007.

48. Touma Z, Gladman DD, Urowitz MB, et al: Mycophenolate mofetil for induction treatment of lupus nephritis: a systematic review and meta-analysis. *J Rheumatol* 38(1):69–78, 2011.

49. Guidance for Industry: Lupus nephritis caused by systemic lupus erythematosus—developing medical products for treatment. http://www.fda.gov/downloads/Drugs/GuidanceComplianceRegulatoryInformation/Guidances/UCM216280.pdf.

50. Petri M, Kasitanon N, Lee SS, et al: Systemic lupus international collaborating clinics renal activity/response exercise: development of a renal activity score and renal response index. *Arthritis Rheum* 58(6):1784–1788, 2010.

51. Albrecht J, Taylor L, Berlin JA, et al: The CLASI (Cutaneous Lupus Erythematosus Disease Area and Severity Index): an outcome instrument for cutaneous lupus erythematosus. *J Invest Dermatol* 125(5):889–894, 2010.

52. Krathen M, Albrecht J, Werth VP: The cutaneous lupus disease activity and severity index as a validated outcome measure for cutaneous lupus erythematosus: comment on the article by Stamm et al. *Arthritis Rheum* 59(4):601–602, 2010.

53. Kuhn A, Meuth AM, Bein D, et al: Revised Cutaneous Lupus Erythematosus Disease Area and Severity Index (RCLASI): a modified outcome instrument for cutaneous lupus erythematosus. *Br J Dermatol* 163(1):83–92, 2010.

54. Ibañez D, Urowitz MB, Gladman DD: Summarizing disease features over time: I. Adjusted mean SLEDAI derivation and application to an index of disease activity in lupus. *J Rheumatol* 30(9):1977–1982, 2010.

55. Ibañez D, Gladman DD, Urowitz MB: Adjusted mean Systemic Lupus Erythematosus Disease Activity Index-2K is a predictor of outcome in SLE. *J Rheumatol* 32(5):824–827, 2010.

56. Ibañez D, Gladman D, Urowitz M: Summarizing disease features over time: II. Variability measures of SLEDAI-2K. *J Rheumatol* 34(2):336–340, 2010.

57. Ibañez D, Gladman DD, Touma Z, et al: Optimal frequency of visits for patients with systemic lupus erythematosus to measure disease activity over time. *J Rheumatol* 38(1):60–63, 2010.

58. Petri M, Buyon J, Skovron ML, et al: Reliability of SELENA SLEDAI and flare as clinical trial outcome measures [abstract]. *Arthritis Rheum* 41:S218, 1998.

59. FitzGerald JD, Grossman JM: Validity and reliability of retrospective assessment of disease activity and flare in observational cohorts of lupus patients. *Lupus* 8(8):638–644, 2010.

60. Petri M, Buyon J, Kalunian KC, et al: Revision of the SELENA Flare Index [abstract]. *Arthritis Rheum* 60:S902, 2009.

61. Petri M, Barr SG, Buyon J, et al: RIFLE: Responder Index for Lupus Erythematosus [abstract]. *Arthritis Rheum* 43:S244, 2000.

62. Burt RK, Traynor A, Statkute L, et al: Nonmyeloablative hematopoietic stem cell transplantation for systemic lupus erythematosus. *JAMA* 295(5):527–535, 2010.

63. Brunner HI, Higgins GC, Klein-Gitelman MS, et al: Minimal clinically important differences of disease activity indices in childhood-onset systemic lupus erythematosus. *Arthritis Care Res (Hoboken)* 62(7):950–959, 2010.

64. Wallace DJ, Kalunian KC, Petri MA, et al: Epratuzumab demonstrates clinically meaningful improvements in patients with moderate to severe systemic lupus erythematosus: results from EMBLEM, a phase IIb study [abstract]. *Arthritis Rheum* 62:S1452, 2010.

65. Touma Z, Gladman DD, Ibanez D, et al: Systemic Lupus Erythematosus Disease Activity Index (SLEDAI-2K) Responder Index (SRI)-50: a valid index for measuring improvement in disease activity [abstract]. *Arthritis Rheum* 62:S1878, 2010.

66. Touma Z, Gladman D, Urowitz M: SLEDAI-2K Responder Index-50 (SRI-50) [abstract]. *Arthritis Rheum* 60:S899, 2009.

67. Touma Z, Gladman DD, Ibañez D, et al: Development and initial validation of the systemic lupus erythematosus disease activity index 2000 responder index 50. *J Rheumatol* 38(2):275–284, 2010.

68. Touma Z, Urowitz MB, Fortin PR, et al: SLEDAI-2K Responder Index (SRI)-50: a reliable index for measuring improvement in disease activity. *J Rheumatol* 38(5):868–873, 2010.

69. Buyon JP, Kalunian KC, Ramsey-Goldman R, et al: Assessing disease activity in SLE patients during pregnancy. *Lupus* 8(8):677–684, 2010.

70. Yee CS, Farewell V, Isenberg DA, et al: The BILAG-2004 index is sensitive to change for assessment of SLE disease activity. *Rheumatology (Oxford)* 48(6):691–695, 2010.

71. Guidance for Industry: Systemic lupus erythematosus—Developing medical products for treatment. http://www.fda.gov/downloads/Drugs/

GuidanceComplianceRegulatoryInformation/Guidances/ucm072063.pdf.

72. Touma Z, Gladman DD, Ibanez D, et al: Retrospective validation of the 3 Laboratory organ systems of Systemic Lupus Erythematosus Disease Activity Index-2000 (SLEDAI-2K) Responder Index (SRI-50) over 10 Years [abstract]. *Arthritis Rheum* 63:S1368, 2011.

73. Urowitz MB, Gladman DD, Tom BD, et al: Changing patterns in mortality and disease outcomes for patients with systemic lupus erythematosus. *J Rheumatol* 35(11):2152–2158, 2008.

74. Gladman D, Ginzler E, Goldsmith C, et al: Systemic lupus international collaborative clinics: development of a damage index in systemic lupus erythematosus. *J Rheumatol* 19(11):1820–1821, 1992.

75. Gladman D, Ginzler E, Goldsmith C, et al: The development and initial validation of the Systemic Lupus International Collaborating Clinics/American College of Rheumatology damage index for systemic lupus erythematosus. *Arthritis Rheum* 39(3):363–369, 1996.

76. Kuriya B, Gladman DD, Ibáñez D, et al: Quality of life over time in patients with systemic lupus erythematosus. *Arthritis Rheum* 59(2):181–185, 2008.

77. Touma Z, Gladman DD, Tulloch-Reid D, et al: Burden of autoantibodies and association with disease activity damage in systemic lupus erythematosus. *Clin Exp Rheumatol* 28(4):525–531, 2010.

78. Gladman DD, Urowitz MB, Goldsmith CH, et al: The reliability of the Systemic Lupus International Collaborating Clinics/American College of Rheumatology Damage Index in patients with systemic lupus erythematosus. *Arthritis Rheum* 40(5):809–813, 1997.

79. Rahman P, Gladman DD, Urowitz MB, et al: Early damage as measured by the SLICC/ACR damage index is a predictor of mortality in systemic lupus erythematosus. *Lupus* 10(2):93–96, 2001.

80. Stoll T, Sutcliffe N, Mach J, et al: Analysis of the relationship between disease activity and damage in patients with systemic lupus erythematosus—a 5-yr prospective study. *Rheumatology (Oxford)* 43(8):1039–1044, 2004.

81. Sutcliffe N, Clarke AE, Gordon C, et al: The association of socioeconomic status, race, psychosocial factors and outcome in patients with systemic lupus erythematosus. *Rheumatology (Oxford)* 38(11):1130–1137, 1999.

82. Maddison P, Farewell V, Isenberg D, et al: The rate and pattern of organ damage in late onset systemic lupus erythematosus. *J Rheumatol* 29(5):913–917, 2002.

83. Brunner HI, Silverman ED, To T, et al: Risk factors for damage in childhood-onset systemic lupus erythematosus: cumulative disease activity and medication use predict disease damage. *Arthritis Rheum* 46(2):436–444, 2002.

84. Costenbader KH, Khamashta M, Ruiz-Garcia S, et al: Development and initial validation of a self-assessed lupus organ damage instrument. *Arthritis Care Res (Hoboken)* 62(4):559–568, 2010.

85. Pons-Estel BA, Sanchez-Guerrero J, Romero-Diaz J, et al: Validation of the Spanish, Portuguese and French versions of the Lupus Damage Index questionnaire: data from North and South America, Spain and Portugal. *Lupus* 18(12):1033–1052, 2009.

86. Panopalis P, Clarke AE: Quality of life in systemic lupus erythematosus. *Clin Dev Immunol* 13(2–4):321–324, 2006.

87. Abu-Shakra M, Mader R, Langevitz P, et al: Quality of life in systemic lupus erythematosus: a controlled study. *J Rheumatol* 26(2):306–309, 1999.

88. Jolly M: How does quality of life of patients with systemic lupus erythematosus compare with that of other common chronic illnesses? *J Rheumatol* 32(9):1706–1708, 2005.

89. Gladman DD, Urowitz MB, Ong A, et al: A comparison of five health status instruments in patients with systemic lupus erythematosus (SLE). *Lupus* 5(3):190–195, 1996.

90. Gladman D, Urowitz M, Fortin P, et al: Systemic Lupus International Collaborating Clinics conference on assessment of lupus flare and quality of life measures in SLE. Systemic Lupus International Collaborating Clinics Group. *J Rheumatol* 23(11):1953–1955, 1996.

91. McElhone K, Abbott J, Shelmerdine J, et al: Development and validation of a disease-specific health-related quality of life measure, the LupusQol, for adults with systemic lupus erythematosus. *Arthritis Rheum* 57(6):972–979, 2007.

92. McHorney CA, Ware JE, Jr, Lu JF, Sherbourne CD: The MOS 36-item Short-Form health survey (SF-36): III. Tests of data quality, scaling assumptions, and reliability across diverse patient groups. *Med Care* 32(1):40–66, 1994.

93. Grootscholten C, Ligtenberg G, Derksen RH, et al: Health-related quality of life in patients with systemic lupus erythematosus: development and validation of a lupus specific symptom checklist. *Qual Life Res* 12(6):635–644, 2003.

94. Leong KP, Kong KO, Thong BY, et al: Development and preliminary validation of a systemic lupus erythematosus-specific quality-of-life instrument (SLEQOL). *Rheumatology (Oxford)* 44(10):1267–1276, 2005.

95. Doward LC, McKenna SP, Whalley D, et al: The development of the L-QoL: a quality-of-life instrument specific to systemic lupus erythematosus. *Ann Rheum Dis* 68(2):196–200, 2009.

96. Panopalis P, Petri M, Manzi S, et al: The systemic lupus erythematosus tri-nation study: longitudinal changes in physical and mental well-being. *Rheumatology (Oxford)* 44(6):751–755, 2005.

97. Touma Z, Gladman DD, Ibáñez, D, et al: Is there an advantage for a lupus specific quality of life measure over SF-36? *J Rheumatol* 38(9):1898–1905, 2011.

98. Hanly JG, Urowitz MB, Jackson D, et al: SF-36 summary and subscale scores are reliable outcomes of neuropsychiatric events in systemic lupus erythematosus. *Ann Rheum Dis* 70(6):961–967, 2011.

99. González-Rodríguez V, Peralta-Ramírez MI, Navarrete-Navarrete N, et al: [Adaptation and validation of the Spanish version of a disease-specific quality of life measure in patients with systemic lupus erythematosus: the lupus quality of life]. *Med Clin (Barc)* 134(1):13–16, 2010.

100. Jolly M, Pickard AS, Wilke C, et al: Lupus-specific health outcome measure for US patients: the LupusQoL-US version. *Ann Rheum Dis* 69(1):29–33, 2010.

101. McElhone K, Castelino M, Abbott J, et al: The LupusQoL and associations with demographics and clinical measurements in patients with systemic lupus erythematosus. *J Rheumatol* 37(11):2273–2279, 2010.

102. Gordon C, Clarke AE: Quality of life and economic evaluation in SLE clinical trials. *Lupus* 8(8):645–654, 1999.

103. Strand V, Gladman D, Isenberg D, et al: Outcome measures to be used in clinical trials in systemic lupus erythematosus. *J Rheumatol* 26(2):490–497, 1999.

104. Aghdassi E, Zhang W, St-Pierre Y, et al: Healthcare cost and loss of productivity in a Canadian population of patients with and without lupus nephritis. *J Rheumatol* 38(4):658–666, 2011.

105. Maetzel A, Tugwell P, Boers M, et al: Economic evaluation of programs or interventions in the management of rheumatoid arthritis: defining a consensus-based reference case. *J Rheumatol* 30(4):891–896, 2003.

106. Karlson EW, Daltroy LH, Rivest C, et al: Validation of a Systemic Lupus Activity Questionnaire (SLAQ) for population studies. *Lupus* 12(4):280–286, 2003.

107. Smolen JS: Clinical and serological features: incidence and diagnostic approach. In Smolen JS, Zielinski CC, editors: *Systemic lupus erythematosus: clinical and experimental aspects*, Germany, 1987, Springer-Verlag: Berlin/Heidelberg, pp 170–196.

MANAGEMENT OF SLE

Principles of Therapy, Local Measures, and Nonsteroidal Medications

Mariko Ishimori, Michael H. Weisman, Katy Setoodeh, and Daniel J. Wallace

FORMULATION OVERVIEW

One of the most difficult and misunderstood aspects of systemic lupus erythematosus (SLE) is its management. Before therapy is initiated, the practitioner must determine which type of lupus is present and, on that basis, formulate a treatment program. Because the prognosis of each clinical subset differs widely, it is essential that the patient database be completed before an educational session is initiated. All blood tests, imaging modalities, and biopsies that provide information and can affect treatment must be performed. Once these prerequisites have been met, the physician should be able to answer the following questions:

1. Does the patient meet the American College of Rheumatology (ACR) criteria for SLE?
   a. If not, does the patient meet the biopsy criteria for discoid lupus, subacute cutaneous lupus, or lupus nephritis? If not, is the physician satisfied that the patient has SLE, despite lacking four criteria? (This distinction is a matter of clinical judgment.)
   b. If not, does the patient have an undifferentiated connective tissue disease (UCTD)? Some patients with clear-cut inflammatory arthritis, a positive antinuclear antibody (ANA) test, and constitutional symptoms are treated similarly to patients with lupus. Approximately 14% of cases of UCTD evolve into classic SLE.
   c. If so, are related disorders such as mixed connective tissue disease, scleroderma, and dermatopolymyositis excluded, or is an overlap syndrome present?
2. If the patient has SLE, is it organ threatening and therefore could potentially shorten lifespan (e.g., cardiopulmonary involvement, renal disease, hepatic involvement, central nervous system vasculitis, thrombocytopenia, or autoimmune hemolytic anemia)? If not, does the patient have non–organ-threatening SLE (e.g., cutaneous, musculoskeletal, serositis, constitutional)?
3. Which subset best describes the disease? Does a particular aspect of the patient's disease require specific considerations, interventions, or counseling (e.g., antiphospholipid syndrome, Sjögren syndrome antigen A [SSA/Ro] positivity, seizures, concurrent fibromyalgia)?

Occasionally, patients who have been labeled as having SLE do not, in fact, have the disease. The implications of telling a patient that he or she has lupus are tremendous. The emotional and psychological effects of receiving this diagnosis open up new worlds of powerful and expensive medications, which will influence career planning and family life, alter one's productivity and lifestyle, and, in the United States, make it difficult to obtain health, life, or disability insurance. Physicians should avoid locking themselves into telling a patient that he or she has lupus if any doubt remains.

EDUCATIONAL SESSION

All patients who are newly diagnosed, as well as those who are new to the treating physician, deserve an educational session that includes concerned family members, friends, and significant others. The session should be supervised by the physician and may involve other health professionals or use audiovisual aids. Several studies have demonstrated that socioeconomic differences account for the widely divergent outcomes in those with SLE (see Chapter 55). It is critical that the patient establish a relationship and rapport with the treating facility or physician, speak a common language, keep appointments, take medication as prescribed, have transportation to the medical office, and have access to medical assistance or advice 24 hours a day. Educational aids, online assistance, and informational literature relating to the various aspects of the disease, including therapy, are available from lupus support organizations such as those listed in the Appendix.

The treatment of SLE includes physical and psychological measures, surgery, and medications. Box 47-1 summarizes the issues that should be discussed with the patient and family during the educational session. (Topics listed in Box 47-1 not covered elsewhere in this textbook are reviewed in the following text, and the reader is also referred to the index.)

GENERAL THERAPEUTIC CONSIDERATIONS
Rest, Sleep, and the Treatment of Fatigue
Fatigue is present in 50% to 90% of patients with SLE and can be its most disabling symptom.[1] Potentially reversible causes of fatigue should first be ruled out. These include active inflammation,

Box 47-1 Curriculum for the Educational Session with a Patient Who Is Newly Diagnosed with Lupus or Is New to the Practice Setting

1. What is lupus? What are its causes?
2. Many types of systemic lupus erythematosus (SLE) exist: cutaneous, mild, drug-induced, and organ-threatening, all of which have a *(fair, good, excellent)* prognosis with treatment.
3. Physical and lifestyle measures to be reviewed:
   a. Diet
   b. Exercise
   c. Rehabilitation (physical, occupational, vocational therapy)
   d. Bone mineralization strategies
   e. Immunizations
   f. Dealing with fevers, infections
   g. Sun protection measures
   h. Smoking cessation, use of alcohol
   i. Climate and barometric pressure
4. Emotional support
   a. Fatigue
   b. Sleep hygiene
   c. Use of mind-body approaches to depression, anxiety, concurrent fibromyalgia, stress reduction
   d. Pregnancy
   e. Genetic counseling
5. Being current with adjunctive measures:
   a. Establishing a regular follow-up system with primary care, gynecologic examinations, mammograms, and colonoscopies, as well as eye examinations for those receiving antimalarial or steroidal medications
   b. Screening for accelerated atherogenesis with intervention as needed
   c. Importance of keeping appointments, taking medications, and following instructions
   d. Managing pain and differentiating inflammatory from non-inflammatory pain
6. Medications
   a. To treat patients with SLE: topical, nonsteroidal, antimalarial, corticosteroid, immune suppressive, biologic agents
   b. To treat lupus subsets (e.g., measures for antiphospholipid syndrome, Raynaud phenomenon, thrombocytopenia, Sjögren syndrome)
   c. To treat lupus-related complications related to the disease or its treatment (e.g., hypertension, hyperlipidemia, glaucoma)
7. Information and access
   a. Who should be called when for what?
   b. Resource listings (e.g., web sites, drug information, lupus advocacy groups)

Box 47-2 Fatigue in Systemic Lupus Erythematosus

1. Present in 50% to 90% of patients according to multiple surveys
2. Causes of fatigue:
   a. Inflammation
   b. Medications (e.g., analgesic, psychotropic, supplemental, antihypertensive agents)
   c. Co-morbidities (e.g., anemia, parenchymal scarring, hypothyroidism in those with concurrent Hashimoto thyroiditis, steroid-induced diabetes)
   d. Fibromyalgia and psychosocial distress
   e. Malnutrition or anorexia, bulimia, or exercise overexertion (observed in 5% of young women)
   f. Infection
   g. Cytokine dysregulation
   h. Hormone imbalances
3. Metrics and fatigue
   a. Statistical associations in SLE: depression, fatigue aerobic insufficiency, disordered sleep, high damage scores, inadequate perceived social support, pain
   b. Measuring fatigue in clinical trials and surveys (fatigue severity scale is the best of 15 validated instruments for rheumatic diseases)
4. Management of fatigue
   a. Treating underlying cause
   b. Pacing activities, providing instruction in sleep hygiene and aerobic exercise
   c. Offering emotional support
   d. Avoiding stimulants unless in a supervised setting

The concept of pacing is paramount in managing fatigue. Total bed rest can worsen fatigue and promote osteoporosis, muscle disuse, atrophy, and contractures. Overexertion and fatigue denial are also counterproductive. Patients are encouraged to pace themselves. Between 1 and 2 hours of morning activity should be followed by a midmorning break. A couple of hours of late-morning activity could be followed by a restful lunch break. Periods of activity followed by periods of rest usually permit most patients with lupus to attain an improved level of functioning and productivity.

Treatment of fatigue requires consideration of the source and contributory factors. Iron deficiency anemia is common because of dietary deficiency, heavy menstrual periods, and/or blood loss resulting from the use of salicylates and nonsteroidal antiinflammatory drugs (NSAIDs). If the fatigue is caused by parenchymal pulmonary disease, then oxygen may be helpful; if it is secondary to inflammation, then antiinflammatory drugs are used. In addition to corticosteroid medications, quinacrine and hydroxychloroquine are cortical stimulants and may decrease fatigue in patients without organ-threatening involvement.[8] Dehydroepiandrosterone (5-DHEA), modafinil (Provigil), armodafinil (Nuvigil), bupropion, and selective serotonin-reuptake inhibitors can be useful. Depression, fibromyalgia, and emotional stress must be excluded as causes. Several surveys have suggested that fibromyalgia and depression are the most common causes of fatigue in patients with SLE.[9] Secondary fibromyalgia with a concomitant sleep disorder is not uncommon. Some physicians empirically prescribe low doses of thyroid, vitamin B12 injections, or amphetamines for nonspecific fatigue of SLE; however, the routine use of these agents should be discouraged. In contrast, the use of anxiolytic agents, especially those that promote restorative sleep, should be considered (Box 47-2).

Exercise, Physical Therapy, and Rehabilitation

Six well-designed studies have evaluated aerobic conditioning in patients with SLE. They concluded that aerobic capacity is decreased by 30% to 40% but does not necessarily correlate with disease activity or damage. However, SLE is associated with fatigue, cardiovascular functioning, obesity, bone mineralization, sleep, and quality of

complications from medication, and co-morbid states such as psychosocial stressors. Occasionally, patients with normal examinations, an absence of acute-phase reactants, and normal chemistry panels (other than a positive ANA test) complain of profound fatigue. The administration of certain cytokines is known to induce fatigue.[2] Reduced muscle aerobic capacity may also play a role.[3] Sleep quality in patients with SLE is impaired.[4] One survey showed that 80% of 172 patients with SLE have disordered sleep, compared with 28% of healthy patients in the control group. Disordered sleep is most likely due to depressed mood, fibromyalgia, steroid therapy, and a lack of exercise.[4,5] Fatigue surveys have statistically associated it with aerobic insufficiency, pain, depression, disordered sleep, altered perceived social support, and a higher Systemic Lupus International Collaborating Clinics (SLICC)/ACR Damage Index (SDI).[6] Fifteen instruments have been evaluated in fatigue-associated SLE in 34 studies, and the fatigue severity scale is regarded as having the best overall results with regard to showing a minimally clinically important difference.[7]

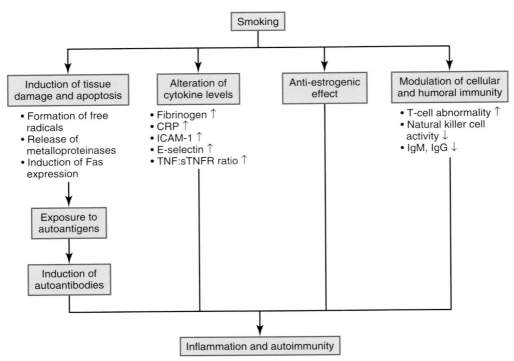

FIGURE 47-1 Effects of smoking on the immune system. CRP, C-reactive protein; ICAM-1, intracellular adhesion molecule 1; Ig, immunoglobublin; sTNFR, soluble tumor necrosis factor receptor; TNF, tumor necrosis factor. *(Reproduced with permission from Harel-Meir M, Sherer Y, Shoenfeld Y: Tobacco smoking and autoimmune rheumatic diseases. Nat Clin Pract Rheumatol 3:707–715, 2007.)*

life.[10,11] Exercise regimens improve physical functioning and fatigue.[12-14] The patient with SLE should remain physically active and avoid excessive bed rest. Exercises that strengthen muscles and improve endurance while avoiding undue stress to inflamed joints are desirable. Activities such as swimming, walking, low-impact aerobics, and bicycling should be encouraged. Recreational activities involving fine-motor movements and placing stress on certain ligamentous and other supporting structures (e.g., bowling, rowing, weight lifting, golf, tennis, jogging) should be considered on an individual basis. Exercises involving sustained isometric contractions increase muscle strength more than isotonic exercises (e.g., stretching, Pilates). Physical measures, such as the use of local moist heat or cold, decrease joint pain and inflammation. Many patients benefit from a whirlpool bath (Jacuzzi), hot tub, or therapy pool or from merely soaking in a tub of hot water.

Physical therapists instruct patients in strengthening and toning exercises, improved body mechanics, and gait training. No specific measures or treatment approaches are unique for patients with lupus. Joint deformities develop in approximately 10% of patients; physical and occupational therapies to minimize deformities are desirable in this group. Splints are useful for most patients with carpal-tunnel syndrome related to SLE. Corrective-tendon surgery and joint replacement are helpful in advanced cases of SLE.

Occupational therapists instruct patients in the principles of energy conservation and joint protection. They evaluate activities of daily living and suggest the use of devices or aids, such as wrist splints, comb handles, and raised toilet seats, when needed.

Vocational rehabilitation may be important in retraining a patient with SLE who can no longer work in the sun (e.g., farmer, construction worker, fisherman) or perform tasks requiring fine hand-motor function (e.g., computer workstation ergonomics).

Tobacco Smoke and Alcohol

Tobacco use can cause tissue damage by inducing apoptosis, altering cytokine and hormone balances, influencing immunogenesis of self-antigens and lymphocyte function that can, in turn, promote autoimmunity.[15] Clinically, smoking impairs oxygenation, raises blood pressure, promotes the formation of autoantibodies, and worsens Raynaud phenomenon, among other adverse actions (Figure 47-1). Numerous reports correlate tobacco use with worse cutaneous lupus or disease activity than among nonsmokers.[16-18] Additional comparisons have confirmed that chronic cutaneous lupus is more common in smokers than in nonsmokers, as is SLE.[19] Two epidemiologic surveys[19,20] associate smoking with 2.3 and 6.69 odds ratios for developing SLE. Because tobacco smoke contains potentially lupogenic hydrazines, abstinence and avoiding second-hand smoke are both important. The efficacy of antimalarial medications may be decreased in smokers, perhaps as a result of the effect of tobacco on the cytochrome P450 enzyme system that metabolizes chloroquines.[21,22]

Although alcohol can worsen reflux esophagitis, which is common in patients with SLE, and is not advised in patients taking methotrexate, approximately 10 studies have addressed the issue with conflicting results. Moderate drinking might be protective for patients with SLE, but a metaanalysis of 7 case-controlled studies and 2 cohort studies found an overall 1.5 odds ratio for developing SLE among those who drink alcohol.[16,17,20,23,24]

Weather and Seasons

Changes in barometric pressure can aggravate stiffness and aching in patients with inflammatory arthritis.[25] In other words, whether the climate is hot or cold or wet or dry, it does not influence joint symptoms; however, changes in the weather do aggravate joint symptoms (e.g., hot to cold or wet to dry). Patients with lupus are counseled to expect some increased stiffness and aching in these circumstances and not to assume that they have done anything wrong. Several surveys of seasonality and weather in patients with SLE have been conducted, but no conclusions have been independently confirmed other than to suggest that more flares and phototoxicity happen in the summer months and weakness, fatigue, and Raynaud phenomenon more often occur in the winter months.[26-28]

Pain Management

Patients with lupus have increased prevalence of problems with pain management.[29,30] Individuals with inflammatory arthritis respond poorly to analgesic medications that have no antiinflammatory effects. The use of morphine and codeine derivatives in patients with SLE should be limited to postoperative management and functionally limiting fixed mechanical deformities. These agents can induce dependence, have short-lived effects, and do not address SLE-related inflammation. Antiinflammatory drugs (e.g., salicylates, NSAIDs, corticosteroids) can be effective in treating pain symptoms in patients with SLE. Some patients with chronic pain that is unresponsive to simple measures should be referred to pain-management centers, which use measures such as acupuncture, electrical stimulation, biofeedback, psychological counseling, and physical therapy to alleviate pain and eliminate narcotic dependence. Anxiolytic measures that work with the mind-body connection are useful as well. Other causes of pain in patients with SLE include avascular necrosis, headache, steroid-induced hyperesthesia, and fibromyalgia.

Role of Stress and Trauma

In a general sense, certain forms of emotional stress, including depression and bereavement, as well as physical trauma can affect the immune system by being associated with decreased lymphocyte mitogenic responsiveness, lymphocyte cytotoxicity, increased natural killer (NK)–cell activity, skin homograft rejection, graft-versus-host response, and delayed hypersensitivity.[31,32] The clinical sequelae of stress are difficult to characterize and quantitate. Could the impairment in T-cell immune functions be responsible for a clinical flare of lupus that is mediated by B-cell hyperreactivity? Acute stress in patients with SLE may correlate with increased urine neopterin levels, interleukin (IL) 4 levels, decreased NK-cell response, and increased numbers of beta-2 adrenergic receptors on mononuclear cells with or without a clinical disease flare.[33,34] However, evidence-based validation of this in a rigorous, reproducible clinical setting is lacking.

Can Stress Induce Lupus?

In 1955, McClary and colleagues[35] first related the onset of disease to significant crises in interpersonal relationships in 13 of 14 patients with SLE. Subsequent reports have reinforced patient perceptions that stress caused their SLE, but the hypothesis remains unproven.

Can Stress Exacerbate Preexisting Systemic Lupus Erythematosus?

Ropes[36] first addressed this question over 50 years ago and observed 45 serious disease flares in her 160-patient cohort study over a 40-year period. Of the 45 patients with serious disease flares, 41 believed that emotional stress precipitated their flare. The development and validation of quality-of-life inventories, fatigue questionnaires, and function scores have correlated disease activity with psychosocial stressors in a general way, but the mechanism by which this correlation may occur has not been elucidated.[37-39] A devastating earthquake was associated with disease improvement in one study, and no change in another.[40,41]

Can Physical Trauma Cause or Exacerbate Systemic Lupus Erythematosus?

No evidence has shown that physical trauma is related to the causation or exacerbation of SLE. Chronic cutaneous lupus erythematosus can develop as a result of physical trauma; King-Smith[42] first observed this response to physical trauma in 1926. Approximately 2% of all chronic cutaneous lesions occur in areas of physical trauma.[43]

In summary, several authors have implicated stress as a factor that can induce or exacerbate SLE. However, a definitive study using a large number of patients and control subjects with similar chronic illnesses is needed before the association can be considered established. Until then, stress reduction is both prudent and important.

HOW IMPORTANT ARE PATIENT COMPLIANCE AND TREATMENT ADHERENCE?

Dr. C. Everett Koop, the former Surgeon General of the United States, is reported to have said, "Drugs don't work in patients who don't take them."[44]

Part of the patient educational session with a new patient with lupus must be a discussion relating to compliance. In the LUMINA Texas and Alabama–based cohort study, nearly one half of the patients were noncompliant. They tended to be young, unmarried, African American, and ill.[45] Adherence to treatment regimens tends to be problematic. One third of 195 patients of Canadian descent with lupus did not participate in mandated annual eye examinations to monitor antimalarial therapies.[46] Compliance problems among 112 patients with lupus in Detroit were related to depression, medication concerns, physical symptoms, short-term memory problems, and the need for child or elder care.[47] Other important factors include previous medication experiences, strong beliefs in alternative methods, communication issues, low educational levels, cultural concerns, very high rates of noncompliance in adolescents, and cost. The failure to comply with physician recommendations was shown to be the cause of renal failure in 5 of the 17 patients in a study conducted at the University of Toronto.[48] In Great Britain, the rate of compliance was treatment specific among 50 women with SLE, ranging from 41% for the use of sun protection to 83% for the use of hydroxychloroquine, 94% for the use of steroids, and 100% for the use of azathioprine therapy.[49] Ninety-five patients at the University of Cincinnati had a similar outcome when pharmacy refill records were examined using a statistically validated compliance metric.[50] Adherence to treatment plans is a critical component in managing SLE, and strategies to address this issue need to be more fully developed and implemented.

SUN AVOIDANCE AND PHOTOTOXICITY

Ultraviolet (UV) light consists of three bands, two of which are important factors in patients with SLE. Ultraviolet A (UVA) light (320 to 400 nm) is responsible for drug-induced photosensitivity (i.e., photoallergic reactions) and delayed tanning, and it is constant during the day. It takes approximately 1 hour of UVA exposure to induce sunburn. Ultraviolet B (UVB) light (290 to 320 nm) is a more significant factor in patients with SLE and more pronounced during midday (10 AM to 4 PM) and causes sunburn readily (i.e., phototoxic reactions).

Hundreds of prescription drugs can cause photoallergic or phototoxic reactions or both. The most common are phenothiazines, tetracyclines, and sulfa-containing agents, as well as piroxicam, methotrexate, amiodarone, psoralens, and phenytoin. Photosensitizing chemicals are found in certain perfumes, mercury-vapor lamps, xenon-arc lamps, tungsten-iodide light sources, halogen lamps, and photocopier machines.[51-53]

Although the majority of patients with lupus have abnormal photosensitivity test results, clinical and self-reported sun sensitivity is recorded in 60% to 70% of patients. Approximately two thirds of these patients observe a significant effect on lifestyle. The mechanism by which this occurs is probably related to the action of UV light on epidermal DNA, which enhances its antigenicity, allowing anti–Sjögren syndrome antigen A (anti-SSA/Ro) antibodies to be exposed to the cell surface, which promotes an inflammatory response, as well as the skin production of cytokines, prostaglandins, and oxygen-free radicals (see Chapter 23). The presence of anti-SSA/Ro antibodies is associated with photosensitivity in more than 90% of Caucasian patients with SLE. Fluorescent lights are a source of UVA and UVB light, but only rarely might their avoidance be beneficial. Clear jacket and bulk covers that control UV emanation without reducing visibility are available and, for all practical purposes, eliminate risks. The introduction of energy-efficient "compact fluorescent lamps" decreases UVA leaks but increases UVB exposure.[54,55]

Which Sunscreen Should Be Used in Lupus?

Although the UV end of the spectrum is the most damaging to lupus skin lesions, heat and infrared exposure can also cause exacerbations. The flares produced by infrared exposure are characterized by a significant increase in erythema of short duration. These are frequently experienced by patients with SLE who work near a hot stove, oven, or furnace for any length of time. One characteristic of discoid lupus erythematosus (DLE) and SLE is that skin burns and scalds can produce localized lesions of DLE at the site of trauma (i.e., Koebner phenomenon) even in apparently normal skin. Sunscreens are UV light–absorbing chemical agents in a cream, oil, lotion, alcohol, or gel vehicle. These chemicals can block UVA, UVB, or both. They include avobenzone (blocks UVA); aminobenzoic-acid esters, cinnamates, and salicylates (block UVB); and benzophenones, anthralite filter systems, and butyl methoxydibenzoylmethanes (block UVA and UVB). Physical sun blocks containing titanium dioxide and zinc oxide scatter light. A sun protection factor (SPF) value is the ratio of the time that is required to produce erythema through a UVB sunscreen product to the time that is required to produce the same degree of erythema without it. The SPF ranges from 2 (provides minimal protection) to 50 (offers the highest protection). Outpatients are advised to use agents with a high SPF value (i.e., at least 15). A sunscreen with an SPF value of 15 will block 93% of UVB light, whereas one with an SPF value of 50 will block only 5% more. The U.S. Food and Drug Administration (FDA) permits sunscreen manufacturers to claim broad-spectrum protection if their products block at least part of UVA-2 light in addition to UVB.[56]

Unfortunately, because of irritation, contact dermatitis, and occasional photosensitivity, patient compliance is poor, and it may be necessary to try several compounds before an acceptable block is found. In particular, the alcohol base in para-aminobenzoic acid (PABA) and PABA esters may sting and dry the skin. Wind, heat, humidity, and altitude can decrease a sunscreen agent's protective effect.

Sunscreens should be applied over active and healed lesions and to areas that may burn, including the cheeks, nose, lips, and arms, approximately 30 minutes before sun exposure. They can be applied over the scalp hair before going outdoors, and cosmetics may be applied over sunscreens.

Sun Protection and Safe Sun Habits

Two aspects of UV light exposure often are overlooked. Skin lesions are frequently more intense on the left cheek and the lateral aspect of the left arm because of UVA exposure while driving an automobile. If the lesions are primarily distributed in these areas, the physician should inquire whether such exposure might be responsible and advise the patient to avoid it.[57] Merely keeping the window closed or tinting the window may sufficiently filter the sunlight. Automotive glass blocks UVB effectively but not UVA light. Another unnoticed source of exposure is UV light that is reflected off the surface of sand, water, cement, or snow, and UV radiation is greater at higher altitudes. For example, the intensity of UV light at 5000 feet is 20% higher than that at sea level. Patients should be cautioned about these sources of danger. In addition, it should be noted that a cloudy day only decreases UV exposure by 20% to 40%. Sunscreens block vitamin D activation in the skin, and oral supplementation may be required. Occasionally, a patient develops eye sensitivity to UV light that is not responsive to the wearing of ordinary sunglasses. Special coated lenses to protect the eyes are available.[58] In patients with SLE and a definite UV sensitivity, walking a few blocks without any protection is usually permitted. If further exposure is necessary, then general measures such as wearing a broad-brimmed hat (4″ or greater is advised) and clothing with long sleeves, as well as using an umbrella, can be beneficial since these measures decrease UV exposure by 30% to 50%. Frequently, otherwise asymptomatic patients have a persistent butterfly erythema that is aggravated by sun exposure, and the use of antimalarial medications and local sunscreens usually controls this condition if it is severe enough to warrant

Box 47-3 Sun Protection and Safe Sun Habits

1. Schedule outdoor activities before 10 AM and after 4 PM.
2. Up to 80% of ultraviolet (UV) rays penetrate cloud cover; therefore sun protection should always be a goal. UV rays can be reflected from water, concrete, sand, snow, tile, and reflective window glass in buildings. (Homes often have UV-blocking plastic films.)
3. Clothing is an excellent form of sun protection, especially loose-fitting, lightweight dark clothing, sunglasses, and 4″-wide brimmed hats.
4. Protective clothing with ultraviolet B (UVB) light with a sun protection factor (SPF) of 30 and higher is commercially available online.
5. Sunscreens (sun blocks) should be applied 15 to 30 minutes before sun exposure and can be liberally applied. They should have broad-spectrum ultraviolet A (UVA) and UVB protection.
6. Sunscreens with at least a 30 SPF (most desirable) and those with avobenzone (blocks UVA1), titanium dioxide, or zinc oxide (which block UVB and UVA1 and are best for very sensitive skin) are recommended. These sunscreens are marketed as creams, lotions, gels, sprays, and lotions, or as a stick; waterproof and sweat-resistant forms are available, as well as lip and eyelid formulations.
7. Adding vitamin D supplements should be considered to ensure that a deficiency of this vitamin does not develop (at least 800 IU/day).
8. Sunscreens should not be applied to broken skin or on rashes.
9. Children with lupus should use sunscreens, but parents are advised to consult their physician before applying these agents. Oil-free sunscreens work best in those who are prone to acne.

therapy. Numerous web sites offer information related to specialized sun-protective clothing, local daily UV indices, and guides for sun protection. The previous points are summarized in Box 47-3, and can also be referenced via the Lupus Foundation of America.

Avoidance of UV exposure has been so overemphasized that many patients are irrational about going out during the day. Unless definite evidence of exacerbations that are provoked by such exposure is noted, normal activities need not be restricted or curtailed. Although cautioning patients that sun exposure may cause increased local erythema or the development of new skin lesions is advisable, the physician should avoid causing a sunlight phobia. The average patient, even one who is photosensitive, can usually walk a few blocks at midday without protection and experience no ill effects. The question of how limited light exposure should be must be determined on an individual basis. The physician must use judgment so that the patient's way of life is interrupted as little as possible. Because sun exposure is greatest at midday, outdoor activities should be undertaken in the morning or later in the afternoon.

Antimalarial therapy increases patients' tolerance to sun exposure, even in those who were extremely sensitive to UV light before taking them. The degree of limitation must be frequently reevaluated, because the tendency to sunlight-induced exacerbation of skin lesions can subside, particularly with disease remissions that are either spontaneous or drug induced.

LOCAL THERAPY FOR CUTANEOUS LUPUS ERYTHEMATOSUS
Topical Corticosteroid Preparations

Local treatment is used for isolated lesions of DLE or for refractory skin lesions in patients with DLE or SLE. The most effective, safe, and least scarring type of local therapy is the use of various steroidal preparations. These can be fluorinated or nonfluorinated, and they may be of low, intermediate, or high potency (Box 47-4). Most nonfluorinated steroids include hydrocortisone cream or ointment and are available as over-the-counter preparations in strengths of less than 1%. These agents are less expensive but also less potent than the fluorinated preparations, which produce more stinging, dermal atrophy, depigmentation, striae, telangiectasia, acne, folliculitis, and *Candida* superinfection. Fluorinated steroids cannot be applied to the face for more than 2 weeks at a time without the expectation of cutaneous side effects (see Box 47-4).

Topical corticosteroid preparations should be used three or four times daily for optimal effectiveness and only applied directly over the lesions. Patients should be warned not to use them on normal skin, because they will induce atrophy. Improvement is usually noted within a few days. Unfortunately, recurrences frequently appear within a few days to weeks after the cessation of treatment, but small lesions can be adequately and indefinitely controlled by the intermittent use of these preparations. Old, indurated, and chronically scaling lesions respond poorly to corticosteroid treatment alone and require occlusive therapy, intracutaneous injections, and/or antimalarial agents. Patients are usually prescribed an intermediate-strength steroid cream or ointment and then high-potency agents for resistant lesions. Ointments are generally used for dry skin and creams for oily skin, but the ointment form is more effective than a cream, gel, or lotion. Fluorocarbon-propelled sprays are the most favored by patients but are the least effective. Thin skin is more permeable to topical steroids as well. Evidence-based studies of topical steroids for the treatment of cutaneous lesions that are less than 40 years old are few in number but support the effectiveness of these approaches.[59]

Other Steroid Delivery Systems: Occlusive Patches and Dressings, Intralesional Therapy, and Intradermal Injections

Newer occlusive patches allows for the improved absorption of high-potency steroids with less irritation. These should complement the use of translucent plastic, steroid-impregnated tape, and occlusive dressings such as plastic wrap, which increase percutaneous absorption by a factor of 100 and have been documented to be effective for those with severe lesions. Airtight occlusion of the skin causes obstruction of the sweat ducts, however, which may exacerbate pruritus and foster bacterial overgrowth on the skin surface. Intralesional therapy is often helpful when topical applications fail. Several studies have shown the value of intradermal injections of steroids in resistant lesions.[60]

Topical Calcineurins for Cutaneous Lupus and Other Approaches

The availability of tacrolimus and pimecrolimus for eczema and allergic dermatitis led to off-label trials for cutaneous lupus. In contrast to fluorinated steroids, these agents have the advantage of being applied facially without fear of inducing cutaneous atrophy, although their penetration is more limited in hypertrophic lesions.[61] Several controlled trials have documented their effectiveness in cutaneous lupus, and they were equivalent to topical corticosteroids in one head-to-head study.[62] Other topical approaches being studied include the beta-2 agonist salbutamol, retinoid, and imiquimod, which is an antiproliferative agent used for skin cancers. The reader is referred to an excellent review of the subject of topical therapies for cutaneous lupus.[57]

Can Patients with Lupus Undergo Topical Cosmetic Procedures?

Lasers, collagen, hyaluronic acid gels, Botox, Thermage, microdermabrasion, and sclerotherapy have been used for butterfly rashes, blemishes, telangiectasias, scars, skin tightening, blemishes, and spider veins in both lupus-related and non–lupus-related purposes. If appropriate precautions are taken (e.g., waiting until steroids are stopped or are at their lowest possible dose, skin testing the patient with collagen first), these procedures can improve a patient's quality of life and appearance.[63]

NONSTEROIDAL ANTIINFLAMMATORY DRUGS FOR THE TREATMENT OF SYSTEMIC LUPUS ERYTHEMATOSUS

Nearly 80% of patients with SLE are treated with NSAIDs for fever, arthritis, serositis, and headaches during the course of their disease. Beginning with phenylbutazone in 1953, indomethacin in 1965, and ibuprofen in 1974, enormous quantities of NSAIDs have been tested, manufactured, and sold worldwide. They are among the most commonly prescribed drugs in the world, with estimates as high as $4 billion spent annually in the United States. Despite the fact that the FDA has not approved a commercial preparation of NSAIDs in the management of SLE, these agents have been widely used for the treatment of SLE-associated arthralgias, myalgias, arthritis, headache, fever, serositis, pleuritis, and pericarditis.[64] Although the number of well-controlled, evidence-based studies in patients with SLE is low, a review by Wallace and associates[64] discusses the role of NSAIDs in the management of patients with lupus and evaluates some of the major side effects associated with their use.

Mechanisms of Action

The cellular membrane bilayer provides the substrate for the synthesis of prostaglandins and thromboxanes. Arachidonic acid is initially produced in response to chemical or mechanical stimuli by the actions of the enzyme phospholipase A. Arachidonic acid is subsequently metabolized either by cyclooxygenase A to form an unstable endoperoxide called prostaglandin H_2 (PGH_2) or by 5-lipooxygenase to produce leukotrienes. PGH_2, in turn, degrades to form prostaglandins PGI_2, PGE_2, and PGD_2, toxic oxygen radicals, and thromboxane A_2. Prostaglandins induce a variety of inflammatory effects such as swelling, erythema, changes in vascular permeability, and neutrophil chemotaxis. Additionally, prostaglandins have a myriad of effects on multiple organ systems, including the renal, gastrointestinal (GI), and musculoskeletal systems.

NSAIDs inhibit the rate-limiting step in the production of prostaglandins by binding to cyclooxygenase A. Three distinct proteins that process cyclooxygenase (COX) activity, known as COX-1, COX-2, and COX-3, are now recognized. COX-1 is ubiquitous throughout the body in the renal-collecting tubules, platelets, endothelial cells, smooth muscle, and gastric mucosa. The COX-2 gene is expressed in a limited number of cells such as neurons, synoviocytes, and smooth muscle cells. COX-3, which is inhibited by high-dose acetaminophen, is constitutively expressed in the brain and heart tissue and thought to be responsible for febrile reactions.[65]

The action of NSAIDs is generally accepted as inhibiting the synthesis of prostaglandins, but this action may not account for all the effects of NSAIDs. NSAIDs inhibit the aggregation of neutrophils in vivo and in vitro and show inhibitory effects additive to those of stable prostaglandins on the generation of the superoxide anion, a product of inflammatory cells.[66] Human T lymphocytes express the COX-2 isoenzyme, where it may serve a role in both early and late events of T-cell activation, such as the production of IL-2, tumor necrosis factor alpha, and interferon gamma. NSAIDs can inhibit experimental skin inflammation, and associated increased prostaglandin synthesis has been demonstrated using the inflammatory response to topical application of tetrahydrofurfuryl nicotinate (Trafuril).[67]

Clinical Efficacy in Systemic Lupus Erythematosus

The number of randomized controlled clinical trials for the use of NSAIDs in patients with lupus is extremely low. The clinical use of NSAIDs in patients with SLE is based primarily on case reports and series, as well as documented efficacy in patients without lupus and patients with other rheumatic diseases such as rheumatoid arthritis and osteoarthritis. Wallace and associates[64] studied patterns of NSAID use by rheumatologists in the treatment of patients with SLE and found that 85% of 12 rheumatologists in private practice caring for 935 patients used NSAIDs. NSAIDs are useful for treating headaches, fevers, serositis, arthralgia, arthritis, myalgias, and generalized pain in patients with SLE.[64] Topically applied NSAIDs (e.g., diclofenac, ketoprofen) have been used for the treatment of arthralgias, arthritis, and myalgias, especially if most of the reported discomfort is local or significant reflux disease is present.

The first report of NSAID use in patients with SLE came from a study by Langhof[68] with phenylbutazone in 1953, and Dubois[69] conducted the first true study with ibuprofen in 1975. (A listing of additional case reports and reviews can be found in the online version of this chapter's bibliography.) However, the only controlled SLE study was performed in 1980 at the National Institutes of Health. This study included 19 patients and was conducted over a period of 10 days. Patients received 2400 mg of ibuprofen versus 3600 mg of aspirin after a placebo washout period.[70] Only 2 of the 8 patients receiving ibuprofen benefited, whereas 7 of the 9 patients who received aspirin improved. Complications including abnormal liver function tests and transient decrease in renal function were observed. The authors of this study concluded that the low incidence of response to ibuprofen and the potential toxicity made the utility of this medication for patients with SLE doubtful. Currently, clinicians routinely use NSAIDs in the treatment of arthralgias and serositis in patients with lupus, despite their potential adverse effects. The literature suggests that indomethacin may improve the nephrotic syndrome.

Cyclooxygenase-2 Inhibition

Immune cells of mice with SLE spontaneously hyperexpress COX-2, and COX-2 inhibitors could cause cell apoptosis. Treatment with COX-2 inhibitors resulted in decreased autoantibody production and the inhibition of the T-cell response to the nucleosome and its presentation by antigen-presenting cells. Lander and associates[71] demonstrated that celecoxib is beneficial and safe in the majority of patients with SLE, in spite of its sulfa moiety. This class of drugs does not interfere with warfarin dosing, unlike conventional NSAIDs (Box 47-5).[72]

Adverse Reactions of Nonsteroidal Antiinflammatory Drugs in Systemic Lupus Erythematosus

Although NSAIDs are frequently used in patients with SLE, risks are associated with their use. Many variables, including co-morbid conditions, concurrent medication use, baseline renal function, and age, may all contribute to the potential toxicity of NSAIDs. Most patients

Box 47-5 Summary Points Relating to the Use of Nonsteroidal Antiinflammatory Drugs in Systemic Lupus

1. No NSAIDs are currently approved by the U.S. Food and Drug Administration (FDA) for SLE.
2. Over 70% of patients with SLE use an NSAID on an intermittent or regular basis, mostly for fever, headache, myalgias, arthralgias or arthritis, and/or serositis.
3. Controlled trial summary: Aspirin is superior to ibuprofen, and celecoxib is effective and safe for musculoskeletal complaints.
4. Patients with lupus have more complications (e.g., transaminitis, sun-sensitized or sun-induced rashes, fluid retention, hypertension, gastrointestinal ulcerations, aseptic meningitis) from using NSAIDs than do healthy persons without SLE. Whether disease activity, disease-related risk factors (e.g., renal disease), or concomitant medications play a supporting role is not completely understood.
5. NSAIDs can be safely prescribed to most patients with lupus, provided they are closely monitored on a regular basis. These drugs should be used with caution in pregnancy.
6. The risks and benefits of NSAIDs must be weighed and discussed. More long-term data are needed to appreciate fully the potential adverse cardiovascular and cerebrovascular events associated with their use. NSAIDs are usually preferable to narcotics for pain.
7. Preferred NSAIDs include aspirin, naproxen, and celecoxib, which have the best efficacy and safety in a review of the lupus and NSAID literature. Topical NSAIDs can be used as a first-line defense for localized inflammation. Consistent dosing minimizes drug interactions, and proton-pump inhibition decreases gastrointestinal perforations, ulcers, and bleeding.

with lupus take NSAIDs on an intermittent basis, whereas the safety data are frequently based on continual use trials; therefore many of the safety concerns do not likely apply to the majority of patients with lupus. The following information is specific for NSAIDs but not necessarily for those with lupus.

Renal System

Renal insufficiency is the most common side effect that typically occurs in patients with additional risk factors such as advanced age, intravascular volume contraction, diabetes, or preexisting renal insufficiency. NSAIDs induce renal side effects by inhibiting prostaglandin synthesis, which plays a key role in vasodilatory regulation, and by reducing creatinine clearance and glomerular filtration rate (GFR). Acute renal failure and acute tubular necrosis have been reported in patients with lupus who are taking ibuprofen, naproxen, and fenoprofen. NSAIDs can lead to chronic renal injury and papillary necrosis, nephrotic syndrome, and acute interstitial nephritis. NSAIDs are therefore generally to be avoided in patients with lupus nephritis.

Gastrointestinal System

GI complications, including dyspepsia, gastric mucosal damage, ulcer risk, and GI bleeding, are thought to be similar in patients, regardless of whether they have lupus. Misoprostol, an H2-receptor antagonist, and a proton-pump inhibitor are used in combination with or in addition to NSAIDs to prevent these side effects. COX-2 inhibitors have shown promise in preventing GI toxicity. Transaminitis is more common in patients with lupus who are taking NSAIDs including aspirin.

Nervous System

Physicians should consider the possibility of NSAID hypersensitivity in patients with SLE whose presentation includes neurologic abnormalities. Although rare and readily reversible, aseptic meningitis in these patients has been reported more frequently with ibuprofen use.[73]

Cutaneous Reactions

Compared with the general population, patients with SLE have higher rates of allergic reactions to all medications, especially antibiotics, and, to a lesser extent, NSAIDs. Sulfonamide-containing medications present problems for some patients with SLE, such as an allergic reaction or precipitating a lupus flare. Celecoxib, a COX-2 inhibitor, contains a sulfonamide moiety but does not contain the arylamine group, which is believed to be responsible for serious sulfa reactions. Therefore, because of the structural differences with sulfonamide antibiotics, the incidence of cross-reactivity resulting in clinically adverse reactions has been rarely seen, and this rarity has been verified in a cohort study. Rare instances have been reported of sun-sensitivity rashes with ibuprofen, indomethacin, sulindac, and piroxicam, as well as with naproxen in subacute cutaneous lupus erythematosus.

Cardiovascular System

Accelerated atherogenesis is an established feature of patients with SLE. Numerous studies indicate that all NSAIDs carry a small increased relative risk for increased hypertension, edema, and myocardial infarction in the range of 1.1 to 2.0. Naproxen is associated with the lowest cardiovascular risk among all NSAIDs and is the first-line agent of choice among individuals who benefit most from daily, high-dose NSAID use.

Hematologic Complications

Patients with lupus are known to be hypercoagulable as a result of complications from inflammation, antiphospholipid syndrome, and nephrosis. Animal models suggest that the suppression of COX-2–derived prostacyclin may increase the risk of myocardial infarction and stroke with selective COX-2 inhibitors (coxibs). Although the suggestion has been made that vascular thrombosis is associated with celecoxib on the basis of four case reports of lupus, a cohort study has shown no supporting evidence.[74,75]

Pregnancy

NSAIDs may be administered during the first two trimesters of pregnancy, if indicated and with the approval of the patient's obstetrician, but they are usually withheld during the third trimester of pregnancy, when their use can lead to the premature closure of the ductus arteriosus. Indomethacin is the most studied NSAID, and studies with ibuprofen have also been reported. Although NSAIDs are generally thought to be safe in the first two trimesters, reports of oligohydramnios, premature closure of the fetal ductus with subsequent persistent pulmonary hypertension of the newborn, fetal nephrotoxicity, and periventricular hemorrhage have been reported. Increased risk of miscarriages associated with exposure to NSAIDs has also been reported. Therefore patients with lupus are advised to consult their high-risk obstetrician before initiating or while taking NSAIDs during pregnancy. Infertility associated with NSAID consumption and cases of infertility have been very rarely reported with NSAID use, secondary to NSAID-induced luteinized unruptured follicle syndrome.

Drug Interactions and Monitoring

Patients with lupus often take multiple medications, increasing the opportunity for potential interactions. NSAIDs have been shown to diminish the antihypertensive effects of thiazide and loop diuretics. NSAID use can increase prothrombin time and the risk for bleeding if taken with warfarin. Methotrexate is used in the treatment of arthritis in patients with SLE. The potential of interference of aspirin, in antiinflammatory doses, with the systemic and renal clearance of methotrexate exists, which will lead to higher methotrexate levels and thus increase the potential for toxicity. Therefore patients taking methotrexate are advised not to vary their daily NSAID use. Since both NSAIDs and corticosteroid medications have potential GI toxicity, they may increase the risk for adverse GI side effects such as

ulcers and bleeding when taken together. The administration of proton-pump inhibitors to patients concurrently taking these two medications may be advisable. Patients with lupus who are taking NSAIDs should be examined at least once every 3 months, at which time a history, physical examination, and laboratory tests should also be performed. The physical examination should screen for hypertension, GI side effects, and edema, and laboratory tests should include a complete blood count and hepatic and renal screening.

References

1. Zonana-Nacach A, Roseman JM, McGwin G, Jr, et al: Systemic lupus erythematosus in three ethnic groups. VI. Factors associated with fatigue within 5 years of criteria diagnosis. LUMINA Study Group. LUpus in MInority populations: Nature vs Nurture. *Lupus* 9:101–109, 2000.
2. Wallace DJ, Margolin K, Waller P: Fibromyalgia and interleukin-2 therapy for malignancy. *Ann Intern Med* 108:909, 1988.
3. Forte S, Carlone S, Vaccaro F, et al: Pulmonary gas exchange and exercise capacity in patients with systemic lupus erythematosus. *J Rheumatol* 26:2591–2594, 1999.
4. Costa DD, Bernatsky S, Dritsa M, et al: Determinants of sleep quality in women with systemic lupus erythematosus. *Arthritis Rheum* 53:272–278, 2005.
5. Greenwood KM, Lederman L, Lindner HD: Self-reported sleep in systemic lupus erythematosus. *Clin Rheumatol* 27:1147–1151, 2008.
6. Iaboni A, Ibañez D, Gladman DD, et al: Fatigue in systemic lupus erythematosus: contributions of disordered sleep, sleepiness, and depression. *J Rheumatol* 33:2453–2457, 2006.
7. Ad Hoc Committee on Systemic Lupus Erythematosus Response Criteria for Fatigue: Measurement of fatigue in systemic lupus erythematosus: a systemic review. *Arthritis Rheum* 57:1348–1357, 2007.
8. Wallace DJ: Antimalarial agents and lupus. *Rheum Dis Clin North Am* 20:243–263, 1994.
9. Bruce IN, Mak VC, Hallett DC, et al: Factors associated with fatigue in patients with systemic lupus erythematosus. *Ann Rheum Dis* 58:379–381, 1999.
10. Sakauchi M, Matsumura T, Yamaoka T, et al: Reduced muscle uptake of oxygen during exercise in patients with systemic lupus erythematosus. *J Rheumatol* 22:1483–1487, 1995.
11. Tench CM, McCarthy J, McCurdie I, et al: Fatigue in systemic lupus erythematosus: a randomized controlled trial of exercise. *Rheumatology* 42:1050–1054, 2003.
12. Strombeck B, Jacobsson LTH: The role of exercise in the rehabilitation of patients with systemic lupus erythematosus and patients with primary Sjögren's syndrome. *Curr Opin Rheumatol* 19:197–203, 2007.
13. Boström C, Dupré B, Tengvar P, et al: Aerobic capacity correlates to self-assessed physical function but to overall disease activity or organ damage in women with systemic lupus erythematosus with low-to-moderate disease activity and organ damage. *Lupus* 17:100–104, 2008.
14. Ayán C, Martin V: Systemic lupus erythematosus and exercise. *Lupus* 16:5–9, 2007.
15. Harel-Meir M, Sherer Y, Shoenfeld Y: Tobacco smoking and autoimmune rheumatic diseases. *Nat Clin Pract Rheumatol* 3(12):707–715, 2007.
16. Costenbader KH, Kim DJ, Peerzada J, et al: Cigarette smoking and the risk of systemic lupus erythematosus: a meta-analysis. *Arthritis Rheum* 50:849–857, 2004.
17. Formica MK, Palmer JR, Rosenberg L, et al: Smoking, alcohol consumption, and risk of systemic lupus erythematosus in the black women's health. *Study J Rheumatol* 30:1222–1226, 2003.
18. Turchin I, Bernatsky S, Clarke AE, et al: Cigarette smoking and cutaneous damage in systemic lupus erythematosus. *J Rheumatol* 36:2691–2693, 2009.
19. Hardy CJ, Palmer BP, Muir KR, et al: Smoking history, alcohol consumption, and systemic lupus erythematosus: a case-control study. *Ann Rheum Dis* 57:451–455, 1998.
20. Nagata C, Fujita S, Iwata H, et al: Systemic lupus erythematosus: a case-control epidemiologic study in Japan. *Int J Dermatol* 34:333–337, 1995.
21. Jewell ML, McCauliffe DP: Patients with cutaneous lupus erythematosus who smoke are less responsive to antimalarial treatment. *J Am Acad Dermatol* 42:983–987, 2000.
22. Rahman P, Gladman DD, Urowitz MB: Smoking interferes with efficacy of antimalarial therapy in cutaneous lupus. *J Rheumatol* 25:1716–1719, 1998.
23. Wang J, Kay AB, Fletcher J, et al: Alcohol consumption is not protective for systemic lupus erythematosus. *Ann Rheum Dis* 68:346–348, 2009.

24. Wang J, Pan HF, Ye DQ, et al: Moderate alcohol drinking might be protective for systemic lupus erythematosus: a systemic review and meta-analysis. *Clin Rheumatol* 27:1557–1563, 2008.

25. Guedj D, Weinberger A: Effect of weather conditions on rheumatic patients. *Ann Rheum Dis* 49:158–159, 1990.

26. Léone J, Pennaforte JL, Delhinger V, et al: Influence of seasons on risk of flare-up of systemic lupus: retrospective study of 66 patients. *Rev Med Intern* 18:286–291, 1997.

27. Amit M, Molad Y, Kiss S, et al: Seasonal variations in manifestations and activity of systemic lupus erythematosus. *Br J Rheumatol* 36:449–452, 1997.

28. Hasan T, Pertovaara M, Yli-Kerttula U, et al: Seasonal variation of disease activity of systemic lupus erythematosus in Finland: a 1 year follow up study. *Ann Rheum Dis* 63:1498–1500, 2004.

29. Líndal E, Thorlacius S, Stefánsson JG, et al: Pain and pain problems among subjects with systemic lupus erythematosus. *Scand J Rheumatol* 22:10–13, 1993.

30. Greco CM, Rudy TE, Manzi S: Adaptation to chronic pain in systemic lupus erythematosus: applicability of the multidimensional pain inventory. *Pain Med* 4:39–50, 2003.

31. Wallace DJ: The role of stress and trauma in rheumatoid arthritis and systemic lupus erythematosus. *Semin Arthritis Rheum* 16:153–157, 1987.

32. Wallace DJ: Does stress or trauma cause or aggravate rheumatic disease? *Baillieres Clin Rheumatol* 8:149–159, 1994.

33. Schubert C, Lampe A, Rumpold G, et al: Daily psychosocial stressors interfere with the dynamics of urine neopterin in a patient with systemic lupus erythematosus: an integrative single-case study. *Psychosom Med* 61:876–882, 1999.

34. Pawlak CP, Jacobs R, Mikeska E, et al: Patients with systemic lupus erythematosus differ from healthy controls in their immunological response to acute psychological stress. *Brain Behav Immun* 13:287–302, 1999.

35. McClary AR, Meyer E, Weitzman EL: Observations on the role of the mechanism of depression in some patients with disseminated lupus erythematosus. *Psychosom Med* 17:311–321, 1955.

36. Ropes MW: *Systemic lupus erythematosus*, Cambridge, MA, 1976, Harvard University Press.

37. Dobkin PL, Fortin PR, Joseph L, et al: Psychosocial contributors to mental and physical health in patients with systemic lupus erythematosus. *Arthritis Care Res* 11:23–31, 1998.

38. Pawlak CR, Witte T, Heiken H, et al: Flares in patients with systemic lupus erythematosus are associated with daily psychologic stress. *Psychother Psychosom* 72:159–165, 2003.

39. Greco CM, Rudy TE, Manzi S: Effects of a stress-reduction program on psychological function, pain, and physical function of systemic lupus erythematosus patients: a randomized controlled trial. *Arthritis Rheum* 51:625–634, 2004.

40. Wallace DJ, Metzger AL: Can an earthquake cause flares of rheumatoid arthritis or lupus nephritis? *Arthritis Rheum* 37:1826–1828, 1994.

41. Chou CT, Hwang CM: Changes in the clinical and laboratory features of lupus patients after the big earthquake in Taiwan. *Lupus* 11:109–113, 2002.

42. King-Smith D: External irritation as a factor in the causation of lupus erythematosus discoides. *Arch Derm Syphilol* 14:547–549, 1926.

43. De Boer EM, Nieboer C, Brunyzeel DP: Lupus erythematosus as an occupational disease. *Acta Derm Venereol* 77:492, 1997.

44. Osterberg L, Blaschke T: Adherence to medication. *N Engl J Med* 353:487–497, 2005.

45. Uribe AG, Alarcón GS, Sanchez ML et al: Systemic lupus erythematosus in three ethnic groups. XVIII. Factors predictive of poor compliance with study visits. *Arthritis Rheum* 51:258–263, 2004.

46. Bernatsky S, Pineau C, Joseph L, et al: Adherence to ophthalmologic monitoring for antimalarial toxicity in a lupus cohort. *J Rheumatol* 30:1756–1760, 2003.

47. Mosley-Williams A, Lumley MA, Gillis M, et al: Barriers to treatment adherence among African American and white women with systemic lupus erythematosus. *Arthritis Rheum* 47:630–638, 2002.

48. Bruce IN, Gladman DD, Urowitz MB: Factors associated with refractory renal disease in patients with systemic lupus erythematosus: the role of patient non adherence. *Arthritis Care Res* 13:406–408, 2000.

49. Chambers SA, Raine R, Rahman A, et al: Why do patients with systemic lupus erythematosus take or fail to take their prescribed medication? A qualitative study in a UK cohort. *Rheumatology* 48:266–271. 2009.

50. Koneru S, Shishov M, Ware A, et al: Effective measuring adherence to medications for systemic lupus erythematosus in a clinical setting. *Arthritis Rheum* 57:1000–1006, 2007.

51. Anonymous. Drugs that cause photosensitivity. *Med Lett Drugs Ther* 28:51–52, 1986.

52. Wildhagen K, Woll R, Deicher H: Case report: systemic lupus erythematosus patients at risk due to unprotected exposure to unsubdued halogen lamps. *Akt Rheumatol* 18:167–169, 1993.

53. Klein LR, Elmets CA, Callen JP: Photoexacerbation of cutaneous lupus erythematosus due to ultraviolet A emissions from a photocopier. *Arthritis Rheum* 38:1152–1156, 1995.

54. Rihner M, McGrath H, Jr: Fluorescent light photosensitivity in patients with systemic lupus erythematosus. *Arthritis Rheum* 35:949–952, 1992.

55. Nuzum-Keim AD, Sontheimer RD: Ultraviolet light output of compact fluorescent lamps: comparison to conventional incandescent and halogen residential lighting sources. *Lupus* 18:556–560, 2009.

56. [No authors listed]: Sunscreens: an update. *Med Lett Drugs Ther* 50:70–72, 2008.

57. Johnson JA, Fusaro RM: Broad-spectrum photoprotection: the roles of tinted auto windows, sunscreens and browning agents in the diagnosis and treatment of photosensitivity. *Dermatology* 185:237–241, 1992.

58. Diddie KR: Do sunglasses protect the retina from light damage? *West J Med* 161:594, 1994.

59. Ting WW, Sontheimer RD: Local therapy for cutaneous and systemic lupus erythematosus: practical and theoretical considerations. *Lupus* 10:171–184, 2001.

60. Callen JP: Intralesional triamcinolone is effective for discoid lupus erythematosus of the palms and soles. *J Rheumatol* 12:630–633, 1985.

61. Wollina U, Hansel G: The use of topical calcineurin inhibitors in lupus erythematosus: an overview, *J Eur Acad Dermatol Venereol* 22:1–6, 2008.

62. Barikbin B, Givrad S, Yousefi M, et al: Pimecrolimus 1% cream versus betamethasone 17-valerate 0.1% cream in the treatment of facial discoid lupus erythematosus: a double-blind, randomized pilot study, *Clin Exp Dermatol* 34:776–780, 2009.

63. Erceg A, Bovenschen HJ, van de Kerkhof PC, et al: Efficacy and safety of pulsed dye laser treatment for cutaneous discoid lupus erythematosus. *J Am Acad Dermatol* 60:626–632, 2009.

64. Wallace DJ, Metzger AL, Klinenberg JR: NSAID usage patterns by rheumatologists in the treatment of SLE. *J Rheumatol* 16:557–560, 1989.

65. Senior K: Homing in on COX-3—the elusive target of paracetamol. *Lancet Neurol* 1:399, 2002.

66. Abramson SB, Weismann G: The mechanisms of action of nonsteroidal antiinflammatory drugs. *Arthritis Rheum* 32:1–9, 1989.

67. Barr RM, Symonds PH, Akpan AS, et al: Culture of human dermal fibroblasts in collagen gels: modulation of interleukin1-induced prostaglandin E2 synthesis by an extracellular matrix. *Exp Cell Res* 198(2):321–327, 1992.

68. Langhof H: Target therapy of the vascular injury in subacute lupus erythematosus Irgapyrin. *Dermatol Wochenschr* 128:877–884, 1953.

69. Dubois EL: Letter: Ibuprofen for systemic lupus erythematosus. *New Engl J Med* 293(15):779, 1975.

70. Karsh J, Kimberly RP, Stahl NI, et al: Comparative effects of aspirin and ibuprofen in the management of systemic lupus erythematosus. *Arthritis Rheum* 23:1401–1404, 1980.

71. Lander S, Wallace DJ, Weisman M: Celecoxib for systemic lupus erythematosus: case series and literature review of the use of NSAIDs in SLE. *Lupus* 11:340–347, 2002.

72. Zhang L, Bertucci AM, Smith KA, et al: Hyperexpression of cyclooxygenase 2 in lupus immune system and effect of cyclooxygenase 2 inhibitor diet therapy in a murine model of systemic lupus erythematosus. *Arthritis Rheum* 56:4132–4141, 2007.

73. Widener HL, Littman BH: Ibuprofen-induced meningitis in systemic lupus erythematosus. *JAMA* 239:1062–1064, 1978.

74. Bresalier RS, Sandler RS, Quan H, et al: Cardiovascular events associated with rofecoxib in a colorectal adenoma chemoprevention trial. *N Engl J Med* 352:1092–1102, 2005.

75. Wallace DJ: Celecoxib for lupus. *Arthritis Rheum* 58(9):2923, 2008.

Chapter 48

Systemic Glucocorticoid Therapy in SLE

Kyriakos A. Kirou and Dimitrios T. Boumpas

Glucocorticoids (GCs), as a result of their powerful antiinflammatory effects, have remained a frontline therapy in rheumatology since Phillip Hench introduced them into clinical medicine in 1949. However, GCs should be used cautiously and at the minimal effective dose, because they may have serious adverse effects. Combination therapies of GCs with other immunosuppressive or antiinflammatory agents can help achieve disease control with less exposure to GCs. Hopefully, future research on both systemic lupus erythematosus (SLE) pathogenesis and the mechanisms of GC action will add safer and more effective therapies to the armamentarium against SLE.

In this chapter, the basic pharmacology of endogenous and synthetic GCs, the mechanisms of their action at the molecular level, and their antiinflammatory and immunosuppressive effects are briefly reviewed. Next, the pharmacokinetics and drug interactions of GCs are discussed, and the authors' opinions regarding their use in patients with SLE are presented. Last adverse effects of GCs with relevance to patients with SLE are reviewed.

ENDOGENOUS AND SYNTHETIC GLUCOCORTICOIDS

Steroidogenesis in the adrenal cortex produces endogenous GCs, mineralocorticoids (MCs), and adrenal androgens. Cortisol (hydrocortisone) is the main human endogenous GC and is secreted primarily in response to adrenocorticotropic hormone (ACTH). Secretion follows a circadian rhythm that achieves maximum plasma concentration at 8 AM (16 µg/dL). However, in the context of stressful stimuli and hypothalamic-pituitary-adrenal (HPA) axis stimulation, these levels can increase to more than 60 µg/dL, losing their diurnal variation. The ability of an organism to maintain appropriate GC levels before and during stress is quintessential for its survival.

Synthetic GCs, more potent and with fewer MC effects than cortisol, have been developed. The biochemical structure of cortisol and synthetic GC is shown in Figure 48-1 and their pharmacologic properties are compared in Table 48-1. Regulatory mechanisms of synthetic GCs, as they apply to binding to the corticosteroid-binding globulin (CBG), tissue-specific metabolism, affinity for GC receptors (GRs), and interaction with transcription factors, may substantially differ from those of native GCs.

The great need for improved synthetic GCs with less adverse effects and intact antiinflammatory and immunosuppressive actions has led to the development of newer synthetic GCs by modifying their pharmacokinetic or pharmacodynamic properties. Budesonide is an example of a GC with high topical activity but low systemic bioavailability as a result of rapid first-pass liver inactivation and has been used by inhalation in asthma and orally in Crohn disease. Of more interest to rheumatology is the development of liposomal formulations of GCs. These agents, which have been successfully used in animal models of arthritis, preferentially target macrophages in tissues, such as the synovium and the spleen, and achieve antiinflammatory effects without the need for repeated administration.[1,2] More recently, modified-release prednisone (PDN) tablets have been designed that release PDN 4 hours after their ingestion at bedtime and before the secretion of interleukin (IL)-6, which normally peaks

at approximately 8:00 AM. This PDN chronotherapy was tested with favorable results against regular PDN therapy in patients with rheumatoid arthritis (RA) in a randomized controlled trial (RCT) with open-label extension.[3]

Yet another strategy proposed for enhanced GC effect with less adverse effects is combination therapy with other drugs that work synergistically or additively. Examples include β-adrenergic agents, phosphodiesterase inhibitors, and nitric oxide–conjugated GCs (nitrosteroids), especially in the treatment of asthma and chronic obstructive pulmonary disease (COPD).[4-6]

MOLECULAR MECHANISMS OF GLUCOCORTICOID ACTION

GC effects are mainly mediated via specific GRs in the cytoplasm that operate as hormone-activated transcriptional regulators.[7] Hydrocortisone and other GCs are also capable of binding MC receptors (MRs) with higher affinity than they bind GRs and mediating aldosterone-like effects (see Table 48-1). GR specificity, at relatively low baseline body cortisol levels, is maintained because of the action of 11 beta–hydroxysteroid dehydrogenase enzyme 2 (11β-HSD_2), a steroid metabolizing enzyme expressed at MC-sensitive tissues (e.g., the kidney) that metabolizes hydrocortisone to the inactive cortisone.

GRs, when inactive, are bound to several receptor-associated proteins, such as the heat shock protein (HSP) 90.[7,8] Upon GC binding, GRs dissociate from these proteins and translocate to the nucleus. There they mediate their effects mainly via either GR homodimerization and direct transactivation/transrepression of genes or indirectly via protein-protein interactions with other transcription factors (Figure 48-2). Indirect transrepression is thought to mediate antiinflammatory effects within a few hours, and direct transactivation/transrepression to mediate both adverse effects and antiinflammatory effects within days. This concept has led to the development of synthetic selective glucocorticoid receptor agonists (SEGRAs) with dissociated activity for indirect transrepression (potent) and direct transactivation (weak) and their successful use in an animal model of skin inflammation.[9] Notably, GCs, by inducing mitogen-activated protein kinase (MAPK) phosphatase 1 (MKP1) and inhibiting p38 MAPK, can downregulate proinflammatory genes, such as cytokines, cyclooxygenase (COX)-2, and inducible nitric oxide synthase (iNOS), as well as via posttranscriptional mechanisms.[6]

Besides having GR-mediated transcriptional genomic effects that depend on new protein synthesis and therefore have a delayed onset (at least 30 minutes and usually several hours), GCs may have more rapid (seconds or minutes) nongenomic effects.[10-13] These GC effects usually occur at relatively large pharmacologic or pulse-GC doses and are mediated by either membranous or cytosolic GRs. Examples include the rapid dissociation of T-cell receptor–associated lymphocyte-specific protein tyrosine kinase (Lck) and Fyn (a Src-family tyrosine kinase) and therefore the inhibition of T-cell signaling.[8] Moreover, GCs, especially at pulse-GC doses, may cause nonspecific physicochemical interactions with cellular membranes and cause immunosuppression by inhibiting calcium and sodium cycling across the plasma membrane of immune cells.[12] A recent

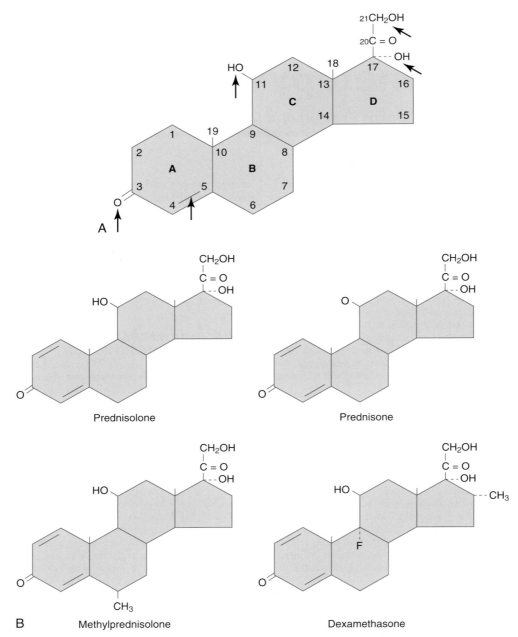

FIGURE 48-1 **A,** Structure of cortisol (hydrocortisone). All Δ^4 double-bond groups, 3-keto group, and 11β-OH groups are essential for glucocorticoid (GC) function, and the first two groups are also required for mineralocorticoid (MC) activity. The hydroxyl group at C21 is required for MC activity and is present on all natural and synthetic GCs. The 17α-hydroxyl group, present on cortisol and synthetic GCs (but not on corticosterone), enhances GC potency. **B,** Structure of selected common synthetic GCs. The addition of a Δ^1 double bond on cortisol (as in all shown GCs) selectively increases GC activity and delays GC metabolism. The methyl group at position 6α (methylprednisolone [MP]) increases GC over MC activity even further. Notably, fluorination at the 9α position (fludrocortisone; *not shown*) greatly enhances GC and MC activity (the latter significantly more than the former). However, when modified with a Δ^1 double-bond group and a methyl group substitution at C16α, fludrocortisone loses all MC activity and becomes dexamethasone (DEX).

study showed that novel GCs, conjugated to glycine or lysine to block genomic effects, were able to rapidly inhibit neutrophil degranulation and immunoglobulin E (IgE)–mediated histamine release from mast cells.[11]

ANTIINFLAMMATORY AND IMMUNOSUPPRESSIVE EFFECTS

The biologic effects of GCs are multiple; they affect all tissues and are essential for body homeostasis during normal or stress conditions. Although GCs are used to suppress inflammation and pathologic immune responses in clinical medicine, a growing number of studies

paradoxically attribute immune-enhancing effects to these agents. It seems that endogenous GCs have an important overall regulatory role in modulating immune responses that develop to such stressors as infections.[13] For example, GCs, on the one hand, act permissively to help immune responses develop adequately and in a timely fashion to fight the invading organisms, and yet, on the other hand, they act suppressively to restrain a potentially deleterious overshoot of these same responses. Parameters that determine the direction of GC-immune effects primarily include the serum levels and timing of GC exposure relative to the initiation of stress. Higher (pharmacologic) levels such as those occurring after the initiation of stress are,

TABLE 48-1 Relative Biologic Potency and Pharmacokinetics of Selected Glucocorticoids

GLUCOCORTICOIDS	GENOMIC ANTIINFLAMMATORY[1]	MINERALOCORTICOID ACTIVITY[2]	HALF-LIFE (MINUTES)	BIOLOGIC HALF-LIFE (HOURS)
Cortisol	20	1	60	8-12
Cortisone	25	0.8	60	8-12
Prednisone (PDN)	5	0.8	180	12-36
Prednisolone	5	0.8	180	12-36
Methylprednisolone (MP)	4	0.5	180	12-36
Triamcinolone	4	0	180	12-36
Dexamethasone (DEX)	0.75	0	220	36-72

[1]Is administered in the form of equivalent doses of various glucocorticoids in milligrams. Therefore 20 mg of cortisol are as potent as 5 mg of PDN and 0.75 mg of DEX, indicating that cortisol is the least potent of the three.
[2]Various glucocorticoids are compared with cortisol, with regard to their mineralocorticoid activity. Thus MP is 0.8 times as potent as cortisol, and DEX has no mineralocorticoid activity.

in general, immunosuppressive, whereas lower (physiologic) levels of GCs present before stress initiation may enhance immune responses. Notably, acute stresses (or a short exposure to GCs) enhance immune responses, whereas long-term exposure to stress or to GCs has the opposite effect.

The antiinflammatory effects of GCs, as shown in Figure 48-2 and Box 48-1, are complex. At the molecular level, GCs act on various cells (e.g., neutrophils, monocytes-macrophages, fibroblasts, endothelial cells) by both genomic and nongenomic effects to inhibit the synthesis and secretion of inflammatory mediators, as well as promote the synthesis and secretion of antiinflammatory proteins (see Figure 48-2). At the cellular level, they not only inhibit the initiation of acute inflammation with the blockade of small-vessel vasodilation and leukocyte (polymorphonuclear neutrophil [PMN] and eosinophil) migration to tissues in response to damage signals, but they also facilitate the nonphlogistic disposal of inflammatory cells and the resolution of inflammation.[14,15]

GLUCOCORTICOID RESISTANCE

Pharmacokinetic causes of resistance to GCs may include impaired oral bioavailability as a result of decreased GC absorption (e.g., by cholestyramine) or increased GC metabolism (e.g., by drugs such as barbiturates). With regard to pharmacodynamic causes, tissue-specific GC resistance has been studied best in steroid-resistant bronchial asthma, in which the lack of GC benefits for airway inflammation contrasts with a high incidence of GC adverse effects from other organs. Cytokines, secreted in the context of such diseases as bronchial asthma, RA, SLE, and depression, are thought to play an important role in mediating tissue-specific GC resistance by inhibiting GR function.[16] In addition and more relevant to patients with SLE, a recent study has shown that signaling via Toll-like receptors (TLRs) 7 and 9 blocks the inhibitory effect of GCs on plasmacytoid dendritic cells (pDCs) with regard to type I interferon (IFN) production by these cells.[17] The authors of the study have proposed that therapy with TLR 7 and 9 inhibitors could work as GC-sparing agents in patients with SLE. Finally, high levels of P-glycoprotein (P-gp) have been noted in lymphocytes of patients with active lupus that was resistant to high doses of prednisolone.[18] GC resistance was reversed after intensive immunosuppressive therapy and/or cyclosporine, which functions as a competitive inhibitor of P-gp.

PHARMACOKINETICS AND DRUG INTERACTIONS

Oral absorption of GCs is excellent whether on an empty or full stomach. Once in the circulation, a large fraction of GCs (90% for hydrocortisone) binds to serum proteins. Only their free fraction is biologically active. Of the two GC-binding proteins, transcortin or CBG binds to GCs with high affinity and low capacity, whereas albumin binds with low affinity and high capacity. Although hydrocortisone and prednisolone bind to both CBG and albumin, their

protein binding is concentration dependent and varies from 90% at lower doses (i.e., with standard oral doses) to 60% at higher doses. In contrast, methylprednisolone (MP) and dexamethasone (DEX) bind almost exclusively (99%) to the high-capacity albumin and therefore have concentration-independent protein-bound fractions (60% to 70%). The 11-keto GC derivatives such as PDN and cortisone are inactive unless reduced by 11-β-HSD$_1$ in the liver to their 11-OH analogs, prednisolone and hydrocortisone (see Figure 48-1). Inactivation of GCs occurs predominantly in the liver and involves the sequential reduction of the Δ^4 double bond (i.e., the rate-limiting step in cortisol metabolism), and the 3-keto group (see Figure 48-1). Glucuronidation and sulfation follow, which confer water solubility and allow for urine excretion. Additionally, 6β-hydroxylation by the cytochrome P450 microsomal enzyme (family 3, subfamily A, polypeptide 4) (CYP3A4) also enhances water solubility and urinary excretion of GC. Serum half-lives of different GCs vary from 60 to 300 minutes. However, biologic half-lives of GCs are dependent on their tissue levels and are much longer than their serum half-lives (see Table 48-1). In addition to the previously mentioned inhibition of enteric GC absorption by cholestyramine, other important drug interactions also exist. Drugs that induce hepatic microsomal enzymes (especially CYP3A4), such as phenobarbital, phenytoin, rifampin, and carbamazepine, increase GC elimination. In contrast, CYP3A4 inhibitors, such as ketoconazole and clarithromycin, increase GC activity.

GENERAL PRINCIPLES OF GLUCOCORTICOID THERAPY

Uncontrolled disease activity in patients with SLE can be both debilitating and life threatening and thus demands rapid and effective intervention. The value of therapy with high doses of GCs in such a setting (e.g., in diffuse proliferative glomerulonephritis [DPGN]) is unquestionable. On the other hand, GCs can have multiple complications that are directly related to the dose and duration of therapy. (See section under "Adverse Effects of Glucocorticoids" later in this chapter.) In fact, Sergent and colleagues[19] have shown increased infection-related mortality in patients with severe neuropsychiatric SLE (NP-SLE) when treated with PDN doses of more than 100 mg/day for an average of 37 days (range, 8 to 68 days).[19] On the other hand, low-dose GC therapy (i.e., a dose equivalent of 7.5 mg or less of PDN per day) appears to be tolerated better but is not free of risks; complications such as growth suppression, osteoporosis (OP), and cataract formation can still occur. Therefore the ultimate goal of therapy should always be the complete cessation of GCs, if possible.

The First European Workshop on GC therapy proposed a standardized nomenclature for GC doses and GC treatment regimens, taking into account the percent saturation of GRs at different doses and clinical practice.[20] The nongenomic effects, which become increasingly important with very high–dose GC and pulse-GC

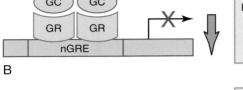

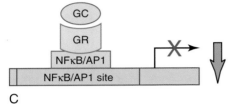

FIGURE 48-2 Mechanisms of genomic effects of GCs. **A,** Direct transactivation of genes through binding of activated GR dimers to GRE on the corresponding gene promoter or enhancer regions. Examples of such transactivated antiinflammatory genes include ANXA1, also known as lipocortin 1, and its receptor; FPR2 or ALXR; IκB, an inhibitor of NF-κB; IL-1Ra, an inhibitor of IL-1β; MAPK phosphatase 1 (MKP1) or DUSP1; SLPI; SLAP 1; neutral endopeptidase; and IL-10. Examples also include enzymes of gluconeogenesis, responsible for hyperglycemic effects of GC7 and GC8. **B,** Direct transrepression of genes (often responsible for GC adverse effects) through binding of activated GR dimers to nGRE on the corresponding gene promoter or enhancer reGC-induced osteonecrosis.[95] Examples include insulin precursor, insulin receptor, POMC, osteocalcin, keratins 5 and 14, cyclin D1, and 11β-HSD₂. **C,** Indirect transrepression through protein-to-protein cross-talk; activated GR monomers interact and inhibit proinflammatory transcription factors, such as NF-κB and AP-1 11, 13. Examples include the following: (1) Cytokines: IL-1, IL-2, IL-4, IL-5, IL-6, IL-12, TNF, and GMCSF, among others. (2) Chemokines: IL-8, MCP-1, MIP-1α, and eotaxin, among others. (3) Proinflammatory enzymes: inducible nitric oxide synthase (iNOS), COX2, and collagenase. (4) Adhesion molecules: ICAM-1 and E-selectin, among others.

Abbreviations: 11β-HSD2, 11 beta–hydroxysteroid dehydrogenase enzyme 2; ALXR, lipoxin A₄ receptor; ANXA1, annexin-A1; AP1, activator protein 1; COX2, cyclooxygenase 2; DUSP1, dual-specificity protein phosphatase 1; FPR2, formyl peptide receptor 2; GCs, glucocorticoids; GMCSF, granulocyte-macrophage colony-stimulating factor; GR, glucocorticoid receptor; GRE, glucocorticoid-responsive elements; ICAM1, intercellular cell adhesion molecule 1; IκB, inhibitor κB; IL, interleukin; IL-1Ra, interleukin 1–receptor antagonist; IL-1β, interleukin-1 beta; iNOS, inducible nitric oxide synthase; MAPK, mitogen-activated protein kinases; MCP-1, monocyte chemoattractant protein-1; MIP-1α, macrophage inflammatory protein–1 alpha; NFAT, nuclear factor of activated T cells; NF-κB, nuclear factor–kappa B; nGRE, negative–glucocorticoid-responsive elements; NO, nitric oxide; POMC, proopiomelanocortin; SLAP, Src-like adaptor protein; SLPI, secretory leukocyte protease inhibitor; TNF, tumor necrosis factor.

Box 48-1 Important Antiinflammatory and Immunosuppressive[1] Effects of Glucocorticoids on Various Cells of the Immune System[4,7,9,76,77]

1. Neutrophils
   Peripheral blood neutrophilia
   Inhibition of neutrophil adhesion to endothelial cells and trans-migration to tissues
   Mobilization of neutrophils from bone marrow to peripheral blood
   Inhibition of apoptosis[78]
   Inhibition of leukoaggregation[79]
2. Eosinophils
   Peripheral blood eosinopenia
   Apoptosis of eosinophils[78]
3. Basophil and mast cells
   Inhibition of mast cell degranulation[11]
   Inhibition of cytokine production
4. Monocytes and macrophages
   Peripheral blood monocytopenia
   Inhibition of monocyte or macrophage activation, secretion of proinflammatory cytokines (e.g., IL-1, IL-6, TNF) and destructive enzymes (e.g., collagenase)
   Inhibition of type I IFN signaling[80]
   Survival and migration of antiinflammatory macrophages to sites of inflammation[81-84]
   Phagocytosis of apoptotic neutrophils; antioxidant function and resolution of inflammation[78,81-83]
5. DC and pDC
   Apoptosis of immature DC
   Inhibition of DC migration to lymph nodes
   Inhibition of DC activation (i.e., reduction of MHC II, co-stimulatory molecules, cytokines) and inflammatory cytokine production
   Induction of tolerogenic DC phenotype associated with IL-10 production[76]
   Inhibition of pDC differentiation and induction of pDC apoptosis,[85] as well as inhibition of type I IL signature in peripheral blood by pulse GC[17,86,87]
6. Lymphocytes
   Lymphopenia—T cells affected more than B cells; CD4 T cells affected more than CD8 T cells (probably due to lymphocyte redistribution, mainly to bone marrow and spleen, and apoptosis)
   T-cell apoptosis[88]
   Blockade of TCR signaling[10,89]
   Inhibition of IL-2 synthesis and signaling
   Inhibition of T-cell migration to tissues[88]
   Direct suppression of both Th1 and Th2 cells, although the effect on the Th1 is greater[2,90,91]
   Suppression of Th17 cells and IL-17—likely indirectly by inhibiting IL-1, IL-6, and IL-23 in macrophages[92]
   Deviation of immune responses toward a Th2-type cytokine formation (by preferentially inhibiting synthesis of IL-12 over that of IL-4 and IL-10)
   Facilitation of development of T-regulatory cells[2,93]
   Possible indirect autoimmune B-cell suppression effect by high-dose dexamethasone via inhibition of BLyS[94]

APC, Antigen-presenting cells; BLyS: B lymphocyte stimulator; CD, cluster of differentiation; DC, dendritic cells; GC, glucocorticoids; IFN, interferon; IL, interleukin; MHC, major histocompatibility complex; pDC, plasmacytoid dendritic cells; TCR, T-cell receptor; Th1, T-helper 1; Th2, T-helper 2; TNF, tumor necrosis factor.
[1]Immunosuppression concerns primarily the cellular and less so the humoral immunity and is more evident with intermediate to high doses of glucocorticoids.
[2]Glucocorticoids also have indirect effects on Th1, Th2, Th17, and T-regulatory cells by modulating the cytokines produced by APC.

---

therapies, were also noted. These definitions have been adopted in this text (Table 48-2). The most effective approach to initiating high-dose or very high–dose GC therapy for severe SLE disease, especially when constitutional symptoms (e.g., high fever, prostration) are present, is to administer it in two to four doses per day. A notable exception is the management of severe focal proliferative glomerulonephritis (FPGN) or DPGN, in which once-a-day regimen is adequate. Should the condition prove GC unresponsive, then the use of pulse-GC or additional immunosuppressive agents or both is

TABLE 48-2 Usual Regimens of Systemic Glucocorticoid Therapy in Patients with Systemic Lupus Erythematosus[1]

GC REGIMEN[2]	REPRESENTATIVE INDICATIONS	COMMON ADVERSE EFFECTS
Pulse GCs: ≥250 mg PDNeq/day for 1-5 days Typically, 0.5-1 g MP/day IV for 1-3 days; monthly as indicated Usually with oral GCs (30-60 mg PDNeq/day)	Life- or organ-threatening complications (RPGN, myelopathy, severe acute confusional state, alveolar hemorrhage, vasculitis, optic neuritis)[3] High-dose GC-refractory disease DPGN or severe FPGN[3]	Same adverse effects as with high-dose GC (see below), but overall incidence of effects may be lower, partly because they may allow more rapid taper of oral GC doses Special considerations, as a result of large doses and route of administration: fluid overload, hypertension, and neuropsychiatric symptoms Rare effects: cardiac arrhythmias or sudden death, myalgias or arthralgias, seizures, intractable hiccups, or GC-anaphylaxis
Very high–dose GCs: >100 mg PDNeq/day, IV or by mouth (start with divided doses)	Life- or organ-threatening complications (as for pulse GC)[3]	Same adverse effects but more severe than with high-dose GCs Psychosis Possible high risk of severe or fatal infection (avoid use for more than 1-2 wk)
High-dose GCs: >30 mg and ≤100 mg PDNeq/day, IV or by mouth	DPGN or severe FPGN (for less than 6-8 wk)[4] Thrombocytopenia or hemolytic anemia Acute lupus pneumonitis Lupus crisis[5]	Same adverse effects for both high and moderate doses of GCs, but lower levels of incidence and severity with the latter HPA axis suppression, Cushing syndrome, hypertension, hypokalemia, hyperglycemia, hyperlipidemia, atherosclerosis, OP, ON, risk of infection, skeletal growth retardation, glaucoma, cataracts, skin fragility, acne, insomnia, steroid psychosis, mood swings
Moderate-dose GCs: >7.5 mg and ≤30 mg PDNeq/day, IV or by mouth	Moderate SLE flares (myositis, severe pleurisy, ophthalmoplegia [except optic neuritis], thrombocytopenia) With pulse GCs; CY or AZA for severe disease	
Low-dose GCs: ≤7.5 mg PDNeq/day, by mouth	Arthritis, mild constitutional symptoms (unresponsive to analgesics, NSAIDs, AM) Generalized LAN Maintenance therapy	Least toxic daily regimen Cataracts, GC-withdrawal symptoms (upon tapering to or below low-dose GCs), possible skeletal growth retardation Infection rates still increased but relatively low compared with higher doses Probably minimal OP, ON, HPA-axis suppression
Alternate-day GCs	Membranous nephritis with nephrotic syndrome (120 mg PDNeq) During tapering-GC dose Maintenance therapy (15 mg PDNeq for GN)	Decreased adverse effects (HPA-axis suppression, skeletal growth retardation, infection, Cushing syndrome), compared with daily regimens Possible OP

[1]All PDNeq doses assume the patient weighs 60 kg; adjustments should be made for different weights.
[2]Adopted from the recommendations of the First European Workshop on GC therapy.[20]
[3]Cyclophosphamide therapy, usually IVCY, is often needed as well.
[4]Is used in combination with IVCY.
[5]Lupus crisis refers to the patient who is acutely and severely ill with an elevated body temperature, extreme prostration, and other symptoms of active SLE (e.g., pleurisy, arthritis, vasculitic rash), who requires large doses of GCs for disease control. Infection has, of course, been excluded as the cause of the symptoms.
AM, antimalarials; AZA, azathioprine; CY, cyclophosphamide; DPGN, diffuse proliferative glomerulonephritis; GC, glucocorticoid; GN, glomerulonephritis; HPA, hypothalamic-pituitary-adrenal; IV, intravenous; IVCY, intravenous cyclophosphamide; LAN, lymphadenopathy; MP, methylprednisolone; NSAIDs, nonsteroidal antiinflammatory drugs; ON, osteonecrosis; OP, osteoporosis; PDNeq, prednisone equivalent; RPGN, rapidly progressive glomerulonephritis; SLE, systemic lupus erythematosus.

necessary. Most disease complications will respond in less than 1 to 2 weeks. However, markers of lupus nephritis (especially proteinuria) may take more than 2 to 6 weeks to improve.

Within 1 to 2 weeks from the initiation of therapy, whether a satisfactory response has occurred or a cytotoxic agent has been added to the regimen for refractory disease, tapering of GC therapy should be initiated.[21,22] The first step is to consolidate the GC regimen into a once-a-day morning dose. The daily dose can then be decreased by 5 mg (or 5% to 10%) per week until a dose of 0.25 to 0.5 mg/kg/day is reached, and more slowly thereafter, aiming for either a complete withdrawal or, if that is not possible, for low-dose GC therapy. Some clinicians prefer to follow an alternate-day GC-tapering regimen, during which the second day's dose is usually first gradually decreased to 0 before further dose decreases are made. Caution should be applied during tapering; too fast- or too slow-dose decrements can lead to disease flares or withdrawal symptoms or increased GC toxicity, respectively. In the event that a flare occurs during the tapering, the dose is increased to the immediate previous effective level for a few weeks, before the next, perhaps slower, tapering is attempted. Less severe SLE manifestations are managed with low- or moderate-dose GCs accordingly. Table 48-2 provides an overview of the suggested GC use in patients with SLE. Finally, some studies have argued for the use of prophylactic GC in patients with SLE and a serologic flare as defined by increases in anti–double stranded DNA (anti-dsDNA) titers or decreases in complement levels.[23,24] In those studies, clinical relapses were prevented without increased cumulative GC doses. The authors of this text believe that in clinical practice, such cases should be followed closely for clinical flares but GC doses should be increased only when new symptoms and signs emerge.

The importance of other immunosuppressive agents (e.g., methotrexate, azathioprine, mycophenolate mofetil, cyclophosphamide) in helping control the disease while allowing safe tapering of GCs (steroid-sparing activity) cannot be overemphasized. Proliferative lupus nephritis is the best-studied SLE complication, and randomized controlled clinical studies have documented the superiority of intravenous (IV) cyclophosphamide (IVCY)-containing regimens over those with GCs or IVCY alone.[25,26] Moreover, with combination therapies, a more effective GC-tapering scheme can be achieved. Additionally, many observational studies, case series, and small trials favor the use of cyclophosphamide (mainly IV) in other life- or organ-threatening SLE complications that may be refractory to GC therapy.[27-29] Severe NP-SLE of nonthrombotic causes (especially acute confusional state, myelopathy, and optic neuritis), pulmonary hemorrhage, interstitial pneumonitis, acute cardiomyopathy, and severe vasculitis of other systems such as the gastrointestinal (GI) are examples. In such grave cases, patients might benefit from the simultaneous administration of GCs and other immunosuppressive agents (mainly IVCY) from the outset of the disease. For less severe disease manifestations such as arthritis, serositis, and mild constitutional symptoms, agents such as hydroxychloroquine, nonsteroidal antiinflammatory drugs (NSAIDs), analgesics, and local GCs (i.e., intraarticular [IA] injections) should be given priority, and systemic GCs used only if necessary and at the lowest effective dose.

This approach to GC use in patients with SLE is based on the assumption that alternative noninflammatory or nonautoimmune diagnoses have been carefully excluded before a patient is committed to prolonged immunosuppressive therapy. Infections hold the first priority, and they can closely mimic many lupus complications, including acute confusional states, aseptic meningitis, lupus nephritis, lupus pneumonitis, arthritis, and GI vasculitis. Acute abdomen (AA) in patients with SLE presents a particularly challenging problem in management and requires the exclusion of common surgical diagnoses and abscesses in patients who are immunosuppressed.[30] Arterial or venous thromboses, without concomitant SLE activity (i.e., cerebrovascular accident [CVA] secondary to the antiphospholipid syndrome), require anticoagulation therapy, and thrombotic thrombocytopenia purpura (TTP) requires plasma exchanges. Seizures or acute confusional states may be the result of hypertension or metabolic or electrolyte abnormalities, whereas psychosis might result from the GC therapy itself. The probability of these alternative diagnoses substantially increases when SLE activity in other systems is low. In such cases of isolated seizures or psychosis, conservative management, which may include anticonvulsant and psychotropic agents, along with careful monitoring, is all that is usually required. Late complications of SLE, such as advanced atherosclerosis (coronary artery disease [CAD]), scarring nephritis (with high chronicity and low-activity indices on kidney biopsy), osteonecrosis, shrinking lung syndrome, and chronic dementia, represent damage and should not be treated with GCs.

When managing certain SLE complications with GCs, aiming for reasonable but not complete resolution of disease activity is often prudent, since often the latter translates into higher and more toxic GC doses. For example, asymptomatic hemolytic anemia or immune thrombocytopenic purpura (ITP) with a hematocrit of more than 30% and the number of platelets between 20,000 and 50,000 per microliter (and no other coagulopathy) do not, per se, warrant increases in GC therapy.[31] In more severe cases that invoke long-term high-dose GC therapy for adequate control, splenectomy or cytotoxic medicines or both should be considered.

Pulse-Glucocorticoid Therapy

Pulse-GC therapy was first used in patients with SLE to treat DPGN. Pulse-GC doses, usually administered as 0.5 to 1 g of MP IV daily for 3 days, is also effective for pneumonitis, serositis, vasculitis, and thrombocytopenia.[27,29] Many published series showed a role of pulse-GC therapy in those with moderate to severe NP-SLE, although an RCT that compared pulse-GC therapy with IVCY clearly demonstrated the superiority of the IVCY.[28] For very severe DPGN (or rapidly progressive glomerulonephritis [RPGN]), pulse-GC doses are generally believed to work faster than standard oral high-dose GC therapy and probably permit the use of both a moderate dose of GCs (0.5mg/kg/day) at therapy initiation and a faster tapering dose of GC.[25] However, two RCTs showed that pulse-GC therapy (monthly for 6 months or for at least 1 year, respectively) was not as effective as an IVCY-containing regimen (monthly for 6 months and then quarterly) for proliferative lupus nephritis.[25,32] The second study and especially another more recent National Institutes of Health (NIH) trial that included 5 years of protocol therapy with IVCY, pulse-GC therapy, or both, and an extended median follow-up of 124 months, have both suggested that the combination can lead to a better renal outcome than therapy with either agent alone.[26] It appears that concurrent use of both agents offers a therapeutic advantage for severe cases of SLE in general, possibly because of a synergistic effect of the two agents. Pulse-GC agents appear to have additional nongenomic effects that may allow for faster and more effective action than conventional high-dose GCs. On the other hand, IVCY has better long-term effects on the scarring consequences of inflammation and a very potent ability to suppress humoral immunity.[33] Advocates of pulse-GC

therapy argue that this therapy may have fewer adverse effects than oral GC alone, partly because it allows for a more rapid tapering of the latter. A more recent 12-month randomized prospective controlled study of patients with RA also reported that pulse-GC therapy did not cause bone loss, in contrast to oral GC, which did.[34] The lipodystrophy and diabetogenic effects of pulse-GC therapy may be less severe as well. However, complications such as GC-induced osteonecrosis, major infections, and mood disorders or psychosis can still occur.[25,35] Seizures, myalgias or arthralgias, dangerous cardiac arrhythmias attributed to potassium deficits, and anaphylaxis have been rarely reported, as well, with this therapy. Badsha and colleagues[36,37] recently published the results of a small retrospective study of 55 patients with very active SLE; this study examined the safety and effectiveness of two pulse-GC regimens for 6 months after therapy. Patients who received 500 mg MP IV daily for 3 days (low dose) had fewer serious infections than (7 out of 26 patients) and the same therapeutic response as those who received the high dose (1 g MP IV daily for 3 days; infections in 17 out of 29 patients). Most infections were due to gram-negative bacteria and occurred within 1 month of administration of pulse-GC agents. Hypoalbuminemia was a risk factor, and the authors of this text recommended low over high pulse-GC therapy, especially for those patients with low serum albumin.

Use of Depot Glucocorticoid Agents

Depot preparations of GCs are designed to have long-lasting effects (3 to 4 weeks) after a single IA or intramuscular (IM) injection. Examples include MP acetate and triamcinolone acetonide. IM injections are used for their potent systemic effects, and IA injections are used for their local action in the affected joint. However, even in the latter case, some systemic absorption and GC toxicity can occur. The use of IM depot GCs can be considered for the treatment of acute mild or moderate flares of the disease.[38]

Glucocorticoid Use During Pregnancy and Lactation

The use of GC therapy during pregnancy is indicated primarily to treat active SLE in the mother and perhaps for incomplete heart block of neonatal lupus in the fetus. Since only fluorinated GCs (e.g., DEX, betamethasone) are able to enter the fetal circulation in significant amounts (they are only partially metabolized by the placental 11β-HSD₂), nonfluorinated GCs (usually PDN) are used for the first indication and fluorinated GCs for the second. According to the PRIDE (PRegnancy and Infant DEvelopment) study, development of third-degree atrioventricular (AV) block in mothers with anti–Sjögren syndrome antigen A (anti-SSA/Ro) antibodies is irreversible.[39] However, DEX may be helpful in some cases of first- or second-degree AV blocks, although at the expense of fetal growth restriction and prematurity.[39]

In treatment of the mother for active SLE, the lowest effective GC dose should be used. Development of cleft lip or palate or both has been associated with the use of GCs early in pregnancy, and high doses should be avoided in the first trimester.[40] Other GC adverse effects on pregnancy outcomes include a high incidence of preterm deliveries, fetal growth restriction, and perhaps behavioral childhood problems.[39,41-43] Maternal complications may include gestational hypertension or diabetes mellitus, edema, and OP. Mothers treated with GCs during pregnancy may need stress GC doses in the peripartum period, especially when prolonged labor or delivery occurs or a caesarean section is required.[43] Hydroxychloroquine should be continued during pregnancy to prevent flares of the disease.[44] Additional immunosuppressive medications that may be safe during pregnancy, such as azathioprine, cyclosporin A, and intravenous immunoglobulin (IVIG), should be considered for moderate to severe SLE disease activity and might help decrease GC doses.[43] The use of PDN at levels below 20 mg per dose in mothers who are breastfeeding is probably safe, because less than 10% of the active drug enters the breast milk. However, waiting 4 hours after GC intake before breast-feeding, especially when higher doses are necessary, is prudent.[43]

Use of Glucocorticoids During Stress

Supplemental GC doses over and above the usual daily GC doses are not routinely recommended for the patient on long-term GC therapy who is about to have surgery.[45] However, clinicians often prefer to use a 24- to 48-hour course of hydrocortisone perioperatively for moderate and severe surgical stress in such patients with SLE.

ADVERSE EFFECTS OF GLUCOCORTICOIDS

Both clinicians and patients should be fully aware that the adverse effects of GC therapy are not uncommon and can be serious.[46,47] Of note, some adverse effects such as skeletal growth inhibition, HPA-axis suppression, GC-induced osteonecrosis, cataracts, acne, skin bruising, and weight gain occur even with low-dose GCs.[47] Other effects (e.g., infection, psychosis, myopathy, hyperlipidemia) usually require large doses of GCs before they occur. Co-morbid conditions and risk factors that may predispose a patient to more severe adverse effects (e.g., hyperlipidemia, hypertension, hyperglycemia–diabetes mellitus (DM), hypokalemia, OP, personal or family history of cataract or glaucoma, prior exposure to tuberculosis) should be identified before institution of GC therapy. Patients and their families should be educated to recognize and promptly report symptoms of such complications as infection (e.g., fever), diabetes, psychosis, and osteonecrosis (joint pain). In parallel, careful clinical and laboratory monitoring for the development of OP, DM, hyperlipidemia, hypertension, and glaucoma should not be neglected. Interventions known to prevent or ameliorate GC adverse effects should be undertaken. This is particularly true for GC-induced osteoporosis (GIOP), infection susceptibility, and atherosclerosis (see "Cardiovascular Effects" later in this chapter). Reversal of some adverse effects (e.g., HPA-axis suppression, Cushing syndrome, psychosis) can be achieved with the cessation of GC therapy or at least a modification into the safer, alternate-day or low-dose GC regimen. Unfortunately, some adverse effects, such as cataract formation, GC-induced osteonecrosis, osteoporotic fractures, growth retardation in children, and atherosclerotic vascular events, are irreversible. GC adverse effects, depending on the dose levels, are also shown in Table 48-2.

GC-induced lipodystrophy (with its characteristic "moon face" or "buffalo hump") is relatively common (in up to 63% of patients taking high-dose GCs) and was the most distressing GC adverse event in a recent cohort study.[46,48] It is associated with features of the metabolic syndrome and can occur in a period of less than 1 month during high-dose GC therapy. GC-induced Cushing syndrome differs from the native disease in that less androgen excess (i.e., androgens are suppressed by GC excess) and less hypertension are evident. On the other hand, GC-induced osteonecrosis, posterior subcapsular cataracts, glaucoma, pseudotumor cerebri, and pancreatitis are more commonly seen.

Recent studies have shown that damage in patients with SLE, as measured by the Systemic Lupus International Collaborating Clinics/ American College of Rheumatology (SLICC/ACR) Damage Index (SDI), is clearly associated with GC use.[49,50] One of these studies described an inception cohort of 73 patients, mostly Caucasian, and noted that although damage related to disease activity occurred early, GC-associated damage accumulated over time to constitute most of the damage at 15 years.[49] This finding was especially true for musculoskeletal damage (55% of patients at 15 years), mainly as the result of osteonecrosis and deforming arthritis, and for ocular damage (32%) caused by cataracts.

Bone Toxicity

GIOP and osteonecrosis are frequent adverse effects of GCs and substantially contribute to the morbidity associated with these agents. GC effects on bone include increased apoptosis of osteocytes and osteoblasts but increased survival of osteoclasts with a reduction in bone formation as the net result, which leads to a loss of bone

marrow density (BMD).[51] Osteocyte apoptosis may also account for the loss of bone strength and osteonecrosis.[51] GIOP predominantly affects cancellous bone and the axial skeleton and affects 30% to 50% of patients undergoing long-term GC therapy. During the first 3 to 6 months of GC therapy, a rapid bone loss (up to 12%) occurs, which slows down thereafter to approximately 3% annually.[51] Of note, however, fractures may occur without BMD loss. Risk factors for GIOP include advanced age, low body mass index (BMI) (less than 24), low BMD, underlying disease, prevalent fragility fractures, smoking, excessive alcohol intake, frequent falls, family history of hip fractures, and high current or cumulative GC doses or long GC therapy duration (or both). Patients with SLE may have additional risk factors for OP, including uncontrolled systemic inflammation; use of sunscreens, which results in inadequate vitamin D formation; inability to exercise as a result of musculoskeletal inflammation or fatigue; hormonal changes, including premature ovarian failure as a result of cyclophosphamide therapy; kidney damage; and medications known to induce OP (e.g., heparin, anticonvulsants, cyclosporine). Careful evaluation of patients with SLE before and after initiation of GC therapy should be performed to identify potentially modifiable OP risk factors and guide further management. Although the 2010 ACR recommendations for the prevention and treatment of GIOP propose the use of the Frax instrument to calculate fracture risk, some authors argue against it.[51,52] Nevertheless, the authors of this text believe that baseline evaluations should be performed for prevalent fragility fractures (including morphometric assessment for asymptomatic vertebral fractures), low BMD, low levels of serum 25-hydroxyvitamin D or secondary hyperparathyroidism, renal insufficiency, and other secondary causes of OP in all patients with SLE about to begin GC therapy or those already receiving it. General measures for OP prevention, including maintaining a well-balanced, low-salt diet, avoiding alcohol and smoking, and performing weight-bearing, muscle-strengthening exercises, should all be encouraged. As a first step to GIOP prevention, low vitamin D levels should be repleted and then calcium and vitamin D intake should be optimized with 1200 to 1500 mg of calcium daily (by diet and supplements) and 800 to 2000 IU of vitamin D daily, unless contraindications exist. The next step of GIOP prevention and therapy calls for pharmacologic intervention and consists of either bisphosphonates or teriparatide. Bisphosphonates are used first with either oral alendronate or risedronate; both decrease the risk of vertebral fractures as secondary outcomes in clinical trials.[53,54] Zoledronic acid has a stronger and more rapid effect in BMD and is preferred for patients with severe GIOP.[55] Because of the lack of adequate safety data and their ability to cross the placenta, these agents are not routinely recommended in young premenopausal female patients. However, physicians should not be discouraged from using them when clinically indicated in such patients.[52] Bisphosphonates should not be used in patients with glomerular filtration rate (GFR) of less than 35 mL per minute, and their discontinuation should be considered when GC doses have been substantially tapered with the stabilization of BMD. Teriparatide, a recombinant polypeptide composed of aminoacids 1-34 of the parathyroid hormone (PTH 1-34), appears to be more potent than bisphosphonates and is usually reserved for patients with the highest risk for GIOP-related fractures.[52,56] Denosumab, a monoclonal antibody that inhibits the receptor activator of nuclear factor–κB ligand (RANKL), is another promising agent that might prove useful in the treatment of GIOP and could be used in patients with renal insufficiency.[51]

GC-induced osteonecrosis occurs in approximately 5% to 40% of patients receiving GCs, and patients with SLE appear particularly vulnerable to this complication. Its presentation usually includes new hip, knee, or shoulder pain, and magnetic resonance imaging (MRI) is required for early diagnosis before the development of bone collapse. Asymptomatic osteonecrosis of the hip, often bilateral, may be detected by MRI as early as 3 months after the initiation of GC therapy, and pulse-GC therapy may augment risk.[57] Although the risk of GC-induced osteonecrosis increases with higher doses and prolonged courses of GCs, it may also occur with short-term exposures to high-dose GCs. Repair of lesions has been observed with stable disease, and aggravation with flares of lupus and increases in GC doses.[58] Hip collapse occurs in approximately 20% to 30% of patients.[57,58] Pediatric patients younger than 14 years of age appear to be protected.[59] Patients should be informed about this GC complication and perhaps be educated on how to recognize symptoms of osteonecrosis (e.g., groin pain with weight-bearing activities). When GC-induced hip osteonecrosis develops at an early stage, relief from weight-bearing activities is recommended and bisphosphonates may be helpful.[60] Advanced disease often requires joint replacement therapy. The roles of statins and warfarin in GC-induced osteonecrosis prevention remain debatable.

Cardiovascular Effects

Hypertension and edema are not uncommon with high-dose GCs, especially in patients with additional risk factors such as lupus nephritis, renal insufficiency, and left ventricular systolic or diastolic dysfunction. Such patients may also develop acute pulmonary edema. Edema may be more likely to occur with GCs of relatively high MC activity such as hydrocortisone and PDN (see Table 48-1). Accelerated atherosclerosis with consequent cardiovascular events is a relatively common complication of patients with SLE (6% to 8%).[61] The prevalence of subclinical atherosclerosis is even higher (35% to 40%).[61,62] In addition to traditional cardiovascular risk factors, SLE-specific variables are also important, including disease activity and damage, proinflammatory high-density lipoproteins (HDLs), as well as GCs.[50,61,63] GC effects are either direct on the cardiovascular system or indirect via metabolic effects on blood lipid and glucose levels and insulin resistance, among others.[48,61,63,64] Finally, GCs may also have prothrombotic effects.[64,65] The clinical significance of this in SLE is not certain, but it might be relevant when treating patients at high risk for thrombosis, such as probable or definite catastrophic antiphospholipid syndrome.[66] In the latter cases, GCs might best be started after the initiation of anticoagulation therapy. In conclusion, both SLE activity and GCs appear to contribute to atherosclerosis in SLE. Therefore management of active SLE should include early aggressive therapy, including the proper use of GCs and other immunosuppressive agents, as well as the timely tapering of GCs as soon as sufficient disease control is achieved. Moreover, other risk factors should be addressed, such as lipid levels, blood pressure, diabetes, smoking, obesity, and lack of exercise. Therapy with hydroxychloroquine and aspirin (81 mg/day) should be encouraged in the absence of contraindications to their use.[61]

Infections

GCs predispose patients to infection and, at the same time, may mask clinical clues of infection as a result of their immunosuppressive and antiinflammatory effects. Infection rates in GC-exposed versus non–GC-exposed patients with RA are higher even with PDN doses less than 5 mg/day and progressively increase with higher GC doses.[67,68] GCs increase the incidence of all types of infections, including bacterial, viral, and invasive fungal infections, as well as increase risk of reactivation of latent tuberculosis and histoplasmosis.[69-72] Of note, active SLE, by itself, increases the risk of bacterial and, more rarely, opportunistic infections, probably as a result of several immune system and genetic perturbations.[73] Therapy with high-dose GCs further augments this susceptibility as well as mortality due to sepsis.[19,73] To reduce the risk of infection in patients with SLE, GC exposure should be minimized to the lowest exposure required to control disease activity. Other protective measures include the following:

a. Prophylaxis for *Pneumocystis* pneumonia in patients receiving high-dose GCs
b. Screening for latent tuberculosis to identify candidates for prophylactic therapy
c. Vaccinations for influenza and pneumococcus (killed vaccines), especially before the initiation of high immunosuppressive

therapy[74] (In contrast, vaccinations with live attenuated viruses, such as in oral poliomyelitis, varicella, and measles-mumps, and rubella [MMR], should be avoided in patients who are immunosuppressed; they may lead to active infection.)

Neuropsychiatric Adverse Effects

Mood changes, including depression or euphoria and insomnia, are relatively common with high-dose GCs and are of particular concern to patients.[46] Severe disease with mania, depression, and aggressiveness was observed in 6 out of 88 patients on high-dose GC therapy in one study.[46] When manic behavior, psychosis, or seizures supervene during therapy, they require differentiation from primary NP-SLE. The distinction can be difficult, but the temporal relationship to increases in GC dosing, along with the lack of focal neurologic signs or cerebrospinal fluid (CSF) abnormalities, suggests the correct diagnosis. Benign intracranial hypertension (pseudotumor cerebri) rarely occurs.

Other Adverse Effects

GC-associated myopathy is not uncommon with high-dose GCs and is usually mild. It improves with physical therapy and the tapering of GC doses. Effects of GCs on protein catabolism, fibroblast function, and collagen metabolism are probably responsible for the suppression of wound healing processes and for skin atrophy and purpura. Of note, long-term GC therapy in patients with SLE has been associated with tendon ruptures. In addition, posterior subcapsular cataract formation is not uncommon with systemic, topical, or inhaled GC use, and children may be more susceptible to this complication. Glaucoma, in contrast to cataracts, often resolves with the discontinuation of GCs. Regular ophthalmologic follow-up examinations for both potential adverse effects are required. No association probably exists between GC use and the development of peptic ulcer disease (PUD) or its complications. However, concomitant use of NSAIDs confers a higher risk of PUD; the same correlation is probably true when other co-morbid conditions (e.g., congestive heart failure, renal failure, old age) are present. A gastroprotective medication is required in such cases. The GC-withdrawal syndrome may occur in patients on long-term GC therapy after attempts to taper GC below physiologic levels (5 to 7.5 mg of PDN) and consist of anorexia, nausea, weight loss, arthralgias, myalgias, lethargy, weakness, and mild orthostatic hypotension and tachycardia. Regarding the management of potential complications of GC therapy, the European League Against Rheumatism (EULAR) has recently published evidence-based recommendations.[75] EULAR recommendations have also been published regarding the monitoring of patients with SLE, including those receiving immunosuppressive medications.[74]

References

1. Rauchhaus U, Schwaiger FW, Panzner S: Separating therapeutic efficacy from glucocorticoid side-effects in rodent arthritis using novel, liposomal delivery of dexamethasone phosphate: long-term suppression of arthritis facilitates interval treatment. *Arthritis Res Ther* 11(6):R190, 2009.
2. Anderson R, Franch A, Castell M, et al: Liposomal encapsulation enhances and prolongs the anti-inflammatory effects of water-soluble dexamethasone phosphate in experimental adjuvant arthritis. *Arthritis Res Ther* 12(4):R147, 2010.
3. Buttgereit F, Doering G, Schaeffler A, et al: Targeting pathophysiological rhythms: prednisone chronotherapy shows sustained efficacy in rheumatoid arthritis. *Ann Rheum Dis* 69(7):1275–1280, 2010.
4. Kvien TK, Fjeld E, Slatkowsky-Christensen B, et al: Efficacy and safety of a novel synergistic drug candidate, CRx-102, in hand osteoarthritis. *Ann Rheum Dis* 67(7):942–948, 2008.
5. Rider CF, King EM, Holden NS, et al: Inflammatory stimuli inhibit glucocorticoid-dependent transactivation in human pulmonary epithelial cells: rescue by long-acting beta2-adrenoceptor agonists. *J Pharmacol Exp Ther* 338(3):860–869, 2011.
6. Newton RR, Leigh R, Giembycz MA: Pharmacological strategies for improving the efficacy and therapeutic ratio of glucocorticoids in inflammatory lung diseases. *Pharmacol Ther* 125(2):286–327, 2010.

7. Rhen T, Cidlowski JA: Antiinflammatory action of glucocorticoids—new mechanisms for old drugs. *N Engl J Med* 353(16):1711–1723, 2005.

8. Perretti M, D'Acquisto F: Annexin A1 and glucocorticoids as effectors of the resolution of inflammation. *Nat Rev Immunol* 9(1):62–70, 2009.

9. Baschant U, Tuckermann J: The role of the glucocorticoid receptor in inflammation and immunity. *J Steroid Biochem Mol Biol* 120(2-3):69–75, 2010.

10. Löwenberg M, Verhaar AP, Bilderbeek J, et al: Glucocorticoids cause rapid dissociation of a T-cell-receptor-associated protein complex containing LCK and FYN. *EMBO Rep* 7(10):1023–1029, 2006.

11. Zhou J, Li M, Sheng CQ, et al: A novel strategy for development of glucocorticoids through non-genomic mechanism. *Cell Mol Life Sci* 68(8):1405–1414, 2011.

12. Song IH, Buttgereit F: Non-genomic glucocorticoid effects to provide the basis for new drug developments. *Mol Cell Endocrinol* 246(1-2):142–146, 2006.

13. Buttgereit F, Burmester GR, Straub RH, et al: Exogenous and endogenous glucocorticoids in rheumatic diseases. *Arthritis Rheum* 63(1):1–9, 2011.

14. Lawrence T, Gilroy DW: Chronic inflammation: a failure of resolution? *Int J Exp Pathol* 88(2):85–94, 2007.

15. Perretti M, Ahluwalia A: The microcirculation and inflammation: site of action for glucocorticoids. *Microcirculation* 7(3):147–161, 2000.

16. Barnes PJ: Glucocorticosteroids: current and future directions. *Br J Pharmacol* 163(1):29–43, 2011.

17. Guiducci C, Gong M, Xu Z, et al: TLR recognition of self nucleic acids hampers glucocorticoid activity in lupus. *Nature* 465(7300):937–941, 2010.

18. Tsujimura S, Saito K, Nakayamada S, et al: Clinical relevance of the expression of P-glycoprotein on peripheral blood lymphocytes to steroid resistance in patients with systemic lupus erythematosus. *Arthritis Rheum* 52(6):1676–1683, 2005.

19. Sergent JS, Lockshin MD, Klempner MS, et al: Central nervous system disease in systemic lupus erythematosus. Therapy and prognosis. *Am J Med* 58(5):644–654, 1975.

20. Buttgereit F, da Silva JA, Boers M, et al: Standardised nomenclature for glucocorticoid dosages and glucocorticoid treatment regimens: current questions and tentative answers in rheumatology. *Ann Rheum Dis* 61(8):718–722, 2002.

21. Boumpas DT, Chrousos GP, Wilder RL, et al: Glucocorticoid therapy for immune-mediated diseases: basic and clinical correlates. *Ann Intern Med* 119(12):1198–1208, 1993.

22. Ad Hoc Working Group on Steroid-Sparing Criteria in Lupus: Criteria for steroid-sparing ability of interventions in systemic lupus erythematosus: report of a consensus meeting. *Arthritis Rheum* 50(11):3427–3431, 2004.

23. Bootsma H, Spronk P, Derksen R, et al: Prevention of relapses in systemic lupus erythematosus. *Lancet* 345(8965):1595–1599, 1995.

24. Tseng CE, Buyon JP, Kim M, et al: The effect of moderate-dose corticosteroids in preventing severe flares in patients with serologically active, but clinically stable, systemic lupus erythematosus: findings of a prospective, randomized, double-blind, placebo-controlled trial. *Arthritis Rheum* 54(11):3623–3632, 2006.

25. Gourley MF, Austin HA, 3rd, Scott D, et al: Methylprednisolone and cyclophosphamide, alone or in combination, in patients with lupus nephritis. A randomized, controlled trial. *Ann Intern Med* 125(7):549–557, 1996.

26. Illei GG, Austin HA, Crane M, et al: Combination therapy with pulse cyclophosphamide plus pulse methylprednisolone improves long-term renal outcome without adding toxicity in patients with lupus nephritis. *Ann Intern Med* 135(4):248–257, 2001.

27. Parker BJ, Bruce LN: High dose methylprednisolone therapy for the treatment of severe systemic lupus erythematosus. *Lupus* 16(6):387–393, 2007.

28. Barile-Fabris L, Ariza-Andraca R, Olguín-Ortega L, et al: Controlled clinical trial of IV cyclophosphamide versus IV methylprednisolone in severe neurological manifestations in systemic lupus erythematosus. *Ann Rheum Dis* 64(4):620–625, 2005.

29. Chatham WW, Kimberly RP: Treatment of lupus with corticosteroids. *Lupus* 10(3):140–147, 2001.

30. Medina F, Ayala A, Jara LJ, et al: Acute abdomen in systemic lupus erythematosus: the importance of early laparotomy. *Am J Med* 103(2):100–105, 1997.

31. Fessler BJ, Boumpas DT: Severe major organ involvement in systemic lupus erythematosus. Diagnosis and management. *Rheum Dis Clin North Am* 21(1):81–98, 1995.

32. Boumpas DT, Austin HA, 3rd, Vaughn EM, et al: Controlled trial of pulse methylprednisolone versus two regimens of pulse cyclophosphamide in severe lupus nephritis. *Lancet* 340(8822):741–745, 1992.

33. Fox DA, McCune WJ: Immunosuppressive drug therapy of systemic lupus erythematosus. *Rheum Dis Clin North Am* 20(1):265–299, 1994.

34. Frediani B, Falsetti P, Bisogno S, et al: Effects of high dose methylprednisolone pulse therapy on bone mass and biochemical markers of bone metabolism in patients with active rheumatoid arthritis: a 12-month randomized prospective controlled study. *J Rheumatol* 31(6):1083–1087, 2004.

35. Wada K, Yamada N, Suzuki H, et al: Recurrent cases of corticosteroid-induced mood disorder: clinical characteristics and treatment. *J Clin Psychiatry* 61(4):261–267, 2000.

36. Badsha H, Kong KO, Lian TY, et al: Low-dose pulse methylprednisolone for systemic lupus erythematosus flares is efficacious and has a decreased risk of infectious complications. *Lupus* 11(8):508–513, 2002.

37. Badsha H, Edwards CJ: Intravenous pulses of methylprednisolone for systemic lupus erythematosus. *Semin Arthritis Rheum* 32(6):370–377, 2003.

38. Danowski A, Magder L, Petri M: Flares in Lupus: Outcome Assessment Trial (FLOAT), a comparison between oral methylprednisolone and intramuscular triamcinolone. *J Rheumatol* 33(1):57–60, 2006.

39. Friedman DM, Kim MY, Copel JA, et al: Prospective evaluation of fetuses with autoimmune-associated congenital heart block followed in the PR Interval and Dexamethasone Evaluation (PRIDE) Study. *Am J Cardiol* 103(8):1102–1106, 2009.

40. Carmichael SL, Shaw GM, Ma C, et al: Maternal corticosteroid use and orofacial clefts. *Am J Obstet Gynecol* 197(6):585e1–e7, 2007.

41. Peltoniemi OM, Kari MA, Hallman M: Repeated antenatal corticosteroid treatment: a systematic review and meta-analysis. *Acta Obstet Gynecol Scand* 90(7):719–727, 2011.

42. French NP, Hagan R, Evans SF, et al: Repeated antenatal corticosteroids: effects on cerebral palsy and childhood behavior. *Am J Obstet Gynecol* 190(3):588–595, 2004.

43. Temprano KK, Bandlamudi R, Moore TL: Antirheumatic drugs in pregnancy and lactation. *Semin Arthritis Rheum* 35(2):112–121, 2005.

44. Clowse ME, Magder L, Witter F, et al: Hydroxychloroquine in lupus pregnancy. *Arthritis Rheum* 54(11):3640–3647, 2006.

45. Marik PE, Varon J: Requirement of perioperative stress doses of corticosteroids: a systematic review of the literature. *Arch Surg* 143(12):1222–1226, 2008.

46. Fardet L, Flahault A, Kettaneh A, et al: Corticosteroid-induced clinical adverse events: frequency, risk factors and patient's opinion. *Br J Dermatol* 157(1):142–148, 2007.

47. McDonough AK, Curtis JR, Saag KG: The epidemiology of glucocorticoid-associated adverse events. *Curr Opin Rheumatol* 20(2):131–137, 2008.

48. Fardet L, Cabane J, Kettaneh A, et al: Corticosteroid-induced lipodystrophy is associated with features of the metabolic syndrome. *Rheumatology* 46(7):1102–1106, 2007.

49. Gladman DD, Urowitz MB, Rahman P, et al: Accrual of organ damage over time in patients with systemic lupus erythematosus. *J Rheumatol* 30(9):1955–1959, 2003.

50. Zonana-Nacach A, Barr SG, Magder LS, et al: Damage in systemic lupus erythematosus and its association with corticosteroids. *Arthritis Rheum* 43(8):1801–1808, 2000.

51. Weinstein RS: Clinical practice. Glucocorticoid-induced bone disease. *N Engl J Med* 365(1):62–70, 2011.

52. Grossman JM, Gordon R, Ranganath VK, et al: American College of Rheumatology 2010 recommendations for the prevention and treatment of glucocorticoid-induced osteoporosis. *Arthritis Care Res* 62(11):1515–1526, 2010.

53. Adachi JD, Saag KG, Delmas PD, et al: Two-year effects of alendronate on bone mineral density and vertebral fracture in patients receiving glucocorticoids: a randomized, double-blind, placebo-controlled extension trial. *Arthritis Rheum* 44(1):202–211, 2001.

54. Reid DM, et al: Efficacy and safety of daily risedronate in the treatment of corticosteroid-induced osteoporosis in men and women: a randomized trial. European Corticosteroid-Induced Osteoporosis Treatment Study. Journal of bone and mineral research. *J Bone Miner Res* 15(6):1006–1013, 2000.

55. Reid DM, Devogelaer JP, Saag K, et al: Zoledronic acid and risedronate in the prevention and treatment of glucocorticoid-induced osteoporosis (HORIZON): a multicentre, double-blind, double-dummy, randomised controlled trial. *Lancet* 373(9671):1253–1263, 2009.

56. Saag KG, Shane E, Boonen S, et al: Teriparatide or alendronate in glucocorticoid-induced osteoporosis. *N Engl J Med* 357(20):2028–2039, 2007.

57. Nagasawa K, Tada Y, Koarada S, et al: Very early development of steroid-associated osteonecrosis of femoral head in systemic lupus erythematosus: prospective study by MRI. *Lupus* 14(5):385–390, 2005.

58. Nakamura J, Harada Y, Oinuma K, et al: Spontaneous repair of asymptomatic osteonecrosis associated with corticosteroid therapy in systemic lupus erythematosus: 10-year minimum follow-up with MRI. *Lupus* 19(11):1307–1314, 2010.

59. Nakamura J, Saisu T, Yamashita K, et al: Age at time of corticosteroid administration is a risk factor for osteonecrosis in pediatric patients with systemic lupus erythematosus: a prospective magnetic resonance imaging study. *Arthritis Rheum* 62(2):609–615, 2010.

60. Agarwala S, Shah S, Joshi VR: The use of alendronate in the treatment of avascular necrosis of the femoral head: follow-up to eight years. *J Bone Joint Surg Br* 91(8):1013–1018, 2009.

61. Skamra C, Ramsey-Goldman R: Management of cardiovascular complications in systemic lupus erythematosus. *Int J Clin Rheumtol* 5(1):75–100, 2010.

62. Roman MJ, Shanker BA, Davis A, et al: Prevalence and correlates of accelerated atherosclerosis in systemic lupus erythematosus. *N Engl J Med* 349(25):2399–2406, 2003.

63. Karp I, Abrahamowicz M, Fortin PR, et al: Recent corticosteroid use and recent disease activity: independent determinants of coronary heart disease risk factors in systemic lupus erythematosus? *Arthritis Rheum* 59(2):169–175, 2008.

64. Hadoke PW, Iqbal J, Walker BR: Therapeutic manipulation of glucocorticoid metabolism in cardiovascular disease. *Br J Pharmacol* 156(5):689–712, 2009.

65. Calvo-Alén J, Toloza SM, Fernández M, et al: Systemic lupus erythematosus in a multiethnic US cohort (LUMINA). XXV. Smoking, older age, disease activity, lupus anticoagulant, and glucocorticoid dose as risk factors for the occurrence of venous thrombosis in lupus patients. *Arthritis Rheum* 52(7):2060–2068, 2005.

66. Cherian J, Duculan R, Amigues I, et al: A 26-year-old white man with a systemic lupus erythematosus flare and acute multiorgan ischemia: vasculitis or thrombosis? *Arthritis Care Res* 63(5):766–774, 2011.

67. Smitten AL, Choi HK, Hochberg MC, et al: The risk of hospitalized infection in patients with rheumatoid arthritis. *J Rheumatol* 35(3):387–393, 2008.

68. Dixon WG, Kezouh A, Bernatsky S, et al: The influence of systemic glucocorticoid therapy upon the risk of non-serious infection in older patients with rheumatoid arthritis: a nested case-control study. *Ann Rheum Dis* 70(6):956–960, 2011.

69. Strangfeld A, Listing J, Herzer P, et al: Risk of herpes zoster in patients with rheumatoid arthritis treated with anti-TNF-alpha agents. *JAMA* 301(7):737–744, 2009.

70. Lionakis MS, Kontoyiannis DP: Glucocorticoids and invasive fungal infections. *Lancet* 362(9398):1828–1838, 2003.

71. Jick SS, Lieberman ES, Rahman MU, et al: Glucocorticoid use, other associated factors, and the risk of tuberculosis. *Arthritis Rheum* 55(1):19–26, 2006.

72. Weng CT, Lee NY, Liu MF, et al: A retrospective study of catastrophic invasive fungal infections in patients with systemic lupus erythematosus from southern Taiwan. *Lupus* 19(10):1204–1209, 2010.

73. Zandman-Goddard G, Shoenfeld Y. Infections and SLE. *Autoimmunity* 38(7):473–485, 2005.

74. Mosca M, Tani C, Aringer M, et al: European League Against Rheumatism recommendations for monitoring patients with systemic lupus erythematosus in clinical practice and in observational studies. *Ann Rheum Dis* 69(7):1269–1274, 2010.

75. Hoes JN, Jacobs JW, Boers M, et al: EULAR evidence-based recommendations on the management of systemic glucocorticoid therapy in rheumatic diseases. *Ann Rheum Dis* 66(12):1560–1567, 2007.

76. Coutinho AE, Chapman KE: The anti-inflammatory and immunosuppressive effects of glucocorticoids, recent developments and mechanistic insights. *Mol Cell Endocrinol* 335(1):2–13, 2011.

77. Barnes PJ, Adcock IM: Glucocorticoid resistance in inflammatory diseases. *Lancet* 373(9678):1905–1917, 2009.

78. Heasman SJ, Giles KM, Ward C, et al: Glucocorticoid-mediated regulation of granulocyte apoptosis and macrophage phagocytosis of apoptotic cells: implications for the resolution of inflammation. *J Endocrinol* 178(1):29–36, 2003.

79. Abramson SB, Dobro J, Eberle MA, et al: Acute reversible hypoxemia in systemic lupus erythematosus. *Ann Intern Med* 114(11):941–947, 1991.

80. Flammer JR, Dobrovolna J, Kennedy MA, et al: The type I interferon signaling pathway is a target for glucocorticoid inhibition. *Mol Cell Biol* 30(19):4564–4574, 2010.

81. Vallelian F, Schaer CA, Kaempfer T, et al: Glucocorticoid treatment skews human monocyte differentiation into a hemoglobin-clearance phenotype with enhanced heme-iron recycling and antioxidant capacity. *Blood* 116(24):5347–5356, 2010.

82. Ehrchen J, Steinmöller L, Barczyk K, et al: Glucocorticoids induce differentiation of a specifically activated, anti-inflammatory subtype of human monocytes. *Blood* 109(3):1265–1274, 2007.

83. McColl A, Bournazos S, Franz S, et al: Glucocorticoids induce protein S-dependent phagocytosis of apoptotic neutrophils by human macrophages. *J Immunol* 183(3):2167–2175, 2009.

84. Barczyk K, Ehrchen J, Tenbrock K, et al: Glucocorticoids promote survival of anti-inflammatory macrophages via stimulation of adenosine receptor A3. *Blood* 116(3):446–455, 2010.

85. Abe M, Thomson AW: Dexamethasone preferentially suppresses plasmacytoid dendritic cell differentiation and enhances their apoptotic death. *Clin Immunol* 118(2-3):300–306, 2006.

86. Bennett L, Palucka AK, Arce E, et al: Interferon and granulopoiesis signatures in systemic lupus erythematosus blood. *J Exp Med* 197(6):711–723, 2003.

87. Kirou KA, Lee C, George S, et al: Activation of the interferon-alpha pathway identifies a subgroup of systemic lupus erythematosus patients with distinct serologic features and active disease. *Arthritis Rheum* 52(5):1491–1503, 2005.

88. Wüst S, van den Brandt J, Tischner D, et al: Peripheral T cells are the therapeutic targets of glucocorticoids in experimental autoimmune encephalomyelitis. *J Immunol* 180(12):8434–8443, 2008.

89. Harr MW, Rong Y, Bootman MD, et al: Glucocorticoid-mediated inhibition of Lck modulates the pattern of T cell receptor-induced calcium signals by down-regulating inositol 1,4,5-trisphosphate receptors. *J Biol Chem* 284(46):31860–31871, 2009.

90. Zhang S, Shen Z, Hu G, et al: Effects of endogenous glucocorticoids on allergic inflammation and T(H)1/T(H)2 balance in airway allergic disease. *Ann Allergy Asthma Immunol* 103(6):525–534, 2009.

91. Liberman AC, Druker J, Refojo D, et al: Glucocorticoids inhibit GATA-3 phosphorylation and activity in T cells. *FASEB J* 23(5):1558–1571, 2009.

92. Deng J, Younge BR, Olshen RA, et al: Th17 and Th1 T-cell responses in giant cell arteritis. *Circulation* 121(7):906–915, 2010.

93. Suárez A, López P, Gómez, J, et al: Enrichment of CD4+ CD25 high T cell population in patients with systemic lupus erythematosus treated with glucocorticoids. *Ann Rheum Dis* 65(11):1512–1517, 2006.

94. Zhu XJ, Shi Y, Sun JZ, et al: High-dose dexamethasone inhibits BAFF expression in patients with immune thrombocytopenia. *J Clin Immunol* 29(5):603–610, 2009.

95. Surjit M, Ganti KP, Mukherji A, et al: Widespread negative response elements mediate direct repression by agonist-liganded glucocorticoid receptor. *Cell* 145(2):224–241, 2011.

Chapter 49

Antimalarial Medications

J. Antonio Aviña-Zubieta and John M. Esdaile

INTRODUCTION

Paine first used quinine for the treatment of discoid lupus erythematosus.[1] It was not, however, until 1951, when Page used quinacrine (Mepacrine) in discoid lupus erythematosus (DLE), rheumatoid arthritis, and systemic lupus erythematosus (SLE), that antimalarial (AM) medications became widely used. The AM compounds hydroxychloroquine (HCQ) and chloroquine (CQ) and, to a lesser extent, quinacrine (also called Atabrine in the United States) remain in use.

PHARMACOKINETICS OF ANTIMALARIAL MEDICATIONS

Hydroxychloroquine

HCQ is a 4-aminoquinoline. Between 75% and 100% is absorbed, and 50% is eventually bound to serum proteins. Excretion occurs in a rapid phase with a half-life of 3 days and a slower phase with a half-life of 40 to 50 days.[2] Approximately 45% is excreted by the kidney, 3% by the skin, and 20% by the bowel. Renal excretion of HCQ can be enhanced by acidification of the urine. Steady-state plasma levels are reached after 6 months of therapy.

High concentrations are stored in the adrenal and pituitary glands, pigmented tissues, liver, spleen, and leukocytes. Epidermal levels are 110 to 200 times the plasma concentrations. Although HCQ and CQ are concentrated in cells throughout the body, the important antirheumatic effect is the result of drug accumulation within the cells of the immune system.

Chloroquine

CQ, another 4-aminoquinoline, is rapidly absorbed after oral administration. Peak plasma levels are reached within 4 to 8 hours. The plasma half-life of CQ ranges from 3.5 to 12 days with plateau plasma levels reached at 4 to 6 weeks. This plateau correlates with CQ's onset of antirheumatic action. Depending of the acidity of the urine, approximately 50% is renally excreted. CQ is detectable in the urine, red blood cells, and plasma up to 5 years after the discontinuation of the medication.

CQ is largely bound by circulating plasma proteins and is eventually deposited into metabolically active tissues. Tissue levels have been reported to be higher for CQ than they are for HCQ, a manifestation that is thought to be responsible for the differences in toxicity between the two compounds.

Quinacrine

Quinacrine, which does not cross-react with HCQ and CQ, is rapidly absorbed after oral administration. Peak plasma levels occur at 8 to 12 hours, and steady-state concentrations happen at 4 weeks.[3]

Approximately 80% to 90% is bound to albumin. Skin deposits are often visible as yellow or blue-black pigmentation, although the latter rarely occurs. Quinacrine also crosses the placenta.

MECHANISMS OF ACTION

In 1993, Fox[2] proposed that AM medications modulate the immune system through their known ability to influence pH in intracytoplasmic vesicles. By increasing the pH, AM drugs inhibit the processing and assembly of self-peptides into complexes with major histocompatibility complex (MHC) class II proteins. This results in decreased stimulation of CD+ T cells that are reactive to autoantigens, decreased release of proinflammatory cytokines and, ultimately, a diminution of autoimmunity (Box 49-1) (Figure 49-1).

A crucial step in the regulation of the immune response is the *processing* of antigens by antigen-presenting cells (APCs) and the *presentation* of antigen-MHC protein complexes to CD4+ T cells. The synthesis of MHC and their assembly into a complex with the antigenic peptide is a pH-sensitive process. Once the antigen is internalized by APCs, it is digested into peptides by proteases, which allows interaction with MHC class II molecules in the cytoplasm of the APC in an acidic vacuole (loading compartment). In this acidic environment, the digested peptides compete with the invariant (I_i) chains (α, and β) to form the complex of peptide-MCH that will be transported to the surface of the cell membrane to interact with CD+ T cells.

AM medications are weak bases that can pass freely across cell membranes. Once inside the acidic vacuole, the AM drug becomes protonated, and the now charged drug (hydroxychloroquine-H) is unable to pass out of the vesicle. The continuous accumulation of hydrogen ions by HCQ leads to a subtle elevation of pH within the acidic vacuole, which decreases the affinity of α-I_i and β-I_i, allowing peptides to displace the I_i and form the $\alpha\beta$-peptide complex (Figure 49-1). When the pH is even slightly elevated, the lower affinity peptide might not be able to displace the I_i. Cryptic autoantigens are characterized by their low affinity for self-MHC. Elevation of the pH in the loading compartment of the endoplasmic reticulum might selectively decrease the loading of autoantigen self-peptides, while leaving the response to exogenous peptides intact. Thus no increase in infections would occur with AM medications.

Increased levels of proinflammatory cytokines are believed to play a role in the pathogenesis of SLE, and AM therapy may influence their release from inflammatory cells.[4,5] For example, Wozniacka and others[4] demonstrated that a significant reduction in the elevated levels of serum interleukin (IL)-1β, IL-6, IL-18, and tumor necrosis factor–alpha (TNF-α) occurred after 3 months of treatment with CQ. IL-18, known as interferon gamma (IFN-γ)-inducing factor, is produced mainly by macrophages during innate immune responses and thus influences adaptive immunity. Contribution of IFN-γ to the pathogenesis of SLE has been demonstrated in animal models and is considered a major effector molecule in SLE.[6] In a separate study, Wozniacka and associates[5] also demonstrated the local inhibitory effect of CQ in the expression of proinflammatory cytokines in the irradiated skin of patients with SLE,[5] and the reduction in human leukocyte antigen (HLA)–DR+ and CD1a+ cell numbers in both unirradiated and ultraviolet-irradiated skin.[7] The latter suggests that CQ reduces the number of APCs in the skin of patients with SLE, thereby explaining the benefits for skin lupus.

Over the last several years, a paradigm shift in understanding the importance of the innate immune system in SLE has been driven by the recognition of a new class of pattern recognition receptors, collectively known as Toll-like receptors (TLRs).[8] Rönnblom and Alm[9] were the first to demonstrate that immune complexes containing DNA or RNA (present in SLE sera) could trigger the production of high levels of IFN-α by plasmacytoid dendritic cells via the Fc-gamma receptor, which is one of the most important receptors for inducing phagocytosis of antibody-coated microbes. Since other kinds of immune complexes did not elicit this kind of IFN-α response, the findings indicated a unique function of nucleic acids in the activation of the innate immune system. Recent evidence suggests that the ability of immune complexes to activate plasmacytoid dendritic cells

---

Box 49-1 Mechanisms of Action of Antimalarial Medications

Immunologic Actions
Inhibit antigen processing and presentation by raising intracytoplasmic pH.
Decrease levels of proinflammatory cytokines in serum and skin (IL-1β, IL-6, IL-18, and TNF-α).
Block of activation of innate and adaptive immunity process mediated by Toll-like receptors.

Antithrombotic Effects
Inhibit platelet aggregation and adhesion.
Inhibit formation of antiphospholipid antibody–β2-glycoprotein 1 complexes.
Prevent antiphospholipid antibody binding of annexin-5.

Cardiovascular Effects
Increase levels of HDL when used alone or in combination with glucocorticoids.
Lower levels of cholesterol and LDL.
Increase large-artery elasticity.
Reduce systemic vascular resistance.
Reduce the risk of diabetes mellitus.

Antimicrobial Effects
Exhibit in vitro activity against bacteria, fungi, and viruses.

Antiproliferative Effects
Promote chemosensitization.
Inhibit cell growth or cell death or both.
Prevent mutations in cells with high mitotic rates.

HDL, high-density lipoproteins; IL, interleukin; LDL, low-density lipoproteins; TNF, tumor necrosis factor.

---

depends on Fc-gamma receptor–mediated delivery to a cellular compartment containing TLR9 or TLR7.[10] The concentration of CQ that is necessary to block TLR9 is in the same range as the concentration of CQ (greater than 1 μg/mL) associated with decreased frequency of SLE flare in vivo.[11,12] Furthermore, in a retrospective study of 130 U.S. military personnel who eventually developed SLE and whose clinical variables in the period before diagnosis were available, James and colleagues[13] found that early HCQ use is associated with the delayed onset of SLE.

TLRs recognize specific patterns of microbial components and regulate the activation of both innate and adaptive immunity. TLR3, TLR7, TLR8, and TLR9 specifically recognize nucleic acid motifs and are also distinct from other TLRs in that they are expressed not on the plasma membrane but intracellularly. This could be of particular relevance in SLE, considering the pathogenic role of anti–double stranded DNA (anti-dsDNA) antibodies. Moreover, signal transduction through these receptors depends on the internalization of the ligand to an acidic intracellular compartment. As a result, agents that interfere with endosome or lysosome acidification, such as AM medications, can block the activation process.[14]

EFFICACY OF ANTIMALARIAL MEDICATIONS
Although AM drugs have been used empirically in SLE since the 1950s, evidence from controlled studies supporting their use is more recent. A systematic review on the clinical efficacy and safety of AM therapy[15] noted that AM medications decreased disease activity in all studies, often by 50%.

Controlled Studies Assessing Efficacy
In 1975, Rudnicki, Gresham, and Rothfield[16] reported the first controlled study of AM medications in SLE. The authors retrospectively studied 43 patients who developed a macular lesion resulting in the discontinuation of AM agents. Every year on AM drugs was matched in consecutive order to a year off AM medications. In total, 76 years could be matched (76 years on AM drugs and 76 years off). Of the 43 patients, 24 (56%) who had received high-dose CQ (500 mg/day) had a significantly lower frequency of constitutional symptoms (e.g., fatigue, weight loss, fever) and skin manifestations during the years they received CQ than the years they did not (Table 49-1). The generalizability of these results is limited because the doses used today are lower. However, because SLE disease activity tends to decrease over time and the years on AM medications always preceded the years off, this pattern biased against demonstrating the efficacy that was identified.

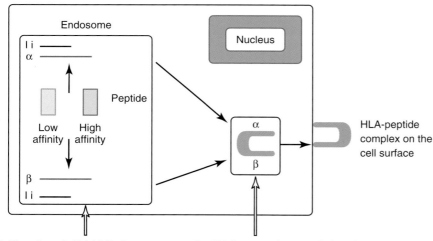

1. Elevation of pH inhibits the dissociation of α-li and β-li.

2. pH influences the association of peptide with αβ li chains. Elevation in pH allows only high-affinity peptides to form trimolecular complex.

FIGURE 49-1 Proposed mechanism of action of antimalarial medications. Because antimalarial drugs elevate the intracytoplasmic pH, the processing of certain self-peptides with low affinity for major histocompatibility complex proteins is diminished, and a lower concentration of this complex will be presented on the cell membrane of the macrophage. (*Adapted with permission from Fox RI: Mechanism of action of hydroxychloroquine as an antirheumatic drug. Semin Arthritis Rheum 23(2 Suppl 1):82–91, 1993.*)

TABLE 49-1 Observational and Controlled Trials Assessing the Efficacy of Antimalarial Medications on Disease Activity in Patients with Systemic Lupus Erythematosus

AUTHOR	STUDY TYPE	ANTIMALARIAL MEDICATION	FOLLOW-UP	MAIN OUTCOME	OBSERVED EFFECTS
Controlled Studies					
Rudnicki et al.[16]	Controlled study	CQ		Constitutional symptoms, flares	Lower rate of constitutional symptoms and flares
Rudnicki et al.[17]	RCT	HCQ	24 weeks	Flares	Lower rate of SLE flare (36% vs 73%, $P = 0.02$) Placebo 2.5 higher risk of flares
Williams et al.[18]	RCT	CQ	48 weeks	Painful and swollen joints	Lower self-assessment of joint pain ($P = 0.02$)
Meinão et al.[19]	RCT	CQ	12 months	Prednisone dose SLE flare (SLEDAI)	Lower rate of flares (18% vs 83%, $P < 0.01$)
Tsakonas et al.[20]	Extended RCT	HCQ	42 months	Time to major flare	Lower rate of major flare (28% vs 50%, $P = 0.08$)
Levy et al.[21]	RCT	HCQ	Pregnancy duration	SLE activity (SLEPDAI) Prednisone dose	Improvement only in patients receiving HCQ ($P = 0.04$)
Observational Studies					
Cortes-Hernandez et al.[22]	Prospective cohort	CQ	Pregnancy duration	SLE flares	CQ discontinuation increased flares ($P = 0.02$)
Clowse et al.[23]	Prospective cohort	HCQ	Pregnancy duration	SLE activity during pregnancy Prednisone use	Women stopping HCQ had higher lupus activity than those never treated and those taking HCQ: Higher rate of flare (55% vs 36% vs 30%, respectively; $P = 0.05$) Maximum dose of prednisone (21 vs 23 vs 16 mg/day, respectively; $P = 0.06$)
Kasitanon et al.[24]	Retrospective cohort	HCQ	12 months	Remission in membranous nephritis treated with MMF	Higher rates of membranous lupus nephritis remission for those receiving HCQ (64% vs 22%, $P = 0.04$)
Costedoat-Chalumeau et al.[11]	Prospective cohort	HCQ	6 months	SLE flare (SLEDAI)	Lower HCQ levels in patients with flare (703 vs 1128, $P = 0.006$)
Wozniacka et al.[4]	Prospective cohort	CQ	3 months	Change in SLAM score	Higher reduction in SLAM score (9.47 vs 4.92, $P < 0.001$)

CQ, Chloroquine; HCQ, hydroxychloroquine; MMF, mycophenolate mofetil; RCT, randomized controlled trial; SLAM, systemic lupus activity measure; SLE, systemic lupus erythematosus; SLEDAI, Systemic Lupus Erythematosus Disease Activity Index; SLEPDAI, Systemic Lupus Erythematosus Pregnancy Disease Activity Index.

A second landmark study was published in 1991 by the Canadian Hydroxychloroquine Study Group, which reported a multicenter, placebo-controlled, double-blind randomized study of the effect of withdrawing HCQ in patients with stable SLE.[17] Forty-seven patients with quiescent SLE were randomized to receive placebo or to continue with HCQ; they were followed for 24 weeks. The HCQ group had significantly fewer disease flares than the placebo group (36% versus 73%, respectively; $P = 0.02$). The time to flare-up was also shorter in the placebo group. Overall, patients randomized to placebo were 2.5 times (95% confidence interval [CI] 1.08-5.58) more likely to have mild clinical flares than those who remained on HCQ. Five of the patients taking placebo (23%) and 1 who continued to take HCQ (4%) had severe exacerbations of disease activity that prompted their withdrawal from the study ($P = 0.06$) (see Table 49-1).

Williams and associates[18] in a 48-week multicenter, placebo-controlled, double-blind randomized study evaluated the efficacy and safety of HCQ in the treatment of articular complaints of 71 patients with SLE requiring less than 10 mg prednisone per day. Only joint pain favored the use of HCQ. As noted by the authors of this study, the small sample size and high dropout rate (41%) limited the power of the study (see Table 49-1).

In certain countries of Latin America and Eastern Europe, CQ is the only AM medication available. In 1996, Meinão and colleagues[19] performed the first prospective, double-blind, randomized trial with CQ in 44 corticosteroid-dependent patients with SLE. At 12 months,

articular involvement was present in 0% of those receiving CQ and in 67% of those receiving placebo ($P = 0.001$). Flares occurred more commonly in those randomized to placebo (10 patients [83%] receiving placebo, 2 [18%] patients receiving CQ). The prednisone dose was decreased in 9 patients (82%) in the CQ group versus 3 (25%) in the placebo group ($P = 0.001$) (see Table 49-1).

Kasitanon and others[24] reported that HCQ therapy predicts complete renal remission at 12 months in patients treated with mycophenolate mofetil for membranous lupus nephritis. This study was the first to demonstrate that concurrent HCQ use has a significant benefit for a severe manifestation of SLE. If this finding is confirmed, AM medications may have a potentially new role as adjunctive therapy in other forms of severe SLE (see Table 49-1).

Wozniacka and associates[5] found that CQ treatment decreased disease activity in SLE. The authors of this study also found that the levels of IL-1, IL-18, and TNF-α decreased significantly after 3 months of CQ use (see Table 49-1).

Efficacy during Pregnancy

In 2001, Levy and others[21] reported the only prospective randomized, placebo, controlled study assessing the efficacy and safety of HCQ in patients with lupus who were pregnant. Twenty patients with SLE or biopsy-proven DLE were randomized to receive HCQ or placebo between 8 and 18 weeks of pregnancy. HCQ use was associated with decreased disease activity scores ($P = 0.04$) and lower prednisone doses at delivery (HCQ, 4.5 mg /day; placebo, 13.7 mg/day; $P = 0.05$). No statistically significant differences, with respect to delivery age or Apgar scores, were observed between the treatment groups. No auditory or other clinical deficits were detected. Ophthalmoscopy was normal in all patients at 12 weeks (see Table 49-1).

In a 2006 prospective study, Cortés-Hernandez and colleagues[22] reported that the discontinuation of CQ significantly predicted disease flares in 103 pregnancies (see Table 49-1).

Clowse and associates[23] assessed 257 pregnancies in 197 women divided into three groups: (1) no HCQ exposure during pregnancy (163 pregnancies), (2) continuous use of HCQ during pregnancy (56 pregnancies), or (3) cessation of HCQ treatment either in the 3 months before or during the first trimester of pregnancy (38 pregnancies). The rates of miscarriage, stillbirth, pregnancy loss, and congenital abnormalities were not statistically different among the three groups. SLE activity during pregnancy was significantly higher in women who discontinued the HCQ, as was the rate of disease flare among women who stopped the medication (55%), compared with those who either continued taking it (30%) and those who never took it (36%). Rates of prednisone use, as well as the prevalence of patients requiring high-dose prednisone (>20 mg/day or pulse therapy), were significantly lower in the group with continuous HCQ therapy (see Table 49-1).

No toxic or developmental delay has been reported in children whose mothers have been exposed to antimalarials during pregnancy or during lactation. Therefore maternal AM use is considered safe during pregnancy and breast feeding.[25]

Antithrombotic Effects

In 1987, Wallace[26] suggested that AM medications protected against clot formation in 92 patients with SLE. Subsequently, several others have confirmed this initial observation (Table 49-2).[27-34]

Because AM drugs are administered in patients with milder disease, the results may be confounded by disease severity and treatment indication. Nevertheless, two studies that adjusted for confounding by indication demonstrated the antithrombotic effects of AM medications.[32,34] The thromboprotective effect of AM agents may arise by effects on platelet aggregation,[35] through formation of antiphospholipid–β_2-glycoprotein 1 complexes with phospholipid bilayers and cells,[36] or by prevention of antiphospholipid antibody binding of annexin-5, a potent anticoagulant believed to play a key role in the thrombophilic effect of antiphospholipid antibodies (see Table 49-2).[37]

Effects on Dyslipidemia and Atherosclerosis

Since the antihyperlipidemic effect of AM medications in SLE was described by Wallace and colleagues,[38] several studies have

confirmed their results.[39,40] Of note, Rahman and others[39] showed that a co-prescription of an AM drug along with corticosteroids is associated with a 9% to 11% reduction in total cholesterol, and AM medications significantly reduce very low–density lipoprotein (VLDL) and low-density lipoprotein (LDL) cholesterol levels.[40] AM medications also appear to increase levels of high-density lipoprotein (HDL) cholesterol when given alone or concomitantly with steroids.[41]

The effect of AM medications on atherosclerosis was recently reviewed.[15] Five studies did not find any effect of current treatment (one study) or past treatment (four studies) with AM medications on the presence of atherosclerosis. The only study specifically designed to analyze the effect of treatment with HCQ on atherosclerosis[42] found increased large-artery elasticity and reduced systemic vascular resistance among patients treated with HCQ, compared with untreated patients and those receiving glucocorticoids alone.

Effects on Diabetes Mellitus

Several authors have reported that AM medications reduce plasma glucose levels in volunteers, patients with malaria, and patients with diabetes. Petri[43] and Penn and others[44] reported that mean glucose levels were significantly less in patients taking HCQ. Although the effect of HCQ on the risk of diabetes has not been studied in SLE, it reduces the risk by 38% (95% CI 0.42-0.92) in patients with rheumatoid arthritis.[45]

Protective Effects on Infections

AM medications demonstrate in vitro activity against bacteria, fungi, and viruses.[46,47] Three recent studies have suggested that AM agents have a protective effect against infection.[48-50] In a study of 249 patients with SLE, Ruiz-Irastorza and associates[48] reported a 93% reduction in the risk of major infection (odds ratio [OR] 0.07, 95% CI 0.03-0.16) among AM users.

Sisó and colleagues[49] reported a lower frequency of infections among those previously treated with AM medications (11% versus 29%, $P = 0.006$). Bultink and colleagues[50] found that treatment with HCQ reduced major infections by 95% (OR 0.05, 95% CI 0.01-0.23). Although confounding by indication may explain the protective effect of AM agents against infection, the very substantial benefit reported is potentially important.

Effects on Cancer

Patients with SLE are at increased risk of cancer.[51,52] Evidence suggests that AM medications could influence cancer risk through several mechanisms, including chemosensitization, inhibition of cell growth, and/or cell death.[53-55] Although a study reported an 85% reduction in the risk of malignancy for patients ever being treated

TABLE 49-2 Studies Assessing the Antithrombotic Effect of Antimalarial Medications

AUTHOR	STUDY TYPE	ANTIMALARIAL MEDICATION	MAIN OUTCOME	OBSERVED EFFECTS IN PATIENTS
Wallace, 1987[25]	Observational	HCQ	Thrombosis	Less thrombosis
Erkan et al. 2002[27]	Cross-sectional	HCQ	Thrombosis	Less thrombosis
Toloza et al. 2004[28]	Observational	HCQ	Arterial thrombosis	No effect
Mok et al. 2005[29]	Observational	HCQ	Thrombosis	No effect
Ho et al. 2005[30]	Observational	HCQ	Thrombosis	47% less risk of thrombosis (95% CI, 6%-70%)
De Leeuw et al. 2006[31]	Cross-sectional	HCQ	Cardiovascular disease	No effect
Ruiz-Irastorza et al. 2006[32]*	Observational	Various AM medications	Thrombosis	72% less risk of thrombosis (95% CI, 10%-92%)
Mok et al. 2007[33]	Observational	HCQ	Arterial thrombosis	No effect
Jung et al. 2010[34]*	Observational	Various AM medications	Thrombosis	68% less risk of thrombosis (95% CI, 26%-86%)

AM, Antimalarial; HCQ, hydroxychloroquine; CI, confidence interval.
*Studies adjusting for confounding by indication using propensity scores.

with AM medications, compared those with never being treated,[56] an earlier study by Sultan and associates,[57] which included risk factors for cancer in the analysis, saw no benefit.

Effects on Damage Accrual and Survival

In 2002, Molad and others[58] reported that HCQ therapy was associated with significantly reduced damage in 151 patients with SLE. Fessler and colleagues[59] examined the impact of HCQ on the accrual of damage in patients in the LUMINA (LUpus in MInorities, NAture versus nurture) cohort. After adjustment for confounders of disease severity using propensity scores, HCQ use was associated with a 27% reduced risk of new damage (hazard ratio [HR] 0.73, 95% CI 0.52-1.0). Patients without damage at baseline had a risk reduction of 45% (HR 0.55, 95% CI 0.34-0.87), whereas patients with damage had no benefit (HR 1.11, 95% CI 0.70-1.74). Using the same cohort, Pons-Estel and associates[60] found a protective effect of HCQ in slowing the occurrence of renal damage (HR 0.12, 95% CI 0.02-0.97).

Considering that damage accrual is a strong predictor of mortality in SLE,[61] one might expect that AM therapy would impact survival. Three studies have analyzed the long-term effects of AM use on the survival of patients with SLE.[32,62,63] Two of these studies adjusted for confounding by indication using propensity scores, and both found decreased mortality.[61,63] The first study was from Spain and reported an 86% (HR 0.14, 95% CI 0.04-0.48) risk reduction, whereas the results from the LUMINA cohort found a 68% (OR 0.32, 95% CI 0.11-0.86) risk reduction on mortality.

ADVERSE EFFECTS OF ANTIMALARIAL THERAPY

A systematic review[15] has reported that AM medications are among the safest drugs used in rheumatology. One study of 940 patients, of whom 178 had SLE,[64] compared the frequency of adverse events among HCQ and CQ users and found that CQ had a higher frequency of adverse events than HCQ (28% versus 15%) (Table 49-3). Among all patients with adverse events, 69% of the patients permanently discontinued the drug.

Gastrointestinal Adverse Effects

Gastrointestinal adverse effects are some of the most common causes of AM discontinuation (see Table 49-3). The most frequent complaints are anorexia, heartburn, nausea, vomiting, diarrhea, and abdominal distention. These symptoms are usually transient and promptly disappear after the drug is stopped or the dose is lowered.

Cutaneous and Pigmentary Adverse Events

Because of its undesirable cutaneous effects, the discontinuation of AM medications occurs in approximately 3% of patients and is more common with CQ.[64] Cutaneous manifestations include urticaria, exfoliative lesions, erythema annulare, and psoriatic flares. These usually disappear after discontinuing the drug. However, hyperpigmentation and hypopigmentation or hair bleaching may not reverse or may do so very slowly after AM discontinuation. Rarely, AM therapy causes Stevens-Johnson syndrome.

Ocular Effects

Ciliary body adverse events are characterized by a disturbance of accommodation with the symptom of blurred vision; they are related to dose and are reversible even with continuation of therapy.

CQ binds more avidly than HCQ to corneal tissues. With slit-lamp examination, 90% of the patients receiving the standard dose of CQ have corneal deposits (i.e., keratopathy), compared with 5% of those on standard doses of HCQ.[65] Keratopathy occurs early, is symptomatic in approximately 50% of patients, and disappears after discontinuation of the drug. Interestingly, though, it does not necessarily reappear after AM therapy is resumed. The most frequent complaint is halos around light sources. Keratopathy does not predict retinal toxicity.

The major adverse event of concern for physicians and patients is retinal toxicity. Although early asymptomatic changes (e.g., premaculopathy) are reversible with discontinuation, the most severe form of retinopathy, maculopathy (bull's eye lesion), can progress even after AM withdrawal and potentially lead to blindness.

Currently, this complication is rare if daily doses are calculated on lean body weight (maximum of 6.5 mg/kg/day lean body weight for HCQ and 3 mg/kg/day for CQ). Among all AM studies reported in patients with SLE, of the 647 patients who were treated with CQ for longer than 10 years, 16 patients (2.5%) were diagnosed with definite retinal toxicity, in comparison with only 2 of 2043 patients (0.1%) taking HCQ for a similar period.[15] Wolfe and colleagues[66] have recently reported an incidence rate of 3 per 1000 within the first 5 years of AM use, increasing to 20 per 1000 between 10 and 15 years of continuous use. The major advantage of quinacrine over HCQ and CQ is its absence of retinal toxicity.

Screening for Ocular Toxicity

Screening seeks to recognize the earliest hints of functional or anatomic change before the toxic damage is well developed. The American Academy of Ophthalmology has recently revised its screening guidelines in light of new data on the prevalence of retinal toxicity.[67] Overall, it recognizes that the risk of toxicity increases toward 1% after 5 to 7 years of use or a cumulative dose of 1000 g or 460 g of HCQ or CQ, respectively. The new guidelines remove the Amsler grid from the list of acceptable screening techniques and strongly advise that sensitive objective tests, such as multifocal electroretinogram, spectral domain optical coherence tomography, and fundus autofluorescence, supplement the Humphrey 10-2 visual fields.

All individuals starting to receive AM drugs should have a complete baseline ophthalmologic examination within the first year of treatment. This should include an examination of the retina through a dilated pupil and the testing of central visual field sensitivity by an automated field tester (Humphrey 10-2). If the results are normal, then no further special ophthalmologic testing is recommended for the next 5 years. The Canadian recommendations call for an assessment every 18 months in low-risk individuals.[68] The most subtle Humphrey 10-2 field changes are now considered serious, and visual fields should always be promptly repeated to determine whether the changes are reproducible. Reproducible changes should trigger further testing with objective procedures. Newer objective tests, such as multifocal electroretinogram, spectral domain optical coherence tomography, and fundus autofluorescence, are considered to be sensitive and are now recommended along with the automated field tester.

TABLE 49-3 Frequency of Adverse Events for Antimalarial Therapy in 938 Patients with Rheumatic Diseases

SIDE EFFECT BY ORGAN	AM N (%)	CQ N (%)	HCQ N (%)
Skin	33 (3)	25 (5)	8 (2)
Rash	31 (2)	23 (4)	8 (2)
Hair bleaching	2 (0.2)	2 (0.4)	0 (0)
Eye	70 (7)	63 (12)	9 (2)
Keratopathy	41 (4)	38 (7)	3 (1)
Blurred vision	26 (3)	21 (4)	5 (1)
Retinal changes*	3 (0.3)	2 (0.3)	1 (0.2)
Gastrointestinal tract	67 (7)	34 (6)	33 (8)
Nausea and vomiting	46 (5)	26 (5)	20 (5)
Diarrhea	14 (2)	5 (1)	9 (2)
Abdominal pain	7 (1)	3 (1)	4 (1)
Neuromuscular	19 (2)	17 (3)	2 (1)
Headache	9 (1)	7 (1)	2 (1)
Nightmares	4 (0.4)	4 (1)	0 (0)
Myopathy	6 (0.6)	6 (1)	0 (0)
Other	23 (2)	16 (3)	7 (2)
Total	212 (23)	153 (28)	59 (14)

*Only one patient was confirmed to have retinopathy as a result of antimalarial therapy.

Neurologic, Muscular, and Cardiac Adverse Effects

Headaches and nightmares are the most frequent neurologic adverse events (see Table 49-3). Insomnia also occurs. These effects stop with the discontinuation of the AM medications.

Tinnitus occurs but disappears after the discontinuation of the drug. One case of sensorineural hearing loss that did not improve with discontinuation has been reported.[69]

Myopathy is another rare adverse event that has been reported mainly with the use of CQ. The reported incidence of myopathy was 1.9 cases in 1000 patient years of HCQ therapy (95% CI 0.2-7.0)[69] and 10 per 1000 person years of CQ (95% CI 2.0-3.0).[70] Clinical presentation is characterized by slow and progressive symmetrical proximal weakness, predominantly in the legs, with no tenderness or soreness of the muscles. Symptoms are usually reversible within 8 weeks of AM discontinuation. Although lactate dehydrogenase may be elevated, the cytokeratin (CK) level is usually normal. Electromyography has low sensitivity for the diagnosis of AM myopathy (eFigure 49-2).[71] Lipid deposits, seen as curvilinear or myeloid bodies or both, and rimmed vacuoles on muscle biopsy in the right clinical context are distinctive but not pathognomonic. Vacuolar myopathy can be observed in other conditions including SLE myopathy, dermatomyositis or polymyositis, and corticosteroid-induced myopathy.

Cardiomyopathy associated with AM therapy has been described in a few cases.[72] Histologic findings are similar to those in skeletal muscle involvement. The clinical presentation is usually as congestive heart failure of short duration or worsening if preexistent, palpitations, or presyncope. The echocardiogram shows a progressive low left-ventricular ejection fraction, myocardial hypertrophy, and sometimes an echodense pattern in the walls and dilation of cavities.

The association of severe cardiac conduction disorders and SLE treated with AM medications is rare.

Adverse Events of Antimalarial Medications during Pregnancy and Breast-Feeding

See "Efficacy during Pregnancy" found earlier in this chapter.

Other Rare Adverse Events

Hematologic adverse effects have been reported, but they are so uncommon that routine assessment is not performed. Agranulocytosis has been reported with very high doses of HCQ. Aplastic anemia has been very rarely reported. Hemolysis and agranulocytosis associated with glucose-6-phosphate deficiency and CQ occurs. Psychosis associated with the use of quinacrine and CQ has been rarely reported.

AM use may worsen some non-SLE disorders (eBox 49-1).

Doses and Dosage Schedule

The dosage schedule used in the management of DLE is slightly different than the one used to treat SLE. DLE usually requires a larger initial dose to achieve a faster response, especially if extensive disease is present. However, the higher dose increases the likelihood of gastrointestinal adverse events, particularly with the use of non–enteric-coated generic HCQ.

In SLE, the recommended dose of HCQ is usually 400 mg, administered either once or in two 200-mg doses/day. As previously mentioned, the dose should be a *maximum* of 6.5 mg/kg/day of lean body weight. An approach used when the maximum dose is between 200 and 400 mg/day is to give 400 mg/day on some days of the week and 200 mg the remaining days to achieve an average weekly dose that is appropriate. This approach is based on the long half-life of AM medications (40 to 50 days and 3.5 to 12 days for HCQ and CQ, respectively). Response to HCQ therapy usually begins between 8 and 12 weeks; however, the drug achieves its peak efficacy in 6 to 12 months. Response to CQ is usually faster because it reaches a plateau plasma level in 4 to 6 weeks.[73]

The maximum dose of CQ should not exceed 3 mg/kg/day of lean body weight.

Quinacrine dose is 100 to 200 mg/day, and response is usually observed in 3 to 6 weeks once steady concentrations have been attained. No cross-reactivity of the 4-aminoquinoline derivatives and quinacrine occurs; therefore an adverse effect with HCQ or CQ does not preclude treatment with quinacrine. Moreover, although based on anecdotal evidence, quinacrine can also be used as an adjunctive therapy in SLE. When needed, it can be administered in doses of 50 to 100 mg/day, in addition to the standard dose of HCQ or CQ.

Evidence suggests that smoking decreases the effectiveness of AM medications, apparently by decreasing absorption, increasing metabolic clearance, and blocking the uptake into lysosomes. These effects of smoking could be additional reasons to encourage smoking cessation.

The dose of an AM medication must be adjusted in patients with renal failure. CQ should be reduced to no more than 50 mg once daily in patients with a glomerular filtration rate (GFR) of 10 to 20 mL/min; further, it is contraindicated in patients with a GFR of less than 10 mL/min.[74] Plasma HCQ levels should be measured in patients with severely compromised function, and the dose adjusted accordingly. HCQ and CQ are extensively sequestered within the tissues; therefore dialysis is not helpful in removing either.

AM drugs have some interactions with other medications that could influence efficacy or toxicity (eTable 49-1). To date, no food interactions with AM medications have been described.

SUMMARY

AM medications are some of the oldest medications used to treat human disease and some of the first disease-modifying antirheumatic drugs. Several factors have favored the wide use of AM therapy in SLE. First, convincing evidence suggests that these agents are effective. Second, the use of low daily doses based on lean body weight has reduced retinal toxicity. Third, effective retinal monitoring strategies are available.

AM drugs have become the first-line therapy in the management of SLE. The future promises many new therapeutic advances, but for now, AM medications are inexpensive, safe, and effective, and they remain a key agent in the management of SLE.

References

1. Wallace DJ: The history of antimalarials. *Lupus* 5(Suppl 1):S2–S3, 1996.
2. Fox RI: Mechanism of action of hydroxychloroquine as an antirheumatic drug. *Semin Arthritis Rheum* 23(2 Suppl 1):82–91, 1993.
3. Wallace DJ: The use of quinacrine (Atabrine) in rheumatic diseases: a reexamination. *Semin Arthritis Rheum* 18(4):282–296, 1989.
4. Wozniacka A, Lesiak A, Narbutt J, et al: Chloroquine treatment influences proinflammatory cytokine levels in systemic lupus erythematosus patients. *Lupus* 15(5):268–275, 2006.
5. Wozniacka A, Lesiak A, Boncela J, et al: The influence of antimalarial treatment on IL-1β, IL-6 and TNF-α mRNA expression on UVB-irradiated skin in systemic lupus erythematosus. *Br J Dermatol* 159(5):1124–1130, 2008.
6. Theofilopoulos A, Koundouris S, Kono D, et al: The role of IFN-gamma in systemic lupus erythematosus: a challenge to the Th1/Th2 paradigm in autoimmunity. *Arthritis Res* 3(3):136–141, 2001.
7. Wozniacka A, Lesiak A, Narbutt J, et al: Chloroquine treatment reduces the number of cutaneous HLA-DR+ and CD1a+ cells in patients with systemic lupus erythematosus. *Lupus* 16(2):89–94, 2007.
8. Rifkin IR, Leadbetter EA, Busconi L, et al: Toll-like receptors, endogenous ligands, and systemic autoimmune disease. *Immunol Rev* 204:27–42, 2005.
9. Rönnblom L, Alm GV: An etiopathogenic role for the type I IFN system in SLE. *Trends Immunol* 22(8):427–431, 2001.
10. Means TK, Latz E, Hayashi F, et al: Human lupus autoantibody-DNA complexes activate DCs through cooperation of CD32 and TLR9. *J Clin Inv* 115(2):407–417, 2005.
11. Costedoat-Chalumeau N, Amoura Z, Hulot J-S, et al: Low blood concentration of hydroxychloroquine is a marker for and predictor of disease exacerbations in patients with systemic lupus erythematosus. *Arthritis Rheum* 54(10):3284–3290, 2006.
12. Lafyatis R, York M, Marshak-Rothstein A: Antimalarial agents: closing the gate on Toll-like receptors? *Arthritis Rheum* 54(10):3068–3070, 2006.

13. James JA, Kim-Howard XR, Bruner BF, et al: Hydroxychloroquine sulfate treatment is associated with later onset of systemic lupus erythematosus. *Lupus* 16(6):401–409, 2007.

14. Macfarlane DE, Manzel L: Antagonism of immunostimulatory CpG-oligodeoxynucleotides by quinacrine, chloroquine, and structurally related compounds. *J Immunol* 160(3):1122–1131, 1998.

15. Ruiz-Irastorza G, Ramos-Casals M, Brito-Zeron P, et al: Clinical efficacy and side effects of antimalarials in systemic lupus erythematosus: a systematic review. *Ann Rheum Dis* 69(1):20–28, 2010.

16. Rudnicki RD, Gresham GE, Rothfield NF: The efficacy of antimalarials in systemic lupus erythematosus. *J Rheumatol* 2(3):323–330, 1975.

17. Canadian Hydroxychloroquine Study Group: A randomized study of the effect of withdrawing hydroxychloroquine sulfate in systemic lupus erythematosus. *N Engl J Med* 324(3):150–154, 1991.

18. Williams HJ, Egger MJ, Singer JZ, et al: Comparison of hydroxychloroquine and placebo in the treatment of the arthropathy of mild systemic lupus erythematosus. *J Rheumatol* 21(8):1457–1462, 1994.

19. Meinão I, Sato E, Andrade L, et al: Controlled trial with chloroquine diphosphate in systemic lupus erythematosus. *Lupus* 5(3):237–241, 1996.

20. Tsakonas E, Joseph L, Esdaile JM, et al: A long-term study of hydroxychloroquine withdrawal on exacerbations in systemic lupus erythematosus. The Canadian Hydroxychloroquine Study Group. *Lupus* 7(2):80-85, 1998.

21. Levy RA, Vilela VS, Cataldo MJ, et al: Hydroxychloroquine (HCQ) in lupus pregnancy: double-blind and placebo-controlled study. *Lupus* 10(6):401–404, 2001.

22. Cortes-Hernandez J, Ordi-Ros J, Paredes F, et al: Clinical predictors of fetal and maternal outcome in systemic lupus erythematosus: a prospective study of 103 pregnancies. *Rheumatology* 41(6):643–650, 2002.

23. Clowse MEB, Magder L, Witter F, et al: Hydroxychloroquine in lupus pregnancy. *Arthritis Rheum* 54(11):3640–3647, 2006.

24. Kasitanon N, Fine DM, Haas M, et al: Hydroxychloroquine use predicts complete renal remission within 12 months among patients treated with mycophenolate mofetil therapy for membranous lupus nephritis. *Lupus* 15(6):366–370, 2006.

25. Østensen M, Khamashta M, Lockshin M, et al: Anti-inflammatory and immunosuppressive drugs and reproduction. *Arthritis Res Ther* 8(3):209, 2006.

26. Wallace DJ: Does hydroxychloroquine sulfate prevent clot formation in systemic lupus erythematosus? *Arthritis Rheum* 30(12):1435–1436, 1987.

27. Erkan D, Yazici Y, Peterson MG, et al: A cross-sectional study of clinical thrombotic risk factors and preventive treatments in antiphospholipid syndrome. *Rheumatology* 41(8):924–929, 2002.

28. Toloza SMA, Uribe AG, McGwin G, et al: Systemic lupus erythematosus in a multiethnic US cohort (LUMINA): XXIII. Baseline predictors of vascular events. *Arthritis Rheum* 50(12):3947–3957, 2004.

29. Mok CC, Tang SSK, To CH, et al: Incidence and risk factors of thromboembolism in systemic lupus erythematosus: a comparison of three ethnic groups. *Arthritis Rheum* 52(9):2774–2782, 2005.

30. Ho KT, Ahn CW, Alarcón GS, et al: Systemic lupus erythematosus in a multiethnic cohort (LUMINA): XXVIII. Factors predictive of thrombotic events. *Rheumatology* 44(10):1303–1307, 2005.

31. De Leeuw K, Freire B, Smit AJ, et al: Traditional and non-traditional risk factors contribute to the development of accelerated atherosclerosis in patients with systemic lupus erythematosus. *Lupus* 15(10):675–682, 2006.

32. Ruiz-Irastorza G, Egurbide MV, Pijoan JI, et al: Effect of antimalarials on thrombosis and survival in patients with systemic lupus erythematosus. *Lupus* 15(9):577–583, 2006.

33. Mok CC, Tong KH, To CH, et al: Risk and predictors of arterial thrombosis in lupus and non-lupus primary glomerulonephritis: a comparative study. *Medicine* 86(4):203–209, 2007.

34. Jung H, Bobba R, Su J, et al: The protective effect of antimalarial drugs on thrombovascular events in systemic lupus erythematosus. *Arthritis Rheum* 62(3):863–868, 2010.

35. Jancinova V, Nosal R, Petrikova M: On the inhibitory effect of chloroquine on blood platelet aggregation. *Thromb Res* 74(5):495–504, 1994.

36. Rand JH, Wu X-X, Quinn AS, et al: Hydroxychloroquine directly reduces the binding of antiphospholipid antibody-beta2-glycoprotein I complexes to phospholipid bilayers. *Blood* 112(5):1687–1695, 2008.

37. Rand JH, Wu X-X, Quinn AS, et al: Hydroxychloroquine protects the annexin A5 anticoagulant shield from disruption by antiphospholipid antibodies: evidence for a novel effect for an old antimalarial drug. *Blood* 115(11):2292–2299, 2010.

38. Wallace DJ, Metzger AL, Stecher VJ, et al: Cholesterol-lowering effect of hydroxychloroquine in patients with rheumatic disease: reversal of deleterious effects of steroids on lipids. *Am J Med* 89(3):322–326, 1990.

39. Rahman P, Gladman DD, Urowitz MB, et al: The cholesterol lowering effect of antimalarial drugs is enhanced in patients with lupus taking corticosteroid drugs. *J Rheumatol* 26(2):325–330, 1999.

40. Tam LS, Gladman DD, Hallett DC, et al: Effect of antimalarial agents on the fasting lipid profile in systemic lupus erythematosus. *J Rheumatol* 27(9):2142–2145, 2000.

41. Borba EF, Bonfa E: Longterm beneficial effect of chloroquine diphosphate on lipoprotein profile in lupus patients with and without steroid therapy. *J Rheumatol* 28(4):780–785, 2001.

42. Tanay A, Leibovitz E, Frayman A, et al: Vascular elasticity of systemic lupus erythematosus patients is associated with steroids and hydroxychloroquine treatment. *Ann N Y Acad of Sci* 1108:24–34, 2007.

43. Petri M: Hydroxychloroquine use in the Baltimore Lupus Cohort: effects on lipids, glucose and thrombosis. *Lupus* 5(1 Suppl):S16–S22, 1996.

44. Penn SK, Kao AH, Schott LL, et al: Hydroxychloroquine and glycemia in women with rheumatoid arthritis and systemic lupus erythematosus. *J Rheumatol* 37(6):1136–1142, 2010.

45. Wasko MCM, Hubert HB, Lingala VB, et al: Hydroxychloroquine and risk of diabetes in patients with rheumatoid arthritis. *JAMA* 298(2):187–193, 2007.

46. Rolain J-M, Colson P, Raoult D: Recycling of chloroquine and its hydroxyl analogue to face bacterial, fungal and viral infections in the 21st century. *Int J Antimicrob Agents* 30(4):297–308, 2007.

47. Savarino A, Boelaert JR, Cassone A, et al: Effects of chloroquine on viral infections: an old drug against today's diseases. *Lancet Infect Dis* 3(11):722–727, 2003.

48. Ruiz-Irastorza G, Olivares N, Ruiz-Arruza I, et al: Predictors of major infections in systemic lupus erythematosus. *Arthritis Res Ther* 11(4):R109, 2009.

49. Sisó A, Ramos-Casals M, Bové A, et al: Previous antimalarial therapy in patients diagnosed with lupus nephritis: influence on outcomes and survival. *Lupus* 17(4):281–288, 2008.

50. Bultink IEM, Hamann D, Seelen MA, et al: Deficiency of functional mannose-binding lectin is not associated with infections in patients with systemic lupus erythematosus. *Arthritis Res Ther* 8(6):R183, 2006.

51. Bernatsky S, Boivin JF, Joseph L, et al: An international cohort study of cancer in systemic lupus erythematosus. *Arthritis Rheum* 52(5):1481–1490, 2005.

52. Moss KE, Ioannou Y, Sultan SM, et al: Outcome of a cohort of 300 patients with systemic lupus erythematosus attending a dedicated clinic for over two decades. *Ann Rheum Dis* 61(5):409–413, 2002.

53. Zheng Y, Zhao Y, Deng X, et al: Chloroquine inhibits colon cancer cell growth in vitro and tumor growth in vivo via induction of apoptosis. *Cancer Invest* 27(3):286–292, 2009.

54. Solomon VR, Lee H: Chloroquine and its analogs: a new promise of an old drug for effective and safe cancer therapies. *Eur J Pharm* 625(1-3):220–233, 2009.

55. Rahim R, Strobl JS: Hydroxychloroquine, chloroquine, and all-trans retinoic acid regulate growth, survival, and histone acetylation in breast cancer cells. *Anticancer Drugs* 20(8):736–745, 2009.

56. Ruiz-Irastorza G, Ugarte A, Egurbide MV, et al: Antimalarials may influence the risk of malignancy in systemic lupus erythematosus. *Ann Rheum Dis* 66(6):815–817, 2007.

57. Sultan SM, Ioannou Y, Isenberg DA: Is there an association of malignancy with systemic lupus erythematosus? An analysis of 276 patients under long-term review. *Rheumatology* 39(10):1147–1152, 2000.

58. Molad Y, Gorshtein A, Wysenbeek AJ, et al: Protective effect of hydroxychloroquine in systemic lupus erythematosus. Prospective long-term study of an Israeli cohort. *Lupus* 11(6):356–361, 2002.

59. Fessler BJ, Alarcon GS, McGwin G, Jr, et al: Systemic lupus erythematosus in three ethnic groups: XVI. Association of hydroxychloroquine use with reduced risk of damage accrual. *Arthritis Rheum* 52(5):1473–1480, 2005.

60. Pons-Estel GJ, Alarcón GS, McGwin G, et al: Protective effect of hydroxychloroquine on renal damage in patients with lupus nephritis: LXV, data from a multiethnic US cohort. *Arthritis Care Res* 61(6):830–839, 2009.

61. Ruiz-Irastorza G, Egurbide M-V, Ugalde J, et al: High impact of antiphospholipid syndrome on irreversible organ damage and survival of patients with systemic lupus erythematosus. *Arch Intern Med* 164(1):77–82, 2004.

62. Hernandez-Cruz B, Tapia N, Villa-Romero AR, et al: Risk factors associated with mortality in systemic lupus erythematosus. A case-control study in a tertiary care center in Mexico City. *Clin Exp Rheumatol* 19(4):395–401, 2001.

63. Alarcon GS, McGwin G, Bertoli AM, et al: Effect of hydroxychloroquine on the survival of patients with systemic lupus erythematosus: data from LUMINA, a multiethnic US cohort (LUMINA L). *Ann Rheum Dis* 66(9):1168–1172, 2007.

64. Avina-Zubieta JA, Galindo-Rodriguez G, Newman S, et al: Long-term effectiveness of antimalarial drugs in rheumatic diseases. *Ann Rheum Dis* 57(10):582–587, 1998.

65. Easterbrook M: The ocular safety of hydroxychloroquine. *Sem Arthritis Rheum* 23(2 Suppl 1):62–67, 1993.

66. Wolfe F, Marmor MF: Rates and predictors of hydroxychloroquine retinal toxicity in patients with rheumatoid arthritis and systemic lupus erythematosus. *Arthritis Care Res* 62(6):775–784, 2010.

67. Marmor MF, Kellner U, Lai TYY, et al, American Academy of Ophthalmology: Revised recommendations on screening for chloroquine and hydroxychloroquine retinopathy. *Ophthalmology* 118(2):415–422, 2011.

68. Canadian Rheumatology Association: Canadian Consensus Conference on hydroxychloroquine. *J Rheumatol* 27(12):2919–2921, 2000.

69. Wang C, Fortin PR, Li Y, et al: Discontinuation of antimalarial drugs in systemic lupus erythematosus. *J Rheumatol* 26(4):808–815, 1999.

70. Avina-Zubieta JA, Johnson ES, Suarez-Almazor ME, et al: Incidence of myopathy in patients treated with antimalarials. A report of 3 cases and review of the literature. *Rheumatology* 34(2):166–170, 1995.

71. Casado E, Gratacós J, Tolosa C, et al: Antimalarial myopathy: an underdiagnosed complication? Prospective longitudinal study of 119 patients. *Ann Rheum Dis* 65(3):385–390, 2006.

72. Baguet JP, Tremel F, Fabre M: Chloroquine cardiomyopathy with conduction disorders. *Heart* 81(2):221–223, 1999.

73. Frisk-Holmberg M, Bergkvist Y, Domeij-Nyberg B, et al: Chloroquine serum concentration and side effects: evidence for dose-dependent kinetics. *Clin Pharmacol Ther* 25(3):345–350, 1979.

74. Thorogood N, Atwal S, Mills W, et al: The risk of antimalarials in patients with renal failure. *Post Med J* 83(986):e8, 2007.

Immunosuppressive Drug Therapy

W. Joseph McCune and Tania Gonzalez-Rivera

Immunosuppressive agents are widely used for serious manifestations of systemic lupus erythematosus (SLE) to minimize irreversible injury and reduce toxicity from corticosteroids. In the past decade, efforts have focused on minimizing the use of cyclophosphamide (CyX) for even the most severe manifestations, particularly nephritis, by (1) using sequential therapy with CyX for induction of remission, followed by maintenance therapy with mycophenolate mofetil (MMF) or azathioprine (AZA); (2) shortening the period of induction with CyX; and (3) substituting MMF for CyX for remission induction in nephritis. The goal of substituting new biologic agents for conventional immunosuppressives for lupus nephritis (LN) has not yet been realized, although rituximab has been successfully substituted for immunosuppression in some patients with cytopenias. MMF and methotrexate (MTX) have been increasingly used for nonrenal lupus in place of AZA.

Most studies of immunosuppressive agents in lupus have been performed on nephritis. The availability of histologic examination and relatively accurate tests of renal function allow for a more accurate estimation of the response to therapy than trials in nonrenal lupus. The duration of nephritis trials (historically up to 20 years) has been significantly shortened by using primary endpoints such as complete remission after 24 weeks of induction treatment, rather than long-term preservation of renal function after many years. The duration of most current clinical trials is therefore much less than the anticipated survival of most patients with lupus.

This chapter focuses on controlled trials of widely used immunosuppressive agents, emphasizing nephritis trials, and reviews the use of the alkylating agents AZA, cyclosporine (CS), tacrolimus (TACRO), MTX, leflunomide, and MMF, and their roles in induction, as well as sequential therapies after treatment with CyX.

ALKYLATING AGENTS

Of the more than 12 alkylating agents that are currently in use, CyX, chlorambucil, and mechlorethamine (nitrogen mustard) have been most widely used to treat patients with SLE. The earliest use of alkylating agents, reported by Osborne and associates[1] in 1947, was the topical application of nitrogen mustard in cutaneous lupus, followed in 1949 with the description by Chasis[2] of rapid and dramatic responses to nitrogen mustard in LN—patients with nephrotic syndrome were sometimes observed to begin diuresing within 1 day of treatment. Mechlorethamine has since been largely abandoned because of toxicity, although it is arguable that those patients with the worst of symptoms might yet benefit even now from such aggressive therapy during initiation of long-term treatment with a better-tolerated compound such as MMF.

CYCLOPHOSPHAMIDE

CyX, despite significant toxicity, particularly gonadal failure, remains a mainstay of treatment of many patients with severe SLE. Its clinical effects, both therapeutic and toxic, vary, depending on the dose, route of administration, duration of administration, and cumulative dose.

CyX is a mechlorethamine derivative that is inactive as administered. It is metabolized by mitochondrial cytochrome P-450 enzymes in the liver to a variety of active metabolites, an increasing number of which have been shown to have both therapeutic and toxic actions. It has been proposed that various genetic polymorphisms of the P-450 enzymes are associated with the toxicity of CyX as well as the clinical response to the drug in patients with LN.

Active metabolites of CyX include 4-hydroxycyclophosphamide, aldophosphamide, phosphoramide mustard, and acrolein, all of which have differing rates of synthesis, half-lives, immunologic effects, and toxicities.[3] Serum levels of these metabolites are not routinely measured; hence, dose adjustment in patients with renal or hepatic failure is largely empiric. Doses should be reduced approximately 30% in patients with a creatinine clearance of less than 30 mL/min. Some investigators have proposed stepwise reduction as renal function declines.[4] Furthermore, CyX is incompletely cleared by dialysis; therefore the dose should be lowered for dialysis patients as well. The effect of hepatic insufficiency on CyX toxicity is incompletely understood, in part because the liver is responsible for both the production of active metabolites and their degradation. CyX is metabolized not only in the liver but also in lymphocytes and transitional epithelial cells in the bladder, which may result in local toxicity or immunosuppression or both. CyX may have toxic and/or therapeutic effects in cells that are not actively dividing, as well as in dividing cells.

CyX is well absorbed orally, and the oral and intravenous doses are equivalent. Large boluses of CyX can be administered orally, achieving comparable serum levels versus intravenous administration. Approximately 20% is excreted by the kidney, and 80% is processed by the liver.

The immunologic effects of CyX have been described. Direct effects of CyX on DNA result in cell death. These effects may occur at any stage during the cell cycle. Direct immunomodulatory effects may also occur and may be responsible for the relatively rapid onset of therapeutic efficacy of CyX (i.e., within 2 to 4 days) that is observed in some patients at a time when attrition of immunocompetent cells would not be expected. Putative mechanisms of action include alteration of macrophage function, increased production of prostaglandin E_2, alteration of gene transcription, and direct functional effects on lymphocytes. Intravenous CyX (IVC) induces suppression of T-cell activation; however, modulation of T-cell function has not been convincingly shown to play an important role in the treatment of lupus.

CyX produces dose-related lymphopenia. IVC reduces the population of cluster of differentiation 4 ($CD4^+$) and cluster of differentiation 8 ($CD8^+$) lymphocytes and B cells, with a more significant reduction of $CD4^+$ lymphocytes and B cells during monthly therapy.[5-7] After the cessation of monthly therapy, B-cell populations rapidly return to baseline, but $CD4^+$ populations remain relatively suppressed during less intensive IVC therapy, resulting in prolonged reduction of the $CD4^+/CD8^+$ ratio.[6]

Persistent reduction of the number of cluster of differentiation 19 ($CD19^+$) lymphocytes 6 months after the completion of therapy has been reported,[8] and specific reduction of B-cell function has been described.[9] Reduction of autoantibody production has been demonstrated in patients with SLE who are treated with both oral CyX and

IVC and in patients with rheumatoid arthritis (RA) who are treated with oral CyX. Despite the reduction of pathogenic autoantibody production, reduction of overall levels of immunoglobulin (Ig) G, IgA, and IgM, and IgG subclasses has not been observed in the authors' patient population. This suggests that specific suppression of autoantibody production is a function of CyX when used in therapeutic doses and may underlie its beneficial action in patients with SLE.

Low doses of CyX in both animals and humans can heighten immune responses. This has been noted in both antibody-mediated and cell-mediated immunity, and it has been theorized that low doses of CyX could enhance antitumor immunity in humans. Low doses of CyX accelerate the production of diabetes in the nonobese, diabetic mouse. The mechanism of action of CyX in these situations is unclear, but it may represent functional alterations, as well as a depletion of lymphocyte subsets. These observations suggest that tapering the dose of CyX may produce unexpected effects, although no clinical data support the hypothesis that during tapering of immunosuppressive drugs, particularly CyX, immunosuppression is supplanted by immunostimulation.

Daily oral CyX, which has been used for induction in some recent nephritis trials, [10,11] is usually initiated at 1 to 2 mg/kg/day. The use of a standard maximum dosage of 2 mg/kg/day, with dose reduction in the presence of leukopenia (white blood cell [WBC] count of less than 3500 cells/mm^3) or neutropenia (WBC count of less than 1000 cells/mm^3), is a common practice. Gradually increasing the dose of CyX with the goal of producing mild leukopenia is another treatment strategy. Although these approaches have not been directly compared in a single trial, it is likely that the avoidance of leukopenia, coupled with prophylaxis against *Pneumocystis carinii*, may significantly reduce morbidity and mortality from infection during daily CyX therapy. Monitoring for toxicity includes weekly complete blood counts (CBCs) initially advancing to monthly when stable, urinalyses to detect hemorrhagic cystitis, and annual urine cytologic studies.

Monthly bolus IVC usually begins with a dose of 500 to 750 mg/m^2 body surface area administered over 1 hour in normal saline. For each subsequent monthly treatment, the dose may be increased 10% to 25% with a goal of achieving a nadir of the WBC count between 2000 and 3000 cells/mm^3. Dose reduction should occur if the nadir of the CBC is a WBC count of less than 2000 cells/mm^3 or a granulocyte count of less than 1000/mm^3. Many physicians limit the maximum CyX dose to 1 g/m^2, with a downward dose adjustment in renal failure. The current evidence-based period of induction using monthly IVC is 6 months. Administering IVC (500 mg) for six doses every 2 weeks, followed by AZA, has also been shown to be effective. Additionally, sodium 2–mercaptoethane sulfonate (MESNA) totaling 80% of the IVC dose (as calculated for intravenous MESNA dosing) is routinely administered in divided doses over 12 hours. The oral dose administered in tablet form is double the intravenous dose; therefore the tablet size of 400 mg is appropriate for patients receiving approximately 1 g IVC. Despite the lack of compelling evidence that this practice is effective in patients with SLE, the use of MESNA has been associated with a very low incidence of IVC-related bladder complications in patients with lupus. Patients unable to empty the bladder completely, such as those with neurogenic bladders, may require catheter drainage or irrigation during treatment. In the authors' institution, two patients with decreased urine output who received IVC without bladder irrigation developed severe hemorrhagic cystitis after treatment. Antiemetic medications, such as granisetron or ondansetron, are also routinely administered; the initial administration of 5 to 20 mg of dexamethasone, 25 to 50 mg of diphenhydramine, and/or 1 mg of lorazepam may also be helpful.

Hemorrhagic Cystitis and Carcinomas of the Bladder

Acrolein, which is directly toxic to the bladder, can cause hemorrhagic cystitis, a premalignant lesion identified in 50% of patients receiving CyX who eventually develop transitional cell carcinoma of the urinary tract; and bladder fibrosis, which has been reported in 5% to 34% of patients receiving daily oral CyX. Hemorrhagic cystitis, which may include either microscopic or gross hematuria (and may be life threatening), mandates permanent discontinuation of CyX, and lifetime annual urologic follow-up. The risk of bladder carcinoma associated with daily CyX therapy is dose dependent and is significantly increased after a total dose of 30 g. In a study of patients with RA, 9 of the 119 patients treated with CyX developed bladder carcinomas after 20 years; of these, 7 received more than 80 g of CyX.[12-15]

In comparison with oral administration, monthly IVC for patients with SLE is rarely complicated by bladder injury except in patients who did not receive intravenous hydration, have urinary tract obstruction, or do not maintain adequate urine output during the 24 hours after treatment. However, IVC cannot be safely administered after bladder complications of daily CyX.

Other Malignancies

Development of malignancies after CyX administration is well described in patients with rheumatic diseases, particularly RA and granulomatosis with polyangiitis (Wegener granulomatosis). Non–urinary tract neoplastic complications of CyX include skin cancers and hematologic malignancies, as well as cervical atypia, which can be observed even in patients who have received cumulative doses of CyX of less than 10 g. In those patients who have received 80 to 120 g cumulative CyX doses, myelodysplastic syndromes are observed, characterized by monozomy-5 or monozomy-7 or both. Long-term follow-up studies by Baltus and associates[13] and Baker and colleagues[14] of patients with RA and treated with oral CyX have established approximately 10% additional incidence of malignancy, compared with age-matched controls after a total dose of 30 g. Doses of less than 10 g are almost certainly safer; doses of 100 g or more are even more likely to produce malignancies. Radis and others[15] reported a 20-year follow-up of the original study by Baker and colleagues[14] and showed continued occurrence of CyX-induced malignancies; after 20 years, only 40% of the original patient population remained free of cancer.

IVC therapy of patients with lupus has not yet been associated with a statistically significant increase in solid tumors, probably because of the lower cumulative doses and the use of intravenous hydration to protect the urinary tract, although a significant increase in cervical intraepithelial neoplasia exists.[16]

Hematologic Toxicity

The acute effects of CyX on the bone marrow are usually benign; stem cells are resistant to CyX. After pulse therapy, the nadir of the lymphocyte count occurs on approximately day 7 to 10 and that of the granulocyte count on approximately day 10 to 14. Usually, a prompt recovery from granulocytopenia occurs after 21 to 28 days. In some patients, the recovery period may be prolonged, necessitating longer dose intervals. Prior use of alkylating agents may be associated with delayed recovery. Immunologically mediated cytopenias often improve after treatment with appropriate doses of IVC, whereas they are more likely to worsen after AZA administration.

Gastrointestinal Toxicity

IVC can be associated with short-term nausea and gastrointestinal (GI) dysmotility during treatment. Occasionally, significant hepatic toxicity may occur with the doses used for autoimmune diseases. With oral or IVC treatment, both anorexia and nausea may occur, particularly with high doses.

Pulmonary Toxicity

Pulmonary toxicity is an infrequent complication during therapy with CyX. Acute interstitial pneumonitis is the most frequently encountered pulmonary involvement of CyX therapy. Pulmonary injury as a result of CyX therapy should be suspected in patients treated with CyX during the previous 6 months before presentation who have bilateral reticular or nodular diffuse opacities on chest x-ray examination or peripheral ground-glass opacities in the upper lung fields on a computed tomographic (CT) scan of the chest. Additionally, a late-onset pneumonitis associated with fibrosis may insidiously develop after months to years of CyX therapy, even with relatively low doses. These late conditions are minimally responsive to corticosteroids, are irreversible, and usually result in terminal respiratory failure or lung transplantation.[17]

Gonadal Toxicity and Teratogenicity

Gonadal failure is an important side effect of CyX in both men and women. CyX is toxic to the granulosa cell and reduces serum estradiol levels and progesterone production, inhibits the maturation of oocytes, and reduces the number of ovarian follicles, ultimately resulting in ovarian failure. Studies in patients with breast cancer receiving CyX show that in women in their 40s, 30s, or 20s, the respective cumulative doses of CyX required to produce ovarian failure were 5, 9, or 20 g, respectively. Amenorrhea or premature ovarian failure is less likely to occur in patients who receive short-term (approximately 6 months) monthly IVC. Some women who develop amenorrhea from CyX subsequently resume menses and are able to bear children.

In addition to minimizing exposure, proposed approaches to fertility preservation include the following: (1) preservation of oocytes, embryos, or ovarian tissue, and (2) the use of depot gonadotropin releasing hormone analogs (GnRH-a) to suppress the metabolism of the ovaries during cytotoxic therapy with CyX. The authors of this text and others have reported favorable results of open trials of depot GnRH-a administration for ovarian protection during monthly IVC therapy. In the authors' study,[18] premature ovarian failure occurred in only 1 of 20 (5%) patients treated with depot GnRH-a, versus 6 of 20 (30%) controls matched for age (mean = 23 years) and cumulative CyX dose (mean = 12 g) (P = <0.05, McNemar test). A metaanalysis has suggested that depot GnRH-a for ovarian protection in women receiving CyX is both safe and effective, and randomized trials are ongoing.[19]

Azoospermia frequently occurs in men after treatment with CyX, and therefore sperm banking should be considered before therapy. In addition, testosterone supplementation has been reported but not proven to offer protection of testicular function in men during CyX therapy.

CyX and its metabolites cross the placenta and appear in breast milk. CyX is a potent teratogen that can cause severe birth defects after administration of as little as 200 mg during early pregnancy. Reported abnormalities included absence of the thumbs, absence of the great toes or all toes, palatal abnormalities, and a single coronary artery.[20] Because fertility is preserved in most patients with lupus, highly effective contraceptive techniques, such as intrauterine devices (IUDs), oral contraceptives, or injected progestins in appropriately selected patients, should be strongly considered. The use of CyX in life-threatening lupus during late pregnancy is controversial but may be appropriate in special circumstances because fetal loss is extremely likely when severe maternal flares are uncontrolled. Major CyX-induced toxicities are believed to occur during the first half of pregnancy.

Infections

The risk of bacterial infections and herpes zoster is increased with CyX therapy, as is the risk of *Pneumocystis carinii* pneumonia (PCP). This risk is further increased when 20 mg/day or more of prednisone or bolus corticosteroids are administered concomitantly. The authors of this text use prophylaxis against PCP, administering either trimethoprim-sulfamethoxazole three times weekly (in patients with lupus already known to tolerate this drug), dapsone (100 mg/day) in patients without glucose-6-phosphate dehydrogenase deficiency, or atovaquone (1500 mg/day). Preexisting or treatment-related hypogammaglobulinemia should be considered in patients who develop

infections. Granulocyte colony–stimulating factor (GCSF) can potentially help decrease the morbidity and mortality associated with accidental severe drug-induced leukopenia during CyX therapy. Although the possibility of inducing lupus flares is a concern, the authors of this text do not use this compound except when the possibility of infection is present. Finally, the syndrome of inappropriate antidiuretic hormone (SIADH) can also occur after administering IVC.

CLINICAL TRIALS ADMINISTERING CYCLOPHOSPHAMIDE FOR LUPUS NEPHRITIS

In this discussion, trials of monthly bolus CyX are emphasized, but many modified regimens have been proposed, such as weekly, biweekly, or a once-every-3-weeks bolus CyX given intravenously, and boluses of CyX given orally. These regimens have been reported to be safe and effective in small series. Results of controlled trials are summarized in eTables 50-1 and 50-2. eTable 50-3 summarizes the results of the controlled trials of sequential therapy using CyX for induction of remission.

In a seminal 20-year clinical trial at the National Institutes of Health (NIH), patients with proliferative nephritis received either prednisone alone or prednisone plus one of the following: AZA (2 mg/kg/day), AZA (1 mg/kg/day) plus CyX (1 mg/kg/day), CyX (2 mg/kg/day), or bolus IVC for approximately 2 to 4 years.[21] Several key findings were revealed: (a) Differences in progression to renal failure were not apparent until more than 5 years had elapsed. After 10 years, however, significant differences in renal survival became apparent, favoring any regimen that included CyX over the administration of prednisone alone. (b) Patients treated with either prednisone alone or with oral CyX had higher death rates than those groups given IVC or AZA plus CyX, which was likely because of the toxicity of daily CyX and the ineffectiveness of prednisone. (c) Oral AZA (1 mg/kg/day) plus CyX (1 mg/kg/day) was equivalent to IVC in terms of preventing renal failure or survival. (d) In serial biopsies, progression of chronic change initially occurred in all patients. Patients who were treated with immunosuppressive agents appeared to stabilize after an initial period of scarring; patients who were treated with prednisone had progressive scarring.

INTRAVENOUS BOLUS CYCLOPHOSPHAMIDE FOR THE TREATMENT OF LUPUS NEPHRITIS

Monthly bolus IVC was first described as a treatment for lupus in the 1980s[6] and for many years was the standard of care for treating severe lupus. Extensive studies have highlighted the issues discussed in the following text.

Relationship of Efficacy and Toxicity to the Effective Dose of Intravenous Cyclophosphamide

In a retrospective study at the NIH,[3] 62 patients with proliferative LN treated with CyX were genotyped for common variant alleles of the P-450 enzyme. Homozygosity or heterozygosity for a particular variant allele (CYP2C19*2) predicted not only lower rates of ovarian toxicity, but also a worse clinical response, including an increased risk of end-stage renal disease and the doubling of serum creatinine, suggesting that efficacy and toxicity were both related to the effective dose given. This study provides the best evidence that higher effective doses of monthly IVC increase both therapeutic response and toxicity.

Advantage of Maintenance Immunosuppression Therapy after Intravenous Cyclophosphamide Induction Therapy

Boumpas and associates[22] confirmed early observations that patients treated with monthly IVC for only 6 months had a high rate of subsequent flares. Seven monthly pulses of IVC, followed by an every-3-month IVC maintenance regimen for 2 years, resulted in significantly fewer flares and fewer doublings of serum creatinine, compared with seven monthly pulses of CyX without maintenance pulses (Figure 50-1). The longer IVC regimens, which became

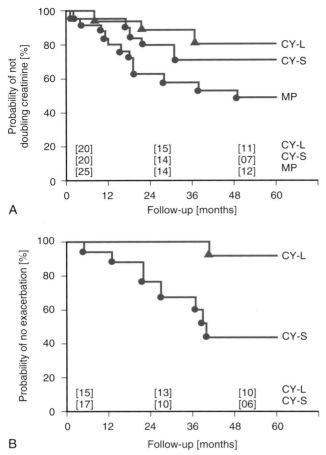

FIGURE 50-1 Treatment of severe lupus nephritis. A, Probability of not doubling serum creatinine levels in 65 patients with severe active lupus nephritis randomly assigned to receive intravenous methylprednisolone (MP) (1.0 g/m² monthly for 6 months); short-course intravenous cyclophosphamide (CY-S) (0.5 to 1.0 g/m² monthly for 6 months); or long-course intravenous cyclophosphamide (CY-L) (0.5 to 1.0 g/m² monthly for 6 months), followed by quarterly infusions for 24 months (Gehan test comparing CY-L with MP, P = .037). **B,** Probability of no exacerbation of lupus activity on completion of monthly pulses in groups randomly assigned to receive CY-L and CY-S (Gehan test, P = .006). Numbers of patients that remain at risk at various times are shown in *brackets* along the abscissa. *(From Boumpas DT, Austin HA, Vaughn EM, et al: Controlled trial of pulse methylprednisolone versus two regimens of pulse cyclophosphamide in severe lupus nephritis. Lancet 340:741–745, 1992. Used with permission.)*

generally accepted as the standard of care for LN, resulted in more toxicity, particularly ovarian failure. It has since been suggested that patients who achieve a complete remission after 6 months may have a lower risk of flare. Nonetheless, prolonged immunosuppression (currently using sequential therapy if IVC is initially used) remains appropriate for the majority of patients.

Concomitant Daily Corticosteroids

All published IVC trials have administered daily oral corticosteroids during induction usually beginning with prednisone (1 mg/kg/day) or equivalent . Administering CyX without corticosteroids for LN (e.g., because of a patient's refusal to take prednisone) is not evidence based and, in the opinion of the authors of this text, unnecessarily exposes patients to a toxic drug using an unproven regimen. One small trial, by Fries and others,[23] addressed this issue in 1973 and compared oral CyX alone with prednisone alone for a mean of 9 weeks in 14 patients with lupus and 10 with nephritis. CyX without prednisone failed to control either minor or major manifestations,

despite the development of leukopenia and significant additional toxicity. Patients who were changed to prednisone from CyX fared better. These results suggest that CyX and prednisone may act synergistically, and CyX without prednisone may be less effective.

Combining Bolus Methylprednisolone with Intravenous Cyclophosphamide

The initial treatment of LN with bolus corticosteroids (e.g., methylprednisolone [MP] [1000 mg/day] for 1 to 3 days) is widely used (including by the authors of this text), especially in patients with severe disease such as crescentic nephritis or acute renal failure. Serial administration of both agents in combination is supported by an NIH study[24] that compared monthly bolus IVC, monthly bolus MP, and the combination of monthly IVC plus bolus MP for LN. During follow-up for a median of 11 years, an intention-to-treat survival analysis revealed the likelihood of treatment failure to be significantly lower in the groups who received CyX (P = 0.04) and combination therapy (P = 0.002) than in the group who received MP alone. Furthermore, the proportion of patients who had doubling of serum creatinine levels was significantly lower in the combination group than in the CyX group. No additional adverse events occurred in the group treated with the combination therapy versus CyX alone, except that patients who received MP pulses had more osteonecrosis.

Racial Differences in Response to Intravenous Cyclophosphamide

Several studies have suggested poorer responses to IVC in African-American versus Caucasian patients. For example, Dooley and associates[25] described poorer renal survival in African Americans during the initial period of monthly IVC administration, with several patients rapidly progressing to renal failure, and further disparity appearing during long-term follow-up studies with renal survival after 5 years at 94.5% for Caucasians and 57% for African Americans. These observations are further supported by the results of trials of induction with MMF versus IVC described in the text that follows.

Sequential Therapy for Lupus Nephritis

In a 2004 study by Contreras and colleagues,[26] 59 patients with LN and the World Health Organization (WHO) class III, IV, or Vb nephritis were treated with monthly IVC for seven doses. Patients were then randomized to maintenance dosing for 1 to 3 years after the initial therapy consisting of quarterly IVC, MMF, or AZA. During maintenance therapy, four deaths occurred in the CyX group and one death was reported in the MMF group; chronic renal failure occurred in three patients in the CyX group, one patient in the MMF group, and one patient in the AZA group. The 72-month, event-free survival, which is defined as no death or progression to hemodialysis, was higher in groups treated with MMF (P = <0.05) and AZA (P = <0.01) versus CyX. The relapse-free survival was also higher in the MMF versus the CyX groups (P = <0.02) (Figure 50-2).

More recently, patients participating in the Aspreva Lupus Management Study (ALMS) were entered into a maintenance phase study that compared maintenance treatment with either MMF or AZA after patients had completed a randomized trial of induction therapy with IVC versus MMF for LN (see the description provided later in this chapter). MMF was superior to IVC in maintaining remissions (Figure 50-3). The data are consistent with the differences observed in the Contreras trial, which showed a statistically significant advantage of MMF but not AZA over IVC administered every 3 months for maintenance. Interestingly, patients who received MMF for maintenance tended to fare better if they had been randomized to receive IVC rather than MMF as induction therapy in the preceding part of the trial.[27]

The intention-to-treat population was made up of 227 patients, of whom 116 were given MMF and 111 were given AZA. Figure 50-3 shows the time to treatment failure (see part A) and the time to renal flare from reference (see part B).[27]

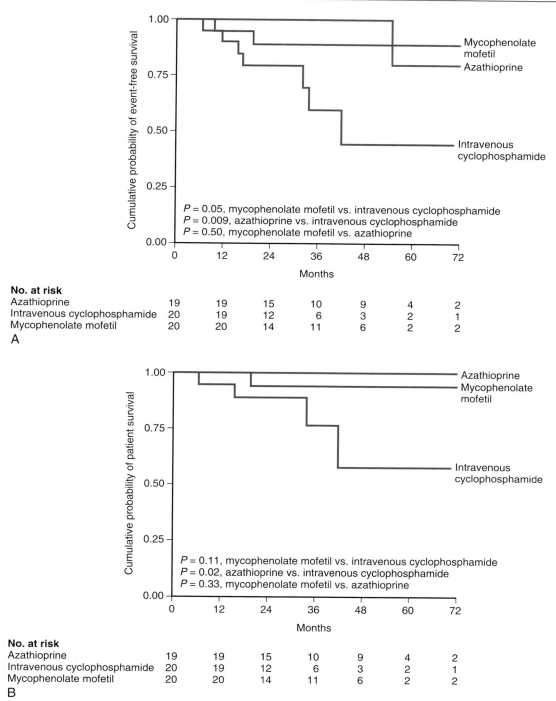

FIGURE 50-2 Mycophenolate mofetil for the treatment of lupus nephritis. *(From Contreras G, Pardo V, Leclercq B, et al: Sequential therapies for proliferative lupus nephritis. N Engl J Med 350:971–980, 2004.)*

Houssiau and associates,[28] on the other hand, did not identify a difference between MMF and AZA as maintenance therapy for LN. Several additional trials have administered daily oral CyX, followed by AZA. For example, Chan and others[29] studied 42 patients with somewhat active diffuse proliferative glomerulonephritis who were randomized to daily CyX for 6 months, followed by AZA versus high-dose MMF for 12 months and then by low-dose MMF for 6 months. At long-term follow-up in the MMF group, 81% experienced a complete remission and 14% experienced a partial remission. In the group randomized to CyX and AZA, 76% experienced a complete remission and 14% experienced a partial remission. Oral CyX appeared to be more toxic than MMF.

As previously noted, the EURO-Lupus study[28] compared high-dose versus low-dose CyX in patients with lupus and proliferative nephritis; they were then switched to maintenance therapy with AZA.

Another group that used sequential therapy, the European League Against Rheumatism (EULAR), conducted a randomized controlled trial of pulse CyX and MP versus continuous CyX and prednisolone, followed by AZA and prednisolone in LN[11]; this study suggested that no significant differences were observed between these two regimens.

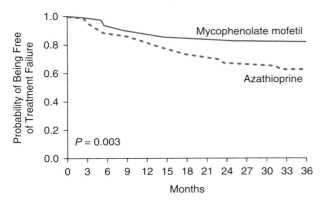

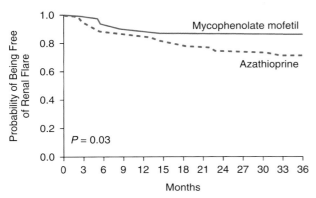

FIGURE 50-3 Kaplan-Meier curves for time-to-treatment failure and time-to-renal flare. *(From Wofsy D, Appel GB, Dooley MA, et al: Aspreva Lupus Management Study maintenance results. Lupus 19:S27, 2010.)*

However, enrollment was difficult, and only 32 patients were treated. The authors encountered cytopenias in the group who received oral CyX (2 mg/kg) and concluded, "…the initial dose of 2 mg/kg oral CyX was felt by the investigators to be too toxic to persist with. The intermittent intravenous pulse regimen appears to be better tolerated than oral continuous treatment, with less severe adverse effects."[11]

INDUCTION THERAPY: COMPARISONS OF INTRAVENOUS CYCLOPHOSPHAMIDE WITH OTHER AGENTS

Intravenous Cyclophosphamide versus Mycophenolate Mofetil

Considerable excitement has been generated by randomized trials that in aggregate have suggested that MMF is either equivalent or superior to IVC as induction therapy for mild to moderately severe LN. Considerable variation in comparative responses to these agents has been demonstrated, both in different racial and ethnic groups and in regions of the world, emphasizing the continuing need to individualize therapy. The following randomized trials have been selected from a larger number to illustrate key points:

Chan and colleagues[29] compared induction with MMF (2 g/day) with long-term MMF maintenance versus daily oral CyX for 6 months, followed by AZA. Patients were from China and had overall moderately active disease. In the MMF group, 81% experienced a complete remission, and 14% experienced partial remission. In the group randomized to CyX followed by AZA, 76% experienced a complete remission and 14% experienced a partial remission. At long-term follow-up, comparable preservation of renal function and reduction of proteinuria were observed.

Ginzler and associates,[30] in a trial that included a high proportion of African-American patients, compared MMF (3 g/day) versus monthly IVC. The higher MMF dose was chosen because of a concern that MMF at 2 g/day was less effective for African Americans than for Caucasians in allogeneic renal transplantation. Patients were required to have creatinine clearances greater than 30 mL/min and serum creatinine levels less than 3.0 mg/dL; overall, they had moderate to very active disease. Patients who did not respond to one regimen were allowed to cross over to the other. At 6 months, the primary endpoint, complete remission, was achieved at a higher rate with MMF than with IVC; however, after 6 months the mean serum creatinine levels and urinary protein excretion were identical when all patients in both groups were considered. A trend revealed that African-American patients responded better to MMF.

Recently, the ALMS trial[31] randomized 370 patients with LN to IVC versus MMF. In contrast to the previously mentioned Ginzler trial,[30] the overall outcomes in terms of both achievement of remission and serious adverse events and mortality were no different in the two groups. However, as detailed in the following text, a significantly higher response rate to MMF than to was achieved in patients of African-American and mestizo descent and individuals of Hispanic origin.[32]

The concern that MMF might not be as effective as IVC in preventing the progression of irreversible renal injury in serial biopsies is addressed in two trials. Ong[33] compared renal biopsies before and after 6 months of MMF (2 g/day) versus IVC and found comparable reduction of NIH activity scores with somewhat greater increases in chronicity scores in the IVC group than in the MMF group.

Hu[34] compared serial renal biopsies in 25 patients treated with MMF versus IVC and showed comparable reductions in activity indices and slight increases in chronicity indices in both groups.

The possibility that brief administration of CyX might be effective in inducing remission was suggested by the Euro-Lupus Nephritis Trial.[35] In this study, 90 patients with proliferative glomerulonephritis were randomized to either high-dose CyX (six monthly and two quarterly pulses, increased according to their WBC nadir) or low-dose CyX (six doses of 500 mg CyX every 2 weeks). Maintenance therapy was with AZA. Renal remission was achieved in 71% of patients receiving low-dose CyX versus 54% of patients who were given high-dose CyX; renal flares were observed in 27% of patients in the low-dose group and 29% of those in the high-dose group.

Pulse Cyclophosphamide versus Intravenous Immunoglobulin

Boletis and others[36] compared IVC with 10 immunoglobulin infusions and found equivalent results over an 18-month period. Proteinuria actually increased slightly in the IVC group.

Oral Cyclophosphamide

Long-term daily CyX has been abandoned for LN, but daily oral CyX continues to be used for induction of remission in some centers.

Daily Oral CyX for Induction

As previously noted, Chan and colleagues[37] randomized 42 patients to either daily CyX for 6 months, followed by AZA for 6 months, or high-dose MMF for 6 months, followed by low-dose MMF. Complete remissions occurred in 81% of those in the MMF group versus 76% of those in the oral CyX group, suggesting that daily CyX is effective for remission induction although it unfortunately results in three times higher cumulative CyX exposure than IVC exposure for a comparable period. In a second study, long-term outcomes in a cohort of patients with lupus and diffuse proliferative nephritis were studied; this cohort received sequential therapy with oral CyX and prednisolone for induction, followed by AZA for maintenance therapy. Of the 66 patients included in the study, 82.4% achieved complete remission, of whom 39.1% experienced relapse during the follow-up period of 91.7 months, ±36.7 months. No end-stage renal failure or death occurred among the patients, although three patients (4.4%) had doubling of baseline creatinine.

Guidelines for Treating Lupus Nephritis

A committee sponsored by the American College of Rheumatology (ACR) has formulated guidelines for the treatment of LN, which should have already been published when this text is available. Either CyX or MMF is considered acceptable first-line therapy. The use of initial bolus MP is encouraged for patients initiating therapy with either CyX or MMF. In the authors' experience, bolus MP will more likely be used in clinical practice in conjunction with IVC rather than with MMF, although the rationale for aggressively initiating corticosteroid treatment is arguably stronger in patients given MMF, since the dose of MMF is gradually increased over 1 to 2 weeks.

Intravenous Cyclophosphamide in Nonrenal Lupus

In general, severe nonrenal manifestations of lupus that result from immune complex disease respond more rapidly and completely to IVC plus corticosteroids than to corticosteroids alone. The required treatment duration and size of the individual IVC boluses vary with different disease manifestations. For example, transverse myelitis may respond to a shorter course of treatment than severe nephritis, and immune-mediated thrombocytopenia may respond to lower than usual doses. During treatment of severe lupus with IVC, improvement of minor manifestations, including constitutional symptoms, fevers, arthralgias, rash, pleurisy, and serologic abnormalities, as well as reduced prednisone requirements, usually occur within 3 months.

Analysis of the recent ALMS trial suggested that nonrenal disease manifestations, in general, responded well to either IVC or MMF and that no significant differences were reported in the responses to one or the other.[38]

Neuropsychiatric Lupus

No clear guidelines exist regarding therapy for neuropsychiatric lupus (NP-SLE) with various modalities, including corticosteroids, CyX, and/or anticoagulation. Distinction among various primary pathogenic mechanisms, such as immune complex–mediated vasculitis, antibody-mediated cerebral injury, microangiopathy, and thrombosis, and secondary causes, such as atherosclerosis or infection, is notoriously difficult and is further complicated by the multifactorial etiologic origin of many events. In many cases, skilled physicians must make a "seat-of-the-pants" decision regarding the use of immunosuppression, anticoagulation, or both, based on clinical, serologic, or magnetic resonance imaging evidence, unless there is biopsy evidence of tissue inflammation or cerebrospinal fluid pleocytosis. In many series, treatment decisions have been made (apparently appropriately) on the basis of clinical judgment rather than on specific inclusion criteria.

Active, steroid-refractory cerebral lupus that is adjudged to be secondary to immunologically mediated injury has responded well to IVC with or without bolus MP in most cases. Anticoagulation has been simultaneously used when distinguishing thrombotic from inflammatory disease has been impossible or to rule out the possibility that vascular inflammation is contributing to the development of thrombosis. Neither the presence of antiphospholipid antibodies nor the involvement of one or more large vessels rules out the use of immunosuppression as opposed to (or in addition to) anticoagulation. Boumpas and associates[39] treated nine patients with monthly doses of IVC, three of whom had transverse myelitis and five of whom had focal neurologic findings, seizures, or both. The duration

of symptoms ranged from 3 to 45 days. All nine patients had findings suggesting an inflammatory process, including anti-DNA antibodies, and five had cerebrospinal fluid pleocytosis. Five of these patients concomitantly had antiphospholipid antibodies. All patients recovered either partially or completely. These observations suggest that in selected patients who have antiphospholipid antibodies that may not be the major cause of their events, IVC administration is associated with clinical improvement.

Other series of IVC in NP-SLE report favorable results. Neuwelt and others[40] retrospectively reviewed 31 patients with NP-SLE who were treated with IVC and in whom a variety of prior therapies had failed, including corticosteroids, warfarin, chlorambucil, and AZA. Indications included organic brain syndrome in 55% of patients, strokes in 35%, peripheral mononeuropathies in 32%, seizures in 29%, and transverse myelitis in 16%. Patients with anticardiolipin antibodies were treated with warfarin. Treatment regimens varied from low-to-high doses of IVC, and plasmapheresis was added in some patients when they appeared not to improve after IVC. Overall, 61% of patients were reported to improve, of whom 26% were not initially improved after 9 months of therapy and appeared to respond to the addition of plasmapheresis. The failure rate for patients with organic brain syndrome was 83%, compared with 37% for other indications. Malaviya and associates[41] treated 14 patients with a variety of focal and diffuse neurologic deficits. All patients except the two with seizures stabilized or improved.

Numerous studies have demonstrated improvement of transverse myelitis with IVC, with or without bolus corticosteroids. Because of the catastrophic nature of transverse myelitis and the importance of prompt therapeutic intervention, it may be appropriate to have a very low threshold for prompt institution of IVC when this syndrome appears suddenly, with or without concomitant high-dose ($1 g/m^2$) MP. In the authors' institution, prompt use of bolus CyX for transverse myelitis has been associated with the preservation of the ability to ambulate in most patients, although many have continued to have neurogenic bladders.

Ten patients with bilateral corticosteroid-refractory optic neuritis and severe visual compromise were treated with bolus IVC for 6 months.[133] Of the 20 patients, the eyes recovered completely in 10 patients and partially in 6, but the eyes of 4 patients did not recover.

Baca[42] treated seven children with NP-SLE (including seizures, focal neurologic deficits, transverse myelitis, and organic brain syndromes) with monthly bolus CyX combined with three initial boluses of MP (30 mg/kg). Three patients had anticardiolipin antibodies but did not undergo anticoagulation. Six patients recovered completely, and one had a minor residual deficit.

Neuromyelitis optica (NMO), which is characterized by antibodies to aquaporin-4, transverse myelitis and optic neuritis, occurs with increased frequency in patients with SLE. In the authors' lupus cohort, transverse myelitis occurred in 23 of 856 patients, and NMO and NMO-spectrum disorders occurred in one third of these patients (unpublished data). Although the neurologic literature encourages the use of AZA or rituximab or both in patients without SLE, the authors of this text have chosen to use IVC plus bolus corticosteroids in their patients, with success comparable to their other patients with transverse myelitis. The increased risk of recurrence in NMO encourages prolonged immunosuppression.

Other Disease Manifestations

Numerous corticosteroid-refractory manifestations of lupus have been reported to benefit from pulse CyX in case reports and uncontrolled series, including systemic vasculitis, GI vasculitis, and pneumatosis intestinalis. Hematologic conditions reported to respond include aplastic anemia, acquired factor VIII deficiency, and acquired von Willebrand disease, as well as lupus-induced cytopenias, particularly thrombocytopenia. Thrombocytopenia in active lupus may possibly respond to lower pulses of CyX than are necessary to control other disease manifestations. Roach and Hutchinson[43] successfully treated steroid-refractory thrombocytopenia on two occasions in one patient with only one 400 mg dose of IVC. Boumpas and colleagues[44] found overall improvement of thrombocytopenia in patients who were treated according to the NIH protocol. Although IVC should not, in the authors' opinion, be substituted for plasmapheresis and plasma exchange in thrombotic thrombocytopenic purpura (TTP) in patients with lupus, it has been added to plasma exchange for this indication. Bolus CyX alone may be ineffective for lupus-related TTP; two of the authors' patients developed TTP during monthly bolus CyX therapy for nephritis, and, despite the prompt addition of plasma exchange, one patient died and the other progressed to renal failure.

Several studies suggest that lupus-related interstitial lung disease and bronchiolitis obliterans may respond to monthly CyX. Fukada and associates[45] also noted a response of pulmonary hemorrhage to IVC. In the authors' experience, IVC is associated with control of pulmonary hemorrhage in the majority of patients with lupus that appears to be steroid refractory. Although cases of idiopathic inflammatory myositis have not uniformly responded well to IVC in the published literature, three patients with SLE were reported by Kono and others[46] to have remission of refractory polymyositis with the addition of IVC. An important caveat is that pulmonary hemorrhage that is the result of co-existent antiphospholipid syndrome may not respond to conventional immunosuppression. Deane and colleagues[47] have reported favorable responses to intravenous immunoglobulin (IVIG), which the authors of this text have also observed.

In summary, these nonrenal manifestations of lupus appear to respond to IVC in most cases when steroid therapy apparently fails. However, these results do not establish the superiority of intravenous over oral CyX for these indications.

Bolus Cyclophosphamide in Children

IVC has been successfully used in children of all ages, including infants. Studies by Lehman and Onel[48] of treatment with IVC for 36 months have shown good disease control and arrest of progression of the chronicity index. This group has also added intravenous MTX to CyX in refractory cases with benefit. Because of its toxicity, daily oral CyX is clearly less desirable in children with lupus, as it is in adults, and it should not be used as first-line therapy instead of bolus CyX.

Aggressive Cyclophosphamide-Containing Regimens

High-dose CyX regimens sufficient to arrest the production of hematopoietic cells are being tried in lupus. Because stem cells are resistant to CyX, the bone marrow recovers after a period, requiring support with cells and colony-stimulating factors. Brodsky and colleagues[49] reported treating patients with severe SLE with CyX (200 mg/kg), with complete responses in one half of the patients; there were no deaths. Another study by Petri and colleagues[50] examined the effect of high-dose CyX in a group of 14 patients with lupus between the ages of 21 and 45 years in whom prior immunosuppressive therapy (5 of 14 had prior CyX) had failed. A complete renal response was achieved in 5 patients, a partial response in 7, and no response in 2, 1 of whom had renal failure. Systemic Lupus Erythematosus Disease Activity Index (SLEDAI) scores significantly improved (pretreatment average score was 6.8, posttreatment average score was 2.7), and prednisone doses were also significantly decreased after treatment (20 mg to 5 mg). A later randomized trial that compared high-dose CyX with monthly IVC in 51 enrolled patients with severe lupus (including 22 patients with LN) found that this regimen was no better than standard IVC treatment. At 6 months, the complete response rate was 52% in the high-dose group versus 35% in the traditional group; at 30 months, the response rate was numerically but not significantly higher in the traditional group (65% versus 48%). The authors noted that some patients crossed over from traditional to high-dose CyX as treatment; five failures appeared to respond to the higher dose regimen.[51]

Autologous stem cell transplantation using high-dose CyX with or without additional immunosuppressives is being evaluated in a number of rheumatic diseases. One study reported enrollment of nine patients in a protocol, of whom one died during induction and seven ultimately underwent transplantation. Fluid overload occurred in all patients; three required dialysis or hemofiltration, and two were intubated. All patients responded clinically and were able to discontinue immunosuppressive medications. The dramatic disease suppression reported appears to exceed that of high-dose CyX regimens. However, the short-term toxicity appears to be greater. Across the world, the mortality of stem cell transplantation for rheumatic diseases exceeds 10%. This figure may improve with modifications of treatment regimens and criteria for patient selection.

Summary of Cyclophosphamide Therapy for Lupus

1. No evidence suggests that IVC is more effective than oral CyX in patients with lupus in the long run, but it is unquestionably less toxic.
2. Prednisone has been used with oral CyX or IVC in all studies showing efficacy. Daily oral CyX without prednisone was not effective in one study.
3. Addition of bolus MP to monthly bolus CyX for LN has the potential to improve efficacy with only modest increased risk of toxicity.
4. The cumulative dose of CyX predicts the risk of gonadal injury and the risk of secondary malignancies. Meticulous surveillance for malignant and premalignant conditions, especially those resulting from human papilloma virus (HPV), is indicated in patients treated with CyX.
5. Maintenance therapy with MMF after remission induction in nephritis may be superior to maintenance with AZA; maintenance with IVC every 3 months is more toxic and is usually less effective; and maintenance therapy with AZA or MMF may provide equivalent or superior protection against flares with reduced toxicity. In the event of a partial but unsatisfactory response, continued monthly treatment after the initial 6 months may be successful. Sequential therapy should be considered in all patients receiving CyX as induction therapy for LN after 6 months.
7. Proteinuria and features of nephrotic syndrome usually improve substantially during the first 6 to 12 months. Although patients who are not in complete remission after 6 months (e.g., proteinuria reduced but not yet less than 1 g) may have continued reduction of proteinuria during less intensive therapy, those in whom remission is not achieved after 6 months have a worse prognosis and presumably require more aggressive therapy than patients in whom remission has been achieved.
8. Patients with renal insufficiency average approximately 30% improvement in creatinine clearance during the first 6 months, but they tend to backslide toward baseline values after 1 to 2 years. It is interesting to speculate that this may be the result of continued glomerular scarring in the apparent absence of inflammation, as described by Chaghac 5 in total lymphoid irradiation–treated patients with LN. However, it is possible that inflammation recurs as immunosuppression is reduced or that other processes such as occult hypertension and hyperfiltration may be important factors.
9. The indications for IVC therapy for neurologic disease are poorly characterized. The possibility that an antiphospholipid antibody syndrome exists is not, in itself, a contraindication to the treatment of apparent inflammatory disease. In catastrophic neurologic disease in which the cause is unclear, combined anticoagulation and immunosuppression should be considered.

CHLORAMBUCIL

Chlorambucil, an alkylating agent with immunosuppressive effects similar to those of CyX, is a potent oncogene and, in this regard more dangerous than CyX. Somatic and germ-cell mutations,[52,53] leukemias, myelodysplastic syndromes, and cutaneous malignancies are increased. Patapanian and others[54] identified significant excess malignancies, compared with controls, in 39 patients with RA and treated with chlorambucil after 5 years of follow-up; three hematologic and eight cutaneous malignancies were identified. Although chlorambucil has been shown to be effective (and toxic) in idiopathic membranous nephritis and the nephrotic syndrome,[55] studies of this potent alkylating agent in patients with SLE are inadequate to permit comparison with other immunosuppressive drugs. Nonetheless, combined with prednisone, chlorambucil is almost certainly effective. Importantly, because chlorambucil is not metabolized to acrolein (in contrast to CyX), no risk of hemorrhagic cystitis exists; it is therefore safer for oral administration than CyX in patients with neurogenic bladders and for patients with prior hemorrhagic cystitis for whom additional CyX is contraindicated.

In 1973, Snaith and associates[56] reported that six female patients with lupus and steroid-resistant disease activity had improvement in their disease after using chlorambucil. Of the six patients, five had biopsy-proven focal proliferative disease, whereas the sixth patient had peripheral vascular lesions and hemolysis. Amenorrhea developed in four patients. Epstein and Grausz[57] reported improved survival in 16 patients with lupus and diffuse proliferative nephritis after receiving chlorambucil in addition to prednisone, compared with 15 patients who were treated with prednisone alone. They also reported serious toxicities, including marrow aplasia in 5 of the 16 patients, which led to the death of 1 patient. In a retrospective study, Sabbour and Osman[58] found that patients with diffuse proliferative nephritis who were treated with a combination of chlorambucil and corticosteroids had resolution or regression of the renal pathologic manifestations, significant improvement of the renal function, and survival.

Summary of Chlorambucil Therapy for Lupus

Chlorambucil has been largely abandoned for the treatment of lupus because of its severe toxicity associated with long-term use. Because short-term use of chlorambucil for remission induction would result in less toxicity, this compound may be valuable for induction in selected cases, such as individuals with neurogenic bladders.

AZATHIOPRINE

AZA has been in use for longer than 50 years for organ transplantation and treatment of rheumatic diseases. Although less potent and slower in onset of efficacy than CyX as a treatment for patients with acute severe SLE, AZA is useful both as a steroid-sparing agent and as a maintenance drug to be used after initial control of LN with CyX.

AZA is inactive as administered and is metabolized intracellularly to the purine antagonists 6-mercaptopurine (6MP) and 6-thioinosinic acid. The immunologic effects of AZA and 6MP differ, despite the fact that 6MP is the major active metabolite of AZA, suggesting that additional metabolites of AZA may also be active. AZA reduces the numbers of T cells, B cells, and natural killer cells, thereby inhibiting both cellular and humoral immunity, suppressing autoantibody formation, and inhibiting prostaglandin synthesis.

In contrast to CyX, AZA has not established itself as an initial therapeutic agent in LN, and it has been sufficiently studied to discourage its use as a single agent for this purpose. Recent studies have emphasized the potential role of AZA as a maintenance drug after induction of remission in LN.

The caveats that apply to older studies of nephritis (e.g., the lack of effective agents to control conditions affecting treatment outcome such as hypertension and hyperlipidemia) apply to the historical evidence regarding AZA as a first-line agent (see eTable 50-1). The following controlled studies of AZA have yielded disparate results, suggesting that AZA is effective in some patients but not all.

In the large NIH trial, low-dose AZA added to low-dose CyX plus prednisone was as effective as IVC (administered every 3 months) plus prednisone, with comparable mortality and toxicity.[59] Compared with oral CyX, renal survival was the same, but there was a trend with the combination regimen that failed to reach statistical significance and association with lower mortality. Thus AZA appears to have a CyX-sparing effect when used in combination with that drug. Overall outcomes in the NIH study of AZA alone plus prednisone were intermediate between prednisone and CyX-containing regimens and failed to achieve significance, although the combinations were better than prednisone alone. In the authors' opinion, the slow onset of action of AZA may be partially responsible for its failure as an initial therapy for active nephritis, and the studies that follow do not necessarily suggest that it will not be effective as an agent either in early, relatively mild nephritis or as a maintenance agent after initial control of severe nephritis has been achieved.

Donadio and colleagues[60] randomized 16 patients to AZA plus prednisone versus prednisone alone. After 6 months, histologic measures of disease activity (e.g., karyorrhexis, proliferation, fibrinoid deposition, hyaline thrombi, necrosis) improved in both groups, but no difference in outcome was achieved after 6 months or after 2 to 3 years.[61] Hahn and others[62] randomized patients with lupus who were severely ill to prednisone with or without AZA over a 2-year period and found no differences in outcomes.

In a study that illustrates the difficulty of distinguishing the toxicity of one drug regimen from the efficacy of alternate therapy, Cade and associates[63] used four different regimens to treat 50 patients with lupus, including prednisone alone, prednisone plus AZA, AZA alone, and AZA plus heparin. Unfortunately, 13 of 15 patients treated with prednisone alone died, with a mean survival of 19 months, after receiving prednisone (60 to 100 mg/day) for 6 months. In the AZA plus prednisone group, which received lower doses of prednisone, 9 of 13 patients survived, with a mean survival of 38 months. Compared with the very-high-dose prednisone regimen AZA alone or in combination with either prednisone or heparin produced superior results. In a double-blind, crossover trial, Ginzler and others[64] compared AZA plus prednisone with prednisone alone for LN and found no benefit.

A recent European trial demonstrated inferiority of induction with AZA versus IVC (see "Cyclophosphamide" earlier in this chapter). The authors of this text do not use AZA as initial therapy in either mild or severe LN.

Esdaile[65] conducted an elegant study of patients who received immunosuppressive agents for LN. Almost all patients who were immunosuppressed were treated with AZA. When patients who received early biopsies and treatment were compared with those who had delayed biopsies and treatment, there was a striking greater preservation of renal function and reduced mortality in the early treatment group. These patients, who were less sick than those reported in earlier trials previously described, appeared to respond to treatment with AZA, suggesting that even weak immunosuppressive agents are more effective for the treatment of LN if promptly begun at the time of onset of LN.

AZA has been used for a variety of nonrenal indications in patients with active SLE. During a controlled trial in patients with active nonrenal lupus, Sztejnbok and colleagues[66] added AZA (2.5 mg/kg/day) to prednisone in one half of the patients. AZA was reported to be unhelpful in controlling acute disease but provided steroid-sparing effects and reduced mortality. A study randomizing patients with well-controlled lupus to continuation or withdrawal of AZA has demonstrated more exacerbations in patients who discontinued the drug.[67]

AZA has been reported to be effective in severe cutaneous lupus in several series[68-70] and to have a steroid-sparing effect. AZA has been reported to be useful in treating chronic active hepatitis complicating lupus, as well as non–virally-mediated chronic active hepatitis in patients without lupus. The relatively slow onset of action and the lack of dramatic responses of disease activity to this drug mandate consummate clinical judgment on the part of the treating physician when decisions are made regarding whether the use of this agent has been effective. The fetal liver lacks the enzyme necessary to convert

AZA into its active form.[71] In a study of pregnant patients with inflammatory bowel disease taking AZA or 6MP, no increase in pregnancy complications or congenital malformations were reported.[72] After conducting a retrospective study of patients at the University of Michigan, the authors of this text recently presented the findings, in abstract form, of the increased likelihood of developmental delays in children of mothers who took AZA for SLE during pregnancy; an unexpected finding mandating further study.

Long-term use of AZA has been variably reported to be associated with the development of lymphomas. There is an increased risk of cutaneous malignancies and HPV–related premalignant and malignant lesions. In the authors' experiences, long-term use of AZA can be associated with cytopenia and it is often difficult to distinguish whether this is the result of AZA toxicity, recurrent lupus, or both.

Summary of Azathioprine Therapy for Lupus

AZA is less effective than either CyX or MMF as initial therapy for proliferative nephritis, although the combination of daily AZA in addition to CyX (1 mg/kg each) was highly effective in one study. AZA is effective as a maintenance drug after induction of remission of LN with IVC or MMF, although recent trials suggest that MMF may be a better initial choice for this purpose. AZA spares both corticosteroids and CyX. Although slow in onset of action, AZA remains a very useful agent in mild to moderately severe SLE. This generic drug has been approved by the U.S. Food and Drug Administration (FDA) for the treatment of lupus and is much less expensive than biologic agents such as belimumab or rituximab, which are agents that have not been shown to be more effective than AZA for the control of corticosteroid-resistant nonrenal lupus. Long-term use of AZA is associated with increased risk of both cutaneous and HPV–related malignancies and possibly with lymphoma.

CYCLOSPORINE AND TACROLIMUS

CS, a calcineurin inhibitor, and TACRO, which binds to FK-binding proteins (FKBP), have complex immunologic effects, including inhibition of T-cell gene activation and inhibition of transcription of genes for interleukin (IL)–2, tumor necrosis factor–alpha (TNF-α), IL-3, IL-4, cluster of differentiation 40 (CD40)–ligand, GCSF, and other cytokines. In addition, they inhibit the recruitment of antigen-presenting cells and antigen presentation, IL-17 production by T-helper (Th)17 cells, and T cell–dependent antibody production by B cells. They do not, however, inhibit growth of bone marrow–derived cell lines.[73]

CS and TACRO are administered orally or intravenously with significant variation in bioavailability after the oral dose. TACRO is also available for topical use. The following discussion focuses on CS, which has been more widely used in the treatment of SLE.

Absorption of CS requires the formation of an emulsion with bile and can be altered by GI conditions, including diarrhea, malabsorption, and delayed gastric emptying. The drug is highly lipophilic, and levels may be increased in patients with hypocholesterolemia. It is eliminated by cytochrome P-450 with the formation of multiple metabolites and excreted in the bile. CS levels are influenced by numerous medications. As a consequence, careful monitoring of CS levels is recommended at currently used doses.

Nephrotoxicity is a major adverse effect. Acute declines in renal function, manifested by increased serum creatinine levels and hypertension, are usually reversible with the discontinuation of CS. Acute toxicity is associated with renal vasoconstriction, is exacerbated by nonsteroidal antiinflammatory agents, and can delay recovery from acute tubular necrosis (ATN), which is often identified in biopsies in acute LN. The associated vasoconstriction can be reduced by calcium channel blockers. Chronic nephrotoxicity contributes to renal failure and death in patients who have undergone renal transplantation and is associated with long-term continuous exposure to either CS or TACRO.[74]

Biopsies reveal an obliterative arteriolopathy, glomerulosclerosis tubular atrophy, and interstitial fibrosis. These changes have been described as appearing in an early, potentially reversible stage at 6 months and progressing to irreversible injury after 3 years. Reduction of glomerular filtration rate (GFR) may be underestimated because of compensatory hyperfiltration, especially in membranous nephritis, and because of the increasing contribution of tubular secretion of creatinine to the measured creatinine clearance as renal function declines. This latter side effect appears to be related to dose, but it is not completely absent even in studies using doses as low as 2 mg/kg. In a population of 192 adults and children, including 152 with diabetes, who were treated with CS for a mean of 13 months before biopsy, 41 had biopsy findings that were consistent with CS-induced nephropathy. Nephropathy is associated with the maximal dose, mean dose, and cumulative dose before biopsy.[75]

Two studies illustrate the risks of CS (5 mg/kg/day) in patients with normal kidneys: Deray and associates[76] evaluated 16 patients with autoimmune uveitis initially treated with CS (5 mg/kg/day). CS was adjusted according to the serum creatinine. A progressive decline of creatinine clearance occurred throughout the study from the baseline of 120 mL/min to 75 mL/min at 24 months. The GFR decreased from 116.8 to 75.3 mL/min, and the total cholesterol levels significantly increased. Altman and others[77] sequentially treated patients with RA with a regimen of: (1) a nonsteroidal antiinflammatory drug (NSAID), (2) CS (5 mg/kg), and (3) both the NSAID and CS. At the end of the study, a significant increase in blood urea nitrogen and creatinine levels in 9 of 11 patients was reported, and an additive effect of the two drugs was postulated. This side effect, in the authors' opinion, is the major potential limiting factor in its use in SLE. Nakamura and associates[78] followed 23 Japanese children treated with CS for lupus or idiopathic nephritis and found that 11 had no toxicity, 7 had reversible toxicity, and 5 had irreversible toxicity. The maintenance dose, blood levels, and duration of treatment were all predictive of toxicity.

Compared with alkylating agents, bone marrow suppression is uncommon with CS. Lymphoproliferative syndromes are frequently observed in patients who have undergone organ transplantation and treatment with CS, but these syndromes are rare in patients with autoimmune disorders. CS appears to have little, if any, ovarian toxicity and has been used in a limited number of pregnancies without obvious birth defects. Hypertension has been observed in 50% to 80% of transplant recipients. CS impairs the excretion of potassium, uric acid, and magnesium, and it is a notorious cause of refractory gout. It can cause hypomagnesemia and has been implicated in central nervous system toxicity, including headache, tremors, and, occasionally, focal neurologic defect. Hirsutism, gingival hyperplasia, and GI disturbances may also occur.

The few controlled trials of CS in patients with SLE suggest overall efficacy in patients with both nephritis and nonrenal lupus.

Induction Therapy of Nephritis

Balletta and colleagues[79] randomized 10 patients with LN to either CS (3 mg/kg/day) plus prednisone or to prednisone alone. After 12 months, no significant change in creatinine or creatinine clearance occurred, but in the CS-treated group, proteinuria declined from 2.7 to 0.3 g/24 hr, whereas in the prednisone-alone group, proteinuria increased from 2.1 to 2.6 g/24 hr.

In an open randomized trial, Fu and associates[80] treated 40 children with WHO class III or IV LN with either CS (2.5 to 5 mg/kg) alone (without corticosteroids) or prednisolone (2 mg/kg) plus CyX (2 mg/kg) orally for 1 year. At entry, all children had growth retardation after 1 year or more of corticosteroids. Subjects received an intense regimen of corticosteroids just before randomization until lupus activity diminished. Comparable control of disease activity and resolution of proteinuria were achieved. Hemolytic complement (CH$_{50}$) and C3 levels were actually lower at the end of treatment in the CS group. The authors concluded that CS controlled clinical but not serologic activity.

Austin[81] randomized 42 patients with class V LN to (1) cyclosporine A (CsA) beginning at 5 mg/kg, (2) alternate-month IVC for six doses, versus (3) prednisone alone (all patients in the study received prednisone). Because of concerns for CsA-induced toxicities, seven patients with a GFR less than 67 mL/min per 1.73 m² body surface area were not randomly assigned to CsA. Both the CS and IVC groups had a higher rate of remission of proteinuria than the prednisone group. The CS group had a higher rate of relapse and relapsed sooner than the IVC group. It is noteworthy that these differences were observed even though IVC is likely less effective when administered in alternate months rather than monthly.

Zavada[82] randomized 40 patients to induction with IVC versus CS. The percent of patients achieving complete and partial responses was comparable in the two groups. Patients treated with CS had significantly more reduction of proteinuria, whereas patients treated with IVC had a significantly greater reduction of serum creatinine.

These studies suggest that CS is effective in reducing proteinuria in LN but may be less effective in improving renal function and/or producing sustained remissions.

Maintenance of Remission after Treatment of Lupus Nephritis with Cyclophosphamide

Moroni and others[83] treated 75 patients with class IV nephritis with bolus corticosteroids, daily prednisone, and daily CyX (2 mg/kg) for 3 months. Patients were then randomized to CS beginning at 4 mg/kg or AZA maintenance starting at 1.6 mg/kg. At 2 and 4 years, substantial reduction in proteinuria and the equivalent prevention of flares were achieved. Although the differences were not statistically significant, after 2 years the mean creatinine clearance declined from 92.5 ± 22 to 82.6 ± 20 mL/min in the CS group and increased from 104.1 ± 46.5 to 109.9 ± 43 mL/min in the AZA group, a trend that is consistent with the hypothesis that long-term CS administration risks the loss of renal function, although 12% of the patients treated with CS had increased levels of creatinine.

Nonrenal Lupus

Griffiths and colleagues[84] randomized 89 patients with active SLE, despite the use of prednisolone (>15 mg/day) to CS (2.5 mg/day) versus AZA (2 mg/kg day). After 12 months the primary outcome, a reduction in the prednisolone dose was similar (CS [9.0 mg]; AZA [10.7 mg/day]). The incidences of adverse outcomes and flares were similar and sustained rises in creatinine were not observed.

TACROLIMUS
Tacrolimus for Induction Therapy of Lupus Nephritis

Although TACRO has not been as extensively studied as CyX, MMF, or AZA, the available studies suggest that TACRO plus corticosteroids is an effective induction regimen for LN.

Chen[85] randomized 81 patients with LN to prednisone plus either TACRO titrated to a trough concentration of 5 to 10 ng/mL or IVC for 6 months. Outcomes were reported to be similar with more rapid reduction of proteinuria in the TACRO group and a numerically higher rate of achieving complete remission (52% versus 39%). Creatinine levels were comparable, and the rate of leukopenia was less in the TACRO group.[85]

Li[86] randomized 60 patients with classes III, IV, and/or V LN to receive MMF (2 g/day), TACRO (trough level 6 to 8 ng/mL) or IVC (0.5 to 0.75 g/m²) in combination with corticosteroids. In this 24-week study the rates of complete and partial remission were comparable in the three groups, although the combined response was lower in the IVC group. Proteinuria decreased more quickly in the TACRO group.[86]

Combined Tacrolimus and Mycophenolate Mofetil Therapy

Bao[87] randomized patients with the combination of class IV plus class V nephritis and creatinine clearances greater than 30 mL/min, presumably representing a group that is difficult to treat, to receive either the combination of MMF adjusted to a target area under the curve of 20 to 45 mg*h/L, plus TACRO (4 mg/day) with a target trough level of 5 to 7 ng/mL or monthly IVC for 6 months. After 6 or 9 months, patients receiving combined therapy had a significantly higher rate of achieving complete remission (50% and 65%, respectively) than those receiving IVC (5% and 15%, respectively). Serial renal biopsies showed no evidence of TACRO-induced nephrotoxicity. Those who achieved a remission had less progression of the NIH chronicity index on serial biopsies. These favorable results encourage further study of this regimen. Targeting the area under the curve of MMF possibly improved the efficacy of this compound, accounting for some of the advantage of MMF in outcome versus IVC.[87]

As a cautionary note, Lanata[88] found that adding TACRO to MMF in cases resistant to careful management of MMF alone was associated with a high failure rate. This suggests that adding TACRO in patients for whom MMF has failed may not be a reliable alternative to switching to CyX.[88]

CALCINEURIN INHIBITORS FOR SKIN DISEASE

Topical preparations of TACRO or pimecrolimus were used alone or in combination with antimalarial medications in 40 patients with cutaneous lupus. Improvement occurred in all groups but was increased when the combination of a topical agent and hydroxychloroquine was used.[89]

Summary of Calcineurin Inhibitors

The available evidence suggests that both CS and TACRO are useful in managing SLE. CS appears to be comparable to IVC administered every other month, a regimen of unknown potency for initial treatment of membranous LN, although its use was associated with an increased likelihood of flare and a shorter time to flare after the cessation of treatment. It also has been reported to be comparable to AZA, both as a maintenance agent after the treatment of proliferative glomerulonephritis and as a steroid-sparing agent in patients with active systemic disease.

The combination of TACRO and extremely carefully titrated MMF as initial therapy of class IV plus V nephritis was notably superior to IVC alone; however, the effectiveness of "rescue" treatment in patients in whom MMF fails has not been established. These agents are attractive because of their lack of bone marrow toxicity and their safety in pregnancy. Although they appear to be particularly effective in reducing proteinuria, they remain less well studied than MMF, AZA, and CyX.

METHOTREXATE

MTX is a folate antagonist that inhibits dihydrofolate reductase. It was synthesized in the 1940s and was initially used for its cytotoxic role against tumor cells. When administered at the doses used in rheumatic diseases, it has more immunomodulatory properties and the cytotoxic effects are less obvious. There is no convincing association of changes in lymphocyte subsets, surface markers, lymphocyte function, or autoantibody levels with the therapeutic effects on rheumatic diseases. MTX appears to have multiple antiinflammatory effects, which have been ascribed to its ability to stimulate adenosine release. In turn, adenosine can suppress the inflammatory functions of neutrophils, macrophages, and lymphocytes.[90] Despite being the cornerstone for treating RA, the exact mechanism by which it works in lupus remains unclear.

MTX is administered orally or subcutaneously with a usual dose range of 10 to 30 mg in adults and up to 0.5 mg/kg/wk in children, in conjunction with folic acid (1 mg/day); adult doses (more than 20 mg/wk) are often administered subcutaneously. Subcutaneous administration is associated with reduced side effects and slightly increased effectiveness. Studies have demonstrated that MTX side effects occurred less frequently in patients with RA who were given 1 mg of folic acid daily; the antiinflammatory effects of MTX were unaltered.[91] Dividing the weekly dose into two doses 12 hours apart and administering folinic acid (5 mg) the day after MTX have been suggested to reduce GI and constitutional side effects.

The side effects of MTX, particularly hepatotoxicity and bone marrow suppression, have been well described. MTX toxicity, especially to the bone marrow, is increased in patients with renal dysfunction, and the risk increases in patients maintained on a stable dose of MTX in the presence of declining renal function[92]; following serum creatinine levels during treatment is prudent. Severe renal dysfunction is a contraindication to MTX use.

MTX-induced lung injury, which has been reported in 2% to 7% of patients with RA, is characterized by cough, bilateral or unilateral pulmonary infiltrates, and dyspnea.[93,94] A nonspecific interstitial inflammatory cell infiltrate and an increased number of T cells are evident in bronchoalveolar lavage fluid.[93] Reported mortality is 17%, with a 50% recurrence rate on rechallenge and up to 50% mortality associated with recurrences. *Pneumocystis jiroveci* prophylaxis for patients receiving MTX plus moderate-to-high doses of corticosteroids should reduce the number of episodes of *Pneumocystis jiroveci* pneumonia (PJP) pneumonitis, requiring distinction from MTX pneumonitis.

MTX is teratogenic and is classified as Category X by the FDA. Women of childbearing age should be alerted, and effective contraception should be instituted. In the authors' center, patients are encouraged to use an IUD as a means of contraception. No conclusive evidence exists regarding fertility and conception in men taking MTX. Several studies suggest that stopping MTX at least 3 months before attempting conception should be recommended to the future father.[95] MTX-induced malignancies appear to be rare. A reversible lymphoproliferative disease can occur and has been reported to evolve into Hodgkin disease.[96]

Since the first report on the use of MTX for the treatment of RA in 1951, multiple controlled trials have proven the efficacy and safety of MTX in the treatment of RA, but a paucity of data is available for patients with SLE. The authors of this text know of only two controlled trials that have evaluated the role of MTX in patients with SLE. In a double-blind, randomized, placebo-controlled trial, Carneiro and Sato[97] treated 41 patients with MTX (15 to 20 mg/wk) versus placebo. Thirty-seven patients completed the study; two patients who received placebo and experienced disease flares dropped out of the study, and two patients who were treated with MTX developed toxicity. After 6 months, in comparison with the placebo group, the MTX-treated group of patients had significantly more resolution of arthritis, rash, and hypocomplementemia, and the mean SLEDAI scores were significantly lower in the MTX arm ($P < 0.01$ for all four observations). Mean prednisone doses at follow-up were increased in the placebo group and significantly decreased in the MTX group.

Fortin and others[98] evaluated the steroid-sparing effects of MTX in patients with SLE in a double-blind, randomized, placebo-controlled trial. They randomized 86 patients—41 patients in the MTX group and 45 in the placebo group. Although 60 participants completed the study, 26 patients terminated early. Patients who were treated with MTX were conferred a significant advantage, compared with placebo in decreasing their steroid dose. The disease activity as measured by the revised Systemic Lupus Activity Measure (SLAM-R) was also significantly reduced.

Further evidence for MTX use in patients with SLE originates from small uncontrolled trials. In an open trial of 10 pediatric patients, Abud-Mendoza and associates[99] added low-dose MTX (5 to 10 mg/dL) to their previous regimens (prednisone or prednisone plus CyX). Eight of the patients were able to taper prednisone and discontinue CyX completely.

Rahman and colleagues,[100] in a retrospective controlled study, concluded that a 60% reduction of the actively inflamed joint count was achieved in patients with antimalarial-resistant synovitis who were treated with MTX versus 12% in the control group. In this study, MTX was not found to have a statistically significant steroid-sparing effect. In an open retrospective trial, Gansauge and others[101] evaluated 22 patients with SLE with no renal or central nervous system involvement. They reported that MTX (15 mg/wk) was effective in reducing disease activity as measured by the SLEDAI and that it had

steroid-sparing effects. These studies are consistent with the authors' clinical experience suggesting that MTX is a relatively rapid-acting, often effective, and overall well-tolerated agent for the treatment of cutaneous and articular SLE. One caution is that patients should be regularly monitored for decline in renal function, in addition to following CBCs and liver function tests.

Summary of Methotrexate Therapy for Lupus

MTX is a relatively safe and well-tolerated alternative for the treatment of lupus, particularly in patients with cutaneous or musculoskeletal manifestations or both. Despite the paucity of controlled trials, the authors of this text frequently use this compound with apparent benefit in patients with moderately severe lupus, particularly patients with arthritis, rash, and/or pleurisy. Monitoring renal function is essential to ensure safety, considering the increased risk of toxicity in the setting of renal dysfunction. To avoid teratogenicity, flawless contraception is mandatory when MTX is used in women at risk of becoming pregnant.

MYCOPHENOLATE MOFETIL

MMF has established itself as a successful immunosuppressive medication in multiple applications. In the United States, it is approved by the FDA for the prevention of renal, cardiac, and hepatic allograft rejection. In the last 20 years, MMF has been the subject of multiple randomized clinical trials in patients with SLE and LN. MMF has a unique mode of action that may be particularly useful to control SLE and its manifestations. MMF is the morpholinoethyl ester of mycophenolic acid (MPA).

MPA was originally isolated from the *Penicillium* species in 1896. It is a potent, noncompetitive, reversible inhibitor of inosine-5′-monophosphate dehydrogenase (IMPDH), a necessary enzyme in the *de novo* pathway of purine synthesis. Although most cells use the salvage pathway of purine synthesis, the *de novo* synthesis pathway is uniquely essential to activated lymphocytes. Not only do lymphocytes primarily depend on this pathway, but activated lymphocytes predominantly use the second isoform of IMPDH against which MPA is most specific.[102] Activities of MPA include the inhibition of antibody formation in humans to equine-derived polyclonal antithymocyte preparation (e.g., ATGAM),[103] the prevention of leukocyte migration by decreasing the expression of endothelial adhesion molecules,[104] the inhibition of both T- and B-lymphocyte proliferation *in vitro* in response to mitogenic stimulation,[105] and the limitation of oxidative damage by suppressing the induction of inducible nitric oxide synthetase (iNOS).[106] MPA's effect on cellular proliferation may also apply to endothelial cells,[107] and it may even play a role in preventing coronary re-stenosis.[108]

MMF is rapidly hydrolyzed to MPA and achieves approximately 94% bioavailability after oral administration. The drug is reversibly converted in the liver into an metabolically inactive compound, 7-0-mycophenolic acid glucuronide (MPAG), and excreted into urine and bile. Much of MPAG is deglucuronidated by intestinal flora and undergoes enterohepatic recirculation. Approximately 97% of MPA is bound to albumin in patients with normal renal and hepatic function.[109]

One cannot overemphasize the high degree of variability in the circulating free MPA levels observed in patients with and without lupus who receive comparable doses of MMF. After the administration of MMF (1000 mg) in patients who have undergone hematopoietic stem cell transplantation, the area under the curve of free MPA varied fourfold for oral administration and sevenfold for intravenous administration; the oral bioavailability ranged from 20% to 170%.[110] It is widely recognized that MPA levels usually increase in renal insufficiency, although the pharmacokinetics are complex.[111] A recent study showed that serum albumin and creatinine clearance both negatively correlated with MPA levels, suggesting levels may increase in nephrotic syndrome.[112] Interestingly, supplemental dietary metals (e.g., magnesium aluminum or iron) appeared to reduce the levels. MMF dosage for LN was initially based on experience in renal transplantation. In transplantation, doses of 2 or 3 g/day were compared with little gain in efficacy but increased toxicity at the 3 g/day dose.[113] The standard 2 g/day dose of MMF for renal transplantation yielded superior graft survival, compared with regimens containing AZA in controlled trials, except in African Americans, which prompted some investigators to use a target dose of 3 g/day in LN trials including African-American patients.

Many patients experience GI distress while taking MMF, with the likelihood related to the peak level attained; hence, three-times-daily dosing is sometimes better tolerated than twice-daily administration of the same total dose. Sustained-release MPA, recently introduced and not yet available as a generic formulation, smooths out blood levels and is better tolerated in some patients. Gradual dose escalation reduces the likelihood of GI toxicity , and most MMF protocols use 500 mg twice a day for the first week, 1000 mg twice a day for the second week, and 1500 mg (when appropriate) for the third week, using caution in patients with renal insufficiency. Although the authors' studies of MMF in nonrenal lupus suggest the usual maximal tolerated dose (from 1 to 2 g), clinical trials in LN showed that, faced with the choice of swallowing 3 g MMF daily or taking CyX, the majority of patients tolerated the larger dose of MMF.

Most MMF studies in LN have enrolled patients with creatinine clearances greater than 30 mL/min or serum creatinine levels less than 3 mg/dL. Data regarding response of patients with fulminant nephritis and renal failure are lacking and will be of great interest when available. Until that time, and because of unpredictable levels in renal failure and the necessity to start MMF gradually, treating the sickest patients initially with bolus MP and IVC remains the practice of the authors of this text.

Animal Studies

In animal models, MMF has proved to be effective far beyond the prevention of allograft rejection. Studies in the Medical Research Laboratory (e.g., Murphy Roths Large–lymphoproliferation strain [MRL/lpr] mice) and the New Zealand black (NZB) × New Zealand white (NZW) F1 mouse models of SLE have shown that MMF-treated mice had suppression of the development of glomerulonephritis, a decrease in glomerular immunoglobulin deposits, and improved survival.[114,115]

In humans, MMF has been established as an effective treatment for LN in numerous controlled trials both for induction and for maintenance of remission. Controlled trials using both MMF and CyX for LN have been reviewed in the CyX section. As noted in this section, the authors' opinions that the relative potency of MMF (as currently administered without monitoring drug levels) and IVC differ in individual patients, as illustrated by the overall greater effectiveness of MMF in African-American and Hispanic participants of clinical trials. Since MMF is less toxic than CyX, especially to reproductive organs, MMF is the initial drug of choice in many patients, particularly in women or men of childbearing age. The following review of additional studies illustrates the use of MMF in LN and the limited data supporting the use of MMF for nonrenal lupus, a practice that the authors of this text encourage.

Nonrenal Lupus

The overwhelming clinical impression that MMF ameliorates nonrenal as well as renal lupus is supported by a post-hoc analysis of the outcome of the ALMS trial (described earlier in this chapter), which showed equivalent effectiveness of MMF versus IVC as induction for LN. In this study, improvement of extrarenal manifestations was believed to be comparable in the two groups. The extents of improvement in assessments of eight organ systems were consistently both significant and similar.[38] Numerous uncontrolled trials support the efficacy of MMF in nonrenal lupus. No controlled trials, however, support the use of MMF in NP-SLE; for truly life-threatening emergencies or transverse myelitis requiring immunosuppression, the preferred initial treatment is CyX. Although MMF may have a promising role as induction therapy, the most recent interest has been directed toward its use as sequential therapy after induction with IVC (see earlier sections on Sequential Therapy for Lupus Nephritis).

Overall, MMF has had lower toxicity than alkylating agents. In controlled trials for the prevention of renal transplant rejection, diarrhea was increased in patients receiving MMF with an incidence of up to 36%, compared with 21% for patients receiving AZA and 14% for patients receiving placebo. Few patients (up to 2%) developed severe neutropenia (absolute neutrophil count less than 0.5×10^3/L). The incidence of malignancies among the patients enrolled who were followed for 1 year was similar to the incidence reported in the literature for renal allograft recipients. A slight increase was reported in the incidence of lymphoproliferative disease in the MMF treatment groups, compared with the placebo and AZA groups. In a study to evaluate the overall tolerability of MMF in patients with SLE,[116] the authors of this text identified 54 patients followed for a mean of 12.4 person-months on MMF. Of the 54 patients, 21 (38.9%) had a total of 28 adverse GI events, 24 (44.4%) had a total of 37 infections, and only 1 patient required hospitalization. Leukopenia occurred three times but never required dose adjustment. Adverse events occurred at a similar rate at all MMF doses. Pisoni and colleagues[117] published a similar report in which they evaluated 93 patients with SLE retrospectively; 37 participants (43%) developed an adverse event; GI intolerance was found in 25 patients and infections in 20. Nonetheless, only 14 patients (16%) discontinued the drug in response to adverse events. Ginzler and associates[118] reviewed the tolerability and toxicity in their randomized trial of MMF versus IVC. Most adverse events were GI- or infection-related; 17 patients in the IVC group had upper GI distress, 6 of whom required hospitalization; 19 patients treated with MMF had mild or moderate GI symptoms. Hematologic toxicity was unusual and seemed to be similar in the two groups with the exception of lymphopenia, which developed in 28 patients treated with IVC versus 18 who were given MMF. The authors reported a trend toward decreased serious infections in patients receiving MMF.

Several studies in animals have demonstrated the teratogenic potential of MMF. It must be used with caution in women of childbearing age because it may cause fetal harm. Effective contraception must be instituted before female patients are started on this agent. Case series have reported several malformations associated with MMF, including cleft palate, microtia, and cardiovascular anomalies.[119,120]

Summary of Mycophenolate Mofetil Therapy for Lupus

1. High-quality controlled trials have established MMF as an effective alternative to CyX for induction therapy of LN. Overall improvements of both clinical parameters and biopsy evidence of inflammation appear to be comparable, although some studies have suggested an advantage for MMF.
2. Genetic factors influence differential responses to MMF versus CyX, as evidenced by improved outcome in African Americans or Hispanics but not Caucasians in MMF-treated groups.
3. MMF is as yet untested in patients with explosive nephritis and renal failure.
4. Bioavailability and area under the curve after MMF administration vary up to sevenfold among patients.
5. Maintenance therapy with MMF or AZA has supplanted quarterly IVC; evidence to date suggests MMF may be superior to AZA for maintenance.
6. The lack of gonadal toxicity of MMF recommends it as a first-line agent in both men and women of childbearing age. Reduced toxicity concerns will likely lead to overall earlier treatment of LN, improving patient outcomes.

LEFLUNOMIDE

Leflunomide is an inhibitor of *de novo* pyrimidine synthesis that is relatively new as a treatment for lupus. It has been extensively used for the treatment of patients with RA and has been shown to be comparable to MTX.[121] Leflunomide is a cytotoxic isoxazole derivative and is structurally unrelated to other immunomodulatory drugs.[122] Leflunomide is rapidly converted to its active metabolite, A77 1726, a malononitrilamide, which is an inhibitor of the mitochondrial enzyme, dihydroorotate dehydrogenase (DHODH), a key enzyme in the *de novo* synthesis pathway of the pyrimidine ribonucleotide uridine monophosphate (rUMP), inhibition of which prevents activated lymphocytes from moving from the G1 to the S phase.[123] A77 1726 has other known antiinflammatory roles as an inhibitor of cyclooxygenase (COX)–2 activity and an inhibitor of leukocyte adhesion. Furthermore, leflunomide may also have antiviral activity and has been proposed as therapy for cytomegalovirus in patients after renal transplantation.[123]

Leflunomide is orally administered at a dose of 10 to 20 mg/day for patients with RA and up to 30 mg/day for patients with SLE or vasculitis. Although early studies with leflunomide use a loading dose of 100 mg/day for 3 days, the practice has been largely abandoned to reduce toxicity. The drug has a relatively long half-life (15 days) and is well absorbed, undergoing extensive enterohepatic recirculation. Before treatment, CBCs and liver function tests should be obtained and monitored at monthly intervals for the first 6 months and at least every 2 months thereafter.

Several controlled trials of leflunomide have been conducted in patients with SLE. One double-blinded placebo controlled study randomized 12 patients with lupus and mild-to-moderate disease activity, who were taking less than 0.5 mg/kg/day of prednisolone, to receive either leflunomide or placebo for 24 weeks.[124] The primary outcome was a change in the SLEDAI, and secondary outcomes included changes in proteinuria, complement levels, anti–double stranded DNA (anti-dsDNA) levels, and prednisolone doses. The results of the study revealed a significant reduction in the SLEDAI in both the leflunomide and placebo groups, but the reduction in the leflunomide group was significantly greater, compared with the placebo group (11.0 ± 6.0 in the leflunomide group and 4.5 ± 2.4 in the placebo group; $P = 0.026$). The secondary endpoints were similar in the two groups.

A second controlled trial was a prospective multicenter study evaluating the safety and efficacy of leflunomide in the treatment of 51 patients with proliferative LN.[125] Patients enrolled in this study had biopsy-confirmed proliferative LN and were divided into three treatment groups. Patients with recent onset nephritis who had never received treatment with immunosuppressive drugs received either leflunomide or IVC. A third group consisted of patients with recurrent nephritis who had received immunosuppressive therapy within 3 months; they were given leflunomide. As reported in the English language abstract, the results of the study after 6 months revealed no differences in the response or remission rates of patients initially treated with either leflunomide or CyX. Furthermore, renal parameters such as proteinuria, serum albumin, and creatinine, as well as SLEDAI, improved similarly in the two groups. Among the 14 patients enrolled with relapsed nephritis, the total response rate was 60% and complete remission rate was 6.7% after treatment with leflunomide. Four patients withdrew from the study because of adverse events, including herpes zoster and severe lung infection.

In a prospective open label study, Tam and others[126] evaluated the safety and efficacy of leflunomide in 19 patients with LN. These patients had a history of previous treatment-related toxicities (e.g., sepsis), contraindications for the use of CyX, or a lack of response to immunosuppressive drugs such as CyX, AZA, or CS. The primary endpoint was the number of patients achieving complete or partial response of nephritis. At the final visit, 29% of patients had achieved a complete response (defined as proteinuria less than or equal to 0.5 g/day, with normal urinary sediment and normal serum creatinine and creatinine clearance). In this study, 47% of patients exhibited a partial response, which was defined as either a reduction of more than 30% in proteinuria or proteinuria less than 2 g/day in a patient who was previously nephrotic. Although long-term follow-up data is lacking, this study suggests that leflunomide is a safe and efficacious treatment in patients with LN whose disease does not respond to or who cannot tolerate conventional therapies.

Wang and colleagues[127] evaluated the efficacy and safety of leflunomide in the treatment of proliferative LN in a prospective multicenter observational trial. Patients with biopsy-proven proliferative LN were assigned (but not randomized) to receive either monthly IVC (500 mg/m²) or leflunomide (30 mg/day) with concomitant prednisone. Of the 110 patients enrolled, 70 were in the leflunomide group and 40 were in the CyX group. Renal parameters improved significantly and similarly in both groups, and complete remission was observed in approximately 20% of each group. Repeat kidney biopsies showed significant reductions in active lesions (but continued activity) after 6 months of leflunomide treatment and overall increase in chronicity indexes. Major adverse events were similar in the two treatment groups. The IVC and leflunomide regimens were comparably, albeit moderately, effective in the induction therapy of proliferative LN. In contrast to this study, Zhang[128] performed renal biopsies at entry and after 1 year in 31 patients and noted no progression of chronicity.

Several potential side effects of treatment associated with leflunomide, including diarrhea, nausea, and alopecia, have been noted to decrease in frequency with continued treatment[129] and when a loading dose is not used.[130] Severe hepatotoxicity has also been reported, although its actual incidence remains controversial. Unacceptably high rates of transaminase elevation, cirrhosis, and liver failure were reported in the initial studies and postmarketing data regarding leflunomide. However, a subsequent FDA review of these data found that most patients with hepatic involvement were concomitantly taking other potentially hepatotoxic drugs such as MTX or had confounding co-morbidities such as viral hepatitis or alcohol abuse. A review of 3325 patients treated with leflunomide found that abnormalities in liver function testing were cited as reasons for drug discontinuation in 5% of patients[131]; furthermore, the review identified no deaths attributable to leflunomide.

An important aspect to consider for the use of leflunomide in patients with lupus, many of whom are young women, is that it is a potent teratogen rated Category X for pregnancy by the FDA and therefore absolutely contraindicated in women who are at risk for becoming pregnant. Leflunomide can persist after administration for up to 2 years[132] and should therefore be used with reluctance in any woman of childbearing age. To ensure safety after discontinuing leflunomide, patients must be instructed to avoid pregnancy until undetectable plasma levels (less than 0.02 µg/mL) are demonstrated. If need be, the drug can be removed from the body by the administration of cholestyramine.[132]

Summary of Leflunomide Therapy for Lupus

1. Improvement of the SLEDAI score with leflunomide has been reported in one controlled trial, and efficacy is comparable to that of standard therapy of proliferative nephritis in another. These findings suggest that leflunomide, currently available as a generic drug, may be useful in situations in which more strongly evidence-based regimens are ineffective or impractical.

2. Persistence of this teratogenic drug in the circulation for years mandates caution with its use in women of childbearing age.

CONCLUSION

Refinement in the use of immunosuppressive agents and the introduction of both sequential therapies and ovarian protection regimens to reduce the toxicity of CyX therapy are taking place in the context of the introduction of new and potentially highly potent biologic agents, such as rituximab, belimumab, and abatacept. These biologic agents may prove to be effective either as monotherapy or in combination with traditional immunosuppressive agents (or each other). The use of these drug combinations has the potential to reduce significantly the reliance on alkylating agents or corticosteroids or both, presumably dramatically decreasing the toxicities associated with conventional agents.

References

1. Osborne ED, Jordon JW: Nitrogen mustard therapy in cutaneous blastomatous disease. *J Am Med Assoc* 135:1123–1128, 1947.
2. Chasis H, Goldring W, Baldwin DS: Effect of febrile plasma, typhoid vaccine and nitrogen mustard on renal manifestations of human glomerulonephritis. *Proc Soc Exp Biol Med* 71:565–567, 1949.
3. Takada K, Arefayene M, Desta Z, et al: Cytochrome P450 pharmacogenetics as a predictor of toxicity and clinical response to pulse cyclophosphamide in lupus nephritis. *Arthritis Rheum* 50:2202–2210, 2004.
4. Stone J: General principles of the use of cyclophosphamide in rheumatic and renal disease. In UpToDate. http://www.uptodate.com/contents/general-principles-of-the-use-of-cyclophosphamide-in-rheumatic-and-renal-disease?source=search_result&selectedTitle=1%7E150. Accessed June 27, 2011.
5. McCune WJ, Fox DA: Immunosuppressive agents: biologic effects in vivo and in vitro. In Kammer GM, Tsokos GC, editors: *Lupus: molecular and cellular pathogenesis*, Totowa, NJ, 1999, Humana Press, pp 612–641.
6. McCune WJ, Golbus J, Zeldes W, et al: Clinical and immunologic effects of monthly administration of intravenous cyclophosphamide in severe systemic lupus erythematosus. *N Engl J Med* 318:1423–1431, 1988.
7. Fox DA, Millard JA, Treisman J, et al: Defective CD2 pathway T cell activation in systemic lupus erythematosus. *Arthritis Rheum* 34:561–571, 1991.
8. Felson DT, Anderson J: Evidence for the superiority of immunosuppressive drugs and prednisone over prednisone alone in lupus nephritis. Results of a pooled analysis. *N Engl J Med* 311:1528–1533, 1984.
9. Takeno M, Suzuki N, Nagafuchi H, et al: Selective suppression of resting B cell function in patients with systemic lupus erythematosus treated with cyclophosphamide. *Clin Exp Rheumatol* 11:263–270, 1993.
10. Chan TM, Tse KC, Tang C, et al: Long-term outcome of patients with diffuse proliferative lupus nephritis treated with prednisolone and oral cyclophosphamide followed by azathioprine. *Lupus* 14:265–272, 2005.
11. Yee CS, Gordon C, Dostal C, et al: EULAR randomised controlled trial of pulse cyclophosphamide and methylprednisolone versus continuous cyclophosphamide and prednisolone followed by azathioprine and prednisolone in lupus nephritis. *Ann Rheum Dis* 63:525–529, 2004.
12. Hoffman GS, Kerr GS, Leavitt RY, et al: Wegener granulomatosis: an analysis of 158 patients. *Ann Intern Med* 116:488–498, 1992.
13. Baltus JA, Boersma JW, Hartman AP, et al: The occurrence of malignancies in patients with rheumatoid arthritis treated with cyclophosphamide: a controlled retrospective follow-up. *Ann Rheum Dis* 42:368–373, 1983.
14. Baker GL, Kahl LE, Zee BC, et al: Malignancy following treatment of rheumatoid arthritis with cyclophosphamide. Long-term case-control follow-up study. *Am J Med* 83:1–9, 1987.
15. Radis CD, Kahl LE, Baker GL, et al: Effects of cyclophosphamide on the development of malignancy and on long-term survival of patients with rheumatoid arthritis. A 20-year followup study. *Arthritis Rheum* 38:1120–1127, 1995.
16. Ognenovski VM, Marder W, Somers EC, et al: Increased incidence of cervical intraepithelial neoplasia in women with systemic lupus erythematosus treated with intravenous cyclophosphamide. *J Rheumatol* 31:1763–1767, 2004.
17. Malik SW, Myers JL, DeRemee RA, et al: Lung toxicity associated with cyclophosphamide use. Two distinct patterns. *Am J Respir Crit Care Med* 154:1851–1856, 1996.
18. Somers EC, Marder W, Christman GM, et al: Use of a gonadotropin-releasing hormone analog for protection against premature ovarian failure during cyclophosphamide therapy in women with severe lupus. *Arthritis Rheum* 52:2761–2767, 2005.
19. Clowse ME, Behera MA, Anders CK, et al: Ovarian preservation by GnRH agonists during chemotherapy: a meta-analysis. *J Womens Health (Larchmt)* 18:311–319, 2009.
20. Greenberg LH, Tanaka KR: Congenital anomalies probably induced by cyclophosphamide. *JAMA* 188:423–426, 1964.
21. Balow JE, Austin HA, 3rd, Muenz LR, et al: Effect of treatment on the evolution of renal abnormalities in lupus nephritis. *N Engl J Med* 311:491–495, 1984.
22. Boumpas DT, Austin HA 3rd, Vaughn EM, et al: Controlled trial of pulse methylprednisolone versus two regimens of pulse cyclophosphamide in severe lupus nephritis. *Lancet* 340:741–745, 1992.
23. Fries JF, Sharp GC, McDevitt HO, et al: Cyclophosphamide therapy in systemic lupus erythematosus and polymyositis. *Arthritis Rheum* 16:154–162, 1973.
24. Illei GG, Austin HA, Crane M, et al: Combination therapy with pulse cyclophosphamide plus pulse methylprednisolone improves long-term renal outcome without adding toxicity in patients with lupus nephritis. *Ann Intern Med* 135:248–257, 2001.
25. Dooley MA, Hogan S, Jennette C, et al: Cyclophosphamide therapy for lupus nephritis: poor renal survival in black Americans. Glomerular Disease Collaborative Network. *Kidney Int* 51:1188–1195, 1997.
26. Contreras G, Pardo V, Leclercq B, et al: Sequential therapies for proliferative lupus nephritis. *N Engl J Med* 350:971–980, 2004.
27. Wofsy D, Appel GB, Dooley MA, et al: Aspreva Lupus Management Study maintenance results. *Lupus* 19:27, 2010.
28. Houssiau FA, D'Cruz D, Sangle S, et al; MAINTAIN Nephritis Trial Group: Azathioprine versus mycophenolate mofetil for long-term immunosuppression in lupus nephritis: results from the MAINTAIN Nephritis Trial. *Ann Rheum Dis* 69:2083–2089, 2010.
29. Chan TM, Li FK, Tang CS, et al: Efficacy of mycophenolate mofetil in patients with diffuse proliferative lupus nephritis. Hong Kong-Guangzhou Nephrology Study Group. *N Engl J Med* 343:1156–1162, 2000.
30. Ginzler EM, Dooley MA, Aranow C, et al: Mycophenolate mofetil or intravenous cyclophosphamide for lupus nephritis. *N Engl J Med* 353:2219–2228, 2005.
31. Appel GB, Contreras G, Dooley MA, et al: Mycophenolate mofetil versus cyclophosphamide for induction treatment of lupus nephritis. *J Am Soc Nephrol* 20:1103–1112, 2009.
32. Isenberg D, Appel GB, Contreras G, et al: Influence of race/ethnicity on response to lupus nephritis treatment: the ALMS study. *Rheumatology (Oxford)* 49:128–140, 2010.
33. Ong LM, Hooi LS, Lim TO, et al: Randomized controlled trial of pulse intravenous cyclophosphamide versus mycophenolate mofetil in the induction therapy of proliferative lupus nephritis. *Nephrology (Carlton)* 10:504–510, 2005.
34. Hu W, Liu Z, Chen H, et al: Mycophenolate mofetil vs cyclophosphamide therapy for patients with diffuse proliferative lupus nephritis. *Chin Med J (Engl)* 115:705–709, 2002.
35. Houssiau FA, Vasconcelos C, D'Cruz D, et al: Immunosuppressive therapy in lupus nephritis: the Euro-Lupus Nephritis Trial, a randomized trial of low-dose versus high-dose intravenous cyclophosphamide. *Arthritis Rheum* 46:2121–2131, 2002.
36. Boletis JN, Ioannidis JP, Boki KA, et al: Intravenous immunoglobulin compared with cyclophosphamide for proliferative lupus nephritis. *Lancet* 354:569–570, 1999.
37. Chan TM, Tse KC, Tang CS, et al: Mofetil as continuous induction and maintenance treatment for diffuse proliferative lupus nephritis. *J Am Soc Nephrol* 16:1076–1084, 2005.
38. Ginzler EM, Wofsy D, Isenberg D, et al; ALMS Group: Nonrenal disease activity following mycophenolate mofetil or intravenous cyclophosphamide as induction treatment for lupus nephritis: findings in a multicenter, prospective, randomized, open-label, parallel-group clinical trial. *Arthritis Rheum* 62:211–221, 2010.
39. Boumpas DT, Yamada H, Patronas NJ, et al: Pulse cyclophosphamide for severe neuropsychiatric lupus. *Q J Med* 81:975–984, 1991.
40. Neuwelt CM, Lacks S, Kaye BR, et al: Role of intravenous cyclophosphamide in the treatment of severe neuropsychiatric systemic lupus erythematosus. *Am J Med* 98:32–41, 1995.
41. Malaviya AN, Singh RR, Sindhwani R, et al: Intermittent intravenous pulse cyclophosphamide treatment in systemic lupus erythematosus. *Indian J Med Res* 96:101–108, 1992.
42. Baca V, Lavalle C, Garcia R, et al: Favorable response to intravenous methylprednisolone and cyclophosphamide in children with severe neuropsychiatric lupus. *J Rheumatol* 26:432–439, 1999.
43. Roach BA, Hutchinson GJ: Treatment of refractory, systemic lupus erythematosus-associated thrombocytopenia with intermittent low-dose intravenous cyclophosphamide. *Arthritis Rheum* 36:682–684, 1993.
44. Boumpas DT, Barez S, Klippel JH, et al: Intermittent cyclophosphamide for the treatment of autoimmune thrombocytopenia in systemic lupus erythematosus. *Ann Intern Med* 112:674–677, 1990.
45. Fukuda M, Kamiyama Y, Kawahara K, et al: The favourable effect of cyclophosphamide pulse therapy in the treatment of massive pulmonary haemorrhage in systemic lupus erythematosus. *Eur J Pediatr* 153:167–170, 1994.
46. Kono DH, Klashman DJ, Gilbert RC: Successful IV pulse cyclophosphamide in refractory PM in 3 patients with SLE. *J Rheumatol* 17:982–983, 1990.
47. Deane KD, West SG: Antiphospholipid antibodies as a cause of pulmonary capillaritis and diffuse alveolar hemorrhage: a case series and literature review. *Semin Arthritis Rheum* 35:154–165, 2005.

48. Lehman TJ, Onel K: Intermittent intravenous cyclophosphamide arrests progression of the renal chronicity index in childhood systemic lupus erythematosus. *J Pediatr* 136:243–247, 2000.

49. Brodsky RA, Petri M, Jones RJ: Hematopoietic stem cell transplantation for systemic lupus erythematosus. *Rheum Dis Clin North Am* 26:377–387, viii, 2000.

50. Petri M, Jones RJ, Brodsky RA: High-dose cyclophosphamide without stem cell transplantation in systemic lupus erythematosus. *Arthritis Rheum* 48:166–173, 2003.

51. Petri M, Brodsky RA, Jones RJ, et al. High-dose cyclophosphamide versus monthly intravenous cyclophosphamide for systemic lupus erythematosus: a prospective randomized trial. *Arthritis Rheum* 62(5):1487–1493, 2010.

52. Steinberg AD: Chlorambucil in the treatment of patients with immune-mediated rheumatic diseases. *Arthritis Rheum* 36:325–328, 1993.

53. Cannon GW, Jackson CG, Samuelson CO Jr, et al: Chlorambucil therapy in rheumatoid arthritis: clinical experience in 28 patients and literature review. *Semin Arthritis Rheum* 15:106–118, 1985.

54. Patapanian H, Graham S, Sambrook PN, et al: The oncogenicity of chlorambucil in rheumatoid arthritis. *Br J Rheumatol* 27:44–47, 1988.

55. du Buf-Vereijken PW, Branten AJ, Wetzels JF: Idiopathic membranous nephropathy: outline and rationale of a treatment strategy. *Am J Kidney Dis* 46:1012–1029, 2005.

56. Snaith ML, Holt JM, Oliver DO, et al: Treatment of patients with systemic lupus erythematosus including nephritis with chlorambucil. *Br Med J* 2:197–201, 1973.

57. Epstein WV, Grausz H: Favorable outcome in diffuse proliferative glomerulonephritis of systemic lupus erythematosus. *Arthritis Rheum* 17:129–142, 1974.

58. Sabbour MS, Osman LM: Comparison of chlorambucil, azathioprine or cyclophosphamide combined with corticosteroids in the treatment of lupus nephritis. *Br J Dermatol* 100:113–125, 1979.

59. Steinberg AD, Steinberg SC: Long-term preservation of renal function in patients with lupus nephritis receiving treatment that includes cyclophosphamide versus those treated with prednisone only. *Arthritis Rheum* 34:945–950, 1991.

60. Donadio JV Jr, Holley KE, Wagoner RD, et al: Treatment of lupus nephritis with prednisone and combined prednisone and azathioprine. *Ann Intern Med* 77:829–835, 1972.

61. Donadio JV Jr, Holley KE, Wagoner RD, et al: Further observations on the treatment of lupus nephritis with prednisone and combined prednisone and azathioprine. *Arthritis Rheum* 17:573–581, 1974.

62. Hahn BH, Kantor OS, Osterland CK: Azathioprine plus prednisone compared with prednisone alone in the treatment of systemic lupus erythematosus. Report of a prospective controlled trial in 24 patients. *Ann Intern Med* 83:597–605, 1975.

63. Cade R, Spooner G, Schlein E, et al: Comparison of azathioprine, prednisone, and heparin alone or combined in treating lupus nephritis. *Nephron* 10:37–56, 1973.

64. Ginzler E, Diamond H, Guttadauria M, et al: Prednisone and azathioprine compared to prednisone plus low-dose azathioprine and cyclophosphamide in the treatment of diffuse lupus nephritis. *Arthritis Rheum* 19:693–699, 1976.

65. Esdaile JM, Joseph L, MacKenzie T, et al: The benefit of early treatment with immunosuppressive agents in lupus nephritis. *J Rheumatol* 21:2046–2051, 1994.

66. Sztejnbok M, Stewart A, Diamond H, et al: Azathioprine in the treatment of systemic lupus erythematosus. A controlled study. *Arthritis Rheum* 14:639–645, 1971.

67. Sharon E, Kaplan D, Diamond HS: Exacerbation of systemic lupus erythematosus after withdrawal of azathioprine therapy. *N Engl J Med* 288:122–124, 1973.

68. Werth V, Franks A Jr: Treatment of discoid skin lesions with azathioprine. *Arch Dermatol* 122:746–747, 1986.

69. Shehade S: Successful treatment of generalized discoid skin lesions with azathioprine. *Arch Dermatol* 122:376–377, 1986.

70. Callen JP, Spencer LV, Burruss JB, et al: Azathioprine. An effective, corticosteroid-sparing therapy for patients with recalcitrant cutaneous lupus erythematosus or with recalcitrant cutaneous leukocytoclastic vasculitis. *Arch Dermatol* 127:515–522, 1991.

71. Polifka JE, Friedman JM: Teratogen update: azathioprine and 6-mercaptopurine. *Teratology* 65:240–261, 2002.

72. Alstead EM, Ritchie JK, Lennard-Jones JE, et al: Safety of azathioprine in pregnancy in inflammatory bowel disease. *Gastroenterology* 99:443–446, 1990.

73. Ishida Y, Matsuda H, Kida K: Effect of cyclosporin A on human bone marrow granulocyte-macrophage progenitors with anti-cancer agents. *Acta Paediatr Jpn* 37:610–613, 1995.

74. Bennett W: Cyclosporine and tacrolimus nephrotoxicity. In UpToDate. http://www.uptodate.com/contents/cyclosporine-and-tacrolimus-nephrotoxicity/contributors. Accessed June 27, 2011.

75. Feutren G, Mihatsch MJ: Risk factors for cyclosporine-induced nephropathy in patients with autoimmune diseases. International Kidney Biopsy Registry of Cyclosporine in Autoimmune Diseases. *N Engl J Med* 326:1654–1660, 1992.

76. Deray G, Benhmida M, Le Hoang P, et al: Renal function and blood pressure in patients receiving long-term, low-dose cyclosporine therapy for idiopathic autoimmune uveitis. *Ann Intern Med* 117:578–583, 1992.

77. Altman RD, Perez GO, Sfakianakis GN: Interaction of cyclosporine A and nonsteroidal anti-inflammatory drugs on renal function in patients with rheumatoid arthritis. *Am J Med* 93:396–402, 1992.

78. Nakamura T, Nozu K, Iijima K, et al: Association of cumulative cyclosporine dose with its irreversible nephrotoxicity in Japanese patients with pediatric-onset autoimmune diseases. *Biol Pharm Bull* 30:2371–2375, 2007.

79. Balletta M, Sabella D, Magri P, et al: Ciclosporin plus steroids versus steroids alone in the treatment of lupus nephritis. *Contrib Nephrol* 99:129–130, 1992.

80. Fu LW, Yang LY, Chen WP, et al: Clinical efficacy of cyclosporin a neoral in the treatment of paediatric lupus nephritis with heavy proteinuria. *Br J Rheumatol* 37:217–221, 1998.

81. Austin HA 3rd, Illei GG, Braun MJ, et al: Randomized, controlled trial of prednisone, cyclophosphamide, and cyclosporine in lupus membranous nephropathy. *J Am Soc Nephrol* 20:901–911, 2009.

82. Zavada J, Pesickova S, Rysava R, et al: Cyclosporine A or intravenous cyclophosphamide for lupus nephritis: the Cyclofa-Lune study. *Lupus* 19:1281–1289, 2010.

83. Moroni G, Doria A, Mosca M, et al: A randomized pilot trial comparing cyclosporine and azathioprine for maintenance therapy in diffuse lupus nephritis over four years. *Clin J Am Soc Nephrol* 1:925–932, 2006.

84. Griffiths B, Emery P, Ryan V, et al: The BILAG multi-centre open randomized controlled trial comparing ciclosporin vs azathioprine in patients with severe SLE. *Rheumatology (Oxford)* 49:723–732, 2010.

85. Chen W, Tang X, Liu Q, et al: Short-term outcomes of induction therapy with tacrolimus versus cyclophosphamide for active lupus nephritis: A multicenter randomized clinical trial. *Am J Kidney Dis* 57:235–244, 2011.

86. Li X, Ren H, Zhang Q, et al: Mycophenolate mofetil or tacrolimus compared with intravenous cyclophosphamide in the induction treatment for active lupus nephritis. *Nephrol Dial Transplant* 27:1476–1472, 2011.

87. Bao H, Liu ZH, Xie HL, et al: Successful treatment of class V+IV lupus nephritis with multitarget therapy. *J Am Soc Nephrol* 19:2001–2010, 2008.

88. Lanata CM, Mahmood T, Fine DM, et al: Combination therapy of mycophenolate mofetil and tacrolimus in lupus nephritis. *Lupus* 19:935–940, 2010.

89. Avgerinou G, Papafragkaki DK, Nasiopoulou A, et al: Effectiveness of topical calcineurin inhibitors as monotherapy or in combination with hydroxychloroquine in cutaneous lupus erythematosus. *J Eur Acad Dermatol Venereol* 2011. [Epub ahead of print.]

90. Cronstein B: How does methotrexate suppress inflammation? *Clin Exp Rheumatol* 28:S21–S23, 2011.

91. Visser K, Katchamart W, Loza E, et al: Multinational evidence-based recommendations for the use of methotrexate in rheumatic disorders with a focus on rheumatoid arthritis: integrating systematic literature research and expert opinion of a broad international panel of rheumatologists in the 3E Initiative. *Ann Rheum Dis* 68:1086–1093, 2009.

92. Chatham WW, Morgan SL, Alarcon GS: Renal failure: a risk factor for methotrexate toxicity. *Arthritis Rheum* 43:1185–1186, 2000.

93. Hargreaves MR, Mowat AG, Benson MK: Acute pneumonitis associated with low dose methotrexate treatment for rheumatoid arthritis: report of five cases and review of published reports. *Thorax* 47:628–633, 1992.

94. Kremer JM, Alarcon GS, Weinblatt ME, et al: Clinical, laboratory, radiographic, and histopathologic features of methotrexate-associated lung injury in patients with rheumatoid arthritis: a multicenter study with literature review. *Arthritis Rheum* 40:1829–1837, 1997.

95. Gromnica-Ihle E, Krüger K: Use of methotrexate in young patients with respect to the reproductive system. *Clin Exp Rheumatol* 28:S80–S84, 2010.

96. Moseley AC, Lindsley HB, Skikne BS, et al: Reversible methotrexate associated lymphoproliferative disease evolving into Hodgkin's disease. *J Rheumatol* 27:810–813, 2000.

97. Carneiro JR, Sato EI: Double blind, randomized, placebo controlled clinical trial of methotrexate in systemic lupus erythematosus. *J Rheumatol* 26:1275–1279, 1999.

98. Fortin PR, Abrahamowicz M, Ferland D, et al; Canadian Network For Improved Outcomes in Systemic Lupus: Steroid-sparing effects of methotrexate in systemic lupus erythematosus: a double-blind, randomized, placebo-controlled trial. *Arthritis Rheum* 59:1796–1804, 2008.

99. Abud-Mendoza C, Sturbaum AK, Vazquez-Compean R, et al: Methotrexate therapy in childhood systemic lupus erythematosus. *J Rheumatol* 20:731–733, 1993.

100. Rahman P, Humphrey-Murto S, Gladman DD, et al: Efficacy and tolerability of methotrexate in antimalarial resistant lupus arthritis. *J Rheumatol* 25:243–246, 1998.

101. Gansauge S, Breitbart A, Rinaldi N, et al: Methotrexate in patients with moderate systemic lupus erythematosus (exclusion of renal and central nervous system disease). *Ann Rheum Dis* 56:382–385, 1997.

102. Allison AC, Eugui EM: Mycophenolate mofetil and its mechanisms of action. *Immunopharmacology* 47:85–118, 2000.

103. Kimball JA, Pescovitz MD, Book BK, et al: Reduced human IgG anti-ATGAM antibody formation in renal transplant recipients receiving mycophenolate mofetil. *Transplantation* 60:1379–1383, 1995.

104. Haug C, Schmid-Kotsas A, Linder T, et al: The immunosuppressive drug mycophenolic acid reduces endothelin-1 synthesis in endothelial cells and renal epithelial cells. *Clin Sci (Lond)* 103(Suppl 48):76S–80S, 2002.

105. Eugui EM, Mirkovich A, Allison AC: Lymphocyte-selective antiproliferative and immunosuppressive effects of mycophenolic acid in mice. *Scand J Immunol* 33:175–183, 1991.

106. Senda M, DeLustro B, Eugui E, et al: Mycophenolic acid, an inhibitor of IMP dehydrogenase that is also an immunosuppressive agent, suppresses the cytokine-induced nitric oxide production in mouse and rat vascular endothelial cells. *Transplantation* 60:1143–1148, 1995.

107. Huang Y, Liu Z, Huang H, et al: Effects of mycophenolic acid on endothelial cells. *Int Immunopharmacol* 5:1029–1039, 2005.

108. Voisard R, Viola S, Kaspar V, et al: Effects of mycophenolate mofetil on key pattern of coronary restenosis: a cascade of in vitro and ex vivo models. *BMC Cardiovasc Disord* 5:9, 2005.

109. Staatz CE, Tett SE: Clinical pharmacokinetics and pharmacodynamics of mycophenolate in solid organ transplant recipients. *Clin Pharmacokinet* 46:13–58, 2007.

110. Jacobson P, Green K, Rogosheske J, et al: Highly variable mycophenolate mofetil bioavailability following nonmyeloablative hematopoietic cell transplantation. *J Clin Pharmacol* 47:6–12, 2007.

111. Neumann I, Haidinger M, Jager H, et al: Pharmacokinetics of mycophenolate mofetil in patients with autoimmune diseases compared renal transplant recipients. *J Am Soc Nephrol* 14:721–727, 2003.

112. Mino Y, Naito T, Shimoyama K, et al: Pharmacokinetic variability of mycophenolic acid and its glucuronide in systemic lupus erythematosus patients in remission maintenance phase. *Biol Pharm Bull* 34:755–759, 2011.

113. No Author: A blinded, randomized clinical trial of mycophenolate mofetil for the prevention of acute rejection in cadaveric renal transplantation. The Tricontinental Mycophenolate Mofetil Renal Transplantation Study Group. *Transplantation* 61:1029–1037, 1996.

114. Van Bruggen MC, Walgreen B, Rijke TP, et al: Attenuation of murine lupus nephritis by mycophenolate mofetil. *J Am Soc Nephrol* 9:1407–1415, 1998.

115. McMurray RW, Elbourne KB, Lagoo A, et al: Mycophenolate mofetil suppresses autoimmunity and mortality in the female NZB x NZW F1 mouse model of systemic lupus erythematosus. *J Rheumatol* 25:2364–2370, 1998.

116. Riskalla MM, Somers EC, Fatica RA, et al: Tolerability of mycophenolate mofetil in patients with systemic lupus erythematosus. *J Rheumatol* 30:1508–1512, 2003.

117. Pisoni CN, Sanchez FJ, Karim Y, et al: Mycophenolate mofetil in systemic lupus erythematosus: efficacy and tolerability in 86 patients. *J Rheumatol* 32:1047–1052, 2005.

118. Ginzler E, Aranow C, Merrill J, et al: Toxicity and tolerability of mycophenolate mofetil (MMF) vs. intravenous cyclophosphamide (IVC) in a multicenter trial as induction therapy for lupus nephritis (LN). *Arthritis Rheum* 48:S586, 2003.

119. Klieger-Grossmann C, Chitayat D, Lavign S, et al: Prenatal exposure to mycophenolate mofetil: an updated estimate. *J Obstet Gynaecol Can* 32:794–797, 2010.

120. Parisi MA, Zayed H, Slavotinek AM, et al: Congenital diaphragmatic hernia and microtia in a newborn with mycophenolate mofetil (MMF) exposure: phenocopy for Fryns syndrome or broad spectrum of teratogenic effects? *Am J Med Genet A* 149A:1237–1240, 2009.

121. Emery P, Breedveld FC, Lemmel EM, et al. A comparison of the efficacy and safety of leflunomide and methotrexate for the treatment of rheumatoid arthritis. *Rheumatology (Oxford)* 39:655–665, 2000.

122. Brazelton TR, Morris RE: Molecular mechanisms of action of new xenobiotic immunosuppressive drugs: tacrolimus (FK506), sirolimus (rapamycin), mycophenolate mofetil and leflunomide. *Curr Opin Immunol* 8:710–720, 1996.

123. John GT, Manivannan J, Chandy S, et al: Leflunomide therapy for cytomegalovirus disease in renal allograft recipients. *Transplantation* 77:1460–1461, 2004.

124. Tam LS, Li EK, Wong CK, et al: Double-blind, randomized, placebo-controlled pilot study of leflunomide in systemic lupus erythematosus. *Lupus* 13:601–604, 2004.

125. Cui TG, Hou FF, Ni ZH, et al: [Treatment of proliferative lupus nephritis with leflunomide and steroid: a prospective multi-center controlled clinical trial]. *Zhonghua Nei Ke Za Zhi* 44:672–676, 2005.

126. Tam LS, Li EK, Wong CK, et al: Safety and efficacy of leflunomide in the treatment of lupus nephritis refractory or intolerant to traditional immunosuppressive therapy: an open label trial. *Ann Rheum Dis* 65:417–418, 2006.

127. Wang HY, Cui TG, Hou FF, et al; China Leflunomide Lupus Nephritis Study Group: Induction treatment of proliferative lupus nephritis with leflunomide combined with prednisone: a prospective multi-centre observational study. *Lupus* 17:638–644, 2008.

128. Zhang FS, Nie YK, Jin XM, et al: The efficacy and safety of leflunomide therapy in lupus nephritis by repeat kidney biopsy. *Rheumatol Int* 29:1331–1335, 2009.

129. Scott DL, Smolen JS, Kalden JR, et al; European Leflunomide Study Group: Treatment of active rheumatoid arthritis with leflunomide: two year follow up of a double blind, placebo controlled trial versus sulfasalazine. *Ann Rheum Dis* 60:913–923, 2001.

130. Cohen SB, Iqbal I: Leflunomide. *Int J Clin Pract* 57:115–120, 2003.

131. Alcorn N, Saunders S, Madhok R: Benefit-risk assessment of leflunomide: an appraisal of leflunomide in rheumatoid arthritis 10 years after licensing. *Drug Saf* 32:1123–1134, 2009.

132. Janssen NM, Genta MS: The effects of immunosuppressive and anti-inflammatory medications on fertility, pregnancy, and lactation. *Arch Intern Med* 160:610–619, 2000.

133. Galindo-Rodriguez G, Avina-Zubieta JA, Pizarro S, et al: Cyclophosphamide pulse therapy in optic neuritis due to systemic lupus erythematosus: an open trial. *Am J Med* 106(1):65–69, 1999.

134. Garancis JC, Piering WF: Prolonged cyclophosphamide or azathioprine therapy of lupus nephritis. *Clin Pharmcol Ther* 14:130, 1973.

135. Sesso R, Monteior M, Sato E, et al: A controlled trial of pulse cyclophosphamide versus pulse methylprednisolone in sever lupus nephritis. *Lupus* 3(2):107–112, 1994.

136. Gourley MF, Austin HA 3rd, Scott D, et al: Methylprednisolone and cyclophosphamide, alone or in combination, in patients with lupus nephritis. A randomized, controlled trial. *Ann Intern Med* 125(7):549–557, 1996.

137. Boletis JN, Ioannidis JP, Boki KA, et al: Intravenous immunoglobulin compared with cyclophosphamide for proliferative lupus nephritis. *Lancet* 354(9158):569–570, 1999.

Chapter 51

Specialized Treatment Approaches and Niche Therapies for Lupus Subsets

Daniel J. Wallace

TREATMENT OF PATIENTS WITH SYSTEMIC LUPUS ERYTHEMATOSUS AND END-STAGE RENAL DISEASE

Incidence and Prevalence

Patients with end-stage renal disease (ESRD) from chronic systemic lupus erythematosus (SLE) represent 1.5% to 2.0% of all patients on dialysis in the United States and 1% of all patients with lupus.[1-3] Between 3000 and 4000 patients with lupus are dialyzed annually, which represents 1000 new patients a year, of whom 10% succumb annually. ESRD is more prevalent among patients with lupus who are African Americans, noncompliant, on Medicaid, and underinsured. Because patients with SLE are surviving longer, the incidence of ESRD is increasing. Between 1982 and 1995, the number of patients with ESRD increased from 1.16 to 3.08 cases per million person years, and again to 4.9 cases per million person years in 2004. Patients with SLE who develop renal failure have improved mental well-being but worse physical functioning and general health, compared with patients with lupus but are not in renal failure.

Uremia and Its Reversibility

Uremia was the major cause of death in patients with SLE until the 1960s when dialysis became available. Up to 20% of all patients with SLE developed ESRD in the 1970s and 1980s, and the rate has decreased to less than 10% since that time.[4-6] Uremia and dialysis are both associated with a decrease in the systemic activity and decreased steroid requirements of SLE in many, but not all, patients. Most disease flares occur during the first year of dialysis. It has been speculated that the toxic effects of uremia on the immune system are responsible for its ameliorative effects on extrarenal disease. The first few months on dialysis appear to be critical. A high mortality rate is observed (approximately 30% to 50%), but many of those who survive either discontinue dialysis or become candidates for transplantation. Patients under 21 years of age have the highest reversibility rates.

Prognosis of End-Stage Renal Disease

The 5-year patient survival rate of those on dialysis has improved from 50% to 70% in the 1970s to 90% in Western Europe at the present time.[7,8] Poorer outcomes are noted in men, those with lower levels of socioeconomic attainment, and African-American women. Most deaths are related to infection and vascular access complications, as well as to thrombotic events in patients with antiphospholipid antibodies.

Hemodialysis versus Peritoneal Dialysis

The success of hemodialysis in ameliorating disease activity may result from its ability to remove circulating pathogenic immune complexes, complement, and other factors.[9-11] Hemodialysis also has anti-inflammatory effects, decreases T-helper lymphocyte levels, and diminishes mitogenic responsiveness. There are a few case reports of new-onset SLE and successful pregnancies in patients with SLE who are on hemodialysis.

Several studies have documented more reactivation of SLE, higher anti–double stranded DNA (anti-dsDNA) levels, more thrombocytopenia, lower albumin levels, and higher steroid and erythropoietin requirements with peritoneal dialysis. In one large study, peritoneal dialysis was associated with poorer survival and more serositis, cytopenias, and serologic activity when compared with hemodialysis. Switching to it from hemodialysis could reactivate lupus. In a gender-matched, controlled study comparing nondiabetic patients with lupus on peritoneal dialysis with those who did not have SLE, the patients with lupus had a higher infection rate. Systemic Lupus Erythematosus Disease Activity Index (SLEDAI) scores are higher in patients with lupus on peritoneal dialysis than in those on hemodialysis.

The experience of the author of this chapter is that hemodialysis is preferable to peritoneal dialysis, barring extenuating or unusual circumstances.

TRANSPLANTATION

Prevalence

Patients with lupus account for 3% of all renal transplantations in the United States.[12-14] Perhaps as a result of medical co-morbidities, patients with lupus and ESRD are less likely than others to be transplanted. Nevertheless, 772 of 32,644 patients who received a kidney transplant in the United States between 1987 and 1994 had lupus nephritis, and 2882 transplant procedures were performed on patients with lupus nephritis between 1995 and 2002; this figure included 254 children.

Graft and Patient Survival

Renal allografts have been performed on a wide scale since 1975. In the 1970s, 2-year graft survival averaged 50%, and now 5-year graft survival averages 70% to 80%.[15-16] These survival averages are approximately 10% lower than those in nonlupus controls. Improved outcomes are related to the introduction of cyclosporine, sirolimus, tacrolimus, mycophenolate, newer antibiotics, and more effective antihypertensive interventions. Allograft rejection in patients with SLE is greater among smokers, indigent populations, recipients of cadaveric (versus related donor) kidneys, patients with antiphospholipid antibodies, low serum complement levels, and human leukocyte antigen (HLA) mismatches. Premature cardiovascular disease is common.[17] Outcomes among pediatric populations are similar to those in adults.

Serologic Features and Disease Recurrence

Patients undergoing transplantation may have persistent elevations of antinuclear antibody and anti-DNA antibody titers, as well as reduced complement levels. These serologic abnormalities are of little

Box 51-1 Dialysis and Transplantation in Systemic Lupus Erythematosus

1. In up to 10% of patients, systemic lupus erythematosus (SLE) evolves to end-stage renal disease. Their 5-year survival with optimal care is 80% to 90%.
2. Hemodialysis has theoretical advantages over peritoneal dialysis and is associated with fewer infections and, perhaps, less lupus activity.
3. The majority of patients with lupus have disease activity improve if uremic before treatment.
4. Graft survival for patients with SLE in the United States at 1 year is less than the 93.9% national average and is usually in the 80% to 90% range.
5. Transplantation is most successful if lupus is not active at the time of surgery.
6. Patients with a history of antiphospholipid antibody–related events have a poor outcome.

importance and do not affect the outcome of the graft.[18-20] Up to one half of transplanted patients with lupus nephritis who undergo biopsy have some evidence for recurrent disease activity, although the activity is usually mild (e.g., mesangial, membranous) and rarely threatens the graft. Isolated case reports of disease recurrence suggest that a disproportionate number of these patients had undergone peritoneal dialysis or had active disease at the time of transplantation. Extrarenal lupus activity is usually quiescent after renal transplantation. One case of de novo SLE in a patient who underwent renal transplantation has appeared.

In conclusion, to achieve the optimal transplant environment, patients should be in remission, be on hemodialysis or no dialysis, and receive an allograft from a living, related donor (Box 51-1).

Pregnancy

According to the National Transplantation Pregnancy Registry, 60 pregnancies were reported among 38 patients with lupus.[21] Although many of the pregnancies were complicated by preeclampsia and hypertension, 77% were successful.

LASER THERAPY

Carbon dioxide lasers have been used to treat discoid lupus lesions and telangiectasias. These lesions can be vaporized, but cellular alterations in nonvaporized cells that are several hundred micrometers away may be responsible for decreased disease activity.[22] Argon lasers also have been used for atrophic facial scars and telangiectasias, although flares have been reported with its use.[23]

APHERESIS AND RELATED TECHNOLOGIES
Lymphocyte Depletion: Thoracic Duct Drainage, Lymphocytapheresis, and Total Lymphoid Irradiation

Evidence has suggested that the lymphocytic actions of alkylating agents, corticosteroids, and radiation were responsible for ameliorating certain disease states, which has led to investigations of the roles of thoracic-duct drainage, total-lymphoid irradiation, and lymphocytapheresis in rheumatic diseases.[24,25] Lymphoid tissue occupies up to 3% of the total body weight; this includes 1% lymphocytes, or 10^{12} lymphocytes per 70 kg. Lymphocytes are widely distributed and consist of both long-lived and short-lived populations. T cells make up roughly 90% of the lymphocytes in the thoracic duct lymph, 65% in the peripheral blood, 75% in the mesentery, and 25% in the spleen; most of these are long-lived lymphocytes. Therefore thoracic duct drainage and localized radiation remove lymphocyte populations in a different manner differently from lymphapheresis. Pioneered by researchers at the University of California at Los Angeles in the early 1970s, cannulation of the thoracic duct, followed by the removal of

billions of lymphocytes, clearly improved disease activity in patients with SLE. The procedure is not practical for clinical use, however, because it is technically difficult, expensive, frequently complicated by infection, and can only be performed once.

One study has demonstrated that lymphocytapheresis can be safely performed along with plasma exchange in patients with SLE. Adacolumn is a membrane that adsorbs granulocytes and monocytes. In pilot studies, it appears to be well tolerated and not associated with an increased infection rate; however, the studies do not adequately address efficacy.[26]

Between 1980 and 1997, a total of 17 patients with lupus nephritis and nephrotic syndrome refractory to conventional drug therapy received 2000 rad of total lymphoid irradiation over a 4- to 6-week period at Stanford University.[27] Clinical responses were achieved within 3 months and sometimes persisted for years. At follow-up ranging from 12 to 79 months, seven patients were off corticosteroids and without nephrosis. However, one patient died, one ultimately required long-term dialysis, and four developed neutropenia; one developed thrombocytopenia, three developed bacterial sepsis, and four developed herpes zoster. T-helper populations (i.e., CD4+ cells) decreased, and selective B-cell deficits were observed. The survival rate at 7.5 years was identical to that of a historical control group treated with steroids and immunosuppressive agents, with an equal prevalence of serious complications. In a long-term follow-up on these patients in 2002, 6 of 21 patients had died, and 4 developed cancer; 57% were dialyzed, and 33% had developed opportunistic infections. Other groups reported similar findings on a smaller scale.

Total lymphoid irradiation and thoracic duct drainage have no place in the management of patients with SLE, and no online lymphocyte depletion method has been shown to be safe and effective in managing lupus.

Photopheresis

In extracorporeal photochemotherapy, commonly known as photopheresis, leukocytes obtained at apheresis are treated with ultraviolet A (UVA) irradiation after the patient has received a photoactivatable drug, 8-methoxypsoralen.[28] Leukocytes reinfused into the patient can function but have diminished responses. Although only 5% of a patient's total circulating lymphocytes are treated, photopheresis is clearly beneficial for treating cutaneous T-cell lymphomas. The literature in lupus is limited to numerous case reports, mostly for cutaneous lupus, and convey modest, if any, benefit.

Plasmapheresis and Plasma Exchange
Basic Science and Clinical Rationale

Apheresis refers to the removal of a blood component (e.g., red-blood cells, lymphocytes, leukocytes, platelets, plasma) by centrifugation or a membrane cell separator, with return of the other components to the patient.[24,29] Removing 1 L of plasma decreases plasma proteins by 1 g/dL; however, because of compartmental equilibration and protein synthesis, 2.5 L of plasma must be exchanged weekly to decrease protein levels. In the intravascular space, 50% of the total immunoglobulin G (IgG) and 67% of the total immunoglobulin M (IgM) are found. Nine exchanges of 40 mL/kg over a 3-week period leave only 5% of the native plasma. The removal rate of plasma proteins and components depends on charge, solubility, avidity to other plasma proteins, configuration, synthesis, and uptake rates. In immunologic disorders, the recovery of immunoglobulin levels can be slowed by the concurrent use of immunosuppressive agents. If none is used, then antibodies rebound, or the tendency of certain antibody levels to rise rapidly above their prepheresis baseline after initially decreasing, is observed; this rebound often correlates with a disease flare. Plasma is usually replaced with a combination of albumin, salt, and water. Certain complications of lupus (e.g., thrombotic thrombocytopenic purpura) necessitate the use of fresh-frozen plasma replacement, because a plasma factor is deficient. When performed by personnel at experienced blood banks or dialysis facilities, plasmapheresis is usually safe; serious complications (e.g., hypotension, arrhythmia, infection) occur less than 3% of the time in this group of sick patients. The reader is referred to detailed reviews of the subject.

The major goals of apheresis in patients with SLE are to remove circulating immune complexes and immune reactants (e.g., free antibody, complement components), alter the equilibrium between free and bound complexes, and restore reticuloendothelial phagocytic function without altering proliferative responses to mitogens or lymphocyte subpopulation percentages.

Clinical Studies in Systemic Lupus Erythematosus

The use of plasmapheresis was reported first by Jones and colleagues in 1976.[30] Follow-up observations concluded that patients who are the most seriously ill and have the highest levels of circulating immune complexes respond the best.[31] Patients who are treated concomitantly with plasmapheresis, prednisone, and cyclophosphamide do better than those who are treated with prednisone and azathioprine, and those who are on prednisone alone may become worse. The procedure is well tolerated in children and pregnant women with SLE.

Lupus Nephritis

Promising case reports and case series led to a National Institutes of Health (NIH)-sponsored multicenter study in which 86 patients with recent-onset proliferative nephritis received oral cyclophosphamide and prednisone, with or without plasmapheresis.[32] Both groups improved, and no differences in the outcomes were noted. Numerous methodologic flaws minimize the value of this study, however.[33] Of the 27 patients with nephrotic syndrome that was resistant to a minimum 3-month trial of steroids and cytotoxic drugs, 10 patients were randomized to continue their therapy, and plasmapheresis was added in 17 of the patients. After 2 years, the apheresis group had statistically improved outcomes that could not be predicted in advance by any of the 30 variables used.[34]

Antiphospholipid Syndrome and Congenital Heart Block

Interest has focused on the removal of anticardiolipin antibody and the lupus anticoagulant by plasmapheresis during pregnancy or in patients who have experienced recurrent thromboembolic episodes.[35] Results have been mixed. Plasmapheresis is safe during pregnancy and can be used weekly for the temporary removal of anticardiolipin. It is especially helpful if large amounts of the IgM isotype are present. The apheretic removal of anti–Sjögren syndrome antigen A (anti-SSA/Ro) in mothers whose fetuses show signs of congenital heart block has been reported, but no conclusions can be made from the small numbers of patients in published studies.[36]

Other Potential Indications

The usefulness of plasmapheresis for cryoglobulinemia, thrombotic thrombocytopenic purpura, pulmonary hemorrhage, central nervous system vasculitis, neuromyelitis optica, and hyperviscosity syndrome complicating SLE is compelling, but the literature has been limited to case series.[37] (The reader is referred to sections of this monograph dealing with these complications.)

Pulse Synchronization Therapy

A group in Germany devised an innovative approach for the treatment of seriously ill patients with SLE.[38] It involves deliberately inducing antibody rebound with plasmapheresis, followed by high-dose intravenous cyclophosphamide to eliminate the increased numbers of malignant clones. Their pulse synchronization technique has resulted in some successes with long-term, treatment-free remissions. However, pulse synchronization did not work using conventional cyclophosphamide doses, neither for lupus nephritis nor for the disease in general; although higher doses of cyclophosphamide may be more effective, such therapy carries much greater risks as well.

Membrane Technologies

Membrane technologies have enabled selective plasmapheresis to be performed.[39] Membranes that remove cryoproteins, anti–single

Box 51-2 Indications for Apheresis in Systemic Lupus Erythematosus

1. Clear-cut evidence that apheresis can be lifesaving when steroids and immunosuppressive agents fail:
   Thrombotic thrombocytopenic purpura
   Cryoglobulinemia
   Neuromyelitis optica
   Pulmonary hemorrhage
   Hyperviscosity syndrome
2. Relative indication—severe organ-threatening disease unresponsive to steroids and immune suppressives, especially central nervous system vasculitis
3. Investigational—antiphospholipid syndrome, anti–Sjögren syndrome antigen A (anti-Ro/SSA) removal in pregnancy
4. Not indicated
   Mild to moderate non–organ-threatening systemic lupus erythematosus (SLE)
   Lymphocyte depletion
   Photopheresis

stranded DNA (anti-ssDNA) IgG containing circulating immune complexes, and anti-dsDNA by immune adsorption have been developed. Unfortunately, membranes activate complement and may present additional risks of hemolysis. Some approaches, such as a complement 1q (C1q) column immunoadsorption, have shown promising clinical effects in early trials.

Summary

At this time, plasmapheresis should be used only for patients with renal disease that is resistant to corticosteroid and cytotoxic drug therapy, specific disease subsets in which its efficacy is established (e.g., those with hyperviscosity syndrome, cryoglobulinemia, or thrombotic thrombocytopenic purpura), and those with acute, life-threatening complications of SLE—in each instance in combination with corticosteroids and cytotoxic therapy (Box 51-2).[40]

ULTRAVIOLET UVA-1 IRRADIATION

A group in Louisiana and another in Germany have reported modest beneficial effects of the longer wavelengths of UVA-1 irradiation (340 nm to 400 nm) in open-label, double-blind, placebo-controlled, and long-term follow-up studies.[41,42] Disease activity indices, cutaneous lesions, and anti-dsDNA levels improved. No side effects were reported. UVA-1 photons may promote DNA repair, cell-mediated immunity, and apoptosis and reduce B-cell function, leading to anti-inflammatory effects. Cold UVA-1 light may be marginally beneficial in selected patients with SLE.

SHOULD RADIATION THERAPY BE AVOIDED?

Although the in vitro intrinsic cell radiosensitivity of patients with SLE is normal, anecdotal reports of disease flares in patients undergoing radiation therapy for cancers are widespread.[43-45] On the other hand, a definitive matched-controlled, prospective evaluation of 61 patients with collagen vascular disorders failed to find an increased incidence of reactions, compared with the nonautoimmune group; this finding has been supported by a smaller survey. Radiation therapy is often inappropriately denied to patients with lupus, who have uniformly tolerated treatments well at the University of Toronto.

Patients with scleroderma seem to tolerate radiation therapy poorly with accelerated cutaneous and systemic fibrosis, and radiation issues with rheumatoid arthritis and other autoimmune diseases have been reviewed.

In summary, unless a patient has lupus with a scleroderma crossover, radiation therapy is infrequently associated with any complications. The author of this text has advised his patients who need radiation therapy to undergo it; these patients have not experienced any problems.

NICHE THERAPIES FOR LUPUS SUBSETS
Antileprosy Drugs
Dapsone

Dapsone, or 4,4-diaminodiphenylsulfone, interferes with folate metabolism and inhibits para-aminobenzoic acid. It also blocks the alternate pathway of complement activation and neutrophil cytotoxicity.[46,47] Small series have reported that dapsone, which has been used in the treatment of lupus since 1978, can ameliorate vasculitis, bullae, urticaria, oral ulcerations, thrombocytopenia, lupus panniculitis, and subacute cutaneous lupus. Dapsone may be steroid-sparing and can be effective in lupus resistant to chloroquine. In the largest study to date, dapsone was given to 33 patients with chronic cutaneous lupus erythematosus (LE)—8 had excellent results and 8 had fair results, but 17 (52%) of the patients had no response. Its use is limited by its toxicity, which includes sulfhemoglobinemia and methemoglobinemia, a dose-related hemolytic anemia, a dapsone-hypersensitivity syndrome, sulfa-related complications, and aplastic anemia.

All patients treated with dapsone should undergo baseline glucose-6-phosphate dehydrogenase levels determination; the drug should not be administered to individuals with low levels. Complete blood counts should be performed every 2 weeks for the first 3 months and then every 2 months thereafter. Dapsone should be started at a dose of 25 mg twice daily and eventually raised to 100 mg daily. Dapsone also interacts with all oxidant drugs, such as phenacetin and macrodantin. Concurrent administration of 800 U of vitamin E daily may decrease the degree of dapsone-induced hemolysis.

In the author's opinion, dapsone has a place in the management of severe bullous lupus or lupus profundus for patients who cannot tolerate corticosteroids or antimalarial medications.

Thalidomide and Lenalidomide

Thalidomide (Thalidomid, Celegene), also known as α-phthalimidoglutarimide, is a highly teratogenic drug with antileprosy and antilupus effects.[48,49] It has no influence on the complement system, but it can stabilize lysosomal membranes, reduce tumor necrosis factor (TNF) activity, antagonize prostaglandin, inhibit neutrophil chemotaxis and angiogenesis, and alter cellular and humeral immunity. Thalidomide inhibits ultraviolet B (UVB)-induced mouse keratinocyte apoptosis in both TNF-dependent and TNF-independent pathways, as well as UVB-induced erythema.

Since its initial use in Mexico in the 1970s, over 20 publications involving hundreds of patients with SLE have shown the following:

a. Between 60% and 70% efficacy is achieved in treating chronic cutaneous, hypertrophic lupus and lupus profundus in doses of 100 mg a day for induction and less for maintenance.
b. Significant irreversible polyneuropathic symptoms are observed in patients receiving doses greater than 100 mg (used for myeloma and myelodysplastic syndrome) along with unacceptable thrombotic risks.
c. Efficacy diminishes rapidly upon discontinuation of the agent.

Thalidomide is available in the United States from physicians who have registered with the Celgene Corporation and comply with stringent monitoring requirements of the System for Thalidomide Education and Prescribing Safety (STEPS) program. Lenalidomide (Revlamid, Celgene) was introduced in 2006 for myeloma and myelodysplastic syndrome as a more potent derivative of thalidomide and is being studied in clinical trials for cutaneous lupus.[50]

Clofazimine

Clofazimine (Lamprene, Novartis) has antileprosy, antibacterial, and antimalarial activity.[51] It is sequestered in macrophages, stabilizes lysosomal enzymes, and stimulates the production of reactive oxidants. Modestly effective for cutaneous lupus in therapeutic doses of 300 mg/day, it produces quinacrine-like pigment stains. Initially approved by the U.S. Food and Drug Administration (FDA) for *Mycobacterium avium* associated with human immunodeficiency virus, it was removed from the market in the United States in 2005 but is available from various international sources and as a compassionate-use intervention.

Novel Immune Suppressive Agents

Most immune-suppressive agents occasionally used to manage SLE are reviewed in Chapter 50. A few additional agents deserve mention here.

Immunophylins: Tacrolimus and Rapamycin

Immunophylins block interleukin (IL)-2, cell-stimulated T-cell proliferation. Cyclosporin, topical tacrolimus, and pinecrolimus are discussed in Chapters 24 and 50.

Tacrolimus (Prograf, FK-506) has been reviewed in several large case series and small controlled trials for proliferative and membranous lupus nephritis.[52-54] In doses of 0.05 mg/kg/day, it has independent ameliorative effects that are not as robust as with mycophenolate (although they can be combined), but it compares favorably with cyclophosphamide when added to corticosteroids. This agent is used when mycophenolate, cyclophosphamide, or azathioprine has either failed or is poorly tolerated.

Rapamycin (Sirolimus, Rapamune, Wyeth-Ayerst) was approved in the United States for renal transplant rejection prevention in 1999. It regulates mitochondrial transmembrane potential and calcium fluxing, and cell–mammalian target of rapamycin (mTOR) signaling, prolongs survival in lupus-prone MRL/lpr mice, and reverses T-regulator (Treg) cell depletion.[55] It has been well tolerated by patients with lupus with renal allografts. A phase II clinical trial is in progress.

Antimetabolites

Mizoribine (4-carbamoyl-1-b-D-ribofuranosylimidazolium) is an oral purine-antagonist immune suppressive similar to azathioprine.[56] It is the only immune suppressive approved for the treatment of lupus nephritis in Japan. Doses of 100 to 300 mg/day of this nucleoside of the imidazole class have been suggested in several studies to be effective for lupus nephritis in children and as a steroid-sparing vehicle, but no controlled trials have been published.[56] It has also been studied in rheumatoid arthritis and renal transplantation.

Fludarabine is a purine antimetabolite that was studied at the NIH, but the study was terminated early as a result of a high rate of bone marrow suppression. The nucleoside analog *2-chlordeoxyadenosine (2-CdA, cladribine)* was given to patients with proliferative nephritis at the NIH with disappointing results. *Cytarabine* has been observed in case reports. These agents do not play a role in SLE.[57-59]

Gold

For practitioners in the 1940s and 1950s, there was no clear-cut classification distinction between rheumatoid arthritis and SLE, and gold was used not infrequently (and sometimes inadvertently) to treat lupus.[57-60] A few case series have documented modest effects of oral and parenteral gold in ameliorating musculoskeletal and cutaneous manifestations of SLE.[60]

Antilymphocyte Globulin

Because antilymphocyte globulin is an immunosuppressive, it has been experimentally tried in a number of patients with SLE and is part of some ongoing stem cell protocols. Treatment has usually been combined with steroids and other agents. Fever, as well as local and hematologic reactions, has been frequent. Results are generally equivocal. In the largest and only controlled study,[61] nine patients given antilymphocyte globulin, azathioprine, and prednisone did no better than those in a prednisone-only treated group.

Beta Carotene and Retinoids

Beta carotene and retinoids are related compounds that may have antilupus actions because of their sun-blocking and antioxidant activities that enhance natural killer–cell activity and mitogenic responsiveness.[62,63] Beta carotene is a vitamin A derivative that has been used to treat polymorphous light eruption, erythrohepatic protoporphyria, and discoid lupus erythematosus (DLE) with modest results at best. Retinoids inhibit collagenase, prostaglandin E2, and rheumatoid synovial proliferation, and they interfere with intracellular binding proteins and interact with kinases, such as cyclic adenosine monophosphate (cAMP). In addition, epidermal antibodies can be altered, and an effect on epidermal cell differentiation may be observed. Three retinoids have been evaluated in cutaneous lupus: (1) *isotretinoin* (*13-cis-retinoic acid*), formerly known as *Accutane* (Roche Laboratories); (2) *etretinate* (*Tegison*, Roche Laboratories), which is no longer available; and (3) the aromatic retinoid *acitretin* (*Soriatene*, Roche Laboratories). Isotretinoin is very effective for refractory subacute cutaneous lupus. It is initiated in doses of 40 mg twice daily and tapered rapidly over several weeks. Unfortunately, its results are rarely sustained, and it may be used as a bridge therapy until other agents become effective. Patients notice increased photosensitivity, arthralgias, and dryness. Because it can induce depression and is teratogenic, a monitoring program for registrants has been mandated by the FDA. An aromatic retinoid, acitretin, is primarily used to manage psoriasis. A literature review documented its efficacy for chronic cutaneous and subacute cutaneous lupus in eight publications, especially with the concomitant use of extra sunscreen.

In summary, patients unable to tolerate or who are nonresponsive to corticosteroids or antimalarial medications may benefit from short courses of isotretinoin or acitretin. However, these drugs are poorly tolerated, potentially toxic, and not intended for long-term use.

Miscellaneous Hormonal Interventions

The use of contraceptive and other menses-altering or menses-regulating hormones is discussed in Chapter 38.

Danazol

Danazol (Danocrine, Sanofi) is an impeded androgen whose effects in patients with SLE are unclear.[64-66] It may decrease Fc-receptor expression and platelet-associated IgG, can reverse protein S deficiency, and may also have a hormonal downregulating action. Danazol displaces steroids by binding to steroid-binding globulin, which frees the latter compound. Its most promising use so far is for the treatment of idiopathic thrombocytopenia purpura (ITP), in which a 67% response rate and steroid-sparing effects are observed; after an initial response, low doses can be administered as maintenance therapy. Unfortunately, the therapeutic dose (up to 800 to 1200 mg daily) greatly exceeds the dose that is well tolerated (no more than 400 mg a day). Isolated cases of cutaneous disease, autoimmune hemolytic anemia, cytopenias, and red-cell aplasias have responded to this agent as well.

In summary, danazol is useful for refractory ITP and possibly hemolytic anemias in patients with SLE as a niche therapy after steroids, rituximab, immunosuppressive agents, and intravenous immunoglobulins (IVIGs) have been used.

Testosterones

In 1948, Lamb[67] gave androgens to five patients with lupus, but the results showed no significant improvement. In 1950, Dubois and others[68] treated several female patients with massive doses of testosterone, both orally and intramuscularly, using as much as 500 to 1000 mg/day for as long as 5 weeks without benefit. After a 30-year hiatus, interest in androgen therapy has resurfaced. Once again, several published trials failed to demonstrate any effect of this hormone.[69]

Dehydroepiandrosterone

Dehydroepiandrosterone (DHEA) is a steroid precursor of androgens and, to a lesser extent, estrogens. It is produced in the adrenal gland, and its levels decline with age. DHEA increases IL-2, soluble-adhesion molecules, and interferon (IFN) while downregulating IL-4, IL-5, and IL-6. Although DHEA is available over the counter as a "dietary supplement," a quality control review of 16 preparations showed that 0% to 150% of what was claimed on the label was actually in the product. Advocates claim that these preparations increase growth-hormone levels and improve bone density, fatigue, libido, and cognitive dysfunction.

Early studies at Stanford University showed that doses of 100 to 200 mg/day (two to three times the available over-the-counter dose) achieved favorable effects in mild to moderate lupus in an open-label study, in a double-blind trial, and at long-term follow-up.[70,71] In patients with severe SLE, bone density improved, but disease activity changes were not statistically significant. Several pivotal trials were ultimately performed. A double-blind, randomized, placebo-controlled trial of 191 female patients with lupus suggested that it was steroid sparing in individuals with a SLEDAI score greater than 2, which was a post-hoc finding. In another trial, 381 patients given 200 mg daily or placebo noted significant improvements in myalgias, oral stomatitis, and serum C3 complement. In a Taiwanese study, 120 women randomized to DHEA versus placebo showed decreased flare rates and improved patient global assessment. IL-10 synthesis was suppressed. The drug was well tolerated with mild acne and hirsutism being common but rarely requiring drug discontinuation. Suggestions that the drug might improve bone mineralization in steroid-dependent patients with lupus led to a controlled trial that failed to reach its primary endpoint. The FDA Advisory Board recommended against recommending approval of DHEA for the treatment of lupus because it objected to a post-hoc analysis by the pharmaceutical company and noted that the drug did not improve sedimentation rate, SLEDAI scores, or anti-DNA. Since the advisory board's vote, subsequent and better-designed studies showed that DHEA had no effect on fatigue, well-being, or biomarkers for atherosclerosis or bone demineralization.[72] DHEA probably has no place in the management of SLE.

Bromocriptine

Prolactin appears to have proinflammatory effects, and its levels are elevated in SLE. Interest has centered on the use of prolactin suppression with bromocriptine in SLE.[73] Two small controlled studies showed slight, if any, benefit.

Gamma Globulin and Intravenous Immunoglobulin

Hypogammaglobulinemia with recurrent infections is a rare event in SLE, and the use of intramuscular gamma globulin to prevent infection in lupus is not uncommon, although no controlled studies have documented its efficacy.

IVIG delays the clearance of antibody-coated autologous red blood cells, competitively inhibits reticuloendothelial Fc-receptor blockade, has antiidiotypic antibody activity, modulates the release and function of proinflammatory cytokines and adhesion molecule expression, and decreases pokeweed mitogen–induced B-cell differentiation.[74,75] Intravenous gamma globulin was first used in a patient with lupus nephritis in 1982. It may be acutely helpful for autoimmune thrombocytopenia secondary to SLE and for the neonatal thrombocytopenia that is seen in children of mothers with SLE. Gamma globulin is thought to be useful for serious disease exacerbations, such as in central nervous system lupus, pericarditis, cardiac dysfunction, acquired factor VIII deficiency, pancytopenia, refractory cutaneous lupus, myelofibrosis, nephritis, polyneuritis, hypoprothrombinemia with the lupus anticoagulant, and pulmonary hemorrhage, as well as to prevent recurrent fetal loss in patients with the antiphospholipid syndrome. In a controlled study, low–molecular-weight heparin was superior to IVIG.[76]

The use of gamma globulin for the treatment of lupus nephritis is controversial. The drug is expensive and potentially dangerous. The reader should appreciate that it is often ineffective or temporarily effective. It can flare disease activity, induce acute renal failure, and promote thromboembolic disease, myocardial infarction, aseptic meningitis, and vasculitic rashes, among other symptoms. Low levels or absence of immunoglobulin A (IgA) (seen in 5% of patients with SLE) is a relative contraindication to its administration.

Evidence-based reviews confirm that IVIG is a first-line therapy for ITP, IgG subclass deficiency, and chronic inflammatory demyelinating polyneuropathy associated with SLE. It may be useful in other serious manifestations of SLE as a second-line therapeutic approach in refractory cases.

Vasodilators as Disease-Modifying Agents

Prostaglandin E1 (PGE), angiotensin-converting enzyme inhibitors and angiotensin-receptor blockers, *pentoxyfylline, bosentan,* 5-phosphodiesterase inhibitors, and other vasodilators can improve renal function by increasing blood flow, lower pulmonary pressures, improve Raynaud syndrome, and heal digital gangrene.[77]

Agents to Avoid and Failed Agents

Numerous reports of disease exacerbation, drug-induced lupus, or the lack of efficacy with *D-penicillamine, sulfasalazine,* and *minocycline,* which may be useful for rheumatoid arthritis, have been written. Extreme caution is advised in the use of these preparations in patients with SLE.

The following agents have a slight effect or no effect in patients with lupus

Levamisole, a T-cell immunostimulant

Antibiotics, which have been evaluated for SLE, including *chloramphenicol, thiamphenicol, penicillin, sulfonamides, tetracycline,* and *streptomycin*

Antiviral agents such as *interferon-alpha* (except perhaps as intralesional injections for cutaneous disease) and *isoprinosine*

Hormonal preparations such as *tamoxifen* and *growth hormone*

Thymosin and *thymectomy,* which have no effect on lupus

Zileuton, methylxanthines, para-aminobenzoic acid, colchicine, aminoglutethimide, 15-deoxyspergualin, transfer factor, phenytoin, hyperbaric oxygen, among other agents, and those listed previously are reviewed in greater detail in previous edition.[78]

Complementary, herbal, and vitamin therapies are discussed in Chapter 52.

References

1. Ward MM: Changes in the incidence of end-stage renal disease due to lupus nephritis, 1982-1995. *Arch Intern Med* 160:3136–3140, 2000.
2. Vu TV, Escalante A: A comparison of the quality of life of patients with systemic lupus erythematosus with and without endstage renal disease. *J Rheumatol* 26:2595–2601, 1999.
3. Ward M: Access to care and the incidence of end stage renal disease due to systemic lupus erythematosus. *J Rheum* 37:1158–1163, 2010.
4. Wallace DJ, Podell TE, Weiner JM, et al: Lupus nephritis. Experience with 230 patients in a private practice from 1950 to 1980. *Am J Med* 72:209–220, 1982.
5. Coplon NS, Diskin CJ, Peterson J, et al: The long-term clinical course of systemic lupus erythematosus in end-stage renal disease. *N Engl J Med* 308:186–190, 1983.
6. Adler M, Chambers S, Edwards C, et al: An assessment of renal failure in an SLE cohort with special reference to ethnicity, over a 25 year period. *Rheumatology* 45:1144–1147, 2006.
7. Ward MM: Changes in the incidence of endstage renal disease due to lupus nephritis in the United States 1996-2004. *J Rheumatol* 36:63–67, 2009.
8. Ward MM: Cardiovascular and cerebrovascular morbidity and mortality among women with end-stage renal disease attributable to lupus nephritis. *Am J Kid Dis* 36:516–525, 2000.
9. Siu YP, Leung KT, Tong MK, et al: Clinical outcomes of systemic lupus erythematosus patients undergoing continuous ambulatory peritoneal dialysis. *Nephrol Dial Transplant* 20:2797–2802, 2005.
10. Huang HW, Hung KY, Yen CJ, et al: Systemic lupus erythematosus and peritoneal dialysis: outcomes and infectious complications. *Perit Dial Int* 21:143–147, 2001.
11. Rodby RA, Korbet SM, Lewis EJ: Persistence of clinical and serologic activity in patients with systemic lupus erythematosus undergoing peritoneal dialysis. *Am J Med* 83:613–618, 1987.
12. Ward MM: Access to renal transplantation among patients with end-stage renal disease due to lupus nephritis. *Am J Kidney Dis* 35:915–922, 2000.
13. Chelamcharla M, Javaid B, Baird BC, et al: The outcome of renal transplantation among systemic lupus erythematosus patients. *Nephrol Dial Transplant* 22:3623–3630, 2007.
14. Tang H, Chelamcharia M, Baird BC, et al: Factors affecting kidney-transplant outcome in recipients with lupus nephritis. *Clin Transplant* 22:263–272, 2008.
15. Stone JH, Amend WJC, Criswell LA: Antiphospholipid antibody syndrome in renal transplantation: occurrence of clinical events in 96 consecutive patients with systemic lupus erythematosus. *Am J Kid Dis* 34:1040–1047, 1999.
16. Stone JH, Amend WJC, Criswell LA: Outcome of renal transplantation in systemic lupus erythematosus. *Semin Arthritis Rheum* 27:17–26, 1997.
17. Norby GE, Leivestad T, Mjoen G, et al: Premature cardiovascular disease in patients with systemic lupus erythematosus influences survival after renal transplantation. *Arthritis Rheum* 63:733–737, 2011.
18. Bartosh SM, Fine RN, Sullivan EK: Outcome after transplantation of young patients with systemic lupus erythematosus: a report of the North American pediatric renal transplant cooperative study. *Transplantation* 72:973–978, 2001.
19. Nyberg G, Blohme I, Persson H, et al: Recurrence of SLE in transplanted kidneys: a follow-up transplant biopsy study. *Nephrol Dial Transplant* 11:1116–1123, 1992.
20. Norby GE, Strom EH, Midtvedt K, et al: Recurrent lupus nephritis after kidney transplantation: a surveillance biopsy study. *Ann Rheum Dis* 59:1484–1487, 2010.
21. McGrory CH, McCloskey LJ, DeHoratius RJ, et al: Pregnancy outcome in female renal recipients: a comparison of systemic lupus erythematosus with other diagnoses, *Am J Transplant* 3:35–42, 2003.
22. Walker SL, Harland CC: Carbon dioxide laser resurfacing of facial scarring secondary to chronic discoid lupus erythematosus. *Br J Dermatol* 143:1101–1102, 2000.
23. Kuhn A, Becker-Wegerich P, Rizicka T: Successful treatment of discoid lupus erythematosus with argon laser. *Dermatology* 201:175–177, 2000.
24. Wallace DJ, Klinenberg JR: Apheresis. *Dis Mon* 30:1–45, 1984.
25. Nyman KE, Bangert R, Machleder H, et al: Thoracic duct drainage in SLE with cutaneous vasculitis. *Arthritis Rheum* 20:1129–1134, 1979.
26. Soerensen H, Schneidewind-Mueller JM, Lange D, et al: Pilot clinical study of Adacolumn cytapheresis in patients with systemic lupus erythematosus. *Rheumatol Int* 26:409–415, 2006.
27. Genovese MC, Uhrin Z, Bloch DA: Long-term follow up of patients treated with total lymphoid irradiation for lupus nephritis. *Arthritis Rheum* 46:1014–1018, 2002.
28. Mayes MD: Photopheresis and autoimmune diseases. *Rheum Dis Clin North Am* 26:75–81, 2000.
29. Kaplan AA: *A practical guide to therapeutic plasma exchange.* Malden, MA, 1999, Blackwell Science, pp. 159–177.
30. Jones JV, Cumming RH, Bucknall RC, et al: Plasmapheresis in the management of acute systemic lupus erythematosus? *Lancet* i:709–711, 1976.
31. Jones JV: Plasmapheresis in SLE. *Clin Rheum Dis* 8:243–260, 1982.
32. Lewis EJ, Hunsicker LG, Lan SP, et al: A controlled trial of plasmapheresis therapy in severe lupus nephritis. *N Engl J Med* 326:1373–1379, 1992.
33. Wallace DJ, Goldfinger D, Savage G, et al: Predictive value of clinical, laboratory, pathologic and treatment variables in steroid/immunosuppressive resistant lupus nephritis. *J Clin Apher* 4:30–34, 1988.
34. Wallace DJ: Plasmapheresis for lupus nephritis (letter). *N Engl J Med* 327:1029, 1992.
35. Neuwelt CM, Daikh DI, Linfoot LA, et al: Catastrophic antiphospholipid syndrome: response to repeated plasmapheresis over three years. *Arthritis Rheum* 40:1534–1539, 1997.
36. Hickstein H, Kulz T, Claus R, et al: Autoimmune-associated congenital heart block: treatment of the mother with immunoadsorption. *Ther Apher Dial* 9:148–153, 2005.
37. Pagnoux C, Korach J-M, Guillevin L: Indications for plasma exchange in systemic lupus erythematosus in 2005. *Lupus* 14:871–877, 2005.
38. Euler HH, Schroeder JO, Harten P, et al: Treatment-free remission in severe systemic lupus erythematosus following synchronization of plasmapheresis with subsequent pulse cyclophosphamide. *Arthritis Rheum* 37:1784–1794, 1994.
39. Stummvoll GH: Immunoadsorption (IAS) for systemic lupus erythematosus. *Lupus* 20:115–119, 2011.
40. Wallace DJ: Apheresis for lupus erythematosus—state of the art. *Lupus* 10:193–196, 2001.
41. Molina JF, Mc Grath H, Jr: Longterm ultraviolet-A1 irradiation therapy in systemic lupus erythematosus. *J Rheumatol* 24:1072–1074, 1997.
42. Polderman MCA, le Cessie S, Huizinga TWJ: Efficacy of UVA-1 cold light as an adjuvant therapy for systemic lupus erythematosus. *Rheumatology* 43:1402–1404, 2004.

43. Carillo-Alascio PL, Sabio JM, Nunez-Torres MI, et al: In-vitro radiosensitivity in patients with systemic lupus erythematosus. *Lupus* 18:645–649, 2009.

44. Ross JG, Hussey DH, Mayr NA, et al: Acute and late reactions to radiation therapy in patients with collagen vascular diseases. *Cancer* 71:3744–3752, 1993.

45. Benk V, Al-Herz A, Gladman D, et al: Role of radiation therapy in patients with a diagnosis of both systemic lupus erythematosus and cancer. *Arthritis Rheum* 53:67–72, 2005.

46. Chang DJ, Lamothe M, Stevens RM, et al: Dapsone in rheumatoid arthritis. *Semin Arthritis Rheum* 25:390–403, 1996.

47. Lindskov R, Reymann F: Dapsone in the treatment of cutaneous lupus erythematosus. *Dermatologica* 172:214–217, 1986.

48. Calabrese L, Fleischer AB: Thalidomide: current and potential clinical applications. *Amer J Med* 108:487–495, 2000.

49. Knop J, Bonsmann G, Happle R, et al: Thalidomide in the treatment of sixty cases of chronic discoid lupus erythematosus. *Br J Dermatol* 108:461–466, 1983.

50. Shah A, Albrecht J, Bonilla-Martinez Z, et al: Lenalidomide for the treatment of resistant discoid lupus. *Arch Dermatol* 145:303–306, 2009.

51. Bezerra ELM, Vilar MJP, Neto PBT, et al: Double-blind, randomized controlled clinical trial of clofaximine compared with chloroquine in patients with systemic lupus erythematosus. *Arthritis Rheum* 52:3073–3078, 2005.

52. Chen W, Tang X, Liu Q, et al: Short-term outcomes of induction therapy with tacrolimus versus cyclophosphamide for active lupus nephritis: a multicenter randomized clinical trial. *Am J Kidney Dis* 57:235–244, 2011.

53. Asamiya Y, Uchida K, Otsubo S, et al: Clinical assessment of tacrolimus therapy in lupus nephritis: one-year follow-up study in a single center. *Nephron Clin Pract* 113:330–336, 2009.

54. Szeto CC, Kwan BCH, Lai FMM, et al: Tacrolimus for the treatment of systemic lupus erythematosus with pure class V nephritis. *Rheumatology* 47:1678–1681, 2008.

55. Fernandez D, Bonilla E, Mizra N, et al: Rapamycin reduces disease activity and normalizes T cell activation-induced calcium fluxing in patients with systemic lupus erythematosus. *Arthritis Rheum* 54:2983–2988, 2006.

56. Yumura W, Suganuma S, Uchida K, et al: Effects of long-term treatment with mizoribine in patients with proliferative nephritis. *Clin Nephrol* 64:28–34, 2005.

57. Illei GG, Yarboro CH, Kuriowa T, et al: Long-term effects of combination treatment of fludarabine and low-dose pulse cyclophosphamide in patients with lupus nephritis. *Rheumatology* 46:952–956, 2007.

58. Yung RL, Richardson BC: Cytarabine for refractory cutaneous lupus. *Arthritis Rheum* 38:1341–1343, 1995.

59. Davis JC, Jr, Austin H, III, Boumpas D, et al: A pilot study of 2-chloro-28-deoxyadenosine in the treatment of systemic lupus erythematosus-associated glomerulonephritis. *Arthritis Rheum* 41:335–343, 1998.

60. Weisman MH, Albert D, Mueller MR, et al: Gold therapy in patients with systemic lupus erythematosus. *Am J Med* 75(Suppl 6A):157–164, 1983.

61. Herreman G, Broquie G, Metzger JP, et al: Treatment of systemic lupus and other collagenoses with antilymphocyte globulins. *Nouv Presse Med* 1:2035–2039, 1972.

62. Newton RC, Jorizzo JL, Solomon AR, et al: Mechanism-oriented assessment of isotretinoin in chronic or subacute cutaneous lupus erythematosus. *Arch Dermatol* 122:170–176, 1986.

63. Ruzicka T, Meurer M, Bieber T: Efficiency of acitretin in the treatment of cutaneous lupus erythematosus. *Arch Dermatol* 124:897–902, 1988.

64. Letchumanan P, Thumboo J: Danazol in the treatment of systemic lupus erythematosus: a qualitative systemic review. *Semin Arthritis Rheum* 40:298–306, 2011.

65. Dougados M, Job-Deslandre C, Amor B, et al: Danazol therapy in systemic lupus erythematosus. A one-year prospective controlled trial on 40 female patients. *Clin Trials J* 24:191–200, 1987.

66. Arnal C, Piette JC, Leone J, et al: Treatment of severe immune thrombocytopenia associated with systemic lupus erythematosus: 59 cases. *J Rheumatol* 29:75–83, 2002.

67. Lamb JH, Lain ES, Keaty C, et al: Steroid hormones, metabolic studies in dermatomyositis, lupus erythematosus and polymorphic light-sensitivity eruptions. *Arch Derm Syphilol* 57:785–801, 1948.

68. Dubois EL, Commons RR, Starr P, et al: Corticotropin and cortisone treatment for systemic lupus erythematosus. *JAMA* 149:995–102, 1952.

69. Gordon C, Wallace DJ, Shinada S, et al: Testosterone patches in the management of patients with mild/moderate systemic lupus erythematosus. *Rheumatology (Oxford)* 47:334–338, 2008.

70. Van Vollenhoven RF, Engleman EG, McGuire JL: Dehydroepiandrosterone in systemic lupus erythematosus. Results of a double-blind, placebo-controlled, randomized clinical trial. *Arthritis Rheum* 38:1826–1831, 1995.

71. Petri MA, Mease PJ, Merrill JT, et al: Effects of prasterone on disease activity and symptoms in women with active systemic lupus erythematosus. *Arthritis Rheum* 50:2858–2868, 2004.

72. Marder W, Somers EC, Kaplan MJ, et al: Effects of prasterone (dehydroepiandrosterone) on markers of cardiovascular risk and bone turnover in premenopausal women with systemic lupus erythematosus: a pilot study. *Lupus* 19:1229–1236, 2010.

73. Walker SE: Treatment of systemic lupus erythematosus with bromocriptine. *Lupus* 10:197–202, 2001.

74. Rauova L, Lukac J, Levy Y, et al: High dose intravenous immunoglobulin for lupus nephritis—a salvage immunomodulation. *Lupus* 10:209–213, 2001.

75. Gonzalez-Gay MA: The pros and cons of intravenous immunoglobulin treatment in autoimmune nephropathy. *Semin Arthritis Rheum* 34:573–574, 2004.

76. Triolo G, Ferrante A, Ciccia F, et al: Randomized study of subcutaneous low molecular weight heparin plus aspirin versus intravenous immunoglobulin in the treatment of recurrent fetal loss associated with antiphospholipid antibodies. *Arthritis Rheum* 48:728–731, 2003.

77. Ooiwa H, Miyaazwa T, Yamanishi Y, et al: Successful treatment of systemic lupus erythematosus and pulmonary hypertension with intravenous prostaglandin I2 followed by its oral analogue. *Intern Med* 39:320–323, 2000.

78. Wallace DJ: Additional therapies used in the management of lupus. In Wallace DJ, Hahn BH, editors: *Dubois' Lupus Erythematosus*, ed 7, Philadelphia, PA, 2007, Lippincott Williams & Wilkins, pp 1298–1310.

Chapter 52

Adjunctive and Preventive Measures

Diane L. Kamen

An improved ability to diagnose and treat systemic lupus erythematosus (SLE) has contributed to longer survival for patients and an increased emphasis placed on the prevention of complications of the disease and its treatments. This chapter reviews common preventive measures, such as immunizations and antibiotic prophylaxis, as well as surrounding issues, including drug allergies, vitamin D, and other supplements. Up to one half of patients with SLE, regardless of access to prescription medications, incorporate some form of complementary or alternative remedies into their treatment regimen. This topic, as well as issues related to adherence to prescribed medications, is reviewed.

IMMUNIZATIONS AND PREVENTION OF INFECTION IN LUPUS

Infection is responsible for approximately 25% of all deaths in patients with SLE, up to 58% in developing countries, making it a leading cause of mortality among patients with SLE.[1-3] Many infections in patients with SLE could be prevented with timely vaccinations, reducing exposure to contagious contacts, screening for latent infections, minimizing exposure to corticosteroids, targeted prophylaxis for high-risk patients, and, unless contraindicated, antimalarial therapy as standards of care.[4] A checklist has been proposed for identifying high-risk patients and identifying prevention opportunities (Table 52-1).[5] Vaccination status, particularly annual inactivated influenza and periodic pneumococcal vaccinations for patients taking immunosuppressants, has been included by expert consensus in the quality indicator set for SLE.[6] Recommendations for specific vaccines in patients with SLE follow guidelines for the general local population, except when the patient is immunosuppressed, in which case the evidence-based guidelines from European League Against Rheumatism (EULAR) provide guidance on vaccines for adult and pediatric patients (Online Supplement 1).[7,8]

A comparison of immunization rates among insured women with SLE, women in the general population, and women with nonrheumatic chronic conditions found similar rates of influenza (59%) and pneumococcal (60%) immunizations among those who were eligible in each group; however, overall rates were low and even lower in those of younger age and lower educational attainment.[9] Not surprisingly, having seen a generalist during the preceding year increased the likelihood of receiving vaccinations, but the overall vaccination rate was still only 61%.

Ruiz-Irastorza and colleagues[10] reported the clinical predictors of major infections found in a prospective cohort of patients with SLE from Spain. The prevalence of life-threatening infections appears to be highest within the first 5 years of disease onset.[1,11] Often, the infections that lead to hospitalization and/or death among patients with SLE are caused by common pathogens such as *Streptococcus pneumoniae* and *Haemophilus influenzae*, for which effective vaccinations exist.[2] Therapy for patients with SLE has shifted to include a greater use of biologics, which, as a class, tend to increase the risk for infection risk, but longer patient exposure is needed to determine whether this shift has altered infection outcomes in those with SLE.[12]

Are There Vaccinations That Should Be Avoided with Systemic Lupus Erythematosus?

More research is needed on the safety and efficacy of live attenuated vaccines (e.g., measles, mumps, rubella, herpes zoster, yellow fever, nasal-spray influenza vaccine) in patients with SLE and other autoimmune diseases who are taking immunosuppressive drugs. Household transmission from someone who has received a live attenuated virus living in close contact with a patient with SLE is rare, and contact precautions during viral shedding (typically 7 to 10 days) are recommended only for those who are severely immunosuppressed.[13]

Should Patients with Systemic Lupus Erythematosus Receive the Varicella Zoster Vaccine?

Reactivation of latent varicella zoster virus is one of the most commonly reported viral infections in SLE and may be complicated by disseminated disease, superinfection, and postherpetic neuralgia. A live attenuated herpes zoster vaccine came to market in 2006, and guidelines from the Centers for Disease Control and Prevention (CDC) Advisory Committee on Immunization Practices recommend vaccination in patients over 60 years of age, 2 to 4 weeks before any anticipated immunosuppression. The immunosuppression threshold, below which the administration of the herpes zoster vaccine is not contraindicated, includes prednisone less than 20 mg/day lasting less than 2 weeks, low doses of methotrexate (≤0.4 mg/kg/wk) or azathioprine (≤3.0 mg/kg/day).[5]

What Is the Risk of a Vaccination Triggering a Lupus Flare or Being Ineffective?

Apprehensions concerning vaccine safety and inefficacy, especially in an immunocompromised host, may be contributing to the low vaccination rates seen among patients with SLE. Despite anecdotal cases of disease exacerbations after vaccinations, multiple studies in different SLE populations have shown vaccinations against influenza, pneumococcal disease, and hepatitis B to be safe but efficacy to be potentially impaired.[14,15]

Several studies have shown that influenza vaccination is safe and does not lead to SLE flares, with the majority of patients developing protective antibodies. In a prospective study of 72 patients with SLE, influenza-specific antibody responses were determined 2, 6, and 12 weeks after vaccination.[16] Compared with high responders, low responders were more likely to have European-American backgrounds, be taking prednisone, have hematologic criteria for SLE, and have evidence of increased disease flares.

Similarly, several small studies have shown the vaccination against *Pneumococcus* to be safe in patients with SLE. The studies to date in SLE involve the 23-valent polysaccharide vaccine that shows good biologic tolerability of the vaccine with approximately 80% having an antibody response.[17] In an efficacy study of 19 patients, titers of antibodies against the polysaccharides are significantly lower at 1, 2, and 3 years after vaccination in patients with SLE, compared with controls.[18] Because reduced antipneumococcal antibody production has

TABLE 52-1 Checklist to Identify Patients with Systemic Lupus Erythematosus at Risk for Preventable Infections

HAS THE PATIENT HAD ...	IF NOT ...
Yearly influenza vaccination	Administer vaccine or recommend to primary care provider.
Pneumococcal vaccination	Administer vaccine or recommend to primary care provider (every 5 years).
Regular Papanicolaou (PAP) smears to screen for cervical dysplasia caused by human papillomavirus (HPV)	Recommend to primary care provider or gynecologist. Consider Gardasil vaccination.
Negative tuberculosis (TB) skin test before starting immunosuppressive agent	Treat with isoniazid for patients with evidence of latent TB infection.
Hepatitis B serologic testing	Obtain baseline serologic findings in all patients.
Hepatitis C serologic testing	Obtain baseline serologic findings in all patients with risk factors.
Human immunodeficiency virus (HIV) serologic testing	Obtain baseline serologic findings in all patients with risk factors.
Screening for *Strongyloides* in patients from endemic areas before starting immunosuppressive therapy	Obtain *Strongyloides* serologic finding, and treat with ivermectin if infected.

From Barber C, Gold WL, Fortin PR: Infections in the lupus patient: perspectives on prevention. *Curr Opin Rheumatol* 23:358–365, 2011.

been reported in patients with SLE, consideration may be made for using the more strongly immunogenic vaccines, although they are not yet studied in SLE.

The hepatitis B vaccine has been shown in both a case-control study of 265 patients and a prospective cohort study of 28 patients not to be associated with the development of SLE or an exacerbation of existing disease.[19,20] No loss of efficacy among patients with SLE is observed, with 93% having adequate anti–hepatitis B surface antigen antibodies after the series of three vaccinations and the remaining 7% having adequate antibody response after a fourth vaccination.[20]

Vaccinations should not be withheld because of misguided fears of precipitating SLE flares. Although the immunologic response may be dampened by concomitant immunosuppressive medications, always addressing the immunization status in patients with SLE is best practice, regardless of their age or other risk factors. Immunogenicity is generally lower among vaccinated patients with SLE, compared with controls, especially for those patients receiving immunosuppressant agents; therefore a booster vaccination later in the influenza season or additional or more frequent vaccinations against other pathogens may be considered.[15]

ANTIBIOTIC PROPHYLAXIS IN LUPUS

The ability of antimicrobial prophylaxis to prevent infection is important for patients with SLE but should be limited to specific, well-supported indications to reduce unnecessary toxicity, costs, and antimicrobial resistance. Indications for the use of antimicrobial prophylaxis and the recommended antibiotic regimens for patients with SLE are consistent with those of the general population,[21] with a few exceptions in which patients with SLE are at a higher risk of opportunistic infections (see detailed text later in this chapter).

Approximately 30% to 38% of patients with SLE will have cardiac vegetations, most of which are asymptomatic but still put them at risk of endocarditis.[22,23] This is especially true for patients with antiphospholipid antibodies, who are at an increased risk of cardiac vegetations.[24] However, the 2007 Antibiotic Prophylaxis Guidelines for preventing endocarditis published by the American

Box 52-1 Cardiac Conditions Associated with the Highest Risk of Adverse Outcomes from Endocarditis for which Prophylaxis with Dental Procedures* Is Reasonable†

Prosthetic cardiac valve or prosthetic material used for cardiac valve repair
Previous infectious endocarditis
Congenital heart disease (CHD), only if one of the following conditions is present:
- Unrepaired cyanotic CHD, including palliative shunts and conduits
- Completely repaired congenital heart defect with prosthetic material or device, whether placed by surgery or catheter intervention, during the first 6 months after the procedure
- Repaired CHD with residual defects at the site or adjacent to the site of a prosthetic patch or prosthetic device, which inhibits endothelialization
Cardiac transplantation recipients who develop cardiac valvulopathy

*Includes all dental procedures that involve manipulation of gingival tissue or the periapical region of teeth or perforation of the oral mucosa.
†Conditions, for which antibiotic prophylaxis is recommended, follow the 2007 Antibiotic Prophylaxis Guidelines for preventing endocarditis and is published by the American Heart Association and the Infectious Diseases Society of America.[25]

Heart Association and the Infectious Diseases Society of America recommend antibiotic prophylaxis for a more limited number of conditions, compared with previous guidelines (Box 52-1). The presence of a murmur or aseptic vegetation alone no longer warrants antibiotic prophylaxis, based on subsequent studies that show a higher risk-to-benefit ratio than previously estimated.[25]

Are There Specific Infections of Concern Requiring Prophylaxis in Patients with Systemic Lupus Erythematosus?

Additional infection risks may also warrant antibiotic prophylaxis in patients with SLE. Patients with latent *Mycobacterium tuberculosis* or with *Strongyloides stercoralis* should be given preventive therapy before starting immunosuppression therapy.[5] Immunosuppressed patients with SLE are also at risk of developing *Pneumocystis jiroveci* pneumonia (PJP), and expert opinion suggests PJP prophylaxis be considered for patients with SLE taking 16 mg or more prednisone or equivalent for 8 weeks or longer with special consideration to those receiving cyclophosphamide.[26] A retrospective study of *Pneumocystis carinii* pneumonia (PCP), which included 119 patients with SLE, estimated the number needed to treat was 14 immunosuppressed patients with trimethoprim-sulfamethoxazole (TMP-SMX) to prevent one case of PJP.[27] They used once daily dosing of single-strength TMP-SMX and found a lower rate of allergic reactions, compared with previous reports, and no increase in SLE flares among those exposed to TMP-SMX. A metaanalysis of randomized controlled trials, including 1245 immunocompromised patients with non–human immunodeficiency virus (HIV), concluded that PJP prophylaxis with TMP-SMX is highly effective at preventing PJP infection, but it was only warranted when the PJP risk was over 3.5%. Based on an estimated PJP rate of 1.0% for the general population of patients with SLE, the number needed to treat ($n = 110$) would be greater than the number needed to harm ($n = 32$) because of adverse reactions and intolerance to TMP-SMX.[28] Similar conclusions came from a review of the literature on PJP in SLE and a survey of U.S. rheumatologists in which investigators found a low incidence of PJP in patients with SLE, yet a high prevalence of rheumatologists routinely prescribing TMP-SMX for patients receiving cyclophosphamide.[29] Until consensus guidelines are in place, the decision to use PJP prophylaxis with TMP-SMX in patients with SLE will depend on the individual assessment of known risk factors for PJP weighed against the potential risks of TMP-SMX. (See detailed discussion later in this chapter.)

Are There Antibiotics That Patients with Systemic Lupus Erythematosus Should Avoid?

Exposure to antibiotics is unavoidable for a majority of patients with SLE, who are more prone to develop infections as a result of disease-related altered immune responses and immunosuppressive medications. However, certain antibiotics carry a higher likelihood for being problematic for patients because of their sun-sensitizing properties, their ability to provoke drug allergies, or their potential to trigger disease flares. Sun-sensitizing antibiotics that can flare cutaneous and occasionally systemic disease include tetracyclines, sulfonamides, and fluoroquinolones. This property alone would not be an absolute contraindication for patients with SLE but would make sun-protective measures (e.g., sun avoidance, sun-protective clothing, broad-spectrum sunscreen) even more of a priority. Minocycline is also associated with causing drug-induced lupus; however, no evidence suggests that these drugs are implicated in drug-induced lupus or precipitate flares in patients with established SLE.[30]

A case-control study of antibiotic allergy in 221 patients with SLE found that patients exposed to antibiotics reported significantly more penicillin and cephalosporin (27% versus 10% and 15%), sulfonamide (32% versus 14% and 12%), and erythromycin (13% versus 3% and 3%) antibiotic allergy, compared with either exposed related or unrelated controls.[31] The increased frequency of tetracycline allergies reported by exposed patients with SLE, compared with either control group (7% versus 4% and 3%), was not statistically significant. Consistent with several previous and subsequent reports, sulfonamide antibiotics were the most likely class of antibiotics to trigger an allergic reaction among patients with SLE[19,32,33] and the most likely to exacerbate SLE with photosensitive rashes and cytopenias being the most common confirmed exacerbations associated with antibiotic exposure.[31,34] Although completely avoiding their use would be unrealistic, they should be used sparingly and with caution, because sulfonamide antibiotics are known to sun-sensitize, provoke allergic reactions, and cause disease flares among patients with SLE.

ALLERGIES IN PATIENTS WITH LUPUS

There is no question that patients with SLE have higher frequencies of antibiotic allergies, compared with healthy controls as previously described in this chapter; however, less is known about the frequency of other allergies in SLE. Studies comparing drug allergies among patients with SLE and other groups, including patients with other rheumatic diseases, have failed to show any higher risk of drug allergies in SLE other than for antibiotics.[33] True allergic reactions were not dissimilar in patients with SLE, compared with controls with inflammatory arthritis, with the exception of cutaneous reactions to sulfonamide antibiotics in patients with SLE.[32] Although sulfonamide nonantibiotic agents are rarely cross-reactive with sulfonamide antibiotics,[35] a relatively high prevalence of sulfonamide nonantibiotic allergic reactions has also been observed among patients with SLE, prompting caution for the entire class of drugs.[36]

Despite an increased family history of allergic disorders, patients with SLE do not appear to have an increased risk of immunoglobulin E (IgE)–mediated and/or associated allergic disorders, such as atopic dermatitis, asthma, allergic rhinitis, and allergic conjunctivitis, compared with controls.[37] Elevated IgE concentrations in patients with active SLE and lupus nephritis have been reported, but the IgE more likely reflects a pathogenic role in SLE rather than the presence of allergic conditions.[37,38]

Should Patients with Systemic Lupus Erythematosus and Allergies Consider Immunotherapy?

For the 30% to 40% of patients with SLE who have environmental allergies,[19,39] the question often arises as to whether immunotherapy

(or "allergy shots") is safe and effective. Immunotherapy for otherwise healthy individuals with allergies carries a small risk of non-specific antibody formation of uncertain clinical meaningfulness. Primarily based on anecdotal experience and small observational studies finding a higher prevalence of antinuclear antibody (ANA) positivity among patients with allergies receiving immunotherapy (which is also seen in asthmatics without immunotherapy),[40,41] the World Health Organization (WHO) Working Group of the International Union of Immunological Sciences formally recommended that patients with autoimmune disease not receive immunotherapy.[42]

VITAMIN D SUPPLEMENTATION IN LUPUS

Vitamin D is an essential steroid hormone with well-established effects on mineral metabolism, skeletal health, and, recently established but still being elucidated, cardiovascular and immune system effects. A high prevalence of vitamin D insufficiency has been found in SLE patient populations around the world, and observational studies suggest that insufficiency contributes to multiple co-morbid conditions and potential complications of SLE.

Despite a growing awareness of vitamin D deficiency and an exponential rise in testing for vitamin D status, deficiency remains a global problem, particularly among pigmented populations living away from the equator.[43] It is important to note that the same ethnic disparities observed in the prevalence of vitamin D deficiency are seen in the prevalence of SLE, with African Americans and Hispanics having a disproportionately high risk for developing SLE and having severe disease manifestations.

Should All Patients with Systemic Lupus Erythematosus Be Screened for Vitamin D Deficiency?

Since the major source of vitamin D is sun exposure and sun protection is advisable for all patients with SLE, the risk of vitamin D deficiency is high and prevalent in up to two thirds of patients worldwide.[44] Other risk factors for vitamin D deficiency include season, latitude, altitude, clothing, sunscreen use, skin pigmentation, and age, which each influences the effectiveness of the photoconversion of 7-dehydrocholesterol in the skin to previtamin D_3, which rapidly isomerizes to vitamin D_3, which is then metabolized in the liver to 25-hydroxyvitamin D (25[OH]D), the best serum measure of overall vitamin D status. Patients taking corticosteroids often require higher daily doses of vitamin D to maintain adequate levels, as do patients who are obese and patients with malabsorption.[45] Genetic polymorphisms in vitamin D hydroxylation enzymes, cholesterol synthesis enzymes, and the vitamin D–binding protein also explain some of the variability in 25(OH)D levels,[46] but they have not been studied specifically in SLE. Studies of vitamin D–binding receptor (VDR) polymorphisms in several populations of patients with SLE, compared with controls, found associations between the VDR BsmI polymorphism and susceptibilities to SLE and nephritis in patients of Asian descent but inconsistent findings in other populations.[47,48]

Considering how common vitamin D deficiency risk factors are among patients with SLE, obtaining a baseline serum 25(OH)D and a follow-up serum 25(OH)D 3 months after a change in vitamin D dosing is recommended. Further studies will provide better-defined thresholds that are needed for certain health outcomes; however, experts recommend a minimum serum 25(OH)D level of 30 ng/mL (75 nmol/L) at this time.[45]

What Are the Consequences of Vitamin D Deficiency for Patients with Systemic Lupus Erythematosus?

In addition to causing rickets in children, vitamin D deficiency accelerates age-related bone loss and increases fall- and fracture-related morbidity. Vitamin D deficiency has also been associated with the presence and exacerbation of multiple chronic diseases, including cancer, cardiovascular disease, metabolic syndrome, and autoimmune diseases including SLE.[45] Metaanalyses of randomized vitamin

D trials have shown a reduction in mortality with vitamin D_3 supplementation, and observational cohorts have shown lower mortality with higher levels of 25(OH)D.[49,50] Several hundred vitamin D–regulated genes have been identified, including many involved with the innate and adaptive immune system. In vitro studies of the active form of vitamin D, 1,25(OH)$_2$D, demonstrate its important role in maintaining of B-cell homeostasis,[51,52] modulating adaptive immune responses, and boosting protective immunity.[53,54]

Multiple studies have examined potential links between vitamin D status and SLE disease activity and disease features (Online Supplement 2) with the largest studies to date showing a significant correlation between higher disease activity and lower 25(OH)D.[53,55-57] Improving vitamin D status among patients with SLE may benefit other common manifestations as well, such as fatigue[58] and subclinical cardiovascular disease.[59,60] Although limited to small numbers of patients with open-label dosing of vitamin D, prospective studies to date have been promising, reporting modest improvements in disease activity and interferon-inducible gene expression.[61] Results from randomized controlled studies to clarify further the understanding of the consequences of deficiency and the potential benefits of repletion are still pending at this time.

What Are the Current Vitamin D Intake Recommendations for Patients with Systemic Lupus Erythematosus?

We are early in our understanding of the role vitamin D plays in health, so specific recommendations for patients with SLE will likely be evolving over the next few years. As knowledge expands, higher thresholds may be needed for optimal health; however, at this time the minimally adequate level of 25(OH)D is 30 ng/mL. To correct vitamin D deficiency with either a daily oral vitamin D_3 (cholecalciferol), 1000 to 2000 IU are recommended; with weekly oral vitamin D_2 (ergocalciferol), 50,000 IU are recommended for 8 weeks, followed by 1000 to 2000 IU of vitamin D_3 daily.[62] The dose required to achieve and maintain adequate levels of 25(OH)D depends on the starting level, with roughly 100 IU of *additional* daily oral vitamin D_3 required to raise the serum 25(OH)D level by 1 ng/mL.[63] It takes approximately 3 months to achieve steady state once supplementation is started; consequently, 25(OH)D should not be rechecked any sooner than 3 months.[64] Individual responses may vary, and known risk factors for deficiency should be taken into account.

COMPLEMENTARY AND ALTERNATIVE MEDICINE IN LUPUS

Many patients with SLE have needs, most common being fatigue management and pain control, that are unmet by current conventional therapies.[65] To satisfy these needs, patients often try complementary and alternative medicine (CAM), defined broadly as treatments, products, and practices that fall outside the mainstream of traditional Western allopathic medicine.[65] The use of CAM is greater among patients with SLE than it is in the general population.[66] Up to 50% of patients with SLE incorporate some form of CAM into their treatment regimen, and the majority use CAM in conjunction with conventional medicine.

A cohort of 752 patients with SLE from Canada, the United States, and the United Kingdom found that CAM users were younger and better educated and exhibited poorer levels of self-related health status and satisfaction with medical care, but they did not have worse disease activity than nonusers.[66] Among patients with SLE, CAM has been associated with poorer physical function, higher cumulative disease damage, and higher self-perception of disease activity, but not necessarily higher objective disease activity.[66,67] A New Zealand cohort study found that CAM was used by 51% of patients with SLE, and 37% of patients believed that these medicines could control their SLE between acute flares.[68] One third of patients believed CAM should substitute for conventional medicines,[68] yet when health resource utilization is examined, the use of conventional medicine by users of CAM exceeds that of nonusers.[66]

What Are the Most Common Types of Complementary and Alternative Therapies Used by Patients with Systemic Lupus Erythematosus?

Patterns of CAM use were found to be similar in Canada, the United States, and the United Kingdom.[66] The most commonly used therapies were relaxation techniques, massage, herbal medicine, and lifestyle diets. Others forms of CAM therapies used among patients with SLE include self-help groups, imagery, folk remedies, spiritual healing, chiropractic manipulation, megavitamin therapy, homeopathic remedies, energy healing, commercial weight loss, biofeedback, acupuncture, and hypnosis.

Supplements that have possible benefit based on limited studies in SLE include dehydroepiandrosterone (DHEA), fish oil, and *Tripterygium wilfordii* Hook. f. (sometimes called the Thunder God Vine).[65,69] A number of studies have shown that yoga, massage, and acupuncture can mitigate pain symptoms; however, effects sizes are typically modest and only the one study of acupuncture focused on patients with SLE.[65,70] Overall, there is a paucity of controlled studies of CAM use in patients with SLE. The use of some specific CAM approaches in SLE is discussed in other sections of this text and includes biofeedback or cognitive behavioral therapy for Raynaud phenomenon and cognitive dysfunction (Chapter 30) and physical measures for fatigue and pain (Chapter 47). Online Supplement 3 summarizes CAM approaches that have been studied for use in patients with autoimmune diseases.

Are There Types of Complementary and Alternative Therapies That Should Be Avoided by Patients with Systemic Lupus Erythematosus?

The use of CAM is widespread among patients with SLE; however, conventional health care providers may have limited knowledge of these therapies. Some may be harmful or may interact with conventional SLE therapies, whereas others may be low risk and potentially beneficial. Dietary supplements and herbal products are not required to meet the same safety, efficacy, and labeling standards as prescription drug products. Herbal products often contain many different active chemical constituents, and the amount of each constituent, bioavailability, and manufacturing quality can be widely variable and possibly unsafe.[71]

Despite many patients' perception that CAM is "natural" and therefore safe, certain therapies may have a negative impact on disease or interfere with other medications. For example, drug-herbal interactions among herbal supplements such as ginkgo, ginseng, garlic, and St. John's wort may potentially interact with warfarin and increase bleeding risk. Some "detoxification regimens" can be dangerous, such as colonic irrigation in patients with bowel wall thinning from corticosteroid use. In SLE, immune-stimulating supplements, such as *Echinacea*, *Astragalus*, and alfalfa, carry theoretical risks. Unfortunately, almost no evidence-based literature is available on the subject of herbal therapies in patients with SLE or other autoimmune diseases.

ADHERENCE ISSUES IN LUPUS

Adherence is critical to the overall management of patients with SLE, and the lack of adherence is directly associated with poor treatment outcomes and high-cost service utilization. In a cohort study of 834 patients with SLE in California, 46% reported problems remembering to take their medications at least some of the time, and medication adherence was an independent predictor of emergency department visits.[72]

What Are the Consequences of Nonadherence in Patients with Systemic Lupus Erythematosus?

A cohort study in New Zealand of 106 patients with SLE receiving at least one immunosuppressive medication examined treatment nonadherence and associations with sociodemographic and disease characteristics, cognitive functioning, and psychosocial factors.[68] This study found 46% of patients were at least occasionally intentionally

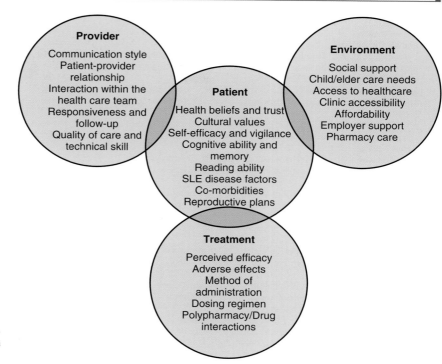

FIGURE 52-1 Model of the complex multifactorial influences on patient adherence, including patient, health care provider, treatment, and environmental factors.

nonadherent, 36% of whom had altered their medication dose, and 59% of patients were at least occasionally unintentionally nonadherent. Prior studies of nonadherence among patients with SLE in the United States and in Mexico found slightly higher percentages, which may in part reflect higher health care costs in these countries. The strongest predictors of nonadherence with medications included self-reported problems with cognitive functioning (specifically with recognition and planning), concerns about medication adverse effects, and younger age. Interestingly, disease activity, disease duration, and the number of medications were not found to influence adherence. In addition, this study did not find the association of education and marital status with adherence that was reported in other studies.[73,74]

Multiple studies convincingly demonstrate the importance that patient perceptions of the role medications play in adherence. In a cross-sectional survey of 102 ethnically diverse patients with SLE, 40% reported stopping medications on their own because of adverse effects.[74] Concern about potential adverse effects was the strongest predictor of intentional nonadherence in the New Zealand study.[68] In addition, although 80% of patients agreed that taking their SLE medications would improve their health, the majority (63%) were concerned about possible adverse effects.[68] One half of the patients used CAM and 25% believed CAM to be more natural and less damaging, but the beliefs about CAM were not associated with SLE medication adherence.

What Strategies Have Been Shown to Improve Adherence?

Improving adherence to complicated medication regimens and lifestyle modifications requires patient, health care provider, and health care system approaches to address the multiple factors behind nonadherence (Figure 52-1). Strategies that target modifiable risk factors identified in observational studies, such as screening for depressive symptoms to identify patients with SLE who may benefit from treatment for depression, have been successful in improving adherence.[72] Breaking down known barriers to adherence by offering enhanced patient education, better explaining the rationale for

interventions, addressing potential medication adverse effects, and simplifying medication regimens to help fit into patient lifestyles are each beneficial when tailored to individual patient needs. The use of adherence aids such as pillboxes are identified by patients as helpful, whereas automatic daily voice mail reminders have not been effective.[73] A study comparing 19 potential adherence barriers in African-American and Caucasian women with SLE found different barriers influenced nonadherence depending on ethnicity, implying that interventions may be more successful if they take ethnicity and cultural beliefs into account.[75]

A common theme across all of the qualitative and quantitative studies of adherence in SLE is the importance of good physician-patient communication. Opportunities exist to improve communication between the health care team and patient, which will enhance understanding of the disease and its treatment and identify barriers to adherence, ultimately having a positive impact on patient adherence and outcomes.

References

1. Cervera R, Khamashta MA, Font J, et al: Morbidity and mortality in systemic lupus erythematosus during a 10-year period: a comparison of early and late manifestations in a cohort of 1,000 patients. *Medicine (Baltimore)* 82:299–308, 2003.
2. Goldblatt F, Chambers S, Rahman A, et al: Serious infections in British patients with systemic lupus erythematosus: hospitalisations and mortality. *Lupus* 18:682–689, 2009.
3. Iriya SM, Capelozzi VL, Calich I, et al: Causes of death in patients with systemic lupus erythematosus in São Paulo, Brazil: a study of 113 autopsies. *Arch Intern Med* 161:1557, 2001.
4. Kamen DL: How can we reduce the risk of serious infection for patients with systemic lupus erythematosus? *Arthritis Res Ther* 11:129, 2009.
5. Barber C, Gold WL, Fortin PR: Infections in the lupus patient: perspectives on prevention. *Curr Opin Rheumatol* 23:358–365, 2011.
6. Yazdany J, Panopalis P, Gillis JZ, et al: A quality indicator set for systemic lupus erythematosus. *Arthritis Rheum* 61:370–377, 2009.
7. Mosca M, Tani C, Aringer M, et al: European League Against Rheumatism recommendations for monitoring patients with systemic lupus erythematosus in clinical practice and in observational studies. *Ann Rheum Dis* 69:1269–1274, 2010.

8. Heijstek MW, Ott de Bruin LM, Biji M, et al: EULAR recommendations for vaccination in paediatric patients with rheumatic diseases. *Ann Rheum Dis* 70:1704–1712, 2011.

9. Yazdany J, Tonner C, Trupin L, et al: Provision of preventive health care in systemic lupus erythematosus: data from a large observational cohort study. *Arthritis Res Ther* 12:R84, 2010.

10. Ruiz-Irastorza G, Olivares N, Ruiz-Arruza I, et al: Predictors of major infections in systemic lupus erythematosus. *Arthritis Res Ther* 11:R109, 2009.

11. Abu-Shakra M, Urowitz MB, Gladman DD, et al: Mortality studies in systemic lupus erythematosus. Results from a single center. I. Causes of death. *J Rheumatol* 22:1259–1264, 1995.

12. Furst DE, Keystone EC, Kirkham B, et al: Updated consensus statement on biological agents for the treatment of rheumatic diseases, 2008. *Ann Rheum Dis* 67(Suppl 3):iii2–iii25, 2008.

13. Block SL, Yogev R, Hayden FG, et al: Shedding and immunogenicity of live attenuated influenza vaccine virus in subjects 5-49 years of age. *Vaccine* 26:4940–4946, 2008.

14. Millet A, Decaux O, Perlat A, et al: Systemic lupus erythematosus and vaccination. *Eur J Intern Med* 20:236–241, 2009.

15. Salemi S, D'Amelio R: Are anti-infectious vaccinations safe and effective in patients with autoimmunity? *Int Rev Immunol* 29:270–314, 2010.

16. Crowe SR, Merrill JT, Vista ES, et al: Influenza vaccination responses in human systemic lupus erythematosus: impact of clinical and demographic features. *Arthritis Rheum* 63:2396–2406, 2011.

17. Elkayam O, Paran D, Burke M, et al: Pneumococcal vaccination of patients with systemic lupus erythematosus: effects on generation of autoantibodies. *Autoimmunity* 38:493–496, 2005.

18. McDonald E, Jarrett MP, Schiffman G, et al: Persistence of pneumococcal antibodies after immunization in patients with systemic lupus erythematosus. *J Rheumatol* 11:306–308, 1984.

19. Cooper GS, Dooley MA, Treadwell EL, et al: Risk factors for development of systemic lupus erythematosus: allergies, infections, and family history. *J Clin Epidemiol* 55:982–989, 2002.

20. Kuruma KA, Borba EF, Lopes MH, et al: Safety and efficacy of hepatitis B vaccine in systemic lupus erythematosus. *Lupus* 16:350–354, 2007.

21. Enzler MJ, Berbari E, Osmon DR: Antimicrobial prophylaxis in adults. *Mayo Clin Proc* 86:686–701, 2011.

22. Luce EB, Presti CF, Montemayor I, et al: Detecting cardiac valvular pathology in patients with systemic lupus erythematosus. *Spec Care Dentist* 12:193–197, 1992.

23. Gabrielli F, Alcini E, Di Prima MA, et al: Cardiac valve involvement in systemic lupus erythematosus and primary antiphospholipid syndrome: lack of correlation with antiphospholipid antibodies. *Int J Cardiol* 51:117–126, 1995.

24. Zuily S, Regnault V, Selton-Suty C, et al: Increased risk for heart valve disease associated with antiphospholipid antibodies in patients with systemic lupus erythematosus: meta-analysis of echocardiographic studies. *Circulation* 124:215–224, 2011.

25. Wilson W, Taubert KA, Gewitz M, et al: Prevention of infective endocarditis: guidelines from the American Heart Association: a guideline from the American Heart Association Rheumatic Fever, Endocarditis, and Kawasaki Disease Committee, Council on Cardiovascular Disease in the Young, and the Council on Clinical Cardiology, Council on Cardiovascular Surgery and Anesthesia, and the Quality of Care and Outcomes Research Interdisciplinary Working Group. *Circulation* 116:1736–1754, 2007.

26. Thomas CF, Jr, Limper AH: *Pneumocystis pneumoniae. N Engl J Med* 350:2487–2498, 2004.

27. Vananuvat P, Suwannalai P, Sungkanuparph S, et al: Primary prophylaxis for *Pneumocystis jirovecii* pneumonia in patients with connective tissue diseases. *Semin Arthritis Rheum* 41:497–502, 2011.

28. Green H, Paul M, Vidal L, et al: Prophylaxis of *Pneumocystis pneumoniae* in immunocompromised non-HIV-infected patients: systematic review and meta-analysis of randomized controlled trials. *Mayo Clin Proc* 82:1052–1059, 2007.

29. Gupta D, Zachariah A, Roppelt H, et al: Prophylactic antibiotic usage for *Pneumocystis jirovecii* pneumonia in patients with systemic lupus erythematosus on cyclophosphamide: a survey of US rheumatologists and the review of literature. *J Clin Rheumatol* 14:267–272, 2008.

30. Mongey AB, Hess EV: Drug insight: autoimmune effects of medications–what's new? *Nat Clin Pract Rheumatol* 4:136–144, 2008.

31. Petri M, Allbritton J: Antibiotic allergy in systemic lupus erythematosus: a case-control study. *J Rheumatol* 19:265–269, 1992.

32. Pope J, Jerome D, Fenlon D, et al: Frequency of adverse drug reactions in patients with systemic lupus erythematosus. *J Rheumatol* 30:480–484, 2003.

33. Aceves-Avila FJ, Benites-Godinez V: Drug allergies may be more frequent in systemic lupus erythematosus than in rheumatoid arthritis. *J Clin Rheumatol* 14:261–263, 2008.

34. Wang CR, Chuang CY, Chen CY: Drug allergy in Chinese patients with systemic lupus erythematosus. *J Rheumatol* 20:399–400, 1993.

35. Strom BL, Schinnar R, Apter AJ, et al: Absence of cross-reactivity between sulfonamide antibiotics and sulfonamide nonantibiotics. *N Engl J Med* 349:1628–1635, 2003.

36. Jeffries M, Bruner G, Glenn S, et al: Sulpha allergy in lupus patients: a clinical perspective. *Lupus* 17:202–205, 2008.

37. Sekigawa I, Yoshiike T, Iida N, et al: Allergic diseases in systemic lupus erythematosus: prevalence and immunological considerations. *Clin Exp Rheumatol* 21:117–121, 2003.

38. Parks CG, Biagini RE, Cooper GS, et al: Total serum IgE levels in systemic lupus erythematosus and associations with childhood onset allergies. *Lupus* 19:1614–1622, 2010.

39. Morton S, Palmer B, Muir K, et al: IgE and non-IgE mediated allergic disorders in systemic lupus erythematosus. *Ann Rheum Dis* 57:660–663, 1998.

40. Phanuphak P, Kohler PF: Onset of polyarteritis nodosa during allergic hyposensitization treatment. *Am J Med* 68:479–485, 1980.

41. Tanaç R, Demir E, Aksu G, et al: Effect of immunotherapy on autoimmune parameters in children with atopic asthma. *Turk J Pediatr* 44:294–297, 2002.

42. [No author]: Current status of allergen immunotherapy (hyposensitization): memorandum from a WHO/IUIS meeting. *Bull World Health Organ* 67:263–272, 1989.

43. Ginde AA, Liu MC, Camargo CA, Jr: Demographic differences and trends of vitamin D insufficiency in the US population, 1988-2004. *Arch Intern Med* 169:626–632, 2009.

44. Kamen DL, Cooper GS, Bouali H, et al: Vitamin D deficiency in systemic lupus erythematosus. *Autoimmun Rev* 5:114–117, 2006.

45. Holick MF: Vitamin D: a d-lightful solution for health. *J Investig Med* 59:872–880, 2011.

46. Wang TJ, Zhang F, Richards JB, et al: Common genetic determinants of vitamin D insufficiency: a genome-wide association study. *Lancet* 376:180–188, 2010.

47. Lee YH, Bae SC, Choi SJ, et al: Associations between vitamin D receptor polymorphisms and susceptibility to rheumatoid arthritis and systemic lupus erythematosus: a meta-analysis. *Mol Biol Rep* 38:3643–3651, 2011.

48. Abbasi M, Rezaieyazdi Z, Afshari JT, et al: Lack of association of vitamin D receptor gene BsmI polymorphisms in patients with systemic lupus erythematosus. *Rheumatol Int* 30:1537–1539, 2010.

49. Bjelakovic G, Gluud LL, Nikolova D, et al: Vitamin D supplementation for prevention of mortality in adults. *Cochrane Database Syst Rev* CD007470, 2011.

50. Zittermann A, Iodice S, Pilz S, et al: Vitamin D deficiency and mortality risk in the general population: a meta-analysis of prospective cohort studies. *Am J Clin Nutr* 95:91–100, 2012.

51. Chen S, Sims GP, Chex XX, et al: Modulatory effects of 1,25-dihydroxyvitamin D3 on human B cell differentiation. *J Immunol* 179:1634–1647, 2007.

52. Linker-Israeli M, Elstner E, Klinenberg JR, et al: Vitamin D(3) and its synthetic analogs inhibit the spontaneous in vitro immunoglobulin production by SLE-derived PBMC. *Clin Immunol* 99:82–93, 2001.

53. Ben-Zvi I, Aranow C, Mackay M, et al: The impact of vitamin D on dendritic cell function in patients with systemic lupus erythematosus. *PLoS One* 5:e9193, 2010.

54. Kamen DL, Tangpricha V: Vitamin D and molecular actions on the immune system: modulation of innate autoimmunity. *J Mol Med (Berl)* 88:441–450, 2010.

55. Amital H, Szekanecz Z, Szücs G, et al: Serum concentrations of 25-OH vitamin D in patients with systemic lupus erythematosus (SLE) are inversely related to disease activity: is it time to routinely supplement patients with SLE with vitamin D? *Ann Rheum Dis* 69:1155–1157, 2010.

56. Mok CC, Birmingham DJ, Leung HW, et al: Vitamin D levels in Chinese patients with systemic lupus erythematosus: relationship with disease activity, vascular risk factors and atherosclerosis. *Rheumatology (Oxford)* 51:644–652, 2012.

57. Ritterhouse LL, Crowe SR, Niewold TB, et al: Vitamin D deficiency is associated with an increased autoimmune response in healthy individuals and in patients with systemic lupus erythematosus. *Ann Rheum Dis* 70:1569–1574, 2011.

58. Ruiz-Irastorza G, Gordo S, Olivares N, et al: Changes in vitamin D levels in patients with systemic lupus erythematosus: effects on fatigue, disease activity, and damage. *Arthritis Care Res (Hoboken)* 62:1160–1165, 2010.
59. Wu PW, Rhew EY, Dyer AR, et al: 25-hydroxyvitamin D and cardiovascular risk factors in women with systemic lupus erythematosus. *Arthritis Rheum* 61:1387–1395, 2009.
60. Reynolds JA, Hague S, Berry JL, et al: 25-Hydroxyvitamin D deficiency is associated with increased aortic stiffness in patients with systemic lupus erythematosus. *Rheumatology (Oxford)* 51:544–551, 2012.
61. Aranow C: Vitamin D and the immune system. *J Investig Med* 59:881–886, 2011.
62. Holick MF: Vitamin D deficiency. *N Engl J Med* 357:266–281, 2007.
63. Heaney RP: Vitamin D in health and disease. *Clin J Am Soc Nephrol* 3:1535–1541, 2008.
64. Kamen DL, Aranow C: The link between vitamin D deficiency and systemic lupus erythematosus. *Curr Rheumatol Rep* 10:273–280, 2008.
65. Haija AJ, Schulz SW: The role and effect of complementary and alternative medicine in systemic lupus erythematosus. *Rheum Dis Clin North Am* 37:47–62, 2011.
66. Moore AD, Petri MA, Manzi S, et al: The use of alternative medical therapies in patients with systemic lupus erythematosus. Trination Study Group. *Arthritis Rheum* 43:1410–1418, 2000.
67. Alvarez-Nemegyei J, Bautista-Botello A, Davila-Velazquez J: Association of complementary or alternative medicine use with quality of life, functional status or cumulated damage in chronic rheumatic diseases. *Clin Rheumatol* 28:547–551, 2009.
68. Daleboudt GM, Broadbent E, McQueen F, et al: Intentional and unintentional treatment non-adherence in patients with systemic lupus erythematosus. *Arthritis Care Res (Hoboken)* 63:342–350, 2011.
69. Chou CT: Alternative therapies: what role do they have in the management of lupus? *Lupus* 19:1425–1429, 2010.
70. Greco CM, Kao AH, Maksimowicz-McKinnon K, et al: Acupuncture for systemic lupus erythematosus: a pilot RCT feasibility and safety study. *Lupus* 17:1108–1116, 2008.
71. Gertner E, Marshall PS, Filandrinos D, et al: Complications resulting from the use of Chinese herbal medications containing undeclared prescription drugs. *Arthritis Rheum* 38:614–617, 1995.
72. Julian LJ, Yelin E, Yazdany J, et al: Depression, medication adherence, and service utilization in systemic lupus erythematosus. *Arthritis Rheum* 61:240–246, 2009.
73. Koneru S, Kocharla L, Higgins GC, et al: Adherence to medications in systemic lupus erythematosus. *J Clin Rheumatol* 14:195–201, 2008.
74. Garcia-Gonzalez A, Richardson M, Garcia Popa-Lisseanu M, et al: Treatment adherence in patients with rheumatoid arthritis and systemic lupus erythematosus. *Clin Rheumatol* 27:883–889, 2008.
75. Mosley-Williams A, Lumley MA, Gillis M, et al: Barriers to treatment adherence among African American and white women with systemic lupus erythematosus. *Arthritis Rheum* 47:630–638, 2002.

INTRODUCTION

Only a very few medications are specifically approved by regulatory agencies for the treatment of systemic lupus erythematosus (SLE), and most of these have been "grandfathered" into the regulatory system on the basis of their established use over many years or decades. The recent regulatory approval of belimumab (Benlysta) for the treatment of SLE may therefore be regarded as a true landmark in the history of therapeutic agents for SLE, raising hopes that more will be approved and become available in the coming years.

However, regulatory approval is not the only factor that guides decisions in clinical practice. For a disease such as SLE, with its limited prevalence and therefore a lesser incentive for industry to develop drugs, it cannot be reasonably expected that all possible therapeutic agents will be tested in large, randomized clinical trials. Furthermore, clinicians have always worked with the off-label use of medications approved for other diseases in the treatment of their individual patients with SLE. For a medication such as methotrexate, with its extensive documentation in other rheumatologic diseases, decades of practical experience, and ample observational documentation of the effects and side effects in the treatment of SLE, such off-label use can hardly be considered controversial. However, when considering the off-label use of relatively novel agents such as the anti–tumor necrosis factor (anti-TNF) biologic medications, abatacept or rituximab, the issues become more contentious. Efficacy and safety are less clearly defined, reported experiences may give a biased view, and cost is a major consideration.

A number of therapeutic agents available to the clinician who is treating patients with SLE are reviewed in this chapter, including the newly approved biologic belimumab as well as several biologic medications that are not approved for the treatment of SLE, but whose off-label use is supported by some published observations or theoretical considerations or both. These data are summarized in Table 53-1. Agents currently in clinical development but not yet available are discussed separately in Chapter 56.

BELIMUMAB

The development of belimumab was based on an improved understanding of the molecular mechanisms leading to B-cell activation[1-3] and the realization that some of the immune abnormalities in SLE might be reversed by the inhibition of the B-lymphocyte stimulator[4] (BLyS); also known as the B cell–activating factor (BAFF), a member of the TNF-ligand family and a key survival cytokine for B cells.[5] An overexpression of BLyS promotes the survival of B cells (including autoreactive B cells), whereas the inhibition of BLyS results in autoreactive B-cell apoptosis. Elevated circulating BLyS levels are common in SLE and correlate with increased SLE disease activity and elevated anti–double stranded DNA (anti-dsDNA) antibody concentrations.[6-9]

Belimumab (Benlysta), formerly LymphoStat-B, is a fully human monoclonal antibody that binds soluble human BLyS and inhibits its biologic activities.[10,11] It is administered in the form of four-weekly infusions. In a phase II study of patients with active SLE who were receiving standard therapies, treatment with belimumab led to modest reductions in the number of circulating CD20+ B lymphocytes and significant reductions in anti-dsDNA antibody titers; in addition, safety and tolerability were good.[12] Although the trial did not meet its prespecified primary endpoint, additional analyses determined that patients with either antinuclear antibodies (ANAs) of 1:80 or greater or anti-dsDNA antibodies of 30 IU/ml or greater had significantly reduced SLE disease activity and fewer flares with belimumab, compared with placebo. From a clinical perspective, focusing on such patients was quite logical, in that patients lacking both antibodies would not generally be considered typical SLE patients. It is also worth noting that from a clinical trials' perspective, performing subanalyses on phase II data to determine the optimal design for phase III is perfectly legitimate.[13]

An additional concern with the phase II data was that the suggestion of efficacy was observed at the 1 mg/kg and 10 mg/kg doses but not at the intermediate 4 mg/kg dose.

In a 5-year, open-label extension of the phase II study, improvement in SLE disease activity was sustained in the seropositive subset remaining on treatment, and rates of adverse events remained stable or decreased.[14]

Subsequently, belimumab was evaluated in two phase III trials, comparing belimumab 1 and 10 mg/kg doses with placebo in patients with seropositive (as previously defined) and active SLE (as defined by the Systemic Lupus Erythematosus Disease Activity Index [SLEDAI] of at least 6 points) and who were receiving stable standard treatment, including glucocorticoids, antimalarial mediations, and/or certain immunosuppressive agents. For these two trials, the following novel outcome, called the SLE Responder Index (SRI), was developed on the basis of the phase II data:

For a patient to be classified as a responder by SRI, he or she must have an improvement in the SLEDAI of at least 4 points, while simultaneously experiencing no worsening of the disease in other organ systems (defined as not having a new British Isles Lupus Assessment Group [BILAG] score of A and not having two new BILAG scores of B) or by physician judgment (defined as not having a worsening of the physician's global assessment [PGA] by 0.3 or more).[15] Both of these trials allowed for changes of glucocorticoid doses on the basis of the clinical course (i.e., increased doses in case of flare, decreased doses in stable situations) and, to a more limited degree, changes in other concomitant medications.

TABLE 53-1 Novel and Clinically Available (but not Necessarily Approved) Targeted Therapies for Systemic Lupus Erythematosus

Therapeutic Agent		Randomized Controlled Trials				APPROVED FOR OTHER RHEUMATIC DISEASE(S)	HIGH-QUALITY OBSERVATIONAL DATA
NAME	MECHANISM	NAME	TYPE	RESULTS	APPROVED FOR SLE		
Belimumab (Benlysta; anti-BLyS monoclonal antibody)	Blocks BLyS or BAFF.		Phase II with long-term extension[12,14]	Failed primary outcome, but significant results in post-hoc analysis of seropositive group. Achieved satisfactory long-term tolerability.	Yes, in seropositive disease (positive for ANAs and/or anti-DNA) and for moderately or highly active disease.	No	N/A
		BLISS-52[16]	Phase III	Met primary and most secondary outcomes.	Unknown efficacy in severe renal or severe CNS disease.		
		BLISS-76[17]	Phase III	Met primary and some secondary outcomes.	Unclear efficacy in African Americans (United States). Considered elevated anti-DNA and low complement as markers for enhanced efficacy (Europe).		
Rituximab (Rituxan, MabThera; anti-CD20 monoclonal antibody)	Depletes CD20-positive B cells.	EXPLORER (nonrenal SLE)[29]	Phase II	Failed primary and most secondary outcomes. Achieved post-hoc efficacy in preventing severe flares.	No	Yes, for RA	Published observations are suggestive of efficacy in patients with lupus nephritis that was refractory to cyclophosphamide and/or MMF. Combination of rituximab with cyclophosphamide has a possible role. Some publications also suggest efficacy in hematologic and CNS disease and, to a lesser extent, in other nonrenal SLE manifestations.[19-28]
		LUNAR (lupus nephritis)[31]	Phase II	Failed primary and most secondary outcomes.			
Abatacept (Orencia; CTLA4-Ig construct)	Blocks second-signal activation of T cells. May bind to CD80/86 positive cells, including B cells.	Nonrenal lupus trial (patients with musculoskeletal, mucocutaneous, or serosal flare)[47]	Phase II	Failed primary and most secondary outcomes. Some improvements in patient-reported outcomes	No	Yes, RA and JIA	
		Lupus nephritis	Phase II	Failed primary outcome, halted*			
Adalimumab, etanercept, and other subcutaneous anti-TNF agents	TNF blockade	*			No	Yes, RA and several other arthritis indications	Efficacy in SLE-related arthritis and for SLE-related proteinuria is suggested in a small series.[42]
Infliximab (anti-TNF monoclonal antibody)	TNF blockade	*			No	Yes, RA and several other arthritis indications	Concerns regarding severe infusion reactions are noted.[43]

ANA, Antinuclear antibody; BAFF, B cell–activating factor; BLyS, B lymphocyte stimulator; CNS, central nervous system; CTLA4-Ig, cytotoxic T-lymphocyte antigen 4–immunoglobulin; EXPLORER, the Exploratory Phase II/III SLE Evaluation of Rituximab; JIA, juvenile idiopathic arthritis; LUNAR, the Lupus Nephritis Assessment with Rituximab; MMF, mycophenolate mofetil; RA, rheumatoid arthritis; SLE, systemic lupus erythematosus; TNF, tumor necrosis factor.

*Two trials, one with etanercept and one with infliximab, in lupus nephritis were both terminated because of recruitment difficulties.

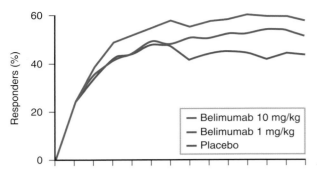

FIGURE 53-1 The effects of belimumab in active, seropositive systemic lupus erythematosus (SLE).[16] Patients were given fourweekly infusions of belimumab or placebo. Percentage responders at each time point were defined by the SLE Response Index (SRI), a compound of the Systemic Lupus Erythematosus Disease Activity Index (SLEDAI), the British Isles Lupus Assessment Group (BILAG), and physician's global assessment. The differences among patient groups were statistically significant at multiple time points, including at the 52-week assessment chosen as the primary outcome of the trial.

A 52-week randomized, controlled clinical trial with 867 patients—a study of Belimumab in Subjects with SLE (BLISS-52)—was conducted primarily in Asia, South America, and Eastern Europe. At several time points, the percentage of patients who achieved the SRI response was significantly greater for patients receiving belimumab, compared with placebo (Figure 53-1).[16] This included the 52-week time point used for the primary outcome of the trial, at which time 44% of patients on placebo were SRI responders and 58% of those who were on belimumab 10 mg/kg ($p = 0.0024$). In addition, significant reductions in SLE disease activity, fewer flares, and reduced glucocorticoid use in patients on belimumab were observed, compared with placebo.

BLISS-76 was a 76-week randomized, controlled clinical trial with 819 patients conducted primarily in North America and Europe. Treatment continued through week 72 with the final evaluation at week 76. In this trial, the primary outcome was the SRI response at week 52, and it was again significantly greater for 10 mg/kg belimumab than for placebo (43% versus 34%, $p = 0.017$). However, in contrast to BLISS-52, the lower belimumab dose did not achieve a significant difference from placebo, and the differences at other time points were likewise not statistically significant. Other outcomes, such as the frequency of flare and the use of concomitant glucocorticoids, were also generally better for the belimumab-treated groups, but statistical significance was more variably achieved.[17]

Subsequent analyses of the pooled data from both trials revealed that the difference between belimumab and placebo was most notable in patients with additional evidence for immune activation in the form of anti-DNA antibodies and/or low complement, as well as in patients who were receiving glucocorticoids at baseline.[18]

In both phase III trials, belimumab was well-tolerated. Infusion reactions were infrequent, and most were mild. Overall, the rates of adverse events and serious adverse events were comparable for the actively treated group versus placebo group, with a possible overrepresentation of common infections with belimumab. Opportunistic infections including tuberculosis and malignancies were not different between the groups.

Based on the results from these trials, both the U.S. Food and Drug Administration (FDA) and the European Medicines Agency approved belimumab for use in seropositive, active SLE. The FDA noted uncertainty regarding the efficacy in patients of African-American descent, an issue that will have to be studied in separate trials in the future. The European agency, in its approval, added the recommendation to consider evidence for immune activation, as evidenced by positive anti-DNA antibodies or low complement.

How then should belimumab be appraised at this time? Undoubtedly, the knowledge of the true benefits and possible risks with belimumab will rapidly multiply, because the drug is going to be used in clinical practice. Based on the clinical trials, however, the efficacy, itself, is not in doubt, but concerns can be expressed about the *effect size*: the difference in response percentage between active drug and placebo is 9% to 14%. This variable could be taken to mean that only 1 in 8 or 10 patients will benefit from the drug, or it could be argued that the drug only improves the average patient by 12%. Neither of those interpretations is completely correct, and two obvious facts must be repeated: (1) some patients will do well without belimumab, and (2) some patients will do poorly despite belimumab. However, the question really revolves around the patients who currently do not do well with available therapies: how many of these patients are likely to do well with belimumab, and how well will they do? Definitively answering these questions is not possible at this time, but two important points must be made, which also have important implications for physicians treating patients with belimumab:

1. In the trials, SLE was measured by complex indices (the SLEDAI and the BILAG) and assessed by a compound based on those indices (the SRI). These measurements are not realistic for clinical practice and, moreover, entail a significant amount of variability or *noise*. Therefore the noise possibly masked the effect of the intervention to some extent, and the true effect is, perhaps, more robust than it seems. In practice, physicians and patients need to have a very clear understanding, when initiating therapy, of what therapeutic goals are going to have to be achieved to motivate continued therapy.

2. Belimumab appears to be most effective in patients who have moderate- or high-clinical SLE activity, who have evidence for serologic immune activation, and who need glucocorticoid medications; each of these patient characteristics increases the likelihood of benefit. Consequently, it would seem sensible to consider belimumab in these types of patients at this time.

RITUXIMAB

Rituximab (Rituxan, MabThera) is a monoclonal anti-CD20 antibody that was originally developed as a therapeutic agent for B-cell lymphoma in the 1990s. After its approval for use in this disease, it rapidly became one of the most widely used biologic agents worldwide, based on its ability to provide benefit for patients with low-grade non-Hodgkin B-cell lymphomas, a patient group for whom few other options are available. It has the ability to synergize with other antineoplastic therapies for the treatment of high-grade lymphoma and, perhaps most importantly for the clinician, it offers a relatively benign side-effect profile, considering the seriousness of the diseases under treatment. In the late 1990s, Dr. Jonathan Edwards in London suggested that rituximab might also benefit patients with rheumatoid arthritis (RA), a suggestion that at the time was not at all intuitive, in that the role of B cells in RA pathogenesis was poorly defined. Despite that fact, subsequent large-scale, randomized clinical trials in RA clearly demonstrated that rituximab had important therapeutic efficacy in the treatment of that disease, and it was subsequently approved for use in patients who had failed anti-TNF agents. Largely based on these encouraging results, various groups of investigators began to explore the possibility of treating other autoimmune diseases with rituximab as well. Because SLE is characterized by a range of autoantibodies, some of which are clearly pathophysiologically important, considering the use of this B-cell agent in SLE was not illogical. Thus Leandro and others[19] initially published data demonstrating important clinical improvements in a group of patients with moderate-to-severe and refractory SLE who were given a single course of rituximab in the dose approved for the treatment of lymphoma (four doses 375 mg/m[2] at weekly intervals). In the author's unit at the Karolinska University Hospital, a large number of patients were treated in this manner, and the results were reported in several publications. Specifically, an initial report of two cases demonstrated dramatic clinical improvements in patients with a prior manifest failure of treatment with cyclophosphamide (CyX)[20] (Figure 53-2).[20] Both patients suffered from lupus nephritis, and biopsies were taken

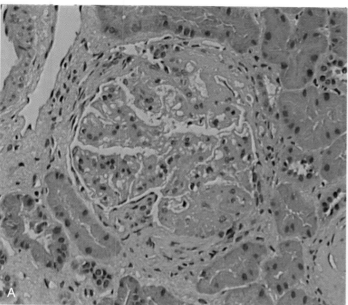
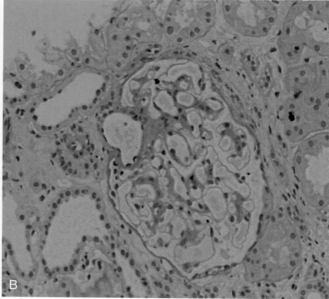

FIGURE 53-2 Effects of rituximab in a patient with refractory lupus nephritis. The patient, in whom a prior biopsy *(not shown)* revealed highly active membranoproliferative glomerulonephritis, received six monthly infusions with cyclophosphamide (CyX) at 0.75 mg/m². After this treatment, a repeat biopsy was performed and revealed ongoing highly active disease *(panel A)*. On the basis of this finding, the patient was given a course of rituximab (four doses at 375 mg/m²) plus CyX (two doses at 500 mg) and methylprednisolone (two doses at 500 mg) over 4 weeks with no further therapy. Three months later, a third biopsy revealed almost complete resolution of the glomerular inflammation (previously unpublished biopsy images from this patient described in reference 18) *(panel B)*. This patient has since remained in a renal remission for more than 8 years without further immunosuppressive therapy.

before and after rituximab treatment in both cases, which demonstrated remarkable improvements in renal histologic findings. Later, a larger group of patients with refractory lupus nephritis demonstrated similar responses, all confirmed by biopsies.[21] It should be noted that these patients were treated with the combination of rituximab in the previously referenced dose plus 500 mg CyX administered twice and glucocorticoids as intravenous boluses and/or a higher oral dose with subsequent tapering. In a separate report from this unit, patients were described with both renal and nonrenal lupus that had remained refractory to conventional immunosuppressive treatments and who were administered rituximab.[22] After rituximab treatment, the vast majority of patients had improvements that were clinically meaningful and relatively long-lasting. The safety profile of rituximab appeared adequate throughout these uncontrolled observations. Additional groups of investigators also reported on the results of rituximab treatment in SLE. Among these reports are the dose-ranging studies in mild SLE by Looney and others,[23] in which some improvements were observed; a large series of patients with lupus nephritis studied in Greece[24]; more follow-up on the large cohort of patients in London[25]; a large cohort of patients in France[26,27]; and other published case series that also supported these general impressions. In a recent metaanalysis, data on 188 cases were included.[28]

Based on the multiple uncontrolled observational data and the *a priori* plausibility of rituximab treatment in SLE, the manufacturers of this drug decided to initiate two relatively large controlled clinical trials of rituximab in SLE: the Exploratory Phase II/III SLE Evaluation of Rituximab (nicknamed EXPLORER) for patients with predominantly nonrenal lupus and the Lupus Nephritis Assessment with Rituximab (LUNAR) study for patients with lupus nephritis. The results of the EXPLORER trial, in which patients with predominantly nonrenal lupus were randomized to receive rituximab versus placebo in addition to standard immunosuppressive background therapy, were published by Merrill and colleagues[29] and did not demonstrate any benefit for the active treatment over placebo. Of note, most patients in EXPLORER had musculoskeletal, mucocutaneous, or generalized lupus, with other lupus manifestations represented in only small or very small numbers. In this trial, despite the lack of positive findings in the primary and secondary outcomes, a robust biologic effect for rituximab was demonstrated (i.e., B cells were depleted and anti-DNA titers were decreased), and some exploratory analyses suggested that certain subsets of patients might have benefitted from treatment. Specifically, in a recent subanalysis the occurrence of severe flares (defined as a new "BILAG A" lupus manifestation) was clearly reduced by rituximab compared to placebo.[30] Nevertheless, the overall findings of that trial must be regarded as negative.

The results of the LUNAR study have also been published.[31] Nevertheless, it is clear that the trial was also negative without a convincing demonstration of clinical benefit for patients who received rituximab versus placebo on a background of immunosuppressive therapy, which in this trial consisted of mycophenolate mofetil (MMF), not CyX.

Consequently, although observational studies and a plausible mechanism made clinicians and clinical scientists confident that rituximab would be a demonstrably effective treatment for SLE, the results of two randomized trials were decidedly negative, which leads to two opposite views on rituximab for SLE. The staunch optimist, choosing to ignore the randomized trial data, could argue that rituximab remains an excellent treatment for SLE because *it depletes autoreactive B cells, decreases autoantibodies, and has been shown to work in observational studies of hundreds of patients.* On the other hand, the more pessimistic but perhaps the more evidence-based reaction would be something similar to *rituximab has failed in two well-controlled randomized clinical trials that represent the highest level of scientific evidence; all have been fooled by the uncontrolled data.*

This argument raises the question whether it is possible for many clinicians to be fooled by appearances when the truth is different. In the specific case of rituximab in SLE, consideration has to be given to the fact that clinicians were perhaps all too eager to embrace apparently positive results and draw conclusions that, although on the face of it reasonable, were in the end not wholly justified.

However, clinicians can also be fooled by data from randomized clinical trials. Even if they are considered to be the highest level of scientific evidence, randomized trials may suffer from various weaknesses that may render the results misleading. Patients are recruited in a strictly regulated fashion according to inclusion and exclusion criteria and therefore may not be representative of the patients for whom the treatment might be of interest. The randomized trial is usually more limited in duration than observational studies. Concomitant medications that do not represent the optimal combinations for the investigational drug may be chosen for the trial. The predefined outcomes for the clinical trial may not present the full picture for a particular intervention. In addition, although clinical trial protocols are typically thoroughly researched and painstakingly designed during a long and tedious process, it is, nonetheless, possible that in the end they do not answer the question about a particular drug that is most relevant for the clinician.

In essence, then, it is clear that a paradox has been presented, and the question is: Did the observational studies trick us into thinking rituximab is effective for SLE while it is not? Or, did the two failed trials mislead us by suggesting rituximab is *not* effective for SLE even though it is?

Rituximab in Nonrenal Systemic Lupus Erythematosus

As indicated in the previous text, treatment with rituximab in most observational studies has led to substantial decreases in anti-DNA antibody titers. Inasmuch as anti-DNA antibodies can have a pathophysiologic role in the treatment SLE, this would lend plausibility to the efficacy claims of rituximab by providing a potential mechanism. Importantly, the ability of rituximab to decrease anti-DNA antibodies was strongly upheld by the results of both EXPLORER and LUNAR. With that said, it should also be recognized that anti-DNA antibodies do not have a proven pathophysiologic role in nonrenal SLE. Antibodies that are more clearly associated with nonrenal lupus manifestations, such as anti–Sjögren syndrome antigen A (anti-SSA/Ro) and anti–Sjögren syndrome antigen B (anti-SSA/La) antibodies in cutaneous lupus, were shown not to be downregulated substantially by rituximab therapy. It is perhaps therefore fair to say that the potential mechanism of rituximab in nonrenal lupus is not as clearly defined as one might hope. This is particularly true for the lupus manifestations that were most widely represented in the EXPLORER trial, namely mucocutaneous, musculoskeletal, and generalized lupus. For patients with hematologic lupus manifestations, prior observational data have suggested very good efficacy of rituximab, which may not be surprising in that such lupus manifestations are typically tied to specific autoantibodies such as antierythrocyte and antiplatelet antibodies. However, as already indicated, these types of patients were present to a limited degree in the EXPLORER trial.

In summary, could the EXPLORER trial have given an incorrect result? This is, of course, always possible. For example, the arguments could be that the trial did not use rituximab in the correct fashion or that the duration of the trial was not long enough; however, neither of these arguments seems particularly strong. It has been argued that patients in EXPLORER were treated with concomitant medications, including glucocorticoids and immunosuppressives, as well as antimalarial drugs, and that a possible therapeutic benefit of the investigational drug could not be demonstrated because of the overwhelming effect of these background medications. However, this criticism fails to be convincing when considering that approximately 70% of patients in the EXPLORER trial were, in the end, classified as nonresponders; consequently, the margin for additional improvement was, in fact, quite large.

Another consideration would be that the outcomes used in EXPLORER were not sufficiently sensitive or robust, which may be said of many outcomes in SLE in general. In EXPLORER, a variety of outcomes were tested; for some of these, including the primary and most of the secondary outcomes, not only was no statistical difference found, but not even the suggestion of a numerical difference

existed, which would argue against the results being misleading because of the noise in the outcome. As mentioned earlier, a recent analysis showed that the occurrence of new BILAG A flares was significantly decreased in patients receiving rituximab versus placebo.[30] Inasmuch as such severe flares are clinically highly relevant and probably easier to measure reliably than milder flares, this conclusion could be an important indication of a relevant treatment benefit for rituximab. On the other hand, the fact that it was a posthoc analysis must make one cautious in embracing this conclusion.

The previously published observational data on rituximab in nonrenal SLE, also tended to be in the minority, compared with lupus nephritis. In the author's own experiences at Karolinska, one patient with severe cutaneous lupus appeared to respond well to combined treatment with rituximab, CyX, and glucocorticoids, but, more recently, several patients with similar clinical disease did not appear to respond at all.

Summarizing the uncontrolled and controlled data on the efficacy of rituximab in generalized nonrenal lupus, it may be fair to conclude at this point in time that perhaps the efficacy, if any, of rituximab in generalized nonrenal SLE is quite modest. The exceptions to this rule might indeed be patients with hematologic lupus and, as has been suggested by others, patients with certain lupus manifestations of the central nervous system (CNS) and possibly patients at risk for severe nonrenal lupus flares.

Rituximab in Lupus Nephritis

Patients, who were reported in observational studies, case series, and case reports of rituximab in SLE, often had lupus nephritis as the dominant disease manifestation. As previously referenced, 25 patients with lupus nephritis class II, III, or IV who had been refractory to CyX in most cases were treated at Karolinska with a "lymphoma course" of four doses of rituximab plus two doses of 500 mg CyX and glucocorticoids; in that experience, all but one patient had a partial renal response and many patients had a complete renal response.[32] Nonetheless, the results of LUNAR were clearly negative as previously indicated. Again, the question can be asked whether this failed trial represents a failure of the drug or a failure of the trial to demonstrate a true benefit. In the case of LUNAR, the answer is more complex than it is for EXPLORER. In LUNAR, patients were treated with concomitant MMF, which might have blunted the ability of rituximab to demonstrate a benefit. Another important concern with LUNAR is the duration of the trial. For renal disease, classical studies at the National Institutes of Health (NIH) have demonstrated that long-term follow-up is needed to be able to discern therapeutic differences among agents.[33] The author's experience at Karolinska suggest that although many patients demonstrate benefits during the first year after rituximab therapy, continuing improvements in the second year of follow-up, during which many patients who preliminarily have a partial response, eventually develop a complete renal response. Because partial clinical responses are hard to assess and are subject to noise in the system, it is possible that such partial responses were missed during the 1-year follow-up in the LUNAR trial. In hindsight, the fact that no longer-term extension was added to that trial is unfortunate.

The fact that the concomitant immunosuppressive medication in the LUNAR trial was always MMF is an additional concern. This is a contrast to the open-label uncontrolled experiences at many centers in which the preferred mode of administration of rituximab is almost invariably in combination with CyX. Based on mechanistic considerations, the possibility certainly exists that CyX would synergize with rituximab in achieving a maximal therapeutic benefit, something that was initially suggested by Edwards and colleagues[34] and, to some extent, supported by the trials in RA.[35] Additional positive therapeutic trials have since then been reported in antineutrophil cytoplasmic antibody (ANCA)–positive vasculitis in which the combination of rituximab plus two low-dose infusions of CyX was demonstrated to be equivalent to standard long-term and high-dose therapy with CyX alone.[36]

Moreover, recent data from a randomized trial in SLE called *BELONG* could also be relevant. In this trial, patients with lupus nephritis were given ocrelizumab or placebo. Ocrelizumab is a humanized anti-CD20 monoclonal antibody with pharmacologic properties and a mechanism of action that is similar to rituximab. In the BELONG trial, ocrelizumab was used on a background of either MMF or CyX (by investigators' choice); although the overall trial results were negative, the suggestion was made that the group who received the anti-CD20 agent in combination with CyX benefited over those receiving placebo plus CyX.[37]

Rituximab in Systemic Lupus Erythematosus: Conclusions

A final conclusion regarding the therapeutic potential of rituximab in SLE cannot yet be conclusively drawn. A compelling mechanism appears to suggest the potential for efficacy in at least some subsets of patients with lupus. These theoretical considerations are, of course, also bolstered by the demonstration of efficacy in the autoimmune diseases RA and ANCA-associated vasculitis. However, the decidedly negative results of the EXPLORER clinical trial would suggest that rituximab is perhaps not a particularly useful drug for the management of generalized nonrenal lupus when mucocutaneous, musculoskeletal, and generalized symptoms predominate. Unless and until a controlled clinical trial demonstrates a benefit for such patients, using this agent in that setting would be distinctly premature. In select circumstances, a possible exception could be made for patients at high risk for severe, nonrenal lupus flares. On the other hand, the data for lupus nephritis from uncontrolled studies are quite convincing, the mechanism in that setting is also more robust, and the criticism at the negative LUNAR trial in various respects is quite solid. Therefore considering the use of rituximab in patients who suffer from lupus nephritis and have manifested therapeutic failure with CyX or MMF or both might still seem clinically reasonable. Some subsets of patients with lupus who were insufficiently represented in either of the randomized clinical trials but whose disease can be pathophysiologically linked to specific autoantibodies that may be downregulated by rituximab might also be considered for off-label use in particularly pressing situations. This category would include patients with severe hematologic lupus manifestations and perhaps certain CNS manifestations.

Recommendations for the Clinician

As previous stated, rituximab should not be considered for the management of generalized lupus at this time. On the other hand, for patients with lupus nephritis who failed to benefit from CyX or MMF or both, the judicious use of rituximab may be considered. For patients with severe or refractory hematologic lupus and perhaps even some CNS manifestations, the off-label use of rituximab can still be advocated under carefully controlled clinical circumstances. The preponderance of the evidence suggests that when rituximab is combined with CyX, an additional benefit might exist. The personal view of the author of this text is that rituximab should, if possible, be combined with CyX and glucocorticoids in regimens such as the ones previously outlined. The specific regimen (two doses of 500 mg CyX) entails so few risks that these should only rarely dissuade the clinician from administering this particular treatment combination.

Safety of Rituximab

Large clinical trials and long-term longitudinal follow-up with patients treated under the indications lymphoma and RA have demonstrated that rituximab is generally well-tolerated and safe in many patients.[38] However, the potential for severe infusion reactions and potentially severe or even life-threatening infections must always be considered. The viral reactivation disease, progressive multifocal leukoencephalopathy (PML), has been documented in a few patients with SLE who had been treated with rituximab, prompting a warning from the FDA. Closer investigations of the literature revealed that the risk for this often fatal infectious complication is elevated in many

autoimmune diseases and linked to a variety of immunosuppressive therapies; whether rituximab confers a uniquely elevated risk remains unclear at this time.[39]

Thus rituximab represents a paradox in lupus management with contradictory data from observational studies and clinical trials. Hopefully with time, newer data will emerge and the discrepancies will be reconciled. Meanwhile, data from the International Registry on Biologics in SLE (IRBIS) demonstrate that rituximab is, by far, the most widely used off-label biologic agent for SLE with considerable cohorts of patients being treated at specialty centers worldwide.

ANTI–TUMOR NECROSIS FACTOR AGENTS

TNF is a proinflammatory and regulatory cytokine that was shown to be elevated in serum from patients with SLE. TNF inhibitors are widely used in rheumatology and have, during the past decade, altered the disease course and prognosis for large groups of patients with RA and other arthritides in a dramatic way. Because some animal experimental studies suggested that treatment with recombinant TNF was beneficial in inducing a delay in nephritis development in at least one animal model of SLE,[40] initial anxieties exist concerning the use anti-TNF agents in patients with SLE. The use of TNF-blocking agents in SLE was also believed to be contraindicated as a result of observations on the development of SLE-related autoantibodies (e.g., ANA, anti-DNA antibodies, anticardiolipin antibodies)[41] and even the development of a drug-induced lupus-like syndrome in some patients with RA who were treated with anti-TNF agents. Thus experiences with anti-TNF agents have only been described for a limited number of patients. Aringer and colleagues[42] first described the use of infliximab in a small cohort of patients with SLE and nephritis or arthritis or both. The arthritis in these patients temporarily improved but required repeated infusion to maintain effect, just as is generally the case in patients with RA. In contrast, in the 4 patients with nephritis, more long-standing reductions of proteinuria were observed but with a concomitant increase in the titers of several autoantibodies. Follow-up data from 13 patients treated with infliximab demonstrated an increase in life-threatening, infusion-related events, including fatal complications after repeated administration of the drug.[43] Subsequently, two randomized controlled trials using TNF inhibitors (infliximab and etanercept) for use in active lupus nephritis have been terminated because of recruitment difficulties. Although anti-TNF medications are used widely in rheumatology, their off-label use in SLE in the IRBIS registry has been limited.

ABATACEPT

Because T cells may play an important role in SLE pathogenesis by supporting B-cell activation, activating macrophages, and/or releasing cytokines, downregulating T cells may have therapeutic benefits in lupus. Indeed, the T cell–specific conventional immunosuppressive cyclosporin A has been effective in some settings in SLE, although potential nephrotoxicity has limited its use. In various animal models of SLE, reducing T-cell activation leads to improvements in the experimental autoimmune disease,[44,45] and one particularly successful strategy was the blockade of the so-called *second signal* of T-cell activation.[46] This principle led to the development for therapeutic purposes of abatacept (Orencia, cytotoxic T-lymphocyte antigen 4–immunoglobulin [CTLA4-Ig]), which is approved for use in RA. It is believed that the drug modulates T-cell co-stimulation by binding to the B7 (CD80/86) molecule on the surface of antigen-presenting cells and B lymphocytes, preventing the mediation of the second signal needed for T-cell activation. However, abatacept may have other mechanisms as well, and it is important to recognize that its binding target is expressed on B cells, not on T cells.

Abatacept has been studied in SLE. In a randomized 1-year placebo-controlled, phase II study on active nonrenal SLE, no statistically significant difference was achieved in primary and secondary outcomes when compared with placebo, but some improvements were observed regarding fatigue, sleep, and quality of life.[47] A recent press release indicated that an additional trial with abatacept in combination with MMF for renal lupus also failed to achieve its primary endpoint, and follow-up treatment was halted. A separate trial is being performed by the NIH Immune Tolerance Network using the CTLA4-Ig molecule in combination with CyX, based on the previously cited promising animal data.[46]

Although theoretical considerations and animal data raised hopes that abatacept would prove beneficial in SLE, clinical trial results to date have been disappointing, and no convincingly encouraging case series or other observational studies have been reported. Data from the IRBIS registry suggest that off-label use of abatacept for SLE is minimal.

References

1. Browning JL: B cells move to centre stage: novel opportunities for autoimmune disease treatment. *Nat Rev Drug Discov* 5:564–576, 2006.
2. Cancro MP, D'Cruz DP, Khamashta MA: The role of B lymphocyte stimulator (BLyS) in systemic lupus erythematosus. *J Clin Invest* 119:1066–1073, 2009.
3. Cancro MP: Signalling crosstalk in B cells: managing worth and need. *Nat Rev Immunol* 9:657–661, 2009.
4. Moore PA, Belvedere O, Orr A, et al: BLyS: member of the tumor necrosis factor family and B lymphocyte stimulator. *Science* 285:260–263, 1999.
5. Avery DT, Kalled SL, Ellyard JI, et al: BAFF selectively enhances the survival of plasmablasts generated from human memory B cells. *J Clin Invest* 112:286–297, 2003.
6. Cheema GS, Roschke V, Hilbert DM, et al: Elevated serum B lymphocyte stimulator levels in patients with systemic immune-based rheumatic diseases. *Arthritis Rheum* 44:1313–1319, 2001.
7. Stohl W, Metyas S, Tan SM, et al: B lymphocyte stimulator overexpression in patients with systemic lupus erythematosus: longitudinal observations. *Arthritis Rheum* 48:3475–3486, 2003.
8. Petri M, Stohl W, Chatham W, et al: Association of plasma B lymphocyte stimulator levels and disease activity in systemic lupus erythematosus. *Arthritis Rheum* 58:2453–2459, 2008.
9. Zhang J, Roschke V, Baker KP, et al: Cutting edge: a role for B lymphocyte stimulator in systemic lupus erythematosus. *J Immunol* 166:6–10, 2001.
10. Baker KP, Edwards BM, Main SH, et al: Generation and characterization of LymphoStat-B, a human monoclonal antibody that antagonizes the bioactivities of B lymphocyte stimulator. *Arthritis Rheum* 48:3253–3265, 2003.
11. Halpern WG, Lappin P, Zanardi T, et al: Chronic administration of belimumab, a BLyS antagonist, decreases tissue and peripheral blood B-lymphocyte populations in cynomolgus monkeys: pharmacokinetic, pharmacodynamic, and toxicologic effects. *Toxicol Sci* 91:586–599, 2006.
12. Wallace DJ, Stohl W, Furie RA, et al: A phase II, randomized, double-blind, placebo-controlled, dose-ranging study of belimumab in patients with active systemic lupus erythematosus. *Arthritis Rheum* 61:1168–1178, 2009.
13. Strand V, Sokolove J: Randomized controlled trial design in rheumatoid arthritis: the past decade. *Arthritis Res Ther* 11:205, 2009.
14. Jacobi AM, Huang W, Wang T, et al: Effect of long-term belimumab treatment on B cells in systemic lupus erythematosus: extension of a phase II, double-blind, placebo-controlled, dose-ranging study. *Arthritis Rheum* 62:201–210, 2010.
15. Furie RA, Petri MA, Wallace DJ, et al: Novel evidence-based systemic lupus erythematosus responder index. *Arthritis Rheum* 61:1143–1151, 2009.
16. Navarra SV, Guzman RM, Gallacher AE, et al: Efficacy and safety of belimumab in patients with active systemic lupus erythematosus: a randomised, placebo-controlled, phase 3 trial. *Lancet* 377:721–731, 2011.
17. Furie R, Petri M, Zamani O, et al: van Vollenhoven RF; BLISS-76 Study Group: A phase III, randomized, placebo-controlled study of belimumab, a monoclonal antibody that inhibits B lymphocyte stimulator, in patients with systemic lupus erythematosus. *Arthritis Rheum* 63(12):3918–3930, 2011.
18. van Vollenhoven RF, Petri MA, Cervera R, et al: Belimumab in the treatment of systemic lupus erythematosus: high disease activity predictors of response. *Ann Rheum Dis* 2012. [Epub ahead of print]
19. Leandro MJ, Edwards JC, Cambridge G, et al: An open study of B lymphocyte depletion in systemic lupus erythematosus. *Arthritis Rheum* 46:2673–2677, 2002.
20. van Vollenhoven RF, Gunnarsson I, Welin-Henriksson E, et al: Biopsy-verified response of severe lupus nephritis to treatment with rituximab (anti-CD20 monoclonal antibody) plus cyclophosphamide after biopsy-documented failure to respond to cyclophosphamide alone. *Scand J Rheumatol* 33:423–427, 2004.
21. Gunnarsson I, Sundelin B, Jonsdottir T, et al: Histopathologic and clinical outcome of rituximab treatment in patients with cyclophosphamide-resistant proliferative lupus nephritis. *Arthritis Rheum* 56:1263–1272, 2007.
22. Jonsdottir T, Gunnarsson I, Risselada A, et al: Treatment of refractory SLE with rituximab plus cyclophosphamide: clinical effects, serological changes, and predictors of response. *Ann Rheum Dis* 67:330–334, 2008.
23. Looney RJ, Anolik JH, Campbell D, et al: B cell depletion as a novel treatment for systemic lupus erythematosus: a phase I/II dose-escalation trial of rituximab. *Arthritis Rheum* 50:2580–2589, 2004.
24. Sfikakis PP, Boletis JN, Lionaki S, et al: Remission of proliferative lupus nephritis following B cell depletion therapy is preceded by down-regulation of the T cell costimulatory molecule CD40 ligand: an open-label trial. *Arthritis Rheum* 52:501–513, 2005.
25. Lu TY, Ng KP, Cambridge G, et al: A retrospective seven-year analysis of the use of B cell depletion therapy in systemic lupus erythematosus at University College London Hospital: the first fifty patients. *Arthritis Rheum* 61:482–487, 2009.
26. Gottenberg JE, Guillevin L, Lambotte O, et al: Tolerance and short term efficacy of rituximab in 43 patients with systemic autoimmune diseases. *Ann Rheum Dis* 64:913–920, 2005.
27. Terrier B, Amoura Z, Ravaud P, et al: Safety and efficacy of rituximab in systemic lupus erythematosus: results from 136 patients from the French AutoImmunity and Rituximab registry. *Arthritis Rheum* 62:2458–2466, 2010.
28. Ramos-Casals M, Soto MJ, Cuadrado MJ, et al: Rituximab in systemic lupus erythematosus: A systematic review of off-label use in 188 cases. *Lupus* 18:767–776, 2009.
29. Merrill JT, Neuwelt CM, Wallace DJ, et al: Efficacy and safety of rituximab in moderately-to-severely active systemic lupus erythematosus: the randomized, double-blind, phase II/III systemic lupus erythematosus evaluation of rituximab trial. *Arthritis Rheum* 62:222–233, 2010.
30. Merrill J, Buyon J, Furie R, et al: Assessment of flares in lupus patients enrolled in a phase II/III study of rituximab (EXPLORER). *Lupus* 20:709–716, 2011.
31. Rovin BH, Furie R, Latinis K, et al: Efficacy and safety of rituximab in patients with active proliferative lupus nephritis: The Lupus Nephritis Assessment with Rituximab study. *Arthritis Rheum* 64(4):1215–1226, 2012.
32. Jonsdottir T, Gunnarsson I, Mourao AF, et al: Clinical improvements in proliferative vs membranous lupus nephritis following B-cell depletion: pooled data from two cohorts. *Rheumatology (Oxford)* 49:1502–1504, 2010.
33. Gourley MF, Austin HA, 3rd, Scott D, et al: Methylprednisolone and cyclophosphamide, alone or in combination, in patients with lupus nephritis. A randomized, controlled trial. *Ann Intern Med* 125:549–557, 1996.
34. Edwards JC, Cambridge G: Sustained improvement in rheumatoid arthritis following a protocol designed to deplete B lymphocytes. *Rheumatology (Oxford)* 40:205–211, 2001.
35. Edwards JC, Szczepanski L, Szechinski J, et al: Efficacy of B-cell-targeted therapy with rituximab in patients with rheumatoid arthritis. *N Engl J Med* 350:2572–2581, 2004.
36. Jones RB, Tervaert JW, Hauser T, et al: Rituximab versus cyclophosphamide in ANCA-associated renal vasculitis. *N Engl J Med* 363:211–220, 2010.
37. Mysler EF, Spindler, AJ, Guzman, RM, et al: Efficacy and safety of ocrelizumab, a humanized antiCD20 antibody, in patients with active proliferative lupus nephritis (LN): results from the randomized, double-blind phase III BELONG study. *Arthritis Rheum* 62:S606–S607, 2010.
38. van Vollenhoven RF, Emery P, Bingham CO, 3rd, et al: Longterm safety of patients receiving rituximab in rheumatoid arthritis clinical trials. *J Rheumatol* 37:558–567, 2010.
39. Molloy ES, Calabrese LH: Progressive multifocal leukoencephalopathy in patients with rheumatic diseases: are patients with systemic lupus erythematosus at particular risk? *Autoimmun Rev* 8:144–146, 2008.
40. Jacob CO, McDevitt HO: Tumour necrosis factor-alpha in murine autoimmune 'lupus' nephritis. *Nature* 331:356–358, 1988.
41. Jonsdottir T, Forslid J, van Vollenhoven A, et al: Treatment with tumour necrosis factor alpha antagonists in patients with rheumatoid

arthritis induces anticardiolipin antibodies. *Ann Rheum Dis* 63:1075–1078, 2004.

42. Aringer M, Graninger WB, Steiner G, et al: Safety and efficacy of tumor necrosis factor alpha blockade in systemic lupus erythematosus: an open-label study. *Arthritis Rheum* 50:3161–3169, 2004.

43. Aringer M, Houssiau F, Gordon C, et al: Adverse events and efficacy of TNF-alpha blockade with infliximab in patients with systemic lupus erythematosus: long-term follow-up of 13 patients. *Rheumatology (Oxford)* 48:1451–1454, 2009.

44. Wu HY, Quintana FJ, Weiner HL: Nasal anti-CD3 antibody ameliorates lupus by inducing an IL-10-secreting CD4+ CD25- LAP+ regulatory T cell and is associated with down-regulation of IL-17+ CD4+ ICOS+ CXCR5+ follicular helper T cells. *J Immunol* 181:6038–6050, 2008.

45. Adachi Y, Inaba M, Sugihara A, et al: Effects of administration of monoclonal antibodies (anti-CD4 or anti-CD8) on the development of autoimmune diseases in (NZW x BXSB)F1 mice. *Immunobiology* 198:451–464, 1998.

46. Finck BK, Linsley PS, Wofsy D: Treatment of murine lupus with CTLA4Ig. *Science* 265:1225–1227, 1994.

47. Merrill JT, Burgos-Vargas R, Westhovens R, et al: The efficacy and safety of abatacept in patients with non-life-threatening manifestations of systemic lupus erythematosus: results of a twelve-month, multicenter, exploratory, phase IIb, randomized, double-blind, placebo-controlled trial. *Arthritis Rheum* 62:3077–3087, 2010.

Chapter 54

Critical Issues in Drug Development for SLE

Ronald F. van Vollenhoven

INTRODUCTION

The development of new drugs for the treatment of systemic lupus erythematosus (SLE) during the first decade of the third millennium has not been uniformly successful. Although expectations were high, based on the dramatic successes of new drug development in rheumatoid arthritis (RA) and other inflammatory joint diseases and the impressive increases in the understanding of the pathophysiology of SLE, a large number of failed clinical trials and aborted development programs attest to the difficulties of designing and implementing appropriate developmental strategies for novel therapeutic agents in the treatment of this disease. Nonetheless, a large number of important lessons have been learnt during the conduct of unsuccessful development programs and clinical trials, and the recent success of phase III trials of belimumab for SLE with the subsequent approval of this biologic agent as the first novel therapeutic in many decades raises hopes that the long period of drought is now coming to an end. However, in order to make maximal use of the insights obtained through the painstaking processes that have evolved over recent years, it will be critical to implement changes in the way clinical trials are designed to achieve maximal outputs and results in the future.

This chapter reviews the critical issues for drug development in lupus from the point of view of (1) SLE disease characteristics that must be considered, and (2) the use of appropriate outcomes, endpoints, and other design features for clinical trials within the regulatory environment in which new drug approval can take place.

SYSTEMIC LUPUS ERYTHEMATOSUS DISEASE CHARACTERISTICS CRITICAL FOR DRUG DEVELOPMENT

SLE has a number of disease characteristics that significantly impact the manner in which drug development has to take place. Among these are the facts that SLE (1) is a chronic, generally nonlethal disease; (2) is associated with significant and incompletely understood detrimental effects on the quality of life; (3) is highly heterogeneous in its clinical expression and probably its underlying pathophysiology; and (4) exhibits a bewildering variation in its long-term course.

Systemic Lupus Erythematosus Is a Chronic Nonlethal Disease

Although a small number of patients suffer from severe and life-threatening complications of SLE, for the vast majority of patients the disease is characterized by chronicity without an immediately life-threatening character. In this regard, the distinctions made by Barr and colleagues,[1] who noted the following three subsets of patients, are important: (1) patients with chronic active disease having continuously smouldering disease activity with or without superimposed flares; (2) patients with a disease characterized by symptom-free periods, punctuated by recurrent flares; and (3) patients exhibiting long quiescence or remission.[2] The same patterns were observed in other large longitudinal studies.[3] Needless to say, the clinical approach to these patients would differ quite significantly, with the first named

group representing the most notable clinical challenges and unmet needs. Remarkably, however, the distinction among these patient profiles has not always been made sufficiently clear in drug development.

In more general terms, developing drugs for chronic, nonlethal diseases invariably leads to the question of therapeutic goals, and these can be formulated in a number of different, mutually nonexclusive ways. In chronic autoimmune diseases with a long and extensive history of clinical trials, such as RA and inflammatory bowel disease (IBD), such goals have been formulated in great detail and the appropriate outcomes for clinical trials have been well established, whereas a greater degree of unclarity remains on these issues for SLE. The following main goals are often addressed in this context:

1. Reduction of the *activity* of the disease
2. Achievement of a satisfactory or acceptable *disease activity state*
3. Reduction of the *risk for flare* of the disease
4. Reduction of the *progression of damage* caused by the disease
5. Improvement in the *health-related quality of life* (as reported by the patient)

Table 54-1 shows these therapeutic goals and ways to measure them in clinical trials for RA, IBD, and SLE.

Systemic Lupus Erythematosus Is Associated with Significant and Incompletely Understood Detrimental Effects on Quality of Life

Both in large registries and during the course of clinical trials performed in recent decades, it has repeatedly been determined that health-related quality of life (HRQoL) is significantly reduced in patients with SLE.[4-8] The decreases observed in trials were often of a magnitude that compares unfavorably with other chronic musculoskeletal diseases but is rather comparable to late-stage disease in chronic pulmonary, cardiac, or infectious conditions. The exact reasons for the striking impact that SLE has on HRQoL is as yet incompletely understood. The persistent activation of immunologic effector mechanisms may give rise to significant subjective symptoms in the form of fatigue, lack of energy, and lassitude; and these mechanisms may also have effects on cognition, mood, and other mental functions.[9] Conversely, it has been suggested that many patients with SLE suffer from fibromyalgia,[10,11] which proposes that these are two separate disease entities that co-exist in such patients. An alternative view has proposed that fibromyalgia may be a manifestation of SLE.[12] Perhaps these distinctions cannot be fully resolved until the nature of the chronic symptoms such as those that occur in fibromyalgia and related conditions are more fully understood. In the individual patient case, it may be impossible to determine whether nonspecific subjective symptoms are due to mechanisms more directly related to the autoimmune process versus those that may be linked to other mechanisms including those at the level of the central nervous system.

For clinical trial design, these observations engender considerable difficulties in determining what outcomes to choose. A treatment

TABLE 54-1 Comparison of Outcomes Dimensions in Three Autoimmune Inflammatory Diseases

THERAPEUTIC GOALS (IN GENERAL TERMS)	*Rheumatoid Arthritis*		*Inflammatory Bowel Disease*		*Systemic Lupus Erythematosus*	
	DISEASE-SPECIFIC THERAPEUTIC GOALS	MEASURES FOR TRIALS	DISEASE-SPECIFIC THERAPEUTIC GOALS	MEASURES FOR TRIALS	DISEASE-SPECIFIC THERAPEUTIC GOALS	MEASURES FOR TRIALS
Reduce disease activity	Reduction of inflamed joints	Reduction of swollen or tender joints Improvement in DAS	Reduction in GI symptoms	Reduction in CDAI, HBI, and among other indices	Reduction in global disease activity	Reduction in SLEDAI, SLAM, ECLAM, and BILAG global scores
Achieve satisfactory disease state	Lower RA disease activity or achieve clinical remission	Defined as threshold values for outcomes such as DAS and SDAI	Low IBD disease activity or (I) clinical remission or clinical remission and biochemical remission (II) biochemical remission (III) endoscopic and histologic remission (mucosal healing)	Defined as: (I) threshold values for outcomes such as CDAI, HBI (II) normal fecal calprotectin (III) no morphologic signs of macroscopic or microscopic inflammation	Low SLE disease activity	Several proposals: SLEDAI score of <4 No BILAG A or B scores
Reduction in the risk for flare	Fewer RA flares	No consensus definition	Fewer IBD flares	Defined by increases in CDAI, HBI, and other indices	Fewer SLE flares	Several proposals: SELENA flare index New BILAG A or B Increase in PGA
Reduction in progression of damage	Reduction in bone and cartilage damage	Assessed by standardized measures on radiographs (modified Sharp score)	Reduction in complications such as strictures and fistulae Obviate need for surgery	Semiquantitative assessments	Reduction in long-term damage from SLE and its treatment	SLICC damage index widely accepted
Improved HRQoL	Improved HRQoL	Disease nonspecifically measured by SF-36, EQ-5D Many disease-specific instruments have been proposed	Improved HRQoL	Disease nonspecifically measured by SF-36, EQ5D Disease-specific instruments have been proposed such as SHS	Improved HRQoL	Disease nonspecifically measured by SF-36, EQ5D Many disease-specific instruments have been proposed

BILAG, The British Isles Lupus Assessment Group; CDAI, Crohn Disease Activity Index; DAS, disease activity score; ECLAM, the European Consensus Lupus Activity Measurement; EQ-5D, generic, disease-nonspecific quality of life instrument; GI, gastrointestinal; HBI, Harvey-Bradshaw Index; HRQoL, health-related quality of life; IBD, inflammatory disease; PGA, physician's global assessment; RA, rheumatoid arthritis; SDAI, the Simplified Disease Activity Index; SELENA, the Safety of Estrogens in Lupus Erythematosus–National Assessment Trial; SF, short form; SHS, the Short Health Scale; SLAM, the Systemic Activity Measure; SLEDAI, the Systemic Lupus Erythematosus Disease Activity Index; SLE, systemic lupus erythematosus; SLICC, the Systemic Lupus International Collaborating Clinics.

expected to have a specific and targeted effect on a component of the autoimmune response, such as an anticytokine- or anticellular-target therapy, would perhaps be analyzed most appropriately in terms of its effect on the measureable immunologic abnormalities. On the other hand, some treatments might be intended primarily for improvements in HRQoL without having a clear immunologic mechanism. It could be said that some established therapies for SLE, such as antimalarial medications, fit the latter bill inasmuch as their mechanisms are incompletely understood. In the end, a therapy that could improve HRQoL by any mechanism would be a major advance. It might be useful therefore to consider clinical trial strategies based primarily on assessments of HRQoL. Unfortunately, the measurement problem in this respect is quite formidable and, from a regulatory point of view, this is not yet possible. (Further discussions provided later in this chapter.)

Systemic Lupus Erythematosus Is Highly Heterogeneous in its Clinical Expression and Probably in its Underlying Pathophysiology

In contrast to diseases such as RA in which the central clinical manifestations are similar among patients and can be defined in terms that are applicable to all patients, SLE is characterized by a bewildering heterogeneity that makes it inevitable that patients have to be assessed

in different ways, depending on a patient's particular clinical situation. From a clinical trials point of view, this characterization presents an exceptionally large challenge. One possible solution to this dilemma is the use of generalized disease activity indices to measure the overall SLE activity, irrespective of the particular disease manifestation from which the patient may be suffering. The instruments developed for this purpose are discussed in the following text and are also discussed Chapter 46. However, approaching SLE trials with a different intention is also possible, namely to investigate patients with similar disease manifestations and focus the assessment on the outcome of that particular organ system or domain. The most well-studied example of this type of approach is lupus nephritis, for which a large number of trials have been performed. In such trials the patients are selected for significant disease activity in the renal system as defined by inclusion and exclusion criteria, and subsequent treatments are then assessed in terms of their ability to control that aspect of the disease. Whether or not other disease manifestations (i.e., in nonrenal organ systems) are also positively impacted is further assessed by appropriately chosen secondary outcome criteria. Although this particular strategy has so far been used almost exclusively for lupus nephritis, it is certainly conceivable that this approach could be used for other organ manifestations as well. For predominantly cutaneous SLE, using the same measures that are employed in dermatology clinical trials, for example, the Cutaneous Lupus Erythematosus Disease Area and Severity Index (CLASI), is possible[13]; and for patients with predominant musculoskeletal disease manifestations in SLE, established arthritis scores such as those employed in clinical trials for RA might be used (e.g., the American College of Rheumatology [ACR] 20 response[14] or responses based on the disease activity score [DAS][15]). The subtle nuances of disease manifestations in SLE and how they differ from other conditions must then, of course, be considered.

Systemic Lupus Erythematosus Exhibits a Bewildering Variation in its Long-Term Course

In addition to the heterogeneity in terms of disease manifestations in each individual patient, a significant heterogeneity in the long-term evolution of the disease also exists. Although this may be true for most chronic diseases, from a clinical perspective it is clear that our ability to predict the medium- and long-term course in SLE is even more limited. All clinicians are aware of patients who, despite initially severe disease activity with dramatic lupus manifestations, had a subsequent course leading to excellent disease control or even remission, whereas other patients who initially appeared to have mild disease subsequently suffered the consequences of grave and sometimes irreversible disease manifestations. It is unfortunately quite likely that many uncontrolled observational studies of therapeutic agents in SLE have led to incorrect conclusions, largely because of these aspects. Although studying every potential new therapy in controlled trials from the outset is not possible, judgment on any new therapeutic option must be suspended until the results of controlled trials are available. In addition, long-term trials and extension studies are needed to determine the precise impact of novel therapeutic agents in the treatment of SLE.

OUTCOMES AND ENDPOINTS FOR CLINICAL TRIALS AND THE REGULATORY ENVIRONMENT

For the purpose of clinical trials, the use of well-characterized and validated outcome measures is critical. It may be of interest to recall the development of such outcome criteria for RA, where, up until the early 1990s, a profusion of outcome measures was used in clinical practice and research. In 1993, Felson and associates[16] analyzed the relative usefulness of many outcome criteria and introduced a condensation of seven important outcomes in RA in the form of the ACR "core set" or response; on these, the ACR 20 response criteria were based.[14] This response in essence requires that out of the seven core outcomes, at least five demonstrate a 20% improvement from baseline; these five must include the swollen joint count and the tender joint count. If the patient demonstrates these improvements in a clinical trial, she or he is considered an ACR 20 responder. Some years later, the European League Against Rheumatism (EULAR) response criteria were also adopted,[17] based on the DAS or on its modification, the DAS 28.[18] Additional modifications, such as the response criteria based on the Simplified Disease Activity Index (SDAI)[19] and other indices, have since been published. Thus without these methodologic innovations, it might have been extremely difficult or even impossible to effectuate the tremendous development of novel biologic therapies for RA during the late 1990s and the past decennium.

This example may underscore the importance of outcome measures for clinical trial development and points to an important need in the field of SLE clinical trials. As of now, a number of instruments are being used, but it is still not entirely clear which, if any of these, will make it possible for investigators to demonstrate efficacy—for drugs that do have true efficacy—in otherwise appropriately designed clinical trials. A number of specific possibilities must be considered.

For trials investigating the overall activity of a given treatment for SLE, the need is most obvious. Several global measures of SLE disease activity have been developed over the past 20 to 30 years, validated, and used in research studies and, to some extent, also in clinical trials.

TABLE 54-2 Comparison of the Most Widely Used Systemic Lupus Erythematosus Disease Activity Indices for Potential Use in Clinical Trials

	SLEDAI	BILAG	SLAM	ECLAM
Validated (face validity, content validity, sensitivity to change)	+++	+++	++	++
Comprehensiveness	+	+++	++	+–
Ease of use	++	–	+	++
Previous experience and use in research setting	+++	+++	++	+
Previous experience and use in clinical trial setting	+++	+++	+–	+–

BILAG, The British Isles Lupus Assessment Group; ECLAM, the European Consensus Lupus Activity Measurement; SLAM, the Systemic Activity Measure; SLEDAI, the Systemic Lupus Erythematosus Disease Activity Index.

Most notable among these are the Systemic Lupus Erythematosus Disease Activity Index (SLEDAI)[20] with its modifications, the Safety of Estrogens in Lupus Erythematosus–National Assessment Trial (SELENA)–SLEDAI[21] and SLEDAI-2K.[22] (For details on these and other lupus activity measures, the reader is referred to Chapter 46). The SLE activity scoring system developed by the British Isles Lupus Activity Group (BILAG) is primarily designed as an organ and system–based assessment, assigning letter codes to indicate the activity in each organ system that can be converted to a numerical global score.[23] Yet other systems, such as the Systemic Lupus Activity Measure (SLAM),[24] the European Consensus Lupus Activity Measurement (ECLAM),[25] the Lupus Activity Index (LAI),[26] and others, have been used somewhat less frequently, although they are validated and have been used in research studies. Key attributes of relevance in clinical trials for each of these measures are listed in Table 54-2.

The SLEDAI and BILAG index have emerged as the most intensively used instruments for clinical trials. An important development was represented by the BLISS phase III clinical trials,[8] for which it was decided, in negotiations between the sponsor (Human Genome Sciences [HGS]) and the U.S. Food and Drug Administration (FDA) to apply a compound outcome measure based on the SELENA-SLEDAI, the BILAG index, and the physician's global assessment (PGA) to arrive at the SLE responder index (SRI). Thus for the patient to be considered a responder in these trials, she or he had to demonstrate an improvement by at least four points on the SELENA-SLEDAI while, at the same time, not having a new BILAG A score (i.e., a significant new level of disease activity necessitating high-dose corticosteroid or immunosuppressive agents) and not either two new BILAG B scores (i.e., somewhat lower new activity in two organ systems) and also no worsening of the PGA by a predefined margin. Needless to say, this outcome measure, being a compound of compound instruments, has raised the concern that it may be far removed from clinical reality. It was therefore of importance to demonstrate in the BLISS trials that, in addition to the former response criteria, improvements in disease activity and control were also achieved in more traditional and clinically understandable outcomes. (See the discussion in greater detail in Chapter 53.)

In recent years, the FDA, working with academicians and in response to the needs of the industry, has developed a guidance document for developing medical products for the treatment of SLE (http://www.fda.gov/downloads/Drugs/GuidanceCompliance RegulatoryInformation/Guidances/ucm072063.pdf). This document was published after the BLISS trials with belimumab were designed but before it was known whether these products were successful. Although the document does not discuss the SRI used in the BLISS trials, it does discuss the pertinent issues relating to an SLE clinical trial and provides a number of key considerations. Most importantly,

TABLE 54-3 FDA Guidance Document Recommendations for Clinical Trials in Systemic Lupus Erythematosus

PRIMARY EFFICACY ENDPOINT	RECOMMENDED INSTRUMENT TO ASSESS	ADDITIONAL RECOMMENDATIONS	COMMENTARY AND CONCERNS
Reduction in disease activity	BILAG (preferred) or other global indices	Restricting and monitoring other therapies, particularly corticosteroidal agents, is important. Provided suggestions on how to define *major* and *partial* clinical responses.	Mixing global with organ-specific activity assessments and other inconsistencies make this section of the guidance document somewhat unclear.
Complete clinical response or remission	Global disease activity indices, including BILAG index and SLEDAI	Zero disease activity (remission) should be sustained for at least 6 months.	May be too high a threshold target to meet in a clinical trial.
Reduction in flare or increase in time to flare	BILAG index or SELENA Flare Index	Both occurrence of flares and time to flare can be used. Other disease activity aspects must also be assessed.	Assessment of mild-to-moderate flare has proven difficult in a recent prospective study (REF.
Reduction in concomitant steroidal agents	Proportion of patients who achieve reduction to ≤10 mg daily prednisolone (or equivalent)	Outcome must be sustained for at least 3 consecutive months and occur in the context of other clinical benefits as well. Corticosteroid-related toxicities should also be evaluated.	
Treatment of serious acute manifestations	Proportion of patients with a lower score in the organ-system score of the involved organ "such that there is no longer a threat to that organ"	Secondary outcomes include: • Time to resolution of acute manifestation • Mortality • Need for retreatment • Use of corticosteroids • Overall disease activity	

BILAG, The British Isles Lupus Assessment Group; FDA, U.S. Food and Drug Administration; REF, recent prospective study; SELENA, the Safety of Estrogens in Lupus Erythematosus–National Assessment Trial; SLEDAI, the Systemic Lupus Erythematosus Disease Activity Index.

it identifies the following potential primary efficacy endpoints for SLE clinical trials (summarized in Table 54-3):
a) Reduction in disease activity
b) Complete clinical response or remission
c) Reduction in flare or increase in time to flare
d) Reduction in concomitant steroidal agents
e) Treatment of serious acute manifestations

With regards to endpoint a, reduction in disease activity, the document specifically states that the "BILAG is the preferred index to study reduction in disease activity in clinical trials." This rather strong endorsement was somewhat unexpected, in that the major strength of the BILAG index lies in its organ-specific nature. The guidance document incorrectly states that the BILAG index is scored "based on the need for therapy," which is not how the BILAG index is scored but how it was developed. This section of the guidance document also mixes the discussion of a reduction in global disease activity with that of a reduction in a specific organ-system manifestation. The discussion also introduces the concepts of major clinical response (MCR) and partial clinical response (PCR), novel concepts that have not yet been tested in any trial and for which no good precedent exists. (The MCR proposed by the FDA for RA clinical trials has had limited usefulness). The discussion on outcome b, a complete clinical response or remission, makes it clear that this outcome would, in practicality, amount to the same outcomes as under a but with a higher threshold for response—in all probability requiring unrealistically large numbers of patients. That being said, these sections leave the reader slightly unsure of what exactly is proposed, and the most useful single advice given is to discuss trial outcomes with the regulator before embarking on one.

In contrast, sections c and d make it clear that flare prevention and corticosteroid reduction can be legitimate primary outcomes for SLE clinical trials, which is gratifying in that these are also clinically important and intuitive features of therapeutic efficacy. Needless to say, these outcomes can only be considered if disease activity is controlled as well. Treatment of acute serious manifestations (section e) is also discussed as a possible primary objective for a trial, but it is acknowledged that this would be a challenging situation in which to perform a registration trial.

Importantly, the FDA guidance document clearly indicates that patient-reported outcomes cannot yet be used as primary outcomes, although they are important and should be included as secondary outcomes in all trials, and neither can biomarkers substitute for clinical outcomes as yet.

Recently, the European Medicines Agency (EMA) announced that a guidance document for SLE clinical trials is being prepared. Thus both large agencies have taken steps to streamline the regulatory pathway for drugs of potential use in SLE; in addition, a climate of openness in reviewing these issues currently exists, raising optimism for the future.

In summary, academic investigators, research leaders in industry, and large regulatory organizations have worked hard to create better frameworks for investigating drugs of potential use in the treatment of SLE. Hopefully, the ongoing interaction among academic investigators, regulators, and industry will lead to further advances in the therapeutic agents of SLE.

References

1. Barr SG, Zonana-Nacach A, Magder LS, et al: Patterns of disease activity in systemic lupus erythematosus. *Arthritis Rheum* 42:2682–2688, 1999.
2. Urowitz MB, Feletar M, Bruce IN, et al: Prolonged remission in systemic lupus erythematosus. *J Rheumatol* 32:1467–1472, 2005.
3. Nikpour M, Urowitz MB, Ibañez D, et al: Frequency and determinants of flare and persistently active disease in systemic lupus erythematosus. *Arthritis Rheum* 61:1152–1158, 2009.
4. Kuriya B, Gladman DD, Ibanez D, et al: Quality of life over time in patients with systemic lupus erythematosus. *Arthritis Rheum* 59:181–185, 2008.
5. Petri MA, Mease PJ, Merrill JT, et al: Effects of prasterone on disease activity and symptoms in women with active systemic lupus erythematosus. *Arthritis Rheum* 50:2858–2868, 2004.
6. Wallace DJ, Tumlin JA: LJP 394 (abetimus sodium, Riquent) in the management of systemic lupus erythematosus. *Lupus* 13:323–327, 2004.
7. Cardiel MH, Tumlin JA, Furie RA, et al: Abetimus sodium for renal flare in systemic lupus erythematosus: results of a randomized, controlled phase III trial. *Arthritis Rheum* 58:2470–2480, 2008.
8. Navarra SV, Guzman RM, Gallacher AE, et al: Efficacy and safety of belimumab in patients with active systemic lupus erythematosus: a randomised, placebo-controlled, phase 3 trial. *Lancet* 377:721–731, 2011.

9. Straub RH: Concepts of evolutionary medicine and energy regulation contribute to the etiology of systemic chronic inflammatory diseases. *Brain Behav Immun* 25:1–5, 2011.

10. Akkasilpa S, Minor M, Goldman D, et al: Association of coping responses with fibromyalgia tender points in patients with systemic lupus erythematosus. *J Rheumatol* 27:671–674, 2000.

11. Akkasilpa S, Goldman D, Magder LS, et al: Number of fibromyalgia tender points is associated with health status in patients with systemic lupus erythematosus. *J Rheumatol* 32:48–50, 2005.

12. Kiani AN, Petri M: Quality-of-life measurements versus disease activity in systemic lupus erythematosus. *Curr Rheumatol Rep* 12:250–258, 2010.

13. Albrecht J, Taylor L, Berlin JA, et al: The CLASI (Cutaneous Lupus Erythematosus Disease Area and Severity Index): an outcome instrument for cutaneous lupus erythematosus. *J Invest Dermatol* 125:889–894, 2005.

14. Felson DT, Anderson JJ, Boers M, et al: American College of Rheumatology. Preliminary definition of improvement in rheumatoid arthritis. *Arthritis Rheum* 38:727–735, 1995.

15. van der Heijde DM, van 't Hof M, van Riel PL, et al: Development of a disease activity score based on judgment in clinical practice by rheumatologists. *J Rheumatol* 20:579–581, 1993.

16. Felson DT, Anderson JJ, Boers M, et al: The American College of Rheumatology preliminary core set of disease activity measures for rheumatoid arthritis clinical trials. The Committee on Outcome Measures in Rheumatoid Arthritis Clinical Trials. *Arthritis Rheum* 36:729–740, 1993.

17. van Gestel AM, Prevoo ML, van 't Hof MA, et al: Development and validation of the European League Against Rheumatism response criteria for rheumatoid arthritis. Comparison with the preliminary American College of Rheumatology and the World Health Organization/International League Against Rheumatism Criteria. *Arthritis Rheum* 39:34–40, 1996.

18. Prevoo ML, van 't Hof MA, Kuper HH, et al: Modified disease activity scores that include twenty-eight-joint counts. Development and validation in a prospective longitudinal study of patients with rheumatoid arthritis. *Arthritis Rheum* 38:44–48, 1995.

19. Smolen JS, Breedveld FC, Schiff MH, et al: A simplified disease activity index for rheumatoid arthritis for use in clinical practice. *Rheumatology (Oxford)* 42:244–257, 2003.

20. Bombardier C, Gladman DD, Urowitz MB, et al: Derivation of the SLEDAI. A disease activity index for lupus patients. The Committee on Prognosis Studies in SLE. *Arthritis Rheum* 35:630–640, 1992.

21. Petri M, Kim MY, Kalunian KC, et al: Combined oral contraceptives in women with systemic lupus erythematosus. *N Engl J Med* 353:2550–2558, 2005.

22. Gladman DD, Ibañez D, Urowitz MB: Systemic lupus erythematosus disease activity index 2000. *J Rheumatol* 29:288–291, 2002.

23. Hay EM, Bacon PA, Gordon C, et al: The BILAG index: a reliable and valid instrument for measuring clinical disease activity in systemic lupus erythematosus. *Q J Med* 86:447–458, 1993.

24. Liang MH, Socher SA, Larson MG, et al: Reliability and validity of six systems for the clinical assessment of disease activity in systemic lupus erythematosus. *Arthritis Rheum* 32:1107–1118, 1989.

25. Bencivelli W, Vitali C, Isenberg DA, et al: Disease activity in systemic lupus erythematosus: report of the Consensus Study Group of the European Workshop for Rheumatology Research. III. Development of a computerised clinical chart and its application to the comparison of different indices of disease activity. The European Consensus Study Group for Disease Activity in SLE. *Clin Exp Rheumatol* 10:549–554, 1992.

26. Petri M, Hellmann D, Hochberg M: Validity and reliability of lupus activity measures in the routine clinic setting. *J Rheumatol* 19:53–59, 1992.

Chapter 55

Socioeconomic and Disability Aspects

Michael M. Ward

Like many other chronic illnesses, systemic lupus erythematosus (SLE) can have a major impact on physical and social functioning and work ability.[1] The costs of care and the economic consequences of illness can be substantial. Fatigue, pain, cardiopulmonary symptoms, cognitive impairment, and neurologic deficits can cause difficulty performing activities of daily living and work tasks.[2] These symptoms and signs, along with the psychological adjustment to illness, can affect how patients manage activities and function at home, school, and work. This chapter examines the impact of SLE on physical and social functioning, schooling, family life, and work ability, as well as the costs of SLE.

Two considerations are important in the evaluation of studies of these outcomes in patients with SLE. First, the source of the patient sample should be considered. Most studies have been performed on samples of patients treated at specialty centers, often ones focused on the treatment of SLE. These samples are convenient but are not representative of all patients with SLE and include higher proportions of patients with more severe illness.[3] Findings are therefore skewed to a more pessimistic appraisal of functioning than is truly the case. To obtain a true assessment of functional status and of the social and economic consequences of SLE, population-based samples should be studied. Population-based studies use all patients in a given locality as the sample, thereby avoiding biases due to selective referral and ensuring that the study includes, in correct proportions, patients across the entire range of severity of illness. Population-based studies are difficult to perform but are valuable sources of information. Community-based studies, which enroll participants from multiple different sources and are not exclusively from clinics, are likely more representative than clinic-based samples. Second, mean results should not be generalized to all patients. All measures have a distribution, and the distribution of results among patients with SLE often overlaps that of healthy individuals. Many patients with SLE have normal functioning and work ability, and impairment should not be viewed as expected or inevitable.

PHYSICAL AND MENTAL FUNCTIONING

Physical functioning refers to an individual's ability to perform basic activities of daily living, such as dressing, bathing, and moving about, and instrumental activities of daily living, such as housework, shopping, and preparing meals. Function is most often measured using patient-reported questionnaires, based on the belief that patients are the most accurate observers of their own abilities. Commonly used measures of physical function, such as the Health Assessment Questionnaire (HAQ) Disability Index and the Medical Outcomes Study short form 36 (SF-36) physical function subscale, include both basic and instrumental activities and integrate them into a single score.[4,5] The physical function subscale of the SF-36 also contributes to the "Physical Component Summary," along with ratings of pain (a symptom rather than a rating of function), general health, and limitations in performing a societal role (e.g., work, housework, schoolwork) as a result of physical health problems. Mental functioning refers to an individual's ability to enjoy life and participate in social interactions. The mental component summary (MCS) of the SF-36 includes ratings of mood, social functioning, fatigue (a symptom),

and limitations in performing an individual's societal role because of psychological concerns.[5] Although the concept of health-related quality of life includes functioning, it also includes symptoms, perceptions, and satisfaction with health.[1]

Physical Functioning

Functional limitations among patients with SLE as measured by the HAQ have generally been reported as mild.[6] In eight cross-sectional studies, all of the patients at referral centers and with samples ranging from 82 to 202 patients, the mean HAQ score ranged from 0.36 to 1.3 (median 0.64) on a 0 to 3 scale, with higher scores indicating greater impairment.[7-14] The variability in scores among patients was high in all studies. Twenty-five percent of patients had an HAQ score of 0.[7,10] The most problematic task was performing errands and chores.[8] Scores were higher among older patients, possibly as a result of co-morbid conditions, and among obese patients.[11,12,15] Scores were also higher among patients with active SLE or permanent organ damage and were correlated with self-reported pain.[7-10,12] Higher scores have also been reported among those with fibromyalgia, depression, and life stresses, indicating associations between mental functioning and perceptions of physical impairments.[9,11,13,16] Studies have not generally reported associations between HAQ scores and the duration of SLE, suggesting that functional limitations are often not progressive.[17]

The SF-36 has been used much more extensively than the HAQ to measure physical functioning in SLE, because functional limitations have been more commonly detected using this measure. Many studies include relatively small samples from single-referral centers, but four studies are notable for their large size. The Tri-Nation study included 708 unselected patients (mean age, 40 years; mean duration of SLE, 10 years) from six referral centers, two each in Canada, the United Kingdom, and the United States.[18] The LUMINA (LUpus in MInorities, NAture versus nurture) study reported data on 346 patients at four referral centers in the United States who enrolled within 5 years of the onset of SLE.[19] Tam and colleagues[20] studied 291 unselected patients (mean age, 42 years; mean duration of SLE, 9.7 years) at a single tertiary center in Hong Kong. Wolfe and colleagues[21] surveyed 1316 patients (mean age, 50 years) in a U.S. nationwide observational study. Results of these studies are generally consistent (Figure 55-1). Mean results for all four physical component subscales—physical functioning, role-physical, bodily pain, and general health—were significantly lower than those of population controls, but values for the physical functioning, role-physical, and bodily pain scales were within 1 standard deviation of the scores in the general population. Scores were lowest on the role-physical subscale, which measures limitations in work or housework as a result of physical problems, and the general health subscale. These scores diverged most from those of the general population, indicating that these subscales are most affected by SLE. The physical component summary (PCS) scores ranged from 37 to 43. These values were slightly more than 1 standard deviation lower than the standardized population score of 50, indicating that SLE has a notable impact on physical health for the typical patient.

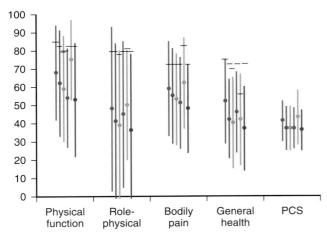

FIGURE 55-1 Scores on the physical health short form 36 (SF-36) subscales and the physical component summary (PCS) by study. Values are means; error bars are standard deviations. Short horizontal bars represent control sample or country-specific population means. Population mean of the PCS is 50 for all studies. Tri-Nation Canada, red; Tri-Nation United States, blue; Tri-Nation United Kingdom, yellow[18]; LUMINA, green[19]; Tam and associates, gray[20]; Wolfe and associates, purple.[21]

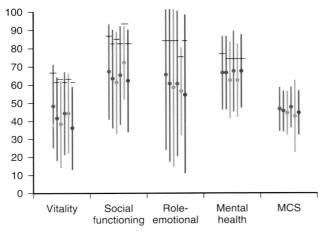

FIGURE 55-2 Scores on the mental health short form 36 (SF-36) subscales and the mental component summary (MCS) by study. Values are means; error bars are standard deviations. Short horizontal bars represent control sample or country-specific population means. Population mean of the MCS is 50 for all studies. Tri-Nation Canada, red; Tri-Nation United States, blue; Tri-Nation United Kingdom, yellow[18]; LUMINA, green[19]; Tam and associates, gray[20]; Wolfe and associates, purple.[21]

Advancing age, lower socioeconomic status, more permanent organ damage, and more co-morbid medical conditions were associated with poorer physical health.[20,21] In the LUMINA study, the presence of fibromyalgia was the most important correlate of the PCS score.[19] Lower self-efficacy, less knowledge about SLE, and less social support have also been associated with poorer physical health as measured by the SF-36.[22]

SF-36 physical function scores have been found to be generally stable over periods up to 8 years in patients with SLE.[19,23-25] Worsening over time was more likely in older patients,[19,23,25] those with fibromyalgia,[19,24] Caucasians,[24] and patients with a recent flare in symptoms.[25]

Mental Functioning

Findings on mental functioning as measured by the SF-36 are remarkably consistent among these four large studies (Figure 55-2).[18-21] Although scores were uniformly lowest on the vitality

(fatigue) subscale, scores on the vitality, social functioning, and role-emotional subscales were equally divergent from those of the general population. The MCS scores ranged from 42 to 47, only slightly lower than the standardized population score of 50. These findings indicate that patients with SLE have less severe impairments in mental functioning relative to the general population than they do in physical functioning. However, one third of patients report being unable to participate in at least one valued life activity, primarily discretionary leisure and social activities.[26]

Lower socioeconomic status, less social support, and the presence of fibromyalgia have been associated with poorer mental functioning,[19,22] as have younger age and more co-morbidities.[21] In longitudinal studies, mental functioning has generally been found to be stable over time.[19,23-25] Predictors of change in mental functioning have been more difficult to identify than predictors of change in physical functioning, but patients of lower socioeconomic status or African-American ethnicity and those with fibromyalgia may be more likely to experience worsening.[19]

Interventions

Educational and cognitive-behavioral interventions have been tested as ways (other than medications) to improve functioning in patients with SLE. In a small short-term trial, patients receiving the Systemic Lupus Erythematosus Self-Help (SLESH) course, an educational intervention modeled after the Arthritis Self-Management Program, had modest improvements in depression and self-efficacy.[27] A 6-month telephone counseling intervention focused on enhancing self-care improved physical function but not pain, fatigue, or affect.[28] A stress management and cognitive restructuring intervention improved physical function but not mental functioning over 15 months in a small trial.[29] In the largest study, an intervention designed to increase self-efficacy and social support improved fatigue and the MCS score of the SF-36 over 12 months, but not physical function.[30] These results support the use of these interventions, but adoption has been limited because of the need for trained counselors.

SCHOOLING AND FAMILY LIFE

SLE most often begins at ages when most people have completed their formal education. However, when SLE begins in childhood or adolescence, patients may experience major effects on schooling. In a cross-sectional study at two referral centers of 41 patients with SLE, ages 9 to 18 years, patients missed a median of 1 day of school per month, either for medical appointments or because of illness.[31] Although some were satisfied with their school performance, two thirds reported difficulty concentrating, remembering, or keeping up with assignments. In studies using the Pediatric Quality of Life Inventory (PedsQL) measures, school was the domain most affected among children with SLE, with scores much lower than in healthy children.[31,32] The school domain asks about problems paying attention, remembering, and keeping up with work, as well as the number of days of school that were missed. Cognitive impairment and mood disorders can interfere with school performance, but the limited data available suggest that SLE does not generally limit educational attainment.[33-35]

The proportion of women with SLE who are married is similar to that in the general population, and most report that SLE had no effect on the relationship with their partner.[35-37] However, concerns about the future course of illness and medication use may affect decisions regarding childbearing.[38] Although women with SLE are as likely as women without SLE to have children, women with SLE are less likely to have several children, suggesting that decisions to limit family size are not uncommon.[38,39]

EMPLOYMENT AND WORK DISABILITY

One of the central roles of adulthood is that of worker. Work provides not only income to purchase material goods, support leisure interests, and generate assets for late life and retirement but also social standing, self-esteem, and opportunities for social interaction. Three

TABLE 55-1 Prevalence of Work Disability in Patients with Systemic Lupus Erythematosus

STUDY	COUNTRY	SAMPLE	NUMBER OF PATIENTS	MEAN AGE (IN YEARS)	MEAN DURATION OF SLE (IN YEARS)	WORK DISABILITY
Partridge, 1997[52]	United States	Referral centers	152	32	3.4	40%
Murphy, 1998[42]	United States	Referral center	46	36	7.4	63%
Sutcliffe, 1999[53]	United Kingdom	Referral center	184	39	9	30%
Boomsma, 2002[37]	Netherlands	Referral center	114	44	13	23%
Bertoli, 2007[54]	United States	Referral centers	273	35	5	19%
Panopolis, 2007[55]	United States	Referral center and community	741	46	13	35%
Mok, 2008[56]	China	Referral center	105	38	10	37%
Utset, 2008[57]	United States	Referral center	143	40	9.2	47%
Al Dhanhani, 2009[58]	Canada	Referral center	210	36	5	27%

SLE, Systemic lupus erythematosus.

work-related outcomes are often examined in patients with chronic illnesses: (1) employment, (2) work disability, and (3) receipt of disability pensions. Employment is the most general and merely considers whether or not the patient is working for pay. Because many factors other than illness influence employment, such as the local job market or the desire for more schooling, and because employment is discretionary for some people, it is less specifically related to disease status than work disability. Work disability refers to the patient-reported inability to work as a result of illness. Estimates of work disability are most appropriately limited to those who were working before the onset of illness. Receipt of disability pensions represents work disability that is certified and compensated by governmental agencies or insurers. Although receipt of disability pensions often signifies a permanent inability to work, this measure underestimates the frequency of work disability, because many patients with SLE who are work disabled do not apply for or are denied disability certification.[40-42] Patient-reported work disability is the work-related outcome that can most directly reflect the impact of medical treatment, because it is ascribed to illness, does not consider those who are electively out of the workforce, and is not influenced by selection factors as are disability pensions.

Employment

In cross-sectional studies of adults with a wide range of durations of SLE and mostly of patients treated at specialty rheumatology clinics, 41% to 55% of patients with SLE were employed.[43-47] In the 1990s, patients with SLE in Germany were only 80% as likely to be employed as those in the general population.[48] Earlier community-based studies reported no relative decrease in employment among patients with SLE.[35,49] In an inception cohort in the United States, 26% of patients stopped working after 3 years of illness, a rate three times higher than that of controls, highlighting the impact of new and perhaps uncontrolled disease on work status.[50] In another large U.S. cohort, employment at 5, 10, and 15 years of SLE duration was estimated at 85%, 64%, and 49%, respectively.[51] Among employed patients with an average duration of SLE of 11 years, the risk of subsequent unemployment was similar to that in matched population controls, suggesting that the time of greatest risk of unemployment is early in the course of SLE. However, patients with SLE who are unemployed are 50% less likely than matched controls to regain employment.[51]

Unemployment is more common among older patients and those with longer durations of SLE and lower educational attainment.[43-46,48,51] Clinical predictors are less clear, because most studies of risk factors have been cross-sectional. Clinical manifestations present at the time of the study may be different from those before the work loss, which may have occurred many years earlier. In two prospective studies, the risk of unemployment was strongly associated with both depression and cognitive impairment.[46,51]

Work Disability

Work disability most often refers to a permanent inability to work, but it can also include a temporary inability to work, sick leave, or reduced work hours. The prevalence of work disability, in samples largely from referral centers, has ranged from 19% to 63%, with most results between 30% and 40% (Table 55-1).[37,42,52-58] These prevalences are quite high, considering that most studies reported on patient groups that are primarily made up of young adults in the first decade of SLE. The prevalence of work disability in the first year of diagnosis was 7% to 9%.[56,58]

In prospective studies, advanced age, longer duration of SLE, lower educational attainment, high SLE activity, and higher scores on the SLE Damage Index have been consistent predictors of future work disability.[52,54,55,58] Of specific clinical features, neuropsychological manifestations, particularly memory deficits and depression, and fibromyalgia and arthritis have each been predictive of a higher likelihood of work disability.[55,58] Although neuropsychological manifestations can be managed, no studies of interventions have been conducted that target cognitive impairment or depression in patients with SLE with the goal of reducing the risk of work disability.[59] The contribution of job characteristics to work loss in patients with SLE has received less attention, although those with more physically demanding jobs are at a greater risk of work loss than those with sedentary jobs.[35,44,52]

Temporary work disability, prolonged sick leave, or a reduction in work hours is also common in patients with SLE. In two U.S. studies, 27% of patients with early SLE had sick leaves of at least 2 months,[50,52] and patients worked on average 5 hours per week less than they had before diagnosis.[44]

COSTS OF ILLNESS

Costs of illness represent the expenses incurred as a consequence of the presence of a disease. Most often, the expenses that are tabulated are those incurred by society, rather than out-of-pocket payments by patients, to achieve a global estimate of costs. These costs can then be compared among patients with different diseases to aid in health planning. Costs can also be compared among patients with the same disease to identify subgroups with high costs, so that the factors contributing to high costs can be learned and interventions might be developed to help reduce costs. Mean costs are often substantially higher than median costs, reflecting the influence of small numbers of patients with very high costs.

Total costs of illness are the sum of direct costs and indirect costs. Direct costs are those related to the provision of care and include the costs of hospitalizations, outpatient visits, medications, diagnostic and laboratory tests, therapy, durable medical equipment, and travel to appointments. Most cost-of-illness studies use a bottom-up approach, in which a broad spectrum of patients is surveyed about their health care. Cost estimates are based on the number of services used (e.g., hospital days, outpatient visits, laboratory tests), to each of which a dollar cost is affixed. This approach standardizes dollar costs so that differences in direct costs among patients represent differences in the sum of medical services used.

In complex multisystem diseases such as SLE, separating costs that are specifically the result of SLE from costs that are the result of co-morbid conditions is difficult, and some co-morbidities, such as osteoporosis or diabetes mellitus, may be complications of SLE treatment. Therefore studies report costs among patients with SLE without attribution to cause. However, even with this approach, costs associated with SLE, per se, can be estimated by comparing the direct costs of an SLE cohort with those of a matched control group without SLE.

Indirect costs are those related to earning potential that is diminished because of illness. For those in the workforce, indirect costs are the wages lost as a result of permanent or temporary work disability. For those not in the workforce, indirect costs represent the costs of household help because of an inability to perform chores or provide child care.

Direct Costs

Nine studies have reported direct cost estimates in patients with SLE, including four studies published within the past 2 years[18,60-67] (Table 55-2). Most studies examined convenience samples of patients treated at tertiary care centers and therefore may disproportionately include patients with more severe SLE. Notable exceptions are the study of Huscher and colleagues,[62] which included data from 24 rheumatology centers across Germany, and the studies of Pelletier and associates[65] and Carls and others,[66] which were based on searches of large insurance databases in the United States for claims of patients with SLE.

Direct cost estimates, expressed in 2008 U.S. dollars, varied widely among studies (see Table 55-2).[68] More recent studies reported high direct costs, as did those studies performed in the United States, possibly as a result of higher price structures in the United States. In most studies, hospitalization costs accounted for the largest proportion of direct costs (one third to one half), with outpatient visits and medications the next most costly categories, each accounting for approximately 10% to 25% of the direct costs.

Direct costs are higher in patients with more severe SLE, whether reflected by the presence of nephritis or neuropsychological manifestations,[60,64-67] functional limitations,[60,62,63] SLE activity,[61-64,69] or permanent organ damage.[61,64,69] Using insurance claims data, Pelletier and colleagues[65] estimated that the direct costs of patients with nephritis were 89% higher than those patients without nephritis, whereas Carls and associates[66] estimated costs to be four times higher in those with nephritis. Patients with end-stage renal disease treated with dialysis or transplantation represent the subgroup of patients with SLE with the highest costs; however, even excluding these patients, the costs of patients with lupus nephritis were 30% higher than those without nephritis.[70] Clearly, the interventions most likely to reduce the direct costs of SLE are those that would prevent or most effectively treat lupus nephritis.

Little consistency exists among studies of predictors of direct costs other than clinical severity. In studies of adults, young age[61,63,64] and a high level of education[61] have been associated with high costs in some studies but not in others.[62-65] Long duration of SLE has been associated with blow[62,64] and high costs.[63] Direct costs of pediatric SLE in the United States have been estimated to be comparable to those of adult SLE.[71]

The direct costs of patients with SLE in the United States were 2.7 times higher than those of matched controls without SLE.[66] The largest differential was due to differences in the frequency of inpatient care, for which costs were over four times higher in patients with SLE. International comparisons suggest that American patients incur higher costs than patients in Canada and the United Kingdom but have similar health status.[18]

Indirect Costs

Indirect costs represent a substantial expense for those with SLE. Indirect costs have been reported to range from 0.62 of direct costs (e.g., 38% lower) to 3.5 times more than direct costs.[60,61-64,72] Stated in another way, indirect costs make up 38% to 78% of the total costs, with total costs ranging from $10,976 to $24,279 per year (in 2008 U.S. dollars).[68] Part of the variability in estimates relates to the differences in the age composition of the samples, the proportion of women employed outside of the home, the estimates used for lost wages, and whether studies included the costs for help with household chores.[72,73] In some studies, indirect costs were higher in men,[60,64] patients of advanced years,[63] and those with functional limitations.[61-63,72] In addition, poorer psychological functioning predicts work loss and higher indirect costs.[60,63] Interventions to improve factors such as mood, job-related stress, and work-life balance may help some patients remain employed and reduce the indirect costs of SLE.

TABLE 55-2 Direct Medical Costs of Patients with Systemic Lupus Erythematosus

STUDY	COUNTRY	NUMBER OF PATIENTS	MEAN ANNUAL COSTS (2008 U.S. DOLLARS)[†]	Components of Direct Costs (as % of Total)*			
				INPATIENT (%)	OUTPATIENT VISITS (%)	MEDICATIONS (%)	LABORATORY AND DIAGNOSTIC TESTS (%)
Clarke, 1993[60]	Canada	164	7244	56	12	11	14
Clarke, 1999[17]	Canada	229	5062	39	17	18	11
	United Kingdom	211	4965	39	16	25	10
	United States	268	5512	26	18	25	14
Sutcliffe, 2001[61]	United Kingdom	105	4852	38	27	17	15
Huscher, 2006[62]	Germany	844	4103	47	7	27	1 (imaging only)
Panopalis, 2008[63]	United States	812	14,410	49	13	26	Not reported
Zhu, 2009[64]	China	306	6788	52	10	4	16
Pelletier, 2009[65]	United States	15,590	13,305	23	7	25	11
Carls, 2009[66]	United States	6269	13,491	41	43	13	Not reported
Aghdassi, 2011[67]	Canada	141	11,711	10	14	36	16

*Proportions total to less than 100% because of several categories contributing smaller costs (e.g., emergency department visits, out-of-pocket expenses, equipment, transportation, rehabilitation stay) were excluded.
[†]After Zhu.[68]

SUMMARY

- The most important health status problems in persons with SLE are fatigue and limitations in performing work, home, or school roles as a result of physical health.
- Functional limitations are often not progressive over long periods.
- Work disability occurs in 30% to 40% of patients, often early in the course of SLE.
- Direct medical costs of SLE, reflecting the amount of care received, are closely associated with the severity of illness and are particularly high for those with nephritis.

ACKNOWLEDGMENTS

This work was supported by the Intramural Research Program, National Institute of Arthritis and Musculoskeletal and Skin Diseases, National Institutes of Health.

References

1. Yazdany J, Yelin E: Health-related quality of life and employment among persons with systemic lupus erythematosus. *Rheum Dis Clin N Am* 36:15–32, 2010.
2. Robinson D, Jr, Aguilar D, Schoenwetter M, et al: Impact of systemic lupus erythematosus on health, family, and work: the patient perspective. *Arthritis Care Res (Hoboken)* 62:266–273, 2010.
3. Ward MM: Severity of illness in patients with systemic lupus erythematosus hospitalized at academic medical centers. *J Rheumatol* 32:27–33, 2005.
4. Fries JF, Spitz P, Kraines RG, et al: Measurement of patient outcome in arthritis. *Arthritis Rheum* 23:137–145, 1980.
5. Ware JE, Jr, Sherbourne CD: The MOS 36-item short-form health survey (SF-36). I. Conceptual framework and item selection. *Med Care* 30:473–483, 1992.
6. Zink A, Fischer-Betz R, Thiele K, et al: Health care and burden of illness in systemic lupus erythematosus compared to rheumatoid arthritis: results from the National Database of the German Collaborative Arthritis Centres. *Lupus* 13:529–536, 2004.
7. Hochberg MC, Sutton JD: Physical disability and psychosocial dysfunction in systemic lupus erythematosus. *J Rheumatol* 15:959–964, 1988.
8. Milligan SE, Hom DL, Ballou SP, et al: An assessment of the Health Assessment Questionnaire functional ability index among women with systemic lupus erythematosus. *J Rheumatol* 20:972–976, 1993.
9. Gladman DD, Urowitz MB, Ong A, et al: A comparison of five health status instruments in patients with systemic lupus erythematosus (SLE). *Lupus* 5:190–195, 1996.
10. Fortin PR, Abrahamowicz M, Neville C, et al: Impact of disease activity and cumulative damage on the health of lupus patients. *Lupus* 7:101–107, 1998.
11. Ward MM, Lotstein DS, Bush TM, et al: Psychosocial correlates of morbidity in women with systemic lupus erythematosus. *J Rheumatol* 26:2153–2158, 1999.
12. Gilboe IM, Kvien TK, Husby G: Health status in systemic lupus erythematosus compared to rheumatoid arthritis and healthy controls. *J Rheumatol* 26:1694–1700, 1999.
13. Akkasilpa S, Goldman D, Magder LS, et al: Number of fibromyalgia tender points is associated with health status in patients with systemic lupus erythematosus. *J Rheumatol* 32:48–50, 2005.
14. Colangelo KJ, Pope JE, Peschken C: The minimally important difference for patient reported outcomes in systemic lupus erythematosus including the HAQ-DI, pain, fatigue, and SF-36. *J Rheumatol* 36:2231–2237, 2009.
15. Oeser A, Chung CP, Asanuma Y, et al: Obesity is an independent contributor to functional capacity and inflammation in systemic lupus erythematosus. *Arthritis Rheum* 52:3651–3659, 2005.
16. Da Costa D, Dobkin PL, Pinard L, et al: The role of stress in functional disability among women with systemic lupus erythematosus: a prospective study. *Arthritis Care Res* 12:112–119, 1999.
17. Gilboe IM, Kvien TK, Husby G: Disease course in systemic lupus erythematosus: changes in health status, disease activity, and organ damage after 2 years. *J Rheumatol* 28:266–274, 2001.
18. Clarke AE, Petri MA, Manzi S, et al: An international perspective on the well being and health care costs for patients with systemic lupus erythematosus. *J Rheumatol* 26:1500–1511, 1999.
19. Alarcón GS, McGwin G, Jr, Uribe A, et al: Systemic lupus erythematosus in a multiethnic lupus cohort (LUMINA). XVII. Predictors of self-reported health-related quality of life early in the disease course. *Arthritis Rheum* 51:465–474, 2004.
20. Tam LS, Wong A, Mok VCT, et al: The relationship between neuropsychiatric, clinical, and laboratory variables and quality of life of Chinese patients with systemic lupus erythematosus. *J Rheumatol* 35:1038–1045, 2008.
21. Wolfe F, Michaud K, Li T, et al: EQ-5D and SF-36 quality of life measures in systemic lupus erythematosus: comparisons with rheumatoid arthritis, noninflammatory rheumatic disorders, and fibromyalgia. *J Rheumatol* 37:296–304, 2010.
22. Karlson EW, Daltroy LH, Lew RA, et al: The relationship of socioeconomic status, race, and modifiable risk factors to outcomes in patients with systemic lupus erythematosus. *Arthritis Rheum* 40:47–56, 1997.
23. Panopalis P, Petri M, Manzi S, et al: The systemic lupus erythematosus tri-nation study: longitudinal changes in physical and mental well-being. *Rheumatology (Oxford)* 44:751–755, 2005.
24. Kuriya B, Gladman DD, Ibañez D, et al: Quality of life over time in patients with systemic lupus erythematosus. *Arthritis Rheum* 59:181–185, 2008.
25. Tamayo T, Fischer-Betz R, Beer S, et al: Factors influencing the health related quality of life in patients with systemic lupus erythematosus: long-term results (2001-2005) of patients in the German Lupus Erythematosus Self-Help Organization (LULA Study). *Lupus* 19:1606–1613, 2010.
26. Katz P, Morris A, Trupin L, et al: Disability in valued life activities among individuals with systemic lupus erythematosus. *Arthritis Rheum* 59:465–473, 2008.
27. Braden CJ, McGlone K, Pennington F: Specific psychosocial and behavioral outcomes from the systemic lupus erythematosus self-help course. *Health Educ Q* 20:29–41, 1993.
28. Austin JS, Maisiak RS, Macrina DM, et al: Health outcome improvements in patients with systemic lupus erythematosus using two telephone counseling interventions. *Arthritis Care Res* 9:391–399, 1996.
29. Navarette-Navarrete N, Peralta-Ramirez MI, Sabio JM, et al: Quality-of-life predictor factors in patients with SLE and their modification after cognitive behavioural therapy. *Lupus* 19:1632–1639, 2010.
30. Karlson EW, Liang MH, Eaton H, et al: A randomized clinical trial of a psychoeducational intervention to improve outcomes in systemic lupus erythematosus. *Arthritis Rheum* 50:1832–1841, 2004.
31. Moorthy LN, Peterson MGE, Hassett A, et al: Impact of lupus on school attendance and performance. *Lupus* 19:620–627, 2010.
32. Brunner HI, Higgins GC, Wiers K, et al: Health-related quality of life and its relationship to patient disease course in childhood-onset systemic lupus erythematosus. *J Rheumatol* 36:1536–1545, 2009.
33. Wyckoff PM, Miller LC, Tucker LB, et al: Neuropsychological assessment of children and adolescents with systemic lupus erythematosus. *Lupus* 4:217–220, 1995.
34. Sibbitt WL, Jr, Brandt JR, Johnson CR, et al: The incidence and prevalence of neuropsychiatric syndromes in pediatric onset systemic lupus erythematosus. *J Rheumatol* 29:1536–1542, 2002.
35. Stein H, Walters K, Dillon A, et al: Systemic lupus erythematosus—a medical and social profile. *J Rheumatol* 13:570–576, 1986.
36. Vinet E, Clarke AE, Gordon C, et al: Decreased live births in women with systemic lupus erythematosus. *Arthritis Care Res (Hoboken)* 63:1068–1072, 2011.
37. Boomsma MM, Bijl M, Stegeman CA, et al: Patients' perceptions of the effects of systemic lupus erythematosus on health, function, income, and interpersonal relationships: a comparison with Wegener's granulomatosis. *Arthritis Rheum* 47:196–201, 2002.
38. Vinet E, Pineau CA, Gordon C, et al: Systemic lupus erythematosus in women: impact on family size. *Arthritis Rheum* 59:1656–1660, 2008.
39. Hardy CJ, Palmer BP, Morton SJ, et al: Pregnancy outcome and family size in systemic lupus erythematosus: a case-control study. *Rheumatology (Oxford)* 38:559–563, 1999.
40. Liang MH, Daltroy LH, Larson MG, et al: Evaluation of Social Security disability in claimants with rheumatic disease. *Ann Intern Med* 115:26–31, 1991.
41. Scofield L, Reinlib L, Alarcón GS, et al: Employment and disability issues in systemic lupus erythematosus: a review. *Arthritis Rheum* 59:1475–1479, 2008.
42. Murphy NG, Koolvisoot A, Schumacher HR, Jr, et al: Musculoskeletal features in systemic lupus erythematosus and their relationship with disability. *J Clin Rheumatol* 4:238–245, 1998.
43. Baker K, Pope J, Fortin P, et al: 1000 Faces of Lupus Investigators: CaNIOS (Canadian Network for Improved Outcomes in SLE): Work disability in systemic lupus erythematosus is prevalent and associated with sociodemographic and disease related factors. *Lupus* 18:1281–1288, 2009.
44. Yelin E, Trupin L, Katz P, et al: Work dynamics among persons with systemic lupus erythematosus. *Arthritis Rheum* 57:56–63, 2007.

45. Bultink IEM, Turkstra F, Bijkmans BAC, et al: High prevalence of unemployment in patients with systemic lupus erythematosus: association with organ damage and health-related quality of life. *J Rheumatol* 35:1053–1057, 2008.

46. Appenzeller S, Cendes F, Costallat LT: Cognitive impairment and employment status in systemic lupus erythematosus: a prospective longitudinal study. *Arthritis Rheum* 61:680–687, 2009.

47. Almehed K, Carlsten H, Forsblad-d'Elia H: Health-related quality of life in systemic lupus erythematosus and its association with disease and work disability. *Scand J Rheumatol* 39:58–62, 2010.

48. Mau W, Listing J, Huscher D, et al: Employment across chronic inflammatory rheumatic diseases and comparison with the general population. *J Rheumatol* 32:721–728, 2005.

49. Jonsson H, Nived O, Sturfelt G: Outcome in systemic lupus erythematosus: a prospective study of patients from a defined population. *Medicine (Baltimore)* 68:141–150, 1989.

50. Campbell R, Jr, Cooper GS, Gilkeson GS: The impact of systemic lupus erythematosus on employment. *J Rheumatol* 36:2470–2475, 2009.

51. Yelin E, Tonner C, Trupin L, et al: Work loss and work entry among persons with systemic lupus erythematosus: comparisons with a national matched sample. *Arthritis Rheum* 61:247–258, 2009.

52. Partridge AJ, Karlson EW, Daltroy LH, et al: Risk factors for early work disability in systemic lupus erythematosus. *Arthritis Rheum* 40:2199–2206, 1997.

53. Sutcliffe N, Clarke AE, Gordon C, et al: The association of socio-economic status, race, psychosocial factors and outcome in patients with systemic lupus erythematosus. *Rheumatology (Oxford)* 38:1130–1137, 1999.

54. Bertoli AM, Fernández M, Alarcón GS, et al: Systemic lupus erythematosus in a multiethnic US cohort LUMINA (XLI): factors predictive of self-reported work disability. *Ann Rheum Dis* 66:12–17, 2007.

55. Panopalis P, Julian L, Yazdany J, et al: Impact of memory impairment on employment status in persons with systemic lupus erythematosus. *Arthritis Rheum* 57:1453–1460, 2007.

56. Mok CC, Cheung MY, Ho LY, et al: Risk and predictors of work disability in Chinese patients with systemic lupus erythematosus. *Lupus* 17:1103–1107, 2008.

57. Utset TO, Chohan S, Booth SA, et al: Correlates of formal work disability in an urban university systemic lupus erythematosus practice. *J Rheumatol* 35:1046–1052, 2008.

58. Al Dhanhani AM, Gignac MA, Su J, et al: Work disability in systemic lupus erythematosus. *Arthritis Rheum* 61:378–385, 2009.

59. Harrison MJ, Morris KA, Horton R, et al: Results of intervention for lupus patients with self-perceived cognitive difficulties. *Neurology* 65:1325–1327, 2005.

60. Clarke AE, Esdaile JM, Bloch DA, et al: A Canadian study of the total medical costs for patients with systemic lupus erythematosus and the predictors of costs. *Arthritis Rheum* 36:1548–1559, 1993.

61. Sutcliffe N, Clarke AE, Taylor R, et al: Total costs and predictors of costs in patients with systemic lupus erythematosus. *Rheumatology (Oxford)* 40:37–47, 2001.

62. Huscher D, Mwerkesdal S, Thiele K, et al: Cost of illness in rheumatoid arthritis, ankylosing spondylitis, psoriatic arthritis and systemic lupus erythematosus in Germany. *Ann Rheum Dis* 65:1175–1183, 2006.

63. Panopalis P, Yazdany J, Gillis JZ, et al: Health care costs and costs associated with changes in work productivity among persons with systemic lupus erythematosus. *Arthritis Rheum* 59:1788–1795, 2008.

64. Zhu TY, Tam LS, Lee VW, et al: Systemic lupus erythematosus with neuropsychiatric manifestation incurs high disease costs: a cost-of-illness study in Hong Kong. *Rheumatology (Oxford)* 48:564–568, 2009.

65. Pelletier EM, Ogale S, Yu E, et al: Economic outcomes in patients diagnosed with systemic lupus erythematosus with versus without nephritis: results from an analysis of data from a US claims database. *Clin Ther* 31:2653–2664, 2009.

66. Carls G, Li T, Panopalis P, et al: Direct and indirect costs to employers of patients with systemic lupus erythematosus with and without nephritis. *J Occup Environ Med* 51:66–79, 2009.

67. Aghdassi E, Zhang W, St. Pierre Y, et al: Healthcare cost and loss of productivity in a Canadian population of patients with and without lupus nephritis. *J Rheumatol* 38:658–666, 2011.

68. Zhu TY, Tam LS, Li EK: Cost-of-illness studies in systemic lupus erythematosus: a systematic review. *Arthritis Care Res (Hoboken)* 63:751–760, 2011.

69. Zhu TY, Tam LS, Lee VW, et al: The impact of flare on disease costs of patients with systemic lupus erythematosus. *Arthritis Rheum* 61:1159–1167, 2009.

70. Li T, Carls GS, Panopalis P, et al: Long-term medical costs and resource utilization in systemic lupus erythematosus and lupus nephritis: a five-year analysis of a large Medicaid population. *Arthritis Rheum* 61:755–763, 2009.

71. Brunner HI, Sherrard TM, Klein-Gitelman MS: Cost of treatment of childhood-onset systemic lupus erythematosus. *Arthritis Rheum* 55:184–188, 2006.

72. Panopalis P, Petri M, Manzi S, et al: The systemic lupus erythematosus tri-nation study: cumulative indirect costs. *Arthritis Rheum* 57:64–70, 2007.

73. Clarke AE, Penrod J, St. Pierre Y, et al: Underestimating the value of women: assessing the indirect costs of women with systemic lupus erythematosus. *J Rheumatol* 27:2597–2604, 2000.

Chapter

56

Investigational Agents and Future Therapy for SLE

Georg H. Stummvoll and Josef S. Smolen

When Moriz Kaposi[1] in 1872 dealt with the therapy of systemic lupus erythematosus (SLE) for the first time in the history of medicine, bed rest, ointments, and plant extracts were the only available remedies for a disease whose cause and pathogenesis were unknown. When Philip Hench[2] introduced glucocorticoids into antirheumatic therapy, their efficacy soon became apparent, and they were then successfully used for SLE—until today.[3] However, pathogenetic insights were still not available and even the prototypic autoantibodies had not yet been characterized. In contrast, in more recent times, the view on SLE became enlightened by an understanding of the final autoantibody- and immune complex–mediated events; and, likewise, by the following developments: (1) the detection of a plethora of cytokines, chemokines, and similar mediators, including the possibly important role of type I interferons[4]; (2) the detection of apoptosis and its regulation[5]; (3) the definition of new cell populations that may be importantly involved; (4) the elucidation of a myriad of signal transduction pathways and transcription factors that regulate gene expression[6]; and (5) the description and sequence determination of SLE susceptibility genes.[7]

As the cause of SLE remains enigmatic and the disease is still incurable in many patients and associated with significant mortality,[8] the insights from basic research activities pave the paths to new therapies. Indeed, although no new drugs for SLE have been licensed for many decades, very recently, belimumab, a biologic agent targeting (no surprise) B cells, has been approved for the treatment of refractory mild and moderate SLE. Many other approaches are still theoretical and will need subtle realization, but others are already in experimental and even in early clinical investigation. In this context, it is important to bear in mind that the life-threatening nature of severe SLE may not allow for traditional blinded controlled clinical trials early in the development of a new therapeutic regimen, but that ultimate proof of efficacy must still be achieved by adhering to established guidance for clinical trials.[9]

The most important therapeutic goal in SLE is the inhibition of inflammation in involved organs and/or the destruction of target cells, usually mediated by complement activation via immune complex formation.

TRIALS AND THEIR DESIGN

New or better remedies are needed, particularly for patients whose disease is refractory to currently available therapies or who are dependent on cytotoxic agents or long-term glucocorticoid medication for disease control, as often seen in patients with renal involvement. These populations are not always easy to be studied in controlled clinical trials because of the heterogeneity of clinical and serologic manifestations of SLE, which may partly behave disparately. However, this is commonly an issue of study design and of reliable outcome measures (see discussion in Chapters 46 and 54), and every new drug tested in patients with SLE will have to be viewed in the context of the trial design and the population selected—with all the potential concerns that have been observed in recent clinical trials.[10]

POTENTIAL NEW THERAPEUTIC TARGETS IN SYSTEMIC LUPUS ERYTHEMATOSUS

For some known and widely used drugs, such as leflunomide, methotrexate, or tacrolimus, new therapeutic opportunities may arise in SLE.[11] However, in this chapter, the focus is primarily on therapeutic principles and drugs that have not yet been licensed; clinical trials in patients with SLE as listed in the U.S.-based Clinical Trials database (*clinicaltrials.gov*) at the time of assembling this review are summarized in eTable 56-1.

Figure 56-1 depicts major pathogenetic pathways believed to be operative in SLE and shows the close interaction of the activated innate and adaptive immune systems, as well as the subsequent inflammatory response. These pathways make up a variety of potential therapeutic targets and promising therapies that are discussed in greater detail in the following text. Table 56-2 summarizes the therapies dealt with in this chapter. The sections in this chapter and in Table 56-2 refer to targets depicted in Figure 56-1, which are numbered correspondingly.

Antigen-Presenting Cells, Dendritic Cells, and Toll-Like Receptors

To summarize the ruling hypothesis on SLE pathogenesis: antigen-presenting cells (APCs), in general, and dendritic cells (DCs), in particular, are key players in initiating the autoimmune process. Although the eliciting antigen(s) are unknown, there has recently been a focus on autoantigens derived from apoptotic cells, since defective apoptosis mechanisms with impaired clearance of apoptotic material have been described,[12] up on which nucleosomes become accessible for APCs. Although they normally have suppressive effects on DCs, they can promote cell activation when bound to the

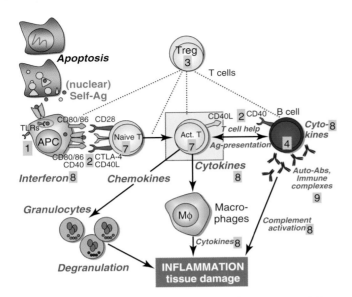

FIGURE 56-1 Overview of major pathogenetic pathways in systemic lupus erythematosus (SLE). The activated innate and adaptive immune systems, as well as the subsequent inflammatory response, offer a variety of potential therapeutic targets and promising therapies. Current strategies aim at interfering with antigen uptake and presentation by dendritic cells (DCs) *(1)* and with the proper co-stimulation *(2)*. Other attempts try to influence function and the numbers of regulatory T (Treg) cells *(3)* or aim to deplete or deactivate B cells *(4)*. Stem cell transplantation *(5, not shown)* tries to eliminate autoreactive lymphocytes and to replace them with newly generated cells originating from undifferentiated stem cells, whereas (oral) tolerogens *(6, not shown)* are designed to induce tolerance in different cell types, thus abrogating autoimmune responses. Targeted therapies also aim at intracellular elements such as kinases and transcription factors *(7)*, whereas several monoclonal antibodies target proinflammatory mediators *(8)*. As a last resort in refractory SLE, extracorporeal procedures *(9)* can remove (pathogenic) autoantibodies and immune complexes. The *(yellow)* numbers in Figure 56-1correspond with those used in Table 56-2.

DNA-binding protein HMGB1 (high-mobility group box–1), during the late apoptotic process. As a consequence, nuclear antigens are internalized by professional APCs and, finally, may be presented to naive T cells along with the respective co-stimulatory molecules, which are also upregulated via Toll-like receptors (TLRs).[13]

Intracellular TLR7 and TLR9, expressed (among others) in endosomes of plasmacytoid DCs, are activated by complexes of self-protein and RNA (TLR7) or DNA (TLR9). Once activated, they promote the production of type I interferons (interferon-alpha [IFN-α]) and proinflammatory cytokines via a MyD88-dependent pathway.[14] Considering the growing emphasis on the role of the interferon signature in SLE pathogenesis and since APCs and TLRs are crucial for initiating the autoimmune response by activating cells of the adaptive immune system, these cells are a tempting target for new therapies.

In contrast to cancer, in which agonists of various TLRs (and those targeting TLR7 and TLR9, in particular) are already in clinical trials,[15] TLR antagonists are sought for in autoimmune disorders. Interestingly, antimalarial medications antagonize TLR9, TLR7, and TLR8, which might partly explain their effectiveness in SLE therapy. The quinazoline derivative CPG-52364 (Pfizer) specifically inhibits TLR7, TLR8, and TLR9 and inhibits SLE progression in animal models; when combined with hydroxychloroquine, it prevented anti–double stranded DNA (anti-dsDNA) antibody formation in SLE-prone mice,[15] but after signals questioning its safety in healthy volunteers, phase 2 of the clinical trial was never started. The TLR7 and TLR9 antagonist IMO-3100 (Idera Pharmaceuticals) is in preclinical evaluation. TLR7 and TLR9 can also be inhibited by short

DNA sequences (immunoregulatory sequences [IRS]); the compound IRS-954 (DV-1079) prevented disease progression in lupus-prone mice and reduced serum levels of nucleic acid–specific serum antibodies.[15]

With the pivotal role of DCs in host defense kept in mind, all strategies aimed at deactivating DCs or at blocking their receptors will have to prove safe with respect to infections.

T Cells and Co-Stimulation

Activated T cells are central players in SLE pathogenesis, since they can support B-cell activation and release cytokines that also enhance granulocyte and macrophage activity (see Figure 56-1). Preventing T-cell activation, deactivating T cells, or (at least) blocking their proinflammatory products are promising paths. Rather rude approaches with antibodies targeting all T cells (anti–cluster of differentiation 3 [anti-CD3] antibodies) have been conducted in type I diabetes and are still in use to treat renal transplant rejection[16]; so far, no trial has been conducted in human SLE. Interestingly, in lupus-prone mice (NZB/NZW F1 [BWF1]), nasal administration of a hamster immunoglobulin G (IgG) anti-CD3 antibody led to a reduced incidence of glomerulonephritis and decreased levels of autoantibodies, most likely by inducing a subtype of Treg cells.[17] Targeting the CD4+ T-cell subtype with anti-CD4 antibodies led to amelioration of lupus in murine models (in contrast to anti-CD8 therapy, which aggravated lupus features)[18] but was not pursued in humans.

Interfering with T-cell activation by blocking co-stimulation has been successfully attempted in rheumatoid arthritis (RA). When studied in SLE, abatacept (cytotoxic T-lymphocyte antigen 4–immunoglobulin [CTLA4-Ig]; Bristol-Meyers Squibb), appeared to improve musculoskeletal signs and symptoms and had a good safety profile,[19] but the primary endpoint was not met, likely because of the high steroid use permitted in this study. A trial in lupus nephritis of abatacept in combination with mycophenolate mofetil (MMF) was halted,[20] and another one is currently being performed by the National Institutes of Health (NIH) Immune Tolerance Network assessing abatacept in combination with cyclophosphamide ([CYC]; EuroLupus regimen) (NCT0077485). Blockade of the CD40L pathway was effective but not safe with anti–CD40 ligand antibody BG9588 (because of thrombotic complications) and safe but not effective with IDEC.[21,22] CDP7657 (UCB), a pegylated Fab′ anti-CD40L compound, may be more promising, since it might not affect thrombocyte activity because of the lack of an Fc portion. In preclinical studies on mice and nonhuman primates, effective interference with the immune response was observed.[23] An inducible co-stimulator (ICOS)–B7-RPI inhibitor (Amgen 557; Amgen) is currently in a phase I trial (NCT00774943) and is planned for a lupus arthritis and a subacute cutaneous lupus erythematosus (SCLE) trial; efalizumab (lymphocyte function–associated antigen [LFA] 1) was tested for cutaneous SLE but was withdrawn because of severe adverse events, namely, the occurrence of progressive multifocal leukoencephalopathy in patients with psoriasis, a disease for which SLE patients are at increased risk.[24,25]

Regulatory T Cells

The role of Treg cells in SLE is still under debate, but recent publications underscore that Treg cells are lower in number and have reduced suppressive capacity in active SLE.[26,27] Treg cells can suppress CD4+ T-helper (Th) cells (Th1, Th2, Th17), CD8+ T cells, B cells, DCs, and a variety of other cells of the immune system. Although new Treg subtypes are continuously described,[28,29] it is not entirely clear, how Treg cells exert their function and to which extent in vitro mechanisms, in fact, mimic in vivo situations or opportunities. Several different ways to suppress have been described, and more than one mechanism may be involved at one time in vivo.[30] Treg cells exert suppression by releasing cytokines such as interleukin (IL)–10, they can act directly on T cells or B cells (e.g., cytolysis), or they interact with antigen presentation.[31]

TABLE 56-2 Overview of Therapies Addressed in This Chapter

SECTION	TITLE	SUMMARY
1	DCs and APCs	As a consequence of specifically encountering activation, exogenous (e.g., virus, bacteria) or endogenous molecules (among those apoptotic nuclear material secondary to defective clearance and potentially present in phagocytosed immune complexes), DCs are activated and/or present autoantigens. TLR7 and TLR9 are activated by RNA and DNA, respectively. Blocking these cells and receptors targets the autoimmune reaction at an early stage.
2	T cells and co-stimulation	T cells are key players in SLE; they activate autoreactive B cells and release proinflammatory cytokines. Blocking the proper co-stimulatory pathways aims at preventing T-cell activation.
3	Treg cells	Treg cells are involved in maintaining peripheral tolerance. Therapeutic strategies aim at increasing their number or functional capacity by applying specific stimuli or by applying extracorporally induced or augmented Treg cells.
4	B cells	As the producers of (pathogenic) autoantibodies, B cells are a major target of therapeutic approaches in SLE. Only a short overview is provided in this chapter.
5	Stem cell transplantation	Self-reactive lymphocytes are eliminated and replaced with newly generated cell originating from undifferentiated stem cells; key aspects of autologous and allogeneic transplantation of HSCs and MSCs are discussed.
6	Tolerogens	Inducing tolerance in DCs, T cells, or B cells might be a promising and safe approach.
7	Intracellular targets and signal transduction molecules	Most conventional immunosuppressive agents aim at intracellular mechanisms but rather nonspecifically. Targeted therapies selectively block kinases or transcription factors, or aim at messenger RNA transcripts.
8	Mediators of inflammation (interleukins, TNF-α, interferons, complement)	Antibodies against proinflammatory mediators are widely used in autoimmune diseases; however, so far, they have not shown convincing efficacy in human SLE.
9	Extracorporeal removal of autoantibodies and immune complexes	Extracorporeal removal of pathogenic autoantibodies or immune complexes is an emergency procedure in highly active SLE.

APC, antigen-presenting cell; DC, dendritic cell; HSC, hematopoietic stem cell; MSC, mesenchymal stem cell; SLE, systemic lupus erythematosus; TNF-α, tumor necrosis factor–alpha; TLR, Toll-like receptor; Treg, T-regulator.

A large body of evidence exists on beneficial effects of Treg cells in experimental models of organ-specific autoimmune diseases such as diabetes or autoimmune gastritis; interestingly, in these diseases, transforming growth factor–beta (TGF-β)–induced antigen-specific Treg cells had a much higher suppressive capacity in vivo than polyclonal (CD4⁺CD25⁺FoxP3⁺) naturally occurring Treg cells; the difference was greatest for suppression of Th17 cells, which are now attributed with the highest autoimmunogenic potential.[32,33] Since an increased antigen specificity appeared to increase the suppressive capacity of Treg cells, interfering with antigen presentation might be a major mechanism of Treg cells in vivo.[31]

Since there is no known specific "lupus antigen" polyclonal Treg cells are the only available Treg population for studies in SLE. In several lupus mouse models, transfer experiments showed promising, beneficial effects; on adoptive transfer, CD4⁺CD25⁺ cells delayed disease onset (BWF1 mice), and in vitro induced polyclonal Treg cells (induction with IL-2 and TGF-β) had protective effects in lupus-like syndromes.[34] In addition, nasal or subcutaneous application of autoantigens or anti-CD3 antibodies led to an increase of some Treg subtypes.[35]

Treg induction in humans has to be approached with caution, since murine and human Treg cells have distinct but functionally important differences. The tempting idea to boost the patients' own Treg cells by applying exogenous triggers that proved effective in murine experiments led to a catastrophic result when a cytokine storm was elicited after the application of an anti-CD28 antibody (TGF1412 trial).[36] The safer and more promising path for the future appears to be an extracorporeal induction or amplification of Treg cells; the respective techniques are already successfully tested in mice and in vitro on human cells.[34]

B Cells

B cells have come to the focus of interest in SLE therapy, especially as a target for biological agents. Some of these biological agents have been designed to deplete B cells, such as the anti-CD20 monoclonal antibodies (mAbs) rituximab and ocrelizumab or the anti-CD22–mAb epratuzumab, which also interferes with proinflammatory pathways.

Despite promising results in observational studies and case series, rituximab has so far failed its endpoints in randomized controlled trials (EXPLORER and LUNAR, respectively); the BELONG trial for ocrelizumab with a design similar to that of LUNAR (renal SLE, in addition to standard of care [SOC] therapy) was halted after showing negative results.[37] Epratuzumab was so far tested in more than 200 patients with moderate to severe SLE and showed higher combined responder index rates than the placebo.[38] Two phase III studies on patients with moderate to severe disease are currently recruiting (EMBODY 1 and 2; NCT01262365 and NCT01261793, respectively).

The B-cell activation blocker belimumab, however, which targets the B cell–activation factor (BAFF), has become the first approved drug for SLE since 1958, thus supporting the concept of B cell–targeted therapies (discussed in greater detail in Chapter 53).

BAFF and a proliferation-inducing ligand (APRIL), both members of the tumor necrosis factor (TNF) superfamily, are produced by macrophages, DCs, and neutrophils, and they target different receptors on B cells. The extracellular domain of one of these receptors, transmembrane activator and calcium modulator and cyclophilin-ligand interactor (TACI), was fused to the constant region of human IgG-1 to form the chimeric molecule atacicept. In contrast to the CD20 and CD22 antibodies, atacicept also has significant effects on plasma cells. Its further use in SLE will have to be considered with caution after the results from the still ongoing trial for nonrenal SLE; one phase II trial in patients with lupus nephritis was stopped because of infections.[10] A-623 (a selective peptibody antagonist of BAFF; PEARL trial) and LY2127399 (an anti-BAFF–mAb) also target BAFF, but not APRIL, and are in phase II clinical trials. In contrast to A-623, LY2127399 binds both soluble and membrane-bound BAFF.

Small modular immunopharmaceutical (SMIP) drug candidates directed against CD20 are in phase I (SBI-087, NCT00714116) or are not further developed because they did not meet the primary endpoint in phase I (TRU-015, NCT00479622; both trials sponsored by Wyeth).

Stem Cell Transplantation

In short, the aim of **hematopoietic stem cell transplantation (HSCT)** is to eliminate self-reactive lymphocytes and replace them with newly generated, unprimed cells originating from undifferentiated stem cells. So far, autologous CD34+ hematopoietic stem cells (HSCs) have been used in the vast majority of trials. As a consequence of the protocols, HSCT also targets long-lived memory plasma cells, which cannot be eliminated by standard immunosuppression with CYC. Protocols vary, but most of them start with (i) the mobilization of HSCs with CYC and granulocyte-macrophage colony-stimulating factor (GMCSF), followed by (ii) leukapheresis and selection of stem cells upon their CD34 expression. In the next step of the procedure (iii), rather than a malignancy-specific myeloablative regimen, the conditioning regimen consists of lymphoablation without complete myeloablation ("nonmyeloablative HSCT", e.g. done with CYC and rabbit-derived antithymocyte globulin [ATG]), which is followed by (iv) transplantation of the previously obtained autologous stem cells and, finally, by the reconstitution of a new, tolerant immune system.[39-41]

Although several patients have achieved long-term remission, the success is confounded by treatment-related serious infections, transplantation-associated mortality, a considerable number of relapses, and the occurrence of secondary autoimmune disorders. So far, HSCT has been used as a "last resort" therapeutic option in negatively selected patients who have been severely ill and whose disease is refractory to therapy; and therefore no control group could be provided. An ongoing multicenter trial in Germany (Autologous Stem Cell Transplantation for Refractory Systemic Lupus Erythematosus [ASSIST], NCT00750971) attempts to deal with this limitation by creating a comparator arm consisting of patients who fulfill the inclusion criteria (i.e., CYC- or MMF-refractory SLE with organ involvement) but do not consent to HSCT. The current status has recently been nicely summarized.[42]

To increase efficacy, some trials include rituximab in the protocol (NCT00278538, phase I) or intensify lymphoablation with rituximab and fludarabine (NCT00076752, phase II); one study in children with refractory disease also added total body irradiation to the protocol (NCT00010335, phase I).

Other trials focus on similar or slightly amended nonmyeloablative concepts but aim at transplanting allogeneic HSCs from matched donors (NCT00849745, NCT00325741, NCT00278590; all are currently recruiting).

In contrast to HSCs, mesenchymal stem cells (MSCs) are pluripotent, can differentiate into multiple mesenchymal cell lines, but can also exert immunomodulatory effects on activated T and B lymphocytes, as well as on natural killer (NK) cells and DCs. MSCs can be found in various tissues, and larger amounts can be isolated from the bone marrow (for autologous transplantation) or from the umbilical cord (for allogeneic transplantation). MSCs express CD29, CD44, CD95, and CD105 but, in contrast to HSCs, not CD34 or human leukocyte antigen (HLA)–DR. MSCs from both bone marrow and the umbilical cord ameliorated lupus nephritis and serologic features in lupus-prone Murphy Roths Large–lymphoproliferation strain (MRL/lpr) mice and also had beneficial effects in human SLE. On transfer of umbilical cord MSCs, Systemic Lupus Erythematosus Disease Activity Index (SLEDAI), antinuclear antibodies (ANAs), and double-stranded DNA (dsDNA) decreased while renal function improved; these improvements were accompanied by an increase of Treg cells (CD4+CD25+FoxP3+) in the peripheral blood.[43] A Chinese trial using allogeneic bone marrow–derived MSCs after immunoablation with CYC is ongoing (NCT00698191, phases I and II).

Tolerogens

The concept of tolerogens is to reestablish a status of peripheral tolerance by exposure to (nucleic) autoantigens or autoantibody peptides. Tolerogens can aim at different cell types (DCs, T cells, B cells) (see Figure 56-1).

So far, tolerogens, which are assumed to interfere with anti-DNA–antibody production, have led to safe but largely ineffective compounds when tried in humans. Worth mentioning are the anti-DNA B-cell tolerogens LJP394 (Riquent; La Jolla Pharmaceutical) and edratide (Teva Pharmaceutical Industries), which have not shown successful results[44]; however, a recent retrospective analysis (performed by Remmunix) revealed that some post-hoc secondary endpoints were met with edratide,[45] and therefore the compound may be further investigated. T-cell tolerogen Lupuzor (IPP-201101; Cephalon) is a spliceosomal peptide of U1 small nuclear ribonucleoprotein (snRNP) that is suggested to promote tolerance by preventing the proliferation of CD4+ T cells. It appeared to decrease IL-10 secretion and anti-dsDNA levels[46]; a phase IIb study is in progress. Laquinimod (quinoline-3-carboxamides by Teva) is currently investigated in arthritis and nephritis trials (NCT01085097) and also in Crohn's disease (NCT00737932) after successful trials in multiple sclerosis.[47]

In mice, however, tolerization and immunization with peptides derived from nuclear autoantigens or from pathogenic anti-dsDNA antibodies were effective and suppressed the development of lupus. A tolerogenic histone H4 peptide (amino acids 471-194) induced the expression of the Treg-typical transcription factor FoxP3 in both CD4 and CD8 cells, leading to TGF-β production and resulting in a delay of glomerulonephritis and in prolonged survival.[48] Interestingly, an anti-CD3 antibody led to an increase of Treg cells (CD4+CD25-LAP+) on nasal application and to a reduction of the clinical signs of lupus.[17]

Finally, nucleosomal antigens (nucleosomal histone peptide epitope H4 [71-94]) showed that plasmacytoid DCs expressed a tolerogenic phenotype upon uptake of the peptide and prolonged survival when injected into lupus-prone mice; they also produced large amounts of TGF-β, which, in turn, might have also increased the number of Treg cells,[48] thus closing the circle between innate and adaptive immunities.

Intracellular Targets and Signal Transduction

When ligands bind to their respective receptors, a series of kinases are activated and initiate a cascade of events. They transduce the original signal and finally activate transcription factors (such as nuclear factor–kappa B [NF-κB]) that induce gene expression and subsequently peptide and protein synthesis. Such kinases are major players in the signaling events of the immune system and in inflammatory processes; some of them have been studied as therapeutic targets during the last decade and may develop into promising targets for modern therapies.

Spleen tyrosine kinase (Syk) is involved in the development of the adaptive immune system and is important for the function of various cell types and in propagating inflammation.[49] In SLE, fragmented, crystallizable gamma receptor (FcγR)–Syk associates with the TCR; this rewiring of the TCR has been claimed to account, at least in part, for the overactive T-cell phenotype observed in SLE. However, Syk is also involved in B-cell activation, which is also a major target in SLE therapy. Fostamatinib (R788; Rigel Pharmaceuticals), an oral Syk inhibitor, has shown efficacy in phase 2 trials of RA.[50] It prevented the development of renal disease and improved the survival of lupus-prone mice.[51] A study in human SLE (Efficacy and Safety Study of R935788 Tablets to Treat Systemic Lupus Erythematosus [SOLEIL]) was withdrawn before enrollment, and the future of the drug in SLE remains unclear (eTable 56-1).

Janus Kinase Inhibitors

Janus kinase inhibitor CP-690550 (tofacitinib; Pfizer) inhibits one third of the activity of the Janus family of protein tyrosine kinases

(JAKs) and has successfully completed phase 2 trials in RA.[52] Considering the involvement of JAKs in the context of cell activation by IL-6, type I interferons, and gamma chain cytokines, it may also constitute a promising compound for SLE.

Proteasome Inhibitor Bortezomib (PS-341; Janssen Cilag)

The selective inhibitor of the 26S proteasome, bortezomib, is approved for the treatment of progressive, relapsing multiple myeloma, a plasma-cell neoplasia. Bortezomib interrupts the NF-κB pathway and suppresses focal adhesion kinase (FAK) expression, as well as modulates tumor microenvironment and cytokine expression. In addition, bortezomib suppresses the activity of plasmacytoid DCs by inhibiting intracellular trafficking of TLRs.[53] Bortezomib efficiently depletes both short- and long-lived plasma cells. It decreased dsDNA-specific antibody production, proteinuria, and kidney damage and drastically prolonged survival in lupus-prone NZB/NZW F1 and MRL/lpr mice.[54] Bortezomib is currently being investigated in World Health Organization (WHO) class III, IV, and V lupus nephritis (NCT01169857). Case reports have shown significant efficacy, which is limited by the neurotoxicity of the drug.[55]

MicroRNAs (miRNAs)

MicroRNAs (miRNAs) can inactivate messenger RNAs (mRNAs) and thus prevent transcription of the respective protein encoded by a specific mRNA. In turn, miRNAs can also be the target of cholesterol-conjugated RNA molecules termed *antagomirs*.[56] In human SLE, a plethora of miRNAs are overexpressed in different types of immune cells (e.g., miRNA-21, 125a, 126, 146a, 148a, 155, 181a); recently miRNA-21 overexpression in T cells was linked with lupus disease activity.[57] MiRNAs are a promising future target in SLE; however, clinical experience in murine or human lupus is lacking so far.

Mediators of Inflammation

Tumor necrosis factor–alpha (TNF-α) blockers are widely used in RA and were the first targeted biological therapy available for treating a rheumatic disorder. Infliximab also improved lupus arthritis and nephritis but was associated with an increase of autoantibodies and adverse events. However, when used only as short-term therapy (four pulses), infliximab induced only a few adverse events and led to long-lasting remissions of lupus nephritis in patients whose renal disease had been refractory to other traditional therapies.[58] A trial using etanercept in lupus nephritis was terminated in phase II (NCT00447265).

Interleukin Blockers

Also originating from RA therapy, anakinra (antagonist to interleukin 1–receptor [anti-IL-1Ra]) was not effective in SLE, tocilizumab (anti–interleukin 6–receptor [anti-IL-6R]) slightly improved activity scores (e.g., SLEDAI) and arthritis, but was not further pursued because of side effects (neutropenia).[59] A trial with CNTO 136 (sirukumab, an anti-IL-6 antibody; Janssen Biotech) for lupus nephritis is currently recruiting (NCT01273389).

In a small trial on six patients with steroid-dependent SLE, anti–IL-10 mAb (B-N10) was safe, and cutaneous lesions and joint symptoms improved after 6 months, but all patients developed antibodies against B-N10.[60] In addition, IL-10 may be a too pleomorphic target, illustrated by the fact that some regulatory cells also secrete IL-10 to accomplish their suppressive actions. In murine SLE, inhibition of IL-12, IL-17, IL-18, IL-21, and IL-23 may be a promising strategy, but so far no trial has been designed for human SLE.[61]

Interferon Blockers

Interferons are thought to play a major role in SLE pathogenesis and are released by plasmacytoid DCs and other cells. Sifalimumab (MEDI-545; Medimmune) and rontalizumab (Roche) are small molecules that bind to IFN-α and can decrease the INF-α signature within days by 90% (protein and gene expression) and decrease skin lesions in biopsies, as shown in phase I studies.[62,63] However, neither phase Ib nor phase IIa trials revealed clinical efficacy beyond that of placebo. Therefore MEDI-545 development has been halted and replaced by the development of MEDI-546, a fully human anti-IFN–α receptor–mAb. It is currently being tested in a scleroderma trial (NCT00930683), and a phase III trial in SLE is planned.

IFN-α–Kinoid (IFN-K; Neovacs) is being tested for safety and clinical impact on SLE disease in mild to moderate SLE (NCT01058343). Novo Nordisk had two anti-IFN agents in development. Their anti-IFNα was recently sold to Argos, which is completing the phase I trial of 40 patients (NCT00960362), whereas the anti–IFN-γ antibody is still in development. Finally, AMG 811 (Amgen) is an anti–IFN-γ mAb that is currently being tested in a lupus nephritis trial (NCT01164917).

Complement

Eculizumab (Solaris; Alexion Pharmaceuticals), an mAb to C5a, was found safe but not overly effective; the agent is effective in and now available for paroxysmal nocturnal hemoglobinuria.[64] A phase I trial on membranous nephritis is ongoing but has stopped recruiting (NCT01221181), and a phase II trial deals with patients suffering from catastrophic antiphospholipid syndrome (CAPS) (NCT01029587). The SLE trial of a newer drug by Novo Nordisk was halted in response to concerns relating to neutropenia.

Extracorporeal Removal of Autoantibodies and Immune Complexes

Historically, plasma exchange (or plasmapheresis) was the only extracorporeal method available, and the fact that it can be applied in any dialysis unit without the need of additional equipment remains its advantage. It is apparently helpful in acute situations such as lung hemorrhage, in which it is still used as a rescue procedure. However, trials on long-term plasmapheresis failed to demonstrate significant benefit, and attempts to increase efficacy by combining plasmapheresis with pulse CYC were associated with severe infections.[65,66]

In contrast, immunoadsorption (IAS) uses specifically coated columns; ligands are either sheep IgG (Miltenyi Biotec), or staphylococcal protein A or the synthetic peptide Gam146 (Fresenius Medical Care) and allows for the specific and nearly complete clearance of circulating immunoglobulins and immune complexes, while neither removing other plasma proteins nor necessitating substitution with fresh-frozen plasma, albumin, or immunoglobulins. Moreover, the plasma volume processed is not restricted, even if patients are maintained on IAS daily. IAS appeared relatively safe with respect to infections and adverse events and can be combined with immunosuppressive medication. IAS reduced proteinuria, global disease activity, and anti-dsDNA antibodies. Therefore IAS is primarily used in those with severe SLE and complicated situations with limited therapeutic options, such as in pregnancy, in the presence of active infections (e.g., tuberculosis), or in patients with antiphospholipid syndrome (APS); as a result, randomized, controlled trials are still lacking.[67] Future therapeutic strategies could combine induction therapy with IAS and CYC (or MMF) with maintenance therapy with MMF or rituximab.

SUMMARY

The expanding knowledge and deeper understanding of the mechanisms behind the phenomenon *autoimmunity* have fueled research on this field in past decades. As in other autoimmune diseases, therapies targeting specific proinflammatory mediators and receptors, as well as intracellular molecules, or at depleting or deactivating certain pathogenic cell types or molecules are the focus of new therapeutic strategies in SLE. With lupus being a prototypic systemic autoimmune disease, which involves both the innate and the adaptive immune systems, approaches to reestablish peripheral tolerance are promising goals but have been difficult to achieve so far. The extracorporeal removal of pathogenic antibodies and immune complexes and the elimination and replacement of immune cells by stem cell transplantation constitute last resorts in refractory cases. Considering the large numbers of trials with a plethora of different agents ongoing (eTable 56-1) and after the first successful introduction of an approved drug for SLE by the U.S. Food and Drug Administration (FDA) and the European Medicines Agency (EMA) since the 1950s, there is hope that more therapeutic options will be found in the near future to establish personalized therapies for the highly heterogeneous population of patients with lupus.

References

1. Kaposi M: Neue Beiträge zur Kenntniss des Lupus erythematosus. *Arch Derm Res* 4:36–81, 1872.
2. Hench PS, Kendall EC: The effect of a hormone of the adrenal cortex (17-hydroxy-11-dehydrocorticosterone; compound E) and of pituitary adrenocorticotropic hormone on rheumatoid arthritis. *Proc Staff Meet Mayo Clin* 24(8):181–197, 1949.
3. Grace AW, Combes FC: Remission of disseminated lupus erythematosus induced by adrenocorticotropin. *Proc Soc Exp Biol Med* 72(3):563–565, 1949.
4. Rossi D, Zlotnik A: The biology of chemokines and their receptors. *Ann Rev Immunol* 18:217–242, 2000.
5. Afford S, Randhawa S: Apoptosis. *Mol Pathol* 53(2):55–63, 2000.
6. Firestein GS, Manning AM: Signal transduction and transcription factors in rheumatic disease. *Arthritis Rheum* 42(4):609–621, 1999.
7. Sestak AL, Förnrohr BG, Harley JB, et al: The genetics of systemic lupus erythematosus and implications for targeted therapy. *Ann Rheum Dis* 70(Suppl 1):i37–i43, 2011.
8. Urowitz MB, Gladman DD: Evolving spectrum of mortality and morbidity in SLE. *Lupus* 8(4):253–255, 1999.
9. Smolen JS, Strand V, Cardiel M, et al: Randomized clinical trials and longitudinal observational studies in systemic lupus erythematosus: consensus on a preliminary core set of outcome domains. *J Rheumatol* 26(2):504–507, 1999.
10. Looney RJ: B cell-targeted therapies for systemic lupus erythematosus: an update on clinical trial data. *Drugs* 70(5):529–540, 2010.
11. Wallace DJ: Advances in drug therapy for systemic lupus erythematosus. *BMC Med* 8:77, 2010.
12. Munoz LE, Gaipl US, Franz S, et al: SLE—a disease of clearance deficiency? *Rheumatology (Oxford)* 44(9):1101–1107, 2005.
13. Santegoets KC, van BL, van den Berg WB, et al: Toll-like receptors in rheumatic diseases: are we paying a high price for our defense against bugs? *FEBS Lett* 585:3660–3666, 2011.
14. Yamamoto M, Takeda K: Current views of toll-like receptor signaling pathways. *Gastroenterol Res Pract* 2010:240365, 2010.
15. Hennessy EJ, Parker AE, O'Neill LA: Targeting Toll-like receptors: emerging therapeutics? *Nat Rev Drug Discov* 9(4):293–307, 2010.
16. Herold KC, Hagopian W, Auger JA, et al: Anti-CD3 monoclonal antibody in new-onset type 1 diabetes mellitus. *N Engl J Med* 346(22):1692–1698, 2002.
17. Wu HY, Quintana FJ, Weiner HL: Nasal anti-CD3 antibody ameliorates lupus by inducing an IL-10-secreting CD4+ CD25− LAP+ regulatory T cell and is associated with down-regulation of IL-17+ CD4+ ICOS+ CXCR5+ follicular helper T cells. *J Immunol* 181(9):6038–6050, 2008.
18. Adachi Y, Inaba M, Sugihara A, et al: Effects of administration of monoclonal antibodies (anti-CD4 or anti-CD8) on the development of autoimmune diseases in (NZW × BXSB)F1 mice. *Immunobiology* 198(4):451–464, 1998.
19. Merrill JT, Burgos-Vargas R, Westhovens R, et al: The efficacy and safety of abatacept in patients with non-life-threatening manifestations of systemic lupus erythematosus: results of a twelve-month, multicenter, exploratory, phase IIb, randomized, double-blind, placebo-controlled trial. *Arthritis Rheum* 62(10):3077–3087, 2010.
20. Lupus nephritis therapeutics—pipeline assessment and market forecast to 2017. 6-3-2011. Available at http://www.companiesandmarkets.com/Market-Report/lupus-nephritis-therapeutics-pipeline-assessment-and-market-forecast-to-2017-529496.asp?prk=0c91637ba39545a71d2eb6e5b cb60fd4 (press release).
21. Boumpas DT, Furie R, Manzi S, et al: A short course of BG9588 (anti-CD40 ligand antibody) improves serologic activity and decreases hematuria in patients with proliferative lupus glomerulonephritis. *Arthritis Rheum* 48(3):719–727, 2003.
22. Kalunian KC, Davis JC, Jr, Merrill JT, et al: Treatment of systemic lupus erythematosus by inhibition of T cell costimulation with anti-CD154: a randomized, double-blind, placebo-controlled trial. *Arthritis Rheum* 46(12):3251–3258, 2002.
23. Wakefield I, Harari O, Hutto D, et al: An assessment of the thromboembolic potential of CDP7657, a monovalent Fab′ PEG anti-CD40L antibody, in Rhesus macaques. [abstract] *Arthritis Rheum* 62 (Suppl 10):1243, 2010.
24. Kothary N, Diak IL, Brinker A, et al: Progressive multifocal leukoencephalopathy associated with efalizumab use in psoriasis patients. *J Am Acad Dermatol* 65(3):546–551, 2011.
25. Molloy ES, Calabrese LH: Progressive multifocal leukoencephalopathy: a national estimate of frequency in systemic lupus erythematosus and other rheumatic diseases. *Arthritis Rheum* 60(12):3761–3765, 2009.
26. Scheinecker C, Bonelli M, Smolen JS: Pathogenetic aspects of systemic lupus erythematosus with an emphasis on regulatory T cells. *J Autoimmun* 35(3):269–275, 2010.
27. Bonelli M, Smolen JS, Scheinecker C: Treg and lupus. *Ann Rheum Dis* 69(Suppl 1):i65–i66, 2010.
28. Shevach EM: From vanilla to 28 flavors: multiple varieties of T regulatory cells. *Immunity* 25(2):195–201, 2006.
29. Sakaguchi S, Sakaguchi N, Asano M, et al: Immunologic self-tolerance maintained by activated T cells expressing IL-2 receptor alpha-chains (CD25). Breakdown of a single mechanism of self-tolerance causes various autoimmune diseases. *J Immunol* 155(3):1151–1164, 1995.
30. Shevach EM: Mechanisms of foxp3+ T regulatory cell-mediated suppression. *Immunity* 30(5):636–645, 2009.
31. DiPaolo RJ, Brinster C, Davidson TS, et al: Autoantigen-specific TGF beta-induced Foxp3+ regulatory T cells prevent autoimmunity by inhibiting dendritic cells from activating autoreactive T cells. *J Immunol* 179(7):4685–4693, 2007.
32. Huter EN, Stummvoll GH, DiPaolo RJ, et al: Cutting edge: antigen-specific TGF beta-induced regulatory T cells suppress Th17-mediated autoimmune disease. *J Immunol* 181(12):8209–8213, 2008.
33. Stummvoll GH, DiPaolo RJ, Huter EN, et al: Th1, Th2, and Th17 effector T cell-induced autoimmune gastritis differs in pathological pattern and in susceptibility to suppression by regulatory T cells. *J Immunol* 181(3):1908–1916, 2008.
34. Horwitz DA: Regulatory T cells in systemic lupus erythematosus: past, present and future. *Arthritis Res Ther* 10(6):227, 2008.
35. Centola M, Wood G, Frucht DM, et al: The gene for familial Mediterranean fever, MEFV, is expressed in early leukocyte development and is regulated in response to inflammatory mediators. *Blood* 95(10):3223–3231, 2000.
36. Stebbings R, Findlay L, Edwards C, et al: "Cytokine storm" in the phase I trial of monoclonal antibody TGN1412: better understanding the causes to improve preclinical testing of immunotherapeutics. *J Immunol* 179(5):3325–3331, 2007.
37. Mysler EF, Spindler AJ, Guzman RM, et al: Efficacy and safety of ocrelizumab, a humanized anti CD20 antibody, in patients with active proliferative lupus nephritis (LN): results from the randomized, double-blind Phase III BELONG study. *Arthritis Rheum* [abstract] 62:606–607, 2010.
38. Wallace DJ, Kalunian KC, Petri MA, et al: Epratuzumab demonstrates clinically meaningful improvements in patients with moderate to severe systemic lupus erythematosus (SLE): results from EMBLEM, a Phase IIb study. [abstract] *Arthritis Rheum* 62(Suppl 10):1452, 2010.
39. Burt RK, Traynor A, Statkute L, et al: Nonmyeloablative hematopoietic stem cell transplantation for systemic lupus erythematosus. *JAMA* 295(5):527–535, 2006.
40. Alexander T, Thiel A, Rosen O, et al: Depletion of autoreactive immunologic memory followed by autologous hematopoietic stem cell transplantation in patients with refractory SLE induces long-term remission through de novo generation of a juvenile and tolerant immune system. *Blood* 113(1):214–223, 2009.
41. Tyndall A, Gratwohl A: Adult stem cell transplantation in autoimmune disease. *Curr Opin Hematol* 16(4):285–291, 2009.
42. Sullivan KM, Muraro P, Tyndall A: Hematopoietic cell transplantation for autoimmune disease: updates from Europe and the United States. *Biol Blood Marrow Transplant* 16(1 Suppl):S48–S56, 2010.
43. Sun L, Wang D, Liang J, et al: Umbilical cord mesenchymal stem cell transplantation in severe and refractory systemic lupus erythematosus. *Arthritis Rheum* 62(8):2467–2475, 2010.
44. Cardiel MH, Tumlin JA, Furie RA, et al: Abetimus sodium for renal flare in systemic lupus erythematosus: results of a randomized, controlled phase III trial. *Arthritis Rheum* 58(8):2470–2480, 2008.
45. Urowitz M, Isenberg D, Wallace DJ: Prelude-Edratide Phase-II study outcome—from predefined analyses to more recent assessment approaches. *Ann Rheum Dis* (Abstract) 70(S3):315, 2011.

46. Page N, Schall N, Strub JM, et al: The spliceosomal phosphopeptide P140 controls the lupus disease by interacting with the HSC70 protein and via a mechanism mediated by gamma delta T cells. *PLoS One* 4(4):e5273, 2009.

47. Comi G, Abramsky O, Arbizu T, et al: Oral laquinimod in patients with relapsing-remitting multiple sclerosis: 36-week double-blind active extension of the multi-centre, randomized, double-blind, parallel-group placebo-controlled study. *Mult Scler* 16(11):1360–1366, 2010.

48. Kang HK, Liu M, Datta SK: Low-dose peptide tolerance therapy of lupus generates plasmacytoid dendritic cells that cause expansion of autoantigen-specific regulatory T cells and contraction of inflammatory Th17 cells. *J Immunol* 178(12):7849–7858, 2007.

49. Pamuk ON, Tsokos GC: Spleen tyrosine kinase inhibition in the treatment of autoimmune, allergic and autoinflammatory diseases. *Arthritis Res Ther* 12(6):222, 2010.

50. Weinblatt ME, Kavanaugh A, Genovese MC, et al: An oral spleen tyrosine kinase (Syk) inhibitor for rheumatoid arthritis. *N Engl J Med* 363(14):1303–1312, 2010.

51. Deng GM, Liu L, Bahjat FR, et al: Suppression of skin and kidney disease by inhibition of spleen tyrosine kinase in lupus-prone mice. *Arthritis Rheum* 62(7):2086–2092, 2010.

52. Tanaka Y, Suzuki M, Nakamura H, et al: Phase 2 study of tofacitinib (CP-690,550) combined with methotrexate in patients with rheumatoid arthritis and inadequate response to methotrexate. *Arthritis Care Res (Hoboken)* 63(8):1150–1158, 2011.

53. Hirai M, Kadowaki N, Kitawaki T, et al: Bortezomib suppresses function and survival of plasmacytoid dendritic cells by targeting intracellular trafficking of Toll-like receptors and endoplasmic reticulum homeostasis. *Blood* 117(2):500–509, 2011.

54. Neubert K, Meister S, Moser K, et al: The proteasome inhibitor bortezomib depletes plasma cells and protects mice with lupus-like disease from nephritis. *Nat Med* 14(7):748–755, 2008.

55. Fröhlich K, Holle JU, Aries PM, et al: Successful use of bortezomib in a patient with systemic lupus erythematosus and multiple myeloma. *Ann Rheum Dis* 70(7):1344–1345, 2011.

56. Czech MP: MicroRNAs as therapeutic targets. *N Engl J Med* 354(11):1194–1195, 2006.

57. Stagakis E, Bertsias G, Verginis P, et al: Identification of novel microRNA signatures linked to human lupus disease activity and pathogenesis: miR-21 regulates aberrant T cell responses through regulation of PDCD4 expression. *Ann Rheum Dis* 70(8):1496–1506, 2011.

58. Aringer M, Smolen JS: Therapeutic blockade of TNF in patients with SLE-promising or crazy? *Autoimmun Rev* 11:321–325, 2012.

59. Illei GG, Shirota Y, Yarboro CH, et al: Tocilizumab in systemic lupus erythematosus: data on safety, preliminary efficacy, and impact on circulating plasma cells from an open-label phase I dosage-escalation study. *Arthritis Rheum* 62(2):542–552, 2010.

60. Llorente L, Richaud-Patin Y, García-Padilla C, et al: Clinical and biologic effects of anti-interleukin-10 monoclonal antibody administration in systemic lupus erythematosus. *Arthritis Rheum* 43(8):1790–1800, 2000.

61. Kunz M, Ibrahim SM: Cytokines and cytokine profiles in human autoimmune diseases and animal models of autoimmunity. *Mediators Inflamm* 2009:979258, 2009.

62. Wallace DJ, Petri M, Olsen N, et al: MEDI-454, an anti-interferon alpha monoclonal antibody, shows evidence of clinical activity in systemic lupus erythematosus. *Arthritis Rheum* (Abstract) 56:S526, 2007.

63. McBride J, Wallace DJ, Morimoto AY, et al: Safety and pharmacodynamic response with administration of single and repeat doses of rontalizumab in a phase 1, placebo controlled, double blind, dose escalation study in SLE. *Lupus* (Abstract) 19:S15, 2010.

64. Kaplan M: Eculizumab (Alexion). *Curr Opin Investig Drugs* 3(7):1017–1023, 2002.

65. Lewis EJ, Hunsicker LG, Lan SP, et al: A controlled trial of plasmapheresis therapy in severe lupus nephritis. The Lupus Nephritis Collaborative Study Group. *N Engl J Med* 326(21):1373–1379, 1992.

66. Aringer M, Smolen JS, Graninger WB: Severe infections in plasmapheresis-treated systemic lupus erythematosus. *Arthritis Rheum* 41(3):414–420, 1998.

67. Stummvoll GH: Immunoadsorption (IAS) for systemic lupus erythematosus. *Lupus* 20(2):115–119, 2011.

Chapter 57

Mortality in SLE

*Sasha Bernatsky, Deborah Levy, Rosalind Ramsey-Goldman,
Caroline Gordon, Anisur Rahman, and Ann E. Clarke*

It is well known that systemic lupus erythematosus (SLE) can be severe and even life threatening. Mortality in SLE may be due to lupus activity (i.e., when vital organs or systems are involved), to complications of treatment (e.g., infections), or to chronic co-morbidity factors (e.g., cardiovascular disease). The literature regarding mortality in SLE has grown considerably over the years; this chapter attempts to consolidate recent findings regarding SLE survival and its predictors.

SURVIVAL RATES IN SYSTEMIC LUPUS ERYTHEMATOSUS
Five-Year Survival
It is generally accepted that survival of patients with SLE has improved significantly. Initially, many studies focused primarily on this parameter, which was calculated as the percent of patients within a cohort who remained alive at least 5 years after the diagnosis date.

The 5-year survival rate for patients with SLE, which was as low as 50% in the report of Merrell and Shulman[1] in 1955, varied between 64% and 87% in the 1980s, and it is fairly consistently reported to be approximately 95% today.[2-4] Some of the increase in the rate of survival is simply a reflection of the improvements in health and survival in developed nations; between 1965 and 2005, mortality rates decreased by at least 70% in the general population.[5] In the United States, the age-standardized death rate from all causes combined decreased from 1242 per 100,000 patients per year in 1970 to 845 per 100,000 patients per year in 2002. The largest percentage decreases have been in death rates from heart disease and stroke, which, as of the turn of the century, remain the two greatest causes of death.

Figure 57-1 illustrates 5-year survival estimates in studies published from the 1950s to the present. These data are consistent with a plateau for short-term survival, at least for patients of European and North American descent. In fact, of the studies featured in Figure 57-1 ($n = 33$), most are from North America ($n = 17$) or Europe ($n = 9$) (two each from Sweden and England and one each from Denmark, Finland, Holland, Norway, and Spain). Only five studies are from south Asia (one each from Malaysia and Singapore and three from India) and two studies from South American centers (one from Chile and one from the multinational Grupo Latinoamericano de Estudio del Lupus [GLADEL] group). The paucity of data from outside North America and Europe makes it hard to judge how comparable 5-year mortality rates are for patients with SLE in less developed parts of the world (e.g., south Asia). In addition, the background variability in average life expectancy should be kept in mind; for example, in a country such as India, the average life expectancy is 65 years, whereas it is 80 years in North America and Europe.

One additional point: even in North America, ethnic factors play a role in SLE survival. This fact is best illustrated in the 5-year survival data from a study published by Alarcón and colleagues in 2001, which studied a cohort with a large proportion of ethnic minorities (i.e., African American, Hispanic) in whom 5-year survival was only 86%. Most alarming is the fact that this lower survival rate was actually less than what had been reported a decade earlier in more predominantly Caucasian SLE cohorts.[6] In general, Caucasians have a better outcome than non-Caucasians, with mortality rates being several times higher in non-Caucasians than in Caucasians.[7-9]

As in patients with SLE of Hispanic descent, the rates of mortality from SLE in African Americans have been shown to be higher than the rates of mortality from SLE in Caucasian Americans on the basis of death statistics, but this is, in part, related to the threefold higher SLE prevalence in African Americans.[10] Rothfield's group reported trends in National Center for Health Statistics data from 1968 to 1991, during which SLE mortality among African Americans rose more than 30% since the late 1970s to a mean annual rate of 18.7 SLE deaths per million.[11] Among female Caucasians, the total SLE mortality was reported to be stable from the late 1970s to 1991, averaging 4.6 deaths per million annually. A limitation of these types of data is that SLE may be underreported as a cause of death on death certificates; in any case, this underreporting is most pronounced in non-Caucasian populations[12]; thus the differences in these trends are likely real.

The interpretation of Rothfield's group was that the observed trends were largely the result of the higher prevalence of SLE among African-American women than had been previously recognized, or the existence of barriers to diagnosis and effective treatment, particularly for young African-American women, or both. These barriers may include the presence of more resistant disease (e.g., lupus nephritis that is more likely to progress to end-stage renal failure [ESRF], regardless of treatment) in African Americans[13]; greater co-morbidity, especially hypertension, diabetes, and obesity; and/or problems with adherence or other social problems that may contribute to poor access to health care and increased mortality (including substance abuse and violence).[14,15]

These concerns are now widely recognized to affect patients from other African backgrounds and patients from other ethnic minorities in many parts of the world. These patients have been shown to have increased incidence and prevalence of lupus and worse outcomes, particularly increased mortality. The underlying reasons are multifactorial in nature and are likely to include genetic predisposition, although at least some of the mortality risk is likely to be modifiable.[16]

Canadian data suggest a similar scenario for patients with SLE of First Nations (i.e., indigenous North American) descent. In Peschken's landmark population-based study from Manitoba, not only was there a twofold increased prevalence of SLE in those of First Nations descent versus Caucasians, but patients with SLE of First Nations descent had higher Systemic Lupus Erythematosus Disease Activity Index (SLEDAI) scores at diagnosis, had more frequent vasculitis and renal involvement, accumulated more damage, and experienced fourfold higher mortality rates, compared with non–First Nations patients with SLE. However, despite Canada's theoretically "universally accessible" health care system for its citizens, First Nations Canadians are known, in general, to have considerable barriers to optimal health outcomes at all levels as a result of the problems with access to care, high co-morbidity (especially hypertension, diabetes, and obesity), and/or the same previously noted problems with adherence and/or other social problems that contribute to mortality,

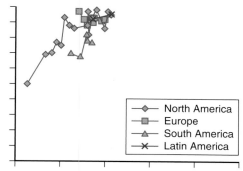

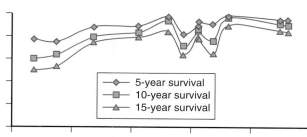

FIGURE 57-1 Calendar trends for 5-year survival is exhibited in those with systemic lupus erythematosus (SLE) and stratified by region. Plot represents studies published from the 1950s to the present.

FIGURE 57-2 Calendar effects for 5-, 10-, and 15-year survival rates in systemic lupus erythematosus (SLE). Plot represents studies published from the 1960s to the present.

especially substance abuse and violence.[17] For these reasons, First Nations patients have a much higher mortality rate than others.

Longer-Term Survival

Data confirming increased long-term survival are important in SLE. A plot representing some of the long-term estimates that are available show that the trends for improvements in survival rates are evident with the passage of calendar years (Figure 57-2).

STANDARDIZED MORTALITY RATES IN SYSTEMIC LUPUS ERYTHEMATOSUS

Of course, life expectancy, in general, has been increasing in the European and North American populations, in which many of the studies have been based. Thus standardized mortality rates (SMRs), which compare the mortality rates of patients with SLE to those in the general population of the same age, sex, and calendar-year period of SLE diagnosis, are better able to determine whether the high mortality risk for patients with SLE is, in fact, decreasing over time, relative to the general population. Reviewing several recent studies that have generated SMRs that compare the death rates in SLE to the mortality rates in the general population is therefore informative. Overall, across these studies, it seems that at least some of the excess death risk in those with SLE, compared with the general population, has been diminishing over time.

In a single-center North American study based in the very large cohort (*n* = 1175), Urowitz and colleagues[18] demonstrated improved mortality risk in patients with SLE over a 36-year period between 1970 and 2005. The age- and sex-adjusted SMR decreased from 12.6 in the 1970s (95% confidence interval [CI] 9.1, 17.4) to 3.5 (95% CI 2.7, 4.4) by the end of the observation interval. In a very large (*n* = 9547) multicenter international SLE cohort, Bernatsky and associates[19] found similar trends for improving mortality in patients with SLE, compared with the general population.

This multicenter international mortality study included adult patients (older than age 16 years) with definite SLE disease activity according to the American College of Rheumatology (ACR) or

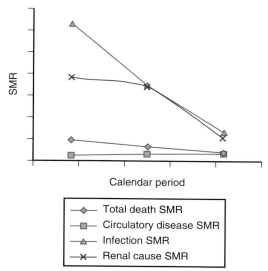

FIGURE 57-3 Unadjusted standardized mortality rate (SMR) estimates by calendar period. *(Data from Bernatsky S, Boivin J, Manzi S, Ginzler E, Gladman DD, Urowitz MB, et al: Mortality in systemic lupus erythematosus. Arthritis Rheum 54(8):2550–2557, 2006.)*

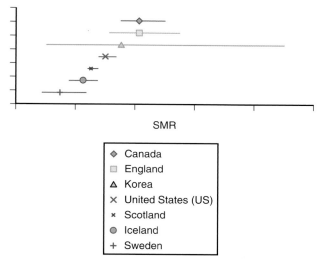

FIGURE 57-4 Unadjusted standardized mortality rate (SMR) estimates, stratified by country.

clinical criteria. The study base encompassed 23 collaborating lupus centers in seven countries across North America (Canada and the United States), the United Kingdom (England and Scotland), Iceland, Sweden, and South Korea.

From this study, the relative risks for death as a result of infection or renal causes in patients with SLE versus the general population were very high in the 1970s (Figure 57-3). These findings emphasize the high relative risks for death related to these causes in those with SLE, which, in the general population, are relatively uncommon. Regarding this multicenter international mortality study, none of the centers contributing data were from developing nations, and, in general, most of the overall SMRs for the period under study did not substantially differ from one country to the next (Figure 57-4).

It should be noted, however, that the rather encouraging findings presented (see Figures 57-1 and 57-2) do not take into consideration that subpopulations of patients with SLE, such as those with serious organ involvement (to be discussed in greater detail later in this chapter), may not enjoy the phenomenon of longer survival that is apparent for SLE overall. In fact, some of the apparent improvement in the 5-year survival rate in SLE (globally, as a disease) may relate to the fact that patients with milder SLE may be more recognized, and therefore more recent estimates arise from patient pools that include such mild cases. Although plausible, this premise is not proven. As discussed in the following text, however, it has been very well demonstrated that patients with more severe SLE most certainly still suffer higher mortality risks, relative to the general population.

CAUSES OF DEATH IN SYSTEMIC LUPUS ERYTHEMATOSUS

Data, to date, emphasize the importance of renal disease, severe lupus disease activity, infection, and cardiovascular disease.[20] Before the advent of effective SLE treatment, progressive disease activity, including renal failure and its associated complications, was one of the most important causes of death for patients with SLE. The exact attribution of lupus as a cause of death can be problematic; most authors have specifically included deaths as a result of renal failure in this category.

The incidence of renal failure was as high as 36% in one dataset from the 1960s,[21] with SLE being the most common cause of death in some early data from North America. Deaths from lupus, although fortunately are considerably less common in at least developed countries, remain a problem. The mortality data from five large pools of patients with SLE published in the past 10 years (the study from Sweden was published in 2003 but the observation interval ended in 1995) show that SLE is still the cause of death for approximately 25% or more of people affected by the disease (Figure 57-5), possibly suggesting an increase in the proportion of deaths attributable to infection, which could reflect a greater use of immunosuppressive agents over time. However, the ability to compare the data is limited by the different methods for outcome ascertainment (e.g., whether it is through chart review or administrative data sources); these methods may be more or less sensitive for the determination of particular causes of death.

Deaths as a result of infections remain a grave concern, because they should be preventable or treatable (see Figure 57-5). The earliest reports of causes of death in those with SLE from 70 years ago noted that most patients died from infections; however, these reports were published during the preantibiotic era. Data actually suggest deaths in SLE as a result of infections have decreased, at least in developed countries, which is best demonstrated by the decrease in SMRs related to infection over time (see Figure 57-3). In the early years,

this improvement probably reflected the increasing availability of antimicrobial medications and the effective recognition and treatment of infectious complications. In recent years, however, this decrease in the relative risk of death in SLE from infection may also be the result of the evolution of strategies that limit the incidence of infections when immunomodulatory therapy is used; for example, by limiting cumulative exposure and ensuring that immunization protocols are used. Although Mok and associates[22] reported a trend to fewer deaths from major infection in patients with SLE of Chinese descent between the years of 2000 and 2006, a recent publication on 5243 patients with SLE assembled from Hong Kong administrative (hospitalization) records reported that infection continued to be an important cause of death.[23]

Infectious disease still contributes greatly to mortality and has been highlighted in other data as well. In a recent update of outcomes in a large multicenter, multinational inception cohort of SLE that began in 2000, 30 patients out of 1593 (89.4% women, average age at SLE diagnosis 34.6 years) died during the mean follow-up of 3.7 years, and the most common causes of death were infections (nine), SLE (nine), and coronary artery disease (CAD) (seven); the cause of death was not established in four patients.[24] Of note, the GLADEL group reported that active disease and infection often co-existed and that both may have contributed to the deaths of some patients with lupus. For all these reasons, physicians should remain aware of the importance of serious infections in SLE-related mortality.

Currently, cardiovascular disease is the other primary cause of death in SLE, although in the large GLADEL (Latin American) group, no deaths were attributed to cardiovascular disease (see Figure 57-3). Demographics may be the reason; the GLADEL patient sample was only 41% Caucasian (compared with the other studies illustrated in Figure 57-3, which were predominantly Caucasian), with an age distribution that was likely younger than the other samples.

Early work by Urowitz and others first drew attention to the importance of mortality as a result of circulatory disease in SLE, particularly late in the disease course. Previous work by Manzi and colleagues[25] has shown a very high incidence of cardiac events (specifically, myocardial infarction and angina) in patients with SLE, compared with those in the general population.

In developed nations like the United States, the greatest contributions to improved mortality in the past 35 years have been decreases in death rates from heart disease and stroke, which still, as of the turn of the century, remain the two greatest causes of death.[5] However, data from the multicenter cohort study of the Systemic Lupus International Collaborating Clinics (SLICC) (see Figure 57-3) show that despite a 60% decrease in the SMR estimates overall, as well as a decrease in deaths related to lupus activity, such as renal disease, the trend for circulatory disease shows no such decline. This finding has been suggested as well by Bjornadal and colleagues.[26]

These findings may reflect, in part, the complex nature of cardiovascular disease in SLE. Classic atherosclerosis risk factors, such as hypertension and hypercholesterolemia, do play a role, although recent work has suggested that additional risk is conferred by some disease-related characteristics, such as SLE duration and, perhaps, severity.[27] However, other elements, such as medication exposures, may alter atherosclerosis risk in those with SLE. The specific role of steroidal drugs in SLE-related mortality is still debated, but hopefully data from currently ongoing large prospective cohorts will offer more insights as time goes on.

Active central nervous system (CNS) lupus is obviously another type of serious organ involvement that can potentially lead to death in SLE and was reportedly a common cause of death in early series, accounting for as much as 26% of the deaths reported by Dubois in the United States in 1956.[28] This is no longer the case. In recent decades, CNS disease accounts for approximately 5% of deaths in SLE,[29] with many of these events being vascular (i.e., hemorrhagic or thrombotic stroke) and not necessarily inflammatory disease in nature. In fact, establishing the underlying pathologic events from mortality reports is often difficult. Vital statistics data from a large

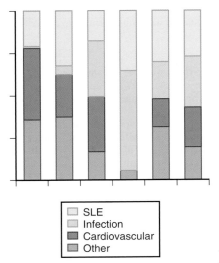

FIGURE 57-5 Comparison of five large recent studies. The contributions of cardiovascular, lupus-related, infectious, renal, and other causes of death in systemic lupus erythematosus (SLE) are portrayed.

Canadian pool of patients with SLE showed a large increase in ill-defined cerebrovascular events, which the authors suggested might represent cases of cerebral vasculitis or other rare forms of CNS disease.[30] However, the alternative view is that this may reflect diagnostic uncertainty regarding the causes of some of the clinical presentations observed in patients with SLE.

Finally, malignancy is a common cause of death in the developed world, and the cancer risk profile in SLE is, of course, very interesting. In the SLICC multicenter international cohort study, a trend toward lower total cancer mortality risk in SLE was actually revealed, relative to the general population (SMR of 0.8, 95% CI 0.6 to 1.0).[19] However, for mortality from hematologic cancers, the risk was elevated in SLE, compared with those in the general population (SMR of 2.1, 95% CI 1.2 to 3.4). This was also true for death from non-Hodgkin lymphoma (NHL) (SMR of 2.8, 95% CI 1.2 to 5.6) and lung cancer (SMR of 2.3, 95% CI 0.6 to 3.0). This apparent discrepancy may be due to the fact that although the incidence of NHL in SLE is known to be elevated, it remains a much less common cancer than other malignancies, such as breast cancer. In fact, new evidence supports the premise that women with SLE actually have a decreased incidence of breast cancer! Thus this decreased risk of a relatively common malignancy, breast cancer, in women with SLE may very well drive the total decreased mortality risk for cancer in SLE.

Co-Morbidities as Predictors of Overall Mortality in Systemic Lupus Erythematosus

In contrast to the preceding section, which discusses death rates in SLE for specific types of mortality, this section discusses co-morbidities as predictors of all-cause mortality.

Cardiac Disease

In the very large multicenter multinational inception SLE cohort, a project begun a decade ago by the SLICC,[31] patients who died had CAD more often at enrollment.[24] Similarly, CAD was a predictor of death (as a result of any cause) in the multivariate hazard ratio (HR) analyses of Urowitz and colleagues,[18] performed on a long-term cohort of prevalent patients with SLE. In this study, the HR for death in patients with CAD, compared with those without CAD, was 1.52, 95% CI 1.02 to 2.26. Of course, patients with CAD are intuitively at a heightened risk for mortality, compared with those who do not have CAD.

In data from the SLICC inception cohort, patients who died had higher SLICC/ACR damage index scores at enrollment, as compared with patients who remained alive at the end of the observation period. In large part, these higher index scores are likely the result of cardiac events, because (as previously mentioned) preexisting cardiac disease and established renal dysfunction are both strongly associated with mortality even in the general population.[32] Recent data from Toronto[18] and California[33] support correlations between both these types of organ damage and the high risk of mortality.

Additional interesting information regarding co-morbidity and death in SLE has been generated from studies focusing on hospitalization data. In one comparison of women with and without SLE who were hospitalized for a cardiovascular event, women with SLE were significantly younger at the time of their hospitalizations. Moreover, of those who died during hospitalization, the patients with SLE were appreciably younger than the comparator group of women who died during hospitalization. This was especially true for African-American women[34] and was interpreted by the authors as emphasizing again the high burden of cardiovascular disease in SLE, which heightens mortality risk.

Interestingly, one study suggested that suboptimal control of infectious complications was a major risk factor for death in patients with SLE undergoing admission into intensive care units.[35] Ward and associates[36-38] have also pointed out that outcomes for such patients were best if the care was provided at a tertiary center, where specialists were familiar with a relatively large volume of patients with SLE.

Renal Disease

Without a doubt, ESRF is also a major risk factor for death in SLE, as is true in the general population.[39] In the University of California Lupus Outcomes Study,[33] with concomitant adjustment for clinical and demographic information, the clinical covariate most associated with increasing risk for mortality was ESRF (HR 2.1, 95% CI 1.1 to 4.0). Based on data from the LUMINA (LUpus in MInorities: NAture versus nurture) multiethnic U.S. cohort, Alarcón's group noted that renal damage was actually the item in the SLICC/ACR damage index that was of greatest predictive value in terms of mortality,[40] although when the regression model included a variable capturing poverty, the finding was attenuated, suggesting that socioeconomic status (SES) may be as important a factor (or more so) or that SES and renal damage are greatly correlated, which, given what is already known of the effects of SES and outcomes in SLE, is likely important.

For patients with ESRF, predialysis co-morbidity (especially cardiovascular disease) is an important predictor of mortality.[41] In fact, even in the general population, cardiovascular disease is recognized as a key element of co-morbidity for patients on dialysis.[42] Thus specialists who care for patients with SLE and ESRF must carefully consider cardiac risk factors and treat these appropriately, although no specific data regarding the impact of such vigilance exist. It has been emphasized that even moderate uncontrolled hypertension worsens the clinical outcome in patients with ESRF, compared with those in the general population, which is often because of a heightened cardiac risk.[43]

Other Important Baseline Factors: Demographics, Organ Involvement, and Medications

Interesting data exist on the influence of demographics, organ involvement, and medication on mortality in SLE.

Demographics: Sex, Age, and Socioeconomic Status

Authors have suggested that mortality rates in SLE vary according to race and ethnicity, as discussed earlier. Considerable literature debating the unique contributions of sex, age, and SES (including income or education or both) also exists.

Several authors have suggested greater mortality in male than in female patients with SLE, when comparing survival rates by sex within the SLE population.[6,7] However, these analyses did not often calculate mortality rates relative to the general population. The longevity of men is generally lower than that of women; thus in a comparison of the effect of sex on mortality in patients with SLE, using a parameter such as the SMR is preferable. In fact, Urowitz and associates[18] in their 2008 publication demonstrated a trend for slightly lower sex- and age-specific SMRs for men with SLE (SMR of 3.96, 95% CI 2.90, 5.40) versus women (4.69, 95% CI 4.04, 5.45).

Similarly, the SMR provides a clearer understanding of which age group of patients with SLE has the greatest increased risk (compared with counterparts in the general population), since mortality rates in the general population increase with age. The study published in 2006 based on the SLICC international multisite cohort calculated a particularly high SMR of 19.2 (95% CI 14.7 to 4.7) for patients with SLE aged 16 to 24 years. In the study's multivariate hierarchical regression models to determine independent effects of the factors examined (e.g., sex, age group, SLE duration, calendar-year period of SLE diagnosis, country) on the relative SMR estimates among patients with SLE, both younger age and female sex were associated with increased risk of death among the patients with SLE, relative to the general population. The longitudinal cohort of 957 adult subjects with SLE from the University of California Lupus Outcomes Study[33] also generated evidence of a high relative risk for death in patients with SLE, aged 19 to 34 years, in whom the SMR was 20.4.

Regarding factors such as SES and education, the longitudinal cohort from the University of California Lupus Outcomes Study also showed that with concomitant adjustment for clinical and demographic information, the demographic covariates most associated with increasing risk for mortality included low education (HR 1.9, 95% CI 1.1 to 3.2).[33] Ward and others[44] also found that, among Caucasians, higher education levels were associated with lower lupus-related mortality.

Studenski and colleagues[45] found that the non-Caucasian race and SES both contributed independently to mortality. In fact, the overall improved survival in Caucasians versus African Americans in one report was primarily attributed to differences in SES, which was lower among the African Americans.[46] A publication from Kasitanon and colleagues[47] in Baltimore demonstrated that patients with an annual family income of less than $25,000 had poorer survival (adjusted HR = 1.7).

Organ Involvement

It seems intuitive that patients with the most severe forms of SLE would have the highest risk of mortality, and significant data substantiate that. In the large Toronto SLE cohort study published in 2000,[48] a multivariate Cox model examined the individual components of disease in predicting risk in SLE and showed that CNS and renal involvement, as well as pleurisy, fever, thrombocytopenia, and leukopenia, each significantly increased the risk of death. In contrast, rash and (perhaps unexpectedly) anti-DNA antibodies conferred relative protective effects. A study from Baltimore published in 2006[47] indicated that in analyses adjusting for demographics, hemolytic anemia and renal disease were significantly associated with poorer survival. When the two clinical characteristics in the same model were compared, hemolytic anemia was more significantly associated with mortality than renal disease.

In an inception cohort of 80 patients with SLE in the United Kingdom, the mean renal SLICC/ACR damage score at 1 year after diagnosis was a significant predictor of ESRF, and the mean pulmonary SLICC/ACR damage score at 1 year significantly predicted death within 10 years of diagnosis.[49] The outcome of 156 patients with lupus nephritis seen at University College Hospital London between 1975 and 2005[50] has been recently reported. The patients were divided into three groups, depending on the date of recognition of renal involvement (1975 to 1985, 1986 to 1995, or 1996 to 2005). The 5-year rate of ESRF remained constant; however, an increasing number of successful renal transplants were performed across the decades. The 5-year mortality rate decreased by 60% between the first and second decades but then remained stable over the third decade. These results suggest that the maximum benefit of conventional therapies may have been achieved and that further improvements may depend on the increasing availability of effective, nontoxic treatments.

In Germany, the 5-year survival rate in patients with SLE improved dramatically during the past four decades to 96.6% but the mortality rate in SLE was still nearly three times as high as age- and sex-matched population controls. At disease onset, risk factors for later death included nephritis and a reduction of creatinine clearance, as well as cardiac and CNS disease. As with other cohorts, an increase in the damage index of two or more points from the first to the third year of disease was the worst prognostic factor.[51]

Administrative data have been used by some researchers to determine predictors of deaths. Ward and others[52] studied in-hospital mortality from 1996 to 2000, focusing on patients with a principal diagnosis of SLE ($n = 3839$), identified from hospitalization data; nephritis and thrombocytopenia were strong predictors of mortality during the hospitalization. Earlier work by Ward and associates[53] emphasized CNS and renal involvement as factors predictive of mortality in SLE.

Other recent data examining clinical characteristics and mortality risk in SLE include a Mexican case-control autopsy study using data from 1958 to 1994, in which each deceased patient was matched by age, calendar-year period of SLE onset, and disease duration. The main clinical predictors of death included kidney, lung, and cardiac involvement, as well as severe thrombocytopenia. In this Mexican study, the overall severity index, based on modified SLEDAI scores,

was associated with mortality, as was the use of steroidal medications and the number of previous admissions and severe infections.[54]

As previously mentioned, despite the fact that survival in SLE has steadily improved overall, many of the deaths are still the result of SLE itself. The risks related to severe disease have been highlighted by studies of patients whose SLE has required hospitalization. In a study performed from 2004 to 2006 in Mexico, 41 patients with SLE requiring hospitalization for SLE and the result of other system and organ involvements (e.g., nephritis, thrombocytopenia, CNS crisis, vasculitis) were assessed. In this fairly young (mean age of 29, ±19 years) group of patients with relatively short mean disease duration (21 ± 9 months), an astounding 39% ($n = 16$) of patients died after a mean follow-up of 9.7 ± 6 months. Predictably, the survival was best (72%) in patients with lower SLEDAI scores (lower than 10) at their first admission and worst (50%) in patients with very high SLEDAI scores (21 or higher). Damage was associated with mortality risk, as was disease activity at the time of admission.[55] Recent data from Toronto[18] and California[33] support this correlation between renal organ damage and a very high risk of mortality.

Drug Use

Recent data from the SLICC inception cohort demonstrated that patients with SLE who died were also more than six times more likely than patients who did not die to have used corticosteroid medications and more than twice as likely to have had early exposure to immunosuppressive drugs (i.e., at enrollment, which was up to 15 months from SLE diagnosis).[24] Data from Mexico also emphasized the higher mortality risk in patients exposed to steroids; however, with these data, differentiating how much of the risk that seems to be conferred by steroid exposure is actually mortality risk related to active SLE is difficult if not impossible, since steroids are not used without active disease or infection, which are both associated with steroid dose and disease activity.[54]

Antimalarial use has been suggested as being protective against death. It remains unknown whether this finding in observational studies reflects some inherent biases; for example, antimalarial medications may be more often used in specific clinical scenarios such as rash, which has been shown (as noted earlier) to correlate inversely with the risk of death.[48,54] Box 57-1 provides a summary of key points regarding survival and mortality in SLE.

MORTALITY IN PEDIATRIC-ONSET SYSTEMIC LUPUS ERYTHEMATOSUS

Although SLE is often observed in women during childbearing years, 15% to 20% of all cases manifest in childhood and adolescence. Although the clinical signs and symptoms are similar to those in adult-onset SLE, pediatric-onset SLE has greater disease activity and severity, with accrual of greater irreversible organ damage in a short period.[56] Like adult-onset SLE, pediatric-onset SLE is more frequent in non-Caucasian populations, especially Hispanic, African-American, Asian, and First Nations populations.[56,57] Unfortunately, long-term outcomes of pediatric-onset SLE are not well described, because predominantly small, tertiary care center, referral-based cohorts have been reported with little more than 5 to 10 years of follow-up.

Moreover, pediatric-onset SLE may have a significantly greater mortality rate than adult-onset SLE. In a recent study,[58] an ethnically mixed pediatric-onset SLE cohort from the United States had a mortality rate of 19% after an average 6.8 years of disease, compared with 10% in the comparable adult-onset SLE cohort. Another recent and large study[26] used the national registers in Sweden and reported on more than 4700 patients with adult-onset SLE and an overall SMR of 3.6, but a significantly greater risk in young adulthood (SMR of 14.3). Despite the publications of these large cohort studies, which include small percentages of patients with pediatric-onset SLE, the majority of pediatric-onset SLE mortality studies are small cohorts that range in size from fewer than 20 to fewer than 220 patients, with most reporting single, tertiary care center retrospective cohorts. Therefore

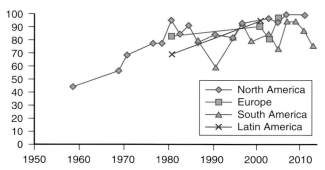

FIGURE 57-6 Calendar trends for 5-year survival in pediatric-onset SLE, stratified by region.

rates in childhood have improved over the past several decades, improved survival for patients with pediatric-onset SLE reflects the availability of both better therapies and medical care. Higher mortality rates are still reported from developing countries; in Thailand a recent report[71] of 213 patients demonstrated a 76% 5-year survival. Reports of short-term survival demonstrate some variation by geographic location (Figure 57-6). Few early reports exist from outside North America and Europe. The North American pediatric-onset SLE studies (see Figure 57-5) are from the United States ($n = 10$)[59-61,63,65,66,69,70,72,73] and Canada ($n = 2$).[67,68] European reports include one each from England,[64] Turkey,[74] as well as Serbia and Montenegro.[75] Included Asian studies originated from Taiwan ($n = 4$),[76-79] Thailand ($n = 2$),[71,80] Hong Kong ($n = 1$),[81] Singapore ($n = 1$),[82] and South Korea ($n = 1$).[83] Only one study was conducted in South America, a multicenter study from Chile that used survival analysis for patients observed during two time periods (50 patients between 1969 and 1980, 31 patients between 1981 and 2000).[84] Although the large GLADEL cohort includes patients with childhood-onset SLE, their analysis does not separate this group and is therefore not included in this text.[57] Only one study from south Asia (India) reports mortality data, with a 63% survival at a mean disease duration of 3.5 years for their cohort of 31 patients treated between 1991 and 2001.

Particular note should be made of a recent study that examined mortality rates in 48,895 patients observed by pediatric rheumatologists at multiple U.S. sites between 1990 and 2001. This study included 1393 patients with pediatric-onset SLE, based on the diagnosis given at their first visit to the pediatric rheumatologist. According to administrative data for death records, the observed 5-year mortality rate for pediatric-onset SLE was 99.5%, the 10-year mortality rate was 98.2%, and the observed SMR for pediatric-onset SLE was 3.0. These numbers contrast with those in other studies, although it is not known what percentage of this cohort had mild versus severe disease.[69]

Comparison of mortality rates over time shows that few pediatric rheumatologists practiced in the 1950s through 1970s; consequently, children with mild symptoms were not likely diagnosed or included in any published cohorts.

Long-Term Survival
Although early 10-year survival rates ranged from 28% to 85%,[61,65,66,72] recent reports demonstrate rates greater than 90% or even 95% in developed countries.[67,69,81] Beyond 10 years, the mortality rate of pediatric-onset SLE has not been well elucidated, because in the few studies that reported 15-year mortality rates (ranging from 28% to 92%), fewer than 20 patients were followed for 15 years.[65-67,70,72,81] Although the 15-year survival is now likely greater than 90%, patients with pediatric-onset SLE are transferred to adult rheumatologists between 16 and 21 years of age; thus accrual of long-term follow-up data poses a significant challenge. Premature cardiovascular disease is a significant morbidity factor and cause of mortality of young adults with SLE; thus patients with pediatric-onset SLE are also

generalizability of any one particular study to another pediatric-onset SLE population is limited.

Evidence of Improved Survival in Pediatric-Onset Systemic Lupus Erythematosus
As in adult-onset SLE, the significantly improved survival rate of patients with pediatric-onset SLE over the decades is an accepted statistic. The initial report by Cook and colleagues[59] from 1960 detailed 44% survival at 2 years' disease duration, whereas studies from the 1960s and 1970s witnessed improvement in the 5-year survival rate from 42% up to 78%.[60-62] The 1980s and 1990s saw significant gains[63-66] with 5-year pediatric-onset SLE survival climbing to the current rates of greater than 95%.[67-70] Although overall mortality

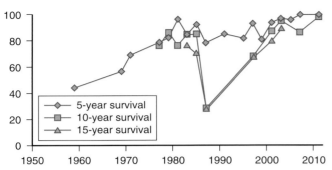

FIGURE 57-7 Calendar effects for 5-, 10-, and 15-year survival rates in pediatric-onset SLE for North America and Europe.

expected to follow a bimodal mortality distribution with the first peak early in the disease course and the second peak during young adulthood. However, as a result of the limitations of long-term study, this expectation has not yet been well demonstrated. Although short-term survival has reached a plateau, the survival rates of patients with pediatric-onset SLE with either renal and CNS involvement (or both) are lower, as is discussed in the next section. Figure 57-7 illustrates the changing survival rates over the decades.

Causes of Death and Risk Factors for Death in Pediatric-Onset Systemic Lupus Erythematosus

Although the cause of death of a patient with pediatric-onset SLE is often multifactorial, the most common reasons include infection, renal failure, and severe SLE disease flares that may encompass neuropsychiatric disease, thrombotic events, cardiopulmonary disease, and severe gastrointestinal events. Few studies have specifically examined risk factors for mortality in pediatric-onset SLE, although renal failure and neuropsychiatric disease are believed to be important.[78,79] Lower SES also likely plays a role, along with the interconnected factors of lower educational status and African-American ethnicity. What is most notable is that childhood-onset SLE is, on its own, an independent mortality risk. In the University of California Lupus Outcomes Study,[33] during the median follow-up period of 48 months, 9 deaths occurred in 98 patients with pediatric-onset SLE (12.5%). With adjustment for age, disease duration, and other covariates, pediatric-onset SLE (versus adult-onset SLE) was independently associated with an increased mortality risk (HR 3.1, 95% CI 1.3 to 7.3).

In addition to a higher prevalence of renal disease in pediatric-onset SLE, compared with adult-onset SLE (up to 80% versus approximately 50%), a greater proportion of patients with pediatric-onset SLE develop diffuse proliferative glomerulonephritis (DPGN), which carries the greatest risk of developing ESRF. Even more concerning is the fact that ESRF is reported in 15% to 50% of patients with pediatric-onset SLE in the limited reports with 10 and 15 years of follow-up.[67,73,76,81] In the United States, a recent analysis of the U.S. Renal Data System (USRDS)[39] observed a 20% mortality rate in 171 patients, 18 years old or younger, with pediatric-onset SLE and ESRF during the period between 1990 and 2004, which carried a threefold greater risk of death, compared with other pediatric patients with ESRF. Almost 75% of the 29 deaths were attributed to cardiovascular disease, and the remaining 25% were attributed to infection (e.g., septicemia). A second study of the USRDS, conducted during the years of 1995 and 2006, identified 583 patients with pediatric-onset SLE associated with ESRF. Of the patients in this study, 51% were African American, and 22% died within 5 years. Mortality was almost double among African-American versus Caucasian patients (odds ratio (OR) 1.83, $P < 0.001$).[85] Consequently, although survival rates of pediatric-onset SLE cohorts that include patients with lupus nephritis are lower than those cohorts that include patients without lupus nephritis, patients with DPGN, in particular, have the greatest

Box 57-2 Mortality in Pediatric-Onset Systemic Lupus Erythematosus

Although long-term outcomes of pediatric-onset SLE are not well described, pediatric-onset SLE may have a significantly greater mortality rate than adult-onset SLE. However, as in adult-onset SLE, it is accepted that survival of patients with pediatric-onset SLE has significantly improved over time. Although the cause of death of a patient with pediatric-onset SLE is often multifactorial, the most common reasons include infection, renal failure, and severe SLE disease flares that may encompass neuropsychiatric disease, thrombotic events, cardiopulmonary disease, and severe gastrointestinal events.

Strategies for Improved Mortality Outcomes in Systemic Lupus Erythematosus
Several domains exist in which improvements in care might be focused; disease control is one of these domains. However, because some have found a positive correlation between the use of immunosuppressive drugs and mortality, the risks and benefits of aggressive treatment must also be considered. Antimalarial medications represent an important option in the drug armamentarium, and heightened attention has been given to improving cardiac risk factors, in the hopes of improving outcomes (including mortality) in SLE. In addition to advances in the diagnosis and treatment of severe infections, vaccinations against influenza viruses, *Streptococcus pneumoniae, Haemophilus influenzae,* and other viral and bacterial infections could represent a major step toward reducing morbidity and mortality associated with infections. Finally, the importance of socioeconomic status cannot be ignored. Although this element is difficult for physicians to tackle, eliminating health disparities in lupus remains an important challenge.

risk of death (in addition to the greatest risk of ESRF), with 5-year survival rates ranging between 67% and 94%.[67,74,76,80]

No systematic analysis of infection as a cause of death in pediatric-onset SLE has been conducted. Certainly, infection is recognized as the ultimate cause of death in more than 50% of deaths in pediatric-onset SLE and these severe infections occur in the setting of immune system dysfunction, especially in patients with ESRF, immunosuppressive medications, and exposure to drug-resistant pathogens during hospital and clinic visits. Box 57-2 provides a summary of the key points regarding mortality in pediatric-onset SLE.

STRATEGIES FOR IMPROVED MORTALITY OUTCOMES IN SYSTEMIC LUPUS ERYTHEMATOSUS

Several domains exist in which improvements in care might be focused; disease control is one of these domains. Urowitz and colleagues[18] showed that over the same interval during which improved survival was documented, average mean disease activity scores also decreased. Mortality was linked to average mean disease activity and organ damage in that study.

Does this mean that aggressive drug treatment may prolong life? The literature is unclear on this point. Urowitz and associates[18] actually found a positive correlation between the use of immunosuppressive drugs and mortality, even with attempts to control analysis for disease activity in patients who were administered these drugs.

Furthermore, co-morbidity may be related to drugs, particularly steroid treatment. Urowitz and colleagues,[18] using data from their Toronto cohort, showed that despite decreasing disease activity, organ damage (e.g., CAD) was on the rise at the same time. One interpretation might be that organ damage such as CAD might be aggravated by steroids. Obviously, a play-off exists between short- and long-term risks and benefits; if patients, as a result of proper treatment, do not die early from active SLE, then they have the opportunity to develop long-term outcomes (e.g., CAD).

Pineau and others[86] have also shown that increasing drug use did not necessarily decrease organ damage over time, although that study did not specifically examine mortality. Although SLE, itself, apparently is still an important cause of death, it remains true that most patients will die of co-morbidity events, particularly CAD, not of SLE. In their large single-center study, Urowitz and others[18] found a strong link between CAD and mortality; this link has been borne out in more recent reports.[24]

The protective effects against mortality related to antimalarial medications (i.e., hydroxychloroquine and the less frequently used chloroquine) seen in observational studies may be, in part, artifact, because these drugs have been traditionally administered to patients with the least severe disease activity; however, considering the very good quality data that suggest long-term antimalarial medications may prevent a relapse in SLE,[87] these drugs represent an important option in the drug armamentarium.

In general, lupus specialists continue to advocate for heightened attention to improving cardiac risk factors in the hopes of improving outcomes (including mortality) in SLE. This advocacy makes sense, considering the data from decades ago that highlighted cardiac risk factors (e.g., hypertension) as independent predictors of mortality.[6]

In addition to the advances in the diagnosis and treatment of severe infections, vaccination against influenza viruses, *Streptococcus pneumoniae, Haemophilus influenzae,* and other viral and bacterial infections, could represent a major step toward reducing morbidity and mortality associated with infections. These vaccinations are believed to be safe and relatively efficacious in SLE.[88] Recent data specifically support the safety and efficacy of H1N1 influenza vaccination in SLE and related diseases.[89,90] When high-dose steroids are used along with other immunosuppressive drugs, prophylaxis against pneumocystis may be of value. Prompt recognition and treatment of infectious complications is additionally important. Here, too, the interplay between disease activity and drug use is important. The association of steroids with infection risk is well known; consequently, emphasis should be placed on reducing steroids as soon as possible. Pulse cyclophosphamide, still useful for some forms of severe SLE, is unfortunately associated with the greatest risks of serious infection, which is one reason alternate strategies—for example, reducing the dose or using alternative drugs such as mycophenolate—are desirable, but again, the risks and benefits need to be weighed. At the same time, it should be kept in mind that active disease with leukopenia and low complement can increase the risk of infection, even without the use of immunosuppressive agents.

The need for hospitalization is a marker for the most severe forms of SLE; for hospitalized patients the risk of later mortality should not be discounted. Instead, physicians should probably take this event as a reminder of the need for very diligent, specialized care. Ward[91] previously showed that patients with SLE in the United States without private insurance had particularly higher risks of mortality if hospitalized at facilities that did not have much specialized experience.

Finally, in an effort to improve outcomes in SLE, the importance of SES cannot be ignored, but this element is difficult for physicians to tackle. Perhaps the best physicians can do on this front is attempt to make available to patients with low SES as many resources and as much education (especially education related to their disease) as possible. Close attention should also probably be paid to ways to heighten adherence, which could be particularly problematic in patients with low SES and low education.[92,93] Here, effective communication is vital.[94,95]

A related issue is access to health care issues. A better understanding of patient beliefs about disease and drugs is needed, which may be important in dealing with some ethnicity and racial issues.[96-98] For additional thoughts on this challenge, readers should consult resources such as the "Lupus Initiative," a new web site on eliminating health disparities in lupus (http://www.thelupusinitiative.org).

References

1. Merrell M, Shulman Le: Determination of prognosis in chronic disease, illustrated by systemic lupus erythematosus. *J Chronic Dis* 1(1):12–32, 1955.
2. Borchers AT, Keen CL, Shoenfeld Y, et al: Surviving the butterfly and the wolf: mortality trends in systemic lupus erythematosus. *Autoimmun Rev* 3(6):423–453, 2004.
3. Trager J, Ward MM: Mortality and causes of death in systemic lupus erythematosus. *Curr Opin Rheumatol* 13(5):345–351, 2001.
4. Uramoto KM, Michet CJ, Jr, et al: Trends in the incidence and mortality of systemic lupus erythematosus, 1950-1992. *Arthritis Rheum* 42(1):46–50, 1999.
5. Therneau TM, Offord J: Expected survival based on hazard rates (updated). 63:1-26, 1999. Rochester, MN, Mayo Clinic–Section of Biostatistics. Available at http://mayoresearch.mayo.edu/mayo/research/biostat/upload/63.pdf.
6. Seleznick MJ, Fries JF: Variables associated with decreased survival in systemic lupus erythematosus. *Semin Arthritis Rheum* 21(2):73–80, 1991.
7. Kaslow RA, Masi AT: Age, sex, and race effects on mortality from systemic lupus erythematosus in the United States. *Arthritis Rheum* 21(4):473–479, 1978.
8. Reveille JD, Bartolucci A, Alarcón GS: Prognosis in systemic lupus erythematosus. Negative impact of increasing age at onset, black race, and thrombocytopenia, as well as causes of death. *Arthritis Rheum* 33(1):37–48, 1990.
9. Alarcón GS, McGwin G, Jr, Bastian HM, et al: Systemic lupus erythematosus in three ethnic groups. VII [correction of VIII]. Predictors of early mortality in the LUMINA cohort. LUMINA study group. *Arthritis Rheum* 45(2):191–202, 2001.
10. Borchers AT, Naguwa SM, Shoenfeld Y, et al: The geoepidemiology of systemic lupus erythematosus. *Autoimmun Rev* 9(5):A277–A287, 2010.
11. Walsh SJ, Algert C, Gregorio DI, et al: Divergent racial trends in mortality from systemic lupus erythematosus. *J Rheumatol* 22(9):1663–1668, 1995.
12. Calvo-Alén J, Alarcón GS, Campbell R, Jr, et al: Lack of recording of systemic lupus erythematosus in the death certificates of lupus patients. *Rheumatology (Oxford)* 44(9):1186–1189, 2005.
13. Korbet SM, Schwartz MM, Evans J, et al: Severe lupus nephritis: racial differences in presentation and outcome. *J Am Soc Nephrol* 18(1):244–254, 2007.
14. Fang J, Madhavan S, Cohen H, et al: Differential mortality in New York City (1988-1992). Part one: Excess mortality among non-Hispanic blacks. *Bull N Y Acad Med* 72(2):470–482, 1995.
15. Caetano R: Alcohol-related health disparities and treatment-related epidemiological findings among whites, blacks, and Hispanics in the United States. *Alcohol Clin Exp Res* 27(8):1337–1339, 2003.
16. Kumar K, Chambers S, Gordon C: Challenges of ethnicity in SLE. *Best Pract Res Clin Rheumatol* 23(4):549–561, 2009.
17. [No authors listed] A statistical profile on the health of First Nations in Canada: determinants of health, 1999 to 2003. Cat.: H34-193/1-2008, 1-62. 2009. Canada, Minister of Health Canada. Available at http://www.hc-sc.gc.ca/fniah-spnia/alt_formats/fnihb-dgspni/pdf/pubs/aborig-autoch/2009-stats-profil-eng.pdf.
18. Urowitz MB, Gladman DD, Tom BD, et al: Changing patterns in mortality and disease outcomes for patients with systemic lupus erythematosus. *J Rheumatol* 35(11):2152–2158, 2008.
19. Bernatsky S, Boivin J, Manzi S, et al: Mortality in systemic lupus erythematosus. *Arthritis Rheum* 54(8):2550–2557, 2006.
20. Ippolito A, Petri M: An update on mortality in systemic lupus erythematosus. *Clin Exp Rheumatol* 26(5 Suppl 51):S72–S79, 2008.
21. Estes D, Christian CL: The natural history of systemic lupus erythematosus by prospective analysis. *Medicine (Baltimore)* 50(2):85–95, 1971.
22. Mok CC, To CH, Ho LY, et al: Incidence and mortality of systemic lupus erythematosus in a southern Chinese population, 2000-2006. *J Rheumatol* 35(10):1978–1982, 2008.
23. Mok CC, Kwok CL, Ho LY, et al: Life expectancy, standardized mortality ratios, and causes of death in six rheumatic diseases in Hong Kong, China. *Arthritis Rheum* 63(5):1182–1189, 2011.
24. Urowitz MB, Gladman D, Ibanez D, et al: Mortality in a multinational inception cohort of SLE [Abstract]. *Arthritis Rheum* (Suppl):S2240, 2011.
25. Manzi S, Meilahn EN, Rairie JE, et al: Age-specific incidence rates of myocardial infarction and angina in women with systemic lupus erythematosus: comparison with the Framingham Study. *Am J Epidemiol* 145(5):408–415, 1997.
26. Björnådal L, Yin L, Granath F, et al: Cardiovascular disease a hazard despite improved prognosis in patients with systemic lupus

erythematosus: results from a Swedish population based study 1964-95. *J Rheumatol* 31(4):713–719, 2004.

27. Roman MJ, Shanker BA, Davis A, et al: Prevalence and correlates of accelerated atherosclerosis in systemic lupus erythematosus. *N Engl J Med* 349(25):2399–2406, 2003.

28. Dubois EL: Systemic lupus erythematosus: recent advances in its diagnosis and treatment. *Ann Intern Med* 45(2):163–184, 1956.

29. Abu-Shakra M, Urowitz MB, Gladman DD, et al: Mortality studies in systemic lupus erythematosus. Results from a single center. I. Causes of death. *J Rheumatol* 22(7):1259–1264, 1995.

30. Bernatsky S, Clarke A, Gladman DD, et al: Mortality related to cerebrovascular disease in systemic lupus erythematosus. *Lupus* 15(12):835–839, 2006.

31. Urowitz MB, Gladman DD: The SLICC inception cohort for atherosclerosis. *Curr Rheumatol Rep* 10(4):281–285, 2008.

32. Elie C, De RY, Jais J, et al: Appraising relative and excess mortality in population-based studies of chronic diseases such as end-stage renal disease. *Clin Epidemiol* 3:157–169, 2011.

33. Hersh AO, Trupin L, Yazdany J, et al: Childhood-onset disease as a predictor of mortality in an adult cohort of patients with systemic lupus erythematosus. *Arthritis Care Res (Hoboken)* 62(8):1152–1159, 2010.

34. Scalzi LV, Hollenbeak CS, Wang L: Racial disparities in age at time of cardiovascular events and cardiovascular-related death in patients with systemic lupus erythematosus. *Arthritis Rheum* 62(9):2767–2775, 2010.

35. Feng PH, Lin SM, Yu CT, et al: Inadequate antimicrobial treatment for nosocomial infection is a mortality risk factor for systemic lupus erythematous patients admitted to intensive care unit. *Am J Med Sci* 340(1): 64–68, 2010.

36. Ward MM: Association between physician volume and in-hospital mortality in patients with systemic lupus erythematosus. *Arthritis Rheum* 52(6):1646–1654, 2005.

37. Ward MM: Hospital experience and expected mortality in patients with systemic lupus erythematosus: a hospital level analysis. *J Rheumatol* 27(9):2146–2151, 2000.

38. Ward MM: Hospital experience and mortality in patients with systemic lupus erythematosus. *Arthritis Rheum* 42(5):891–898, 1999.

39. Sule S, Fivush B, Neu A, et al: Increased risk of death in pediatric and adult patients with ESRD secondary to lupus. *Pediatr Nephrol* 26(1):93–98, 2011.

40. Danila MI, Pons-Estel GJ, Zhang J, et al: Renal damage is the most important predictor of mortality within the damage index: data from LUMINA LXIV, a multiethnic US cohort. *Rheumatology (Oxford)* 48(5):542–545, 2009.

41. Liang CC, Lin HH, Wang IK, et al: Influence of predialysis comorbidity and damage accrual on mortality in lupus patients treated with peritoneal dialysis. *Lupus* 19(10):1210–1218, 2010.

42. Sidhu MS, Dellsperger KC: Cardiovascular problems in dialysis patients: impact on survival. *Adv Perit Dial* 26:47–52, 2010.

43. Foley RN, Parfrey PS, Harnett JD, et al: Impact of hypertension on cardiomyopathy, morbidity and mortality in end-stage renal disease. *Kidney Int* 49(5):1379–1385, 1996.

44. Ward MM: Education level and mortality in systemic lupus erythematosus (SLE): evidence of underascertainment of deaths due to SLE in ethnic minorities with low education levels. *Arthritis Rheum* 51(4):616–624, 2004.

45. Studenski S, Allen NB, Caldwell DS, et al: Survival in systemic lupus erythematosus. A multivariate analysis of demographic factors. *Arthritis Rheum* 30(12):1326–1332, 1987.

46. Ward MM, Pyun E, Studenski S: Long-term survival in systemic lupus erythematosus. Patient characteristics associated with poorer outcomes. *Arthritis Rheum* 38(2):274–283, 1995.

47. Kasitanon N, Magder LS, Petri M: Predictors of survival in systemic lupus erythematosus. *Medicine (Baltimore)* 85(3):147–156, 2006.

48. Cook RJ, Gladman DD, Pericak D, et al: Prediction of short term mortality in systemic lupus erythematosus with time dependent measures of disease activity. *J Rheumatol* 27(8):1892–1895, 2000.

49. Stoll T, Seifert B, Isenberg DA: SLICC/ACR damage index is valid, and renal and pulmonary organ scores are predictors of severe outcome in patients with systemic lupus erythematosus. *Br J Rheumatol* 35(3):248–254, 1996.

50. Croca SC, Rodrigues T, Isenberg DA: Assessment of a lupus nephritis cohort over a 30-year period. *Rheumatology (Oxford)* 50(8):1424–1430, 2011.

51. Manger K, Manger B, Repp R, et al: Definition of risk factors for death, end stage renal disease, and thromboembolic events in a monocentric cohort of 338 patients with systemic lupus erythematosus. *Ann Rheum Dis* 61(12):1065–1070, 2002.

52. Ward MM, Pajevic S, Dreyfuss J, et al: Short-term prediction of mortality in patients with systemic lupus erythematosus: classification of outcomes using random forests. *Arthritis Rheum* 55(1):74–80, 2006.

53. Ward MM, Pyun E, Studenski S: Mortality risks associated with specific clinical manifestations of systemic lupus erythematosus. *Arch Intern Med* 156(12):1337–1344, 1996.

54. Hernández-Cruz B, Tapia N, Villa-Romero AR, et al: Risk factors associated with mortality in systemic lupus erythematosus. A case-control study in a tertiary care center in Mexico City. *Clin Exp Rheumatol* 19(4):395–401, 2001.

55. Zonana-Nacach A, Yanez P, Jiménez-Balderas FJ, et al: Disease activity, damage and survival in Mexican patients with acute severe systemic lupus erythematosus. *Lupus* 16(12):997–1000, 2007.

56. Kamphuis S, Silverman ED: Prevalence and burden of pediatric-onset systemic lupus erythematosus. *Nat Rev Rheumatol* 6(9):538–546, 2010.

57. Pons-Estel BA, Catoggio LJ, Cardiel MH, et al: The GLADEL multinational Latin American prospective inception cohort of 1,214 patients with systemic lupus erythematosus: ethnic and disease heterogeneity among "Hispanics." *Medicine (Baltimore)* 83(1):1–17, 2004.

58. Tucker LB, Uribe AG, Fernandez M, et al: Adolescent onset of lupus results in more aggressive disease and worse outcomes: results of a nested matched case-control study within LUMINA, a multiethnic US cohort (LUMINA LVII). *Lupus* 17(4):314–322, 2008.

59. Cook CD, Wedgwood RJ, Craig JM, et al: Systemic lupus erythematosus. Description of 37 cases in children and a discussion of endocrine therapy in 32 of the cases. *Pediatrics* 26:570–585, 1960.

60. Meislin AG, Rothfield N: Systemic lupus erythematosus in childhood. Analysis of 42 cases, with comparative data on 200 adult cases followed concurrently. *Pediatrics* 42(1):37–49, 1968.

61. Walravens PA, Chase HP: The prognosis of childhood systemic lupus erythematosus. *Am J Dis Child* 130(9):929–933, 1976.

62. Fish AJ, Blau EB, Westberg NG, et al: Systemic lupus erythematosus within the first two decades of life. *Am J Med* 62(1):99–117, 1977.

63. Abeles M, Urman JD, Weinstein A, et al: Systemic lupus-erythematosus in the younger patient: survival studies. *J Rheumatol* 7(4):515–522, 1980.

64. Caeiro F, Michielson FM, Bernstein R, et al: Systemic lupus erythematosus in childhood. *Ann Rheum Dis* 40(4):325–331, 1981.

65. Platt JL, Burke BA, Fish AJ, et al: Systemic lupus erythematosus in the first two decades of life. *Am J Kidney Dis* 2(1 Suppl 1):212–222, 1982.

66. Glidden RS, Mantzouranis EC, Borel Y: Systemic lupus erythematosus in childhood: clinical manifestations and improved survival in fifty-five patients. *Clin Immunol Immunopathol* 29(2):196–210, 1983.

67. Hagelberg S, Lee Y, Bargman J, et al: Longterm followup of childhood lupus nephritis. *J Rheumatol* 29(12):2635–2642, 2002.

68. Miettunen PM, Ortiz-Alvarez O, Petty RE, et al: Gender and ethnic origin have no effect on longterm outcome of childhood-onset systemic lupus erythematosus. *J Rheumatol* 31(8):1650–1654, 2004.

69. Hashkes PJ, Wright BM, Lauer MS, et al: Mortality outcomes in pediatric rheumatology in the US. *Arthritis Rheum* 62(2):599–608, 2010.

70. Candell Chalom E, Periera B, Cole R, et al: Educational, vocational and socioeconomic status and quality of life in adults with childhood-onset systemic lupus erythematosus. *Pediatr Rheumatol Online J* 2:207–226, 2004.

71. Vachvanichsanong P, Dissaneewate P, McNeil E: Twenty-two years' experience with childhood-onset SLE in a developing country: are outcomes similar to developed countries? *Arch Dis Child* 96(1):44–49, 2011.

72. McCurdy DK, Lehman TJA, Bernstein B, et al: Lupus nephritis: prognostic factors in children. *Pediatrics* 89(2):240–246, 1992.

73. Baqi N, Moazami S, Singh A, et al: Lupus nephritis in children: a longitudinal study of prognostic factors and therapy. *J Am Soc Nephrol* 7(6):924–929, 1996.

74. Emre S, Bilge I, Sirin A, et al: Lupus nephritis in children: prognostic significance of clinicopathological findings. *Nephron* 87(2):118–126, 2001.

75. Bogdanović R, Nikolić V, Pasić S, et al: Lupus nephritis in childhood: a review of 53 patients followed at a single center. *Pediatr Nephrol* 19(1): 36–44, 2004.

76. Yang LY, Chen WP, Lin CY: Lupus nephritis in children—a review of 167 patients. *Pediatrics* 94(3):335–340, 1994.

77. Lo JT, Tsai MJ, Wang LH, et al: Sex differences in pediatric systemic lupus erythematosus: a retrospective analysis of 135 cases. *J Microbiol Immunol Infect* 32(3):173–178, 1999.

78. Wang LC, Yang YH, Lu MY, et al: Retrospective analysis of mortality and morbidity of pediatric systemic lupus erythematosus in the past two decades. *J Microbiol Immunol Infect* 36(3):203–208, 2003.

79. Yu HH, Lee JH, Wang LC, et al: Neuropsychiatric manifestations in pediatric systemic lupus erythematosus: a 20-year study. *Lupus* 15(10):651–657, 2006.

80. Pattaragarn A, Sumboonnanonda A, Parichatikanond P, et al: Systemic lupus erythematosus in Thai children: clinicopathologic findings and outcome in 82 patients. *J Med Assoc Thai* 88(Suppl 8):S232–S241, 2005.

81. Wong SN, Tse KC, Lee TL, et al: Lupus nephritis in Chinese children—a territory-wide cohort study in Hong Kong. *Pediatr Nephrol* 21(8):1104–1112, 2006.

82. Lee BW, Yap HK, Yip WCL, et al: A 10 year review of systemic lupus-erythematosus in Singapore children. *Aust Paediatr J* 23(3):163–165, 1987.

83. Lee BS, Cho HY, Kim EJ, et al: Clinical outcomes of childhood lupus nephritis: a single center's experience. *Pediatr Nephrol* 22(2):222–231, 2007.

84. González B, Hernández P, Olguin H, et al: Changes in the survival of patients with systemic lupus erythematosus in childhood: 30 years experience in Chile. *Lupus* 14(11):918–923, 2005.

85. Hiraki LT, Lu B, Alexander SR, et al: End-stage renal disease due to lupus nephritis among children in the US, 1995-2006. *Arthritis Rheum* 63(7):1988–1997, 2011.

86. Pineau CA, Bernatsky S, Abrahamowicz M, et al: A comparison of damage accrual across different calendar periods in systemic lupus erythematosus patients. *Lupus* 15(9):590–594, 2006.

87. Tsakonas E, Joseph L, Esdaile JM, et al: A long-term study of hydroxychloroquine withdrawal on exacerbations in systemic lupus erythematosus. The Canadian Hydroxychloroquine Study Group. *Lupus* 7(2):80–85, 1998.

88. Millet A, Decaux O, Perlat A, et al: Systemic lupus erythematosus and vaccination. *Eur J Intern Med* 20(3):236–241, 2009.

89. Lu CC, Wang YC, Lai JH, et al: A/H1N1 influenza vaccination in patients with systemic lupus erythematosus: safety and immunity. *Vaccine* 29(3):444–450, 2011.

90. Ori E, Sharon A, Ella M, et al: The efficacy and safety of vaccination against pandemic 2009 influenza a (H1N1) virus among patients with rheumatic diseases. *Arthritis Care Res (Hoboken)* 63(7):1062–1067, 2011.

91. Ward MM: Hospital experience and mortality in patients with systemic lupus erythematosus: Which patients benefit most from treatment at highly experienced hospitals? *J Rheumatol* 29(6):1198–1206, 2002.

92. Chambers S, Raine R, Rahman A, et al: Factors influencing adherence to medications in a group of patients with systemic lupus erythematosus in Jamaica. *Lupus* 17(8):761–769, 2008.

93. Garcia-Gonzalez A, Richardson M, Garcia Popa-Lisseanu M, et al: Treatment adherence in patients with rheumatoid arthritis and systemic lupus erythematosus. *Clin Rheumatol* 27(7):883–889, 2008.

94. Chambers SA, Raine R, Rahman A, et al: Why do patients with systemic lupus erythematosus take or fail to take their prescribed medications? A qualitative study in a UK cohort. *Rheumatology (Oxford)* 48(3):266–271, 2009.

95. Koneru S, Kocharla L, Higgins GC, et al: Adherence to medications in systemic lupus erythematosus. *J Clin Rheumatol* 14(4):195–201, 2008.

96. Kumar K, Gordon C, Barry R, et al: "It's like taking poison to kill poison but I have to get better": a qualitative study of beliefs about medicines in rheumatoid arthritis and systemic lupus erythematosus patients of South Asian origin. *Lupus* 20(8):837–844, 2011.

97. Kumar K, Gordon C, Toescu V, et al: Beliefs about medicines in patients with rheumatoid arthritis and systemic lupus erythematosus: a comparison between patients of South Asian and White British origin. *Rheumatology (Oxford)* 47(5):690–697, 2008.

98. Demas KL, Costenbader KH: Disparities in lupus care and outcomes. *Curr Opin Rheumatol* 21(2):102–109, 2009.

Lupus Resource Materials

Compiled by Jenny Thorn Palter on Behalf of the Lupus Foundation of America, Inc.

WHAT ORGANIZATIONS PROVIDE PATIENT SUPPORT IN THE UNITED STATES?

Many such organizations exist. Only those with a budget of over $1 million are listed.

Lupus Foundation of America, Inc. (LFA)

2000 L. St. NW, Suite 410, Washington, DC 20036; (202) 349-1155, toll-free (800) 558-0121; e-mail: lupusinfo@lupus.org for health education information; info@lupus.org for general information; lupusnow@lupus.org for magazine information; web site: www. lupus.org.

The LFA is the nation's foremost nonprofit voluntary health organization dedicated to finding the causes of and the cure for lupus and to providing support, services, and hope to all people affected by lupus. The LFA and its network of chapters, branches, and support groups conduct programs of research, education, and advocacy. The LFA publishes patient education materials and a national magazine, *Lupus Now.*

Arthritis Foundation

PO Box 7669, Atlanta, GA 30357; toll-free (800) 283-7800; web site: www.arthritis.org for general information and for magazine information.

The Arthritis Foundation is the only national not-for-profit organization that supports the more than 100 types of arthritis and related conditions. With multiple service points located throughout the country, the Foundation helps people take control of arthritis by providing public health education, pursuing public policy and legislation, and conducting evidence-based programs to improve the quality of life for those living with arthritis. The Arthritis Foundation publishes patient education materials and a national magazine, *Arthritis Today.*

American Autoimmune Related Diseases Association (AARDA)

National office: 22100 Gratiot Ave. E., Detroit, MI 48021; (586) 776-3900; *Washington D.C. office:* 750 17th Street, NW; Suite 1100, Washington, DC 20006; (202) 466-8511; literature request line (800) 598-4668; web site: www.aarda.org.

The AARDA is the only national nonprofit health agency dedicated to bringing a national focus to autoimmunity, the major cause of serious chronic diseases. The AARDA publishes a national newsletter, *InFocus.*

Sle Lupus Foundation

New York City office: 330 Seventh Ave., Suite 1701, New York, NY 10001; (212) 685-4118; toll-free (800) 74LUPUS (5-8787); e-mail: lupus@lupusny.org; web site: www.lupusny.org. *Los Angeles office:* 8383 Wilshire Blvd., Suite 232, Beverly Hills, CA, 90211; (310) 657-LOOP (5667); email: info@lupusla.org; web site: www.lupusla.org.

With headquarters in New York City and Los Angeles, the Foundation promotes early diagnosis of lupus and provides support to people with the illness—especially in disadvantaged neighborhoods of New York City and Los Angeles—through public service campaigns, public education programs, and community outreach efforts.

IN ADDITION TO THESE ORGANIZATIONS, WHERE CAN RELIABLE INFORMATION ABOUT LUPUS BE OBTAINED?

American College of Rheumatology (ACR) and the Association of Rheumatology Health Professionals (ARHP)

2200 Lake Boulevard NE, Atlanta, GA 30319; (404) 633-3777; web site for both organizations: www.rheumatology.org.

The ACR is the professional organization to which nearly all U.S. and many international rheumatologists belong. The ARHP is a division of the ACR.

National Institute of Arthritis and Musculoskeletal and Skin Diseases (NIAMS), National Institutes of Health

31 Center Drive, Room 4C02, MSC 2350, Rockville Pike, Bethesda, MD 20892. NIAMS Information Clearinghouse, National Institutes of Health, 1 AMS Circle, Bethesda, MD 20892; (301) 495-4484, toll-free (877) 22NIAMS; TTY (301) 565-2966; e-mail: NIAMSInfo @mail.nih.gov; web site: www.niams.nih.gov.

The NIAMS funds lupus research at the Bethesda campus and elsewhere in the country and also offers a wide variety of free information on rheumatic diseases, including lupus. (Information is also available in Spanish.)

IN ADDITION TO THESE ORGANIZATIONS, WHAT OTHER ORGANIZATIONS FUND LUPUS RESEARCH?

Many such organizations exist. The following list is restricted to those that give more than $1 million a year to lupus-related research at more than one institution.

Lupus Foundation of America, Inc. (LFA)

2000 L. St. NW, Suite 410, Washington, DC 20036; (202) 349-1155, toll-free (800) 558-0121; web site: www.lupus.org/research.

The LFA provides direct funding for researchers at universities and medical institutions nationwide through its National Research Program, *Bringing Down the Barriers,* which is dedicated to addressing research issues that have for decades obstructed basic biomedical, clinical, epidemiologic, behavioral, and translational lupus research.

Alliance for Lupus Research

28 West 44th Street, Suite 501, New York, NY 10036; (212) 218-2840, toll-free (800) 867-1743; e-mail: info@lupusresearch.org; web site: www.lupusresearch.org.

The Alliance for Lupus Research was founded in 1999 with the mission to support research into the cause, cure, treatment, and prevention of systemic lupus erythematosus.

Lupus Research Institute

330 Seventh Avenue, Suite 1701, New York, NY 10001; (212) 812-9881; e-mail: lupus@lupusresearchinstitute.org; web site: www.lupusresearchinstitute.org.

The Lupus Research Institute fosters and supports the highest-ranked new science to prevent, treat, and cure lupus.

ACR Research and Education Foundation (REF)

2200 Lake Boulevard NE, Atlanta, GA 30319; (404) 633-3777; e-mail: ref@rheumatology.org; web site: www.rheumatology.org/ref.

REF, the research funding arm of the American College of Rheumatology (ACR), promotes and advances the field of rheumatology by funding research, training, and education opportunities for clinicians, students, health professionals, researchers, and academic institutions.

HOW CAN I FIND OUT ABOUT LUPUS SUPPORT OUTSIDE OF THE UNITED STATES?
Lupus Canada

3555 14th Avenue, Unit #3, Markham, Ontario L3R 0H5, Canada; (905) 513-0004, toll-free (800) 661-1468; e-mail: info@lupuscanada.org; web site: www.lupuscanada.org (in French and English).

Lupus Canada is Canada's national voluntary organization dedicated to improving the lives of people living with lupus through advocacy, education, public awareness, support, and research.

Lupus Europe

Web site: www.lupus-europe.org.

Lupus Europe is the umbrella association of 23 national lupus groups from 21 member countries throughout Europe. Affiliate groups are located in Belgium (Flemish), Belgium (French), Cyprus, Denmark, Finland, France, Germany, Hungary, Iceland, Ireland, Italy, Malta, the Netherlands, Norway, Portugal, Romania, Slovenia, Spain, Sweden, Switzerland, and the United Kingdom.

Lupus UK

St. James House, Eastern Road, Romford, Essex RM1 3NH England; (00 44) (0) 1708-731251, e-mail: headoffice@lupusuk.org.uk; web site: www.lupusuk.org.uk.

Lupus UK supports people with systemic and discoid lupus, and assists those approaching diagnosis.

Pan American League of Associations for Rheumatology

E-mail: panlar@panlar.org; web site: www.panlar.org.

The Pan American League is made up of the scientific societies of rheumatology health professionals and rheumatic patient associations of all countries in the Americas.

HOW CAN I FIND OUT ABOUT ORGANIZATIONS THAT SERVE PATIENTS WITH LUPUS-RELATED DISORDERS?

Fibromyalgia Network: PO Box 31750, Tucson, AZ 85751; (520) 290-5550; toll-free (800) 853-2929; e-mail: inquiry@fmnetnews.com; web site: www.fmnetnews.com.

Raynaud's Association: 94 Mercer Ave., Hartsdale, NY 10530; toll-free (800) 280-8055; e-mail: info@raynauds.org; web site: www.raynauds.org.

Scleroderma Foundation: 300 Rosewood Drive, Suite 105, Danvers, MA 01923; (978) 463-5843, toll-free (800) 722-HOPE (4673); e-mail: sfinfo@scleroderma.org; web site: www.scleroderma.org.

Sjogren's Syndrome Foundation: 6707 Democracy Boulevard, Suite 325, Bethesda, MD 20817; (301) 530-4420, toll-free (800) 475-6473; e-mail: tms@sjogrens.org; web site: www.sjogrens.org.

WHAT ARE THE BEST BOOKS ON LUPUS WRITTEN BY NONPHYSICIANS?

Phillips RH: *Coping with lupus,* ed 3, New York, 2001, Avery/Penguin Putnam. (The anticipated publication date for the 4th edition is April 2012). Learn how to live your best life with lupus in this book written by psychologist Phillips, founder of the "Center for Coping."

Phillips RH: *Successful living with lupus: an action workbook,* Hicksville, NY, 2005, Balance Enterprises. Learn to improve your emotional and social well-being by emphasizing the positive.

Hospital for Special Surgery (HSS), Department of Patient Care and Quality Management: *For inquiring teens with lupus: our thoughts, issues & concerns,* 2003, HSS. This colorful teen-speak booklet is available free of charge by calling the Charla de Lupus (Lupus Chat) Program toll-free at (866) 812-4494.

Hospital for Special Surgery (HSS), Department of Patient Care and Quality Management: *What Chinese-Americans and their families should know about lupus,* 2003, HSS. This bilingual booklet is available free of charge by calling the Lupus Asian Network (LANtern) toll-free at (866) 505-2253.

Lupus Foundation of America: *Loopy lupus helps tell Scott's story about a disease called lupus,* Washington, DC, 2002, The LFA. Written by third-grade students and their teacher after a classmate was diagnosed with lupus, this book is charmingly illustrated by the boy's sister and includes information on lupus and Scott's story in his own words.

ARE THERE OTHER BOOKS ABOUT LUPUS AND RELATED DISEASES WRITTEN BY PHYSICIANS?

Quintero del Rio A: *Lupus: a patient's guide to diagnosis, treatment, and lifestyle,* Munster, IN, 2007, Hilton Publishing Company. Dr. Quintero del Rio discusses at length how lupus is detected, its many symptoms and complications, the most successful and current treatments available, and ongoing research. Personal stories throughout this book lend a warm touch and illustrate how people with lupus are crafting solutions to the many challenges of living with this complex and unpredictable disease.

Wallace DJ: *The new Sjögren's syndrome handbook*, NY/London, 2011, Oxford University Press. This comprehensive and authoritative guide illuminates the major clinical aspects of the syndrome in a readable and understandable manner and is loaded with practical tips and advice.

Wallace DJ: *The lupus book: a guide for patients and their families,* NY/London, 2012, Oxford University Press. This book is ideal for the motivated patients who wanting a concise and practical overview of their disease. It contains detailed information on how lupus affects the different organ systems of the body, as well as sections relating to genes and environment, the immune system, economic impact of the disease, medications biologic agents and other new drugs, and proactive lifestyle strategies.

Pellegrino MJ: *Fibromyalgia: up close and personal,* Columbus, OH, 2005, Anadem Publishing. Written by a physician who has fibromyalgia, this book offers information on the diagnosis, treatment, and research, as well as living with the challenges of the disease.

Lahita RG, Phillips RH: *Lupus Q & A: everything you need to know,* New York, 2004, Avery Press. Written is an easy-to-read question-and-answer format, this book combines the vast experience of a renowned lupus physician-researcher and a highly experienced psychologist.

Lehman TJA: *It's not just growing pains: a guide to childhood muscle, bone, and joint pains, rheumatic diseases, and the latest treatments,* New York, 2004, Oxford University Press. In this comprehensive resource guide for parents and professionals, distinguished pediatric rheumatologist Dr. Lehman offers easy-to-understand information on the causes, symptoms, tests, and treatments for a variety of rheumatic diseases and childhood pain.

Pratt M, Hallegua D: *Taking charge of lupus,* New York, 2002, New American Library/Penguin Group–USA. Co-written by Pratt who is a lupus patient and rheumatologist Hallegua, this book seeks to help the person with lupus understand and manage all the aspects of lupus. Topics include coping with the side effects of medications, picking the right physician, and coping with finances.

WHAT ABOUT RHEUMATOLOGY OR LUPUS TEXTBOOKS?

The best and most current general rheumatology textbooks are the following:

Hochberg MC, Silman A, Smolen JS, et al: *Rheumatology,* ed 5, St Louis, 2010, Mosby–Elsevier.

Coblyn JS, Weinblatt M, Helfgott S, Bermas B: *Brigham and Women's experts' approach to rheumatology,* Sudbury, MA, 2010, Jones & Bartlett Publishers.

Tsokos G, Buyon J, Koike T, Lahita RG: *Systemic lupus erythematosus,* ed 5, Waltham, MA, 2010, Academic Press–Elsevier.

Ginzler E: *Systemic lupus erythematosus, an issue of rheumatic disease clinics,* Philadelphia, 2010, Saunders–Elsevier.

Firestein GS, Budd RC, Harris ED, et al: *Kelley's textbook of rheumatology,* ed 8, Philadelphia, 2008, Saunders–Elsevier.

Index

Page numbers followed by "f" indicate figures, "t" indicate tables, and "b" indicate boxes. **Boldface** terms indicate supplemental online material.